MW00846031

GRABB AND SMITH'S
PLASTIC SURGERY

Eighth Edition

GRABB AND SMITH'S
PLASTIC SURGERY

EIGHTH EDITION

Editor-In-Chief

KEVIN C. CHUNG, MD, MS

Chief of Hand Surgery, Michigan Medicine
Director, University of Michigan Comprehensive Hand Center
Charles B.G. de Nancrede Professor of Surgery
Professor of Plastic Surgery and Orthopaedic Surgery
Assistant Dean for Faculty Affairs
Associate Director of Global REACH
University of Michigan Medical School
Ann Arbor, Michigan

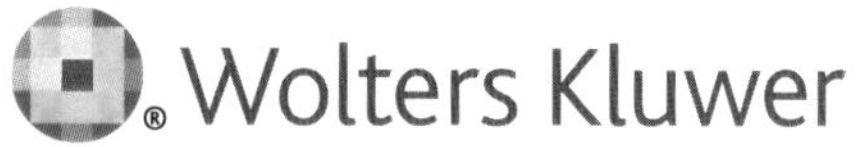

Philadelphia • Baltimore • New York • London
Buenos Aires • Hong Kong • Sydney • Tokyo

Acquisitions Editor: Brian Brown
Product Development Editor: Ashley Fischer/ Grace Caputo
Editorial Assistant: Jeremiah Kiely
Marketing Manager: Julie Sikora
Production Project Manager: Barton Dudlick/ Linda Van Pelt
Design Coordinator: Stephen Druding
Artist/Illustrator: Jen Clements
Manufacturing Coordinator: Beth Welsh
Prepress Vendor: TNQ Technologies

9 8 7 6 5 4 3

Printed in the United States of America

Library of Congress Cataloging-in-Publication Data

Names: Chung, Kevin C., editor.
Title: Grabb and Smith's plastic surgery / editor-in-chief, Kevin C. Chung.
Other titles: Plastic surgery
Description: Eighth edition. | Philadelphia : Wolters Kluwer, [2020] | Includes bibliographical references and index.
Identifiers: LCCN 2019015649 | ISBN 9781496388247
Subjects: | MESH: Reconstructive Surgical Procedures | Cosmetic Techniques | Surgery, Plastic
Classification: LCC RD118 | NLM WO 600 | DDC 617.9/5–dc23
LC record available at https://lccn.loc.gov/2019015649

shop.lww.com

To the memory of Dr. William C. Grabb
To the Faculty, Residents, and Fellows at the University of Michigan

To Chin-Yin and William

CONTRIBUTORS

Joshua M. Adkinson, MD
Assistant Professor of Surgery
Chief of Hand Surgery
Division of Plastic Surgery
Department of Surgery
Indiana University School of Medicine
Indianapolis, Indiana

Jayant P. Agarwal, MD
Chief, Division of Plastic Surgery
Associate Professor of Surgery
University of Utah School of Medicine
Salt Lake City, Utah

Shailesh Agarwal, MD
Section of Plastic Surgery
Department of Surgery
University of Michigan Medical School
Ann Arbor, Michigan

Rachel E. Aliotta, MD
Department of Plastic and Reconstructive Surgery
Cleveland Clinic
Cleveland, Ohio

Oluseyi Aliu, MD, MS
Assistant Professor
Department of Plastic Surgery
Johns Hopkins Hospital
Baltimore, Maryland

Ashley N. Amalfi, MD
Assistant Professor of Surgery
Division of Plastic Surgery
University of Rochester School of Medicine and Dentistry
Rochester, New York

R. Rox Anderson, MD
Professor of Dermatology
Harvard Medical School
Director, Wellman Center of Photomedicine
Department of Dermatology
Massachusetts General Hospital
Boston, Massachusetts

Anne Argenta, MD
Assistant Professor
Medical College of Wisconsin
Milwaukee, Wisconsin

Mohammed Asif, MD
Clinical Instructor
Department of Plastic Surgery
Johns Hopkins Burn Center
Johns Hopkins School of Medicine
Baltimore, Maryland

William G. Austen, JR, MD, FACS
Division Chief
Plastic and Reconstructive Surgery
Burn Surgery
Massachusetts General Hospital
Boston, Massachusetts

Deniz Basci, MD
Aesthetic Fellow
Department of Plastic Surgery
University of Texas Southwestern Medical Center
Dallas, Texas

John H. Bast, MD
Clinical Assistant Professor of Surgery
Penn Medicine Lancaster General Hospital
Lancaster, Pennsylvania

Omar E. Beidas, MD
Department of Plastic Surgery
University of Pittsburgh Medical Center
Pittsburgh, Pennsylvania

Nicholas L. Berlin, MD, MPH
Resident, Section of Plastic Surgery
Department of Surgery
University of Michigan Medical School
Ann Arbor, Michigan

Jessica I. Billig, MD
Resident, Section of Plastic Surgery
Department of Surgery
University of Michigan Medical School
Ann Arbor, Michigan

Gregory H. Borschel, MD, FAAP, FACS
Associate Professor
Institute of Biomaterials and Biomedical Engineering
Associate Scientist
SickKids Research Institute Program in Neuroscience and Mental Health
Sickkids Hand, Nerve and Microsurgery
Nerve Regeneration Laboratory
The Hospital for Sick Children
Division of Plastic and Reconstructive Surgery
Toronto, Ontario, Canada

James P. Bradley, MD
Professor, Vice Chairman
Department of Surgery
Zucker School of Medicine at Hofstra/Northwell
New York, New York

Gerald Brandacher, MD
Associate Professor of Surgery
Scientific Director, Reconstructive Transplantation Program
Department of Plastic and Reconstructive Surgery
Johns Hopkins University School of Medicine
Baltimore, Maryland

David A. Brown
Assistant Professor
Plastic and Reconstructive Surgery
Duke University Medical Center
Durham, North Carolina

David L. Brown, MD
Professor of Surgery
Section of Plastic Surgery
University of Michigan Medical School
Ann Arbor, Michigan

Steven R. Buchman, MD, FACS
M. Haskell Newman Professor of Plastic Surgery
Professor of Neurosurgery
Professor of Surgery
Program Director, Craniofacial Surgery Fellowship
University of Michigan Medical School
Chief, Pediatric Plastic Surgery
CS Mott Children's Hospital
Director, Craniofacial Anomalies Program
University of Michigan Medical Center
Ann Arbor, Michigan

Grant W. Carlson, MD
Chief, Division of Plastic Surgery
Emory University School of Medicine
Emory Aesthetic Center
Atlanta, Georgia

Christi M. Cavaliere, MD, MS
Medical Director of Wound Care
Staff Plastic Surgeon
Cleveland Clinic
Cleveland, Ohio

Rodney Chan, MD, FACS, FRCSC
Chief, Plastic and Reconstructive Surgery
Clinical Division and Burn Center
U.S. Army Institute of Surgical Research
San Antonio Military Medical Center
Associate Professor, Department of Surgery
Uniform Services University of the Health Sciences
San Antonio, Texas

James Chang, MD
Chief, Division of Plastic and Reconstructive Surgery
Johnson & Johnson Distinguished Professor of Surgery (Plastic Surgery) and Orthopaedic Surgery
Stanford University Medical Center
Palo Alto, California

Edward I. Chang, MD, FACS
Associate Professor
Department of Plastic Surgery
University of Texas MD Anderson Cancer Center
Houston, Texas

Ming-Huei Cheng, MD, MBA, FACS
Professor
Division of Plastic Reconstructive Microsurgery
Department of Plastic and Reconstructive Surgery
Chang Gung Memorial Hospital
Kweishan, Taiwan

Ernest S. Chiu, MD
Director and Associate Professor of Plastic Surgery
Institute of Reconstructive Plastic Surgery
Helen L. & Martin S. Kimmel
Hyperbaric and Advanced Wound Healing Center
New York University Langone Medical Center
New York, New York

Carrie K. Chu, MD
Assistant Professor
Department of Plastic Surgery
University of Texas MD Anderson Cancer Center
Houston, Texas

Kevin C. Chung, MD, MS
Chief of Hand Surgery, Michigan Medicine
Director, University of Michigan Comprehensive Hand Center
Charles B.G. de Nancrede Professor of Surgery
Professor of Plastic Surgery and Orthopaedic Surgery
Assistant Dean for Faculty Affairs
Associate Director of Global REACH
University of Michigan Medical School
Ann Arbor, Michigan

Mark W. Clemens II, MD, FACS
Associate Professor
Department of Plastic Surgery
University of Texas MD Anderson Cancer Center
Houston, Texas

Amy S. Colwell, MD
Associate Professor
Harvard Medical School
Massachusetts General Hospital
Boston, Massachusetts

Carisa M. Cooney, MPH
Assistant Professor
Director of Education Innovation
Clinical Research Manager
Department of Plastic and Reconstructive Surgery
Johns Hopkins University School of Medicine
Baltimore, Maryland

Damon S. Cooney, MD, PhD
Assistant Professor
Associate Program Director
Johns Hopkins/University of Maryland
Plastic Surgery Residency Training Program
Department of Plastic and Reconstructive Surgery
Johns Hopkins University School of Medicine
Baltimore, Maryland

Wendy L. Czerwinski, MD, PhD
Associate Professor
Division of Plastic Surgery
Department of Surgery
Baylor Scott & White Medical Center
Texas A&M University College of Medicine
Dallas, Texas

Leahthan F. Domeshek, MD
Fellow, Division of Plastic and Reconstructive Surgery
The Hospital for Sick Children
Toronto, Ontario, Canada

Matthias B. Donelan, MD
Chief of Staff
Shriners Hospital for Children
Visiting Surgeon
Massachusetts General Hospital
Associate Professor of Surgery
Harvard Medical School
Boston, Massachusetts

A. Samandar Dowlatshahi, MD
Instructor, Harvard Medical School
Division of Hand Surgery
Department of Orthopaedics
Division of Plastic Surgery
Department of Surgery
Beth Israel Deaconess Medical Center
Boston, Massachusetts

Katherine E. Duncan, MD
Ophthalmologist/Oculoplastic Surgeon
Greater Baltimore Medical Center
Baltimore, Maryland

Paul D. Durand, MD
Chief Resident, Department of Plastic Surgery
Cleveland Clinic
Cleveland, Ohio

William W. Dzwierzynski, MD
Professor and Program Director
Department of Plastic Surgery
Medical College of Wisconsin
Milwaukee, Wisconsin

Kyle R. Eberlin, MD
Assistant Professor of Surgery
Division of Plastic Surgery
Massachusetts General Hospital
Harvard Medical School
Boston, Massachusetts

Kate E. Elzinga, MD, FRCSC
Section of Plastic Surgery
University of Calgary
Calgary, Alberta, Canada

Benjamin P. Erickson, MD
Assistant Professor
Department of Ophthalmology
Stanford University School of Medicine
Palo Alto, California

William B. Ericson, Jr., MD, FACS, FAAOS
Orthopaedic Hand Surgeon
Ericson Hand and Nerve Center
Seattle, Washington

Russell E. Ettinger, MD
Chief Resident, Section of Plastic Surgery
Department of Surgery
University of Michigan Medical School
Ann Arbor, Michigan

Kenneth L. Fan, MD
Department of Plastic and Reconstructive Surgery
MedStar Georgetown University Hospital
Washington, DC

Frank Fang, MD
Assistant Professor
Division of Plastic Surgery
Department of Surgery
Icahn School of Medicine at Mount Sinai
Attending Physician
Division of Plastic Surgery
Department of Surgery
The Mount Sinai Hospital
New York, New York

Jeffrey B. Friedrich, MD, FACS
Professor of Surgery and Orthopaedics
Division of Plastic Surgery
University of Washington
Seattle, Washington

Natalia Fullerton, MD
Plastic and Reconstructive Surgery
New York-Presbyterian Hospital of Columbia and Weille Cornell Medicine
New York, New York

Warren L. Garner, MD, FACS
Professor of Plastic Surgery
University of Southern California
Los Angeles, California

Michael S. Gart, MD
Fellow, Hand and Upper Extremity Surgery
OrthoCarolina Hand Center
Charlotte, North Carolina

Katherine M. Gast, MD, MS
Assistant Professor
Division of Plastic Surgery
University of Wisconsin School of Medicine and Public Health
Madison, Wisconsin

Aviram M. Giladi, MD, MS
Hand Surgery and Plastic Surgery
Research Director
The Curtis National Hand Center
MedStar Union Memorial Hospital
Baltmiore, Maryland

Justin Gillenwater, MD, MS
Assistant Professor
Plastic and Reconstructive Surgery
Burn and Critical Care
University of Southern California
LAC+USC Burn Center
Los Angeles, California

Robert H. Gilman, MD, DMD
Clinical Assistant Professor
Section of Plastic Surgery
University of Michigan Medical School
Ann Arbor, Michigan

Jesse A. Goldstein, MD
Associate Professor, Department of Plastic Surgery
Children's Hospital of Pittsburgh
University of Pittsburgh Medical Center
Pittsburgh, Pennsylvania

Arun K. Gosain, MD
Professor and Chief, Division of Pediatric Plastic Surgery
Lurie Children's Hospital of Chicago
Northwestern Feinberg School of Medicine
Chicago, Illinois

Amanda A. Gosman, MD
Professor and Interim Chief of Plastic Surgery
Residency Program Director
Craniofacial Fellowship Director
Director of Craniofacial and Pediatric Plastic Surgery
Division of Plastic Surgery
University of California San Diego
Chief of Plastic Surgery
Rady Children's Hospital San Diego
San Diego, California

Arin K. Greene, MD. MMSc
Department of Plastic and Oral Surgery
Boston Children's Hospital
Associate Professor of Surgery
Harvard Medical School
Boston, Massachusetts

Buket Gundogan, BSc (Hons), MBBS
East and North Hertfordshire NHS Trust
Hertfordshire, United Kingdom

Jeffrey A. Gusenoff, MD
Associate Professor of Plastic Surgery, Clinical and Translational Science
Co-Director, Life After Weight Loss Program
Department of Plastic Surgery
University of Pittsburgh Medical Center
Pittsburgh, Pennsylvania

Steven C. Haase, MD
Associate Professor
Section of Plastic Surgery
Department of Surgery
Department of Orthopaedic Surgery
University of Michigan Medical School
Ann Arbor, Michigan

Warren C. Hammert, MD
Professor of Orthopaedic Surgery and Plastic Surgery
Chief, Division of Hand Surgery
Department of Orthopaedics and Rehabilitation
University of Rochester Medical Center
Rochester, New York

Matthew M. Hanasono, MD
Professor
Department of Plastic Surgery
University of Texas MD Anderson Cancer Center
Houston, Texas

Chelsea A. Harris, MD
Research Fellow, Section of Plastic Surgery
Department of Surgery
University of Michigan Medical School
Ann Arbor, Michigan

Asra Hashmi, MD
Craniofacial Surgery Fellow
Division of Plastic Surgery
University of San Diego
San Diego, CA

Lydia A. Helliwell, MD
Division of Plastic Surgery
Instructor of Surgery
Brigham and Women's Hospital
Harvard Medical School
Boston, Massachusetts

Gwendolyn Hoben, MD, PhD
Hand Surgery Fellow
Department of Plastic Surgery
Medical College of Wisconsin
Milwaukee, Wisconsin

Scott T. Hollenbeck, MD, FACS
Associate Professor
Plastic and Reconstructive Surgery
Duke University Medical Center
Durham, North Carolina

Ian C. Hoppe, MD
Craniofacial Surgery Fellow
Division of Plastic Surgery
Children's Hospital of Philadelphia
Perelman School of Medicine at the University of Pennsylvania
Philadelphia, Pennsylvania

Henry C. Hsia, MD, FACS
Associate Professor of Surgery
Section of Plastic Surgery, Department of Surgery
Yale University School of Medicine
Director, Yale Regenerative Wound Healing Program
Yale New Haven Hospital
New Haven, Connecticut

Katherine M. Huber, MD
Chief Resident
Division of Plastic Surgery
Department of Surgery
University of South Florida Morsani College of Medicine
Tampa, Florida

C. Scott Hultman, MD, MBA, FACS
Professor and Vice Chair
Department of Plastic and Reconstructive Surgery
Johns Hopkins University
Director, Johns Hopkins Bayview Medical Center Burn Center
Department of Plastic and Reconstructive Surgery
Johns Hopkins Hospitals
Baltimore, Maryland

Paul F. Hwang, MD
Chief of Breast Reconstruction
Assistant Professor of Surgery
Department of Surgery
Division of Plastic and Reconstructive Surgery
Walter Reed National Military Medical Center
Bethesda, Maryland

Paul H. Izenberg, MD
Clinical Instructor
Section of Plastic Surgery
Department of Surgery
University of Michigan Medical School
Medical Director Outpatient Surgical Center
Department of Surgery
St. Joseph Mercy Hospital
Ann Arbor, Michigan

Oksana A. Jackson, MD
Associate Professor of Surgery
Division of Plastic Surgery
Perelman School of Medicine at the University of Pennsylvania
Surgical Associate, Division of Plastic Surgery
The Children's Hospital of Philadelphia
Philadelphia, Pennsylvania

Jeffrey E. Janis, MD, FACS
Professor of Plastic Surgery, Neurosurgery, Neurology, and Surgery
Executive Vice Chairman, Department of Plastic Surgery
Chief of Plastic Surgery, University Hospitals
Ohio State University Wexner Medical Center
Columbus, Ohio

Reza Jarrahy, MD, FACS, FAAP
Associate Clinical Professor of Surgery, Neurosurgery, and Pediatrics
Division of Plastic and Reconstructive Surgery
David Geffen School of Medicine at UCLA
Los Angeles, California

Christine M. Jones, MD
Assistant Professor
Division of Plastic Surgery
Temple University Hospital
Lewis Katz School of Medicine
Philadelphia, Pennsylvania

Neil F. Jones, MD, FRCS, FACS
Chief of Hand Surgery
Professor of Orthopaedic Surgery
Professor of Plastic and Reconstructive Surgery
University of California Irvine
Irvine, California

Loree K. Kalliainen, MD, MA
Associate Professor
Division of Plastic Surgery
University of North Carolina
Chapel Hill, North Carolina

Sirichai Kamnerdnakta, MD, FRCST
Associate Professor
Division of Plastic Surgery
Department of Surgery
Faculty of Medicine
Siriraj Hospital
Bangkok, Thailand

Steven J. Kasten, MD
Section of Plastic and Reconstructive Surgery
University of Michigan Medical School
Ann Arbor, Michigan

Brian P. Kelley, MD
Surgeon
Institute of Reconstructive Plastic Surgery of Central Texas
Dell Seton Medical Center of the University of Texas
Austin, Texas

Jeffrey Kenkel, MD
Professor and Chair
Department of Plastic Surgery
UT Southwestern Medical Center
Dallas, Texas

Jason H. Ko, MD
Associate Professor
Division of Plastic and Reconstructive Surgery
Department of Orthopaedic Surgery
Northwestern University Feinberg School of Medicine
Chicago, Illinois

Stephen J. Kovach, MD
Associate Professor of Surgery
Divisions of Plastic Surgery and Orthopaedic Surgery
University of Pennsylvania
Perelman Center for Advanced Medicine
Philadelphia, Pennsylvania

Carrie A. Kubiak, MD
House Officer
Department of Surgery
Section of Plastic and Reconstructive Surgery
University of Michigan Medical School
Ann Arbor, Michigan

Theodore A. Kung, MD
Assistant Professor of Surgery
Section of Plastic and Reconstructive Surgery
University of Michigan Medical School
Ann Arbor, Michigan

William M. Kuzon, Jr., MD
Reed O. Dingman Collegiate Professor of Surgery
Section of Plastic and Reconstructive Surgery
University of Michigan Medical School
Chief of Surgery
VA Ann Arbor Healthcare
Ann Arbor, Michigan

Alvin C. Kwok, MD, MPH
Division of Plastic and Reconstructive Surgery
University of Utah
Salt Lake City, Utah

W. P. Andrew Lee, MD
The Milton T. Edgerton, MD, Professor and Chairman
Department of Plastic and Reconstructive Surgery
Johns Hopkins University School of Medicine
Baltimore, Maryland

Justine C. Lee, MD, PhD
Associate Professor
Bernard G. Sarnat Endowed Chair
Department of Plastic and Reconstructive Surgery
University of California Los Angeles
Los Angeles, California

Benjamin Levi, MD
Director, Burn/Wound and Regenerative Medicine Laboratory
Director, Burn/Scar Rehabilitation Program
Associate Burn Director
Assistant Professor in Surgery
University of Michigan Medical School
Ann Arbor, Michigan

L. Scott Levin, MD, FACS
Paul B. Magnuson Professor of Bone and Joint Surgery
Chairman, Department of Orthopaedic Surgery
Professor of Surgery (Plastic Surgery)
University of Pennsylvania
Philadelphia, Pennsylvania

Howard Levinson, MD, FACS
Director of Plastic Surgery Research
Associate Professor of Plastic and Reconstructive Surgery
Division of Surgical Sciences
Associate Professor of Pathology and Dermatology
Departments of Surgery, Pathology, and Dermatology
Duke University Medical Center
Durham, North Carolina

Samuel J. Lin, MD, MBA
Program Director, Aesthetic Plastic Surgery Fellowship
Associate Professor of Surgery
Division of Plastic and Reconstructive Surgery
Beth Israel Deaconess Medical Center
Boston, Massachusetts

Joseph E. Losee, MD
Ross H. Musgrave Endowed Chair in Pediatric Plastic Surgery
Associate Dean for Faculty Affairs
University of Pittsburgh School of Medicine
Professor and Executive Vice Chair
Department of Plastic Surgery, UPMC
Division Chief, Pediatric Plastic Surgery
UPMC Children's Hospital of Pittsburgh
Pittsburgh, Pennsylvania

David W. Low, MD
Professor of Surgery
Division of Plastic Surgery
Perelman School of Medicine at the University of Pennsylvania
Surgical Associate, Division of Plastic Surgery
The Children's Hospital of Philadelphia
Philadelphia, Pennsylvania

Michele Ann Manahan, MD
Associate Professor
Department of Plastic and Reconstructive Surgery
Johns Hopkins Medical Institution
Johns Hopkins Hospital
Baltimore, Maryland

Ernest K. Manders, MD
Professor of Plastic Surgery
University of Pittsburgh Medical Center
Pittsburgh, Pennsylvania

Malcolm W. Marks, MD
Wake Forest University Baptist Medical Center
Department of Plastic and Reconstructive Surgery
Medical Center Boulevard
Winston Salem, North Carolina

Alan Matarasso, MD, FACS, PC
Clinical Professor of Plastic Surgery
Zucker School of Medicine at Hofstra/Northwell
President, Executive Committee and Board of Directors
American Society of Plastic Surgeons
Past President, Board of Trustees
Chairman, 2016-2017 Traveling Professor
The Rhinoplasty Society
Past President, Board of Trustees
Chairman
New York Regional Society of Plastic Surgeons
New York, New York

Evan Matros, MD, MPH
Associate Attending
Memorial Sloan Kettering Cancer Center
Weill Cornell Medical College
New York, New York

Alexander F. Mericli, MD
Assistant Professor
Department of Plastic Surgery
University of Texas MD Anderson Cancer Center
Houston, Texas

Brett F. Michelotti, MD
Assistant Professor of Surgery
Division of Plastic and Reconstructive Surgery
University of Wisconsin – School of Medicine and Public Health
Madison, Wisconsin

Nathanial R. Miletta, MD, FAAD
Board-Certified Dermatologist and Fellowship-Trained Dermatologic Surgeon
Chief, Laser Surgery and Scar Center
San Antonio Military Medical Center
Assistant Professor
Uniformed Services University of the Health Sciences
San Antonio, Texas

Erin A. Miller, MD
Department of Plastic and Reconstructive Surgery
University of Washington
Seattle, Washington

Gabriele C. Miotto, MD, MEd
Assistant Professor of Surgery
Division of Plastic and Reconstructive Surgery
Emory University School of Medicine
Atlanta, Georgia

Adeyiza O. Momoh, MD
Associate Professor of Surgery
Program Director, Integrated Plastic Surgery Residency
Department of Surgery
University of Michigan Medical School
Ann Arbor, Michigan

Brian A. Moore, MD, FACS
Chair, Otorhinolaryngology and Communication Sciences
Director, Ochsner Cancer Institute
Ochsner Health System
New Orleans, Louisiana

Neal Moores, MD
Division of Plastic Surgery
University of Utah School of Medicine
Salt Lake City, Utah

Terence M. Myckatyn, MD, FACS, FRCSC
Professor, Plastic and Reconstructive Surgery
West County Plastic Surgeons
Washington University School of Medicine
Saint Louis, Missouri

Maurice Y. Nahabedian, MD
Professor and Section Chief
Department of Plastic Surgery
MedStar Washington Hospital Center
Georgetown University
Washington, DC

Foad Nahai, MD
Marice J. Jurkiewicz Chair in Plastic Surgery
Professor of Surgery
Emory University School of Medicine
Atlanta, Georgia

Anne C. O'Neill, MBBCh, MMedSci, FRCS(Plast), MSc, PhD
Assistant Professor
Division of Plastic and Reconstructive Surgery
Department of Surgery
University of Toronto
Toronto, Ontario, Canada

Dennis P. Orgill, MD, PhD
Medical Director, The Wound Care Center
Brigham and Women's Hospital
Professor of Surgery
Harvard Medical School
Boston, Massachusetts

Wayne Ozaki, MD, DDS
Clinical Professor
Director of Craniofacial Surgery
Chief of Pediatric Plastic Surgery
Division of Plastic and Reconstructive Surgery
UCLA David Geffen School of Medicine
Los Angeles, California
Chief of Plastic Surgery
Olive View-UCLA Medical Center
Sylmar, California

Christopher J. Pannucci, MD, MS
Division of Plastic and Reconstructive Surgery
University of Utah
Salt Lake City, Utah

Julie E. Park, MD, FACS
Stephan R. Lewis Professor of Surgery
Division of Plastic Surgery
University of Texas Medical Branch
Galveston, Texas

Sabrina N. Pavri, MD, MBA
Chief Resident
Section of Plastic Surgery
Department of Surgery
Yale University School of Medicine
Yale New Haven Hospital
New Haven, Connecticut

Wyatt G. Payne, MD
Professor of Surgery
Division of Plastic Surgery
University of South Florida
Tampa, Florida
Chief, Plastic Surgery
Bay Pines VA Healthcare System
Bay Pines, Florida

Chad A. Perlyn, MD, PhD
Chief, Division of Plastic Surgery
Florida International University College of Medicine
Attending Surgeon
Nicklaus Children's Hospital
Miami, Florida

Ivo A. Pestana, MD
Wake Forest University Baptist Medical Center
Department of Plastic and Reconstructive Surgery
Medical Center Boulevard
Winston-Salem, North Carolina

Mitchell A. Pet, MD
Fellow, Curtis National Hand Center
MedStar Union Memorial Hospital
Baltimore, Maryland

Nicole A. Phillips, MD
Senior Resident, Division of Plastic Surgery
Harvard Medical School
Massachusetts General Hospital
Boston, Massachusetts

Brett T. Phillips, MD, MBA
Division of Plastic, Maxillofacial, and Oral Surgery
Department of Surgery
Duke University Medical Center
Durham, North Carolina

Julian J. Pribaz, MD
Professor of Surgery
Morsani College of Medicine
University of South Florida
Tampa, Florida

Brian C. Pridgen, MD
Division of Plastic and Reconstructive Surgery
Stanford University Medical Center
Stanford, California

Mark E. Puhaindran, MBBS, MRCS, MMed
Senior Consultant
Department of Hand and Reconstructive Microsurgery
National University Hospital
Singapore

Xuan Qiu, MD, PhD
Hand Surgery Fellow
Section of Plastic Surgery
Department of Surgery
University of Michigan Medical School
Ann Arbor, Michigan

Ali A. Qureshi, MD
Washington University in St Louis
Barnes-Jewish Hospital
St Louis, Missouri

Paymon Rahgozar, MD
Hand Surgery Fellow
Section of Plastic Surgery
University of Michigan Medical School
Ann Arbor, Michigan

Kavitha Ranganathan, MD
Resident, Section of Plastic Surgery
Department of Surgery
University of Michigan Medical School
Ann Arbor, Michigan

Patrick L. Reavey, MD, MS
Assistant Professor
Department of Surgery
Section of Plastic and Reconstructive Surgery
Department of Orthaepedic Surgery and Rehabilitation Medicine
University of Chicago Medicine
Chicago, Illinois

Christine Hsu Rohde, MD, MPH
Associate Professor of Surgery
Vice Chair of Faculty Development and Diversity
Department of Surgery
Columbia University Medical Center
New York-Presbyterian Hospital
New York, New York

Jessica F. Rose, MD
Microsurgery Fellow
Division of Plastic Surgery
University of Pennsylvania
Philadelphia, Pennsylvania

J. Peter Rubin, MD, FACS
UPMC Endowed Professor and Chair
Director, Life After Weight Loss Surgical Body Contouring Program
Department of Plastic Surgery
University of Pittsburgh
Pittsburgh, Pennsylvania

Ara A. Salibian, MD
Resident Physician
Hansjörg Wyss Department of Plastic Surgery
New York University Langone Health
New York, New York

Ian C. Sando, MD
Plastic and Reconstructive Surgeon
Ascension St. Vincent
Indianapolis, Indiana

Sarah E. Sasor, MD
Hand Surgery Fellow
Section of Plastic Surgery
University of Michigan Medical School
Ann Arbor, Michigan

Jesse C. Selber, MD, MPH
Professor
Department of Plastic Surgery
University of Texas MD Anderson Cancer Center
Houston, Texas

Akhil K. Seth, MD
Division of Plastic and Reconstructive Surgery
NorthShore University HealthSystem
Clinical Assistant Professor of Surgery
University of Chicago Pritzer School of Medicine
Evanston, Illinois

Sammy Sinno, MD
Private Practice
Chicago, Illinois

Sheri Slezak, MD
Professor
Division of Plastic Surgery
University of Maryland School of Medicine
Baltimore, Maryland

David J. Smith, MD
Professor of Surgery
Chief, Division of Plastic Surgery
University of South Florida Monsani School of Medicine
Tampa, Florida

Darren M. Smith, MD
Voluntary Faculty
Department of Plastic Surgery
Manhattan Eye, Ear, and Throat Hospital
Lenox Hill Hospital
New York, New York

Alison K. Snyder-Warwick, MD
Assistant Professor of Surgery
Division of Plastic and Reconstructive Surgery
Washington University School of Medicine
St. Louis, Missouri

Nicole Z. Sommer, MD
Associate Professor of Surgery
Director of SIU Cosmetic Clinic
Institute for Plastic Surgery
Southern Illinois University School of Medicine
Springfield, Illinois

Mark W. Stalder, MD
Assistant Professor of Plastic and Reconstructive Surgery
Department of Surgery
Louisiana State University Health Sciences Center School of Medicine
New Orleans, Louisiana

Jill P. Stone, MD
Microvascular Reconstructive Surgery Fellow
Department of Plastic Surgery
Johns Hopkins Hospital
Baltimore, Maryland

Christopher C. Surek, DO
Aesthetic Surgery Fellow
Department of Plastic Surgery
Cleveland Clinic
Cleveland, Ohio

Amir H. Taghinia, MD, MPH, MBA
Staff Surgeon
Boston Children's Hospital
Assistant Professor of Surgery
Harvard Medical School
Boston, Massachusetts

Jesse A. Taylor, MD
Mary Downs Endowed Chair of Craniofacial Surgery
Division of Plastic Surgery
Children's Hospital of Philadelphia
University of Pennsylvania School of Medicine
Philadelphia, Pennsylvania

Peter W. Thompson, MD
Assistant Professor of Plastic Surgery
Emory University Hospital
Atlanta, Georgia

Matthew D. Treiser, MD, PhD
Assistant Professor
Department of Surgery
Albert Eistein College of Medicine
Faculty
Department of Surgery, Division of Plastic and Reconstructive Surgery
Montefiore Medical Center
Bronx, New York

Sergey Y. Turin, MD
Resident Physician
Division of Pediatric Plastic Surgery
Lurie Children's Hospital of Chicago
Northwestern Feinberg School of Medicine
Chicago, Illinois

John A. van Aalst, MD
Chief, Division of Plastic Surgery
Cincinnati Children's Hospital Medical Center
Cincinnati, Ohio

Christian J. Vercler, MD, MA
Associate Professor
Section of Plastic Surgery, Department of Surgery
University of Michigan Medical School
Ann Arbor, Michigan

Jennifer F. Waljee, MD, MPH, MS
Associate Professor
Section of Plastic Surgery, Department of Surgery
University of Michigan Medical School
Ann Arbor, Michigan

Derrick C. Wan, MD
Associate Professor, Department of Surgery
Director of Maxillofacial Surgery
Lucile Packard Children's Hospital
Endowed Faculty Scholar
Child Health Research Institute at Stanford University
Hagey Family Faculty Scholar in Stem Cell Research and Regenerative Medicine
Stanford University Medical Center
Stanford, California

Jeremy Warner, MD, FACS
Associate Professor
Section of Plastic and Reconstructive Surgery
University of Chicago
Chicago, Illinois

Robert A. Weber, MD
Professor and Vice Chair of Surgery
Chief, Section of Hand Surgery
Baylor Scott & White Medical Center
Texas A&M University College of Medicine
Temple, Texas

Thomas D. Willson, MD
Assistant Professor of Surgery
Larner College of Medicine at the University of Vermont
Director of the Cleft/Craniofacial Program
Vermont Children's Hospital
Burlington, Vermont

Alex K. Wong, MD, FACS
Associate Professor of Surgery
Director, Basic, Translational, and Clinical Medicine
Director, Microsurgery Fellowship and Medical Student Education
Division of Plastic and Reconstructive Surgery
Keck School of Medicine of University of Southern California
Los Angeles, California

Sang Hyun Woo, MD, PhD
President
W Institute for Hand and Reconstructive Microsurgery
W Hospital
Daegu, Korea

Akira Yamada, MD, PhD
Professor of Surgery
Northwestern University Feinberg School of Medicine
Department of Plastic Surgery
Ann & Robert H. Lurie Children's Hospital of Chicago
Chicago, Illinois

Guang Yang, MD
Associate Professor
Department of Hand Surgery
China-Japan Union Hospital of Jilin University
Changchun, People's Republic of China

Peirong Yu, MD
Professor
Department of Plastic Surgery
University of Texas MD Anderson Cancer Center
Houston, Texas

Frank Yuan, MD
General Surgery Resident
Department of Surgery
University of Massachusetts Medical School
Worcester, Massachusetts

Toni Zhong, MD, MHS, FRCS
Associate Professor
Departments of Surgery and Surgical Oncology
University of Toronto
Clinical and Scientific Director
UHN Breast Reconstruction Program
Fellowship Director
Division of Plastic and Reconstructive Surgery
University of Toronto
Toronto, Ontario, Canada

James E. Zins, MD
Chairman, Department of Plastic Surgery
Cleveland Clinic
Cleveland, Ohio

Terri A. Zomerlei, MD
Resident
Department of Plastic Surgery
Ohio State University Wexner Medical Center
Columbus, Ohio

I am honored and most excited to present to you the 8th edition of this classic textbook in plastic surgery. With any historic textbook, at a certain time the content needs complete rejuvenation. In celebration of this 8th edition, I took the liberty of inviting new authors to rewrite every chapter to reflect the innovative spirit of plastic surgery. The authors are some of the best in our specialty, who impart knowledge in a clear and succinct style that is the hallmark of this book. I have also included additional content by presenting annotated classic articles so that the reader can refer to these foundation papers to gain even more insight. Furthermore, the authors have shared select questions and discussed the answer choices in an interactive format.

This edition is illustrated richly with artistic drawings to highlight the anatomy and surgical approaches. This textbook is not meant to be an encyclopedic textbook, but serves as an essential reference by striving to "get to the facts" in this era of rapid dissemination of information. As I traveled in the United States and around the world, I am struck by how much this textbook is revered by trainees and senior surgeons during their formative years of becoming a plastic surgeon. The Grabb and Smith textbook strives to bind the plastic surgery family all over the world, even in remote regions where plastic surgery is not yet recognized as a specialty.

I want to acknowledge all of the authors who understood the gravity and honor of contributing to this classic textbook. They have done a magnificent job in distilling the essence of plastic surgery, for which I am grateful. I want to recognize Brian Brown, the publisher of Grabb and Smith, for his confidence in me after serving as a section editor for many years. I appreciate my team at the University of Michigan, Jennifer Sterbenz and You Jeong Kim, who toiled intensely to help me and our authors ensure timely delivery of the chapters and a quality product. Finally, I would like to thank Grace Caputo, who was relentless in her attention to detail, and her dedication to deliver this textbook one year early.

I welcome Grabb and Smith back to the University of Michigan, for Dr. Grabb was the second chairman of plastic surgery at our historic program. Through the legacy of Dr. Grabb and his trainees, they laid the foundation for our current success. Lastly, I should thank all of the readers of this textbook. Just because one has purchased previous editions does not mean that this edition is no longer worthwhile. This invigorated 8th edition will certainly set the standard in the publishing world for its educational excellence in synthesizing the encyclopedic plastic surgery specialty into a single textbook. I am grateful and proud to present to you the 8th Edition of *Grabb and Smith's Plastic Surgery*.

Kevin C. Chung, MD, MS
Chief of Hand Surgery, Michigan Medicine
Director, University of Michigan Comprehensive Hand Center
Charles B.G. de Nancrede Professor of Surgery
Professor of Plastic Surgery and Orthopaedic Surgery
Assistant Dean for Faculty Affairs
Associate Director of Global REACH
University of Michigan Medical School
Ann Arbor, Michigan

FOREWORD

It is a distinct privilege for me as the Chief of Plastic Surgery at the University of Michigan to write the Foreword for the 8th Edition of *Grabb and Smith's Plastic Surgery*, edited by Kevin C. Chung, MD, MS. What an honor for Dr. Chung to be able to edit this landmark textbook which has its roots at the University of Michigan where William C. Grabb, MD, served as Professor and Chief of the Section of Plastic Surgery. Dr. Grabb was a consummate clinician, surgeon, educator, and innovator whose legacy has lived on through this book. Dr. Grabb, along with his Co-Editor Dr. Smith, has educated a generation of plastic surgeons, helping to prepare plastic surgery residents for the in-service examination, helping to prepare recent graduates for their written examination, and most importantly, helping plastic surgeons care for patients operatively and nonoperatively. Grabb and Smith has always been a great source of information for plastic surgeons during training and many years thereafter.

The 8th Edition of Grabb and Smith has been designed by Dr. Chung to build on this important legacy of education. Reviewing the Table of Contents will quickly demonstrate to you that the list of authors reads like a "Who's Who in Plastic Surgery." At the same time, the best and brightest young minds in plastic surgery have also contributed to the book. It is this mix of authors that provides a healthy diversity of opinion, viewpoint, and presentation style, which will undoubtedly enhance the value of the material to all readers. The topics may be similar to prior editions of Grabb and Smith, but the chapters have all been completely rewritten. In fact, some of the authors who have contributed chapters to Grabb and Smith in the past have been asked to write new chapters, on different topics, to keep the material fresh, interesting, contemporary, and educational. Additionally, there are many new authors who have not previously contributed to this book, ensuring that the content is current, presented in a way that is relevant to the modern day learner, and yet still maintains the high quality of information necessary to be valuable to all plastic surgeons.

The world around us is changing and the only thing that is constant is change. If we are not adapting to this changing world, we will be falling behind. As a result, the 8th Edition has been completely redesigned to optimize its value and to ensure that all of the critical elements of our rapidly changing specialty are captured. The chapters are written in a consistent style to provide the basic knowledge, fundamental principles, and crucial information needed to become a plastic surgeon and to assist those pursuing lifelong learning. The book is formatted in such a way that the information can be gathered quickly through clear and concise writing, visually pleasing full color figures, photographs, expertly crafted decision algorithms, tables, and flowcharts. The days of reading long chapters have gone. The information is provided in a style well suited for in-service examination or written board exam preparation. More importantly, the information is provided in a style that is well suited for plastic surgeons as they provide high-quality, thoughtful, and compassionate care for their patients.

The pedagogy of the book has been specifically designed by Dr. Chung with the needs and interests of the plastic surgery resident, young practicing plastic surgeon, or the plastic surgeon who needs rapid access to information "at point of care" with a patient. Each chapter begins with 5 to 7 key points, which have been carefully selected by the authors to be the most critical elements of the chapter. An in-depth discussion of each of these bullet points is performed in the body of the chapter where the learner can find as much depth and breadth of information as they desire. At the conclusion of each chapter, there are 5 to 10 multiple-choice questions, which have been designed to reinforce the learning that has occurred throughout the chapter. This chapter construction follows a very traditional and highly successful model of learning: (1) Tell them what you are going to teach them; (2) Teach them; (3) Tell them what you taught them; and (4) Test them on their new knowledge. This approach has worked for decades in the classroom and works very nicely here as well. Additionally, each question includes a detailed description of why the correct answer is correct and even more importantly, why the incorrect answer is incorrect. Lastly, for those who wish to collect the classic articles in plastic surgery, each chapter includes 5 to 10 classic articles, which have been appropriately cited, highlighted, and briefly annotated for historical perspective.

It is such a pleasure to have the 8th Edition of *Grabb and Smith's Plastic Surgery* return home to the University of Michigan with Kevin C. Chung, MD, MS, as the Editor, and so many of our faculty as contributing authors. The book has been expertly designed, beautifully executed, and will be an outstanding addition to any library. It is written in a clear and concise way with easy access to all information. At the same time, the book is sufficiently comprehensive to provide lifelong learning from the very infancy of someone's plastic surgery career to their mature practice. Most of all, this book will help to make us all better physicians and surgeons. I credit the 1st Edition of *Grabb and Smith's Plastic Surgery* for teaching me what I needed to know to be a good plastic and reconstructive surgeon. I am sure many will be able to say the same thing about the 8th Edition of this landmark book.

Paul S. Cederna, MD
Chief, Section of Plastic Surgery
Robert Oneal Professor of Plastic Surgery
Professor, Department of Biomedical Engineering
University of Michigan

CONTENTS

PART VIII
HAND

PART IX
TRUNK AND LOWER EXTREMITY

PART I

■ PRINCIPLES, TECHNIQUES, AND BASIC SCIENCE

CHAPTER 1 Fundamental Principles of Plastic Surgery

Theodore A. Kung and Kevin C. Chung

KEY POINTS

- Plastic surgery is a diverse surgical specialty and its practice is guided by a set of fundamental principles.
- There is an inexorable connection between cosmetic surgery and reconstruction surgery because every plastic surgery operation aims to restore both form and function.
- Elective surgeries should be pursued only after considering whether the benefits of surgery will outweigh the risks.
- Outcomes in plastic surgery can be enhanced by addressing modifiable patient factors, adequately preparing wounds prior to reconstruction, replacing lost structures with tissues of similar quality, ensuring optimal vascularity, minimizing donor site morbidity, and deliberately protecting the surgical site.
- A plastic surgeon is always prepared to confront complications with a series of surgical backup plans.
- Plastic surgeons must continually innovate new solutions to clinical problems and will remain at the vanguard of surgical innovation.

Plastic surgery is an incredibly diverse specialty that is challenging to define because its scope cannot simply be characterized by patient age, gender, organ system, or pathology. The purview of plastic surgery extends from neonatal to end-of-life care and is inclusive of a myriad of conditions that affect every single area of the human body. Plastic surgeons possess unique and versatile skills for reconstructing defects relating to cancer extirpation, cosmetically enhancing normal anatomy, salvaging limbs after trauma, rehabilitating burn patients, ameliorating childhood deformities, and performing autotransplantation as well as allotransplantation. This expertise is also critical in devising creative solutions to a variety of problems faced by other physicians, and for this reason, plastic surgeons are frequently consulted by their colleagues in other specialties. How is it possible for one surgical specialty to encompass this enormous breadth and depth of practice?

The unifying trait of all plastic surgeons is a comprehensive understanding of a set of important fundamental principles. Every plastic surgeon abides by these principles to successfully execute the many complex assessments, judgment calls, and technical decisions in the daily practice of plastic surgery. Therefore, the specialty of plastic surgery is exceptional because it is distinguished not by its association to a particular patient population or anatomic region, but by a dedication to imperative principles that enable plastic surgeons to provide effective and individualized care. These principles were conceptualized through centuries of plastic surgery evolution and formalized in recent history by Gillies and Millard, who outlined a collection of philosophical yet practical principles in their text *The Principles and Art of Plastic Surgery*.[1] Years later, Millard published an expanded set of tenets in *Principalization of Plastic Surgery*.[2] This chapter modernizes and expounds on 10 of the most essential fundamental principles of plastic surgery and provides relevant examples of how plastic surgeons utilize these principles in a wide range of clinical scenarios.

PRINCIPLE I: MAKE AN INFORMED DECISION TO OPERATE OR NOT OPERATE

Some types of plastic surgery are mandatory. A wound resulting from resection of a sarcoma with exposed bone requires a reconstructive operation that provides soft tissue coverage over the defect durable enough to withstand the infliction of adjuvant radiation therapy. However, in many situations, the plastic surgeon must make an informed decision whether to perform an operation or not based on a thorough evaluation of the potential benefits against the potential risks. Although this is conspicuously germane to cosmetic surgery, the same thought process is necessary for reconstructive surgery. For example, a large but clean traumatic wound on a patient's thigh could be treated reasonably with one of several options, from nonsurgical strategies such as dressing changes to surgical intervention such as local tissue rearrangement. A multitude of factors must be carefully pondered to select the most appropriate treatment. If dressing changes are used, the wound may be healed eventually but at what burden to the patient? Does the patient have the patience or ability to perform satisfactory dressing changes? Would a definitive surgery result in a healed wound more efficiently? How feasible is the surgery, and what is the likelihood of specific complications? Ultimately, the surgeon must decide if the benefits of surgery will outweigh the risks and predict that the expected outcomes of surgery will enhance the patient's overall health status.

This determination is made more difficult because of the inherently subjective nature of plastic surgery outcomes. Success in plastic surgery is not measured solely on binary scales, such as patency versus occlusion or union versus nonunion. Instead, success is also subjectively gauged by patient satisfaction and is influenced by patient expectations.[3] Consider a consultation between a plastic surgeon and a woman interested in postmastectomy breast reconstruction, an elective operation with substantial psychosocial advantages. In a relatively short amount of time, the plastic surgeon needs to educate the patient regarding the available surgical choices for breast reconstruction and provide an individualized assessment of her candidacy for each option. To guide the patient to the most suitable decision for her, the surgeon must shrewdly evaluate the patient's expectations and her level of understanding of the desired reconstructive surgery. Are her expectations consistent with what is possible from a technical standpoint? Does the patient seem ready to make this decision amidst the other stresses associated with a breast cancer diagnosis? Does the patient understand the possible setbacks that may occur with the surgery? The answers to these types of questions will greatly affect the patient's perception of the success of reconstruction and her reported satisfaction with both the surgery and the plastic surgeon.

PRINCIPLE II: OPTIMIZE MODIFIABLE PATIENT FACTORS

Deliberate identification and management of patient risk factors will decrease the chances of complications and increase the likelihood of successful surgical outcomes. For example, smoking is a commonly encountered modifiable risk factor. Nearly 20% of Americans are smokers and cigarette smoking remains the leading cause of preventable disease and death in the United States.[4,5] The noxious components of cigarette smoke are known to cause vasoconstriction, induce endothelial injury, cause thrombogenesis, diminish oxygen transport, and hinder cellular repair mechanisms.[6] Together, these detrimental processes work synergistically to impair wound healing and will directly confer additional risk to plastic surgery patients. Other modifiable medical risk factors that also exacerbate poor wound healing include uncontrolled diabetes, obesity, infection, steroid use, certain homeopathic medications, and malnutrition.[7] These treatable comorbidities should be recognized during preoperative screening and sufficiently addressed prior to any operation. Social risk factors should also be carefully considered during the preoperative evaluation. After surgery, patients will frequently need assistance with their activities of daily living and comply with strict restrictions. The plastic surgeon should inquire about the social support available to the patient and ensure that the patient's postoperative safety is entrusted to either family members or a rehabilitation center.

The importance of risk factor optimization is demonstrated in the care of body contouring patients. During the preoperative consultation, a thorough history is taken to solicit all modifiable risk factors that would impair the patient's ability to heal long incisions and wide dissection planes.[8] For a majority of plastic surgeons, smoking is an absolute contraindication to any body contouring operation. Cessation of smoking for at least 4 weeks and confirmation with a urine cotinine test is a common requirement before surgery is scheduled. Frequently, collaboration with the patient's primary care physician is critical in correcting hyperglycemia, anemia, or vitamin deficiencies. Patients who would benefit from additional weight loss may be referred to a nutritionist or a bariatric surgeon. After the operation, the patient will have considerable activity restrictions and will need to care for the wounds; therefore, a detailed preoperative discussion with the patient about postoperative care and limitations will serve to set expectations and to establish a social support system for the patient.

PRINCIPLE III: PERFORM ADEQUATE DEBRIDEMENT PRIOR TO RECONSTRUCTION

Debridement is performed to physically remove any barriers to tissue growth, such as infection, biofilm, and senescent cells.[9] The plastic surgeon may choose one of many forms of debridement, from dressing changes to operative excision of the wound, but the critical concept is that the debridement must be adequate to remove all elements hindering wound healing. In many instances, this objective is accomplished only after the wound is debrided serially in the operating room. Chronic wounds are often associated with some degree of necrotic tissue that must be sharply and completely debrided away before definitive reconstruction can be performed. Failure of reconstruction is often attributed to inadequate debridement of the wound. Although *adequate debridement* is usually a term associated with the management of chronic wounds, this essential principle also applies to acute wounds. Acute traumatic wounds, such as open fractures of the lower extremity or lacerations from bite injury, are notoriously contaminated, and adequate debridement in this setting is also critical to the success of reconstruction. In fact, this principle of adequate debridement is so relevant to all forms of plastic surgery that it may even be applied to clean surgical wounds. For example, during reduction mammoplasty, there is often a widespread accumulation of devitalized globules of fat and clots scattered throughout the surgical field. Prior to closure, meticulous removal of this biologic debris facilitates wound healing by decreasing the risks of fat necrosis and infection.

Certain situations will complicate the plastic surgeon's ability to perform adequate debridement. For example, in some traumatic wounds, exposed orthopedic hardware cannot be removed because doing so would result in unacceptable fracture instability.[10] In these challenging cases, debridement serves to decrease the microbial burden of the wound, and deep tissue cultures are taken to help guide antimicrobial therapy. However, the persistent presence of contaminated material will be a major risk factor for infection, and therefore the patient may need suppressive antibiotic therapy until the hardware can be removed. This necessary adaptation of the principle of adequate debridement is also exemplified in the treatment of pressure ulcers with underlying osteomyelitis. These chronic wounds exhibit many deleterious factors that impede wound healing.[11] The first step in surgical treatment is completely excising the soft tissue bursa surrounding the wound. If the osteomyelitis is limited to a small focus of bone at the base of the pressure ulcer, it is possible to remove the area of bone infection entirely during debridement. However, if the osteomyelitis is extensive, complete resection of this bone is not feasible, and the patient will often need suppressive antibiotic therapy guided by intraoperative bone cultures. In this situation, aggressive excision of the bursa is still beneficial because this promotes healing of the soft tissues after surgery and results in a smaller, cleaner, and more manageable chronic wound.

PRINCIPLE IV: IF POSSIBLE, REPLACE LIKE WITH LIKE; IF NOT POSSIBLE, CREATE IT

One of the most famous plastic surgery principles is that lost tissues should be replaced in kind. The plastic surgeon examines the defect carefully and determines the best donor tissues necessary to optimally achieve both a durable reconstruction and an optimal aesthetic outcome. For instance, when primary skin closure is not possible after excision of a cutaneous tumor from an upper eyelid, a frequently chosen donor site is full-thickness skin from the opposite upper eyelid.[12] This option is elegant because it replaces the missing tissue with tissue of the same thickness, color match, pliability, and elasticity. In addition, donor site morbidity is acceptably low when relatively excess skin from one eyelid is used to reconstruct the other eyelid. When such an ideal donor site is unavailable, the next most similar tissue substitute is selected; in this example, skin for eyelid reconstruction can be harvested from postauricular skin or supraclavicular skin. This principle can also be applied to substantially more challenging wounds. An extensive mandibular tumor may necessitate the removal of bone, muscle, mucosa, and skin, and successful reconstruction is predicated on the replacement of these tissues with appropriately similar donor tissues. In these complex cases, reconstruction often requires the use of free flaps that are transferred to the defect, such as a fibula bone flap with associated skin based on the peroneal vascular system.[13]

In some cases, no suitable donor sites exist, and innovative strategies must be employed to create sufficient replacement tissues of similar quality. One example of this is the use of tissue expanders to induce growth of tissues through cellular proliferation.[14] Tissue expansion has revolutionized the treatment of various conditions and given plastic surgeons another tool to better replace *like with like* in clinical scenarios that were previously impossible because of the severity of tissue deficiency. Tissue expanders now serve a critical role in the replacement of hair-bearing skin for large scalp defects, the creation of additional abdominal wall tissue for the closure of large hernias, the expansion of mastectomy skin for breast reconstruction, and the resurfacing of skin affected by giant congenital nevi. This concept of cellular response to force is also the mechanism behind distraction osteogenesis in craniofacial surgery.[15] This technique leverages the natural processes of fracture healing to yield outcomes superior to those achievable through other means such as nonvascularized bone grafting or free tissue transfer. For example, distraction osteogenesis is an excellent strategy for treating micrognathia in children with Pierre Robin sequence.[16] Internal or external distractors are placed surgically around the site of mandibular osteotomies, and a tensile force is slowly delivered to gradually elongate the intervening callus. One major advantage of distraction osteogenesis is that during the process of new bone formation, the overlying soft tissue envelope is also expanded incrementally. This reduces the constrictive effects of the soft tissue on the growing bone and consequently results in a stable reconstruction that is less prone to relapse. These powerful techniques to grow living structures outside of the laboratory setting have completely transformed the plastic surgeon's ability to replace missing tissues and are often principal options for many complex clinical problems.

PRINCIPLE V: OPTIMIZE VASCULARITY AT EVERY OPPORTUNITY

Plastic surgeons are obsessed with blood supply. Vascularity is paramount to tissue viability and therefore to the success of healing. The plastic surgeon must possess an unparalleled comprehension of the blood supply to various types of tissues and methods to preserve this blood supply during surgery. For example, knowledge of the vastness of the subdermal plexus allows a plastic surgeon to reliably raise thin flaps of skin during a facelift operation. In reconstructive surgery, donor tissues must remain well-vascularized to transfer from one location to another. A detailed understanding of the vascular anatomy of these flaps permits their use for definitive closure of any wound. When vascularity to a surgical site is insufficient, the plastic surgeon must strive to improve it. For instance, surgery may be postponed to await smoking cessation or time may be given for other specialists to help optimize blood flow. An illustration of the latter is when a patient with arterial insufficiency and a chronic lower extremity wound is referred to a vascular surgeon for revascularization prior to surgical treatment of the wound. Vascularity of a particular flap may also be enhanced by performing a delay procedure, which is a staged operation whereby the plastic surgeon partially raises the flap and then waits 1 to 2 weeks before fully elevating the flap for reconstruction. A delay period allows choke vessels to physiologically dilate within the flap and results in greater flap reliability.[17]

This respect for blood supply is also evident in many intraoperative decisions that are made by plastic surgeons. Judicious placement of incisions, especially in the context of unfavorable previous incisions, requires a careful consideration of blood supply. Additionally, at many points during an operation, the plastic surgeon will tailor numerous surgical techniques to maximize vascularity. For example, when a local flap such as a V-Y flap or a rotational flap is used for closure of a wound, minimal undermining is performed during flap elevation to reduce disruption of the flap's underlying blood supply. Any sizable perforating vessels that are encountered during dissection of these local flaps are deliberately preserved if possible. During flap inset, pickups and retractors are handled thoughtfully to prevent iatrogenic tissue injury, and undue tension of the closure is avoided to minimize tissue ischemia. Even the selection of sutures and suturing technique is weighed against the effects on vascularity. For instance, placement of too many deep dermal sutures may cause relative ischemia of the edge of a cutaneous flap, and the choice of horizontal mattress suturing may lead to more ischemia compared with vertical mattress suturing. Each of these intraoperative decisions may influence the quality of the blood supply to the closure and may make a meaningful difference in the functional or cosmetic outcome of the surgery.

PRINCIPLE VI: PRESERVE FORM AND FUNCTION

Every plastic surgery operation seeks to restore and preserve form and function. In many instances, the goals of surgery are both cosmetic and reconstructive. Patients with excess upper eyelid skin, for example, may describe dissatisfaction with their appearance as well as visual field deficits. During the preoperative consultation, the plastic surgeon must establish that the objectives of upper lid blepharoplasty are to both rejuvenate the upper eyelids and expand the visual field. A more challenging consideration of form and function occurs in children presenting with congenital facial nerve paralysis. In these patients, abnormalities of the facial nerve result in severe facial asymmetry that leads to devastating psychological consequences such as social isolation and difficulties with eating, speech articulation, emotional expression, and control of saliva. Frequently, the optimal solution for these cases is facial reanimation using a microsurgical transfer of an innervated muscle.[18] This reconstruction elevates the corner of the mouth and nasal ala on the paralyzed side to enhance resting facial symmetry and improve the dynamics of mastication, speech, and oral competence. Furthermore, because the muscle is innervated by a functional donor nerve at the recipient site, this operation can achieve animation of the paralyzed face, and in many instances, continued rehabilitation will result in spontaneous smiling.[19]

In some situations, restoration of form and function is accomplished through a surgical solution that replaces multiple tissue deficiencies. An illustrative example of this is reconstruction after pelvic exenteration for advanced colorectal cancer.[20] Removal of organs such as the bladder and rectum will result in a void in the pelvis, and occasionally, the extent of tumor invasion mandates resection of other structures such as the vagina and perianal skin. The goals of reconstruction in these cases are to recreate normal anatomy, obliterate dead spaces within the pelvis, and supply additional vascularity to a surgical site that often is subject to neoadjuvant radiation. One exceptionally suitable choice that fulfills many of these reconstructive needs is the oblique rectus abdominis myocutaneous (ORAM) flap.[21] The ORAM flap has long reach for a pedicled flap, comprises a large amount of soft tissue bulk, and possesses a highly reliable blood supply. Furthermore, the flap is capable of supporting a large skin paddle that can be used for resurfacing vaginal defects as well as perianal skin deficits. With proper surgical planning, the ORAM flap can achieve excellent form and function by filling the pelvic dead space with vascularized tissue after tumor resection, providing sufficient lining for vaginal reconstruction, and decreasing the tension of closure in the perineum to optimize wound healing.

PRINCIPLE VII: MINIMIZE DONOR SITE MORBIDITY

When donor tissues are required, the plastic surgeon must focus on minimizing the functional and cosmetic sacrifices to the patient. Each operation already possesses inherent risks relating to the surgical site, such as hematoma, infection, or abnormal scarring. The donor site adds an additional anatomic area where complications may arise, and the plastic surgeon must weigh the possibility of donor site morbidity against the benefits of the use of that tissue for reconstruction. Often, several suitable donor sites exist, and a surgeon's ultimate decision will be based upon careful consideration of the potential complications with each site. For example, during a rhinoplasty operation, structural support can be augmented by performing autologous cartilage grafting to the nasal framework.[22] Cartilage grafts can be harvested from the nasal septum, from the conchal bowl of the ear, or from the cartilaginous portion of a rib. The nasal septum would be an ideal donor site if septoplasty is also being performed, but use of this cartilage may cause further destabilization of the nasal framework and has a small risk of septal perforation. Harvest of conchal cartilage can provide adequate grafting material but may be complicated by hematoma, keloid formation, or ear asymmetry. The rib donor site offers an abundance of high-quality cartilage, but its indications must warrant the additional scar and added potential for pneumothorax. Ultimately, the plastic surgeon must choose the most appropriate donor site for reconstruction and justify the unique risks associated with that donor site.

To reduce donor site morbidity, plastic surgeons avoid unnecessary sacrifice of important adjacent anatomic structures. This focus on preservation of function during the harvest of donor tissues contributed to the advent of perforator flaps. For example, breast reconstruction using transverse rectus abdominis myocutaneous flaps commonly results in considerable abdominal wall morbidity, including bulges, hernias, and the need for mesh placement.[23] This morbidity is directly related to the removal of one or both rectus abdominis muscles from their native position, which weakens core strength and the integrity of the anterior abdominal wall. In contrast, the use of deep inferior epigastric perforator flaps for breast reconstruction is associated with lower morbidity to the abdominal donor site. During harvest of a deep inferior epigastric perforator flap, the perforating vessels supplying the skin and fat overlying the abdominal wall are meticulously dissected out of the rectus abdominis muscle, and every effort is made to maintain the continuity of the muscle. Segmental nerves are identified and protected whenever possible to preserve innervation to the rectus abdominis muscle, and a minimal amount of fascia is taken to reduce the tension of fascial closure. A continued ambition to limit donor site morbidity and extensive recent experience with perforator flap techniques have now led to the widespread use of many other workhorse perforator flaps for reconstruction, such as the anterolateral thigh (ALT) flap, the superior gluteal artery perforator flap, the thoracodorsal artery perforator flap, and the internal mammary artery perforator flap.[24]

PRINCIPLE VIII: PROTECT THE SURGICAL SITE POSTOPERATIVELY

In plastic surgery, an operation cannot be deemed fully successful at the time of its completion; instead, this evaluation can only be made several weeks to months after the operation. This interval allows for preliminary healing to occur, subsidence of postsurgical swelling, initiation of rehabilitation therapy, and management of any complications. During this critical time, the surgical site must be protected diligently to facilitate recovery and to prevent injury to the healing tissues. The plastic surgeon must actively counsel patients to follow strict activity restrictions and help patients understand the rationale behind the necessary postoperative protocols. Strenuous activity, for example, may increase the likelihood of bleeding, seroma, or wound dehiscence and should be avoided for a period of time that commensurates with the magnitude of the operation and its associated risks. Clear postoperative instructions are provided to patients and may include customized information on various relevant issues such as wound care, splinting, compression garments, weight-bearing status, or limb elevation. Regular follow-up visits are also necessary to ensure that wounds are healing appropriately and to recognize the development of any complications. All of these efforts are directed at protecting the surgical site. Failure to do so may jeopardize the final outcome.

Complex lower extremity reconstruction exemplifies the importance of this principle.[25] An open tibial fracture with a large soft-tissue defect can be reconstructed with a free muscle flap and skin grafting to provide durable coverage of the underlying bone and orthopedic hardware. However, postoperative protection of the surgical site is as influential to successful salvage of the limb as the reconstructive surgery itself.[26] After surgery, the free flap is safeguarded from compression, especially when the muscle extends posteriorly where it would be crushed by the weight of the limb without proper elevation. This can be done using pillows, blankets, or foam; alternatively, if the patient has an external fixator in place, attachments can be added to prop up the leg much like the kickstand of a bicycle. Limb elevation also opposes venous congestion and facilitates the resolution of postsurgical edema. Immobilization is also a critical component of the postoperative protocol because it safeguards the reconstruction from any shearing forces that might disrupt either the muscle or the skin graft. Plaster or plastic splints are useful adjuncts to aid in immobilization of joints after surgery. Although each clinical scenario is unique, soft tissues generally require several weeks of protected healing time before being able to sustain any significant challenges. Therefore, once this initial healing period has occurred, a gradual and supervised release of these restrictions is commenced until complete return to normal activities is possible.

PRINCIPLE IX: HAVE A BACKUP PLAN (AND A BACKUP PLAN FOR THAT BACKUP PLAN)

Complications will always arise, and the prepared plastic surgeon will be ready with multiple contingency plans. Most commonly, complications such as wound infection, marginal flap necrosis, or dehiscence can be successfully managed with straightforward and standardized treatment protocols. However, occasionally, the first operative plan fails to adequately address the goals of surgery, and a new plan is necessary. In reconstructive surgery, an old paradigm known as the *reconstructive ladder* advocates for a linear, stepwise approach to surgical problems whereby less-complicated surgical techniques are initially attempted, and progression up the ladder to more complex strategies is pursued only when needed. More recently, significant advancements in the field of plastic surgery have led to a shift away from this paradigm in favor of a treatment algorithm that encourages selection of the most definitive method for reconstruction even if it means picking a more complex one first.[27] If a backup plan is necessary, the plastic surgeon may either choose an alternative surgical plan from another rung of the reconstructive ladder or decide to try the previous plan again. Despite the antiquated adage in plastic surgery that instructs: "Make sure that plan B is not the same as plan A," the same approach may in fact be attempted if careful consideration is given to the reasons why the prior surgery resulted in a failed reconstruction. If these factors can be readily identified and appropriately corrected, the same operative strategy may be performed another time and a successful outcome can be expected.

Reconstruction of upper extremity defects frequently exemplifies this fundamental principle. For example, a dorsal hand wound from a full-thickness burn injury with several exposed extensor tendons and metacarpal bones can be reconstructed by numerous techniques.[28] Although less-sophisticated approaches such as dermal substitutes and skin grafting may ultimately result in a closed wound, these options would not provide sufficiently durable soft tissue coverage over gliding tendons and therefore would result in unacceptable hand stiffness. A superior first choice for reconstruction might be a reverse radial forearm flap from the ipsilateral extremity or another regional flap. Should the plastic surgeon encounter insurmountable complications with the reverse radial forearm flap, a reasonable backup plan might entail the use of a free gracilis muscle flap. If the free flap reconstruction fails, the next backup option might be another free tissue transfer as long as the problems that led to loss of the previous flap are elucidated and the surgeon is confident that these issues can be sufficiently overcome prior to performing another free flap. Alternatively, the plastic surgeon might choose to reconstruct the dorsal hand wound with a pedicled groin flap. This fundamental principle of having a series of sensible backup plans guides the plastic surgeon to prepare for any number of potential setbacks during the reconstructive process and serves to optimize the chances of successful surgical outcomes.

PRINCIPLE X: INNOVATE NEW SOLUTIONS TO OLD PROBLEMS

Innovation drives the practice and progress of plastic surgery. Plastic surgeons possess an inherent ambition to improve surgical approaches to existing clinical problems. For this reason, rarely is the exact same operation ever performed twice. Each surgery is individualized according to the clinical situation and specific patient needs. Thus, the plastic surgeon must strive to tailor every operation and often makes numerous adjustments to the accepted *standard techniques*. For example, a cleft lip repair for one child is never precisely the same as that for another child.[29] Although the basic tenets are constant, such as restoring continuity of the orbicularis oris and re-establishing labial subunits, the surgeon must remain flexible during the operation and modify the repair technique to account for the unique abnormalities present in each patient.

This spirit of adaptation and creative problem-solving is a large part of what distinguishes plastic surgery from other surgical disciplines and contributes to the constant evolution of the specialty. Over the course of the last century, plastic surgery has undergone enormous cycles of change that has resulted in significant paradigm shifts in patient care. One of the most profound examples is the advent of microsurgery. Previously, wounds resulting from tumor extirpation, infection, or trauma were reconstructed with either devascularized grafts that were often too thin to provide reliable soft tissue coverage or pedicle flaps that were frequently limited in reach or size. With the development of the operating microscope in the 1960s and a concomitant surge in our understanding of the vascular anatomy of muscle and myocutaneous flaps,[30-33] plastic surgery experienced an explosion of innovation and growth. The ability to raise and transfer a variety of tissue types as free flaps opened an entire realm of reconstructive solutions for problems that were once deemed impossible. For instance, distal third injuries of the lower extremity that commonly resulted in amputation could now be reconstructed with a free flap. Free tissue transfer quickly became the primary reconstructive choice after head and neck cancer resection. Hand surgery was completely revolutionized by the ability to replant amputated parts and reconstruct challenging defects of the upper extremity through the use of free flaps consisting of a variety of tissues including skin, muscle, fascia, and bone. More recently, microsurgical techniques have made vascularized composite allotransplantation a reality, and replacement of an entire complex anatomic structure such as a face, hand, or abdominal wall is now being performed at multiple centers around the world.[34-36]

Plastic surgery will no doubt continue to be at the vanguard of innovating solutions to surgical problems. Plastic surgeons are spearheading ongoing research and development in a variety of emerging fields that are gaining increasing momentum, including tissue engineering,[37] transplant immunosuppression,[38] supermicrosurgery,[39] prosthetic interfaces,[40] perforator flap surgery,[41] and robotic surgery.[42] The ensuing chapters of this textbook will illustrate the persistent evolution of plastic surgery and demonstrate how numerous critical innovations in the field have completely transformed the care of our patients. Additionally, while each chapter will focus on a different aspect of plastic surgery, the reader will appreciate frequent allusions to the themes presented in this introduction and understand that plastic surgery is truly a specialty characterized by a devotion to a set of fundamental principles that guides its practice.

ACKNOWLEDGMENT

This work was supported by the American Association of Plastic Surgeons Academic Scholar Program to Theodore A. Kung and a Midcareer Investigator Award in Patient-Oriented Research (2 K24-AR053120-06) to Kevin C. Chung. The content is solely the responsibility of the authors and does not necessarily represent the official views of the American Association of Plastic Surgeons or the National Institutes of Health.

REFERENCES

1. Gillies HD, Millard DR. *The Principles and Art of Plastic Surgery*. Boston: Little, Brown & Co; 1957.
   Ambroise Pare is often credited as the first to publish a set of five plastic surgery principles in 1564. However, this classic text by Gilles and Millard modernized the idea that the practice of plastic surgery is guided by fundamental principles. The principles compiled in this book reflect Gilles' distinguished career, including his experience treating countless wounded patients during World War I.
2. Millard DR. *Principalization of Plastic Surgery*. Boston, MA: Little Brown & Co; 1986.
   Three decades after the publication of The Principles and Art of Plastic Surgery, *Millard published this second text, elaborating on 33 principles of plastic surgery. This collection of principles was organized in various categories and included innovational principles as well as inspirational principles.*
3. Waljee J, McGlinn EP, Sears ED, Chung KC. Patient expectations and patient-reported outcomes in surgery: a systematic review. *Surgery*. 2014;155(5):799-808.
4. *The Health Consequences of Smoking – 50 Years of Progress: A Report of the Surgeon General*. Atlanta, GA: US Department of Health and Human Services, Centers for Disease Control and Prevention, National Center for Chronic Disease Prevention and Health Promotion, Office on Smoking and Health; 2014. https://www.cdc.gov/tobacco/data_statistics/sgr/50th-anniversary/index.htm. Accessed February 22, 2018.
5. Centers for Disease Control and Prevention. Current cigarette smoking among adults—United States, 2016. *MMWR*. 2018;67(2):53-59.
6. Rinker B. The evils of nicotine: an evidence-based guide to smoking and plastic surgery. *Ann Plast Surg*. 2013;70(5):599-605.
   This is an excellent review of the detrimental effects of nicotine on wound healing and summarizes the known effects of smoking on plastic surgery patients. The article also discusses smoking cessation methods and emphasizes the importance of quitting at least 4 weeks prior to a planned operation.
7. Harrison B, Khansa I, Janis JE. Evidence-based strategies to reduce postoperative complications in plastic surgery. *Plast Reconstr Surg*. 2016;137(1):351-360.
8. Rubin JP, Nguyen V, Schwentker A. Perioperative management of the post-gastric-bypass patient presenting for body contour surgery. *Clin Plast Surg*. 2004;31(4):601-610, vi.
9. Anghel EL, DeFazio MV, Barker JC, et al. Current concepts in debridement: science and strategies. *Plast Reconstr Surg*. 2016;138(3 Suppl):82S-93S.
10. Leland HA, Rounds AD, Burtt KE, et al. Soft tissue reconstruction and salvage of infected fixation hardware in lower extremity trauma. *Microsurgery*. 2018;38(3):259-263.
11. Kwok AC, Simpson AM, Willcockson J, et al. Complications and their associations following the surgical repair of pressure ulcers. *Am J Surg*. 2018;216(6):1177-1181.
12. Patel SY, Itani K. Review of eyelid reconstruction techniques after Mohs surgery. *Semin Plast Surg*. 2018;32(2):95-102.
13. Largo RD, Garvey PB. Updates in head and neck reconstruction. *Plast Reconstr Surg*. 2018;141(2):271e-285e.
14. Razzak MA, Hossain MS, Radzi ZB, et al. Cellular and molecular responses to mechanical expansion of tissue. *Front Physiol*. 2016;7:540.
15. Buchman SR, Muraszko K. Frontoorbital reconstruction. *Atlas Oral Maxillofac Surg Clin North Am*. 2002;10(1):43-56.
16. Lee JC, Bradley JP. Surgical considerations in Pierre Robin sequence. *Clin Plast Surg*. 2014;41(2):211-217.
17. Lucas JB. The physiology and biomechanics of skin flaps. *Facial Plast Surg Clin North Am*. 2017;25(3):303-311.
18. Kim J. Neural reanimation advances and new technologies. *Facial Plast Surg Clin North Am*. 2016;24(1):71-84.
19. Dong A, Zuo KJ, Papadopoulos-Nydam G, et al. Functional outcomes assessment following free muscle transfer for dynamic reconstruction of facial paralysis: a literature review. *J Craniomaxillofac Surg*. 2018;46(5):875-882.
20. Nelson RA, Butler CE. Surgical outcomes of VRAM versus thigh flaps for immediate reconstruction of pelvic and perineal cancer resection defects. *Plast Reconstr Surg*. 2009;123(1):175-183.
21. Lee MJ, Dumanian GA. The oblique rectus abdominis musculocutaneous flap: revisited clinical applications. *Plast Reconstr Surg*. 2004;114(2):367-373.
22. Sajjadian A, Rubinstein R, Naghshineh N. Current status of grafts and implants in rhinoplasty: part I. Autologous grafts. *Plast Reconstr Surg*. 2010;125(2):40e-49e.
23. Shubinets V, Fox JP, Sarik JR, et al. Surgically treated hernia following abdominally based autologous breast reconstruction: prevalence, outcomes, and expenditures. *Plast Reconstr Surg*. 2016;137(3):749-757.
24. Geddes CR, Morris SF, Neligan PC. Perforator flaps: evolution, classification, and applications. *Ann Plast Surg*. 2003;50(1):90-99.
   This comprehensive review describes the advent, advantages, and disadvantages of perforator flaps. In addition, it provides a discussion of the most commonly used perforator flaps in reconstructive surgery.
25. Soltanian H, Garcia RM, Hollenbeck ST. Current concepts in lower extremity reconstruction. *Plast Reconstr Surg*. 2015;136(6):815e-829e.
26. Rohde C, Howell BW, Buncke GM, et al. A recommended protocol for the immediate postoperative care of lower extremity free-flap reconstructions. *J Reconstr Microsurg*. 2009;25(1):15-19.
27. Gottlieb LJ, Krieger LM. From the reconstructive ladder to the reconstructive elevator. *Plast Reconstr Surg*. 1994;93(7):1503-1504.
28. Bashir MM, Sohail M, Shami HB. Traumatic wounds of the upper extremity: coverage strategies. *Hand Clin*. 2018;34(1):61-74.

29. Greives MR, Camison L, Losee JE. Evidence-based medicine: unilateral cleft lip and nose repair. *Plast Reconstr Surg*. 2014;134(6):1372-1380.
30. Jacobson JH, Suarez EL. Microvascular surgery. *Dis Chest*. 1962;41:220-224.
31. Buncke HJ, Schulz WP. Experimental digital amputation and replantation. *Plast Reconstr Surg*. 1965;36:62-70.
32. Buncke HJ, Schulz WP. Total ear reimplantation in the rabbit utilising microminiature vascular anastomoses. *Br J Plast Surg*. 1966;19(1):15-22.
The pioneering work of Buncke, among others, provided the essential foundation that led to an incredible transformation in the field of microsurgery. This study presents the use of specially designed microsurgical instruments to anastomose vessels less than 1 mm in diameter in a rabbit ear model.
33. Mathes SJ, Nahai F. Classification of the vascular anatomy of muscles: experimental and clinical correlation. *Plast Reconstr Surg*. 1981;67(2):177-187.
This landmark publication by Mathes and Nahai classifies muscle flaps into five distinct categories based on patterns of vascular anatomy. An increased comprehension of the blood supply of muscle flaps expanded the reconstructive utility of these flaps in various clinical scenarios and contributed to the subsequent development of perforator flaps.
34. Siemionow M. The decade of face transplant outcomes. *J Mater Sci Mater Med*. 2017;28(5):64.
35. Shores JT, Malek V, Lee WPA, Brandacher G. Outcomes after hand and upper extremity transplantation. *J Mater Sci Mater Med*. 2017;28(5):72.
36. Patel NG, Ratanshi I, Buchel EW. The best of abdominal wall reconstruction. *Plast Reconstr Surg*. 2018;141(1):113e-136e.
37. Levi B, Longaker MT. Concise review: adipose-derived stromal cells for skeletal regenerative medicine. *Stem Cells*. 2011;29(4):576-582.
38. Chang J, Graves SS, Butts-Miwongtum T, et al. Long-term tolerance toward haploidentical vascularized composite allograft transplantation in a canine model using bone marrow or mobilized stem cells. *Transplantation*. 2016;100(12):e120-e127.
39. Badash I, Gould DJ, Patel KM. Supermicrosurgery: history, applications, training and the future. *Front Surg*. 2018;5:23
40. Kung TA, Bueno RA, Alkhalefah GK, et al. Innovations in prosthetic interfaces for the upper extremity. *Plast Reconstr Surg*. 2013;132(6):1515-1523.
41. Koh K, Goh TLH, Song CT, et al. Free versus pedicled perforator flaps for lower extremity reconstruction: a multicenter comparison of institutional practices and outcomes. *J Reconstr Microsurg*. April. 34(8):572-580. doi:10.1055/s-0038-1639576.
42. Selber JC. Robotic surgery. *J Reconstr Microsurg*. 2012;28(7):433-434.

QUESTIONS

1. A 55-year-old woman with long-standing bilateral symptomatic macromastia presents to the office to discuss breast reduction surgery. Her medical history is significant for hypertension and obesity with a body mass index of 39. During the consultation, the plastic surgeon notices a faint smell of cigarette smoke in the room. The patient states she quit smoking 6 months ago but her husband still smokes in the house. What course of action will result in the most favorable patient outcomes?

a. Perform the surgery after thoroughly discussing the risks of the operation.
b. Refer the patient to another plastic surgeon.
c. Defer the operation until modifiable risk factors are addressed.
d. Refuse to perform the operation because it will not benefit the patient.
e. Perform the surgery but remove as little breast tissue as possible.

2. A 45-year-old man with vascular disease presents with a nonhealing wound on the medial ankle. Workup is negative for underlying infection, and a reverse sural artery flap is planned for reconstruction to provide durable soft tissue coverage over the wound. The plastic surgeon is concerned about the blood supply to this flap. What can be done to optimize vascularity?

a. Keep the foot in a dependent position after reconstruction.
b. Perform a delay operation first and then the definitive operation 2 weeks later.
c. Apply nitroglycerin ointment to the proximal lower extremity to dilate the vasculature.
d. Apply compression wraps to the lower extremity after the flap is inset.
e. Place the patient on a high-protein diet to improve preoperative nutrition.

3. A 65-year-old woman undergoes abdominoperineal resection followed by reconstruction using a pedicled ORAM flap. On postoperative day 1, the plastic surgeon examines the skin paddle of the ORAM flap within the perineum and notes that the flap is mottled with several areas of blistering. It is noted that the patient has been in an upright sitting position since she arrived to the floor after her operation. Which fundamental plastic surgery principle was most likely not heeded?

a. Make an informed decision to operate or not operate.
b. Perform adequate debridement prior to reconstruction.
c. If possible, replace like with like.
d. Protect the surgical site postoperatively.
e. Have a backup plan.

4. An 8-year-old boy presents with a 5 cm × 4 cm full-thickness burn of the plantar foot. After adequate debridement and dressing changes, the wound is now ready for reconstruction. There is healthy granulation tissue throughout, and there are no exposed critical structures such as bone or tendon. Which of the following reconstructive options is the best choice for this patient?

a. Letting the wound heal secondarily with dressing changes
b. Free ALT flap
c. Applying a negative pressure device to expedite secondary healing
d. Split-thickness skin from the thigh
e. Full-thickness skin from the lower abdomen

5. A 50-year-old woman undergoes excision of a large squamous cell carcinoma from the scalp. The resultant defect is approximately 40% of the total area of the hair-bearing scalp. A temporary dressing is placed on the wound until final negative margins are confirmed by pathology. The open wound is now ready for reconstruction. There is no exposed calvarium, and the wound consists of healthy granulation tissue and galea aponeurotica. The patient desires a reconstruction that will optimize the appearance of the scalp. Which of the following reconstructive options is the best choice for this patient?

a. Elevate multiple rotation-advancement flaps from the remaining scalp to close the wound with one operation.
b. Apply a negative pressure device now and then perform split-thickness skin grafting in a separate operation.
c. Perform a free latissimus dorsi muscle flap with split-thickness skin grafting.
d. Close the wound with a split-thickness skin graft now and then place tissue expanders in a separate operation to expand the remaining hair-bearing scalp.
e. Apply a dermal substitute now, and then perform full-thickness skin grafting in a separate operation.

1. Answer: c. The plastic surgeon should make an informed decision to defer the operation until a later date. This patient has several modifiable risk factors that significantly increase the likelihood of postoperative complications. Patients who are obese have a higher risk of wound healing complications after breast reduction surgery. In addition, she is living with an active smoker, and therefore the second-hand smoke will further contribute to wound healing difficulties. Preoperative interventions such as weight loss, smoking cessation, and control of hypertension will reduce her risks of experiencing complications.

2. Answer: b. During a delay operation, the plastic surgeon partially raises a flap and then waits 1 to 2 weeks before fully elevating the flap. This results in opening of choke vessels within the tissues and enhances the vascularity of the flap. The other answers do not directly improve the inherent vascularity of a flap.

3. Answer: d. Postoperative protection of the surgical site can be as important as the reconstruction itself. The patient has been sitting immediately after perineal reconstruction, and this is causing vascular compromise of the ORAM flap. Once this problem is identified, safeguards must be in place to offload the flap to avoid further tissue injury or else the entire reconstruction may be jeopardized. The other fundamental principles that are listed may very well have been followed during the patient's perineal reconstruction.

4. Answer: e. When selecting a donor site to close a wound, the plastic surgeon must choose the most reliable tissue for reconstruction while minimizing donor site morbidity. Plantar wounds that demonstrate healthy granulation tissue without exposure of critical structures can be resurfaced with a skin graft. In this location, a full-thickness skin graft is preferable to a split-thickness skin graft because it results in a more durable reconstruction on the weight-bearing surface of the foot. Letting the wound heal secondarily (choices a and c) would result in more scarring and possibly contractures of the toes. A free ALT flap may be considered for more complex wounds with exposed critical structures.

5. Answer: d. The primary goals in this case are to close the wound and to optimize the appearance of the scalp. The best tissue to replace lost hair-bearing scalp is the patient's own hair-bearing scalp, but in this case the size of the wound precludes the success of local flap options (choice a). Because the base of the wound consists of healthy granulation tissue and galea aponeurotica, a split-thickness skin graft is an appropriate choice to close the wound. Subsequently, after the skin graft is well healed, tissue expanders are placed to slowly grow the hair-bearing scalp. When sufficient growth has been achieved, an operation is performed to remove the implants and excise the split-thickness skin graft, and then the expanded hair-bearing scalp is used to resurface the wound. Scalp defects up to approximately 50% of the hair-bearing scalp can be reconstructed in this manner. A free flap operation (choice c) is not indicated in this scenario because there are no exposed critical structures and because it does not provide hair-bearing tissue. Choices b and e are incorrect because there is no need to delay skin grafting because the wound already consists of healthy vascularized tissue.

CHAPTER 2 Basic Science of Wound Healing and Management of Chronic Wounds

Buket Gundogan and Dennis P. Orgill

KEY POINTS

- Wounds present with a discontinuity of tissue and rely on complex processes for healing to occur. Most wound healing research focuses on molecular and cellular pathways, but we now appreciate the importance of the extracellular matrix (ECM) and mechanical forces. Classically, wound healing has been summarized into four phases: (1) hemostasis, (2) inflammation, (3), proliferation, and (4) remodeling.
- Aberrant wound healing occurs when normal pathways are disrupted, most commonly in the inflammatory or proliferative phases leading to chronic wounds.
- The most common chronic wounds are arterial ulcers, pressure injuries, venous stasis ulceration, and diabetic foot ulcers.
- Other factors that adversely affect wound healing include radiation therapy, nutrition, and microorganisms.
- Healing strategies involve keeping the wound moist, platelet-derived wound healing techniques, biological skin equivalents, topical growth factors, stem cells, scaffolds, and the application of biophysical forces.

BASIC SCIENCE OF WOUND HEALING

Wound healing is a complex and highly coordinated biological process. A sound understanding of the traditional stages of wound repair underpins many aspects of wound healing research. The four phases of wound healing—hemostasis, inflammation, proliferation, and remodeling—do not follow a simple and linear chronological order but overlap in time and are densely interconnected. Importantly, increasing research has demonstrated the importance of mechanical forces and the extracellular matrix (ECM) in wound healing biology (**Figure 2.1**).

Classic Stages of Wound Healing

Hemostasis

Tissue injury and the consequent damage to capillary blood vessels initiates the coagulation cascade through the activation of fibrinogen. This activation results in the formation of platelet aggregation and fibrin scaffold that stems blood loss and allows for the migration of cells. Platelets play a critical role in the stages of wound healing and in particular are the chief effector cells during hemostasis. In addition to contributing to the hemostatic plug, their cytoplasm contains α-granules that release several growth factors and cytokines, such as platelet-derived growth factor (PDGF) and transforming growth factor-β (TGF-β), which facilitate wound healing by attracting neutrophils, macrophages, and fibroblasts.[1,2] Platelets are also responsible for releasing several proangiogenic and antiangiogenic growth factors that are critical for revascularization of wounds, such as vascular endothelial growth factor (VEGF) and platelet-derived stromal cell–derived factor 1 (SDF-1).

Inflammation

The coagulation cascade, the activation of complement, and bacterial degradation facilitate and trigger the inflammatory phase, which typically lasts 48 hours.[3] These pathways produce various chemotactic factors (such as TGF-β) and complement components (such as C3a and C5a) to attract inflammatory cells to the scaffold. Neutrophils invade the wound and phagocytose foreign debris, followed by monocytes that eventually differentiate into macrophages and further consume debris in their paths.[2] Macrophages are responsible for releasing a whole host of mediators primarily through binding to integrin receptors on the ECM, such as tumor necrosis factor α and interleukin-1 (IL-1)[4] (**Figure 2.2**). These proinflammatory cytokines stimulate fibroblast infiltration from the surrounding healthy ECM. It is important to note that macrophage invasion is critical to the inflammatory phase because macrophage-defective or macrophage-depleted animals undergo abnormal wound healing.[5]

Proliferation

From approximately 48 hours to 10 days after tissue injury, healing enters the proliferation phase (**Figure 2.3**). Keratinocytes migrate to eventually proliferating enough to create an epithelial layer that covers the wound. This is directly stimulated by epidermal growth factors, heparin-binding epidermal growth factor (HB-EGF), and transforming growth factor-alpha (TGF-α), which are the main members of the epidermal growth factor family involved in wound healing.[6] Fibroblasts are also critical to this stage of wound healing, as they produce collagen that acts as a scaffold for a vascular network. The hypoxic environment increases expression of hypoxia-inducible factor 1 (HIF-1α) protein to serve as the primary stimulus of angiogenesis.[7] HIF-1α activates several target genes such as VEGF and SDF-1 to induce neovascularization.[7] Fibroblasts and macrophages replace the fibrin mesh to form granulation tissue. Granulation tissue, also known as new stroma, consists of new connective tissue (specifically hyaluronic acid, procollagen, elastin, and proteoglycan) and blood vessels. It owes its granular appearance to the new capillary network.[1] The formation of blood vessel networks increases oxygen supply to the wound surface. Finally, fibroblasts that have differentiated into myofibroblasts have contractile ability to assist in bringing the wound edges together in a process known as wound contraction.[8]

Remodeling

The fourth and final stage of wound healing is the remodeling phase, which starts at approximately 2 weeks and can last for years. Throughout this stage, many of the cells contained in the wound undergo apoptosis or exit the wound, to eventually leave collagen and ECM proteins. This entire matrix is remodeled and strengthened from type III collagen into mainly type I collagen by matrix metalloproteinases (MMPs). MMPs are produced by fibroblasts as well as other cell types. The wound eventually forms scar tissue and never fully regains complete strength comparable to undamaged skin, at approximately 80% normal strength.[9] The ECM is also implicated in the formation of scarring. Cutaneous scar tissue is composed of the same ECM macromolecules as normal tissue but contains different ratios of these macromolecules and typically an absence of hair follicles or fat.[10] Increased levels of TGF-β1 have been implicated in hypertrophic adult scars.[11]

Mechanical Forces in Wound Healing

Human cells and tissues are subjected to many biophysical forces such as electrical, magnetic, and mechanical forces. These forces have various biological effects, and here we specifically discuss mechanical forces. Mechanical forces on cells include but are not limited to tension, shear force, gravity, and osmosis.[12] It is now clear that all phases of wound healing are affected by mechanical forces. In a process known as mechanotransduction, cells have the ability to detect mechanical stimuli in its microenvironment and respond by activating specific cellular pathways. These pathways can modulate cell functions such as proliferation, migration, and differentiation.

Focal adhesion (FA) complexes that are transmembrane proteins to anchor the cell cytoskeleton to other cells or the ECM are key to understanding mechanotransduction. FA complexes contain integrins, which act as primary receptors for the ECM.[13] This process of anchorage generates intracellular mechanical tension and serves not only to sense the wound microenvironment but also to modify its behavior and the surrounding ECM.

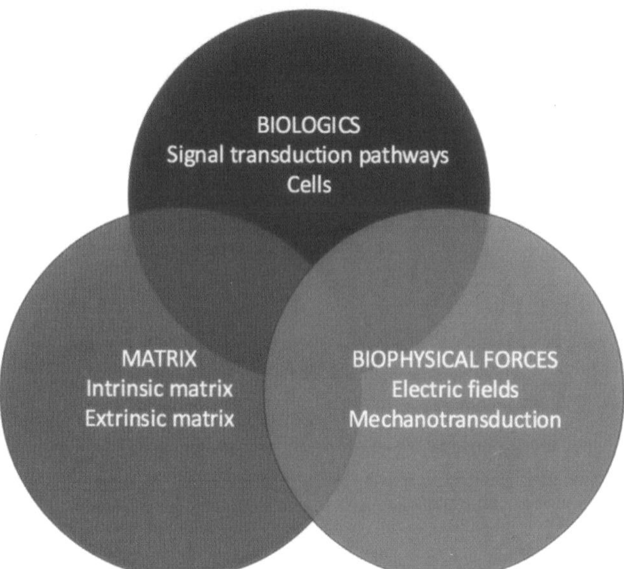

FIGURE 2.1. Factors involved in wound healing. Wound healing strategies involve the use of biologics (in particular cells and signal transduction pathways influenced by growth factors), matrix (intrinsic extracellular matrix proteins and extrinsic mechanical forces), and biophysical forces (electric fields and mechanotransduction). These domains have considerable overlap.

Cell migration is of critical importance in wound healing and mechanical forces are key to this. Tension generated by the cytoskeleton-integrin connections pulls the cell cytoplasm of the leading edge forward in a process known as protrusion. At the same time protein complexes of the trailing edge must disconnect from the ECM, resulting in the entire cell body moving forward and the cell producing traction forces.[13] Fibroblasts are thought to generate cell traction forces that are much greater than needed for cell migration, and this excess force deforms the ECM contributing to collagen reorganization in wound healing.[14] Similarly, mechanical forces involved in cellular migration also occur during epithelial repair and restoration.

It is also known that cell proliferation is influenced by mechanical stress, which can be defined as the force per unit area. Keratinocytes respond to mechanical stress by changing morphology, such as stretching, and these mechanotransduction pathways regulate cell proliferation. For example, cells without mechanical stress or stimuli adopt a spherical shape and enter cell-cycle arrest and apoptosis.[15]

Electric fields also play an important role in wound healing. Transepithelial electric potentials are created by the movement of ions across pumps in the epithelium, termed the *skin battery*. Damage to the continuous epithelium generates a current of injury whereby electric potential is directed toward the wound to signal cell migration, termed *electrotaxis*.[16] Studies have demonstrated that influencing such electric fields can alter wound healing in vivo.[16]

The effect of mechanical stimuli on the wound microenvironment is utilized by treatments, such as negative-pressure wound therapy (NPWT) and extracorporeal shock wave therapy (ESWT), which are explained in later sections.

Extracellular Matrix in Wound Healing

The ECM is a meshlike dynamic structure composed of different macromolecules and proteolytic enzymes. These macromolecules include collagen, elastin, glycosaminoglycans, glycoproteins, and proteoglycans. The ECM plays an important role in wound healing. Its function includes providing organization for cells as a physical scaffold, storage for growth factors, controlling cell shape, cell metabolism, and influences many cell behaviors such as migration, proliferation, and differentiation (**Figure 2.4**).

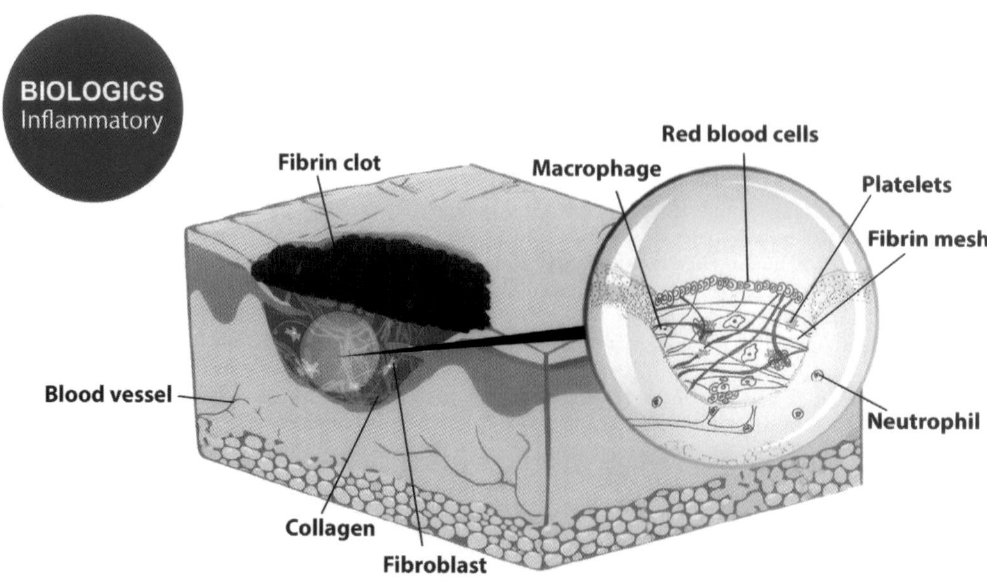

FIGURE 2.2. Inflammatory phase of wound healing. The inflammatory phase typically lasts 48 hours. Neutrophils invade the wound and phagocytose foreign debris, followed by monocytes that eventually differentiate into macrophages, which further consume debris in their paths.

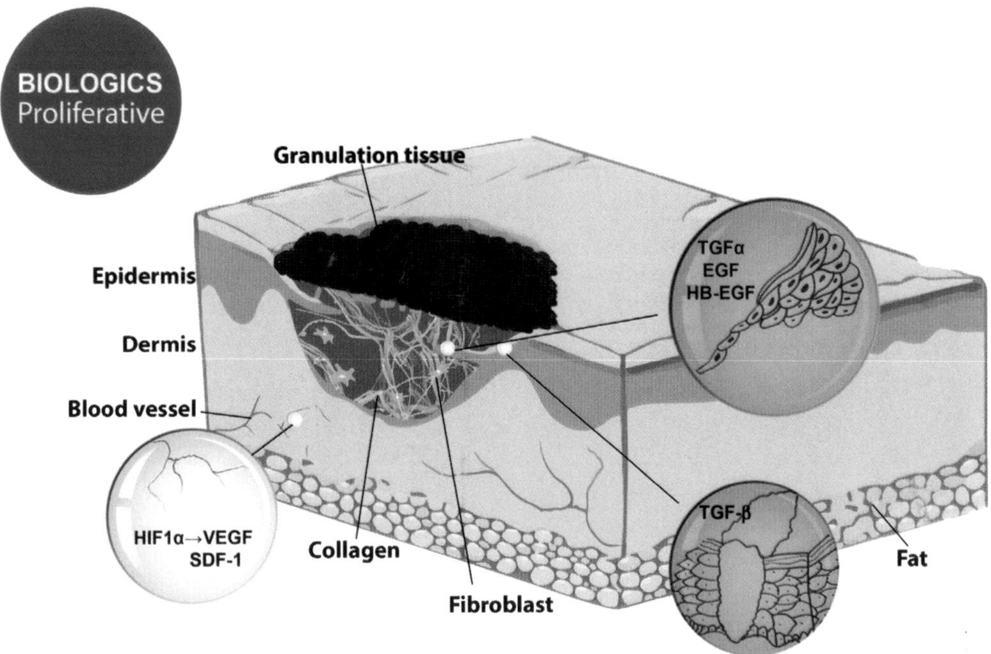

FIGURE 2.3. Proliferative phase of wound healing. During the proliferative phase, the hypoxic environment increases expression of hypoxia-inducible factor 1 (HIF-1α) protein, which is the primary stimulus of angiogenesis. Further downstream growth factors influencing the vascular network include vascular endothelial growth factor (VEGF) and platelet-derived stromal cell–derived factor 1 (SDF-1). Keratinocytes also migrate eventually proliferating enough to create an epithelial layer that covers the wound. This is directly stimulated by epidermal growth factors (EGFs), heparin-binding epidermal growth factor (HB-EGF), and transforming growth factor-alpha (TGF-α), which are the main members of the EGF family involved in wound healing. Factors such as transforming growth factor-β (TGF-β) facilitate wound healing by attracting neutrophils, macrophages, and fibroblasts.

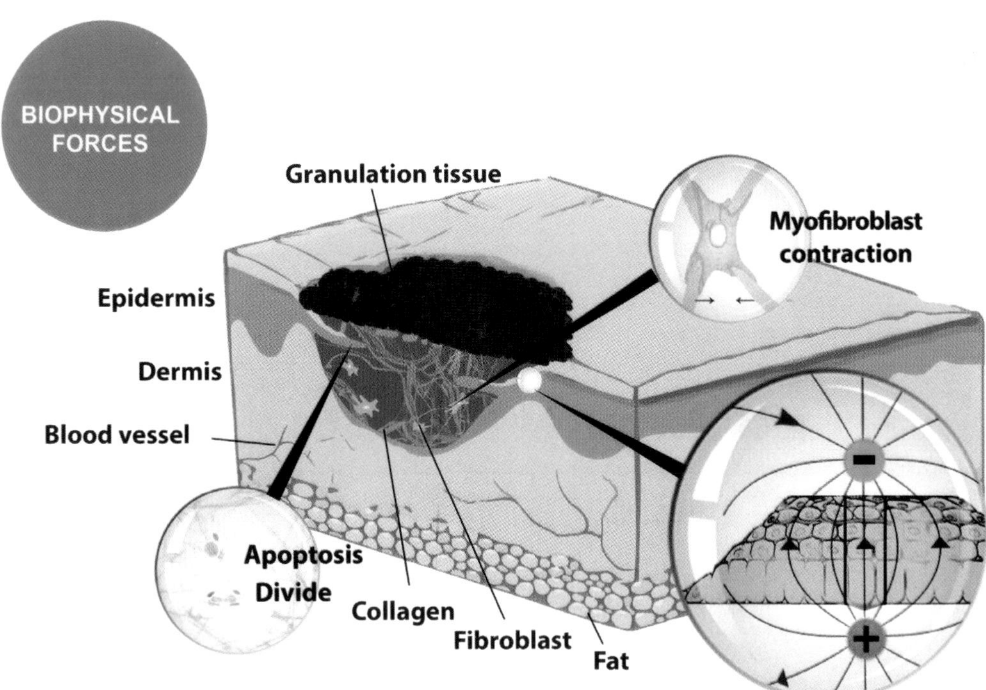

FIGURE 2.4. Biophysical forces in wound healing. Several biophysical forces influence wound healing. In a process known as mechanotransduction, cells have the ability to detect mechanical stimuli in its microenvironment and respond by activating specific cellular pathways. For example, cells without mechanical stress or stimuli adopt a spherical shape and enter cell-cycle arrest and apoptosis. Myofibroblasts also contract and exert tension on the extracellular matrix. Damage to the continuous epithelium generates a current of injury whereby electric potential is directed toward the wound, which has been shown to signal cell migration, termed *electrotaxis*.

The composition, density, and stiffness of the ECM influence the wound microenvironment. In newly injured tissue, ECM is soft and fibrin-rich and this change initiates a repair process of fibroblast differentiation into myofibroblasts that contract and exert tension on the surrounding ECM.

After cutaneous tissue injury, mechanical forces activate the focal adhesion kinase pathway. This pathway is known to be the main regulator of FAs. The focal adhesion kinase pathway has been shown to potentiate the secretion collagen, as well as monocyte chemoattractant protein-1, which has been linked to human fibrosis.[17,18]

The most prominent glycosaminoglycan, hyaluronic acid (hyaluronan) is known to interact with cell surface receptors, mainly CD-44 and RHAMM (*r*eceptor for *h*yaluron*a*n-*m*ediated *m*obility) to trigger a cascade of processes involved in wound healing, such as modulation of inflammation, chemotaxis, cell migration, collagen secretion, and angiogenesis.[19]

ABERRANT WOUND HEALING

Chronic Wounds

Chronic wounds can be defined as a loss of continuity of the skin secondary to injury that persist for longer than 6 weeks. Chronic wounds are classified into vascular ulcers (arterial and venous), diabetic ulcers, and pressure ulcers. Despite each type of wound having different underlying pathologies, they all share common features such as an excessive and persistent inflammatory phase, impaired cell proliferation, abnormal cell migration, microbial colonization, the presence of biofilms, and ultimately an inability to complete all four phases of wound healing within the normal timeframe. However, they each have distinct pathophysiologies, which are further discussed in this section.

Vascular Ulcers

Vascular ulcers include venous, arterial, or mixed etiology. It has been reported that ulcers related to venous insufficiency constitute 70%, arterial disease 10%, and ulcers of mixed etiology 15% of leg ulcer presentations. The remaining 5% of leg ulcers result from less common pathophysiological causes.

Venous Ulcers

Chronic venous leg ulceration is common and is thought to occur in up to 5% of the population older than 65 years.[20] Venous ulcers are classically distributed in the *gaiter area* on the medial aspect between the knee and ankle. They occur secondary to venous insufficiency where there is valvular incompetence in veins, and the resulting backflow of blood results in increased venous pressure. This leads to capillary leakage of plasma constituents into the surrounding perivascular area, such as fibrin, which is known to decrease collagen production.[21]

The primary pathological events leading to venous disease and therefore venous ulceration are changes in the vein wall and vein valve environment. Elevated venous pressures change shear stress and mechanical forces, which are then detected by endothelial cell intercellular adhesion molecule-1 (ICAM-1, CD54) and the mechanosensitive transient receptor potential vanilloid channels. The endothelial cells respond by secreting vasoactive molecules to begin an inflammatory cascade, ultimately leading to the progression of venous disease.[22]

Arterial Ulcers

Arterial ulcers occur because of arterial insufficiency where there is narrowing of the arterial lumen most commonly secondary to atherosclerosis. They are classically located over bony prominences including the toes, heels, and ankles. Apart from atherosclerosis, other conditions that cause arterial obstruction include embolism, diabetes mellitus, vasculitis, pyoderma gangrenosum, and hematological disorders of sickle cell disease and thalassemia.

Diabetic Foot Ulcers

The prevalence of diabetic foot ulcers in individuals with diabetes mellitus is common and occurs in approximately 15% of patients over their lifetime.[23] There are several pathophysiological factors that contribute to aberrant healing in diabetic individuals. These include abnormal and chronic inflammatory response, hyperglycemia, microvascular abnormalities, hypoxia, and changes of the ECM scaffold. Peripheral neuropathy, peripheral arterial disease, and trauma also contribute to diabetic ulceration.

Chronic inflammation and an impaired inflammatory response is also the hallmark of diabetic wounds. Studies have demonstrated persistent and raised levels of proinflammatory cytokines, such as IL-1, IL-6, and tumor necrosis factor α.[24] Wounds also typically have imbalances in protease production and their inhibitors, which stop normal matrix synthesis and remodeling.[25]

Hyperglycemia leads to nonenzymatic binding of sugar residues to proteins through free amino acid groups, and further alterations lead to advanced glycation end-products. Advanced glycation end-products are known to decrease the solubility of the ECM and exacerbate the inflammatory changes.[26] Glycation of the ECM is linked to cell apoptosis and disruption of normal wound healing processes such as angiogenesis, cell migration, and proliferation.[27] High levels of glucose induce expression of MMP by fibroblasts, endothelial cells, and macrophages to break down the matrix.

Oxygen supply to a wound is also essential for healing, and hypoxic environments adversely affect wound healing. Chronic hyperglycemia prolongs inflammation and delays wound healing by increasing the levels of free radicals.[26]

Pressure Injuries

The pathophysiology underlying pressure injury is a combination of pressure, friction, shearing forces between tissue planes, and moisture. Pressure exceeding arteriolar pressure results in tissue hypoxia, the creation of free radicals, an ischemic reperfusion injury, and consequent tissue necrosis.[28] Factors contributing to the development of pressure ulcers include prolonged immobility, patient position, neuropathy, and existing arterial or venous insufficiency.[28] The National Pressure Ulcer Advisory Panel (NPUAP) staging system defines four stages of severity to pressure injuries: stage 1 pressure injury is nonblanchable erythema of intact skin (**Figure 2.5A**), stage 2 pressure injury is a partial-thickness skin loss with exposed dermis (**Figure 2.5B**), stage 3 pressure injury involves full-thickness skin loss (**Figure 2.5C**), and stage 4 pressure injury involves full-thickness skin and tissue loss (**Figure 2.5D**).[29]

Factors That Adversely Affect Wound Healing

Radiation Therapy

Radiation therapy such as those used as part of oncologic therapies disrupts the complex pathways of wound healing. Ionizing radiation produces both acute and late effects on tissues. Acutely, basement membrane is damaged, and increased vascular permeability introduces edema to reduce neovascularization of wounds.[30] During the inflammatory phase, there is excess expression of several growth factors, leading to tissue fibrosis. Fibroblasts are also injured and contribute to the late effects of radiation injury such as fibrosis and contraction.[30]

Nutrition

Nutrition has long been known to affect wound healing and chronic wounds. This includes a general malnutrition state, inadequate caloric intake, and deficiencies in vitamins, micronutrients, and macronutrients. Malnutrition is known to prolong the inflammatory phase of wound healing through reducing the proliferation of fibroblasts and the formation of collagen.[31] It can also increase the risk of infection of wounds by altering the function of immune cells, such as reducing phagocytosis and decreasing complement levels.[31]

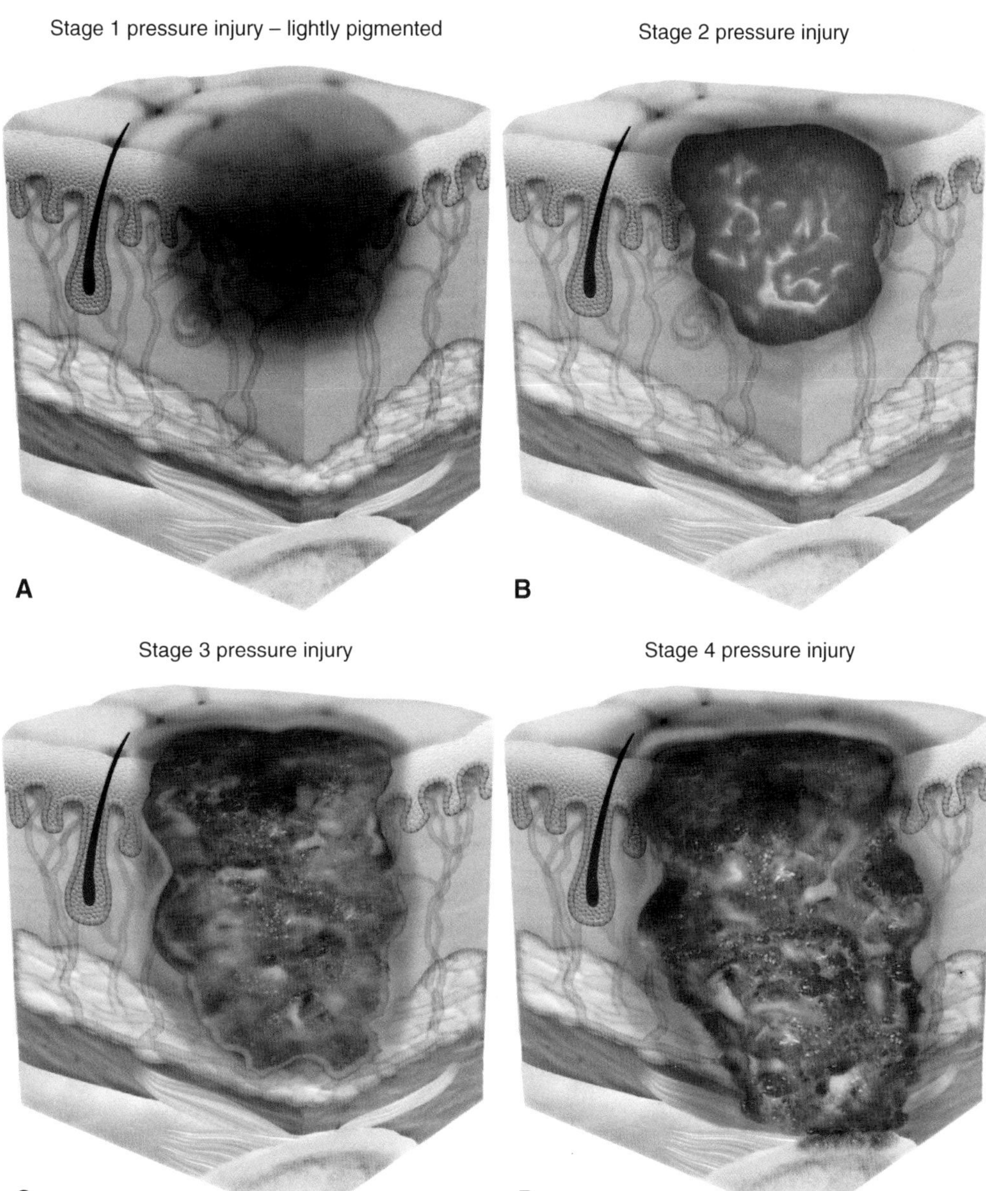

FIGURE 2.5. Pressure injury staging. **A.** Stage 1 is the least severe according to NPUAP staging system. It is defined as nonblanchable erythema of intact skin. **B.** Stage 2 is defined as a partial-thickness skin loss with exposed dermis. **C.** Stage 3 involves full-thickness skin loss. **D.** Stage 4 is the most severe stage of pressure injury. It involves full-thickness skin and tissue loss. Reproduced with permission from National Pressure Ulcer Advisory Panel, European Pressure Ulcer Advisory Panel, Pan Pacific Pressure Injury Alliance. Prevention and treatment of pressure ulcers: quick reference guide. In: Haesler E, ed. Cambridge Media: Osborne Park, Western Australia; 2014.

Micronutrients such as copper, zinc, and magnesium are elements and minerals that are essential to bodily chemical processes and, in particular, in wound healing. Deficiencies in these micronutrients can adversely affect wound healing, for example, in copper deficiency.

Macronutrients include protein, amino acids, carbohydrates, fiber, water, and fats. These are required at sufficient levels to promote optimal wound healing. Significantly reduced protein intake is associated with increased rates of wound infection and wound strength.[31] Similarly, lipid deficiencies are associated with altered wound healing.[31]

Microorganisms

Microorganisms have long been known to influence the healing of chronic wounds, and all open wounds contain microbes. Bacteria predominantly exist in biofilms in clinical and natural settings, as opposed to planktonic states (single organisms/free-floating). Biofilms describe adherent populations of microbes that form three-dimensional populations and are organized on extracellular polymers. Over time, chronic wounds are known to develop biofilms, as complex interactions between the host wound microenvironment and heterogeneous bacterial populations mean they are able to proliferate unchecked.

Biofilm bacterial populations delay and inhibit wound healing by not only producing toxins and damaging enzymes, but also promoting the complex chronic inflammatory pathways.[32] Proteases released from bacteria impede growth factors and wound healing proteins. Large levels of microbial exudate have also been shown to affect cell proliferation and wound healing.[32]

Biofilm-infected chronic wounds are clinically challenging to manage and are resistant to elimination by antimicrobials and by the immune system. The current mainstay management of dealing with microorganism-related complications in chronic wounds includes pressure off-loading, appropriate dressings, systemic antibiotics, tissue debridement, and the instillation of NPWTs such as vacuum-assisted closure devices.

Similarly, antiseptic dressings such as those containing chlorhexidine, silver, or iodine and topical antimicrobials (e.g., fusidic acid creams) have been developed over the years to a limited degree of success. Topical antimicrobials have promoted bacterial resistance, and several studies concluded that antiseptic dressings are not significantly better than saline gauze alone.[33] However, there are special situations when topical antimicrobials are proven beneficial. They are particularly useful in burn injuries (especially second-degree burn injuries) to treat infection and therefore prevent sepsis.[34]

Systemic antibiotics are beneficial in infected chronic wounds but are not indicated for most chronic wounds that are merely colonized with bacteria. Antibiotics should have high tissue bioavailability and should be targeted to the specific organisms from deep wound cultures. Studies demonstrate that superficial cultures do not represent the diverse populations of bacteria of the biofilm.[33]

Debridement involves the removal of necrotic tissue and debris at the wound edges and is often surgical, although other mechanical modes and enzymatic and autolytic methods are also utilized. The current theory is that debridement reduces biofilm. It is thought to promote wound healing and decrease the biofilm load. Recolonization of the wound after debridement is common, and often sequential debridements are required for successful healing.

NPWTs, such as vacuum-assisted closure devices, are known to aid wound healing. Several studies have investigated their effect on the microorganisms within chronic wounds, and observational data of NPWT with adjunctive topical dressings have demonstrated decreased biofilm load.[33] A recent small randomized trial (n = 20) of NPWT with instillation and adjunctive sodium hypochlorite solution was effective at reducing both planktonic and nonplanktonic (biofilm) microorganisms.[35]

Obesity and Metabolic Syndromes

Obesity is correlated with increased rates of wound complications such as wound infection, impaired wound healing, pressure injuries, venous ulcers, hematoma, and seroma formation. Hypovascularity, difficulty in repositioning, and friction between skin-to-skin contact points in skin folds are all known to contribute to the formation of pressure injuries in obese individuals.

On a molecular level, obesity is related to lower levels of lymphocyte proliferate, altered cytokine levels and peripheral immune function which improves upon weight loss.[23]

ADVANCED WOUND HEALING STRATEGIES

Nonsurgical, advanced would healing strategies can briefly be categorized into those that employ biological therapeutics, use or enhance the matrix, and exploit biophysical forces (see Figure 2.1). Although these modalities are important, basic and simple strategies still form the foundation of wound care. These measures are manifold and include optimizing the management of primary pathological conditions that lead to wound formation, such as optimal lifestyle measures (e.g., nutrition), medication, and patient education. Other measures include debridement of necrotic tissue, local ulcer care, mechanical off-loading, mechanical compression (for venous ulcers), and infection control.

Biological Therapies

Biological therapies have been of great interest in wound healing therapies, and we specifically discuss the use of cadaveric skin and xenografts, placental constructs, growth factors, hyperbaric oxygen therapy (HBOT), biological skin equivalents, and stem cells (see Figure 2.1).

Growth Factors

Growth factor–related wound repair has been of immense interest in wound healing science. Commercially marketed growth factors currently available include recombinant human fibroblast growth factor, recombinant human platelet-derived growth factor, and recombinant human epidermal growth factor. Several other growth factors are also being developed.

Recombinant human epidermal growth factor is a well-known growth factor that can be applied topically or injected and has been shown to improve wound healing in small clinical trials worldwide.[36] Fibroblast growth factor has also shown promising results, in particular an isoform known as recombinant human keratinocyte growth factor-2 to be applied as a topical spray. The trial showed significantly increased wound healing compared with placebo.[37]

Platelet-Derived Growth Factors and Platelet-Rich Plasma

Several studies shown the efficacy of platelet-rich plasma (PRP) and PDGFs obtained from centrifugation of blood.[38]

PDGF has been demonstrated to be effective when compared with placebo, with 7 studies totaling 685 patients that showed a statistically significant percentage of ulcers healed compared with sham therapy.[39] The first commercially available topical PDGF in the United States is becaplermin gel (Regranex®), which was studied in chronic diabetic foot ulcers. It is important to note that becaplermin gel contains the US Food and Drug Administration (FDA) black box warning, whereby consumers are cautioned to the increased risk of rate of mortality secondary to malignancy if several tubes are used.[40]

Conversely, the evidence for PRP has been scant, with randomized controlled trial (RCT) data showing no significant difference in the percentage of ulcers healed when compared with placebo or platelet-poor plasma therapy.[39]

Stem Cells

There has been significant interest in the use of stem cells to address the defective pathways in aberrant wound healing. Stem cells are undifferentiated cells that possess the ability to mature into differentiated cells of either one embryonic germ layer (multipotent) or all three embryonic germ layers (pluripotent).[41]

Perhaps one of the most widely studied multipotent adult stem cells in wound healing research has been mesenchymal stem cells (MSCs). In several animal-based studies, MSCs have demonstrated the ability to migrate to areas of cutaneous injury, secrete angiogenic and immune-mediating factors, and differentiate into skin cells.[41] There are now several ongoing and published clinical trials using MSCs in wound healing as well as a few commercial products.[41] Multiple clinical trials have shown promising outcomes with regard to wound closure rates; however, they have been limited by small sample sizes and lack of controls.[41] At the time of writing, several clinical trials in the United States are recruiting patients to study the use of MSCs in healing cutaneous wounds.[41]

However, challenges remain with stem cell technologies. Firstly, there are numerous ethical concerns surrounding its use, in particular, pluripotent stem cells; hence, much of the research has focused on multipotent stem cells.[41] Secondly, there are still many questions that need to be answered in the field. Two important questions posited by Sorice et al are which population of stem cells are the most effective in healing wounds and what is the best method to deliver stem cells into a wound?[41] These are important considerations if stem cells are to move into clinical translation.

Hyperbaric Oxygen Therapy

HBOT utilizes compression chambers to deliver high levels of oxygen concentration at raised atmospheric pressures. HBOT aims to promote oxygen-dependent wound healing pathways and has particularly been a treatment strategy when revascularization in vascular insufficiency has been unsuccessful.[42] Systematic review evidence of four long-term studies totaling 233 patients concluded that there was a significant difference in percentage of healed ulcers compared with sham therapy when HBOT was used adjunctively, with one short-term study finding no significant difference. However, strength of evidence was deemed low for all studies. One study of poor quality found HBOT less effective compared with ESWT (n = 84).[39]

Cell Cultured Products

Cell cultured products, also known as tissue-engineered constructs, include Apligraf, Epicel, and Dermagraft. Apligraf (Organogenesis, Canton, MA) utilizes a bovine collagen matrix incorporated with human neonatal fibroblasts and neonatal keratinocytes to act as a scaffold as well as providing cells that produce growth factors and ECM components. Similarly, Dermagraft (Organogenesis, Canton, MA) comprises a polyglactin scaffold with dermal neonatal fibroblasts. A large Apligraf RCT (n = 309) found a significant increase in the number of healed ulcers and a reduced length of time to complete healing compared with standard therapy with compression.[39] Furthermore, cultured epithelial autografts using patients' own keratinocytes, such as Epicel, have been utilized to treat large burns and take 2 to 3 weeks in culture to grow.[43] Genetic manipulation of keratinocytes has recently been reported to regenerate an entire fully functional epidermal layer in junctional epidermolysis bullosa.[44]

Scaffolds

Scaffolds act as a platform for cell migration and angiogenesis and are a key therapeutic modality. Scaffolds can be of human origin (donated tissue or cadaveric) and nonhuman origin (porcine or synthesized through extraction and cross-linking). Several such scaffolds are commercially available. Integra™ (Integra LifeSciences) is a bilayer matrix of bovine collagen and glycosaminoglycan derived from shark skin that is lyophilized to form a highly porous scaffold. Integra™ has been used with considerable success in burns, and clinical trial data have attested its use in the healing of chronic wounds, specifically decreasing time to wound closure in diabetic foot ulcers.[45] Allopatch®, which is a decellularized scaffold derived from human cadaveric tissue, has demonstrated efficacy in closure of nonhealing diabetic foot ulcers.[46] Placental constructs, such as Grafix, which is a cryopreserved placental membrane, have shown to significantly improve diabetic foot ulcer healing and reduce related complications.[47]

Biophysical Forces

Negative-Pressure Wound Therapy

NPWT effectively ensures wound drainage, aids granulation tissue development, and expedites wound contraction.[48] RCT data have shown improved healing of ulcers as well as reduced second amputations.[39]

Extracorporeal Shock Wave Therapy

ESWT delivers high-energy acoustic pulses to tissues and is the standard of care in treating nephrolithiasis and various musculoskeletal conditions. It has been reported to improve cutaneous wound healing through increasing cell proliferation and stimulating angiogenesis.[49]

Electromagnetic Therapies

Electromagnetic therapies, such as pulsed electromagnetic field therapy, have effectively been used in orthopedic practice, and numerous in vitro and animal studies have demonstrated improved cutaneous wound healing. These therapies are thought to interact with endogenous electric fields in the skin to increase expression of growth factors and nitric oxide and also promote angiogenesis[50] (see Figure 2.4). However, RCT data showed mixed results, with one showing no difference between placebo and electromagnetic therapy and another reporting a significant increase in the percentage of healed ulcers between the two groups.[39]

Knowledge Gaps

There has been an explosion in therapeutic options for wound healing in the last 30 years, as the number of wounds has increased because of our aging population, increases in the incidence of type 2 diabetes, and increases in obesity. Currently, there is a lack of clinical data in well-controlled prospective studies to document the clinical efficacy of several of the modalities now used clinically including HBOT, PRP, antimicrobial dressings, topical oxygen therapy, and pulsed electromagnetic stimulation. There is also almost a complete lack of comparative studies on advanced wound healing modalities. Prospective RCTs are challenging in wound healing because of the difficulty in binding both the patient and practitioner as well as the desire by both to achieve a healed wound. Registry studies may provide a powerful method to look at comparative advanced healing modalities and also allow us to better assess the cost-effectiveness of these therapies.

ACKNOWLEDGMENT

We would kindly like to acknowledge Mr. Ilya Shiltsin for the artwork in this chapter.

REFERENCES

1. Diegelmann RF, Evans MC. Wound healing: an overview of acute, fibrotic and delayed healing. *Front Biosci*. 2004;9:283-289.
2. Velnar T, Bailey T, Smrkolj V. The wound healing process: an overview of the cellular and molecular mechanisms. *J Int Med Res*. 2009;37(5):1528-1542.
3. Gurtner GC, Werner S, Barrandon Y, Longaker MT. Wound repair and regeneration. *Nature*. 2008;453(7193):314-321.
   Review article highlighting the basics of wound repair and wound regeneration biology.
4. Singer AJ, Clark RA. Cutaneous wound healing. *N Engl J Med*. 1999;341(10):738-746.
   Similar key review paper highlighting the stages of wound healing, reviewing pathways in abnormal wound healing and a review of skin substitutes.
5. Enoch S, Leaper DJ. Basic science of wound healing. *Surgery (Oxford)*. 2005;23(2):37-42.
6. Oda K, Matsuoka Y, Funahashi A, Kitano H. A comprehensive pathway map of epidermal growth factor receptor signaling. *Mol Syst Biol*. 2005;1:2005.0010.
7. Ahluwalia A, Tarnawski AS. Critical role of hypoxia sensor: HIF-1alpha in VEGF gene activation. Implications for angiogenesis and tissue injury healing. *Curr Med Chem*. 2012;19(1):90-97.
8. Olsen L, Sherratt JA, Maini PK. A mechanochemical model for adult dermal wound contraction and the permanence of the contracted tissue displacement profile. *J Theor Biol*. 1995;177(2):113-128.
9. Levenson SM, Geever EF, Crowley LV, et al. The healing of rat skin wounds. *Ann Surg*. 1965;161:293-308.
10. Profyris C, Tziotzios C, Do Vale I. Cutaneous scarring: pathophysiology, molecular mechanisms, and scar reduction therapeutics Part I. The molecular basis of scar formation. *J Am Acad Dermatol*. 2012;66(1):1-10.
11. O'Kane S, Ferguson MW. Transforming growth factor beta and wound healing. *Int J Biochem Cell Biol*. 1997;29(1):63-78.
12. Ingber DE. Tensegrity II. How structural networks influence cellular information processing networks. *J Cell Sci*. 2003;116(Pt 8):1397-1408.
13. Bokel C, Brown NH. Integrins in development: moving on, responding to, and sticking to the extracellular matrix. *Dev Cell*. 2002;3(3):311-321.
14. Ehrlich HP, Rajaratnam JB. Cell locomotion forces versus cell contraction forces for collagen lattice contraction: an in vitro model of wound contraction. *Tissue Cell*. 1990;22(4):407-417.
15. Huang S, Ingber DE. The structural and mechanical complexity of cell-growth control. *Nat Cell Biol*. 1999;1(5):E131-E138.
   Article outlining the importance of extracellular matrix and cytoskeletal tension in cell signalling and cell growth.
16. Hunckler J, de Mel A. A current affair: electrotherapy in wound healing. *J Multidiscip Healthc*. 2017;10:179-194.
17. Wong VW, Rustad KC, Akaishi S, et al. Focal adhesion kinase links mechanical force to skin fibrosis via inflammatory signaling. *Nat Med*. 2012;18(1):148-152.
   Key research paper that concluded the importance of mechnical forces in inflammatory pathways, particularly through focal adhesion kinase signalling.
18. Wynn TA. Common and unique mechanisms regulate fibrosis in various fibroproliferative diseases. *J Clin Invest*. 2007;117(3):524-529.
19. Prosdocimi M, Bevilacqua C. Exogenous hyaluronic acid and wound healing: an updated vision. *Panminerva Med*. 2012;54(2):129-135.
20. Lautenschlager S, Eichmann A. Differential diagnosis of leg ulcers. *Curr Probl Dermatol*. 1999;27:259-270.
21. Pardes JB, Takagi H, Martin TA, et al. Decreased levels of alpha 1(I) procollagen mRNA in dermal fibroblasts grown on fibrin gels and in response to fibrinopeptide B. *J Cell Physiol*. 1995;162(1):9-14.
22. Schmid-Schonbein GW, Takase S, Bergan JJ. New advances in the understanding of the pathophysiology of chronic venous insufficiency. *Angiology*. 2001;52(suppl 1):S27-S34.
23. Guo S, DiPietro L. Factors affecting wound healing. *J Dent Res*. 2010;89(3):219-229.

24. Ochoa O, Torres FM, Shireman PK. Chemokines and diabetic wound healing. *Vascular*. 2007;15(6):350-355.
25. Pierce GF. Inflammation in nonhealing diabetic wounds: the space-time continuum does matter. *Am J Pathol*. 2001;159(2):399-403.
26. Blakytny R, Jude E. The molecular biology of chronic wounds and delayed healing in diabetes. *Diabet Med*. 2006;23(6):594-608.
27. Kuo PC, Kao CH, Chen JK. Glycated type 1 collagen induces endothelial dysfunction in culture. *In Vitro Cell Dev Biol Anim*. 2007;43(10):338-343.
28. Thomas DR. Does pressure cause pressure ulcers? An inquiry into the etiology of pressure ulcers. *J Am Med Dir Assoc*. 2010;11(6):397-405.
29. National Pressure Ulcer Advisory Panel, European Pressure Ulcer Advisory Panel and Pan Pacific pressure injury Alliance. Prevention and treatment of pressure ulcers: quick reference guide. In: Haesler E, ed. Osborne Park, Western Australia: Cambridge Media; 2014.
30. Tibbs MK. Wound healing following radiation therapy: a review. *Radiother Oncol*. 1997;42(2):99-106.
31. Stechmiller JK. Understanding the role of nutrition and wound healing. *Nutr Clin Pract*. 2010;25(1):61-68.
32. Percival SL, McCarty SM, Lipsky B. Biofilms and wounds: an overview of the evidence. *Adv Wound Care (New Rochelle)*. 2015;4(7):373-381.
33. Gompelman M, van Asten SA, Peters EJ. Update on the role of infection and biofilms in wound healing: pathophysiology and treatment. *Plast Reconstr Surg*. 2016;138(3 suppl):61s-70s.
34. Neely AN, Gardner J, Durkee P, et al. Are topical antimicrobials effective against bacteria that are highly resistant to systemic antibiotics? *J Burn Care Res*. 2009;30(1):19-29.
35. Yang C, Goss SG, Alcantara S, et al. Effect of negative pressure wound therapy with instillation on bioburden in chronically infected wounds. *Wounds*. 2017;9(8):240-246.
36. Fernandez-Montequin JI, Valenzuela-Silva CM, Diaz OG, et al. Intra-lesional injections of recombinant human epidermal growth factor promote granulation and healing in advanced diabetic foot ulcers: multicenter, randomised, placebo-controlled, double-blind study. *Int Wound J*. 2009;6(6):432-443.
37. Robson MC, Phillips TJ, Falanga V, et al. Randomized trial of topically applied repifermin (recombinant human keratinocyte growth factor-2) to accelerate wound healing in venous ulcers. *Wound Repair Regen*. 2001;9(5):347-352.
38. Driver VR, Hanft J, Fylling CP, Beriou JM. A prospective, randomized, controlled trial of autologous platelet-rich plasma gel for the treatment of diabetic foot ulcers. *Ostomy Wound Manage*. 2006;52(6):68-70.
39. Greer N, Foman N, Dorrian J, et al. Advanced wound care therapies for non-healing diabetic, venous, and arterial ulcers: a systematic review. VA-ESP Project #09-009. *Ann Intern Med*. 2013;159(8):532-542.
40. *Regranex Gel post Market Drug Safety Information*; 2008. https://www.fda.gov/downloads/drugs/drugsafety/postmarketdrugsafetyinformationforpatientsand-providers/ucm142821.pdf.
41. Sorice S, Rustad KC, Li AY, Gurtner GC. The role of stem cell therapeutics in wound healing: current understanding and future directions. *Plast Reconstr Surg*. 2016;138(3 suppl):31s-41s.
42. Kranke P, Bennett M, Roeckl-Wiedmann I, Debus S. Hyperbaric oxygen therapy for chronic wounds. *Cochrane Database Syst Rev*. 2004(2):Cd004123.
43. Carsin H, Ainaud P, Le Bever H, et al. Cultured epithelial autografts in extensive burn coverage of severely traumatized patients: a five year single-center experience with 30 patients. *Burns*. 2000;26(4):379-387.
44. Hirsch T, Rothoeft T, Teig N, et al. Regeneration of the entire human epidermis using transgenic stem cells. *Nature*. 2017;551(7680):327-332.
Recent seminal research paper demonstrating that genetic manipulation of keratinocytes can regenerate an entire fully functional epidermal layer in junctional epidermolysis bullosa.
45. Driver VR, Lavery LA, Reyzelman AM, et al. A clinical trial of Integra Template for diabetic foot ulcer treatment. *Wound Repair Regen*. 2015;23(6):891-900.
46. Zelen CM, Orgill DP, Serena T, et al. A prospective, randomised, controlled, multicentre clinical trial examining healing rates, safety and cost to closure of an acellular reticular allogenic human dermis versus standard of care in the treatment of chronic diabetic foot ulcers. *Int Wound J*. 2017;14(2):307-315.
47. Lavery LA, Fulmer J, Shebetka KA, et al. The efficacy and safety of Grafix((R)) for the treatment of chronic diabetic foot ulcers: results of a multi-centre, controlled, randomised, blinded, clinical trial. *Int Wound J*. 2014;11(5):554-560.
48. Saxena V, Hwang CW, Huang S, et al. Vacuum-assisted closure: microdeformations of wounds and cell proliferation. *Plast Reconstr Surg*. 2004;114(5):1086-1096.
49. Contaldo C, Hogger DC, Khorrami Borozadi M, et al. Radial pressure waves mediate apoptosis and functional angiogenesis during wound repair in ApoE deficient mice. *Microvasc Res*. 2012;84(1):24-33.
50. Callaghan MJ, Chang EI, Seiser N, et al. Pulsed electromagnetic fields accelerate normal and diabetic wound healing by increasing endogenous FGF-2 release. *Plast Reconstr Surg*. 2008;121(1):130-141.

? QUESTIONS

1. **A 65-year-old woman with diabetes mellitus presents with a heel ulceration not involving the calcaneus. She has palpable pulses. Which therapy has the best published efficacy for healing?**
   a. HBOT
   b. Silver alginate dressings
   c. NPWT
   d. Pulsed electromagnetic therapy

2. **A 25-year-old man with paraplegia presents with a large ulcer over his right ischium that probes to bone. What stage of pressure injury would this be considered?**
   a. Stage 1
   b. Stage 2
   c. Stage 3
   d. Stage 4
   e. Unstageable

3. **A patient presents with a heavy scar 3 weeks following a stab wound to the back. What phase of wound healing would this be considered?**
   a. Hemostasis
   b. Inflammatory
   c. Proliferation
   d. Remodeling

4. **Which of the following wound care modalities would mechanical forces be considered a major factor in the mechanism of action?**
   a. Platelet-derived growth factor
   b. Placental-derived constructs
   c. Negative-pressure wound therapy
   d. Saline wash

5. **Which of the following would be considered a chronic wound?**
   a. A 67-year-old man with a 2-cm heel ulceration for 1 month who just completed external iliac angioplasty
   b. A 75-year-old woman with a prosthetic heart valve on Coumadin who presents with severe bruising of her anterior tibial area 3 weeks after injury
   c. A 30-year-old man with Crohn disease on steroids presents with a dehisced laparotomy wound 1 month following surgery
   d. A 45-year-old woman with breast cancer who has severe desquamation of her skin at the end of her radiation therapy
   e. A 24-year-old man paraplegic with an ischial stage 4 pressure injury for 3 months

1. **Answer: c.** Although all of these modalities have been proposed for use in this patient population, NPWT has the most published high-level studies in wounds.

2. **Answer: d.** Pressure injuries that go to bone are considered stage 4.

3. **Answer: d.** Although there are components of inflammation and proliferation that are still occurring, 3 weeks after an injury, the wound is being actively remodeled and would generally be considered to be in the remodeling phase.

4. **Answer: c.** Negative-pressure wound therapy. This therapy is commonly used by placing an open-pore polyurethane sponge directly over the wound and connecting this to suction. This induces deformations to the wound surface and draws the wound together.

5. **Answer: e.** Wounds should be present for 6 weeks to be considered chronic. Although the severe bruising and the radiation injury cases could turn into chronic wounds, at this point these patients do not have an actual wound.

CHAPTER 3 Management of Scars

Wyatt G. Payne and David J. Smith

KEY POINTS

- Keloids: Heaped scars that extend beyond the margins of the original wound; rarely spontaneously regress; frequently result from minor trauma; familial predisposition common.
- Hypertrophic scar: Raised; erythematous; pruritic; remains confined to the limits of the original wound.
- Fibroproliferative scars/healing describe a state of excessive healing with collagen formation imbalance.
- TGF-beta excess contributes to fibroproliferative scar formation (keloids and hypertrophic scar).
- A combination of treatment modalities may be required for scar improvement management.

With the exception of fetal healing,[1,2] the end result of wound healing is a scar. In terms of evolution, this process developed as a necessity to traumatic injury and as a response to the alternative—failure to survive.

Scars can pose numerous problems and complications: seizures (brain scar), intestinal obstruction (bowel scar), loss of range of motion (soft tissue, skin, muscle, joint scar), etc. Although *normal* scarring is beneficial, as it achieves a healed wound, the site and extent of scar, as related to plastic surgery, may pose both aesthetic and/or functional problems.

Normal wound healing is a complex series of dynamic interactive processes that begin at the moment of wounding and involves soluble mediators, many cell types, and extracellular matrices. The process follows a specific time sequence and includes coagulation, inflammation, deposition and differentiation of extracellular matrix, fibroplasia, epithelialization, contraction, and remodeling with the end result—formation of a healed wound, by scar.[3,4] The end result of *normal* scar is an equilibrium between collagen synthesis/deposition and collagen lysis/degradation; the *mature scar*, which has approximately 80% of the tensile strength of normal unwounded skin, occurs between 6 and 18 months after wounding.[5]

Proliferative healing has been described by Dvorak as a spectrum with normal healing on one end and tumor cell proliferation at the other.[6] Proliferative scar formation describes a series of events resulting in *overhealing* as if an equilibrium point between collagen deposition and collagen lysis has never been reached.[3,7]

Types of proliferative scar formation include the following:

- Keloids[3,5,8] **(Figure 3.1)**
  - Familial predisposition
  - Enlarged *heaped-up* scar that extends beyond the margins of the original wound
  - Rarely regress
  - Frequently result from relatively minor injury or insult
  - Elevated TGF-beta
- Hypertrophic scars[3,5,8-10] **(Figure 3.2)**
  - Raised
  - Erythematous
  - Pruritic
  - Remain at the site or confines of the original wound
  - Partial or total resolution or regression can spontaneously occur
  - Result from trauma, incision, burns
  - Result from prolonged wound healing
  - Increased epidermal/dermal thickness
  - Lack of epithelial ridges
  - Random orientation of collagen fibrils
  - Decreased collagen content
  - Elevated TGF-beta
  - Increased number of mast cells
  - Decreased collagen production

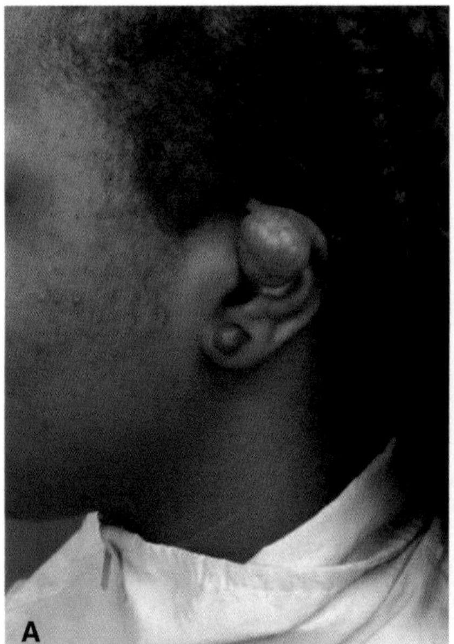

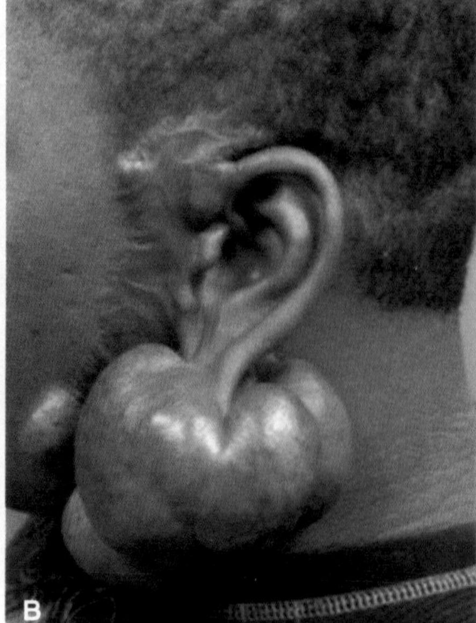

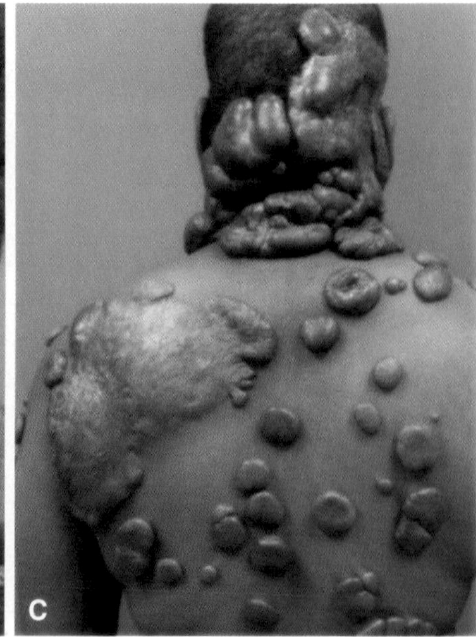

FIGURE 3.1. A. Keloid scarring of the ear after ear piercing. **B.** Massive keloid scarring of the ear. **C.** Extreme keloid formation on the back and neck. (Photos courtesy of Matthew Hiro, MD.)

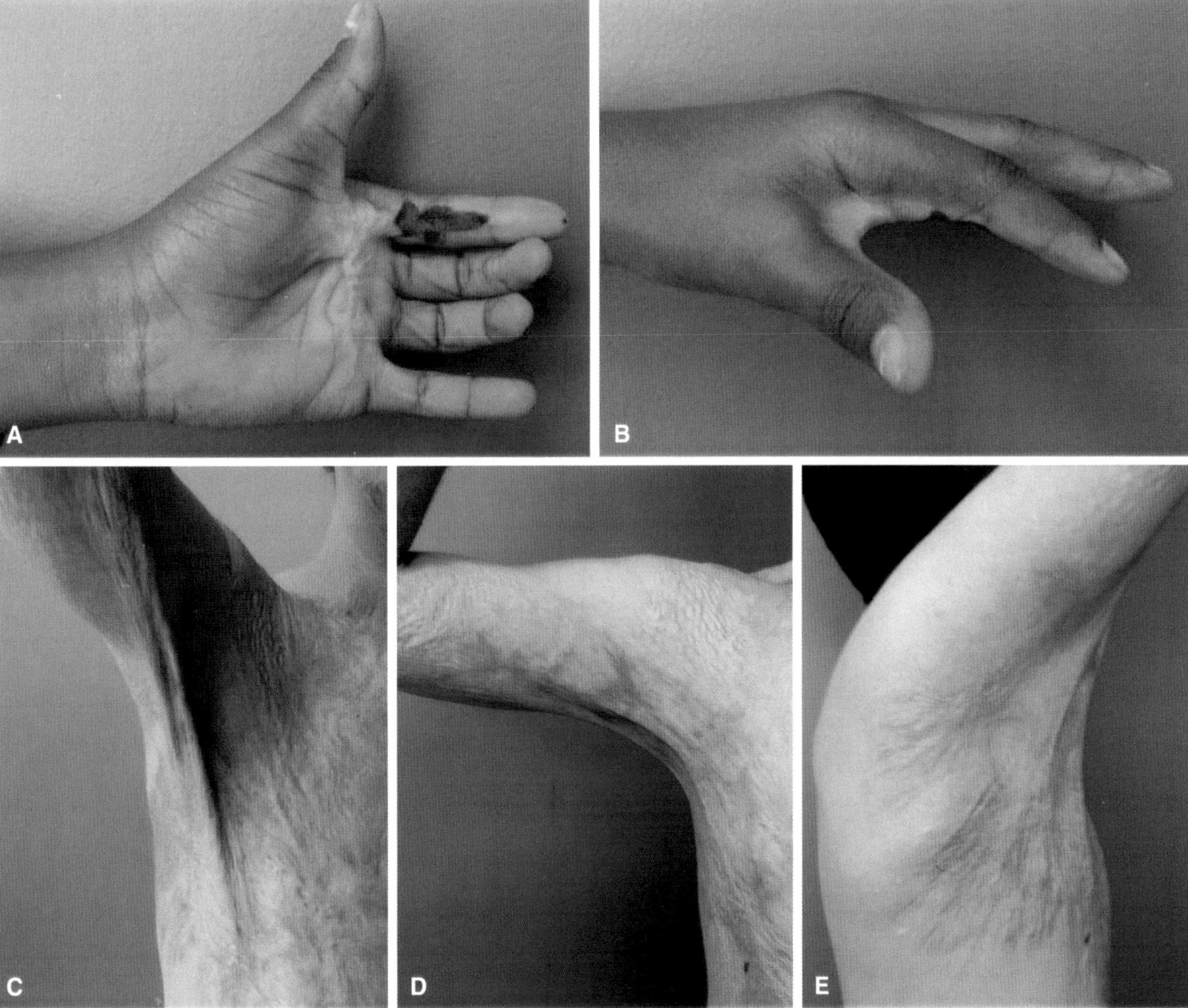

FIGURE 3.2. **A,B.** Hypertrophic burn scar of the hand with thumb web space contracture. **C** to **E.** Hypertrophic burn scar of the axilla with axillary contracture. (Photos courtesy of Matthew Hiro, MD.)

Related fibroproliferative disorders, all of which demonstrate similarities to proliferative scar[3,11-13]:

- Periprosthetic capsules—capsular contracture
- Dupuytren contracture—palmar fascia contractures
- Rhinophyma—tissue fibrosis

THE PROBLEM

Aesthetic Problems

Scarring may create a variably noticeable *abnormality* because of the direction, quality, position, size, or orientation of the scar. Beauty is in the eye of the beholder. Assessing scars can be problematic, and subjective measures sometimes determine the aesthetic problem for the patient, significant others, professionals, or casual observers. Validated scar measures are described and used; however, what one may declare acceptable, another may deem unsightly and unacceptable.[14-20] The displeasing scar is no less problematic for some patients as functionally impairing scars.

Functional Problems

Scarring can limit functional capability, and the mere presence of scar can be symptomatic, in and of itself. Pain and pruritus are common symptomatic complaints. Scar contractures leading to diminished range of motion at joints, or other structures dependent upon mobility for their function, can cause variable disability. Scar bulk can also lead to pain, decreased function, and aesthetic concerns (as with keloids).

PREVENTION

As with most problems, an ounce of prevention is worth a pound of cure. The use of sound, meticulous surgical wound closure technique to optimize operative incisional and traumatic wound closures to minimize tension, adequately debride nonviable tissue, remove foreign bodies, approximate layers, fill dead space, prevent hematoma and seroma, and prevent infection, and removing sutures at appropriate time intervals, can contribute to minimizing scarring.[21-23] Adequate undermining with deep dermal suturing creating wound edge eversion can aid to reduce wound tension and diminish/minimize scar width.[21,24-26]

Reducing chronic inflammation by alleviating foreign bodies, infection, and/or prolonged time to healing can improve eventual wound/scar outcomes.[27] Adequate debridement, minimization of foreign materials (including sutures), and wound closure timing (especially as with burn wound grafting) are all advantageous to improve scarring outcomes.[28]

Incision placement and orientation are of prime concern to eventual scar formation/noticeability and also to relieve incisional tension. The noticeable scar is a function of light reflection that catches attention. Placing scars in natural creases, in junctions between contours, and at the edges of hair-bearing skin can camouflage to produce more inconspicuous scar lines. Working within the relaxed skin tension lines, as described by Borges, Kraissl, and Langer, allows scars to lie in planes and directions of less obvious orientation, and reduces the tension on incisions to produce less widened scars.[29-31]

SCAR MANAGEMENT

Medical Management

Massage

Frequently advised for postoperative scarring, this noninvasive, inexpensive method of scar manipulation/reduction does have evidence of effectiveness.[27,28] Although its usefulness is generally limited, massage can aid in the flattening and softening of scars and limiting some scar contractures (e.g., after lower eyelid procedures). Reported to be of benefit in the scenario of burn scarring, improvements in scar appearance, pruritic pain, and psychologic effects have been shown.[32] Professional massage therapists appear to be of benefit in scarring related to burn.[32]

Silicone Gel

Application of silicone gel has been shown to benefit the appearance of hypertrophic scar, keloids, and surgical incisions.[33-38] The mechanism of action appears to be the occlusive nature of silicone dressing and epithelial hydration, not that of temperature increase, nor by any chemical effects of absorbed silicone.[36,39,40] Likely the effect is an influence in the collagen remodeling phase of wound healing. There is differing evidence as to the efficacy of silicone gel as a preventative treatment measure as compared with good evidence to indicate effective management after scarring.[21,23,33,41] Recommendation for treatment is to wear the silicone gel dressing for 12 to 24 hours per day for 2 to 3 months at the onset of visible scar abnormality.

Compression, Pressure, and Mechanomodulation

Pressure garments are commonly utilized after burn injury/treatment to aid in hypertrophic scar control.[28,42] Compression garments are recommended prophylactically in burn injury after extensive skin grafting and/or if spontaneous wound healing requires longer than 10 to 14 days.[27,28,43] The exact mechanism that pressure garments influence hypertrophic scarring is not completely understood; however, influence on collagen synthesis and remodeling is a likely effect.[43] Pressure requirements for effectiveness have not been established, although 15 to 25 mm Hg is the target pressure reported by many authors.[9,43,44] The appearance, discomfort, texture, and heat reflection/generation (especially in warm climates) of pressure garments limit patient compliance and therefore their effectiveness.

Pressure therapy is also effective for keloid treatment/therapy, generally as a postoperative adjunctive measure.[9,45] Compression earrings (for ear lobe keloids) are commercially available for postoperative application but require patient compliance. Effectiveness may be up to 80% following complete surgical excision.[9,21,22,45,46]

Significant wound tension leads to widened scarring.[24-26,45] Mechanomodulation to relieve scar tension at the time of incision closure can positively affect incisional scar formation and improve scar appearance.[23,25,26] Available as a commercial device and placed to redistribute and relieve tension across an incision line, the device is well tolerated by patients, is effective, and has a minimal complication rate.[23,25] This device is recommended for truncal incisions such as abdominoplasty.

Corticosteroids

Injection of steroids (triamcinolone) is widely used as an initial treatment for keloids and hypertrophic scars and is commonly applied in conjunction with other modalities including surgical excision to decrease scar recurrence rates.[5,9,21,23,33,45] Dosage may range from 2.5 to 40 mg either as primary solo treatment or prior to surgical excision and can be injected with a mixture of xylocaine + epinephrine to diminish local pain and to decrease steroid dispersion, to maximize its effect.[22,46] Solo steroid therapy for hypertrophic scars can be repeated at 4-week to 6-week intervals until the desired effect is observed, side effects are observed, or if surgical excision is expected. Steroid pretreatment for keloids followed by surgical excision and follow-up postoperative injections produce reported cure rates of up to 80%.[45,47-51]

Complications and side effects arising from the use of injectable corticosteroids include skin atrophy, hypopigmentation, and pain with injection.[45,47]

Radiation Therapy

Radiation therapy can be utilized as an adjunct therapeutic with surgical excision in the treatment of keloids. Keloid excision followed by radiation therapy within 24 to 48 hours either as a single dose or as multiple doses can reduce recurrence and lead to cure rates between 67% and 98%, depending on the anatomic area. Although there is no overwhelming prospective evidence to indicate definitive effectiveness of radiation therapy after surgical excision in keloid treatment, retrospective data from relatively large clinical patient series indicate it as a worthwhile treatment.[52-55] Radiation damages keloid fibroblasts, affecting collagen production and structure.[45,53,56] Radiation monotherapy is not effective. Concern for generation of malignancy due to radiation therapy is advisable, especially in the pediatric age patient or in areas prone to radiation-induced carcinomas, such as thyroid and breast.[57] The reported rates for carcinogenesis are low, with few cases associating radiation therapy for treatment of keloids with malignant tumor generation. Recommendations are for adequate shielding of vulnerable areas from radiation and careful patient selection.[58]

Radiation therapy for refractory/intractable hypertrophic scarring has been reported as effective; however, there are few data to support its use.[53]

Side effects of hyperpigmentation, hypopigmentation, and transient erythema have been reported. Few wound healing problems have been attributed to the low-dose radiation, and soft tissue fibrosis as encountered with higher doses of radiation therapy is not likely.[53]

Cryotherapy

Topical cryotherapy may achieve initial positive results in hypertrophic scars and keloid treatment; subsequent recurrence rates are high, making this therapy less than optimal, unless repetitive treatments/sessions are utilized.[58] Intralesional cryotherapy requiring a specialized cryoprobe does show effectiveness, but this method is not widely used.[58]

Molecular Therapies

There is experimental (and some clinical) evidence to indicate that treatment of hypertrophic scar and/or keloids with agents such as 5-fluorouracil, bleomycin, mitomycin C, tamoxifen, paclitaxel, methotrexate, TGF-beta 3, and interferon may be of benefit. Likely the mechanisms of antiscarring action are due to their interaction with TGF-beta receptors and downregulation of fibroblast function.[59-63] The current utility of these agents is limited because of a lack of adequate clinical evidence.

Botulinum Toxin

Botulinum toxin has recently been reported to improve surgical incisional scars.[64] Although only reported as a small case series, final scar outcome improved with intraoperative injection of botulinum toxin type A, 10 U/cm in a split-scar randomized trial. The presumed mechanism of action of botulinum toxin is inhibition of TGF-beta 1 and cell cycle interaction, diminishing fibroblast cell functions/regulation.[64]

Other Modalities

Vitamin E and onion extract have little clinical evidence to recommend their use for treatment.[21,65] Reviews of over-the-counter products with claims to scar treatment and scar improvement provide little evidence for these products' effectiveness beyond the earlier discussions.[66,67]

Surgical Management

Scar revision surgery can vary from excision (re-excision) and closure to more complex modalities and combinations of modalities. The type of scar, extent of scarring, size, orientation, location, etiology, symptomatology, and patient preferences are all factors to consider when planning surgical scar treatments. Surgical adjuvants (corticosteroid injection, laser therapy, radiation therapy) deserve consideration in planning scar treatment/management for their possible benefits (versus risks and side effects).

Excision and Direct Closure

Considered in instances where local tissue conditions warrant, minimal/no tension and optimal orientation would be prime considerations. The etiology of unsatisfactory scar in this instance should be considered so that results similar to the initial scarring problem are not repeated.

Excision and Z-Plasty or W-Plasty Closure

Redirecting the orientation and tension of the scar to a more favorable or more optimal direction can produce less tension, more proper alignment, and improved appearance. Borges[29,30] described extensively the relaxed skin tension lines and the utilization of Z-plasty and W-plasty for the revision of scars to improve their appearance as well as to describe the placement of incisions in orientations for improved primary outcomes.

Z-plasty can be considered to realign tissue in instances of scar creating functional deficits such as joint contracture. Functional reorientation and scar lengthening may improve limitation of motion and decrease scar tension. A standard Z-plasty with equivalent length sides and an angle of 60 degrees provides lengthening along the central limb of approximately 75% of its original length. A longer central limb provides (theoretical) linear increase, as does increasing the Z-plasty angle.[29] Multiple in-series Z-plasties can be used for longitudinal gain and reorientation. Adequate skin laxity lateral to the original scar is necessary for adequate Z-plasty flap closure. W-plasty serves to *break up* the scar outline and camouflage the appearance, producing less light reflection and less noticeability.

Excision and Skin Grafting

This is helpful in instances of hypertrophic/widened scars with poor appearance and/or scars causing functional limitations, such as with cicatricial ectropion of the eyelid or minor axillary contracture with minimal linear banding. Attention to recreating the original tissue deficiency with adequate scar release to the point of allowing full range of motion and *overgrafting* the original area of scarring can help to minimize tension on the newly created site. Once skin grafting is complete, compression garments, range of motion therapy, and scar massage may contribute to eventual improved outcomes.

Excision, Dermal Replacement, and Grafting

Recent reports of improved scar revision outcomes have described the use of dermal replacement after scar excision as a basis for secondary skin grafting as an adjuvant to scar and keloid surgical revisions.[68-72] Acellular dermal matrix products allow for vascular ingrowth from contact of matrix edges with normal tissue. These matrices are used over nonvascularized and minimally vascularized structures such as exposed bones and tendons. As opposed to the time-limited nature of skin autografts, which require relatively immediate revascularization for survival, dermal matrices time line of wound bed preparation are longer but provide immediate wound coverage until second-stage grafting can be successfully accomplished.

Excision/Flap Closure

Flap closure after scar excision is worthy of consideration. Flaps including cutaneous, myocutaneous, and fasciocutaneous, whether local, random, pedicled, perforator, or a free tissue transfer, can serve to relieve tension in the area of original scar, fill dead space, and improve aesthetics and/or function. The more severe the scar contracture, especially across major joints such as the knee, elbow, and axilla, the more likely flap closure is indicated and beneficial. Maximal scar release, dead space filling, and tension-free closure are required for adequate results.

Combination Surgical Revision With Adjuvants

Excision with radiation therapy, excision with corticosteroids, and excision with pressure garments have been discussed earlier.

Laser Treatment

Laser has been successfully utilized and shown to improve scar appearance, although further investigations are warranted.[72-75] Much of the positive supporting data are reported for hypertrophic burn scarring utilizing pulsed dye 585/595-nm wavelength as treatment for pruritus and erythema.[72,76,77] Treatments for scar prevention as well as established hypertrophic scar therapy indicated response rates in the range of 70%.[72,74] Other hypertrophic scarring etiologies such as median sternotomy and inframammary scars have been reported to respond to, with good results.[78,79] Results concerning the timing of pulsed dye laser treatments on hypertrophic burn scars appear to indicate that earlier treatment with pulsed dye laser may lead to improved outcomes.[75,80] Hypertrophic scars, treated when early, less than 1-year while still erythematous, responded better than those of more mature age.

Pulsed dye laser therapy works by destruction of scar microvasculature via photothermolysis, and possibly collagen modulation by reducing TGF-beta expression.[75,76] CO_2 laser is ablative, causing tissue vaporization due to selective absorption by water in the tissues.[76]

Fat Grafting

Recent enthusiasm for fat grafting as scar treatment appears to have merit and effectiveness. Effects of fat grafting include filling and elevating of depressed scars, improvement in the quality and pliability of scar, and improvement and pliability in radiated soft tissue.[81-86] The exact effects and mechanism of action on scars and scarring are unknown. There appears to be more effects than simple volumetric filling, and a tissue regenerative effect may occur.[82-86] Adipose-derived stem cells may stimulate local cytokine growth factors leading to increased vascularization, collagen remodeling, and inflammatory response modulation.[82,83] Positive results in studies using fat grafting in the treatment of scar and fibrosing entities are found, although there are few controlled trial and quantitative data. There is growing subjective evidence to suggest that fat grafting may become a mainstay for scar treatment.

CONCLUSION

Scar tissue is the end result of the normal healing process. Abnormal scarring is *enhanced* healing or *overhealing*, usually with resulting aesthetic unacceptability and/or functional impairment. Exact mechanisms of unfavorable scarring are not well elucidated, although excess TGF-beta receptor activity appears to have a major molecular influence. Many treatment options are available either surgically or in combination; however, problematic recurrence remains high. There is no single good therapeutic option in all situations, and individual treatment is advised based on the clinical scenario, available modalities, and patient preference.

REFERENCES

1. Walmsley GG, Maan ZN, Wong VW, et al. Scarless wound healing: chasing the holy grail. *Plast Reconstr Surg*. 2015;135:907-917.
2. Ferguson MWJ, O'Kane S. Scar-free healing: from embryonic mechanisms to adult therapeutic intervention. *Pil Trans R Soc Lond*. 2004;359:839-850.
3. Robson MC, Steed DL, Franz MG. Wound healing: features and approaches to maximize healing trajectories. *Curr Prob Surg*. 2001;38(2):61-140.
A comprehensive monograph on wound healing including abnormal wound healing and fibroproliferative/scarring entities. Discussion on the molecular biology of scarring.
4. Robson MC, Stenberg BD, Heggers JP. Wound healing alterations caused by infection. *Clin Plast Surg*. 1990;17(3):485-492.
5. Tredget EE, Nedelec B, Scott PG, Ghahary A. Hypertrophic scars, keloids and contractures. *Surg Clin North Amer*. 1977;77(3):701-730.
6. Dvorak HF. Tumors that do not heal-similarities between tumor stroma generation and wound healing. *N Engl J Med*. 1986;315(26):1650-1659.
7. Como CB. Scars and keloids. In: Jurkiewicz MJ, Krizek TJ, Mathes SJ, Ariyan S, eds. *Plastic Surgery: Principals and Practice*. St Louis, MO: CV Mosby; 1990:1411-1428.
8. Kisher CW, Bunce H, Shetlar MR. Mast cell analysis in hyphic scars, hypertrophic scars treated with pressure, and mature scars. *J Invest Dermatol*. 1978;70(6):355-357.
9. Ogawa R. The most current algorithms for the treatment and prevention of hypertrophic scars and keloids. *Plast Reconstr Surg*. 2010;125:557-568.
Recent review of hypertrophic scar and keloid treatment by a long-time scar researcher.
10. Polo M, Ko F, Busillo F, Cruse CW, Krizek TJ, Robson MC. The 1997 Moyer Award. Cytokine production in patients with hypertrophic burn scars. *J Burn Care Rehibil*. 1997;18:477-482.
11. Kuhn A, Singh S, Smith PD, et al. Periprosthetic breast capsules contain the fibrogenic cytokines TGF-beta 1 and TGF-beta 2, suggesting possible new treatment approaches. *Ann Plast Surg*. 2000;44:387-391.
12. Kuhn MA, Payne WG, Kierney PC, et al. Cytokine manipulation of explanted Dupuytren's affected human palmar fascia. *J Surg Invest*. 2001;2(6):443-456.
13. Pu LL, Smith PD, Payne WG, et al. Overexpression of transforming growth factor beta-2 and its receptor in rhinophyma: an alternative mechanism of pathobiology. *Ann Plast Surg*. 2000;45:515-519.
14. Brown BC, McKenna SP, Solomon M, et al. The patient-reported impact of scars measure: development and validation. *Plast Reconstr Surg*. 2010;125:1439-1449.
15. Trong PT, Lee JC, Soer B, et al. Reliability and validity testing of the patient and observer scar assessment scale in evaluating linear scars after breast cancer surgery. *Plast Reconstr Surg*. 2007;119(2):487-494.
16. Kerrigan CL, Homa K. Visual assessment of linear scars: a new tool. *Plast Reconstr Surg*. 2009;124(5):1513-1519.
17. Thompson CM, Sood RF, Honari S, Carrougher GJ, Gibran NS. What score on the Vancouver scar scale constitutes a hypertrophic scar? Results from a survey of North American burn-care providers. *Burns*. 2015;41(7):1442-1448.
18. Bae SH, Bae YC. Analysis of frequency of use of different scar assessment scales based on the scar condition and treatment method. *Arch Plast Surg*. 2014;41:111-115.
19. Fearmonti R, Bond J, Erdmann D, Levinson H. A review of scar scales and scar measuring devices. *EPlasty*. 2010;10:354-363.
20. Draaijers LJ, Tempelman FRH, Botman YAM, et al. The patient and observer scar assessment scale: a reliable and feasible tool for scar evaluation. *Plast Reconstr Surg*. 2004;113:1960-1965.
21. Khansa I, Harrison B, Janis JE. Evidence-based scar management: how to improve results with technique and technology. *Plast Reconstr Surg*. 2016;138;165S-178S.
Recent comprehensive review of clinical scar therapies.
22. Wolfram D, Tzankov A, Pulzl P, Piza-Katzer H. Hypertrophic scars and keloids: a review of their pathophysiology, risk factors, and therapeutic management. *Dermatol Surg*. 2009;35:171-181.
23. Perez JL, Rohrich RJ. Optimizing postsurgical scars: a systemic review on best practices in preventive scar management. *Plast Reconstr Surg*. 2017;140:782e-793e.
Recent comprehensive, evidenced-based treatment review of scar prevention. Useful algorithms for treatment.
24. Wray RC. Force required for wound closure and scar appearance. *Plast Reconstr Surg*. 1983;72(3):380-382.
25. Longacre MT, Rohrich RJ, Greenberg L, et al. A randomized controlled rial of the embrace advanced scar therapy device to reduce incisional scar formation. *Plast Reconstr Surg*. 2014;134(3):536-546.
Excellent study design and execution showing benefits of tension reduction to reduce scarring in high-tension abdominoplasty incisions.
26. Lim AF, Weintraub J, Kaplan EN, et al. The embrace device significantly decreases scarring following scar revision surgery in a randomized controlled trial. *Plast Reconstr Surg*. 2014;133(2):398-405.
27. Atiyeh BS. Nonsurgical management of hypertrophic scars: evidence-based therapies, standard practices, and emerging methods. *Aesth Plast Surg*. 2007;31:468-492.
28. Bloemen MCT, van der Veer WM, Ulrich MMW, van Zuijlen PPM, Niessen FB, Middelkoop E. Prevention and curative management of hypertrophic scar formation. *Burns*. 2009;35:463-475.
29. Borges AF. *Elective Incisions and Scar Revision*. Boston, MA: Little, Brown & Co; 1973.
Classic textbook with definitive explanations of relaxed skin tension lines, Z-plasty, and incision placement to reduce or minimize scarring.
30. Borges AF. Relaxed skin tension lines (RTSL) versus other skin lines. *Plast Reconstr Surg*. 1984;73(1):144-150.
31. Wilhelmi BJ, Blackwell SJ, Phillips LG. Langer's lines: to use or not to use. *Plast Reconstr Surg*. 1999;104:208-214.
32. Ault P, Plaza A, Paratz J. Scar massage for hypertrophic burn scarring: a systematic review. *Burns*. 2018;44:24-38.
33. Mustoe TA, Cooter RD, Gold MH, et al. International clinical recommendations on scar management. *Plast Reconstr Surg*. 2002;110(2):560-571.
34. Mustoe TA. Evolution of silicone therapy and mechanism of action in scar management. *Aesth Plast Surg*. 2008;32:82-92.
A comprehensive review of silicone and its benefits and mechanism of action on scars.
35. Li-Tsang CWP, Zheng PY, Lau JCM. A randomized clinical trial to study the effects of silicone gel dressing and pressure therapy on posttraumatic hypertrophic scars. *J Burn Care Res*. 2010;31(3):448-457.
36. Tandara AA, Mustoe TA. The role of the epidermis in the control of scarring: evidence for the mechanism of action for silicone gel. *J Plast Reconstr Aesth Surg*. 2008;61:1219-1225.
37. Ahn ST, Monafo WW, Mustoe TA. Topical silicone gel for the prevention and treatment of hypertrophic scar. *Arch Surg*. 1991;126:499-504.
38. Gold MH, Foster TD, Adair MA, et al. Prevention of hypertrophic scars and keloids by the prophylactic use of topical silicone gel sheets following a surgical procedure in an office setting. *Dermatol Surg*. 2001;27:641-644.
39. Quinn KJ, Evans JH, Courtney JM, Gaylor JD, Reid WH. Non-pressure treatment of hypertrophic scars. *Burns Incl Therm Inj*. 1985;12(2):102-108.
40. Mustoe TA, Gurjala A. The role of the epidermis and the mechanism of action of occlusive dressings in scarring. *Wound Rep Reg*. 2011;19:S16-S21.
41. O'Brien L, Pandit A. Silicon gel sheeting for preventing and treating hypertrophic and keloid scars. *Cochrane Database Syst Rev*. 2006;9:1-77.
42. Kisher CW, Shetlar MR, Shetlar C. Alteration of hypertrophic scars induced by mechanical pressures. *Arch Dermatol*. 1975;111:60-64.
43. Macintyre L, Baird M. Pressure garments for use in the treatment of hypertrophic scars: a review of the problems associated with their use. *Burns*. 2006;32:10-15.
44. Van den Kerckhove E, Stappaerts K, Fieuws S, et al. The assessment of erythema and thickness on burn related scars during pressure garment therapy as a preventive measure for hypertrophic scarring. *Burns*. 2005;31:696-702.
45. Al-Attar A, Mess S, Thomassen JM, Kauffman CL, Davison SP. Keloid pathogenesis and treatment. *Plast Reconstr Surg*. 2006;117:286-300.
46. Agrawal K, Panda N, Arumugam A. An inexpensive self-fabricated pressure clip for the ear lobe. *Br J Plast Surg*. 1998;51:122-123.
47. Brissett AE, Sherris DA. Scar contractures, hypertrophic scars, and keloids. *Facial Plast Surg*. 2001;17(4):263-271.
48. Roques C, Teot L. The use of corticosteroids to treat keloids: a review. *Int J Lower Ext Wounds*. 2008;7(3):137-145.
49. Ketchum LD, Robinson DW, Masters FW. Follow-up on treatment of hypertrophic scars and keloids with triamcinolone. *Plast Reconstr Surg*. 1971;48(3):256-259.
50. Ketchum LD, Smith J, Robinson DW, Masters FW. The treatment of hypertrophic scar, keloid and scar contracture by triamcinolone acetonide. *Plast Reconstr Surg*. 1966;38(3):209-218.
51. Griffith BH, Monroe CW, McKinney P. A follow-up study on the treatment of keloids with triamcinolone acetonide. *Plast Reconstr Surg*. 1970;46(2):145-150.
52. Ogawa R, Mitsuhashi K, Hyakusoku H, Miyashita T. Postoperative electron-beam irradiation therapy for keloids and hypertrophic scars: retrospective study of 147 cases followed for more than 18 months. *Plast Reconstr Surg*. 2003;111:547-553.
Extensive retrospective look at a large series of patients treated by scar excision with postoperative radiation therapy, indicating benefit of the combined therapy.
53. Ogawa R, Miyashita T, Hyakusoku H, et al. Postoperative radiation protocol for keloids and hypertrophic scars – statistical analysis of 370 sites followed for over 18 months. *Ann Plast Surg*. 2007;59(6):688-691.
54. Norris JEC. Superficial x-ray therapy in keloid management: a retrospective study of 24 cases and literature review. *Plast Reconstr Surg*. 1995;95(6):1051-1055.
55. Kim K, Son D, Kim J. Radiation therapy following total keloidectomy: a retrospective study over 11 years. *Arch Plast Surg*. 2015;42:588-595.
56. Sclafani AP, Gordon L, Chadha M, Romo T. Prevention of earlobe keloid recurrence with postoperative corticosteroid injections versus radiation therapy. *Dermatol Surg*. 1996;22:569-574.
57. Ogawa R, Yoshitatsu S, Yoshida K, Miyashita T. Is radiation therapy for keloids acceptable? The risk of radiation-induced carcinogenesis. *Plast Reconstr Surg*. 2009;124(4):1196-1201.
58. Har-Shai Y, Amar M, Sabo E. Intralesional cryotherapy for enhancing the involution of hypertrophic scars and keloids. *Plast Reconstr Surg*. 2003;111(6):1841-1852.
59. Uberti MG, Pierpont YN, Bhalla R, et al. Down regulation of scar fibroblasts by antineoplastic drugs: a potential treatment for fibroproliferative disorders. *Surg Sci*. 2016;7:258-271.
60. Shridharani SM, Magarakis M, Manson PN, et al. The emerging role of antineoplastic agents in the treatment of keloids and hypertrophic scars. *Ann Plast Surg*. 2010;64(3):355-361.
61. Gragnani A, Warde M, Furtado F, Ferreira LM. Topical tamoxifen therapy in hypertrophic scars or keloids in burns. *Arch Dermatol Res*. 2010;302:1-4.
62. Uppal RS, Khan U, Kakar S, et al. The effects of a single dose of 5-flurouracil on keloid scars: a clinical trial of timed wound irrigation after extralesional excision. *Plast Reconstr Surg*. 2001;108(5):1218-1224.
63. Haurani M, Foreman K, Yang JJ, Siddiqui A. 5-Flurouracil treatment of problematic scars. *Plast Reconstr Surg*. 2009;123(1):139-148.
64. Hu L, Zou Y, Chang S, et al. Effects of botulinum toxin on improving facial surgical scars: a prospective, split-scar double-blind, randomized controlled trial. *Plast Reconstr Surg*. 2018;141(3):646-650.
Recent study describing improvement of scars treated intraoperatively with botulinum toxin. A split-scar study demonstrating efficacy.
65. Curran JN, Crealey M, Sadadcharam G, et al. Vitamin E: patterns of understanding, use, and prescription by health professionals and students at a university teaching hospital. *Plast Reconstr Surg*. 2006;118(1):248-252.

66. Shih R, Walzman J, Evans GRD. Review of over-the-counter topical scar treatment products. *Plast Reconstr Surg.* 2007;119(3):1091-1095.
67. Morganroth P, Wilmot AC, Miller C. Over-the-counter scar products for postsurgical patients: disparities between online advertised benefits and evidence regarding efficacy. *J Am Acad Dermatol.* 2009;61:e31-47.
68. Moiemen NS, Staiano JJ, Ojeh NO, et al. Reconstructive surgery with a dermal regeneration template: clinical and histologic study. *Plast Reconstr Surg.* 2001;108(1):93-103.
69. Frame JD, Still J, Lakhel-LeCoadou A, et al. Use of dermal regeneration template in contracture release procedures: a multicenter evaluation. *Plast Reconstr Surg.* 2004;113(5):1330-1338.
70. Bloemen MCT, van Leeuwen MCE, van Vucht NE, et al. Dermal substitution in acute burns and reconstructive surgery: a 12-year follow up. *Plast Reconstr Surg.* 2010;125(5):1450-1459.
71. Clayman MA, Clayman SM, Mozingo DW. The use of collagen-glycosaminoglycan copolymer (Integra) for the repair of hypertrophic scars and keloids. *J Burn Care Res.* 2006;27:404-409.
Comprehensive review describing current evidence for the use of laser therapy for hypertrophic burn scars.
72. Hultman CS, Fredstat JS, Edkins RE, et al. Laser resurfacing and remodeling of hypertrophic burn scars. *Ann Plast Surg.* 2014;260(3):519-532.
73. Friedstat JS, Hultman CS. Hypertrophic burn scar management: what does the evidence show? A systematic review of randomized controlled trials. *Ann Plast Surg.* 2014;72:S198-S201.
74. Jin R, Huang X, Li H, et al. Laser therapy for prevention and treatment of pathologic excessive scars. *Plast Reconstr Surg.* 2013;132(6):1747-1758.
75. Brewin MP, Lister TS. Prevention or treatment of hypertrophic burn scarring: a review of when and how to treat with the pulsed dye laser. *Burns.* 2014;40:797-804.
76. Al Harithy R, Pon K. Scar treatment with lasers: a review and update. *Curr Derm Rep.* 2012;1:69-75.
77. Kim DH, Ryu HJ, Choi JE, et al. A comparison of the scar prevention effect between carbon dioxide fractional laser and pulsed dye laser in surgical scars. *Dermatol Surg.* 2014;40:973-978.
78. Alster TS, Williams CM. Treatment of keloid sternotomy scars with 585-nm flashlamp-pumped pulsed dye laser. *Lancet.* 1995;345:1198-1200.
79. Alster T. Laser scar revision: comparison study of 585-nm pulsed dye laser with and without intralesional corticosteroids. *Dermatol Surg.* 2003;29(1):25-29
80. Goldman MP, Fitzpatrick RE. Laser treatment of scars. *Dermatol Surg.* 1995;21:685-687.
81. Negenborn VL, Groen J, Smit JM, et al. The use of autologous fat grafting for treatment of scar tissue and scar-related conditions: a systematic review. *Plast Reconstr Surg.* 2016;137(1):31e-43e.
82. Conde-Green A, Marano AA, Lee ES, et al. Fat grafting and adipose-derived regenerative cells in burn and wound healing and scarring: a systematic review of the literature. *Plast Reconstr Surg.* 2016;137(1):302-312.
83. Klinger M, Caviggioli F, Klinger FM, et al. Autologous fat in scar treatment. *J Craniofac Surg.* 2013;24:1610-1615.
84. Coleman SR. Structural fat grafting: more than a permanent filler. *Plast Reconstr Surg.* 2006;118(3 suppl):108S-120S.
85. Kan HJ, Selles RW, van Nieuwenhoven CA, et al. Percutaneous aponeurotomy and lipofilling (PALF) versus limited fasciectomy in patients with primary Dupuytren's contracture: a prospective, randomized, controlled trial. *Plast Reconstr Surg.* 2016;137(6):1800-1812.
86. Khouri RK, Khouri RK. Current clinical applications of fat grafting. *Plast Reconstr Surg.* 2017;140(3):466e-486e.
Review of a broad spectrum of fat-grafting indications including the utility in scar and fibroproliferative disease treatment.

QUESTIONS

1. **Radiation therapy is useful for treatment of keloids:**
   a. Preoperatively
   b. Infrequently
   c. As a sole modality
   d. At high doses
   e. In the immediate postoperative period

2. **Common complications from corticosteroid injection for scar treatment include:**
   a. Skin atrophy
   b. Cushing disease
   c. Hypopigmentation
   d. a, b, and c
   e. a and c

3. **Definitive scar improvement has been demonstrated with randomized controlled trials for which of the following modalities?**
   a. Mechanomodulation
   b. Laser therapy
   c. Fat grafting
   d. Pressure therapy
   e. Excision and XRT

4. **A 60-degree angle Z-plasty theoretically lengthens the central limb of the method by:**
   a. 50%
   b. 60%
   c. 75%
   d. 100%

5. **Concerning laser therapy for hypertrophic burn scars:**
   a. Pulsed dye laser is indicated for scar erythema.
   b. CO_2 laser is indicated for scar erythema.
   c. CO_2 laser is indicated for scar texture treatment.
   d. Pulsed dye laser is indicated for scar texture treatment.
   e. a and c
   f. b and d

1. **Answer: e.** Radiation therapy is an effective, frequently used treatment as an adjunct to surgical excision in a relatively low dose, usually in divided multiple sessions, immediately postoperatively. Radiation therapy is not effective preoperatively, or as a solitary treatment, as recurrence rates of keloids are high.

2. **Answer: e.** Corticosteroid injection for scar management is an effective management, usually requiring multiple interval injections. Pain, skin atrophy, and hypopigmentation are common side effects encountered. Cushing disease as a result of local corticosteroid injection would be very unusual, because of the relative low doses and minimal systemic absorption of the drug.

3. **Answer: a.** Although evidence exists to consider laser therapy, fat grafting, pressure therapy, and excision plus radiation therapy, the majority of reports utilizing these modalities are case series, retrospective studies, and comparative studies. Only mechanomodulation with a device to alleviate tension at the time of surgical incision has shown improvement in randomized controlled trials.

4. **Answer: c.** Theoretical geometric lengthening of the central limb of a Z-plasty with flaps incised at 60 degrees is 75%.

5. **Answer: e.** Pulsed dye laser at 585/595-nm wavelength is used to treat scar erythema. CO_2 laser works by tissue ablation and water vapor absorption and is indicated for scar texture treatment.

CHAPTER 4 Principles of Flap Design and Application

Julian J. Pribaz and Katherine M. Huber

KEY POINTS

- A flap is a body of tissue with its own inherent blood supply that can be elevated and moved to reconstruct defects.
- Thorough knowledge of blood supply to tissue is critical for safe and reliable flap elevation and transfer.
- Use of two- and three-dimensional templates will assist with proper flap design.
- Attempt to minimize residual donor site deformity. Consider the consequences of scar contracture, contour deformity, and functional loss.
- For a complex defect, consider staged reconstruction with methodical planning of each stage. Always have a backup plan.
- The primary goal of flap reconstruction is to maintain adequate flap vascularity. Plan for secondary revisions to improve contour and appearance.

The word *principle* stems from the Latin *princeps* meaning *a beginning*. Tenets of practice should begin with the principles, yet these should be subject to change as knowledge of the subject increases.[1] There has been significant evolution of our knowledge of flaps in recent years, primarily due to improvements in the understanding of vascular anatomy. This has led to noteworthy advances in the reconstructive options available.

The simplest definition of a flap is a body of tissue with its own original inherent blood supply that can be elevated and moved to repair and reconstruct defects. In this way, a flap differs from a graft, which does not carry its own blood supply. Flaps, in one form or another, serve as the basis of reconstructive surgery.

FLAP BLOOD SUPPLY AND PHYSIOLOGY

A thorough knowledge of blood supply to the skin and accompanying tissue is critical in safe and reliable flap elevation and transfer of flaps. The skin, because of its role in thermoregulation to maintain homeostasis and its immunological function, has a rich blood supply, far greater than what is needed for its own inherent metabolic demand. This is an important fact in facilitating skin flap survival. The blood reaches the skin from deeper named vessels, via multiple perforating arteries and their accompanying veins that course through overlying muscles, septa, and fascia to supply the more superficial vascular plexuses, creating a continuous three-dimensional (3D) network of vessels supplying all layers of tissues. For the skin, the blood supply is concentrated at the suprafascial and subdermal levels, from which smaller vessels branch to supply the intervening tissues[2] (**Figure 4.1**).

In 1987, Taylor and Palmer rediscovered and further elaborated on the work of Manchot and Salmon on the blood supply of the skin and underlying tissue, and proposed the concept of the *angiosome*, which they defined as a 3D body of tissue supplied by a source (segmental or distributing) artery and its accompanying vein(s) that span between the skin and bone.[3] Each angiosome could be subdivided into a matching arteriosome (arterial territory) and venosome (venous territory). Angiosomes can vary in size and interdigitate with adjoining angiosomes via true small anastomotic bidirectional arterioles and venules by reduced-caliber choke (retiform) anastomotic vessels.[4]

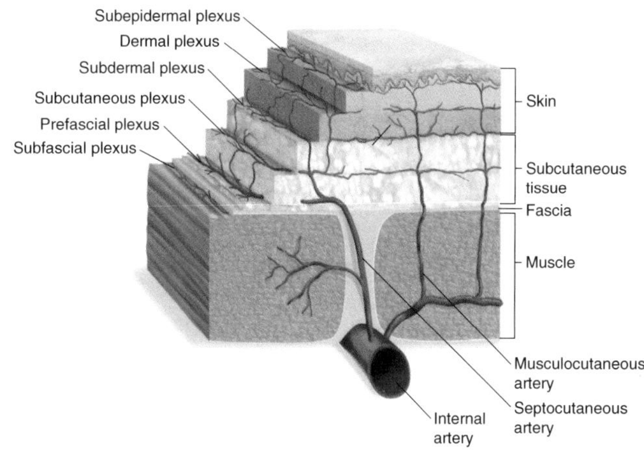

FIGURE 4.1. Vascular plexuses of the skin and subcutaneous tissue.

More recent work by Saint-Cyr et al.[5] advanced the angiosome concept to provide additional and more practical insight into vascular territory and flow characteristics that are important in flap design. They studied both 3D (static) and 4D (dynamic) blood flow through multiple single perforators and mapped out the territory supplied, calling this a *perforasome* (**Figure 4.2**). They found greater complexity and variability than was initially anticipated, and they confirmed that each perforasome is connected to an adjacent perforasome by both direct (fascial) and indirect (subdermal) linking vessels (**Figure 4.3**).

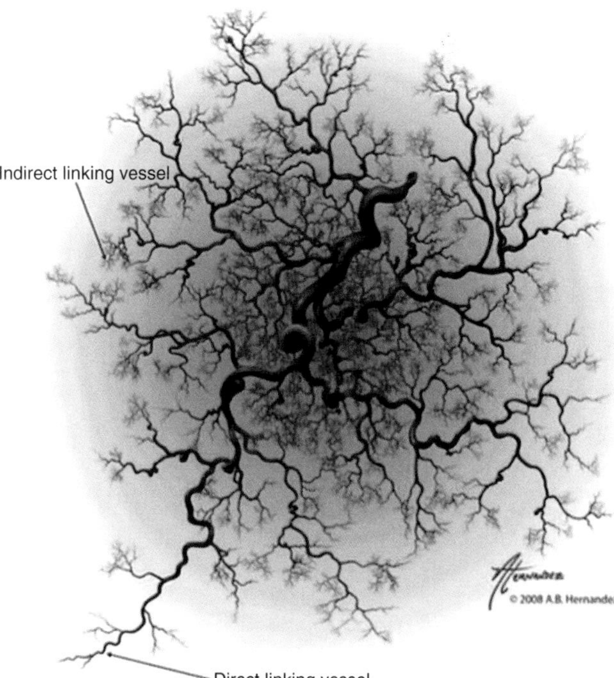

FIGURE 4.2. Perforators have a distinct arterial and venous vascular territory. This image depicts the vascular arterial anatomy of a perforasome. Note the dense vascular network centered around the perforator that decreases progressively toward the periphery. Large linking vessels branch peripherally in multiple directions away from the perforator origin. From Saint-Cyr M, Wong C, Schaverien M, Mojallal A, Rohrich RJ. The perforasome theory: vascular anatomy and clinical implications. *Plast Reconstr Surg.* 2009;124(5):1529-1544; with permission.

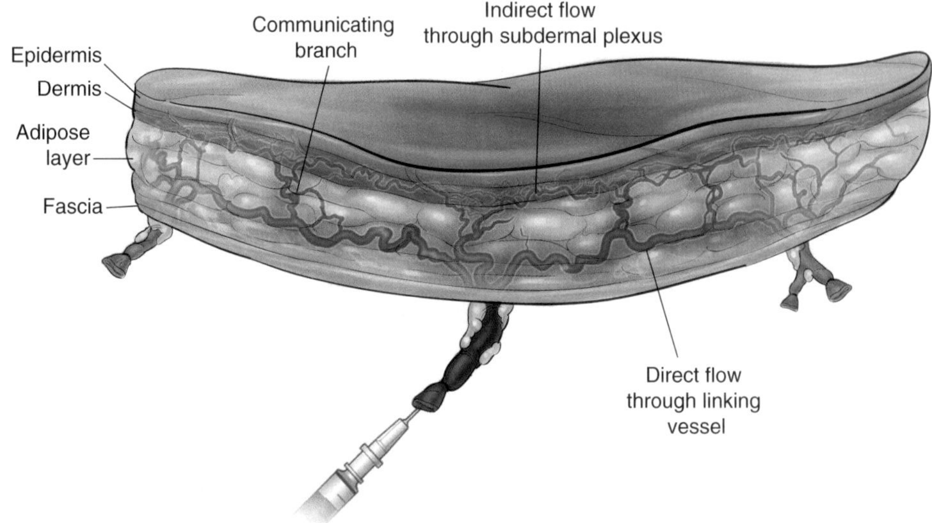

FIGURE 4.3. Interperforator flow occurs by means of direct and indirect linking vessels. Direct linking vessels communicate directly with an adjacent perforator to maintain perfusion, and travel within the suprafascial and adipose tissue layers. Indirect linking vessels communicate with adjacent perforators by means of recurrent flow through the subdermal plexus. Communicating branches between direct and indirect linking vessels are also seen and help maintain vascular perfusion in case of injury. From Sur YJ, Morsy M, Michel Saint-Cyr M. The pedicled perforator (propeller) flap in lower extremity defects. In: Strauch B, Vasconez LO, Herman CK, Lee BT, eds. *Grabb's Encyclopedia of Flaps: Upper Extremities, Torso, Pelvis, and Lower Extremities*. 4th ed, vol. 2. Philadelphia, PA: Wolters Kluwer; 2016:1420-1425.

NOMENCLATURE AND CLASSIFICATION

The nomenclature of flap classification is somewhat imperfect and fluid. As Converse stated, "There is no simple and all-encompassing system which is suitable for classifying skin flaps."[6] This is true for skin flaps as well as flaps of other tissue types. Although the nomenclature is imperfect and overlapping, it is important to develop a vocabulary of terms to describe flaps for improved understanding and communication with other medical professionals.

Flaps can be classified in multiple ways. Classification occurs according to flap content and tissue type, mechanics of movement or transfer, blood supply, and manipulation prior to harvest.

Flap Content

Flap classification begins with the content of the planned flap. The simplest flap contains skin and subcutaneous tissue. These are referred to as *cutaneous* flaps. Cutaneous flaps can be harvested relatively thinly to fit a similar defect. Generally, the blood supply in a cutaneous flap is random in nature and located within the subdermal plexus.

As defects become more complex, so can the harvested flap. Flaps containing skin, subcutaneous tissue, and fascia are referred to as *fasciocutaneous* flaps.[7] Fascial flaps devoid of the overlying skin can also be harvested if a very thin flap that is easily contoured is desired. These are known as *fascial* and *adipofascial* flaps and are usually accompanied by an overlying skin graft to maintain a thin contour. Fasciocutaneous flaps were described and further classified by their pattern of blood supply by Cormack and Lamberty in 1984[8] (**Table 4.1**). The temporoparietal and anterolateral thigh fasciocutaneous flaps are excellent examples.

Muscle flaps are a staple of reconstructive surgery. They may be used in stand-alone fashion, or with an overlying skin graft. These flaps can be harvested with overlying skin and soft tissue for added bulk and are called *myocutaneous* flaps. Muscle and myocutaneous flaps were classified by Mathes and Nahai in 1981 based on their inherent blood supply[9] (**Figure 4.4**). Often in cases of lower extremity trauma with exposed bone or hardware, well-vascularized muscle tissue is desired for coverage and has the advantage of conforming to an irregular wound bed to minimize dead space. However, recent literature shows that muscle and fasciocutaneous flaps achieve comparable rates of limb salvage and functional recovery.[10]

When structural support at the defect is required, flaps containing bone can be used. Vascularized bone flaps, or *osseous* flaps, can be harvested free from surrounding tissue. For example, a bone-only free fibula can be harvested on the peroneal artery and is a workhorse of head and neck bony reconstruction. Conversely, overlying soft tissue and skin can be included. In this case, the flap is categorized as *osteomyocutaneous* and *osteocutaneous*.

In a separate category are omental and intestinal flaps. The omental flap can be raised on the gastroepiploic vessels and utilized in pedicled fashion to fill sternal or other chest wall defects. The omentum has angiogenic and immunogenic properties that make it ideal for reconstruction of sternal wound infections. As a free flap, it is extremely useful as thin vascularized tissue that can be covered with skin grafts for defects in the head and neck or lower extremity.[11] Various intestinal flaps can be harvested to reconstruct laryngopharyngeal and esophageal defects.[12]

TABLE 4.1. CORMACK AND LAMBERTY CLASSIFICATION OF FASCIOCUTANEOUS FLAPS

Type	Description	Example
A	A pedicled fasciocutaneous flap dependent on multiple fasciocutaneous perforators at the base and orientated with the long axis of the flap	Lateral arm flap
B	A pedicled or a free flap depending on a single sizeable and consistent fasciocutaneous perforator feeding a plexus at the level of the deep fascia	Parascapular fap
C	The blood supply of the skin is dependent upon the fascial plexus that is supplied by multiple small perforators along its length, which reach it from a deep artery by passing along the fascial septum between muscles.	Radial forearm flap
D	The fascial septum is taken in continuity with adjacent muscle and bone which derive their blood supply from the same artery	Free fibula flap

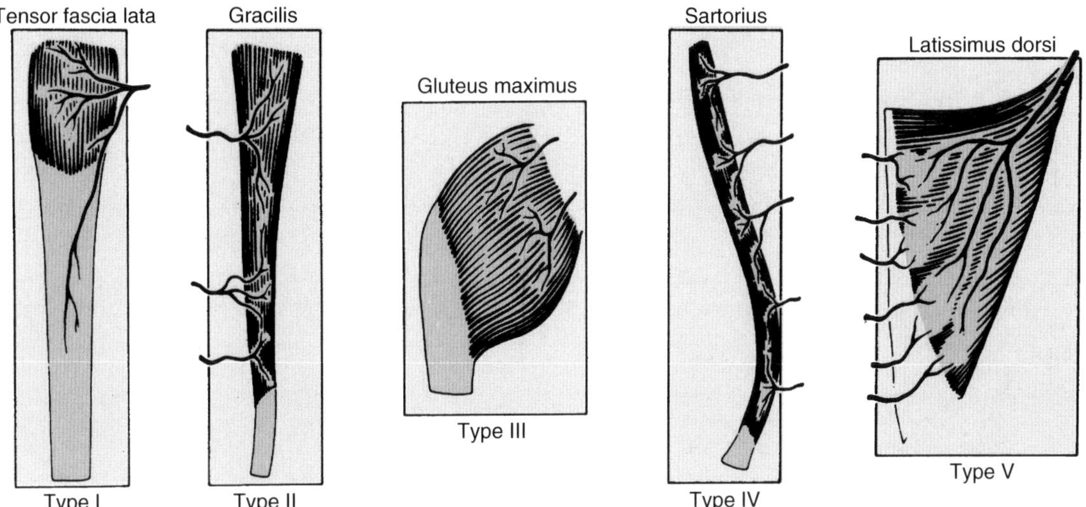

FIGURE 4.4. Mathes and Nahai classification. Patterns of vascular anatomy: type I, one vascular pedicle; type II, dominant pedicle(s) and minor pedicles; type III, two dominant pedicles; type IV, segmental vascular pedicles; type V, one dominant pedicle and a secondary segmental pedicle. Reproduced with permission from Mathes SJ, Nahai F. Classification of the vascular anatomy of muscles: experimental and clinical correlation. *Plast Reconstr Surg.* 1981;67(2):177-187.

Composites of any of the above categories are used frequently and can include other local tissue such as cartilage, tendon, or mucosa.

Movement and Proximity to Defect

The type of movement or transfer required to inset a flap provides an additional system of classification. Based on proximity to the defect to be reconstructed, flaps are described as *local*, *regional*, or *distant*. Local flaps are moved into an adjacent defect by a process of advancement, transposition, rotation, and interpolation, or combinations of these basic movements (**Table 4.2**).

Regional flaps such as pedicled muscle flaps require larger movements than those seen in local flaps. These often still include rotations (**Figure 4.5**), advancements (**Figure 4.6**), and transpositions (**Figure 4.7**). Distant flaps include tubed flaps and free flaps. Tubed flaps are the oldest known type of flaps, first described in the literature in 1917 by Filatov.[13,14] These involve harvest of a pedicled flap followed by a series of transpositions known as *walking*. After inset of each transposition, the flap obtains new blood supply from the surrounding tissue by neovascularization and vessel ingrowth. At the subsequent stage, the opposite end is transposed, allowing for movement of the flap and maintenance of blood supply. In this way, the flap is *walked* or *waltzed* to its final destination for inset, often necessitating several stages. The advent of free tissue transfer has reduced the use of tubed flaps; however, a distant tubed flap may still play a role in patients who are poor candidates for free tissue transfer.

Blood Supply

A flap can be further classified by the orientation of its blood supply. The pattern of blood supply to cutaneous flaps is generally described as either *axial* or *random*. An axial pattern flap has a known or named artery coursing along its longitudinal axis. A random-pattern flap is designed without a known vessel at its core and relies on the random subdermal plexus for perfusion.[15] Random-pattern flaps must generally be limited to a 3:1 length to width ratio to remain viable at the tip.[16,17] Axial pattern flaps can be designed with a longer length to width ratio and may carry a random extension with the same limitations described earlier.

Flaps containing muscle or fascia can also be classified further by the type of blood flow that supplies them. The Mathes and Nahai classification of muscle flaps and the Cormack and Lamberty classification of fascial flaps are mentioned above (see Figure 4.4 and Table 4.1).

The blood supply of a flap can additionally be classified as either *pedicled* or *free*. Pedicled flaps remain attached to a known native vascular pedicle and are limited to the arc of rotation or advancement that these vessels afford. The pedicle can be dissected free from surrounding tissues and the flap *islandized* for maximizing transfer distance. Conversely, a free flap is one that is raised on a known vascular pedicle that is transected and anastomosed to a new blood supply at the recipient site, largely requiring microsurgical techniques.[18] Free flaps allow for true freedom of tissue transfer. A flap harvested in one location can reconstruct a defect that is distant from it, assuming adequate blood flow exists at the recipient site.

Perforator flaps are those based on a perforating artery from a named vessel and include the surrounding 3D area of tissue perfused by that perforator, also known as the *perforasome*[5,19] (see earlier). Perforating vessels can be thought to travel in a plane perpendicular to that of the skin surface and the axial vessels beneath. Perforators are frequently identified by use of a handheld Doppler on the skin, and one or more perforators can be included in any given flap. Blood flow then arborizes and fills vessels linking one perforasome to the next (see Figure 4.2). Flaps designed around a perforator often also include proximal dissection of the named vessel from which the blood flow originates, and this allows for longer pedicle length or larger caliber of vessels for free tissue transfer. Perforator flaps have become increasingly popular as local flaps for reconstructing both difficult small and larger defects that previously had required a free tissue transfer.

The keystone perforator island flap was described by Behan and has been used throughout the body as an island flap designed adjacent to a defect, and typically based on one or more smaller perforators. The flap has the shape of a keystone-like arch that is designed parallel to the defect and is at least as wide as the defect. It extends beyond each end of the defect, completing the archlike design (**Figure 4.8**). The dissection extends through the skin, subcutaneous tissue, and fascia, thus mobilizing the flap to advance into the defect. The closure borrows tissue from all directions, as each end is repaired as a V-Y advancement.[20]

Another local use of a perforator flap is as a *propeller* flap. This was first described by Hyakusoku et al. in 1991[21] and is based on a single large perforating vascular pedicle close to the defect that is rotated up to 180°. The main perforator is identified with a handheld Doppler

TABLE 4.2. CLASSIFICATION OF FLAPS BY MOVEMENT TYPE

Flap Movement	Subtypes	Illustration
Rotation	Rotation	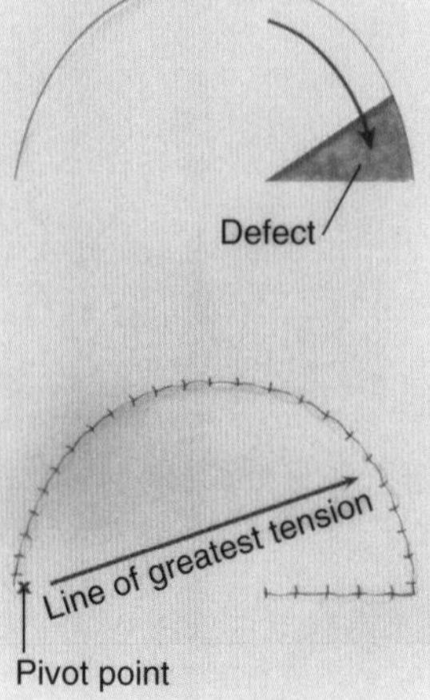 Defect; Line of greatest tension; Pivot point
Advancement	V-Y Bipedicled Keystone	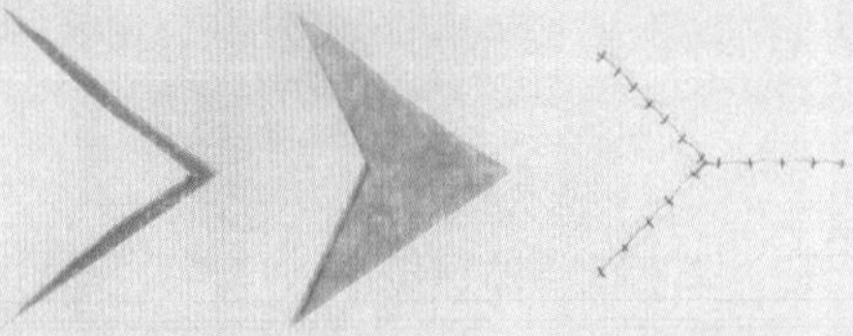
Transposition	Z-plasty Rhomboid Bilobed	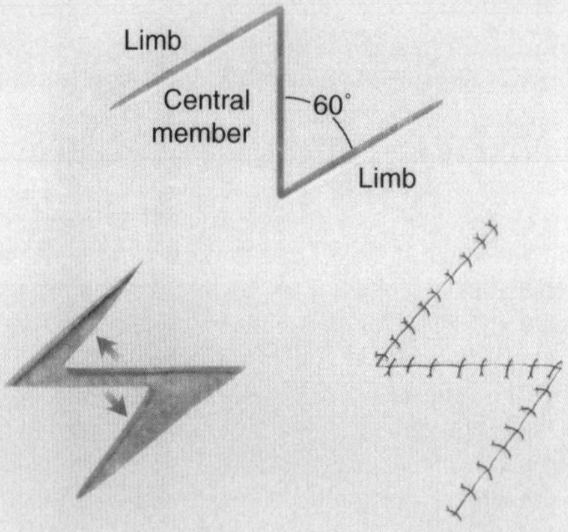 Limb; Central member; 60°; Limb
Islandization	Propeller Pedicled	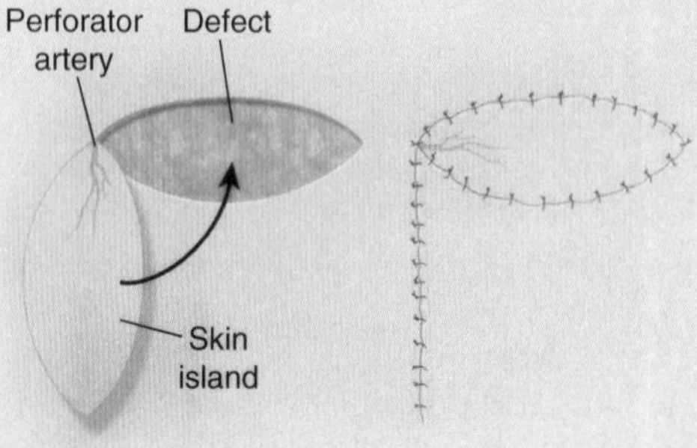 Perforator artery; Defect; Skin island

and will be the pivot point for flap rotation. Careful measurement and precise flap design to reach the distal end of the defect is mandatory. The perforator can be visualized early in the dissection and the flap design confirmed prior to circumscribing the island flap. It is important to dissect the perforator through the fascia and free up the adventitia so that there is no venous kinking[21,22] (**Figure 4.9**).

Modifications to flap blood flow have resulted in added classifications such as the *reverse-flow* flap, the *venous* flap, and the *supercharged* flap. A reverse-flow flap is one in which the native direction of flow through the main pedicle is reversed at inset. An example is the reverse radial forearm flap, in which the radial artery is transected proximally, and the flap must rely on reverse blood flow in the radial artery across the palmar arch[23] (**Figure 4.10**). A venous flow-through flap is composed of skin, subcutaneous tissue, and a plexus of veins. It is devoid of arterial tissue within the flap. A linear vein is anastomosed to an artery proximally and a vein

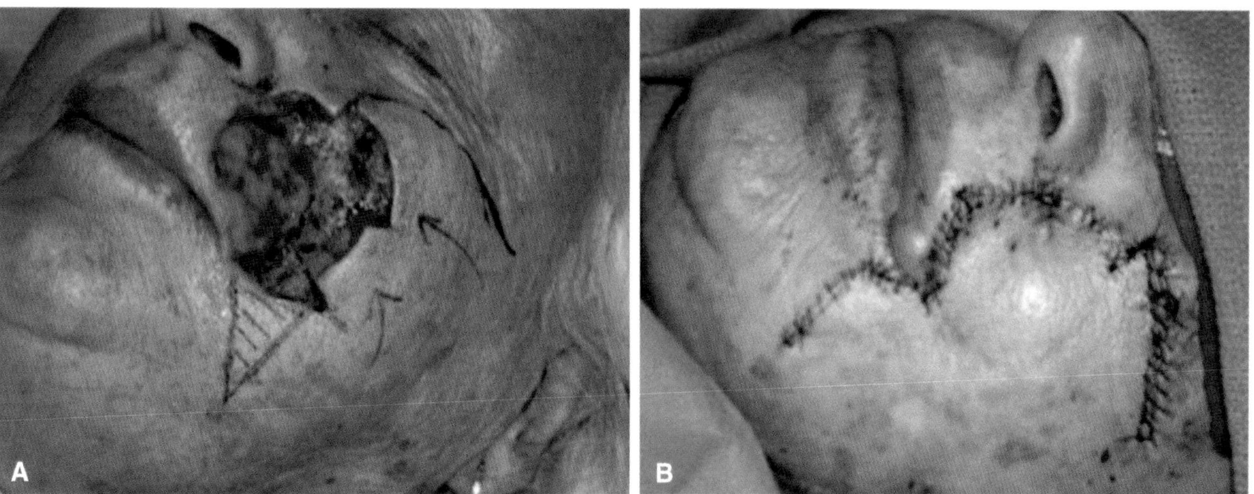

FIGURE 4.5. Rotation flap. **A.** Cheek defect after excision of a basal cell cancer with plans for a cheek rotation flap and excision of dog-ear. **B.** Scars are placed along natural crease lines to maximize cosmesis.

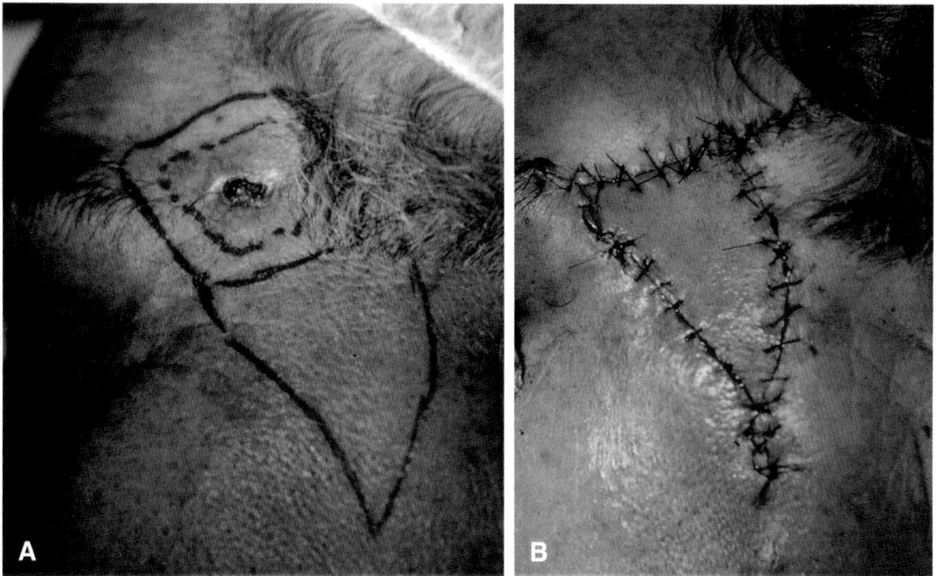

FIGURE 4.6. V-Y advancement flap. **A.** Left temple basal cell carcinoma showing planned excision and design of V-Y flap. This type of advancement flap causes minimal distortion to surrounding tissues and replaces *like with like*. **B.** Final result includes a well-vascularized flap without alteration of brow position.

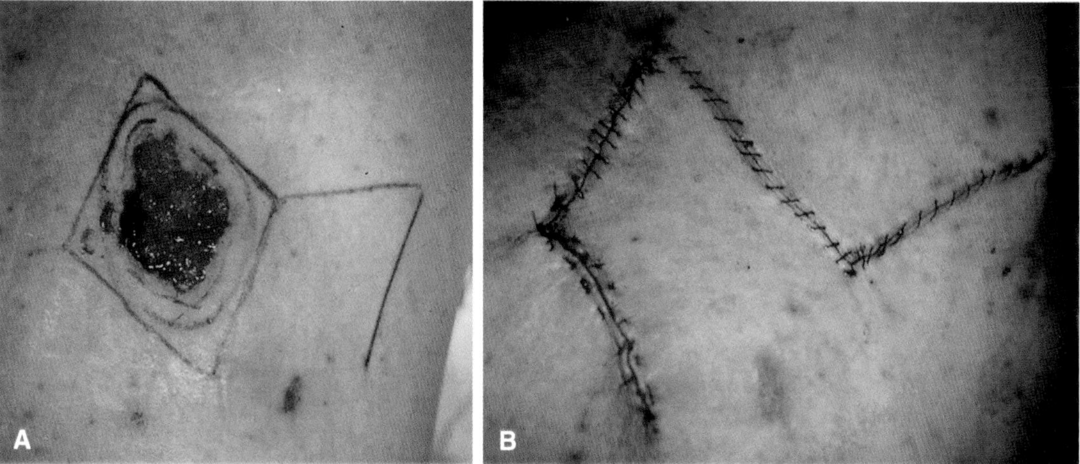

FIGURE 4.7. Transposition flap. **A.** Ulcerated lesion with planed excision and rhomboid flap. **B.** Transposed flap closes defect while distributing tension along the planes of the donor site.

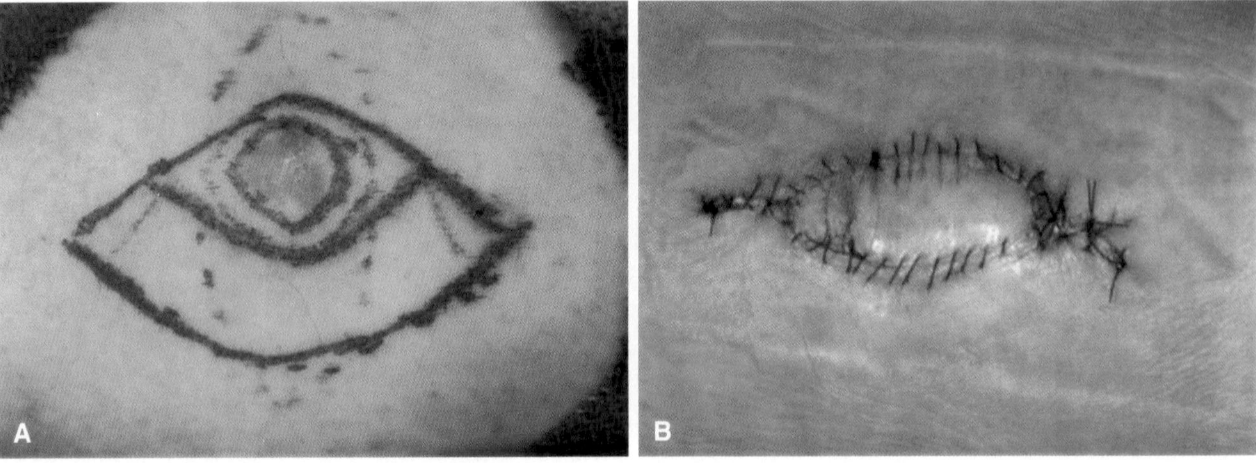

FIGURE 4.8. Keystone flap. **A.** Lower extremity lesion with planned excision and keystone flap design. **B.** Resulting flap redistributes tension as each end is closed in V-Y fashion.

distally, allowing for both inflow and outflow. These are generally small flaps and can be prone to congestion and partial necrosis.[24] A supercharged flap is one in which the arterial inflow or venous outflow is augmented by using microsurgical techniques to perform a second anastomosis, bringing in an additional inflow or outflow capabilities.[25]

Manipulation

A discussion of classification of flaps would be incomplete without mention of the different types of flap manipulation that can occur prior to harvest. First, tissue that is desired for a planned flap can undergo tissue expansion. An *expanded* flap allows for

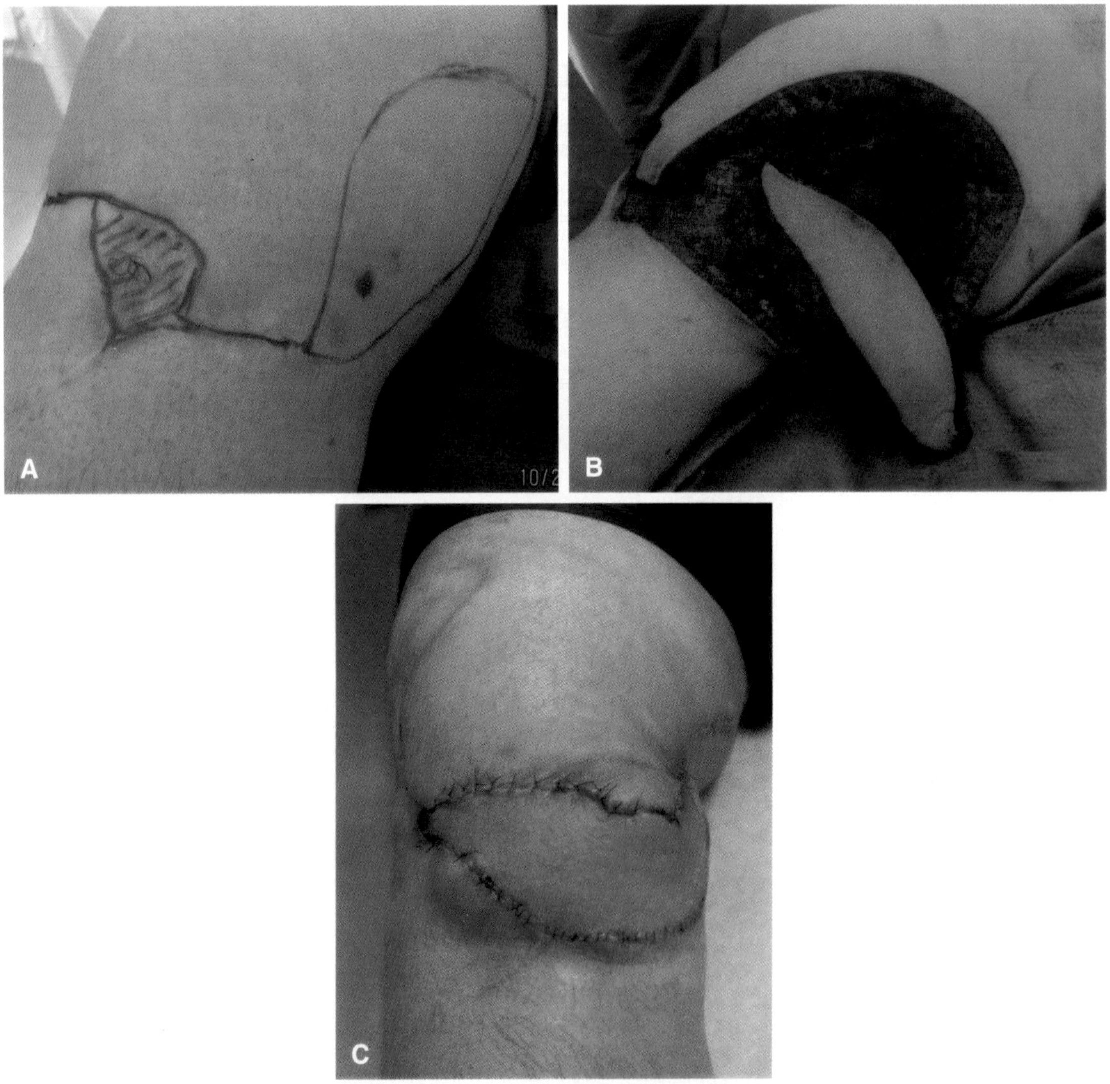

FIGURE 4.9. Propeller flap. **A.** Unstable scar in patient undergoing total knee replacement. Perforator marked with red dot is used as center of rotation. **B.** Flap elevation includes dissection of perforator. **C.** Rotation and final inset offers excellent coverage of hardware and primary closure of donor site.

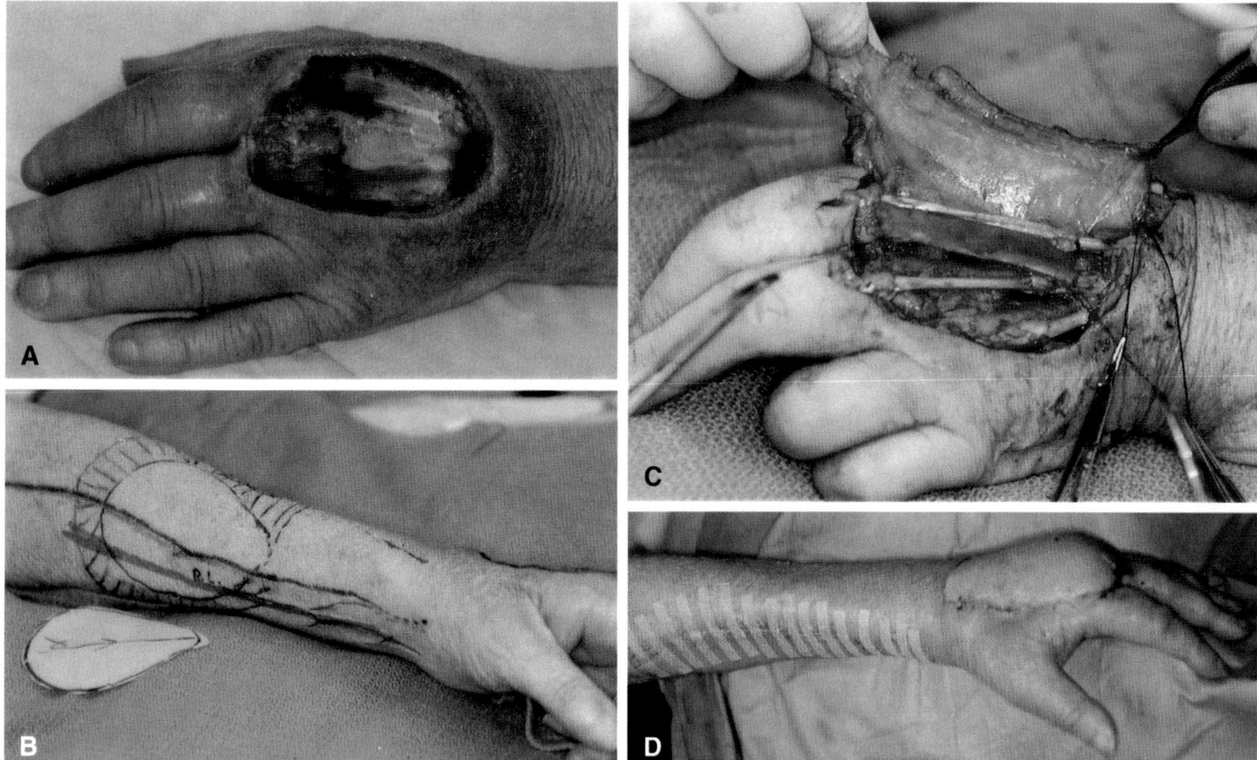

FIGURE 4.10. Reverse radial forearm flap. **A.** 70-year-old woman with a left dorsal hand wound after intravenous extravasation injury. **B.** Reverse radial forearm flap is designed based on retrograde flow across the palmar arch. Note the inclusion of palmaris longus tendon for extensor tendon reconstruction. **C.** An added layer of antebrachial fascia is utilized to wrap the tendon reconstruction for improved glide. **D.** Routine inset and healing with primary closure of the donor site.

greater reach and coverage and can minimize the donor site defect.[26] Furthermore, the mechanical force of stretching tissues has also been shown to enhance tissue neovascularity,[27] and the accompanying thinning of the flap can be an additional bonus in reconstruction.

In situations where there is concern for the ultimate perfusion of the flap, flap delay can be employed. A *delayed* flap is one in which a preliminary surgical stage is planned to partially raise the flap and divide a portion of the blood supply, delivering a sublethal ischemic insult that stimulates vessel dilation, ischemic preconditioning, and neovascularization. This allows for axialization of blood flow and conditioning of the flap tissues to lower oxygen levels in anticipation of flap transfer at a second stage[28] (**Figure 4.11**).

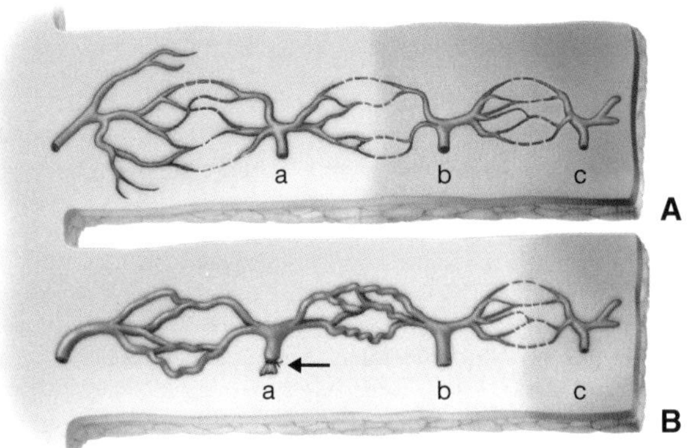

FIGURE 4.11. Diagrammatic representation of the same flap raised with and without a surgical delay to illustrate the necrosis line and the changes in the choke vessels between *a* and *b*. In **B**, vessel a has been delayed by a previous operation before raising the flap. Note the dilation of choke vessels and the more distal site of the necrosis line.

The techniques of flap prefabrication and prelamination are other more recent additions to our armamentarium and can greatly expand the functional capacity of the flap. These will be discussed in more detail later in this chapter.

FLAP DESIGN AND APPLICATION

The reconstructive surgeon must be familiar with the full spectrum of reconstructive options and select the flap or method of repair that will give the best outcome. The optimal reconstructive strategy may involve multiple modalities of treatment and/or multiple staged procedures. One must take care not to burn bridges and compromise the final result.

The flap options available have increased greatly in recent years, and the focus has shifted from ensuring flap survival to limiting the number of flaps required to close a defect and ultimately to enhanced flap selection and refinements. Refinements are achieved by careful preoperative and intraoperative assessment of the defect, determining the reconstructive requirements, and then selecting the donor tissue that gives the best functional and aesthetic result.

Assessing the Defect

For successful flap reconstruction, an accurate diagnosis of the defect, its underlying causes, and reconstructive requirements is needed. The surgeon should consider what tissues are missing (e.g., skin, functional muscle, bone). Precise measurements of shape and size should be taken, including consideration of the 3D depth of the defect for appropriate contour restoration. Photos, templates, and 3D moulages are of great assistance in defect assessment and should be used liberally[29] (**Figure 4.12**). Modern image-guided planning, especially in planning bony flaps, is also advantageous and can reduce operative time.[30]

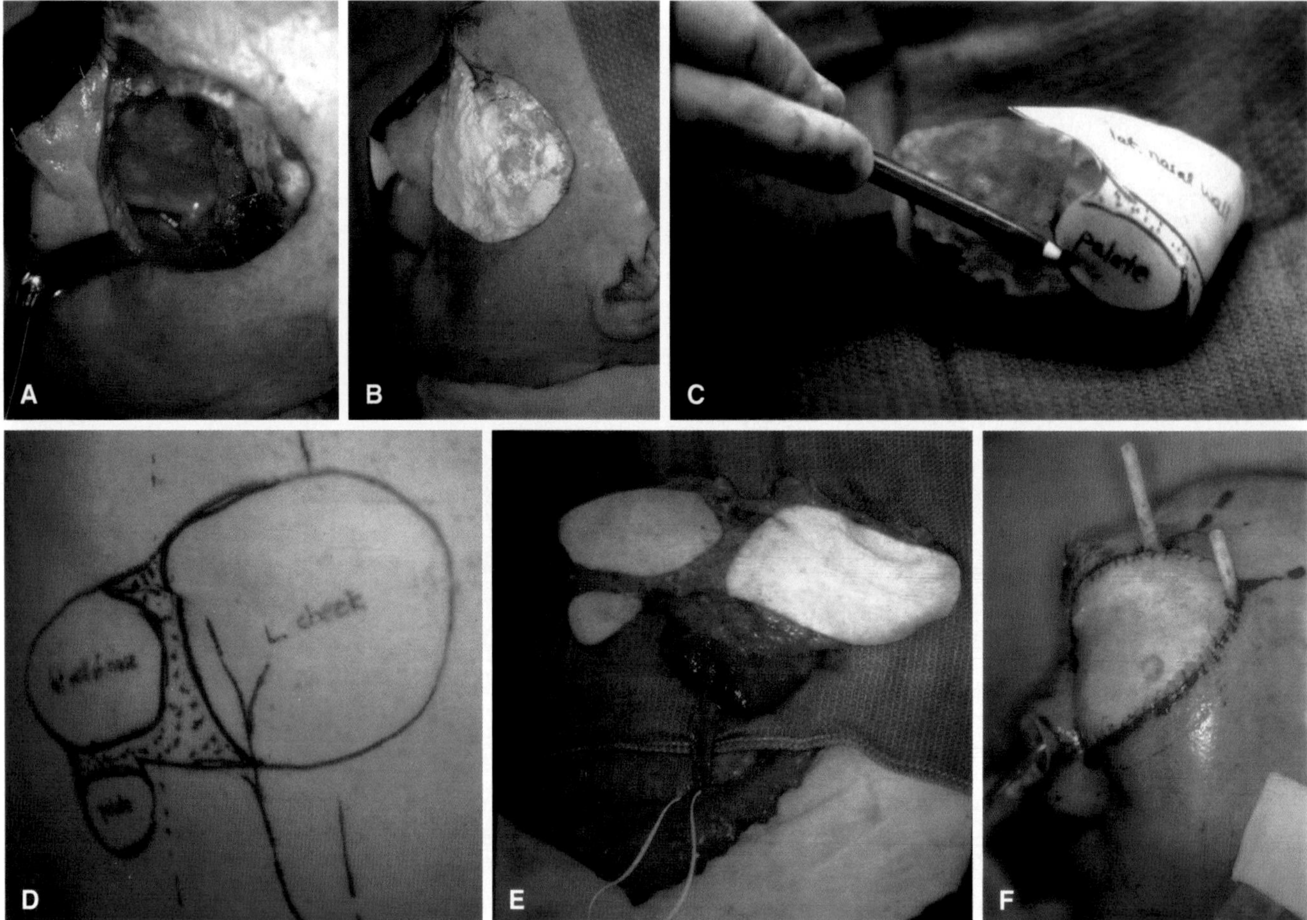

FIGURE 4.12. **A.** A 67-year-old woman had a complex defect of the left orbit with palatal and nasal defect after cancer resection. **B.** Three-dimensional alginate moulage is used for on-table flap planning. **C.** Moulage is wrapped with a template to represent flap folding. **D.** Template is used to create flap outline overlying the deep inferior epigastric vessels on the abdomen. **E.** Flap elevation including a portion of rectus abdominis for filling of dead space. **F.** Final inset with complete reconstruction of internal lining and excellent external contour.

One of the most important steps in reconstruction is satisfactory preparation of the defect. The wound bed should be debrided of necrotic material, granulation tissue, and attenuated or scarred tissue. In some cases, quantitative cultures are beneficial to verify the wound is free from infection and bacterial balance has been achieved.[31] In oncologic defects, pathology should ensure clear margins prior to reconstruction. Despite excellent flap selection and harvest technique, inadequate preparation of the wound can lead to flap compromise and reconstructive failure.

Patient selection is also a consideration when planning reconstruction. Inherent patient factors such as diabetes, clotting disorders, and poor compliance can hamper flap success. Modifiable factors such as smoking and patient weight should also be contemplated. If risk factors for flap failure are high, a simple method of wound closure may be better than complex multistage reconstruction.

In free tissue transfer, the presence of recipient vessels must be evaluated. Ideal recipient vessels are in close proximity (either deep or adjacent) to the wound to be reconstructed. The quality of these vessels should be assessed. If the planned recipient vessels appear injured either on preoperative angiogram or during direct inspection intraoperatively, consider use of different vessels. Use of vessels outside the zone of injury during free flap reconstruction leads to increased rates of lower extremity limb salvage.[32] Additionally, recipient vessels should be of adequate caliber to anastomose easily to the flap vessels and provide adequate perfusion. If there are no adequate recipient vessels near the defect, consideration can be given to vein grafts or creation of an AV loop from a regional blood supply source.[33] In the extremities, flow-through flaps should be considered if perfusion of the hand or foot would otherwise be compromised by anastomosis of a flap.

Selection and Management of the Donor Site

The full extent of the reconstructive ladder is contemplated for each wound, preferably from simplest to most complex. Local tissue will often provide better color match and appearance but may be limited depending on the location of the wound. Many local, regional, and distant donor sites are available. Consider the suitability of each donor site to fulfill the goals of reconstruction and the logistics and positioning on the operating table, avoiding positional changes if possible. Attempt to minimize residual donor site deformity.

Site and Content Selection

In selecting the appropriate donor site, first consider the skin surrounding the defect. Color match, texture, thickness, and special characteristics such as hair growth should be taken into account. Design the flap to be slightly larger than the defect for adequate skin coverage. This will help account for the thickness of the flap, avoid tight closure over the vascular pedicle, and facilitate donor site closure. Often significant edema of the flap occurs during the procedure that will make closure tight if some excess tissue is not included in flap design. After assessment of skin requirements, flap thickness and content can be selected. Can adequate thickness be reconstructed with skin and subcutaneous fat? Is muscle bulk needed to fill the defect, or is a functional muscle needed to restore movement? Is bone or cartilage support of the soft tissues necessary? For complex reconstructions of the head and neck, lining may be required in addition to external skin coverage. Mucosal lining can be fashioned from skin, skin graft, mucosa, or raw muscle surface, which will mucosalize with time.

Pedicle Considerations

Once content requirements of the flap have been determined, decisions can be made concerning the pedicle. The surgeon should consider both caliber and length required, especially in the case of free tissue transfer. The caliber should approximate that of the recipient vessels; however, if significant size mismatch exists, end-to-side anastomosis is an option.[34] Concerning pedicle length, the surgeon should consider the ergonomic constraints of microsurgical vessel anastomosis. Free tissue transfer can be made significantly easier with slight slack in the pedicle for creation of a tension-free anastomosis that occurs in an orientation that is comfortable for the operating surgeon's hands. Appropriate length can be obtained either by initial selection or by dissection proximally on the flap pedicle to its origin.

Manipulation of Donor Site Tissue

Manipulation of donor site tissue at the time of flap transfer is utilized for complex reconstruction to provide a better-tailored flap and minimize donor defects. For a complex wound, two (or more) flaps can be carried on one pedicle. These flaps are known as compound or chimeric flaps.[35] An example is the latissimus dorsi, parascapular, scapular bone, serratus anterior flap, which can be one complex compound flap based on the subscapular vascular system (**Figure 4.13**).

Conversely, a very large flap may benefit from a double pedicle. A simple example of this is the bipedicled advancement flap. However, in more complex cases, very large flaps, such as double pedicle TRAM (transverse rectus abdominis myocutaneous) flaps, may be raised and left pedicled, or transferred as a double pedicle free flap if the volume of tissue required exceeds the amount that can be transferred on a single pedicle.[36,37]

Flaps can be designed to be folded on themselves to create added bulk or can be employed in reconstruction of a lamellar surface such as the lower lip. In this case, a donor site with a thin subcutaneous layer should be selected.[38] Complex central facial defects often require reconstruction of the multiple external and internal epithelial surfaces. As mentioned earlier, the use of a 3D intraoperative alginate moulage to facilitate flap planning and folding to accurately repair the multiple epithelial defects has been found to be very useful (see Figure 4.12).

Management of the Donor Site

Inherent in flap design is management of residual donor site defects. Commonly the donor site of a flap is repaired primarily, or in cases of undue tension, skin grafted. Attempts should be made to minimize donor site deformity as much as possible. Consider the consequences of scar contracture such as decreased range of motion and pain. When possible, orient incisions within resting skin tension lines. Contour deformity may be considered cosmetic; however, functional issues with hygiene may occur in severe cases. Functional loss from muscle or nerve transfer must be contemplated preoperatively and discussed with the patient. Choose muscle flaps that have redundant function when possible. Revision of donor site deformities should be offered when a functional problem exists and a solution is apparent.

Staging Reconstruction in Complex Defects

Staged reconstructions are often required for complex defects. In such cases, it is important to plan ahead and perform the best possible surgery at each stage, keeping in mind the opportunity cost of additional procedures and time for maturation at each stage. Avoid burning bridges and consider adjunct techniques, including delay, expansion, prelamination, and prefabrication.

Delay of a flap involves a preliminary surgical stage to partially raise the flap and divide a portion of the blood supply. This allows for axialization of blood flow and conditioning of the flap tissues to low oxygen levels in anticipation of flap transfer at a second stage. Delay can increase survival of a larger surface area on a given pedicle.[28]

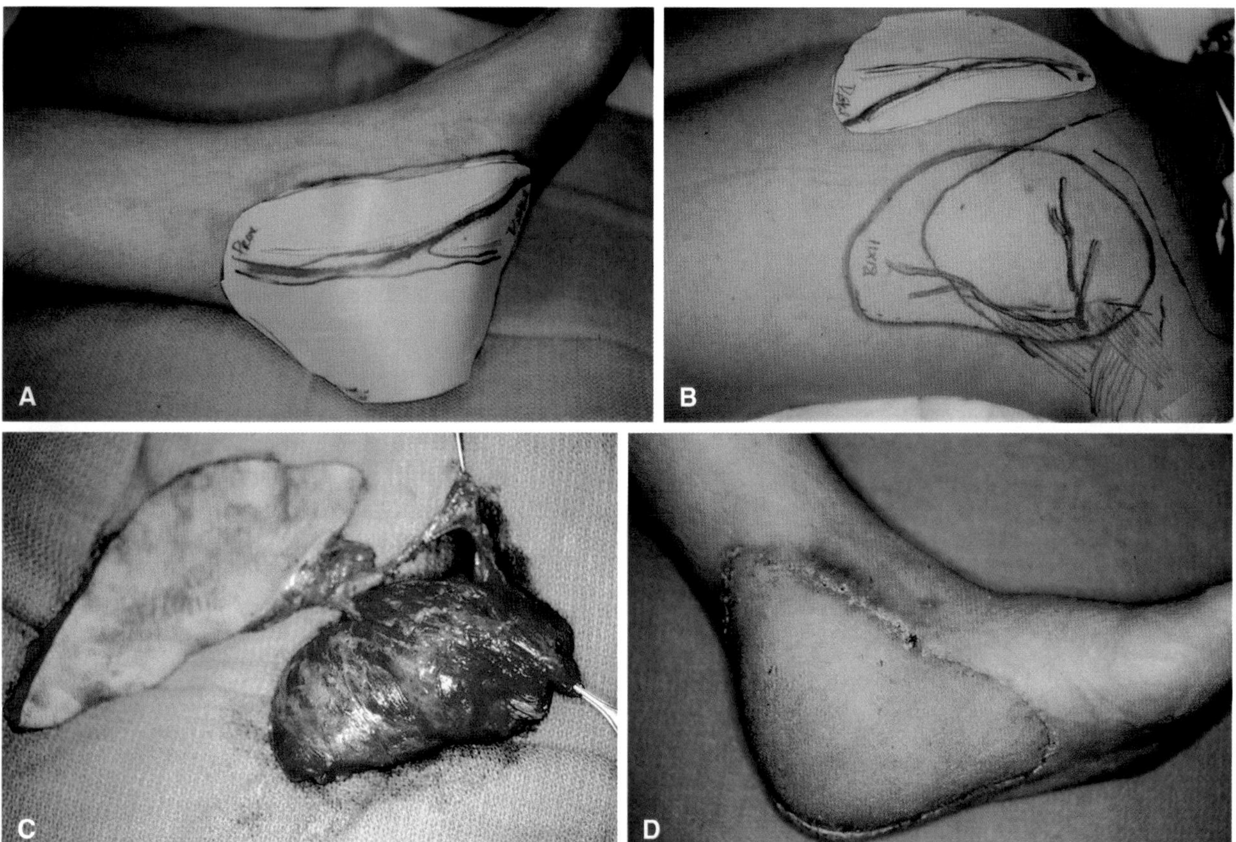

FIGURE 4.13. Compound chimeric flap to heel defect. **A.** A young man with a medial foot wound with exposed calcaneus after osteomyelitis. **B.** Compound flap design using the teres major muscle and fasciocutaneous parascapular flap harvested on the subscapular vascular system. Note the intraoperative use of templates for better planning reconstruction of this three-dimensional defect. **C.** The harvested flap. **D.** After inset and healing.

As discussed previously, tissue expansion of the donor flap provides more tissue and a thinner flap and alleviates tension at the donor site, resulting in easier closure and improved scarring.

Prefabrication of a flap involves transferring a vascular pedicle into a desired block of tissue, then waiting 8 weeks for spontaneous neovascularization, thus creating a new vascular territory not previously found in nature.[39] After maturation, the neovascularized tissue is transferred based on the implanted pedicle. This technique has been used to provide thin axial flaps and to transfer tissue with enhanced color and texture match (**Figure 4.14**).

The technique of *prelamination* involves implantation of tissue (usually bone or cartilage) or an alloplastic device into a vascular territory prior to transfer. It has been used mainly for reconstruction of complex defects in the central third of the face.[40]

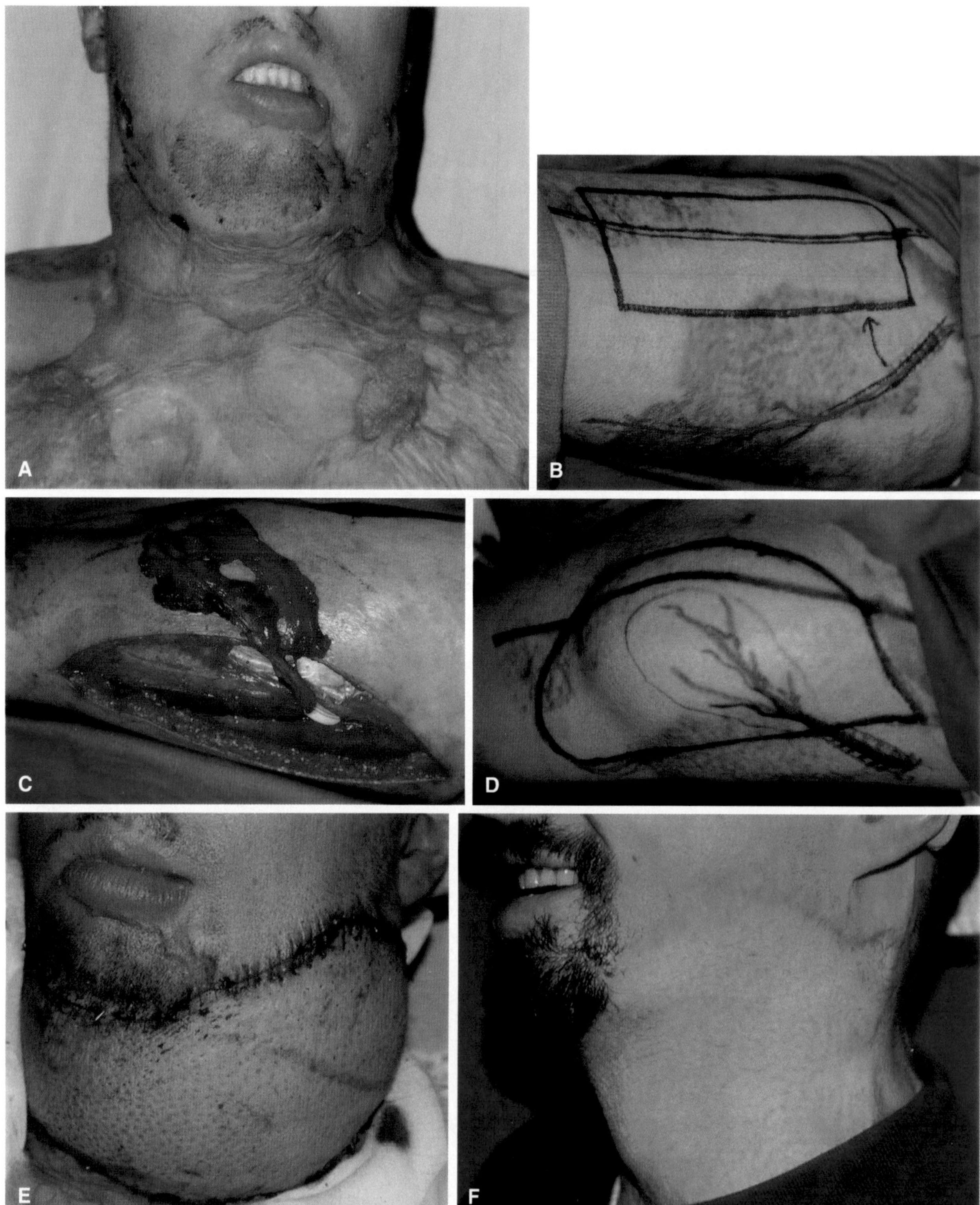

FIGURE 4.14. Flap prefabrication. **A.** A 40-year-old man with hypertrophic burn scar contracture of the anterior neck. **B.** To avoid areas of scarring on the thigh, a prefabricated flap is designed on the anteriomedial thigh using the descending branch of the lateral femoral circumflex vessels. **C.** Vessels are transposed to the desired area; a tissue expander is also placed to expand the new flap. **D.** After expansion and neovascularization of the tissue around the new pedicle. **E.** Flap inset. **F.** After flap debulking the patient is left with a thin, pliable flap, excellent color match, functional improvement, and minimal scarring.

Options in Case of Flap Compromise

Despite the surgeon's best efforts, some flaps will inevitably experience decreased arterial perfusion or venous congestion after elevation and inset. In pedicled or free flaps, inadequate arterial flow is usually recognized early and may be the result of poor flap design or pedicle kinking. In a free flap, the arterial insufficiency represents thrombosis of the new anastomosis until proven otherwise. These cases require revision on the table or urgent return to the operating room to revise the anastomosis.

Venous insufficiency of a flap is more common and the onset more insidious than that of arterial insufficiency. This phenomenon is multifactorial. In elevating a flap, longitudinal venous channels in the flap are disconnected. Additionally, the low pressure in the venous system is more vulnerable to extrinsic pressure because of compression from inset and flap edema. Numerous methods have been described to improve flap survival in the case of venous congestion. First, the surgeon should attempt to release insetting sutures causing tension or kinking. The flap may be pricked with a needle serially to reduce the venous burden. Deepithelialization of a portion of the flap, or removal of the nail plate in the case of a digit, with periodic application of heparin solution may increase venous outflow. Use of *Hirudo medicinalis* or medicinal leeches can ensure ongoing flap outflow until venous microanastomoses form. Finally, augmenting outflow by cannulation of a vein with an angiocatheter and periodically draining the flap may be useful.[41]

CONCLUSION

Flaps are the mainstay of reconstructive surgery. In the words of Gillies, always consider "blood supply before beauty."[1] Remember to maintain adequate flap vascularity and plan for secondary revision to improve contour and appearance. When performing staged reconstructions for complex defects, plan ahead and do not burn bridges.

REFERENCES

1. Gillies H, Millard D. *The Principles and Art of Plastic Surgery*. Boston: Little and Brown; 1957.
2. Daniel RK, Kerrigan CL. Skin flaps: an anatomical and hemodynamic approach. *Clin Plast Surg*. 1979;6(2):181-200.
3. Taylor GI, Palmer JH. The vascular territories (angiosomes) of the body: experimental study and clinical applications. *Br J Plast Surg*. 1987;40(2):113-141.
4. Taylor GI, Corlett RJ, Ashton MW. The functional angiosome: clinical implications of the anatomical concept. *Plast Reconstr Surg*. 2017;140(4):721-733.
The authors review data from experimental work of other researchers on vascular imaging of skin flaps in various animal models. The study then used a rabbit model to focus on the role of anastomotic vessels between angiosome territories in tissue perfusion. Using fluorescein infusion, rabbit perforator flaps showed conversion of choke vessels to true anastomoses by 7 days, allowing distal territory survival in 95% of flaps. This highlights the dynamic, functional nature of anastomotic vessels as they can control flow between territories. The functional angiosome is thereby defined as the volume of tissue that clinically can be isolated on a source vessel. The area extends beyond its anatomical territory to capture an adjacent territory if connections are by choke anastomoses, or more if they are by true anastomoses.
5. Saint-Cyr M, Wong C, Schaverien M, et al. The perforasome theory: vascular anatomy and clinical implications. *Plast Reconstr Surg*. 2009;124(5):1529-1544.
6. Converse JM. *Introduction to Plastic Surgery. Reconstructive Plastic Surgery*. 2nd ed, vol. 1. Philadelphia, PA: WB Saunders; 1977:3-68.
7. Cormack GC, Lamberty BG. Fasciocutaneous vessels. Their distribution on the trunk and limbs, and their clinical application in tissue transfer. *Anat Clin*. 1984;6(2):121-131.
8. Cormack GC, Lamberty BG. A classification of fascio-cutaneous flaps according to their patterns of vascularisation. *Br J Plast Surg*. 1984;37(1):80-87.
9. Mathes SJ, Nahai F. Classification of the vascular anatomy of muscles: experimental and clinical correlation. *Plast Reconstr Surg*. 1981;67(2):177-187.
The authors summarize data from previous studies involving vascular injections of latex solutions into muscle of cadavers. They determine the pattern of blood supply to each muscle establishes the extent of safe transposition and usefulness in reconstruction. A classification system is suggested based on the blood supply of each muscle. This classification of vascular anatomy is shown clinically to predict arcs of rotation and ultimate muscle flap survival after elevation.
10. Cho EH, Shammas RL, Carney MJ, et al. Muscle versus fasciocutaneous free flaps in lower extremity traumatic reconstruction: a multicenter outcomes analysis. *Plast Reconstr Surg*. 2018;141(1):191-199.
11. McLean DH, Buncke HJ. Autotransplant of omentum to a large scalp defect, with microsurgical revascularization. *Plast Reconstr Surg*. 1972;49(3):268-274.
12. Moradi P, Glass GE, Atherton DD, et al. Reconstruction of pharyngolaryngectomy defects using the jejunal free flap: a 10-year experience from a single reconstructive center. *Plast Reconstr Surg*. 2010;126(6):1960-1966.
13. Filatov V. Plastic procedure using a round pedicle. McDowell F, trans. *Vestnik Oftalmol*. 1917;34:149-158.
14. Gillies H. The tubed pedicle in plastic surgery. *N Y Med J*. 1920;111:1.
15. Stell PM. The viability of skin flaps. *Ann R Coll Surg Engl*. 1977;59(3):236-241.
16. Milton SH. Pedicled skin-flaps: the fallacy of the length: width ratio. *Br J Surg*. 1969;56(5):381.
17. McGregor IA, Morgan G. Axial and random pattern flaps. *Br J Plast Surg*. 1973;26(3):202-213.
18. Taylor GI, Daniel RK. The free flap: composite tissue transfer by vascular anastomosis. *Aust N Z J Surg*. 1973;43(1):1-3.
19. Morris SF, Tang M, Almutari K, Geddes C, Yang D. The anatomic basis of perforator flaps. *Clin Plast Surg*. 2010;37(4):553-570, xi.
20. Behan FC. The keystone design perforator island flap in reconstructive surgery. *ANZ J Surg*. 2003;73(3):112-120.
21. Hyakusoku H, Yamamoto T, Fumiiri M. The propeller flap method. *Br J Plast Surg*. 1991;44(1):53-54.
22. Teo TC. The propeller flap concept. *Clin Plast Surg*. 2010;37(4):615-626, vi.
23. Timmons MJ. The vascular basis of the radial forearm flap. *Plast Reconstr Surg*. 1986;77(1):80-92.
24. Fukui A, Inada Y, Maeda M, et al. Venous flap: its classification and clinical applications. *Microsurgery*. 1994;15(8):571-578.
25. Tan O, Atik B, Bekerecioglu M. Supercharged reverse-flow sural flap: a new modification increasing the reliability of the flap. *Microsurgery*. 2005;25(1):36-43.
26. Zhou XT. Effects of tissue expansion on the ratio of length to width of random-pattern skin flaps. *Zhonghua Wai Ke Za Zhi*. 1989;27(7):417-418, 445.
27. Leighton WD, Russell RC, Feller AM, et al. Experimental pretransfer expansion of free-flap donor sites: II. Physiology, histology, and clinical correlation. *Plast Reconstr Surg*. 1988;82(1):76-87.
The authors endeavor to evaluate the changes in blood flow and tissue histology that occur with tissue expansion. Using pig models, flaps are designed, expanded, and elevated. Blood flow and angiography were recorded and tissue samples were examined and compared with a nonexpanded control site. The authors found the vascular trees within flaps enlarge following expansion, and pronounced neovascularization is seen in the papillary dermis and capsular layers. There is thinning of all the tissue layers except for the epidermis. Successful clinical application of these principles in humans is depicted.
28. Taylor GI, Corlett RJ, Caddy CM, Zelt RG. An anatomic review of the delay phenomenon: II. Clinical applications. *Plast Reconstr Surg*. 1992;89(3):408-416.
29. Kane WJ, Olsen KD. Enhanced bone graft contouring for mandibular reconstruction using intraoperatively fashioned templates. *Ann Plast Surg*. 1996;37(1):30-33.
30. Toto JM, Chang EI, Agag R, et al. Improved operative efficiency of free fibula flap mandible reconstruction with patient-specific, computer-guided preoperative planning. *Head Neck*. 2015;37(11):1660-1664.
31. Breidenbach WC, Trager S. Quantitative culture technique and infection in complex wounds of the extremities closed with free flaps. *Plast Reconstr Surg*. 1995;95(5):860-865.
32. Stranix JT, Lee ZH, Jacoby A, et al. Not all Gustilo type IIIB fractures are created equal: arterial injury impacts limb salvage outcomes. *Plast Reconstr Surg*. 2017;140(5):1033-1041.
33. Atiyeh BS, Sfeir RE, Hussein MM, Husami T. Preliminary arteriovenous fistula for free-flap reconstruction in the diabetic foot. *Plast Reconstr Surg*. 1995;95(6):1062-1069.
34. Ikuta Y, Watari S, Kawamura K, et al. Free flap transfers by end-to-side arterial anastomosis. *Br J Plast Surg*. 1975;28(1):1-7.
35. Hallock GG. Simultaneous transposition of anterior thigh muscle and fascia flaps: an introduction to the chimera flap principle. *Ann Plast Surg*. 1991;27(2):126-131.
The authors endeavor to differentiate a chimeric flap from the previously described compound or composite flaps. A chimeric flap is defined as a flap in which more than one tissue type is linked together, but tissue components may be independently maneuvered while remaining attached by a common regional source vessel. They describe specific surgical dissection technique of the ALT and rectus femoris muscle chimeric flap and offer a case report of a patient treated with this method.
36. Wagner DS, Michelow BJ, Hartrampf CR Jr. Double-pedicle TRAM flap for unilateral breast reconstruction. *Plast Reconstr Surg*. 1991;88(6):987-997.
37. Agarwal JP, Gottlieb LJ. Double pedicle deep inferior epigastric perforator/muscle-sparing TRAM flaps for unilateral breast reconstruction. *Ann Plast Surg*. 2007;58(4):359-363.
38. Jeng SF, Kuo YR, Wei FC, et al. Total lower lip reconstruction with a composite radial forearm-palmaris longus tendon flap: a clinical series. *Plast Reconstr Surg*. 2004;113(1):19-23.
39. Khouri RK, Upton J, Shaw WW. Prefabrication of composite free flaps through staged microvascular transfer: an experimental and clinical study. *Plast Reconstr Surg*. 1991;87(1):108-115.
40. Pribaz JJ, Fine NA. Prelamination: defining the prefabricated flap: a case report and review. *Microsurgery*. 1994;15(9):618-623.
41. Talbot SG, Pribaz JJ. First aid for failing flaps. *J Reconstr Microsurg*. 2010;26(8):513-515.
The authors present a descriptive article on the possible etiologies of arterial and venous insufficiency in flaps. Based on their experience and expertise, they highlight surgical techniques that can prevent blood flow compromise before it occurs. Citing other studies, they propose an algorithm for assessing and treating a flap that is experiencing venous insufficiency or congestion.

42. Pallua N, Machens HG, Rennekampff O, et al The fasciocutaneous supraclavicular artery island flap for releasing postburn mentosternal contractures. *Plast Reconstr Surg.* 1997;99(7):1878-1884; discussion 1885-1876.
43. Ross RJ, Baillieu CE, Shayan R, Leung M, Ashton MW. The anatomical basis for improving the reliability of the supraclavicular flap. *J Plast Reconstr Aesthet Surg.* 2014;67(2):198-204.
44. Vijayasekaran A, Mohan AT, Zhu L, et al. Anastomosis of the superficial inferior epigastric vein to the internal mammary vein to augment deep inferior artery perforator flaps. *Clin Plast Surg.* 2017;44(2):361-369.
45. Lee KT, Mun GH. Benefits of superdrainage using SIEV in DIEP flap breast reconstruction: a systematic review and meta-analysis. *Microsurgery.* 2017;37(1):75-83.
46. Leedy JE, Janis JE, Rohrich RJ. Reconstruction of acquired scalp defects: an algorithmic approach. *Plast Reconstr Surg.* 2005;116(4):54e-72e.
47. Simsek T, Engin MS, Yildirim K, et al. Reconstruction of extensive orbital exenteration defects using an anterolateral thigh/vastus lateralis chimeric flap. *J Craniofac Surg.* 2017;28(3):638-642.
48. D'Arpa S, Cordova A, Pignatti M, Moschella F. Freestyle pedicled perforator flaps: safety, prevention of complications, and management based on 85 consecutive cases. *Plast Reconstr Surg.* 2011;128(4):892-906.
49. Maciel-Miranda A, Morris SF, Hallock GG. Local flaps, including pedicled perforator flaps: anatomy, technique, and applications. *Plast Reconstr Surg.* 2013;131(6):896e-911e.

QUESTIONS

1. A 62-year-old man with squamous cell cancer of the ear is treated with total auriculectomy including burring of the mastoid bone. Flap reconstruction to close the wound is planned with a pedicled supraclavicular flap. The blood supply to the supraclavicular flap is considered which of the following?

a. Random
b. Free
c. Reverse flow
d. Axial
e. Perforator

2. A 45-year-old woman with recurrent breast cancer undergoes mastectomy and free deep inferior epigastric artery perforator flap. Routine anastomoses of one artery and one vein are completed, and the flap is inset. On the table, the flap appears congested. Insetting sutures are released with no improvement. The arterial and venous anastomoses are visualized and noted to be patent. What is the next best step to resolve the congestion?

a. Anastomose the superficial inferior epigastric vein (SIEV).
b. Revise the venous anastomosis.
c. Start leech therapy.
d. Administer systemic TPA.
e. Revise the arterial anastomosis.

3. A 70-year-old man is involved in a motor vehicle collision. A large portion of his scalp was avulsed and could not be salvaged. After multiple debridements, the resultant defect comprises 70% of the scalp with exposed calvarium at the base. Reconstruction is best achieved with which of the following?

a. Split-thickness skin graft
b. Free omental flap with split-thickness skin graft
c. Wet-to-dry dressing changes with healing by secondary intention
d. Tissue expansion with staged advancement of flaps
e. Scalp flap with skin graft to the donor defect

4. A 13-year-old girl is diagnosed with rhabdomyosarcoma of the left orbit and face. Orbital exenteration and radical en bloc resection including bone is planned followed by chemotherapy and radiation. Which of the following best reconstructs the resulting 3D defect?

a. Dermal substitute
b. Skin graft
c. Local advancement flap including skin and subcutaneous fat
d. Free anterolateral thigh (ALT) flap including skin, subcutaneous fat, and fascia
e. Free ALT flap including skin, subcutaneous fat, fascia, and vastus lateralis muscle

5. A 65-year-old man is evaluated for reconstruction of a chronic wound to the lateral malleolus. Because of medical comorbidities, he is a poor candidate for free tissue transfer. Reverse sural flap is planned. On the evening of postoperative day zero, the patient has mild hypotension, and the flap is noted to be dark and congested distal to a line of tension created by insetting sutures. What is the next best step?

a. Apply moisturizer cream to the affected area.
b. Release insetting sutures at area of maximum tension.
c. Administer a fluid bolus.
d. Elevate extremity.
e. Observe and reassure that this will likely improve with time.

6. An otherwise fit 30-year-old man, following a compound fracture of the distal third of the tibia, previously treated by the orthopedist with open reduction and internal fixation, presents with a small open wound breakdown (4 × 3 cm) with exposed hardware. He has good pulses. After further debridement and removal of hardware and application of an external fixator, the soft tissue defect is repaired with a local propeller perforator flap, based on a posterior tibial artery perforator. During flap dissection and inset, the flap becomes progressively more congested along its entire length. Which of the following is the most appropriate next step in management?

a. Observation
b. Application of nitropaste
c. Postoperative leech therapy
d. Proximal perforator dissection to source vessel
e. Free flap salvage

1. **Answer: d.** The supraclavicular flap is an axial flap based on axial blood flow through the supraclavicular artery.[42] It is not considered a random flap, although random-pattern extensions can be added to the distal aspect.[43] Blood flow in the supraclavicular artery is antegrade and not considered a reverse-flow flap. As the flap is based on a named axial vessel, it is not a perforator flap. A supraclavicular flap is typically left pedicled and rotated to fill defects of the head and neck. It is particularly useful in patients who are not good candidates for free flaps. In this question, a pedicled flap is desired and therefore the tissue is not harvested as a free flap.

2. **Answer: a.** In this case, the best course of action is to locate the SIEV at the edge of the flap and create a second venous anastomosis, thereby supercharging venous outflow.[44,45] Some surgeons routinely preserve the SIEV during dissection in case of need for added venous drainage. Revision of the existing venous and arterial anastomoses would likely provide no benefit if each is already a visibly patent anastomosis, as mentioned in the question stem. Leech therapy is useful in smaller, thin flaps; however, in this bulky high-flow flap, the small amount of venous outflow leech therapy provides would be negligible. Systemic use of tissue plasminogen activator would not improve venous outflow and could increase the risk of hemorrhagic complications.

3. **Answer: b.** The omental free flap is an excellent option in large defects of the calvarium and can be easily skin grafted for ultimate coverage. A skin graft alone would be inadequate coverage for exposed bone as graft ***take*** would be limited because of a poorly vascularized wound bed. Wet-to-dry dressing changes may be considered as a temporizing measure to help debride devitalized tissue and prepare the wound for coverage; secondary intention healing would progress very slowly and leave the patient at risk for infection and desiccation of bone. Tissue expansion is an appropriate option for defects comprising up to 50% of the hair-bearing scalp, but would be insufficient for a 70% defect. A scalp flap with skin grafting of the donor defect is also not appropriate for near total scalp loss.[46]

4. **Answer: e.** Three-dimensional contour deformities are best reconstructed using a flap that contains muscle, which can conform to the defect and fill dead space. The same flap without muscle would not be the best option.[47] A skin graft would likely not vascularize over exposed bone. Dermal substitutes would likewise be unsatisfactory coverage in this complex defect. Local flaps may play a role in coverage of a large wound; however, insufficient local tissue exists to fill a defect this large and would likely lead to unsightly scarring and additional deformity.

5. Answer: b. The flap described is likely suffering from impaired venous outflow distal to the area of tension. Release of insetting sutures in this area will likely improve outflow at this site.[41] Moisturizing cream is unlikely to improve venous outflow. Mild hypotension postoperatively is not ideal for flap survival and would be more likely to impair arterial inflow. Augmentation of blood pressure with a fluid bolus would not reliably improve venous outflow. Elevation of the extremity may decrease flap edema and offer some mild improvement in venous outflow but would not solve the issue of a specific line of tension across the flap. Observation is incorrect, as the congestion will likely progress if left unrevised.

6. Answer: d. Propeller flaps, which are single perforator flaps, are being used more commonly in reconstruction of small defects that had previously been treated with free flaps. However, proper dissection of the pedicle is mandatory in this type of flap which usually has to rotate 180°. The most common complication associated with propeller flap dissection is venous congestion. This is usually due to impaired venous outflow through the very thin and fragile comitant veins running with the perforating artery. This is more likely to happen if there is a bulky pedicle due to additional soft tissue and fascia, which makes kinking of these small veins more likely when the flap and pedicle is twisted 180°. The best way to minimize this is to fully dissect the pedicle and free it from surrounding soft tissue and fascia.[48,49] If venous congestion persists, this suggests injury to the draining veins; the flap can be returned to its initial position, and venous leeching from a distended vein within the flap may be used to salvage the flap. This is much more effective than topical leech therapy. Nitropaste therapy is not effective with venous congestion. Traditionally, free flap salvage was the preferred choice of treatment for distal third leg defects and may be required should the perforator flap fail, but one should try to salvage the problem at hand before proceeding to another method of repair.

CHAPTER 5 Principles of Microsurgery

Sarah E. Sasor and Kevin C. Chung

KEY POINTS

- Microsurgical techniques are used to repair blood vessels, nerves, and lymphatics; applications include free tissue transfer, nerve repair, replantation, and transplantation.
- Surgical precision is the key factor in anastomotic patency.
- There is no difference in patency rate based on suture technique (simple interrupted versus continuous) or anastomotic technique (end-to-end versus end-to-side).
- Routine use of antithrombotic agents in the postoperative period is optional.
- Thrombosis is most common within 24 hours of surgery. Early failure is often related to anastomotic imperfections or pedicle positioning. If a problem is detected early, the flap can be salvaged by exploration and revision of the anastomosis.

Microsurgery is a discipline that requires magnification, precision instruments, and specialized surgical techniques. Magnification, using surgical loupes or an operating microscope, makes it possible to repair tiny, delicate structures that exceed the limits of normal human eyesight. Microsurgical techniques are used to repair blood vessels, nerves, and lymphatics; transplant tissue from one area of the body to another; and reattach amputated parts.

HISTORY

The origin of microsurgery can be traced back to the late 1890s when surgeons began repairing blood vessels both in laboratory animals and humans without the use of magnification. The first successful end-to-end anastomosis was performed on the carotid artery of a sheep in 1889 by Jassinowski.[1] In 1902, Carrel described the triangulation method of anastomosis that is still routinely used today.[2] The following year, Höpfner performed the first experimental extremity replantation on a canine hind limb.[3]

The introduction of the operating microscope in Sweden by Nylen[4] and Holmgren[5] in the early 1920s revolutionized the field of microsurgery; it was used successfully in ear and eye procedures in centers throughout Europe. Fine surgical instruments specifically designed for use under magnification were adapted from those used by watchmakers and jewelers. The development of fine sutures swaged on suitably fine needles followed thereafter.

Jacobson and Suarez are credited with the first successful microsurgical anastomosis using an operating microscope on a canine carotid artery in 1960.[6] They encountered significant difficulty while attempting the procedure with the unaided eye, and after trying multiple forms of magnification, were successful with a microscope previously used in otology.

Throughout the 1960s, Buncke experimented with replantation and transplantation in laboratory animals. In 1966, he performed rabbit ear replantation with the anastomosis of vessels approximately 1 mm in diameter. Buncke developed many important principles and techniques and is often called the *founding father of microsurgery*.[7]

Technological improvements such as coaxial illumination, motorized and optical zoom, binocular viewing, and independent focus controls made small anastomoses more reliable. With flap failure rates less than 2%,[8] microsurgical techniques are now used with confidence.

BASIC SCIENCE CONCEPTS IN MICROSURGERY

To optimize outcomes, microsurgeons must understand the basic mechanisms of vessel injury and regeneration, the clotting mechanism, and how tissues respond to ischemia and reperfusion.

Vessel Injury and Regeneration

Microvascular anastomoses disrupt all three layers of a vessel wall. Exposure of subendothelial collagen to the bloodstream results in platelet aggregation and the formation of thrombotic plugs. Full-thickness sutures provide intimal continuity at the anastomosis site and result in the highest rates of patency.[9] Soon after anastomosis, a layer of platelets adhere to the denuded endothelium at the suture line—provided there is no exposed media or extensive vessel damage, fibrin deposition and thrombosis will not occur. Platelets gradually dissipate over the next 24 to 72 hours. As the vessel wall heals, a pseudointima forms. Dissipation of platelets in the vessel lumen and formation of the pseudointima correlates clinically with the critical period of thrombus formation within the first 3 to 5 days.[10]

Clotting Mechanism

Platelet adherence and aggregation is the first step in thrombus formation. Platelets do not adhere to undamaged endothelium; however, collagen within the subendothelium is highly thrombogenic. If the intima is damaged, exposed collagen within the media triggers platelet adhesion to the vessel wall. Platelets contain alpha and dense granules that secrete von Willebrand factor, fibrinogen, ADP (adenosine diphosphate), calcium, and serotonin. Together, these factors promote the recruitment and adherence of additional platelets through the formation of proteinaceous bridges. Activated platelets stimulate the conversion of fibrinogen to fibrin to strengthen the growing clot. Eventually, a critical mass is reached, resulting in thrombus formation by either occlusion of the vessel lumen or activation of the extrinsic pathway of coagulation.[11]

Antithrombotic drugs intervene at various steps in the clotting cascade with the aim to reduce platelet aggregation and clot formation. Heparin increases antithrombin-3 activity, which inactivates thrombin. Aspirin causes irreversible inactivation of cyclooxygenase (COX) and, subsequently, blocks the formation of thromboxane A_2. Dextran decreases red blood cell aggregation through both antiplatelet and antifibrin effects; its exact mechanism of action is unknown. Despite widespread use, evidence on the benefit of antithrombotics in microsurgery is equivocal.[12] Dextran has been shown to have no effect on flap survival but a 3.9- to 7.2-fold increase in systemic complications including renal failure, pulmonary edema, and congestive heart failure.[13] Heparin and aspirin continue to be commonly used.

Tissue Response to Ischemia and Hypoxia

Free tissue transfer requires a period of flap ischemia while the vascular anastomosis is performed. The main mechanism of ischemic injury is hypoxia, which leads to anaerobic glycolysis. Cellular acidosis is particularly severe because the absence of blood flow results in the accumulation of local metabolic by-products (lactic acid). Coagulative necrosis will ensue if ischemia is not promptly reversed.

Tissues have varying levels of tolerance to ischemia based on their composition and metabolic requirements. Skin and subcutaneous tissue remain viable for approximately 24 hours.[14] Muscle is less tolerant; irreversible damage to the microcirculation occurs at approximately 6 hours without blood flow.[15] Connective tissue has very low metabolic requirements and can withstand prolonged periods of hypoxia.[16] Cooling prolongs tolerance to ischemia for all types of tissues.[17]

Restoration of blood flow to ischemic tissues may cause additional damage owing to the production of free radicals and reactive oxygen species. The localized inflammatory response leads to leakage of intravascular fluid into the interstitial space and cellular swelling. Despite excellent anastomotic technique, it may be difficult or impossible to restore flow in flaps subjected to prolonged ischemia. Brisk inflow immediately after the anastomosis is followed by a sharp decline in flow rate shortly thereafter. The low flow state triggers intravascular thrombosis and flap ischemia. The process is termed the *no-reflow* phenomenon.[18]

TECHNICAL FACTORS

Many variables contribute to the success of a microvascular anastomosis: patient selection, operative planning, and technical setup, including magnification, instrumentation, and exposure. Meticulous technique and surgeon experience play the greatest role in success.

Equipment

Instrumentation

Basic microsurgical instruments include jeweler's forceps, smooth-tipped dilating forceps, micro needle drivers, straight and curved microscissors, and single and double microvascular clamps. Instruments should be of the highest quality—glare-free, nonmagnetic, and ergonomic. Heparinized saline irrigation should be available in a 3 mL syringe with a 26-gauge angiocatheter tip. A microsurgical background of contrasting color (yellow, blue, or green) provides improved visualization. Additional necessary instruments include bipolar electrocautery, micro clips and appliers, suction, and a sterile Doppler ultrasound (**Figure 5.1**).

Magnification

Magnification in the form of surgical loupes or an operating microscope is required for microsurgical anastomoses; the choice depends on the clinical scenario, availability of equipment, and individual surgeon preference.

The operating microscope provides wide-field, adjustable magnification with excellent depth perception. A halogen or xenon light source projects bright, even light throughout the field, and cool fiber optic systems prevent tissue desiccation. Beam-splitting devices and multiple eyepieces allow surgeons to operate together with the same, full stereoscopic view. Video capability enables the operative field to be displayed on a large monitor, which is helpful for the scrub team. Magnification ranges from 6× to 40×. Low magnification (6–12×) may be used for vessel preparation and suture tying; medium magnification (10–15×) is used for suture placement; and high magnification (>15×) is helpful in performing small-caliber anastomosis and for careful inspection at the completion of the procedure.

Surgical loupes range from 2 to 8× magnification and are available in expanded viewing field options. Generally, 3.5× or higher magnification is recommended for microsurgery. Loupes offer an ergonomic advantage when the anastomosis is performed in a deep cavity or at an odd angle. Loupes-only microsurgery reduces operative time (microscope setup is eliminated),[19] provides an opportunity to perform microsurgery when a scope is not available, and results in equally high patency rates in vessels over 1 mm diameter.[20,21]

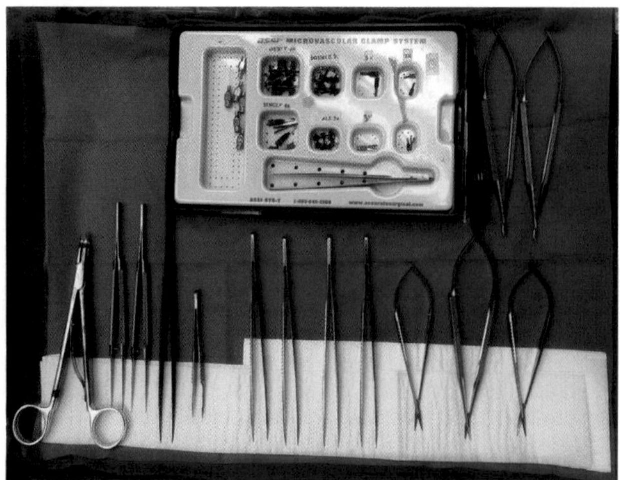

FIGURE 5.1. Microinstrumentation.

Suture

Nonabsorbable, monofilament suture (prolene or nylon) is used to perform anastomoses. Suture size depends on vessel caliber and typically ranges from 8-0 to 11-0. Microneedles are 50 to 130 μm in diameter with a sharp, tapered tip to pierce the tissue and a flat body to improve stability when held in the needle driver.

Automatic Suturing Devices

Anastomotic couplers are commonly used to simplify and expedite end-to-end venous anastomoses. Patency rates are equivalent to hand-sewn anastomoses.[22] After matching the bushel size to the vessel diameter, vessel ends are passed through a polyethylene ring, everted, and evenly secured on pins. Once both donor and recipient vessels are prepared, the coupling device is used to approximate the vessel ends and the rings are held together by interdigitating pins. The result is an automated anastomosis that is stented open by a soft, plastic ring (**Figure 5.2**). This technique provides flexibility in tailoring the anastomosis when vessel size mismatch is present by differential placement of the everted vessel wall on the pins. Coupling devices may also be used on soft-walled arteries over 1 mm in diameter[23] but should not be used on irradiated vessels.

PREOPERATIVE PLANNING

A multitude of flap options are available to the skilled microsurgeon. Donor site choice is dependent on the size, location, and type of defect; the availability of recipient vessels; and functional needs of the patient. Donor site morbidity should be considered and minimized.

Preoperative angiography (traditional or image-based) is sometimes required at the defect or donor site; it is particularly helpful when physical examination findings are abnormal or if diseased or injured vessels are suspected. When microsurgical reconstruction is needed for traumatic or infected wounds, adequate debridement of the recipient site is required. Ideally, patients should be medically and nutritionally optimized prior to free tissue transfer.

Patient Considerations

It is essential to consider the patient's general state of health and mindset when considering microsurgical options. Patients must be fit enough to tolerate prolonged general anesthetic and willing to participate in the lengthy recovery process. Active comorbidities, such as diabetes mellitus (DM), obesity, and nicotine use, should be documented and optimized.

Age alone is not a contraindication for microsurgical reconstruction. Studies show that microsurgery can be safely performed in children[24] and elderly patients[25] without an increase in flap failure or surgical complications.

Macrovascular and microvascular diseases are known sequelae of diabetes; however, it is controversial as to whether DM affects free flap outcomes. Animal models show poor intimal healing at the anastomotic site and reduced venous patency,[26–28] but clinical studies

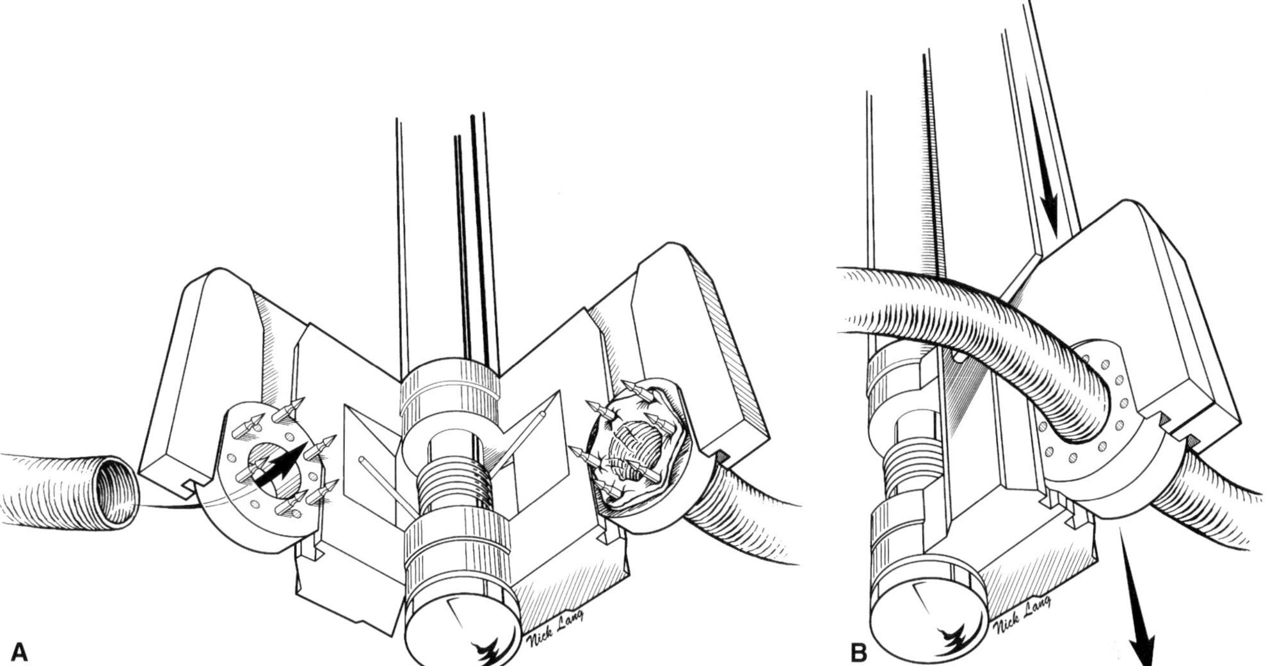

FIGURE 5.2. Use of an anastomotic coupling device. **A.** With the device's lateral wings open, each vessel is passed through a plastic ring, and the vessel walls are everted and impaled on pins mounted on the rings. **B.** After both vessels are mounted, the knob is turned to close the wings and secure the rings with the vessels in opposition. The rings are securely attached to each other by the pins of one ring interlocking with the opposite plastic ring. After the anastomosis, the coupled rings are released in the direction of the arrow by continuing to turn the knob. Copyright held by, and used with permission of, The University of Texas M.D. Anderson Cancer Center.

show no difference in the rate of flap failure.[29] Strict perioperative glycemic control reduces overall surgical complications in diabetic patients.

Obesity is a known risk factor for flap and donor site complications. Free flaps in obese patients are twice as likely to fail[30]; however, the overall rate of flap failure is still very low,[31] especially when compared with nonmicrosurgical alternatives (i.e., implant-based breast reconstruction).[32] The risks of seroma, delayed wound healing, and mastectomy flap necrosis increase in obese patients.[30,33]

Patients should be advised to quit smoking at least 4 weeks before surgery to reduce perioperative complications.[34] Smoking impairs oxygenation, causes vasoconstriction, and introduces free radicals.[35,36] Studies indicate that smoking does not reduce anastomotic patency but does affect wound healing, skin graft take over flaps, infection risk, flap necrosis, hernia formation, and length of hospital stay.[33,36,37]

MICROSURGICAL TECHNIQUES

Surgical precision is the key factor in anastomotic patency. Ergonomic setup is the first step to success.

The surgeon should be seated or standing in a comfortable position with the shoulders and neck relaxed and the forearms and wrists adequately supported. Ideally, the surgeon should position his or her body parallel to the long axis of the vessel to allow for ergonomic intubation of the vessel lumen and forehand suture placement. Wide surgical exposure is important; it may be necessary to extend the incision, further mobilize recipient vessels, or reposition retractors to avoid operating in a hole.

Recipient vessels are prepared prior to division of the flap pedicle to minimize ischemia time. Adventitia and periadventitial tissue is sharply excised to prevent it from becoming interposed between the donor and recipient vessels, which is highly thrombogenic (**Figure 5.3**). Side branches are sealed with bipolar electrocautery or micro clips. The vessels are then clamped, divided, and irrigated with heparinized saline to remove intraluminal clot.

The flap pedicle is likewise prepared and divided. Immediately after division, the flap is flushed through with heparinized saline and transferred to the recipient site. It is positioned and secured in close proximity to the defect, paying careful attention to the pedicle to ensure that it is not twisted, kinked, compressed, or under tension. Both donor and recipient arteries are dilated by inserting smooth-tipped forceps into the lumen. Repeated dilation is avoided, as it weakens the vessel wall and causes vasospasm.

A forward-flow test is performed by releasing the clamp on the recipient artery to check inflow. This is often done in replantation

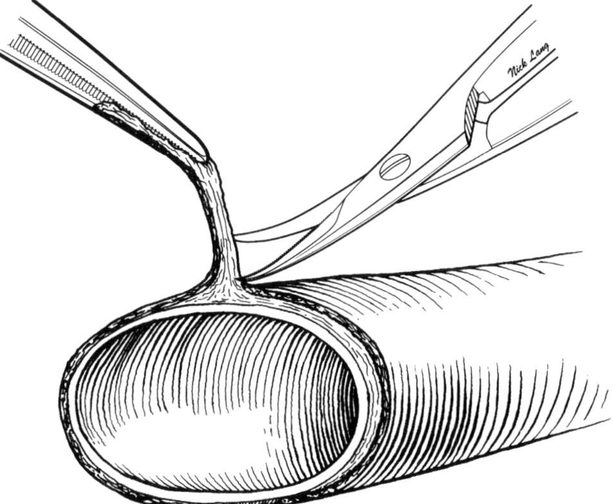

FIGURE 5.3. Donor and recipient vessel preparation. The excess adventitial tissue near the cut edge of the vessel is removed with dissecting scissors to prevent intrusion into the lumen during the anastomosis. Care is taken to avoid excessive thinning, which can result in vessel tears during the placement of sutures. Copyright held by, and used with permission of, The University of Texas M.D. Anderson Cancer Center.

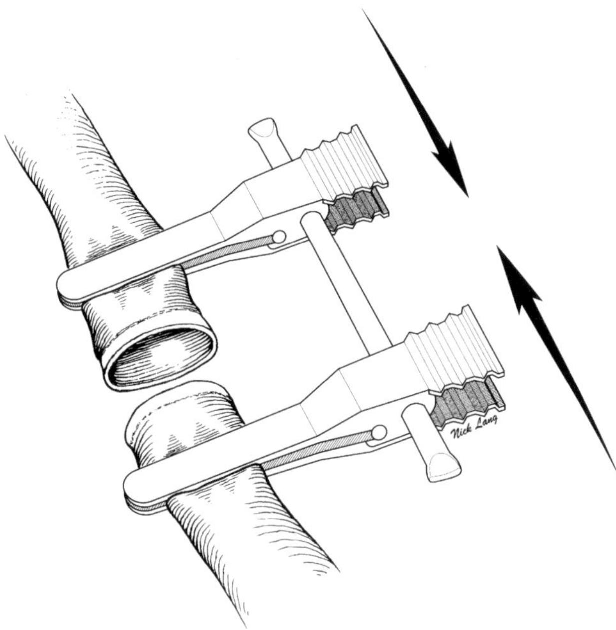

FIGURE 5.4. Use of double-approximating microvascular clamps. The donor and recipient vessels are placed within the clamps, and the vessel ends are approximated along the direction of the arrows. This technique maintains the correct orientation of the vessels and facilitates suture placement. After the anterior suture line is complete, the clamps are turned over to allow access to the posterior suture line. Copyright held by, and used with permission of, The University of Texas M.D. Anderson Cancer Center.

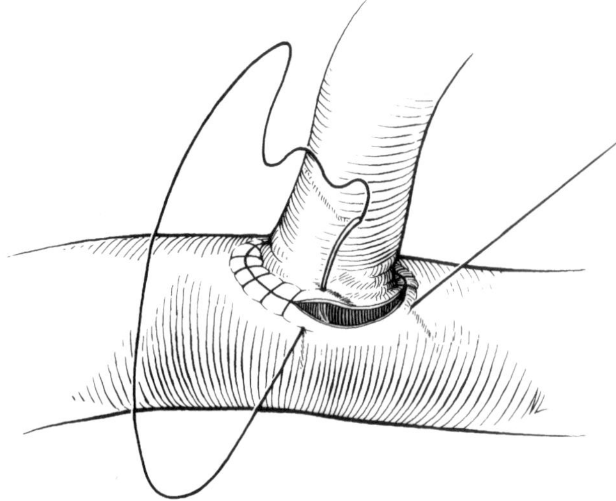

FIGURE 5.5. End-to-side anastomosis using continuous (running) sutures. An elliptical opening is created on the recipient vessel wall, and the end of the donor vessel is anastomosed to this opening. The end-to-side technique maintains distal flow in the recipient vessel and is frequently performed when there is a donor and recipient vessel diameter mismatch. Copyright held by, and used with permission of, The University of Texas M.D. Anderson Cancer Center.

when vasospasm in injured vessels leads to the loss of the spurt sign in which the blood flows intensely from the cut end of the vessel. The clamp is then replaced and the vessel end is irrigated with heparinized saline. A double-opposing clamp is applied to approximate the donor and recipient vessels. Vessels should be positioned for tension-free, intima-to-intima apposition (**Figure 5.4**). Vascular grafts may be necessary if a tension-free anastomosis cannot be achieved.

Never start the anastomosis until you are satisfied with the setup.

Anastomotic Technique

Variations on technique exist. Recent literature suggests no difference in patency rate based on suture technique (simple interrupted versus continuous)[38] or anastomotic technique (end-to-end versus end-to-side).[39] Surgeon preference and clinical scenario prevail.

Interrupted sutures are preferred when there is significant vessel size discrepancy. Continuous sutures require less knot tying and are more time efficient. Continuous sutures have the added advantage of equally distributing tension along the suture line, providing less opportunity for leakage. In practice, interrupted sutures are commonly used for arterial anastomoses and continuous sutures for venous anastomoses.

End-to-end anastomosis is appropriate for most arterial and venous anastomoses. End-to-side anastomosis may be necessary in limb reconstruction to maintain distal perfusion, or when significant size mismatch exists (**Figure 5.5**). End-to-side anastomoses are technically more difficult, evidenced by longer mean ischemia times.[40]

Regardless of the anastomotic technique used, the following technical principles are critical:

- The needle should be held halfway along its length.
- The most difficult sutures should be placed first.
- Suture must enter the vessel perpendicular to the vessel wall and include all three layers of the wall (**Figure 5.6**).
- The distance from the cut end of the vessel to the needle entry point should be slightly greater than the thickness of the vessel wall.
- The tip of the needle should be visualized at all times within the vessel lumen.
- Bisecting or trisecting sutures should be used for orientation (**Figure 5.7**).
- Sutures should be placed equidistant from each other.
- Between sutures, the needle should be placed within the visual field of the microscope to facilitate retrieval for the next stitch.
- The suture should not be tied if there is any concern that it has caught the back wall.

Throughout the procedure and prior to placement of the last suture, the vessel lumen is irrigated with heparinized saline. After completion of the both arterial and venous anastomoses, clamps are removed. Venous clamps are removed first to restore outflow. The distal arterial clamp is then removed, backflow is checked, and leaks are repaired. The proximal arterial clamp is removed last.

At this point, vessel handling should be limited. Topical lidocaine or papaverine and warm saline are applied to reduce spasm. If bleeding occurs near the anastomotic site, the vessels are inspected for unligated side branches, a second outflow vein from the flap, and leakage from the anastomosis itself.

After 3 to 5 minutes, the anastomoses are examined for patency. The artery should be pulsatile distal to the anastomosis. Patent veins appear full and maroon in color. The flap is inspected for return of color and bleeding from the edges. If doubt exists, a patency test (**Figure 5.8**) is performed as follows:

1. Jeweler's forceps are used to gently occlude the vessel distal to the anastomosis.
2. A second pair of jeweler's forceps is used to empty blood for several millimeters downstream.
3. The proximal forceps is then released while maintaining distal compression.
4. If patent, the empty segment fills with blood.

This test is traumatic and should be performed only when necessary.

For nonflowing anastomoses, the artery and vein are inspected for twists, kinks, and points of compression. The vessels are left alone for an additional 15 minutes. If the anastomosis is still not patent or has thrombosed, the suture line is excised and the anastomosis redone. Excessive manipulation of thrombosed vessels is avoided to prevent showering clot downstream. In the case of repeated thrombosis despite a technically sound anastomosis, thrombolytic agents may be administered within the flap.

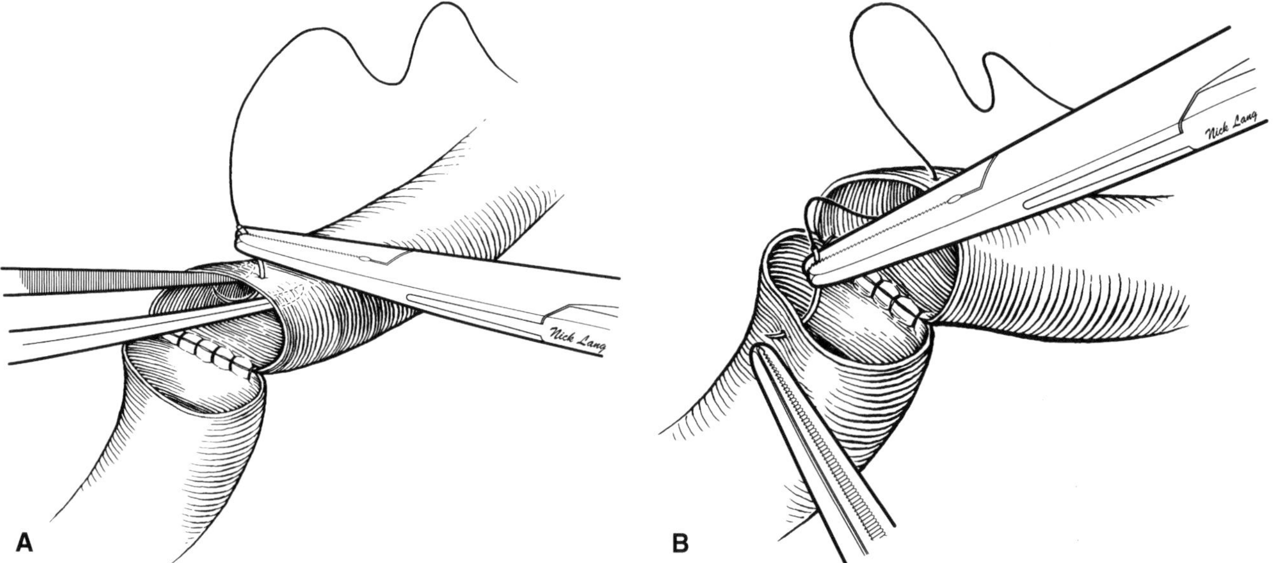

FIGURE 5.6. Forceps countertraction to facilitate needle placement and penetration. **A.** In select cases, partially open blunt jeweler's forceps tips are placed into the vessel lumen to evert the vessel wall, avoid inclusion of the back wall in sutures, and provide countertraction for needle penetration. Extreme care must be taken to avoid traumatizing the vessel intima; some microsurgeons avoid this technique for this reason. **B.** When the needle is passed from inside the vessel lumen to outside the lumen, it is often useful to use the tips of the forceps to provide countertraction on the adventitial surface of the vessel to facilitate needle penetration. Copyright held by, and used with permission of, The University of Texas M.D. Anderson Cancer Center.

Secondary Microsurgical Techniques

When it is not possible to perform tension-free, primary anastomosis of the donor and recipient vessels, interposition grafts are used; this is often the case in replantation and extremity trauma when recipient vessels must be outside the zone of injury. Autogenous vein grafts are readily available and are the most common conduit used. They should be placed directionally for spanning vein gaps and reversed for arterial gaps. The diameter of the graft should approximate that of the donor and recipient vessels—small grafts are harvested from the volar wrist or forearm, and medium grafts from the dorsal foot. The saphenous veins are often used when large-diameter vessels are required. Grafts should be harvested at least 35% longer than the measured gap to accommodate for contraction; redundancy disappears with time.[41] Long-term patency rates for vein grafts approach 100%, regardless of the length of the graft required.[41] When used to bridge arterial gaps, histologic changes occur in vein grafts over time. A neointima is formed by the ingrowth of smooth muscle cells from the recipient vessel, and the wall thickens.[42]

Arterial grafts are similarly reliable but less frequently used. Use of the radial, thoracodorsal, and branches of the lateral femoral circumflex arteries has been described.

Synthetic grafts are not common in microsurgery. Animal models using fibrous polyurethane (PU) and microporous polytetrafluoroethylene (PTFE) grafts show adequate early patency in high-flow,[43] short segment conduits, but long-term anastomotic narrowing due to neointimal hyperplasia.[44] Significant thrombosis and occlusion occur early in low-flow flaps.[45]

Microsurgery on Irradiated Vessels

Extreme care must be taken if the recipient vessels have been previously irradiated. Radiated vessels are fragile, atherosclerotic, and fibrotic. It is difficult to recognize the junction between adventitia and media. When the media is damaged during dissection, the vessel wall is weakened and at higher risk for leakage and thrombosis. The intima is also more likely to be disrupted during vessel preparation, and sections may lift away from the underlying media, which is highly thrombogenic. If any layer of the vessel wall is injured, the vessel should be trimmed back proximal to the site of injury.

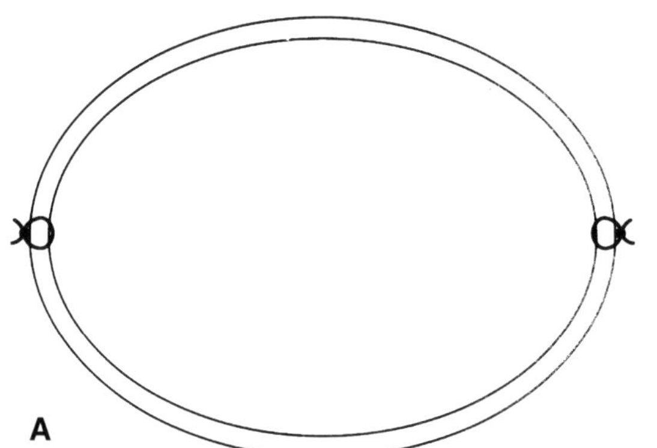

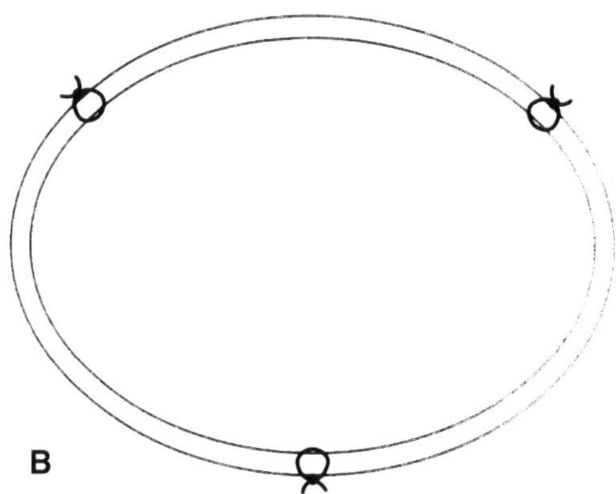

FIGURE 5.7. Orientation sutures. **A.** Bisecting interrupted sutures are placed 180° apart, dividing the vessel circumference into half. This technique is particularly useful when there is a vessel size mismatch. **B.** Triangulating interrupted sutures are placed 120° apart, dividing the vessel circumference into thirds. This technique helps prevent inadvertent inclusion of the opposite wall of the vessel in the remaining sutures; the surgeon applies gentle downward traction on the posterior orientation suture while the other two sutures are gently retracted upward and laterally during placement of the remaining anastomotic sutures. Copyright held by, and used with permission of, The University of Texas M.D. Anderson Cancer Center.

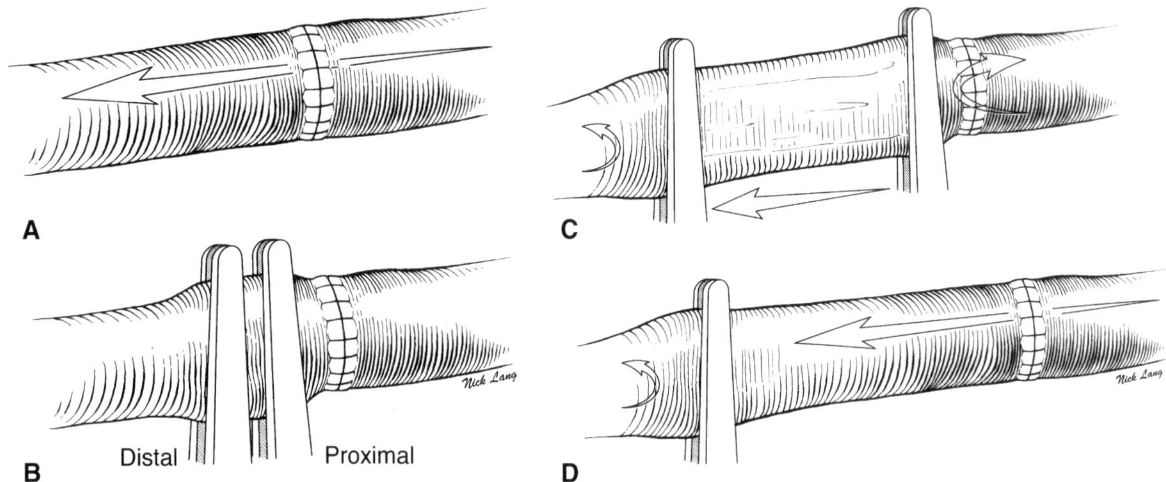

FIGURE 5.8. Use of the Acland test to confirm antegrade vascular flow through an anastomosis. **A.** The direction of blood flow is indicated by the arrow. **B.** Two jeweler's forceps are used to gently occlude the vessel distal to the venous anastomosis. **C.** Blood is milked out of the vessel between the two forceps by gently sliding the distal forceps along the vessel without injuring it. This results in a segment of collapsed vessel between the proximal and distal forceps. **D.** Releasing the proximal forceps allows the collapsed vessel segment to be filled by antegrade flow if the anastomosis is patent. The distal forceps prevent retrograde filling of the collapsed segment. This test should be performed sparingly to minimize potential trauma to the vessel intima. Copyright held by, and used with permission of, The University of Texas M.D. Anderson Cancer Center.

Evidence on the patency of microvascular anastomoses in irradiated tissue beds is conflicting; some studies show higher rates of free flap failure,[46] whereas others show no effect on flap-related complications.[47–49]

Anesthetic Considerations

Anesthesia is important in maximizing success in microsurgery. Basic intraoperative goals include supporting circulatory volume, avoiding peripheral vasoconstriction, and maintaining normal body temperature.

Adequate mean arterial pressure and cardiac output is required for flap perfusion. A combination of crystalloid and colloid is appropriate for volume replacement with the goal of maintaining urine output at 0.5 mL/kg/h. Adequate blood pressure promotes flap perfusion by increasing regional blood flow, enhancing microvascular patency, and maintaining the fluidity of the blood in the microcirculation.

Anecdotally, vasopressors are avoided in microsurgery; however, multiple studies show no increase in flap loss with intraoperative use of vasoactive medications.[50,51] Some studies even suggest that pressors may be beneficial in microsurgery by increasing blood flow to skin flaps.[52] It is thought that the rise in blood pressure overcomes any vasospastic effect of the medication. Adventitial stripping leads to denervation of the donor and recipient vessels during dissection, further supporting this theory.

Temperature control during and after microsurgery is critical. Hypothermia causes vasoconstriction and increases hematocrit and plasma viscosity because of erythrocyte and platelet clumping. Large body surface areas may be exposed in microsurgical cases, making maintenance of temperature difficult. Patients can be warmed by forced-air blankets, warmed IV fluids, humidified and warmed anesthetic gases, and increased ambient room temperature.

POSTOPERATIVE MANAGEMENT

Postoperatively, efforts are made to offload pressure from flap and prevent vasospasm. Dressings are minimized so that the whole flap is easily evaluated. Circumferential dressings and ties are avoided. Patients are positioned to prevent direct pressure on the flap; this may include application of an external fixator for extremity reconstruction. The room is warmed. Fluids are managed to maintain adequate urine output and systolic blood pressure and keep hematocrit at 25% to 35%. Pain control is optimized. Caffeine and nicotine are prohibited.

Antithrombotics

The routine use of antithrombotic agents in the postoperative period remains controversial. Multiple studies show that postoperative antithrombotic use of any type offers no protection from microvascular thrombosis and increases complication rates.[12,13] However, in a recent survey, 84% of surgeons who routinely perform lower extremity reconstruction reported using at least one form of antithrombotic before, during, or after surgery.[53] The most common antithrombotic agents used in routine postoperative care are aspirin and heparin. Further investigation is required.

Postoperative Monitoring

Thrombosis is most common within 24 hours of surgery. Early failure is often related to anastomotic imperfections or pedicle positioning. If a problem is detected early, the flap can be salvaged by exploration and revision of the anastomosis. The success rate of flap salvage is inversely related to the time interval from the onset of ischemia to restoration of blood flow. Prompt recognition and timely intervention is required. Overall, approximately 50% of ailing free flaps can be salvaged.[8]

Clinical evaluation is standard for flap monitoring. Color, capillary refill, turgor, and temperature are evaluated. A flap without inflow will be cool, be pale, and lack capillary refill. Rapid capillary refill, swelling, or purple discoloration may indicate venous thrombosis.

Many adjuncts to clinical evaluation exist. Hand-held Doppler ultrasound is commonly used to monitor both arterial and venous waveforms. Perforators to the skin are identified intraoperatively, and their location is marked with a fine suture on the skin surface for future localization. Implantable, ultrasonic Doppler probes can be used for flaps without a skin paddle or completely buried flaps. Surface temperature measurements and pulsoximetry are helpful in digital replantation. Other monitoring systems include transcutaneous oxygen tension, near-infrared spectroscopy, intravenous fluorescein angiography, pH measurement, interstitial fluid pressure, and reflection plethysmography. There is no consensus on which method is most effective.

Regardless of the monitoring technique, flap checks should be performed by an experienced observer at least once every hour for the first 48 hours following surgery. After 48 hours, flap monitoring is spaced out to every 2 hours until postoperative day 5 and then decreased to every 4 hours until discharge. The rate of successful flap salvage is highest in the early postoperative course.[8]

MANAGEMENT OF THE AILING FREE FLAP

At the first sign of a problem, the flap and patient are inspected to detect any easily correctable issues—patient positioning, flap dependency, constrictive dressings, etc. Flap inset sutures are released if external pedicle compression is suspected. The threshold to return to the operative room is low. Exploration should proceed immediately if there is any clinical suspicion for thrombosis. Doppler signals may persist for several hours despite venous thrombosis.

During a take-back procedure, the flap is elevated and the anastomosis inspected. Intravenous heparin (5000 units) is administered and the anastomosis is taken down. If clot is present, mechanical thrombectomy is performed with a Fogarty catheter. The goal is to remove the thrombus in its entirety—residual clot may be a nidus for additional thrombus or the source of microemboli. Both the donor and recipient vessels are trimmed back to pristine intima. Vein grafts may be required if primary anastomosis cannot be performed without tension. A thrombolytic agent (streptokinase, urokinase, or tissue plasminogen activator) is infused while the flap is occluded from systemic circulation. If there is no longer inflow from the recipient vessels, a different recipient site is chosen.

There is no indication for routine anticoagulation when conditions are optimal; however, in the case of postoperative thrombosis, intraoperative, local fibrinolytic therapy and postoperative anticoagulation may be indicated in situations where mechanical and vascular factors are unfavorable.

Leeches

Leeches are a useful adjunct for flaps with signs of venous congestion despite a patent venous anastomosis. They are only indicated when a flap has good inflow but limited drainage, and should not replace reexploration of the venous anastomosis if patency is in question. Leeches are applied directly to the flap. They consume several milliliters of blood at each meal and fall off at satiety. Prophylaxis against *Aeromonas hydrophila* is necessary because this organism routinely inhabits the digestive tract of leeches.

Flap Failure

Salvage attempts are abandoned when there is no return of perfusion after reexploration. Tissue type and warm ischemia time are also considered. Obviously necrotic flaps should be debrided promptly to reduce inflammation. After removal of a failed free flap, dressings or skin grafts can be used to temporize a wound. Local or regional flap options or a second free flap may be considered.

APPLICATIONS OF MICROSURGERY

Free Tissue Transfer

Free flaps are used to close wounds and restore form and function in patients with traumatic, oncologic, or congenital defects. Multiple types of flaps exist and selection is based on the type of defect and the goals of reconstruction.

Muscle flaps are useful when bulk is required or a dead space exists. A skin paddle may be included depending on the contour requirements of the defect, or a skin graft may be placed over the bare muscle. Functional free muscle transfer is also possible; it involves transfer of a muscle with microvascular anastomosis and microsurgical reinnervation at the recipient site.

Skin and fascia flaps can be derived from any perforating blood vessel using the angiosome concept. These flaps provide versatile, thin, well-vascularized soft tissue coverage. If desired, bulk may be provided by including subcutaneous tissue. Donor site morbidity is minimal because muscle is spared. Fascia-only flaps have the added advantage of providing a gliding surface for tendon reconstruction.

Osseous flaps are used less frequently than soft tissue flaps but are helpful to reconstruct bony defects of the mandible, midface, and extremities. Vascularized bone autografts are superior to nonvascularized bone graft in defects over 5 centimeters in regard to early incorporation, bone hypertrophy, mechanical strength, and osseous mass retention.[54]

Microvascular transfer of bowel segments (proximal jejunum or colon) is used to reconstruct the oral cavity, pharynx, and esophagus. The greater omentum is an excellent source of well-vascularized tissue. It is commonly used for sternal and scalp reconstruction. Laparoscopic harvest is possible.

Nerve Repair

Peripheral nerves have some capacity to regenerate after injury; however, poor functional results are common. Microsurgical techniques are required to optimize outcomes. Microdissection, identification and resection of injured nerve segments, fascicular matching, and tension-free epineurial or grouped fascicular repair are prudent. Recent advances in nerve surgery include end-to-side repairs and nerve transfers. In an end-to-side repair, the distal end of an injured nerve is coapted to the side of an uninjured donor nerve. Nerve transfers use redundant or unimportant fascicles from a donor nerve to innervate critical motor or sensory branches close to their target end organ. Techniques such as these improve functional results and reduce morbidity after peripheral nerve injury.

Lymphatic Surgery

Refinements in magnification, equipment, and technique have revolutionized the treatment of lymphedema. Lymphatic surgery is an exciting application of supermicrosurgery, defined as the anastomosis of structures less than 0.5 mm in diameter. Vascularized lymph node transfer and lymphaticovenous bypass offer physiologic solutions for restoration of lymphatic flow.

Vascularized lymph node transfer involves transplanting functioning lymph nodes to an area affected by lymphedema. Donor sites include supraclavicular, submental, groin, or gastroepiploic nodes. The exact mechanism of action in vascularized lymph node transfer is unknown; however, two theories exist: (1) transplanted lymph nodes provide growth factors that induce lymphangiogenesis in the affected limb; and (2) transplanted lymph nodes act as a lymphatic pump, driven by high-pressure arterial inflow and low-pressure venous outflow.

In lymphaticovenous bypass, obstructed lymphatic channels are identified and their flow is redirected into a nearby low-pressure venule. Restoration of unimpeded flow reduces lymphedema severity, particularly in patients with early-stage upper extremity disease.

Replantation

Microsurgical techniques are used to primarily repair amputations of extremities, genitalia, and facial structures. Replantation is most successful in patients who sustain sharp injuries and seek medical attention immediately. Crush or avulsion-type mechanisms cause a significant zone of injury and replantation is less likely to succeed. Patients with segmental or multilevel injuries are also poor replant candidates. When successful, replantation can help patients avoid disabling or disfiguring defects and complex, multistage reconstructive procedures.

CONCLUSION

Microsurgical techniques have forever changed the face of plastic surgery. Modern microsurgery has progressed far beyond the simple tenet of keeping a vessel patent. Refined techniques focus on maximizing function, restoring near-normal form, and minimizing donor site morbidity.

ACKNOWLEDGMENT

The work was supported by a Midcareer Investigator Award in Patient-Oriented Research (2 K24-AR053120-06) to Kevin C. Chung. The content is solely the responsibility of the authors and does not necessarily represent the official views of the National Institutes of Health.

REFERENCES

1. Jassinowski A. Die Artiennhat: eine experimentelle Studie. *Inaug Diss Dorpat.* 1889.
2. Carrel A. La technique operatoire des anastomoses vasculaires et la transplantation des visceres. *Lyon Med.* 1902;98:859-863.
3. Hopfner E. Uber Gefassnhaht, Gefasstransplantationen und Replantation von amputierten Extremitaten. *Arch Klin Chir.* 1903;70:417-471.
4. Nylen CO. The microscope in aural surgery: its first use and later development. *Acta Otolaryngol Suppl.* 1954;116:226-240.
5. Holmgren G. Some experiences in surgery of otosclerosis. *Acta Otolaryngol.* 1923;5:460-466.
6. Jacobson JH, Suarez EL. Microsurgery in the anastomosis of small vessels. *Surg Forum.* 1960;11:243-245.
7. Tamai S. History of microsurgery. *Plast Reconstr Surg.* 2009;124(suppl 6):e282-e294.
8. Mirzabeigi MN, Wang T, Kovach SJ, et al. Free flap take-back following postoperative microvascular compromise: predicting salvage versus failure. *Plast Reconstr Surg.* 2012;130(3):579-589.
   This article provides recent data on microsurgical success rates from a high-volume center.
9. Harashina T, Fujino T, Watanabe S. The intimal healing of microvascular anastomoses. *Plast Reconstr Surg.* 1976;58(5):608-613.
10. Hayhurst JW, O'Brien BM. An experimental study of microvascular technique, patency rates and related factors. *Br J Plast Surg.* 1975;28(2):128-132.
11. Chang WH, Petry JJ. Platelets, prostaglandins, and patency in microvascular surgery. *J Microsurg.* 1980;2(1):27-35.
12. Lighthall JG, Cain R, Ghanem TA, Wax MK. Effect of postoperative aspirin on outcomes in microvascular free tissue transfer surgery. *Otolaryngol Head Neck Surg.* 2013;148(1):40-46.
   This article reviews a large case series of patients treated with various combinations of antithrombotic agents and concludes that postoperative thromboprophylaxis with aspirin does not increase the odds of flap survival and may be associated with a higher complication rate.
13. Disa JJ, Polvora VP, Pusic AL, et al. Dextran-related complications in head and neck microsurgery: do the benefits outweigh the risks? A prospective randomized analysis. *Plast Reconstr Surg.* 2003;112(6):1534-1539.
   This study evaluates morbidity associated with dextran administration in head and neck microsurgery patients and concludes that there is no effect on overall flap survival and a significantly increased risk of systemic complications.
14. Serafin D, Lesesne CB, Mullen RY, Georgiade NG. Transcutaneous PO2 monitoring for assessing viability and predicting survival of skin flaps: experimental and clinical correlations. *J Microsurg.* 1981;2(3):165-178.
15. Eriksson E, Anderson WA, Replogle RL. Effects of prolonged ischemia on muscle microcirculation in the cat. *Surg Forum.* 1974;25(0):254-255.
16. Berggren A, Weiland AJ, Dorfman H. The effect of prolonged ischemia time on osteocyte and osteoblast survival in composite bone grafts revascularized by microvascular anastomoses. *Plast Reconstr Surg.* 1982;69(2):290-298.
17. Cooley BC, Hansen FC, Dellon AL. The effect of temperature on tolerance to ischemia in experimental free flaps. *J Microsurg.* 1981;3(1):11-14.
18. May JW, Chait LA, O'Brien BM, Hurley JV. The no-reflow phenomenon in experimental free flaps. *Plast Reconstr Surg.* 1978;61(2):256-267.
19. Ross DA, Ariyan S, Restifo R, Sasaki CT. Use of the operating microscope and loupes for head and neck free microvascular tissue transfer: a retrospective comparison. *Arch Otolaryngol Head Neck Surg.* 2003;129(2):189-193.
20. Pannucci CJ, Kovach SJ, Cuker A. Microsurgery and the hypercoagulable state: a hematologist's perspective. *Plast Reconstr Surg.* 2015;136(4):545e-552e.
21. Shenaq SM, Klebuc MJ, Vargo D. Free-tissue transfer with the aid of loupe magnification: experience with 251 procedures. *Plast Reconstr Surg.* 1995;95(2):261-269.
22. Cope C, Lee K, Stern H, Pennington D. Use of the vascular closure staple clip applier for microvascular anastomosis in free-flap surgery. *Plast Reconstr Surg.* 2000;106(1):107-110.
23. Spector JA, Draper LB, Levine JP, Ahn CY. A technique for atraumatic microvascular arterial coupling. *Plast Reconstr Surg.* 2007;119(6):1968-1969.
24. Momeni A, Lanni M, Levin LS, Kovach SJ. Microsurgical reconstruction of traumatic lower extremity defects in the pediatric population. *Plast Reconstr Surg.* 2017;139(4):998-1004.
25. Serletti JM, Higgins JP, Moran S, Orlando GS. Factors affecting outcome in free-tissue transfer in the elderly. *Plast Reconstr Surg.* 2000;106(1):66-70.
26. Barr LC, Joyce AD. Microvascular anastomoses in diabetes: an experimental study. *Br J Plast Surg.* 1989;42(1):50-53.
27. Cooley BC, Hanel DP, Anderson RB, et al. The influence of diabetes on free flap transfer: I. Flap survival and microvascular healing. *Ann Plast Surg.* 1992;29(1):58-64.
28. Colen LB, Stevenson A, Sidorov V, et al. Microvascular anastomotic thrombosis in experimental diabetes mellitus. *Plast Reconstr Surg.* 1997;99(1):156-162.
29. Miller RB, Reece G, Kroll SS, et al. Microvascular breast reconstruction in the diabetic patient. *Plast Reconstr Surg.* 2007;119(1):38-45.
30. Kroll SS. Necrosis of abdominoplasty and other secondary flaps after TRAM flap breast reconstruction. *Plast Reconstr Surg.* 1994;94(5):637-643.
31. Seidenstuecker K, Munder B, Mahajan AL, et al. Morbidity of microsurgical breast reconstruction in patients with comorbid conditions. *Plast Reconstr Surg.* 2011;127(3):1086-1092.
32. Garvey PB, Villa MT, Rozanski AT, et al. The advantages of free abdominal-based flaps over implants for breast reconstruction in obese patients. *Plast Reconstr Surg.* 2012;130(5):991-1000.
33. Selber JC, Kurichi JE, Vega SJ, et al. Risk factors and complications in free TRAM flap breast reconstruction. *Ann Plast Surg.* 2006;56(5):492-497.
34. Rohrich RJ. Cosmetic surgery and patients who smoke: should we operate? *Plast Reconstr Surg.* 2000;106(1):137-138.
35. Kaufman T, Eichenlaub EH, Levin M, et al. Tobacco smoking: impairment of experimental flap survival. *Ann Plast Surg.* 1984;13(6):468-472.
36. Chang LD, Buncke G, Slezak S, Buncke HJ. Cigarette smoking, plastic surgery, and microsurgery. *J Reconstr Microsurg.* 1996;12(7):467-474.
37. Spear SL, Ducic I, Cuoco F, Hannan C. The effect of smoking on flap and donor-site complications in pedicled TRAM breast reconstruction. *Plast Reconstr Surg.* 2005;116(7):1873-1880.
38. Alghoul MS, Gordon CR, Yetman R, et al. From simple interrupted to complex spiral: a systematic review of various suture techniques for microvascular anastomoses. *Microsurgery.* 2011;31(1):72-80.
39. Tsai YT, Lin TS. The suitability of end-to-side microvascular anastomosis in free flap transfer for limb reconstruction. *Ann Plast Surg.* 2012;68(2):171-174.
40. Apostolides JG, Magarakis M, Rosson GD. Preserving the internal mammary artery: end-to-side microvascular arterial anastomosis for DIEP and SIEA flap breast reconstruction. *Plast Reconstr Surg.* 2011;128(4):225e-232e.
41. Mitchell GM, Zeeman BJ, Rogers IW, et al. The long-term fate of microvenous autografts. *Plast Reconstr Surg.* 1988;82(3):473-479.
42. Biemer E, Holzmann T, Wriedt-Lubbe I, et al. Autologous vein grafts as artery replacement in microsurgery. An experimental study of micro- and macro-morphologic changes 3 weeks to 12 months postoperatively. *Handchirurgie.* 1981;13(1-2):108-113.
43. van der Lei B, Wildevuur CR. Microvascular polytetrafluoroethylene prostheses: the cellular events of healing and prostacyclin production. *Plast Reconstr Surg.* 1988;81(5):735-741.
44. Hess F, Jerusalem C, Braun B, Grande P. Evaluation of the patency rate of fibrous microvascular polyurethane prostheses after implantation in the rat aorta. *Microsurgery.* 1983;4(3):178-181.
45. Shen TY, Mitchell GM, Morrison WA, O'Brien BM. The use of long synthetic microvascular grafts to vascularise free flaps in rabbits. *Br J Plast Surg.* 1988;41(3):305-312.
46. Khouri RK, Cooley BC, Kunselman AR, et al. A prospective study of microvascular free-flap surgery and outcome. *Plast Reconstr Surg.* 1998;102(3):711-721.
   This study reviews outcomes from a large group of microsurgeons and concludes that reconstruction of an irradiated recipient site and the use of a skin-grafted muscle flap were the only statistically significant predictors of flap failure. Flap recipient site, indication for surgery, patient factors, anastomosis technique, and thromboprophylaxis did not have a significant effect on flap outcome.
47. Kroll SS, Schusterman MA, Reece GP, et al. Choice of flap and incidence of free flap success. *Plast Reconstr Surg.* 1996;98(3):459-463.
48. Shaari CM, Buchbinder D, Costantino PD, et al. Complications of microvascular head and neck surgery in the elderly. *Arch Otolaryngol Head Neck Surg.* 1998;124(4):407-411.
49. Chow WB, Rosenthal RA, Merkow RP, et al. Optimal preoperative assessment of the geriatric surgical patient: a best practices guideline from the American College of Surgeons National Surgical Quality Improvement Program and the American Geriatrics Society. *J Am Coll Surg.* 2012;215(4):453-466.
50. Chen C, Nguyen MD, Bar-Meir E, et al. Effects of vasopressor administration on the outcomes of microsurgical breast reconstruction. *Ann Plast Surg.* 2010;65(1):28-31.
51. Harris L, Goldstein D, Hofer S, Gilbert R. Impact of vasopressors on outcomes in head and neck free tissue transfer. *Microsurgery.* 2012;32(1):15-19.
   This study reviews intraoperative vasopressor administration during microsurgical cases and concludes that they are frequently used and do not adversely affect flap outcomes.
52. Cordeiro PG, Santamaria E, Hu QY, Heerdt P. Effects of vasoactive medications on the blood flow of island musculocutaneous flaps in swine. *Ann Plast Surg.* 1997;39(5):524-531.
53. Xipoleas G, Levine E, Silver L, et al. A survey of microvascular protocols for lower-extremity free tissue transfer I: perioperative anticoagulation. *Ann Plast Surg.* 2007;59(3):311-315.
54. Weiland AJ, Phillips TW, Randolph MA. Bone grafts: a radiologic, histologic, and biomechanical model comparing autografts, allografts, and free vascularized bone grafts. *Plast Reconstr Surg.* 1984;74(3):368-379.

QUESTIONS

1. **Which of the following conditions is a risk factor for free flap failure?**
   a. Age less than 18 years
   b. Age greater than 65 years
   c. Active nicotine use
   d. Obesity
   e. DM

2. **Which of the following is a proven benefit of using a coupler device?**
   a. Decreased anastomosis time
   b. Improved anastomotic patency
   c. Increased intima-to-intima apposition
   d. Reduced cost
   e. Decreased vessel kinking

3. **A 23-year-old man with a traumatic wound involving the distal third of the leg is scheduled to undergo soft-tissue reconstruction with an anterolateral thigh free flap. Which of the following is most likely to have the greatest effect on anastomotic patency?**
   a. Anastomotic technique
   b. Magnification type
   c. Surgical precision
   d. Antithrombotic use
   e. Suture technique

4. **A 62-year-old woman with invasive ductal carcinoma undergoes mastectomy and reconstruction with a deep inferior epigastric artery free flap. Intraoperatively, the patient experiences hypotension and norepinephrine is administered. Which of the following is the most likely effect of this treatment on the outcome of the flap?**
   a. Microvascular thrombosis
   b. Partial flap loss
   c. Delayed wound healing
   d. Fat necrosis
   e. No effect

5. **Systemic dextran administration is associated with which of the following effects?**
   a. Improved anastomotic patency
   b. Protection from ischemia reperfusion injury
   c. Neutropenia
   d. Hypokalemia
   e. Increased systemic complications

6. **A 73-year-old man undergoes resection of an 8 × 10 cm invasive squamous cell carcinoma of the scalp and immediate reconstruction with a radial forearm free flap. Flap monitoring is planned. Vascular compromise is most likely to occur during which of the following postoperative time periods?**
   a. 0 to 1 days
   b. 2 to 3 days
   c. 4 to 5 days
   d. 6 to 7 days
   e. 8 to 9 days

7. **A 43-year-old woman is evaluated 6 hours after undergoing delayed breast reconstruction with profunda artery perforator flaps. Arterial signals are present bilaterally on Doppler examination. Capillary refill time is 3 seconds on the right and 1 second on the left. The left flap appears mottled and darker in color compared with the right side. Which of the following is the most appropriate management of the left breast?**
   a. Observation
   b. Administration of systemic heparin
   c. Application of nitroglycerin paste
   d. Application of leeches
   e. Return to the operating room

8. **A 46-year-old women undergoes bilateral breast reconstruction using deep inferior epigastric artery free flaps. On evaluation of the flaps 6 hours later, the right breast appears mottled and engorged. Administration of which of the following is contraindicated in this patient?**
   a. Thrombolytics to the flap vessels
   b. Systemic thrombolytics
   c. Heparinized saline irrigation to the flap vessels
   d. Systemic heparin
   e. Papaverine to the flap vessels

9. **A 17-year-old girl is evaluated 18 hours after undergoing soft-tissue coverage of Gustilo Grade III distal tibia fracture with a latissimus dorsi free flap. The flap appears dark and swollen and Doppler signals are absent. On reexploration in the operating room, thrombus is noted within the artery and vein. Which of the following is the most appropriate treatment to salvage this flap?**
   a. Aspirin
   b. Heparinized saline to flap vessels
   c. Systemic dextran
   d. Systemic thrombolytic
   e. Mechanical thrombectomy

1. **Answer: d.** Age is not a contraindication for microsurgical reconstruction. Microsurgery can be safely performed in children and elderly patients without an increase in flap failure.

Patients should be advised to quit smoking at least 4 weeks before surgery to reduce perioperative complications. Smoking does not reduce anastomotic patency but does affect wound healing, skin graft take over flaps, infection risk, flap necrosis, hernia formation, and length of hospital stay. Vascular disease is a known sequela of diabetes; however, studies show no difference in the rate of flap failure in diabetic patients. Obesity is a known risk factor for flap and donor site complications. Free flaps in obese patients are twice as likely to fail.

2. **Answer: a.** Anastomotic couplers expedite end-to-end venous anastomoses. Patency rates are equivalent to hand-sewn anastomoses. The other options have not been proven as benefits of a coupler device over other techniques.

3. **Answer: c.** Surgical precision is the key factor in anastomotic patency. Magnification in the form of surgical loupes or an operating microscope is acceptable. Studies show equal patency rates in vessels over 1 mm in diameter. Postoperative antithrombotic use offers no protection from microvascular thrombosis and increases complication rates. There is no difference in patency rate based on suture technique (simple interrupted versus continuous) or anastomotic technique (end-to-end versus end-to-side).

4. **Answer: e.** Vasopressors are typically avoided in microsurgery because of the concern that vasospasm of the anastomosis will result in thrombosis. Volume resuscitation is the first-line treatment for hypotension, when possible. Despite this, multiple studies show that intraoperative use of vasoactive agents has no effect on postoperative flap outcomes.

5. Answer: e. Dextran is an antithrombotic agent sometimes used in microsurgical procedures. It decreases red blood cell aggregation through both antiplatelet and antifibrin effects. Dextran has no effect on flap survival but a 3.9- to 7.2-fold increase in systemic complications including renal failure, pulmonary edema, and congestive heart failure. Protection from ischemia reperfusion injury, neutropenia, and hypokalemia are not associated with dextran.

6. Answer: a. Thrombosis is most common within 24 hours of surgery. Early failure is often related to anastomotic imperfections or pedicle positioning. If a problem is detected early, the flap can be salvaged by exploration and revision of the anastomosis. Vascular thrombosis can occur at later times, but such events are generally infrequent.

7. Answer: e. The left flap shows signs of venous insufficiency—brisk capillary refill, mottled and dark appearance. Doppler signals may persist for several hours despite venous thrombosis. The most appropriate management is emergent reexploration. If a problem is detected early, the flap can be salvaged by revision of the anastomosis. The success rate of flap salvage is inversely related to the time interval from the onset of ischemia to restoration of blood flow. Observation is unacceptable. Systemic heparin may prevent further clot formation but will not dissolve acute clot or resolve pedicle kinking. Nitroglycerin paste can improve venous congestion in pedicled flaps but does not obviate the need for reexploration in a microsurgical flap. Application of leeches will drain excess blood from the flap but will not address the underlying problem.

8. Answer: b. Heparin may be used locally or systemically during flap salvage to irrigate existing thrombus and discourage clot propagation. Topical papaverine is routinely applied to flap vessels to reduce spasm. Thrombolytic agents, such as tissue plasminogen activator (tPA) or streptokinase, may be used within the flap but should not be administered systemically.

9. Answer: e. The most important treatment in this patient is mechanical thrombectomy of the flap artery and vein, which reduces clot burden and may restore flow. Intraflap tPA is also commonly used during flap salvage to dissolve microthrombi.

Systemic thrombolytic administration carries a high risk of distant complications and is unlikely to dissolve clot within the flap. Administration of intraflap heparin will prevent further clot formation but will not dissolve the clot in the flap pedicle. Dextran has mild thrombolytic properties but it is not as effective as tPA in lysing clot within the flap and carries a high risk of systemic complications. Aspirin has no thrombolytic properties and has a slow onset of action.

CHAPTER 6 Concepts of Skin Grafts and Skin Substitutes

Sabrina N. Pavri and Henry C. Hsia

KEY POINTS

- Split-thickness skin grafts contain epidermis and a portion of underlying dermis, whereas full-thickness skin grafts contain epidermis and the entire dermis.
- Split-thickness skin grafts, when compared with full-thickness skin grafts, experience less primary contracture, more secondary contracture, may experience more pigment changes, be more susceptible to trauma, and have a lower metabolic demand of the recipient site wound bed.
- Skin grafts heal by a process of imbibition and revascularization through angiogenesis. Graft healing is associated with swelling of the graft, increased mitotic activity leading to desquamation, and eventual reepithelialization over a span of about 4 weeks.
- Common causes of graft failure include hematoma, infection, seroma, shear forces, and a poorly vascularized wound bed.
- Skin substitutes come in a variety of forms and can be considered as biologic dressings that provide clinicians more options in complex wound management, either as an alternative to traditional dressings or as a bridge to more definitive treatment such as surgical closure.

Providing wound coverage for a patient through the application and grafting of skin harvested from a distinct or separate region located elsewhere on that patient's body is a key foundational technique in the armamentarium of the plastic surgeon. Skin grafting originated in India approximately 3000 years ago, where full-thickness grafts comprising the entire dermis and epidermis layers of the skin harvested from the gluteal region were used by the Koomes tilemaker caste for nasal reconstruction after amputation, a common punishment for criminals.[1] The knowledge of this surgical technique did not make its way into Western medicine until the early 19th century. In 1817, Sir Astley Cooper used a full-thickness skin graft from a man's amputated thumb to provide coverage for the remaining stump. This was followed by a successful nasal reconstruction using a skin graft, performed by Buenger in 1823.

However, because of the difficulties his European contemporaries encountered while attempting to replicate his technique, skin grafting did not become widely popular until 1869, when Reverdin published his landmark paper reporting successful pinch grafts. Thin split-thickness grafts were popularized in the late 19th century by Ollier (1871) and Thiersch (1874), as a method to cover defects with a large surface area, becoming known as Ollier-Thiersch grafts. However, the drawbacks of these grafts quickly became evident, with several reports in the 1890s detailing the subsequent wound contractures and graft susceptibility to trauma. During the same period, surgeons and ophthalmologists were using full-thickness skin grafts to correct cases of ectropion. The technique of full-thickness skin grafting was published by Wolfe in 1874 and popularized by Krause, with full-thickness skin grafts becoming known as *Wolfe-Krause* grafts.[2,3]

Despite the development of more advanced surgical techniques, autologous skin grafting remains a mainstay of wound coverage reconstruction, especially for burn trauma. However, the relative lack of donor site availability in patients with extensive burns and the suboptimal aesthetic and functional outcomes commonly associated with autologous skin grafts drive a search for alternatives and led to the development of skin substitutes in recent decades. Although initially intended for primary coverage, skin substitutes have been found to have a salutary impact on wounds even when they fail as permanent wound coverage options. In contemporary applications, skin substitutes have been used more commonly as biologic dressings and bridging therapies to eventual definitive closure via autologous skin grafts or other conventional plastic surgical techniques. Nonetheless, much ongoing work continues in efforts to develop an alternative to autologous skin grafts that would promote regenerative healing of wounds in a definitive fashion.

ANATOMY OF SKIN GRAFTS

The skin is the largest organ in the body, accounting for 15% of total adult body weight, with a layered structure (**Figure 6.1**) that assists in its functions of protection, sensation, thermoregulation, control of evaporation, and absorption.[4] The epidermis, or the outermost layer of the skin, is of ectodermal origin; and its cells undergo continuous differentiation, migration, and eventual shedding. 90% to 95% of epidermal cells are keratinocytes, with the remainder including Langerhans cells, melanocytes, and Merkel cells. The epidermis is substratified into five layers (from superficial to deep)—stratum corneum, stratum lucidum, stratum granulosum, stratum spinosum, and stratum basale. The epidermis has an average thickness of 100 μm, but this can range widely, from 50 μm on the eyelids to 1 mm on the glabrous skin of the hands and feet.

The dermis is a structure of mesodermal origin comprised of collagen and elastin fibers, ground substance, and the deeper portions of the epithelial appendages (eccrine and apocrine sweat glands, and pilosebaceous follicles). Although fibroblasts are the dominant cell type in the dermis, it also contains mesenchymal dermal dendrocytes and mast cells. The papillary dermis is the thin uppermost layer of the dermis composed of loosely arranged collagen fibers, which contains a capillary network that provides nutrients to the epidermis and acts as a mechanism of heat exchange and regulation. The reticular dermis lies below the papillary dermis and is composed of dense irregular collagen fibers. It also contains most of the dermal elastin, as well as the pilosebaceous units and sweat glands.

Within the dermis layer, there exist two horizontal plexuses of vessels connected by bridging vessels that traverse the dermis vertically. The superficial plexus lies at the interface of the papillary and reticular dermis, whereas the deep plexus lies adjacent to the deep border of the dermis. These plexuses are closely associated with nerve bundles and structures that help mediate sensations such as pain, temperature, itch, touch, and pressure. Below the dermis lies the hypodermis or subcutis, which is composed of adipocytes separated by fibrous septa containing fibroblasts, dendrocytes, and mast cells, and into which extend the deepest parts of the epithelial appendages, as well as vessels and nerves that contribute to the overlying dermal plexuses. In structural continuity with the underlying subcutaneous fat, this layer provides thermoregulation, insulation, energy, and mechanical protection for the skin.

Split-thickness skin grafts are defined as grafts involving the epidermis and any part of the dermis, and range in thickness from approximately 0.005 to 0.030 inches. They are classified as thin (0.005–0.012 inches), medium (0.012–0.018 inches), or thick (0.018–0.030 inches) grafts, depending on the amount of dermis included.[1] Full-thickness skin grafts are defined as grafts composed of the epidermis and the entire dermis.

Many factors play into the choice between a split- and full-thickness skin graft for wound coverage. Primary contraction of a skin graft is due to elastin fibers within the dermis and occurs

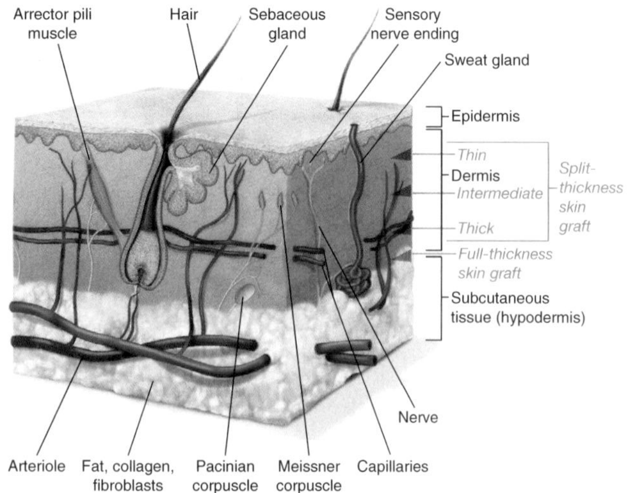

FIGURE 6.1. The anatomy of autologous skin grafts. Human skin is a layered structure comprised of several elements. Split-thickness skin grafts include the epidermis and the superficial portion of the dermis, whereas full-thickness skin grafts include the epidermis and the entire dermis layers.

immediately after harvest. The amount of primary contraction that a graft experiences is proportional to the amount of dermis in the graft; therefore full-thickness grafts exhibit more primary contraction than split-thickness grafts harvested from the same site.[5] By comparison, secondary contraction is a myofibroblast-mediated process that occurs during graft healing and is more likely to occur in grafts with a thinner dermal component. Secondary contraction can cause significant limitations in the stretch and mobility of the healed graft, and therefore, full-thickness grafts are favored in areas such as wounds over joint surfaces where mobility affects function. Although both split-thickness and full-thickness grafts are vulnerable to shear forces during the healing process, once healed, grafts with a larger dermal element are less fragile to subsequent trauma.

One must also take into account the size of the graft needed, as the harvest of a split-thickness graft heals the donor site by secondary intention with minimal morbidity, whereas the donor site for a full-thickness graft usually necessitates primary closure for optimal mitigation of donor site morbidity (thereby limiting the size and potential donor sites for a full-thickness skin graft). Split-thickness grafts are also more amenable to size expansion via meshing techniques, making them more suitable for large wounds. Thicker skin grafts place greater metabolic demands on the wound bed during healing because of the larger tissue component needing nutrients and eventual revascularization, with full-thickness grafts having a slightly lower chance of complete survival and healing than split-thickness grafts on an equivalent wound bed. Because they include only the most superficial portions of the dermis, split-thickness skin grafts also generally do not contain intact accessory skin structures such as hair follicles and sweat glands.

MECHANISMS OF SKIN GRAFT HEALING

A healthy ungrafted wound bed will typically undergo healing by secondary intention—granulation, contraction, and reepithelialization. Placing a skin graft on a wound bed fundamentally alters these processes. Skin grafts become incorporated into the wound bed by a process known as graft *take*, a loosely defined term generally accepted to imply graft healing and survival. This process is largely dependent on the reestablishment of vascular perfusion to the graft within a critical time frame.

Skin graft take has historically been broken down into three classic phases of engraftment—imbibition (0–48 hours), inosculation (48–72 hours), and revascularization (>96 hours). Much of our knowledge in this area relies on decades-old research based largely on in vitro models and histologic analysis, and there remain several competing theories of the exact mechanisms of graft revascularization. However, the recent development of in vivo models has proven enlightening in repetitive intravital microscopic analyses of the microcirculation and revascularization of a skin graft within the wound beds of live organisms.[6]

With all other factors being equal, graft survival has been shown to be dependent on the vascularity of the donor site (with grafts harvested from a highly vascular area healing better than a graft from a poorly perfused area), as well as the metabolic activity of the graft at the time of placement. Freshly harvested grafts have also been shown to attract blood vessel ingrowth more rapidly than grafts that have been frozen and subsequently thawed, but they are also less tolerant of the ischemic period because of increased metabolic activity.[7]

Imbibition

The first stage of skin graft healing is an ischemic phase known as plasmatic or serum imbibition, a concept first developed by Huebscher in 1888,[8] who theorized that grafts were initially nourished by fluid from the wound bed prior to restoration of perfusion. The exact duration of this phase is variable and depends on the characteristics of the wound bed. It lasts approximately 24 hours in a proliferative wound and 48 hours in a fresh wound and can last up to several days in a poorly perfused wound bed. Although it is widely accepted that imbibition allows the graft to survive the initial ischemic period until perfusion is restored, the exact effects on the skin graft of this stage are unclear. Some believe that the graft is nourished by the serum absorbed from the wound bed,[9,10] whereas others believe that the serum has no metabolic function and only serves to keep the graft moist and its vessels patent in the initial period following grafting.[8,11,12]

During imbibition, plasma leaks from recipient capillaries into the wound bed-graft interface, and fibrinogen in the plasma is converted into fibrin, which serves to adhere the graft to the wound bed. As the grafts absorb serum, they become edematous and gain as much as 40% of their initial weight in the first 24 hours, starting to decrease in weight after 96 hours, as lymphatic and venous return develop.[8] During imbibition, metabolism within the graft becomes anaerobic and the pH level falls, reaching a pH of 6.8 as determined by Rous.[13] The metabolic demands of the graft also fall, with ATP levels falling 70% and glucose levels falling 80%.

Historically, the second stage of skin graft healing was thought to be a process called inosculation, by which blood vessels from the underlying wound bed connect with existing vessels in the skin graft at the graft interface. This mechanism in its traditional definition is no longer considered truly valid, as it would require close approximation of the cut ends of the wound bed and graft vessels. While connections between the wound bed vessels and graft vasculature do occur, they are through the process of angiogenesis and new vessel ingrowth in a unidirectional fashion from the wound bed into the graft. Additionally, these new vascular connections do not necessarily occur at the wound interface with the graft, as inosculation would infer. Recent animal studies have shown that after 48 to 72 hours, microvascular growth of capillary-sized vessels (averaging 10–11 μm in diameter) from the wound bed into the graft has been established in the fibrin interface of the wound. A peak in vessel density is seen at postgraft day 7, with the vascular density at the interface increasing 2.5-fold between postgraft days 3 and 7 before returning to levels near those of postgraft day 3 by day 10.[14]

Revascularization

Historically, there have been three theories laid out to explain graft revascularization. The first proposes that anastomoses are formed between the capillaries of the wound bed and the native vessels in the skin graft, and that circulation is restored in the original skin graft vessels.[12,15-17] The second theory involves new vessels originating from the wound bed growing into the skin graft and establishing a new circulation after the initial reperfusion, implying angiogenesis and vasculogenesis, with the native graft vessels eventually degenerating.[18-20] The third theory also suggests reperfusion by angiogenesis from the wound bed but hypothesizes that recipient-derived endothelial cells migrating into the graft use the skin graft's intrinsic preexisting vascular network as a conduit for ingrowth, with eventual replacement of the graft's endothelial structure.[21] Recent development of in vivo animal models supports the third theory of skin graft healing.

In 2010, an in vivo mouse model was developed by Lindenblatt et al. to model skin graft revascularization, allowing for analysis of the microcirculation of the graft and wound bed using fluorescein and intravital fluorescence microscopy during healing.[6] Microcirculatory analysis included the determination of vessel diameter, red blood cell velocity, and functional capillary density defined as length of perfused capillaries per area of observation. During the first 72 hours after grafting, there were a progressive widening of the wound bed capillaries (from 10.6 ± 0.1 μm to 15.9 ± 0.2 μm) and the development of small capillary protrusions representing early bud formation and angiogenesis, although the skin graft still lacked reperfusion of the dermal plexus. At 72 hours, a sluggish blood flow within the graft appeared in a pattern comparable to the original skin microcirculation at the donor site prior to graft harvest, likely representing reperfusion of preexisting graft capillaries. After 96 hours, both the wound bed and the skin graft demonstrated increased capillary diameter and functional capillary density, indicating continued angiogenesis in the wound bed, and ingrowth of newly formed vessels into the graft tissue. At 120 hours, capillary diameter and functional capillary density within the wound bed began to decrease, while still increasing within the graft. By 10 days after grafting (240 hours), the skin graft was fully revascularized, with the wound bed vessels still showing a slightly increased diameter (but without signs of ongoing angiogenesis), and the capillary diameter and functional capillary density of the graft at baseline.

This model supports the theory that angiogenesis is the primary factor in skin graft revascularization, beginning as early as 24 hours after grafting, leading to vessel growth through the fibrin wound bed-graft interface, eventually leading to reperfusion of the graft's native microcirculation within 48 to 72 hours, predominantly within the center of the skin graft. These findings are supported by previously demonstrated dermal graft vessel growth of 5 μm/h, which would mean that a skin graft 200 to 300 μm in thickness would be fully traversed by new microvessels within 48 to 72 hours.[21] Additional research by Lindenblatt et al. has demonstrated that the graft vessels demonstrate an angiogenic response to reperfusion between 3 and 8 days post grafting, suggesting that they are more than simply mechanical conduits. Buds visualized within the grafts at capillary junctions contained endothelial cells and pericytes on histology, indicating a temporary angiogenic response within the skin graft.[22]

Matrix metalloproteinases MT1-MMP and MMP-2 are associated with the initiation of angiogenesis, by promoting the degradation of the endothelium and interstitial matrix. MT1-MMP enables endothelial cells to form invading tubular structures and to lyse the existing capillaries, as these invading structures connect the graft and wound bed vasculature. The temporary angiogenic buds of the graft showed increased expression of MT1-MMP on their surface and served in vivo as docking points for ingrowing capillaries. MMP-2 expression was concentrated around the vessel sprouts of ingrowing vessels as they advanced toward the deep dermal layer of the skin graft.[23]

Using a crossover wild-type/green fluorescent protein (WT/GFP) skin transplantation mouse model (where WT skin was grafted onto GFP mice), GFP-positive structures appeared within the graft vessels starting 48 to 72 hours after transplantation. Preexisting vascular channels in the periphery of the skin graft were 100% replaced by vessel ingrowth from the wound bed by day 10, whereas those in the center of the graft were replaced to a much lesser extent (50%–60%).[24] This may be because the hypoxic stimulus for angiogenesis is no longer present after subsequent revascularization and nutrient supply in the center of the graft where the revascularization process started.[25]

In conclusion, skin graft healing is a process of imbibition and revascularization, which represents a combination of angiogenic vessel outgrowth originating in the wound bed, reperfusion of the preexisting graft vasculature, and partial replacement of the existing graft vessels.

Histology of the Healing Skin Graft

During the first 4 days after grafting, the epidermis of the graft doubles in thickness. This has been hypothesized to be due to multiple processes, including swelling of the nuclei and cytoplasm of epidermal cells, epidermal cell migration to the surface of the graft, and accelerated mitosis of follicular and glandular cells.[26] Between the fourth and eighth days after grafting, the epithelium continues to proliferate and starts to desquamate. This increased cellular turnover does not return to baseline until 4 weeks after grafting.[27,28]

The dermis of a healing skin graft also demonstrates considerable turnover of its cellular and noncellular structures. It is generally accepted that fibroblasts within the dermis of a healing skin graft are not native graft fibroblasts. In a rat model, Converse and Ballantyne noted decreased fibrocyte populations in the first 3 days after grafting, with the appearance of new fibroblast-like cells after day 3, which would also coincide with graft reperfusion.[18] Collagen turnover in the dermis parallels that of the epidermal hyperplasia, peaking at 2 to 3 weeks after grafting at three to four times faster than the collagen turnover rate for normal skin. Approximately, 85% of the original collagen in a skin graft is replaced within 5 months of grafting, although split-thickness grafts replace only half as much of their original collagen compared with full-thickness grafts of the same size.[29,30] Elastin within the graft is also replaced, with degeneration from postgraft day 3, and regeneration starting 4 to 6 weeks after grafting.

Graft Contraction

Graft contraction occurs in both split-thickness and full-thickness grafts. Primary contraction occurs immediately after graft harvest and is a result of the recoil of elastin fibers in the dermis. A full-thickness graft loses approximately 40% of its surface area after harvest because of primary contraction, whereas a split-thickness graft loses 10% to 20% of its area. Secondary contraction occurs during the healing of a skin graft and is a myofibroblast-mediated process that is inversely proportional to the amount of dermis in the graft.[31]

The mechanism behind the inhibition of wound contraction by the presence of dermal elements in the graft is unclear, although multiple hypotheses have been proposed. Rudolph had suggested that increased dermis causes more rapid turnover and elimination of the myofibroblasts that mediate wound contraction.[32] However, further studies by Oliver et al. demonstrated that grafts without dermal cells and other noncollagenous dermal proteins, but possessing a collagen matrix, in fact behave much like full-thickness skin grafts in terms of inhibiting wound contraction.[33] Once wound contraction is complete, full-thickness grafts are able to grow with the surrounding tissue, whereas split-thickness grafts remain fixed.[5]

SKIN GRAFTING TECHNIQUES

Choosing a Donor Site

A skin graft donor site is selected based on several factors. Split-thickness grafts are commonly taken from the lateral thigh to minimize difficulties during harvest and dressing changes, although patients may prefer donor sites with less visible scarring such as the buttocks. Split-thickness grafts taken from the scalp are also successful with minimal donor morbidity and no visible scarring once hair has regrown, but are less commonly used because of the need to shave the donor area prior to taking the graft. Common full-thickness graft donor sites include the inguinal creases, the postauricular region, and the supraclavicular area. Consideration must also be taken to obtain an appropriate color match, especially with head and neck skin graft reconstruction, with grafts optimally taken from donor sites above the clavicles.

Graft Fixation

Adherence of the skin graft to the wound bed during the revascularization process is critical for graft survival. During imbibition, the graft adheres to the wound bed by a thin fibrin layer. Once revascularization begins, vascular ingrowth from the wound bed into the graft reinforces this bond. Shear forces, fluid collections (hematoma/seroma), and infection all decrease the chances of graft adherence and take. For these reasons, optimal graft fixation methods minimize movement, and gently compress the graft to reinforce hemostasis and minimize the chance of fluid collections. Tie-over bolsters using a xeroform sheet filled with mineral oil–soaked cotton balls are common, especially for the fixation of smaller grafts.

For larger skin grafts, grafts in mobile areas, or grafts in areas that are difficult to bolster (e.g., the hand and axilla), negative-pressure dressing techniques such as vacuum-assisted closure therapy (KCI, San Antonio, TX) have become increasingly popular as an alternative bolster dressing for meshed skin grafts. Negative-pressure therapy allows the patient to maintain mobility; however, it does require the patient to carry and recharge the negative-pressure device unit, and the attachment of the dressing to the unit may prove to be cumbersome, especially in patients at increased risks for falls. Spray fibrin sealants such as Evicel (Ethicon, Somerville, NJ) and Artiss (Baxter Healthcare, Deerfield, IL) are also gaining popularity for both securing the edges of the graft (instead of sutures or staples) and increasing adherence of the graft surface. They offer the benefit of immediate mobility, minimal dressings, and ease of application. However, these products may be cost prohibitive in certain settings and also work optimally on thin split-thickness grafts without much primary contraction.

The initial dressing over a skin graft is usually removed approximately 1 week following grafting, once adherence of the graft to the wound bed is more secure and the revascularization process has begun. However, adherence does not imply full graft survival and healing, and local wound care (typically with xeroform and gauze to keep the wound moist and minimize shear forces) is necessary in the postacute phase following the removal of the initial dressing until the skin graft has had the opportunity to mature and become more durable, usually by 3 to 4 weeks following grafting.

Causes of Graft Failure

In addition to mechanical factors in the fibrin interface between the wound bed and graft that interfere with revascularization (such as hematoma, seroma, or shear forces), other causes of graft failure include infection, medical comorbidities of the patient (such as diabetes mellitus, peripheral arterial disease, or a history of radiation), and inherent properties of both the wound bed and the graft. Meshing (performed using a hand-driven roller instrument that creates uniform slits throughout the graft) and pie-crusting (using a scalpel to create multiple small fenestrations in the graft) are common techniques intended to avoid fluid buildup under the skin graft.

Skin grafts in diabetic patients with associated comorbidities often demonstrate delayed healing, with one study showing skin grafts take approximately 2 weeks longer to heal in diabetic patients than in nondiabetic patients.[34] Diabetic patients are also at increased risk for wound dehiscence, infection, and the need for revision surgery. Lower extremity peripheral vascular disease (PVD) also plays an important role in the ability of the wound bed to support a healing graft needing revascularization. In patients whose clinical pictures suggest PVD, a low threshold should be maintained for obtaining noninvasive vascular studies and arteriography. These patients may be candidates for surgical bypass or endovascular angioplasty techniques to optimize blood flow to the wound bed.

A wound bed with necrotic tissue that is poorly perfused, is grossly infected, or has chronically exposed bone or tendon (without periosteum or paratenon) is not appropriate for a graft and will need to be optimized prior to graft placement to maximize the chance of graft survival. Robson and Krizek found that skin grafts are likely to fail if bacterial loads on quantitative culture are greater than 10^5 organisms per gram of tissue.[35] Additionally, inherent properties of the graft may also play a role in graft failure. A thin split-thickness graft will have a greater chance of engraftment than a full-thickness graft taken from the same area, because the metabolic demands of the graft are less and a thinner graft requires a shorter distance of new vessel ingrowth for full revascularization.

Management of the Skin Graft Donor Site

The optimal dressing for the split-thickness skin graft donor site continues to be a matter for debate, as multiple options exist and there are no comprehensive studies comparing all materials in a standardized manner. Generally speaking, the ideal donor site dressing encourages rapid reepithelialization, minimizes pain, decreases the risk of infection, and curtails scarring. In general, dressings that promote a moist wound environment until reepithelialization occurs (at least 7 days) have been shown to improve rates of healing and pain control.

A 2013 multicenter randomized clinical trial compared six common donor site dressings and assessed both primary outcomes (time to reepithelialization and pain scores) and secondary outcomes (itching, scarring, and adverse events such as infection, allergic reaction, and hypergranulation).[36] Patients were randomly allocated to an alginate (Kaltostat; ConvaTec, Skillman, NJ; Algisite; Smith & Nephew, London, UK; or Melgisorb; Mölnlycke Health Care, Gothenburg, Sweden); a semipermeable film (Tegaderm; 3M, St Paul, Minnesota; or Opsite; Smith and Nephew); a gauze dressing (Adaptic; Acelity, San Antonio, TX; or Jelonet; Smith & Nephew); a hydrocolloid (DuoDERM; ConvaTec); a hydrofibre (Aquacel; ConvaTec), or a silicone dressing (Mepitel; Mölnlycke Health Care). Time to complete reepithelialization was 7 days (30%) shorter when hydrocolloid dressings were used (median 16 days) than with any other dressing (median 23 days). Pain scores were lowest in the semipermeable film group, but the difference did not reach statistical significance. Gauze dressings had the highest infection rates.

This trial's protocol prescribed the uniform use of gauze-based secondary dressings; therefore, the effects of other secondary dressings (such as semipermeable film) used in clinical practice could not be studied. Additionally, in clinical practice, other factors such as cost, patient compliance with wound care, and availability must be considered. Skin graft donor site dressings continue to be a matter of surgeon preference with no strong evidence directed to any one option. However, it is generally accepted that the dressing should maintain a moist wound environment for at least 1 week.

EMERGING ALTERNATIVES TO CONVENTIONAL SKIN GRAFTS

Cultured epidermal grafts have been used clinically since the 1980s, when burn patients were successfully grafted with cultured allografts,[37] and Phillips et al. treated refractory chronic lower extremity wounds with both cultured autografts and cultured allografts.[8] Although it seems intuitive that cultured epithelial autografts would heal on a wound, the successful engraftment of cultured epithelial allografts in the setting of complete lack of immunosuppression needed further explanation. In the 1990s, several studies demonstrated that all donor cells in the graft were replaced by recipient keratinocytes by as early as 1 week following grafting,[38–40] leading to the subsequent conclusion that cultured epidermal allografts provide growth factors that lead to rapid wound healing despite the technical failure when the graft fails to survive. This concept of an epithelial graft as a pharmacologic agent to aid wound healing rather than a technical replacement of the epithelium was an important development in understanding how skin substitutes and similar products may be used to promote wound closure.

The clinical applications of cultured epidermal autografts (Epicel; Genzyme, Cambridge, MA) have been limited because of variable graft take rate, limited mechanical resistance, hyperkeratosis, scar contracture, ulceration, and blister formation because of reactions to foreign fibroblasts in feeder media, as well as the lengthy culture time (3–4 weeks) required and the high cost. Recently, there has been development of several modifications of skin grafting technique to address the drawbacks of traditional skin grafting, including dermal-epidermal grafts, fractional skin harvesting, and epidermal grafts.[41,42]

In epidermal grafting, harvesting systems provide continuous negative pressure to separate the epidermis from the dermis at the dermal-epidermal junction while preserving the histological architecture of the epidermis. Although it has been used to treat vitiligo for decades, it has only recently been evaluated as a possible treatment for wound healing. Healing of epidermal grafts is associated with keratinocyte activation, growth factor secretion, and reepithelialization from the wound edge, more akin to cultured keratinocytes than full- or split-thickness grafts.[42]

Dermal-epidermal grafting creates micrografts of approximately 0.8 mm × 0.8 mm in size from a split-thickness skin graft using the Xpansion Micrografting system (ACell, Colombia, MD). This increases the border area and regenerative capacity of the grafts, and allows expansion by a factor of 1:100 (instead of the typical 1:5 expansion of a full-thickness skin graft and 1:9 expansion of a meshed split-thickness skin graft). Micrografts also do not need to retain their dermal orientation, thereby decreasing the procedural complexity. This minimizes the size of the skin graft required and resultant donor site morbidity, allowing the procedure to take place under local anesthetic in an outpatient setting.[41]

Fractional skin harvesting requires harvesting a large number of full-thickness microscopic skin tissue columns measuring approximately 700 μm in diameter using customized hypodermic needles. The extracted skin columns are placed randomly in the wound without maintaining the dermal orientation. Advantages of this technique include minimal morbidity, faster healing of the donor site without scarring, and lack of the expanded mesh graft pattern of the healed graft. Although this is still a new technique currently only being used in experimental animal models, it shows promise for future commercial development.[41]

Autologous noncultured cell therapy such as ReCell (Avita Medical, Royston, UK) isolates cells from the dermal-epidermal junction of a thin split-thickness skin graft using trypsin incubation, followed by mechanical agitation to separate the cells, and immediate suspension in a lactate solution, which then undergoes spray application on the wound. Benefits of this system include quick application and a large expansion ratio (1:80). Drawbacks include poor attachment and loss of cells secondary to mechanical pressure while spraying, as well as high cost. One promising application of this technique is potential one-stage creation of an epidermal layer when used concurrently with dermal matrices. In a pilot study,[43] ReCell was combined with the dermal substitute Integra (Integra LifeSciences Corp., Plainsboro, NJ) to treat full-thickness wounds in a porcine model. Cells isolated with the ReCell system were sprayed on the underside of the dermal matrix prior to application. The study indicated that cells stay viable, migrate through the dermal substitute, and self-organize into a differentiated epidermis.

SKIN SUBSTITUTES

The scarcity of donor site availability in patients with extensive burns and the suboptimal aesthetic and functional outcomes commonly associated with autologous skin grafts have prompted the search for viable substitutes for skin grafts. The earliest skin substitutes were allografts of cadaveric human skin used to treat patients with extensive burns and limited donor sites for autograft harvest. The high antigenicity of skin allografts, in particular the epidermal layer, with subsequent graft sloughing and rejection led to the combination of cultured epidermal autografts over dermal allografts in the 1980s.[44] Observation that the formation of a *neodermis* comprised of healthy connective tissue is stimulated in the wound bed even though the allograft does not successfully survive, as well as concerns about disease transmission from donors and persistent scarring and contractures, has spurred continued efforts to develop bioengineered skin substitutes.[45]

In 1984, Pruitt and Levine[46] detailed the attributes of an ideal skin substitute:

- Little or no antigenicity
- Tissue compatibility
- Lack of toxicity, either local or systemic
- Permeability to water vapor just like normal skin
- Impenetrability to microorganisms
- Rapid and persistent adherence to a wound surface
- Porosity for ingrowth of fibrovascular tissue from the wound bed
- Malleability to conform to an irregular wound surface
- Elasticity for motion of underlying tissues
- Structural stability to resist linear and shear stresses
- A smooth surface to discourage bacterial proliferation
- Sufficient tensile strength to resist fragmentation
- Biodegradability
- Low cost
- Ease of storage
- Indefinite shelf life

Although the intervening decades have seen the development of a broad range of products that attempt to embody many of these attributes, the term *skin substitute* belies how these products are currently used in complex wound management. Furthermore, inconsistency in terminology and how these products are applied can make consistent classification challenging, but skin substitutes and related products may be categorized in several ways: composition of source material (e.g., synthetic versus biologic; human versus animal), intended duration (permanent versus temporary), intended tissue to be replaced (epidermal versus dermal), and number of layers (single versus bilaminate). Many products do not neatly fit into these categories, however. For example, Biobrane (Smith & Nephew) is a biosynthetic composite containing both synthetic elements comprised of silicone and a nylon mesh along with a biologic element derived from porcine collagen. Another composite product, Dermagraft (Organogenesis, Canton, MA) is created by seeding neonatal foreskin fibroblasts onto a biodegradable polyglycolic acid mesh. The fibroblasts are cryopreserved at −80°C and regain their viability once the product is applied on the wound, which must be done within 30 minutes after thawing.[45]

Marketed under a variety of terms including artificial skin equivalent, dermal regeneration template, wound matrix, biologic dressing, tissue scaffold, or some other permutation of these words, these bioengineered products share the similar purpose of promoting wound closure, and contrasts are only found on whether the emphasis of a product is placed on acting as an in situ replacement of skin tissue that is eventually incorporated into the recipient wound bed, or on promoting endogenous tissue repair processes within the wound bed to achieve a more optimal healing outcome. In fact, rather than evaluating these products as true substitutes for native skin and treating them as equivalent to autologous skin grafts, it is more useful when deciding whether to use them for clinical purposes to regard the role of these bioengineered skin products as constructs that may deliver growth factors and extracellular matrix components, or attract cells to the wound bed, that can stimulate endogenous healing processes to help promote wound closure and assist in preparing the wound bed for definitive surgical treatment, especially for patients with wounds such as diabetic foot ulcers that can be extremely challenging to treat.[45]

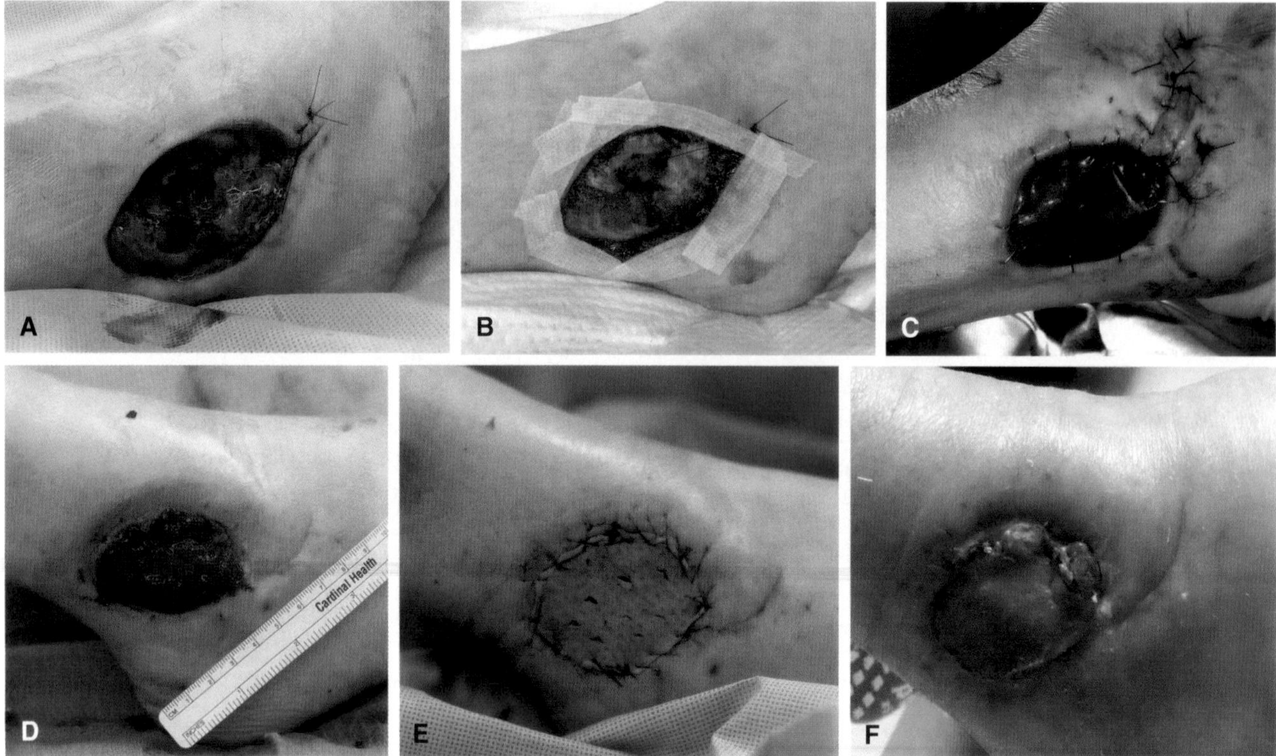

FIGURE 6.2. Using skin substitutes as a bridging therapy. **A.** This patient sustained an open fracture to his left lateral ankle after a motor vehicle collision. **B.** After open reduction and internal fixation by the orthopedic surgeon, the patient underwent debridement and was left with a significant soft tissue deficit with exposed bone and hardware (visible near posteroinferior wound border). Lengthy surgical intervention with conventional flap reconstruction techniques was deemed inadvisable because of cardiac issues. **C.** To provide temporary coverage, Integra was applied over the wound. **D.** Negative-pressure wound therapy was initiated over the Integra and continued for 8 weeks, at which point viable revascularized neodermis had fully filled the 2-cm deep cavity, provided coverage of the bone and hardware, and was flush with the surrounding skin. **E.** This allowed placement of a split-thickness skin graft. **F.** The skin graft demonstrated good take, with near-complete reepithelialization 3 weeks after application.

One product mentioned more frequently on plastic surgery examinations is Integra, a bilaminar membrane system consisting of a porous coprecipitate of bovine tendon type I collagen and shark glycosaminoglycan (chondroitin-6-sulfate), covered by a temporary silicone epidermal substitute. The silicone layer prevents excessive moisture loss and formation of granulation tissue on the matrix surface. Chondroitin-6-sulfate provides elasticity to the matrix, controls the biodegradation rate, and maintains an open pore structure that allows cell migration into the matrix.[49] Integra heals in phases similar to skin graft healing, progressing through (1) imbibition, (2) fibroblast migration, (3) neovascularization, and (4) remodeling and maturation. During imbibition, the interstices of the matrix fill with wound fluid containing red blood cells, and the fibrin in the wound exudate fosters adherence of the matrix to the wound bed. By day 7, myofibroblasts start migrating into the matrix and start producing collagen by the beginning of week 3. The silicone epidermal layer has usually sloughed or been removed by this point in time. New blood vessels can be seen in the deep portion of the matrix by day 12 and reach the superficial surface by day 28, at which point a thin split-thickness skin graft may be applied.

Recent data showed clinical effectiveness using Integra to help achieve eventual wound closure with successful skin grafting performed as early as 1 week after Integra application in combination with negative-pressure therapy.[50] However, neovascularization of the matrix at that early time point has yet to be demonstrated at the histological level. Integra can also be used without the silicone layer as a filler for contour deformities, although this does require a lengthier period of neovascularization for vessel ingrowth through a thicker matrix. Though not uniform, empiric observations that use of this product, especially in combination with other modalities such as negative-pressure wound therapy, can often generate granulation tissue even over challenging surfaces, such as bone, tendon, and hardware, have led to its off-label application for clinical situations where other methods of reconstruction are not feasible as illustrated in the accompanying case (**Figure 6.2**).

Each year sees the introduction of new or modified products intended as *advanced wound therapy*. However, high-level clinical evidence, rigorous cost-benefit analyses, and other research supporting their routine use remain incomplete, with many of the products not uniformly available because of lack of regulatory approval or restrictive reimbursement and formulary policies. Nonetheless, the use of skin substitutes and related products has entered the mainstream of contemporary clinical practice. Recent reviews summarizing these products with extensive lists and tables can be found in the existing medical and scientific literature,[47,48] and therefore will not be duplicated here, given the constant flux and changes in available products and evidence. Although the full potential of skin substitutes remains yet to be achieved, with their ability to promote wound closure and act as important temporizing bridges to definitive treatment, skin substitutes and their related brethren products have become an important adjunct in complex wound management for the plastic surgeon.

CONCLUSION

Autologous skin grafts are a key foundational technique of plastic surgeons and remain a mainstay of reconstructive surgery for wounds despite the development of more advanced surgical techniques. Surgeons may choose between split-thickness and full-thickness skin grafts depending on various factors including graft characteristics (color match, size, amount of primary and secondary contraction), donor site availability and morbidity, and recipient site requirements. Once applied to a wound bed, skin grafts heal by a process of imbibition and revascularization, which is a combination of angiogenic vessel outgrowth originating in the wound bed, reperfusion of the preexisting graft vasculature, and partial replacement of the existing graft vessels. To minimize shear forces and fluid collecting at the interface, both of which can lead to graft loss, skin grafts are typically immobilized during the postoperative period with bolster dressings, which in recent years are more frequently comprised of negative-pressure wound dressings. Limitations of conventional skin grafts spur the development of biologic and synthetic skin substitutes. Although the goal of using skin substitutes for definitive wound coverage remains elusive, skin substitutes and similar products have established a role in providing temporary wound coverage and assisting in the healing and preparation of wound beds until definitive coverage can be obtained.

REFERENCES

1. Ratner D. Skin grafting: from here to there. *Dermatol Clin*. 1998;16(1):75-90.
2. Hauben DJ, Baruchin A, Mahler A. On the history of the free skin graft. *Ann Plast Surg*. 1982;9(3):242-245.
3. Chick LR. Brief history and biology of skin grafting. *Ann Plast Surg*. 1988;21(4):358-365.
4. Kanitakis J. Anatomy, histology and immunohistochemistry of normal human skin. *Eur J Dermatol*. 2002;12(4):390-399; quiz 400-391.
5. Corps BV. The effect of graft thickness, donor site and graft bed on graft shrinkage in the hooded rat. *Br J Plast Surg*. 1969;22(2):125-133.
6. Lindenblatt N, Calcagni M, Contaldo C, et al. A new model for studying the revascularization of skin grafts in vivo: the role of angiogenesis. *Plast Reconstr Surg*. 2008;122(6):1669-1680.
   This 2008 study detailed the development of a mouse model that allowed repeated intravital microscopy to assess the microcirculation during skin graft healing. They determined that capillary widening in the wound bed appeared at day 1 after grafting and increased until day 4, while capillary buds and sprouts first appeared at day 2. Blood filling of autochthonous graft capillaries occurred at day 3, resulting in almost complete restoration of the original skin microcirculation on day 5 through interconnections between the microvasculature of the wound bed and the skin graft through a temporary angiogenic response.
7. O'Donoghue MN, Zarem HA. Stimulation of neovascularization: comparative efficacy of fresh and preserved skin grafts. *Plast Reconstr Surg*. 1971;48(5):474-478.
8. Converse JM, Uhlschmid GK, Ballantyne DL. "Plasmatic circulation" in skin grafts. The phase of serum imbibition. *Plast Reconstr Surg*. 1969;43(5):495-499.
   This classic 1969 paper by Converse et al. defined the phase of serum imbibition, *referring to the absorption of serum from the wound bed after grafting, which replaced the previously accepted* plasmatic circulation. *Full-thickness skin grafts were excised in rats, weighed prior to grafting, and re-weighed 1 to 11 postoperative days after grafting. The grafts had a characteristic increase in weight in the first 48 to 72 hours, followed by a steady decrease, which they hypothesized was due to serum absorption from the wound bed, which was followed by the resolution of the edema once the graft microcirculation was reestablished.*
9. Pepper FJ. Studies on the viability of mammalian skin autografts after storage at different temperatures. *Br J Plast Surg*. 1954;6(4):250-256.
10. Hinshaw, Miller ER. Histology of healing split-thickness, full-thickness autogenous skin grafts and donor sites. *Arch Surg*. 1965;91(4):658-670.
11. Clemmesen T. The early circulation in split skin grafts. *Acta Chir Scand*. 1962;124:11-18.
12. Peer LA, Walker JC. The behavior of autogenous human tissue grafts: a comparative study. 1. *Plast Reconstr Surg (1946)*. 1951;7(1):6-23.
13. Rous P. The relative reaction within living mammalian tissues. VI. Factors determining the reaction of skin grafts; a study by the indicator method of conditions within an ischemic tissue. *J Exp Med*. 1926;44(6):815-834.
14. Wu X, Kathuria N, Patrick CW, Reece GP. Quantitative analysis of the microvasculature growing in the fibrin interface between a skin graft and the recipient site. *Microvasc Res*. 2008;75(1):119-129.
15. Clemmesen T. Experimental studies on the healing of free skin autografts. *Dan Med Bull*. 1967;14(suppl 2):1-73.
16. Haller JA, Billingham RE. Studies of the origin of the vasculature in free skin grafts. *Ann Surg*. 1967;166(6):896-901.
17. Birch J, Branemark PI. The vascularization of a free full thickness skin graft. I. A vital microscopic study. *Scand J Plast Reconstr Surg*. 1969;3(1):1-10.
18. Converse JM, Ballantyne DL. Distribution of diphosphopyridine nucleotide diaphorase in rat skin autografts and homografts. *Plast Reconstr Surg Transpl Bull*. 1962;30:415-425.
19. Converse JM, Rapaport FT. The vascularization of skin autografts and homografts: an experimental study in man. *Ann Surg*. 1956;143(3):306-315.
20. Wolff K, Schellander FG. Enzyme-histochemical studies on the healing-process of split skin grafts. I. Aminopeptidase, diphosphopyridine-nucleotide-diaphorase and succinic dehydrogenase in autografts. *J Invest Dermatol*. 1965;45:38-45.
21. Zarem HA, Zweifach BW, McGehee JM. Development of microcirculation in full thickness autogenous skin grafts in mice. *Am J Physiol*. 1967;212(5):1081-1085.
22. Lindenblatt N, Platz U, Althaus M, et al. Temporary angiogenic transformation of the skin graft vasculature after reperfusion. *Plast Reconstr Surg*. 2010;126(1):61-70.
23. Knapik A, Hegland N, Calcagni M, et al. Metalloproteinases facilitate connection of wound bed vessels to pre-existing skin graft vasculature. *Microvasc Res*. 2012;84(1):16-23.
   Skin graft vasculature in this mouse model demonstrated a temporary angiogenic response to reperfusion, which was pruned after several days and exhibited a different morphology than regular sprouting angiogenesis present within the wound bed. Matrix metalloproteinases were found to be involved in capillary ingrowth and regression, with MT1-MMP expressed predominantly on sprout tips imparting vessel-to-vessel connections, and MMP-2 around vessel sprouts during sprouting angiogenesis facilitating the degradation of the extracellular matrix.
24. Calcagni M, Althaus MK, Knapik AD, et al. In vivo visualization of the origination of skin graft vasculature in a wild-type/GFP crossover model. *Microvasc Res*. 2011;82(3):237-245.
   To determine the origin of skin graft vasculature once healed, a crossover wild-type/GFP skin transplantation model was created, in which each animal carried the graft from the other strain. This demonstrated a replacement of existing graft capillaries with vessels from the wound bed in 68% of the vessels overall, with vessel replacement in almost 100% of graft vessels at the periphery of the graft. These data indicate an early ingrowth of angiogenic bed vessels into the existing vascular channels of the graft and subsequent partial to full centripetal replacement.
25. Cassavaugh J, Lounsbury KM. Hypoxia-mediated biological control. *J Cell Biochem*. 2011;112(3):735-744.
26. Smahel J. The healing of skin grafts. *Clin Plast Surg*. 1977;4(3):409-424.
27. Medawar PB. The behaviour and fate of skin autografts and skin homografts in rabbits: a report to the War Wounds Committee of the Medical Research Council. *J Anat*. 1944;78(Pt 5):176-199.
28. Medawar PB. A second study of the behaviour and fate of skin homografts in rabbits: a report to the War Wounds Committee of the Medical Research Council. *J Anat*. 1945;79(Pt 4):157-176 154.
29. Rudolph R, Klein L. Isotopic measurement of collagen turnover in skin grafts. *Surg Forum*. 1971;22:489-491.
30. Ohuchi K, Tsurufuji S. Degradation and turnover of collagen in the mouse skin and the effect of whole body x-irradiation. *Biochim Biophys Acta*. 1970;208(3):475-481.
31. Brown D, Garner W, Young VL. Skin grafting: dermal components in inhibition of wound contraction. *South Med J*. 1990;83(7):789-795.
32. Rudolph R. Inhibition of myofibroblasts by skin grafts. *Plast Reconstr Surg*. 1979;63(4):473-480.
33. Oliver RF, Grant RA, Kent CM. The fate of cutaneously and subcutaneously implanted trypsin purified dermal collagen in the pig. *Br J Exp Pathol*. 1972;53(5):540-549.
34. Ramanujam CL, Han D, Fowler S, et al. Impact of diabetes and comorbidities on split-thickness skin grafts for foot wounds. *J Am Podiatr Med Assoc*. 2013;103(3):223-232.
35. Robson MC, Krizek TJ. Predicting skin graft survival. *J Trauma*. 1973;13(3):213-217.
36. Brolmann FE, Eskes AM, Goslings JC, et al. Randomized clinical trial of donor-site wound dressings after split-skin grafting. *Br J Surg*. 2013;100(5):619-627.
37. Kirsner RS, Falanga V, Eaglstein WH. The biology of skin grafts: skin grafts as pharmacologic agents. *Arch Dermatol*. 1993;129(4):481-483.
38. Gielen V, Faure M, Mauduit G, Thivolet J. Progressive replacement of human cultured epithelial allografts by recipient cells as evidenced by HLA class I antigens expression. *Dermatologica*. 1987;175(4):166-170.
39. Burt AM, Pallett CD, Sloane JP, et al. Survival of cultured allografts in patients with burns assessed with probe specific for Y chromosome. *BMJ*. 1989;298(6678):915-917.
40. Phillips TJ, Bhawan J, Leigh IM, et al. Cultured epidermal autografts and allografts: a study of differentiation and allograft survival. *J Am Acad Dermatol*. 1990;23(2 Pt 1):189-198.
41. Singh M, Nuutila K, Kruse C, et al. Challenging the conventional therapy: emerging skin graft techniques for wound healing. *Plast Reconstr Surg*. 2015;136(4):524e-530e.
42. Kanapathy M, Hachach-Haram N, Bystrzonowski N, et al. Epidermal grafting for wound healing: a review on the harvesting systems, the ultrastructure of the graft and the mechanism of wound healing. *Int Wound J*. 2017;14(1):16-23.
43. Hammer D, Rendon JL, Sabino J, et al. Restoring full-thickness defects with spray skin in conjunction with dermal regenerate template and split-thickness skin grafting: a pilot study. *J Tissue Eng Regen Med*. 2017;11(12):3523-3529.
44. Cuono C, Langdon R, McGuire J. Use of cultured epidermal autografts and dermal allografts as skin replacement after burn injury. *Lancet*. 1986;1:1123-1124.
45. Lazic T, Falanga V. Bioengineered skin constructs and their use in wound healing. *Plast Reconstr Surg*. 2011;127(suppl 1):75S-90S.
46. Pruitt BA, Levine NS. Characteristics and uses of biologic dressings and skin substitutes. *Arch Surg*. 1984;119(3):312-322.
47. Nyame TT, Chiang HA, Leavitt T, et al. Tissue-engineered skin substitutes. *Plast Reconstr Surg*. 2015;136(6):1379-1388.
48. Vig K, Chaudhari A, Tripathi S, et al. Advances in skin regeneration using tissue engineering. *Int J Mol Sci*. 2017;18(4).
49. Moiemen NS, Vlachou E, Staiano JJ, et al. Reconstructive surgery with Integra dermal regeneration template: histologic study, clinical evaluation, and current practice. *Plast Reconstr Surg*. 2006;117(suppl 7):S160-S174.
   The healing of the Integra dermal regeneration template was assessed in 20 human patients using weekly punch biopsies. Four stages of dermal regeneration could be demonstrated histologically: imbibition, fibroblast migration, neovascularization, and remodeling, and maturation. Full vascularization of the neodermis occurred at 4 weeks.
50. Molnar JA, DeFranzo AJ, Hadaegh A, et al. Acceleration of Integra incorporation in complex tissue defects with subatmospheric pressure. *Plast Reconstr Surg*. 2004;113(5):1339-1346.

QUESTIONS

1. **Which option correctly describes the properties of split-thickness skin grafts compared with full-thickness skin grafts?**
   a. More primary contracture, less secondary contracture, more metabolic demand from the graft bed
   b. Less primary contracture, more secondary contracture, more metabolic demand from the graft bed
   c. More primary contracture, less secondary contracture, less metabolic demand from the graft bed
   d. Less primary contracture, more secondary contracture, less metabolic demand from the graft bed

2. **Which combination of biologic events characterizes the stage of plasma imbibition of skin graft healing?**
   a. Aerobic metabolism of graft cells, increased metabolic demand of the graft, plasma leak into the wound bed, and increased graft weight secondary to edema
   b. Plasma leak into the wound bed, increased metabolic demand of the graft, microvascular ingrowth into the graft, and increased graft weight secondary to edema
   c. Anaerobic metabolism of graft cells, decreased metabolic demand of the graft, plasma leak into the wound bed, and acidic pH
   d. Anaerobic metabolism of graft cells, acidic pH, decreased weight of the graft secondary to evaporative losses, and fibrinogen conversion to fibrin at the graft interface

3. **What is the primary mechanism by which blood flow is reestablished in a skin graft?**
   a. Reperfusion of existing graft vasculature by inosculation, a process by which blood vessels from the underlying wound bed connect end-to-end with existing vessels in the skin graft at the graft interface
   b. Microvascular ingrowth from the wound bed, with a temporary angiogenic response from the preexisting graft vasculature, which also acts as a conduit for capillary ingrowth
   c. Revascularization from the wound bed, with formation of entirely new vascular channels via angiogenesis within the graft and obliteration of preexisting vessels
   d. Temporary angiogenic response within the graft, leading to capillary budding within the graft, increased expression of matrix metalloproteinases MT1-MMP and MMP-2, and microvascular growth from the graft to the wound bed

4. **A 23-year-old man presents to the emergency department after sustaining full-thickness burns to the volar fingers of his dominant hand. After debridement, the tendons are exposed, with viable paratenon. The patient wants to minimize his number of surgeries and time out of work. What is the best option for resurfacing?**
   a. Split-thickness skin graft from the anterolateral thigh
   b. Application of Integra, with staged application of a split-thickness skin graft from the buttock
   c. Application of Alloderm
   d. Full-thickness skin graft from the inguinal crease
   e. Split-thickness skin graft from the scalp

5. **A 65-year-old man with PVD, congestive heart failure, and well-controlled type 2 diabetes is evaluated for a chronic lower extremity wound. The wound appears to have a well-granulating bed, and it is not debrided before a split-thickness skin graft from the anterior thigh is applied. What is the factor most likely to lead to graft failure in this patient?**
   a. Peripheral edema secondary to congestive heart failure
   b. PVD
   c. Type 2 diabetes
   d. Quantitative wound bacterial count greater than 10^5 organisms per gram of tissue

1. **Answer: d.** Split-thickness skin grafts (containing epidermis and a portion of dermis) experience less primary contracture, experience more secondary contracture, may experience more pigment changes, are more susceptible to trauma, and have a lower metabolic demand of the recipient site wound bed, when compared with full-thickness skin grafts (which contain epidermis and the full dermis).

2. **Answer: c.** The first stage of graft healing, the stage of plasma imbibition, is characterized by fibrinogen conversion to fibrin at the graft interface to facilitate adherence, plasma leak from wound bed capillaries, increased weight of the graft secondary to edema, anaerobic metabolism and decreased metabolic demands of graft cells, and an acidic pH of approximately 6.8. Microvascular ingrowth does not occur until the stage of revascularization.

3. **Answer: b.** After the stage of plasma imbibition, blood flow to the healing graft is established by revascularization. Angiogenesis begins within the wound bed, with capillary budding and the ingrowth of newly formed vessels into the graft tissue. A temporary angiogenic response within the graft also occurs, with increased expression of matrix metalloproteinases MT1-MMP and MMP-2 allowing lysis of the existing capillaries to connect the graft and wound bed vasculature, leading to reperfusion of parts of the existing graft vasculature. Preexisting graft vasculature acts as a conduit for capillary ingrowth and is replaced either partially or fully by host endothelial cells by 10 days after grafting.

4. **Answer: d.** To receive a skin graft, a wound bed must have healthy vascularized tissue at its base. A skin graft is less likely to heal over exposed tendon or bone without paratenon or periosteum. The increased secondary contraction of split-thickness skin grafts mean that they are not ideal for resurfacing the flexor surfaces of joint, as they can cause joint contracture and limited range of motion. This patient wants to minimize his number of surgeries and time out of work; therefore a staged reconstruction with Integra and a split-thickness skin graft would be more time-consuming than a one-stage procedure. Alloderm can be used as temporary wound coverage but is only a dermal skin substitute and the wound would likely still need to be definitively covered with an autologous skin graft at a later time point.

5. **Answer: d.** Skin grafts are likely to fail if bacterial loads on the quantitative culture are greater than 10^5 organisms per gram of tissue. Although peripheral edema, PVD, and type 2 diabetes are all factors than can contribute to delayed skin graft healing, adequate debridement of the wound leading to decreased bacterial counts is necessary for successful graft healing.

CHAPTER 7 Principles of Flap Reconstruction: Muscle Flaps, Myocutaneous Flaps, and Fasciocutaneous Flaps

Michele Ann Manahan

KEY POINTS

- Understand the definition of the term flap.
- Understand classifications of types of flaps.
- Become familiar with elements of essential clinical decision-making with regard to flaps as treatment options.
- Understand basic procedural elements associated with common flaps.
- Increase awareness of and vigilance for pitfalls of flap use.

An understanding of surgical manipulation of vascularized tissue or *flaps*, and the ability to employ this, could be considered the defining core competency of plastic surgery. A chapter dedicated to flaps can only ever be a starting point from which to build a lifetime of learning. This chapter could never be considered completely comprehensive, because an understanding of flaps requires a thorough knowledge of basic principles as well as a working knowledge of current popular and successful surgical techniques, balanced with awareness of more historical flap designs that may still be called into use in salvage situations. This chapter will begin with a review of high points in the historical chronology of surgical transfer of vascularized tissue, or *flaps*. Principles will then be explained as they relate to the broad categories of flaps. Pertinent clinical examples will be reviewed in these areas as well.

PATIENT AND TECHNIQUE SELECTION

Although the remainder of the chapter will serve to highlight the vast number of *flap* choices available for reconstruction, several unifying tenets regarding patient and technique selection remain important. One must always consider patient factors such as comorbidities, nicotine dependence, and local tissue history (e.g., radiation, trauma, previous surgery) in preoperative planning because these may all affect intraoperative and postoperative outcomes.[1] Optimize nutrition when possible.

Consideration of the reconstructive ladder is also essential. The great variety of flap techniques, and modern facility with these, makes flap use appealing. One should remember, however, that healing by secondary intention, primary closure, skin grafting, and other techniques continue to have valid places in modern reconstruction. Flap selection should also be considered in terms of the size of the flap, recipient site needs, location of donor site, and potential associated morbidities. Muscle flaps are generally believed to fill dead space effectively, potentially owing to bulk, blood supply, and *stickiness* of tissue, although many authors believe that fasciocutaneous flaps are fully capable of these tasks.

A healthy flap does not obviate the need for appropriate surgical timing, in terms of both overall patient condition and local wound readiness. Proper debridement and control of infection must be balanced with the need for coverage of critical structures when considering flap coverage timing. One must also remember to consider temporizing measures for wound control in situations when preparation of the donor site is necessary. For example, prefabrication of flaps with pretransfer tissue expansion can increase the surface area of the transferred tissue, decrease donor site closure difficulty, and thin flaps for better fit into recipient areas.[1]

Understanding of the flap itself is insufficient for adequate use of flaps as surgical treatments. One must also understand the recipient site needs and interactions between flaps and recipient sites. For example, recipient site vessel size, orientation, and flow must be considered prior to free tissue transfer. Techniques including end-to-end anastomoses, end-to-side anastomoses, surgical delays (selective ligation of some vascularity to augment remaining vascularity), vein grafting and/or loops, retrograde vessel properties, supercharging, and many others can salvage a suboptimal situation. Alternative techniques need to be considered preoperatively should an intraoperative failure of the planned flap occur. Patients should be counseled about the potential use of alternative treatments before they become necessary.

HISTORICAL CLASSIFICATIONS

The key defining feature of transfer of a vascularized segment of soft tissue, the most basic definition of a *flap*, is maintenance of blood supply. There are many types of vascularity.[2] Esser characterized the necessity of vascular inflow as well as outflow.[3] McGregor and Morgan defined random versus axial patterns of blood supply. They described random pattern flaps as without bias in vascular pattern compared with axial pattern flaps with an arteriovenous system oriented along the long axis.[4] Taylor and Palmer defined angiosomes, or segments of skin reliably supplied by single source vessels. They further described that these vessels can approach the skin directly or indirectly through fascial septae (septocutaneous perforators), perforating through muscle (musculocutaneous perforators), and via choke vessels between cutaneous and fascial networks.[5] Free tissue transfer with microvascular anastomosis was described as a separate method of moving tissue by pedicled transfer in the early 1970s.[6,7] Separation of the target tissue from bulky underlying soft tissue serving as a conduit for the source vessel was first described as *perforator* surgery in 1989.[8] Increasing variety of designs based not only on known, named vessels but also on a *free style* fashion by deriving vessels from and to nearly any part of the body.[2]

We will now review some of the more widely accepted flap classifications pertinent to current practice.

CONTEMPORARY CLASSIFICATION SYSTEMS

Muscle Flap Classification

Mathes and Nahai created the most widely used classification for muscle flaps based on pedicle type. Their classification is reproduced in Table 7.1. These anatomical variations affect arc of rotation, skin island design, survival of more distal portions of the muscle flap, microvascular utility, and need for consideration of surgical delay techniques (partial harvest separated by a period of weeks from completion of harvest of tissue).[9]

TABLE 7.1. MATHES AND NAHAI CLASSIFICATION OF MUSCLE FLAPS[9]

Type	Vascular Pedicle	Examples	Considerations
I	One dominant	Gastrocnemius, rectus femoris, tensor fascia lata	One main blood supply for flap
II	One dominant, minor supplemental	Biceps femoris, gracilis, platysma, peroneus longus/brevis, soleus, temporalis, trapezius, vastus lateralis	One main blood supply for flap
III	Two dominant	Semimembranosus, rectus abdominis, gluteus maximus	Two, often equivalent, blood supplies for flap
IV	Multiple segmental	Tibialis anterior, sartorius	One main blood supply, necessary to maintain pedicle for each transferred segment
V	One dominant, multiple segmental	Pectoralis major, latissimus dorsi	May be based on dominant or multiple segmental sources

Myocutaneous Flap Classification

Myocutaneous flaps are most easily considered in a similar fashion to the underlying muscle that serves as the bridge of vascularity to the overlying skin and subcutaneous tissue. For myocutaneous flaps, the reliability of the main pedicle is quite important as is the likelihood of musculocutaneous perforators arising from this pedicle. As Mathes and Nahai also describe in their landmark paper, skin islands most distal from the vascular source are least likely to be reliable, and certain patterns (types II and IV, particularly) are known to have the least reliable skin paddles, most particularly distally.[9]

Fasciocutaneous Flap and Perforator Flap Classifications

Thorough understanding of muscle flaps and their vascular anatomy stands as an essential base for understanding fasciocutaneous flaps. Over time, the evolution of perforator flaps from basic fasciocutaneous flaps has decreased sacrifice of muscle. The ability to transfer substantial pieces of skin and subcutaneous tissue on single submillimeter diameter vessels perforating into flap substances from underlying source vessels has allowed a nearly uncategorizable plethora of flaps to become useful and popular in modern reconstruction.

Perforator flaps provide greater variety and reliability of skin paddle design because individual perforators are now routinely able to be identified and dissected as they enter fasciocutaneous islands. This versatile flap uses tissue from adjacent areas for good color and structural match to the recipient site. These techniques have made classifications of fasciocutaneous flaps less essential and prone to overgeneralization, but an understanding of the core anatomical variations as initially described can be helpful in designing modern flaps. Historically, Cormack and Lamberty described four categories, as shown in **Table 7.2.**[10]

As discussed in this section, the concept of fasciocutaneous flaps has progressed well beyond this more basic classification schema.

TABLE 7.2. CORMACK AND LAMBERTY HISTORICAL FASCIOCUTANEOUS FLAP CLASSIFICATION[10]

Type	Vascular Anatomy	Examples
A	Multiple, codominant fasciocutaneous perforators	Sartorius, upper arm
B	Single, dominant fasciocutaneous perforator	Supraclavicular
C	Single or multiple septocutaneous perforators	Radial forearm flap
D	Inclusion of other structures like bone and muscle along the source vessel	Radial forearm with radius

Much debate has occurred in the effort to better classify modern flap usages.[11-15] Building upon the perforator concept, chimeric flaps can be designed to incorporate various flaps and flap substances (bone, muscle, fascia, skin/subcutaneous fat) based on different perforators coalescing to a single source vessel.

LOCAL TISSUE REARRANGEMENT

Understanding of perforator flap anatomy expands the standard random pattern local tissue rearrangement techniques (e.g., bilobed flaps, rhomboids) for wound closure. More recently defined propeller flaps and keystone flaps utilize perforator anatomy for local tissue rearrangement. Greater flexibility of flap design allows for accommodation of local tissue laxity and availability.

Insider tip:

- *Design the skin paddle over perforator* hot spots *to incorporate dominant or multiple perforators.*[1]

Propeller Flap

Described by Hyakusoku et al. in 1991, the propeller flap is an island flap that reaches the recipient site through an axial rotation.[1,16,17] The propeller flap technique creates a wide exploratory incision near expected perforator vessel sites, followed by selection of the dominant perforator (supra- or subfascially) at the optimal pivot point. Perforator location closest to the defect is preferred for wider angle of rotation to minimize tension on the pedicle. Dissection toward and along the source vessel is performed until adequate length is obtained for a lazy S-turn without kinking. The flap perfusion should be confirmed prior to inset with handheld Doppler evaluation. The remainder of the flap skin island can be incised after perforator dissection to optimize flap rotation.[1,18]

Insider tips:

- *Skeletonizing the pedicle toward the flap can increase pedicle length.*[1]
- *Design the skin paddle larger than the defect for tension-free closure, even with postoperative edema.*[1]

Keystone Flap

The keystone flap, described in 2003 by Behan,[19] is designed as two opposing V-Y flaps oriented parallel to the longitudinal axis of the defect, elevated as a single multiperforator fasciocutaneous advancement flap. Several variations have been described. Centering the flap over the perforators expands the undermining, and circumferential incision of the deep fascia at the flap margin can increase mobility. Larger flaps may increase donor site morbidity but may be necessary to accommodate difficult local tissue environments (e.g., inflammation, previous irradiation/undermining).[1]

FREE-STYLE FLAPS AND SUPERMICROSURGERY

By applying basic perforator flap techniques, transfer of fasciocutaneous, fascia only, or cutaneous only components may be accomplished in nearly any part of the body. Technical mastery of the following critical steps will open the entire anatomy to consideration for tissue transfer as a flap with over 350 known potential perforators for use.[1,11]

The technique begins with prediction of existence of perforating blood vessels into the superficial soft tissue of choice. Certain locations have fairly predictable perforating blood supply (e.g., periumbilical perforators from the deep inferior epigastric vessel, through the rectus abdominis muscle, and into a vertical or transversely designed lower abdominal skin island). In these areas, and in areas with less interpatient reliability of the presence of these perforators, imaging techniques can optimize preoperative predictability of skin island design. These include handheld Doppler, color duplex scanning, magnetic resonance angiography, multidetector-row helical computed tomography, and laser angiography.[2]

Dissection through the soft tissue of the flap is usually followed by elevation of the underlying soft tissue known to contain the source vessel. After identification of the perforator or perforators, selective inclusion of one or several is decided, and these are followed proximally to larger and larger caliber vessels, considered the source. Depending on the unique characteristics of the recipient site needs, the proximal dissection can proceed until sufficient pedicle length and size for anastomosis is obtained.[2]

Supermicrosurgery is becoming more popular as the aforementioned techniques are considered for shorter pedicles and smaller-diameter anastomoses with increased magnification and refinement of microsurgical instruments and skills. Anastomoses of vessels well under 1 mm in diameter permit preservation of deep fascia and minimize risk to underlying soft tissues such as muscles that require dissections through their substance to trace to the larger source vessel.[2,20]

Donor site size, texture, color, thickness, and pliability can all be optimized with freedom to design flaps over virtually any part of the body. It is expected that in the future, these techniques may be considered routine; however, it is still worth noting that at this point, these are considered technically demanding and best attempted after mastery of more basic perforator flap techniques.[2]

Insider tips:

- *Assessment of perforator adequacy can be determined by preoperative imaging, intraoperative imaging and Doppler assessment, visual inspection for size and pulsation, and differential temporary vessel clamping with assessment of end-organ (flap) viability.*
- *Incorporating potential* lifeboats *such as possible backup perforating vessels, backup skin paddle designs, and backup flaps and* burning bridges *to these options as late as possible in the dissection may allow salvage in the event of an unforeseen and undesirable intraoperative circumstance.*[2]

CLINICAL EXAMPLES

Lateral Arm Flap

This flap is most commonly used when thin, pliable tissue is needed and may be harvested as a chimeric flap with bone. Most of the time, primary closure of the donor site is possible (particularly with skin paddles less than 5-7 cm in width). Some surgeons consider it a workhorse, whereas others express concerns about inconsistent perforator anatomy, short pedicle length, small vessel caliber, and challenging dissection.[21]

Surgical Technique

With the arm across the torso, the deltoid insertion and lateral epicondyle may be palpated and connected by a line along which septal perforators from the radial collateral artery between the biceps brachii and triceps can be found with handheld Doppler probe. After marking a skin paddle centered over these, the posterior incision is usually made first, followed by subfascial dissection and identification of the perforators that may then be followed proximally. The skin island dissection can then be completed.[21]

Insider tips:

- *Identify and protect the radial nerve during dissection.*[21]
- *The deltoid insertion may also be divided to increase pedicle length as the radial collateral artery courses toward the brachial artery.*[21]
- *The posterior antebrachial cutaneous nerve must be divided but can be used to create a sensate flap.*[21]

Radial Forearm Flap

This fasciocutaneous flap provides thin, pliable tissue in most types of bodies. It has been used for many reconstructive needs (e.g., intraoral, penile/urethral, extremity). Its popularity arises from the ease of dissection; robust, reliable vascularity; malleability; and ability to support associated tissues such as bone, tendon, and nerve.[22] The donor site is difficult to hide and may be associated with stigma in certain populations as it often needs a skin graft (meshed or sheet, with or without dermal support) for closure. This flap can be used as a sensate flap, in a reversed fashion, as a flow-through flap, as an adipofascial flap, or with a short segment of partial thickness radius. When harvested with the palmaris longus tendon, the flap can also be used for functional purposes. Some of the versatility arises from the multiple venous drainage options, including the superficial system based on the larger cephalic vein and/or the deep system based on the paired venae comitantes of the radial artery, which are considered to more reliably drain the radial forearm tissue.[22-24]

Surgical Technique

The skin paddle is outlined on the volar, distal, radial forearm. Incision through the skin, adipose tissue, and fascia may be performed, elevating these toward the radial artery that runs between the brachioradialis and flexor carpi radialis in the distal forearm, sending multiple septocutaneous perforators to the overlying soft tissue.[25] Lateral antebrachial cutaneous nerve, palmaris longus tendon, and superficial veins may be incorporated in the harvest and followed along their courses prior to transection. The radial nerve should be protected as should the vascularity of the tendon sheaths so that a skin graft may be applied.[25]

Insider tips:

- *Check the Allen test prior to flap harvest to confirm a* complete arch *communication between the ulnar and radial artery to protect distal perfusion.*
- *A tourniquet is useful, but keep in mind tourniquet times.*
- *Nearby upper extremity flaps to know: Medial arm (introduced by Tagliacozzi in the 1600s),*[26] *ulnar artery (less hairy, better postoperative donor site appearance than radial), digital flaps*

Rectus Abdominis, Deep Inferior Epigastric, and Superficial Inferior Epigastric Flaps

The abdomen, specifically the rectus abdominis muscle and the skin supplied by its musculocutaneous perforators, is a common donor site. Because of its type II, dual blood supply, a superiorly based rectus flap can be pedicled for upper trunk reconstruction. The more reliable blood supply is the deep inferior epigastric system entering the inferior aspect of the muscle. This reliably supplies perforators, most commonly to the periumbilical area, which can be pedicled or free transfer of muscle, muscle and skin island, or skin and subcutaneous tissue alone. The skin is usually oriented either vertically as a VRAM (vertical rectus abdominis myocutaneous) flap or transversely as a TRAM (transverse rectus abdominis myocutaneous) flap. These orientations are also appropriate when used as a perforator flap without muscle or fascial sacrifice.[27]

Sensation can be restored with harvest of branches of thoracolumbar spinal nerves.[28] Skin and adipose tissue of a large surface area can also be based on the superficial inferior epigastric system, although reliability of adequate blood vessels in this area is less assured. Flaps are usually harvested as a unilateral single unit based on blood supply from one rectus muscle or as two flaps, each based on its ipsilateral blood supply. These flaps are popular for breast and perineal reconstruction, among other uses.[27]

Surgical Technique

Incision of one side of the planned flap is usually accomplished through the subcutaneous fat, and the tissue is elevated superficial to the anterior rectus fascia (if starting in midline) or fascia of the external oblique (if starting laterally). Perforators are identified and followed through the fascia and rectus muscle toward the inferior epigastric vessels' origins in the groin. When a muscle flap is used, the borders of the rectus muscle are identified rather than perforators, and the anterior fascia is resected with the muscle. Care should be given to identification and ligation of the opposite epigastric system (superior epigastric if deep inferior epigastric vessels are harvested as the pedicle).[27]

With perforator flaps, the anterior rectus fascia can often be closed primarily. Some authors choose to reinforce this with prosthetic mesh or biologic matrix. Harvest of a portion of the rectus fascia and/or muscle may require more formal abdominal wall reconstruction using the many available techniques discussed elsewhere in this text. These are important considerations, as abdominal weakness, bulge, and hernia are the most specific complications associated with this flap.[28]

Insider tips:

- *Islandization of the umbilical stalk provides a more aesthetic donor site, but patients should understand that harvest of a vertical unilateral skin island may distort the midline.*
- *Preservation of portions of the multiple superficial and deep blood supplies to this tissue (e.g., contralateral deep system, ipsi or contralateral superficial system) can salvage clinically marginal tissue noted during flap harvest through additional venous drainage or supercharging.*
- *Nearby trunk flaps to know: Superficial circumflex iliac artery , groin, Rubens flaps (deep circumflex iliac artery flaps)*[29]

Latissimus Dorsi and Thoracodorsal Artery Perforator Flaps

The latissimus muscle flap may be harvested based on multiple medial posterior thoracic intercostal or lumbar perforators or on the laterally based thoracodorsal pedicle. This arises as a terminal branch of the subscapular artery off the axillary artery (or occasionally directly from the axillary artery).[30] The latissimus is a broad, fan-shaped muscle (originating from the posterior iliac crest and lower six vertebrae and inserting into the humerus to form the posterior axillary fold)[30] that can be useful for many defects extending as a pedicled flap to the head and neck and anterior trunk and as free tissue transfer anywhere on the body.[31,32] Its versatility arises from the ease of harvest, large surface area, and long vascular pedicle.[30] Skin islands may be designed in multiple orientations to address reconstructive needs or to minimize donor site morbidity. Using perforator techniques similar to that described earlier for deep inferior epigastric artery perforator flaps, a thoracodorsal artery perforator flap (TDAP) may be harvested with dissection from the desired skin island, along the preferred perforator and more proximally along the thoracodorsal source vessel.[30] The TDAP can still provide a long vascular pedicle and large surface area but decreases potential morbidity and unnecessary bulk.[33] Additionally, the muscle or perforator flap can be harvested with more than one soft tissue island, splitting the tissue based on the transverse and vertical branches of the thoracodorsal, or including bone based on the angular branch to the tip of the scapula.

Surgical Technique

Positioning is often via lateral decubitus for unilateral harvest and prone for bilateral harvest, but some authors advocate supine harvest for a TDAP.[30] Technique depends on skin island design and perforator- or muscle-harvesting technique. Key points include identification of the vascular pedicle when using the muscle and dissection of this as proximal as possible for greater pedicle length, useful either for pedicled or free indications. Closure of the donor site with careful use of percutaneous drains, quilting sutures, or other techniques to minimize seroma is necessary as this donor site has risk for seroma formation. Shoulder function may be impaired, but many authors support preservation of ability to engage in activities of daily living.[30]

Insider tips:

- *Consider previous treatment that might interrupt the thoracodorsal pedicle such as axillary dissection. In this situation, this flap can still be used by relying on blood flow through the serratus branch.*
- *When used in breast reconstruction, it often requires volume supplementation with an implant.*
- *Consider denervating the muscle flap by transecting the thoracodorsal nerve.*
- *Nearby posterior trunk flaps to know: Paraspinous muscle, trapezius, scapular/parascapular flaps*

Gluteal and Superior Gluteal Artery Perforator Flaps

Early descriptions of the gluteal myocutaneous flap occurred in the 1970s, and the perforator flap based on the superior gluteal artery became widely recognized two decades later.[34,35] The superior gluteal artery perforator flap harvest is considered technically difficult by many. Lateral decubitus or supine positioning is recommended. The buttock tissue yields firmer, more septated, and less malleable flaps than most other areas. Donor scars can be positioned horizontally or obliquely with a lateral translocation in some patients who demonstrate appropriate perforator anatomy for a better lift of the inferior buttock and hip.[36] Concern exists regarding donor site scarring, contour, and possible impact on ambulation, but those who perform many of these flaps report high success.[36-39]

Surgical Technique

Markings and skin island design may be approached variably. One method uses Doppler identification of perforators one-third to two-thirds of the distance between the posterior superior iliac spine and greater trochanter with skin island design centered on a line from coccyx to anterior superior iliac spine (ASIS). Dissection can be beveled away from the flap, particularly deep to superficial fascia to capture more tissue. The gluteus maximus fascia is incised and either the muscle flap is harvested or the fascia is elevated off the gluteal muscle (with cautery action parallel to direction of muscle fascicles) to identify the perforator. Deep to the gluteal muscle, a venous plexus requires exacting dissection.[36]

Insider tips:

- *Careful hemostasis is required deep to the gluteal muscle within the vascular plexus to avoid damage to surrounding structures or pedicle.*
- *Be prepared for a shorter pedicle or smaller vessel size than with some other flaps.*
- *Nearby gluteal flaps to know: Inferior gluteal artery perforator, lumbar artery perforator flap*

Upper Thigh Flaps: Gracilis, Transverse/Diagonal Upper Gracilis, Profunda Artery Perforator

The gracilis is a versatile muscle that can be used alone (e.g., to fill perineal defects), with branch of obturator nerve (e.g., facial reanimation), or with overlying skin (e.g., breast reconstruction). Soft tissue can be limited, and the flaps necessitate careful management near the femoral triangle to avoid donor site morbidity, damage to nearby structures, or lymphatic disruption.[27] One must consider potentially poor donor site scar appearance/position and sensory disturbance,[40] which may be mitigated with careful technique.

Surgical Technique

Frog leg positioning is usually adequate. The gracilis is expected to run 2 to 3 cm posterior to the palpable adductor longus in this position. If required, the cutaneous island is designed transversely from adductor tendon posteriorly to the buttock crease with the superior incision in the groin/buttock crease (transverse upper gracilis flap). This can also be designed diagonally (diagonal upper gracilis flap). Slight posterior translocation and use of a perforating branch of the profunda femoris vessels (usually through adductor magnus) without use of the gracilis can also be performed (PAP). Width is determined by pinch test. The skin island may be elevated traveling posteriorly in the subfascial plane to identify the intermuscular septum between adductor longus and gracilis and its perforators. These vessels may be followed from the gracilis (usually entering 10 cm distal to the ischium) toward the source medial femoral circumflex vessels off the profunda femoris vessels, sacrificing the branches to the other thigh musculature. The gracilis muscle can be isolated, its distal, minor pedicle divided, and the flap harvested. If muscle only is used, a vertical incision may be used to identify the muscle posterior to the adductor tendon. The scar can be short, with harvest performed through a tunnel with a counterincision near the tendon at the knee.[40]

Insider tips:

- *Avoid damaging the greater saphenous vein.*[27]
- *Resuspend fascia to avoid labial distortion.*[27]
- *If performing a PAP flap, superficial dissection posteriorly may help decrease damage to the posterior femoral cutaneous nerve to the thigh.*

Anterolateral Thigh Perforator Flap

The thigh is a versatile donor site for many types of reconstruction. Muscle, myocutaneous, adipofascial, fascial, and fasciocutaneous flaps can all be harvested. Functional limitations can be concerning if they occur, as lower extremity function is important. Techniques should be considered to minimize this. A common flap with many indications and usually minimal impact on donor site function is the anterolateral thigh (ALT) flap.

Surgical Technique

With the patient supine, a line can be drawn from the ASIS to the superolateral border of the patella (overlying the septum between vastus lateralis and rectus femoris). Another line from the midpoint of this line to the midpoint of the distance from ASIS to pubic symphysis will approximate the source vessels' course (descending branch of lateral circumflex femoral). The perforators are expected at the midpoint of the vertical line (or between 1/3 and 2/3 of the distance along the line), usually within a 3-cm radius, and spaced superiorly and inferiorly apart by about 5 cm.[41] The skin island can be designed two-thirds posterior to the vertical line. Dissection from the anterior flap margin can proceed, initially supra- or subfascially and then subfascially as the junction between the muscles is approached. The septum can be divided distally and the muscles retracted away from each other. The descending branch and perforators are identified; perforators are selected and dissected through the vastus lateralis and followed proximally. The remainder of the skin island can then be harvested.[41] Skin pinch can be used to determine skin island, but often recipient needs exceed this, necessitating skin graft donor site closure.

Insider tips:

- *In the absence of perforators, the same initial incision can become the posterior border of a newly designed skin island based on perforators through rectus femoris.*[41]
- *Preserve motor branches of the femoral nerve, but the posterior femoral cutaneous nerve of the thigh can be harvested to provide a sensate flap.*[41]
- *A proximal perforator is usually larger, adequate in length, and less intramuscular.*[41]
- *Nearby lower extremity flaps to know: Sartorius, rectus femoris, vastus lateralis, tensor fascia lata, anteromedial thigh, posterior thigh, gastrocnemius, soleus, fibula flaps*

Pectoralis Flap

The pectoralis muscle and/or myocutaneous flap was first described in 1968 by Hueston and McConchie for sternal reconstruction.[42] Ariyan described its uses in head and neck reconstruction in 1979.[43] Although it has remained as the top choice for anterior sternal reconstruction since its description (sternal wound dehiscence following cardiac surgery), it experienced increased popularity prior to the advent of routine microvascular head and neck reconstruction; however, its values remain in head and neck indications as a fast, versatile, and reliable salvage option.[16]

The pectoralis muscle is divided into a clavicular portion (originating from clavicle, inserting into humerus) and the sternocostal portion (originating from sternum and costal cartilages 1-6, inserting into external oblique aponeurosis). Its blood supply is a Mathes and Nahai type V through the thoracoacromial artery and perforators of the internal thoracic, intercostal, and lateral thoracic arteries.[9,44]

Surgical Technique

Sternal defects can be covered with unilateral or bilateral advancement based on the thoracoacromial vessel with routine dissection of the superior, medial, inferior, and lateral borders. This is often necessary when the intercostal vessels have been used for cardiac bypass grafts or through extensive sternal debridement. Additional medial translocation can be accomplished through disinsertion from the humerus, which can usually be accomplished from the midline sternal wound but may require a counterincision over the humeral head. Often the reconstruction will be performed with dissection of the muscle from the anterior skin and subcutaneous fat and closure of the muscle flap layer within the midline bony defect and disparate closure of the skin and subcutaneous fat. However, this anterior dissection can be spared, allowing for advancement of the muscle, subcutaneous fat, and skin as a single unit toward midline. Alternatively, a turnover flap based on multiple medial intercostal perforators may be used to introduce bulky muscle into the anterior sternal wounds. This requires anterior and posterior undermining, as well as superior, inferior, and complete lateral release of the muscle borders.[16]

Insider tip:

- *Position the arms by the side to facilitate muscle advancement.*

For head and neck reconstruction the muscle is usually rotated based on the thoracoacromial pedicle (should be visualized and protected on the superior/posterior surface of the muscle) and may include a skin paddle of a variety (over 10 different described approaches) of different designs based medially or inferiorly, particularly along the inframammary fold.[16] The flap is inset most often using a subcutaneous tunnel.

Special manipulations can be accommodated. These include double skin paddles, extension based on inclusion of the rectus fascia and overlying skin, fascial release, clavicular manipulation, or division of the sternal portion of the flap. This can also be harvested in concert with a deltopectoral flap.[16]

Insider tips:

- *Include a portion of the fifth rib or avascular bone graft for mandibular reconstruction.*
- *Denervation of the muscle can decrease bulk over time.*[16]
- *Prepare for distortion of the breast and difficulty with hair growth if used for esophageal or pharyngeal reconstruction.*[16]
- *Nearby flaps to know: Serratus, deltopectoral flaps*

CONCLUSION

Flaps are essential reconstructive modalities frequently used by plastic surgeons. As techniques evolve, infinite varieties of tissue transfer emerge. Thorough understanding of basic principles, ability to apply these in unique situations, and careful assessments of all aspects of patients and their reconstructive needs are necessary for successful use of this tool.

REFERENCES

1. Mohan AT, Sur YJ, Zhu L, et al. The concepts of propeller, perforator, keystone, and other local flaps and their role in the evolution of reconstruction. *Plast Reconstr Surg*. 2016;138(4):710e-729e.
   Classic article describing this area.
2. Wallace CG, Kao HK, Jeng SF, Wei FC. Free-style flaps: a further step forward for perforator flap surgery. *Plast Reconstr Surg*. 2009;124(6):e419-426.
   Classic article describing this area.
3. Esser J. General rules used in simple plastic work on Austrian war-wounded soldiers. *Surg Gynecol Obstet*. 1917;34:737.
4. McGregor IA, Morgan G. Axial and random pattern flaps. *Br J Plast Surg*. 1973;26:202-213.
5. Taylor GI, Palmer JH. The vascular territories (angiosomes) of the body: experimental study and clinical applications. *Br J Plast Surg*. 1987;40:113-141.
6. Taylor GI, Daniel RK. The free flap: composite tissue transfer by vascular anastomosis. *Aust N Z J Surg*. 1973;43:1-3.
7. Daniel RK, Taylor GI. Distant transfer of an island flap by microvascular anastomoses: a clinical technique. *Plast Reconstr Surg*. 1973;52:111-117.
8. Koshima I, Soeda S. Inferior epigastric artery skin flaps without rectus abdominis muscle. *Br J Plast Surg*. 1989;42:645-648.
9. Mathes SJ, Nahai F. Classification of the vascular anatomy of muscles: experimental and clinical correlation. *Plast Reconstr Surg*. 1981;67(2):177-187.
   Classic article describing this area.
10. Cormack GC, Lamberty BG. A classification of fascio-cutaneous flaps according to their patterns of vascularization. *Br J Plast Surg*. 1984;37(1):80-87.
11. Wei FC, Mardini S. Free-style free flaps. *Plast Reconstr Surg*. 2004;114:910-916.
12. Hallock GG. Direct and indirect perforator flaps: the history and the controversy. *Plast Reconstr Surg*. 2003;111:855-865.
13. Kim JT. New nomenclature concept of perforator flap. *Br J Plast Surg*. 2005;58:431-440.
14. Blondeel PN, Van Landuyt KH, Monstrey SJ, et al. The "Gent" consensus on perforator flap terminology: preliminary definitions. *Plast Reconstr Surg*. 2003;112:1378-1383.
15. Wei FC, Jain V, Suominen S, Chen HC. Confusion among perforator flaps: what is a true perforator flap? *Plast Reconstr Surg*. 2001;107:874-876.
16. Teo KG, Rozen WM, Acosta R. The pectoralis major myocutaneous flap. *J Reconstr Microsurg*. 2013;29(7):449-456.
17. Hyakusoku H, Yamamoto T, Fumiiri M. The propeller flap method. *Br J Plast Surg*. 1991;44:53-54.
18. Pignatti M, Ogawa R, Hallock GG, et al. The "Tokyo" consensus on propeller flaps. *Plast Reconstr Surg*. 2011;127:716-722.
19. Behan FC. The keystone design perforator island flap in reconstructive surgery. *ANZ J Surg*. 2003;73:112-120.
20. Koshima I, Inagawa K, Urushibara K, Moriguchi T. Paraumbilical perforator flap without deep inferior epigastric vessels. *Plast Reconstr Surg*. 1998;102:1052-1057.
21. Chang EI, Ibrahim A, Papazian N, et al. Perforator mapping and optimizing design of the lateral arm flap: anatomy revisited and clinical experience. *Plast Reconstr Surg*. 2016;138(2):300e-306e.
   Classic article to describe this area.
22. Patel SA, Pang JH, Natoli N, et al. Reliability of venous couplers of microanastamosis of the venae comitantes in free radial forearm flaps for head and neck reconstruction. *J Reconstr Microsurg*. 2013;29(7):433-435.
23. Futran ND, Stack BC. Single versus dual venous drainage of the radial forearm free flap. *Am J Otolaryngol*. 1996;17(2):112-117.
24. Cha YH, Nam W, Cha IH, Kim HJ. Revisiting radial forearm free flap for successful venous drainage. *Maxillofac Plast Reconstr Surg*. 2017;39(1):14.
25. Ho AM, Chang J. Radial artery perforator flap. *J Hand Surg*. 2010;35:308-311.
26. Xue B, Liu Y, Zhu S, et al. Total cheek reconstruction using the pre-expanded medial arm flap with functional and aesthetic donor site closure. *J Craniofac Surg*. 2018;29(3):640-644.
27. Patel NG, Ramakrishnan V. Microsurgical tissue transfer in breast reconstruction. *Clin Plast Surg*. 2017;44:345-359.
   Classic article describing this area.
28. Rozen WM, Ashton MW, Kiil BJ, et al Avoiding denervation of rectus abdominis in DIEP flap harvest II: an intraoperative assessment of the nerves to rectus. *Plast Reconstr Surg*. 2008;122(5):1321-1325.
29. Elliott LF, Hartrampf CR. The Rubens flap: the deep circumflex iliac artery flap. *Clin Plast Surg*. 1998;25(2):283-291.
30. O'Connell JE, Bajwaa MS, Schachea AG, Shaw RJ. Head and neck reconstruction with free flaps based on the thoracodorsal system. *Oral Oncol*. 2017;75:46-53.
31. Quillen CG, Shearin JC, Georgiade NG. Use of the latissimus dorsi myocutaneous island flap for reconstruction in the head and neck area. *Plast Reconstr Surg*. 1978;62:113-117.
32. Maxwell GP, Stueber K, Hoopes JE. A free latissimus dorsi myocutaneous flap. *Plast Reconstr Surg*. 1978;62:462-466.
33. Yang LC, Wang XC, Bentz ML, et al. Clinical application of the thoracodorsal artery perforator flaps. *J Plast Reconstr Aesthet Surg*. 2013;66(2):193-200.
   Classic article describing this area.
34. Fujino T, Harasina T, Aoyagi F. Reconstruction for aplasia of the breast and pectoral region by microvascular transfer of a free flap from the buttock. *Plast Reconstr Surg*. 1975;56:178-181.
35. Allen RJ, Tucker C. Superior gluteal artery perforator free flap for breast reconstruction. *Plast Reconstr Surg*. 1995;95:1207-1212.
   Classic article describing this area.
36. Hunter C, Moody L, Luan A, et al. Superior gluteal artery perforator flap: the beauty of the buttock. *Ann Plast Surg*. 2016;76(3):S191-S195.
   Classic article describing this area.
37. Yaghoubian A, Boyd JB. The SGAP flap in breast reconstruction: backup or first choice? *Plast Reconstr Surg*. 2011;128:29e-31e.
38. DellaCroce FJ, Sullivan SK. Application and refinement of the superior gluteal artery perforator free flap for bilateral simultaneous breast reconstruction. *Plast Reconstr Surg*. 2005;116:97-103.
39. Hur K, Ohkuma R, Bellamy JL, et al. Patient-reported assessment of functional gait outcomes following superior gluteal artery perforator reconstruction. *Plast Reconstr Surg Glob Open*. 2013:1(5):1-6.
40. Locke MB, Zhonga T, Mureauc MAM, Hofer SOP. Tug 'O' war: challenges of transverse upper gracilis (TUG) myocutaneous free flap breast reconstruction. *J Plast Reconstr Aesth Surg*. 2012;65:1041e-1050e.
   Classic article describing this area.
41. Saint-Cyr M, Oni G, Lee M, et al. Simple approach to harvest of the anterolateral thigh flap. *Plast Reconstr Surg*. 2012;129(1):207-211.
   Classic article describing this area.
42. Hueston JT, McConchie IH. A compound pectoral flap. *Aust NZ J Surg*. 1968;38(1):61-63.
43. Ariyan S. The pectoralis major myocutaneous flap: a versatile flap for reconstruction in the head and neck. *Plast Reconstr Surg*. 1979;63(1):73-81.
44. Wei WI, Lam KH, Wong J. The true pectoralis major mycocutaneous island flap: an anatomical study. *Br J Plast Surg*. 1984;37(4):568-573.

QUESTIONS

1. The vascular surgery team requests an inpatient consult on a debilitated 74-year-old woman with a recent history of uncontrolled diabetes who was incidentally noted to have a cold foot upon admission for mental status changes associated with diabetic ketoacidosis. Past medical history includes hypertension, hypercholesterolemia, and myocardial infarction treated with three stents 9 months ago. The vascular surgery team completed an urgent femoral popliteal bypass graft with PTFE graft 9 days ago, but the patient's wound has separated and dressing changes are currently being performed with exposed vessels and PTFE with minimal redundancy of soft tissue at the margins. What is the optimal next step in management?

a. Continue dressing changes, optimize nutrition and glucose control, and allow wound to heal secondarily.
b. Perform operative debridement and place split thickness skin graft to wound base.
c. Perform operative debridement and perform primary closure with extensive undermining to decrease tension.
d. Perform operative debridement and perform gracilis muscle rotational flap with split thickness skin graft.
e. Perform operative debridement and perform latissimus dorsi myocutaneous free tissue transfer.

2. The orthopedic surgery team requests an inpatient consult for a 24-year-old otherwise healthy man, 6 days after Gustilo IIIB distal third of the tibia and fibula fractures treated with hardware at the fracture site. He returned to the operating room for a *second look* washout procedure 3 days after injury, and the wound was found to be stable and clean. Free tissue transfer is deemed necessary, but the patient is extremely concerned about visible scars outside of the ankle from flap reconstruction when he is at the pool. Which of the following flaps represents the best option in this circumstance?

a. ALT free flap
b. Latissimus dorsi free flap
c. Vertical rectus abdominis myocutaneous free flap
d. Radial forearm free flap
e. Lateral arm free flap

3. A 50-year-old woman is undergoing autologous tissue breast reconstruction at the time of bilateral skin-sparing mastectomy for breast cancer. As abdominal skin and subcutaneous flaps are being raised in the abdomen in preparation for a deep inferior epigastric perforator flap, the internal mammary vein is noted to be extremely small on the left despite proximal dissection. Which of the following is least likely to allow salvage of abdominal-based reconstruction?

a. Use of thoracodorsal vessels as recipients rather than the internal mammary vessels
b. Use of a rotational transverse rectus abdominis myocutaneous flap based on the superior epigastric vessels
c. Use of the right distal internal mammary vein in a retrograde fashion as a recipient vein
d. End-to-side anastomosis of the flap vein end into the internal mammary vein
e. Surgical delay of the internal mammary vessels

4. A 65-year-old man with an anterior chest wall defect due to liposarcoma resection undergoes latissimus dorsi rotational flap reconstruction. Postoperatively, he reports unsightly and uncomfortable motion of his flap when moving the ipsilateral arm. This result is most likely due to which of the following?

a. Absence of postoperative complete shoulder immobilization
b. Failure to divide the thoracodorsal nerve during flap dissection
c. Inadequate security of inset into recipient site
d. Maintenance of insertion into the humerus
e. Fracture of underlying ribs during sarcoma resection

5. A trainee is working on preoperative planning and is marking landmarks and planned incisions for a gracilis muscle flap harvest for use in facial reanimation. The patient is placed in a frog leg position and the most prominent longitudinal medial thigh structure palpable through the skin is which of the following?

a. Gracilis muscle
b. Rectus femoris muscle
c. Adductor longus muscle
d. Sartorius muscle
e. Tensor fascia lata muscle

1. **Answer: d.** The clinical scenario represents a common situation in which suboptimal patient factors (i.e., increased age, uncontrolled diabetes, cardiac disease) exist in the setting of exposure of critical structures (in this case, prosthetic material and large vessels). Careful consideration of all aspects and weighing of the risks and benefits improves treatment planning for each unique situation. A gracilis muscle flap would provide bulk to fill dead space, cushioning against external trauma, and increased quantity of healthy tissue to combat bacterial contamination or infection in the groin. Risk of prosthetic infection, anastomotic failure, and difficult-to-control, potentially life-threatening bleeding from femoral vessels would argue against ongoing dressing changes or skin grafting directly over exposed structures although optimization of patient factors is always ideal. Although some patients with risk factors for wound healing complications have redundancy for primary closure, this patient's ***minimal redundancy*** makes this choice less favorable. A debilitated patient with active, significant medical comorbidities would not be as good a candidate for a free tissue transfer procedure with likely increased operative length and complexity when a less complex, good option exists.

2. **Answer: a.** Any flap donor site will result in a scar. Some donor sites are able to be closed primarily and are likely less visible than those that require, for example, skin grafting. In this male patient concerned about pool activities, the ALT donor site can be closed primarily if the size of the skin island is not large and is most likely to be covered by clothes compared to the other options, i.e., latissimus dorsi, VRAM, radial forearm, and lateral arm flaps.

3. **Answer: e.** Understanding of flap harvest is insufficient for successful use of flaps in surgical treatment of patients. One must also understand recipient site dynamics and the interactions between the flap and the recipient site. A surgical delay is not likely a useful technique for internal mammary vein size augmentation as there is not an alternate blood flow to ligate for increased flow through the internal mammary vessels. Internal mammary vessels as well as thoracodorsal vessels are recipient vessels of appropriate reliability and proximity for anastomosis to the usually long deep inferior epigastric vessel pedicle. Vein grafting could also be used if length is insufficient. The nature of the blood supply to the rectus muscle uses the superior blood supply in a rotational fashion for breast reconstruction. Use of retrograde flow in vessels is an established and often successful technique of flap manipulation. End-to-side anastomoses manage size mismatch between donor and recipient vessels.

4. Answer: b. The thoracodorsal nerve supplies motor innervation to the latissimus dorsi muscle and may be divided during pedicle dissection to decrease muscle activity. Complete shoulder immobilization is not a standard practice after latissimus dorsi flap use. Inadequate inset may move the flap out of the ideal position in the recipient site over time but is less likely to impact muscle activity itself. Division of the muscle tendon to the humerus may be performed, but this is also less likely to affect motor activity of the muscle itself. Soft tissue tumor resection is not likely to cause unrecognized fracture of underlying osseous structures.

5. Answer: c. It is important to understand the relationship of the gracilis muscle and adductor longus muscle as the more prominent structure is the adductor longus; however, the gracilis is more commonly used for reconstruction as its function is less essential to the lower extremity. The sartorius, while existing in the medial thigh for a portion of its course, does not run longitudinally through the thigh's length and is not a contributor to the main palpable structure. The rectus femoris and tensor fascia lata muscles do not travel longitudinally along the medial thigh.

CHAPTER 8 Transplantation Biology and Applications to Plastic Surgery

Gerald Brandacher and W. P. Andrew Lee

KEY POINTS

- Advances in transplant immunology and microsurgical techniques enabled reconstructive transplantation to evolve from an experimental idea to a clinical reality over the past 2 decades
- For select patients, transplantation of vascularized composite allografts (VCA) provides a means to replace *like with like* tissue and thus represents the best restorative modality currently available
- Both functional and immunological outcomes after upper extremity and face transplantation have exceeded initial expectations
- Minimization of immunosuppression (single drug) and use of alternative regimens have been successfully realized in favoring the risk-benefit equation
- Innovative immunomodulatory and cell-based tolerance protocols have been proven feasible in translational large animal VCA models and are about to enter the clinical arena
- Indications for reconstructive transplantation are rapidly expanding including pediatric patients, transplantation of functional subunits, and urogenital reconstructive transplants

The idea of transplanting tissues, organs, or even whole-body parts seems to have always been a dream and one of the wild fantasies of mankind that eventually has developed into one of the greatest success stories in Medicine of the last century. In particular, in the field of plastic and reconstructive surgery, transplantation of tissue from one location of the body to another to restore tissue defects is a fundamental concept. Thus, it is not surprising that the first successful application of this technique to transplant tissue from one person to another in the form of allogeneic kidney transplant was first performed by a plastic surgeon. Dr. Joseph E. Murray on December 23, 1954, at the Brigham and Women's Hospital in Boston helped usher in the dawn of a new field of organ transplantation.[1] The constant and new developments in surgical techniques and more potent, sophisticated types of immunosuppressive agents have enabled us to perform more and more complex types of transplants over the past 60 years. As a consequence, transplantation has become the treatment of choice for end-stage organ failure of the liver, heart, lung, pancreas, and kidney, thus allowing longer and better lives for thousands of patients. These advances also enabled us to continuously improve graft survival rates to highly acceptable levels across the board for all types of transplants. According to a recent report by Rana et al. more than 2 million years of lives could be saved in just 25 years of organ transplantation in the United States alone.[2]

It is fitting that these techniques have now more than half a century later returned to the field of plastic surgery with the development of reconstructive transplantation as the next chapter and a new era in transplant medicine. However, it is only within the last 2 decades that transplantation of VCAs such as hand/upper extremity, face, abdominal wall, as well as urogenital organs including penis and uterus transplants have become a clinical reality and viable treatment option. These modalities represent the transplantation of composite structures of the human form for reconstructive surgery to fulfill the prime mandate of Plastic and Reconstructive Surgery to replace and restore devastating tissue defects using *like with like* tissue.[3–5] The ability to transfer VCAs through microvascular surgical techniques, restoring form and function for complex cutaneous and musculoskeletal defects, is revolutionizing the field of reconstructive surgery to add another rung to the *reconstructive ladder*. However, despite all those advancements, long-term allograft survival in reconstructive transplantation can only be achieved, as for any other type of solid organ transplant, through the use of systemic immunosuppression with its associated sequela of organ toxicity, opportunistic infections, and potential for malignant transformation. Current research on immunomodulation and tolerance induction holds great promise to reduce the need for long-term high-dose immunosuppression.[6,7] Although reconstructive allotransplantation in humans is a relatively new area with small numbers of patients, there are reasons to think that new innovations in immunomodulation and tolerance may come from the field of VCAs. For example, reconstructive transplant patients are usually not suffering from life-threatening illness or comorbidities, and therefore the ethical impetus to minimize side effects from immunosuppressive medications is stronger. Also, the ability to directly and continuously observe a graft that includes a skin component allows for the use of novel experimental protocols, as rejection will be seen earlier and potentially could be reversed by topical agents. Finally, the presence of a vascularized bone marrow niche in many VCAs raises the possibility of unique immunomodulatory strategies, as will be discussed.

HISTORICAL PERSPECTIVE

Transplantation of allogeneic tissues has captivated human imagination since antiquity and began as the medicine of mythology with a timeline that spans three millennia. Indeed, Greek mythology and religious texts are rich with examples of xeno- and allotransplantation. Of note, the concept of transplantation transcended temporospatial boundaries and has been reported in Egyptian, Chinese, Indian, and early Christian mythology as early as 2000 BC.[8] Probably the most famous legend highlighting transplantation is the *miracle of the black leg* in the third century AD by the two Saints Cosmas and Damian—twin brothers who replaced the gangrenous leg of a parishioner with the leg of a deceased Ethiopian Moor. This legend, in particular, describes for the first time a new concept: cadaveric transplantation—where the body of the dead can help the living.

Experimentation with various types of transplants continued in the following centuries. Although proper surgical techniques were not available to facilitate successful performance of solid organ transplantation in those days, the procedure of skin grafting had already been performed for many centuries. In the second century BC, the Indian surgeon Sushruta pioneered skin grafting and rotational pedicle flaps for nasal reconstruction and described over a dozen ways to reconstruct ears and lips. His forward-thinking concepts were compiled in the *Sushruta Samhita*, which served as the primary treatise on plastic and reconstructive surgery for centuries.[9] In the 16th century, Gaspare Tagliacozzi emerged as a popular figure in transplantation, and he, like Sushruta, was a specialist in rhinoplasty. Tagliacozzi successfully performed nasal reconstruction on a patient who had lost his nose using a flap from the patient's upper arm, which represents one of the earliest records of a human autograft. In 1804, the Milanese surgeon Giuseppe Baronio claimed to perform successful autogenous and xenogeneic skin transplants as well as free tendon allografts in sheep. Baronio's contributions are considered fundamental to the field of plastic surgery and laid the groundwork for research in the fields of both skin grafting and transplant immunology. Reports of successful allografts began to circulate around the turn of the 19th century, when the Scottish surgeon, John Hunter, successfully transplanted the testes of a chicken into a hen *without altering the disposition of the hen.*[10] These experiments led Hunter to conclude that *transplantation is founded on a disposition in all living substances to unite when brought into contact with each other*, one of the earliest revelations regarding chimerism and allograft acceptance.

At this point organ transplantation was still not technically feasible owing to limitations in suturing techniques for vascular anastomosis. This obstacle was overcome in 1902 when Alexis Carrel introduced his vascular anastomosis technique, which unlocked a continuum of research in experimental organ transplantation. Within the same year, Austrian surgeon Emerich Ullmann performed the first experimental kidney transplantation in animals in Vienna, which was followed a few years later by reports of unsuccessful attempts in humans by Mathieu Jaboulay.[8,11]

The earliest reliable, documented outcomes of allogeneic and xenogeneic skin grafts in human recipients were published by Schone in 1912 and Lexer in 1914. Schone and Lexer demonstrated that these grafts did not survive more than 3 weeks after transplantation. Padgett provided further evidence in 1932, when he reported rejection of all skin allografts within 35 days in 40 patients. However, Padgett also demonstrated that skin grafts exchanged between identical twins survived indefinitely. World War II accelerated progress in allotransplantation. Gibson, a plastic surgeon at the Glasgow Royal Infirmary, described the accelerated rejection of allogeneic tissue due to the presence of humoral antibodies from prior exposure to the same allogeneic source, also known as *second set rejection*, of skin allografts when treating pilots with burn injuries. Medawar joined Gibson to investigate this phenomenon and, in combination with Billingham and Brent, laid the foundation of modern immunology. Medawar concluded that the rejection of human skin allografts is a result of actively acquired immune reactions—work that was later summarized by Billingham, Brent, and Medawar in their manuscript *Actively Acquired Tolerance*, which became the preeminent treatise on modulating the immune system for transplantation.[12] In this manuscript, the authors discuss the importance of chimerism for tolerance induction, noting the development of donor-specific tolerance by injection of donor cells into neonatal animals. This knowledge of immunology ultimately facilitated the advent of successful solid organ transplantation.

Prior to the 1950s, outcomes after organ transplantation were poor. However, the incorporation of Medawar's findings led Dr. Joseph Murray to perform the first successful living-related kidney transplantation between identical twins in 1954.[1] Shortly thereafter, a rapid development of new chemical immunosuppressive agents occurred. The use of drugs such as azathioprine (AZT), 6-mercaptopurine, and steroids in the 1960s allowed for the success of cadaveric renal transplants in 1962 and paved the way for a new era in solid organ transplantation.[13] Thereafter, many organs were successfully transplanted for the first time. In 1963, Dr. James Hardy transplanted the first lung at the University of Mississippi; 1966, the first successful pancreas transplant was performed at the University of Minnesota; Dr. Thomas E. Starzl performed the first liver transplant in the following year on a 3-year old child; the first successful heart transplant was carried out by Christian Barnard in 1967, followed by the first successful bone marrow transplant by E. Donnall Thomas in 1968.[14] A 4-month-old boy who had Wiskott-Aldrich syndrome received a bone marrow transplant from his sibling that effectively restored his immune system duplicating Medawar's animal findings that had previously resulted in immune tolerance in chimeric mice. In 1972, Jean-François Borel discovered cyclosporine, which further improved survival outcomes after transplantation enabling the first successful small bowel transplant in 1988 by Goulet et al. Since then, many potent and more selective immunosuppressive agents have been developed that controlled acute rejection and prolonged the survival of transplanted organs, which enabled transplantation to become the standard of care for patients with end-stage organ disease.

Out of these immunologic and surgical innovations, the idea of reconstructive transplantation was being formulated and as a result human hand transplantation was first attempted in Ecuador in 1964.[8,15] Although the procedure was a surgical technical success, the available immunosuppressive agents at the time were insufficient to prevent rejection, and the graft was eventually lost.

This failure underscored the previously described immunological challenges of skin transplants between genetically disparate individuals. As a result, it was felt that the transplantation of any skin-bearing allograft would be an insurmountable hurdle and another attempt was not carried out for over 3 decades. During this hiatus, accumulating evidence suggested that the skin of a VCA behaved differently than an isolated skin graft and, therefore, would not be rejected as vigorously. In addition, animal models of VCAs designed to investigate newer generations of immunosuppressive agents such as calcineurin inhibitors (CNIs) (e.g., tacrolimus) and antiproliferative agents (e.g., mycophenolate mofetil [MMF]) indicated that the loss of VCAs could now be prevented.[16] These findings paved the way to preforming the first successful unilateral hand transplantation in September 1998 by a French team led by Prof. Jean Michel Dubernard.[17] This was followed shortly thereafter by the first US hand transplant in January 1999 and many more around the world since then.[3,5] In the past decade, over 140 hand and upper extremity transplants have been performed with encouraging functional and immunologic outcomes that have exceeded all initial expectations.[18] The success of clinical hand transplantation heralded other new eras for reconstructive transplantation. In November 2005, Dubernard and Devauchelle performed the first successful face transplant in Amiens, France.[19] Since then almost 40 face transplants have been performed at multiple centers around the world.[20,21] In addition, many other types of VCAs have successfully been carried out with highly encouraging outcomes including the transplantation of larynx, trachea, vascularized knee, femur, abdominal wall, tongue, penis, uterus, as well as individual tissue components such as peripheral nerve, flexor tendon, and skin.[8,22-25] Although the surgical techniques to perform these complex procedures have been optimized, broad application of this reconstructive modality is still hampered by the risks of life-long, high-dose, multidrug, immunosuppression needed to prevent rejection.[7] Thus, continued progress in the field of transplant immunology is critical to the continued success of reconstructive transplantation, as minimization or elimination of immunosuppressive agents is a key goal in bringing this life-changing procedure to routine clinical applicability.[6] The field of reconstructive transplantation will become ubiquitous once transplant tolerance can be reliably achieved. Currently great strides are being made in experimental large animal studies and first clinical trials, moving ever closer to elucidating the immunological processes that will help overcome these barriers.

NOMENCLATURE AND DEFINITIONS

A brief note on nomenclature will help clarify further discussions of transplantation techniques outlined in this chapter. Certain terms such as transplant, flap, and graft are often loosely used to refer to a VCA. However, these terms should be used carefully with knowledge of their specific meaning to ensure clear communication.

Transplantation can be defined as the transfer of tissue or solid organs to another person or to a different anatomical location in the same person. According to this definition much of what reconstructive surgeons do can be classified as a type of transplant. However, in its usual medical usage the term transplantation is used to describe an allotransplant or tissue transferred from a living or deceased human donor to another genetically not identically human patient. Within this chapter, our discussion of transplantation will be focused mostly on the topic of allotransplantation, as the transfer of autologous tissue locally or distantly is covered elsewhere in the text.

A *graft* is tissue completely separated from its donor bed and moved to a separate recipient bed, with its survival relying on ingrowth of new vessels from the surrounding recipient tissue. A *vascularized graft* or *flap* either remains attached to its native blood supply or becomes revascularized via microvascular anastomoses to recipient vessels (aka, free flap). An *autograft* refers to tissue transplanted from one anatomical location to another within the same individual. An *isograft* is tissue transplanted between genetically identical individuals, such as transplants between syngeneic animals or human monozygotic twins. An *allograft* or *homograft* is tissue transplanted between unrelated individuals of the same species. A *xenograft* or *heterograft* is tissue transplanted between different species.

Transplantation can also be described according to the anatomical site into which the tissue is transferred. An *orthotopic* transplant is transferred into an anatomically similar site, whereas a *heterotopic* transplant is transferred into a different site from its donor origin. The term *reconstructive transplantation* is used to differentiate the transfer of composite tissues such as the hand or face from more traditional solid organ transplants. However, the issuance of a Final Rule in July 2013 by the United States Secretary of Health has redefined VCAs as organs rather than tissues and thereby acknowledged the importance of reconstructive transplantation as a vital treatment option as well as opened up the potential to formalize policies and procedures, under the auspices of the Organ Procurement and Transplantation Network, that can improve VCA donation and procurement practices, develop allocation algorithms, and provide transparent oversight equal to solid organ transplantation.[26]

TRANSPLANT IMMUNOLOGY

Three-Signal Model of Alloimmunity

Transplantation of organs or tissues between genetically disparate individuals of the same species leads to recognition and rejection of the allogeneic tissue by the recipient's immune system. This *alloimmune response* that discriminates between self- and nonself tissues remains the main barrier to successful transplantation.

The key initiators of an alloimmune response are genetically encoded polymorphic proteins that constitute graft antigens referred to as major histocompatibility complex (MHC) or in humans are known as human leukocyte antigens (HLA). The MHC complex is a cell surface molecule (glycoprotein) that is common to a polymorphic multigene cluster located on chromosome 6 in humans. There are two classes of MHC molecules, class I and II, that differ in their structure, function, and tissue distribution. MHC class I antigens consist of two polypeptide chains, an α-chain with a transmembranous domain and the β_2-microglobulin chain that is expressed on all nucleated cells. MHC class II antigens consist also of two polypeptide chains an α- and a β-chain; however, their expression is restricted to antigen-presenting cells (APCs) such as dendritic cells (DCs), monocytes, macrophages, some endothelial cells, thymic epithelial cells, and B lymphocytes.[27] Each MHC has an inherited group of HLA genes or haplotypes: HLA class I genes known as HLA-A, -B, and -C and HLA class II genes known as HLA-DR, -DP, and -DQ. The HLA determines the compatibility of all organ and tissue transplants. The primary function of MHC molecules is to bind short peptides that are derived from proteins processed by the cell. Such non–self-protein-MHC complexes coordinate the interaction of lymphocytes during the acute and chronic alloimmune response.

There are two main pathways by which host T cells recognize donor alloantigens (**Figure 8.1**). Following transplantation, donor APCs migrate toward host lymphoid tissues and can directly activate naïve recipient T cells. Once T cells are activated, they become effector T cells and migrate to the graft and mediate rejection. This is aptly named the *direct pathway* of allorecognition. In contrast to the direct pathway, recipient APCs play a significant role in the *indirect pathway* of allorecognition where they take up, process,

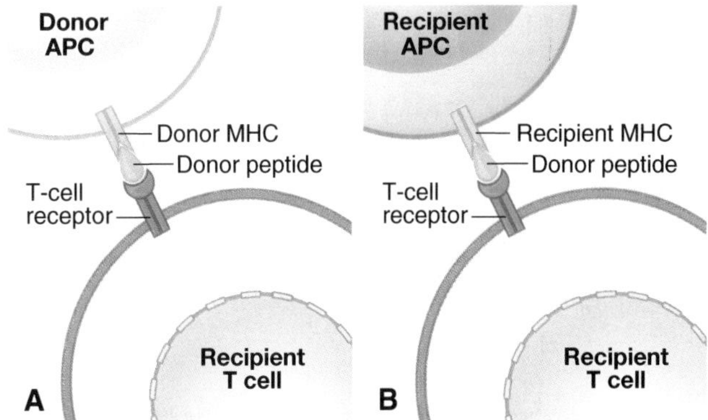

FIGURE 8.1. T cell recognition of alloantigens. **A.** Direct pathway, recipient T cells interact with intact allogeneic major or minor histocompatibility peptide complexes presented by donor APCs. **B.** Indirect pathway, recipient T cells interact with processed allogeneic major or minor histocompatibility peptide complexes presented by recipient APCs. APC, antigen-presenting cell; MHC, major histocompatibility complex.

and present donor antigens to host T cells. Both pathways of allorecognition are important in mediating graft rejection; however, the direct pathway is considered to be the main initiator of acute rejection, whereas the indirect pathway is thought to be of greater significance in the physiology of chronic graft rejection in the long term.[28]

The initiation of an alloimmune response is a well-orchestrated and choreographed interplay of various different players of the immune system including DCs, naïve and memory T cells, and B cells. DCs are key players in the initiation of an alloimmune response post transplant, as they express high levels of MHC class II and costimulatory molecules essential for T cell activation.[29] Upon activation, DCs of both donor and recipient origin migrate to the T cell areas of secondary lymphoid organs of the host where they encounter naive CD4+ T cells and central memory T cells, which recirculate within the lymphoid tissues. Within the secondary lymph nodes, T cells encounter the MHC alloantigen that is expressed on the surface of the DCs with their specific T cell receptors (TCRs) combined with the CD3 complex that facilitates signal transduction. This interaction of MHC, TCR, and CD3 complex is referred to as *signal 1* (**Figure 8.2**). Typically, MHC class I molecules present antigen peptides derived from intracellular sources to CD8+ T cells, whereas MHC class II molecules present antigen derived from endolysosomal compartments to CD4+ T cells.

In addition to signal 1, APCs provide so called costimulatory signals to fully activate T cells. These costimulatory signals are also referred to as *signal 2* during T cell activation. Two of the best-characterized costimulatory signals/pathways in transplantation are the B7/CD28 and the CD40/CD154 pathways. In addition, there are a multitude of other second signals including 4-1BB (CD137) and 4-1BBL, inducible costimulator and ligand of inducible costimulator, OX40/OX40L, LFA1/ICAM-1, or PD-1/PDL-1/2[29,30] (see Figure 8.2).

Once a naïve T cell receives both signal 1 and signal 2 through a single specific APC, three intracellular signal transduction pathways are activated including the calcium-calcineurin pathway, RAS-mitogen-activated protein kinase pathway, and the NF-κB pathway. Through those pathways, several transcription factors such as NFAT, AP-1, and NF-κB are activated, which subsequently leads to the expression of cytokine-encoded genes for IL-2, CD154, and CD25. These cytokines, in particular IL-2 and IL-15, then act via autocrine mechanisms to initiate T cell proliferation and expansion. This final step is also referred to as *signal 3*.

Types of Rejection

Based on the timing of allograft, transplant rejection has been divided into three major categories: hyperacute, acute, and chronic.[31]

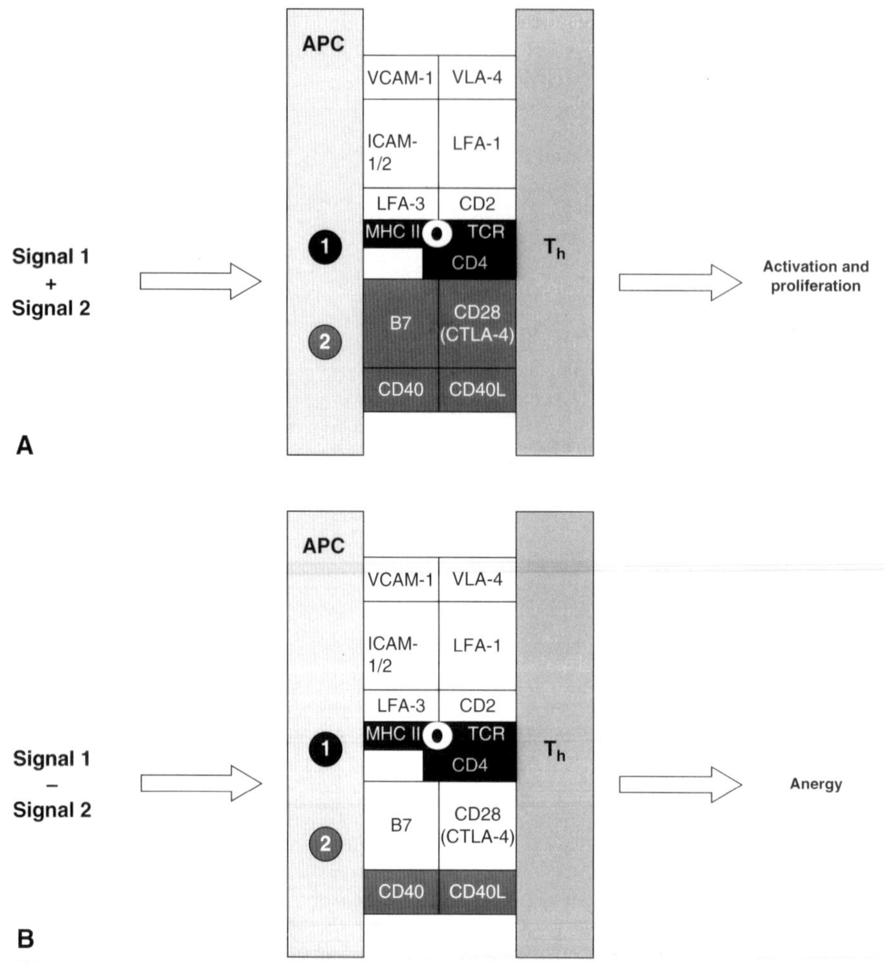

FIGURE 8.2. Costimulatory blockade. **A.** Antigen-specific T cell activation depends on T cell receptor-ligand interaction (signal 1) and costimulatory signals (signal 2) for full activation and proliferation. **B.** Blocking of T cell costimulatory pathways (signal 2) results in T cell anergy and thus prevents allograft rejection, promotes long-term graft survival, and induces tolerance in various rodent and nonhuman primate transplant models. APC, antigen-presenting cells; MHC, major histocompatibility complex; TCR, T cell receptor.

Hyperacute Rejection

This type of rejection is a *peracute* form with a very rapid onset that occurs within minutes to hours after transplantation and can destroy the allograft in an equally short period of time. It is mediated through preexisting antibodies against HLA or ABO antigens which have been acquired as a result of pretransplant blood transfusions, pregnancies, or previous transplants. These antibodies bind to their corresponding antigen expressed on endothelial cells of the transplant and subsequently can activate the coagulation and complement cascade. This leads to the formation of microthrombi, vascular occlusion, and ultimately necrosis of the allograft. However, blood type matching, HLA typing of donor and recipient, and pretransplant routine clinical cross-matching, whereby preformed anti-HLA antibodies are screened for have virtually eliminated hyperactive rejection episodes in both solid organ as well as reconstructive transplantation.

Acute Rejection

Acute rejection episodes typically manifest within a period of days or weeks after transplant but can occur also at much later time points (months or years) if the immune system is *awakened* either by infection or by a significant reduction in immunosuppression. The primary mediator of acute rejection episodes are effector T cells that infiltrate the graft and lead to inflammatory damage and parenchymal necrosis. About 30% of all cases of acute rejection, however, are mediated by antibodies (donor-specific IgG antibodies) and are referred to as humoral or vascular rejection episodes. These antibodies bind to endothelial cells and activate the complement cascade which in turn leads to deposition of complement factors C3d and C4d that trigger endothelial inflammation and cellular infiltration resulting in vascular damage and occlusion. Given the advances in modern immunosuppression, acute rejection episodes for most type of organ transplants are ranging between 3% and 10% and can usually be successfully reversed with either steroid bolus therapy, antibody treatment (thymoglobulin or alemtuzumab), or with plasmapheresis and high-dose IVIG.

Chronic Rejection

Chronic rejection is the leading cause affecting long-term outcomes after transplantation. This type of rejection is a slow form of rejection that primarily targets the graft vasculature (concentric vascular stenosis also referred to as graft vasculopathy) and causes graft fibroses. The onset of chronic rejection is usually beyond 1 year post transplant and most often progresses gradually over several years, eventually leading to a gradual decline in organ function and ultimately graft loss. Mechanistically both humoral as well as cellular responses, including DTH reactions and proinflammatory cytokines (IFN-g, fibroblast growth factor, or TGF-b), are involved in the onset and progression of chronic rejection. In addition, residual scarring from episodes of acute rejection contributes to chronic graft failure. Alloreactive T cells are infiltrating the transplant and release cytokines and chemokines such as CCL5 which in turn recruit monocytes that differentiate into macrophages. The second phase of this chronic inflammatory process is dominated by macrophages which release IL-1, TNF-a, and MCP-1 and thereby perpetuate the chronic inflammatory state, ultimately leading to graft fibrosis and sclerosis and loss of function. In addition to these antigen-specific mechanisms, antigen-independent factors such as ischemia-reperfusion injury, chronic toxicity of maintenance immunosuppression, and infectious complications such CMV can contribute to the development of chronic rejection and graft vasculopathy.

IMMUNOSUPPRESSION

In addition to advances in surgical techniques, the development of potent and targeted immunosuppressive agents has probably contributed the most to the success story of organ transplantation.[29,32,33] Today, there is a whole armamentarium of pharmacological agents available that can be used to prevent and control allograft rejection[32] (**Figure 8.3**; **Table 8.1**). Based on their mode of action, there are six major categories of immunosuppressive drugs: induction agents (e.g., mono- and polyclonal antibodies), antiproliferative agents, CNIs, mTOR inhibitors, corticosteroids, and biologic agents.

Induction Agents

Polyclonal antithymocyte globulin or antilymphocyte globulin reagents can be distinguished from each other by the cells used for the immunization and the animal species from which they are produced. The mechanism by which antithymocyte globulins achieve their immunosuppressive action is by peripheral blood lymphocyte depletion through antibody-dependent cell-mediated cytotoxicity or Fas-dependent apoptosis. Alemtuzumab (Campath-1H) is an anti-CD52 monoclonal antibody that similarly depletes T cells, B cells, and NK cells by antibody-dependent cellular-mediated lysis. Basiliximab is a recombinant monoclonal antibody that binds to and blocks the IL-2 receptor on the surface of T cells. Induction therapy with lymphodepleting agents has allowed for a significant reduction in the incidence of acute allograft rejection and to a diminution of maintenance immunosuppression to promote CNI reduction and steroid avoidance or withdrawal.

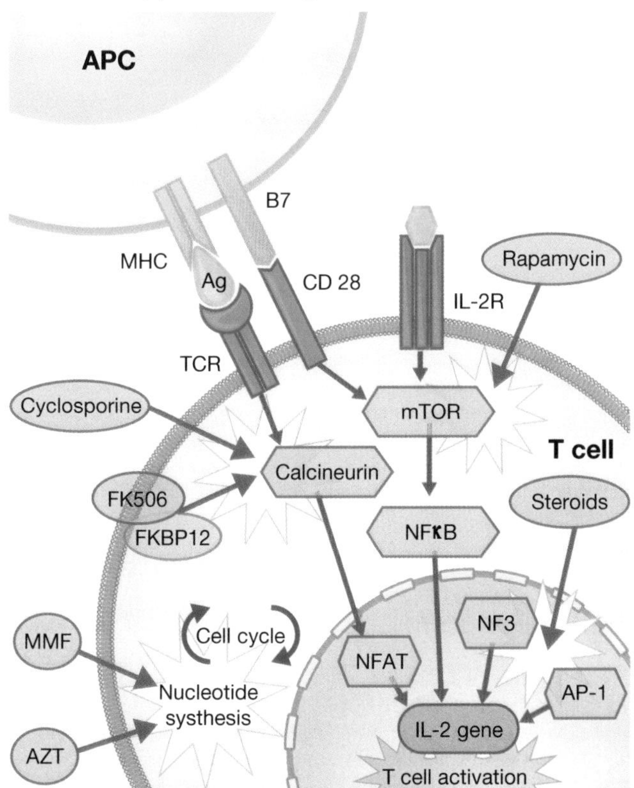

FIGURE 8.3. Targets of immunosuppressants during T cell activation. Immunosuppressive medications interrupt T cell activation at various pathways. CsA and tacrolimus interrupt the TCR signaling cascade by blocking calcineurin activation, the latter by interaction with FK-binding proteins. RAPA blocks mTOR signaling from both IL-2 receptor activation and from TCR coreceptors interrupting the *second signal* pathway. Steroids alter gene transcription by modulating the effects of transcription factors including several necessary for T cell activation. AZT and MMF inhibit the production of nucleotides in lymphocytes blocking the cell cycle and proliferation. APC, antigen-presenting cells; AZT, azathioprine; MMF, mycophenolate mofetil; TCR, T cell receptor.

Antiproliferative Agents

Cytotoxic/antiproliferative drugs include cyclophosphamide, methotrexate, AZT, and MMF. These agents interfere with DNA replication and arrest proliferating alloreactive lymphocytes. Earlier nonspecific antiproliferative agents such as AZT had many side effects and unwanted toxicities. MMF has replaced these agents in many protocols due to its ability to selectively block purine synthesis in T and B cells, which dramatically improves the side effect profile.

Calcineurin Inhibitors

Cyclosporine A (CsA) and tacrolimus both inhibit the signaling pathways of T cell activation by interfering with calcineurin activation and IL-2 gene transcription. CsA is a metabolic extract from the fungus *Tolypocladium inflatum* Gams first described in 1976. Its discovery revolutionized the field of solid organ transplantation by significantly increasing survival of kidney, heart, and liver allografts. CsA has been shown to prolong limb allograft survival in various experimental animal models and thereby significantly encouraged to pursue clinical VCA in the 80s and 90s. Tacrolimus is a macrolide lactone antibiotic isolated from soil fungus and also inhibits the calcineurin/IL-2 pathway of T cell activation, although at a different point in the pathway from cyclosporine. It has a favorable side effect profile as compared with CsA and less transplant-associated malignancy potential, although it has significant nephrotoxicity when used for long periods of time. Tacrolimus has replaced cyclosporine in many protocols in solid organ and has been the backbone of all the clinical reconstructive transplantation treatment regimens. A beneficial side effect of immunosuppression with tacrolimus in the setting of VCA is its dose-dependent acceleration of axonal regeneration, which promotes functional recovery after reconstructive transplantation.

mTOR Inhibitors

The unfavorable toxicity profile of CNIs, in particular its considerably high nephrotoxicity, has led some centers to switch to the mTOR inhibitor rapamycin (sirolimus, everolimus). Rapamycin and other mTOR inhibitors act downstream of signal 3, inhibiting the response to IL-2 (as well as IL-4, IL-7, IL-12, and IL-15), thereby effectively inhibiting T cell proliferation. Rapamycin is a very attractive alternative to CNIs, as it has a significantly different side effect profile in particular with regard to its nephrotoxicity and having antiproliferative and antineoplastic properties. It does, however, suffer the drawback of having profound negative effects on wound healing that may preclude its use in the early postoperative period.

Corticosteroids

One of the first available immunosuppressants for transplantation was steroids with broad anti-inflammatory actions (i.e., prednisone, prednisolone). These medications inhibit activation of several transcription factors, thus modifying gene expression, inhibiting cellular activation, and cytokine production. Prednisolone was one of the first pharmacological agents used in allogeneic organ transplantation. Despite the well-known side effects of long-term use, steroids are still widely utilized today in combination with other immunosuppressive

TABLE 8.1. IMMUNOSUPPRESSIVE AGENTS IN CURRENT USE

Class of Drug	Agents	Mode of Action	Main Adverse Effects
Induction agents	Antithymocyte globulin (ATG), alemtuzumab	Antibody-dependent cell-mediated cytotoxicity	Cytokine release syndrome, leukopenia, anemia, bleeding, hypertension
Antiproliferative agents	Azathioprine Mycophenolate mofetil (MMF)	Blockade of DNA synthesis and replication	Gastrointestinal (GI) complaints, diarrhea, viral reactivation, myelosuppression/leukopenia
Calcineurin inhibitors	Cyclosporine A (CsA) Tacrolimus	Inhibition of IL-2 gene transcription	Nephrotoxicity, hypertension, hyperglycemia, tremor, hirsutism, gingival hyperplasia, acne
mTOR inhibitors	Rapamycin Everolimus	Inhibits signal transduction	Hyperlipidemia, wound-healing problems, thrombocytopenia, anemia, peripheral edema, ulceration of oral mucosa
Steroids	Methylprednisolone Prednisolone	Inhibition of multiple transcription factors anti-inflammatory	Diabetes, fluid retention, weight gain, dyslipidemia, hip necrosis, acne, glaucoma
Biologics	Cytotoxic T-lymphocyte–associated antigen-4 immunoglobulin (CTLA4-Ig) (Belatacept)	Blocks costimulatory pathway B7-CD28	Cytokine release syndrome, fever, leukopenia, anemia
	Basiliximab	IL-2 receptor antagonism	Tremor, bleeding, fever, chills
	Rituximab	CD20 binding on B cells	Infusion reaction, cytokine release syndrome
	Infliximab	TNF-a inhibition	Infection, tuberculosis reactivation, drug-induced lupus

agents in most solid organ and VCA protocols. However, steroid avoidance, minimization, and withdrawal had been common practice even from the beginning of transplantation. Short courses of high-dose bolused steroids continue to be the frontline treatment for acute rejection episodes in all types of transplantation.

Biologic Agents

Biologic agents such as cytotoxic T-lymphocyte–associated antigen-4 immunoglobulin (CTLA4-Ig) (e.g., abatacept, belatacept), which block T cell costimulation, were developed to overcome the limitations of conventional immunosuppressants and represent a new paradigm in immunosuppression—biological therapy for maintenance immunosuppression devoid of the toxicities associated with CNIs. CTLA4-Ig is an engineered fusion protein comprised of the extracellular human domain of CTLA4 and the hinge CH2 and CH3 domains of a human or mouse IgG1 that binds to B7 molecules with high affinity thus preventing CD28-B7 engagement and leading to partial T cell activation and T cell anergy. Multiple groups have demonstrated potent immunosuppressive properties of CTLA4-Ig in vivo using rodent models of transplantation and autoimmunity. Recently a novel mutant of CTLA4-Ig (LEA29Y, belatacept) with increased binding affinity to B7 has been generated and successfully introduced into human trials with favorable results. These phase II and III studies in renal transplantation demonstrated that belatacept-based immunosuppression is an effective alternative to CNIs.[34]

Other biologic agents used for immunosuppression in transplantation include *rituximab*, a chimeric murine/human monoclonal antibody that reacts with the CD20 antigen on B cells, *infliximab* a high-molecular-weight (149 kDa) chimeric monoclonal antibody against TNF-a, *CFZ533* a new, fully human, Fc-silenced, nondepleting, IgG1 mAb preventing CD40 pathway signaling and activation of CD40 + cell types, and the IL-2 receptor antagonists also referred to as anti-CD25 monoclonal antibodies, *basiliximab* and *daclizumab*.[32]

Despite this plethora of immunosuppressive agents, there is currently no standard immunosuppressive protocol established for either solid organ or reconstructive transplantation.

The current immunosuppressive protocols applied to hand, upper extremity, and face transplantation are extrapolated from various different regimens and protocols used in solid organ transplantation. The overall amount of immunosuppression required to ensure graft survival is comparable or even slightly higher than it is for kidney transplantation.

TRANSPLANTATION TOLERANCE

Sir Peter Medawar's seminal experiments with skin transplantation laid the foundation for Transplant Immunology; subsequent experimentation by his group in animal models led to the first documentation of *acquired immune tolerance*. This phenomenon was defined as *a state of donor-specific hyporesponsiveness, in the absence of immunosuppression*, while maintaining adequate immune responses to third party antigens.[12] This definition is still valid today and implies that a state of tolerance must coexist with general immune competence, including normal immune responses to pathogens and cancer risks no different than the general population. During development, one of the critical functions of the immune system is to prevent responses directed toward self-antigens and thereby preventing autoimmune disease. This vital ability of the immune system to distinguish between self- and foreign antigens is controlled by two main mechanisms referred to as *central* and *peripheral* tolerance. Central tolerance is facilitated in the thymus whereas peripheral tolerance is induced in extrathymic secondary lymphoid tissues. The mechanism of T cell tolerance in the thymus is based on the deletion of self or alloreactive T cells upon interaction with bone marrow–derived APCs. In general, during T cell development, the majority of T cells found in the thymus have undesirable reactivities and are therefore deleted via negative selection. T cells that recognize foreign antigen in the context of self-MHC are positively selected and allowed to circulate in the peripheral blood. Another widely researched approach for the induction of tolerance is the use of hematopoietic stem cell transplantations to induce mixed chimerism.[35]

Mixed chimerism refers to a state in which donor and recipient cells coexist within the recipient. This state can be established in clinical practice via donor hematopoietic stem cells, which are mobilized from the donor bone marrow, collected from peripheral blood, and then administered to the recipient. Donor HSCs engraft into the recipient's bone marrow and, in conjunction with recipient HSCs, ensure the constant production of myeloid and lymphoid cell lineages: the recipient's immune system is now composed by cells both of donor and of recipient origin. Immune tolerance was achieved via mixed chimerism in a variety of animal models; clonal deletion was demonstrated as one of the primary mechanism in this process. In humans, mixed chimerism was achieved, in the vast majority of cases, only as a transient state; however, in certain patients, immune tolerance persists long after the loss of mixed chimerism: this indicates that mechanisms other than clonal deletion might be at play. A remaining major challenge to achieving tolerance routinely through the induction of mixed chimerism is the need for intense preconditioning regimens with considerable toxicities.[35,36]

Peripheral tolerance in contrast is maintained by a number of mechanisms, including clonal deletion, anergy (e.g., nonresponsiveness), and suppression/regulation. The induction of T cell anergy has been demonstrated by blockade of costimulatory signals (signal 2) using monoclonal antibodies during T cell activation (see Figure 8.2). Anergic T cells are incapable of producing IL-2 and are unresponsive to repeat antigen stimulation unless exogenous IL-2 is added. The induction of T regulatory/suppressor cells is another mechanism to induce T cell tolerance specific to donor antigens. T regulatory cells (CD4+CD25+Foxp3+ T regs) play a key role in the maintenance of tolerance to both self- and foreign antigens.[37] Furthermore, studies in recent years have demonstrated the potential role for particular subtypes of DCs such as plasmacytoid to promote and maintain peripheral tolerance to transplantation antigens. Another mechanism leading to peripheral tolerance is clonal exhaustion and deletion, which is due to chronic or overwhelming antigen exposure/stimulation under suboptimal conditions.

TRANSPLANTATION APPLICATIONS IN PLASTIC SURGERY

Skin

Skin allografts are the most commonly performed human allotransplant and were the basis of the first transplantation research. Pioneering experiments by Giuseppe Baronio, as outlined above, on auto- and allografts in sheep laid the groundwork for research in the fields of both skin grafting and transplant immunology.[8] The most frequent clinical use for skin allografts is in the treatment of extensive burns. The ability to place temporary skin grafts without jeopardizing limited autogenous donor sites in these patients has resulted in dramatic improvements in survival of high total body surface area burn wounds. In some patients who are immunosuppressed either through medications or through severe illness, skin allografts have been shown to be tolerated with continued immunosuppression. Anecdotal reports of patients who have undergone slow withdrawal of immunosuppression have not required regrafting either through permanent tolerance of the graft or more likely through slow substitution of the allograft with recipient cells.[38] Future research developments that enable prolonged graft survival in the absence of immunosuppression would precipitate a significant paradigm shift in the treatment of severe wounds and burns.

Skin Xenograft

Porcine xenograft has been used as a temporary dressing for large burns. It is applied with a technique similar to that used for human allograft, with seeding of autologous grafts beneath it. The application of xenogeneic dermis has also been found valuable in preparing a wound for subsequent grafting by stimulation of granulation tissue formation. Xenogeneic tissue has limited uses in skin grafting at present, and its cellular components are susceptible to hyperacute rejection typical of all xenograft materials.

Bone Allograft

Reconstruction of large bony defects in the axial and peripheral skeleton with nonvascularized allogeneic bone has been widely practiced. Well-organized tissue banks and improved methods of bone sterilization and preservation have made this possible. Very few of the donor cells, if any, in the nonvascularized bone allograft survive. These donor cells express antigens similar to other allogeneic tissues and are susceptible to rejection. The remaining bone acts as a scaffold for ingrowth of recipient mesenchymal stem cells (osteocyte precursors), which repopulates the donor by *creeping substitution*. Although technically an allogeneic tissue transplant, these grafts are essentially totally replaced by recipient cells once the healing process is complete and no immunosuppression is given. Owing to slow union, long-term fixation is required of bone allograft, which is prone to stress fracture and loosening of fixation hardware. In studies of retrieved human allografts, however, union was seen at the graft-host interface.

Vascularized bone allograft on the other hand contains living donor cells and is susceptible to immunologic rejection. The humoral and cellular response generated to transplanted bone was found to be similar in intensity and timing as that generated by other vascularized allogeneic limb tissues such as the skin and muscle. Although individual bone cells express antigens, the predominant antigenic stimulus in a bone allograft is thought to be derived from the marrow. Removal of bone marrow by irradiation or replacement with recipient marrow has been shown experimentally to prolong allograft survival. Like any other allogeneic tissue, this rejection process can be ameliorated with immunosuppression, and long-term survival of orthotopic vascularized skeletal allograft has been achieved in animal models. However, the adverse effects of prolonged immunosuppression required for survival of a vascularized bone allograft preclude its clinical application currently as an autologous sources of vascularized bone. Non-vascularized allografts are usually sufficient to reconstruct most simple bone defects.

Cartilage Allograft

Cartilage is composed of chondrocytes within lacunae dispersed throughout a water-laden matrix. The matrix is composed predominantly of proteoglycans and type II collagen. Water is important as cartilage has no intrinsic blood supply and relies on diffusion of nutrients and oxygen through this matrix. The combination of water and proteoglycans imparts the characteristic of viscoelasticity depending on the relative concentrations of both elements. The variable water content in the matrix causes a balanced tension within it and helps maintain its three-dimensional shape. The viscoelastic property of the matrix confers *memory* such that cartilage returns to its original shape after deformation. Surgical manipulation or scoring disrupts this equilibrium. In contrast to osteocytes, chondrocytes have little reparative ability and heal by forming fibrous scar tissue. There are histologically three types of cartilage: hyaline, elastic, and fibrocartilage. Chondrocytes express HLA antigens on their surface and are thus immunogenic in isolation. Cartilage, however, is immunologically privileged owing to the shielding of chondrocytes by its matrix, which is only weakly antigenic. Surgical scoring or dicing of cartilage allograft with resultant exposure of allogeneic cells has been shown to hasten cartilage resorption. Cartilage allografts have been used successfully for similar applications as autologous cartilage. Allogeneic cartilage can be either preserved or fresh. Preserved cartilage has the advantage of a more abundant supply and decreased risk of infection in comparison to fresh cartilage. Although immunologically privileged, cartilage allografts are still susceptible to loss of volume through resorption. Whether this is due to immunologic rejection or lack of viable cells following preservation is a matter for debate.

Cartilage Xenograft

Some authors have advocated the use of bovine-derived cartilage xenografts. However, both chondrocytes and matrix are subject to xenogeneic mechanisms of rejection with a generally poorer outcome in comparison to autologous or allogeneic cartilage grafts. Attempts to modify these xenogeneic responses by altering the graft's immunologic stereotactic structure have been reported as being beneficial.

Nerve Allograft

The best clinical outcome following nerve transection is achieved with primary repair. More extensive injuries or a delay in repair may result in a nerve gap following debridement of damaged nerves, and a nerve graft may be necessary to achieve neurorrhaphy without tension. The nerve graft undergoes the same degenerative process as in the distal nerve after division. The myelin sheath remains with Schwann cells that act as a biological conduit for the regenerating axons. Vascularized nerve grafts are theoretically advantageous particularly in scarred beds. Other *conduits* used as nerve grafts have included autologous vein, silicone tubes seeded with Schwann cells, and freeze-fractured autologous muscle. Autologous nerve grafts with acceptable donor site morbidity are limited, and extensive nerve reconstruction may require other sources such as nerve allografts. Immunological rejection of nerve allograft can be ameliorated experimentally with immunosuppressive drugs, and axons were found to traverse the allogeneic nerve graft in rodents. A similar result has also been demonstrated in primates. Immunosuppression was necessary during axonal regeneration but could be terminated afterward in some studies with satisfactory nerve functions. In the only clinical experience, Mackinnon reported return of motor and sensory functions in the upper or lower limbs of six out of seven patients following nerve allograft reconstruction.[39]

RECONSTRUCTIVE TRANSPLANTATION

Reconstructive transplantation or, as it is also referred to, vascularized composite allotransplantation (VCA) has become a valid therapeutic and restorative option for patients with severe tissue defects not amendable to conventional reconstruction.[3–5,20,21] Significant advances in both basic science and translational research related to transplant immunology paired with the development of more potent and targeted immunosuppressive agents over the past 2 decades as well as highly encouraging functional and immunological clinical outcomes have led VCA to transition from an experimental and sometimes controversial procedure to an accepted and rapidly expanding field with great promise.

Upper Extremity Transplantation

It has been well documented that reconstructive transplants can be maintained on conventional triple drug immunosuppression at levels similar to that used in solid organ transplantation.[40,41] Patients after upper extremity transplantation have functional motor and sensory recovery similar to that seen with replantation. Since the beginning of the modern era of hand transplantation in 1998, there have been over 140 hand and upper extremity transplants performed worldwide in centers across the United States, Europe, and Asia. In general, and as reported in the International Registry on Hand and Composite Tissue Transplantation, results have been highly satisfactory with very few grafts lost, on average good hand function, and relatively few major side effects and complications.[3,5,18] Immunosuppressive side effects included predominately opportunistic infection (i.e., CMV), metabolic complications such as diabetes and hypertension, nephrotoxicity (requiring renal transplantation in some cases), avascular necrosis of the hip, and the occurrence of posttransplant malignancy such as PTLD. Although the risk/benefit equation of placing a patient on long-term immunosuppressive medications for a nonlifesaving type of transplant must always be considered, advances such as minimization protocols using donor bone marrow infusion and monotherapy maintenance have been successfully developed in large animal models and are currently being studied in humans.[6,7,42–44] Such innovative alternative protocols are anticipated to favorably alter this balance in the future. Thus, the consensus among many patients is that VCA delivers considerable improvements in function, independence, and quality of life. Such functional gains allow these patients to perform a variety of daily activities such as eating, writing, driving, grasping, shaving, while, in some cases, dramatically improving their social life and enabling them to return to work full time (**Figure 8.4**). As a consequence, upper extremity transplantation is increasingly being seen as another alternative in the reconstructive armamentarium used to treat patients with upper extremity amputations. Hand and upper extremity transplantation has demonstrated the ability to restore the structure and function of the hand in a way not possible with any other reconstructive technique by truly replacing *like with like* (**Figure 8.5**). Hence, it appears that reconstructive transplantation will continue to play an increasing role in the treatment of patients with upper limb amputations. However, balancing the

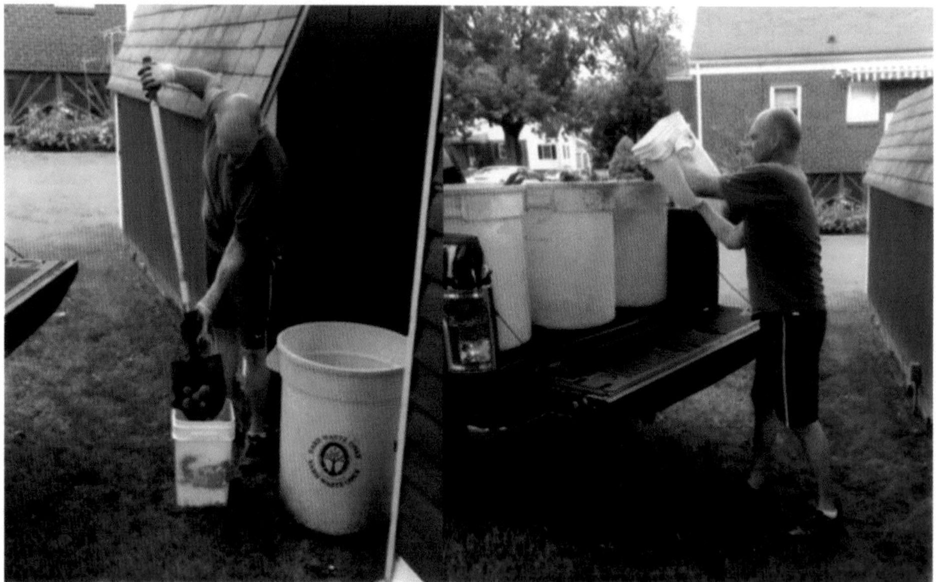

FIGURE 8.4. Functional outcome after bilateral upper extremity transplantation. Demonstration of excellent functional outcome in a patient more than 8 years after bilateral upper extremity transplantation (left side at wrist level and right side above elbow at mid humerus level).

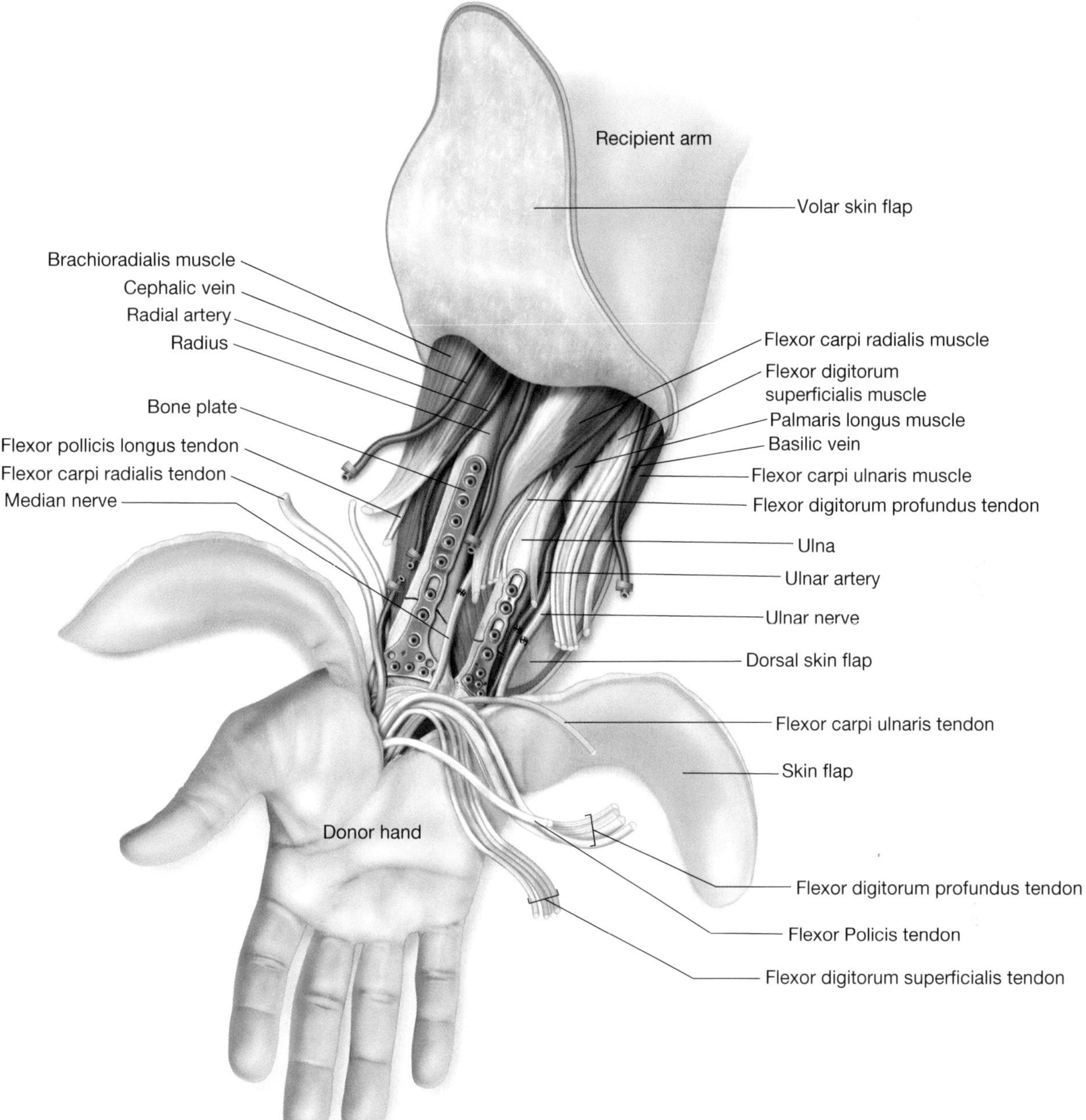

FIGURE 8.5. Upper extremity transplantation. Schematic diagram showing the technique of mid-forearm hand transplantation. All structures are prepared and labeled prior to transplantation and osseous fixation. Note the opposing, interdigitating skin flap design.

risk/benefit ratio in particular the risks of and toxicities of systemic immunosuppression against all the improving in function, patient autonomy, and quality of life will remain the prime task of this field for the foreseeable future.

Face Transplantation

No other area of reconstructive transplantation captures the imagination of patients, clinicians, and the public like face transplantation. Especially because human beings' perception of *self* is intimately tied to one's facial appearance. In addition, the face provides information not only about self-identity, but also age, gender, and ethnicity of an individual and thus affects social interactions, integration, and perception of body image. For patients with severe and devastating injuries to the craniofacial skeleton and soft tissues of the face, there is currently no other acceptable, effective restorative option using standard reconstructive techniques. For these patients, transplantation of allogeneic cadaveric facial structures has shown to be the only viable option of regaining normal facial appearance and being able to reintegrate into society in a meaningful way.

Since the first partial face transplantation has been carried out in 2005 by Drs. Dubernard and Devauchelle in France, a total of 40 cases of craniofacial transplantation have been performed worldwide and thereby shown technical feasibility and promising immunological, functional, psychological, and aesthetic results.[20,21,45] Transplanted grafts have consisted of just soft tissue (the nose and lips) up to and including all facial soft tissue and portions of facial bones and the tongue (entire face, maxilla, anterior portion of the mandible, and tongue). Indications for these procedures have included ballistic trauma sustained by military personnel and civilians, animal bites, tumor resection, neurofibromatosis, and burns. All of the facial allografts have included either portions of the orbicularis oris or oculi; loss of the sphincter function of the mimetic muscles of the face is generally considered to be one of the indications for facial transplantation. In general, patients have been maintained on immunosuppression similar to that used for upper extremity or solid organ transplantation with all patients receiving induction therapy followed by triple drug immunosuppression. Tacrolimus has been the cornerstone of nearly the majority of immunosuppression protocols used in face transplantation with target trough levels of 10 to 15 ng/mL for the first 6 months with most patients subsequently lowering to a maintenance level of 8 to 10 ng/mL. Corticosteroids have been safely tapered after a few months, with complete withdrawal possible within a year in some cases, depending on the immunosuppression regimen. Overall, immunological and functional patient outcomes have been highly satisfactory. All patients receiving facial transplantation have dramatically improved their aesthetic appearance allowing them to be reintegrated into society and have a normal and productive social life. However, functional outcomes are difficult to quantify uniformly owing to the complexity of facial functions and the wide range of extend of injures across face transplantation recipients. All patients for whom outcomes have been reported in the literature have developed nearly normal sensory function with return of two-point discrimination and temperature differentiation between 3 and 8 months after transplantation. Motor recovery has been slightly slower but all patients have recovered some degree of motor function allowing for oral competence, the ability to breathe, eat, taste, smell, and speak, and for facial expression. Typical motor recovery is detectable as early as 6 to 8 months post transplant with maximum recovery around 18 months after transplant. Unfortunately, there have now been first cases of chronic rejection reported for face transplantation which resulted in subsequent graft loss, including the very first French patient. In addition, as of the time of this writing and to the best of the author's knowledge, there have been five mortalities associated with facial transplantation. Two perioperative deaths occurred when combined VCA face + upper extremity was attempted. One case of mortal tumor recurrence in an HIV + recipient, one case of de novo posttransplant lung cancer, and one case due to noncompliance, resulting in an 86% patient survival rate after face transplantation. Other known risks include the development of systemic infections, metabolic complications, or the chance to develop cancer due to long-term immunosuppression.[20,21] Although technically highly demanding and the potential for serious and eventually life-threatening complications, facial transplantation has the unique potential to restore patients to normalcy and save them from social death. There is a clear indication that for carefully selected patients, facial transplantation offers a procedure that, although not lifesaving, is potentially life restoring.

OTHER AREAS AND LATEST DEVELOPMENTS IN RECONSTRUCTIVE TRANSPLANTATION

Developments in reconstructive transplantation have clearly been led by upper extremity and facial transplantation. However, there have been smaller series of patients treated with transplantation of several other composite structures including vascularized knee joints, lower extremities, trachea, larynx, abdominal wall, and reproductive organs. With the exception of vascularized knee joints (which have failed in five of the six patients attempted owing to chronic vascular complications), reconstruction with these varied types of transplants has met with some qualified success. Although these less common types of transplants continue to be highly experimental, they demonstrate the possibilities that reconstructive transplantation offers. Traditional plastic surgery techniques are unable to restore complex tissues and anatomical structures with the fidelity equal to that of reconstructive transplantation as evidenced by recipients' functional and aesthetic outcomes.

Uterus Transplantation

Given the highly encouraging outcomes seen in upper extremity and face transplantation, indications for VCA to reconstruct other devastating tissue defects or organ losses are rapidly expanding. One such example is uterus transplantation, which has now emerged as the first therapy for women with absolute uterine factor infertility, who have traditionally been regarded as unconditionally infertile. Two isolated cases of uterine transplantation were reported in 2000 and 2011 by teams in Saudi Arabia and in Turkey. Although both surgeries were initially successful, the first patient lost the graft at 3 months due to uterine artery thrombosis and the second patient suffered two early miscarriages after embryo transfer. In 2014, a team in Sweden reported the first birth of a child to a uterine transplant recipient, who had undergone single embryo transfer 1 year after transplantation.[46] Several more successful live births have been reported since then from the nine women who have entered this initial Swedish trial. The field of uterus transplantation is expanding at a staggering pace, with active centers being established all around the world. At least 10 new clinical trials have just started or are in the process to start as of 2018.

Of note, uterine transplantation represents the first *ephemeral* type of transplantation.[47] As hysterectomy can be performed after successful pregnancy, concerns about long-term side effects from immunosuppression would not apply. Although uterus transplantation has been shown to be a highly effective and successful treatment for absolute uterine factor infertility, it also raises a series of ethical questions. For instance, Huet et al. reviewed potential candidates for transplantation: some presented with complete androgen insensitivity syndrome.[48] These patients are phenotypically and psychosocially female but genetically male; the question that has been posed was should they be considered eligible? This question can further be extended to transgender individuals and will require further sensitive discussion.

Penile Transplantation

Penile transplantation is another emerging option for patients with severe genital defects not amenable to traditional reconstructive techniques.[49] Patients with penile defects frequently suffer from debilitating physical and psychosocial impairments, including inability to have sexual intercourse or urinate while standing, feelings of emasculation, disruption of interpersonal relationships, and profound loss of quality of life. Although traditional phalloplastic reconstruction can produce satisfactory outcomes in many cases, it is limited by a high rate of complications involving prosthesis extrusion and urinary strictures and fistulae. Furthermore, there is a growing cohort of patients with traumatic penile loss and concomitant extremity injuries who are not candidates for autogenous reconstruction because they lack adequate donor sites. For patients who have either failed autogenous reconstruction or are not appropriate candidates, penile allotransplantation may offer a viable alternative.

The first penile transplant was performed in 2006 by a team in Guangzhou, China: a patient who sustained traumatic amputation received a transplant from a deceased donor. The surgery involved microsurgical anastomoses of the urethra, deep and superficial dorsal veins, dorsal arteries, and dorsal nerves, as well as of the corpus spongiosum and corpora cavernosa. Despite encouraging early results, the graft was explanted 2 weeks later at the recipient's request because of *severe psychological problem of the patient and his wife*. The second and third cases were performed in 2014 and 2016 in South Africa and in the United States, respectively. The South African patient was a 21-year-old man who suffered partial loss of his penis as a complication of ritual circumcision.[50] The Boston patient was a 64-year-old man who, 4 years earlier, underwent penectomy to treat penile squamous cell carcinoma.[51] In March 2018, a team at Johns Hopkins University performed the world's first entire penis and scrotum transplantation in a wounded warrior who had sustained a devastating injury several years earlier from an improvised explosive device while serving in Afghanistan. These three successful transplants provide proof of principle that penile transplantation is technically feasible with encouraging functional outcomes (urination, erogenous sensation, and erectile function) and thus constitutes a promising option for repair of extensive urogenital tissue loss. Given that penile transplantation is still in its infancy, implementing a successful penile transplantation program will require development of de novo protocols that take into account a number of important immunological, diagnostic, logistical, procedural, and ethical considerations. To maximize the utility and viability of penile transplantation as a reconstructive option, careful attention must be given to these important aspects pertaining to penile transplantation.

Novel Technologies and Future Outlook

Novel technologies such as tissue engineering and regenerative medicine will play a significant role in the future development of reconstructive transplantation. Regenerated nerves, vessels, bone, etc., will further expand indications to full arm and lower extremity and to eventually perform transplants in a more rapid, safer, and successful fashion. Along those lines, three-dimensional bioprinting could help to further optimize outcomes by enhancing the graft or advancing rehabilitation strategies and approaches currently in use for upper extremity transplantation. Ultimately, bioengineering technologies, which are currently developed in advanced prosthetic programs, could further help to improve outcomes and efforts and even augment or enhance function after VCA in the future. As clinical experience with these techniques is accumulated and immunosuppressive and immunomodulatory protocols are optimized, the risk-benefit ratio of reconstructive transplantation will continue to shift in favor of these procedures, making these techniques an increasingly available and important part of plastic surgeons' reconstructive options for treating these crippling defects.

REFERENCES

1. Guild WR, Harrison JH, Merrill JP, Murray J. Successful homotransplantation of the kidney in an identical twin. *Trans Am Clin Climatol Assoc*. 1956;67:167-173.
2. Rana A, Gruessner A, Agopian VG, et al. Survival benefit of solid-organ transplant in the United States. *JAMA Surg*. 2015;50(3):252-259.
3. Shores JT, Brandacher G, Lee WP. Hand and upper extremity transplantation: an update of outcomes in the worldwide experience. *Plast Reconstr Surg*. 2015;35(2):351e-360e.
   This review provides a comprehensive overview of the current status and outcomes after upper extremity transplantation globally.
4. Brandacher G. Composite tissue transplantation. *Methods Mol Biol*. 2013;1034:103-115.
5. Petruzzo P, Lanzetta M, Dubernard JM, et al. The International Registry on hand and composite tissue transplantation. *Transplantation*. 2010;90(12):1590-1594.
6. Fryer M, Grahammer J, Khalifian S, et al. Exploring cell-based tolerance strategies for hand and face transplantation. *Expert Rev Clin Immunol*. 2015;11(11):1189-1204.
7. Brandacher G, Lee WP, Schneeberger S. Minimizing immunosuppression in hand transplantation. *Expert Rev Clin Immunol*. 2012;(7):673-683.
8. Brandacher G, Khalifian S, Lee WPA. *Reconstructive transplantation: from scientific dream to clinical reality. The Science of Reconstructive Transplantation*. New York, NY: Humana Press; 2015.
9. Bhishagratna KL. Sushruta Samhita. Vol 1. 1907. Forgotten Books.
10. Martin C. John Hunter and tissue transplantation. *Surg Gynecol Obstet*. 1970;131(2):306.
11. Schultheiss D, Bloom DA, Wefer J, Jonas U. Tissue engineering from Adam to the zygote: historical reflections. *World J Urol*. 2000;18(1):84-90.
12. Billingham RE, Brent L, Medawar PB. Actively acquired tolerance of foreign cells. *Nature*. 1953;172(4379):603-606.
13. Merrill JP, Murray JE, Takacs FJ, et al. Successful transplantation of kidney from a human cadaver. *JAMA* 1963;185:347-353.
14. Starzl TE. History of clinical transplantation. *World J Surg*. 2000;24(7):759-782.
15. Gilbert R. Transplant is successful with a cadaver forearm. *Med Trib Med News*. 1964;5:20.
16. Jones JW Jr, Ustuner ET, Zdichavsky M, et al. Long-term survival of an extremity composite tissue allograft with FK506-mycophenolate mofetil therapy. *Surgery*. 1999;126(2):384-388.
17. Dubernard JM, Owen E, Herzberg G, et al. Human hand allograft: report on first 6 months. *Lancet*. 1999;353:1315-1320.
18. Shores JT, Malek V, Lee WPA, Brandacher G. Outcomes after hand and upper extremity transplantation. *J Mater Sci Mater Med*. 2017;(5):72.
19. Devauchelle B, Badet L, Lengele B, et al. First human face allograft: early report. *Lancet*. 2006;368(9531):203-209.
20. Khalifian S, Brazio PS, Mohan R, et al. Facial transplantation: the first 9 years. *Lancet*. 2014;384(9960):2153-2163.
21. Tasigiorgos S, Kollar B, Krezdorn N, et al. Face transplantation-current status and future developments. *Transpl Int*. 2018;(7):677-688.
   This review provides a comprehensive overview of the current status and outcomes after upper extremity transplantation globally. This review provides an excellent summary of the current status and latest developments of the field of face transplantation.
22. Strome M, Stein J, Esclamado R, et al. Laryngeal transplantation and 40-month follow-up. *N Engl J Med*. 2001;344:1676-1679.
23. Delaere P, Vranckx J, Verleden G, et al. Tracheal allotransplantation after withdrawal of immunosuppressive therapy. *N Engl J Med*. 2010;362(2):138-145.
24. Hofmann GO, Kirschner MH. Clinical experience in allogeneic vascularized bone and joint allografting. *Microsurgery*. 2000;20(8):375-383.
25. Levi DM, Tzakis AG, Kato T, et al. Transplantation of the abdominal wall. *Lancet*. 2003;361(9376):2173-2176.
26. McDiarmid SV. Donor and procurement related issues in vascularized composite allograft transplantation. *Curr Opin Organ Transpl*. 2013;(6):665-671.
27. Ali JM, Bolton EM, Bradley JA, Pettigrew GJ. Allorecognition pathways in transplant rejection and tolerance. *Transplantation*. 2013;96(8):681-688.
28. DeWolf S, Sykes M. Alloimmune T cells in transplantation. *J Clin Invest*. 2017;127(7):2473-2481.
29. Halloran PF. Immunosuppressive drugs for kidney transplantation. *N Engl J Med*. 2004;351(26):2715-2729.
30. Borges TJ, Murakami N, Riella LV. Current status of alloimmunity. *Curr Opin Nephrol Hypertens*. 2016;(6):556-562.
31. Etra JW, Raimondi G, Brandacher G. Mechanisms of rejection in vascular composite allotransplantation. *Curr Opin Organ Transpl*. 2018;(1):28-33.
32. Wiseman AC. Immunosuppressive medications. *Clin J Am Soc Nephrol*. 2016;11(2):332-343.
   An excellent overview of immunosuppressive agents in current use in transplantation and their individual mode of action.
33. Agarwal A, Ally W, Brayman K. The future direction and unmet needs of transplant immunosuppression. *Expert Rev Clin Pharmacol*. 2016;(7):873-876.
34. Schwarz C, Mahr B, Muckenhuber M, Wekerle T. Belatacept/CTLA4Ig: an update and critical appraisal of preclinical and clinical results. *Expert Rev Clin Immunol*. 2018;(7):583-592.
35. Zuber J, Sykes M. Mechanisms of mixed chimerism-based transplant tolerance. *Trends Immunol*. 2017;(11):829-843.
   A comprehensive discussion of the principles and underlying mechanisms of mixed chimerism-based tolerance induction in solid organ transplantation.
36. Mahr B, Granofszky N, Muckenhuber M, Wekerle T. Transplantation tolerance through hematopoietic chimerism: progress and challenges for clinical translation. *Front Immunol*. 2017;8:1762.
37. Vaikunthanathan T, Safinia N, Lombardi G. Optimizing regulatory T cells for therapeutic application in human organ transplantation. *Curr Opin Organ Transpl*. 2018;23(5):516-523. doi: 10.1097/MOT.0000000000000561.
38. Wendt JR, Ulich TR, Ruzics EP, Hostetler JR. Long-term survival of human skin allografts in patients with immunosuppression. *Ann Plast Surg*. 2004;113(5):411-417.
39. Mackinnon SE, Doolabh VB, Novak CB, Trulock EP. Clinical outcome following nerve allograft transplantation. *Plast Reconstr Surg*. 2001;107(6):1419-1429.
40. Howsare M, Jones CM, Ramirez AM. Immunosuppression maintenance in vascularized composite allotransplantation: what is just right? *Curr Opin Organ Transpl*. 2017;(5):463-469.
41. Schneeberger S, Khalifian S, Brandacher G. Immunosuppression and monitoring of rejection in hand transplantation. *Tech Hand Up Extrem Surg*. 2013;17(4):208-214.
42. Kueckelhaus M, Fischer S, Seyda M, et al. Vascularized composite allotransplantation: current standards and novel approaches to prevent acute rejection and chronic allograft deterioration. *Transpl Int*. 2016;(6):655-662.
43. Cetrulo CL Jr, Drijkoningen T, Sachs DH. Tolerance induction via mixed chimerism in vascularized composite allotransplantation: is it time for clinical application? *Curr Opin Organ Transplant*. 2015;(6):602-607.
44. Vyas KS, Mohan AT, Morrison SD, et al. Cell-based therapies in vascularized composite allotransplantation. *J Reconstr Microsurg*. 2018;34(8):642-650. doi:10.1055/s-0038-1661336.
45. Giatsidis G, Sinha I, Pomahac B. Reflections on a decade of face transplantation. *Ann Surg*. 2017;5(4):841-846.
46. Brännström M, Johannesson L, Bokström H, et al. Livebirth after uterus transplantation. *Lancet*. 2015;385(9968):607-616.
   Seminal report of the pioneering efforts and the first livebirth after uterus transplantation.
47. Brännström M. Womb transplants with live births: an update and the future. *Expert Opin Biol Ther*. 2017;17:1105-1112.
48. Huet S, Tardieu A, Filloux M, et al. Uterus transplantation in France: for which patients? *Eur J Obstet Gynecol Reprod Biol*. 2016;205:7-10.
49. Tuffaha SH, Cooney DS, Sopko NA, et al. Penile transplantation: an emerging option for genitourinary reconstruction. *Transpl Int*. 2017;(5):441-450.
50. van der Merwe A, Graewe F, Zühlke A, et al. Penile allotransplantation for penis amputation following ritual circumcision: a case report with 24 months of follow-up. *Lancet*. 2017;390(10099):1038-1047.
   Seminal report of the first successful penis allotransplanation.
51. Cetrulo CL Jr, Li K, Salinas HM, et al. Penis transplantation: first US experience. *Ann Surg*. 2018;7(5):983-988.

QUESTIONS

1. **Which of the following immunosuppressive agents belongs to the class of CNIs?**
   a. Rapamycin
   b. Belatacept
   c. Tacrolimus
   d. Thymoglobulin

2. **The initiation of an alloimmune response is a well-orchestrated and choreographed interplay of various different players of the immune system. Alloreactive T cells require three distinct signals for full activation. What constitutes signal 2?**
   a. The NF-κB pathway
   b. Costimulatory pathways (B7-CD28, CD40-CD154)
   c. The interaction of MHC and TCR
   d. None of the above

3. **What cell type is predominantly driving an acute alloimmune response?**
   a. B cells
   b. Macrophages
   c. T regulatory cells
   d. CD4+ and CD8+ T cells
   e. DCs

4. **Most upper extremity and face transplant patients experience episodes of acute rejection during the first year post transplant. In which tissue component of the graft does acute rejection predominately manifest in VCA?**
   a. Muscle
   b. Vasculature
   c. Bone
   d. Skin
   e. Nerves

5. **Technical limitations with regard to the feasibility of performing vascular anastomosis have hampered the development of organ transplantation for centuries. This obstacle was finally overcome when which surgeon introduced his vascular anastomosis technique?**
   a. Joseph E. Murray
   b. Alexis Carrel
   c. Giuseppe Baronio
   d. Gaspare Tagliacozzi
   e. Thomas E. Starzl

1. **Answer: c.** Tacrolimus and CsA are CNIs and are the most widely used maintenance immunosuppressive agents for both solid organ and reconstructive transplantation. Both agents inhibit the calcineurin/IL-2 pathway of T cell activation and due to their potent immunosuppressive activity have revolutionized the field of solid organ transplantation by significantly increasing survival of kidney, heart, and liver allografts in the 80s and 90s. Belatacept is a biologic agent (monoclonal antibody CTLA-Ig) and inhibits the costimulatory signal B7-CD28. Rapamycin is an mTOR inhibitor and acts downstream of signal 3 inhibiting the response to IL-2. Thymoglobulin is a polyclonal antithymocyte antibody primarily used as induction agent to deplete peripheral blood lymphocytes through antibody-dependent cell-mediated cytotoxicity.

2. **Answer: b.** In addition to signal 1, APCs provide so called costimulatory signals to fully active T cells. These costimulatory signals are also referred to as signal 2 during T cell activation. Two of the best-characterized costimulatory signals/pathways in transplantation are the B7/CD28 and the CD40/CD154 pathways. The NF-κB pathway is activated as part of the intracellular signal transduction cascade referred to as signal 3 during T cell activation. Within the secondary lymph nodes, T cells encounter the MHC alloantigen that is expressed on the surface of the DCs with their specific TTCRs combined with the CD3 complex that facilitates signal transduction. This interaction of MHC, TCR, and CD3 complex is referred to as signal 1.

3. **Answer: d.** The primary mediators of acute rejection episodes are CD4+ and CD8+ T cells that upon activation infiltrate the graft and lead to inflammatory damage and parenchymal tissue necrosis. B cells are involved in the production of donor-specific antibodies and late antibody-mediated rejection. These antibodies bind to endothelial cells and activate the complement cascade, which in turn leads to deposition of complement factors C3d and C4d that trigger endothelial inflammation and cellular infiltration resulting in vascular damage and occlusion. T regulatory cells (CD4+CD25+Foxp3+ T regs) play a key role in the maintenance of peripheral tolerance to both self- and foreign antigens. DCs are key players in the initiation of an alloimmune response and serve as APCs to T cells but do not have effector function. Macrophages contribute to both the innate and acquired arms of the alloimmune response and play pluripotent roles during allograft rejection. They can induce allograft injury but, conversely, can also promote tissue repair in ischemia-reperfusion injury and acute rejection.

4. **Answer: d.** Acute rejection remains a considerable challenge in reconstructive transplantation. Notably, 85% of all hand, upper extremity, and face allograft recipients have experienced at least one episode of acute rejection within the first year after transplant, and as much as 56% experienced multiple episodes. The skin is the most antigenic component of a vascularized composite allograft and thus represents the primary manifestation of acute rejection. The high antigenicity of the skin can in part be related to the high proportion of potent APCs (Langerhans cells) and keratinocytes which express MHC I constitutively and MHC II, ICAM-I, and proinflammatory cytokines upon stimulation. Skin rejection usually manifests clinically with maculopapular skin lesions restricted to small areas or spread over the whole allograft, varying in color and location and presenting with or without edema. While skin rejection is most frequently observed after human hand and face allotransplantation, an immune response toward tissues other than the skin such as muscle, nerves, and bone has been documented, however, to a much lesser extend and usually only during very advanced stages of untreated rejection. More recent findings, furthermore, indicate that also the vasculature of the graft may be affected and proliferation of the myointima can occur as a sign of chronic rejection.

5. **Answer: b.** The obstacle of vascular anastomosis was overcome in 1902 when Alexis Carrel introduced his vascular anastomosis technique, which unlocked a continuum of research in experimental organ transplantation. Within the same year, Austrian surgeon Emerich Ullmann performed the first experimental kidney transplantation in animals in Vienna. Dr. Joseph E. Murray performed the first successful living-related kidney transplantation between identical twins in 1954 and was awarded the Nobel Prize for this pioneering effort in 1990. Giuseppe Baronio's (1758–1814) contributions are considered fundamental to the field of plastic surgery, and he laid the groundwork for research in the fields of both skin grafting and transplant immunology. Gaspare Tagliacozzi was a surgeon in the 16th century who emerged as a popular figure in transplantation and was a specialist in rhinoplasty. Thomas E. Starzl performed the first human liver transplant in 1967 at the University of Colorado in Denver and has often been referred to as ***the father of modern transplantation***.

CHAPTER 9 Principles of Prosthetics in Plastic Surgery

Ara A. Salibian and Ernest S. Chiu

KEY POINTS

- Prosthetics, when used appropriately, can successfully provide a variety of restorative functions including permanent reconstruction of osseous and soft tissue defects, reinforcement of complex wound closures, stabilization of bony discontinuities, optimization of autologous tissue for reconstruction, and augmentation of aesthetic features.
- The ideal prosthetic should minimize foreign body reactions, incorporate into the surrounding tissues, resist infection, retain its shape, easily be implanted and manipulated, and be permanent.
- Implantation of prosthetics requires strict sterile technique, minimization of handling by multiple personnel, use of antibiotic solutions, and limitation of contact with skin or other potential sources of infection.
- Facial prosthetics can provide excellent cosmetic results, alone or in combination with autologous techniques for skeletal augmentation as well as bony and soft tissue reconstruction with the appropriate implant choice, incision design with respect for aesthetic subunits, and proper implant placement in the subperiosteal plane.
- Success with temporary implants for tissue expansion relies on good soft tissue coverage, appropriate implant shape and position, controlled expansion, patient counseling, and patience.
- The use of prosthetics for skeletal and soft tissue augmentation requires balancing the requests of the patient with the surgeon's understanding of what is medically appropriate for each individual patient.
- The most common complications with prosthetics are infection and extrusion, which can be minimized by adherence to the aforementioned principles but must be addressed promptly if present for eventual reconstructive salvage.
- A thorough preoperative discussion of the potential risks of prosthetics is crucial, including the need for explantation as well as other rare and serious complications such as implant-associated neoplasm.

BACKGROUND

Prosthetics are a subset of biomaterials or substances used to support, augment, or replace a particular tissue or group of tissues of function in the body.[1] Prosthetics have a variety of critical functions as an adjunct to or a replacement of autologous methods of reconstruction and augmentation. Lack of availability of adequate autologous material for reconstruction may require the use of synthetic compounds. At other times, an implant can enhance the reconstructive capabilities of autologous tissue, as with mechanical and biologic creep,[2,3] or can support the healing of autologous structures, as with titanium internal fixation of fractures. Implants can also be used in aesthetic surgery to augment the appearance of the facial skeleton, or enhance volume and soft tissue contours throughout the body.

The utilization of prosthetic implants requires adherence to basic guidelines, many of which parallel general plastic surgery principles. All implants should be meticulously handled using strict sterile technique and limited contact with personnel, skin and external surfaces. Implantation requires creation of an adequate pocket in the appropriate tissue planes that provides a well-vascularized environment to prevent infection and extrusion and minimize palpability and visibility. Along the same lines, infected, irradiated, and poorly vascularized tissue must be avoided.

The ideal prosthetic implant has long been sought after and unfortunately has still not been developed. There is a commonality of important characteristics to minimize complications from prosthetics and maximize their benefits. These central traits were outlined by Cumberland[4] and Scales[5] in the 1950s. They can be summarized as principles pertaining to the utility of an implant such as its ability to be adaptable but still resist mechanical strain as well as requirements for safety and compatibility such as minimizing inflammation and cellular foreign body responses (**Table 9.1**). Considering these characteristics when determining the need for a prosthetic can help guide the appropriate utilization of implants.

HISTORY

The search for adequate replacements of damaged or missing bodily structures is not a recent phenomenon. Implantable materials have been traced back to the use of suture over 32,000 years ago and later to the ancient Egyptians.[6] Dental fillings made of beeswax have been found in Neolithic mandibles that are 6500 years old.[7] Trephination defects from Peru dating to 3000 BC have been found to be filled with various materials from gold and silver to shells.[8]

Limitations of early prosthetic implantation were several, and included the nature of materials utilized as well as the handling of these items that would inevitably lead to breakdown, infection and failure. The concept of aseptic technique, introduced in the 19th century,[9] was a critical scientific advancement for the successful utilization of implants. The development of radiography in the late 19th century[10] was also a major milestone, as many of the initial modern implants consisted of metal internal fixation hardware for fractures since introduced in 1895.[11]

The 20th century marked the transition from the reliance on natural materials for implants to the development of metal alloys, ceramics, and polymers. The infamous accidental discovery of the suitability

TABLE 9.1. CHARACTERISTICS OF IDEAL PROSTHETIC IMPLANTS[4,5]
■ Allow for tissue ingrowth
■ Nonallergenic
■ Noncarcinogenic
■ Sterilizable
■ Permanence (when indicated)
■ Minimize foreign body reaction
■ High tolerance for mechanical stress
■ Easily fabricated at low cost
■ Adaptable
■ Easy to manipulate and handle
■ Resistant to infection

of a plastic polymer as a prosthetic after the traumatic implantation of the material led Harold Ridley to utilize PMMA for artificial lenses in 1949.[6] Soon thereafter Arthur Voorhees used fabric grafts to develop arterial prostheses,[12] and Cumberland described nylon mesh for ventral hernia.[4] Major strides continued in the mid-20th century as scientists worked to improve the applicability and biocompatibility of implants, an effort that persists today.

THE FOREIGN BODY RESPONSE

The foreign body reaction is the body's immunologic response to implantation of a nonhost material. The reaction is mediated by a cascade of molecular factors initiated by platelets, fibrinogen, and complement proteins that results in a chronic inflammatory state with the recruitment of macrophages, the formation of foreign body giant cells, and the persistence of inflammation and eventually fibrosis.[13] The extent of this response is influenced by the nature of the implant.

Biocompatibility of an implanted prosthetic characterizes the ability of the device to coexist within the host. This concept has migrated away from describing an inert material in isolation from the body to representing a mutual but favorable interaction between the implant and the host. With regard to implantable devices, biocompatibility can be redefined as the *ability of the device to perform its intended function, with the desired degree of incorporation in the host, without eliciting any undesirable local or systemic effects in that host.*[1]

The long-term implications of the foreign body response can be practically divided into two end points: fibrous encapsulation versus tissue incorporation. Fibrous encapsulation of an implant results in a dense scar plate around the foreign, whereas tissue incorporation results in more random extracellular matrix deposition, cellular infiltration, and neovascularization.[14] The characteristics of a particular implant, such as pore size, can significantly impact which pathway predominates.[15] Macroporous mesh will allow tissue to cross pores and promote mesh incorporation whereas microporous mesh prevents cell migration and results in mesh encapsulation.

IMPLANT MATERIALS

Different prosthetic materials have different reconstructive implications with regard to physical properties, interaction with the surrounding tissues, management of complications, and long-term retention. Although many different implant materials have been used historically, this review will summarize only the most commonly used synthetic materials (**Table 9.2**).

TABLE 9.2. COMMON PROSTHETIC IMPLANT MATERIALS

Metals
Stainless steel
Titanium
Gold
Platinum
Ceramics
Hydroxyapatite
Tricalcium phosphate
Calcium phosphate cement
Polymers
Polyester
Polyethylene
PMMA
Polypropylene
Expanded polytetrafluoroethylene
Polyurethane urea
Silicone
Biodegradable polymers

Metals

Initial metal implants, typically for fracture fixation, suffered from corrosion.[11] It was not until the refinement of different combination of metals, or alloys that promoted the more widespread applicability of metal implants. Key characteristics of biocompatible metal implants include nontoxicity, resistance to corrosion, ability to osseointegrate (when needed), appropriate mechanical properties and high wear resistance, or resistance to loss of surface material secondary to mechanical forces.[16]

Stainless Steel

Stainless steel refers to a number of iron-based alloys that usually contain a high percentage of chromium and varying amounts of nickel. Stainless steel has a high tensile strength and elastic modulus as well as low cost and was one of the earlier alloys to be utilized for medical implants. Stainless steel, however, is limited by its poor resistance to fatigue as well as corrosion, which has resulted in premature failure of these implants. Stainless steel also has poor wear resistance that results in debris that can induce inflammation and allergic reactions. In addition, leaching of nickel and chromium from the alloy has been shown to be toxic. These characteristics limit the utility of this alloy in long-term applications. Currently, stainless steel is most often used for temporary implants such as surgical wires and arch bars for maxillomandibular fixation.

Titanium

Titanium is utilized as a pure low-density chemical element or a stronger but less malleable alloy usually combined with aluminum and vanadium. This alloy was developed more recently and has replaced many of its prior counterparts such as stainless steel and vitallium. The most important properties of titanium include its low density, high strength-to-density ratio, inert character, and high resistance to corrosion secondary to formation of a protective stable oxide layer.[17] It is therefore considered to be the most biocompatible of metals, which has led to its widespread use in implantable medical devices.

Titanium also has a lower modulus of elasticity than stainless steel and cobalt-chromium alloys.[16] This modulus more closely matches that of bone and therefore decreases stress shielding, allowing for more loading of bone. Titanium integrates with bone without formation of an intervening fibrous capsule, which allows it to be used for osseointegrated implants. Furthermore, titanium is nonferromagnetic and therefore does not preclude patients from undergoing magnetic resonance imaging. In the realm of plastic surgery, titanium is primarily utilized for osteosynthesis plates and screws (**Figure 9.1**), maxillofacial implants, and cranioplasty.

Gold

Gold has been used for medicinal purpose since ancient civilization. It is a useful metal implant owing to its resistance to corrosion and nontoxic and highly inert character. Pure gold does not react with any known substances in the body. Although gold is very malleable, it lacks strength, limiting its applications. The most common use of gold implants is for upper eyelid weight in the treatment of lagophthalmos secondary to facial nerve palsy. These implants typically are purer 24-carat gold alloys to maximize nonreactivity and biocompatibility.

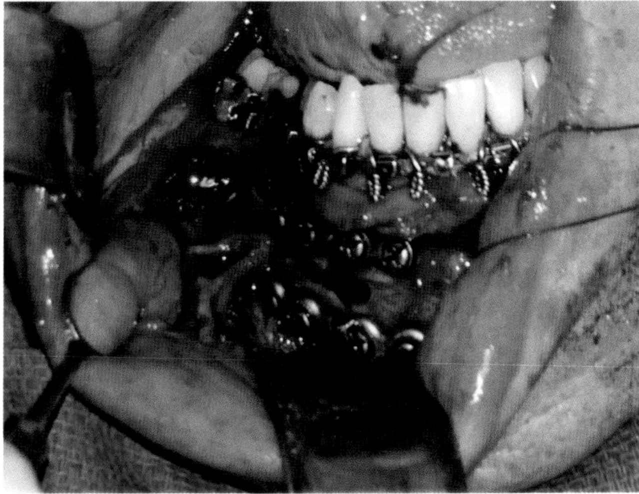

FIGURE 9.1. Titanium mandible plate and mini-plate with screws to provide rigid fixation of a comminuted parasymphyseal fracture. Also pictured are stainless steel arch bars and wire for placement in temporary maxillomandibular fixation.

Platinum

Platinum is a dense and malleable chemical element. Plastic Surgery applications are primarily for eyelid weights for treatment of paralytic lagophthalmos. The higher density of platinum than gold allows for the use of smaller, lower profile implants. The high malleability of platinum is also beneficial when molding of an implant is needed. Platinum is also used in the cross-linking of medical-grade silicone or poly(dimethylsiloxane) (PDMS) in silicone breast implants.

Calcium Ceramics

Ceramics are inorganic compounds with a spectrum of crystalline structures. The most commonly used ceramic implants in plastic surgery are calcium phosphate–based ceramics typically utilized as alloplastic bone substitutes. These materials are typically porous, allowing for tissue ingrowth and osteoconductive. A critical limitation of the widespread application of calcium phosphates is their mechanical properties. These cements have low impact resistance and low tensile strength and are brittle, limiting their use in any load-bearing areas. They are therefore typically used for reconstruction, and less so, augmentation of the craniofacial skeleton. The most common ceramics are hydroxyapatite, $Ca_{10}(PO_4)_6(OH)_2$; tricalcium phosphate, $Ca_3(PO_4)_2$; and derivatives of calcium phosphate cement pastes.

Hydroxyapatite

Hydroxyapatite is formed from naturally occurring calcium carbonate coral and has organized porous channels. It is available in particulate and block forms that can be carved to fit a cranioplasty defect, as well as bone cement pastes that set isothermally and have decreased radiologic scatter. These cement pastes (Mimix [Walter Lorenz Surgical, Inc., Jacksonville, FL]; BoneSource [Stryker Leibinger, Portage, MI]) have been widely use in craniofacial reconstruction, usually for cranioplasty[18,19] but also for interpositional bone grafts in orthognathic surgery. Hydroxyapatite is osteoconductive, but as a microporous cement, direct bony and vascular ingrowth is limited, and bony replacement tends to occur by resorption and turnover of hydroxyapatite to bone at the periphery of the implant.

Tricalcium Phosphate

Tricalcium phosphate is a synthetic, porous ceramic that, like hydroxyapatite, provides a scaffold for tissue ingrowth. It has more random pore structure and is more quickly resorbed and replaced by bone than hydroxyapatite. It is also available both in block and particulate form.

Carbonated Calcium Phosphate Cement

Carbonated calcium phosphate pastes have also been developed from calcium phosphate and calcium carbonate. Dahllite, a carbonated apatite (Norian Cranial Repair System, Synthes, Paoli, PA), has higher tensile and compressive strength and a composition that closely resembles bone.[20] This carbonated apatite cement has been shown to have a greater resistance to fracture when compared with hydroxyapatite cement products.[21] The solubility of dahllite at a lower pH has been suggested to increase resorption and replacement by natural bone.

Polymers

Polymers are a broad category of synthetic and naturally occurring macromolecules that are composed of repeating subunits. Unlike metals and ceramics, they have widespread indications in both hard and soft tissue reconstruction and augmentation. There are a wide variety of different polymers used as prosthetic implants; the most common synthetic materials are covered here.

Polyester

Polyesters are polymers containing an esther group and usually refer to the compound polyethylene terephthalate. This material is a high-molecular-weight polymer that is primarily used as knitted mesh such as Mersilene mesh (Ethicon, Inc., Somerville, NJ) for hernia repair. Mersilene is a nonabsorbable mesh with high tensile strength that allows for tissue ingrowth and has also been used for chin and nasal augmentation. Certain polyesters such as poly-4-hydroxybutyrate are bioderived, in that they are produced by microorganisms and have been used in biodegradable mesh products such as Phasix (Bard Davol, Warwick, RI).[22]

Polyethylene

Polyethylene is the most commonly produced plastic. There are multiple different types of this polymer differentiated primarily by their density and branching. The molecular weight of polyethylene influences its mechanical properties, which can range from 40,000 daltons (low density) resulting in a ductile material used for bags, to ultra-high-molecular-weight polyethylene (2–6 million daltons) used for orthopedic hip implants. Importantly, the material is inert and has low tissue reactivity and long-term structural stability when used as implants.

Polyethylene implants are typically used for facial reconstruction and augmentation. These are usually high-density porous implants (e.g., Medpor, Stryker, Kalamazoo, MI), which permit vascularization as well as soft tissue and bony ingrowth with pore sizes ranging from 100 to 250 μm in diameter.[23] This porosity results in incorporation of the implant and prevention of migration, though simultaneously makes incorporated implants difficult to remove. High-density porous polyethylene implants are utilized in cranioplasty, ear reconstruction, and orbital implants as well as reconstruction and augmentation of the mandible, malar eminence, nose, and frontal bone among others areas.[24] Complications with these implants include infection, exposure, extrusion, and visibility, which are highly reliant on the vascularity of the surrounding tissues and the placement technique.[25]

PMMA

PMMA is a nondegradable acrylic resin formed by mixing liquid methyl methacrylate monomer with the accelerator, PMMA powder. The resulting strong but light high-molecular-weight polymer is chemically inert, rigid, nonconductive, and easily handled. The material is not porous, and therefore does not allow of tissue ingrowth and osteoconduction when utilized on its own. PMMA is most commonly used for cranioplasty owing to its rigidity and lack of significant movement or mechanical stress in this region.[26] This material can be molded in situ or can be preformed as a custom implant. PMMA is also used for stabilization of chest wall. It can be added to or sandwiched between mesh reinforcement for some tissue incorporation and durability.

A significant exothermic reaction occurs during curing of PMMA that can reach temperatures of 40 to 56°C. Active cooling of the surrounding tissues with saline is therefore required to prevent thermal tissue necrosis. Furthermore, curing in vivo can results in a small amount of shrinkage that must be accounted for and can also release the unbound monomer systemically, which is toxic.

Polypropylene

Polypropylene is similar to the chemical structure of polyethylene but with the inclusion of a methyl group. Polypropylene is most widely used as a high-tensile, nonabsorbable suture and mesh. Polypropylene mesh is typically used for bridging repair of fascial defects or reinforcements of hernia repairs as well as chest wall reconstruction. These meshes are macroporous and therefore allow for tissue ingrowth, but also can have an increased risk of adhesions if placed intraperitoneally.

Expanded Polytetrafluoroethylene

Expanded polytetrafluoroethylene (ePTFE) or Gore-Tex (W.L. Gore, Flagstaff, AZ) is created by expanding a linear polymer of fluorine and carbon molecules to create a microporous structure. ePTFE is a modification of PTFE that is a more lightweight and pliable material with good biocompatibility, a high strength-to-weight ratio, and a similarly low coefficient of friction. Owing to its microporous structure, the material has significantly less tissue ingrowth compared with macroporous mesh and a higher propensity for encapsulation.[14]

ePTFE products have a variety of applications in plastic surgery. Woven microporous meshes are used in abdominal and chest wall reconstruction. Solid blocks can be carved and adapted for volume restoration in facial reconstruction and augmentation such as with malar, chin, and nasal implants.

Polyurethane Urea

Polyurethane urea is a multiblock copolymer with good mechanical properties and biocompatibility. These polymers have been modified to form slow-degrading, filament-based meshes that serve as scaffolds for tissue ingrowth. The Artelon CMC Spacer (Artimplant, Vastra Frolunda, Sweden) is a fabric of the polymer designed for interposition between the metacarpal and trapezium for treatment of basal joint arthritis by stabilizing the carpometacarpal joint by augmentation of the capsule and joint resurfacing.[27]

Silicone

Medical-grade silicone is formed from PDMS, a polymer of organosilicone. Silicone is biologically inert, does not dissolve in the environment found within the body, and is nontoxic. The mechanical properties of silicone, most practically its viscosity, are altered by changing the length of the polymer and its molecular weight. Cross-linking of PDMS chains has also become a clinically useful chemical alteration that creates a firmer gel used for form-stable, highly cohesive implants.

Silicone is a widely used material across multiple different specialties in medicine and is used as components of thousands of medical products. Short polymer chains of PDMS result in a low-viscosity liquid form of silicone. Liquid silicone has been used extensively as a soft tissue filler but causes several adverse effects including ulceration, cellulitis, abscesses, foreign body migration, and granulomas.[28] Liquid silicone injections are not Food and Drug Administration approved and must be avoided.

The polymerization of Dimethyl sulfoxide into longer chains is used to form silicone gels for implants. Silicone has had a tumultuous past in the field of Plastic Surgery owing to the temporary restriction on silicone gel implants by the Food and Drug Administration over concerns on toxicity and association with connective tissue disease in 1992. Since then, however, studies have demonstrated the safety of silicone breast implants with regard to a lack of toxicity and association with connective tissue disease[29] with a cessation of the ban in 2006. Silicone implants are now utilized for a wide spectrum of indications in Plastic Surgery including breast reconstruction, breast augmentation, facial reconstruction and augmentation, ear reconstruction, gluteal augmentation, and joint and flexor tendon reconstruction.

Because silicone implants are not porous, they become encapsulated with scar tissue. This foreign body reaction can have significant consequences for the long-term implications of silicone implants as fibrosis, and encapsulation can result in contracture of surrounding tissues, aesthetic distortion, and pain.

Biodegradable Polymers

Biodegradable polymers are designed to break down into natural byproducts such as water and carbon dioxide. The most common biodegradable polymers include poly (lactic acid), poly (glycolic acid) (PGA), and poly (lactic-co-glycolic acid), which are degraded into lactic or glycolic acid.

Formulations of these materials and their combinations, such as Vicryl mesh (Polyglactin 910; Ethicon, Inc., Somerville, NJ) are used for support in abdominal and chest wall reconstruction as well as breast reconstruction. Biodegradable plates and screws consist of similar polymers and are useful in craniofacial surgery and fracture fixation in pediatric patients in whom bone growth limits the use of permanent devices.[30] Other devices such as biodegradable suture anchors (e.g., Endotine, Coapt Systems, Inc., Palo Alto, CA) consist of a mix of poly (lactic acid) and PGA.

INDICATIONS BY BODY REGION

Prosthetic implants have a wide range of indications for both reconstructive and aesthetic purposes. The following sections summarize the most common uses of prosthetic implants in plastic surgery by body region and indication (**Table 9.3**).

Facial Reconstruction

Bony Skeleton

Osteosynthesis of the facial skeleton is usually performed with different titanium hardware consisting of load-bearing and load-sharing plates, secured with screws to provide rigid or semirigid fixation. In the setting of pediatric reconstruction, hardware composed of biodegradable polymers may be chosen for facial growth without having to remove hardware. Temporary implants in the form of internal and external titanium distraction devices are also commonly used in craniofacial surgery for manipulation of the skeleton after osteotomies.

Implants to restore the devoid facial skeleton are commonly used in orbital blowout fractures to reconstruct the orbital floor. These implants usually consist of titanium, porous polyethylene, or a combination of both and can be custom fabricated to the individual defect. A variety of other implants, typically porous polyethylene, can also be used to restore bony contours in the face such as the mandible, malar eminence, and zygoma.[24] These implants are placed in the subperiosteal plane to prevent disruption of the overlying structures, visualize skeletal contours, maximize soft tissue coverage, and ensure a well-vascularized environment.

Ear

Reconstruction of the cartilaginous framework of the ear is most commonly required for defects and malformations secondary to anotia, microtia, and trauma such as burns. Cited benefits of

TABLE 9.3. COMMON PROSTHETIC IMPLANT INDICATIONS AND MATERIALS IN PLASTIC SURGERY

Facial Reconstruction
Skeletal reconstruction (titanium, porous polyethylene, ePTFE, silicone)
Osteosynthesis hardware (titanium, biodegradable polymers)
Arch bars (stainless steel)
Ear reconstruction (polyethylene, silicone)
Eyelid weights (gold, platinum)
Facial Augmentation
Solid implants (porous polyethylene, ePTFE, silicone)
Mesh (polyester)
Anchoring devices (titanium, biodegradable polymers)
Calvarial Reconstruction
Osteosynthesis hardware (titanium, biodegradable polymers)
Cranioplasty (titanium, calcium phosphate ceramics, PMMA, polyethylene)
Breast Reconstruction and Augmentation
Breast implants (silicone)
Tissue expanders (silicone)
Support scaffolds (titanium, biodegradable polymers)
Chest Wall Reconstruction
Mesh (polypropylene, ePTFE, polyglycolic acid, biodegradable polymers)
Rigid reconstruction (PMMA)
Abdominal wall reconstruction
Mesh (polyester, polypropylene, ePTFE, biodegradable polymers)
Lower Extremity
Gluteal implants (silicone)
Hand
Osteosynthesis hardware (titanium, stainless steel)
Joint replacement (polyurethane urea, silicone, pyrolytic carbon, polyethylene)
Tendon reconstruction (polyester/silicone)
Skin
Tissue expanders (silicone)

ePTFE, expanded polytetrafluoroethylene.

alloplastic reconstruction include limitless material, age independence, decreased patient discomfort, and improved ear definition.[31] Moldable implants usually consist of porous polyethylene, which have been revolutionized by the utilization of a temporoparietal fascial flap to provide well-vascularized coverage of the implant and minimize complications of infection and extrusion.

Eyelid

Eyelid weights are commonly used for treatment of paralytic lagophthalmos secondary to facial nerve palsy. Original implants were stainless steel,[32] which were later replaced with gold[33] and platinum. The implant is typically placed in a pocket deep to the orbicularis oculi and can be secured to the tarsal plate, without disrupting the insertion of the levator apparatus. Complications include implant migration, extrusion, skin ulceration, capsule formation, implant visibility, over/undercorrection, and infection. Platinum has been suggested to be superior, as its higher density allows for a smaller, thinner profile implant, with potentially lower rates of extrusion.[34]

Facial Augmentation

Aesthetic augmentation of the facial skeleton is typically performed with alloplastic prosthetic implants. Similar to reconstruction, implants are fixated to the underlying bone in the subperiosteal plane to minimize injury to nerves and directly visualize bony contours. The most common implants are porous polyethylene, ePTFE, and silicone; the last does not allow for tissue ingrowth and heals with fibrous encapsulation. Common areas of augmentation include the malar eminence, infraorbital rim, and paranasal regions in the midface, as well as almost all anatomic areas of the mandible including the mentum, body, angle, and ramus.[35]

Calvarial Reconstruction

Calvarial reconstruction often utilizes titanium plates and screws for osteosynthesis of traumatic fractures or for fixation of osteotomy sites. Osteosynthesis of the skull in pediatric patients may utilize biodegradable hardware to allow for skull growth. Temporary stainless steel hardware has also been utilized in infants such as the use of stainless steel springs to promote outward expansion of the skull in sagittal craniosynostosis.[36]

Prosthetic implants have proven to be valuable in large calvarial defects given the lack of adequate autologous replacements. Alloplastic cranioplasty materials most commonly are calcium phosphate ceramics including hydroxyapatite and derivatives of calcium phosphate cement pastes. Use in large quantities in areas with potential bacterial contamination has been associated with an increased risk of complications.[37] Customizable cranial implants with both PMMA and polyethylene, as well as titanium implants, have also been described for adult cranioplasty with low major complication rates (**Figure 9.2**).[38] Preoperative radiation has been shown to be the strongest independent predictor of postoperative complications.[39]

Breast

Implants

First generation Cronin-Gerow implants from 1963 had a teardrop-shaped silicone rubber shell filled with silicone gel and a posterior Dacron patch for fixation. Subsequent generations of implants have progressively improved to provide more natural results while

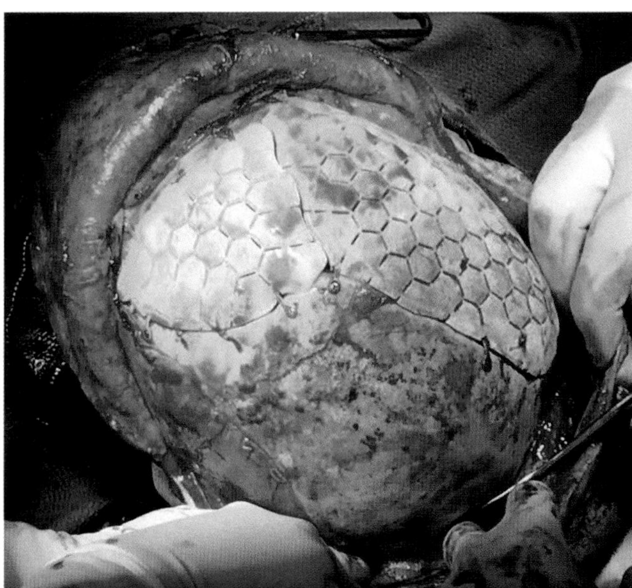

FIGURE 9.2. Cranioplasty with custom prefabricated 3D-printed implant made of titanium mesh and calcium phosphate tiles designed with virtual surgical planning (OssDsign AB, Uppsala, Sweden) and secured with titanium mini-plates.

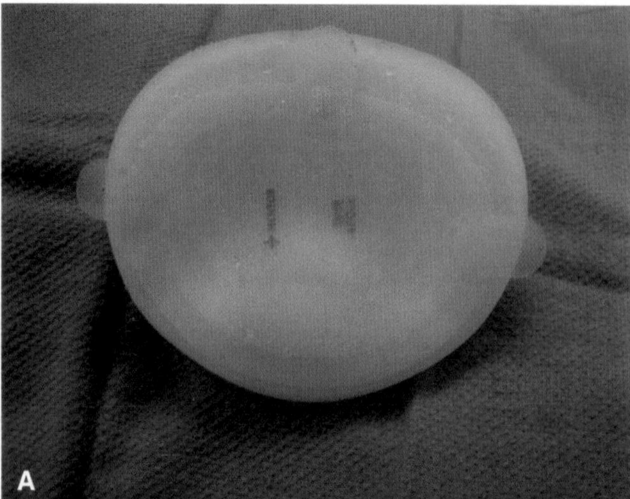

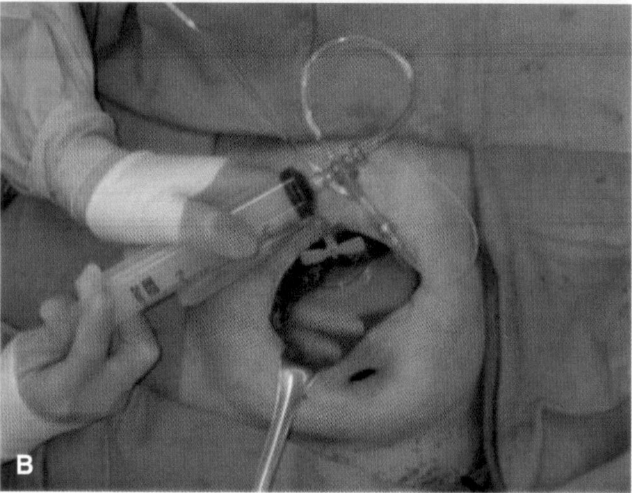

FIGURE 9.3. Tabbed tissue expander (**A**; Mentor, Irvine, CA) being filled with saline (**B**) during first stage of two-stage breast reconstruction.

minimizing complications such as silicone leakage, capsular contracture, palpability, and visibility. Modern day implants consist of an elastic silicone shell and highly cohesive silicone gel filling or a hard outer shell filled with saline (**Figure 9.3**).

Silicone implants are approved for breast augmentation in patients age 22 years or older or for breast reconstruction in women of any age. Complications of silicone breast implants include capsular contracture, infection, extrusion, rippling, double-bubble deformity, and rupture.[29] Implants with textured surfaces have lower rates of capsular contracture; however, only when placed in the subglandular and not submuscular plane.[40] Fifth generation cohesive gel implants have increased cross-linking allowing for the production of anatomic implants that retain their shape. These highly cohesive implants tend to have lower rates of contracture and rippling but higher rates of malposition and seromas.

Capsular Contracture

As silicone breast implants are not porous, the foreign body reaction to these implants is one of fibrous encapsulation. Capsular contracture is an exaggeration of this response with the immune system playing a central role believed to be triggered by multiple factors including subclinical infection and biofilm. This response can have significant clinical implications with severe cases resulting in aesthetic deformities and pain secondary to contracture, which requires total capsulectomy and implant exchange. Several risk factors have been identified including smooth implants, periareolar incisions, subglandular placement, and postoperative hematoma, among others.[41]

Breast Implant–Associated Anaplastic Large Cell Lymphoma

Breast implant–associated anaplastic large cell lymphoma (BIA-ALCL) is a rare T cell lymphoma associated with primarily textured breast implants.[42] Patients most commonly present with a delayed-onset seroma (>1 year) and less commonly a capsular mass. Any suspicious cases require aspiration of periprosthetic fluid and/or biopsy of masses sent for cytology, histology, flow cytometry, and CD30+ immunohistochemistry. Most localized cases have a good prognosis with complete capsulectomy and implant removal. Successful management of this disease is highly reliant on identification, treatment, and proper reporting by plastic surgeons.

Support: Polypropylene and Vicryl Mesh

Various synthetic materials have also been described to provide implant support in dual-plane reconstruction. These include polypropylene-based (TiLoop Bra [pfm medical, Köln, Germany]) and biodegradable polymer–based (Polyglactin 910 [Ethicon, Inc., Somerville, NJ]) products as cheaper alternatives to biologic materials such as acellular dermal matrix. Superiority in outcomes between biologic and synthetic products has yet to be determined in large, prospective studies.

Chest Wall

Prosthetic implants can be useful tools in reconstruction of chest wall owing to the strength, rigidity, and adaptability of certain materials to the three-dimensional contours of the thoracic cage. Proposed criteria for the need for skeletal reconstruction of the chest wall include the absence of four or more ribs or a defect greater than 5 cm in size owing to the potential for developing a flail chest.[43]

Several types of implantable materials have been utilized in chest wall reconstruction. Polypropylene meshes such as Marlex (CR Bard, Murray Hill, NJ) and Prolene (Ethicon Inc., Somerville, NJ) are commonly used for tissue ingrowth whereas ePTFE (Gore-Tex, Gore, Flagstaff, AZ) can be used to provide a watertight closure.[44] Multiple other polymers such as PGA and poly (lactic acid) serve the same purpose. PMMA can be used to create a rigid, moldable reconstruction and can be sandwiched between layers of macroporous mesh for tissue incorporation.

Abdominal Wall

Mesh plays a critical role in abdominal wall reconstruction by providing support for primary repair of the musculofascial wall or serving as a bridging material. Reinforcement of primary midline repairs with mesh has been shown to significantly decrease the rate of recurrence in ventral hernia repair in a multicenter, randomized controlled trial.[45]

Synthetic mesh materials can be divide into three categories: (1) macroporous mesh (e.g., polypropylene; **Figure 9.4**), which allows for tissue ingrowth but also has a high risk for adhesions of placed intraperitoneally; (2) microporous mesh (e.g., ePTFE), which does not have tissue-growth and heals with a capsule; and (3) composite mesh that contains an additional coating such as cellulose or collagen to decrease adhesions when placed intraperitoneally. Recently developed biosynthetic meshes are made of fully absorbable synthetic polymers (Bio-A [Gore], Phasix [Bard/Davol], TIGR [Novus Scientific]) and are aimed at providing better support of the abdominal wall than biologic matrices while still undergoing tissue ingrowth and resorption.

Lower Extremity and Gluteal Region

Augmentation

Silicone implants have been utilized for augmentation of different lower extremity structures. Gluteal augmentation with silicone implants is the most well-studied region. A variety of different

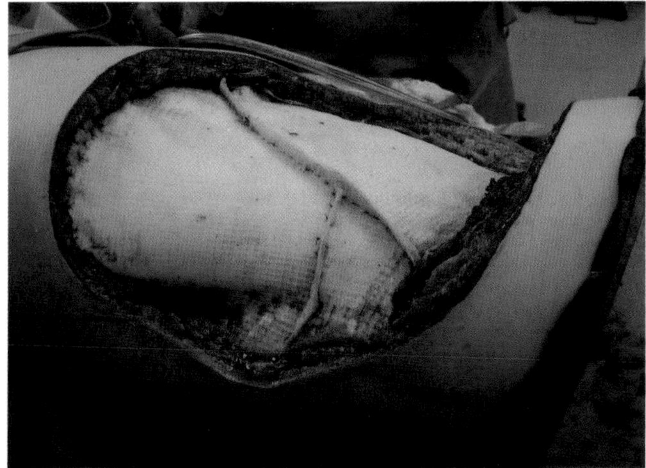

FIGURE 9.4. Abdominal reconstruction with synthetic macroporous polypropylene mesh (©Ethicon, Inc. Reproduced with permission).

placement techniques exist, usually differing in plane of placement with the most common approaches being intramuscular or subfascial implant placement.[46]

Hand

Osteosynthesis

A variety of different titanium plates and screws are available for rigid fixation of phalangeal, metacarpal, and carpal fractures. Stainless steel Kirschner wires are also frequently used in hand surgery for percutaneous pin fixation of bone fragments.

Joint Replacement

Sequelae of rheumatoid arthritis, osteoarthritis, trauma, and even infection may necessitate the replacement of joints in the hand. Arthroplasty is most often performed in the basal joint (osteoarthritis) and the metacarpophalangeal and interphalangeal joints (rheumatoid arthritis). Traditional alloplastic arthroplasty has utilized silicone joint replacement, though complications include synovitis, displacement, and giant cell reactions. Polyurethane urea joint replacements (Artelon CMC Spacer; Artimplant, Vastra Frolunda, Sweden) have also been introduced; however, evidence is still lacking on the superiority of outcomes among different materials. Other implant materials include pyrolytic carbons and polyethylene-based products.

Tendon Reconstruction

Two-stage tendon reconstruction involves the placement of temporary tendon implants. The use of a prosthetic implant overcomes the problem of a scarred tendon bed through the foreign body response to the implant that results in a well-organized pseudosheath, allowing for tendon graft gliding. These implants consist of variations silicone rods with different cores, such as polyester. Permanent tendon implants have also been described but are limited owing to unreliable fixation to the bone distally and native tendon proximally.

Skin (Tissue Expanders)

Tissue expanders are used frequently throughout the body owing to the benefits of mechanical and physiologic creep in providing adequate skin for closure of a defect. Two-stage breast reconstruction utilizes tissue expanders that consist of an outer silicone shell and internal port to allow the breast pocket to reach the appropriate size for implant placement without placing excess stress on the breast skin envelope. Other common locations for tissue expansion are the scalp, forehead, neck, and back. Tissue expansion is particularly useful in infants with lesions that have a high size-to-body surface area ratio such as congenital nevi and vascular malformations.

The success of tissue expansion relies on a thorough knowledge of appropriate incision for insertion,[47] planes of implant placement, use of correct expanders, appropriate expansion timing, design of expanded skin flaps, and management of complications. Tissue expansion often initially causes skin erythema and mottling without fever or signs of infection in which expansion should be continued. On the other hand, pain and erythema may suggest the need for fluid removal whereas fever, purulence, and signs of infection require expander removal.

FUTURE DIRECTIONS

There is still a significant need to continue to improve the characteristics of implantable prosthetics. Although creating an autologous equivalent is the standard, today's products are still by no means the *ideal* implant first outlined in the 1950s. Recent research advances in prosthetics aim at creating new materials while utilizing well-known products for different indications. As technology moves forward, research must be focused on further understanding the interaction between the implant and the host at the macroscopic and molecular level to continue to work toward optimizing the biocompatibility of implants.

REFERENCES

1. Williams DF. On the nature of biomaterials. *Biomaterials*. 2009;30:5897-5909.
2. De Filippo RE, Atala A. Stretch and growth: the molecular and physiologic influences of tissue expansion. *Plast Reconstr Surg*. 2002;109:2450-2462.
3. Cherry GW, Austad E, Pasyk K, et al. Increased survival and vascularity of random-pattern skin flaps elevated in controlled, expanded skin. *Plast Reconstr Surg*. 1983;72:680-687.
4. Cumberland VH. A preliminary report on the use of prefabricated nylon weave in the repair of ventral hernia. *Med J Aust*. 1952;1:143-144.
5. Scales JT. Tissue reactions to synthetic materials. *Proc R Soc Med*. 1953;46:647-652.
6. Ratner BD, Bryant SJ. Biomaterials: where we have been and where we are going. *Annu Rev Biomed Eng*. 2004;6:41-75.
7. Bernardini F, Tuniz C, Coppa A, et al. Beeswax as dental filling on a neolithic human tooth. *PLoS One*. 2012;7:e44904.
8. Verano JW, Andrushko VA. Cranioplasty in ancient Peru: a critical review of the evidence, and a unique case from the Cuzco area. *Int J Osteoarchaeol*. 2010;20:269-279.
9. Miller JT, Rahimi SY, Lee M. History of infection control and its contributions to the development and success of brain tumor operations. *Neurosurg Focus*. 2005;18:e4.
10. Scatliff JH, Morris PJ. From Roentgen to magnetic resonance imaging: the history of medical imaging. *N C Med J*. 2014;75:111-113.
11. Lane WA. Some remarks on the treatment of fractures. *Br Med J*. 1895;1:861-863.
12. Voorhees AB. The development of arterial prostheses. A personal view. *Arch Surg*. 1985;120:289-295.
13. Major MR, Wong VW, Nelson ER, et al. The foreign body response: at the interface of surgery and bioengineering. *Plast Reconstr Surg*. 2015;135:1489-1498.
   A review of the mechanisms behind the foreign body response to implants and the current strategies to manipulate these pathways.
14. Bellon JM, Bujan J, Contreras L, Hernando A. Integration of biomaterials implanted into abdominal wall: process of scar formation and macrophage response. *Biomaterials*. 1995;16:381-387.
15. Jordan SW, Fligor JE, Janes LE, Dumanian GA. Implant porosity and the foreign body response. *Plast Reconstr Surg*. 2018;141:103e-112e.
16. Chen Q, Thouas GA. Metallic implant biomaterials. *Mater Sci Eng R*. 2015;87:1-57.
17. Healy KE, Ducheyne P. A physical model for the titanium-tissue interface. *ASAIO Trans* 1991;37:M150-M151.
18. David L, Argenta L, Fisher D. Hydroxyapatite cement in pediatric craniofacial reconstruction. *J Craniofac Surg*. 2005;16:129-133.
19. Burstein FD, Williams JK, Hudgins R, et al. Hydroxyapatite cement in craniofacial reconstruction: experience in 150 patients. *Plast Reconstr Surg*. 2006;118:484-489.
20. Constantz BR, Ison IC, Fulmer MT, et al. Skeletal repair by in situ formation of the mineral phase of bone. *Science*. 1995;267:1796-1799.
21. Miller L, Guerra AB, Bidros RS, et al. A comparison of resistance to fracture among four commercially available forms of hydroxyapatite cement. *Ann Plast Surg*. 2005;55:87-92.
22. Deeken CR, Matthews BD. Characterization of the mechanical strength, resorption properties, and histologic characteristics of a fully absorbable material (poly-4-hydroxybutyrate-phasix mesh) in a porcine model of hernia repair. *ISRN Surg*. 2013;2013:238067.
23. Spector M, Flemming WR, Sauer BW. Early tissue infiltrate in porous polyethylene implants into bone: a scanning electron microscope study. *J Biomed Mater Res* 1975;9:537-542.

24. Yaremchuk MJ. Facial skeletal reconstruction using porous polyethylene implants. *Plast Reconstr Surg*. 2003;111:1818-1827.
25. Rubin JP, Yaremchuk MJ. Complications and toxicities of implantable biomaterials used in facial reconstructive and aesthetic surgery: a comprehensive review of the literature. *Plast Reconstr Surg*. 1997;100:1336-1353.
26. Zanotti B, Zingaretti N, Verlicchi A, et al. Cranioplasty: review of materials. *J Craniofac Surg*. 2016;27:2061-2072.
27. Nilsson A, Wiig M, Alnehill H, et al. The Artelon CMC spacer compared with tendon interposition arthroplasty. *Acta Orthop*. 2010;81:237-244.
28. Singh M, Solomon IH, Calderwood MS, Talbot SG. Silicone-induced granuloma after buttock augmentation. *Plast Reconstr Surg Glob Open*. 2016;4:e624.
29. Spear SL, Murphy DK, Allergan Silicone Breast Implant USCCSG. Natrelle round silicone breast implants: core study results at 10 years. *Plast Reconstr Surg*. 2014;133:1354-1361.
Ten-year results of Allergan core study on silicone implants used in breast reconstruction and breast augmentation. The study provides important data on rates of common complications after these procedures such as infection, malposition, capsular contracture and need for implant removal/replacement.
30. Eppley BL, Morales L, Wood R, et al. Resorbable PLLA-PGA plate and screw fixation in pediatric craniofacial surgery: clinical experience in 1883 patients. *Plast Reconstr Surg*. 2004;114:850-856; discussion 857.
31. Reinisch J, Tahiri Y. Polyethylene ear reconstruction: a state-of-the-art surgical journey. *Plast Reconstr Surg*. 2018;141:461-470.
Detailed summary of the author's evolution of technique for polyethylene ear reconstruction from experience with over 1500 patients.
32. Sheehan JE. Progress in correction of facial palsy with tantalum wire and mesh. *Surgery*. 1950;27:122-125.
33. Illig KM. A new method of lagophthalmos surgery. *Klin Monbl Augenheilkd Augenarztl Fortbild*. 1958;132:410-411.
34. Silver AL, Lindsay RW, Cheney ML, Hadlock TA. Thin-profile platinum eyelid weighting: a superior option in the paralyzed eye. *Plast Reconstr Surg*. 2009;123:1697-1703.
35. Yaremchuk MJ. Improving aesthetic outcomes after alloplastic chin augmentation. *Plast Reconstr Surg*. 2003;112:1422-1432.
36. van Veelen MC, Kamst N, Touw C, et al. Minimally invasive, spring-assisted correction of sagittal suture synostosis: technique, outcome, and complications in 83 cases. *Plast Reconstr Surg*. 2018;141:423-433.
37. Gilardino MS, Cabiling DS, Bartlett SP. Long-term follow-up experience with carbonated calcium phosphate cement (Norian) for cranioplasty in children and adults. *Plast Reconstr Surg*. 2009;123:983-994.
38. Wolff A, Santiago GF, Belzberg M, et al. Adult cranioplasty reconstruction with customized cranial implants: preferred technique, timing, and biomaterials. *J Craniofac Surg*. 2018;29(4):887-894.
39. Reddy S, Khalifian S, Flores JM, et al. Clinical outcomes in cranioplasty: risk factors and choice of reconstructive material. *Plast Reconstr Surg*. 2014;133:864-873.
40. Liu X, Zhou L, Pan F, et al. Comparison of the postoperative incidence rate of capsular contracture among different breast implants: a cumulative meta-analysis. *PLoS One*. 2015;10:e0116071.
41. Calobrace MB, Stevens WG, Capizzi PJ, et al. Risk factor analysis for capsular contracture: a 10-year Sientra study using round, smooth, and textured implants for breast augmentation. *Plast Reconstr Surg*. 2018;141:20S-28S.
42. Clemens MW, Brody GS, Mahabir RC, Miranda RN. How to diagnose and treat breast implant-associated anaplastic large cell lymphoma. *Plast Reconstr Surg*. 2018;141:586e-599e.
CME article summarizing diagnostic criteria for BIA-LCL, appropriate workup for suspected cases of BIA-ALCL, and proper treatment and reporting of documented cases.
43. McCormack PM. Use of prosthetic materials in chest-wall reconstruction: assets and liabilities. *Surg Clin North Am* 1989;69:965-976.
44. Arnold PG, Pairolero PC. Chest-wall reconstruction: an account of 500 consecutive patients. *Plast Reconstr Surg*. 1996;98:804-810.
A large case consecutive case series of chest wall reconstruction using both autologous and alloplastic materials. The study outlines basic principles of chest wall reconstruction and highlights reconstructive options.
45. Luijendijk RW, Hop WC, van den Tol MP, et al. A comparison of suture repair with mesh repair for incisional hernia. *N Engl J Med*. 2000;343:392-398.
A multicenter randomized controlled trial of mesh reinforcement versus primary repair only of primary and first recurrent ventral hernias less than 6 cm in length or width. Mesh reinforcement of repairs was found to have a 75% lower recurrence rate irrespective of hernia size.
46. Mofid MM, Gonzalez R, de la Pena JA, et al. Buttock augmentation with silicone implants: a multicenter survey review of 2226 patients. *Plast Reconstr Surg*. 2013;131:897-901.
47. Zide BM, Karp NS. Maximizing gain from rectangular tissue expanders. *Plast Reconstr Surg*. 1992;90:500-504.

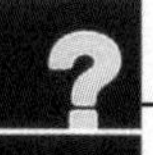

QUESTIONS

1. A 13-month-old child with a giant congenital nevus of the flank undergoes uncomplicated placement of a 10 × 15 cm subcutaneous rectangular tissue expander in preparation for subsequent reconstruction with adjacent tissue. After initiation of expansion in the following weeks, the parents of the child are worried that the skin over the expander looks red. Upon examination, there is slight erythema of the skin overlying the expander without warmth or surrounding skin changes and with no palpable fluid collections. The child is afebrile and well appearing and does not appear to be in pain. The next appropriate step in management of this patient involves

a. Starting intravenous antibiotics
b. Removing the tissue expander
c. Continuing with expansion
d. Starting oral antibiotics
e. Aspirating fluid from the tissue expander to send for culture

2. A 24-year-old patient presents with dissatisfaction of his facial appearance. Examination reveals a retruded chin, and alloplastic chin augmentation is planned. Compared with porous polyethylene implants for facial augmentation, silicone implants have

a. Lower infection rate
b. Decreased concern for migration
c. Better contour to the facial skeleton
d. Easier removal
e. Increased visibility

3. A 23-year-old woman presents for consultation regarding breast augmentation. The patient has small, symmetric breasts, without breast ptosis. She desires to be at least two bra sizes larger. Breast augmentation with form-stable anatomic implants is planned with placement in the subglandular plane. Which of the following answer choices best describes the advantages of using textured, anatomic implants compared with smooth, round implants in this patient?

a. Decreased risk of malrotation
b. Decreased risk of postoperative capsular contracture
c. Superior cosmetic result
d. Decreased risk of seroma
e. e. Increased risk of rippling

4. A 56-year-old man undergoes resection of a large left anterior chest wall sarcoma, and you are consulted intraoperatively for reconstruction. The resection includes the full-thickness chest wall with five ribs and the left half of the sternum. Intraoperative defect size is 10 × 20 cm. He has not received any other neoadjuvant treatments. Which of the following is the best choice for reconstruction?

a. PMMA sandwiched in polypropylene mesh and left latissimus dorsi flap
b. PMMA sandwiched in polypropylene mesh and left vertical rectus abdominis myocutaneous (VRAM) flap
c. Polypropylene mesh and left latissimus dorsi flap
d. Polypropylene mesh and left VRAM flap
e. Acellular dermal matrix and left latissimus dorsi flap

5. A 60-year-old woman with a history of right breast cancer and bilateral mastectomy and implant-based reconstruction 6 years ago presents to your office complaining of right breast discomfort. The patient initially had a two-staged reconstruction with placement of highly cohesive textured implants. She denies any changes in size of her breasts, skin changes, fever, or recent trauma to her breasts. On examination, she has no significant abnormalities. A magnetic resonance image is obtained, which reveals a moderately sized right periprosthetic fluid collection. Which of the following is the most appropriate next step in management?

a. Fine-needle aspiration of the collection to send for culture
b. Fine-needle aspiration of the collection to send for CD30+ immunohistochemistry
c. Explantation of bilateral breast implants and total capsulectomy
d. Admission to the hospital and intravenous antibiotics
e. Observation

1. Answer: c. Skin undergoing tissue expansion can often become slightly hyperemic upon initial expansion. Although skin erythema should always raise suspicion for infection with an underlying foreign body, the absence of other signs of infection in this case including surrounding cellulitis, pain, warmth, or fever makes infection unlikely. If the erythema persists or is worsening, further workup for an infection is warranted. However, mild skin changes are expected, and expansion should proceed normally in the absence of other symptoms. Starting antibiotics would be the correct choice if an early infection was suspected. Although the traditional dogma for any tissue expander infection entails explantation, more recent studies have shown that mild cellulitis without exposure can be salvaged with oral antibiotic regimens.[1] In these cases, aspiration of fluid for culture can also help guide antibiotic therapy. Severe infection, impending implant exposure or extrusion, requires explantation of the expander, washout of the pocket, antibiotic therapy, and delayed reimplantation after the infection has cleared.

2. Answer: d. Polyethylene and silicone implants are commonly used in facial augmentation. Both implants are usually placed subperiosteally to maximize soft tissue coverage, minimize damage to overlying neurovascular structures, and directly visualize bony contours. Both implants are contoured to the facial skeleton and have different profiles that can be selected and adjusted as needed. Porous polyethylene allows for tissue ingrowth and therefore is theoretically better vascularized and has less of a risk of migration than silicone implants if not secured to bone. Because silicone implants are not porous, they do not allow for tissue ingrowth and therefore are easier to remove.

3. Answer: b. Fifth generation breast implants have increased cross-linking that results in a highly cohesive implant that maintains this shape. Textured implants have been shown to have decreased rates of capsular contracture than smooth implants; however, only when placed in the subglandular plane. This difference is not significant in implants placed in the submuscular plane. Textured anatomic implants have not been demonstrated to have superior cosmetic outcome. In fact, evaluation by both plastic surgeons and nonmedical professional has not been able to identify anatomic versus round patients in photographs of patients with breast augmentation. Anatomic implants have a higher rate of malposition than round implants owing to their asymmetric shape, which is visible with rotation. Highly cohesive fifth generation implants have also been shown to have higher rates of seroma and decreased rates of rippling.

4. Answer: a. The patient has undergone a large chest wall resection that involves five ribs and a portion of the sternum. He has a composite defect that includes the skin, soft tissue, and bone. Patients who undergo resection of four or more ribs or have a bony defect greater than 5 cm are at a higher likelihood of developing flail chest. Therefore, mesh and dermal allograft alone will not provide adequate rigidity in this patient. PMMA is frequently used in chest wall reconstruction as a polymer that can be molded but cures into a rigid structure. In certain cases, rigidity of the chest wall secondary to fibrosis after radiation therapy may preclude the need for rigid chest wall reconstruction, as flail chest is less prevalent in this cohort. However, this is not the situation in this patient who has not previously received radiation. As the patient had resection of the sternum as well as ribs on either side, there is likely compromise of the internal mammary vessels, which would prevent the use of a flap based on the superior epigastric vessels. Therefore, the best answer choice provides a rigid reconstruction with PMMA sandwiched in macroporous mesh to allow for some tissue ingrowth as well as durable soft tissue coverage with a latissimus dorsi myocutaneous flap.

5. Answer: b. More than 500 worldwide cases of BIA-ALCL have been reported. This rare T cell lymphoma is primarily associated with textured implants and usually presents with a delayed-onset seroma and less commonly a capsular mass. Patients who present with a seroma greater than 1 year postoperatively should raise suspicion for BIA-ALCL. Appropriate steps in diagnosis include sending periprosthetic fluid for CD30+ immunohistochemistry. Additional diagnostic tests from fluid aspirate include cytology, flow cytometry, and histology. If a mass is present, it should also be biopsied and sent for pathology. Observation is not correct, as the presentation of seroma greater than 1 year postoperatively in a patient with textured implants is highly suggestive of BIA-ALCL.

Although explantation of implants and total capsulectomy is the treatment for BIA-ALCL localized to the implant pocket, this would be premature without a diagnosis of BIA-ALCL. This patient does not report any symptoms concerning for infection and the examination is otherwise benign. An indolent infection is possible but unlikely this later postoperatively.

CHAPTER 10 Principles of Nerve Repair and Reconstruction and Neuroma Management

Carrie A. Kubiak, David L. Brown, and Theodore A. Kung

KEY POINTS

- Appropriate management of nerve injuries is dictated by correct identification of the degree of nerve injury and the time since injury.
- Acute nerve transection injuries are best treated with primary, tensionless repair.
- Restoring appropriate alignment of corresponding fascicles in the proximal and distal nerve segments is important for optimizing outcomes in primary neurorrhaphy.
- In crush or avulsion nerve lesions where the zone of nerve injury is unclear, the viability of injured nerve should be allowed to demarcate before definitive reconstruction is attempted.
- Electrodiagnostic studies (EMG/NCV) can be used to help diagnose nerve injuries as well as track nerve regeneration.
- Autologous nerve grafts are the most reliable method to reconstruct segmental nerve gaps.
- Nerve transfers should be considered in proximal injuries and when there is concern that degradation of neuromuscular junctions will occur prior to reinnervation.

Peripheral nerve injuries result in a myriad of symptoms, ranging from minor sensory disturbances to devastating loss of function. Debilitating chronic pain can be difficult to manage even with surgical intervention. The mechanism, level, and severity of the trauma directly contribute to the expected morbidity, prognosis, and recommended treatment following peripheral nerve injury. Recent advances in microsurgical techniques, graft materials, and nerve transfer strategies have greatly improved our ability to address peripheral nerve injuries, but reliable restoration of sensation and motor function can still be difficult to achieve. Outcomes following nerve repair or reconstruction can be optimized by ensuring a timely diagnosis and treatment, performing meticulous alignment of nerve ends during surgery, and following appropriate rehabilitation protocols. This chapter discusses the pathophysiology of nerve injury and summarizes the various operative strategies that are employed after trauma to peripheral nerves.

PERIPHERAL NERVE ANATOMY

Peripheral nerves consist of three main cell types. Neurons facilitate the transfer of information to and from the central nervous system, conveying both afferent sensory stimuli as well as efferent motor signals. Axons are extensions from the neuron cell bodies that reside in the spinal cord and spinal ganglia. Axons are either myelinated or unmyelinated and are grouped together spatially in bundles known as fascicles. Anterograde and retrograde axonal transport transfers structural proteins, as well as communicate between the cell body and the target end organ through cycling of neurotransmitters.[1] Supportive glial and stromal cells play an important role in the support and function of peripheral nerves. Schwann cells are the principal glial cells of the peripheral nervous system and produce the myelin sheath to myelinated axons. Myelin acts as an insulating coating to axons, efficiently augmenting the propagation of action potentials and increasing the conduction velocity in a process known as saltatory conduction. Stromal cells form the connective tissue scaffold around neurons and glial cells.[2]

The endoneurium is the innermost layer of loose connective tissue that surrounds individual axons and their supporting Schwann cells to provide nourishment through microvessels. The perineurium serves to bundle axons together to form fascicles and is a major contributor to peripheral nerve tensile strength. A *fascicular group* consists of two or more fascicles surrounded by perineurium. The internal epineurium is the connective tissue that envelops individual fascicles and group fascicles. The epineurium is the outermost layer and is the tissue that defines an anatomically distinct peripheral nerve. Finally, the mesoneurium is a thin layer of loose areolar tissue that connects the peripheral nerve to surrounding structures and permits smooth gliding during bodily movements (**Figure 10.1**).

Peripheral nerves are supplied by a series of segmental nutrient arteries that feed into a network of blood vessels within the nerve. The vasa nervorum vessels run superficially and longitudinally along the epineurium. These vessels send branches to intraneural vessels located within the interfascicular perineurium and in turn join a multitude of capillaries that extend into the endoneurium. This extensive communication maximizes the blood supply within the nerve and permits mobilization of a segment of a nerve for a length up to 45 times its diameter.[3]

PHYSIOLOGY OF PERIPHERAL NERVE INJURY

Loss of axonal continuity leads to an irreversible cascade of cellular and inflammatory events known as Wallerian degeneration.[4] This process begins within 24 to 48 hours of injury and involves complete axonal degeneration distal to the site of injury. Additionally, axonal degeneration occurs for a short distance proximally. An influx of calcium and sodium ions triggers the sequence of axonolysis. Disruption of both anterograde and retrograde transport systems leads to a buildup of proteins and subsequent swelling of the nerve on both sides of the injury.[5] Schwann cells transform into a more dedifferentiated and reactive phenotype[6] and begin to break down their own myelin, phagocytose debris, and recruit macrophages to the site of injury.[7] These macrophages in turn promote a positive feedback

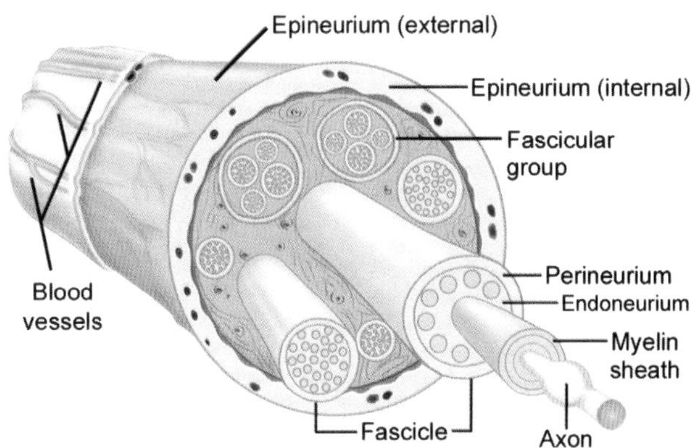

FIGURE 10.1. The normal peripheral nerve consists of myelinated and unmyelinated axons organized into bundles of fascicles. Peripheral neural tissue is supported by three major connective tissue sheaths: the endoneurium, perineurium, and epineurium.

loop that further stimulates Schwann cell proliferation through the release of growth factors.[8] Wallerian degeneration proceeds until empty endoneurial tubes remain, devoid of axonal or myelin material. In the proximal nerve segment, Wallerian degeneration halts at the closest intact node of Ranvier, which also serves as the site of subsequent axonal growth.[9]

To begin regeneration, dedifferentiated Schwann cells proliferate along the residual endoneurial tubes and create columns known as Bands of Büngner. These longitudinally aligned Schwann cells provide a supportive microenvironment and serve to guide regenerating axons to their appropriate distal target organs.[10] For this reason, superior clinical outcomes are observed when endoneurial tube remains intact.[11] Schwann cells further support regenerating axons via release of cytokines and neurotrophic factors that stimulate axonal growth.[12] Axonal regeneration is mediated by a host of neurotrophic factors that are released from local tissue including sensory and motor targets.[13] A divided neuron may form up to 50 to 100 axonal sprouts in an effort to reinnervate its target tissue. Each regenerating axon forms a *growth cone* consisting of multiple filopodia that guide outgrowth during regeneration. Proteases are also released from the growth cone to aid in the removal of any physical barriers hindering its path. Clinically, the site of axonal regeneration can be localized by tapping along the course of the peripheral nerve. A positive Tinel sign occurs when an *electric shock* or *pins and needles* sensation is produced. Elongation proceeds until the axons reach intact endoneurial tubes within the distal nerve segment that serve to guide growth towards the end organ. When functional connections are not made in a timely fashion, axons can degenerate in a process known as pruning. Axons that continue to grow aimlessly will form a disorganized and painful mass known as a neuroma.[14] Studies have shown that more severe nerve injuries lead to greater scarring and disordered axonal regeneration.[15]

Axonal regeneration occurs at a rate of approximately 1 to 3 mm per day or just slightly more than an inch per month.[16] Therefore, when the location of nerve injury is known, one can predict the amount of time regenerating axons will take to reach their end organ. In distal peripheral nerve transections, regenerating axons will need to grow a relatively short distance. However, with more proximal peripheral nerve injuries, the time for regenerating axons to reach their targets can be estimated at many months to several years, resulting in Schwann cells losing their ability to facilitate nerve regeneration and distal endoneurial sheaths collapsing.[17] This precludes successful reinnervation even with the most optimal surgical techniques. For this reason, the level of peripheral nerve injury is critically relevant to the expected functional outcome. Muscle fibers will undergo irreversible loss of neuromuscular junctions and progressive fibrosis if not reinnervated with 1 to 2 years. In contrast, sensory end organs do not undergo such degeneration and can be reinnervated many years later with satisfactory results.

CLASSIFICATION OF NERVE INJURY

In 1943, Seddon described three degrees of peripheral nerve injury: neuropraxia, axonotmesis, and neurotmesis.[18] Sunderland later expanded this classification to five degrees based on histologic and structural changes seen within the nerve after injury[19] (**Table 10.1**, **Figure 10.2**).

Neuropraxia is equivalent to Sunderland first-degree nerve injury. In this condition, the axons within the nerve remain intact, but a temporary, localized conduction block results from segmental demyelination. Acutely, neuropraxia can ensue after stretching injuries or blunt force trauma, whereas chronic etiologies of neuropraxia include longstanding compression neuropathies at locations where peripheral nerves pass through tight anatomic spaces (e.g., carpal tunnel syndrome). Axonal integrity is preserved, neurons maintain their connections to end organs, and Wallerian degeneration with subsequent axonal regeneration is not required for restoration of function. Electrodiagnostic studies (EDS) will show normal electromyographic (EMG) findings with decreased nerve conduction velocities and increased latencies. Recovery time is dependent on remyelination of the axons by Schwann cells and requires approximately 6 to 8 weeks.

TABLE 10.1. CLASSIFICATION OF PERIPHERAL NERVE INJURIES IS BASED ON THE LEVEL OF ANATOMIC DISRUPTION

Seddon Classification	Sunderland Classification[a]	Nerve Anatomy[b]					Recovery	Surgery
		Myelin	Axon	Endoneurium	Perineurium	Epineurium		
Neurapraxia	First degree	–	+	+	+	+	Full spontaneous recovery within days to months	None
Axonotmesis	Second degree	–	–	+	+	+	Full spontaneous recovery; regenerates at a rate of 1–3 mm per day	None
	Third degree	–	–	–	+	+	Partial spontaneous recovery; regenerates at a rate of 1–3 mm per day	None
	Fourth degree	–	–	–	–	+	No spontaneous recovery; regenerates at a rate of 1–3 mm per day after appropriate surgical intervention	Nerve repair, graft, or transfer
Neurotmesis	Fifth degree	–	–	–	–	–	No spontaneous recovery; regenerates at a rate of 1–3 mm per day after appropriate surgical intervention	Nerve repair, graft, or transfer
	Sixth degree	–	+/–	+/–	+/–	+/–	Recovery depends on combination of degrees of nerve injury	Variable

[a]Degree of nerve injury determines likelihood of spontaneous recovery and/or need for surgical intervention.
[b]+ Indicates structure is intact; – indicates structure is injured.

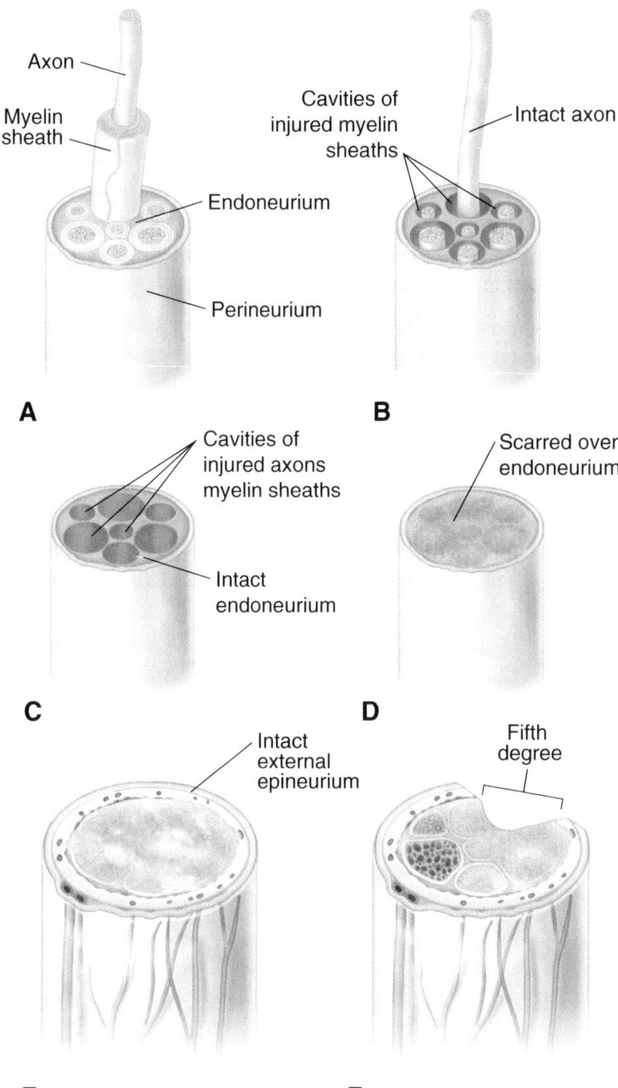

FIGURE 10.2. Classification of nerve injuries. **A.** Uninjured nerve consists of myelinated axons surrounded by endoneurium. **B.** In first-degree injury, axons are demyelinated but intact. **C.** In second-degree injury, axons are injured and undergo degeneration. **D.** A third-degree injury includes damage to axons, myelin, and endoneurium. **E.** A fourth-degree is a complete scar block that prevents regeneration. **F.** A fifth-degree injury is a division of the nerve. **G.** A sixth-degree injury is a combination of any of the five levels of injury within the same nerve.

In axonotmesis, there is focal demyelination as well as axonal injury with Wallerian degeneration. Axonotmesis is a component of Sunderland second-, third-, and fourth-degree injuries and is usually caused by severe traction or crush injuries. Second-degree injury is characterized by the disruption of the continuity of axons but with preservation of intact endoneurial tubes. Regenerating axons are guided by their original endoneurial tubes that lead them directly to their target tissues, and therefore full functional recovery can be expected. Third-degree injury involves damage to the axon, myelin sheath, and endoneurium. The perineurium is intact, and the fascicular structure remains patent. Because the endoneurial sheaths are violated, scarring may serve as a physical barrier to regenerating axons. Functional recovery is variable and often incomplete. In fourth-degree injury, there is injury to the myelin, axon, endoneurium, and perineurium, and only the epineurium remains intact. Common causes of fourth-degree nerve injury include traction and iatrogenic nerve injection. Spontaneous recovery does not occur due to interposed fibrosis, and surgical intervention is required.

Sunderland fifth-degree injury is equivalent to Seddon neurotmesis. This type of injury is the complete transection of axons and all connective tissue layers, commonly due to a sharp laceration. Surgical intervention is required, and functional outcomes are more unpredictable. Although the Sunderland classification is a useful paradigm for organizing peripheral nerve injuries into differing severities, it does have limited clinical utility. For instance, there is no diagnostic test to distinguish between second-, third-, and fourth-degree injuries, as these can only be diagnosed histologically.[20] Therefore, Mackinnon and Dellon introduced a sixth-degree category, which represents a mixed injury pattern.[21] Sixth-degree injury represents a combination of any of the previous five levels of injury within the same nerve. Sixth-degree injury results in variable recovery that is dependent on an accurate diagnosis and timely intervention.

DIAGNOSIS

A critical factor in the management of peripheral nerve injuries is the timeliness of both diagnosis and surgical treatment. Therefore, a thorough clinical assessment and history is performed to establish the location, nature, and severity of the injury. This includes testing motor, sensory, and pain fibers of the suspected injured nerves. When possible, muscles innervated by the nerve should be evaluated individually. The extent of motor nerve injury is determined by assessment of muscle strength, range of motion, and atrophy. Sensory impairments can be identified by decreased sensation, hypersensitivity, or allodynia in the distribution of the nerve territory. In the classic *ten test*, patients rank the magnitude of sensation in the affected region compared with that in the contralateral region using a scale from 0 to 10. Quantitative sensory testing can also be performed as a means to detect the perception threshold for mechanical stimuli in patients with injured peripheral nerves.[22] This approach utilizes the pressure-specified sensory device[22] to objectively quantify sensory innervation by measuring pressure thresholds for perception of static and moving one- and two-point discrimination of the skin in the distribution of the injured nerve. Vibration instruments and Semmes-Weinstein monofilaments are also used to evaluate the sensory innervation and are most useful in evaluating chronic compressive neuropathies.

The exact site of nerve injury can be identified by clinical examination or through the use of electrodiagnostic or imaging studies. The progress of axonal regeneration can be localized by tapping along the course of the peripheral nerve. This finding is known as a positive Tinel sign and is experienced as an *electric shock* or *pins and needles* sensation. Over the course of several weeks, distal migration of a Tinel sign demonstrates ongoing regeneration and suggests that functional improvements may be expected as long as the distance from the site of nerve injury to the target end organs is not exceedingly long. Nerve block may also play an important role in establishing a diagnosis and discerning the location of injury. Blocks are performed by injecting local anesthetic to anesthetize specific peripheral nerves to identify the source of pain or allodynia. Symptomatic improvement after injection helps to isolate the affected nerve, but the test is fairly nonspecific.[23]

Electrodiagnostics

The term *electrodiagnostic studies* (EDS) encompasses both nerve conduction studies (NCS) and EMG. These tests are often performed together and provide useful information about the location of nerve injury as well as severity and prognosis. NCS are used to assess both motor and sensory function by measuring the conduction velocity of action potentials traveling through a nerve. To measure conduction velocity in motor axons, a transcutaneous electrical stimulus is given and subsequently compound muscle action potentials (CMAPs) from the corresponding distal muscle are recorded. For sensory axons, recording skin electrodes are placed within the cutaneous territory of a sensory nerve to record the transmission of the stimulus.

Slower conduction velocities or increased latencies indicate the presence of demyelination and reflect at least a first-degree Sunderland nerve injury. The position of the distal recording electrodes can be repositioned at various places over the length of the peripheral nerve to localize the conduction block. Amplitude of the recorded CMAPs provides an estimate of the number of intact motor axons activating muscle fibers. Small or absent CMAP amplitudes indicate that some degree of axon loss has occurred. The amplitude of the recorded compound sensory nerve action potential similarly provides a reflection of the number of intact sensory axons.

The addition of needle EMG studies provides further insight regarding the condition of peripheral nerves. In this test, a needle is inserted into a target muscle to measure muscle activity at rest and during voluntary contraction.[24] Fibrillations and positive sharp waves (PSWs) on needle EMG indicate axonal loss and therefore at least second-degree Sunderland injury, but these findings may not be apparent for several weeks depending on how proximal the lesion is.[25] PSWs can be observed as early as 3 weeks after nerve injury, whereas fibrillations are typically observed around 6 weeks after nerve injury. The presence of fibrillations and PSWs on EMG are significant to the prognosis because they reveal that the distal motor plates in the target muscle fibers are still available for reinnervation. The size, shape, and recruitment pattern of motor unit potentials (MUPs) on needle EMG is helpful in determining the duration of nerve injury and the expected potential for functional recovery. Immediately after denervation, the number of motor units is reduced to a level that is commensurate with injury severity. The reappearance of MUPs on EMG about 12 weeks after injury reflects the collateral sprouting of adjacent, uninjured nerve fibers and thus represents second- and third-degree Sunderland nerve injuries. These findings can become evident before any clinical signs of recovery are apparent. Owing to the extensive nature of intraneural damage and scarring seen in fourth- or fifth-degree Sunderland injuries, MUPs are not typically seen on EMG because all of the axons have lost continuity with their target muscle fibers.

Electrodiagnostic studies may be obtained immediately after significant trauma to help determine the presence and degree of nerve injury (**Table 10.2**). However, these studies are unable to distinguish between severe axonotmetic and neurotmetic injuries in the acute setting. Total division of a peripheral nerve may be better diagnosed with imaging studies such as ultrasound or magnetic resonance imaging. NCS and EMG do play an important role in the timing of surgical intervention. For example, after a suspected injury to a peripheral nerve, the presence of at least some motor units under voluntary control shows that the lesion is incomplete, which implies a more favorable prognosis. On the contrary, the lack of any signs of recovery on NCS or EMG after 3 to 6 months is usually an indication for surgical exploration. Even when functional recovery is identified, these electrodiagnostic tests can also be performed serially over time to help follow the progress of axonal regeneration and end organ reinnervation.

MANAGEMENT OF ACUTE NERVE INJURIES

The management of acute traumatic peripheral nerve injuries is largely dependent of the severity of injury, the mechanism of trauma, and the distance from the injury to the target end organs. Intact but contused nerves can often be expected to recover. Continued observation with close follow-up may be appropriate before surgical intervention is warranted. However, with a more severe injury, prompt surgical exploration and nerve repair may be the more suitable course of action.

In acute closed injuries, such as from blunt force trauma and blast mechanisms, peripheral nerves usually suffer a contusion but remain structurally intact. Frequently, these are first-, second-, and third-degree Sunderland injuries that are treated expectantly with sufficient time before surgery is considered. For several weeks following the injury, patients should be seen frequently and serial examinations are performed to look for any signs of recovery, such as a progressing Tinel sign and electrodiagnostic evidence of recovery. These clinical findings help distinguish axonotmetic lesions that may recover spontaneously from neurotmetic lesions that require surgical intervention. If there is confirmation of return of function clinically or electrophysiologically, the patient should continue to be followed expectantly, as recovery is still possible. If there is no return of function or if functional improvement plateaus, nerve exploration may be considered. During this observation period, if none of these signs are noted, it is more likely the patient sustained a higher grade injury (e.g., at least third degree) such that axons either cannot find their way into distal endoneural tubes or their passage is blocked by intervening scar tissue. Nerve exploration should be pursued and definitive surgical management will be dictated by intraoperative findings. For example, neurolysis is indicated to excise pathologic scarring around and within the substance of the peripheral nerve whereas a neuroma-in-continuity that is discovered is often excised and reconstructed.

In contaminated wounds with acute crush or avulsion nerve injuries, the type and zone of injury can be difficult to determine. In these scenarios, it is better to first debride any devitalized tissue and tack the two nerve ends to a surrounding structure to prevent retraction. The wound and injured nerve are then allowed to heal for at least 3 weeks for demarcation of the zone of injury. At the time of reexploration, the extent of nerve injury will be more evident. The neuroma located at the proximal nerve segment must be excised in bread-loaf fashion until a healthy fascicular pattern is seen. A similar technique is

TABLE 10.2. ELECTRODIAGNOSTIC FINDINGS BY DEGREE OF PERIPHERAL NERVE INJURY

Sunderland Classification of Nerve Injury	Acute Nerve Injury		Chronic Nerve Injury	
	Fibrillations/PSWs	MUPs	Fibrillations/PSWs	MUPs
First degree	No	Normal	No[a]	Normal
Second degree	Yes[b]	Present: secondary to collateral sprouting	No[a]	Present: secondary to axonal regeneration
Third degree	Yes[b]	Present: secondary to collateral sprouting	No[a]	Present: secondary to axonal regeneration
Fourth degree	Yes[b]	No	No[a]	No
Fifth degree	Yes[b]	No	No[a]	No
Sixth degree[c]	Yes[b]	Variable	No[a]	Variable

[a]Fibrillations and PSWs disappear after a period of chronic denervation.
[b]Fibrillations and positive sharp waves (PSWs) are not identifiable until 3 to 6 weeks after nerve injury.
[c]Electrodiagnostic findings vary depending on the mixed severity and location of damage in sixth degree nerve injuries.
PSWs, positive sharp waves; MUPs, motor unit potentials.

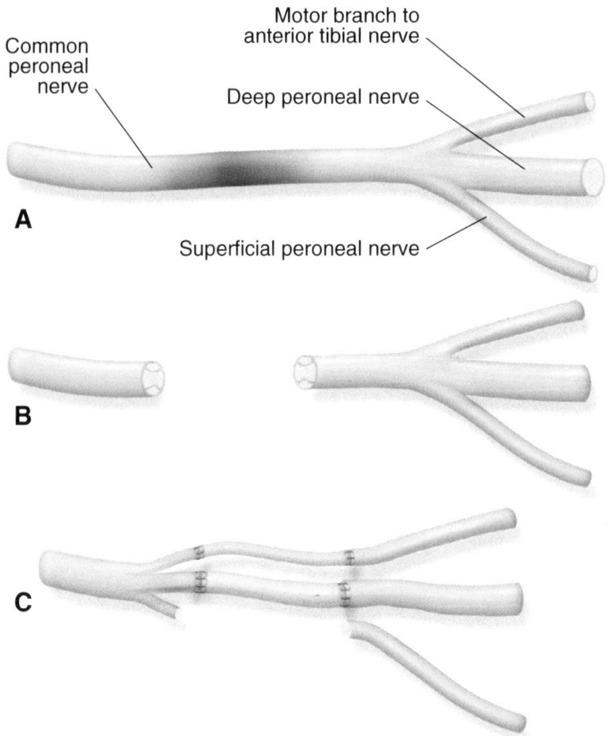

FIGURE 10.3. Management of severe crush or avulsion injuries. **A.** When the zone of nerve injury is unclear, the nerve should be allowed to demarcate for at least 3 weeks before definitive debridement of devitalized tissue is performed. **B.** Neuroma and scar must then be excised in *bread-loaf* fashion until a healthy fascicular pattern is seen in both proximal and distal nerve stumps. **C.** Only upon sufficient debridement should the nerve defect be repaired or reconstructed.

used for the distal nerve segment, although there will be no neuroma present in this location. The resultant defect will require either direct nerve repair or nerve reconstruction using a graft (**Figure 10.3**).

Primary Repair

Acute, clean peripheral nerve lacerations are best repaired immediately. If the wound bed is well vascularized and end-to-end approximation is possible, tension-free primary repair should be performed within the first 2 to 3 days following injury. Transposition or mobilization of the nerve may be required to minimize tension and facilitate repair. Excessive tension at the suture line results in compromise of endoneurial blood supply, causing necrosis, fibrosis, and scar blockage of nerve regeneration.[3] This diminishes the potential for successful functional recovery. Restoring appropriate alignment of corresponding fascicles in the proximal and distal segment is similarly important for optimizing regenerative outcomes in primary neurorrhaphy. Epineurial vascular landmarks are useful to ensure optimal alignment of fascicles. If performed within 72 hours after injury, direct stimulation of distal motor fascicles can further aid in mapping fascicular arrangements in the distal nerve stump.[26] After this amount of time, the distal nerve segment is depleted of neurotransmitters, and direct stimulation will not reliably result in muscle contractions. Intraoperative histologic staining of proximal and distal nerve ends has been described as a means to align motor and sensory fascicles, although this process can take up to an hour in even experienced hands.[27]

Direct epineurial nerve coaptation with microsutures remains the standard surgical treatment for peripheral nerve lacerations that can be repaired without undue tension. Microsutures (9-0 or 10-0) are loosely placed through the external epineurium such that nerve ends and fascicular groups are *kissing* and not bulging to the sides. Should bulging occur, trimming of the fascicles with microscissors

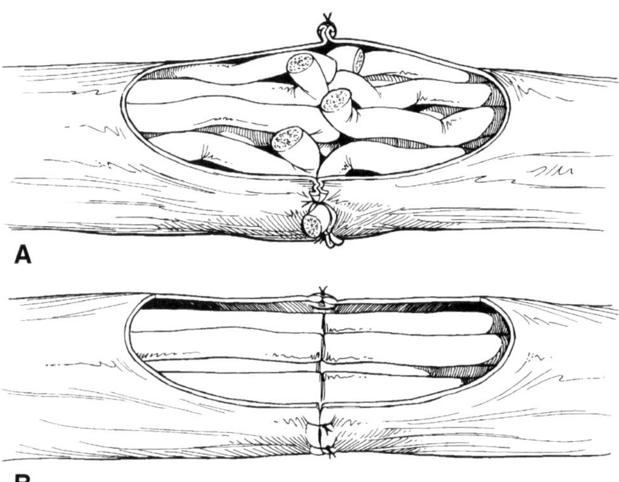

FIGURE 10.4. Primary nerve repair. **A.** In an epineural repair, the fascicles must be appropriately trimmed so that they do not buckle, which will result in misdirection of the regenerating fibers. **B.** Well-performed nerve repairs will result in good alignment of fascicles without the need for fascicular sutures.

will facilitate end-to-end approximation within the endoneurial sheath (**Figure 10.4**). The fewest number of epineurial sutures should be used for the repair to decrease iatrogenic harm to the nerve. In contrast, in a *fascicular repair* technique, intraneural dissection is performed at the edges of the cut nerve and then individual fascicles are realigned with microsutures. Adjunctive epineurial sutures may be placed or may be omitted. However, the advantages that might be gained from direct alignment of individual fascicle segments may be offset by the higher chances of axonal injury during the procedure and increased foreign body reaction caused by the greater suture material burden within the nerve. A more conservative method of controlling the alignment of fascicles is known as *group fascicular repair*, whereby identifiable groups of fascicles are aligned before a standard epineural repair is performed. Although this modification is conceptually logical, clinical studies have not shown a clear superiority of one technique over another.[28]

An alternative repair technique utilizes tissue adhesives such as fibrin glue or poly(ethylene glycol) hydrogel to supplement or replace epineurial sutures. Advantages of using adhesives for nerve repair include its ease of use, reduced operative times, less tissue trauma, and less intraneural scarring compared with using microsutures.[29] However, concerns remain about the lack of adequate tensile strength after the application of these strategies alone.[30] Although animal studies have reported superiority or at least equivalency to suture repair,[31] there are limited clinical data to support a complete shift away from traditional microsurgical repair of nerve transection injuries.

Autografts

When tensionless primary repair is not possible, an autologous nerve graft is preferred for nerve gap reconstruction. A nonvascularized graft can be harvested from an expendable sensory nerve and is interposed in the segmental nerve defect. The harvested nerve graft undergoes Wallerian degeneration but maintains the supportive scaffold (i.e., endoneurium, perineurium, and epineurium) with Schwann cell basal laminae, neurotrophic factors, and adhesion molecules to support regenerating axons. Axonal regeneration through the nerve graft proceeds in a manner identical to that following primary neurorrhaphy.

Utilization of a nerve autograft requires the sacrifice of a healthy, functioning nerve (usually sensory) for reconstruction of a more important injured nerve (often motor). Autogenous nerve grafts can be harvested from several sites, the most common being the sural nerve, medial antebrachial cutaneous (MABC) nerve, and lateral antebrachial cutaneous (LABC) nerve. A sural nerve graft offers 30 to

40 cm of graft length from each leg, whereas the medial antebrachial cutaneous nerve provides up to 20 cm of length and the LABC up to 8 cm. These nerves are selected as donors because the sensory deficit is either negligible owing to sensory innervation overlap or is considered acceptable compared to the potential gain in motor function by using that nerve. The distal stump of the donor nerve can be sewn end-to-side to an adjacent normal nerve to restore improved sensation to the donor dermatome. Expendable motor nerves that can be harvested for autogenous grafting have a much more limited availability owing to increased donor site morbidity. Harvest of motor nerves grafts are thus reserved for instances where no sensory donors are available and nerve transfers would not provide a better option. A nerve innervating a free muscle transfer can be considered as a possible graft (e.g., thoracodorsal nerve to the latissimus dorsi muscle).

Autografts should be approximately 10% to 20% longer than the segmental defect in anticipation of fibrosis-related graft shortening to ensure a tension-free repair. The autograft should be placed in reversed orientation at the repair site to prevent loss of regenerating axons down side branches. If the nerve graft diameter matches that of the segmental defect, the autograft can be simply interposed between the two cut ends. Reconstruction of large diameter nerves often requires cable grafts. By aligning multiple smaller caliber grafts (i.e., cable grafts) in parallel between corresponding fascicular groups, the entire diameter of the large caliber nerve can be reconstructed. Autografts are associated with a number of disadvantages including a separate donor site for the nerve graft harvest, the potential for neuroma formation at the donor site, and occasionally insufficient donor nerve availability. Still, nerve autografts are considered the standard for reconstruction of any segmental nerve defect.

Allografts

When there is a paucity of autologous nerve donor tissue available, human cadaveric allografts can be utilized in nerve reconstruction. Clinical implementation of allograft nerve reconstruction is hampered by the substantial immunogenic response elicited from resident Schwann cells present in the allograft.[24] Recipients of cadaveric allografts must therefore be immunosuppressed (e.g., with tacrolimus) for up to 2 years until the donor nerve graft has been repopulated with host Schwann cells.[32]

Allografts can be decellularized to avoid the need for immunosuppression. A chemical detergent process with enzyme degradation and irradiation removes all cellular and immunogenic material from the graft, including residual nerve material and donor Schwann cells. This technique preserves the natural extracellular matrix and physical architecture (e.g., endoneurial tubes, basal lamina) that facilitate axonal regeneration but eliminates the need for immunosuppression.[33] The decellularized allograft can then serve as a scaffold to be repopulated by host axons and Schwann cells over time. These conduits confer the beneficial characteristics inherent to autograft nerve tissue while avoiding donor site morbidity, having unlimited *off-the-shelf* availability, and being associated with decreased surgical time. However, there remain significant costs with their use.[34]

Nerve Conduits

A prodigious amount of research has focused on the development of synthetic nerve guidance conduits designed to facilitate axonal regeneration across segmental nerve gaps. An ideal nerve conduit needs to be widely available, have low antigenicity, and be biocompatible. Currently commercially available conduits are constructed from biocompatible materials such as collagen, polyglycolic acid (PGA), poly-DL-lactide-co-caprolactone, polyvinyl alcohol, and N-fibroin (silk protein).[35] These materials have varying degrees of permeability for diffusion of supportive nutrients while providing adequate structural scaffolding for regenerating axons. The absorbable nature of these conduits limits the associated foreign body reaction that can result in scar tissue encapsulation and subsequent inhibition of axonal growth.[36]

The newest tissue-engineered conduits incorporate structural elements for delivery of molecular- or cellular-based therapies to optimize regeneration potential.[37] Stem cells and Schwann cells seeded into nerve conduits have demonstrated significantly better functional outcomes compared with empty conduits.[38] Controlled release of regenerative neurotrophic factors (e.g., nerve growth factor [NGF], brain-derived neurotrophic factor [BDNF], neurotrophin-3 [NT3], neurotrophin-4-5 [NT4-5] others) from conduits has also been shown to be beneficial for axonal growth.[39] There is mounting evidence to support synthetic nerve conduit reconstruction of short defects in sensory nerves. Specifically, these constructs have been shown to support successful nerve regeneration across small diameter nerves with gaps up to 3 cm or with large diameter nerves with gaps less than 0.5 cm. In fact, all alternatives to autologous nerve grafts, including decellularized allografts and tissue-engineered conduits, demonstrate similar efficacy in reconstruction of sensory nerve defects of less than 3 cm. However, for motor defects or nerve defects that span more than 3 cm, autologous nerve grafting is still considered the standard of care.

Nerve Transfers

In proximal nerve defects, functional outcomes following nerve repair or reconstruction at the site of injury are poor due to the extended length of time and distance until regenerating axons can be expected to reach their distal targets. The effect of prolonged denervation results in target muscle fibrosis with loss of motor end plates[40] and senescence of Schwann cells that normally provide trophic support to regenerating axons. In these cases, nerve transfers can provide regenerating axons from a donor nerve to the distal aspect of the injured nerve by considerably shorten the time until reinnervation of important muscles and to preserve function.[41] When done properly, donor site morbidity is minimal and the procedure can produce predictably good outcomes.[42,43]

Nerve transfers are traditionally reserved for restoration of muscle function, but the technique has also been used in the reconstruction of critical sensory nerves. The most common applications of motor nerve transfers include the restoration of elbow flexion, shoulder abduction, ulnar-innervated intrinsic hand function, forearm pronation, and radial nerve function.[44] For example, the thoracodorsal nerve transferred to the musculocutaneous nerve can restore elbow flexion after brachial plexus injury. This nerve transfer purposefully sacrifices the motor function to the latissimus dorsi muscle, for which action can be compensated by other shoulder muscles, to power the more critical contraction of the biceps brachii, brachialis, and coracobrachialis muscles. The choice of optimal donor nerve for motor transfer is based on factors such as the quantity of motor axons, proximity to the target muscle, and synergy of muscle function.[44] Motor fascicles that can be readily separated from a mixed nerve (e.g., the flexor carpi ulnaris fascicle of the ulnar nerve) can also serve as ideal donor nerves.[44]

Sensory nerve transfers are more frequently performed at the level of the distal forearm or palm to restore critical digit sensation, such as the contact surfaces of the thumb and index finger. For sensory transfers, suitable donor nerves should innervate noncritical sensory distribution, contain a large number of purely sensory axons, and be located close in proximity to the target sensory end organs. If possible, the distal end of a transferred sensory nerve can be coapted end-to-side to an adjacent sensory nerve for some recovery of sensation in the donor territory. When an end-to-end repair is planned, the donor nerve is ideally transected as distally as possible and the recipient nerve is transected as proximally as possible to optimize a tension-free coaptation.

RECOVERY

Functional outcomes following nerve repair and reconstruction depend on the degree of nerve injury, level of injury, and time since injury, as well as number of patient and surgical factors. In 1990, Sunderland summarized 40 years of clinical experience highlighting the principles of peripheral nerve repair and expected outcomes[16]: early repairs are better than late; nerve coaptation is better than interposing nerve grafts; and sharp transection injuries have better outcomes than crush or avulsion injuries. Younger patients also have better prognosis and distal nerve repairs do better than proximal repairs. Furthermore, pure sensory or pure motor nerve repairs do better than mixed nerve repairs.[16]

After surgical intervention, functional recovery is monitored with serial physical examinations and electrodiagnostic studies. The most widely used grading system for nerve recovery is the Medical Research Council Grading System for Nerve Recovery. This system is grades sensory recovery from S0 to S5 and motor recovery from M0 to M5 based on physical examination findings.[24] The greater the numerical grade, the greater the functional recovery.

NEUROMAS

Any peripheral nerve injury involving transection of axons is at risk for neuroma formation.[45] Neuromas result from failure of the regenerative growth cone to reach peripheral targets. Sprouting axons that are unable to reach the distal endoneurial tube will continue to elongate at the site of injury, forming a mass of disorganized fibroneural tissue containing axons, connective tissue, and scar.[45] Neuromas can form at the site of axonal disruption along the course of a peripheral nerve (i.e., neuroma-in-continuity) or at the end of a transected peripheral nerve (i.e., terminal bulb or end neuromas). Neuromas signify the presence of unsuccessful reinnervation and can often be associated with disabling neuropathic pain.

Efforts to prevent neuroma formation should be considered during management of any nerve injury. Even small sensory nerves can produce debilitating neuroma pain after transection. Therefore, when these minor nerves are identified during surgery, formal repair is recommended to prevent aberrant axonal sprouting and subsequent neuroma formation. When a painful neuroma does develop, a course of desensitization therapy is warranted as first-line treatment. When the pain is refractory to conservative measures or if functional recovery is poor, surgical intervention is indicated. Surgery may entail neurolysis or neuroma resection and interposition nerve graft reconstruction.[46] If the nerve is expendable (e.g., a noncritical sensory nerve), neurectomy may be considered. Numerous methods have been explored to prevent neuroma formation, yet there remains no standard for treatment or prevention. Several surgical approaches utilizing epineurial closure, nerve transposition with muscle implantation, and neurorrhaphy techniques have all been employed with inconsistent results.[47]

Traditional neuroma prevention methods are all aimed at minimizing or masking aberrant nerve regeneration. However, these methods do not seek to prevent neuroma formation but instead place the anticipated recurrent neuroma in a less symptomatic location. Newer strategies for neuroma management provide functional connections for regenerating axons and consequently prevent neuroma formation. Both targeted muscle reinnervation[48] and regenerative peripheral nerve interface[49] techniques provide distal physiologic targets (i.e., denervated muscle fibers) for regenerating axons for new neuromuscular junctions. The number of axons from a regenerating nerve without a functional connection is greatly reduced, and this results in significantly lower chances of neuroma formation.

CONCLUSION

Significant advances in strategies for peripheral nerve repair and reconstruction have improved our ability to optimize functional outcomes after various types of nerve injury. Accurate diagnosis of the level and severity of nerve injury is paramount to the selection of the most appropriate treatment. Whenever possible, direct end-to-end repair of a transected nerve is performed. Nerve autografts remain the standard option for reconstruction of segmental nerve defects. Continuing research will elucidate the roles of allografts and nerve conduits in nerve repair, and further development of techniques to diminish symptomatic neuroma formation will greatly improve functional recovery following peripheral nerve injury.

ACKNOWLEDGMENT

This work was supported by the American Association of Plastic Surgeons Academic Scholar Program to Theodore A. Kung. The content is solely the responsibility of the authors and does not necessarily represent the official views of the American Association of Plastic Surgeons.

REFERENCES

1. Lundborg G, Dahlin L, Danielsen N, Zhao Q. Trophism, tropism, and specificity in nerve regeneration. *J Reconstr Microsurg.* 1994;10(5):345-354.
2. Dellon AL, Mackinnon SE. Basic scientific and clinical applications of peripheral nerve regeneration. *Surg Annu.* 1988;20:59-100.
3. Lundborg G. Structure and function of the intraneural microvessels as related to trauma, edema formation, and nerve function. *J Bone Joint Surg Am.* 1975;57(7):938-948.
   Dr. Göran Lundborg describes the extrinsic and intrinsic microvascular anatomy of peripheral nerves and associated structural changes following peripheral nerve trauma. Any interference with intraneural microcirculation will cause disturbances in nerve function. The structure and function of the vasa nervorum are of great interest to surgeons who need to know to what extent a peripheral nerve can withstand various kinds of trauma without loss of blood supply.
4. Bittner GD, Schallert T, Peduzzi JD. Degeneration, trophic interactions, and repair of severed axons: a reconsideration of some common assumptions. *Neuroscientist.* 2016;6(2):88-109.
5. Lunn ER, Brown MC, Perry VH. The pattern of axonal degeneration in the peripheral nervous system varies with different types of lesion. *Neuroscience.* 1990;35(1):157-165.
6. Bosse F, Hasenpusch-Theil K, Küry P, Müller HW. Gene expression profiling reveals that peripheral nerve regeneration is a consequence of both novel injury-dependent and reactivated developmental processes. *J Neurochem.* 2006;96(5):1441-1457.
7. Taskinen HS, Röyttä M. The dynamics of macrophage recruitment after nerve transection. *Acta Neuropathol.* 1997;93(3):252-259.
8. Brück W. The role of macrophages in wallerian degeneration. *Brain Pathol.* 1997;7(2):741-752.
9. Burnett MG, Zager EL. Pathophysiology of peripheral nerve injury: a brief review. *Neurosurg Focus.* 2004;16(5):1-7.
10. Bhatheja K, Field J. Schwann cells: origins and role in axonal maintenance and regeneration. *Int J Biochem Cell Biol.* 2006;38(12):1995-1999.
11. Campbell WW. Evaluation and management of peripheral nerve injury. *Clin Neurophysiol.* 2008;119(9):1951-1965.
12. Lundborg G, Dahlin LB, Danielsen N, Nachemson AK. Tissue specificity in nerve regeneration. *Scand J Plast Reconstr Surg.* 1986;20(3):279-283.
13. Lee SK, Wolfe SW. Peripheral nerve injury and repair. *J Am Acad Orthop Surg.* 2000;8(4):243-252.
14. Menorca RMG, Fussell TS, Elfar JC. Nerve physiology: mechanisms of injury and recovery. *Hand Clin.* 2013;29(3):317-330.
15. Pan YA, Misgeld T, Lichtman JW, Sanes JR. Effects of neurotoxic and neuroprotective agents on peripheral nerve regeneration assayed by time-lapse imaging in vivo. *J Neurosci.* 2003;23(36):11479-11488.
16. Sunderland SS. The anatomy and physiology of nerve injury. *Muscle Nerve.* 1990;13(9):771-784.
   In this report, Sir Sydney Sunderland summarizes forty years of clinical experience managing peripheral nerve injuries. Salient peripheral nerve anatomy is reviewed with focus on microstructure, fascicular distribution and blood supply. The manner in which anatomical features at the suture line influence the outcome of axon regeneration is also described.
17. Dedkov EI, Kostrominova TY, Borisov AB, Carlson BM. Survival of Schwann cells in chronically denervated skeletal muscles. *Acta Neuropathol.* 2002;103(6):565-574.
18. Seddon HJ. Three types of nerve injury. *Brain.* 1943;66(4):237-828.
   This seminal article by Sir Herbert Seddon in 1943 describes three types of peripheral nerve injuries – neurapraxia, axonotmesis, and neurotmesis – based on the severity of tissue injury, prognosis and time for recovery. Peripheral nerve surgeons still use this nerve injury classification system today.
19. Sunderland S. A classification of peripheral nerve injuries producing loss of function. *Brain.* 1951;74(4):491-516.
   In this 1951 classic paper by Sir Sydney Sunderland, a more complex and specific classification scheme of peripheral nerve injury is introduced. This classification system stratifies nerve injuries into one of five categories according to severity of injury based on the level of anatomic nerve disruption.
20. Pfister BJ, Gordon T, Loverde JR, et al. Biomedical engineering strategies for peripheral nerve repair: surgical applications, state of the art, and future challenges. *Crit Rev Biomed Eng.* 2011;39(2):81-124.

21. Dellon AL, Mackinnon SE. *Nerve repair and nerve grafts*. In: *Surgery of the Peripheral Nerve*. New York, NY: Thieme Medical Publishers; 1988.
22. Dellon AL. Management of peripheral nerve problems in the upper and lower extremity using quantitative sensory testing. *Hand Clin*. 1999;15(4):697-715.
23. Lipinski LJ, Spinner RJ. Neurolysis, neurectomy, and nerve repair/reconstruction for chronic pain. *Neurosurg Clin N Am*. 2014;25(4):777-787.
24. Griffin JW, Hogan MV, Chhabra AB, Deal DN. Peripheral nerve repair and reconstruction. *J Bone Joint Surg Am*. 2013;95(23):2144-2151.
25. Robinson LR. Traumatic injury to peripheral nerves. *Muscle Nerve*. 2000;23(6):863-873.
26. Chaudhry V, Cornblath DR. Wallerian degeneration in human nerves: serial electrophysiological studies. *Muscle Nerve*. 1992;15(6):687-693.
27. He YS, Zhong SZ. Acetylcholinesterase: a histochemical identification of motor and sensory fascicles in human peripheral nerve and its use during operation. *Plast Reconstr Surg*. 1988;82(1):125-132.
28. Lundborg G. A 25-year perspective of peripheral nerve surgery: evolving neuroscientific concepts and clinical significance. *J Hand Surg Am*. 2000;25(3):391-414.
29. Tse R, Ko JH. Nerve glue for upper extremity reconstruction. *Hand Clin*. 2012;28(4):529-540.
30. Cruz NI, Debs N, Fiol RE. Evaluation of fibrin glue in rat sciatic nerve repairs. *Plast Reconstr Surg*. 1986;78(3):369-373.
31. Martins RS, Siqueira MG, Da Silva CF, Plese JPP. Overall assessment of regeneration in peripheral nerve lesion repair using fibrin glue, suture, or a combination of the 2 techniques in a rat model: which is the ideal choice? *Surg Neurol*. 2005;64:S10-S16.
32. Mackinnon SE, Doolabh VB, Novak CB, Trulock EP. Clinical outcome following nerve allograft transplantation. *Plast Reconstr Surg*. 2001;107(6):1419-1429.
33. Karabekmez FE, Duymaz A, Moran SL. Early clinical outcomes with the use of decellularized nerve allograft for repair of sensory defects within the hand. *Hand*. 2009;4(3):245-249.
34. Moore AM, Ray WZ, Chenard KE, et al. Nerve allotransplantation as it pertains to composite tissue transplantation. *Hand*. 2009;4(3):239-244.
35. Gaudin R, Knipfer C, Henningsen A, et al. Approaches to peripheral nerve repair: generations of biomaterial conduits yielding to replacing autologous nerve grafts in craniomaxillofacial surgery. *Biomed Res Int*. 2016;2016(13):1-18.
36. Lundborg G, Dahlin LB, Danielsen N. Ulnar nerve repair by the silicone chamber technique. *Scand J Plast Reconstr Surg Hand Surg*. 2009;25(1):79-82.
37. Kubiak CA, Kung TA, Brown DL, Cederna PS, Kemp SWP. State of the art techniques in treating peripheral nerve injury. *Plast Reconstr Surg*. 2018;141(3):702-710.
38. Georgiou M, Golding JP, Loughlin AJ, et al. Engineered neural tissue with aligned, differentiated adipose-derived stem cells promotes peripheral nerve regeneration across a critical sized defect in rat sciatic nerve. *Biomaterials*. 2015;37:242-251.
39. Cui Q. Actions of neurotrophic factors and their signaling pathways in neuronal survival and axonal regeneration. *Mol Neurobiol*. 2006;33(2):155-180.
40. Nath RK, Mackinnon SE. Nerve transfers in the upper extremity. *Hand Clin*. 2000;16(1):131-139.
41. Lee SK, Wolfe SW. Nerve transfers for the upper extremity: new horizons in nerve reconstruction. *J Am Acad Orthop Surg*. 2012;20(8):506-517.
42. Novak CB, Mackinnon SE. Distal Anterior interosseous nerve transfer to the deep motor branch of the ulnar nerve for reconstruction of high ulnar nerve injuries. *J Reconstr Microsurg*. 2002;18(6):459-464.
43. Teboul F, Kakkar R, Ameur N, et al. Transfer of fascicles from the ulnar nerve to the nerve to the biceps in the treatment of upper brachial plexus palsy. *J Bone Joint Surg Am*. 2004;86A(7):1485-1490.
44. Dvali L, Mackinnon S. Nerve repair, grafting, and nerve transfers. *Clin Plast Surg*. 2003;30(2):203-221.
    This article presents a detailed overview of principles and techniques in peripheral nerve repair and management of segmental nerve gaps. Autogenous nerve grafts, vascularized nerve grafts, conduits, and allografts are all reviewed. The prinicples and techniques of nerve transfers are also discussed with numerous transfer procedures described.
45. Ide C. Peripheral nerve regeneration. *Neurosci Res*. 1996;25(2):101-121.
46. Capek L, Clarke HM, Curtis CG. Neuroma-in-continuity resection: early outcome in obstetrical brachial plexus palsy. *Plast Reconstr Surg*. 1998;102(5):1555-1562.
47. Ives GC, Kung TA, Nghiem BT, et al. Current state of the surgical treatment of terminal neuromas. *Neurosurgery*. 2017;89(3):422.
48. Souza JM, Cheesborough JE, Ko JH, et al. Targeted muscle reinnervation: a novel approach to postamputation neuroma pain. *Clin Orthop Relat Res*. 2014;472(10):2984-2990.
49. Kubiak CA, Kemp SWP, Cederna PS. Regenerative peripheral nerve interface for management of postamputation neuroma. *JAMA Surg*. 2018;153(7):681-682.

QUESTIONS

1. **1. A 23-year-old man is brought to the emergency department 6 hours after sustaining a single gunshot to the right upper arm. Physical examination shows an open wound and a high radial nerve palsy. Which of the following is the most appropriate first step in management of potential nerve injury?**
   a. Immediate surgical exploration and primary nerve repair if the nerve is lacerated
   b. Immediate surgical exploration and repair with a nerve graft if the nerve is lacerated
   c. Immediate surgical exploration, resection of devitalized nerve, and suture tagging of the nerve ends for delayed repair
   d. Observation with EMG 6 months after injury followed by exploration and repair if no return of function

2. **A 45-year-old woman is brought to the emergency department after a rollover motor vehicle accident. Physical examination shows significant soft tissue loss and a median nerve injury at the wrist. The patient is taken immediately back to the operating room where a 5 cm segmental nerve gap is observed. Which of the following treatment options is most likely to provide the best long-term functional outcome for this patient?**
   a. PGA conduit
   b. Acellular allograft reconstruction
   c. Collagen conduit reconstruction
   d. Peripheral nerve autograft
   e. Primary nerve repair

3. **A 37-year-old woman presents to clinic with nerve compression of her right ulnar nerve at the elbow. Both NCS and EMG are planned. Which of the following best indicates loss of motor axons?**
   a. Decreased distal motor latency
   b. Presence of fibrillation potentials
   c. Absent PSWs
   d. Increased amplitudes
   e. Increased conduction velocity

4. **A 25-year-old woman presents to clinic 8 months after sustaining a stab wound to her right forearm with complaints of weakness of grip strength in her right hand. Physical examination reveals a Tinel sign present over the ulnar aspect of the mid-volar forearm adjacent to a well-healed laceration. She is taken to the operating room where a neuroma-in-continuity is identified along her right ulnar nerve. The neuroma is resected, and a 3 cm nerve gap remains. Which of the following is the most appropriate next step in management?**
   a. Nerve reconstruction with synthetic nerve conduit
   b. Mobilize nerve both proximally and distally and perform primary neurorrhaphy
   c. Nerve reconstruction with LABC nerve graft
   d. Sural nerve cable grafting
   e. Perform tendon transfers to assist with grip

5. **A 21-year-old man presents to the emergency department after sustaining a deep laceration to his left elbow. Physical examination shows decreased function of the ulnar nerve, and the patient is taken for urgent operative exploration. Following proximal and distal dissection, a 1 cm gap persists between the proximal and distal nerve ends. Which of the following is the most appropriate next step in management?**
   a. Nerve transfer
   b. Primary neurorrhaphy
   c. PGA nerve conduit
   d. Nerve transposition
   e. Sural nerve grafting

6. **A 27-year-old man comes to clinic after sustaining a brachial plexus injury in a motorcycle accident. Nerve transfer to the biceps for restoration of elbow flexion is planned. Which of the following fascicles or nerves is the most appropriate donor?**
   a. Distal spinal accessory nerve
   b. Medial pectoral nerve
   c. Thoracodorsal nerve
   d. Palmaris longus fascicle of the median nerve
   e. Flexor carpi ulnaris fascicle of the ulnar nerve

7. **A 7-year-old girl is brought to the emergency department after sustaining an injury to the left upper extremity, 3 cm proximal to the antecubital fossa. Which of the following factors is associated with improved functional outcomes following peripheral nerve repair?**
   a. Proximal nerve injury
   b. Young patient age
   c. Increased time between injury and repair
   d. Tension at nerve repair
   e. Few suture strands used in nerve repair

1. **Answer: c.** In general, nerve injuries associated with open wounds should be explored and, if appropriate, repaired early. For example, if the nerve injury resulted from a relatively clean laceration or wound, it should be explored and repaired immediately. However, in the case of crush or significant soft tissue injury, like in the case of a gunshot wound, nerve repair should be delayed until the extent of devitalized tissue can be determined and the soft tissue repair is stable.

2. **Answer: d.** Peripheral nerve autografts are the most reliable choice for reconstruction of nerve gaps greater than 3 cm. Autograft use is limited by availability and donor site morbidity from additional incisions, loss of sensation, and possible neuroma formation. Nerve conduits, such as PGA conduits, collagen conduits, and acellular allografts are limited in their use in short gaps (<3 cm). Beyond 3 cm, there is no clinically meaningful regeneration. Lastly, even with extensive mobilization of the nerve, it is unlikely tensionless primary repair could be performed in a 5 cm nerve gap.

3. **Answer: b.** There are numerous electrodiagnostic findings suggestive of axonal loss: decreased CMAP/compound sensory nerve action potential amplitudes, slowed conduction velocity, prolonged latency, and the presence of fibrillations and PSWs. It should be noted that fibrillations and PSWs do not become evident for 3 to 6 weeks following an acute nerve injury.

4. **Answer: d.** Synthetic nerve conduit reconstruction of nerve has not proven effective in gaps longer than 2 cm and is less effective in motor nerve defects. A tension-free repair is always the goal for nerve anastomoses but is likely not attainable with a nerve gap of 3 cm. The LABC nerve is the distal continuation of the musculocutaneous nerve. Given the size of the defect and the need for at least two cable grafts, this nerve would not be an appropriate donor. The sural nerve is a more appropriate donor, as it provides sufficient length of graft to enable cable graft reconstruction. Tendon transfers are a last-resort means of restoring function.

5. Answer: d. Primary neurorrhaphy is performed whenever possible, provided that the repair is free of any tension at the suture site. Performing primary repair in the setting of a 1 cm segmental nerve defect would likely result in undue tension at the repair site. Fortunately, the ulnar nerve at the elbow is unique in that anterior nerve transposition allows significant shortening of the distance between nerve ends, making tension-less, primary repair possible. Nerve transfers are indicated in very proximal nerve injuries where primary repair and grafting are unavailable, or there is concern that target muscle denervation might occur prior to nerve regeneration. PGA nerve conduits represent an option for nerve reconstruction without any associated donor site morbidity; however, recovery outcomes are inferior to that of primary repair and autograft reconstruction. Autologous nerve grafts are the gold standard for reconstruction of nerve gaps, but nerve mobilization/transposition and primary repair is preferable if possible.

6. Answer: e. The fascicle of the largest caliber and with the greatest number of motor axons should be selected as the donor nerve. The other suggested nerve transfers are also possibilities, but the flexor carpi ulnaris fascicle of the ulnar nerve to biceps (Oberlin procedure) is the most preferable for this reason.

7. Answer: b. Recovery after peripheral nerve injuries is affected by several patient factors. Younger patients have better outcomes than older patients. Earlier repairs have also been shown to have better outcomes than those attempted at later time points. The more distal the injury, the better the prognosis in terms of functional recovery. Minimal tension and an increasing number of suture strands crossing the repair site are both associated with improved function.

CHAPTER 11 Principles of Tissue Expansion

Paul F. Hwang and Samuel J. Lin

KEY POINTS

- Tissue expansion is a simple technique which has wide-range soft tissue coverage capabilities.
- These prosthetics provide broader coverage through changes at the histologic level as well as altering physiologic properties of the skin.
- The epidermal layer thickens in reaction to tissue expansion, whereas the dermal layer becomes thinner.
- Up to 50% of the scalp can be reconstructed utilizing tissue expansion.
- Extremities have the highest level of complications when tissue expanders are placed in these anatomic regions.

Tissue expansion is a simple yet effective tool in one's armamentarium to reconstruct adjacent cutaneous and soft tissue defects. This technique takes advantage of the viscoelastic properties of the skin to create donor material that can truly replace like tissue with like. Its applicability to almost all parts of the body and even the most complexity of wounds makes this a valuable technique that should be familiar to all reconstructive surgeons.

HISTORY

The foundation for tissue expansion technique actually has its derivation from distraction osteogenesis. At the turn of the 20th century, Codvilla applied the principles of external distraction directly to bones and used this to shortened limbs in stages with traction of medium intensity, thus enabling to overcome the resistance with a lesser force to distract the bony component.[1] In 1921, Putti continued the work on refining femur-lengthening technique by pinpointing the need for continuous and elastic forces to overcome the resistance of the soft tissues.[2] This expansion of soft tissue accommodates newfound limb lengthening.

One of the earliest descriptions of skin expansion came several years later in 1957 when Neumann became the pioneering surgeon to first use gradual distention of a rubber balloon through an externally exposed tube with a stopcock to expand local skin and subcutaneous tissue to reconstruct a partial ear defect.[3] This technique was revolutionary in that we now have the ability to secure skin that was high in quality in regard to color and texture with tissue immediately adjacent to the defect, avoiding the need for harvesting from a remote donor site.

Unfortunately, this case report on tissue expansion did not receive the enthusiastic fervor and legitimacy as a potential option in reconstructive surgery. More than two decades later, Radovan reinvigorated the concept of expansion through the use of an internally placed port.[4] Further work by Austad and Rose elucidated much of the physiology behind tissue expansion through the use of an osmotically driven, self-inflating expander in a guinea pig model.[5]

Since then tissue expansion is now widely accepted and considered a familiar technique for any reconstructive surgeon. Although a simple technique, understanding of the physiology behind tissue expansion and special considerations in design make it more intricate in nature. Appreciation of these concepts is critical to the widespread application of this method to areas all over the body that may not have been previously possible.

BIOLOGICAL EFFECTS OF TISSUE EXPANSION

At the molecular level, tissue expansion is possible secondary to elaborate intrinsic signaling. The principle of strain-induced cellular growth involves a network of several integrated cascades that include growth factors, cytoskeletal structures, and protein kinases.[6] Growth factors such as platelet-derived growth factor and angiotensin II have been implicated in cell growth.[7,8] Not only are there implications on cell growth, but also there are other growth factors such as epidermal growth factor (EGF) and transforming growth factor (TGF) that are involved in cell migration, differentiation, and wound healing.[9,10] Protein kinase C is known to play a crucial role in signal transduction through a cascade of events through its activation of other proteins by an unknown mechanism.[11]

Despite an unknown mechanism, these molecular activities created by mechanical stress translate into the creep phenomenon. Creep is defined as stretching of a material under a constant load over time.[12] With regard to tissue expansion, it comes in the form of mechanical and biologic creep. Mechanical creep relies on the skin's ability to acutely stretch and increase in surface area during immediate intraoperative tissue expansion.[13] It is explained by the displacement of fluids out of the collagen network leading to dehydration of tissues, collagen fiber realignment in a parallel fashion, elastic fibers microfragmentation, and adjacent tissue migration into the expanded field as a result of the stretching force.[13,14]

Biologic creep, on the other hand, derives its significant gain in tissue from increased fibroblast and collagen synthesis, increased myofilaments, increased mitotic activity, and neovascularization.[13] It is very much dependent on the chronicity of controlled tissue expansion, as the imposed deformation allows for stress-relaxation in preventing the tissue from retracting back into its pre-expansive form because of the formation of new tissue.[15] Essentially, the force required to maintain tissue elongation decreases with time as the tissue expansion is maintained.

Many of the predictable changes to the layers of the skin and soft tissue are listed in **Table 11.1**.[11,16,17] Of special note is the increased vascularity associated with an expanded flap with increased number and caliber of vessels when compared with a nonexpanded counterpart.[17] This can be attributed to increased angiogenic factors such as vascular endothelial growth factor (VEGF) expressed in expanded tissues.[18] These factors may also have the same effect seen in delayed flaps. In fact, skin flap viability and capillary blood flow were similar between expanded flaps and delayed flaps as well as significantly higher than those of acute random skin flaps raised on the normal skin.[11] In principle, expanded tissues are a form of a delayed flap.

TYPES OF TISSUE EXPANSION DEVICES

Through technological advances, the modern day tissue expander has changed tremendously since the initial inflatable balloon and external tubing with a stopcock apparatus that was used by Neumann.[3] Currently, there are a multitude of tissue expanders of different types that are available from a variety of manufacturers (**Figure 11.1**). The type of expander chosen will depend on the clinical scenario at hand.

Each type of tissue expander will have specific characteristics that make them more advantageous to use in different anatomic sites and situations. The shape of tissue expander will be the first distinction to make. In general, they can be round, rectangular, or crescent shaped.

TABLE 11.1. CHANGES IN SKIN AND SOFT TISSUE AFTER TISSUE EXPANSION

Location	Change
Epidermis	Increased mitotic activity
	No significant decrease in thickness
Dermis	Dermal thinning
	Collagen synthesis markedly increased
	Increase fibroblasts and myofibroblasts
	Realignment of collagen fibers
	Decreased hair follicle density
Muscle	Increased thinning
	Function unchanged
	Myofibril and myofilament disorganized arrangement
	Increased size and number of mitochondria
Fat	Permanent decrease in fat cells and thickness
	Fat necrosis and fibrosis may occur with aggressive expansion
Blood vessels	Proliferation of blood vessels with increase venules and arterioles

They can also be further subcategorized, depending on the manufacturer, into specific types such as angled, ellipsoid, oval, etc. In addition to shape, the texture of the tissue expander can come into play when deciding which one to choose. Some studies have shown that capsular formation quality may be better with texture versus smooth tissue expanders, thus affecting capsular contracture rates when replaced with definitive implants in breast reconstruction.[19] Finally, the size of the tissue expander will help determine choice between the different types. Although obvious that a larger expander will accommodate a large eventual flap, one may be limited in size because of the internal characteristics of the tissues or amount of cutaneous coverage needed in the end.

Another important feature of the tissue expansion apparatus is the route of expansion needed. Tissue expanders are typically accessed through self-sealing, single ports that can serve as a point for injectable flow in or out, allowing for serial expansions in addition to the fill placed intraoperatively. However, the port can also be distal to the expander itself or integrated within the apparatus itself. Distal ports have the advantage of minimizing risk of iatrogenic rupture by accidental puncture. However, they have their own faults such as manipulation of the port itself (e.g., flipping, migration) if not placed into a proper pocket as well as obstruction of the tubing in between the port and the expander. Integrated ports have the obvious advantage of not having the need to make a separate dissection for the port along with any mechanical issues one would find with the distant ports. However, one has the main issue of iatrogenic injury to the tissue expander itself with the integrated port. Also, an integrated port is less ideal if there is lack of coverage secondary to the thinning of overlying soft tissue.

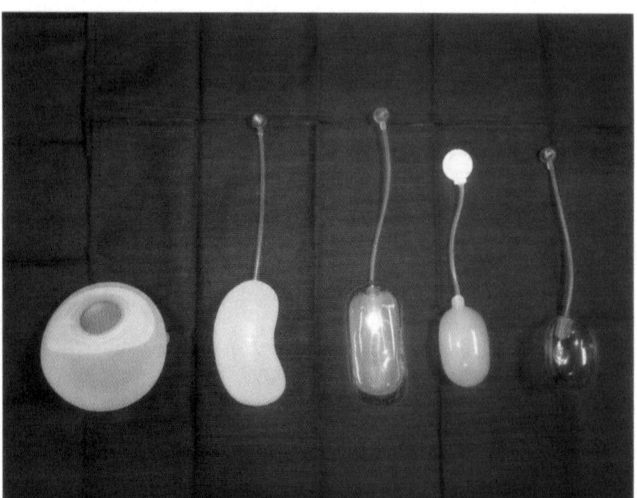

FIGURE 11.1. Tissue expanders of various shapes (breast specific, curvilinear, rectangular, oval) and port integration versus nonintegration.

There has been a renewed interest in self-expanding tissue expanders because of logistical considerations. As tissue expander technology has evolved, so have the logistics for expansion. To decrease clinic time, costs for travel, and stress on patients, some clinical situations provide for self-expansion at home through self-injection, and it is proven to be safe and reliable.[20] More recently, the Food and Drug Administration had cleared for the use of carbon dioxide–filled, remote-controlled tissue expanders for further convenience of home expansion and obviating the need for percutaneous saline injections in breast reconstruction.[21] If this technology is applied to tissues expanders of all shape and sizes, this may eliminate the complications of both distant and integrated ports entirely.

SURGICAL DESIGN AND CONSIDERATIONS

Tissue expansion not only involves the surgery to place the expander, expansion, and then subsequent flap placement or permanent implant exchange, but preoperative conditions must be considered. Patient selection is crucial if a clinician chooses this form of reconstruction. The patient will require a maturity level and need to demonstrate emotional stability to withstand the pain or discomfort associated with the expansion as well as temporary additional aesthetic disfigurement. Smoking, radiation, and infections have a higher risk of wound complications both during the expansion process and afterward. We would also not consider tissue expansion as a viable option in the need for acute coverage of a defect. If home self-injectable expansions will be done, adequate education and training must be given to non–health care attendants.

Even before an incision is made, flap design incorporating placement of incisions in regard to final scars, direction of flap movement, and proper placement of the prosthesis itself are all critical factors leading to a successful tissue expander reconstruction. Incisions are typically made at the border of the defect needing coverage or lesion needing excision. Flaps can be of any type such as advancement, rotation, or interpositional flaps, but the incision must take into account that the direction of movement will be perpendicular to the incision placed to maximize flap coverage and minimize tension during expansion. Proper placement of the expander will be important and what type of port will factor into this. When placing a distant filling port, one needs to ensure a separate pocket is created that will accommodate the port, minimize manipulation resulting in migration or flipping, and be placed typically with a posterior backing with stiff skeletal support if possible to accommodate ease of injection. The injectable port should be superficial enough to be palpable, not be in an area of pressure or sensitivity, and not be in the line of a healing incision. Expanders with integrated ports will require a pocket that will account for the port and its added projection as well as still have durable overlying tissue in anticipation of some of it thinning during the expansion process. This is important because there are certain integrated tissue expanders with a significant height/thickness of the expander with the integrated port requiring careful planning for adequate soft tissue coverage over the expander. During placement, the expander should also be partially filled to unravel any folds in the device. This allows for a snug fit with the surrounding tissue envelope and allows for the closure of any dead space. This will help to minimize seroma formation along with placement of drains. Clinical evaluation of the skin is necessary to ensure that the expander is not overfilled to compromise the tissues from the start. The incisions made to place the expanders are closed in layers.

Once the tissue expander has been placed and wounds have healed for 3 weeks, serial expansion can begin. The expansion schedule will have to be geared toward the individual on a case-by-case basis to expand with smaller increments on a daily basis. However, realistically, owing to coordination of clinic schedules and patient transport issues, expansion is typically done on a weekly or biweekly basis until the goal is met. After each expansion, the skin and subcutaneous tissues should be checked for tightness and vascularity. The patient should be asked to report pain or discomfort during and after completion of the serial expansion. If the patient is in any discomfort, the expansion could be stopped and/or fluid can be taken out until comfortable again. Once the goal is met, it is best to wait 3 to 4 weeks before the second-staged reconstruction. The second stage may be for permanent implant exchange or flap placement and to take advantage of the stress-relaxation effect from prolonged positioning after the final serial expansion.

INDICATIONS BY ANATOMIC REGION

Head and Neck

Scalp

Scalp defects can occur secondary to tumor excision, infection, traumatic injury, burns, radiation injury, or excision of a congenital lesion. Reconstructive goals are to obtain coverage over a reconstructed scalp (**Figure 11.2**) as well as realignment of hair-bearing areas if alopecia is involved (**Figures 11.3** and **11.4**). Tissue expansion has been widely accepted and used by plastic surgeons in reconstruction of these medium to large scalp defects. One can use this technique to cover large defects involving up to 50% of the scalp without significant thinning of the hair-bearing areas.[22] The robust vascular nature of the scalp along with incorporation of a dominant vessel in the flap design will ensure a durable flap of good hair-bearing quality. Even though expansion brings upon a decrease in hair density, this is usually unnoticeable.[23] The expander is typically placed in the subgaleal plane under hair-bearing area. The expansion process takes weeks to months depending on patient characteristics. Afterward, the expander is taken out through the initial incision, and the flap is designed in such a way to avoid transection of any dominant vessels. Capsulectomies are avoided, as they may devascularize the flap. Galeotomies may also devascularize the flap, but if carefully done, one may preserve the galeal blood supply for easier and faster expansion of the scalp with fewer expander extrusion complications.[24] There were initial concerns for cranial skeletal morphology changes; however, studies have shown that temporary cranial molding occurs with correction in 3 to 4 months.[19] Nonetheless, the rates of extrusion of the tissue expansion of the scalp in the general adult population is not insignificant, and careful planning must be undertaken at each step of the way. Tissue expanders that become exposed during the expansion process may be successfully exchanged with a smaller amount of volume with closure of the wound with subsequent expansion over time.

Forehead

Forehead reconstruction with tissue expanders is a particular challenge as goals are required to incorporate aesthetic units involving the brow as well as anterior and lateral hairline symmetries. Resurfacing of the forehead without distortion of these structures will depend upon the size of the defect. Expansion with direct advancement of tissues can be used to reconstruct 25% to 70% of forehead defects.[25] Anything less may just require serial excisions, and anything more may require going up the reconstructive ladder to an expanded full-thickness skin graft or even a free flap. Adjacent scalp and cheek sometimes need to be mobilized to obtain improved symmetry. Brow symmetry and ptosis should be assessed simultaneously with any flap advancement.

Face and Neck

The face and neck are obviously highly visible and therefore aesthetically demanding in regard to reconstructive resurfacing. Tissue expanders can be used and are usually placed in the lateral facial areas such as in the cheek and neck. Areas such as the neck are ideal donor sites, as they are optimal in quality similar to the facial skin.[26]

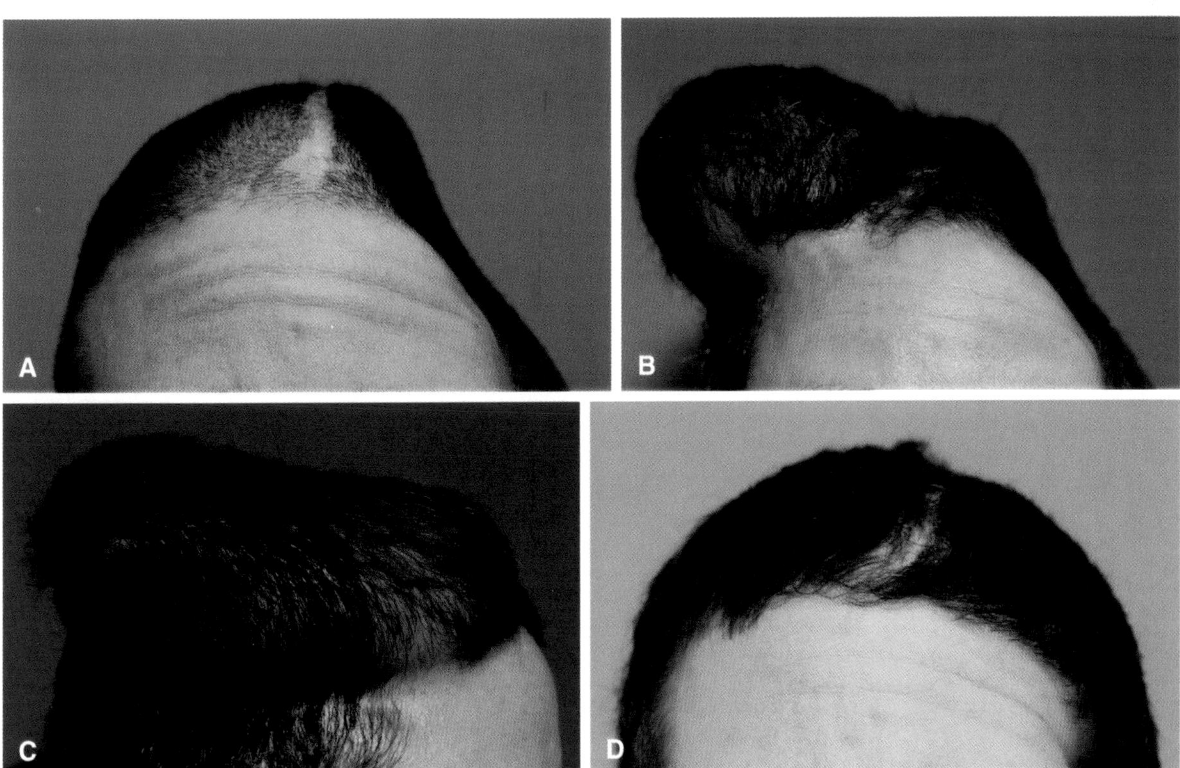

FIGURE 11.2. Tissue expansion after cranial reconstruction. **A.** Preoperative expansion. **B.** Expansion phase, front profile. **C.** Expansion phase, right lateral profile. **D.** Postoperative expansion.

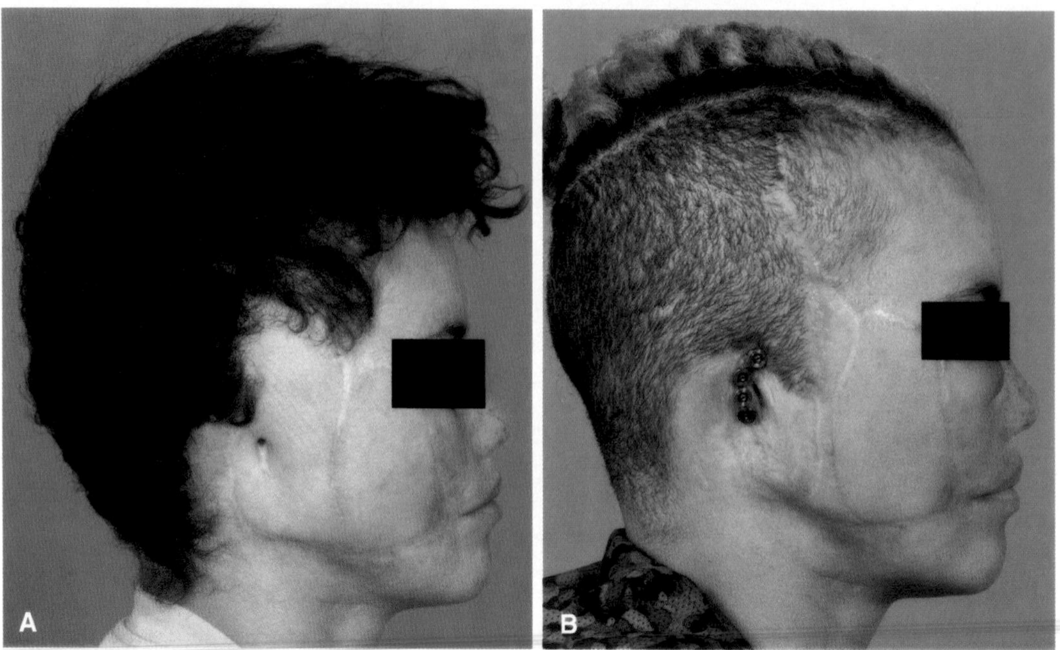

FIGURE 11.3. Tissue expansion for hairline restoration. **A.** Preoperative expansion. **B.** Postoperative expansion. (Courtesy of Kerry Latham, M.D.)

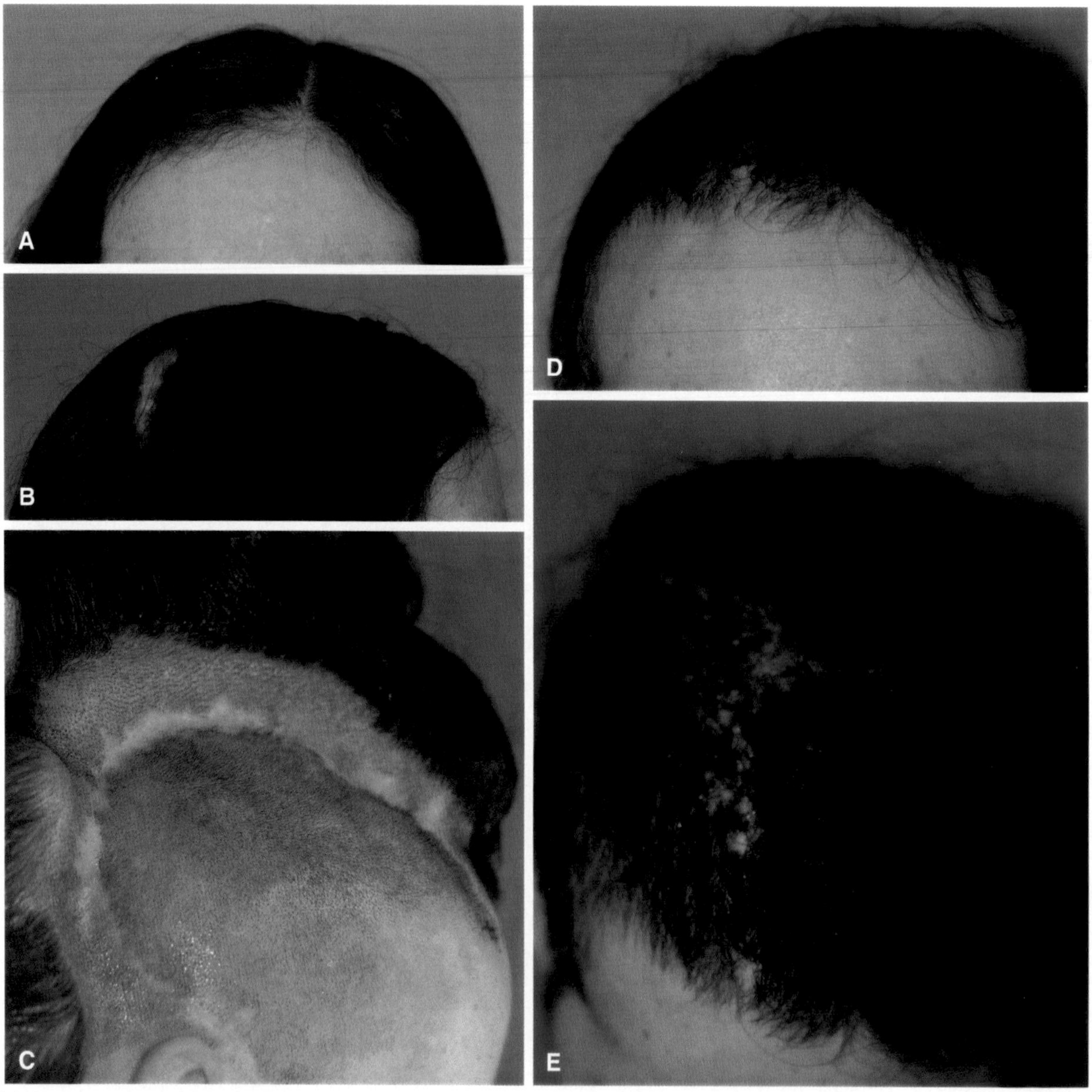

FIGURE 11.4. Tissue expansion for scar alopecia. **A.** Preoperative expansion, front profile. **B.** Preoperative expansion, right lateral profile. **C.** Intraoperative. **D.** Postoperative expansion, front profile. **E.** Postoperative expansion, birds-eye view.

Care is taken to maintain intact aesthetic facial subunits and to keep incisions in aesthetically compliant locations. Typically, an incision is made in a preauricular facelift-type incision and placement of the expander above the platysma or submuscular aponeurotic system. A distal port is commonly used and can be placed postauricularly or within the neck. Once the flap is elevated and rotated into position, careful suture techniques will be needed to maintain the tissue in the area of defect but also avoid unnecessary tension that would lead to iatrogenic distortion such as lower lid dropping, oral incompetence, and facial mimetic asymmetry.

Breast

Postmastectomy Breast Reconstruction

Breast reconstruction using tissue expanders is a common technique that all plastic surgeons are familiar with. Implant-based reconstruction accounts for almost 65% of all breast reconstructions in the United States because of its safety, cost-effectiveness, and reliability.[27] In general, after mastectomy, tissue expanders are placed in a subpectoral or more recently prepectoral position in conjunction with acellular dermal matrix for supplemental or total coverage. The surgical wounds are allowed to heal, and expansion is commenced in 2 to 3 weeks on a weekly or biweekly basis until goal breast volume. An exchange procedure is undertaken to replace the tissue expander with a similar-sized permanent implant.

Although the majority of plastic surgeons in the United States most likely practice placement of tissue expanders in a subpectoral pocket, prepectoral placement with total acellular dermal matrix coverage has gained interest, as it foregoes the need to detach the pectoralis muscle. This translates into quicker postoperative recovery and decreased operative duration for reconstruction. Although long-term studies are necessary to determine and compare outcomes, some early studies show this technique to be effective with comparable complication rates to the subpectoral technique.[28] The topic of breast reconstruction using prosthetic techniques is covered in more detail in Chapter 59.

Special Considerations: Congenital Anomalies, Gender Identity Disorder (Male to Female)

Congenital anomalies of the breast consist of Poland syndrome, idiopathic unilateral breast hypoplasia, or tuberous breast deformity. Although not congenital, breast asymmetry can also be secondary to trauma or iatrogenic injuries to the breast bud at a young age, leading to an abnormal growth pattern. Regardless of the etiology, timing of reconstruction and expansion is what that differs between these cases and in postmastectomy breast reconstruction. One can place the tissue expander once the patient has stopped growing so there is a goal in mind (i.e., size and shape of the contralateral normal side); however, this would be a long time for a young adolescent female to live with this unilateral deformity. Tissue expanders can be used as a temporary but prolonged measure to incrementally expand the size of the breast as the patient continues to grow. This can continue until the patient reaches the age of maturity at which time definitive reconstruction with a permanent prosthesis or autologous reconstruction can be done. Congenital breast anomalies are covered in more detail in Chapter 62.

Male-to-female transgender patients desiring breast augmentation may need tissue expanders to expand their skin and soft tissues to fit the size of implant they desire. The Endocrine Society recommends transgender females to delay breast augmentation until at least 2 years of estrogen therapy, as the breasts continue to grow during that time period.[29] This may not necessarily negate the need for a tissue expander but would overall allow for the development of a more suitable soft tissue envelope for the final prosthetic implant.

Trunk

There is a wide variety of cases for the trunk such as burns, congenital anomalies, traumatic injuries, and large hernia defects that require reconstruction. Unless it is amenable to excision in three stages or less, tissue expansion is the reconstructive option of choice when it comes to the back, abdomen, and chest.[30] Expansion of the skin, with or without the underlying fascia, allows for primary closure when necessary. Subcutaneously placed expanders are used for defects with minimal fascial tension, whereas intermuscularly placed expanders can close large defects involving the fascia and abdominal musculature.[31] Although they are uncomfortable and can interfere with daily activities of living, tissue expansion of the trunk is associated with low rates of morbidity and mortality and high rates of primary fascial closure and incisions, while hernia recurrences rates appear to be low.[32]

Tissue expanders can also be used to expand truncal donor flaps in preparation for use at a different recipient site. Pre-expanding the flap increases the flap dimension and reduces the flap thickness and donor site morbidities. Reports of this method of expanding the donor site have been used to create donor sites that were large enough to fill the defects of various regions such as the lower extremity, abdominal wall, perineum, and hand.[33-35]

Extremities

Using an extremity as a donor site with tissue expansion is not ideal. They are typically known to have a disproportionately higher rate of complications when compared with using expanders in other regions of the body.[36] Most algorithms for tissue expansion to treat upper extremities rely upon the use of tissue expansion in regional areas such as the back, shoulder, and flank.[37] Lesions of the proximal arm to elbow, if noncircumferential, do well with expanded transposition flaps from the back or shoulder. If large and requiring more soft tissue, an expanded free transverse rectus abdominus muscle flap can be an option. Expanded flaps from the flank and abdomen can serve as good donor sites for lesions of the forearm and hands, respectively. For the lower extremity, limited mobility of the tissues results in the need for using more complex reconstructive approaches even for smaller lesions.[38] Expanded transposition flaps, local flaps, and even free flaps are the mainstream treatments for these difficult cases.

COMPLICATIONS

Several factors play a role in complications from tissue expansion. These factors depend on patient characteristics, technique, site of expansion, and the aggressiveness of expansion schedule and volume. One study showed complications necessitating some form of revision to the original treatment plan in as high as 39% of cases.[36] However, enough tissue was generated from the expansion itself to complete the reconstructive plan without affecting final outcomes. Fortunately, most complications from tissue expansion are minor, consisting of things such as seroma formation, widened scar, discomfort from the expansion itself, bone resorption, neuropraxia, remnant excessive soft tissue, and other aesthetic concerns.[11,39,40]

Major complications consist of hematoma, infection, implant exposure, implant failure or iatrogenic injury, and overlying tissue compromise (**Table 11.2**). Hematomas would require reoperation and possible explantation, although salvage is an option if found early on. Infections, if minimal, can be treated with intravenous and oral antibiotic therapy. Persistent and purulent infections may necessitate explantation. Colonization of the prosthesis can occur with each injection so sterile technique is mandatory for each expansion. Implant failure can be secondary to the internal failure in the manufacturing of the device itself or iatrogenic injury. It is important to use a proper-sized needle such as 23 gauge and to access the port at a 90-degree angle to minimize injury to the self-sealing port where saline can leak from. Finally, it is important to reevaluate the overlying soft tissues every time one expands the tissue expander. One should check that the skin is not too taut, that capillary refill is present, and that it is not too uncomfortable for the patient. Rapid expansion is possible but that should not compromise the vascularity to the flap that can lead to early extrusion.

TABLE 11.2. COMPLICATIONS FROM TISSUE EXPANSION
Major
■ Infection
■ Implant exposure
■ Implant failure
■ Soft tissue compromise
■ Hematoma formation
Minor
■ Seroma formation
■ Widened scar
■ Patient discomfort/pain
■ Excess soft tissue
■ Aesthetic concerns

REFERENCES

1. Codvilla A. On the means of lengthening, in the lower limbs, the muscles and tissues which are shortened through deformity. *Am J Orthop Surg*. 1905;2:353-357.
2. Putti V. The operative lengthening of the femur. *JAMA*. 1921;77:934-935.
3. Neumann CG. The expansion of an area of skin by progressive distention of a subcutaneous balloon. *Plast Reconstr Surg*. 1957;19:124-130.
   This article describes the use of a buried inflatable rubber balloon that was gradually distended to supply soft tissue coverage of a subtotally avulsed ear. At 2 months, this allowed for a 50% increase from its original surface area. Although just a case report, this article laid the foundation for future acceptance of tissue expansion as a legitimate form of reconstruction.
4. Radovan C. Breast reconstruction after mastectomy using the temporary expander. *Plast Reconstr Surg*. 1982;69:195-208.
   The author describes his operative technique which laid the foundation for current day two stage immediate breast reconstruction. In this article, he reviews his experience in reconstructing 68 patients.
5. Austad ED, Rose GL. A self-inflating tissue expander. *Plast Reconstr Surg*. 1982;70:588.
   The authors developed a silicone expandable implant that used differential osmotic gradients to drive self-inflation of the expander. This work was essential to fully understanding the physiological properties behind tissue expansion.
6. De Filippo RE, Atala A. Stretch and growth: the molecular and physiologic influences of tissue expansion. *Plast Reconstr Surg*. 2002;109:2450-2562.
7. Wilson E, Mai Q, Sudhir K, et al. Mechanical strain induces growth of vascular smooth muscle cells via autocrine action of PDGF. *J Cell Biol*. 1993;123:741.
8. Sudhir K, Wilson E, Chatterjee K, et al. Mechanical strain and collagen potentiate mitogenic activity of angiotensin II in rat vascular smooth muscle cells. *J Clin Invest*. 1993;92:3003.
9. Sporn M, Roberts A. Transforming growth factor-B: recent progress and new challenges. *J Cell Biol*. 1992;119:1017.
10. Mustoe TA, Pierce GF, Thomason A, et al. Accelerated healing of incisional wounds in rats induced by transforming growth factor-B. *Science*. 1987;237:1333.
11. Takei T, Mills I, Azai K, et al. Molecular basis for tissue expansion: clinical implications for the surgeon. *Plast Reconstr Surg*. 1998;102:247-258.
12. Gibson T. Physical properties of skin. In: McCarthy J, ed. *Plastic Surgery*. Philadelphia, PA: WB Saunders; 1990:209-211.
13. Johnson TM, Lowe L, Brown MD, et al. Histology and physiology of tissue expansion. *J Dermatol Surg Oncol*. 1993;19:1074-1078.
   This is a review of the histological and physiological changes that occur during tissue expansion. Expansion is shown to result in epidermal hypertrophy, decrease in dermis, muscle and adipose thickness, and bone resorption. This article attempts to define tissue expansion at the microscopic level in order to better understand the properties behind tissue expansion and its subsequent effect grossly.
14. Wilhelmi BJ, Blackwell SJ, Mancoll JS, et al. Creep vs. stretch: a review of the viscoelastic properties of skin. *Ann Plast Surg*. 1998;41:215-219.
15. Wee SS, Logan SE, Mustoe TA. Continuous versus intraoperative expansion in the pig model. *Plast Reconstr Surg*. 1992;90:808-814.
16. Sasaki GH, Pang CY. Pathophysiology of skin flaps raised on expanded pig skin. *Plast Reconstr Surg*. 1984;74:59-67.
17. Cherry GW, Austad E, Pasyk K, et al. Increased survival and vascularity of random pattern skin flaps elevated in controlled, expanded skin. *Plast Reconstr Surg*. 1983;72:680.
18. Lantieri LA, Martin-Garcia N, Wechsler J, et al. Vascular endothelial growth factor expression in expanded tissue: a possible mechanism of angiogenesis in tissue expansion. *Plast Reconstr Surg*. 1998;101:392-397.
19. Kuriyama E, Ochiai H, Inoue Y, et al. Characterization of the capsule surrounding smooth and textured tissue expanders and correlation with contracture. *Plast Reconstr Surg Glob Open*. 2017;5:e1403.
20. Mohmand MH, Sterne GD, Gowar JP. Home inflation of tissue expanders: a safe and reliable alternative. *Br J Plast Surg*. 2001;54:610-614.
21. Morrison KA, Asherman BM, Asherman JA. Evolving approaches to tissue expander design and application. *Plast Reconstr Surg*. 2017;140:23S-29S.
22. MacLennan SE, Corcoran JF, Neale HW. Tissue expansion in head and neck burn reconstruction. *Clin Plast Surg*. 2000; 27:121-132.
23. Kabaker SS, Kridel RW, Krugman ME, et al. Tissue expansion in the treatment of alopecia. *Arch Otolaryngol Head Neck Surg*. 1986;112:720-725.
24. El Sakka DM. Tissue expanders in post-burn alopecia: with or without galeotomies? *Ann Burns Fire Disasters*. 2015;28:210-214.
25. Gosain AK, Zochowski CG, Cortes W. Refinements of tissue expansion for pediatric forehead reconstruction: a 13-year experience. *Plast Reconstr Surg*. 2009;124:1559-1570.
26. Hu X, Zeng G, Zhou Y, Sun C. Reconstruction of skin defects on the mid and lower face using expanded flap in the neck. *J Craniofac Surg*. 2017;28:e137-e141.
27. Bertozzi N, Pesce M, Santi P, et al. Tissue expansion for breast reconstruction: methods and techniques. *Ann Med Surg (Lond)*. 2017;21:34-44.
28. Jafferbhoy S, Chandarana M, Houlihan M, et al. Early multicenter experience of pre-pectoral implant based immediate breast reconstruction using Braxon®. *Gland Surg*. 2017;6:682-688.
   Pre-pectoral placement of tissue expanders in breast reconstruction is a relatively new technique. This article is a prospective study of 78 immediate breast reconstructions showing this to be an effective technique with complication rates comparable to subpectoral placement. Further long-term studies will be necessary to validate these results.
29. Meyer WJ, Webb A, Stuart CA, et al. Physical and hormonal evaluation of transsexual patients: a longitudinal study. *Arch Sex Behav*. 1986;15:121-138.
30. Arnja JS. Gosain AK. Giant congenital melanocytic nevi of the trunk and an algorithm for treatment. *J Craniofac Surg*. 2005;16:886-893.
31. Wooten KE, Ozturk CN, Ozturk C, et al. Role of tissue expansion in abdominal wall reconstruction: a systematic evidence-based review. *J Plast Reconstr Aesthet Surg*. 2017;70:741-751.
32. Alam NN, Narang SK, Pathak S, et al. Methods of abdominal wall expansion for repair of incisional herniae: a systematic review. *Hernia*. 2016;20:191-199.
33. Monsivais SE, Webster ND, Wong S, et al. Pre-expanded deep inferior epigastric perforator flap. *Clin Plast Surg*. 2017;44:109-115.
34. Wang C, Zhang J, Yang S, et al. Pre-expanded and prefabricated abdominal superthin skin perforator flap for total hand resurfacing. *Clin Plast Surg*. 2017;44:171-177.
35. Liu Y, Zang M, Zhu S, et al. Pre-expanded paraumbilical perforator flap. *Clin Plast Surg*. 2017;44:99-108.
36. Antonyshyn O, Gruss JS, Mackinnon SE, et al. Complications of soft tissue expansion. *Br J Plast Surg*. 1988;41:239-250.
37. Margulis A, Bauer BS, Fine NA. Large and giant congenital pigmented nevi of the upper extremity: an algorithm to surgical management. *Ann Plast Surg*. 2004;52:158-167.
38. Kryger ZB, Bauer BS. Surgical management of large and giant congenital pigmented nevi of the lower extremity. *Plast Reconstr Surg*. 2008;121:1674-1684.
39. Bennett RH, Hirt M. A history of tissue expansion: concepts, controversies and complications. *J Dermatol Surg Oncol*. 1993;19:1066-1073.
40. Casanova D, Bali D, Bardot J, Legre R, Magalon G. Tissue expansion of the lower limb: complications in a cohort of 103 cases. *Br J Plast Surg*. 2001;54:310-316.

QUESTIONS

1. **A 13-year-old girl comes to the office 16 months after a scalding hot oil–burn injury to the scalp. At the time of injury, the patient was treated with debridement and skin grafting. On examination, the patient had an area of well-healed skin graft encompassing approximately 45% of the scalp total surface area. Which of the following is the best approach to reconstruction the scalp to effectively address the area of alopecia?**
   a. Free tissue transfer with latissimus muscle flap
   b. Serial excision and closure
   c. Tissue expansion
   d. Rotational flap
   e. Hair transplantation
2. **Which layer of the soft tissue thickens during tissue expansion?**
   a. Muscle
   b. Epidermis
   c. Dermis
   d. Subcutaneous fat
3. **What factor is responsible for the increased vascularity and angiogenesis found in animal studies following tissue expansion?**
   a. VEGF
   b. EGF
   c. TGF
   d. Angiotensin II
4. **What is true of prepectoral breast reconstruction with tissue expanders/implants when compared with submuscular placement?**
   a. Prepectoral tissue expansion results in less acute and chronic pain
   b. It leads to lower aesthetic outcomes and patient satisfaction
   c. Overall complications are higher in prepectoral breast reconstruction.
   d. Animation deformity is a common complaint after this technique.
5. **Flaps developed from expanded skin**
   a. Have thickening of the dermis
   b. Have thinning of the epidermis
   c. Decrease in collagen density
   d. Decrease angiogenesis
   e. Act as flaps that underwent a delay phenomenon

1. **Answer: c.** Replacing like with like, in this case scalp tissue with scalp tissue, would be most ideal because of the hair-bearing qualities of scalp tissue. Tissue expansion can effectively reconstruct up to 50% of scalp tissue loss. Free tissue transfer with a latissimus muscle flap would give a more durable coverage; however, the lack of hair would resemble the previous alopecia defect. If this were a smaller wound, serial excision and closure may have been an option. A rotational flap with the remaining scalp will not be able to fully cover the entire defect in regard to anatomic landmarks, borders, and zones of normal hair-bearing scalp. Hair transplantation works in pathology such as male pattern baldness as the recipient site is ready to receive follicular units in a fresh bed of tissue for growth. In this patient, the skin graft site is a terrible recipient bed to accept follicular units.

2. **Answer: b.** Out of all the soft tissue layers, only the epidermal layer has been found to reliably increase in thickness. Examination at the microscopic level showed this to be primarily due to the hyperkeratosis that was present within this layer. Studies have also shown there to be increased mitotic activity within the epidermis. This was not seen in the dermis along with thinning of this layer as well. Fatty tissue and muscle decrease in thickness considerably with some permanence.

3. **Answer: a.** Temporary hypoxia caused by the pressure of the expander leads to an increase in vascularity and angiogenesis. This was associated with an increased expression of VEGF. EGF has been shown to lead to actin depolymerization and the formation of membrane ruffles to eventually induce cell proliferation through the microfilament system. TGF has been reported to eventually manipulate morphology, migration, and wound healing by enhancing fibroblast growth and stimulation of extracellular matrix production. Angiotensin II has been reported to play a role in strain-induced cell growth.

4. **Answer: a.** Prepectoral tissue expander placement leads to decreased acute pain, as it negates the need for a submuscular dissection of the pectoralis muscle. Subsequently, pain is also decreased as the tissue expansion occurs above the muscle. Aesthetic outcomes and patient satisfaction have been relatively the same despite prepectoral or submuscular breast reconstruction. Overall complications including flap necrosis, implant exposure, implant infection and total explantation rates have been shown to be similar as well. Animation deformity is actually less in this patient population.

5. **Answer: e.** Random flaps developed on tissues that were expanded undergo a delay phenomenon. These flaps have an increased likelihood of survival because of this. The dermis actually thins because of tissue expansion and conversely the epidermis thickens. Collage density remains the same and increased angiogenesis occurs.

CHAPTER 12 Principles of Procedural Sedation and Local and Regional Anesthesia

Neal Moores and Jayant P. Agarwal

KEY POINTS

- Local anesthetics differ widely in potency, toxicity, and duration of action.
- Epinephrine can be used in digits and end organs, if used safely.
- Local anesthetic dosing differs significantly when used in tumescent solution, relative to standard use as a soft tissue infiltrate.
- Regional blockade techniques facilitate conduct of complex procedures without the need for general anesthesia.
- Sedation is an important tool for the plastic surgeon.

Local anesthetics may be applied topically, injected subcutaneously, or injected in the area of major peripheral nerves. There are a variety of local anesthetics available, which differ in onset, duration, allergenicity, and toxicity. For office-based procedures, peripheral nerve blocks and sedation that may be administered without the need of endotracheal intubation are increasingly relevant in contemporary plastic surgery practice.

PHARMACOKINETICS

Mechanism of Action

Local anesthetic drugs enter the neuronal cell by passive diffusion in the nonionic state. Once inside the cell, they inhibit sodium channel function and thereby prohibit the cell from achieving threshold potential and thus preventing signal transduction. It is important to note that the aforementioned reliance on passive diffusion has significant ramifications in clinical practice. The highly acidic (and charged) nature of inflamed wounds severely inhibits the diffusion of local anesthetics into nerve cells. For this reason, infiltrative anesthesia may be much less effective in inflamed tissue, and alternate methods may be required.[1-3]

Pharmacology

Local anesthetics are classified as either amides or esters. The different chemical behavior (metabolism, allergenicity) of the drugs depends on the presence of this amide or ester linkage. Esters include procaine (novocaine), chloroprocaine, tetracaine, and cocaine. Amides include lidocaine, mepivacaine, prilocaine, bupivacaine (Marcaine), and etidocaine.[2,3]

Metabolism

Esters are metabolized by hydrolysis in the plasma by pseudocholinesterase. Amide anesthetics are metabolized in the liver.[3]

Allergenicity

A true allergic reaction to local anesthetic is extremely rare. In a Danish case series, over 5 years, no patients referred for allergy testing relating to local anesthetics tested positive for a true allergy.[4] Patients with allergic reactions to local anesthetics are more likely reacting to preservatives in the preparations such as para-aminobenzoic acid.[3] In patients who do demonstrate allergy to local anesthetics, allergy to esters are far more common than to amides.

Potency

Local anesthetic potency is determined primarily by the degree of lipid solubility of the drug. This is because the local anesthetic molecule must enter and traverse the neuronal cell membrane to take effect. In clinical settings, however, other factors such as vasodilatory activity, addition of epinephrine, and the tissue redistribution properties of the different local anesthetics also have some effect on potency.[3]

Duration of Action

Duration of action is largely determined by the rate at which the infiltrated local anesthetic is cleared to the intravascular space away from the desired target tissue. This is determined by the vasodilatory activities of the various drugs. The more vasodilation the drug causes, the faster the drug is cleared from the interstitial space and the shorter the duration of action.

The addition of vasoconstrictors (epinephrine) helps to significantly prolong the duration of action of local anesthetics. Epinephrine causes vasoconstriction and thus delays the clearance of the local anesthetic from the interstitium. Epinephrine is most commonly added to local anesthetics in concentrations of 1:100,000 to 1:200,000. The addition of epinephrine to a plain lidocaine solution will augment the duration of action from 30 to 60 minutes to 1.5 to 6 hours. See **Table 12.1** for the effect of additional epinephrine on various local anesthetics.[3]

CLINICAL APPLICATION

Peripheral Nerve Blocks

Blockade of a single targeted nerve is generally referred to as a minor nerve block, whereas blockade of two or more nerves or a nerve plexus is referred to as a regional block.

Examples of common minor nerve blocks include infraorbital, mental, median, and ulnar nerve blocks. These are commonly utilized in plastic surgery for minor office procedures and for laceration repair in the emergency department. Examples of regional nerve blocks include brachial plexus block, femoral nerve block, and transversus abdominis plane block (TAP block). These may be utilized to anesthetize entire limbs or body regions with a single cutaneous puncture. Regional nerve blocks are most commonly performed by anesthesia providers under ultrasound guidance. **Tables 12.2** and **12.3** show the maximal dose, onset, and duration of action of the commonly used local anesthetics for minor and major nerve blocks.

Topical Anesthesia

Topical anesthesia is used by many surgeons to lessen the discomfort of injectables such as hyaluronic acid filler or Botox. These topical agents will provide dermal anesthesia if applied far enough in advance and in sufficient aliquots, although clinical experience with these drugs may at times be disappointing. Topical anesthesia is commonly utilized in the pediatric population to lessen the pain associated with cutaneous puncture associated with intravenous (IV) placement or local anesthetic administration.

TABLE 12.1. DOSAGE AND DURATION CHARACTERISTICS OF THE LOCAL ANESTHETICS WHEN USED FOR INFILTRATION ANESTHESIA (E.G., INFILTRATION AROUND THE PERIPHERY OF A SKIN LESION BEFORE EXCISION)

	Plain Solution			Epinephrine-Containing Solution	
Drug	Concentration (%)	Maximal Dose (mg)	Duration (min)	Maximal Dose (mg)	Duration (min)
Duration					
Procaine					
Chloroprocaine	1.0–2.0	800	15–30	1,000	30–90
Moderate Duration					
Lidocaine	0.5–1.0	300	30–60	500	120–360
Mepivacaine	0.5–1.0	300	45–90	500	120–360
Prilocaine	0.5–1.0	500	30–90	600	120–360
Long Duration					
Bupivacaine	0.25–0.5	175	120–240	225	180–420
Etidocaine	0.5–1.0	300	120–180	400	180–420

Reprinted with permission from Strichartz GR, Covino BG. Local anesthetics. In: Miller RD, ed. *Anesthesia*. 4th ed. New York, NY: Churchill Livingstone; 1994.

TABLE 12.2. DOSAGE AND DURATION CHARACTERISTICS OF THE LOCAL ANESTHETICS WHEN USED FOR MINOR NERVE BLOCKS (E.G., MEDIAN NERVE BLOCK AT THE WRIST)

	Plain Solutions				Epinephrine-Containing Solutions
Drug	Usual Concentration (%)	Usual Volume (mL)	Dosage (mg)	Average Duration (min)	Average Duration (min)
Procaine	2	5–20	100–400	15–30	30–60
Chloroprocaine					
Lidocaine					
Mepivacaine	1	5–20	50–200	60–120	120–180
Prilocaine					
Bupivacaine	0.25	5–20	12.5–50	180–360	240–480
Etidocaine	0.5	5–20	25–100	120–240	180–420

Reprinted with permission from Strichartz GR, Covino BG. Local anesthetics. In: Miller RD, ed. *Anesthesia*. 4th ed. New York, NY: Churchill Livingstone; 1994.

TABLE 12.3. DOSAGE AND DURATION CHARACTERISTICS OF THE LOCAL ANESTHETICS WHEN USED FOR MAJOR NERVE BLOCKS (E.G., AXILLARY BLOCK OF THE BRACHIAL PLEXUS)

Drug With Epinephrine 1:200,000	Usual Concentration (%)	Usual Volume (mL)	Maximal Dose (mg)	Usual Onset (min)	Usual Duration (min)
Lidocaine	1–1.5	30–50	500	10–20	120–240
Mepivacaine	1–1.5	30–50	500	10–20	180–300
Prilocaine	1–2	30–50	600	10–20	180–300
Bupivacaine	0.25–0.5	30–50	225	15–30	360–720
Etidocaine	0.5–1.0	30–50	400	10–20	360–720
Tetracaine	0.25–0.5	30–50	200	20–30	300–600

Reprinted with permission from Strichartz GR, Covino BG. Local anesthetics. In: Miller RD, ed. *Anesthesia*. 4th ed. New York, NY: Churchill Livingstone; 1994.

Eutectic mixture of local anesthetics is a combination of 25 mg lidocaine and 50 mg prilocaine per gram. The drug is best applied 30 to 60 minutes prior to the procedure and may be serially reapplied to keep the skin saturated, or it is often applied and then covered with an occlusive dressing to assist in absorption.[5]

Infiltration of Local Anesthetics

Most often, local anesthesia is achieved by simple subcutaneous infiltration of local anesthetic. Here, local anesthetic is infiltrated into the tissues immediately adjacent to the wound or planned incision. Specific nerves are not targeted, only those sensory nerve endings immediately surrounding the surgical field. The addition of epinephrine in this setting is invaluable for hemostasis in vascular tissue beds and for prolonging the effect of the drug by preventing clearance to the intravascular space.

Because of the drug's acidity, infiltration of local anesthetic can itself be a painful experience. Anesthetics are prepared in a range of pH from 3.5 to 7.0, which serves to lengthen the drug's shelf life. It is known that hydrogen ions stimulate peripheral nociceptors, and thus the infiltrated acid causes pain.[6] It is hypothesized that the time required for the body to alkalinize the solution to a physiologic pH that will facilitate diffusion into the neuron prolongs the duration to efficacious anesthesia.[6] Furthermore, alkalinization may serve to augment the amount of nonionized drug available for neuronal cell uptake.[7] Buffered lidocaine solutions have been demonstrated to improve patient comfort and satisfaction in double-blind randomized controlled trials.[8] Table 12.1 shows the maximal dose and duration of local anesthetics when used for infiltrative anesthesia.

Toxicity of Local Anesthetics

Toxicity of local anesthetic is related to the specific anesthetic being utilized, as well as the tissue it is utilized in. Tissues that are more vascular may carry higher risk of intravascular injection, or the local anesthetic may be more efficiently cleared to the intravascular space thereby inducing systemic toxicity. Clinically, when toxic reactions occur, it is often the result of inadvertent intravascular injection or administration of too large a dose. Furthermore, intravascular injection of epinephrine may cause its own complications or confuse the presentation of local anesthetic toxicity. It is essential that the syringe be aspirated prior to injection to confirm that the needle tip is not intravascular. Repeat aspirations should be performed serially during infiltration to further avoid this complication.

Local anesthetics induce both central nervous system (CNS) and cardiovascular system (CVS) toxicities. CNS toxicity occurs at a lower dose range than CVS toxicity. Although CNS toxicity is more common, CVS toxicity is more dangerous and more challenging to treat.

CNS toxicity includes light-headedness, tinnitus, tremors, numbness of the lips or tongue, restlessness and CNS depression, seizures, apnea, and loss of consciousness at high doses. Benzodiazepines, which alter the seizure threshold for lidocaine, may be used either as treatment for these symptoms or as pretreatment when large doses are anticipated.[9]

Although rarely observed in the clinical setting, CVS toxicity of local anesthetics can be life-threatening and difficult to treat. Local anesthetics depress myocardial activity by acting directly on the myocardium as well as the conduction system of the heart. Local anesthetic also acts on vascular smooth muscle to induce vasodilation. Hypotension, tachycardia, bradycardia, arrhythmias, or cardiac arrest may be observed as a result. The longer acting local anesthetics such as bupivacaine (Marcaine) may induce very difficult-to-treat cardiac complications owing to the drugs' special affinity for myocardial tissue and long half-life. Protracted periods of resuscitation have been observed resulting from bupivacaine cardiac toxicity.[10]

Epinephrine Infiltration and End Organ Perfusion

It was previously believed that epinephrine should be omitted from anesthetic solutions injected in proximity to end arteries (e.g., fingers, toes, and penis) because of the danger of ischemic necrosis. Recent experience and research contradicts this notion. It is now accepted that epinephrine is safe for infiltration in proximity to end arteries such as in the digits and in fact may improve visualization in the surgical field and reduce painful tourniquet use. Infiltrated epinephrine in end organ anesthesia is now considered safe, and a number of studies to date have demonstrated the safety and efficacy of this intervention in digital anesthesia.[11,12] In cases where epinephrine has been infused in the digit and concern persists, the epinephrine effect may be reversed with phentolamine, but most often this is unnecessary because simple observation will suffice and perfusion will gradually return as the epinephrine wears off.

Tumescent Technique for Liposuction

Clinical experience with tumescent technique for local anesthetic infiltration has cast new light on toxicity associated with local anesthetic infiltration. The tumescent technique uses highly dilute concentrations of local anesthetic with epinephrine (1:500,000–1:100,000) in normal saline or lactated Ringer solution. Contrary to long-accepted maximum safe doses of 7 mg/kg lidocaine, in the tumescent technique, doses of up to 35 mg/kg lidocaine are routinely safely administered.[13] However, these dose parameters are dependent on the tissues subjected to the infiltration. For example, in the face, which is considerably more vascular than the abdomen, clearance of tumescent doses of lidocaine to the intravascular space occurs much more quickly and toxicity may be faster. Peak serum lidocaine levels may occur as late as 10 to 14 hours after initial injection, as it has been demonstrated that only approximately 20% of infiltrated local anesthetic is removed along with the lipoaspirate.[14,15] Although large local anesthetic doses are routinely utilized in practice with the tumescent technique in the trunk and extremities, until a safe maximum dose is more completely defined, the recommended dose by the manufacturer is no more than 7 mg/kg.

Treatment of Local Anesthetic Toxicity

The initial treatment of a patient suffering local anesthetic toxicity is supportive. This includes airway control and oxygenation with 100% FiO2. Hypercarbia can worsen CNS toxicity, and in the convulsing patient, hyperventilation with 100% oxygen may alter the seizure threshold and terminate the seizure. If needed, the patient may also be intubated. If seizure activity persists, diazepam (0.1 mg/kg) or thiopental (2 mg/kg) have also proven effective.[9,16]

In the case of hypotension resulting from local anesthetic toxicity, interventions are again initially supportive. IV fluids should be started and, if needed, vasopressors (phenylephrine) or inotropes to maintain the blood pressure. In the case of cardiac collapse, in addition to supportive measures, a lipid rescue protocol should be initiated, as resuscitative measures may be prolonged owing to the long half-life of the local anesthetic drugs.[16]

Intralipid, an infusible 20% lipid emulsion developed for IV nutrition (total parenteral nutrition), is now a studied and efficacious intervention in local anesthetic overdose. It has been incorporated since 2008 into safety protocol guidelines in the United States for the management of local anesthetic–induced cardiotoxicity. During the resuscitative effort, a 20% lipid emulsion infusion can initially be bolused (1.5 mL/kg) and subsequently infused. The mechanism is not well understood, but it is hypothesized that augmenting the intravascular lipid concentration creates a *lipid sink* and acts to draw the lipid-avid local anesthetic out of the myocardial tissue to the intravascular space, where it may be metabolized by the liver or circulating plasma esterases.[17]

Cocaine

Cocaine is the only local anesthetic that induces a vasoconstrictive, rather than vasodilatory response. It is uncommonly used in clinical practice today owing to its CNS stimulant effects including euphoria, behavioral stimulation, and arousal. The drug is readily absorbed through the mucous membranes. Numerous deleterious side effects are associated with the drug including tachycardia, hypertension, mydriasis, tremors, and perspiration. Cocaine is known to simultaneously augment cardiac output while also inducing coronary vasoconstriction, which may increase the risk of myocardial infarction.[18] Cocaine has in the past been utilized in nasal surgery for its vasoconstrictive properties. The safe maximum dose for nasally administered cocaine solution is 1.5 mg/kg.[18,19]

Liposomal Bupivacaine

A liposomal bupivacaine formulation is now Food and Drug Administration (FDA) approved for use in postsurgical analgesia. Marketed under the name Exparel by Pacira Pharmaceuticals, it uses *DepoFoam* technology to encapsulate bupivacaine in multivesicular liposomal particles. These liposomes are slowly degraded, gradually releasing local anesthetic for up to 72 hours after injection. FDA approval of the drug was based on several early placebo-controlled trials in bunionectomy and hemorrhoidectomy for which improved pain control was demonstrated in hours 0 to 24 after injection. However, no significant benefit was observed in either trial in the hours 24 to 72.[20,21]

Applications of liposomal bupivacaine are now broad. Exparel is commonly used for postoperative analgesia in abdominoplasty, peripheral nerve blockade, pharyngoplasty, and any application where extended analgesia is desired following surgical intervention. The drug is FDA approved for local infiltration to improve postoperative pain control and for interscalene brachial plexus blockade following shoulder surgery.[22]

PERIPHERAL NERVE BLOCKS

Minor nerve blockade generally refers to the infiltration of local anesthetic adjacent to singular peripheral nerves to achieve distal analgesia. Minor peripheral nerve blockades are incredibly common in the practice of plastic surgery and are used frequently in both the operating room (OR) and in office- and emergency room (ER)–based interventions. Applications are as wide ranging as infraorbital and mental nerve blockade for facial laceration repair or filler injection, to blockade of peripheral nerves in the digits, wrist, or elbow for hand surgeries, to intercostal nerve blockade for abdominal procedures. These blockades may serve as an independent anesthetic modality, obviating the need for anesthesia providers, or may serve as meaningful adjuncts to pain management in conjunction with general anesthesia or procedural sedation.

Face

In the face, infiltrative anesthesia is most often employed because of the generalized application of epinephrine and benefit of diffuse vasoconstriction in such a vascular tissue bed; however, minor peripheral nerve blockade may provide targeted and sufficient analgesia when diffuse vasospasm is unnecessary or undesirable or in addition to infiltrative anesthesia.[23]

In the setting of cosmetic filler injection, facial nerve blockade functions well in the sensitive skin of the midface and mouth. Perforation of the oral mucosa with a small-bore needle is generally less painful than the highly innervated skin of the face. The infraorbital and mental nerves may be easily approached via mucosal puncture to achieve analgesia of the entire lower and midface (**Figure 12.1**).

Although less commonly used, blockade of the supraorbital and supratrochlear nerves may be utilized for procedures on the forehead and scalp. The supraorbital nerve may be infiltrated on the supraorbital rim in the mid-pupillary line.

Auricular blockade is an important adjunct in the repair of ear trauma both in the ER and OR. This is especially true in the mangled ear where small flaps of potentially threatened skin must have their viability serially assessed during repair for which infiltrative anesthesia would prove unacceptable. Blockade of the ear may be accomplished by serial infiltration of the greater auricular and lesser occipital nerves in the neck along the posterior border of the sternocleidomastoid muscle. Blockade of the auriculotemporal nerve may be accomplished just anterior to the tragus. However, the ear cannot be completely blocked in this manner, as terminal branches of cranial nerve ten and Arnold nerve will require infiltrative anesthesia in the otic canal and conchal bowl if intervention is required in the central ear (**Figure 12.2**).

Hand

In the hand, minor nerve blockade is the cornerstone of procedural anesthesia. Here tourniquets may be applied for procedural hemostasis and directed local anesthetic may be utilized to completely anesthetize a single digit or the entire hand. Depending on the level of injury, anesthetics can be applied at multiple levels of the hand, wrist, and arm to facilitate ER- or office-based hand procedures or to facilitate hand surgery in the OR without the need of endotracheal intubation. In the OR, tourniquets are easily applied to facilitate

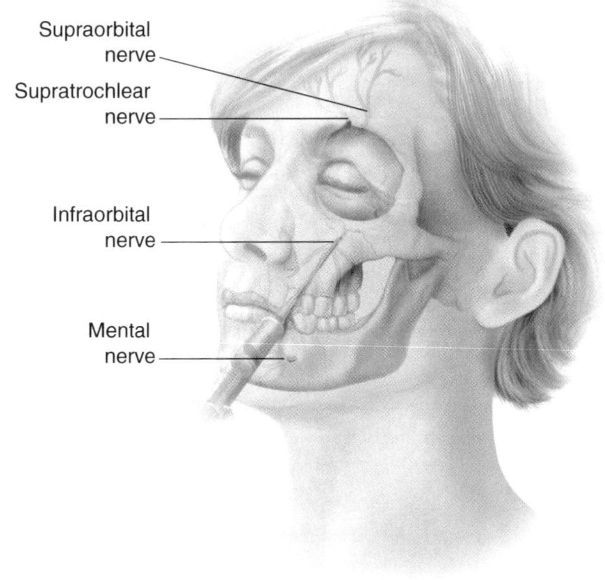

FIGURE 12.1. The infraorbital nerve is generally found at the intersection of a vertical mid-pupillary line and a horizontal line drawn from the lateral margin of the ala. The mental nerve may be reliably infiltrated along the anterior mandible just inferior and anterior to the first mandibular premolar. Each of these locations may be sufficiently anesthetized with 3 to 5 cc of local anesthetic. The supratrochlear nerve is commonly blocked at the same time and is found along the supraorbital rim 1 to 2 cm medial to the supraorbital nerve. Both nerves may be blocked with the same injection in a supraperiosteal plane (2–5 cc).

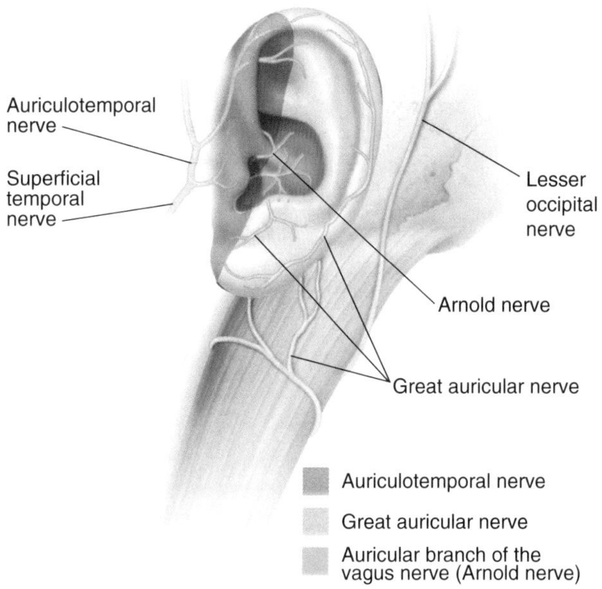

FIGURE 12.2. The ear, its sensory nerves, and cutaneous dermatomes.

hemostasis in this very vascular tissue bed; however, when undesired, or when in the ER or performing office-based procedures, the addition of epinephrine to infiltrated anesthetic in the hand and digits has been proven safe and efficacious.[11,12]

Complete digital anesthesia may be induced by infiltration of each individual digital nerve at the level of the proximal phalanx on the volar-lateral surface of the digit (**Figure 12.3A**). Alternatively, the digits may be blocked at the level of the metacarpophalangeal joint at their bifurcation. When a longer needle is passed across the metacarpal heads, multiple fingers may be blocked with a single cutaneous puncture.

The median nerve is approached on the ulnar side of the palmaris longus at the proximal wrist crease (**Figure 12.3B**). This approach avoids direct puncture of the median nerve, which typically lies immediately below or radial to the palmaris longus tendon. Should the patient complain of lancinating pain in the median nerve distribution, concern for direct nerve puncture should be raised and the needle removed and reinserted in a more ulnar location. The needle is advanced in line with the axis of the arm, where 5 to 10 cc of long- or short-acting anesthetic may be infiltrated into the carpal tunnel.

The ulnar neurovascular bundle is located immediately deep to the flexor carpi ulnaris tendon and proximal to the hook of the hamate (**Figure 12.3C**). Both structures are readily palpated on examination. The needle is advanced horizontally, in an ulnar to radial direction under the flexor carpi ulnaris tendon. Care must be taken to aspirate before infiltration to avoid intravascular injection in the ulnar artery. When in the appropriate location 1 to 3 cc of local anesthetic may be infiltrated.

The superficial radial nerve emerges from the deep fascia of the arm along the lateral aspect of the radius 6 to 9 cm proximal to the radial styloid (**Figure 12.3D**). After this, it runs in the subcutaneous plane and may be anesthetized by diffusely infiltrating the dorsoradial aspect of the wrist from the ulnar styloid dorsally to the mid-dorsal wrist (3–10 cc).

The entire hand may be blocked at the level of the wrist by infiltration of the median, ulnar, and superficial radial nerves with three cutaneous punctures.

REGIONAL NERVE BLOCKS

Regional nerve blockade can provide significant anesthesia to an entire region of the body such as the entire arm or leg. Some of the most common examples include brachial plexus block, femoral nerve block, TAP block, and spinal and/or epidural blockade. These procedures are most commonly performed by anesthesia providers with the assistance of ultrasound guidance. These similarly may be used to provide procedural anesthesia without the requirement of sedation but are generally associated with procedures performed in the OR.

Transversus Abdominis Plane Block

Transversus abdominis plane (TAP) block is a powerful adjunct for abdominal wall procedures ranging from hernia repair to abdominoplasty and deep inferior epigastric artery perforator flap (DIEP) flap harvest. Deep vein thrombosis (DVT) risk is theoretically augmented

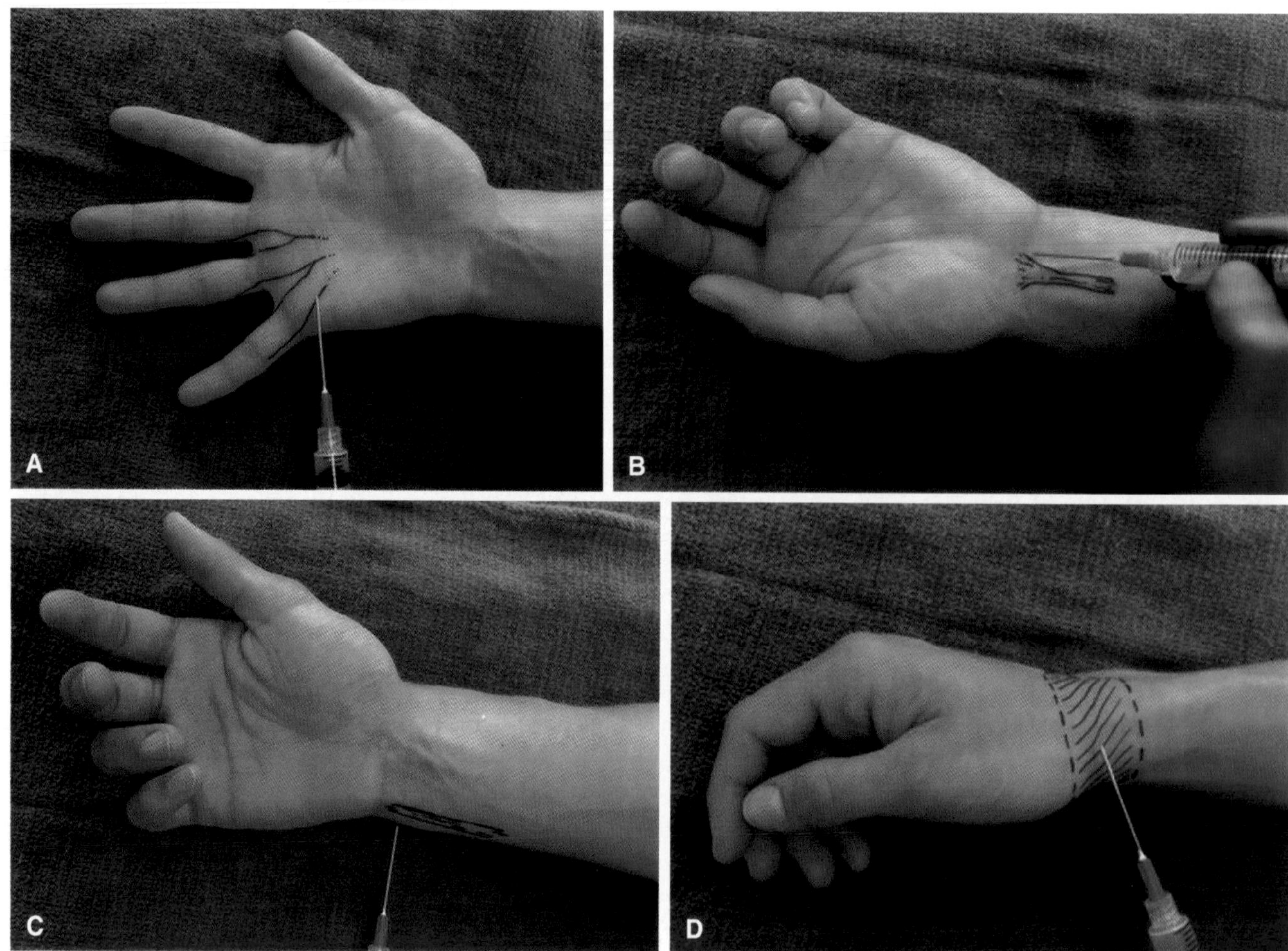

FIGURE 12.3. The course and relative location of the nerves of the hand. **A.** Expected locations and course of common and proper digital nerves at the level of the metacarpophalangeal joint. **B.** Location of palmaris longus tendon in the wrist. **C.** Anatomic location of the flexor carpi ulnaris tendon in the wrist. **D.** Area of superficial infiltration that would reliably block the superficial branch of the radial nerve.

in abdominal wall procedures by pain, which may inhibit postoperative mobility, and also augment pressure in the inferior vena cava, which may lead to venous stasis in the legs and pelvis.[24,25]

TAP block is commonly performed either preoperatively or intraoperatively for the management of post-op abdominal pain. The abdominal wall is innervated by the branches of the intercostal nerves, which run in the lateral abdominal wall on the superficial surface of the transversus abdominis muscle before perforating the posterior rectus sheath at its lateral margin. These nerves may be blocked with ultrasound guidance by infiltration of local anesthetic in the plane between the internal oblique muscle and the transversus muscle. This important adjunct has been shown to improve postoperative pain control and augment early mobilization protocols in reconstructive procedures involving the abdomen.[26,27]

Pectoral Nerve Block

Blockade of the medial and lateral pectoral nerves is a powerful pain control adjunct for breast surgery and has been shown to decrease length of stay and narcotic utilization in the postoperative period.[28] The pectoral muscle may be anesthetized via the medial and lateral pectoral nerves. These may be approached in the plane between pectoralis major and minor just medial to the acromion. For cutaneous anesthesia, the intercostal nerves may be accessed in the intercostal spaces of ribs 2 to 5. Blocking the intercostal nerves lateral to the anterior axillary line will effectively anesthetize both the lateral and medial intercostal perforating cutaneous nerves. These blocks may be performed under ultrasound guidance by anesthesia providers or may be accomplished intraoperatively by the surgical team.[29] Pectoral block has been suggested by some authors as sufficient anesthesia for breast procedures without the requirement of general anesthesia.[30]

SEDATION

Sedatives that do not require endotracheal intubation are useful in plastic surgery. Plastic surgery includes many procedures that may be carried out with local anesthesia alone or with the addition of a sedative.[31] This is especially true in the care of pediatric patients in the ER setting where a sedative such as midazolam (Versed) or ketamine may alleviate a great deal of unnecessary psychological distress for smaller procedures that do not mandate progress to the OR. Sedation is also successfully used as a preoperative adjunct to alleviate procedural anxiety.

The most common drugs utilized for sedation are midazolam, diazepam, fentanyl, and ketamine. Propofol may also be used in the nonoperative setting in lower doses, but it is less commonly used without the assistance of an anesthesia provider. The most common benzodiazepines, midazolam and diazepam, differ chiefly in the duration of action. Midazolam is much shorter acting, lasting approximately 3 hours. Diazepam is longer acting, 6 to 12 hours. These drugs are often utilized to diminish patient anxiety during minor office-based procedures as an adjunct to local anesthesia. For more involved procedures, they are sometimes combined with IV fentanyl for an additional analgesia effect. The combination of infiltrative local anesthesia with the addition of a benzodiazepine and possibly also a narcotic such as fentanyl are successfully used for myriad procedures both in and out of the OR. These procedures range from the closure of simple lacerations to scar revision, smaller liposuction cases, a wide variety of hand procedures, and even facelifts.[31]

Ketamine is a powerful neuroleptic drug that at lower doses is used as an analgesic and at higher doses induces a dissociative type of anesthesia. It is safe when administered in the appropriate setting. Ketamine is a unique anesthetic because it does not depress the respiratory drive. Instead, the CNS stimulant properties of ketamine may induce agitation and/or hypertension as side effects. Ketamine is relatively contraindicated in hypertensive patients, though it is a good anesthetic in the hypotensive patient. The chief advantage of ketamine anesthesia is that patients may be anesthetized without the need for endotracheal intubation.[32]

Onset of the drug when administered IV is immediate, and duration of up to 25 minutes may be expected. Ketamine induces a dissociative (trancelike) state but also has analgesic and amnestic properties. Anesthetic onset is often marked by the initiation of horizontal nystagmus. Hallucinations and attendant verbalizations are also common which may be distressing to parents when the drug is administered in the pediatric setting for ER-based procedures. If the parents of a pediatric patient are to be present, it is recommended that these effects of the drug be explained in advance.

It is advisable that the surgical provider employ the assistance of a dedicated health care provider to continuously monitor the airway and vital signs when anesthetic doses of ketamine are utilized. A patient who has received anesthetic doses of ketamine is not able to protect their own airway. Nausea is a known side effect of the ketamine, and these factors may culminate in a devastating aspiration event. An appropriate period of NPO must be observed, and antiemetics may be administered prior to ketamine dosing for prophylaxis.

REFERENCES

1. Ueno T, Tsuchiya H, Mizogami M, Takakura K. Local anesthetic failure associated with inflammation: verification of the acidosis mechanism and the hypothetic participation of inflammatory peroxynitrite. *J Inflamm Res*. 2008;1:41-48.
2. Swerdlow M, Jones R. The duration of action of bupivacaine, prilocaine and lignocaine. *Br J Anaesth*. 1970;42(4):335-339.
3. Miller RD, Miller RD, Eriksson LI. *Miller's Anesthesia*. 7th ed. Philadelphia, PA: Churchill Livingstone/Elsevier; 2010.
4. Kvisselgaard AD, Mosbech HF, Fransson S, Garvey LH. Risk of immediate-type allergy to local anesthetics is overestimated-results from 5 years of provocation testing in a Danish allergy clinic. *J Allergy Clin Immunol Pract*. 2018;6(4):1217-1223.
5. Hallen B, Uppfeldt A. Does lidocaine-prilocaine cream permit painfree insertion of IV catheters in children? *Anesthesiology*. 1982;57(4):340-342.
6. Bunke J SR, Hult J, Malmsjo M. Buffered local anesthetics reduce injection pain and provide anesthesia for up to 5 hours. *J Plast Reconstr Aesthet Surg*. 2018;71(8):1216-1230.
7. Best CA, Best AA, Best TJ, Hamilton DA. Buffered lidocaine and bupivacaine mixture - the ideal local anesthetic solution? *Plast Surg (Oakv)*. 2015;23(2):87-90.
8. Cepeda MS, Tzortzopoulou A, Thackrey M, Hudcova J, Arora Gandhi P, Schumann R. Adjusting the pH of lidocaine for reducing pain on injection. *Cochrane Database Syst Rev*. 2010;(12):CD006581.
9. De Jong RH, Heavner JE. Diazepam prevents local anesthetic seizures. *Anesthesiology*. 1971;34(6):523-531.
10. Marwick PC, Levin AI, Coetzee AR. Recurrence of cardiotoxicity after lipid rescue from bupivacaine-induced cardiac arrest. *Anesth Analg*. 2009;108(4):1344-1346.
Important analysis of the long duration of bupivicane induced cardiovascular depression, which can recur even after successful resuscitative effort.
11. Lalonde D, Bell M, Benoit P, et al. A multicenter prospective study of 3,110 consecutive cases of elective epinephrine use in the fingers and hand: the Dalhousie Project clinical phase. *J Hand Surg Am*. 2005;30(5):1061-1067.
The largest and most rigorous study to date documenting the excellent safety profile of epinephrine in digital anesthesia.
12. Chowdhry S, Seidenstricker L, Cooney DS, et al. Do not use epinephrine in digital blocks: myth or truth? Part II. A retrospective review of 1111 cases. *Plast Reconstr Surg*. 2010;126(6):2031-2034.
13. Klein JA. Tumescent technique for local anesthesia improves safety in large-volume liposuction. *Plast Reconstr Surg*. 1993;92(6):1085-1098.
Posits that does up to 35 mg/kg lidocaine, much higher than manufacturer recommended doses are likely safe when administered in highly dilute tumescent solution formulations in liposuction cases.
14. Rubin JP, Bierman C, Rosow CE, et al. The tumescent technique: the effect of high tissue pressure and dilute epinephrine on absorption of lidocaine. *Plast Reconstr Surg*. 1999;103(3):990-996.
15. Swanson E. Prospective study of lidocaine, bupivacaine, and epinephrine levels and blood loss in patients undergoing liposuction and abdominoplasty. *Plast Reconstr Surg*. 2012;130(3):702-722.
Case series evaluating blood levels and toxicity associated with local anesthetic infiltration in liposuction cases finding that, though the technique is safe, only 20% of infiltrated local anesthetic is removed with the lipoaspirate.
16. Lynch C III. Depression of myocardial contractility in vitro by bupivacaine, etidocaine, and lidocaine. *Anesth Analg*. 1986;65(6):551-559.
17. Ciechanowicz S, Patil V. Lipid emulsion for local anesthetic systemic toxicity. *Anesthesiol Res Pract*. 2012;2012:131784.
18. Kelton PL. Local anesthetics, cocaine, and CPR. *Select Read Plast Surg*. 1992;7(5).
19. Fleming JA, Byck R, Barash PG. Pharmacology and therapeutic applications of cocaine. *Anesthesiology*. 1990;73(3):518-531.
20. Golf M, Daniels SE, Onel E. A phase 3, randomized, placebo-controlled trial of DepoFoam(R) bupivacaine (extended-release bupivacaine local analgesic) in bunionectomy. *Adv Ther*. 2011;28(9):776-788.

21. Gorfine SR, Onel E, Patou G, Krivokapic ZV. Bupivacaine extended-release liposome injection for prolonged postsurgical analgesia in patients undergoing hemorrhoidectomy: a multicenter, randomized, double-blind, placebo-controlled trial. *Dis Colon Rectum*. 2011;54(12):1552-1559.
Along with reference 19, the basis for FDA approval of Exparel. Though the drug elutes over 48 hours, improvement in pain control was not seen beyond 24 hours.
22. Rabin T. *FDA in Brief: FDA Approves New Use of Exparel for Nerve Block Pain Relief Following Shoulder Surgeries*. 2018.
23. Diepenbrock RM, May JR, Cone WR, Ehland EL. Patient preference for preprocedural anesthetic prior to facial cosmetic injectable fillers. *Am J Cosmet Surg*. 2017;34(3):143-149.
24. Willenberg T, Clemens R, Haegeli LM, et al. The influence of abdominal pressure on lower extremity venous pressure and hemodynamics: a human in-vivo model simulating the effect of abdominal obesity. *Eur J Vasc Endovasc Surg*. 2011;41(6):849-855.
25. Pannucci CJ, Alderman AK, Brown SL, et al. The effect of abdominal wall plication on intra-abdominal pressure and lower extremity venous flow: a case report. *J Plast Reconstr Aesthet Surg*. 2012;65(3):392-394.
26. Sforza M, Andjelkov K, Zaccheddu R, et al. Transversus abdominis plane block anesthesia in abdominoplasties. *Plast Reconstr Surg*. 2011;128(2):529-535.
27. Araco A, Pooney J, Araco F, Gravante G. Transversus abdominis plane block reduces the analgesic requirements after abdominoplasty with flank liposuction. *Ann Plast Surg*. 2010;65(4):385-388.
28. Shah A, Rowlands M, Krishnan N, et al. Thoracic intercostal nerve blocks reduce opioid consumption and length of stay in patients undergoing implant-based breast reconstruction. *Plast Reconstr Surg*. 2015;136(5):584e-591e.
29. Lanier ST, Lewis KC, Kendall MC, et al. Intraoperative nerve blocks fail to improve quality of recovery after tissue expander breast reconstruction: a prospective, double-blinded, randomized, placebo-controlled clinical trial. *Plast Reconstr Surg*. 2018;141(3):590-597.
30. Moon EJ, Kim SB, Chung JY, et al. Pectoral nerve block (pecs block) with sedation for breast conserving surgery without general anesthesia. *Ann Surg Treat Res*. 2017;93(3):166-169.
31. Iverson RE. Sedation and analgesia in ambulatory settings. American Society of Plastic and Reconstructive Surgeons Task Force on Sedation and Analgesia in Ambulatory Settings. *Plast Reconstr Surg*. 1999;104(5):1559-1564.
32. Ersek RA. Dissociative anesthesia for safety's sake: ketamine and diazepam: a 35-year personal experience. *Plast Reconstr Surg*. 2004;113(7):1955-1959.

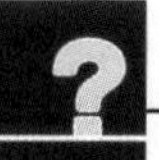

QUESTIONS

1. 30 minutes after digital injection with a solution of lidocaine and epinephrine for removal of a small foreign body from the distal pad of the index finger that was otherwise untraumatized. The digit remains cool, pale in color, and without capillary refill. What is the appropriate course of action at this time?

a. Infiltration of phentolamine
b. Administer aspirin
c. Elevation of the extremity
d. Operative exploration for possible vascular injury

2. TAP block is a powerful anesthetic technique for abdominal procedures, wherein local anesthetic is administered in the plane between these two muscles in the abdominal wall.

a. Internal and external obliques
b. Internal oblique and transversus abdominis
c. Transversus abdominis and peritoneum
d. Rectus abdominis and posterior sheath

3. You are operating at a local outpatient surgery center, and one of the other surgeons is preparing to perform a liposuction case. She states that she has just administered a dilute local anesthetic formulation to the entire subcutaneous surface of the abdomen and flanks with a total lidocaine dose of 30 mg/kg. What do you do next?

a. Inform the surgical team that a dangerously high dose of lidocaine has been administered.
b. Suggest that liposuction begin as soon as possible to quickly aspirate the local anesthetic overdose.
c. Say nothing, as this is an acceptable dosage of subcutaneous lidocaine in this setting.

4. A patient informs you that they have an allergy to local anesthetics that causes diffuse hives and sometimes even wheezing and shortness of breath. Which of the following are they most likely having the allergic reaction to?

a. A preservative in the local anesthetic preparation
b. An amide moiety
c. An ester moiety

5. A patient undergoing facelift is administered a preoperative local anesthetic formulation of 0.25% bupivacaine, 1% lidocaine and epinephrine. Shortly after subcutaneous infiltration, but before incision, the patient goes into cardiac arrest. Anesthesia begins supportive measures with 100% FiO2 administered endotracheally, diazepam is administered, and chest compressions are commenced. It is hypothesized that the cardiac arrest is due to the local anesthetic administered, and the anesthesiologist is concerned about the duration of bupivacaine prolonging the resuscitative effort. Lipid rescue is begun with a 20% IV lipid emulsion. What is the appropriate dose of this medication in this setting?

a. 150 mL/kg
b. 500 mL/kg
c. 1.5 mL/kg
d 5 mL/kg

1. **Answer: c.** 30 minutes following infiltration of lidocaine and epinephrine into the digit, the digit should not yet be expected to have robust capillary refill. Elevation of the extremity will most often suffice for resolution of drug effect in digital epinephrine injection, as it aids in removal of the drug from the tissues of the digit. Phentolamine, although an option, would not yet be indicated in this clinical scenario. Aspirin would not assist with this clinical scenario, as there is not a concern for thrombosis of the digital arteries. Operative exploration would also not be indicated as in an otherwise untraumatized digit, and in the presence of a known vasoconstrictor, the cause is both known and temporary.

2. **Answer: b.** TAP block is administered by blockade of the intercostal nerves, as they run in the lateral abdominal wall before they pierce the rectus sheath. At this level, they are found between the transversus abdominis muscle and the internal oblique. This block is most often administered under ultrasound guidance, by the anesthesia team.

3. **Answer: c.** It is not necessary to say anything in this setting. It is now well documented that doses of 30 mg/kg administered in tumescent formulation is a safe and acceptable clinical practice. This dose of lidocaine, administered in this manner, would be highly typical in today's clinical practice.

4. **Answer: a.** True allergic reactions to local anesthetics are exceedingly rare. When allergic reactions to infiltrated local anesthetics are seen in clinical practice, it is most often an allergy to para-aminobenzoic acid, which is used as a preservative in the solutions. In the very rare case that a patient does suffer a true allergy to local anesthetic, it is more often an allergy to ester local anesthetics than amides.

5. **Answer: c.** Accepted dosage for lipid rescue in the treatment of local anesthetic toxicity consists of an initial 1.5 mL/kg bolus of lipid infusion. This is then followed by continuous infusion. The exact mechanism of lipid rescue is unknown; however, it is hypothesized that the intravascular lipid functions as a ***lipid sink***. In this way, lipid infusion draws the lipid-avid local anesthetic to the intravascular space and away from the intracellular space of the vascular and cardiac tissues.

CHAPTER 13 Concepts of Tissue Engineering

Matthew D. Treiser and William G. Austen

KEY POINTS

- Tissue engineering is defined as the application of the principles and methods of engineering and life sciences toward the fundamental understanding of structure-function relationships in normal and pathological mammalian tissues and the development of biological substitutes for the repair or regeneration of tissue or organ function.
- Regenerative medicine seeks to use the natural regenerative properties of cells to repair the body, whether by direct tissue formation or by the release of trophic factors to induce endogenous healing.
- Tissue engineering and regenerative medicine currently employ three main strategies:
  - Implantation of isolated or cultured cells for injection and subsequent healing
  - In situ directed tissue regeneration
  - Implantation of *ex vivo* assembled constructs containing cells and scaffolds
- The main cell sources utilized in tissue engineering are cultured somatic cells lines, embryonic stem cells, adult stem cells, and induced pluripotent stem cells.
- Tissue engineering may provide solutions to commonly encountered clinical challenges in plastic surgery; however, to date, few devices and/or products have gained wide clinical use.

TISSUE ENGINEERING AND REGENERATIVE MEDICINE

Tissue loss, chronic disease and end organ failure present an enormous social and economic strain on the afflicted individuals and society at large. In the United States, the treatment of these patients costs over $400 billion per year with over eight million surgical procedures performed annually to treat these disorders.[1] Although tissue loss, chronic disease, and end organ failure encompass a heterogeneous grouping of pathologic conditions ranging from liver failure to musculoskeletal injury, current surgical interventions often fail to provide curative solutions. Traditional treatment strategies depend on extracorporeal devices, such as kidney dialysis machines, or operative interventions, such as the allografting of organs from living/cadaveric donors and free tissue transfer. Although these approaches have provided positive patient outcomes for some, many patients fail to receive viable long-term cures. Unfortunately, current transplantation approaches suffer from extreme shortages in donor organs and not all patients with organ failure are candidates. In 2017, 125,737 patients were registered for organ transplants, while only 34,771 organs were transplanted.[2] These data underestimate the true need, as studies have demonstrated that there are about 730,000 deaths in the United States annually from end organ disease.[3] Non–transplantation-based surgical reconstructions also frequently fail owing to their associated postoperative complications and further suffer from donor site morbidity. For these reasons and others, current surgical and mechanical interventions often fail to provide adequate curative solutions to tissue loss and organ failure. The ideal solutions would recreate whole organ function in corporeal devices that are biocompatible and easily integrated into the patient's anatomy.

Tissue engineering and regenerative medicine seek to facilitate the healing of tissues and organs lost to pathological processes via the development of devices/biologics that stimulate, supplement, or act in lieu of the body's natural regenerative abilities. The term *tissue engineering* was defined at an National science foundation meeting in 1988 as, the "application of the principles and methods of engineering and life sciences toward the fundamental understanding of structure-function relationships in normal and pathological mammalian tissues and the development of biological substitutes for the repair or regeneration of tissue or organ function."[4] Although the terms *tissue engineering* and *regenerative medicine* are often used synonymously, it is important to note that although they share the same end purpose, the terms imply subtly different approaches. Tissue engineering focuses on the creation and formation of biological substitutes, whereas regenerative medicine seeks to utilize the natural regenerative properties of cells to repair the body, whether by direct tissue formation or by the release of trophic factors to induce endogenous healing.[5] To clarify, regenerative medicine functions by stimulating cells to repair damaged tissue, whereas tissue engineering utilizes engineered constructs to reform solid tissues or organs. These strategies are not mutually exclusive and often a given approach for tissue repair represents a combination of both tissue engineering and regenerative medicine. Proponents of these strategies believe they can address the clinical needs of patients suffering from organ or tissue loss by developing biologically derived constructs that maintain the functionality of the original organ or tissue. These constructs would reduce the need for whole organ donation and surgical repair by providing artificial surrogates that are nonimmunogenic and effectively perform the functions of endogenous tissues.

STRATEGIES IN TISSUE ENGINEERING AND REGENERATIVE MEDICINE

Historically, attempts by physicians to artificially induce tissue regeneration date back to 1500 BC.[6] These early attempts at nasal reconstruction utilized autologous grafted skin in conjunction with wood scaffolds to reform the nose. In its modern formulation, tissue engineering and regenerative medicine currently employ three main strategies[7] (**Figure 13.1**):

- Implantation of isolated or cultured cells for injection and subsequent healing
- In situ directed tissue regeneration
- Implantation of *ex vivo* assembled constructs containing cells and scaffolds

Injectable Cell Therapies

The interest in injectable cell therapies, particularly injectable stem cell therapies, derives from their avoidance of a surgical procedure and associated complications, the enormous availability of cell sources in the form of aspirates from donors, and the replacement of only damaged cells rather than whole organs.[5] Studies have shown some success in both animal models and clinical applications with this strategy for repair of cardiac function in heart disease.[8] However, the true feasibility and effectiveness of this approach remains unclear. Although injection of stem cells appears to improve cardiac function, a clinical review published by Collins et al. indicates that few of the injected cells are retained in the heart and that most improvements in cardiac function are more likely a result of stimulated angiogenesis via secreted cytokines rather

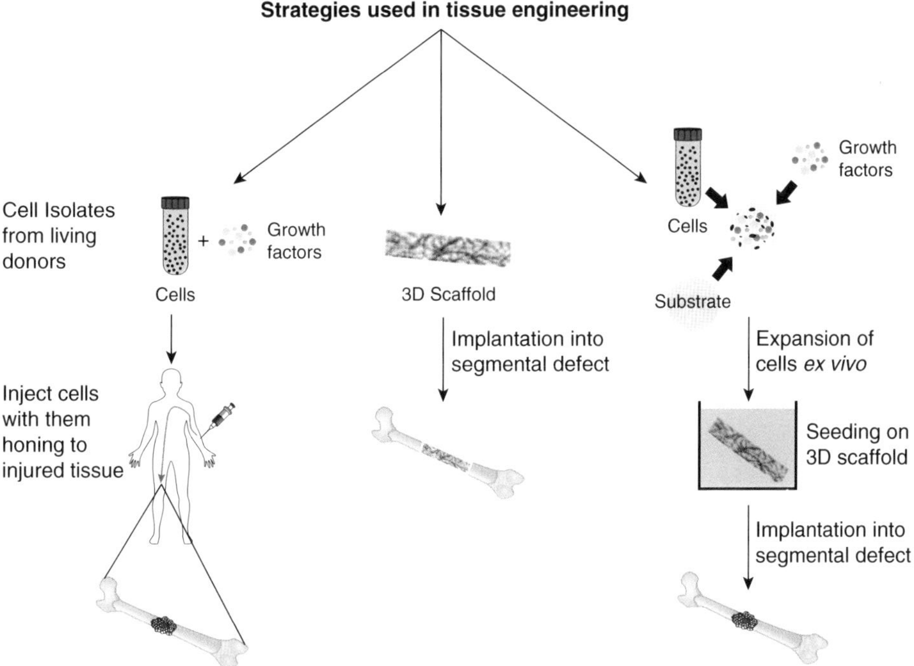

FIGURE 13.1. The three main strategies in tissue engineering: (1) implantation of isolated or cultured cells for injection and subsequent healing; (2) in situ directed tissue regeneration; and (3) implantation of *ex vivo* assembled constructs containing cells and scaffolds.

than via reparation of cardiac tissue.[9] This review highlights some of the greatest criticisms of the injectable approach. First, although some cells may localize to the wound site, the lifetime of those cells and the location and consequences of the remainder of the injected cells within the body remain concerns. Second, the benefit of injecting stem cells may be artifact, with the greatest benefit derived from secreted soluble factors as opposed to tissue reformation.[8] Finally, even though this approach may be adequate for the repair of focally damaged tissue, it is not expected to provide restoration of whole organ failure because it is believed that isolated cells cannot themselves form new tissues in the absence of a supporting material.

In Situ Tissue Regeneration

In situ tissue regeneration depends on the ability of the native cells within the body to synergize with an acellular implanted device. This device may be permanent or degradable, and the material may be natural (e.g., fibrin, gelatin, thrombin, collagen, cadaveric decellularized matrices) or synthetic. In contrast to prostheses for which the ultimate goal is to provide an artificial replacement, here the device acts as a scaffold for endogenous cell repair. The scaffold provides the mechanical support necessary to maintain functional form. The material may include bioactive or biomimetic factors to promote cellular attachment, proliferation and/or differentiation thereby promoting tissue regeneration. In situ tissue engineering devices have shown clinical promise in applications such as sutures, orthopedic devices, tissue sealants, and hernia repair devices. Interestingly, most of the work performed involving in situ tissue regeneration focuses on the repair of focal defects in connective tissues (i.e., bone, cartilage, tendons, and skin). Investigators focus on focal defects because, in situ, avascular scaffolds only allow cells to penetrate 100 μm owing to oxygen diffusion limitations.[10] Although some work has been attempted to simultaneously promote cell migration and angiogenesis within a scaffold, to date, the creation of microvasculature networks in situ remains suboptimal.[11] Therefore, in the absence of a previously established vascular network or an angiogenic material, tissue engineering strategies that utilize acellular constructs focus on applications in which oxygen diffusion is nonlimiting.

Cell-Material Hybrids

The final tissue engineering strategy uses cells seeded within a porous implant to create a cell-material hybrid (**Figure 13.2**). In these constructs, cells are isolated from donors (autologous or allogeneic) and seeded onto biomaterial scaffolds in vitro. The cells are cultured on the scaffolds within a bioreactor until they assemble an organized tissue similar to that of the damaged tissue the device is intended to repair. Once implanted, this artificially engineered organ functions as native tissue. This approach interests researchers because it addresses many of the weaknesses of the other two. Unlike both the injectable and in situ regeneration paradigms, the cell-material hybrid strategy, in theory, allows for the construction of a whole living organ *ex vivo*.

Assembling the tissue *ex vivo* allows researchers to construct complex structures that mimic the natural biology of endogenous tissue. For example, utilizing micro patterning and machining, vascular networks can be assembled and combined with the cell-material hybrid to provide adequate perfusion of the construct. Additionally, as opposed to in situ differentiation, the *ex vivo* approach assembles spatially controlled tissue analogues of multiple cell types within scaffolds that are seeded uniformly with viable cells. Finally, the cell-material hybrid approach provides the testing of the engineered tissue before implantation to ensure that it functions properly. This technique has been clinically demonstrated in the fabrication and implantation of a tissue-engineered bladder device as described by Atala et al.[12] They reported on the isolation and *ex vivo* expansion of bladder cells on collagen/polyglycolic acid scaffolds with clinical implantation in cystoplasty candidates. Although this approach shows much promise, it is not without its current limitations. The cell-material hybrid approach suffers from the complexity of the system and the difficulty in correctly tuning the multiple facets of the approach. Creating scaffolds that promote cell differentiation while maintaining mechanical integrity is challenging, but in conjunction with directing cell phenotypic behaviors, these constructs often do not produce desired outcomes. This complexity is evident by the dearth of clinical products to date that have employed these techniques.

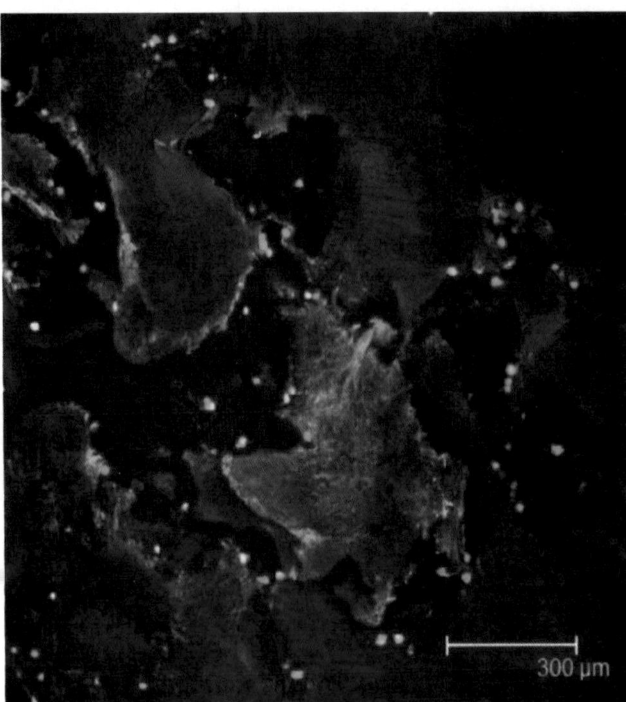

FIGURE 13.2. Osteoblasts seeded on a porous, three-dimensional poly (polymer carbonate) scaffold. Cells are imaged at 72 hours and stained with calcein AM for living cells (green) and ethidium homodimer-1 for dead cells (red). The scaffold (blue) was imaged in reflection mode. The image is a maximum projection image from 50 individual slices taken every 10 microns (100×).

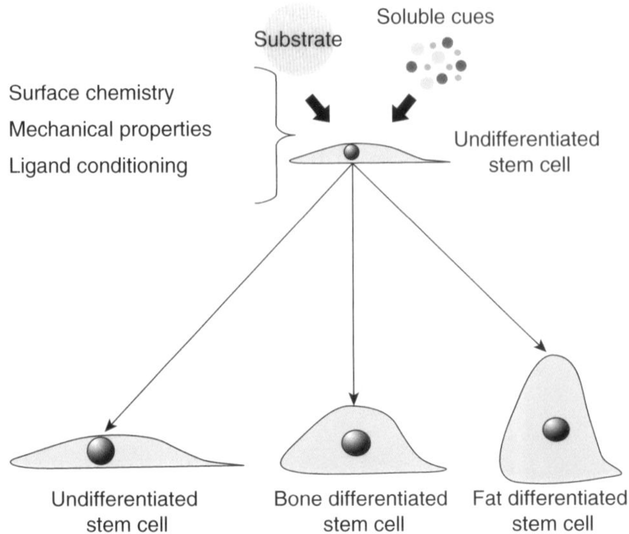

FIGURE 13.3. Stem cells in the presence of external stimuli have the potential for differentiation to somatic cell types or self-renewal and expansion with maintenance of their stem-like state.

CELL SOURCES FOR TISSUE ENGINEERING

Fully Differentiated Somatic Cell Lines

Fully differentiated somatic cells and stem cells represent the two most commonly used cell sources for tissue engineering. Somatic cells demonstrate the potential for tissue regeneration when seeded in artificial scaffolds. Examination of review articles within the literature shows that these cells have been applied in organs such as the cartilage,[13] pancreas,[14] bone,[15] skin,[16] and liver.[17] Although these reviews highlight the potential terminally differentiated cells provide, these cells suffer from difficulty in balancing differentiation with proliferative ability. Cell proliferation provides the cell numbers that are critical for tissue construction. Ideally, a small amount of donor cells expand to homogenously populate the scaffold. Unfortunately, as explained by Strehl and coauthors, terminally differentiated somatic cells often lose their ability of self-renewal.[18] Although methods exist to reinitiate cell proliferation in these cells, this process may result in the downregulation of differentiation behaviors. Thus although these cells are terminally differentiated and therefore should demonstrate the desired cell phenotypes, obtaining adequate cell numbers to create constructs of adequate size and cell density often perturbs their desired phenotypes. Furthermore, somatic cells are often difficult to culture *ex vivo*, limiting their utility.

Stem Cells for Tissue Engineering

In an attempt to find a cell source that maintains both proliferative and differentiation potentials, researchers have turned to stem cells. Stem cells are pluripotent cells (i.e., have the ability to differentiate into a number of terminal cell types) that display self-renewal in their stem-like states (**Figure 13.3**). These stem cells may be isolated from human embryonic tissues or from niches within adult tissues such as, but not limited to, the bone marrow, liver, skin, adipose tissue, and brain. Other sources of these stem cells use techniques to derive them from human somatic cells lines via genetic manipulation creating induced pluripotent stem cells (iPSCs).[19,20] These techniques induce both pluripotency and self-renewal capabilities in fully differentiated somatic cells. All of these stem cell types require either the downregulation of immunogenic markers or the isolation of these cell sources from the ultimate recipient, as the elicitation of an immune response results in destruction of the construct. Stem cells are of great interest because their immunogenicity can be tailored so as to provide little to no response promoting integration into the recipient. Stem cells provide the abilities of self-renewal, pluripotency, and immune tolerance that make them ideal cell source candidates for tissue engineering and regenerative medicine approaches.

Adult Stem Cells

Adult stem cells represent a readily obtainable class of potential stem cells. Adult stem cells are multipotent progenitor cells isolated from adult donors. They can be derived from a number of tissues; however, the most extensively used in cell therapies are those derived from the bone marrow or adipose tissues, also known as human mesenchymal stem cells (hMSCs). hMSCs have gained interest in the scientific community because of their multipotency, specifically their ability to differentiate into a multitude of mesenchymal cell phenotypes including, but not limited to, smooth muscle cells, chondrocytes, osteoblasts, and adipocytes. Bone marrow or fat aspirates from donors provide a readily available supply of these stem cells, with a number of isolation and propagation procedures to enrich this population.[21] hMSCs are a self-renewing cell population allowing for their use in both injectable cell approaches and strategies that utilize the *ex vivo* expansion and seeding of cells onto scaffold materials intended for implantation. The successful creation of constructs that integrate scaffold materials and hMSCs requires the expression of the appropriate differentiated cellular phenotypes post seeding. Unlike other cell sources that will be discussed below, the differentiation potential of hMSCs are somewhat limited in their abilities to become cell phenotypes that are not of the mesenchymal lineages (i.e., difficulty forming ectodermal and endodermal derived tissues).

Embryonic Stem Cells

Human embryonic stem cells (hESCs) are a cell source extracted from human embryonic tissues that maintain the abilities of self-renewal and differentiation to multiple cellular phenotypes. James Thomson and his colleagues first identified these cells from the blastocysts of in vitro fertilization–donated human embryos in 1998.[22] hESCs immediately garnered interest owing to their pluripotent capabilities that promote differentiated phenotypes of all derivatives including ectodermal, endodermal, and mesenchymal lines. Cell types that have been demonstrated in vitro to arise from hESCs include neurons, skin, hematopoietic cells, hepatocytes, pancreatic cells, endothelial cells, cardiac and skeletal muscle cells, chondrocytes, adipocytes, and osteoblasts.[23] These immortalized cell lines provide a foundation for the understanding of the cellular mechanisms driving cellular proliferation and cell fates. The versatility of the cells in terms of near limitless proliferation in conjunction with unrestricted differentiation thrust this cell source to the forefront of early tissue engineering and regenerative medicine efforts. However, the use of human embryos to derive these cell lines has generated ethical concerns that have limited public funding and use of these lines.

Induced Pluripotent Stem Cells

In an effort to create cells that have the same pluripotency and self-renewal capabilities without the ethical concerns, iPSCs were created. Using research derived from hESC research, Yamanaka et al. identified factors (Oct3/4, Sox2, c-Myc, and Klf-4) whose expression resulted in dedifferentiation of somatic cells to the stem cell phenotype.[19,24] These iPSC-generated cell lines had self-renewal and pluripotency similar to hESCs but without the ethical concerns. However, iPSC cells and hESCs are not identical, as they share only approximately 4% of their gene expression profile.[19] The expression of these *Yamanaka factors* is produced via viral transfection and subsequent expression by the somatic cells. This raises concerns for possible mutagenesis and teratogenesis in clinical applications. The potential for tumorogenesis is present for all stem cells, as the potential for unrestricted growth is the hallmark of both stem cells and oncogenic cells.

Stem Cell Differentiation

The paradigm for the use of stem cells (regardless of the type of stem cell used) in tissue engineering and regenerative medicine involves the expansion of a cell population that can then be steered to differentiate to the desired cell phenotype. Methods for steering this differentiation can involve the application of soluble factors, the application of mechanical stimuli, or the binding of specific ligands. Although the process of differentiation is different for individual cell types, as an example, the process of stem cell differentiation toward bone is discussed to demonstrate the concepts involved (**Figure 13.4**). The process of osteoblastic differentiation is believed to proceed largely via stimulation with soluble factors. In vitro, osteogenic induction of stem cells is generally achieved via application of media containing dexamethasone, ascorbate, and β-glycerophosphate. This combination of soluble factors can achieve high levels of bone differentiation.[25] It is believed that osteoblastogenesis proceeds via transcription and subsequent activation of the osteoblast-specific core-binding factor a1 (Cbfa1), also commonly referred to in the literature as runt-related transcription factor 2 (RUNX2). Cbfa1 is the earliest and most specific marker of osteoblastogenesis and induces cells to produce type I collagen and alkaline phosphatase, both early markers of osteoblastic differentiation, signifying the preosteoblastic stage. Although soluble factors play a dominant role in osteoblastogenesis, they are not the only signals involved. Cell adhesion molecules such as integrins, selectins, cadherins, the arginylglycylaspartic acid polypeptide–binding sequence found in collagen, fibronectin, osteopontin, thrombospondin, bone sialoproteins, and vitronectin have all been shown to be required for differentiation.[26–28] Finally, material mechanics can influence stem cell differentiation toward the osteoblastic phenotype, with the greatest osteoblastogenesis occurring when stem cells are cultured on stiffer materials.[29,30] Thus, the production of differentiated cell phenotypes from a stem cell represents a complicated and robust process requiring a number of chemical and mechanical cues.

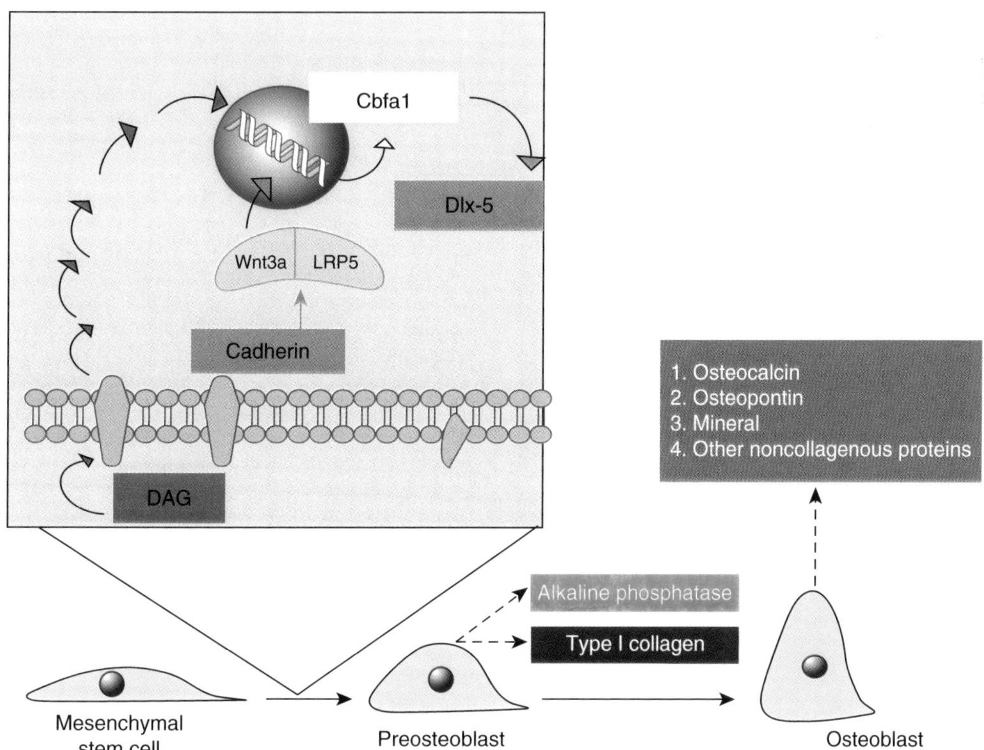

FIGURE 13.4. Human mesenchymal stem cells, in vitro, differentiate to osteoblasts via application of dexamethasone, ascorbate and β-glycerophosphate (DAG). DAG activates a cascade resulting in the upregulation of the earliest osteoblastic marker, Cbfa1. Osteoblastogenesis has also been shown to act via the Wnt pathway, in which Wnt3a, an active form of β-catenin, forms a complex with LRP5, which also results in upregulation of Cbfa1. Upregulation of Cbfa1 induces the expression of Dlx-5, which coincides with differentiation to the preosteoblastic stage signified by production of alkaline phosphatase and type I collagen. Terminal differentiation to the osteoblastic phenotype is characterized by production of late osteoblastic markers including mineral, osteocalcin, osteopontin, and other noncollagenous proteins.

Tissue engineering and regenerative medicine strategies all utilize some combination of soluble factors, mechanical cues and/or scaffolds to direct cell (somatic and stem) fates in predictable manners as described in the example above. It is this interplay that remains essential to the understanding and creation of viable constructs.

SCAFFOLDS FOR TISSUE ENGINEERING

Many of the strategies in tissue engineering utilize biomaterials as tissue scaffolds. A degradable and resorbable material is desired so that once the defect is repaired, only native/implanted tissue remains. Optimally, the degradation and resorption rate of such a scaffold should be tuned so that the falloff in scaffold strength is compensated with an increase in tissue growth. Naturally occurring matrices such as collagen, hyaluronic acid, and decellularized complete extracellular matrices (ECMs) have all been seeded with cells to create tissue engineering constructs.[31] Furthermore, polymeric scaffolds are promising candidates for engineering new tissues because they offer a wide array of materials with three-dimensionality, tunable surface chemistry and degradation rates, an assortment of physical parameters, incorporation of bioactive substances (i.e., growth factors, cytokines, adhesive proteins), and various scaffold architectures (**Figure 13.5**).[32]

Polymeric biomaterials utilized for clinical needs today, like the poly(α-hydroxy ester)s, were not created explicitly for tissue engineering but were adapted from preexisting materials. Unfortunately, the implementation of biomaterials that were not designed a priori to meet biologic applications often results in materials that have nonspecific or unidentified reactions with tissues, decreasing the efficacy of the implant. The ability to tailor endogenous or synthetic materials to promote cellular functions such as motility, proliferation, and stem cell differentiation provides the prospect of composing complex multicellular tissues in vitro and represents one of the first steps in the realization of engineered whole organ regeneration. To date, the ideal materials have not been identified, and there remains no consensus on whether synthetic or natural occurring scaffolds hold more promise.

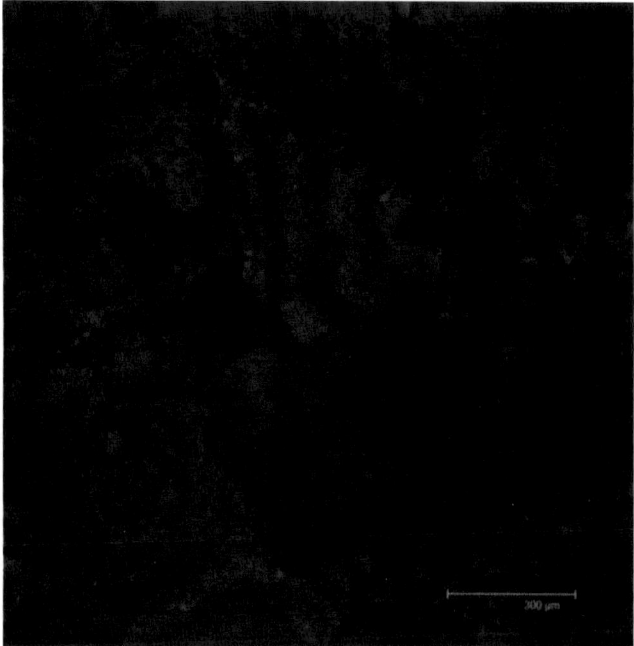

FIGURE 13.5. Alizarin red mineral staining of poly(polymer carbonate) scaffold. This scaffold is made to form a porous material that allows fluid and nutrient flow along with architecture conducive to cell seeding.

PLASTIC SURGERY AND TISSUE ENGINEERING

Plastic surgery uses tissues and materials in conjunction for reconstructive purposes. If tissue engineering focuses on *the creation of biological substitutes for the repair or regeneration of tissue or organ function*, then plastic surgery, with its focus on tissue manipulation techniques (e.g., composite tissue allotransplantation and free tissue transfer), may be described as the *clinical practice of tissue engineering*. For these reasons, plastic surgeons have often been at the forefront of the development and adoption of tissue engineering and regenerative medicine strategies. Some tissue engineering applications that are pertinent to plastic surgeons are discussed below. This list is not meant to be exhaustive but to highlight some of the areas in clinical medicine utilizing tissue engineering solutions with pertinence to plastic surgeons.

Skin Substitutes and Chronic Wounds

Chronic wounds represent a debilitating injury to patients, and the treatment of these conditions remains difficult and costly. Local tissue rearrangement and serial debridement strategies are the mainstay of treatment but often suffer from recurrence and eventual wound breakdown. Commercial products that use tissue engineering and regenerative medicine approaches that are currently available for wound healing generally fall into three categories: acellular products for structural matrices, cellular products, and growth factor products. Currently there are approximately 27 commercially available acellular products.[33] These products are constructed using a combination of synthetic and naturally occurring materials (e.g., collagen in conjunction with silicone sheeting, decellularized matrices, fibrin) without cells. These products promote wound healing by improving the wound microenvironment and/or providing temporary coverage to protect the wound from contamination. Unfortunately, as these products lack a cellular component, they are entirely dependent on the synergy with endogenous tissue for healing. In situations when recipient-site tissue healing capacity may be impaired, these products do not provide long-term solutions. Cellular products typically utilize cultured keratinocytes with synthetic scaffolds. Some products include fibroblasts along with the keratinocytes and scaffolds. Currently, they are nine commercially available cellular products for skin and chronic wound treatment.[33] Skin substitutes, to date, stimulate wound healing by the production of matrix proteins and other soluble factors that influence cell migration and angiogenesis.[33] These constructs lack sources of progenitor cells and are, therefore, self-limited.[34] Thus, healing with these products is via augmentation of natural healing rather than recapitulation. Growth factor products simply use soluble factors to promote healing in a regenerative medicine capacity. There are two products on the market that seek to increase wound healing via the delivery of platelet-derived factors. Although all of these devices hold promise, none has been able to mimic the healing capacity of native skin. The difficulty in skin and wound healing tissue engineering stems from the complex interplay between multiple cell types and even tissues that promote skin homeostasis. The need for a device that fulfills the barrier functions of skin but maintains the ability for cellular proliferation and renewal represents the greatest barrier to whole skin tissue engineering.[34]

Fat

Interest in adipocyte or fat tissue engineering stems from its relevance to disease models for obesity, diabetes, and other lipodystrophic disorders,[35] as well as from recent cosmetic and reconstructive advances to address volume depletion and soft tissue loss. Autologous fat grafting techniques have been developed to isolate adipocytes and fat-derived stem cells.[36] However, these autologous tissue transfer techniques suffer from graft loss and scarring. Plastic surgeons and tissue engineers alike have investigated cells harvested in lipoaspirates as cell sources for tissue-engineered constructs.[37] Adipocytes are harvested from the lipoaspirate and expanded on three-dimensional scaffolds that hope to maintain form and volume. Early work has demonstrated retention of form for up to 4 weeks after implantation through adipogenesis.[34,37] Further work has examined the *ex vivo* expansion of the fat-derived stem cells with subsequent reimplantation. These studies have demonstrated potentially improved volume retention with engineered fat as compared with traditional aspirates.[38] To date, tissue-engineered fat has remained largely experimental; however, the abundance of adipocyte cell source has made fat tissue engineering one of the most investigated tissue constructs.

Cartilage

Cartilage consists of a largely avascular arrangement of chondrocytes within a dense ECM. This lack of vascularity results in decreased healing and self-repair. Pathologic conditions of cartilage include decreased joint function and tissue deformities. For these reasons and others, commercial tissue-engineered cartilage products have been developed and tested clinically. These products hope to address the lack of endogenous healing potential of cartilage and promote healing and repair. Commercial products have been developed using implantation of isolated or cultured cells for injection and subsequent healing and implantation of *ex vivo* assembled constructs containing cells and scaffolds. Autologous chondrocytes have been harvested, expanded *ex vivo*, and reimplanted in cartilaginous lesions. These approaches depend on the ability to create chondrocytes and increase cell numbers utilizing soluble factors in both two-dimensional and three-dimensional cultures. Techniques have been developed utilizing both scaffold- and non–scaffold-based constructs. The non–scaffold-based strategies focus on cell expansion to deliver viable chondrocytes to the diseased tissue. Unfortunately, these approaches often lack the mechanical stability needs of load-bearing cartilage. In terms of scaffold-based approaches, hydrogels, decellularized xenogeneic matrices, freeze-dried scaffolds, woven and nonwoven microfiber meshes, and 3D-printed scaffolds have all been investigated.[39] These scaffolds can be based on naturally occurring ECM molecules (e.g., collagen and hyaluronic acid) or new synthetic molecules. Clinical indications for these products include the treatment of pathologic conditions of articular surfaces secondary to trauma and osteoarthritis for orthopedic purposes and in ear and tracheal reconstruction.

Bone

Musculoskeletal injuries cost Americans over $215 billion yearly, with fractures representing more than half of the injuries. The loss of bony tissue secondary to trauma, cancer, or primary bone disease results in significant mortality, morbidity, and socioeconomic loss. Current surgical techniques to address large volume bony loss focus on reparation via autologous tissue transfer with either bone grafting or free tissue transfer or bone transport mechanisms. Tissue engineering approaches have been developed and investigated to address these injuries without the donor site morbidity or lengthy process for bone transport. Most of these devices use synthetic polymer and processed biologic materials to provide acellular osteoconductive scaffolds with and without osteoinductive ligands. For example, previously tested constructs used human decellularized bone allograft doped with bone morphogenetic protein 2 to promote osteoinduction and osteoconduction.[40] However, more recent work has focused on the creation of *ex vivo* assembled constructs seeded with endothelial cells and hMSCs.[41] The goal of these devices is to provide a load-bearing construct that, when implanted, maintains a rich vascular network with a preformed lattice of viable osteoblast and osteocytes. Although these devices show promise, they have yet to obtain wide acceptance clinically. To date, an integrated tissue engineering solution providing structural, vascularized bone constructs for large bone defects remains to be clinically translated.

CONCLUSION

Regardless of the strategy or tissue, tissue engineering, in its current form, has not delivered as billed. In 1995, US-based market analysts predicted that tissue engineering would generate $3 billion by 2002. In reality, the total tissue engineering market in 2002 was less than $50 million.[42-45] In 2016, the tissue engineering still only reached $2.2 billion in sales. Although many factors contribute to the current inability for tissue engineering to provide *off-the-shelf* tissues, perhaps the greatest is the lack of fundamental understanding regarding cells, materials, and how they interact. Because the two main components of tissue-engineered constructs are the cells and scaffolding material, these two factors and their interactions must be understood and optimized to maximize the efficacy of the approach.[7] A 2007 study performed by Johnson et al. surveyed 24 leaders of the tissue engineering field to determine the best paths to obtain clinically viable products.[46] Their findings indicated that one of the most needed areas is the understanding and control of stem cell behavior by measuring responses at the molecular level. Using these structure-function responses of stem cells probed at the molecular level may enable the identification of biomarkers for guidance in the design of tissue-engineered products. To that end, a strategic assessment of the field from the US Government Multi-Agency Tissue Engineering Science group of federal agencies provided a list of the critical priorities to identify these structure-function relationships, including[47]

- Understanding the cellular machinery
- Identifying and validating biomarker and assays
- Advancing imaging technologies
- Defining cell/environment interactions
- Establishing computational modeling systems

The US Government Multi-Agency Tissue Engineering Science assessment indicates that these five priorities are essential to accomplishing what they consider the four overarching goals of the field[46,47]:

- Understanding and controlling the cellular response
- Formulating biomaterial scaffolds and the tissue-matrix environment
- Developing enabling tools (i.e., high-throughput assays, instrumentation, imaging modalities, and computational modeling)
- Promoting scale-up, translation, and commercialization

Therefore, current efforts have focused on the fundamental science driving tissue engineering. It is hoped that with new developments tissue engineering may become an essential and valued tool to the reconstructive surgeon.

REFERENCES

1. Niklason LE, Langer R. Prospects for organ and tissue replacement. *JAMA*. 2001;285(5):573-576.
2. OPTN. *Transplant: Organ by diagnosis*; 2018. http://www.optn.org/latestData/rptData.asp. Accessed March 11, 2018.
3. Israni AK, Zaun D, Rosendale JD, et al. OPTN/SRTR 2012 annual data report: deceased organ donation. *Am J Transpl*. 2014;14(suppl 1):167-183.
4. Skalak R, Fox CF. *Tissue Engineering: Proceedings of a Workshop Held at Granlibakken. February 26–29, 1988; Lake Tahoe, CA*; 1988.
5. Langer R, Vacanti JP. Tissue engineering. *Science*. 1993;260(5110):920-926.
6. Singh G, Kelly M. Origins of the "Indian method" of nasal reconstruction. *Plast Reconstr Surg*. 2005;116(4):1177-1179.
7. Griffith LG, Naughton G. Tissue engineering: current challenges and expanding opportunities. *Science*. 2002;295(5557):1009-1014.
8. Reffelmann T, Konemann S, Kloner RA. Promise of blood- and bone marrow-derived stem cell transplantation for functional cardiac repair: putting it in perspective with existing therapy. *J Am Coll Cardiol*. 2009;53(4):305-308.
9. Collins JM, Russell B. Stem cell therapy for cardiac repair. *J Cardiovasc Nurs*. 2009;24(2):93-97.
10. Nose Y, Okubo H. Artificial organs versus regenerative medicine: is it true? *Artif Organs*. 2003;27(9):765-771.
11. Morrison WA. Progress in tissue engineering of soft tissue and organs. *Surgery*. 2009;145(2):127-130.

12. Atala A, Bauer SB, Soker S, et al. Tissue-engineered autologous bladders for patients needing cystoplasty. *Lancet*. 2006;367(9518):1241-1246.
First study to demonstrate the clinical use of a tissue-engineerined product. An autologous bladder was created via seeding scaffolds in vitro with bladder cells and implanted in patients.
13. Iwasa J, Engebretsen L, Shima Y, Ochi M. Clinical application of scaffolds for cartilage tissue engineering. *Knee Surg Sports Traumatol Arthrosc*. 2008;17(6):561-577.
14. Ohgawara H, Edamura K, Kawakami M, Umezawa K. Diabetes mellitus: rational basis, clinical approach and future therapy. *Biomed Pharmacother*. 2004;58(10):605-609.
15. Hutmacher DW. Scaffolds in tissue engineering bone and cartilage. *Biomaterials*. 2000;21(24):2529-2543.
16. Priya SG, Jungvid H, Kumar A. Skin tissue engineering for tissue repair and regeneration. *Tissue Eng B Rev*. 2008;14(1):105-118.
17. Ohashi K. Liver tissue engineering: the future of liver therapeutics. *Hepatol Res*. 2008;38:S76-S87.
18. Strehl R, Schumacher K, de Vries U, Minuth WW. Proliferating cells versus differentiated cells in tissue engineering. *Tissue Eng*. 2002;8(1):37-42.
19. Takahashi K, Tanabe K, Ohnuki M, et al. Induction of pluripotent stem cells from adult human fibroblasts by defined factors. *Cell*. 2007;131(5):861-872.
First study to use the expression of certain factors to induce pluripotency in adult stem cells. This effectively created the ability to take somatic cells without the concerns of embryonic stem cells and induce pluripotency. The factors identified are deemed essential to cell stemness *and have been termed the Yamanaka factors.*
20. Yu J, Vodyanik MA, Smuga-Otto K, et al. Induced pluripotent stem cell lines derived from human somatic cells. *Science*. 2007;318(5858):1917-1920.
21. Beyer Nardi N, da Silva Meirelles L. Mesenchymal stem cells: isolation, in vitro expansion and characterization. *Handb Exp Pharmacol*. 2006(174):249-282.
22. Thomson JA, Itskovitz-Eldor J, Shapiro SS, et al. Embryonic stem cell lines derived from human blastocysts. *Science*. 1998;282(5391):1145-1147.
Landmark publication for the identification of embryonic stem cell lines and their pluripotency. This publication demonstrated that embryonic cells maintain the ability of self-renewal and pluripotency.
23. Behr B, Ko SH, Wong VW, et al. Stem cells. *Plast Reconstr Surg*. 2010;126(4):1163-1171.
24. Chhabra A. Derivation of human induced pluripotent stem cell (iPSC) lines and mechanism of pluripotency: historical perspective and recent advances. *Stem Cell Rev*. 2017;13(6):757-773.
25. Pittenger MF, Mackay AM, Beck SC, et al. Multilineage potential of adult human mesenchymal stem cells. *Science*. 1999;284(5411):143-147.
This study identifies the multipotency potential of adult stem cells. Previously, only embryonic stem cells were believed to have self-renewal and multilineage potential. This study demonstrated that cells derived from adult tissue can maintain these abilities.
26. Grzesik WJ, Robey PG. Bone matrix RGD glycoproteins: immunolocalization and interaction with human primary osteoblastic bone cells in vitro. *J Bone Miner Res*. 1994;9(4):487-496.
27. McBeath R, Pirone DM, Nelson CM, et al. Cell shape, cytoskeletal tension, and RhoA regulate stem cell lineage commitment. *Dev Cell*. 2004;6(4):483-495.
28. Ross FP, Chappel J, Alvarez JI, et al. Interactions between the bone matrix proteins osteopontin and bone sialoprotein and the osteoclast integrin alpha v beta 3 potentiate bone resorption. *J Biol Chem*. 1993;268(13):9901-9907.
29. Engler AJ, Sen S, Sweeney HL, Discher DE. Matrix elasticity directs stem cell lineage specification. *Cell*. 2006;126(4):677-689.
30. Discher DE, Janmey P, Wang YL. Tissue cells feel and respond to the stiffness of their substrate. *Science*. 2005;310(5751):1139-1143.
This article demonstrated that in the presence of all soluble cues, the mechanical properties of the scaffolds steers stem cell differentiation. Stiffer materials promoted bone differentiation, and softer materials promoted differentiation toward soft tissues. This article supports the hypothesis that stem cells respond to the mechanical cues of their substrate environment to steer determine lineage fates.
31. Yesmin S, Paget MB, Murray HE, Downing R. Bio-scaffolds in organ-regeneration: clinical potential and current challenges. *Curr Res Transl Med*. 2017;65(3):103-113.
32. Dee KC, Bizios R. Proactive biomaterials and bone tissue engineering. *Biotechnol Bioengin*. 1996;50(4):438-442.
33. Ho J, Walsh C, Yue D, et al. Current advancements and strategies in tissue engineering for wound healing: a comprehensive review. *Adv Wound Care (New Rochelle)*. 2017;6(6):191-209.
34. Wong VW, Rustad KC, Longaker MT, Gurtner GC. Tissue engineering in plastic surgery: a review. *Plast Reconstr Surg*. 2010;126(3):858-868.
35. Park KW, Halperin DS, Tontonoz P. Before they were fat: adipocyte progenitors. *Cell Metab*. 2008;8(6):454-457.
36. Ogura F, Wakao S, Kuroda Y, et al. Human adipose tissue possesses a unique population of pluripotent stem cells with nontumorigenic and low telomerase activities: potential implications in regenerative medicine. *Stem Cells Dev*. 2014;23(7):717-728.
37. Stosich MS, Mao JJ. Adipose tissue engineering from human adult stem cells: clinical implications in plastic and reconstructive surgery. *Plast Reconstr Surg*. 2007;119(1):71-83; discussion 84-75.
38. Bashir MM, Sohail M, Bashir A, et al. Outcome of conventional adipose tissue grafting for contour deformities of face and role of ex vivo expanded adipose tissue-derived stem cells in treatment of such deformities. *J Craniofac Surg*. 2018; 29(5):1143-1147.
39. Huang BJ, Hu JC, Athanasiou KA. Cell-based tissue engineering strategies used in the clinical repair of articular cartilage. *Biomaterials*. 2016;98:1-22.
40. Jones AL, Bucholz RW, Bosse MJ, et al. Recombinant human BMP-2 and allograft compared with autogenous bone graft for reconstruction of diaphyseal tibial fractures with cortical defects: a randomized, controlled trial. *J Bone Joint Surg Am*. 2006;88A(7):1431-1441.
41. Ren L, Kang Y, Browne C, et al. Fabrication, vascularization and osteogenic properties of a novel synthetic biomimetic induced membrane for the treatment of large bone defects. *Bone*. 2014;64:173-182.
42. Kohn J, Welsh WJ, Knight D. A new approach to the rationale discovery of polymeric biomaterials. *Biomaterials*. 2007;28(29):4171-4177.
43. Lysaght MJ, Hazlehurst AL. Tissue engineering: the end of the beginning. *Tissue Eng*. 2004;10(1-2):309-320.
44. Lysaght MJ, Nguy NA, Sullivan K. An economic survey of the emerging tissue engineering industry. *Tissue Eng*. 1998;4(3):231-238.
45. Lysaght MJ, Reyes J. The growth of tissue engineering. *Tissue Eng*. 2001;7(5):485-493.
46. Johnson PC, Mikos AG, Fisher JP, Jansen JA. Strategic directions in tissue engineering. *Tissue Eng*. 2007;13(12):2827-2837.
47. U.S. Government Multi-Agency Tissue Engineering Science (MATES) Integracy Working Group. Advancing tissue science and engineering: a foundation for the future: a multi-agency strategic plan. *Tissue Eng*. 2007;13(12):2825-2826.

QUESTIONS

1. **Strategies used in tissue engineering and regenerative medicine include which of the following (choose all that are correct)?**
   - i. Implantation of isolated or cultured cells for injection and subsequent healing
   - ii. Autologous tissue transfer
   - iii. In situ directed tissue regeneration
   - iv. Implantation of *ex vivo* assembled constructs containing cells and/or scaffolds

   a. i
   b. i and iv
   c. ii
   d. i, iii, and iv
   e. All of the above

2. **Cell sources that maintain the ability to differentiate to all germ cell lines utilized in tissue engineering and regenerative medicine include which of the following?**
   - i. Somatic cell lines
   - ii. Adult stem cell lines
   - iii. Embryonic stem cell lines
   - iv. Induced pluripotent cell lines

   a. i
   b. ii and iii
   c. iii
   d. iii and iv
   e. All of the above

3. **Which of the following scaffold materials represents a synthetic rather than a naturally occurring cell matrix?**

   a. Collagen
   b. Poly-α-hydroxy esters
   c. Hyaluronic acid
   d. Fibronectin
   e. Decellularized human tissues

4. **Stem cell differentiation to the osteoblastic phenotype is influenced by which of the following factors in vitro?**

   a. Soluble cues
   b. ECM proteins and cell adhesion molecules
   c. Mechanical properties of the scaffolds
   d. None of the above
   e. Answers a, b, and c

1. **Answer: d.** Tissue engineering and regenerative medicine currently employ three main strategies: (1) implantation of isolated or cultured cells for injection and subsequent healing; (2) in situ directed tissue regeneration; and (3) implantation of *ex vivo* assembled constructs containing cells and scaffolds. Autologous tissue transfer is traditionally utilized by plastic surgeons to treat tissue loss but is not used in tissue engineering strategies. The goal of tissue engineering is to create biologic devices that act ***in lieu*** of traditional treatment modalities, such as autologous tissue transfer.

2. **Answer: d.** Somatic cell lines represent terminally differentiated cells that are unable to change cell lines. They are traditionally limited to the cell phenotype from which they are derived. For example, somatic neurons do not possess the ability to differentiation to muscle and other nonneuronal cells. Adult stem cells are cells that maintain the ability of self-renewal and have the ability to differentiate to certain but not all germ cell lines. For example, bone marrow–derived stem cells typically can differentiate to any mesenchymal stem cell lineages including bone, muscle and fat but not ectodermal tissues such as neurons. Embryonic stem cell lines and iPSC lines have the ability to become any of the germ cell lines. The induced pluripotent cells are reengineered with the Yamanaka factors to allows the cells to become stem cell like.

3. **Answer: b.** Poly-α-hydroxy esters are synthetic polymers derived from the monomer of lactic acid. It is synthesized through the ring-opening polymerization of the lactone. Common materials in the family include poly(L-lactic acid) and poly(glycolic acid). These polymers are degradable but have acid breakdown products (lactic acid) with their degradation. Collagen, hyaluronic acid, fibronectin, and decellularized human tissues are all naturally occurring. They can be processed into multiple forms including hydrogels, meshes, and porous scaffolds.

4. **Answer: e.** In vitro, osteogenic induction of stem cells is generally achieved via application of media containing dexamethasone, ascorbate, and β-glycerophosphate. This combination of soluble factors can achieve high levels of bone differentiation. Cell adhesion molecules such as integrins, selectins, cadherins, the arginylglycylaspartic acid polypeptide–binding sequence found in collagen, fibronectin, osteopontin, thrombospondin, bone sialoproteins, and vitronectin have all been shown to be required for osteoblastic differentiation. Finally, material mechanics can influence stem cell differentiation toward the osteoblastic phenotype, with the greatest osteoblastogenesis occurring when stem cells are cultured on stiffer materials.

CHAPTER 14 Standardization of Photography and Videography in Plastic Surgery

Frank Yuan and Kevin C. Chung

KEY POINTS

- High-quality photography is critical in the presentation of surgical outcomes, assurance of standards, and advancement of surgical education.
- Maintaining a high level of consistency requires several factors to be tightly controlled—camera equipment, lighting, patient positioning, background, patient clothing, and magnification/size.
- Defining and promoting a standardized set of guidelines when shooting different areas of interest on the body promotes effective analyses and comparison of outcomes.
- An important goal of preoperative and postoperative videos is to capture the functional changes in specific areas of interest that result from different operative techniques to facilitate evaluation of outcomes.
- High-quality intraoperative videos capture the dynamic aspects of surgery and add important context to facilitate understanding of scientific presentations.
- An effective video operator must know and understand the procedure being performed, as well as all the pertinent steps and relevant anatomy; thus no time is wasted by the operating surgeon during the critical steps of an operation.

IMPORTANCE OF MEDICAL PHOTOGRAPHY

High-quality photographic documentation is essential in plastic surgery. Not only are they useful for scientific presentations and manuscripts, but more importantly, preoperative and postoperative photographs are used as tools to evaluate and track surgical outcomes, and often serve as benchmarks for quality standards.[1,2] Intraoperative photographs of procedures can also document operations and outcomes for educational and medicolegal purposes, as well as providing context for communication among residents and attending surgeons.[2] Lastly, these photographs are essential in shaping public perception.[3] In the age of social media, patients are often inundated with online *before and after* images of other patients, particularly on cosmetic practice websites. Consequently, plastic surgeons and their practice groups are often judged before ever meeting the patient.[4,5]

Thus, maintaining standardization and optimizing photographic quality establishes the perception of quality for a surgeon. Even minuscule oversights in the photographing process by the plastic surgeon (e.g., photographs that are blurry, or contain extraneous surgical instruments or anatomy with no pertinence to the subject of the photograph) will detract attention from the theme they are trying to depict and, consequently, diminish the photograph's educational value (**Figure 14.1**).[2]

MAINTAINING CONSISTENCY

The key to great medical photography is consistency—taking every photograph the exact same way every time. To maintain a high level of consistency, several factors have to be tightly controlled, e.g., camera equipment, lighting, patient positioning, background, patient clothing, and magnification/size.[6] Fortunately, as technology continues to improve and modern-day cameras become more advanced, several parameters, such as aperture, shutter speed, and the sensitivity of the image sensor to light (i.e., ISO), which were once manually adjusted, are now set according to an installed algorithm. Each of the different automatic camera settings (e.g., sport, portrait, landscape) represents a different exposure algorithm, optimized to achieve the best combination of these parameters.[6] Thus, the quality of photographs with most of today's cameras will be excellent. Nevertheless, several considerations in the photographic process are operator dependent and should still be thoroughly considered to maintain a high level of quality and consistency.

Equipment

When ensuring high-quality photographic documentation in plastic surgery, two main camera types should be considered—a digital single-lens reflex (SLR) 35 mm camera or a point and shoot digital camera.[7,8] The digital SLR 35 mm camera offers the possibility of a variation of lenses. We recommend having one lens with a short focal length range of 50 to 60 mm, which is ideal for body contouring and photographs that use a large area, and a lens with a longer focal length range of 90 to 105 mm, which is ideal for closer photographs of the face and head (**Figure 14.2**). These high-quality lenses assure a maximum depth of field and minimal alteration of colors. Additionally, these lenses produce minimal distortion, whereby creating a flat field and, ultimately, an accurate depiction of the body area photographed without the *bulging* that occurs with wide-angle lenses. Whichever the lens selected, all lenses should have macro capabilities, which helps the photographer focus on objects close to the camera lens.[7,8]

Aside from SLR cameras, some surgeons recommend the use of point and shoot cameras, particularly for intraoperative photographs. The point and shoot camera offers the advantages of not being too cumbersome, is practical and easy to operate (even for first-time users), and is cheaper on average, while still being able to provide high-quality images that satisfy the stringent requirements necessary for medical photography.[2]

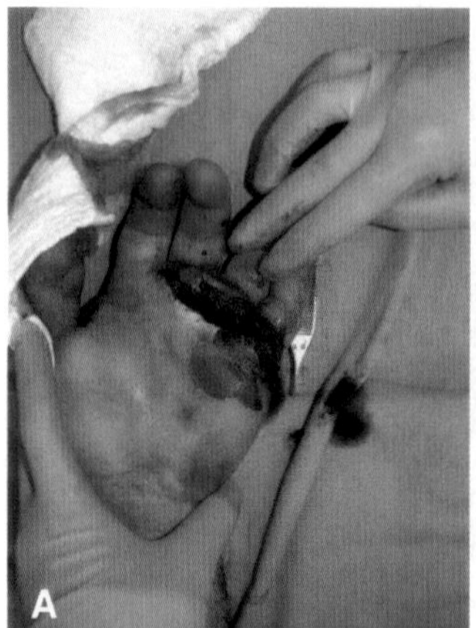

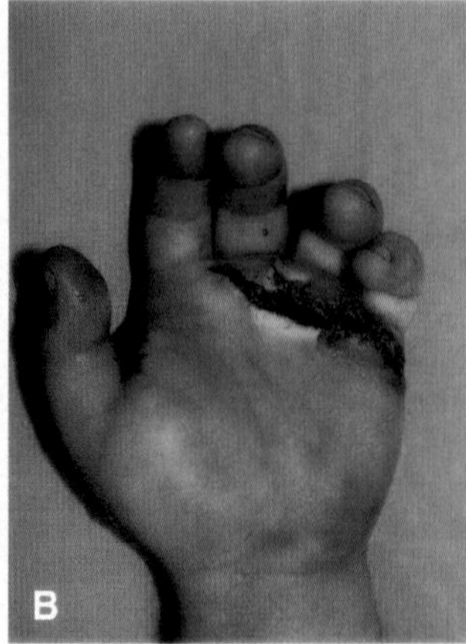

FIGURE 14.1. A. Example of a bad surgical photo. The surgeon's and assistant's hands, excess blood, and misplaced gauze and surgical instruments all distract from the focus of the picture. **B.** Example of a good surgical photo. The view is unobstructed and allows the viewer to be drawn to the focal point of the picture.

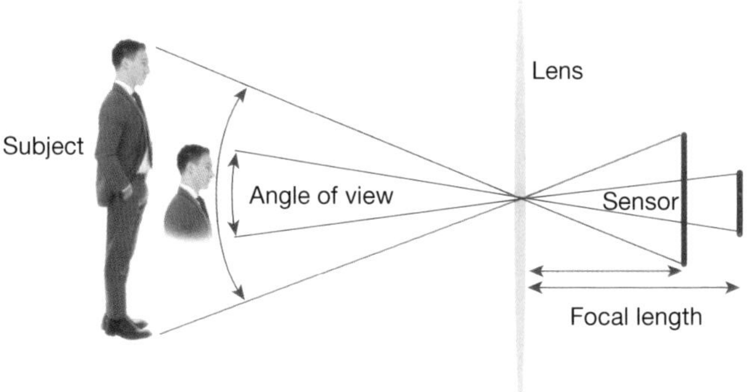

FIGURE 14.2. A shorter focal length produces a wider angle of view, whereas a longer focal length produces a narrower angle of view.

Regardless of the camera type, we highly recommend using a camera that has the capability to project a grid screen in its viewfinder, which can ensure that patients are properly aligned within the viewfinder frame. Precise framing of anatomic landmarks both preoperatively and postoperatively will guarantee consistency and reproducibility.[7-9] Additionally, it is beneficial for the camera to have a swivel screen so the operator is able to shoot a wide array of angles, particularly for intraoperative photographs where it may be difficult to position oneself over a sterile field.[2]

Background

The choice of background and maintenance is extremely important and has a significant impact on the quality of medical photographs. It is essential that the background is even, nonreflecting, and monochromatic.[2,7,9] Any degree of unevenness or clutter will detract from the focus of the image and diminish its value. After multiple tests of different background colors, the Clinical Photography Committee has decided that a sky blue background is the most visually pleasing, independent of whether the photograph is taken in black-and-white or in color. Furthermore, a sky-blue background provides a sufficient color contrast to various skin tones and diminishes the appearance of shadows.[7,10,11] Black, white, and even green have all been used as background colors. However, a white background tends to produce harsh shadows, whereas a black background tends to provide less contrast for darker-skinned patients.[2,7,9]

Lighting

Lighting is one of the most crucial aspects of medical photography when it comes to maintaining consistency. Thus, using different types of lighting for preoperative and postoperative photographs is unacceptable. Classically, there are three main types of light sources that may be used—a ring light, a mounted strobe light, and a studio light.[12] The ring light, located circumferentially around the lens, is the simplest and most foolproof source of light. Although it is technically impossible to alter the angle of the light source to the patient, the drawbacks to the ring light are its availability and flat lighting (i.e., little or no contrast or gradients of light to define shapes). A camera-mounted strobe light has the advantage of producing side lighting and negates the problem of flat lighting. However, maintaining consistent preoperative and postoperative lighting with the mounted strobe light relies heavily on the photographer's ability to keep it positioned in a constant relationship to the patient at all times. Perhaps, the most effective form of lighting is studio lighting. However, it requires that photographs are taken with the same lighting at consistent angles every time. Otherwise, for instance, underexposed side lighting will emphasize contour irregularities, whereas overexposed front lighting will de-emphasize contour irregularities.[12] Maintaining specific lighting arrangements for each corresponding body area of interest should be facilitated with labels throughout the studio to better direct the patient, as well as the camera operator.[12,13] If equipment is not available, it is acceptable to use the built-in flash on a camera, as long as it is in a well-lit room; poor lighting conditions create shadows and uneven lighting.[2]

AREAS OF INTEREST

To maintain accuracy and consistency between preoperative and postoperative photographs, patient and camera positions must be kept constant. Thus, a standardized set of guidelines for each of the various areas of the body should be utilized.[14] Not only are standardized guidelines important when comparing one's own preoperative and postoperative photographs, they are important when comparing preoperative and postoperative photographs among different surgeons as well.

A comprehensive set of guidelines were established in 2006 by the American Society of Plastic Surgeons (ASPS) and the Plastic Surgery Foundation (PSF).[14] Despite the significance of these published guidelines, only approximately 66% of ASPS and ASAPS plastic surgeons adhered to these guidelines. It is unclear if this discrepancy was attributed to surgeon preference, technique, or unclear patient instructions.[5] And although it may not be possible for all plastic surgeons to exactly conform to a set of guidelines owing to inexperience or availability of equipment or studio space, promoting and striving to adhere to a standardized set of guidelines will facilitate surgeons to critically analyze and compare outcomes, and review results and ensure quality standards.

Guidelines for Photographs

Head (Figure 14.3)

- Patient should have their hair pulled away from the face and tucked behind the ears with a headband or clip. All jewelry and eyewear, as well as heavy makeup and lipstick, should be removed.
- Patient should be seated on a stool and positioned at a premarked area in the examination room. The patient should rotate the entire body (shoulder and feet) when turning for oblique and lateral views.
- Facial expressions must be controlled so that they do not distort the surgical outcomes or the deformities of interest.
- Close-up face (Figure 14.3A): Eyebrows should be positioned at the top of the frame. The nose should be centered horizontally in all views. For basal views, the tip of the nose should be aligned with the upper eyelid crease.
- Full face (Figure 14.3C): Ears should be centered vertically in all views. The head should be centered horizontally for frontal and oblique views. The front of the patient's face should be placed a quarter frame from the edge for lateral views.
- Ears (Figure 14.3D): The head should be centered horizontally in anterior and posterior views. Ears should be centered in the frame for close-up views.
- Mouth (Figure 14.3B): The mouth should be centered vertically in all views and horizontally for anterior views. Lips should be positioned a quarter frame from the edge for oblique and lateral views.

Breasts (Figure 14.4)

- Patient should have all jewelry and gown completely removed and be given a photo garment to wear.
- Patient should stand comfortably with arms to the side and positioned at a premarked area in the examination room. Distal arms should be moved back slightly for oblique views.
- Clavicles should be positioned at the top of the frame. The torso should be centered horizontally for frontal and oblique views. The proximal breast should be centered horizontally for lateral views; the distal breast should no longer be visible.

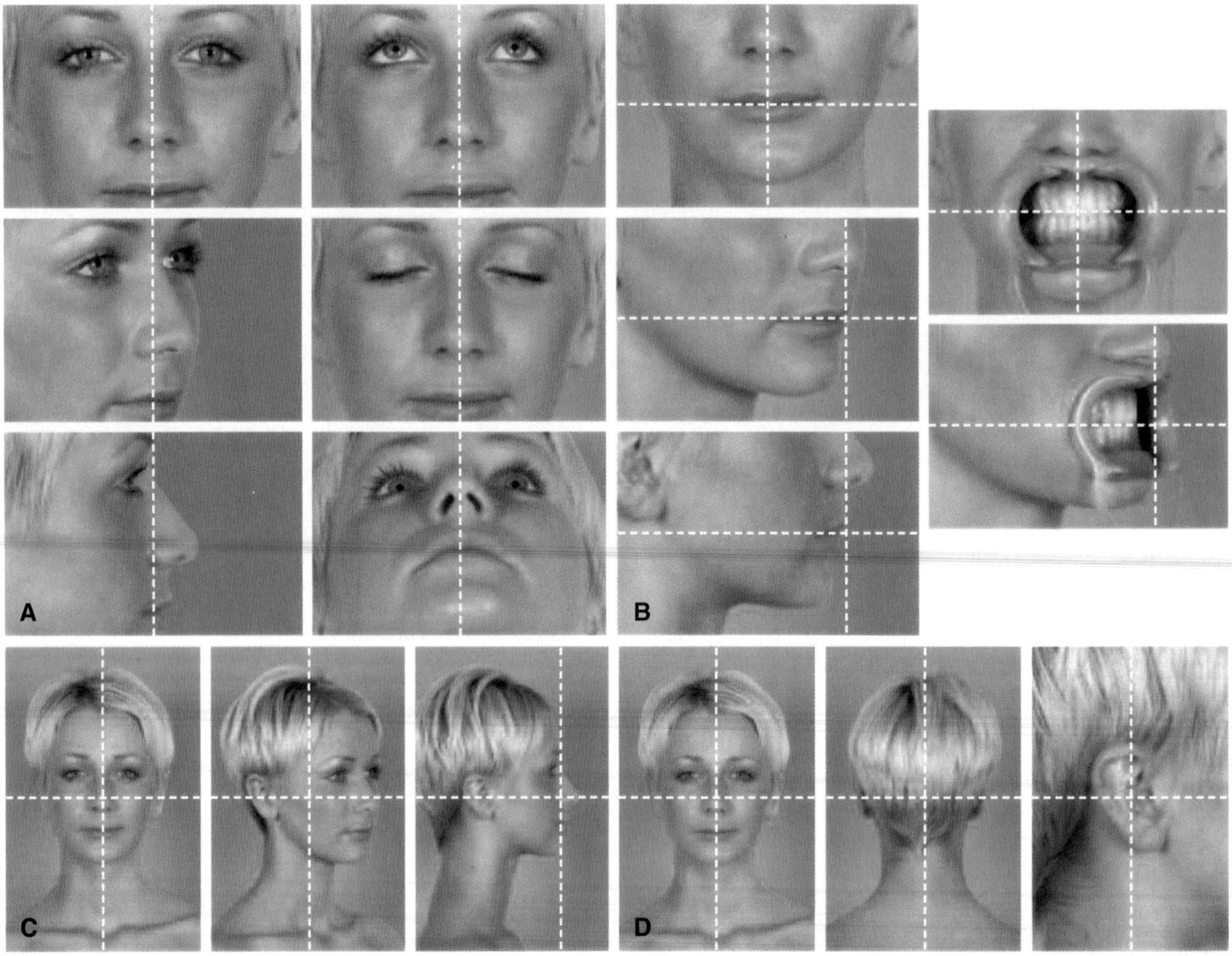

FIGURE 14.3. **A.** Standard positioning and up close views of the face. Eyebrows positioned at the top of the frame; nose centered horizontally in all views. **B.** Standard positioning and views of the mouth. The mouth centered vertically in all views and horizontally in anterior views. **C.** Standard positioning and views of the full face. Ears centered vertically in all views. **D.** Standard positioning and views of the ears. The head centered horizontally in anterior/posterior views; ears centered in close-up views. (Used with permission of the American Society of Plastic Surgeons.)

Abdomen (Figure 14.5)

- Patient should have the gown completely removed and be given a photo garment to wear.
- Patient should stand comfortably with arms folded above the breasts and positioned at a premarked area in the examination room.
- The inframammary folds should be positioned at the top of the frame. The torso should be centered horizontally.

Hips/Thighs (Figure 14.6)

- Patient should have their gown completely removed and given a photo garment to wear.
- Patient should stand comfortably with arms folded above the breasts and positioned at a premarked area in the examination room.
- Knees should be positioned at the bottom of the frame, with the hips centered horizontally. The distal leg should not be visible in the lateral view.

Hand and Forearm (Figure 14.7)

- Patient should have all jewelry and nail polish removed.
- Patient should be seated on a stool and directly face the camera operator. Both hands should be held a few inches above a table/background; the patient should avoid touching the background to prevent distortion of the natural finger posture.
- Patient's hands should be lined up at the fingertips.
- A set of six standard views of both hands should be photographed.

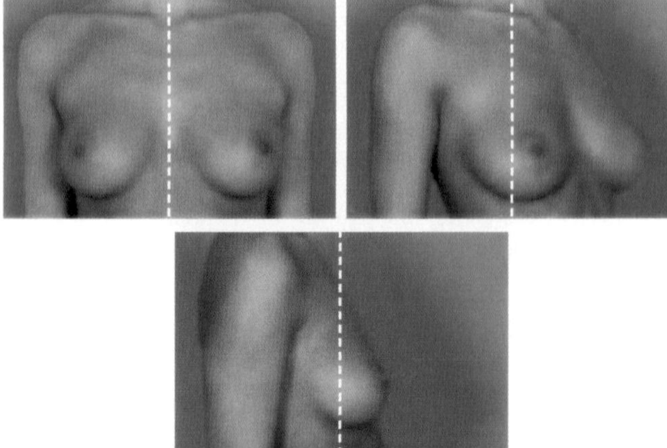

FIGURE 14.4. Standard positioning and views of the breasts. Clavicles positioned at the top of the frame; torso centered horizontally for frontal/oblique views. (Used with permission of the American Society of Plastic Surgeons.)

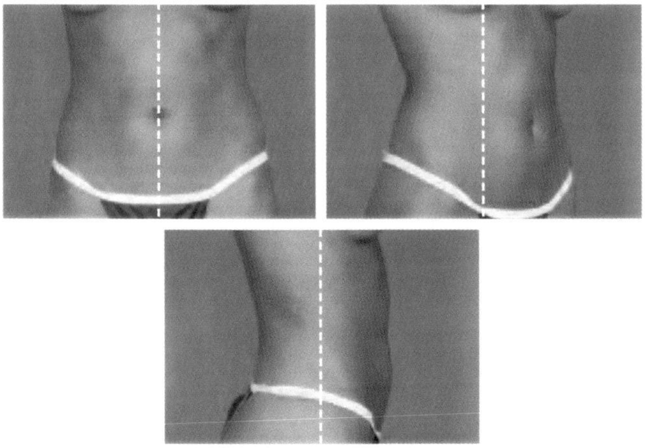

FIGURE 14.5. Standard positioning and views of the abdomen. Inframammary folds positioned at the top of the frame; torso centered horizontally. (Used with permission of the American Society of Plastic Surgeons.)

Lower Extremity (Figure 14.8)

- Patient should have all clothes and jewelry below the waist completely removed; nail polish should also be removed.
- Patient should stand on a step stage with feet at shoulder width.
- Toes should be positioned at the bottom of the frame, with feet centered horizontally. The distal leg should not be visible in the lateral view.

APPLICATION OF VIDEOGRAPHY IN PLASTIC SURGERY

In recent times, videography has quickly become an important adjunct not only in the documentation of patient outcomes for scientific presentations and research, but in facilitating effective surgical education and physician-to-physician communication as well. High-quality videos are able to capture all stages of the surgery (if needed), while still ensuring enough detail to adequately demonstrate the pertinent surgical anatomy. Thus, videography adds context for scientific presentations to be more understandable in comparison to the use of figures or schematics.[15-20] Furthermore, owing to the increasing use of social media outlets by plastic surgeons (e.g., YouTube, Facebook, Instagram, Twitter, SnapChat), high-quality videos can successfully augment plastic surgeons' online repertoire when presenting their techniques and outcomes to prospective patients.

Well-shot videos promote effective comparison and evaluation of surgical outcomes not only across different operative techniques, but also among their peers as well.[15-20] Additionally, it is important to understand that unlike photographs, which capture patients' preoperative and postoperative conditions, videos have the advantage of capturing dynamic aspects of an operation. Thus,

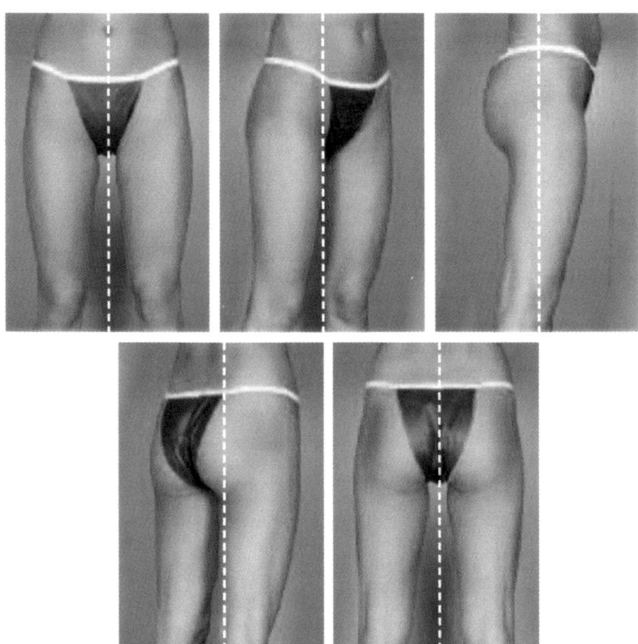

FIGURE 14.6. Standard positioning and views of the hips and thighs. Knees positioned at bottom of frame; hips centered horizontally. (Used with permission of the American Society of Plastic Surgeons.)

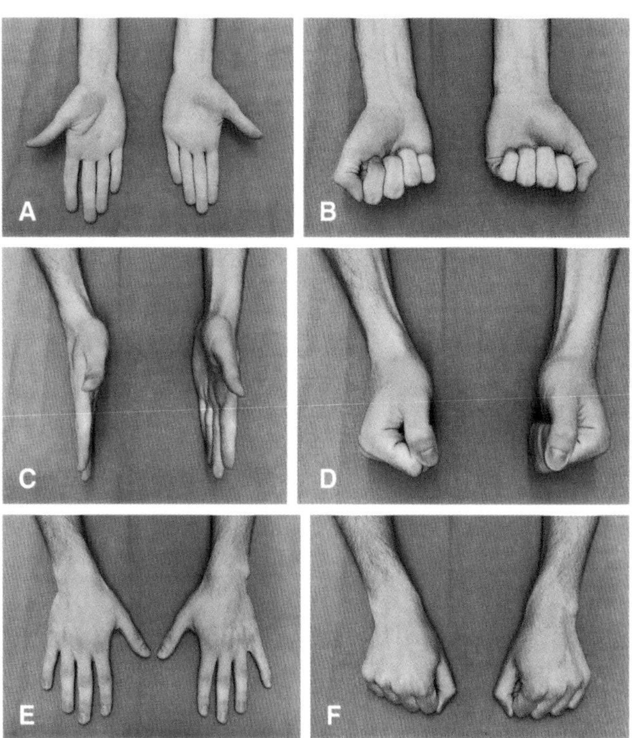

FIGURE 14.7. A. Fingers straight in palmar view. **B.** Clenched fist in palmar view. **C.** Fingers straight in lateral view. **D.** Clenched fist in lateral view. **E.** Fingers straight in dorsal view. **F.** Clenched fist in dorsal view.

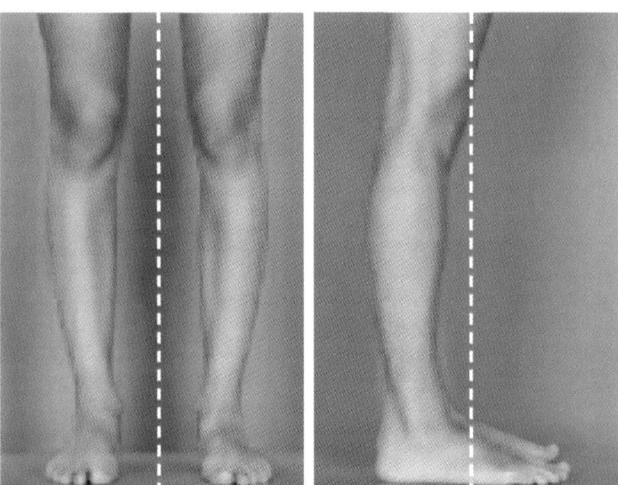

FIGURE 14.8. Standard positioning and views of the lower extremity. Toes positioned at bottom of frame; feet centered horizontally. (Used with permission of the American Society of Plastic Surgeons.)

compared with photography, videography is much more difficult to standardize, because no two operations in plastic surgery are performed the exact same way; it is challenging to compare key components of one operation with key components of another operation (even if they are the same operation). Despite these challenges, certain aspects of videography in plastic surgery can be standardized, such as camera type, positioning, and video editing. Maintaining consistency in videography can prove extremely useful, particularly when comparing preoperative and postoperative functional outcomes.[15,16]

GENERAL CONCEPTS OF VIDEOGRAPHY

Equipment

Many types of cameras exist for video recording, from remote-controlled cameras mounted on tripods and handheld camcorders with swivel screens to operating room light handle cameras, and even newer generation wearable or head-mounted devices.[15,17-19] Despite the many available options, the majority of video cameras will be precalibrated to capture the highest-quality images; technical aspects, such as aperture size and light exposure, will generally be automatic depending on which mode is selected. Thus, it is less important which device is used when recording videos, and more important that whichever device one uses, it should be the same device every time to maintain consistency.

Background

Backgrounds should be kept consistent, particularly when recording a series of videos of the same patient at different time intervals (e.g., hand function at different periods of follow-up). We recommend either a sky blue or green background when recording surgical videos, as they are optimal for a wide variety of skin tones and minimize shadows.[15] Additionally, the surgical field should be cleared of unused equipment (e.g., retractors, gauze, scissors), as well as any bloodstains or debris, as to not distract viewers from the important details of the operation.

Lighting

Whether in the clinic or in the operating room, it is important to use a uniform light source when recording videos, as nonuniform light can create unnecessary shadows and diminish the image quality. Thus, ambient operating room fluorescent lights, surgical LED lights, or even flood lights (if in a clinic studio) should be used to maximize uniformity.[15,16] With improved technology, automatic white balance capabilities will better compensate for varying light intensities and prevent over-exposure of images.

GUIDELINES FOR VIDEOGRAPHY

When recording preoperative and postoperative videos, the goal is to capture functional changes in the specific areas of interest (e.g., facial movements, extremity range of motion). Therefore, to effectively compare preoperative and postoperative videos, several things should be considered. The patient's body area of interest should be positioned the same way each time. The angles at which a video is recorded and the positioning of certain body areas of interest should be consistent across all recording sessions. Clear instructions should be given to patients before video recording regarding how they should position themselves or what motions need to be captured.

For instance, for patients undergoing hand procedures, the hand should be positioned with its longitudinal axis going from left to right across the screen, as opposed to up and down. The patient should be asked to slowly move the joint or area of interest at least three times and in three different views (i.e., dorsal, medial, and palmar).[15] Similarly, if a patient is undergoing cleft surgery, the patient's face should be positioned within the field of view consistently each time. The same video angles should be used during each session, and the patient should be asked to repeat the same phrases and make the same series of lip movements during each view.[16] Only by carefully coordinating these details will it allow the surgeon to effectively compare and evaluate surgical outcomes and ensure quality.

When recording intraoperative videos, the goal is to capture and illustrate the dynamic aspects of an operation. Thus, the video operator should know and understand the procedure being performed, as well as all the pertinent steps and relevant anatomy. Having a full understanding of these key aspects of an operation guarantees that no unnecessary video memory is wasted and, more importantly, that no time is wasted by the operating surgeon trying to communicate the critical steps of the operation at hand.[15]

If using a handheld camcorder, it is essential that the camera operator always position himself or herself directly behind the operating surgeon to capture video from the surgeon's point of view. Alternating perspectives from the operating surgeon to the assistant is disruptive to the viewers in understanding the pertinent anatomy in the operation. The videographer should take the pictures and videos from the operating surgeons' vantage point. It is also critical to maintain good ergonomics when recording video in order to minimize user fatigue and motion. For instance, the videographer's elbows should be tucked in to the body instead of in an outstretched position to avoid excessive arm movement while recording and fatigue. A poorly recorded video footage can be detrimental to the final product and often cannot be salvaged later during the editing process.[15] Additionally, the videographer should avoid zooming in and out with the camera, which can make the video appear haphazard.[15] Of note, these considerations may not be as relevant when using mounted devices, such as GoPro cameras. However, there are apps that are available for certain mounted cameras that allow an assistant to remotely control the recording process.[18,19]

CONCLUSION

Photography and videography are important aspects of plastic surgery, aiding in surgical education, medicolegal documentation, and most importantly, assessment of patient outcomes to gauge quality. In this age of quality metrics and rating systems, it is important for surgeons to document carefully and learn from past mistakes. The guidelines set forth in this chapter provide direction in the best way to standardize photography and to record videos. As always, before capturing any photographs or videos, it is important to obtain patient informed consent to use the recorded material in order to comply with Health Insurance Portability and Accountability Act (HIPAA) regulations. Patient identifiers, such as name, address, or medical record numbers, should be excluded from all forms of media.

REFERENCES

1. Henderson JL, Larrabee WF Krieger BD. Photographic standards for facial plastic surgery. *Arch Facial Plast Surg*. 2005;7(5):331-333.
2. Wang K, Kowalski EJ, Chung KC. The art and science of photography in hand surgery. *J Hand Surg Am*. 2014;39(3):580-588.
3. Hamilton GS, Carrithers JS, Karnell LH. Public perception of the terms "cosmetic," "plastic," and "reconstructive" surgery. *Arch Facial Plast Surg*. 2004;6(5):315-320.
4. Szychta P, Zielinski T, Rykala J, Kruk-Jeromin J. The internet as a source of information for patients prior to rhinoplasty. *Clin Exp Otorhinolaryngol*. 2011;4(3):131-136.
5. Sanniec KJ, Velazco CS, Macias LH, et al. Adherence to Photographic Standards: a review of ASPS and ASAPS member surgeons' websites. *J Aesthet Reconstr Surg*. 2016;2:11.
This article evaluated how closely ASPS and ASAPS members adhered to the published photographic standards set forth by the Plastic Surgery Educational Foundation (PSEF) in 2006. The authors evaluated members' websites and reported that only approximately 66% of members adhered to PSF standards.

6. Hagan KF. Clinical photography for the plastic surgery practice: the basics. *Plast Surg Nurs*. 2008;28:188-192.
7. DiBernardo BE, Adams RL, Krause J, et al. Photographic standards in plastic surgery. *Plast Reconstr Surg*. 1998;102(2):559-568.
Among the first definitive guidelines published on photographing patients using specific anatomic landmarks and standardized views for the general plastic and reconstructive practice.
8. Ettorre G, Weber M, Schaaf H, et al. Standards for digital photography in cranio-maxillo-facial surgery. Part I: basic views and guidelines. *J Craniomaxillofac Surg*. 2006;34(2):65-73.
This article proposes a European-wide set of standards for the range of photographic views for craniomaxillofacial surgery, including both intraoral and facial photographs. It also provides important assistance on selecting the proper software and equipment necessary to ensure high-quality photographic documentation.
9. Gherardini G, Matarasso A, Serure AS, et al. Standardization of photography for body contour surgery and suction-assisted lipectomy. *Plast Recontr Surg*. 1997;100(1):227-237.
10. Neff LL, Humphrey CD, Kriet JD. Setting up a medical portrait studio. *Facial Plast Surg Clin North Am*. 2010;18(2):231-236.
11. Yavuzer R, Smirnes S, Jackson IT. Guidelines for standard photography in plastic surgery. *Ann Plast Surg*. 2001;46(3):293-300.
12. Zarem HA. Standards in photography. *Plast Reconstr Surg*. 1984;74(1):137-146.
13. Archibald DJ, Carlson ML, Friedman O. Pitfalls of nonstandardized photography. *Facial Plast Surg Clin North Am*. 2010;18(2):253-266.
14. Plastic Surgery Educational Foundation. *Photographic Standards in Plastic Surgery*. American Society of Plastic Surgeons; 2006.
This guide was developed by the Plastic Surgery Educational Foundation (PSEF) to maintain consistency when taking preoperative and postoperative photographs in the clinic/studio setting. The guide standardizes camera settings, background, lighting, framing, and patient positioning and poses across various body areas of interest.
15. Rehim AR, Chung KC. Education video recording and editing for the hand surgeon. *J Hand Surg Am*. 2015;40(5):1048-1054.
This article outlines the key considerations involved in choosing the necessary software and hardware, as well as the technical aspects of recording, editing, and archiving videos in hand surgery.
16. Morrant DG, Shaw WC. Use of standardized video recordings to assess cleft surgery outcomes. *Cleft Palate Craniofac J*. 1996;33(2):124-142.
17. Sandri A, Hunt D, Rhobaye S, Juma A. Video recording of surgery to improve training in plastic surgery. *J Plast Reconstr Aesthet Surg*. 2013;66(4):e122-
18. Vara AD, Wu J, Shin AY, et al. Video recording with a GoPro in hand and upper extremity surgery. *J Hand Surg Am*. 2016;41(10):e383-e387.
19. Graves SN, Shenaq DS, Langerman AJ, Song DH. Video capture of plastic surgery procedures using the GoPro HERO 3+. *Plast Reconstr Surg Glob Open*. 2015;3(2):e312.
20. Kucuker I, Keles MK, Aydoğdu IO. An easy and applicable method for capturing high-quality rhinoplasty videos: handle banded camcorder. *Plast Reconstr Surg*. 2013;132(6):1082e-1084e.

QUESTIONS

1. **Which of the following are enhanced as a result of standardizing photography and videography in plastic surgery?**
   a. Effectively tracking, evaluating, and comparing surgical outcomes
   b. Gauging quality and learning from mistakes
   c. Aid in medicolegal documentation
   d. All of the above

2. **A 44-year-old woman presents to your clinic in consultation for a TRAM flap. When taking her preoperative and postoperative photographs, a lens of what focal length would be most appropriate?**
   a. 50 to 60 mm
   b. 60 to 70 mm
   c. 80 to 90 mm
   d. 90 to 105 mm

3. **What color background has been proven to be the most effective and visually pleasing?**
   a. Black
   b. White
   c. Sky blue
   d. Green

4. **Which of the following are examples of uniform light sources?**
   a. Ambient operating room fluorescent lights
   b. Surgical LED lights
   c. Studio flood lights
   d. All of the above

5. **You are using a handheld camcorder in the operating room to record the attending surgeon perform a trapeziectomy with ligament reconstruction. Where is the best place to stand when shooting this video?**
   a. Directly behind the first assistant at all times
   b. Directly behind the operating surgeon at all times
   c. Alternating between standing behind the operating surgeon and the first assistant depending on the operative step
   d. Wherever will give you the best image

1. **Answer: d.** Maintaining a high level of consistency when capturing photographs or recording videos will enhance all of the abovementioned. Thus, it is essential to establish standardized guidelines for photography and videography in plastic surgery.

2. **Answer: a.** Lenses with a short focal length range of 50 to 60 mm are ideal for body contouring and photographs that use a large area (e.g., breast and abdomen). Lenses with a longer focal length range of 90 to 105 mm are ideal for closer photographs (e.g., face and head).

3. **Answer: c.** Sky blue background has been studied extensively and deemed by the Clinical Photography Committee to be the most visually pleasing background color, independent of whether the photograph is taken in black and white or in color; it provides sufficient color contrast to various skin tones and diminishes the appearance of shadows. Black background tends to provide less contrast for darker-skinned patients, whereas white background tends to produce harsh shadows.

4. **Answer: d.** Ambient operating room fluorescent lights, surgical LED lights, and flood lights (if in a clinic studio) are all examples of uniform light sources. Using uniform light sources minimizes unnecessary shadows and maximizes image quality.

5. **Answer: b.** It is essential that the camera operator always position himself or herself directly behind the operating surgeon to capture video from the surgeon's point of view. Alternating perspectives from the operating surgeon to the assistant confuses the viewers and impairs proper understanding of the pertinent anatomy.

CHAPTER 15 Principles of Psychology for Aesthetic and Reconstructive Surgery

Sergey Y. Turin and Sammy Sinno

KEY POINTS

- Psychological nuances must be considered when caring for both aesthetic and reconstructive patients.
- Surgeons tend to underestimate the prevalence of psychiatric disorders in their patients, yet these comorbid conditions can place the patient at a high risk for postoperative dissatisfaction.
- Strong data show positive effects on psychologic well-being and quality of life for breast reconstruction, congenital and acquired deformity correction, as well as for addressing aesthetic concerns.
- Surgeons should always consider the psychologic facets of the patients' complaints and the treatment options offered, both to improve the patient-doctor relationship and to enhance satisfaction rates, as well as to identify the patients with psychiatric comorbidities who may be poor surgical candidates.

Both *aesthetic* and *reconstructive* procedures aim to restore congruency between the patient's own body image and the corporeal self. Accomplishing this hinges equally on the surgeon's operative results as well as on patients successfully adapting their body image to this result. The importance of the psychological aspect should not be underestimated, as psychologic complications may be more frequent than surgical or medical complications and can have a detrimental impact on the overall outcome, including time to return to work, quality of life, and satisfaction with the surgical result.[1]

Concepts particular to aesthetic or reconstructive surgery will be discussed separately only for the sake of clarity in organization, because the psychological framework underpinning patient attitudes and motivations is very much the same. Although the etiology of the presenting complaints may be different, the magnitude of its impact on the patient and the amount of expected improvement are similar: aesthetic patients report similar levels of dissatisfaction with their overall appearance and concern for the feature in question as reconstructive patients.[2]

A comprehensive understanding of the psychologic aspects of the patient's complaint is key to ensuring a shared mindset when discussing surgery and will build a stronger patient-surgeon relationship as well as improve the likelihood of patient satisfaction with the end result. This process is rooted in identifying three variables: (1) the presenting complaint (e.g., dorsal hump, unfavorable scar, or mastectomy defect); (2) the patient's attitude toward this feature (i.e., his or her level of concern and impact on quality of life, as well as source of concern—pressure from significant other, professional expectations, or self-motivated); and (3) amount of motivation for surgery. These variables can then be evaluated in the context of the surgeon's objective assessment of the defect and his or her skill set to determine the likelihood of delivering a satisfying result.

PRINCIPLES OF PSYCHOLOGY IN PLASTIC SURGERY

Psychology in plastic surgery often focuses on the congruence of the patient's body image and the objective appearance, as the idea of body image is pivotal to the concept of the patient's relationship with his or her body. Body image, simplistically, may be thought of as the individual's subjective experience of his or her body, and it includes all facets of that experience: functional (e.g., dysphagia, loss of limb function, or ability to perform a task), sensory (e.g., pain, paresthesia, anesthesia), and outward appearance (e.g., deformity, scarring). It is important to always recognize that body image is subjective, and therefore must be understood in a social context.[3,4] These concepts can explain the seeming disconnect between an objectively *minor* deformity and the great level of distress it causes to the patient, or the drive toward the currently en vogue appearance or *look*. If a patient's body image and appearance are aligned, then changes in his or her appearance due to injury, age, or disease may cause distress if the body image does not change accordingly. Similarly, a patient can suffer the same distress if his or her body image and physical appearance are never aligned, as in the scenario of a congenital malformation or body feature that is never incorporated into the body image.

Another key concept applicable specifically to any intervention is patient expectations. It is incumbent on the surgeon to verify what the patient expects as a result of the surgery, and that the surgeon is able and willing to deliver that result. Again, the body image the patient is seeking may be subjective, so an excellent result in the surgeon's eyes may be a failure for the patient if he or she was not pursuing the same goal. With this in mind, the term defect, as used in this text, will be used to denote the deficiency perceived by the patient, whether it may be a disfiguring feature or a lack of the desired aesthetic feature, as they are, in principle, psychologically the same.

It has been said that satisfaction is result divided by expectation, and when the expectations are well defined, this relationship holds.[5] Clarity and openness in communication is key, and this dovetails with the concepts of informed consent—a well-defined goal and an honest discussion of the risks are not only the basic foundation of informed consent, but also set up a healthy relationship in case of complications.

The last general principle is that a surgeon can deliver a surgical result but cannot always deliver the emotional effects the patient desires—his or her well-being, self-perception, and satisfaction will all be derived from the relationship between the result and the patient's goals. The more direct and strong that relationship, the more likely the patient is to be satisfied. To illustrate the concept, consider a patient with a single painful neuroma who only desires relief from the pain, and delivering this result will almost certainly guarantee satisfaction. This is in contradistinction to a patient desiring any surgery the surgeon considers appropriate to *improve the looks* in the hope of attaining a promotion at work. The surgeon does not have a clearly defined result to deliver, and the patient is seeking a vague improvement for a secondary gain, setting both parties up for disappointment.

THE PSYCHOLOGY OF AESTHETIC SURGERY

Multiple studies provide evidence that aesthetic procedures have high satisfaction rates and improve patients' quality of life and sexual well-being, and help them look younger, more attractive, healthy, and successful.[6-8] However, these positive outcomes can depend as much on the patient as upon the surgical result. As an extreme example, a patient with body dysmorphic disorder (BDD) is unlikely to be satisfied regardless of how excellent the surgical result may be.[9-11]

Patient Perspective

Goals and Expectations

The patient's goals and expectations must be clearly delineated as they may not be one and the same. For example, a patient presenting for breast augmentation may be expecting an increase in her breast size with no complications and an acceptable scar, yet the goal may be to salvage a troubled relationship. In this scenario, meeting the expectations for the surgical result has no guarantee of the patient achieving her goals. Unless this is clarified and understood, she may still risk dissatisfaction with her surgery despite a good surgical result.

Clarity and shared understanding should be the guiding principles when discussing the defect and the intended surgical result. Although surgeons and patients usually agree in their general assessment of the body part in question, perception of the details and their relative importance may be different.[12] Surgeons' assessment tends to be comprehensive in the sense of understanding the defect, the available interventions, their risks, and likely outcomes. On the other hand, the patient will almost always be limited in his or her understanding of surgical concepts relevant to the etiology of the defect and its treatment, such as focusing on the *protuberant* mandible without appreciating a concave midface. It has been shown that patients are reliably able to understand the basics of a procedure, but an in-depth understanding is usually lacking.[13] It falls to the surgeon to bring both parties to consensus on all of these points.

Instruments have been proposed to introduce a systematic method to assessing patient suitability for surgery (both subjective and objective),[14] yet none have gained wide acceptance at this time. An empathetic, individualized approach still remains the cornerstone of patient counseling, and there is yet no substitute for time spent in consultation.

Confounding Factors

Probably more so than any other area of health care, aesthetic surgery is governed by the laws of demand and supply, with sensitivity to price and behavior akin to a luxury good.[15] Although many aesthetic practices are forced to compete on the basis of cost, the surgeon is well advised to prioritize excellent patient care instead of discounts to expand the practice.[16] Moreover, pricing can be a confounding factor in patient decision-making, and extra care must be taken that the patient is well informed and has appropriate and organic motivations for surgery as opposed to being financially motivated to take advantage of a special offer.

Psychiatric or Personality Disorders

Multiple studies have shown a relatively high prevalence of psychiatric diagnoses in the plastic surgery population, reaching as high as 48% to 70%,[17,18] with up to 50% of patients receiving psychotropic medication. This has prompted the question of whether standardized psychological screening tests should be incorporated into the routine plastic surgery patient evaluation,[19] but no consensus exists on the topic at this time. Disorders such as BDD or bipolar personality disorder (BPD) have an extreme impact on patients' postoperative recovery and mental acceptance of the result. In these patients, the psychiatric process may have a greater bearing on the patient's satisfaction than the actual surgical outcome and may put the surgeon at risk for an unhappy, adversarial patient regardless of the result. We will discuss BDD and BPD as these are the more common diagnoses the surgeon will encounter that also carry the highest risk.

Body Dysmorphic Disorder

Epidemiology

The prevalence of BDD in adults in the general population is estimated at 1.9% but is reported to be as high as 6% to 33% in patients presenting for cosmetic surgery, with some of the higher numbers seen in rhinoplasty patients.[11,20-22] Plastic surgeons are aware of this disorder but tend to underestimate its prevalence in their own practice[23]: in one multicenter study, 9.7% of all patients screened positive for BDD using a validated screening tool, but only 4.0% raised the surgeon's suspicion.[24]

Presentation

Per the DSM-5, BDD is defined as an obsessive-compulsive or related disorder, with the diagnostic criteria detailed in **Table 15.1**.[25]

The most common complaints are perceived defects of the skin, hair, eyes, nose, and teeth, explaining why these patients seek treatment by dermatologists, cosmetic dentists, orthodontists, and plastic surgeons.[26]

Impact

BDD patients experience dissonance between their body image and their appearance primarily because their body image is distorted, even as their appearance may not change. The nature of this disorder makes it impossible to deliver a surgical result that will satisfy the patient, exactly because the patient's complaint is a psychiatric one disguised as a physical feature. Failure to recognize BDD and treat the patient correctly incurs not only a very high risk of an unhappy patient, but also legal liability even if the objective result is satisfactory, as the BDD patient dissatisfied with surgery falls into the category of *victim*[11] because of his or her underlying psychiatric condition.

Management

There is no consensus on the optimal method of screening for BDD in the plastic surgery practice. Routine screening with existing psychiatric surveys[27] may be the ideal approach, but the limitations of a busy practice have led to poor adoption of routine screening outside of cases raising suspicion for BDD. Surgery for the presenting complaint is ill-advised, if not contraindicated,[9-11] as multiple series have shown that cosmetic surgery in patients with BDD provides no benefits and may even cause an exacerbation of the condition, resulting in a patient who is beyond unhappy, sometimes resorting to litigation,[10] attacks on the surgeon's reputation and practice, or even violence.[28] However, there may be patients who can be successfully treated with a multidisciplinary approach combining psychiatric and surgical care,[29] thus suggesting that BDD may not always be a hard contraindication to surgery.

TABLE 15.1. DIAGNOSTIC PRINCIPLES FOR BODY DYSMORPHIC DISORDER[25]
There are four main elements to making a diagnosis of body dysmorphic disorder:
■ The patient is preoccupied with one or multiple more subjective flaws in his or her appearance that would be objectively considered minimal or within the range of normal by others.
■ This preoccupation hinders patient functioning in some way (social, professional, etc.).
■ This preoccupation is or has been associated with repetitive behaviors, such as frequent mirror checking, manipulation of the body feature in question, etc.
■ There is no other better-suited diagnosis that would explain the patient's symptoms. For example, concerns regarding body habitus in a patient who is suffering from an eating disorder would be best attributed to the eating disorder rather than BDD.
Patients may exhibit excellent to poor insight into their condition and the correlation of their beliefs with the objective truth. While pertinent to future psychotherapy, neither situation changes the mainstays of diagnosis as described above.

SUMMARY

The prevalence of BDD in an aesthetic practice is likely higher than clinically suspected, and these patients require very different care. Although presenting with a physical complaint, the true pathology is psychiatric and must be treated as such. Surgical intervention is associated with a prohibitively high rate of dissatisfaction, so identifying these patients early is crucial to ensure they receive appropriate care.

Bipolar Personality Disorder

EPIDEMIOLOGY

BPD is a common mental disorder characterized by impulsive behavior and instability of emotions, interpersonal relationships, and self-image, with a prevalence of up to 9% in plastic surgery population.[18,30]

DIAGNOSIS

One of the notable features of BPD as opposed to BDD is the concern with multiple features. It has been suggested that such patients may be more precisely diagnosed with BPD and comorbid BDD, as opposed to the opposite. Splitting is also a core feature of BPD. Signs and features of BPD that should raise suspicion in a plastic surgery patient include[30]:

- Female gender (dominant)
- Age early 20 to 30s
- History of other psychiatric disorders (especially depressions and other personality disorders)
- History of adverse events during childhood
- History of multiple aesthetic procedures with *doctor shopping*
- Self-harm behavior (e.g., cutting, burning) or suicidal ideation
- Tattoos and multiple body-piercings
- Psychosocial impairment (but some individuals show good psychosocial adjustment)
- Dissatisfaction or anger toward the previous surgeon
- Splitting phenomenon toward the surgeon or clinic staff
- Concern with one or more body parts, which is less profound and shifts from one to another over time

MANAGEMENT

Operating on a patient with BPD predictably runs a high risk of extremely poor patient satisfaction,[11,18] with some patients directing anger or disappointment at family, friends, clinic staff, or the surgeon, going so far as litigation or even violence such as self-mutilation.[30,31] The surgeon is advised to be empathetic and understanding in the counseling process, enabling the patient to be aware that surgery without an appropriate indication will not only fail to solve the problem, but may exacerbate it.

SUMMARY

BPD patients tend to focus on multiple issues, request multiple revisions due to fear of abandonment, are quick to split, and have disproportionally worse postoperative satisfaction. As in BDD, the principal complaint is most likely actually psychiatric, rather than physical, and recognizing this prior to any surgery will help the surgeon avoid the poor postoperative outcomes so prevalent in these patients.

Many screening tools are available for personality disorders, but there is not one that has shown itself to be the optimal solution.[32] At this time, surgeons are still best advised to use their own judgment and refer to the many available questionnaires when suspicion for psychopathology is raised. The surgeon should be exceedingly weary of any surgical intervention in these patients as the risks of dissatisfaction and adverse outcomes are very high.

External Influences

When considering the patient's motivation for surgery, it is important to recognize the presence and magnitude of extrinsic influences. The stereotypical example is a patient presenting for a procedure to satisfy his or her significant other's preferences, as opposed to desiring alteration of a body feature to conform to the patient's own body image. The pervasive role of mass and social media in our everyday lives has expanded the influence of social trends and beauty standards, and patient attitudes reflect this.[33] The majority of patients will thus request their actual appearance align both with their self-image and with the prevailing social concepts of beauty and attractiveness.

Intuitively, meeting the expectations of the patient is easier to accomplish than additionally meeting those of the significant other or some other social group. It is, of course, imperative to avoid any intervention in a patient that may be coerced into seeking it against his or her will, but the surgeon must otherwise be the judge in determining what is or is not an appropriate mix of intrinsic or extrinsic motivation. Some warning signs of external influences inappropriately affecting patient judgment include:

- A controlling or overbearing spouse or significant other that drives the consultation—in this scenario, if able, interview the patient alone (or with a chaperone if there is any suspicion of abuse or harmful manipulation) to clarify his or her own attitudes and goals to more appropriately evaluate the suitability for surgery
- A secondary goal as the main driving factor, such as expecting the surgery to salvage or change a personal relationship, results in workplace advancement or some other aspirations that are ultimately not under the patient's control. The risk here lies in the possibility of failing to achieve this secondary goal despite a good surgical outcome, ultimately leading to patient dissatisfaction. The stereotypical example is a patient requesting a facelift or breast augmentation with the goal of salvaging a relationship—the real goal is not a rejuvenated face and neck or enhanced breast contour and size, but changing the behavior of another person—something that no surgeon can promise
- A desire to comply with a social trend against their own preferences, again an example of attempting to fulfill the desires or expectations of someone other than the patients themselves

The surgeon must always exercise his or her judgment in evaluating each patient individually—as social beings, the majority of the decisions we make are guided by the desire to please others as much as ourselves, but the patients too strongly influenced by external factors must be evaluated thoroughly to minimize the chance of disappointment on their part.

Physician Perspective

Adverse Outcomes

Complications, however rare, can happen even in the best of hands and can weigh heavily on the surgeon. The emotional toll of an adverse outcome can be high in aesthetic cases, which by definition is elective and makes a well person temporarily unwell in the hope of an eventual improvement.[34]

The nonoperative management of poor outcomes hinges on the principles described earlier, customized to each patient and founded on empathetic care. Frequent postoperative visits, time spent face-to-face, and honest efforts to rectify the situation can salvage patient expectations and even result in overall positive reviews despite experiencing a surgical complication. The patient with a personality disorder or unrealistic expectations that were not clear preoperatively is treated in the same fashion, focusing on treating the underlying psychiatric issue. These cases may be distressing and disruptive to the practice, yet no clear algorithm or protocol exists for addressing such concerns, except that involving a mental health professional sooner rather than later and thorough documentation. Empathetic care postoperatively can sometimes allow the patient to still walk away with an overall positive appreciation of his or her care.[35]

Litigious and Adversarial Patients

The burden of litigation, when encountered, weighs heavily on the physician and its costs are not insignificant, even though the majority of cases are still won by the physician.[36] Documentation of good surgical practices and informed consent are of prime importance in dealing with a litigious patient, as these activities are integral to the defense. Moreover, after claims for poor outcomes due to lack of expertise, lack of informed consent is a frequent cause for legal action, again underscoring its importance.[37] Because the decay of the patient-physician relationship cannot always be foreseen ahead of time, it is important to practice these good habits proactively.

Given the evidence for surgeons underestimating the prevalence of psychiatric disease in their patients, there should be a low threshold to involve mental health professionals. Unfortunately, that may often come too late, as patients with factitious disorders are liable to continually switch surgeons when psychiatric evaluation is suggested, only undergoing the formal psychiatric evaluation when forced to do so for a trial.

THE PSYCHOLOGY OF RECONSTRUCTIVE SURGERY

Patient Perspective

Goals and Expectations

The breadth of reconstructive surgery presents many unique psychological scenarios. Patients who acquire a deformity tend to seek a return to their baseline state to restore harmony with their established body image. Patients with congenital deformities would align psychologically with many aesthetic patients, in that their body image and appearance were not congruent at baseline. In either scenario, the goal for these patients is restoration of their normal/baseline selves to fit in their social environment, and surgery may be the best option as psychotherapy is often ineffective.[38] As in aesthetics, the patient's psychological state has a great impact on recovery and attitude toward the results of the surgery, as shown by the strong correlation between preoperative life satisfaction and coping ability and postoperative recovery course.[39]

Oncologic Reconstruction

As in aesthetic surgery, it is key to understand that the psychologic burden may not correlate to the degree or type of deformity: some scar revision patients report levels of dissatisfaction with their body appearance and preoccupation that could be consistent with BDD.[2,4,40]

Breast Reconstruction

Mastectomy is known to inflict a psychological burden upon the patient, altering the patient's perception of her feminity, cascading into mood and interpersonal relationship sequelae.[41] Fortunately, breast reconstruction can ameliorate and reverse some of the negative impact of mastectomy. Specifically, immediate breast reconstruction appears to impose a lower overall psychological burden on the patient than delayed reconstruction, potentially sparing the patient from some of the psychological burden of mastectomy.[42] Contrary to some previous notions, it appears the patients do not *appreciate* the reconstruction more or feel like there is relatively more improvement after having to live with their deformity in cases of delayed reconstruction.[43] Multiple studies have shown a benefit to quality of life and subjective well-being after breast reconstruction, such that the issue in question is now access to reconstruction, as opposed to any argument over its value in restoring not only the physical body feature but the patient's self-image and social function. Moreover, even when postoperative complications are encountered, reconstruction is still beneficial as patients tend to recover predictably from the psychological burden of the complications experienced.

Amputation and Neuroma Pain

Aside from the well-known functional impact of amputation, many patients develop chronic pain due to neuromas at the amputation stump, leading to significant secondary morbidity due to this constant painful stimulus. Chronic pain affects the patient on many levels and can result in fatigues, sleep disturbance, alteration of social function, and mood disorders due to the constant stressor effect it creates in the patient. Intervention can be efficacious in treating these secondary effects, as successful surgical treatment of neuroma pain has been shown to have a positive impact on self-reported depression and quality of life.[44]

Congenital Anomalies and Orthognathic Surgery

The wide variety of congenital anomalies corresponds to an equally wide variety of patient attitudes toward them. When discussing surgical intervention, the patient who is more satisfied with the appearance preoperatively is likely also be satisfied with the appearance postoperatively, demonstrating the ability to adapt the self-image to the appearance in a healthy fashion. In general, evidence shows improved adaptation to social functioning after reconstruction or correction of congenital deformities, as illustrated by patients with microtia reporting improvement in body image and life satisfaction after ear reconstruction,[45] similar to cleft lip/palate patients after undergoing delayed repair.[46] Many patients adapt their self-image and show good coping with the deformity. For example, patients with cleft lip/palate report a high prevalence of teasing focused on the cleft stigmata, but the majority grow up to be well-adjusted and well-functioning adults[47] despite some persistence of social and psychologic stigmata of the cleft.[48] Other craniofacial deformities demonstrate the same pattern.[49]

Physician Perspective

As reconstructive techniques continue to advance, surgeons are able to salvage and reconstruct increasingly more complex defects. Taking care of patients with challenging problems often results in a close relationship between the surgeon and patient, as both become invested in each step of the process and the eventual outcome. Surgeons know firsthand the importance of clear thinking and mental fortitude in the face of complications and difficulties in the operating suite. The patient's state of mind and attitudes can be just as important, but inadequate psychologic preparation may only become apparent postoperatively when the patient is unable to comply with the rigorous demands of rehabilitation. Anticipating stressful scenarios and situations that may cause psychologic strain on the patient and addressing these issues ahead of time will pay dividends in these scenarios. In both aesthetic and reconstructive scenarios, patient expectations and self-image are a key factor in their satisfaction and success of the surgical process. The surgeon should have a low threshold to offer psychological help and counseling to patients undergoing prolonged or complex reconstruction to maximize the chances of the patients being in the optimal state of mind before and after the surgery.

CONCLUSION

Psychology is a key component of plastic and reconstructive surgery because it can determine the patient's acceptance and satisfaction with the operative result independently of the objective outcome. Failure to account for this variable may result in an unhappy patient despite a well-planned and executed surgical plan. This concept applies both to healthy patients presenting for aesthetic surgery and patients with congenital or acquired defects presenting for reconstructive surgery, as the driving motivation is the same in both groups: correction of some defect (whether subjective or objective) to restore congruity between the patient's body image and the corporeal self.

The plastic surgeon should be aware of warning signs for patients with personality disorders, unrealistic expectations, or poor coping skills that would place them at risk for a poor psychological outcome. These psychological factors present in the minority of patients but can have disproportionately large effects and thus are important to bear in mind during patient evaluations.

REFERENCES

1. Borah G, Rankin M, Wey P, Borah G. Psychological complications in 281 plastic surgery practices. *Plast Reconstr Surg.* 1999;104(5):1241.
2. Sarwer DB, Whitaker LA, Pertschuk MJ, et al. Body image concerns of reconstructive surgery patients: an underrecognized problem. *Ann Plast Surg.* 1998;40(4):403.
   This is one of the high-quality articles dealing with self-image in the reconstructive population, showing the parallels to the aesthetic patient.
3. Pruzinsky T. Who chooses to undergo reconstructive surgery? Empirically confirming the subjectivity and social basis of body image. *J Burn Care Rehabil.* 1997;18(4):372.
4. Heinberg LJ, Fauerbach JA, Spence RJ, Hackerman F. Psychologic factors involved in the decision to undergo reconstructive surgery after burn injury. *J Burn Care Rehabil.* 1997;18(4):374.
   This is an important study showing that psychosocial factors were far better correlated with burn victims undergoing reconstructive surgery, as compared with the severity of their deformity
5. Morselli P, Micai A, Boriani F. Eumorphic plastic surgery: expectation versus satisfaction in body dysmorphic disorder. *Aesthet Plast Surg.* 2016;40(4):592.
6. Stofman GM, Neavin TS, Ramineni PM, Alford A. Better sex from the knife? an intimate look at the effects of cosmetic surgery on sexual practices. *Aesthet Surg J.* 2006;26(1):12.
7. Shridharani SM, Magarakis M, Manson PN, Rodriguez ED. Psychology of plastic and reconstructive surgery: a systematic clinical review. *Plast Reconstr Surg.* 2010;126(6):2243.
8. Bater KL, Ishii LE, Papel ID, et al. Association between facial rejuvenation and observer ratings of youth, attractiveness, success, and health. *JAMA Facial Plast Surg.* 2017;19(5):360 367.
9. Crerand CE, Franklin ME, Sarwer DB. Body dysmorphic disorder and cosmetic surgery. *Plast Reconstr Surg.* 2006;118(7):167e.
10. Sarwer DB, Crerand CE, Didie ER. Body dysmorphic disorder in cosmetic surgery patients. *Facial Plast Surg.* 2003;19(1):7.
11. Honigman RJ, Phillips KA, Castle DJ. A review of psychosocial outcomes for patients seeking cosmetic surgery. *Plast Reconstr Surg.* 2004;113(4):1229.
12. Shipchandler TZ, Sultan B, Ishii L, et al. Aesthetic analysis in rhinoplasty: surgeon vs. patient perspectives: a prospective, blinded study. *Am J Otolaryngol Head Neck Surg.* 2013;34(2):93.
13. Hoppe IC, Ahuja NK, Ingargiola MJ, Granick MS. A survey of patient comprehension of readily accessible online educational material regarding plastic surgery procedures. *Aesthet Surg J.* 2013;33(3):436.
14. Rees L, Myers S, Bradbury E. A comprehensive screening, education, and training tool for the psychological assessment of patients seeking aesthetic surgery: "desirable op?" *Aesthet Plast Surg.* 2012;36(2):443.
15. Alsarraf R, Alsarraf NW, Larrabee WF, Johnson CM. Cosmetic surgery procedures as luxury goods: measuring price and demand in facial plastic surgery. *Arch Facial Plast Surg.* 2002;4(2):105.
16. Rohrich RJ. The market of plastic surgery: cosmetic surgery for sale: at what price? *Plast Reconstr Surg.* 2001;107(7):1845.
17. Ishigooka J, Iwao M, Suzuki M, et al. Demographic features of patients seeking cosmetic surgery. *Psychiatry Clin Neurosci.* 1998;52(3):283.
18. Napoleon A. The presentation of personalities in plastic surgery. *Ann Plast Surg.* 1993;31(3):193.
19. Meningaud JP, Benadiba L, Servant JM, et al. Depression, anxiety and quality of life among scheduled cosmetic surgery patients: multicentre prospective study. *J Craniomaxillofac Surg.* 2001;29(3):177.
20. Picavet VA, Prokopakis E, Gabriels L, et al. High prevalence of body dysmorphic disorder symptoms in patients seeking rhinoplasty. *Plast Reconstr Surg.* 2011;128(2):509.
21. Veale D, Gledhill LJ, Christodoulou P, Hodsoll J. Body dysmorphic disorder in different settings: a systematic review and estimated weighted prevalence. *Body Image.* 2016;18:168.
22. Sarwer DB, Wadden TA, Pertschuk MJ, Whitaker LA. Body image dissatisfaction and body dysmorphic disorder in 100 cosmetic surgery patients. *Plast Reconstr Surg.* 1998;101(6):1644.
23. Sarwer DB. Awareness and identification of body dysmorphic disorder by aesthetic surgeons: results of a Survey of American Society for Aesthetic Plastic Surgery Members. *Aesthet Surg J.* 2002;22(6):531.
24. Joseph AW, Ishii L, Joseph SS, et al. Prevalence of body dysmorphic disorder and surgeon diagnostic accuracy in facial plastic and oculoplastic surgery clinics. *JAMA Facial Plast Surg.* 2017;19(4):269-274.
25. American Psychiatric Association. *Obsessive-compulsive and related disorders.* In: *Diagnostic and Statistical Manual of Mental Disorders.* 5th ed. American Psychiatric Association; 2012.
26. Phillips K. *The Broken Mirror: Understanding and Treating Body Dysmorphic Disorder.* New York, NY: Oxford University Press; 1996.
   This is a landmark publication from Dr. Phillips on BDD, comprehensively describing its diagnosis and treatment.
27. Claiborn C, Perdick C. *The BDD Workbook.* New Harbinger Publications; 2002.
   While perhaps not easily available, this is a good example of a BDD screening tool.
28. Sweis I, Spitz J, Barry D, Cohen M. A review of body dysmorphic disorder in aesthetic surgery patients and the legal implications. *Aesthet Plast Surg.* 2017;41(4):949.
   Dr. Sweis et al. provide a very concise and updated review of the evidence available regarding BDD in the aesthetic surgery population.
29. Edgerton MT, Langman MW, Pruzinsky T. Plastic surgery and psychotherapy in the treatment of 100 psychologically disturbed patients. *Plast Reconstr Surg.* 1991;88(4):594.
30. Morioka D, Ohkubo F. Borderline personality disorder and aesthetic plastic surgery. *Aesthet Plast Surg.* 2014;38(6):1169.
   This is an outstanding reference comprehensively covering all aspects of BPD in the aesthetic patient population.
31. Davis RE, Davis RE, Bublik M. Psychological considerations in the revision rhinoplasty patient. *Facial Plast Surg.* 2012;28(4):374.
32. Wildgoose P, Scott A, Pusic AL, et al. Psychological screening measures for cosmetic plastic surgery patients: a systematic review. *Aesthet Surg J.* 2013;33(1):152.
33. Crockett RJ, Pruzinsky T, Persing JA. The influence of plastic surgery "reality TV" on cosmetic surgery patient expectations and decision making. *Plast Reconstr Surg.* 2007;120(1):316.
34. Gorney M. Recognition and management of the patient unsuitable for aesthetic surgery. *Plast Reconstr Surg.* 2010;126(6):2268.
35. Dorfman RG, Purnell C, Qiu C, et al. Happy and unhappy patients: a quantitative analysis of online plastic surgeon reviews for breast augmentation. *Plast Reconstr Surg.* 2018;141(5):663e-673e
36. Svider PF, Blake DM, Husain Q, et al. In the eyes of the law: malpractice litigation in oculoplastic surgery. *Ophthal Plast Reconstr Surg.* 2014;30(2):119.
37. Kandinov A, Mutchnick S, Nangia V, et al. Analysis of factors associated with rhytidectomy malpractice litigation cases. *JAMA Facial Plast Surg.* 2017;19(4):255.
38. Bessell A, Moss TP. Evaluating the effectiveness of psychosocial interventions for individuals with visible differences: a systematic review of the empirical literature. *Body Image.* 2007;4(3):227-238.
39. Kopp M, Bonatti H, Haller C, et al. Life satisfaction and active coping style are important predictors of recovery from surgery. *J Psychosom Res.* 2003;55(4):371.
40. Fingeret MC, Nipomnick S, Guindani M, et al. Body image screening for cancer patients undergoing reconstructive surgery. *Psychol Oncol.* 2014;23(8):898.
41. Mendelson BC. The psychological basis for breast reconstruction following mastectomy. *Med J Aust.* 1980;1(11):517.
42. Zhong T, Hu J, Bagher S, et al. A comparison of psychological response, body image, sexuality, and quality of life between immediate and delayed autologous tissue breast reconstruction: a prospective long-term outcome study. *Plast Reconstr Surg.* 2016;138(4):772-780.
43. Wellisch DK, Schain WS, Noone RB, Little JW. Psychosocial correlates of immediate versus delayed reconstruction of the breast. *Plast Reconstr Surg.* 1985;76(5):713.
44. Domeshek LF, Krauss EM, Snyder-Warwick AK, et al. Surgical treatment of neuromas improves patient-reported pain, depression, and quality of life. *Plast Reconstr Surg.* 2017;139(2):407.
45. Awan B, Samargandi O, Aldaqal S, Sehlo M. Life satisfaction and quality of life in adolescents with grade III microtia: the effect of improved body image disturbance after ear reconstructive surgery. *Eur Psychiatry.* 2014;29:1.
46. Kapp-Simon KA. Psychological issues in cleft lip and palate. *Clin Plast Surg.* 2004;31(2):347.
47. Crocker EC, Clifford E, Pope BA. *The Cleft Palate Child Grows Up an Analysis of the Adulthood of Former Patients.* Portland, Oregon: American Cleft Palate Association; 1970.
48. Tobiasen JM, Hiebert JM. Clefting and psychosocial adjustment: influence of facial aesthetics. *Clin Plast Surg.* 1993;20(4):623-631.
49. Endriga MC, Kapp-Simon KA. Psychological issues in craniofacial care: state of the art. *Cleft Palate Craniofac J.* 1999;36(1):3.

QUESTIONS

1. A 24-year-old woman comes to the office requesting rhinoplasty. She is bothered by the appearance and asymmetry in her nose. She spends several hours each day looking in the mirror at her *huge hump and wide tip*. On examination, she has excellent symmetry, a 1 mm hump, well-defined dorsal aesthetic lines, and tip defining points. What is the most appropriate next step?

   a. Scheduling the patient for septoplasty
   b. Scheduling the patient for rhinoplasty
   c. Psychiatric referral
   d. Injectable fillers to camouflage the dorsal hump

2. A 45-year-old man is presenting to your office requesting correction for gynecomastia. He has had a negative medical workup for it and reports that the appearance of his chest has bothered him since childhood. When discussing his social history, he reveals that he and his spouse have been *going through a rough patch* and a few months ago decided to separate for a year. He eats a healthy diet and exercises four times a week but has stayed the same weight for more than a decade. On examination, he is a slightly overweight male with bilateral breast enlargement that is mostly adipose with little glandular tissue. What is the appropriate next step?

   a. Schedule the patient for gynecomastia correction with liposuction.
   b. Ask the patient to return at the end of the separation period with the spouse.
   c. Refer the patient to a psychiatrist for more thorough evaluation.
   d. Ask the patient to lose more weight prior to surgery.

3. A 21-year-old woman presents to the office for breast augmentation. She is accompanied by her boyfriend, who states that he will be paying for the procedure, and they are interested in a promotion for saline implants that your practice has advertised recently. She reports that her breast size has been stable "around a B cup" for 3 or 4 years and that she "wouldn't mind if they were bigger, maybe even as much as a DD cup that he [the boyfriend] wants." On examination, she has fairly symmetric breasts with no ptosis, masses, or other anomalies. What is the next step?

   a. Counsel the patient on saline versus silicone implants and then discuss sizing.
   b. Ask the patient to obtain a psychiatric evaluation prior to further discussion.
   c. Tell the patient that she must be the one to pay for surgery.
   d. Ask to examine her with a chaperone, without the boyfriend present, to clarify her own motivation and expectations for surgery.

4. A 35-year-old woman presents to your office for a scar revision consultation. She suffered a deep laceration to the left thigh in a motor vehicle collision during her childhood and has been unhappy with the scar ever since. She finds herself unable to go out in public for fear of people ostracizing her because of the scar and worries about it constantly. She has tried all available scar creams and therapies and has had four revisions in the past. She reports that her previous surgeons had treated her poorly and discriminated against her because of her multiple tattoos and piercings, which is why they took out the sutures too early, causing scar widening. On examination, the left lateral thigh has a 10 cm linear scar, which is widened to about 5 mm and is slightly raised. There are also multiple narrow linear scars on her thighs and forearms that are tattooed over. What is the next step?

   a. Tell the patient that after four revisions, the likelihood of improvement is minimal and that you would advise against surgery.
   b. Confront the patient about her doctor shopping.
   c. Suggest to the patient that surgical intervention is unlikely to make her feel better about her appearance, and suggest counseling with a possible surgical reevaluation afterward.
   d. Schedule the patient for scar revision.

5. A 35-year-old right hand–dominant male steelworker presents with pain in the left forearm after a traumatic amputation 2 years ago at work. He reports pain at the distal end of the stump with pressure and touch. He has not been fitted for a prosthetic of any kind and has not been participating in any rehabilitation as he has compensated with his right hand. His spouse, who accompanies him, reports that he lost motivation after the accident and has been in a poor mood, withdrawing from social activities and spending all his time at home. On examination, he has a mid-forearm amputation with two points distally that elicit severe pain with percussion, but it otherwise appears well healed. The spouse asks you what they can expect if surgery to treat the neuromas is successful?

   a. He will be able to be fitted for a prosthesis and improve his function.
   b. His pain will improve, reducing the amount of pain medications necessary, but counseling and rehabilitation will likely be needed to restore his functional capacity.
   c. He will be able to take advantage of rehabilitation services to retrain for a new position at work.
   d. Even though the pain will be addressed, the psychologic morbidity of the amputation will likely persist as a permanent disability.

1. **Answer: c.** Although this may not provide enough data to make a definitive diagnosis of BDD, two warning signs are listed: preoccupation with what is described as a minor deformity and repetitive behavior (mirror checking). Surgical intervention is not indicated until a more thorough psychiatric evaluation of the patient is carried out either by the surgeon or by a mental health provider.

2. **Answer: a.** This patient reports a long-standing concern with his chest, with a negative hormonal workup and a stable weight. He does not exhibit any signs of disproportionate concern with the deformity. He does not indicate that he is trying to change his appearance for a secondary gain. Given that he is otherwise a good surgical candidate, surgery would be an appropriate next step.

3. **Answer: d.** Although many patients will be seeking their significant others' advice or support when considering surgery, it is important to recognize when these external influences become overbearing or inappropriate. In this scenario, the boyfriend appears to be the primary motivator for the patient seeking surgery. The surgeon should investigate the patient's own attitudes and desires to ensure that she will be happy with the result as well.

4. **Answer: c.** Multiple clues should raise the suspicion of bipolar disorder in this patient—splitting behavior, doctor shopping, signs of self-harm, etc. Leaving aside the idea of whether a fifth scar revision can be indicated, the patient's psychologic status makes her a poor candidate for a surgical intervention. Although mostly anecdotal, existing literature supports avoiding a direct

confrontation, which will usually lead to an angry patient who will then move on to the next practice. Although it may get the patient out of the office in the short term, it does not help address the real issue at hand. A sensitive approach and steering the patient toward mental health care instead of an outright refusal to treat is the more compassionate and diplomatic way of dealing with this patient.

5. **Answer: b.** Treatment of neuromas can address the painful sensory symptoms, both from the neuromas being directly stimulated and due to phantom pains. There can be secondary positive change after relief of these pains such as improvement in function with or without prosthesis fitting, improvement in quality of life due to reduction in pain medications, and maybe return to work. However, these do not directly result from a successful surgery—accomplishment of these goals will depend on the patient and so cannot be guaranteed (although relief of chronic pain does improve the chances of the patient improving in other areas). Similar to an aesthetic surgery not guaranteeing a promotion at work, the relief of pain does not guarantee an improvement in other areas of life.

CHAPTER 16 Patient Safety in Plastic Surgery

Omar E. Beidas and Jeffrey A. Gusenoff

KEY POINTS

- Patient selection is important in reducing perioperative risk and postoperative complications
- DVT prophylaxis should be considered based on Caprini score
- Careful attention should be paid to patient positioning on all cases
- Patients should be kept warm before, during, and after surgery
- Early ambulation, adequate hydration, and reduced narcotic use can ease postoperative recovery
- Patient education of warning signs can aid in avoiding severe complications

Patient safety is perhaps the most important aspect of surgery and begins from the moment the patient-physician relationship is established. It is the duty of every member of the health care team but ultimately the responsibility of the surgeon. Attention to detail must be maintained throughout the preoperative, perioperative, and postoperative periods. This chapter provides the most recent guidelines at the time of writing. The reader is encouraged to use the online resources referenced herein to adhere to the most up-to-date recommendations.

PREOPERATIVE CARE

Patient Selection and Evaluation

Patient Expectations

With any surgical procedure, it is of utmost importance to manage patient desires and expectations. A patient's expectations of the outcome should be aligned with results that the surgeon can reasonably deliver. If a patient has unrealistic or idealistic expectations, or the surgeon does not believe he or she can deliver the result expected, then it is best to avoid operating on such a patient.

Medical Comorbidities

It is critical for a surgeon to tease out certain details of a patient's history to determine their overall health and risk for general anesthesia. A quick set of questions to screen for any red flags during the initial history and physical examination follows. If a patient answers *yes* to any of the following questions, it should prompt further questioning and possible testing or referral to the patient's primary care physician (PCP) or specialist.

- Have you ever had a heart attack or stroke?
- Do you get short of breath climbing one flight of stairs?
  - In nonambulatory patients: if surgery is high risk, consider pharmacologic stress test
- Do you use any nicotine products? Do you vape, dip, or use cessation products?
- Do you or anyone in your family have a history of abnormal bleeding or clotting?

The complexity of the planned surgical procedure must be considered, as a blepharoplasty will have a different risk profile compared with that of a free fibula osteocutaneous flap for mandible reconstruction after resection of a floor of mouth tumor. For surgery involving more than minimal risk, a preanesthesia unit—if one is available—should assess the patient's suitability for general anesthesia and order any necessary tests prior to surgery. Electrocardiograms and/or chest X-rays may be required by anesthesia personnel; however, this is institution specific. Alternatively, a PCP or other medical specialist familiar with the patient may provide clearance for the suggested procedure. Management of any medical comorbidity such as hypertension and diabetes should be left to these physicians. Communication is key to assure patient safety.

A useful online resource is the American College of Surgeons National Surgical Quality Improvement Program's risk calculator (http://www.riskcalculator.facs.org). The calculator considers patient factors—such as age, functional status, American Society of Anesthesia class, medical comorbidities—and the procedure to determine a percent risk of common complications. The surgeon may even increase the estimated risk based on patient factors that are not accounted for by the calculator.

Cardiac History

Patients should be asked about their history of coronary artery disease, peripheral vascular disease, and stent or bypass surgery. For patients with cardiac disease or risk factors, perioperative risks can be reduced by following accepted American College of Cardiology (ACC) and American Heart Association guidelines[1] as follows:

No cardiac preoperative testing is required in

- Patients undergoing low-risk surgery (regardless of functional capacity)
- Patients who can perform ≥ 4 metabolic equivalents (METs) (regardless of procedural risk level)
  - 1 MET
    - Self-care
    - Activities of daily living
    - Walking on level ground at 2 to 3 mph
  - 4 METs
    - Light housework
    - Walking up a flight of stairs
    - Walking on level ground at 4 to 5 mph
    - Running a short distance
  - >10 METs
    - Strenuous sports (i.e., swimming, tennis, football, basketball, skiing)

Plastic surgery is generally considered low-risk surgery, having less than 1% risk of major adverse cardiac event.[2] However, long, complex reconstructive procedures may pose additional risk. Patients unable to achieve 4 METs, a measure of functional capacity, have an increased cardiac risk. No preoperative cardiac testing is needed in patients undergoing low-risk surgery or in patients who can perform greater than 4 METs, irrespective of other factors.[1] Similarly, no routine testing is required on a patient who can perform greater than 4 METs, even if undergoing high-risk surgery.

Patients with a history of cardiac disease or previous percutaneous cardiac interventions are at an increased risk of cardiac events if medications are managed inappropriately. Discontinuation of dual antiplatelet therapy (DAPT) within weeks after percutaneous cardiac intervention is one of the strongest risk factors for stent thrombosis. One must weigh this risk against the risk of delaying surgery or performing surgery while the patient remains on DAPT. Decisions regarding management are best made with the interventionist who performed the procedure or physician managing the medications.

ACC recommendations for patients undergoing elective noncardiac surgery on DAPT are summarized in **Table 16.1**. If a patient requires an urgent procedure within the minimum duration of DAPT,

TABLE 16.1. MANAGEMENT OF PATIENTS WITH PREVIOUS CARDIAC INTERVENTION

	Minimum Duration of DAPT	
Previous Cardiac Intervention	SIHD (Stable Angina or Low-Risk Unstable Angina)	ACS (NSTE-ACS or STEMI)
Medical therapy*	N/A	1 y
Balloon angioplasty	2 wk	1 y
Bare-metal stent	1 mo	1 y
Drug-eluting stent	6 mo	1 y
Coronary artery bypass graft	1 y	1 y

*P2Y12 platelet inhibitors include clopidogrel (Plavix), prasugrel (Effient), and ticagrelor (Brilinta).
This table summarizes 2016 ACC recommendations regarding the minimum duration of DAPT depending on cardiac intervention and timing of noncardiac surgery. It is advised to communicate the decision to perform surgery and the associated risks with the physician managing the patient's medications.
DAPT, dual antiplatelet therapy; *NSTE-ACS*, non–ST-elevation acute coronary syndrome; *SIHD*, stable ischemic heart disease; *STEMI*, ST-segment elevation myocardial infarction.

the ACC recommends continuing DAPT unless the relative risk of bleeding outweighs the benefit of prevention of stent thrombosis. If the risk of bleeding is too high, the patient is to continue aspirin but hold the $P2Y_{12}$ platelet receptor inhibitor (i.e., clopidogrel [Plavix]) and restart it as soon as possible. For obvious reasons, emergency surgeries will have to proceed on DAPT and therapy-related decisions made postoperatively. Guidelines by the ACC/American Heart Association are routinely updated,[3] and the most recent recommendations are published online (http://www.acc.org/guidelines).

Anemia and Blood Disorders

Preoperative anemia is associated with increased morbidity and mortality.[4,5] The World Health Organization (WHO) and Centers for Disease Control (CDC) define anemia as <13 g/dL in a male and <12 g/dL in a female.[6] The most common cause for anemia is iron deficiency, and this is treated with oral or intravenous (IV) iron supplementation.

Most blood disorders can be ruled out by simple, but focused, history-taking and does not necessitate workup if no pertinent findings are uncovered.[7] Screening laboratory studies are ill-advised and may yield false positive results, leading to unnecessary additional workup and delaying surgery.[8,9] Therefore, routine preoperative testing is not only of little clinical benefit but costly in healthy patients undergoing elective procedures.[10]

Clotting disorders are estimated at 5% to 10% in the general population. The most common hypercoagulable state is factor V Leiden, whereas other common disorders include hyperhomocysteinemia, lupus anticoagulant, and deficiencies in protein C, protein S, or antithrombin. To screen for serious hypercoagulability disorders, one must inquire about a patient's history of venous thromboembolism (VTE) and, in a female, spontaneous abortions or miscarriages. Patients already on an oral anticoagulant should be sent back to the physician managing their medication or referred to a hematologist to formulate a plan for bridging pre- and postoperatively. A patient who has suffered a VTE within the last month may require placement of an inferior vena cava filter, especially if resumption of anticoagulation could be delayed more than 12 hours postoperatively. A prophylactic inferior vena cava filter may be considered in newly diagnosed cancer patients who cannot afford to delay surgery but require a complex resection and reconstruction, as these patients are at high risk of VTE.

On the other spectrum of the coagulation cascade, an estimated 1% of patients have a bleeding disorder, most commonly some form of hemophilia or von Willebrand disease.[11] To rule out any issues with coagulopathy, one should ask about personal or family history of bruising or bleeding tendencies after dental extractions, minor trauma, or previous surgery. In women, a history of menorrhagia or excessive postpartum bleeding should warrant further investigation. Patients known or discovered to have a bleeding abnormality should be referred to a hematologist for perioperative management.

Summary of recommendations for preoperative screening for coagulation disorders:

- History should guide preoperative testing for bleeding or coagulation disorders
- Routine screening laboratory tests do not necessarily correlate with clinical findings and therefore may only confound the picture
- A history of bruising, bleeding, or thromboembolism should prompt further investigation
- Patients with a known hypocoagulable or hypercoagulable disorder should be referred to a hematologist

Diabetes

Uncontrolled or poorly controlled diabetes is a risk factor for overall complications, especially wound healing problems. If indicated, a hemoglobin A1c can verify that the patient's 3-month average blood glucose is within an acceptable range for the proposed surgery. Studies have shown an increase in postoperative complications in patients with a hemoglobin A1c >6.5%.[12,13] Concern for elevated blood glucose or hemoglobin A1c preoperatively should prompt a referral to an endocrinologist or PCP.

Modifiable Risk Factors

Modifiable risk factors include body mass index (BMI), tobacco use, and nutrition status, among other things. The surgeon should not agree to any procedure until these factors have been optimized to his or her satisfaction. The patient should be held accountable for meeting these expectations before any consent is signed. Ideally, BMI should be optimized preoperatively, as several studies have demonstrated an increased risk of complications in patients with a BMI above 35 kg/m^2; this is mostly true for chest and trunk procedures[14-17] but has not held true in hand surgery.[18]

The most easily modifiable risk factor is the use of nicotine products. With smokeless tobacco products becoming more popular, surgeons should specifically ask about whether patients vape, dip, or use other sources of nicotine including cessation products, as they will never volunteer this information. Although there is no agreed upon consensus on the optimal time to abstain from nicotine prior to a surgical procedure, most would agree that at least 4 weeks is best to decrease the risk of complications. If patient noncompliance is suspected, a urine cotinine test can be checked prior to surgery.

A thorough history and examination must elucidate a patient's past surgeries, especially those pertinent to the anatomic site in question. The surgeon must pay attention to previous scars and be mindful of disrupted vascular connections that could lead to untoward outcomes.[19,20] Additionally, one must rule out a history of postoperative wound infection or known colonization with methicillin-resistant *Staphylococcus aureus*. High-risk patients should be screened for MRSA colonization and a decolonization protocol used preoperatively, as this has shown a significant reduction in surgical site infection (SSI).[21,22] A typical treatment regimen includes 5 days of nasal mupirocin ointment and chlorhexidine baths.

Psychiatric History

Patients seeking elective plastic surgery may harbor a psychiatric diagnosis, most commonly narcissistic personality, histrionic personality, or body dysmorphic disorder.[23,24] Many surgeons consider body dysmorphic disorder a clear contraindication to any surgical procedure, as the results will never be satisfactory to the patient. The acronym SIMON (single, immature, male, overly expectant, and narcissistic) should be in the back of a surgeon's mind, especially when evaluating rhinoplasty patients, as those who fit these criteria generally have worse outcomes and lead to malpractice claims.[25] Referral to a mental health specialist may be indicated should the mental stability of a patient be uncertain.

Surgical Planning

Informed Consent

It behooves the surgeon to conduct a proper informed consent, reviewing all risks, benefits, and alternatives to the planned surgical procedure. An appropriate informed consent process requires a face-to-face discussion with the patient, providing ample time to ask and answer questions. Early education of potential complications can decrease postoperative patient dissatisfaction if an adverse event occurs. The surgeon should discuss alternatives—surgical and nonsurgical—available to the patient, even if the surgeon does not offer all options. As is the case with any elective procedure, it is the physician's duty to educate the patient that not undergoing said operation is an option.

The legal definition of a minor, or one who cannot sign a binding contract or consent, is governed by each state, but in most states, the minimum age is 18 years. However, each state also has a set of circumstances whereby a minor may become emancipated and provide his or her own consent. Legally, only one parent of a minor needs to sign a consent for it to be valid.

Surgery Location/Certification

Although some procedures can be performed in more than one setting—office, outpatient, or inpatient—patient and procedural factors must be taken into consideration when choosing the surgical location. Patient safety should be the top priority when making this decision and should not be compromised for any reason. Accreditation of both staff and surgical setting is required. Several agencies provide certification for hospitals or surgery centers, including the Joint Commission on Accreditation of Healthcare Organizations, Accreditation Association for Ambulatory Health Care, and American Association for Accreditation of Ambulatory Surgery Facilities.

Medications

Management of patient medications in the perioperative period:[1]

Take on day of surgery

- Statin
- Pulmonary medication
- Cardiovascular medication except those listed below

Stop on day of surgery

- Angiotensin-converting enzyme inhibitor and angiotensin-receptor blocker
- Diuretic medication
- Diabetic medication

Stop 1 to 2 weeks before surgery

- Blood thinner
- Monoamine oxidase inhibitor
- Herbal medication

Site-Specific Considerations

For any patient undergoing an elective breast procedure, the surgeon should at minimum follow the most recent mammography guidelines.[26] Certain patients under the age of 40 years may warrant a screening mammogram based on personal or family history.[27] When planning tissue transfer procedures, one must ensure that vessels sacrificed during harvest of the flap will not compromise the blood supply to the remaining tissue, as this could lead to disastrous consequences.[28]

Operating Room Time

Increased surgery time is correlated with greater morbidity and linked to increased rates of hypothermia, SSI, thrombotic events, and hospital admission.[29-31] Patients presenting for elective surgery may desire multiple anatomic sites addressed simultaneously. Staging procedures may have to be done to minimize operative time, blood loss, and surgeon fatigue. Reconstructive procedures involving more than one anatomic site should include more than one team, when feasible, to carry out the operation more expeditiously.

PERIOPERATIVE CARE

Appropriate patient preparation includes attention to VTE prophylaxis, body temperature, antibiotic timing and duration, fluid shifts, and positioning in the operating room. In any female capable of childbearing, a day-of-surgery pregnancy test[32] should be obtained to rule out an unknown pregnancy.

Communication

Clear, timely communication before, during, and after surgery is essential to deliver good patient care. The surgeon must communicate with the patient's PCP and other medical specialists as needed during the perioperative period. Intraoperatively, communication between members of the operating room team—nursing, anesthesia, and surgical staff—is critical for any procedure to be executed well and without complications. When there is a breakdown in communication, there is bound to be a problem.

Universal Protocol

It is imperative that the nationally mandated Joint Commission Universal Protocol be followed and proper *time-out* be performed prior to the start of any surgical procedure. This process protects the patient by requiring the health care team to agree that the procedure about to be performed is on the correct patient, site, and side, if applicable.

Deep Vein Thrombosis Prophylaxis

Intermittent pneumatic compression devices must be on and functioning at least 30 minutes prior to induction of anesthesia. If not contraindicated, patients should be encouraged to ambulate with assistance postoperatively on the day of surgery. The 2005 Caprini risk-assessment model for VTE[33] is a validated tool for plastic and reconstructive surgery,[34] and surgeons should refer to recommendations for appropriate mechanical and chemical prophylaxis.

Antibiotics and Skin Preparation

Shaving the surgical site the day before a procedure is associated with an increased risk of SSI. Patients should be advised to shave at least 2 days preoperatively; if not, clippers should be used to trim the surgical site before the skin site preparation in the operating room. Chlorhexidine-alcohol is preferred as the surgical skin antiseptic of choice, as it has been shown to be more efficacious than povidone-iodine.[35]

TABLE 16.2. COMMON ANTIBIOTICS USED FOR PREOPERATIVE SURGICAL PROPHYLAXIS[a]

Antibiotic	Timing (Before Skin Incision)	Pediatric Dose	Adult Dose	Half-Life ($t_{1/2}$)
Cefazolin	30–60 min	30 mg/kg	2 g (3 g for ≥120 kg)	2 h
Clindamycin	60 min	10 mg/kg	900 mg	3 h
Vancomycin	2 h	15 mg/kg	15 mg/kg	6 h

[a]Dose should be repeated for every two half-lives or blood loss exceeding 1500 mL. Cefazolin is the agent of choice, and if a patient has a true allergy to cephalosporins, the second-line antibiotic is clindamycin. Vancomycin is not recommended except in patients who are colonized with or have a history of infection with methicillin-resistant *Staphylococcus aureus*.

Preoperative IV antibiotics should be based on the surgical procedure being performed, taking into consideration any patient allergies. Patients who claim to have an allergy to penicillin should be further questioned regarding whether the allergy is life-threatening. Antibiotic prophylaxis should be administered according to the surgical care improvement project guidelines.[36] A list of common options is provided in **Table 16.2**. Redosing is indicated for every two half-lives ($t_{1/2}$) elapsed, or blood loss is greater than 1500 mL. No data justify continued prophylactic use beyond 24 hours, despite widespread practice to continue postimplant placement or until drains are removed. To the contrary, prolonged use of antibiotics may promote resistant strains of bacteria. Minor procedures being performed in the operating room do not require preoperative antibiotics.

Fluid Balance

Fluid balance is critical in many plastic surgery procedures, especially with increasing operating time. Anesthesia studies show improved outcomes with balanced fluid management rather than restrictive or traditional liberal fluid administration.[37] If a Foley catheter is in place, an output of 30 to 50 mL/h is a reasonable goal for the anesthesia team to maintain, as fluid overload can have disastrous consequences.

Warming

Hypothermia, defined as body temperature less than 36°C, is an independent risk factor for bleeding and postoperative wound healing complications.[38] The most effective method of maintaining normothermia is by prewarming the patient with forced warm air for at least 15 minutes prior to the procedure.[39] Several intraoperative techniques can be used to prevent or combat hypothermia: covering regions outside of the surgical site, using forced warm air and/or a warming blanket, maintaining of an ambient room temperature of at least 21°C, and using of warm IV and irrigation fluids. Although cutaneous temperature monitoring is frequently used, it is less accurate than other methods such as esophageal, bladder, or rectal temperature monitoring.

Patient Positioning

Intraoperative positioning is important in the prevention of VTE, as well as in avoiding nerve and ocular damage. Bony prominences should be appropriately padded to prevent a pressure nerve injury. Knees should be gently flexed to 15° and shoulders abducted no more than 90°. When prone, eyes should be well protected against pressure and the neck should be comfortably positioned in neutral alignment. If the surgical procedure necessitates an intraoperative position change, this should be well coordinated and executed to prevent patient injury.

POSTOPERATIVE CARE

Blood and Fluid Monitoring

Blood transfusions are indicated for all patients with a hemoglobin level below 7 g/dL and are indicated above this threshold for certain patients, such as those with symptomatic anemia or a cardiac history.[40] Fluid shifts are common in the postoperative period, and a Foley catheter can be helpful to guide resuscitation and monitor urine output. If a Foley catheter is present, it should be removed as soon as possible, preferably within 48 hours postoperatively unless justified for longer.

Ambulation

Ambulation postoperatively is the best preventative measure against VTE. Patients should be encouraged to ambulate as early as the evening after surgery if it will not compromise the outcome of the procedure.

Warning Signs/Complications

Knowledge of how to prevent and manage complications for the procedure in question is paramount, and the inexperienced surgeon should not tackle a case without experience. The surgical site can develop several issues, including but not limited to erythema, cellulitis, deep tissue infection, seroma, hematoma, vascular compromise, or wound dehiscence. Hematoma incidence is higher in breast procedures, combined procedures, and male patients.[41] An expanding hematoma in any location is an indication to return to the operating room as soon as possible to evacuate the clot and control the source of bleeding. Drains can indicate an evolving hematoma if output remains sanguineous, especially with bright red drainage. A drain that is no longer holding suction may indicate a wound dehiscence or drain extrusion from the wound.

Systemic warning signs include fevers, lower extremity edema, diarrhea, and sustained or increased need for supplemental oxygen. Although temperature spikes may be common postoperatively, a sustained fever or alternating fevers and chills is a cause for investigation. Lower extremity edema can be a sign of VTE or heart failure. An inability to wean off oxygen postoperatively should raise suspicion in an otherwise healthy patient who underwent a minor procedure.

Follow-Up

Patients are seen postoperatively within a week of surgery after a major procedure or within 2 weeks after a minor procedure. It is best to leave the initial postoperative dressing in place until seen in clinic, although the patient may remove an outer layer to allow for showering 1 or 2 days after surgery. If drains are used, patients are seen weekly until all have been removed; a common criterion is output less than 30 mL/d. If a major procedure was performed, lifting is restricted to 5 kg for 6 weeks to decrease the risk of wound dehiscence. As long as the procedure performed does not interfere with the ability to drive, then a patient can drive once no longer taking narcotic medication.

REFERENCES

1. Fleisher LA, Fleischmann KE, Auerbach AD, et al. 2014 ACC/AHA guideline on perioperative cardiovascular evaluation and management of patients undergoing noncardiac surgery: a report of the American College of Cardiology/American Heart Association Task Force on practice guidelines. *J Am Coll Cardiol*. 2014;64(22):e77-e137.

These are the latest guidelines for preoperative workup of patients undergoing non-cardiac surgery. It is important to review this document (or the most up-to-date document at the time) to assure that patients are being appropriately evaluated before surgery. As always, institutional policies may vary and may not be in line with the guidelines here.

2. Jordan SW, Mioton LM, Smetona J, et al. Resident involvement and plastic surgery outcomes: an analysis of 10,356 patients from the American College of Surgeons National Surgical Quality Improvement Program database. *Plast Reconstr Surg*. 2013;131(4):763-773.
3. Levine GN, Bates ER, Bittl JA, et al. 2016 ACC/AHA guideline focused update on duration of dual antiplatelet therapy in patients with coronary artery disease: a report of the American College of Cardiology/American Heart Association Task Force on Clinical Practice Guidelines. *J Am Coll Cardiol*. 2016;68(10):1082-1115.
4. Clark JR, McCluskey SA, Hall F, et al. Predictors of morbidity following free flap reconstruction for cancer of the head and neck. *Head Neck*. 2007;29(12):1090-1101.
5. Musallam KM, Tamim HM, Richards T, et al. Preoperative anaemia and post-operative outcomes in non-cardiac surgery: a retrospective cohort study. *Lancet*. 2011;378(9800):1396-1407.
6. report*Assessing the Iron Status of Populations: Report of a Joint World Health Organization/Centers for Disease Control and Prevention Technical Consultation on the Assessment of Iron Status at the Population Level*. 2nd ed. Geneva, Switzerland: World Health Organization; 2007. Available at http://www.who.int/nutrition/publications/micronutrients/anaemia_iron_deficiency/9789241596107.pdf.
7. Kaplan EB, Sheiner LB, Boeckmann AJ, et al. The usefulness of preoperative laboratory screening. *JAMA*. 1985;253(24):3576-3781.
8. Peterson P, Hayes TE, Arkin CF, et al. The preoperative bleeding time test lacks clinical benefit: College of American Pathologists' and American Society of Clinical Pathologists' position article. *Arch Surg*. 1998;133(2):134-139.
9. Dumanian GA, Bontempo FA, Johnson PC. Evaluation and treatment of the plastic surgical patient having a potential to bleed. *Plast Reconstr Surg*. 1995;96(1):211-218.
10. Fischer JP, Shang EK, Nelson JA, et al. Patterns of preoperative laboratory testing in patients undergoing outpatient plastic surgery procedures. *Aesthet Surg J*. 2014;34(1):133-141.
    A study examining data from ambulatory plastic surgery procedures over 5 years from the NSQIP database. 8645 patients were analyzed, and the results showed that preoperative laboratory analysis is of little benefit in this patient population.
11. Mensah PK, Gooding R. Surgery in patients with inherited bleeding disorders. *Anaesthesia*. 2015;70(suppl 1):112-120.
12. Endara M, Masden D, Goldstein J, et al. The role of chronic and perioperative glucose management in high-risk surgical closures: a case for tighter glycemic control. *Plast Reconstr Surg*. 2013;132(4):996-1004.
13. Galdyn I, Lewis P, Gupta S. Retrospective analysis of hemoglobin A1C levels in plastic surgery patients with postoperative morbidity: a call to action. *Plast Reconstr Surg*. 2014:134(4S-1):103.
14. Fischer JP, Nelson JA, Kovach SJ, et al. Impact of obesity on outcomes in breast reconstruction: analysis of 15,937 patients from the ACS-NSQIP datasets. *J Am Coll Surg*. 2013;217(4):656-664.
15. Nelson JA, Fischer JP, Chung CU, et al. Obesity and early complications following reduction mammaplasty: an analysis of 4545 patients from the 2005-2011 NSQIP datasets. *J Plast Surg Hand Surg*. 2014;48(5):334-339.
16. Gupta V, Winocour J, Rodriguez-Feo C, et al. Safety of aesthetic surgery in the overweight patient: analysis of 127,961 patients. *Aesthet Surg J*. 2016;36(6):718-729.
17. Fischer JP, Basta MN, Wink JD, et al. Optimizing patient selection in ventral hernia repair with concurrent panniculectomy: an analysis of 1974 patients from the ACS-NSQIP datasets. *J Plast Reconstr Aesthet Surg*. 2014;67(11):1532-1540.
18. Lipira AB, Sood RF, Tatman PD, et al. Complications within 30 days of hand surgery: an analysis of 10,646 patients. *J Hand Surg Am* 2015;40(9):1852-1859.
19. Laporta R, Longo B, Sorotos M, et al. Tips and tricks for DIEP flap breast reconstruction in patients with previous abdominal scar. *Microsurgery*. 2017;37(4):282-292.
20. Losee JE, Caldwell EH, Serletti JM. Secondary reduction mammaplasty: is using a different pedicle safe? *Plast Reconstr Surg*. 2000;106(5):1004-1008.
    A retrospective study of 10 women undergoing secondary breast reduction. Seven out of 10 women had a reduction using a different pedicle from the primary reduction. This is important because the surgeon does not need to rely on operative reports of a previous reduction before proceeding with repeat surgery.
21. van Rijen M, Bonten M, Wenzel R, Kluytmans J. Mupirocin ointment for preventing *Staphylococcus aureus* infections in nasal carriers. *Cochrane Database Syst Rev*. 2008;(4):CD006216.
22. Humphreys H, Becker K, Dohmen PM, et al. Staphylococcus aureus and surgical site infections: benefits of screening and decolonization before surgery. *J Hosp Infect*. 2016;94(3):295-304.
23. Shridharani SM, Magarakis M, Manson PN, Rodriguez ED. Psychology of plastic and reconstructive surgery: a systematic clinical review. *Plast Reconstr Surg*. 2010;126(6):2243-2251.
24. Picavet VA, Prokopakis EP, Gabriëls L, et al. High prevalence of body dysmorphic disorder symptoms in patients seeking rhinoplasty. *Plast Reconstr Surg*. 2011;128(2):509-517.
25. Gorney M, Martello J. Patient selection criteria. *Clin Plast Surg*. 1999;26(1):37-40.
26. US Preventive Services Task Force. Screening for breast cancer: U.S. Preventive Services Task Force recommendation statement. *Ann Intern Med*. 2009;151(10):716-726.
27. Sharabi SE, Bullocks JM, Dempsey PJ, Singletary SE. The need for breast cancer screening in women undergoing elective breast surgery: an assessment of risk and risk factors for breast cancer in young women. *Aesthet Surg J*. 2010;30(6):821-831.
28. Saydam FA, Basaran K, Ceran F, Mert B. Foot ischemia after a free fibula flap harvest: immediate salvage with an interpositional sapheneous vein graft. *J Craniofac Surg*. 2014;25(5):1784-1786.
29. Gold BS, Kitz DS, Lecky JH, Neuhaus JM. Unanticipated admission to the hospital following ambulatory surgery. *JAMA*. 1989;262(21):3008-3010.
30. Fogarty BJ, Khan K, Ashall G, Leonard AG. Complications of long operations: a prospective study of morbidity associated with prolonged operative time. *Br J Plast Surg*. 1999;52(1):33-36.
31. Hardy KL, Davis KE, Constantine RS, et al. The impact of operative time on complications after plastic surgery: a multivariate regression analysis of 1753 cases. *Aesthet Surg J*. 2014;34(4):614-622.
32. Apfelbaum JL, Connis RT, Nickinovich DG, American Society of Anesthesiologists Task Force on Preanesthesia Evaluation. Practice advisory for preanesthesia evaluation: an updated report by the American Society of Anesthesiologists Task Force on Preanesthesia Evaluation. *Anesthesiology*. 2012;116(3):522-538.
33. Caprini JA. Thrombosis risk assessment as a guide to quality patient care. *Dis Mon*. 2005;51(2-3):70-78.
34. Pannucci CJ, Bailey SH, Dreszer G, et al. Validation of the Caprini risk assessment model in plastic and reconstructive surgery patients. *J Am Coll Surg*. 2011;212(1):105-112.
    A landmark article that examined the 2005 Caprini for the purposes of plastic surgery patients and validated the results from that original study. When performing outpatient plastic surgery procedures, this is the model that should be used to stratify VTE risk and guide prophylaxis.
35. Darouiche RO, Wall MJ, Itani KM, et al. Chlorhexidine-alcohol versus povidone-iodine for surgical-site antisepsis. *N Engl J Med*. 2010;361(1):18-26.
36. Rosenberger LH, Politano AD, Sawyer RG. The surgical care improvement project and prevention of postoperative infection, including surgical site infection. *Surg Infect (Larchmt)*. 2011;12(3):163-168.
    The Surgical Care Improvement Project (SCIP) has been revolutionary in guiding many facets of the perioperative care of patients. This paper gives recommendations regarding postoperative infection prophylaxis. Readers should refer to other articles on SCIP guidelines as the data are high evidence.
37. Shin CH, Long DR, McLean D, et al. Effects of intraoperative fluid management on postoperative outcomes: a hospital registry study. *Ann Surg*. 2018;267(6):1084-1092.
38. Kurz A, Sessler DI, Lenhardt R. Perioperative normothermia to reduce the incidence of surgical-wound infection and shorten hospitalization: study of Wound Infection and Temperature Group. *N Engl J Med*. 1996;334(19):1209-1215.
39. Horn EP, Bein B, Böhm R, et al. The effect of short time periods of preoperative warming in the prevention of perioperative hypothermia. *Anaesthesia*. 2012;67(6):612-617.
40. Carson JL, Duff A, Poses RM, et al. Effect of anaemia and cardiovascular disease on surgical mortality and morbidity. *Lancet*. 1996;348(9034):1055-1060.
41. Kaoutzanis C, Winocour J, Gupta V, et al. Incidence and risk factors for major hematomas in aesthetic surgery: analysis of 129,007 patients. *Aesthet Surg J*. 2017;37(10):1175-1185.

QUESTIONS

1. **A 45-year-old woman is referred for immediate breast reconstruction after mastectomy scheduled in 12 days. She has had two vaginal deliveries and desires autologous breast reconstruction. She smokes seven cigarettes a day and is otherwise healthy. What is the best approach?**
   a. Ask her to quit immediately and proceed with surgery
   b. Delay her reconstruction until she is nicotine free for at least 4 weeks
   c. Deny her surgery for her smoking habit
   d. Proceed with surgery, as this is a cancer-related procedure
   e. Refer her to another physician willing to operate on smokers

2. **A 67-year-old male presents for correction of ptotic skin after a 60-kg weight loss 2 years after his Roux-en-Y gastric bypass. Current BMI is 29.5 kg/m^2 and has been stable for 6 months. Medical history is significant for ST-elevation myocardial infarction 4 months ago treated with a drug-eluting stent. What is the evidence-based approach to the management of this patient with respect to surgery?**
   a. Proceed with surgery with the patient on all his medications
   b. Have the patient hold his antiplatelet medications for 2 weeks prior to surgery
   c. Have the patient hold his antiplatelet medications 2 days prior to surgery
   d. Delay surgery for at least 2 months
   e. Tell the patient he is too high risk to have surgery given his cardiac history

3. **On a busy clinic day with many patients, you see a new patient referred to you by a local orthopedic surgeon for coverage of a leg defect after planned melanoma resection. The anticipated defect on the anterior calf includes skin and subcutaneous tissue down to fascia, leaving a wound with 5 cm diameter. What is the best course of action?**
   a. Ask the medical assistant in the clinic to carry out the consent process and move on to the next patient because you are running behind
   b. Have an informed consent with the patient and explain all options and risks
   c. Offer the patient a free flap reconstruction because you completed a microsurgery fellowship
   d. Tell the patient that his best option is a skin graft and have him sign the consent form

4. **A 14-year-old girl presents desiring correction of mammary hypertrophy. She is accompanied by her father. Her history includes a rapid 1-year history of breast growth, and recently she complains of difficulty fitting in a bra and playing lacrosse, which she has done since 9 years of age. What is the appropriate management of this patient who desires a breast reduction?**
   a. Have the father sign the consent form
   b. Have the patient sign the consent form
   c. Refuse to perform the procedure until the patient is at 18 years of age so she can sign her own consent
   d. Require the patient to return with both parents so that they may both sign the consent form
   e. Require the patient to return with the mother to sign the consent form

1. **Answer: b.** Smoking is a modifiable risk factor that can increase complications after surgery. Nicotine can lead to vasoconstriction and reduced oxygenation of healing tissues, leading to increases in wound healing problems and infection. The best option is to counsel the patient to stop and agree to perform her reconstruction—an elective portion of her cancer treatment—once she is off nicotine for at least 4 weeks. If noncompliance is suspected, a urine cotinine test can be checked. It can take up to 10 days to get the results back, so it should not be performed close to the surgical date. Having a smoking policy in place can avoid postoperative complications.

2. **Answer: d.** Current guidelines after cardiac stenting recommend at least 6 months of DAPT: aspirin and clopidogrel or equivalent. Stopping or holding either or both medications is associated with a high risk of stent thrombosis. Any elective noncardiac surgery should be delayed until after the patient has completed the minimum duration of therapy. Additionally, the surgeon should ideally obtain clearance from a cardiologist before proceeding with surgery.

3. **Answer: b.** The purpose of informed consent is to have a face-to-face discussion between a physician and patient. Critical to the discussion is an unbiased presentation of possible risks, benefits, and alternatives. The person performing the informed consent process must be able to perform the procedure in question, so this task should not be left to a medical assistant. Furthermore, a patient should be offered all reasonable treatment options, not just simply the option that puts a physician's specialty/subspecialty training to use. Even though a skin graft may be the best option for coverage, a surgeon should do his or her due diligence to go through the R/B/A rather than make the patient sign the consent form.

4. **Answer: a.** Either parent, or a legal guardian, of a minor may consent to a surgical procedure. The patient in question is 14 years old, and in no state is that of legal age to provide consent. It is not necessary to have the mother, or both parents, sign the consent. Given the severity of the symptoms, it is appropriate to proceed with a breast reduction and there is no need to wait until the patient's 18th birthday.

CHAPTER 17 Ethics in Plastic Surgery

Christian J. Vercler

KEY POINTS

- The patient-surgeon relationship is fiduciary in nature and cannot be reduced to merely an exchange of goods and services.
- Surgeons should not operate on family members.
- Relationships with industry introduce inherent biases into research and practice that must be acknowledged and thoughtfully managed.
- Using patient images on social media is rife with ethical pitfalls that the plastic surgeon must avoid.
- Innovation is inherent in plastic surgery, and the surgeon has the duty to responsibly conduct research in a way that balances scientific rigor and at patient's best interests.
- Promoting the autonomy of a patient in decision-making requires understanding their values and interpreting them in the context of the surgical options.
- Informed consent is a process, not just a signature on a form.

The right or wrong course of action can sometimes be unclear in the practice of plastic surgery. There is no one universally accepted account of what constitutes *the good life* in our secular pluralist society—in fact, there are many competing ideas. Ethics involves disciplined reflection on these moral ambiguities. Laws, policies, and published guidelines can assist in drawing the boundaries beyond which we should not go, but these things alone do not define what is ethical. Certainly, unethical behavior persists despite a myriad of laws, policies, and guidelines intended to prevent it. Unlike in science, where data illuminate what *is* factual, ethics deals with values, where a factual statement does not carry with it a moral imperative. Generally, there are three approaches in moral inquiry: What kind of *person* do you become by doing this? Is this *act* itself ethical (and the intentions that justify it)? What are the *outcomes*? This chapter will not fully articulate the philosophical rationale for the positions put forth. These are provided in many of the references. Understanding basic principles in ethics can help one to deal with a myriad of ethical issues as they arise, just as understanding the basic principles of plastic surgery prepares one for a host of difficult surgical problems.

ETHICS AND PROFESSIONALISM

Professionalism refers to behaviors that are expected from individuals who take on the mantle of a profession in a way that holds them to a higher standard and sets them apart from nonprofessionals. Professionalism among plastic surgeons is extremely important, given the nature of the patient-surgeon relationship, which is one of inherent power and knowledge imbalance. This must be a fiduciary relationship, that is, the health, well-being, and best interests of the patient must always be prioritized.[1] This is the foundational principle of surgical ethics. Although there is not a bright line that separates ethics from professionalism, the general understanding is that the particular professional standards inherent to the practice of plastic surgery may change, but that ethical principles are more broadly based concepts that are less mutable.[2]

Both the American Society of Plastic Surgeons (ASPS) and the American Board of Plastic Surgeons (ABPS) have a code of ethics that members must follow (**Tables 17.1** and **17.2**). These are concepts that every plastic surgeon must know. A recent survey of plastic surgery program directors[3] identified interpersonal communication, informed consent, and billing as the issues within ethics and professionalism that are the most important to teach residents. Inappropriate billing is certainly a professionalism issue, but it also may constitute fraud. This chapter will not cover billing further other than to note that ignorance of the law generally is not a valid excuse. Surgeons who lack good communication skills may find themselves in a situation when their behavior is being understood as *unprofessional*, but that will also not be discussed further in this chapter. Informed consent for an operation is the critical activity that must precede an operation and will be discussed at length, in addition to several other topics that are important in daily practice.

TRUTHFULNESS AND ERROR DISCLOSURE

Most specific principles in the ASPS Code of Ethics relate directly to transparency and truthfulness. For example, misleading patients through deceptive advertising, failing to report licensing sanctions, fraudulent billing, etc. are all forbidden. Deception and subterfuge are clearly outside the bounds of acceptable behavior for a plastic surgeon, but the profession calls to an even higher level of transparency.

Surgical errors are devastating to both the patient and the surgeon. Although it goes against our impulse to save face, disclosing these errors is essential for several reasons. At the interpersonal level, the harm-causing error threatens the trustworthiness of the surgeon, particularly if it remains undisclosed. Paradoxically, a growing body of evidence supports that patients are less likely to sue when an error is accompanied by disclosure, apology, and an offer to *make it right*. Disclosure of error also facilitates improvement of systems issues at the institutional level.[4]

OPERATING ON FAMILY MEMBERS

Emergencies aside, the plastic surgeon should avoid operating on family members when possible.[5] Interestingly, Slavin and Goldwyn found that 88% of plastic surgeons surveyed said that they would perform aesthetic surgery on a family member and 84% said that they had.[6] However, familial relationships and interpersonal dynamics are fundamentally different than the patient-surgeon relationship, which at the very least assumes that the patient is free to refuse the operation or seek a second opinion. Prudence and judgment come with experience, and the wisdom of the surgical community for generations has continued to admonish surgeons to avoid operating on family members.[7]

PRIVACY AND CONFIDENTIALITY

This issue is tightly regulated by the Health Insurance Privacy and Accountability Act (HIPAA), and several issues around privacy and confidentiality are referenced in the ASPS Code of Ethics. Patient's health information should not be shared with anyone except those directly involved in the care of that patient. This is particularly relevant in the practice of plastic surgery, as patient photos are routinely taken on phones and shared over unsecured networks. To ensure patient privacy, photos should be taken on devices that are encrypted, shared over secure networks, and shown only to those individuals involved in the care of the patient. Consent for the use of photos beyond patient care, such as for education and advertising, requires explicit written consent.[8]

TABLE 17.1. AMERICAN BOARD OF PLASTIC SURGERY CODE OF ETHICS—GENERAL PRINCIPLES

I.	Medical professionals shall provide their services with respect for human dignity. Physicians should merit the confidence of patients entrusted to their care, and render to each a full measure of service and devotion.
II.	Physicians shall strive to improve their medical knowledge and skills, and avail their patients and colleagues of the benefit of their professional attainments. Physicians have an affirmative duty to disclose new medical advances to patients and colleagues.
III.	The honored ideals of the medical profession imply that the responsibility of the physician extends both to the individual patient and to society. Activities that improve the health and well-being of the individual, as well as the community, deserve the interest and participation of the physician.
IV.	Plastic surgeons shall provide competent and scientifically sound medical and surgical services, while respecting the rights and privacy of their patients.

American Board of Plastic Surgery. ABPS Code of Ethics. Available at https://www.abplasticsurgery.org/media/2654/abps-code-of-ethics-11-2011.pdf. Revised May 18, 2018.

ADVERTISING AND SOCIAL MEDIA

The ASPS has guidelines for the use of advertising that reflect professional values of truthfulness and privacy. Photos used in advertising must show results as truthfully as possible. Showing atypical results with the claim that the results are typical is prohibited, also are the claims about being the *best plastic surgeon* and so on. The use of models who idealize standards of beauty and are not patients is commonplace. This skirts the admonition by ASPS to avoid language and images that induce insecurities and a desire for the operation. Advertising has moved from print, to web-based, to now more ephemeral app-based platforms such as Twitter, Instagram, and Snapchat. The utmost respect for our patients must guide the use of these mediums.[9,10]

RELATIONSHIPS WITH INDUSTRY AND CONFLICTS OF INTEREST

Plastic surgery is an innovative field, and relationships with industry facilitate that innovation.[11] Financial relationships with companies that are motivated by profit rather than the best interests of the patient constitute a conflict of interests that the plastic surgeon must address. These conflicts of interest affect not only patient care but also research findings.[12] For the innovating plastic surgeon, these inevitable conflicts of interest are not to be avoided at all costs, but rather to be actively and thoughtfully managed. The Physician Payments Sunshine Act (PPSA) requires all payments made by biomedical companies to physicians to be openly reported via the Open Payments Program (OPP). The idea is that greater transparency will potentially mitigate the effects the payments might have on the surgeon's decision-making.[13]

INFORMED CONSENT

Justice Benjamin Cardozo's words from the 1914 decision in *Schloendorff v. Society of New York Hospital* set the backdrop for any discussion of informed consent: "a surgeon who performs an operation without his patient's consent commits an assault for which he is liable in damages"—hence the contemporary practice of having a patient sign a consent form before any procedure. The form is a legal document. Actual informed consent, however, requires that (1) the patient is a *competent adult* with *decision-making capacity*, and (2)

TABLE 17.2. AMERICAN SOCIETY OF PLASTIC SURGEONS CODE OF ETHICS—GENERAL PRINCIPLES

I.	The principal objective of the medical profession is to render services to humanity with full respect for human dignity. Members should merit the confidence of patients entrusted to their care, rendering to each a full measure of service and devotion.
II.	Members should strive continually to improve medical knowledge and skill, and make available to their patients and colleagues the benefits of their professional achievements. Members have an affirmative duty to disclose new medical advances to patients and colleagues.
III.	Members should practice a method of healing founded on a scientific basis and should not voluntarily associate professionally with anyone who violates this principle.
IV.	Members should observe all laws, uphold the dignity and honor of the profession, and accept its self-imposed disciplines. They should expose, without hesitation, illegal or unethical conduct of fellow members of the profession.
V.	Members may choose whom to serve. In emergency situations, however, members should render service to the best of their ability. Having undertaken the care of a patient, a member may not neglect the patient, and until the patient has been discharged, a member may discontinue services only after giving adequate notice.
VI.	Members should provide services under the terms and conditions that permit the free and complete exercise of sound medical judgment and skill.
VII.	A member should seek consultation upon request, in doubtful or difficult cases, or whenever it appears that the quality of medical service may be enhanced thereby.
VIII.	A member may not reveal a patient's confidence, any observed characteristics of the patient, or any information obtained from the patient in a professional capacity, without such patient's consent or unless required to do so by law or unless it becomes necessary to protect the welfare of the patient or of the community.
IX.	The honored ideals of the medical profession imply that the responsibilities of the member extend not only to the patient but also to society. Activities that have the purpose of improving both the health and well-being of the patient and the community deserve the interest and participation of the member.
X.	To assist the public in obtaining medical services, members are permitted to make their services known through advertising. Advertising, however, entails the risk that the member may employ practices that are false, fraudulent, deceptive, or misleading. Regulation is, therefore, necessary and in the public interest. Subsection II of the Specific Principles permits public dissemination of truthful information about medical services, while prohibiting false, fraudulent, deceptive, or misleading communications, and restricting direct solicitation.
XI.	In their public and private communications with or concerning patients and colleagues made in a professional capacity or environment, members shall strive to use accurate and respectful language and images.

Code of Ethics of the American Society of Plastic Surgeons. Reproduced with permission from American Society of Plastic Surgeons. Available at https://www.plasticsurgery.org/documents/Governance/asps-code-of-ethics.pdf.

that the patient understands the risks, benefits, and alternatives to the proposed operation. *Competency* is a legal designation and is task specific. A patient is *incompetent for making medical decisions* when a judge declares it and that judgment is permanent. At this point, a legal guardian is appointed and is recognized as the authorized decision-maker.

Decision-making capacity, on the other hand, waxes and wanes. For example, a patient who is drunk, or sedated, or uremic, may lack decision-making capacity for a time but may regain it later. This is a clinical determination that does not need to be made by a psychiatrist, although his or her expertise is helpful in difficult cases. When a patient lacks decision-making capacity, a surrogate decision-maker must make decisions for the patient based on *substituted judgment*. Substituted judgment requires that the surrogate knows the patient's values well and can use them to apply to the situation at hand to try to make the decision the patient would make if they were able. These issues become especially difficult around the end of life because most people lose decision-making capacity as part of the dying process. Fortunately, most plastic surgery patients are not terminal, but many patients may have fluctuating levels of cognition that require a working understanding of these concepts. Surrogates may be named in a living will, or assigned as a durable power of attorney for health care (DPOA-H). If these legally appointed individuals are not available, then spouses and family are turned to for consent to treatment.

Ensuring that the patient understands the risks, benefits, and alternatives to the proposed operation is a difficult but necessary task. Even though many patients implicitly trust their surgeons, the act of discussing risks, benefits, and alternatives demonstrates respect for the individual personhood of the patient. By showing respect for the patient's autonomy in this way, the plastic surgeon is fulfilling a significant ethical duty. However, when a patient refuses an indicated operation, things become more complicated. Simply accepting a refusal of an operation can lead to patient harm and loss of the proposed benefit. In certain cases, the surgeon must also ensure that the patient is giving an *informed dissent*. That is, that the refusal of the proposed operation is not based on a misunderstanding of the facts (e.g., "the implant is not infected") or on false beliefs (e.g., "magic will heal this"). If a competent adult with decision-making capacity understands the risks, benefits, and alternatives of an operation and refuses the procedure, then the surgeon must follow that decision, even if the outcome for the patient is loss of life or limb.

The right of a competent adult to refuse any operation offered by a surgeon does not extend to a positive right to demand any operation a patient desires. Surgeons are given the responsibility to refuse to perform operations that do more harm than good, that are physiologically futile, or that do not meet the overall goals of care or best interests of the patient. Also, a parent may not refuse an operation for a child if the refusal will bring harm to the child.[14] These are some of the limits to autonomy.

SUMMARY

Although there are many individual topics within plastic surgery ethics, the foundational principles are as follows: (1) respect the individual personhood of the patient, (2) prioritize the interests of the patient over your own, and (3) shoulder the responsibility of maintaining an honest relationship with the patient and society.

REFERENCES

1. Vercler CJ. Surgical ethics: surgical virtue and more. *Narrat Inq Bioeth*. 2015;5(1):45-51.
   Brief introduction to a series of articles written by surgeons about ethical dilemmas they have encountered. It introduces the idea that surgeons have unique ethical responsibilities to their patients.
2. Preminger BA, Hansen J, Reid CM, Gosman AA. *Plast Reconstr Surg*. 2018;141(4):1071-1072.
3. Bennett KG, Ingraham JM, Schneider LF, et al. The teaching of ethics and professionalism in plastic surgery residency: a cross-sectional survey. *Ann Plast Surg*. 2017;78(5):552-556.
4. Vercler CJ, Buchman SR, Chung KC. Discussion harm-causing errors with patients: an ethics primer for plastic surgeons. *Ann Plast Surg*. 2015;74(2):140-144.
   Introduction to ethical reasoning and to applying different approaches to a case where an error occurred resulting in harm to a patient. The ethical arguments for disclosing harm-causing medical errors to patients are summarized, including a review of data that support better outcomes in cases where full disclosure and apology occurs. Practical recommendations on how to do it are also discussed.
5. Gold KJ, Golman EB, Kamil LH, et al. No appointment necessary? Ethical challenges in treating friends and family. *N Engl J Med*. 2014;371(13):1254-1258.
6. Slavin SA, Goldwyn RM. A family operation: plastic surgeons who perform aesthetic surgery on spouses or other family members. *Plast Reconstr Surg*. 2010;125(3):1018-1023.
7. Jones JW, McCullough LB, Richman BW. The ethics of operating on a family member. *J Vasc Surg*. 2006;42(5):1033-1035.
8. Bennett KG, Bonawitz SC, Vercler CJ. Guidelines for the ethical publication of facial photographs and review of the literature. *Cleft Palate Craniofac J*. 2019;56(1):7-14. doi:10.1177/1055665618774026.
9. Bennett KG, Vercler CJ. When is posting about patients on social media unethical medutainment? *Am Med Assoc J Ethics*. 2018;20(4):384-391.
10. Bennett KG, Berlin NL, MacEachern MP, et al. Ethical and professional use of social media in surgery: a systematic review of the literature. *Plast Reconstr Surg*. 2018;142(3):388e-398e.
    Engagement in social media is part of contemporary plastic surgery practice. This systematic review summarizes published guidelines of the ethical and professional use of social media, draws upon well-established principles in ethics and professionalism, and provides a set of guidelines to follow to ensure compliance with the tenets of the Code of Ethics of the American Board of Plastic Surgery and American Society of Plastic Surgeons.
11. Wang Y, Kotsis SV, Chung KC. Applying the concepts of innovation strategies to plastic surgery. *Plast Reconstr Surg*. 2013;132(2):483-490.
12. Lopez J, Lopez S, Means J, et al. Financial conflicts of interest: an association between funding and findings in plastic surgery. *Plast Reconstr Surg*. 2015;136(5):690e-697e.
13. Ahmed R, Lopez J, Bae S, et al. The dawn of transparency: insights from the physician payment sunshine act in plastic surgery. *Ann Plast Surg*. 2017;78(3):315-323.
14. Diekama D. Parental refusals of medical treatment: the harm principle as threshold for state intervention. *Theor Med Bioeth*. 2004;25(4):243-264.

QUESTIONS

1. A 65-year-old man with 15% TBSA (total body surface area) flame burns on his upper extremity is intubated for smoke inhalation. His daughter refuses excision and grafting for his burns and requests that the patient be taken off the ventilator and allowed to die, citing a discussion with him that he would *never want to live on a ventilator*. What should you do?

a. Honor her request; she is the appropriate surrogate decision-maker.
b. Ask to see paperwork (e.g., DPOA-H or living will) to confirm her statements, and then remove the ventilator.
c. Seek a court-appointed guardian to approve the operation and ongoing critical care interventions.
d. Continue to treat the patient and call the ethics committee.
e. Have another MD sign the consent along with you and document in the chart that the operations are an emergency and must be performed.

2. A father brings his 1-year-old son with a left unilateral complete cleft lip and palate to your clinic for evaluation. He states that he does not want to have his son's cleft lip or palate repaired and is in your office only because his pediatrician coerced him to come. He thinks that operating on his baby to *force society's standards of beauty on him* is barbaric. He also has been applying an herbal balm on the lip and palate and believes that it is getting better with this treatment. What do you do?

a. Tell him that you have to fix his palate because that is a functional operation for speech but that he does not need to have his lip repaired.
b. Tell him that the lip and palate both need to be repaired and that you will report him to Child Protective Services if he refuses to let the operations occur.
c. Call hospital security to escort the child to the operating room for immediate lip repair.
d. Take some photos to document the child's appearance and thank him for coming to your office. Have him follow-up in 6 months.

3. Which of the following must you do to maintain patient privacy when using photos of them?

a. Obtain informed consent for all intended uses.
b. Take the photos on an encrypted device.
c. Store photos on an encrypted drive.
d. All of the above.

4. You are performing an abdominoplasty and inadvertently *buttonhole* the flap with the Bovie and burn the skin. You notice that the Bovie is set to 85. The defect is large enough that you decide to excise it and close it primarily. In follow-up, the patient asks what the incision is. She seems to think you removed a mole from the area (you did not). What did you tell her?

a. "I'm sorry, but that's an area where I inadvertently burned through your skin. The electrocautery was set much higher than I usually use it and we are investigating as to why that occurred."
b. "Yes, don't worry about that mole. You are better off without it."
c. "That's from an equipment malfunction. It could have been much worse. You're lucky."
d. "That's nothing. Don't worry about it."

5. You maintain a professional Instagram account where you post before and after photos of your patients, who have all given written informed consent for this specific purpose. One of your patients on whom you did a facelift, blepharoplasty, and laser resurfacing posts a *selfie* and tags you, giving you credit for her look. She messages you and asks you to repost her photo on your page. You notice that she has used a filter to alter the photo giving her skin a much smoother appearance than your procedure did and the angle from which the photo is taken gives her neckline a more defined angle than you achieved with your facelift. Which of the following violates the ASPS Code of Ethics?

a. Repost the photo to your account. There are no privacy or confidentiality concerns as she has already posted the photo to her account identifying as her surgeon.
b. Repost the photo, but in the description state *results not typical* and note that a filter was used to enhance the appearance of the skin.
c. Have her come back to your office for a set of postoperative photos that adhere to the photographic standards of the ASPS, sign a consent for use of images on social media, and post as a *before and after* in the same style as the other images on your account.
d. Ask her to continue to post photos of herself using these same techniques while *tagging* you, and additionally to add #bestplasticsurgeonever to the post.
e. Answers a and d.
f. Answers b and c.

1. **Answer: d.** Choice a is incorrect because it is ***not*** clear that her daughter is the appropriate surrogate decision-maker. She could be if she was designated by a DPOA-H document, or if there was no other available next-of-kin. Choice b is incorrect because even if documentation was produced confirming that the patient would ***not want to live on a ventilator***, it is imprudent to make a hasty decision in the acute setting, as it is not clear that the patient will need to ***live on the vent*** and may be weaned expeditiously. Choice c is incorrect because the patient has a next-of-kin who is available to aid with decisions, using substituted judgment (i.e., speaking to what the patient would want for himself if he could speak). Choice e is also incorrect—the ***two-MD consent*** is a misnomer that refers to cases where an urgent or emergent procedure is needed and delaying the procedure would result in significant harm to the patient. This is more accurately characterized as ***presumed consent*** (where it is presumed that most reasonable people would prefer the urgent operation), and some hospitals have a policy that the urgency of the situation has to be documented by a second MD. This concept does not apply in this scenario. Choice d is the correct answer because it facilitates a more in-depth assessment of the values that seemingly conflict in this case. The issues that require clarifying are: whether the daughter is the appropriate surrogate decision-maker; if she is, whether she is truly making judgments that reflect the patient's values. Living wills are documents that are executed by persons to guide end-of-life care. They are helpful in guiding decisions when a patient has a terminal diagnosis, which is not the case in this scenario. In most cases, it is not necessary to consult a hospital ethics committee; their expertise can help guide cases or mediate disputes when there is a conflict in values.

2. **Answer: b.** Parents are not allowed to make decisions that will harm their child. Articulation errors continue to worsen when palates are not repaired by 12 months. So, d is incorrect because it would allow his palate to go unrepaired until 18 months. Getting Child Protective Services involved can be the ***encouragement*** that a family might need to adhere to surgical recommendations so that a situation as in c is not needed.

3. **Answer: d.** Identifying patient information, including photos, should be handled in a manner compliant with HIPAA, and if photos are used to do anything other than direct patient care, such as education or in a promotional way on social media, specific consent for those uses must be obtained.

4. **Answer: a.** Apologizing, being honest, and discussing steps that are being taken to prevent the error from occurring again in the future is the best way to approach errors. The other answers involve deception.

5. **Answer: e.** The ASPS Code of Ethics specifically addresses deceptive or misleading practices in advertising and these tenets apply to posts on social media accounts as well. Choice a is incorrect because even if the patient has given tacit consent by putting her image online, the image uses ***different light, poses, or photographic techniques to misrepresent the results achieved by the individual***, which is forbidden. Choice d violates that same principle and but also violates the admonition to not claim superiority over other surgeons with similar training. Only answers b and c adhere to the guidelines set forth by the ASPS.

CHAPTER 18 Principles of Research Designs and Outcomes Research

Chelsea A. Harris and Kevin C. Chung

KEY POINTS

- How to develop and evaluate a research question
- Defining populations and sampling techniques
- Major statistical terms and concepts
- Prominent study designs
- Sources of bias

Statistical thinking will one day be as necessary a qualification for efficient citizenship as the ability to read and write.

H.G. Wells

Medical knowledge is expanding at exponential rates. In 1950, scholars estimated that it would take 50 years for medical knowledge to double; by 2010, this period had shrunk to just 3.5 years. If trends continue, by 2020, medical knowledge will double in a mere 73 days. In this climate of ever-increasing information, being able to design impactful studies and interpret the medical literature is essential to being an effective academic plastic surgeon. This chapter will review the fundamental principle of research design.

DEVELOPING YOUR RESEARCH QUESTION

Answering the *Who Cares?* Question

Formulating a good research question is at the core of performing excellent research (**Figure 18.1**). Without an impactful question, researchers risk wasting time and effort on a problem no one cares about solving. In fact, selecting meaningless research topics may actually make it harder for others to obtain relevant, quality data by forcing them to sift through more low-quality data in what is often an already crowded field. Thus, when beginning a project, researchers must first be able to make a strong case to potential readers why they should care. For more experienced researchers, a reminder to answer the *Who cares?* question may seem obvious. However, habitually evaluating topics through this lens will help the team make broader connections and prevent embarking on projects whose sole aim is to produce a published manuscript.

As a corollary, researchers should also carefully consider whether answering a particular question requires a scientific process. Take, for example, surgery residents' emotional well-being at work. As demonstrated by multiple randomized trials, this is a growing area of scientific interest and easily passes the *Who cares?* test. However, a study that examines whether throwing scalpels at residents damages their emotional well-being is not needed. Besides being unethical, the question is readily answerable with some common sense. Although this is clearly an extreme example, there are many instances when clinical knowledge and rational thought are sufficient, and further scientific examination is not warranted.

Finally, a focus on the *Who cares?* question should not preclude research on rare diseases or highly specific topics. Often insight derived from an esoteric project can be applied to multiple conditions or problems. Rather, investigators should begin by addressing the *Who cares?* question to help structure their approach and maximize impact. At the very least, a clearly defined case for why their work matters will facilitate later efforts to publish and disseminate their work.[1,2]

Steps to Formulating an Impactful Research Question

Once the team has selected an impactful issue, the next step is to appropriately narrow the question. For example, everyone can agree that cancer is an important topic; however, the question *What causes cancer?* is clearly too broad. Adapting the PICOS criteria (**Figure 18.2**), which were first developed in the context of structuring systematic reviews, can be helpful in systematically defining the scope of your question.[3] Of course, investigators should also be wary of narrowing their question too much, as undue restrictions can actually make performing the research more difficult and may reduce some of the potential *Who cares?* factors.

As investigators move through the PICOS criteria, they should also begin to evaluate whether their developing question is answerable with their available resources. Do they have access to the population in question? Has the relevant exposure variable been measured with enough accuracy and consistency that it can be used to generate meaningful results? Would the outcome manifest in the relevant timeframe? Prematurely attempting to answer the research question without carefully considering study feasibility is a setup for wasted effort.

Finally, prior to commencing investigation, prudent researchers must ensure that their question has not already been answered.

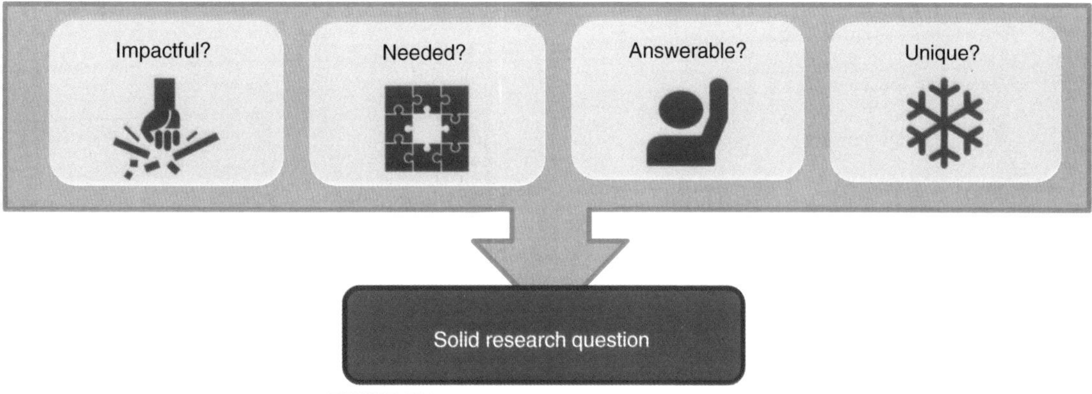

FIGURE 18.1. Developing quality research questions.

PICOS criteria	
P	Patient or population
I	Intervention
C	Comparison
O	Outcome
S	Study design

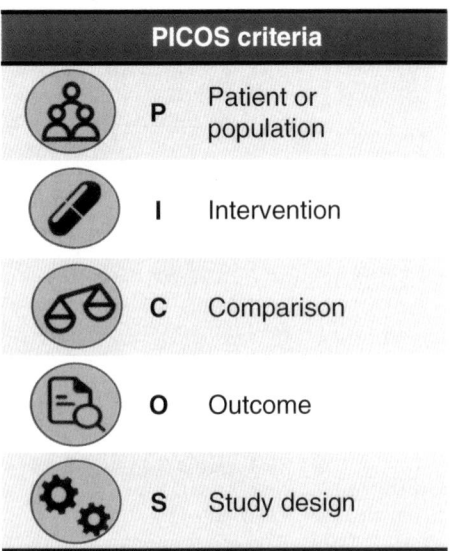

FIGURE 18.2. PICOS criteria.

A systematic literature review should readily reveal pertinent studies; however, similar publications do not necessarily mean the research team should abandon their project. Substantial differences between the published study population and the current target population, small sample sizes, serious methodologic flaws, or long time lapses all leave room for additional study. However, if the current literature fully addresses the query, it is time to come up with a new question.

SELECTING A POPULATION AND SAMPLING TECHNIQUE

Defining the population and the study sample is an important first step in beginning your research. This should begin by creating inclusion criteria (the conditions prospective subjects must meet to be relevant to the outcome) and exclusion criteria (the characteristics that disqualify prospective subjects). The pool of people who meet these clearly defined criteria represents the study population. The study sample is the subset that you will assess in the study.

Effect Size and Generalizability

How well the study sample represents the larger population from which they were drawn speaks to how generalizable the study is. In other words, the degree to which study findings apply to the greater population will depend on how closely the sample and the population match. If researchers include 100% of the parent population in their sample, their findings (assuming the study is done well) will be perfectly generalizable. If the sample is narrowed to 63-year-old men named Steve currently admitted to room 612, the findings are unlikely to be broadly applicable.

When weighing how restrictive it is to make inclusion and exclusion criteria, researchers also have to consider the anticipated effect size among different subsets of the population. Prioritizing generalizability may dilute the strength of a proposed association. For example, if a pharmacist is trying to test the benefits of a weight loss drug, including people with only 2 or 3 pounds of excess body weight may make it more difficult to demonstrate an effect than testing the drug in patients with body mass indices above 40. Although, as we will detail later, there are some statistical methods that can overcome this issue, it remains an important upfront consideration.

There are some additional nuances to note when considering population and study sample (**Figure 18.3**). First, the defining inclusion/exclusion criteria should actually be a two-staged process. When authors report inclusion and exclusion criteria in academic journals, they often include practical considerations such as the ability to speak English or ability to consent. These sorts of logistical concerns should only be applied when selecting the study sample from the population, not in defining the population itself. The goal in defining the population is to establish the boundaries of all possible study candidates based on exposures and disease potential.

Researchers must also be mindful of the *de facto* exclusion criteria they introduce in how they recruit their sample. For example, if they invite individuals to join their study through e-mail, they may unintentionally exclude people with low literacy and those with no access to a computer. As will be discussed in greater detail in the section explaining bias, researchers must carefully consider how the exclusion criteria and sampling techniques they employ may stand to alter their results.[4]

Understanding the Sampling Unit

Most data exist in some sort of structure; thus, researchers must decide at what level they wish to study. For example, if the team is interested in obesity, they could decide to study neighborhoods, families, or individuals (**Figure 18.4**). The source material (e.g., a list of all the individuals in a neighborhood) is called the *sampling frame*. The level at which subjects are enrolled (e.g., family) is called the *primary sampling unit*. If researchers then perform additional sampling that either goes into finer details (the individual) or aggregates to broader categories (neighborhood), this level is the *secondary sampling unit*.[5]

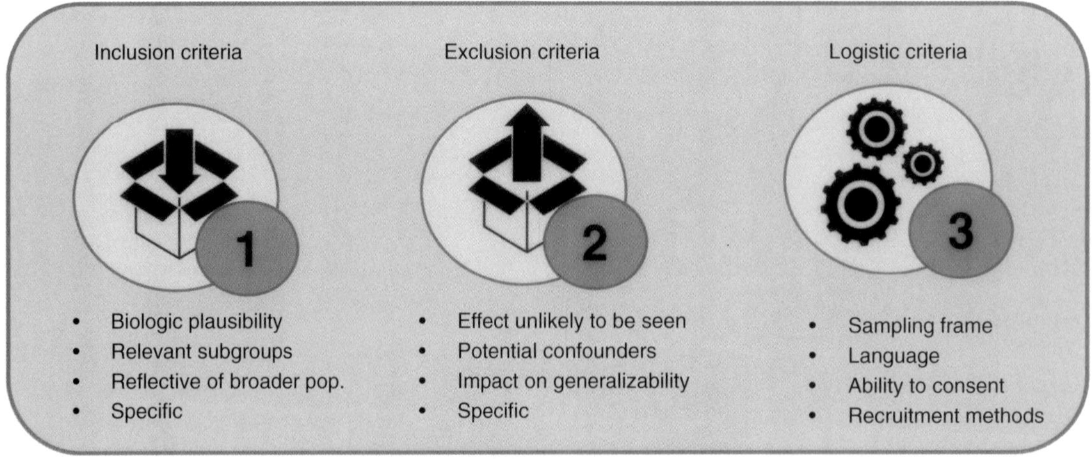

FIGURE 18.3. Steps in determining a study sample.

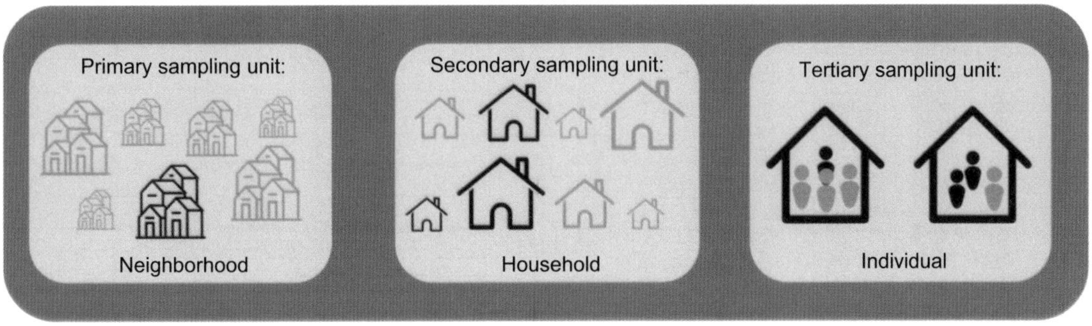

FIGURE 18.4. Examples of different sampling units.

SAMPLING TECHNIQUES

Once you have determined who should be in your study sample, the next step is to determine who you are and how you are going to assemble them. There are multiple ways researchers can create a study sample, each with distinct benefits and drawbacks (**Table 18.1**). Researchers must carefully evaluate how these features will affect their ability to answer the question of interest. Sampling only deals with how you include people in your sample; it is not synonymous with randomization, meaning if the study protocol has two arms, sampling does not describe who gets intervention (more on this distinction later).[6]

Nonprobability Sampling

Convenience sampling is probably the most common form of nonprobability sampling. As the name suggests, this sampling method basically says, "Well, this is the group to which we have access so let's examine them." Convenience samples often tap into existing clusters or structures. Common examples include patients at a given clinic, members of a specific residency program, or conference attendees. The benefit of this method (and why it is usually employed) is that it is easy: a group of individuals with appropriate demographic characteristics are already assembled, and researchers can often leverage existing relationships to encourage participation. The drawback of this approach is that factors that caused this group to assemble in the first place may cause the study sample to be substantially different than the general population, which introduces bias and limits generalizability. Patients with diabetes who attend a clinic in an affluent area may differ substantially from those in a resource-poor location; residents at urban programs may have different attitudes than those in rural programs; conference attendees may be more attuned to medical developments than those in community practice. Convenience trade-offs may have direct impact on study results.

Probability Sampling

Simple Random Sampling

Simple random sampling describes randomly drawing a subset of individuals from a broader population. Statisticians have developed many different ways to perform simple random sampling, but the most straightforward way is to assign each unit or individual a number and then use a random number generator to select them.

In addition, simple random sampling can be done with or without replacement. This can be understood by picturing a bunch of numbered balls in a jar. To draw the sample, a ball is randomly pulled from the jar and its number is noted. If the study protocol does not include replacement, the ball is taken out of the jar permanently; if replacement is allowed, the ball is returned to the jar, meaning it can be selected multiple times before enrollment is complete. Simple random sampling with replacement is not often used in creating real-world samples of individuals but is often used to build hypothetical samples in complex statistical models.

TABLE 18.1. SUMMARY OF SAMPLING TECHNIQUES

Sampling Type	Method	Benefits	Drawbacks
Convenience sampling	Drawn from a population to which you have easy access	■ Fast, easy	■ Often not representative
		■ Existing relationship with subjects	■ Subject to volunteer bias
			■ Difficult to generalize
Simple random sampling	Subject are pooled together and randomly selected, can be with or without replacement	■ Does not require detailed knowledge of population at start	■ Difficult to achieve in large populations
		■ Decreases sampling bias	■ May not include members of small subgroups due to chance
		■ If done well, findings are generalizable	■ Can have unequal group size
Systematic sampling	Subjects are grouped based on important characteristics first, then random sampling within subgroups	■ Ensures sample reflects parent population	■ Labor-intensive
		■ With oversampling can target important subgroups	■ Requires detailed knowledge of parent population
Block sampling	Randomly enrolls subjects in equal-sized blocks	■ Ensures equal group sizes	■ May not evenly distribute confounders
		■ Can be fixed or random blocks	■ May be predictable, which allows investigators to *game* results

Systematic Sampling

To perform systematic sampling, researchers must first select their sampling frame or the source from which participants will be identified. They then proceed through the sampling frame in a systematic way. The Framingham Study is perhaps the most famous example of systematic sampling. In it, researchers listed every household in Framingham, Massachusetts, alphabetically and then selected every third household for long-term follow-up.[7]

Sources of bias from systematic sampling come from how the sampling frame is selected and from ordering of subjects, for example, say researchers decide to recruit every 10th person listed in the phone book. Their sampling frame (phone book) will cause a selection bias because they may exclude young people who are unlikely to have landlines and individuals who cannot afford phones. Additionally, their sampling technique may lead to nonrandom selection as last names are more likely to begin with certain letters.

Stratified Sampling

Stratified random sampling is used when the research team does not want to leave the distribution of a certain characteristic in their study to chance. This process starts by dividing the population into groups based on the demographic characteristic of interest (e.g., race, age, BMI). Simple random sampling is then used to select a subset within each group to make up the overall study sample.

Researchers can also decide whether they want their stratified sample to be representative, with sample proportions matching those seen in the greater population. For example, if people with blood groups AB, A, B, and O make up 1%, 5%, 20%, and 74% of the population, a representative stratified sample of 100 people would include 1 person with AB type blood, 5 with A, 20 with B, and 74 with O, each of whom was randomly selected from a group of people with the same blood time. If researchers are particularly interested in a certain group, they may elect to oversample. For example, if researchers believe that posttransfusion complications are most likely to occur in people with blood group A, they may elect to create a sample with 50 blood group A individuals and only 44 blood group O.

Block Sampling

Block sampling combines concepts from several previously discussed samples. In this approach, researchers define demographic categories of interest (blocks), the number of subjects they want in each block, and then proceed with their sampling technique. To illustrate how this works, we will say the researchers want a sample with three white subjects, three black subjects, and three Asian subjects, and they plan on using simple random sampling. Sampling commences, and the first few draws are black, white, Asian, Asian, white, white. At this point, the investigators have met target enrollment for the white block, so even if the next randomly selected subject is white, that person will be excluded, and they will continue drawing until the system selects a black or Asian subject. This process continues randomly drawing over and over until each category is filled.

This technique may be used if when the research team has a good theoretic reason to suspect the demographic characteristic will affect the study outcomes (meaning they want to include enough subjects to adequately power subgroup analyses), but they do not have enough accurate data to divide the population *a priori* and perform stratified random sampling.

CREATING THE ANALYTIC PLAN

Now that the research team has defined the study population and sampling techniques, it is time to determine the analytic plan. To do this, the team must systematically think through the kind of data they want to collect, define their variables, and create a clear map of how variables affect one another. These steps will ensure rigorous data collection and will also determine the analytic techniques used to interpret the data.

Understanding Variable Types

- *Dichotomous variables:* variables have only two possible outcomes: yes/no, positive/negative, complete/incomplete.
- *Categorical variables:* as the name suggests, *categorical* denotes a variable that can have a limited (usually fixed) number of values (i.e., it can fall into one of several categories).
  - *Ordinal variables:* are categorical variables that have a specific and consistent order. For example, scales assessing frequency (often [1], sometimes [2], rarely [3], never [4]) represent four response categories in which the lower number always means higher frequency.
  - *Nominal variables:* are categorical variables with no intrinsic value. Color is a classic example. Unlike ordinal variables where progression matters, ordinal variable coding is arbitrary.
- *Continuous variables:* variables that have an infinite number of possible values and unit increase is consistent across all parts of the spectrum (i.e., an increase in 1 degree Fahrenheit means the same temperature increase whether the system moves from 20 to 21 degrees or 83 to 84 degrees). Standard arithmetic can be performed on continuous variables, in this case, calculating the average temperature.
- *Count variables:* similar to continuous variables in that one unit increase denoted the same amount across the entire spectrum; however, count variables are finite because they take up time or space. Take, for example, the cigarettes smoked per day. At low amount numbers, this variable behaves exactly like a continuous variable: moving from three cigarettes smoked per day to four is exactly the same unit increase as moving from six to seven. However, unlike continuous variables, which progress uniformly to infinity, count variables have an upper limit. Because it takes time to smoke a cigarette, there comes a point when the number of cigarette smoked per day simply cannot get higher, and this can change the analytic techniques used to describe these variables.

Building Your Conceptual Model: Assigning Variables

Next, researchers should build a simple conceptual model to clearly define their outcome of interest, the predictors of the outcomes, and other variables that may affect their results (**Figure 18.5**). Because the terminology here is often challenging, we will walk through this step using wound healing.

Predictor Variables

If you moved through the PICOS process thoughtfully, you should have already identified variable predictor variables (often called independent variables or exposure variables; the value is plotted on

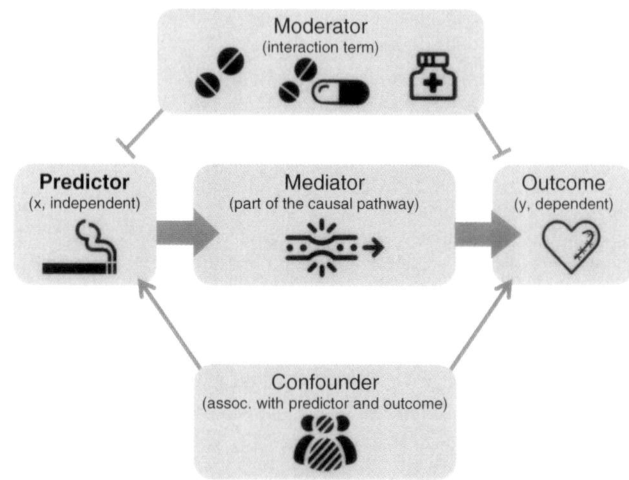

FIGURE 18.5. Relationship of study variables.

the x-axis): this is the factor that you believe drives the outcomes of interest (wound healing). For the purpose of this example, we will use smoking status. Now, based on your data, you may have to make some decisions as to how to approach this variable. Smoking status could be a dichotomous (smoker versus nonsmoker), ordinal (daily, weekly, monthly, never), or count variable (note: This is *not* a continuous variable because unless patients are smoking more than one cigarette at a time, the time it takes to smoke each one puts an upper limit on how many they could possibly smoke per day). Variable type will have an impact on how you power your study so this is important to consider early on.

Confounding Variables

Once you have your predictor, you must then identify the confounding variables. To be a confounder, each candidate variable must meet two conditions. First, it must be independently associated with the main exposure (predictor variable). Additionally, although this may seem obvious, confounders must be present before the exposure in question. For instance, smokers who develop lung disease may eventually take oral steroids, which are known to delay wound healing. However, steroid usage would not qualify as a confounder if the patient started taking them months after they developed a wound.[8]

Second, to qualify as a confounder, the variable must be associated, but not a product of, the outcome. For example, although decreased quality of life may be correlated with poor wound healing, it is more likely to be a result of an open wound rather than a predicting factor, and therefore would not qualify. A useful thought experiment to check if a candidate variable is indeed a confounder is to ask if it is predictive of the outcome independent of its association with the predictor.

Mediators

Mediators are variables that are directly part of the causal pathway. In this example, tissue ischemia would qualify because smoking causes vasoconstriction leading to tissue ischemia, which then produces poor wound healing. Often mediators are difficult to measure directly, so the predictor acts as a surrogate variable. There are no empiric tests that differentiate mediators from confounders; the distinction is based purely on the research team's theoretical framework.

Moderators

Moderators (also called interaction terms) are factors *that change the magnitude* or the direction of the effect the predictor has on the outcome. In contrast to mediators, which you can identify by asking "How does smoking cause poor wound healing?" you can identify moderators when the answer to "Does smoking cause ischemia?" is "It depends on the circumstance." This relationship can be difficult to conceptualize, so we will offer several ways to think about it. First, imagine that you plot the number of cigarettes smoked per day for everyone in your sample on the *x* axis, and the number of days it takes for their wound to heal on the *y*. You make a line of best fit and note a positive linear relationship between daily cigarette number and length of wound healing. Now, to identify moderators, you start trying to pinpoint factors that could increase or decrease the effect smoking has on wound healing.

In this case, you hypothesize that anticoagulation will change the effect smoking has on wound healing by lessening the negative effects of vasoconstriction. To test this, you divide your sample based on intensity of anticoagulation regimen: no medication, aspirin alone, aspirin plus clopidogrel, warfarin. You still plot cigarettes smoked per day on the *x* axis and days to healing on the y, but instead of a single line for the whole sample, each medication subgroup gets its own line (**Figure 18.6**). In this hypothetical example, you can see that cigarette number has a big impact on people who are not on anticoagulation (steep slope), but almost no effect on patients taking warfarin (the line is essentially flat). This demonstrates that moderators change the strength of the association between the predictor and the outcome.[9]

HYPOTHESIS TESTING

Now that we have covered how to design a research question, identify and sample the study population, and define variables, the next step is to understand how you can test your hypothesis. Here we will review the basics of inferential statistics.

The Null and Alternative Hypotheses

The *null hypothesis* (H_0) is the basis of formal statistical significance testing. It is essentially a default hypothesis that states "there is no effect" or "there is no difference between these two populations." By using the null hypothesis as a starting point, statistical tests can then estimate the probability that an association of the magnitude seen in the study is due to chance. Conversely, the *alternative hypothesis* (H_1) states that there is an effect or a difference between study populations. To indicate that an association between the predictor variable and the outcome variable exists, one can either reject the null hypothesis or accept the alternative hypothesis. The significance testing methodology differs slightly between rejecting the null hypothesis and accepting the alternative, but a general discussion is enough for our purposes.[10]

Effect Size

Effect size is a numerical representation of the magnitude of the association between the predictor and the outcome variable. In other words: how big was the impact of the intervention. As will be discussed in more depth later, effect size is important because it affects power calculations. This makes intuitive sense: if the effect size is big, like that seen with a pill that causes patients to lose 30 pounds in 2 weeks, the research team will not need to enroll many people in their study before they see an impact. If the effect size is smaller, say 1 or 2 pounds over a year, the team will have to enroll many more people to overcome the noise of everyday weight fluctuation to show a consistent trend toward decreased weight.

In reality, it is difficult to know exactly what the effect size will be prior to the trial. It should therefore be estimated using both existing data and a determination of what a meaningful difference should be. It may be possible to complete a study that shows a diet pill produces a 1- or 2-pound yearly weight loss, but if the effect is not clinically meaningful, completing the study may not be a good use of resources.

Significance Testing: Alpha and *P* Values

To test whether study results are statistically significant, that is, if a real difference is indeed present, researchers must first set their alpha (commonly reported in the medical literature as a *P* value). Alpha (α) is the

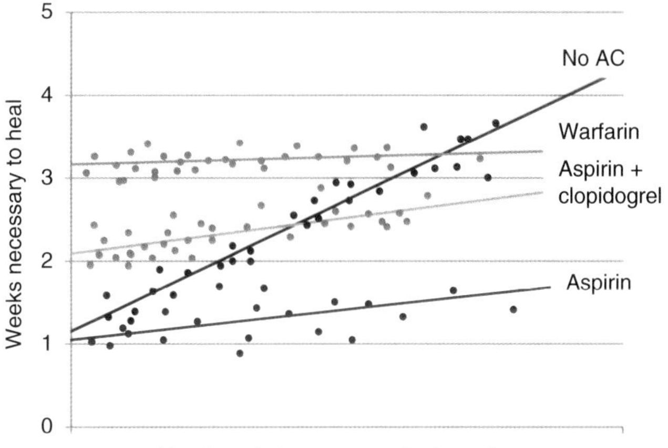

FIGURE 18.6. Representation of interaction terms. Example shows relationship between smoking and wound healing by anticoagulation regimen.

probability that you would find an effect size (or a difference between populations) of the same magnitude or larger, if the null hypothesis was true. In medicine, alpha is commonly set to 5% ($P = 0.05$).

A useful way to think about this operationally is in the context of a trial comparing the effects of identical drugs, where we know the null hypothesis is true. For example, say the research team drew up a sample and randomized half to get a blood pressure medication as a square pill, and the other half to get an identical dose, only in a round form. Both study groups faithfully take the drug for a month, and then come back to have their blood pressure measured. We would expect that because the drug is identical, it would have exactly the same effect in both groups. This is indeed true most of the time, but because blood pressure fluctuates, some people may have a higher or lower reading just by chance. If the people with a higher reading are randomly concentrated in group A and the people with a lower reading are randomly concentrated in group B, it will appear as though the round pill worked better. Setting the alpha at 5% means that if the study team repeated the experiment 100 times, there would be five instances where low blood pressure people are randomly clustered together because of chance alone. Incorrectly stating that there is a difference when none exists is a *type 1 error*.[11]

Power and Beta

Beta (β) describes the probability of accepting the null hypothesis (reporting that the drug did not work, or there was no difference between populations) when a difference truly does exist. In medical literature, beta is commonly set at 0.20; however, like alpha this is a theoretical not an absolute distinction. In cases for which the outcome is particularly dire, such as deaths secondary to consuming contaminated drinking water, a 20% chance of missing a mortality difference between a population consuming clean and contaminated water may be unacceptable. Thus, cutoffs must be tailored to the clinical question.

In study design, power equals [1 − beta], and it represents the probability of correctly rejecting the null hypothesis if the actual effect size is equal to or greater than the one specified in the study. Setting a certain power does not mean it is impossible to detect an effect size smaller than the one specified, it just makes it less likely. Incorrectly accepting the null hypothesis, that is, saying that there is no difference between populations when one truly exists, is a *type II error*.[12]

Normal Distribution

Another important step in evaluating study results is looking at the distribution of your data. Many statistical models are built around the normal (Gaussian) distribution. The normal distribution is a continuous probability distribution in which the mean and variance are not dependent on each other, meaning you can increase or decrease one without changing the other's value. Data that are normally distributed are symmetrical, and the mean, median, and mode are identical. Researchers have to understand whether their data are normally distributed because parametric statistics, such as t-tests and ANOVA (described in the next section), include assumptions that the data are normal.

In addition to the eyeball test (*do my data look normal?*), there are several tests including evaluating skewness and kurtosis that can more formally quantify normality, but those are beyond the scope of the discussion here. Additionally, if sample size is below 30, this usually means you cannot assume data are normally distributed.[13]

Basic Statistics

Comparing Populations

Understanding these basic tenets allows us to perform statistical tests to evaluate whether the differences we observe between populations in our study are due to chance alone. This section is meant to provide a brief overview and is in no way a comprehensive report of all statistical options. Comparison tests are summarized in **Table 18.2**.[14]

- *t-test:* used to compare means and thus requires normally distributed data so the means are not skewed by extreme outliers. Standard t-tests are used to describe two unrelated groups (the average GPAs of premedical students versus engineers), whereas paired t-tests are used to compare the same group at different times (the average GPAs of a group of premedical students their first, second, and third years of school).
- *Analysis of variance (ANOVA):* works like a t-test but compares multiple rather than two groups (the average GPA of premedical students, engineers, and political scientists). ANOVA can be one-way like in the example just described, or two-way where we would compare GPA not just across major but also by gender. Importantly, if ANOVA is statistically significant, it doesn't say which groups are different from one another, just that they are different.[15]
- *Chi-square tests:* used when comparing dichotomous or categorical data expressed as a proportion. For example, a chi-square could be used to compare the proportion of women across residency programs. Like ANOVA, this test can be used to compare multiple groups but does not specify where the difference between groups resides.
- *Fisher's exact test:* also compares dichotomous or categorical data expressed as a proportion but is used in instances where there are very few observations (often <30).

TABLE 18.2. STATISTICAL TEST EVALUATION

Predictor (Independent) Variable	Outcome (Dependent) Variable	Example	Parametric Tests (Assumes Normal Distribution)	Nonparametric Tests
Dichotomous	Continuous	Mean exam score of two classrooms	t-test	Wilcoxon Rank Sum
Pre-post test	Continuous	Mean exam score before and after a new study technique	Paired t-test	
Dichotomous, Categorical Ordinal	Categorical	Proportion of women in class	Chi-square	N/A
Categorical	Continuous	Mean exam score of different college majors	ANOVA	Kruskal-Wallis
Continuous	Dichotomous	Active smokers by age	Logit or probit function	N/A
Continuous	Continuous	Age and weight	Pearson correlation or ordinary least squares regression	Spearman correlation

Evaluating Tests

Learners should also be able to use 2 × 2 tables, a favorite in many medical standardized tests, to evaluate screening tests and population impact (**Figure 18.7**). These values are sensitive to changes in disease prevalence, which makes intuitive sense. If a disease is enormously rare, a positive test is more likely to be a false positive than a true positive.[16]

- *Sensitivity*: the ability of the test to detect the disease: A/(A + C)
- *Specificity:* the ability of the test to correctly identify true negatives: D/(D + B)
- *Positive predictive value:* if the test is positive, how likely is it to be a true positive: A/(A + C)
- *Negative predictive value:* if the test is negative, how likely is it to be a true negative: D/(D + C)

Risk and Incidence

Incidence describes the number of new cases over a set period, whereas *prevalence* describes the number of existing cases at a single point in time. The risk of developing a condition can then be described using the same 2 × 2 table, except that, instead of test positivity, the left column now denotes exposure positivity.

- *Relative risk (RR):* compares the incidence of disease (for example, new cases of thyroid cancer) between two populations (e.g., people living near Chernobyl versus Americans). Note, because this is based on incidence, relative risk is appropriate for studies that follow up people over time, but cannot be used for those that simply provide a snapshot in time.

$$RR = \frac{(\#\text{ cases in exposed population / total exposed population})}{(\#\text{ cases in unexposed population / total unexposed population})}$$

or

$$RR = [A / (A + C)] / [C / (C + D)]$$

- *Absolute risk reduction:* quantifies how much the risk for the disease goes down if you were able to eliminate the exposure.

$$ARR = (\text{incidence in exposed}) - (\text{incidence in unexposed})$$

$$ARR = [A / (A + C)] = [C / (C + D)]$$

- *Number needed to treat (NNT):* indicates the number of people we would need to treat who would derive no benefit, in order to prevent one person from developing the disease.

$$NNT = 1 - ARR$$

- *Odds ratio (OR):* compares the prevalence of the disease across populations. It is the odds that the outcome will occur after a given exposure, that is, the odds of disease in exposed versus odds of disease in unexposed (e.g., if you are exposed to radiation, what are your odds of developing thyroid cancer).

$$OR = \frac{(\#\text{ cases in exposed population / }\#\text{ non - cases in exposed population})}{(\#\text{ cases in unexposed / }\#\text{ non - cases in unexposed population})}$$

or

$$[(A / B)] / (C / D) \longrightarrow AD / BC$$

	Disease (+)	Disease (−)
Test (+)	A True positive	B False positive (type I error, α)
Test (−)	C False negative (type II error, β)	D True negative

FIGURE 18.7. 2 x 2 contingency table of possible test results and disease status.

STUDY DESIGN

Finally, all these come together in the overall study design (**Table 18.3**).

Observational Studies

Observational studies are used when sufficient randomization is not possible. They can either characterize the distribution of relevant predictor and outcome variables in a study (descriptive) or seek to quantify the relationship between the predictor and outcome variable (analytic).

Cross-sectional studies are studies that perform one-time measurements to offer a single snapshot in time. The strengths of this approach include that they are often relatively easy to perform and they can be used to examine multiple predictors and outcomes. These studies are primarily descriptive. Although they can be used to examine associations between predictor and outcome variables, they risk missing broader trends that more robust study designs would detect.

For example, suppose researchers wanted to examine the effects of a handwashing intervention on central line–associated bloodstream infection (CLABSI) rates. To test their intervention, they tally the CLABSI rate for October, make all the hospital staff attend a handwashing seminar on October 31, and then tally the CLABSI rate at the end of November. If the rate goes down, they might conclude that their seminar worked. However, by only measuring two points, the researchers may be missing broader trends. If instead they performed a *time series analysis* and plot the CLABSI rate for the last 12 months, it becomes evident that the trend was already moving toward decreased infection, and the handwashing seminar did nothing to change the slope of the trajectory.

Case-Control Studies

In conditions where an outcome is rare, it can be difficult to generate meaningful information using a cross-sectional approach because a massive sample is needed to generate even a few cases. In these instances, case-control studies are appropriate. Here, individuals with the known outcome are identified (cases), and their values for potentially relevant observable variables are obtained. Cases are then matched to individuals with similar characteristics who did not have the outcome (controls). The samples are compared to see if there is a common thread in the cases group that is not present in the control group that may explain the outcome. Case-control subjects can be matched proportionately (1:1) or disproportionately (1:2, 1:3). To be even more precise in establishing an effect, having several control groups is prudent to be sure that the effect detected is still seen with different control groups. However, at some point, adding more controls does not improve power to detect an effect.

This study design is good for hypothesis generation: the research team identified characteristics they think are associated with an outcome and can test this relationship in prospective studies. The

TABLE 18.3. STUDY DESIGNS

Sampling Type	Method	Benefits	Drawbacks	Analysis
Cross sectional	Measurements are drawn for a single instance in time. Design can be improved by taking multiple measurements over time	■ Less labor-intensive than other designs	■ Cannot establish sequence of events	■ Descriptive statistics
		■ Determines prevalence	■ Cannot calculate incidence	■ Time-series
		■ Can examine multiple factors	■ Hard to study rare outcomes	■ Difference-in-difference
Case-control	Matches known cases to similar control to compare predictor variables	■ Good for rare outcomes	■ Subject to recall bias	■ Descriptive statistics
		■ With oversampling can target important subgroups	■ Can be difficult to appropriately match controls	■ Odds ratio
Cohort	Longitudinal study, enrolls subjects tracks outcomes over time	■ Better way to examine causality	■ Expensive, time-intensive	■ Incidence
		■ Unbiased measurement of predictor variables	■ Inefficient for rare outcomes	■ Relative risk
			■ Loss-to-follow-up is a major potential confounder	■ Cumulative incidence ratio
Randomized control trial	Gold standard. Subjects are randomly allocated to receive intervention or control, and outcomes are measured	■ Balances measured and unmeasured confounders	■ Expensive, time-intensive	■ Per-protocol
		■ Ability to make casual inference	■ Strict selection may limit generalizability	■ As-treated
			■ Loss-to-follow-up is a major threat	■ Intention-to-treat

weaknesses of this approach are that it is a retrospective design (the outcomes must be known at the start of the study) and there is substantial potential for recall bias. Case subjects may be highly attuned to factors that caused their outcomes, whereas controls may not remember exposures in as much detail. Additionally, it may be difficult to find appropriately matched controls.

Cohort Studies

Cohort studies are studies that examine a group of people and follow them up over time. Cohort studies can be prospective, meaning a group of people are identified at the study outset and they are followed up for relevant outcome or they can be retrospective, where baseline characteristics and follow-up data have already been collected. One of the major advantages of prospective cohort studies, the most famous of which is probably the Framingham Study, is that because they are longitudinal, they can establish incidence. In addition, establishing time sequences between predictors and outcomes helps establish causality.

The major drawbacks of cohort studies come from their logistical challenges. It is often costly and labor-intensive to follow up people for long periods. As noted previously, if an outcome is rare, researchers must enroll large samples in order to achieve adequate power. In addition, loss-to-follow up is a common problem, and because it is often nonrandom (meaning people drop out of the study for specific reasons), assessing relevant confounders can prove difficult. Some of these can be overcome with a retrospective design, but there are usually trade-offs in data quality because the team may not have had oversight in what data were collected or how rigorous the approach was.[17]

Randomized Controlled Trials

Randomized controlled trials are the gold standard for study design. The strength of this approach rests on adequate randomization, as this ensures that both measured and unmeasured confounders are equally distributed in both study arms. Once confounding is balanced, it is easier to attribute observed effects to the intervention and suggest causality.

Randomization

Randomization is distinct from sampling and describes the process of determining who gets the intervention, not who is included in the study. This can be confusing as the terminology is similar. Simple randomization involves sorting participants into the intervention or control group using some randomizer (coin flip, dice roll, envelope draw). Where possible, research personnel should be blinded to the randomization to prevent unintentional biases from contaminating the effects and to prevent attempt to *game* the system and enroll certain participants in a given arm. A problem with some simple randomization methods is that they do not always produce even groups (e.g., three heads, seven tails). This can be overcome by block randomization. Here participants are randomly assigned to the heads (intervention) or tails (control) arm based on a coin flip until the heads block is filled, at which point the remaining participants are assigned to the control.

It is also important to distinguish stratified random *sampling* from stratified *randomization,* as these processes are two distinct steps (**Figure 18.8**). As previously described, in stratified random sampling, the parent population is divided into subgroups based on a certain characteristic (e.g., race, age, income), and participants are randomly selected within those categories. This process has no bearing on what treatment a given individual gets, rather it simply describes how the group eligible for randomization is assembled. In fact, if the study sample is created by stratified random sampling, but simple randomization is used to determine who gets treatment, the intervention and control arms could be highly unbalanced.

Stratified randomization ensures that important covariates are evenly distributed between study arms. This technique is especially helpful in small trails where chance is more likely to lead to demographic imbalance between arms. Stratified sampling works by dividing the already selected study sample into groups based on known predictors. Group members are then block-randomized separately, ensuring that the proportion of individuals with a given characteristic is equal in both arms. Stratified randomization can be used to account for multiple covariates, but this adds significant logistical complexity.

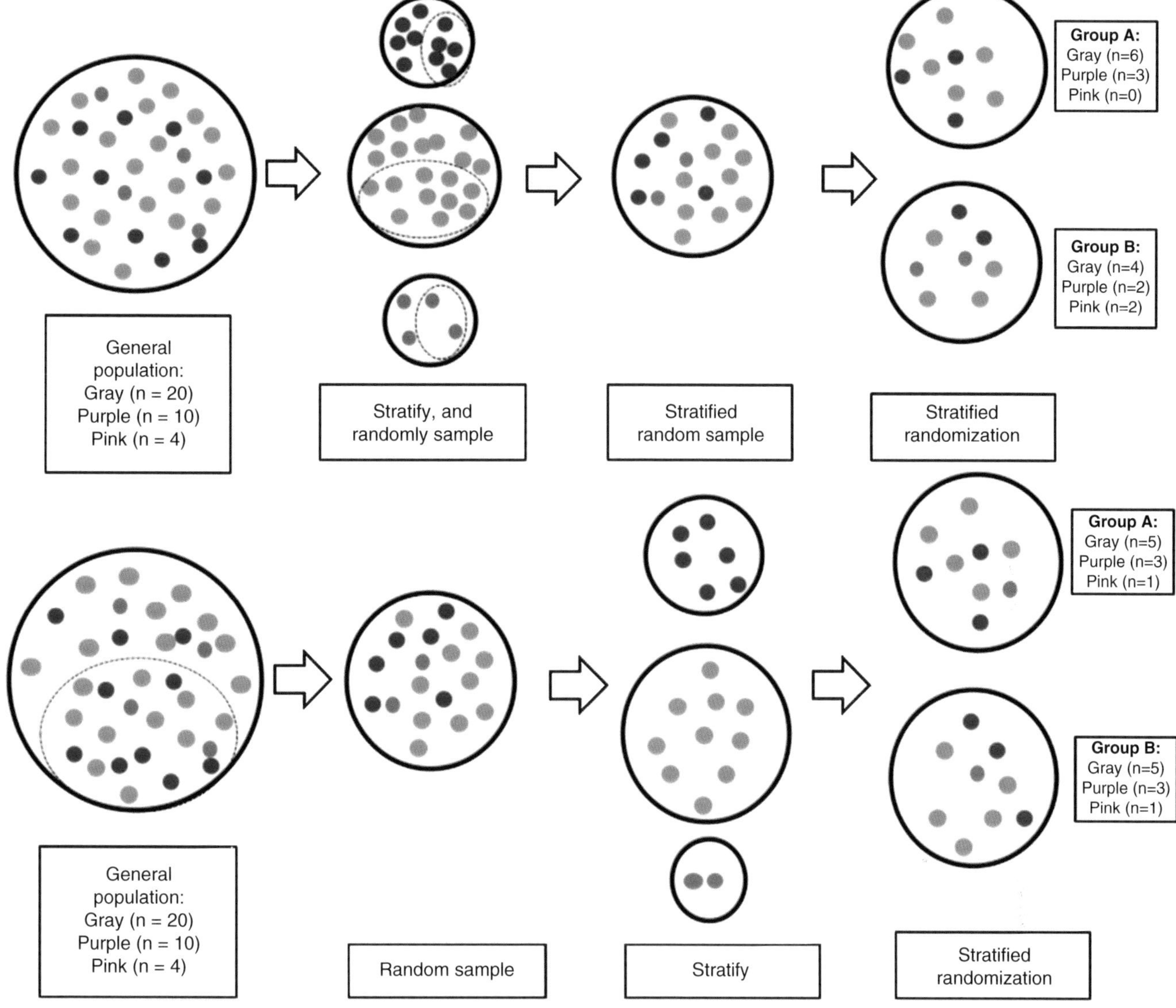

FIGURE 18.8. Stratified random sampling versus stratified randomization.

CONCLUSION

Understanding study design and basic statistics is fundamental to being able to evaluate the medical literature. This chapter should provide a solid overview of these topics and assist budding researchers in designing and evaluating future studies.

REFERENCES

1. Burns PB, Chung KC. Developing good clinical questions and finding the best evidence to answer those questions. *Plast Reconstr Surg*. 2010;126(2):613-618.
   This article methodically reviews the necessary steps in formulating and evaluating good research questions for evidence-based medicine. This is a fundamental first step in engaging in and evaluating scholarly work. The authors review the types of research questions scholars may ask, the PICO framework, and hierarchies of evidence.
2. Boynton PM, Greenhalgh T. Selecting, designing, and developing your questionnaire. *Br Med J*. 2004;328(7451):1312-1315.
3. Liberati A, Altman DG, Tetzlaff J, et al. The PRISMA statement for reporting systematic reviews and meta-analyses of studies that evaluate healthcare interventions: explanation and elaboration. *Br Med J*. 2009;339:b2700.
4. Ferguson CJ. An effect size primer: a guide for clinicians and researchers. *Prof Psychol Res Pract*. 2009;40(5):532-538.
5. Lavrakas P. *Encyclopedia of Survey Research Methods*. Sage Publishing; 2008.
6. Hulley SB, Newman TB, Cummings SR. *Choosing the study subjects: specification, sampling and recruitment*. In: *Designing Clinical Research*. Philadelphia, PA: Lippincott Williams & Wilkins; 2007.
   This chapter outlines the core principles in subject selection, sampling, and recruitment. Understanding how to define and build a study cohort is an integral part of health services research. This text reviews the benefits and drawbacks of various sampling and recruitment techniques and clearly demonstrates how sampling decisions will affect the conclusions study teams may draw from their results.
7. *Epidemiological Background and Design: The Framingham Study*. 2018. https://www.framinghamheartstudy.org/fhs-about/history/epidemiological-background/. Accessed April 26, 2018.
8. Maldonado G, Greenland S. Simulation study of confounder-selection strategies. *Am J Epidemiol*. 1993;138(11):923-936.
9. Baron RM, Kenny DA. The moderator mediator variable distinction in social psychological-research: conceptual, strategic, and statistical considerations. *J Pers Soc Psychol*. 1986;51(6):1173-1182.
10. Kass RE, Raftery AE. Bayes factors. *J Am Stat Assoc*. 1995;90(430):773-795.
11. George BJ, Beasley TM, Brown AW, et al. Common scientific and statistical errors in obesity research. *Obesity (Silver Spring, Md)*. 2016;24(4):781-790.
12. Chung KC, Kalliainen LK, Hayward RA. Type II (beta) errors in the hand literature: the importance of power. *J Hand Surg Am*. 1998;23(1):20-25.
13. Salkind N. *Encyclopedia of Research Design*. Sage Publishing; 2010.
14. Song JW, Haas A, Chung KC. Applications of statistical tests in hand surgery. *J Hand Surg*. 2009;34(10):1872-1881.
    This article provides an introduction to basic statistical concepts necessary for interpreting medical literature. The authors describe hypothesis testing, review different types of data, and explain how parametric and nonparametric statistical tests can be used to compare groups.
15. Lakens D. Calculating and reporting effect sizes to facilitate cumulative science: a practical primer for t-tests and ANOVAs. *Front Psychol*. 2013;4:12.
16. Aliu O, Chung KC. Assessing strength of evidence in diagnostic tests. *Plast Reconstr Surg*. 2012;129(6):989e-998e.
17. Song JW, Chung KC. Observational studies: cohort and case-control studies. *Plast Reconstr Surg*. 2010;126(6):2234-2242.

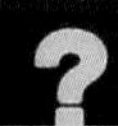

QUESTIONS

1. **Stratified random sampling does which of the following?**
   a. Ensures that sample demographics in a study's treatment arm and intervention arm are identical
   b. If sampling is proportional, ensures that study sample demographics are reflective of the larger population
   c. Always oversamples the population subset of interest
   d. Requires investigators to weight summary statistics such as sample means
   e. All of the above

2. **Sensitivity refers to:**
   a. The ability to detect all the true negatives in a population
   b. The ratio of the true negatives to true positives
   c. The probability that if a test is positive, this represents a true positive
   d. The ability of the test to detect every instance where disease is present

3. **If you are conducting a case-control trial and you discover that cases tended to eat higher-fat diets, you should convey this information using:**
   a. An odds ratio
   b. The relative risk of a high-fat diet
   c. The absolute risk reduction of a low-fat diet
   d. The incidence of a high-fat diet

4. **Disproving the null hypothesis means that:**
   a. The results are not statistically significant
   b. The observed effect size is not clinically significant
   c. The chances that you would observe an effect size equal to or greater than the one observed are below alpha
   d. The chances that you would observe an effect size equal to or greater than the one observed are below beta

5. **To be considered a confounder, a variable must:**
   a. Be part of the causal pathway
   b. Change the strength of the effect size
   c. Be present in both comparison groups
   d. Be independently associated with the main exposure

1. **Answer: b.** Stratified random sampling only concerns how a study sample is generated; it has no impact randomization (i.e., whether a given individual is in the intervention or control arm). Stratified random sampling involves breaking the population of interest into groups based on a relevant demographic, such as race or age, and then creating the study sample by randomly selecting participants within each of those groups. Randomization occurs as a second and distinct process. In simple randomization (exemplified by a coin flip), each individual in the sample population has a 50/50 chance of being in the control versus the intervention arms. This means that even though the starting study sample may have been the representative of the general population, the control and intervention arms may be significantly different from one another because of chance. Stratified randomization refers to the process whereby a randomly selected sample population is stratified to ensure that the intervention and control groups are as identical as possible for a characteristic.

2. **Answer: d.** Sensitivity refers to the ability of a diagnostic test to detect disease and is equal to the number of true positives/(true positives + false negatives). In fact, one could make a test 100% sensitive by setting it to be positive no matter what—in this case, it would detect every single positive case and there would be no false negatives. Obviously, this is not very useful in real life, but it can be helpful to remember to keep the terminology straight. This is also the basis of many screening programs: you administer a highly sensitive test first accepting that there may be some false negatives, in order not to miss anyone, and then ask people who screen positive to take a second more specific test.

3. **Answer: a.** Odds ratio is the appropriate calculation for a case-control study and would be set up as (# case high fat/# noncases high fat)/(# cases regular diet/# noncases regular diet). If the 2 × 2 table looked as follows:

	Disease + (Case)	Disease − (Control)
High fat	25	40
Regular diet	5	30

OR = (25/40)/(5/30) = 0.625/.166 = 3.8, meaning having a high-fat diet increases the odds of the outcome by 3.8 times.

4. **Answer c.** Rejecting the null hypothesis means that you are saying that the chances that you would observe an effect size equal to or greater than the one observed in the study are below your threshold for statistical significance (alpha). In real-world terms, if you were evaluating the impact of a blood pressure drug, you would first define a meaningful effect size, say a drop in systolic blood pressure of 10 mmHg. You would then perform a power calculation to determine how many people you would need to enroll in your study to see an effect that size (by convention beta is often set at 0.8). Next you set your threshold for statistical significance (alpha), which by convention is usually set to 0.05. You then administer the drug to one group and a placebo to the other and compare the results. If group A (received drug) had an 11 mmHg drop in blood pressure, group B (placebo) was unchanged, and $P < 0.05$, you could reject the null hypothesis, saying that the chances you would find a difference between group A's and group B's blood pressure equal to or greater than 11 mmHg due to chance alone are less than 5%.

5. **Answer: d.** To be a confounder, a variable must be independently associated with the main exposure and associated but not a product of the outcome. Additionally confounders must be present before the outcome of interest manifests. A variable that is part of the causal pathway is a mediator. A variable that changes the strength of the effect size is a modifier. Confounders do not have to be present in both comparison groups.

CHAPTER 19 Basic Statistics for the Practicing Physician

Damon S. Cooney and Carisa M. Cooney

KEY POINTS

- Appropriate estimation of the effect size is vital to establishing sample size and sufficiently powering a study.
- A priori (planned) analyses are considered *purest*, although post hoc (decided after the experiment and reviewing the data) analyses are acceptable so long as this is clearly stated.
- Beware of unnecessary adjustment and overadjustment when performing controlled analyses.
- Statistical significance does not necessarily indicate importance, clinical significance, or relevance of a finding.
- Consult a statistician during the study design phase to establish sample size, run a power calculation, and design the statistical plan.

USING STATISTICS TO READ AND WRITE RESEARCH STUDIES

Statistics are a growing presence affecting the practicing physician. We are increasingly surrounded by statistics in the course of the workday. Consenting patients for surgery requires a review of various risks and the likelihood with which they may occur. Educating patients about different ways to repair a defect includes outlining what can be subtle differences in postoperative quality of life or relative complication rates. Five-year survival, short- and long-term outcomes, incidence versus prevalence, *P*-values: how do all these numbers relate back to the patient in the gown and the counseling you provide? How do you know how to interpret a recent publication's findings and integrate it into your patient consultation?

Statistics can be confusing, overwhelming, and if employed incorrectly, misleading and potentially harmful. It is important not only for researchers but also for busy clinicians to have a basic understanding of how statistics should be and are used in the medical literature. This chapter is intended to provide basic guidance for clinically oriented practitioners to be able to tell when a scientific publication has employed the correct test and to provide basic information regarding statistical designs for those interested in writing grants, papers, and conducting clinical research.

Basic Terminology Helpful to This Chapter

Null hypothesis (H_0): The notion that there is no difference in the average values of the different groups being compared.

Alpha: The probability that the null hypothesis will be rejected when it is true (*false positive*).

Beta: The probability that the null hypothesis will be accepted (not rejected) when a true difference exists between the control and treatment groups (*false negative*).

Type I error: Incorrect rejection of the null hypothesis (rejecting the null hypothesis when it is true, aka, an incorrect claim of statistical significance). Also called *alpha error*.

Type II error: Incorrect acceptance of the null hypothesis (failing to reject the null hypothesis when it is false). Also called *beta error*.

Statistical power (1-beta): The likelihood with which a study can distinguish an actual effect from that which occurs by chance. Also called *sensitivity*.

Sample size (n): The total number of patients/participants included in the study.

Control group: Group to which all other comparisons will be made. May be thought of as the group most representative of *normal* (e.g., *untreated*) population.

Experimental group: Any group subjected to an intervention that could change an outcome.

Continuous variable: A variable with a numeric value that has an infinite number of possible values. This includes both infinitely large or small values and the difference between two numbers if that difference can be infinitely subdivided (e.g., age, time).

Discrete variable: A variable with a numeric value that has a finite number of possible values.

Categorical variable: A variable that contains a finite number of possible categories or distinct groups (e.g., race/ethnicity, sex). Continuous and discrete variables may be reclassified into categorical variables (e.g., BMI class, age group) to facilitate more meaningful analyses.

Dichotomous variable: A type of categorical variable that has only two possible values (e.g., yes/no, right/left).

Confidence level: The likelihood that the value of a parameter falls within a range of values (i.e., margin of error). Usually calculated at 95% or 99%.

Confidence interval (CI): Calculated from a data set: the estimated range of values likely to include an unknown variable's value (the parameter) based on the selected confidence level. The smaller the range of a CI, the more convincing the result (demonstrates less sample variability). CIs that include or cross 1 demonstrate insufficient evidence to conclude that your study groups are statistically significantly different.

Bias: A systematic error that causes one to over- or underestimate an outcome in a population. It may be introduced into one's results through sampling or measuring errors or through an unrepresentative sample.

CONSORT (Consolidated Standards of Reporting Trials): A published statement developed and refined by experts in clinical research to guide investigators toward best practices when designing and conducting clinical trials.[1] This statement is widely endorsed by leading medical journals and international editorial groups.

Absolute difference: A sum arrived at by subtracting the intervention's event rate from the baseline or expected event rate.

Relative reduction: Ratio that expresses the percent change between the absolute difference (numerator) and the baseline or expected event rate (denominator). Sometimes used because it *feels* bigger than an absolute difference; however, these ratios alone do not supply specific information about the baseline or expected event rate.

Skewedness: Non-normal data that cluster around a zero value or other natural limit. When mapped out in a histogram, the distribution may appear to lean or trail off to one side or the other.

Sample average: Value measured from sample or expected sample.

Test value: Value to which the sample average will be compared.

STATISTICAL SIGNIFICANCE

What Is and Is Not Meaningful

The most frequent way statistics tend to be used in plastic surgery is to compare two or more treatments to determine if differences exist between them. Is treatment A better than treatment B? How much better? What differences in outcomes exist between the two groups?

Between-groups differences are studied by performing repeated assessments of a chosen outcome. After selecting a way to assess potential differences, you then use statistical methods to describe and compare the groups. Unless your groups' measurements are identical, there will be a difference between them; the crucial question is whether the difference is *significant*.

Significance can be *statistical* or *clinical*. *Statistical significance* is when the difference in the between-groups measurement can be reliably reproduced and is not the result of a random data distribution that will disappear when further measured. The most frequent way in which this is determined is the *P*-value. This number indicates the probability that the between-groups difference in the data set is *not real* and that the population the groups and data represent are not different (the null hypothesis [H_0]). Therefore, the smaller the *P*-value, the more likely the between-groups difference in the data represents a true difference in the population. *Clinical significance* is when the difference in the between-groups measurement can have an impact on patient care. Interestingly, clinical significance can be present when findings are *not* statistically significant. Conversely, statistically significant findings may not be clinically significant. When putting findings in the context of clinical significance, it is important to frame the discussion using the published literature.

An increasing number of biomedical research studies are using *P*-values and placing value on results that are statistically significant. However, one must address the possibility of alpha error, the influence of sample size in determining statistical significance, and whether statistically significant findings are clinically significant.

P-Values: 0.05 and 0.01

First we should review exactly what a *P*-value means because, as was pointed out by Ioannidis in his 2018 *JAMA* article, "*P*-values are misinterpreted, over trusted, and misused in biomedical research."[2]

A *P*-value is a measurement of the strength of the evidence against a null hypothesis; the smaller the *P*-value, the stronger the evidence that you should reject the null hypothesis. Importantly, it does not represent a percent (%) value that the null hypothesis is either right or wrong. This is a subtle but important difference on how one should consider this piece of data in view of one's results.

Statistical significance is reached when a *P*-value falls below your predetermined significance level. Per convention, significance levels are commonly set at 5% ($P = 0.05$) or 1% ($P = 0.01$). Importantly, just because a finding is statistically significant does not mean it is clinically relevant, or that it has real-world significance. It simply means the two groups may be differentiated statistically. (This becomes increasingly important in the world of *big data* because merely increasing sample size increases your chances of between-group differences becoming *statistically significant*.[3]) Additional considerations for calculating significance must be made when including interim analyses in your study design.

Although you may think *P*-values only come in at the end of a study, they should be considered during the study design phase. This is because the significance level is one of the key pieces of information needed to perform power calculations and determine your study's sample size.

Note: Some debate exists within the American Statistical Association (ASA) regarding appropriate levels of significance, and a proposal has been made to lower *P*-value thresholds by an order of magnitude.[2] This may be more than what the typical plastic surgeon cares to know (particularly if it causes you to question all your previous research findings or the data on which you have been basing your practice). However, if you are concerned about this issue, the ASA's position statement on *P*-values raises some interesting arguments of which it may be helpful to be aware.[4]

POWER CALCULATIONS AND SAMPLE SIZES

Assessing differences between groups in meaningful ways can be tricky. *P*-values are a way of expressing how confident you are that the between-group differences you detected accurately represent the between-groups differences in the population from which your samples are drawn. Increasing the sample size will increase the significance of the *P*-value. The relationship of *P*-value to sample size is described by the power calculation.

Power calculations are an important way of assessing the adequacy of your proposed study sample size. For example, the smaller the difference you try to detect, the more subjects you will need to enroll. This raises the question of whether a study has enough samples, subjects, or measurements to be able to say that a statistically significant difference between groups does or does not exist.

To determine this, one has to calculate the sample size needed to *sufficiently power* the study to prove or disprove the null hypothesis. *Sufficient power* is a way of stating that based on the number of subjects enrolled, you can say with a given level of confidence that your findings are true. That being said, power calculations and determining sample size go hand-in-hand and can pose a *chicken-or-the-egg* dilemma. Whatever your approach, good research practices dictate that you must be able to describe how your sample size was determined, justify your methods (e.g., choice of population used to determine event rate, *see next section*), and include explanations of any planned interim analyses and stopping rules.[1] In short, your description should be sufficient to enable study replication.

Establishing an Anticipated Effect Size

Sample size is often calculated by a statistician and usually requires computing power. Alternatively, many sample size calculators are available on the Internet. Regardless, several specific pieces of information are needed to calculate sample size[5]:

Event rate: Estimate of the frequency of your outcome of interest in the control group by extrapolating from a population similar to the population in your study. One way to determine differences is based on how often the anticipated condition or event occurs in a given population. This can be done by ascertaining rates in the published literature or assessing rates in a local or similar population.

Note: If event rates vary widely within the published literature, you may have identified another study you can perform using either a local patient population or a population available through a previously collected database.

Smallest clinically important difference: Determine, for the primary outcome, the smallest difference that will be of clinical importance. Sometimes what is considered a clinically significant difference may not be statistically significant, and vice versa. There are several ways to determine the smallest clinically significant difference; absolute difference (found by subtracting the intervention event rate from the expected event rate) is one way to make this estimate. *Absolute difference* should not be confused with *relative reduction* (a ratio of the absolute difference divided by the event rate), which usually seems larger, may be used to make a more dramatic statement about a treatment difference than its real-world clinical reality, and provides no data regarding your starting place (the baseline or expected rate).

Power: The ability to detect a true difference between the control arm and experimental arm of a study. Power is usually determined by convention, such as 80%. Eighty percent power means there is a 20% chance that the study will not detect a true difference (*false negative* or *beta error*) between the control and experimental arms.[5] Power can be raised to 90% if desired, reducing the false-negative rate to 10%. However, increasing the study's power will increase its sample size and very likely its costs and time-to-completion.

Significance level: The likelihood of detecting a treatment effect when no effect exists (*false positive* or *alpha error*). Typically set at 5% ($P = 0.05$) or 1% ($P = 0.01$).

Additional Terms Helpful to Know[1,5,6]

Allocation ratio: The number of participants assigned to each of the study arms. Most commonly assigned in a one-to-one ratio in randomized trials, although other allocation ratios (e.g., two-to-one, three-to-two) may be used. Not relevant to retrospective studies.

Lack of compliance calculation: Adjustment made to the calculated sample size for the expected level of noncompliance participants will have with treatment. Similar to, but different from, *lost-to-follow-up adjustment*.

Lost-to-follow-up adjustment: Adjustment made to the calculated sample size in anticipation of the loss of participants (failure to complete) during the study. Similar to, but different from, *lack of compliance calculation*.

Intention-to-treat (ITT): Analysis that includes all originally enrolled participants in the final analysis even though some participants may not have provided measurements for all outcome variables. In ITT analysis, imputation using observed values is used to estimate missing data. This is recommended as the standard practice per CONSORT guidelines.[1] ITT analysis may dilute an intervention's true effect; however, its use is important to eliminate potential post hoc or selection bias.

Doing Your Homework Can Be Cost-Effective

Calculating the correct sample size for a study has important monetary and ethical consequences. Monetarily, it can be incredibly frustrating to complete a study only to realize your study was underpowered, meaning your sample size was insufficient to demonstrate statistically significant results. In addition to having insufficient funds to recruit additional participants, adding on participants at the end of the study can be viewed as methodologically questionable, potentially invalidating the entire study. Ethically, it may be unethical to enroll participants into a study that is unlikely to demonstrate statistical differences or meaningful results.[5] Either way, the result is poor.

UNDERSTANDING YOUR DATA AND APPROPRIATE ANALYSES

Getting to Know Your Data

To make informed decisions on how to analyze your data, it is vital that you familiarize yourself with your data set. When designing a study, there are certain assumptions you make a priori about the data you intend to collect. These assumptions need to be explored once you have the data to ensure that you use the correct statistical tests and adjust your analyses, if warranted.

Sociodemographic Tables

Many manuscripts include comprehensive sociodemographic tables describing the study population. These are often most informative when they compare sociodemographic characteristics between the groups. Although this may seem like a waste of journal space, it serves at least two important functions:

- *Acquaints the audience (and the authors) with the study population.* Reviewing demographic tables can inform the reader as to how similar or different the study population is from his or her own patient or study populations. This can be an indication of whether the study findings may translate to the reader's patient population and may affect the relative value the reader places on the article.
- *Provides important information regarding potential bias.* Demonstrating that many sociodemographic factors are statistically similar between study groups provides a reasonable justification for not needing to control for those factors in subsequent analyses. This is helpful because depending on your sample size, there are a limited number of variables you may reasonably include in an adjusted analysis before you increase your likelihood of obtaining false positive results (alpha or type I error). These tables also show that you have asked the correct or relevant questions pertaining to your population to see what you *should* control for in your analysis.

With the increasing use of parallel online publication and online appendices, comprehensive tables can be available online only to provide proof of summary descriptions of study group similarities or differences within a publication's text. In short, creating sociodemographic tables is a worthwhile exercise that should not cost you publication space and can strengthen your study.

Assessing Normality: Parametric versus Nonparametric Data

Determining the *normality* of your data is critical to selecting the correct statistical tests. *Normality* is often expressed in relation to how well the data fits a bell-shaped curve. It is categorized in one of two ways: parametrically (*normally*) distributed or nonparametrically (*non-normally*) distributed.

Parametric: Data that assume a *normal* distribution. Parametric data fit a bell-shaped curve that, if split down the middle, is nearly symmetrical. Large data sets (e.g., hundreds to thousands of patients) often are parametrically distributed because, at least in theory, enough values are collected to reasonably represent the true variation of values that exist in the general population. However, you should never assume: always assess your data's distribution.

Nonparametric: Data that have a *non-normal* distribution. Nonparametric data make no assumptions about their distribution. Non-normal data can result from several causes including extreme values (outliers), overlap of two or more processes (multimodal data), insufficient data discrimination (measures made by imprecise tools), sorted data (assessing data after they have been sorted, not the original data), values close to zero or a natural limit (results in skewedness), and data that follow a different distribution.[7] Sometimes nonparametric data can be mathematically transformed (e.g., by using a variable's logarithm) to force the data into a normal distribution.[7,8] If transformation successfully converts non-normal data distributions into normal ones, then you may use parametric tests for your analysis. However, you must (1) confirm that transformation has resulted in a normal distribution, (2) transform all data in the same way prior to analysis, and (3) document your data transformation process as a part of your methods.

You should always know your data's distribution before performing any statistical analyses because different tests are needed to control for the data's variability. For example, using parametric tests to analyze nonparametric data is much more likely to result in falsely statistically significant results (alpha error), not to mention a rejection notice from a journal or grant review for employing inappropriate methods.

Fortunately, various statistical programs enable researchers to efficiently determine if their data are normal or non-normal through functions that *check data normality*. A longer-hand version may be used to generate pictorial representations (histograms) of the various values.

Skewedness

When checking normality in statistical programs, responses will include if the data are approximately normally distributed (parametric), positively skewed (data are shifted to the right side of the anticipated bell-shaped curve), or negatively skewed (data are shifted to the left side of the anticipated bell-shaped curve). But then you also have to determine what this skewedness may mean and explain it to your audience.

Because the data are not *normal* in a skewed distribution, it is helpful to provide more information about your data so the audience can better understand your study population. The following are some first-line examples of measures of central tendency:

Mean and standard deviation (±SD): The mean is the mathematical average of your data values. It is typically reported with the standard deviation, which tells you how spread out the values in your data are. The smaller your SD, the less variability you have within your data; the larger the SD, the more variability. In normal data distributions, about 68% of all values in a data set are captured within one ±SD of the mean, about 95% within two ±SDs, and about 99.7% in three ±SDs.[9]

Mode: The most common value in a data set. It can be helpful to report the mode with the lowest and highest values of your data set (the range). *Note*: It is possible for a data set to have more than one mode (2 modes = bimodal, >2 = multimodal), or to have no mode. If you have >1 mode, you should determine whether your data are truly multimodal or if you have two or more overlapping data sets that can be separated.

Median and interquartile range (IQR): The median is the middle value of a data set, or the value at which exactly half of the data values are to the right and the other half are to the left. Median is most informative when it includes the IQR. The IQRs are the median values for the left half of your data range (1%–50%, or the 25th percentile [Q_1]) and the right half of your data (51%–100%, or the 75th percentile [Q_3]). IQR can be written as the values (Q_1:Q_3), or as a single number representing the range ($Q_3 - Q_1$ = IQR). By definition, the IQR will contain 50% of your data set's values. The smaller the IQR, the less variability present in the data values.

Why does this matter? Importantly, the mean (±SD) may not be meaningful in skewed data sets. One example of this is hospital length-of-stay (LOS). Outliers are common for this variable and can cause the standard deviation to be large, pushing the left side of your LOS SD range into negative days (e.g., LOS = 3 days ± 7 days, range = (−)4 days through (+)10 days), which is nonsensical. In such cases it is better to choose a different measure of your data's central tendency. Finally, you may characterize your data using more than one of these measures as each provides additional information regarding your data's distribution.

One-Tailed versus Two-Tailed Tests

When looking for differences in your data, it is important to understand how the value of interest in the experimental group may differ from the value of interest in the control or comparison group. For example, can the experimental group's value *only* be greater than the comparison group's value? *Only* less? Or is the answer merely anticipated to be different, with the direction of the anticipated difference unknown? Answers to these questions determine whether you should use a one-tailed or two-tailed test.

One-tailed test: Used when the value you are testing in the experimental group would only be anticipated to be more *or* less (change in value is one-directional) than the comparable value in the control group. Generally, your evidence of only needing a one-tailed test should be very strong to choose this test type.[8]

Two-tailed test: Used when the value you are testing in the experimental group is anticipated to be different from (change in value may be more or less than) the comparable value in the control group.

A common question may be, *To what does* tail *refer in these tests?* The tail or tails are the extremes of the data distribution.[8] When picturing the bell-shaped curve, the tails are the small areas to the far left and/or right of your histograms. In a one-tailed test, the area not covered by the certainty of your *P*-value is all in the one tail of your distribution. In a two-tailed test, the area of uncertainty is evenly divided between both the left and right tails.

Choosing Statistical Tests

Statistics, much like plastic surgery, is as much an art as a science: although there is a formal structure, there is room for interpretation and some creativity. Approaches to the same study can vary between statisticians or with the same statistician asked at different points in time. Keeping this in mind, it is important to make sure your research is reproducible, meaning that all methods including the details of your analysis are meticulously recorded.

The statistical tests you choose may depend on your statistical expertise. If you are inexperienced with statistics, it is recommended that you use simple, straightforward, less flexible yet robust analyses.[3] Although such tests may slightly minimize any real effect present in your data, they are more likely to yield meaningful results (avoid false-positive findings). We review some relatively simple statistical tests in the following sections, starting with the relatively simple t-test and progressing through ANOVA and regression analyses.

t-Test

The t-test, also known as student's t-test, compares the means of two samples to tell you if the means differ, and how much they differ from each other (if difference is significant). There are three primary types of t-tests:

Independent t-test: Compares the means of two different (independent) samples (e.g., 6-month postintervention scores in two different treatment groups).

Paired t-test: Compares the means of two related (dependent) samples (e.g., repeated measures of a value in the same group, like pre-to-post-intervention). Also called the paired samples t-test, dependent samples t-test, or repeated measures t-test.

Note: When using a paired t-test, the repeated measures tested should be from the same source, such as the exact same patients, for both variables. Using data collected from slightly different pre-to-post patient groups is unlikely to represent your sample's true pre-to-post change. Although it is tempting to include as many patients as possible in these types of analyses, this is a misuse of the paired t-test. If your samples differ slightly, you may be able to use the comparable nonparametric Wilcoxon signed-rank test.[10]

One-sample t-test: Compares the mean of a single group against a known or hypothesized mean (which you provide and should justify in your methods). It may also be used to find the statistical difference between the sample mean and the sample midpoint. Also called the single sample t-test.[11]

ANOVA or Analysis of the Variance

When determining if differences exist between the means of ≥2 independent groups, ANOVA, or analysis of the variance, can be used. ANOVA expresses this difference through the F statistic, a ratio of the between-groups and within-groups variances. (Interestingly, the ANOVA can be used instead of the independent t-test to compare two independent samples, with the resulting ANOVA F statistic equal to t^2 from the independent t-test.)

There are several data requirements you should check in order to use the one-way ANOVA correctly (including confirming that your data are normally distributed).[12] Here we briefly address two: *variance* and *balanced sample size*.

Variance: The amount of variability or range of values within a group. The within-groups variance and between-groups variance should be approximately equal; otherwise, ANOVA results may not be trustworthy. To analyze data with unequal variances between groups, it is better to use tests that do not assume equal variances among populations, such as the Brown-Forsythe or Welch statistics.[13] *Note*: The Brown-Forsythe and Welch statistics are not nonparametric correlates to the ANOVA, that is, the Kruskal-Wallis test, used for non-normal data distributions. Brown-Forsythe or Welch statistics are intended for use in parametric data sets with unequal variances.

Balanced sample size: When performing a one-way ANOVA, you should have at least six subjects (and hopefully more) in each group; it is best to have balanced sample sizes in each comparison group, as extremely unbalanced group comparisons increase the possibility of decreasing the validity of the ANOVA's F statistic.

We briefly describe four types of ANOVA tests here:

One-way ANOVA: Also called *one-factor ANOVA*, *one-way analysis of variance*, or *between-subjects ANOVA*, the one-way ANOVA will tell you if there is a significant difference between the means of any of the included groups. However, it will not tell you which group(s) is/are significantly different. Additional post hoc testing (after running the ANOVA), such as with Dunnett C or the Tukey test, is needed to determine this.[12,14] Dunnett C test compares each sample mean to a control mean (hence the C) that you provide. If you do not have a control mean for comparison purposes, then the Tukey or another post hoc test can be used.

Two-way ANOVA: A two-way ANOVA can be used to efficiently compare the impact ≥2 independent variables may have on one dependent variable. This test provides information about the effect of each independent variable by itself as well as the interaction between the two variables (e.g., effect modification). *Note*: ANOVA techniques can be extended to three-way, four-way, and beyond, provided your sample size is large enough.

Repeated measures ANOVA: The repeated measures ANOVA is used for variables measured more than once for the same subject, like those that change over time. (In this case use of the standard ANOVA is inappropriate because it does not account for the correlation between repeated measures of the same variable.) The repeated measures ANOVA is used frequently in longitudinal studies when subjects are measured repeatedly in regard to some outcome.

Multivariate analysis of variance (MANOVA): This test is essentially an ANOVA with several continuous dependent variables.[14] It combines the selected dependent variables into a weighted combination or composite variable to see how the new composite variable differs by groups or levels of the independent variable.

Regression Analysis

Regression analyses allow one variable (a dependent variable) to be predicted or estimated from one or more other variables (independent variables). These mathematical models are one-directional, meaning that the independent variable(s) can be used to predict the dependent (outcome) variables, but not the other way around. Regression analysis is a useful tool in medical research and clinical practice because it helps researchers determine who might be at risk for various illnesses, behaviors, etc., based on different exposures. An example is predicting who may be at risk for postoperative complications based on their preoperative comorbidities.

Several pieces of data are derived from regression analyses to describe the predictive relationship between your independent and dependent variables. Three of these are slope, correlation coefficient, and *P*-value:

Slope: Indicates where different patients may be mapped in your predictive model. In univariate regression analyses, the slope indicates how much your dependent variable will change with each unit change in your independent variable. In multiple linear regression analyses, the slope indicates how much your dependent variable will change as a result of the combined influence of all your independent variables.

Correlation coefficient (r): Also called r value, or Pearson product-moment correlation coefficient. This indicates the strength of a predictive relationship. Values for r range from (+)1 to (−)1, where (+)1 represents a perfect positive correlation, (−)1 represents a perfect negative correlation, and zero represents a perfect lack of any correlation. Correlation coefficients of ≥(+)0.7 or ≤(−)0.7 may be considered strong.[15]

P-value: Determines how likely it is that the correlation between your independent and dependent variables is due to chance. *P*-values should always accompany the r values.

Several types of regression analyses are commonly used in biomedical studies. We briefly describe them here with the goal of illustrating when each can be used.

Univariate or simple linear regression: Also called *linear regression*. Analysis performed using one independent variable to predict the variable of interest (dependent variable).[15,16] In simple linear regression, the outcome (dependent) variable is continuous.[16] These analyses are often performed first to determine which independent variables warrant further investigation using more complex and realistic regression models (e.g., multiple linear regression).

Multiple linear regression: Also called *multivariable linear regression*. Analysis performed using ≥2 independent variables (also called covariables or covariates) to predict the variable of interest (dependent variable).[15] In multiple linear regression, the outcome (dependent) variable is continuous.[16]

Multivariate regression: Differs from *multiple* or *multivariable* linear regression in that it deals with multiple *dependent* variables (e.g., repeated measures or clustered data) to predict an outcome.[16]

Multiple logistic regression: Useful for identifying potential confounders. This differs from multiple linear regression in that the outcome (dependent) variable of interest is dichotomous. In these models, the independent variables are called covariates and can be categorical, ordinal, or continuous.

Despite its implication of a directional influence, regression in of itself does not prove causality.[15]

It is important to note that *multivariate* regression and *multivariable* regression are not the same. This can be confusing as the two terms are sometimes used interchangeably although they represent two different analyses.

Survival Analysis

Understanding how long patients may remain disease-free following treatment or survive given certain predisposing factors, or how long an intervention may be effective, can be very informative for patients and physicians. Survival analysis, or what is now more often referred to as Kaplan-Meier curves, are one way to perform such analyses.

Kaplan-Meier curves were developed to help account for incomplete observations and differing survival times.[17,18] This type of analysis is also called *time-to-event* analysis as successful survival (the *event*) does not need to be limited to the absence of mortality. Instead, the event of interest can be any of many different outcomes including a complication, the efficacy of an intervention, or resolution of an adverse event, with the analysis observing the time it takes for the variable of interest to develop, occur, or resolve.[17,18]

Although there are a few methods to conduct survival analyses, the Kaplan-Meier method is generally preferred. When used, data that should be included are the time-to-event (expressed as the median, not the mean) confidence limits (as a measure of variability) and the number of patients who are included at each point of survival (e.g., censoring versus duration of known survival). It should be noted that the further away in time the results are from the beginning of the study, the greater the censoring (attrition/dropout, death) rate and the more approximate the curve calculation becomes. Finally, when comparing two or more survival curves, a suitable rank test should be used.[17]

Summary of Simple Parametric and Nonparametric Tests

There are some straightforward situations in which a nonparametric test can be substituted for a parametric test. These are included in **Table 19.1**. However, when exploring options for more complex ANOVAs and regression analyses, several additional factors, such as variable type, factor into the type of test that should be used.

Now that we have reviewed several commonly performed types of analyses, we will review when you should develop your statistical plan within the context of your protocol or study design.

ANALYTIC APPROACHES: A PRIORI VERSUS POST HOC

The time at which you design your statistical plan, meaning before conducting the study or after all data are collected, is important in identifying the presence or absence of true effects within your data

TABLE 19.1. PARAMETRIC AND NONPARAMETRIC TESTS USED FOR VARIOUS STATISTICAL COMPARISONS[8]

Analysis You Want to do	Example	Parametric Test	Nonparametric Test
Compare means between two independent samples or groups	Group A versus group B	Independent t-test (one-tailed or two-tailed)	Mann-Whitney U test
Compare two quantitative measures taken from the same individual	Pre-to-post-intervention differences	Paired t-test	Wilcoxon signed-rank test
Compare means between three or more samples	Group A versus group B versus group C	Analysis of variance (ANOVA), or one-way ANOVA	Kruskal-Wallis test, or one-way ANOVA on ranks
Compare the distributions of a discontinuous variable in two or more independent samples	Is *x* more likely to occur given *y*?	Chi-square test	Fisher exact test

set. We review best practice guidance for including appropriately performed a priori and post hoc analytical designs to ensure your findings are as trustworthy and meaningful as possible.

A Priori Analyses

Definition

Best practices for research recommend designing your data analysis plan beforehand (a priori), or when you plan the project or write up a proposal. This is considered the purest type of analysis and is intended to achieve several goals:

- Provide evidence regarding whether your hypotheses should be accepted or rejected.
- Demonstrate the least amount of bias in the results obtained.
- Prevent inappropriate use of statistics to obtain statistically significant results.
- Help determine sample size and study power sufficient to detect an effect size, if present.
- Help inform appropriate budget development based on determination of number of subjects needed.

Appropriate Use

A priori analyses are designed in parallel with protocol development. Details of the analysis should be included in a dedicated section of the protocol document (or grant proposal). The analysis should then be completed according to this description following collection of the necessary data (e.g., interim analysis, final analysis). Being faithful to your statistical approach is vital to minimizing bias and producing reproducible results.

One concern when following a strictly outlined data analysis plan for which the results are not statistically significant is that the study was meaningless (or worse: *not publishable*). However, this is not necessarily the case. If you have carefully designed the study, meaning that it was appropriately powered and you used appropriate statistical tests, your negative results are likely important and should be shared with the field.[a] Certainly, you should not panic and turn your analysis into a fishing expedition intended to identify statistically significant results. Although this is tempting given the time and costs to conduct research, it is an inappropriate use of statistics, will potentially introduce false data into the literature and clinical practice, and may ultimately hurt patient care. However, in certain circumstances performing exploratory, post hoc analyses on an existing data set can be informative.

[a]The scientific community is becoming increasingly aware of the bias against publishing and citing negative results in biomedical journals.[19] For more information on this topic and potential solutions, see the review by Carroll et al. (2017), "The perceived feasibility of methods to reduce publication bias".[20]

Post Hoc Analyses

Definition

Post hoc analyses are any statistical analyses not described previously (a priori) in the protocol and performed after data collection has been completed. Generally, these analyses do not address the study's primary or secondary aims. Instead, they help generate future hypotheses. Importantly, these results do not provide proof regarding these newly generated hypotheses.[21]

Appropriate Use

Certain post hoc analyses are an integral part of your a priori analysis plan. Examples include post hoc testing following ANOVA to determine which means differ significantly from each other, or conducting a Bonferroni correction.[22] Although these types of tests technically meet the definition of post hoc analysis, chances are you were able to plan for these prior to study implementation. This section is intended to address unplanned analyses researchers would like to perform based on the collected data after the study has been finished.

Researchers can conduct post hoc analyses and include these in publications, provided that this is clearly stated in the study methods, results, and discussion of these results.[1] After completing a study and reviewing your data, additional questions may arise. These may have been anticipated based on the literature and included as exploratory study aims, or they may arise from the data itself. In these situations, it is acceptable to perform exploratory analyses. The objectives of conducting post hoc analyses include the following[21]:

- Identification of unsuspected findings or associations
- Development of new hypotheses
- Informing the design of future prospective studies (e.g., inclusion/exclusion criteria, study design, statistical power)

Additionally, retrospective studies, meta-analyses, and secondary analysis of existing data sets are all subject inherently to post hoc analysis. Authors need to acknowledge the limitations of their data sets or source data used (e.g., existing data sets, retrospective studies) and level of evidence of included studies (e.g., meta-analyses), as relevant. This knowledge helps readers determine how much weight to give to such studies. Finally, just as with your a priori analysis, meticulous documentation of your post hoc analysis to demonstrate your process and facilitate reproducibility helps readers determine the relative impact of your study.

ADJUSTED ANALYSES: TO CONTROL OR NOT TO CONTROL

Despite the best planning, it is not always possible or practical to design a study to minimize your between-groups variation. In these situations, adjusted analyses may be used. Study results may be expressed as *unadjusted* (aka, crude) or *adjusted*. *Adjusted* refers to controlling for potential overestimation of the influence of any single independent variable on your outcome when several variables may be at work. This can also be thought of as controlling for bias. In addition to adjustment, we address a few factors that can influence your findings and make adjustment necessary, such as confounding, effect modification, and interaction.

Adjustment

Adjustment is needed when several independent variables may be influencing your outcome of interest. To perform an adjusted analysis, you first need to know how to choose the independent variables to include. This can be done by (1) reviewing the literature to determine what variables have been identified in other similar studies (*the usual suspects*) and (2) performing a preliminary unadjusted or univariate analysis to help identify variables that may be affecting the outcome variable. Because unadjusted analyses are prone to alpha (type I) error (overestimating significance), it is normal for certain variables that looked promising after unadjusted analysis (have significant *P*-values) to become statistically insignificant after an adjusted analysis.

Adjusted analyses reduce the combined alpha value to mitigate the chance for alpha error. This provides more realistic estimations of the relationships between variables. One example of such a multiple-comparison correction is the Bonferroni correction.[23]

Adjusted analysis can be very helpful when comparing two different groups. Here *different* means *unmatched*. The advantages of these analyses are you may use them on groups with nonidentical sample sizes and to account for characteristics you were unable to match based on study design, recruitment, or your source data.

Overadjustment and Unnecessary Adjustment

When faced with many interesting variables, it can be challenging to limit the number to include for an adjusted analysis. However, selecting too many variables by which to adjust your analysis can result in overadjustment and/or unnecessary adjustment. Although they differ slightly and their influence is relative,[b] both can introduce bias.[24,25].

Overadjustment: Occurs when your controlling variable introduces, rather than eliminates, bias.[25] It can also cause problems by subsetting your groups to such an extent that the results are not meaningful and can put researchers at risk for beta error (false-negative results).[24] Simple first steps to help prevent overadjustment are (1) taking care to select independent variables based on knowledge (e.g., those substantiated by the literature or indicated by your data set via univariate analysis) and (2) having ≥10 subjects for each dependent variable included in a multivariate adjusted analysis.[24]

Unnecessary adjustment: Similar to but different from overadjustment. It is unlikely to introduce additional bias (aka, *bias-neutral adjustment*) but can affect precision, here meaning a clear understanding of the influence of the exposure on the outcome.[24,25] Unnecessary adjustment occurs when the variable used to control an analysis is a variable (1) unrelated to the relationship being investigated, (2) that only causes the exposure, (3) that is created as a result of the exposure but is not involved in the causal (exposure-to-outcome) pathway, or (4) that causes the outcome but is not involved in the causal (exposure-to-outcome) pathway.[24] Importantly, its role is relative,[b] can be subtle, and may go unnoticed.

Confounding, Effect Modification, and Interaction

Confounding, effect modification, and interaction are three similar yet different events in which two (or more) variables influence the outcome of interest in a way that makes the resulting apparent association inaccurate.

Confounding bias: Comes from a variable that influences both the outcome of interest and the independent variable (or exposure) being assessed, but is not involved in the pathway between the two. This confounding factor makes an inaccurate association between the exposure and the outcome. An example is breast cancer treatment assignment and postoperative complications. As patients' cancer stage increases, they are more likely to receive more aggressive treatment. Such patients would have more complications due to both their more aggressive treatment and their advanced cancer stage, not merely treatment alone.

Although not a statistical panacea, adjusted analyses help control for potential confounders.[26] Another way to minimize confounding is by using propensity scores.[26,27] Propensity scores are intended to replace many different pieces of baseline data with one summary score and are calculated using a specific type of logistic regression model.[27] The propensity scores can then be used to help match patients between your groups, or as an independent variable for which you can adjust your analysis. In other words, propensity score analysis attempts to retrospectively recreate randomization.[27] However, these potential solutions only work for known confounders and cannot address unknown confounders.[27]

Effect modification: Comes from a variable that influences the outcome but not the exposure and occurs when an exposure has a different effect in different subgroups. This third variable can potentially mask (conceal) or increase (sometimes multiplicatively) the true impact of the exposure on the outcome. In this situation, analysis of pooled data can be misleading. Effect modification can be checked using multivariable analysis or stratification to control for the potential effect modifier. Tools that can be used to measure the impact of effect modification include risk ratio, odds ratio, and risk difference.[28]

Interaction: Occurs when two exposures or interventions influence an outcome.[29] Although similar, interaction and effect modification are different; while they often are, the two terms should not be used interchangeably.[29]

Stratification

Another method by which you may control your comparative analyses between populations is stratification. It allows you to further subdivide your comparison groups to better match control and treatment groups.[27] Although stratification can work well in large populations with a few variables (and thus, a few strata), it rapidly falls apart when there are many baseline characteristics for which you want to stratify. One way you may address the problem of excessive population subsetting is to stratify by propensity scores.[27]

PRESENTING DATA

After you have designed your analysis; selected your tests; completed the study, data collection, and analysis; and assessed your results for bias, you get to the final reward: presenting your hard-earned data for publication. When presenting data, it is helpful to remember a few things:

- You or your team is the expert on the study you just completed, so be sure to present your audience with a complete picture of the study.
- Keep in mind the most important or interesting finding(s) and how to present them in the most meaningful way.
- Use simple language, particularly if you are presenting something complex; your audience will thank you for it.

We have included some tips here for how you can present a comprehensive view of your findings in concise and meaningful ways.

Formatting Findings

Statistical results tend to be most meaningful when several measures describing the same finding are presented together. This provides a

[b]If you are interested in this topic, more information can be found in the article by VanderWeele (2009): "On the Relative Nature of Overadjustment and Unnecessary Adjustment".[25]

more comprehensive picture of your sample, its relative heterogeneity or homogeneity, and the potential strength of the effect you found. Some recommended formats for presentation of statistical findings follow:

Mean ± SD, n = __ (95% CI:_-_), *P*-value = __

Median (IQR), (95% CI:_-_), *P*-value = __

Odds ratio (OR), (95% CI:_-_), *P*-value = __

Writing your findings in this way or including these data in a well-conceived table can improve your use of journal space and be more effective than wordier verbal descriptions. This efficiency can also enable you to share more information about your findings by freeing up your word count.

Correlation Versus Causation

When discussing findings there is some confusion surrounding the terminology used to indicate relationships between variables. Here we briefly clarify correlation and causation.

Correlation (or association): This term indicates that there appears to be a relationship between your exposure (independent variable) and outcome of interest (dependent variable), but that you are unable to determine if one causes the other. Correlation and association are important when conducting studies in which it is not possible to collect every variable that could affect an outcome and to help indicate what variables should be investigated further through more vigorous studies (e.g., controlled clinical trials).

Causation: This term indicates that there is a quantifiable relationship between your exposure (independent variable) and outcome of interest (dependent variable), and that you can prove that one is causing the other. Causation is difficult to prove in complex interactions, such as situations in which many different exposures may contribute to an outcome over many years.

A WORD ABOUT DATA COLLECTION

When discussing statistics, it is necessary to touch upon data collection, or considerations regarding your source data set. For one thing, your findings can only ever be as good as the data used to derive them. An example of this is a beautifully designed meta-analysis of level 3 evidence papers; regardless of how perfectly the meta-analysis is performed, the resulting paper's level of evidence cannot exceed that of its source material (per this example, level 3 evidence).

The old term still applies: *garbage in, garbage out*. Therefore, collecting good data and understanding what your data can or cannot tell you are vital to understanding what you can ask of it.

Potential Database Tools

Research can be more expensive than anticipated, whether conducting a relatively small retrospective review or a phase 3 clinical trial. This causes many people to make use of free (or prepaid) resources for the purposes of storing data. Though understandable, researchers must be aware of the strengths and weaknesses of commonly used tools. We provide a summary of some commonly used electronic data collection tools and their strengths and weaknesses in **Table 19.2**. This is not intended to be comprehensive; rather, this table touches upon points meant to help researchers in selecting the tool most appropriate for them.

Regardless of the tool used, some forethought and design need to go into creating your data collection tool. Once created, it should be tested. You can do this by entering data using a few sample or test cases. This step can be very helpful in the long-term as it will illustrate any problems that may exist (e.g., missing or redundant data fields, imprecise prompts or descriptors, forms that do not work correctly) and the changes that may be needed.[30] It is much more efficient and cost-effective to recognize and correct any potential problems early than after all your data have been collected.

Finally, although it can be challenging to identify funding on the front end of a project, it may be more cost-effective to pay for a database that is unlikely to corrupt data or that can provide structure to enable easy and uniform data entry by individuals of varying medical or research knowledge. Realizing halfway through or at the end of a project that your source data and/or analyses are corrupted or flawed is enough to make anyone give up research.

Data Collection

Like other disciplines, there is a science to data collection to ensure accuracy, completeness, and patient privacy.

Good practices for data collection for industry, as published in the Food and Drug Administration's good laboratory practice, follow the acronym ALCOA to identify elements of data quality.[34] ALCOA stands for:

Attributable: Data entries and any changes can be traced back to the person who made the entries or changes.

Legible: Data entries and any changes are easily read, even after being corrected. This pertains to hard copies (paper) and electronic records (entry history).

Contemporaneous: That data collection and entry occurs as close in time as possible to the observation.

Original: The first and therefore generally considered to be the most accurate and reliable recording of data.

Accurate: The recorded data correctly reflect the observation.

Following these principles puts you on the right track for high-quality data collection that you can trust months or years later.

TABLE 19.2. STRENGTHS AND WEAKNESSES OF SOME COMMON DATA COLLECTION TOOLS

Data Collection Tool	Strengths	Weaknesses
Excel[30,31]	Inexpensive or free, easily accessible, nearly universal across operating systems and versions, can be password-protected.	Easily corrupted (e.g., missorted), users have to create their own data dictionary.
REDCap[32]	Web-based for easy access between team members, has tiered access for users, inexpensive or free, easily updated by study team if changes need to be made to DB design, creates data dictionary for users. Designed for research use. Can be HIPAA-compliant.	Flat (not relational) database, will need to pay for database design/setup if no team members know how to do this.
Access[33]	Included in many MS Office packages, has capacity to hold relatively large amounts of data, creates data dictionary for users.	Designing queries can be taxing, not inherently HIPAA-compliant.
FileMakerPro	Has tiered access for users, DB can be changed easily by study team if needed, can be made to create data dictionary for users.	Paid licenses are needed for all users. Will need to pay for database design/setup if no team members know how to do this.

Preexisting Data Sets

There can be great value in secondary analysis of preexisting data sets. Some examples are:

- Access to sample sizes to which you might not otherwise have access
- Leverages preexisting resources making research more affordable
- May consist of data from more than one institution, state, or country
- Larger sample size may make study population more comparable to general population

However, researchers must be aware of the potential drawbacks of preexisting data sets. Some examples are:

- Potential for missing data
- Data collected may change from year to year, making multiyear comparisons challenging or infeasible
- May require significant data preparation and cleaning prior to analysis
- May not include variables most informative for testing your hypothesis

When using a preexisting data set, you must familiarize yourself with the data, how it was collected, and obtain and review the user's guide or primary protocol documenting how the data were collected. Taking these steps will educate you as to what questions you can ask appropriately of the data set. Design of an appropriate research question, thoughtful design of a post hoc analysis plan, and transparency in stating how the study was conducted are important parts of reporting findings for studies conducted using these resources.

Data Preparation

Although it is best to proactively prevent data entry errors, some entry errors are inevitable. Data preparation, also called *data cleaning*, is a crucial and potentially time-consuming part of ensuring your data are as amenable to analysis as possible.

Data preparation is when you review and format your data in a spreadsheet to make it compatible with the program the statistician will use.[30,35] This is intended to enable direct importing of the data from a shared spreadsheet into the statistical software program without any unintended changes being performed automatically by the analysis software on your data. It can include many different levels of review, from formatting to editing abnormalities. Importantly, this is not manipulation of your data: corrections may be made, but data values should not be changed. Changes should be tracked such that it is possible to compare the originally exported data set with the cleaned version.[35] Some examples of data cleaning activities:

- *Indicating missing data versus zero values.* Blank fields can present problems during analysis. Therefore, missing data may have a specific entry such as a "." (period) instead of remaining blank. Fields whose values are left unaddressed may be assigned values by the analysis software and are likely to yield inaccurate results.
- *Variable name length.* Software programs often have character limits for their field names. This can cause some overly long names to be cut off and potentially unrecognizable. Checking, editing names down, and tracking changes in your data dictionary can prevent this from occurring.
- *Data accuracy.* Ensuring that data are correctly and consistently displayed (no typographical errors, use of letters in number fields, revisiting abnormal values to ensure they are real results, etc.).
- *Additional variable categorization.* Although data were collected on a precise level, it can be helpful to recategorize certain variables into larger classes prior to analysis (e.g., BMI into BMI classes). Such choices may be made based on the literature.

It is important for the study team to complete this work because (1) it can be time-consuming and (2) you are more likely than your statistician to be an expert on your data and how it should be included in analyses.

To best streamline the data preparation process, ask your statistician about desired formatting or formatting requirements before preparing and sharing your data.

Data Dictionaries

A data dictionary is a comprehensive document that includes the full and abbreviated names of all of your data fields, the possible answers for coded or categorized data, and indications for which fields are labeled as free-text fields. This document acts as a translation book to ensure you and your statistician are referring to and using the same field(s) when discussing your study and performing analyses.

You must be aware when selecting a data management tool which ones will and will not generate a data dictionary. Importantly, if your data management tool does not create a data dictionary, you will need to create one and keep it updated. This can require a considerable amount of effort and should not be underestimated.

WHEN TO CONSULT A STATISTICIAN

Many individuals new to research ask when they should consult a statistician. To misquote a phrase, you should consult one early and often. As previously stated, a carefully designed study including an a priori statistical plan is vital to producing meaningful results or convincing a review committee to fund your project.[36]

Finding a Knowledgeable Statistician

Though not necessary, it is helpful to work with statisticians who understand your area of study or who can understand it based on similar work in a different field. Familiarity often means that the statistician will be able to apply his or her time more efficiently to your project. If the statistician is unfamiliar with your area of study, be prepared to orient him or her. This will go into how much time you need to spend with the individual during the planning phase.

First, there may be several types of statisticians who are available to you:

- Academics (master's or PhD level)
- Students studying statistics (earning their MPH, PhD)
- Students formally overseen by PhD-level statisticians
- Private or ad hoc personnel
- A member of the team who is comfortable with statistics

The complexity of your study, importance of results, and availability of funding may dictate the level of statistician you approach. It may also be advisable to obtain references for their work and/or to look up past publications to determine if the statistician's past experience aligns with your research needs. There are advantages and drawbacks to each of the aforementioned individuals: be aware that going with the inexpensive option may require more oversight and knowledge on your part, whereas going with a highly qualified individual may require significant wait-time prior to gaining assistance and payment for their time.

Keeping the Statistician On-Board

There are several approaches researchers can take to engage a statistician. It is best to ask directly regarding the relative importance of hourly compensation, documentation of utility across an organization, and authorship as any of these may apply.

Compensation for Time

As with all skilled positions, hourly rates for statisticians can vary depending on their level of education and years of experience. If you are looking for a less costly but reasonably reliable option, blended rates may be available for students who are overseen by a PhD-level statistician. It is important to understand how skilled a statistician you need for your project so that your efforts are adequately supported.

Authorship

Depending on whether your statistician is an academician interested in the area of your study, you may be able to offer authorship for their involvement. Certain types of studies rely heavily on the statistician and warrant prominent authorship. Such studies include secondary analyses of preexisting databases (e.g., NSQIP, NIS) or in-depth meta-analyses of multiple studies. In these cases, the statistician's authorship may need to be as high as co-first authorship. If the statistical consultation is used to confirm your statistical plan, you may only need to include the statistician's contribution in the acknowledgments section. It is important to fully understand the effort request you are making of the statistician so that you can make an appropriate offer of authorship.

Documenting Organization Utility or Benefit

In certain academic environments, biostatistics core facilities are available. These can be funded in any number of ways (indirect costs, federal grants, etc.) and often include reporting metrics to justify ongoing funding. If this is the case, a certain number of in-kind hours may be available to faculty, students, or staff. (In the case of grant design, these free hours are also intended to assist with budgeting for future use of the statistician's time when data collection is complete.) In these situations, a combination approach that includes compensation and authorship in published articles may be needed: be sure to ask.

Statistical Plans: Get Them in Writing

Research, and particularly prospective clinic trials in human subjects, can take much longer than anticipated to complete. For example, delays in IRB approvals, start-up, and recruitment; dropout or lost-to-follow-up rates; and stringent inclusion/exclusion criteria can all contribute to slower study completion timelines. Given all the other details to which one must pay attention during a research study or clinical trial, it is easy to forget one's analysis plan.

If you have not written out your a priori analysis plan, chances are you will not remember it when you finally have data to analyze. Additionally, you need to have the analysis plan in writing in case the original biostatistician is no longer available to you at the time the study is completed. Because statistics can be somewhat open to interpretation, different statisticians may create different yet valid approaches for analyzing the same set of data. This is fine unless it renders your collected data inappropriate.

REFERENCES

1. Moher D, Hopewell S, Schulz KF, et al. CONSORT 2010 explanation and elaboration: updated guidelines for reporting parallel group randomised trials. *Int J Surg.* 2012;10(1):28-55.
   A published statement developed and refined by experts in clinical research to guide investigators toward best practices when designing and conducting clinical trials. This statement is widely endorsed by leading medical journals and international editorial groups.
2. Ioannidis JPA. The proposal to lower P value thresholds to .005. *JAMA.* 2018;319(14):1429-1430.
3. Leek J. On the scalability of statistical procedures: why the p-value bashers just don't get it. Simply Statistics, A Statistics Blog by Rafa Irizarry, Roger Peng, and Jeff Leek. https://simplystatistics.org/2014/02/14/on-the-scalability-of-statistical-procedures-why-the-p-value-bashers-just-dont-get-it/. Published February 14, 2014. Accessed May 9, 2018.
4. Wasserstein RL, Lazar NA. The ASA's statement on p-values: context, process, and purpose. *Am Stat.* 2016;70(2):129-133.
   The American Statistical Association's statement articulates in nontechnical terms a few select principles that could improve the conduct or interpretation of quantitative science, according to widespread consensus in the statistical community.
5. Kirby A, Gebski V, Keech AC. Determining the sample size in a clinical trial. *Med J Aust.* 2002;177(5):256-257.
6. Sedgwick P. What is intention to treat analysis? *BMJ.* 2013;346:f3662.
7. AButhman. Dealing with non-normal data: strategies and tools. iSixSigma. https://www.isixsigma.com/tools-templates/normality/dealing-non-normal-data-strategies-and-tools/. Accessed May 7, 2018.
8. Greenhalgh T. How to read a paper. Statistics for the non-statistician. I: different types of data need different statistical tests. *BMJ.* 1997;315(7104):364-366.
   The first in a series of articles excerpted from the book, How to Read a Paper: The Basics of Evidence-Based Medicine. This article provides clinicians with a checklist of preliminary questions to help assess the statistical validity of a scientific publication.
9. Mean and Standard Deviation. BMJ. https://www.bmj.com/about-bmj/resources-readers/publications/statistics-square-one/2-mean-and-standard-deviation.
10. Statistical Consulting, Kent State University Libraries. SPSS Tutorials: Paired SamplestTest. https://libguides.library.kent.edu/SPSS/PairedSamplestTest. Updated May 24, 2018. Accessed May 25, 2018.
11. Statistical Consulting, Kent State University Libraries. SPSS Tutorials: One Sample t Test. https://libguides.library.kent.edu/SPSS/OneSampletTest. Updated May 25, 2018. Accessed May 25, 2018.
12. Statistical Consulting, Kent State University Libraries. SPSS Tutorials: One-Way ANOVA. https://libguides.library.kent.edu/SPSS/OneWayANOVA. Updated May 25, 2018. Accessed May 25, 2018.
13. Reed JF III, Stark DB. Robust alternatives to traditional analysis of variance: Welch W*, James J I*, James J II*,Brown-Forsythe BF*. *Comput Methods Progr Biomed.* 1988;26(3):233-237.
14. Bird KD. Simultaneous contrast testing procedures for multivariate experiments. *Multivariate Behav Res.* 1975;10(3):343.
15. Greenhalgh T. How to read a paper: statistics for the non-statistician. II: "Significant" relations and their pitfalls. *BMJ.* 1997;315(7105):422-425.
    The second in a series of articles excerpted from the book, How to Read a Paper: The Basics of Evidence-Based Medicine. This article provides clinicians with a checklist of preliminary questions to help assess the statistical validity of a scientific publication.
16. Hidalgo B, Goodman M. Multivariate or multivariable regression? *Am J Public Health.* 2013;103(1):39-40.
17. Mathew A1, Pandey M, Murthy NS. Survival analysis: caveats and pitfalls. *Eur J Surg Oncol.* 1999;25(3):321-329.
18. Rich JT, Neely JG, Paniello RC, et al. A practical guide to understanding Kaplan-Meier curves. *Otolaryngol Head Neck Surg.* 2010;143(3):331-336.
19. Duyx B, Urlings MJE, Swaen GMH, et al. Scientific citations favor positive results: a systematic review and meta-analysis. *J Clin Epidemiol.* 2017;88:92-101.
20. Carroll HA, Toumpakari Z, Johnson L, Betts JA. The perceived feasibility of methods to reduce publication bias. *PLoS One.* 2017;12(10):e0186472.
21. Elliott HL. Post hoc analysis: use and dangers in perspective. *J Hypertens Suppl.* 1996;14(2):S21-S24.
22. EWWeisstein. "Bonferroni correction." From MathWorld – A Wolfram Web Resource. http://mathworld.wolfram.com/BonferroniCorrection.html.
23. Guyatt G, Walter S, Shannon H, et al. Basic statistics for clinicians: 4. Correlation and regression. *CMAJ.* 1995;152(4):497-504.
24. Schisterman EF, Cole SR, Platt RW. Overadjustment bias and unnecessary adjustment in epidemiologic studies. *Epidemiology.* 2009;20(4):488-495.
25. VanderWeele TJ. On the relative nature of overadjustment and unnecessary adjustment. *Epidemiology.* 2009;20(4):496-499.
26. Cook JA, Ranstam J. Statistical models and confounding adjustment. *Br J Surg.* 2017;104(6):786-787.
27. Adamina M, Guller U, Weber WP, Oertli D. Propensity scores and the surgeon. *Br J Surg.* 2006; 93: 389-394.
28. VanderWeele TJ, Robins JM. Four types of effect modification: a classification based on directed acyclic graphs. *Epidemiology.* 2007;18(5):561-568.
29. VanderWeele TJ. On the distinction between interaction and effect modification. *Epidemiol.* 2009;20(6):863-871. Errata in: Epidemiology. 2011;22(5):752, and 2010;21(1):162.
30. Juluru K, Eng J. Use of spreadsheets for research data collection and preparation: a primer. *Acad Radiol.* 2015;22(12):1592-1599.
31. Elliott AC, Hynan LS, Reisch JS, Smith JP. Preparing data for analysis using Microsoft Excel. *J Investig Med.* 2006;54(6):334-341.
32. Harris PA, Taylor R, Thielke R, et al. Research electronic data capture (REDCap): a metadata-driven methodology and workflow process for providing translational research informatics support. *J Biomed Inform.* 2009;42(2):377-381.
33. Schneider JK, Schneider JF, Lorenz RA. Creating user-friendly databases with microsoft access. *Nurse Res.* 2005;13(1):57-75.
34. TJKuhn. ALCOA: a standard for evidence. GxP zone: good practice for the pharmaceutical industry from the quality assurance perspective. https://tjkuhn.wordpress.com/2008/07/23/alcoa/. Posted July 23, 2008. Accessed June 28, 2018.
35. Van den Broeck J, Cunningham SA, et al. Data cleaning: detecting, diagnosing, and editing data abnormalities. *PLoS Med.* 2005;2(10):e267.
36. De Muth JE. Preparing for the first meeting with a statistician. *Am J Health Syst Pharm.* 2008;65(24):2358-2366.

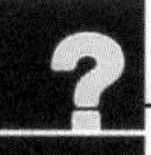

QUESTIONS

1. **PRS has published a study examining the pre-to-post change in patient satisfaction with breast reconstruction comparing a new implant sling technique (n = 13) with conventional implant placement (n = 28). What is the most appropriate test to use to determine if a statistically significant difference in satisfaction exists between groups?**

   a. Paired t-test
   b. Independent t-test
   c. Wilcoxon signed-rank test
   d. One-way ANOVA

2. **Which of the following scenarios would require an increase in the sample size?**

   a. Changing the significance level from 0.05 to 0.01
   b. Changing the power of the study from 90% to 80%
   c. Determining that the difference in the means is less than originally calculated
   d. Determining that the standard deviation of the means is less than originally calculated

3. **A *P*-value of 0.05 indicates which of the following?**

   a. 5% chance the null hypothesis is correct
   b. 5% chance the null hypothesis was incorrectly rejected
   c. 95% chance the null hypothesis was correctly accepted
   d. 95% chance the null hypothesis is correct

4. **A study is performed to determine the outcomes between two different breast reconstruction techniques. One technique is performed by surgeon A at hospital X and the second technique is performed by surgeon B at hospital Y. Surgeon A has significantly better patient satisfaction scores based on a *P*-value of less than 0.01. Which type of bias is at risk for affecting the data?**

   a. Skewing
   b. Post hoc analysis
   c. Confounding bias
   d. Overadjustment

5. **A study team conducts a prospective, randomized, placebo-controlled trial designed to determine the effect of an experimental medication on flap necrosis rates. While completing the analysis of the study aims, the team notices an apparent correlation between participant BMI and postoperative infection rates. After conferring with the protocol principal investigator, the team decides to publish these additional findings in a separate manuscript. Which type of bias is at risk for affecting the data?**

   a. Skewing
   b. Post hoc analysis
   c. Stratification
   d. Overadjustment

1. **Answer: c.** The sample size is small indicating that a nonparametric analysis should be performed because it cannot be assumed that the data are normally distributed. The pre-to-post change in patient satisfaction indicates that the data are dependent (repeated measurements in the same patients) and should be analyzed as such.

2. **Answer: a.** When performing a power calculation four pieces of information are needed: the event rate, the smallest clinically important difference, power (to detect the difference), and significance level. Decreasing power (answer b) reduces the sample size needed but increases the chance of beta error. Lowering the significance level (answer a) decreases the likelihood of alpha error and increases the number of subjects needed in the study. This is because you are seeking a greater level of confidence with which to correctly reject the null hypothesis (a 99%, or 99 in 100, chance).

3. **Answer: b.** A *P*-value is a measurement of the strength of the evidence against a null hypothesis; the smaller the *P*-value, the stronger the evidence that you should reject the null hypothesis. However, the *P*-value indicates the percent (%) chance that the null hypothesis would be incorrectly rejected, in this case a 5%, or a 1 in 20, chance.

4. **Answer: c.** Many different factors may be influencing differences in patient satisfaction between the two groups of patients being compared, including the surgeon's skill level and interpersonal skills, the breast reconstruction technique employed, the hospital, the clinic and nursing staff, and more. Although this may serve as an initial hypothesis-generating study to help indicate how to better ascertain what precisely is causing these differences, this study alone is not very informative.

5. **Answer: b.** The analysis exploring a correlation between participant BMI and postoperative infection rates was not a part of the originally approved protocol's specific aims or a priori statistical plan. By definition, this analysis was done post hoc and is subject to all the shortcomings inherent to post hoc analyses. Although it can be acceptable to publish post hoc findings, the study team needs to clearly state this fact and may not assume that a post hoc finding has ***proven*** a true correlation. Instead, post hoc findings can be considered hypothesis-generating and informative to future study designs.

PART II

SKIN AND SOFT TISSUE

CHAPTER 20 Skin Care and Benign and Malignant Dermatologic Conditions

John H. Bast and Alex K. Wong

KEY POINTS

- Understand the role of Fitzpatrick skin types and their role when choosing a chemical peel regimen or laser treatment
- Understand the spectrum of dermatitis and be able to distinguish eczema from psoriasis
- Identify risk factors for development of NMSCs
- Be able to formulate a surgical treatment plan for melanoma

The skin serves as an important interface to the external environment as both a physical and an immunologic barrier. Over the course of a lifetime, the skin undergoes characteristic changes as a result of aging and the constant damage and remodeling that takes place. Plastic surgeons will frequently encounter patients with concerns regarding the skin because it is the most visible of all the organs. It also plays an important role in the manifestation of disease processes through dermatologic symptoms. An example of a well-established form of external insult is ultraviolet (UV) radiation. UV radiation has been implicated as a strong risk factor for the development of both nonmelanoma skin cancers (NMSCs) and melanoma skin cancer, but also contributes to other benign skin lesions that develop. Latitude plays an important part in UV radiation exposure with lower latitudes having more direct and greater UV radiation exposure.[1] Although an external stimulus is often required, phenotypes of an individual also play a factor in the development of diseases affecting the skin. Inadequate DNA repair mechanism (xeroderma pigmentosum), those lacking melanin (albinism and lower Fitzpatrick score [I-IV]), and immune deficiency have all been implicated in increased risk for skin cancer. In the United States, a significant portion of health care dollars is spent managing the effects of UV damage to the skin in the form of skin rejuvenation therapies as well as skin cancer treatment.[2] Skin cancer has the highest incidence worldwide of all cancers.[3] There is also significant expenditure in the prevention strategies in the form of sunscreen and other agents for skin resurfacing to reverse the effects of sun damage. This chapter will review the effects of UV damage on the skin as well as go over some benign skin conditions that may present to the clinician for evaluation. It will also cover the most common skin cancers and the treatment strategies around those cancers.

SKIN

Anatomy

The skin is composed of two distinct layers—the epidermis, which is the most superficial layer, and the dermis, which is the deeper layer. Below this is a layer of subcutaneous fat. Glabrous skin is found on the palm and soles. It is without hair and has much thicker layer than the other skin of the body (Figure 20.1). Hair-bearing skin is found throughout the body.

There are four layers of epidermis in the skin, and the glabrous has an additional fifth layer. The epidermis is primarily composed of keratinocytes along with melanocytes, Langerhan cells, and Merkel cells. The dermis is divided into two layers, with the more superficial papillary dermis and the deeper reticular dermis. The dermis holds its integrity through a dense matrix composed of collagen and elastin fibers that give both strength and elasticity. The dermis also houses the other skin appendages such as hair follicles, sebaceous glands, and the apocrine and eccrine sweat glands.

With photoprotection, the skin will become thin, dry, smooth, and unblemished with aging. Aging photodamaged skin is characterized by fine and course wrinkles, roughness, laxity, scaling, dryness, telangiectasia, and dyschromia with an increase in the frequency of both benign and malignant lesions. Solar elastosis describes the photodamaged extracellular matrix of the dermis with abnormal elastin and decreased, disorganized collagen fibrils.

Fitzpatrick Skin Type

Fitzpatrick skin type classifies the skin into six phenotypes based on the melanin content of the skin (color), the inherent pigmentation of the skin, and the sensitivity of the skin to sun damage.[4] Lower Fitzpatrick score indicates less melanin in the skin and hence a greater sensitivity to sun damage. This leads to an increased risk for skin cancer in these individuals. The Fitzpatrick classification system has also been applied to other modalities of skin resurfacing such as chemical peels and laser resurfacing as a guide to how the skin will respond and the propensity for pigmentation damage and scarring after resurfacing procedures.[4,5]

Sunscreen

There has been a clear and consistent link of sun exposure history (UV) and skin cancer. UV radiation that reaches the earth's surface is UVA and UVB. 95% is in the form of UVA; however, UVB is the most carcinogenic through direct photochemical damage to cellular DNA and to the DNA repair mechanism of the cell. Primary means of preventing damage from UV include ways that minimize the UV that can penetrate the skin and cause photodamage, especially at a young age. Avoiding UV radiation exposure at peak times (10 AM–4 PM) and wearing protective outer clothing are examples of primary prevention. Sunscreens protect the skin either chemically or physically. Chemical sunscreens absorb UV (usually UVB) radiation with the most common sunscreen ingredient being para-aminobenzoic acid (PABA), benzophenones, and cinnamates. Physical sunscreens work by reflecting UV radiation and producing a protective barrier. They are usually opaque and include agents such as zinc oxide and titanium dioxide. Sunscreens that block both UVA and UVB are best; however, the UV protection listed on the sunscreen is for the UVB only, and many do not effectively block the UVB. Appropriate application ensures the protective effect of the sunscreen.

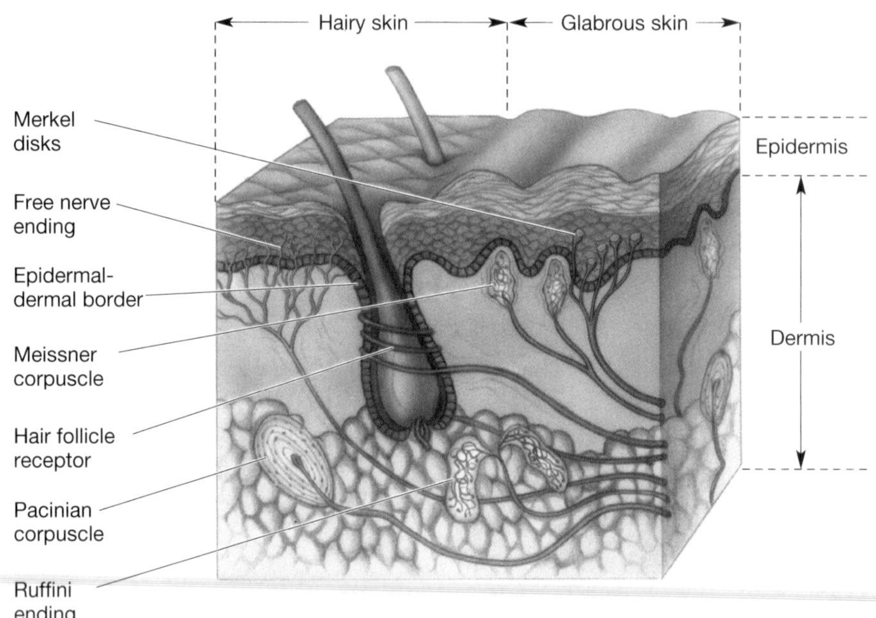

FIGURE 20.1. Glabrous versus nonglabrous (hair-bearing) skin layers. Reproduced with permission from Bear MF, Connors BW, Paradiso WA. The somatic sensory system. In: Bear MF, Connors BW, Paradiso WA, eds. *Neuroscience: Exploring the Brain*. 4th ed. Philadelphia, PA: Wolters Kluwer; 2016:415-482. Figure 12-1.

Retinoids

Retinoids (derivative of vitamin A) are well studied for the protective effects in the skin and reversal of photoaging. They work by binding to nuclear receptors and modulating cellular gene expression. Clinically, this leads to epidermal thickening and increased collagen in the dermis because of decreased breakdown and increased collagen synthesis in the dermis.[6] They are available as topical (e.g., tretinoin or Retin-A) and can be used to treat areas of actinic damage. Retinoids are also available systemically (e.g., isotretinoin) and can be used to treat acne and rosacea; however, they are known teratogen and thus must be used under close monitoring in women of childbearing years. Side effects such as pruritus, burning, erythema, and peeling are usually seen with onset of treatment and can lead to noncompliance, especially in patients with a history of sensitive skin. Photosensitivity is another common side effect of topical therapies, and patients are advised to avoid sun exposure when starting therapy.

Chemical Peels

Chemical peel strength is typically classified based on the depth of effect with deeper peels having longer-lasting effects: superficial, medium, or deep. Superficial peels cause exfoliation of the epidermis without deeper penetration. Medium peels affect the epidermis and penetrate into the papillary dermis, and deep peels penetrate into the reticular dermis where they cause realignment of collagen. Peels are used for a wide variety of skin conditions ranging from management of photodamage and melasma to hyperpigmentation, rosacea, and acne. Deeper peels tend to have more profound and longer-lasting effect compared with superficial peels. Common superficial peels include glycolic acid and salicylic acid, whereas TCA (20%–35%) and Jessner's are considered medium peels. Phenol and TCA (45%–50%) are examples of deep peels. Peels are commonly used in conjunction with other skin resurfacing modalities for improved outcomes.[7]

Laser Resurfacing

Laser resurfacing relies on the principles of selective thermal destruction (photothermolysis) to disrupt damaged areas of skin and to induce remodeling. Ablative laser resurfacing causes wounding of the skin to the dermis and then allows wound healing from dermal regenerative cells. Examples include the CO_2 laser and erbium:yttrium-aluminum-garnet laser. Fractional lasers create microthermal zones of injury that are spatially confined rather than confluent. This preserves some epidermis and shortens the recovery time and diminishes the side effects. Healing occurs from the surrounding unaffected follicular units.[8]

EVALUATION AND MANAGEMENT OF COMMON SKIN DISORDERS

Skin and Soft-Tissue Infections

Bacterial Infections

As a barrier to the external environment, the skin is in constant balance with the external bacteria. When this balance is shifted, as in an open wound, bacteria proliferate, which can manifest as cellulitis and/or an abscess. Cellulitis is caused by a break in the skin barrier that allows bacteria access to the deep dermis. It manifests as spreading erythema and warmth. 85% of the time, no bacteria are cultured from cellulitis, and treatment should cover the staph and strep of the skin flora with consideration of methicillin-resistant *Staphylococcus aureus* (MRSA) in certain at-risk groups.[9] An abscess is a collection of pus in the dermis/subcutaneous space. In the immunocompetent patient, the most common cause of abscess is *S. aureus* but can be multifloral. In the immunocompromised patient, other more atypical bacteria and fungi need to be considered.

Bites and Stings

Bites and stings from mammals, spiders, reptiles, ticks, and insects are a common source of bacterial infection. By causing a break in the normal protective skin barrier and inoculation of bacteria into the deeper layers, the skin flora invades into the dermis. When treating bites from mammals and reptiles, the oral flora of the animal should be considered for targeting therapy. Tetanus is also a risk, and appropriate treatment is warranted depending on immunization history. Bites can also deliver toxins that can produce both local and systemic effects. The brown recluse spider, for example, causes wide local tissue destruction from the enzyme sphingomyelinase D.[10] Systemic toxicity from envenomation includes neurotoxicity and coagulopathy and can be quickly fatal. Early treatment with respiratory management, treatment of shock, and antivenom administration can be lifesaving.

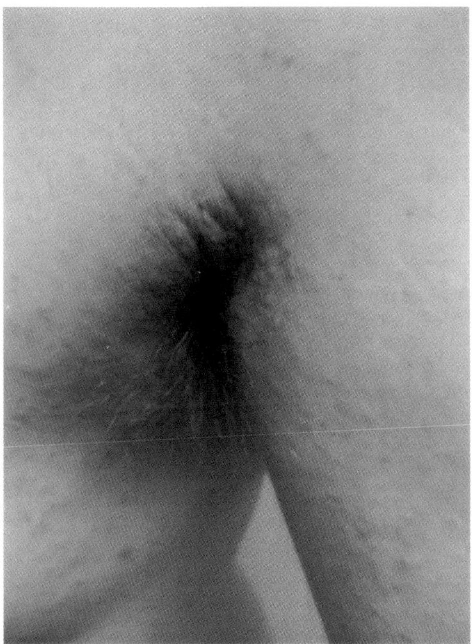

FIGURE 20.2. Scabies of the axillary fold. (Courtesy of Henry K. Wong, MD, PhD.)

Infestations

Infestations including pediculosis (from lice [e.g., *Pediculus humanus capitis, Pediculus humanus humanus, and Phthirus pubis*]), scabies, infection from bedbugs, schistosome cercarial dermatitis, and myiasis are another source of skin lesion/irritation. Lice present with excoriated erythematous papules along with pruritus and regional lymphadenopathy. Permethrin is first-line treatment for the condition. Scabies (*Sarcoptes scabiei* var *homonis)* involves female mites living within epidermal burrows that create a hypersensitivity reaction after 3 to 4 weeks (Figure 20.2). Usually the web space, wrists, and/or genitalia are pruritic and erythematous. Topical permethrin 5% is the treatment of choice. Schistosomiasis is manifested by pruritic erythematous plaques after the larvae penetrate the skin. Typically treatment is symptomatic because most are animal schistosomes.

Cutaneous Viral Infections and Exanthems

Viral infections are well studied for the effect they can have on the skin by both direct infection of the skin and mucus membranes and the cutaneous manifestations of a viral illness through exanthemas. Human papillomaviruses (HPVs) are DNA viruses that often induce benign papillomas or warts but have the potential to cause cancerous lesions in the skin. The virus is passed by person-to-person contact or by contact with a contaminated surface. The virus affects basal keratinocytes. Anogenital HPV infections represent the most common sexually transmitted infection in the United States and include high-risk types such as HPV 16 and 18, which have been implicated in cervical and anal cancers.[11] These high-risk strains are the target of prophylactic HPV vaccines and have been shown to protect from the target-specific HPV types when given prophylactically.[12]

Herpes virus represents a large family of DNA viruses that are known to have a clinical history of infection, latency period, and reactivation. Common examples include herpes simplex, which presents with vesicular eruptions usually in the orolabial and genital regions (Figure 20.3), varicella-zoster virus (chicken pox/shingles; Figure 20.4), Epstein-Barr virus (EBV), and cytomegalovirus. Topical and systemic antiviral therapies have been helpful in modifying the disease presentation.

Viruses can also present with clinical manifestations, especially in the juvenile population. Some of these exanthemas (a skin eruption occurring as a sign of a general disease) can be pathognomonic for a virus, whereas others are more generalized. Diagnosis is aided by identification of other symptoms, including low-grade fever, malaise, GI complaints, and rhinorrhea to help suggest it is the manifestation of viral illnesses. Some common examples include hand, foot, and mouth (Coxsackie virus), measles (rubeola), German measles (rubella), Fifth disease (parvovirus B19). Generally, treatment is supportive; however, some of these can pose a significant health risk if left untreated.

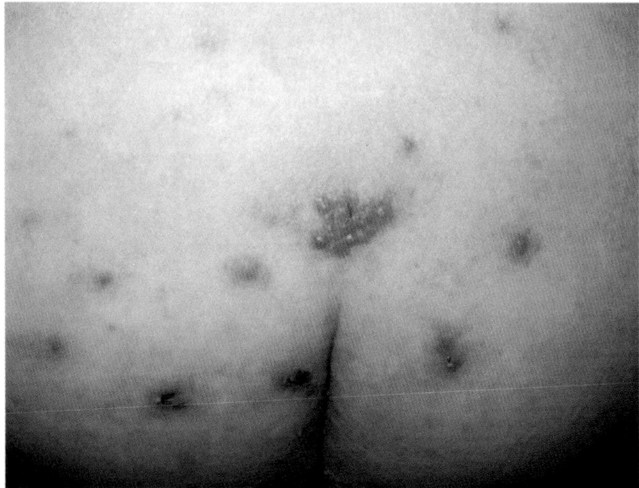

FIGURE 20.3. Herpes simplex virus infection of the gluteal area. (Courtesy of Henry K. Wong, MD, PhD.)

Fungal Infections

Fungal skin infections are also common and classified based on depth and extent of involvement. Superficial infections include dermatophytoses and tinea versicolor along with cutaneous candidiasis. Deeper infections include sporotrichosis and result from the organism being deposited in the dermis or subcutaneous tissue. They can have a prolonged course and are often treated with topical agents to avoid the side effects of systemic antifungals. Diagnosis is usually clinical but can be made with scrapings.

Dermatologic Manifestations of Sexually Transmitted Diseases

The most common sexually transmitted diseases (STDs) with skin changes include syphilis, gonorrhea, chancroid, and lymphogranuloma venereum. Syphilis has mucocutaneous manifestations that range from a chancre typically in the genital (sometimes oral) area in the primary stage of the disease to widespread papulosquamous eruptions (Figure 20.5) in the secondary stage and in the last stage may present with granulomatous nodules called gummas. The lesions of the primary and

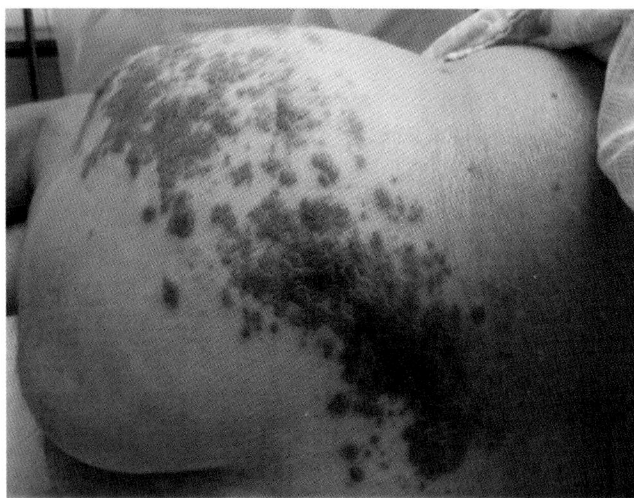

FIGURE 20.4. Varicella-zoster virus infection of the hip in a dermatomal distribution. (Courtesy of Henry K. Wong, MD, PhD.)

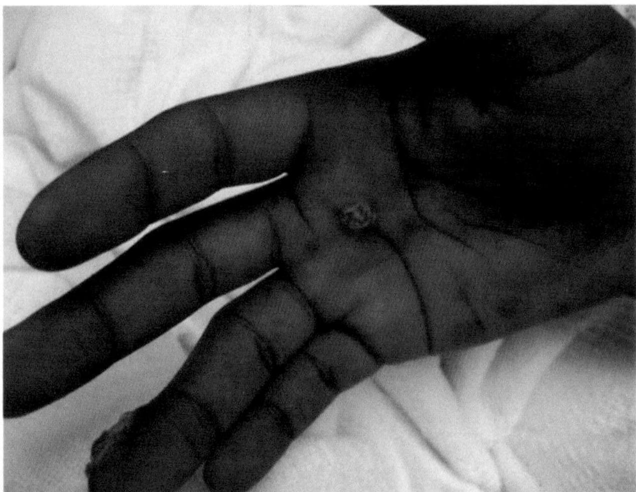

FIGURE 20.5. Syphilis of the palm and ring finger. (Courtesy of Henry K. Wong, MD, PhD.)

secondary stage are highly contagious, and care must be taken when examining patients suspected of having the disease.

Gonorrhea is an STD that can manifest with cutaneous pustules along with arthritis and fever. Disseminated gonococcal infections should be treated with IV ceftriaxone. Chancroids are another STD, causing genital ulcers and inguinal lymphadenopathy. Treatment is with antimicrobials.

Benign Skin Lesions

Contact Dermatitis

Contact dermatitis is a common condition that is caused by a delayed hypersensitivity reaction (type IV) within the skin that clinically presents with pruritus and a well-demarcated, erythematous, sometimes vesicular patch (**Figure 20.6**). It is typically localized to the area of contact by the allergen. Common allergens include poison ivy and nickel. Patch testing remains the standard for identification where allergens are placed on the skin and the patient is monitored for a response to identify causative agents after 48 hours. Treatment starts by avoiding the offending allergen. If there is a reaction, corticosteroids are the treatment of choice and have many formulations that can be administered depending on severity of reaction, with topical being the most common form for milder presentations.[13,14]

Eczema (Atopic Dermatitis)

Eczema (atopic dermatitis) is a benign condition that often develops in infancy and childhood with relapsing curse of pruritus that may become chronic. It may be accompanied by other disorders such as allergic rhinitis, asthma, food allergies, and more rarely eosinophilic esophagitis. There is usually an age-specific distribution pattern affecting extensor surfaces, face, and neck in infants and then flexor surfaces later. Management typically involves patient education, daily use of moisturizers, and use of anti-inflammatory medications (topical corticosteroids) during a flare up. Severe disease may require the use of systemic medications.[15]

Nevi (Benign Melanocyte Proliferation)

Congenital nevi are present at birth or appear in infancy and are classified based on their size (small, medium, large, and giant). Common acquired melanocytic nevi include:

Junctional nevi: where there is proliferation of the melanocytes at the dermal-epidermal junction

Intradermal nevi: with the melanocytes being located in the dermis

Compound nevi: with both intraepidermal and intradermal complexes of melanocytes

Differentiating these from melanoma can be difficult, and often the ABCDE pneumonic—asymmetry, border irregularity, color variation, diameter >6 mm, enlarging or evolving—is used as a guide for when to intervene with biopsy and further workup (**Figure 20.7**, **Table 20.1**).[16]

Rosacea

Rosacea is a common chronic inflammatory facial dermatosis usually affecting lighter-skinned individuals and typically appearing in middle age. Clinically, it has variable presentation from facial flushing and telangiectasias to papules and pustules. There are four subtypes, and treatment includes patient education on skin care and need for maintenance therapy along with the use of topical and oral antibiotics such as doxycycline and topical ivermectin.[17]

Seborrheic Dermatitis

Seborrheic dermatitis is characterized by sharply demarcated patches or plaques that can range from pink-yellow to red-brown and may have flaky greasy scales. It typically affects areas high in sebaceous glands including the face, scalp, ears, parasternal region, and sometimes intertriginous areas. It may present in infancy *cradle cap* where it tends to have a more limited course or in adults typically presents as a chronic relapsing course and often affects the scalp. Treatment

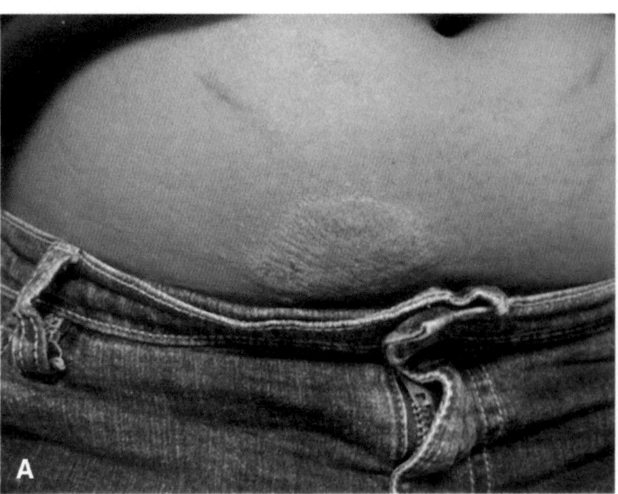

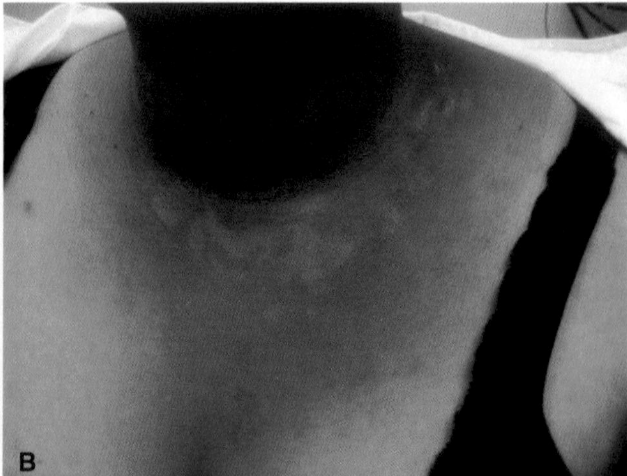

FIGURE 20.6. Contact dermatitis due to nickel **(A)** and necklace **(B)**. (Courtesy of Henry K. Wong, MD, PhD.)

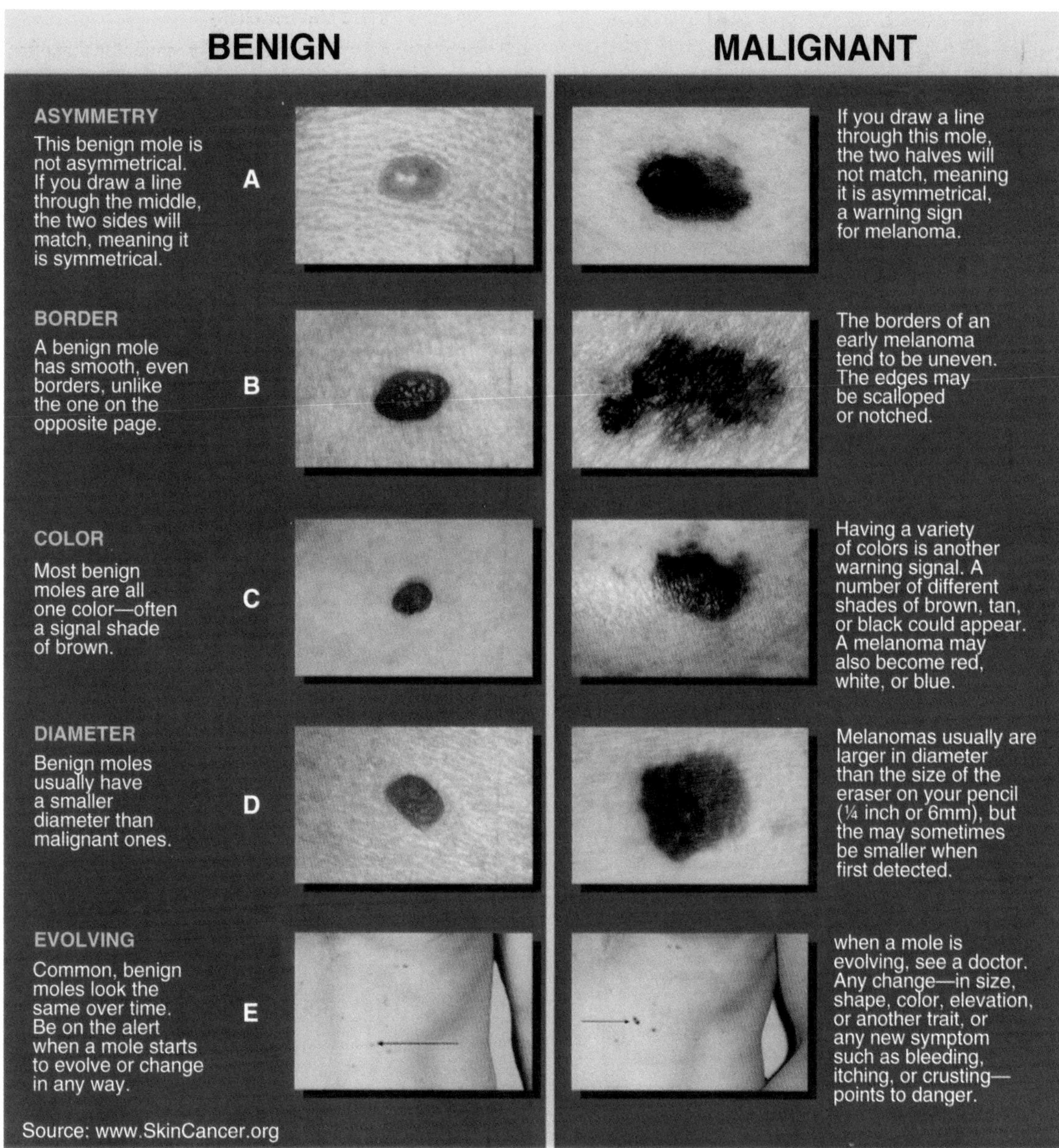

BENIGN
MALIGNANT
ASYMMETRY
This benign mole is not asymmetrical. If you draw a line through the middle, the two sides will match, meaning it is symmetrical.
A
If you draw a line through this mole, the two halves will not match, meaning it is asymmetrical, a warning sign for melanoma.
BORDER
A benign mole has smooth, even borders, unlike the one on the opposite page.
B
The borders of an early melanoma tend to be uneven. The edges may be scalloped or notched.
COLOR
Most benign moles are all one color—often a signal shade of brown.
C
Having a variety of colors is another warning signal. A number of different shades of brown, tan, or black could appear. A melanoma may also become red, white, or blue.
DIAMETER
Benign moles usually have a smaller diameter than malignant ones.
D
Melanomas usually are larger in diameter than the size of the eraser on your pencil (¼ inch or 6mm), but the may sometimes be smaller when first detected.
EVOLVING
Common, benign moles look the same over time. Be on the alert when a mole starts to evolve or change in any way.
E
when a mole is evolving, see a doctor. Any change—in size, shape, color, elevation, or another trait, or any new symptom such as bleeding, itching, or crusting—points to danger.
Source: www.SkinCancer.org

FIGURE 20.7. ABCDE mnemonic as a guide for assessing pigmented lesions. (From www.skincancer.org.)

in infants is often satisfactory with emollients, with more extensive cases requiring ketoconazole and low-potency steroids to suppress inflammation. In adults, the condition usually responds well to topical azoles (e.g., ketoconazole along with emollients).

Psoriasis

Psoriasis is a common inflammatory disease affecting the skin that causes characteristic silver scaly, erythematous plaques that are often well demarcated (Figure 20.8). It typically affects the scalp, extensor surface of elbow and knees, and intergluteal folds. It can also affect the nails, hands, and trunk. The disease is thought to be caused by T-cells interacting with dendritic cells and other innate cells of immunity. The pathognomonic pathologic finding is accumulation of neutrophils as spongiform pustules in the epidermis. Other associated manifestations include arthritis but also some cardiovascular diseases and depression. Treatment of the condition depends on disease severity with mild forms being treated with topical steroids and other topical agents such as vitamin D analogues. Patients with more advanced disease can be treated with phototherapy and immunomodulators, which have shown to be effective in more severe disease forms. Treatment of the disease should focus on managing acute flares as well as maintenance when not having flares because it is a chronic disease process.[18]

Urticaria (and Drug Eruptions)

Urticaria, commonly referred to as hives, welts, or wheals, is typically a well-circumscribed intensely raised pruritic plaque. It is usually caused by a trigger, such as food, insect bites, or drugs. Urticaria may also present with angioedema, representing deeper swelling in the skin and typically affecting the face and lips, extremities, and genitals. It is mediated by mast cells and basophils releasing mediators that include histamine. A majority of new acute urticaria lesions are self-limiting, but in severe cases, chronic cases, and cases that include angioedema, H1 blockers and glucocorticoids can be considered for treatment.[19]

Acne

Acne represents a common dermatologic condition affecting the pilosebaceous units and typically presents in adolescence. Commonly affected areas include the face and upper trunk. Clinical manifestations can vary but are generally broken down into inflammatory (papules, pustules, and nodules) and noninflammatory (open and closed comedones). Clinical presentation varies in severity, and many factors are known to play a

TABLE 20.1. INDICATION FOR MOHS EXCISION IN PRIMARY LESIONS

■ Areas with high rate of treatment failure (periorbital, periauricular, Nose, paranasal)
■ Tumor with poorly delineated clinical borders or arising from scar tissue
■ Tumors with aggressive malignant features
■ SCC: Breslow depth >2 mm, poorly differentiated or undifferentiated, spindle cell, acantholytic, sclerosing, small cell, clear cell, lymphoepithelioma-like, sarcomatoid
■ BCC: Morpheaform (sclerosing), micronodular, basosquamous(metatypical), infiltrating
■ Location in critical structures such as the eyelid or where desirable to preserve as much uninvolved tissue as possible
■ Perineural invasion
■ Dermatofibrosarcoma protuberans
■ Microcystic adnexal carcinoma

Reprinted from Connolly SM, Baker DR, Coldiron BM, et al. AAD/ACMS/ASDSA/ASMS 2012 appropriate use criteria for Mohs micrographic surgery: a report of the American Academy of Dermatology, American College of Mohs Surgery, American Society for Dermatologic Surgery Association, and the American Society for Mohs Surgery. *J Am Acad Dermatol.* 2012;67(4):531-550. Copyright © 2012 American Academy of Dermatology, Inc. and the American Society for Dermatologic Surgery, Inc. With permission.
BCC, basal cell carcinoma; SCC, squamous cell carcinoma.

role in disease manifestation including genetics, hormones, and environmental factors. Treatments are typically geared toward reducing the predisposing risk factors and include facial cleansers, hormone therapy and vitamin A analogues, and antibiotic therapy (both oral and topical).

Alopecia and Hair Disorders

Alopecia can be the result of hair follicle loss, loss of the hair shaft, or a combination of both. There are three phases of hair growth: anagen, telogen, and catagen. Identifying hair follicles in their phases and any disruption in this cycle can help lead to a diagnosis and treatment.

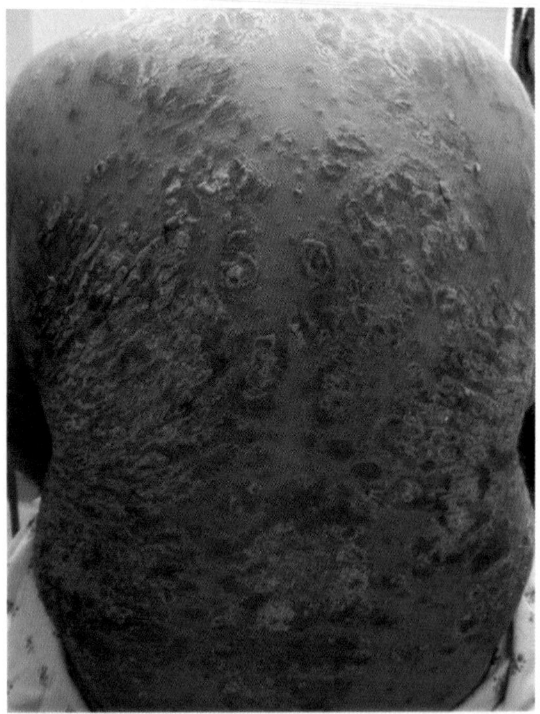

FIGURE 20.8. Psoriasis of the back. (Courtesy of Henry K. Wong, MD, PhD.)

Androgenic alopecia represents one of the most common acquired forms of hair loss and is known to be genetically driven in the presence of androgen. In genetically susceptible hair follicles, there is miniaturization of hairs in a symmetric pattern (on the crown, vertex, or frontal region) in response to normal levels of circulating androgens. Antiandrogen medications have been helpful in treating this condition.

Telogen effluvium represents an increase in shedding of otherwise normal telogen hairs in response to a pathologic or physiologic change. This is, for example, seen in the postpartum period, after some medications, and there will be time of shedding usually around 3 months after the event.

Alopecia areata is a form of noncicatricial alopecia that is thought to be from hair-specific autoimmune disorder. Clinically, there are often circular patches of hair loss but can involve the entire scalp in some cases. Topical and intralesional steroids are often first-line therapy in smaller areas.

Nail Disorders

The nail serves many purposes including protection of the finger, counterpressure for the pulp, and utility in fine object manipulation and scratching. The nail is composed of the nail bed (germinal and sterile matrices), hyponychium, and the nail plate. The nail matrix produces the nail plate through keratinization and this is occurs continuously. The nail grows approximately 0.1 mm/d. Nail disorders are a wide range of clinical disorders, and presentations vary depending on what part of the nail is affected and how it manifests. Trauma to the underlying matrix can lead to a wide assortment of disorders depending on the severity of damage to the nail bed (e.g., nail ridge, split nail, onycholysis [nonadherence]). Pitting and clubbing represent two aberrant nail presentations that can be indicative of systemic processes.

Melanonychia is caused by melanin production of nail matrix melanocytes. It presents as a longitudinal pigmented band starting at the proximal nail fold, and in adults without a history of trauma, the clinician should consider a matrix biopsy to rule out melanoma.

Infections are also common and can be acute as in a paronychial infection usually bacterial in origin or chronic with bacterial and often fungal.

Hyperpigmentation and Hypopigmentation

Hypopigmentation is a general term to describe lightening of the skin, which is most often from a decreased melanin content in the skin. It may be localized or diffuse depending on the underlying cause. This decreased melanin production (e.g., albinism) can be from the melanocytes not synthesizing melanin or from destruction of the melanocytes, which may be hereditary or the result of trauma or autoimmune attack (e.g., vitiligo). Inflammation can also cause a state of hypomelanosis that may resolve once the cause of inflammation is treated. Tyrosinase inhibitors and hydroquinone work by preventing tyrosinase, which is essential in melanogenesis, and have been used to prevent hyperpigmentation in patients seeking resurfacing procedures.

Hyperpigmentation disorders are usually the result of increase in melanin production but rarely can be from an increase in the melanocyte number. It may be diffuse, circumscribed, linear, or more rarely reticulated. If the hyperpigmentation is acquired, removal of the inciting stimulus may help ameliorate the issue.

NONMELANOMA SKIN CANCERS (KERATINOCYTE CANCERS)

NMSCs are the most common form of cancer in the United States with the incidence estimated to be 5.5 million in 2012.[3] The most important risk factor for NMSC is the skin phenotype, but it is also influenced by UV radiation exposure. For basal cell carcinoma (BCC), especially, intermittent intense episodes of UV exposure appear to increase the risk, whereas a history of childhood sunburns, especially severe burns, gives an increased risk for actinic keratosis (AK) and squamous cell carcinoma (SCC). Another well-established risk factor is immunosuppression. Patients with human immunodeficiency syndrome are known to have a 1.8- and 5.4-fold increase in the risk for developing BCC and SCC, respectively, compared with the general population.[20] Patients on immunosuppressive therapy also exhibit a greater incidence of NMSC development.

The standard for diagnosis of NMSC remains a thorough physical examination followed by conventional biopsy with histopathology for definitive diagnosis. Dermoscopy and confocal microscopy, cross-polarized light, and fluorescence photography have all been used as adjunct screening tools to identify at-risk lesions before proceeding with biopsy. In terms of biopsy technique, there are several techniques but no one standard method. Options for biopsy include shave, excisional, incisional, and punch biopsy. All have advantages and disadvantages with the goal of identifying cancerous cells for eventual destruction without significant tissue distortion.

Basal Cell Carcinoma

Basal cell cancer represents the most common form of skin cancer and malignancy in the Caucasian population. They arise from the pluripotent stem cells within the epidermis and hair follicles. BCC is well known to be locally aggressive, and the biggest risk for recurrence is locally rather than with metastasis. Because of its propensity to occur in sun-exposed areas, particularly on the face, head, and neck, they can cause great disfigurement. There is no role for lymph node sampling in BCC because it stays local. Factors in BCC that are known to be prognostic include location with high-risk regions being on the face, forehead, scalp, neck, and pretibial regions, where lesions in these areas that are >10 mm are considered high risk. Other factors that increase the risk for recurrence include poorly defined borders, recurrent cancer, perineural invasion, immunosuppression, and prior XRT at the site.

There are 26 listed subtypes of BCC. A general schematic for breakdown include dividing them based on their histopathologic pattern, which is more important than the differentiation. The two subtypes are circumscribed BCC and the diffuse subtypes of BCC. In the circumscribed group, nodular represents the most common form of BCC and accounts for about 50% of all BCC. Its appearance is a pink/red papule that has a pearly appearance. Other examples that would fall in the circumscribed group include adenoid cystic, keratotic, fibroepithelioma of Pinkus.

Diffuse basal cell cancers include superficial, micronodular, infiltrating, and morpheaform (sclerosing). Morpheaform is the most aggressive type and typically has the appearance of a firm depressed plaque in a scar. Typically, there is invasion beyond the visible edges of the lesion that will often extend into the deep dermis.

Treatment of BCC can be broken down into three categories: surgical, destructive, and medical. Surgical is either primary surgical excision or Mohs surgical excision. Surgical margins in primary excision depend on risk factors including location, tumor size, and histologic subtype. Mohs surgical incision uses saucer-like layers to remove all tumor, creating a map for the surgeon to mark areas of tumor for further excisions. Mohs excision is recommended for most recurrent basal cell and squamous cell cancers (see Table 20.1). Mohs has the advantage of preserving normal tissue, and this technique is used in the face or for other lesions that may be more aggressive. Destructive therapy aims to destroy the tissue and is only indicated for superficial lesions. Techniques include electrodissection, cryotherapy, and radiotherapy. Medical therapy includes 5-FU and imiquimod but is inferior to surgical and destructive techniques.

Squamous Cell Carcinoma

AK represents an intradermal early stage SCC and is most commonly seen in areas of prolonged UV exposure in fair-skinned and elderly patients. It has a rough erythematous papule appearance and is typically located in sun-exposed areas (helices of ear, upper forehead, nasal bridge, bald scalp, etc.). Lesions may be small or very large and broad. They are characterized as *precancerous* because they have atypical keratinocytes confined to the epidermis. Their risk of transformation to invasive carcinoma is up to 0.06% per year.[21]

SCC in situ is commonly referred to as Bowen disease. It typically presents as a scaly elevated plaque often in sun-exposed areas but in younger patients, may be in sun-protected sites. SCC in situ and AK can be difficult to distinguish from psoriasis papules and plaques that may resemble these processes.

Keratoacanthomas are considered by many to be a variant of SCC. They typically present as rapidly enlarging papules over a few months that are sharply circumscribed and have a keratotic core. Sometimes, they spontaneously resolve, but this can take months and given similar appearance to SCC most advocate excision.[22] They often present as a solitary lesion but may be in multiple locations as part of a syndrome.

Invasive SCC often develops in sun-exposed areas such as the scalp, face, neck, dorsal hands, skin and extensor forearms, with the risk factor being more related to the cumulative effect. It can have a variable presentation with some becoming hyperkeratotic and having crusting, erosions, and ulcerations. The growth history is variable, but signs of paresthesia, anesthesia, and pain are indicative of perineural invasion (at least T3). Diagnosis of SCC is with tissue biopsy and also clinical examination of draining lymph node basins.

SCC is staged using the AJCC TNM with recent changes in 2017 to reflect the clinicohistopathologic features that increase the risk for recurrence. Sites where the tumor behaves more aggressively include the ear, lips, and mucosal sites. When evaluating patients, palpation of regional lymph nodes should be performed to assess for the presence of palpable nodes as well as the size. Any palpable nodes should be biopsied with fine needle aspiration. Risk factors that increase risk for metastasis are listed in **Table 20.2**.

Treatment of SCC depends on the stage of SCC, with some low-risk cancers being amenable to destructive therapy similar to BCC. Direct surgical excision (primary or with Mohs) can be used for both low- and high-risk lesions.

TABLE 20.2. HIGH-RISK FEATURES OF SQUAMOUS CELL CARCINOMA

Features on History and Physical
■ Borders: poorly defined
■ Diameter: Area L ≥ 20 mm; Area M ≥ 10 mm
■ Recurrent
■ Arising within a scar, prior RT site or other chronic inflammatory process
■ Immunosuppression
Features on Pathology
■ Poorly differentiated or undifferentiated, developing within Bowen disease
■ Acantholytic, adenosquamous, desmoplastic, or metaplastic subtypes
■ Tumor thickness: ≥2 mm or Clark IV, V
■ Perineural, lymphatic, or vascular involvement

Adapted with permission from the NCCN Clinical Practice Guidelines in Oncology (NCCN Guidelines®) for Squamous Cell Carcinoma V.2.2018. To view the most recent and complete version of the NCCN Guidelines, go online to NCCN.org. The NCCN Guidelines are a work in progress that may be refined as often as new significant data become available.

SKIN AND SOFT TISSUE

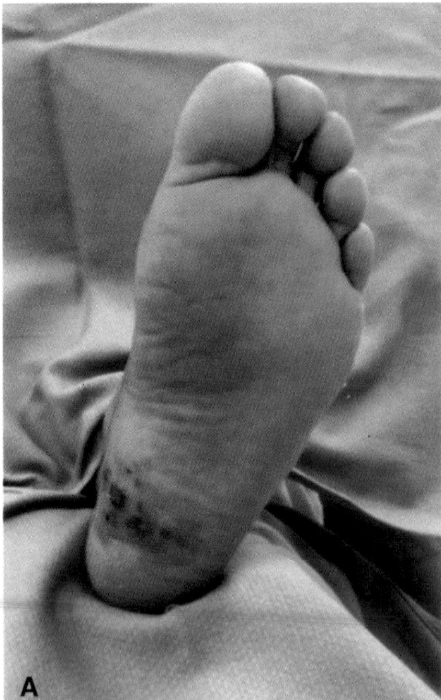

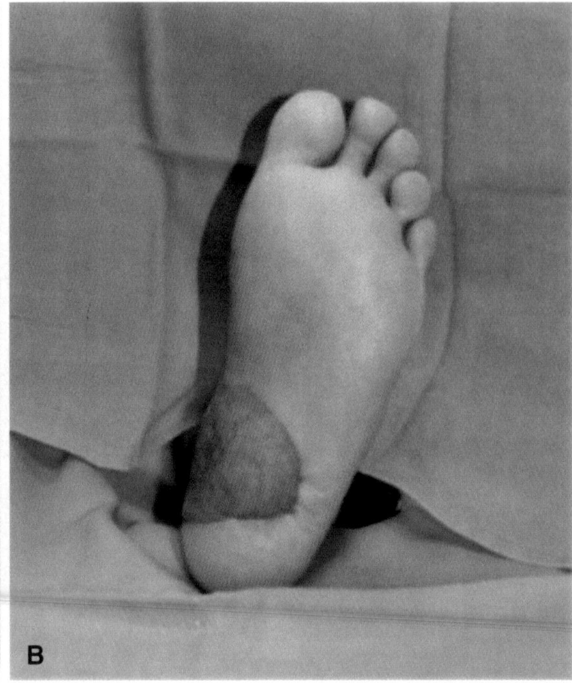

FIGURE 20.9. **A.** Melanoma of the heel. **B.** Result after wide local excision and reconstruction with free radial forearm fasciocutaneous flap.

MELANOMA

Melanoma is the most deadly of all the skin cancers and accounts for 75% of all the deaths related to skin cancer whereas only accounting for less than 5% of skin cancer diagnosis. Trends suggest that its incidence continues to rise. Melanocytes that undergo a malignant transformation are most commonly in the skin but may also be present in the eye or mucus membranes.

Melanomas arise from the melanocyte that is a dendritic cell located in the basal layer of skin. It is responsible for producing the melanin pigment that gives the skin phenotypes. Melanocyte numbers are equal among all skin colors; however, the production of melanin varies. Melanomas can grow in both a radial and vertical growth pattern. The radial pattern is usually in the epidermis and some melanomas can stay in this radial growth pattern for a long time. In the vertical growth, the growth shifts down into the dermis and indicates a worse prognosis.

Melanomas can be broken down into five clinical and histological growth patterns. Superficial spreading is the most common. This can occur anywhere but often occurs in regions of sun exposure. As the name might suggest, it typically has a prolonged radial growth pattern before transforming into a more vertical. Nodular melanoma is the second most common type and has a classic presentation of a singular lesion with a domed-shaped dark appearance that can resemble a blood blister. It tends to develop in a vertical growth pattern more quickly and often occurs on the trunk, and head and neck regions. Because of the growth pattern, it is often more advanced at the time of diagnosis. Lentigo melanoma is a rare form that presents as large tan lesions with convoluted patterns and amelanotic patterns. It has a low malignancy potential and is more common in women, typically on the head, face, and neck. Acral-lentiginous melanoma is the rarest in Caucasians but accounts for greater than 30% of all melanomas that occur in dark-skinned individuals.[16] This often occurs on the palms, on soles of feet (**Figure 20.9**), and beneath the nail beds. In the subungual presentation, they commonly cause a longitudinal line in the nail plate known as Hutchinson sign. Amelanotic melanomas are responsible for 2% to 8% of invasive cases and characterized by malignant cells that lack pigment, making them clinically difficult to identify and leading to later identification. Desmoplastic melanomas are another rare melanoma form that typically has an aggressive local growth pattern but less propensity to metastasize.

Diagnosis of a melanoma starts with clinical examination. The ABCDE mnemonic (see Figure 20.7) can be used as a guide for assessing pigmented lesions and can guide a clinician on when to biopsy a lesion.[23] Definitive diagnosis of melanoma is with incisional biopsy. The two classic staging classifications are the Clark and Breslow classifications. The Clark classification is based on the anatomic level of local invasion. Breslow classification is based on vertical depth of the invasion in millimeters. The AJCC is what is used for staging, but part of the staging related to depth is similar to the Breslow classification because it was a better prognosticator of disease severity and risk recurrence.[24] As part of staging workup, it is important that the specimen is viewed with standard stains rather than frozen sectioning to prevent specimen distortion and allow for adequate assessment of Breslow depth, which is calculated using ocular micrometer and is in reference to the greatest depth of invasion of the tumor measured down from the granular layer of the epidermis. This has been shown to be one of the best prognostic values for tumor prognosis as well as lymph node metastasis.[25]

Management of the primary tumor is with wide excision of the primary tumor site. Excision should include skin and subcutaneous fat down to but not including the fascia. The National Comprehensive Cancer Network (NCCN) has recommended surgical margins based on Breslow depth, which are listed in **Table 20.3**.

In addition to tumor depth, ulceration and mitotic rate also play a role in staging. Mitotic rate has also been identified as an independent predictor of survival and so is also a part of the AJCC staging.[26] The thickness correlates with prognosis with modifications in each T category if there are mitotic figures or ulceration indicating worse prognosis.

The sentinel lymph node is the first lymph node in the draining basin from the primary tumor site. Because this node is usually involved, if there is regional nodal metastasis it can be used as a selective sample marker to see if the rest of the nodal basin is affected. Sentinel lymph node sampling is advocated in patients with stage I/II melanoma with tumor thickness 1.0 to 4.0 mm Breslow depth, or those with depth of 0.76 to 1.0 mm with other high-risk factors, including ulceration, lymphovascular invasion, significant vertical growth phase, and increased mitotic rate. Additionally patients with tumor >4.0 mm depth and clinically negative nodes also benefit from SLN biopsy.

TABLE 20.3. NCCN GUIDELINES FOR TUMOR MARGIN BASED ON BRESLOW THICKNESS

Tumor Microstage	Thickness	Margin
Melanoma in situ (Tis)		0.5 cm
Thin (T1)	≤1.0 mm	1.0 cm
Intermediate (T2)	1.0–2 mm	1.0–2.0 cm
Intermediate (T3)	2.0–4.0 mm	2.0 cm
Thick (T4)	>4 mm	2.0 cm

Adapted with permission from the NCCN Clinical Practice Guidelines in Oncology (NCCN Guidelines®) for Squamous Cell Carcinoma V.2.2018. To view the most recent and complete version of the NCCN Guidelines, go online to NCCN.org. The NCCN Guidelines are a work in progress that may be refined as often as new significant data become available.

Complete surgical lymphadenectomy is recommended for any patient with clinically involved nodes diagnosed via examination, FNA, or SLN biopsy. Node status is the most important prognostic factor in staging melanoma.

Clinically advanced (stage IV) melanoma carries a poor prognosis, with only 10% to 15% of patients living past 5 years.

MERKEL CELL CARCINOMA

Merkel cell carcinoma is a rare form of skin cancer typically affecting older (>50) fair-skinned individuals in sun-exposed areas. It usually presents as a solitary erythematous nodular lesion in sun-exposed areas of the head and neck. It commonly spreads to lymph nodes with 25% to 30% of initial presenting patients having positive nodes. It is aggressive like melanoma, and like melanoma staging depends on node involvement with SLN biopsy. Primary surgical excision with wide margins or Mohs is standard treatment. Local recurrence is 40% to 45%. Radiation can be used as adjuvant therapy.[27]

REFERENCES

1. Lomas A, Leonardi-Bee J, Bath-Hextall F. A systematic review of worldwide incidence of nonmelanoma skin cancer. *Br J Dermatol*. 2012;166:1069-1080.
2. Guy GP, Machlin SR, Ekwueme DU, Yabroff KR. Prevalence and costs of skin cancer treatment in the U.S., 2002–2006 and 2007–2011. *Am J Prev Med*. 2014;104(4):e69-e74.
   Using data obtained from the Medical Expenditure Panel Survey from 2002 to 2011, this study looked to estimate the trends in NMSC prevalence and treatment costs. Although limited by relying on self or household-reported survey data, this study suggests a significant rise in skin cancer incidence as well as the cost associated with the treatment of skin cancer.
3. Rogers HW, Weinstock MA, Feldman SR, Coldiron BM. Incidence estimate of nonmelanoma skin cancer (keratinocyte carcinomas) in the US population, 2012. *JAMA Dermatol*. 2015;151(10):1081-1086.
   Using the Center for Medicare & Medicaid Services Physicians' Claims database (to calculate total skin cancer procedures performed) and the National Ambulatory Medical Care Survey database (to estimate the NMSC-related office visits), these authors attempt to estimate the incidence of keratinocyte carcinomas in the United States and compared it with numbers from 2006 to 2011.
4. Fitzpatrick TB. The validity and practicality of sunreactive skin types I through VI. *Arch Dermatol*. 1988;124:869.
5. Fitzpatrick TB. Soleil et peau [Sun and skin]. *J Méd Esthétique*. 1975;2:33-34.
6. Farmer KL, Goller M, Lippman SM. Prevention of nonmelanoma skin cancer. *Clin Plast Surg*. 1997;24(4):663.
7. Weissler JM, Carney MJ, Carreras Tartak JA, et al. The evolution of chemical peeling and modern-day applications. *Plast Reconstr Surg*. 2017;140(5):920-929.
   This review article starts with a historical perspective of chemexfoliation in ancient times and the progress to present-day practices. The mechanism of the peel is briefly reviewed, and there is a chemical peel classification table that offers some common peels. Indications are listed as well as options for prepeel skin care regimens to maximize chemical peel effects. The article reviews peel application as well as posttreatment care with a supplemental video. Through a better understanding of the mechanism of the chemical peel agents as well as modifications to the solutions, clinicians are able to offer safe and effective resurfacing options to the patient with aesthetic concerns. Potential side effects are reviewed for peels at the end of the paper.
8. Alexiades-Armenakas MR, Dover JS, Arndt KA. The spectrum of laser skin resurfacing: nonablative, fractional, and ablative laser resurfacing. *J Am Acad Dermatol*. 2008;58:719-737.
9. Raff AB, Kroshinsky D. Cellulitis: a review. *JAMA*. 2016;316(3):325-337.
10. Binford GJ, Wells MA. The phylogenetic distribution of sphingomyelinase D activity in venoms of Haplogyne spiders. *Comp Biochem Physiol B Biochem Mol Biol*. 2003;135(1):25.
11. Hariri S, Unger ER, Sternberg M, et al. Prevalence of genital human papillomavirus among females in the United States, the National Health and Nutrition Examination Survey, 2003–2006. *J Infect Dis*. 2011;204:566-573.
12. Paavonen J, Naud P, Salmerón J, et al. Efficacy of human papillomavirus (HPV)-16/18 AS04-adjuvanted vaccine against cervical infection and precancer caused by oncogenic HPV types (PATRICIA): final analysis of a double-blind, randomized study in young women. *Lancet*. 2009;374:301-314.
13. Clark SC, Zirwas MJ. Management of occupational dermatitis. *Dermatol Clin*. 2009;27:365.
14. Mowad CM, Anderson B, Scheinman P, et al. Allergic contact dermatitis: patient diagnosis and evaluation. *J Am Acad Dermatol*. 2016;74:1029-1040.
15. Eichenfield LF, Tom WL, Berger TG, et al. Guidelines of care for the management of atopic dermatitis. Section 2: management and treatment of atopic dermatitis with topical therapies. *J Am Acad Dermatol*. 2014;71:116-132.
16. Bradford PT, Goldstein AM, McMaster ML, Tucker MA. Acral lentiginous melanoma incidence and survival patterns in the United States, 1986-2005. *JAMA Dermatol*. 2009;145(4):427-434.
17. Powell FC. Rosacea. *N Engl J Med*. 2005;352(8):793-803.
18. Boehncke WH, Schon MP. Psoriasis. *Lancet*. 2015;386(9997):983-994.
19. Kaplan AP. Clinical practice: chronic urticaria and angioedema. *N Engl J Med*. 2002;346:175-179.
20. Omland SH, Ahlström MG, Gerstoft J, et al. Risk of skin cancer in HIV-infected patients: a Danish nationwide cohort study. *J Am Acad Dermatol*. 2018;79(4):689-695. pii:S0190-9622(18) 30475-4.
21. Siegel JA, Korgavkar K, Weinstock MA. Current perspective on actinic keratosis: a review. *Br J Dermatol*. 2017;177:350-358.
   AK is a health concern with over $1 billion US dollars in annual cost in diagnosis and management; however, there is no universally agreed-upon diagnostic gold standard. AK can cause significant disfigurement making it a cosmetic issue in addition to the possibility of malignant transformation. The natural history of AK is spontaneous remission, stable existence, or malignant transformation to keratinized carcinoma with variable reported rates of 0% to 21%. Some of the discrepancy in the malignant transformation in the reported studies may be related to different definitions for AK. Further study is needed for more universal diagnostic criteria of AK, further understanding of malignant progression and therapeutic strategies to better manage AK.
22. Schwartz RA. Keratoacanthoma. *J Am Acad Dermatol*. 1994;30:1-19.
23. Abbasi NR, Shaw HM, Rigel DS, et al. Early diagnosis of cutaneous melanoma. *JAMA*. 2004;292:2771-2776.
24. Breslow A. Thickness, cross-sectional areas and depth of invasion in the prognosis of cutaneous melanoma. *Ann Surg*. 1970;172:902-908.
   In this sentinel publication, Alexander Breslow described a technique of using an ocular micrometer to measure the depth of invasion from the skin surface to the maximal depth of invasion. He studied 98 patients and performed 5 years of follow-up. He also looked at cross-sectional area and diameter but found that the tumor thickness was the most significant variable and best for predicting a patient's outcome. He also postulated it could guide which patients should have prophylactic lymph node dissections and which group would not need them (stages I and II and stage III with thickness <0.76 mm).
25. Dzwierzynski WW. Managing malignant melanoma. *Plast Reconstr Surg*. 2013;132:446e-460e.
26. Allen PJ, Bowne WB, Jaques DP, et al. Merkel cell carcinoma: prognosis and treatment of patients from a single institution. *J Clin Oncol*. 2005;23(10):2300-2309.
27. Amin M, Edge SB, et al, eds. *AJCC Cancer Staging Manual*. 8th ed. American Joint Committee on Cancer; 2017.

QUESTIONS

1. **Sentinel lymph node biopsy (SLNB) would have the most benefit in which of the following patients?**
   a. A 50-year-old man with a 4.0 cm diameter BCC with lymphovascular invasion
   b. A 80-year-old woman with a 1.0 cm diameter melanoma with thickness of 1.0 mm and a palpable 2 cm lymph node in the affected extremity
   c. A 4-year-old boy with a 10.0 cm diameter congenital melanocytic nevus
   d. A 67-year-old man with a 0.5 cm diameter melanoma with a thickness of 1.5 mm

2. **Choose the most correct statement regarding retinoids.**
   a. Derived from vitamin C, they work by binding to nuclear receptors and modulating gene expression.
   b. Derived from vitamin A, they work by binding to transmembrane receptors and modulating gene expression.
   c. Common side effects include of topical retinoids include pruritus, peeling, photosensitivity, and erythema.
   d. Treatment results in epidermal thinning and decreased collagen in the dermis.

3. **Clinically, psoriasis is a characterized by silver scaly, erythematous plaques that are often well demarcated. Histologically, psoriasis is characterized by:**
   a. Vacuolar alteration of basal keratinocytes
   b. Accumulation of neutrophils as spongiform pustules in the epidermis
   c. Dermal changes consisting of interstitial mucin deposition and a sparse lymphocytic infiltrate
   d. Basement membrane degeneration

4. **Which Fitzpatrick skin type rarely burns and tans dark easily?**
   a. II
   b. III
   c. IV
   d. V

5. **Patients with which systemic disease are known to have a significantly increased risk for developing a primary NMSC compared with the general population?**
   a. Rheumatoid arthritis
   b. Hyperlipidemia
   c. EBV infection
   d. Human immunodeficiency syndrome

1. Answer: d. SLNB is useful in the prognostic evaluation of patients with melanoma who have stage IB/II lesions. It allows these patients with tumor of 1 to 4 mm Breslow depth (0.8–1 mm plus ulceration) to be evaluated for nodal spread without doing a full nodal dissection. Patients with tumors <0.8 mm and no ulceration are not likely to have nodal involvement. Patients who have clinically palpable lymph nodes (stage III) should have complete therapeutic lymph node dissection in addition to wide excision of the primary tumor. There is no role or SLNB in BCC as it invades locally and not through lymphovenous spread. Giant congenital nevi are excised for their potential risk of malignancy and so removal of nodes is not necessary.

2. Answer: c. Retinoids are a derivative of vitamin A and are well studied for the protective effects in the skin and reversal of photoaging. They work by binding to nuclear receptors and modulating cellular gene expression. Clinically, this leads to epidermal thickening and increased collagen in the dermis because of decreased breakdown and increased collagen synthesis in the dermis. Side effects such as pruritus, burning, erythema, and peeling are usually seen with onset of treatment and can lead to noncompliance, especially in patients with a history of sensitive skin. Photosensitivity is another common side effect of topical therapies, and patients are advised to avoid sun exposure when starting therapy.

3. Answer: b. Psoriasis is a common inflammatory disease affecting the skin that causes characteristic silver scaly, erythematous plaques that are often well demarcated. It typically affects the scalp, extensor surface of elbow and knees, and intergluteal folds. It can also affect the nails, hands, and trunk. The disease is thought to be caused by T-cells interacting with dendritic cells and other innate cells of immunity. The pathognomonic pathologic finding is accumulation of neutrophils as spongiform pustules in the epidermis. Treatment of the condition depends on disease severity with mild forms being treated with topical steroids and other topical agents such as vitamin D analogues. Patients with more advanced disease can be treated with phototherapy and immunomodulators, which have shown to be effective in more severe disease forms.

4. Answer: d. Fitzpatrick skin type classifies the skin into six phenotypes based on the melanin content of the skin (color), the inherent pigmentation of the skin, and the sensitivity of the skin to sun damage. Lower Fitzpatrick score indicates less melanin in the skin and hence a greater sensitivity to sun damage. Type I always burns and does not tan. Type II burns easily and tans poorly; type III tans after an initial burn. Type IV burns minimally, tans easily. Type V rarely burns and tans dark easily. Type VI never burns and always tans darkly.

5. Answer: d. In a matched, nationwide population-based cohort study, Omland et al. studied 4280 HIV-infected patients from a HIV cohort study with a background population cohort and found that HIV-infected patients had an increased risk ratio of 1.79 for BCC and 5.40 for SCC compared with the background population.[20] There was no increased risk of melanoma. Rheumatoid arthritis and hyperlipidemia are not associated with NMSC. EBV is associated with development of nasopharyngeal cancer and Burkitt lymphoma but not with skin cancer.

CHAPTER 21 Thermal, Chemical, and Electrical Injuries

Justin Gillenwater and Warren L. Garner

KEY POINTS

- Burn depth and size are predictive of outcomes and guide initial and definitive management.
- The goal of resuscitation is maintaining tissue perfusion, specifically the skin.
- Burn wounds that will not heal within 3 weeks usually should be excised and autografted.
- Burn care is best provided by a multidisciplinary team working with a committed patient.

EPIDEMIOLOGY

Burn injury represents a significant burden of disease. Most recent estimates indicate 486,000 people in the United States receive medical treatment for burn injuries each year. Of these, 40,000 require inpatient hospital admission and 3275 are fatal.[1] Burn survivors can develop lifelong deformities as a result of their cutaneous injury with ensuing health care needs including corrective surgical procedures, therapy sessions, and scar management. A recent systematic review estimates the average total health care cost per burn patient is $88,218 in high-income countries.[2]

PATHOPHYSIOLOGY

Local

A burn injury occurs when a thermal insult on the skin causes acute changes in its composition, killing cells and denaturing proteins. Initially, burn depth is based on two extrinsic factors: intensity of heat and duration of contact. The hotter the source or the longer the duration of contact, the deeper the burn injury. In the area of direct thermal injury, cellular and matrix proteins are irreversibly damaged, causing a release of cytokines such as IL-1, IL-8, and tumor necrosis factor alpha. This inflammatory cascade causes a secondary reaction and results in local cellular apoptosis, loss of endothelial vascular integrity, transmigration and degranulation of leukocytes, and complement activation. Although evolutionarily advantageous from an anti-infective and hemostatic perspective, this area of inflammation causes decreased tissue perfusion and may lead to conversion of burn wounds from smaller, superficial injuries to larger, deeper wounds. Appropriate resuscitation and local wound care are central to limiting reversible tissue loss and are the goal of initial burn care.

Systemic: Burn Shock

Burns greater than 20% of total body surface area (TBSA) cause a system-wide inflammatory response and lead to a systemic inflammatory response syndrome, sometimes called burn shock. As the local events become systemic, the release of inflammatory mediators into the central circulation leads to leaky microvasculature, vasodilation, decreased cardiac output, tissue hypoperfusion, and ultimately, if left unresuscitated, death.

Similar to within burned tissue, capillary integrity becomes compromised systemically. Osmotic pressure generated by transudate of proteins and electrolytes in addition to the low-flow state results in loss of intravascular volume into the interstitium. Decrease in the intravascular volume causes an increase in hematocrit and higher blood viscosity. Cell membrane alteration leads to movement of fluid into the intracellular space. Total body edema and intravascular volume depletion is the result. Maximal fluid shifts occur around 12 hours after burn.[3]

Within 24 hours after a large burn, capillary integrity in non-burned tissue returns to near normal and transudation of colloids out of the vascular space diminishes. By this time, the loss of plasma proteins into burned tissue is significant enough to decrease vascular oncotic pressure. Water continues to collect in the interstitial space even after restoration of capillary integrity and further perpetuates global tissue edema.

Burn shock results from loss of intravascular volume, cardiac dysfunction, and vascular changes. Prior to initiation of resuscitation when capillary leak predominates, relative hypovolemia and increased systemic vascular resistance predominates. As resuscitation occurs and circulating blood volume is restored, vascular tone diminishes and the systemic vascular resistance drops. Cardiac function is dynamic and unpredictable; cytokine release and current intravascular volume status affect preload, contractility, and afterload.[4,5] The kidney is particularly susceptible to damage from hypoperfusion, and acute kidney injury can be perpetuated by increased blood viscosity from elevated hematocrit and myoglobinemia from deeper tissue damage.[6,7]

INITIAL MANAGEMENT OF BURNS

Treatment of burn injuries, especially large burns, is resource intensive and best done by a dedicated multidisciplinary team (**Table 21.1**).

ABCs

Burn injuries are traumatic injuries, and treatment should adhere to the airway, breathing, and circulation (ABCs) of standard trauma care. An upper airway inhalation injury can lead to early edema formation and airway obstruction. In the event of suspected inhalation

TABLE 21.1. MULTIDISCIPLINARY TEAM FOR THE TREATMENT OF BURNS

Burn Team Member	Role in Team
The acute burn surgeon	Surgical management of burn wounds
A critical care physician	Medical management of burn shock, multiple system failure, and organ dysfunction
A reconstructive surgeon	Manage the aesthetic and functional deformities resulting from burn scars
Specially trained burn nurses	Comprehensive daily burn wound debridement and dressing changes
Physical and occupational therapists	Prevent functional disabilities and limit contracture formation Fabricate splints
Clinical nutritionists	Assess for adequate caloric supplementation
Social workers, clinical psychologists	Manage psychosocial factors, prevent posttraumatic shock disorder
Clinical pharmacists	Manage drug dosing and interactions

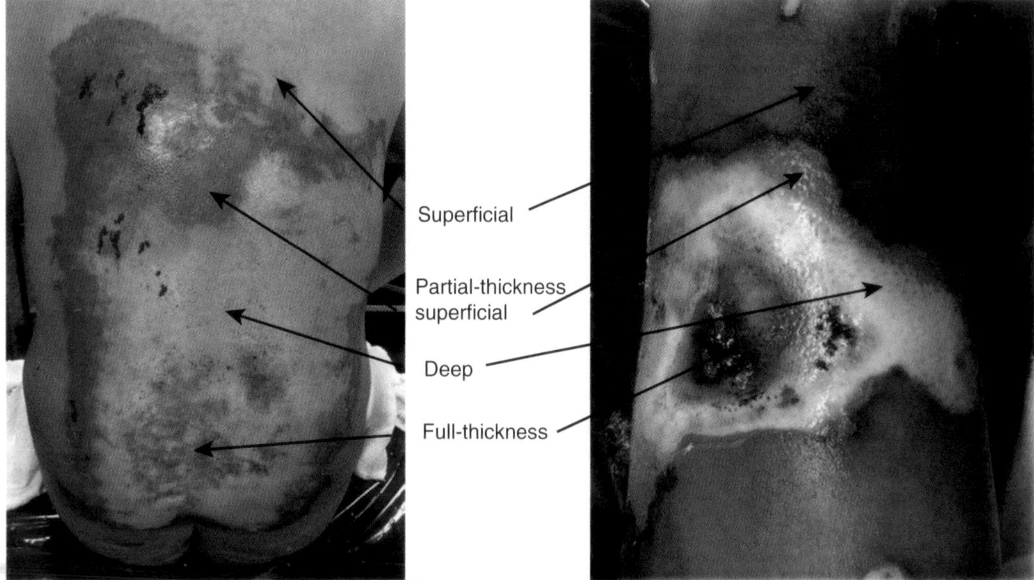

FIGURE 21.1. Superficial, partial-thickness (superficial and deep), and full-thickness burns.

injury, securing airway patency with endotracheal intubation is the critical first step. Patients with suspected inhalation injury that do not exhibit signs or symptoms of impending airway obstruction may be carefully monitored in an intensive care unit (ICU) setting. Consultation to otolaryngologist may be indicated for serial fiber optic laryngoscopic examinations.

Patients with circumferential torso burns may need escharotomies to improve their thoracic compliance and promote adequate ventilation—breathing—to occur. Similarly, patients with circumferential extremity burns may need escharotomies to restore circulation distally. Although escharotomies are best done by an experienced provider, they should not be delayed if a prolonged transport is anticipated.

Once the patient is stabilized, a full and detailed history should be obtained to determine the etiology of the injury, obtain medical comorbidities, etc. If the patient is obtunded, then family members, emergency medical technician providers, or witnesses can be valuable sources of information. Tetanus immunization status should be assessed and prophylaxis administered as indicated.

Determination of Burn Depth

After assessing for ABCs and providing initial stabilization, burn size and depth are evaluated. Quantifying the severity of injury guides resuscitation and determines further management, including prognosis. Nomenclature for burn wounds can be confusing, but descriptive terminology—superficial, partial-thickness, full-thickness instead of first, second, and third degree—is advocated by the International Society for Burn Injuries, is most represented in the burn literature, and is generally preferred.[8] On the contrary, ICD-10 codes quantify burn depth in degrees instead of descriptive terms.[9] The clinician should be familiar with both descriptive terminology and how it corresponds to degree of burn depth (**Figure 21.1**).

Superficial (first-degree) burns affect the epidermis only. These are dry, erythematous, blanch with pressure, and painful without blistering or ulceration of the skin. Sunburn is a common presentation. They require no further management or treatment and do not lead to a systemic inflammatory response requiring resuscitation. These can be managed as an outpatient with adequate nonopioid analgesia.

Partial-thickness (second-degree) burns extend into the dermis and are the most challenging to treat from the perspective of the surgeon. Their appearance can be varied, and a correct diagnosis is necessary for correct surgical management. Superficial partial-thickness burns limited to the upper layers of the dermis will often heal without the need for grafting, whereas those extending into the deeper dermis and involving the dermal appendages may require excision and autografting for best results. Therefore, determining the exact depth of the partial-thickness burn on initial examination requires experience and is important for prognostic and therapeutic reasons. Superficial partial-thickness burns generally present with blisters that, when unroofed, reveal a pink, moist, edematous, painful blanching base (see Figure 21.1). In contrast, deep partial-thickness burns are whiter, have varying degrees of sensation and edema, and often do not demonstrate blanching or capillary refill. Finally, it is important to remember that any patient may have mixed areas of injury that will require different treatment.

Full-thickness (third-degree) burns are obvious in their presentation and appearance. The skin is contracted, dry, leathery, and insensate and can be brown, black, white, or dark red in color. There is no moisture or exudate, and subcutaneous thrombosed veins may be visible through translucent dermis. In most cases, full-thickness burns will require excision of the burn and grafting to achieve wound closure.

New technologies have been used to assist in assessing burn wound depth. Ultrasound, laser Doppler, and fluorescein all attempt to assess perfusion of the burn wound and thus its depth.[10] These technologies have not found widespread routine use yet, but they may show potential for determining regenerative potential with more investigation.

Assessing Burn Size

An accurate assessment of burn size is critical because triage and resuscitative efforts are based on the TBSA affected. Overestimation or underestimations of burn size can lead to inappropriate transfers or poor resuscitation. The Lund-Browder chart is the oldest but historically most accurate method of assessing burn size. The *rule of nines* is generally the most frequently used strategy because of its simplicity (**Figure 21.2**). Alternatively, the *palmar method* utilizes the patient's own palm as an estimate of 1% TBSA. Computer-based applications such as the SAGE diagram can give more precise assessments. More recently some mobile applications have been validated and can provide rapid and precise estimations of TBSA.

Age and body habitus affect burn size estimation. Children have disproportionately larger heads than their legs, and this should be taken into consideration by using a pediatric chart. Obese patients have a relatively larger proportion of skin on their trunks.

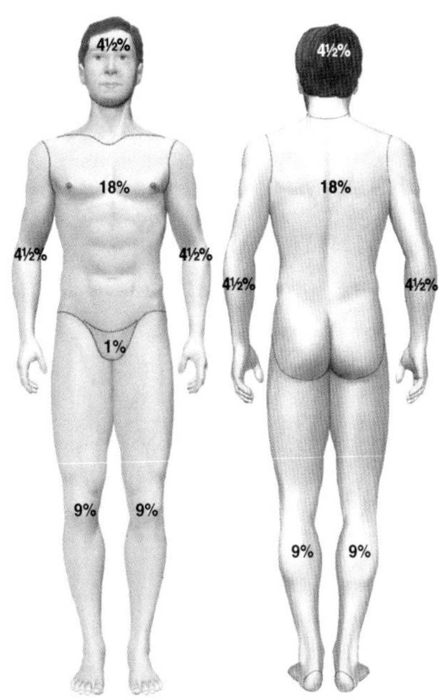

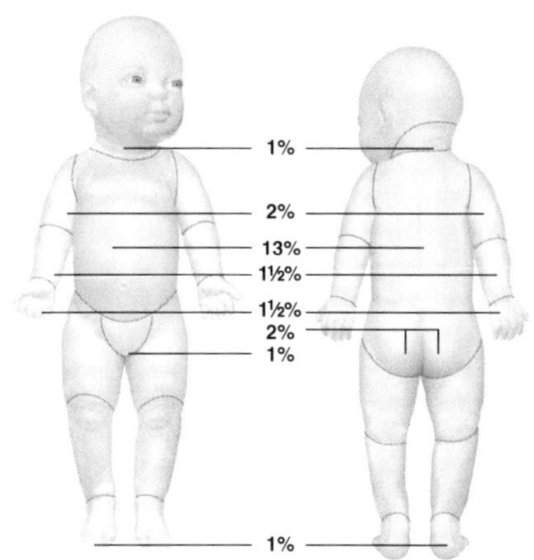

A Rule of nines

AREA	PERCENT OF BURN					SEVERITY OF BURN		TOTAL PERCENT
	0–1 Year	1–4 Years	5–9 Years	10–15 Years	Adult	2°	3°	
Head	19	17	13	10	7			
Neck	2	2	2	2	2			
Ant. Trunk	13	13	13	13	13			
Post. Trunk	13	13	13	13	13			
R. Buttock	2½	2½	2½	2½	2½			
L. Buttock	2½	2½	2½	2½	2½			
Genitalia	1	1	1	1	1			
R. U. Arm	4	4	4	4	4			
L. U. Arm	4	4	4	4	4			
R. L. Arm	3	3	3	3	3			
L. L. Arm	3	3	3	3	3			
R. Hand	2½	2½	2½	2½	2½			
L. Hand	2½	2½	2½	2½	2½			
R. Thigh	5½	6½	8½	8½	9½			
L. Thigh	5½	6½	8½	8½	9½			
R. Leg	5	5	5½	6	7			
L. Leg	5	5	5½	6	7			
R. Foot	3½	3½	3½	3½	3½			
L. Foot	3½	3½	3½	3½	3½			
Total				**Total**				

B Lund and Browder chart

FIGURE 21.2. Common methods of estimating burn size. (Reproduced with permission from Stout LR. Burns and common integumentary disorders. In: Morton PG, Fontaine DK, eds. *Critical Care Nursing: A Holistic Approach*. 11th ed. Philadelphia, PA: Wolters Kluwer; 2018:1031. **A.** Adapted from *Anatomical Chart Company: Atlas of Pathophysiology*. 3rd ed. Springhouse, PA: Springhouse; 2010:385. Figure 32-1A and Figure 32-1B.)

There are currently no consensus guidelines from major burn organizations to guide burn size estimation. Consequently, the treating clinician should use the most familiar method, while understanding the limitations of each.

Patient Triage

Triage of the burn patient depends on the severity of the injury and the resources available to the initial treatment team. **Table 21.2** gives criteria for burn center referral from the American Burn Association (ABA).[11]

Patients meeting criteria for transfer should have large-bore intravenous access to begin resuscitation and be placed in clean, dry dressings. Further wound care will complicate initial management and is unnecessary because a comprehensive evaluation will be performed when the patient arrives at the burn unit. Normothermia must be maintained, especially for larger burns, because thermoregulation can be impaired.

Patients who do not meet burn center referral criteria may be managed at the referring facility at the discretion of the treating surgeon. For these patients, bedside mechanical debridement should be performed under appropriate sedation to fully assess the depth and extent of burn injury. Blisters should be unroofed, and broad-spectrum topical antimicrobials should be placed over the wound depending on its depth and extent. Systemic antibiotics have no role in treated uninfected burns.

Superficial partial-thickness burns or small full-thickness burns may be taken care of as an outpatient provided the patient meet certain criteria: One, the ability to provide adequate local wound care at home. Two, adequate analgesia does not interfere with wound care. Three, adequate oral intake and thus nutritional support and hydration. Four, compliance with therapeutic instructions to prevent stiffness across joints or loss of range of motion. If these criteria are met, the patient can have close follow-up on an outpatient basis.

If the patient does not fully satisfy criteria for management as an outpatient then consider admission to the hospital for provision of local wound care, analgesia, hydration, nutrition, and physical therapy.

As per ABA criteria, burns greater than 20% or greater than 10% in a child should be admitted to the ICU for additional resuscitation and hemodynamic monitoring. ICU admissions will in general require placement of a central venous catheter, an arterial line, a Foley catheter, and a nasogastric tube.

TABLE 21.2. BURN CENTER REFERRAL CRITERIA
■ Partial-thickness burns greater than 10% total body surface area (TBSA)
■ Burns that involve the face, hands, feet, genitalia, perineum, or major joints
■ Third-degree burns in any age-group
■ Electrical burns, including lightning injury
■ Chemical burns
■ Inhalation injury
■ Burn injury in patients with preexisting medical disorders that could complicate management, prolong recovery, or affect mortality
■ Any patient with burns and concomitant trauma (such as fractures) in which the burn injury poses the greatest risk of morbidity or mortality. In such cases, if the trauma poses the greater immediate risk, the patient may be initially stabilized in a trauma center before being transferred to a burn unit. Physician judgment will be necessary in such situations and should be in concert with the regional medical control plan and triage protocols
■ Burned children in hospitals without qualified personnel or equipment for the care of children
■ Burn injury in patients who will require special social, emotional, or rehabilitative intervention

Survivable Injuries

When treating large burn injuries, like any other devastating traumatic injury, the physician must first consider *primum non nocere* or first, do no harm. Aggressively treating a patient with a nonsurvivable injury leads to undue pain, anxiety, and suffering by the patient, family, and the treating team. In some extreme cases, the best management may be simply keeping the patient comfortable and not pursuing resuscitation. The historic prognostic indicator for burn mortality is the Baux score: the patient's age plus TBSA is equal to the likelihood of mortality. Twenty percent is added for inhalational injuries. Currently, with advances in modern burn critical care and early excision of burn wounds, mortality rates have decreased. The revised Baux score and associated nomogram are more accurate reflections of current mortality rates.[12] The physician should work hand-in-hand with the severely burned patient's family or medical decision-maker in the cases of a severe burn to determine how best to proceed according to the patient's wishes. Preinjury designations for the patient's desired care, such as do not resuscitate or do not intubate, should be meticulously adhered to, based on the patient's advanced directives.

RESUSCITATION

The goal of burn resuscitation is to maintain adequate tissue perfusion—especially to the skin—during the first 24 to 48 hours after a large burn (>20% TBSA) injury. Resuscitation must proceed carefully because the consequences of both over or under resuscitation can be devastating. Under resuscitation leads to hypoperfusion of critical tissues and can result in ischemic burn wounds by converting to deeper injuries and ischemia of other organs. Over resuscitation leads to excess edema formation and its sequelae: compartment syndromes of the extremities and abdomen, as well as organ dysfunction including worsening respiratory function. Onset of intra-abdominal hypertension requires prompt treatment including systemic paralysis and ultimately decompressive laparotomy if progression to abdominal compartment syndrome develops.

Although many different formulas exist to guide burn resuscitation, all are based on the patient's initial weight and the size of the burn. The Parkland (4 cc × weight [kg] × % TBSA) and ABA consensus formula (2 cc × weight [kg] × % TBSA for adults) are two common methods used to estimate the total amount of fluids needed during the first 24 hours after a large burn injury and to set initial fluid infusion rates.[13] A sample calculation for the Parkland formula is as follows.

$$\text{Parkland formula} = 4\,\text{cc} \times \text{weight (kg)} \times \%\,\text{TBSA}$$

$$50\%\text{ over first 8 hours (from time of injury)}$$

$$50\%\text{ over next 16 hours}$$

$$100\text{ kg patient with }60\%\text{ TBSA burn}: 100 \times 60 \times 4$$

$$12\text{ liters first 8 hours}: 1500\text{ cc lactated Ringer solution / hour}$$

$$12\text{ liters next 16 hours}: 750\text{ cc lactated Ringer solution / hour}$$

Balanced, isotonic crystalloid solutions such as lactated Ringer solution are preferred, as they limit diffusion into the interstitial space. Normal saline is generally avoided because it provides excess chloride load and can perpetuate a metabolic acidosis. Glucose should be added when resuscitating smaller children. There is no evidence to support the use of colloid over or in addition to crystalloid in the first 24 hours after burn injury, although this topic is still intensely debated. Early administration of colloid may worsen burn wound edema, as large molecules leak from the intravascular space to increase the oncotic gradient. Given the lack of evidence for its benefit, colloids have a narrow role in acute burn resuscitation and are limited to instances when the volume of resuscitation is exceeding predicted levels.

Whatever formula is used to begin fluid infusion, adequacy of resuscitation is assessed using vital signs and hourly urine output as a surrogate for end organ perfusion. The standard of resuscitation is to maintain 0.5 to 1.0 mL of urine output per kilogram per hour and mean arterial pressure greater than 65 mm Hg. The kidney is susceptible to changes in perfusion pressure, so consistent urine output indicates globally adequate end organ perfusion. Complex algorithms to assess the end points of resuscitation have been developed based on advanced physiologic parameters (such as central venous pressure, pulmonary capillary wedge pressure, end diastolic volume, stroke volume variation) and biomarkers (such as lactate, hemoglobin, base deficit, creatinine). However, there are no evidence to demonstrate improved outcomes with these parameters over tracking urine output and vital signs.

Medically complex patients with premorbid systemic disease, for example, chronic kidney disease or congestive heart failure, is a challenge from a resuscitative standpoint and may benefit from other methods of goal-directed therapy such as provided with a Swan-Ganz or other cardiac monitoring device. Initiation of vasopressor or inotropic support may be indicated, especially in the setting of fluid resuscitation exceeding predicted amounts. Care of these patients is best left to the experienced burn intensivist.

In a randomized controlled trial comparing ascorbic acid (vitamin C) to lactated Ringer solution alone, Tanaka et al. in 2000 found ascorbic acid at a dose of 66 mg/kg/h for 24 hours decreased overall volume requirements for resuscitation.[14] The authors posit vitamin C acts as an oxidative scavenger and may also limit tissue damage from the inflammatory process of the burn. In our Unit, patients with greater than 30% TBSA are treated with ascorbate as an adjunct during the first 24 hours after burn injury.

Analgesia and Sedation

Appropriate analgesia and sedation are critical to the care of the burn patient. From the time of presentation to ultimate wound closure, optimizing these parameters may provide many clinical challenges. Given the density of cutaneous nerve endings, most burn injuries are very painful and require multiple painful procedures such as dressing changes or surgeries to treat. Moreover, many burn patients present with substance dependence or abuse disorders that complicate the adequate provision of analgesia or sedation.

Analgesia

First-line agents are opioid-based analgesics such as morphine or fentanyl. These may be given orally or intravenously depending on the circumstance and should be titrated for the desired effect. Oral administration has, in general, a longer duration of effect and thus is preferred if possible. Analgesia in a newly burned patient should be intravenous, as small frequent doses to define needs. Opioid side effects, such as respiratory depression, should be balanced against inadequate analgesia. Background pain can often be treated with a sustained-release opioid analgesic such as OxyContin or MS Contin. Breakthrough or procedural pain can be treated with more acute agents such as morphine sulfate immediate release or oxycodone. Nonsteroidal anti-inflammatory drugs have a role in burn pain control but are associated with bleeding risks (both gastrointestinal and postsurgical) which can limit their use.

Sedation

Sedation, in the form of anxiolysis, should be used in burn patients as a procedural or background adjunct to analgesia. Although benzodiazepine use has been associated with longer ICU stays and worse outcomes, these drawbacks may be unavoidable in a patient with a large burn undergoing frequent anxiety provoking procedures. Other agents such as propofol or dexmedetomidine can be considered for sedative purposes but also have drawbacks to long-term use. Ketamine is a useful alternative that does not contribute to hemodynamic depression but may cause transient hypertension.

In the patient with a large burn and a long hospital stay, care must be taken to prevent dependence, tolerance, and withdrawal to analgesic and anxiolytic agents.

Wound Care and Initial Debridement

Once patients have been adequately sedated and their pain is managed, initial mechanical debridement of their wounds should be performed to remove any debris. Blister on partial-thickness burns should be unroofed (Table 21.3). The serum beneath the blister can become infected and causes infection of the underlying burn wound with subsequent conversion to a deeper injury.

After debridement, dressings are applied, which should be individualized based on the qualities of the wound and patient. The goal of these dressings is to prevent wound desiccation, limit further trauma, and control microbial growth. Topical antimicrobials are the standard of care for all burn wounds that lack an epidermal barrier. The thermal injury destroys the normal skin flora, which opens the door for opportunistic flora to propagate in the wound leading to infection.

There are many broad-spectrum topical antimicrobials effective over a broad range of microbes, including bacteria, viruses, and fungi. The traditional dressing of daily silver sulfadiazine and gauze is always reasonable, especially for an evolving burn wound or if there is need for removal of eschar, pseudoeschar, or necrotic burn tissue by daily mechanical debridement. Silver-releasing dressings are widely available and fabricated in numerous formats. Many of these silver dressings have sustained activity for up to 7 days after placement. This has the advantage of limiting multiple painful debridements, an important consideration for more stable wounds. Many of these products are especially suitable for superficial partial-thickness wounds that meet criteria for outpatient management. This is particularly true for pediatric scald burns.

Escharotomy

In patients with full-thickness burns, practitioners should evaluate patients for swelling of the underlying tissues, beneath a nonexpanding, inflexible eschar. Such situations can limit distal extremity perfusion or torso expansion. Neurovascular checks are indicated for any partial-thickness or full-thickness near-circumferential burn of the extremities. A palpable radial pulse and audible Doppler signals in the palmar arch and digits indicate adequate perfusion to the hand. Any change or decrease in the neurovascular examination should prompt the clinician to consider performing emergent escharotomies on the involved extremity. Similarly, limited chest expansion with hypoventilation or elevated intra-abdominal pressures indicate the need for torso release.

The escharotomy procedure may be performed at bedside under adequate sedation. Electrocautery is used to divide through the burn wound into deeper uninjured tissue, thereby releasing the pressure that has been building up underneath the inelastic burned skin. After escharotomies are completed, a follow-up neurovascular examination should document adequate release and return of pulses and distal perfusion.

Incision patterns follow mid-axial lines, except over the hand, where they continue over the dorsal hand (Figure 21.3). Care is needed to prevent damage to underlying superficial structures, including the radial artery at the wrist, the ulnar nerve at the medial epicondyle of the elbow, and the common peroneal nerve as it crosses the fibular neck.

TABLE 21.3. KEY POINTS FOR SUCCESSFUL SURGICAL TREATMENT OF A FULL-THICKNESS BURN
1. Complete removal of all abnormal tissue
2. Quality skin graft from a donor site approved by patient
3. Limit blood loss with injectable and topical epinephrine
4. Dressing (with or without splints) that prevents shear
5. Early motion to maintain function

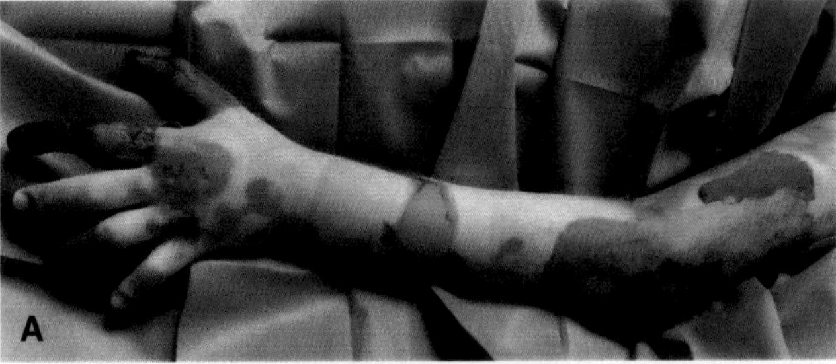

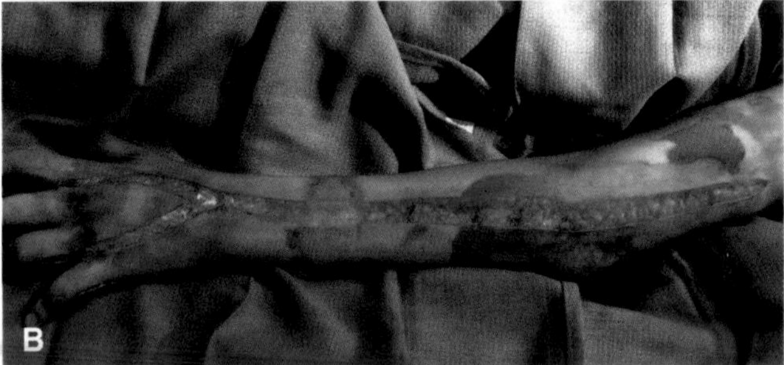

FIGURE 21.3. Full-thickness flame burns of the left arm and hand. **A.** Before escharotomy. **B.** After escharotomy.

In severe burns that have a large volume resuscitation or in crush or electrical injuries, fasciotomies may be indicated in addition to escharotomies. If distal vascular examinations do not improve after adequate escharotomies, if there appears to be muscle bulging through the fascia, or if compartment pressures are elevated, then fasciotomies should be performed in the usual manner. Additionally, rhabdomyolysis and accompanying metabolic and physiologic derangements should be identified and addressed with special attention to maintaining adequate flow through the kidneys.

Nutrition and Mediation of Hypermetabolism

The inflammatory cascade generated by large burn wounds causes a systemic hypermetabolic response with enhanced gluconeogenesis, insulin resistance, and protein catabolism. Initiation of early enteral feeding is a central component of burn care with the goal of full caloric support within 24 hours after admission. Patients can be started on a regular diet and should be provided with proteinrich nutrition supplements. Patients unable to eat for reasons such as age, painful hand or facial burns, or noncompliance may require placement of an enteral feeding tube.

Consultation with a dietician or nutritionist should be considered for every burn patient. Various nutritional formulas are available for use to guide caloric requirements, although the Curreri formula is the most popular:

$$\text{Adult}: 25\ \text{kcal} \times \text{weight (kg)} + 40\ \text{kcal} \times \%\text{TBSA}$$

$$\text{Children}: 60\ \text{kcal} \times \text{weight (kg)} + 35\ \text{kcal} \times \%\text{TBSA}$$

Protein and multivitamin supplementation are indicated as well. Serial measurements of prealbumin, an acute phase reactant with a half-life of 3 days, allow monitoring the nutritional status over time. Enteral nutrition is superior to parenteral nutrition, with gastric feeds preferred over small bowel feeding. Early feeding provides nourishment of intestinal mucosa and prevents its atrophy and bacterial translocation.

Gastroparesis is common, and prokinetic agents such as metoclopramide and erythromycin are helpful in promoting gastric emptying. If gastric feeding intolerance occurs, the tube should be advanced to a post pyloric position. Hemodynamically unstable patients requiring increasing amounts of vasopressor support may require reduction of enteral feeds to trophic levels to prevent intestinal ischemia.

The response to inadequate enteral nutrition is controversial. We believe adequate nutrition is essential. In our Unit, parenteral nutrition is indicated in patients with open wounds who fail full enteral feeding.

In a randomized, placebo-controlled trial, Demling and Orgill evaluated the effects of oxandrolone, a testosterone analogue, in 20 patients with between 40% and 70% TBSA.[15] They found patients receiving the medication demonstrated decreased muscle loss and improved donor site wound healing compared with controls. Hepatic dysfunction may develop with long-term or higher dosages, so liver function tests should be followed and the drug stopped if elevations occur. Oxandrolone should be used cautiously in children less than 4 years of age.

Beta-blockers can mediate the cholinergic response and also help blunt hypermetabolism by decreasing the resting heart rate. In a seminal article from 1988, Herndon et al. demonstrated that propranolol decreased myocardial work (heart rate, left ventricular work, and rate pressure product) in pediatric patients.[16] Further work in adults substantiated their findings.[17] Propranolol or metoprolol are commonly used agents.

Prophylaxis

Burn patients are hypercoagulable and are at an overall higher risk for deep vein thrombosis. Chemical thromboprophylaxis is generally indicated but must be balanced against bleeding risk from wounds or after surgery. There is no clear benefit for either unfractionated heparin or low-molecular-weight heparin, but dosing must be adjusted for the hypermetabolic state. In our Unit, we use subcutaneous heparin three times daily.

Last, critically ill burn patients are at risk for stress gastritis or upper gastrointestinal stress ulcers (Curling ulcer). Prophylaxis with an H2 blocker or a PPI is recommended, although intragastric continuous feeds are protective as well.[18]

Extremes of Age

Pediatric and geriatric patients require special consideration. Their physiology may be different from the standard healthy adult. Moreover, these are vulnerable patients who are often burned as a consequence from abuse. This must be ruled out during the initial evaluation. If concern for abuse exists, the appropriate child protective services or other legal entity should be contacted immediately. This will vary by hospital policy provider and local laws.

Inhalation Injury

After the size of the burn, inhalation injury is the most critical determination for survival.[19] Stigma of inhalation injury include tachypnea, wheezing, singed nasal hair or facial burns, soot in the oropharynx, increasing oxygen requirements, or dropping transcutaneous saturations. Inhalation injury may be supraglottic, subglottic, or both. Upper airway inhalation injury is defined by injury to the supraglottic airway from breathing in hot air. Damage to the supraglottic epithelium can result in edema formation and potential for obstruction of the airway. This is treated by early endotracheal intubation and supportive mechanical ventilation until such time when the airway edema resolves, usually in 48 to 72 hours, which can be determined by a cuff leak around the endotracheal tube or endoscopy by an experienced upper airway endoscopist.

Subglottic inhalation injury is characterized by inhaling the *toxic products of combustion* and results in a chemical pneumonitis similar to acute respiratory distress syndrome. Diagnosis is confirmed by bronchoscopy, and findings may not be immediately evident on chest X-ray. The treatment is also supportive with mechanical ventilation until the acute lung injury resolves, in this case usually over 5 to 10 days. The high-flow percussive ventilator is a useful adjunct that works by recruiting alveoli with low pressures and by removing debris from the lower airways. When the percussive ventilator is used, inhaled heparin and acetylcysteine are helpful to avoid airway desiccation and bleeding.

Carbon monoxide (CO) poisoning should be suspected with any inhalation injury. The CO molecule competes with oxygen at the binding site on hemoglobin and is not detectible by pulse oximetry. Carboxyhemoglobin level is measured at time of presentation, and if elevated, treatment is initiated with inhaled oxygen either by non-rebreather mask or endotracheal tube. Application of 100% oxygen can reduce the half-life of carbon monoxide in the circulation from 4 hours to 40 to 60 minutes.[20]

At all times, established protective ventilatory strategies should be employed as possible to prevent progressive pulmonary damage. After treatment of CO poisoning, low FiO_2 should be attempted to prevent oxidative damage to the pulmonary parenchyma.

Infection

Large burn injuries result in systemic immunocompromise, and infectious complications are commonplace after large burn injuries. Many of these patients are admitted for extended periods of time and are exposed to pathogenic, hospital-acquired, drug-resistant organisms. Thus, the judicious use of broad-spectrum antibiotics is required to prevent the emergence of multidrug-resistant pathogens.

The most common sites for infection in burn patients are the respiratory tract, the burn wound, and imparted devices such as central line–associated bloodstream infections and catheter-associated urinary tract infections. Differentiating secondary infection and sepsis from the hypermetabolic response of the burn injury is challenging and should be made with thoughtfulness. Changes in clinical condition such as worsening or new-onset hyper- or hypothermia, tachycardia, hypotension, insulin resistance, leukocytosis or leukopenia, rising lactates, or base deficits should prompt a head to toe examination of the patient for signs of secondary infection and a culture of any suspicious areas.

Broad-spectrum antibiotics can be initiated after cultures are sent but should be de-escalated when the culture's sensitivities are returned. Pneumonias are treated with supportive mechanical ventilation until it resolves. Bloodstream infections are treated by exchanging infected central venous catheters and evaluating the source of septicemia. Burn wound infections are treated with topical antimicrobial and broad-spectrum intravenous antibiotics targeting gram-positive organisms and pseudomonas if it appears the infection has spread outside of the burn wound and into the surrounding soft tissues.

SURGICAL MANAGEMENT OF BURNS

Indications

Superficial partial-thickness thermal injuries that will heal in less than 3 weeks should be managed nonoperatively. This means local wound care (which may include superficial surgical debridement), good nutrition, and optimization of medical comorbidities. By not autografting these patients, the burn care provider limits a painful and deforming donor site while optimizing the appearance and functional outcomes of the burned tissue. Mixed or indeterminate depth burns should be followed closely for 5 to 7 days to allow possible healing to occur, deeper areas to declare, and surgical plans to be confirmed.

Deep partial-thickness or full-thickness burn wounds are best treated with early excision and autografting to avoid wound sepsis, decrease systemic inflammation, and achieve best wound healing outcomes.[21-23] Burke et al. in 1974 were the first to promote early excision and grafting in a series of 200 patients. They found that patients with early (<14 days) excision had improvements in mortality (4% versus 11%) and faster wound closure. Now, *early excision* generally refers to removal of all nonviable burn tissue within 7 to 10 days, and there are data to indicate that *ultra-early excision* within 72 hours after injury may lead to better results overall.[23]

Burn wound excision and grafting can be staged or concurrent. Depth of excision depends on the depth of the burn wound. Injured tissue must be completely excised if grafting is being considered. If complete excision will expose critical, ungraftable structures, leaving questionable tissue in place for 2 or 3 days is a reasonable temporizing step.

Surgical Steps

Operative Planning and Communication

There should be careful communication between the burn surgeon and the anesthesiologist at all phases of the case. Blood loss during excision is expected and can be difficult to quantify. Communication about transfusions is critical. Similarly, maintaining intraoperative normotension and normothermia is important to prevent poor postoperative outcomes. Similarly, postoperative hypertension from inadequate pain control can cause hematomas beneath the skin grafts.

Debridement and Wound Bed Preparation

The excision of burn wounds occurs by either of two common techniques. The first method, tangential excision, requires stepwise sharp excision of burned tissue to a level deep to the level of thermal injury. Serial excision occurs using a Weck or Watson blade until healthy tissue is found, indicated by petechial bleeding or normal tissue morphology. Benefits to this method are that it preserves as much healthy tissue as possible, sometimes deep dermis, often subcutaneous tissue. This results in better functional and aesthetic outcomes. Care must be taken to avoid excessive blood loss during tangential excision, especially when removing large areas of burn or when operating more than a week after injury. Preoperative injection of dilute epinephrine solution or extremity tourniquets are useful to decrease blood loss during excision but may make assessment of the underlying wound bed more difficult. Tangential excision may not be suitable for a hemodynamically unstable patient who could not tolerate the blood loss or in cases where the burn is third degree and extends into subcutaneous tissue.

An alternative method of excision is prefascial excision. In this method, the surgeon removes all of the skin and subcutaneous tissue to the level of the deep investing fascia. This method is quick and reliable, with less blood loss than with tangential excision. However, by removing all dermis and subcutaneous tissue, there are significant long-term functional and aesthetic deformities. In general, tangential excision is preferred to prefascial excision for this reason. Prefascial excision is indicated only in critically ill patients who would not tolerate long operations or large volume blood loss.

Hemostasis

After adequate debridement has occurred, meticulous hemostasis must be achieved prior to grafting. Topical epinephrine soaked sponges may be placed immediately after debridement. Wound bed irrigation and electrocautery should be used to precisely achieve hemostasis. The use of the electrocautery device should be judicious so as not to re-create deep and diffuse thermal injury to the healthy wound bed. If the wound is to be grafted at the same stage, as is most common, meticulous hemostasis at this point is critical to prevent postoperative graft loss from hematomas.

Wound Closure

After the wound bed has been adequately prepared, the wound should be closed. Plastic surgery principles are followed. If primary closure or local flaps can be used, they should be considered. Most commonly, because of the size of most burn wounds, the wound is closed using autograft or a skin substitute. If the wound bed is reliable with healthy vascular tissue and the patient is medically stable, then autografting can be performed in a single stage. If there is doubt as to the integrity of the wound bed to support an autograft, then skin substitutes should be prioritized and autografting delayed until a suitable wound bed can be developed. If the procedure is staged and autografting is delayed, there should be a plan for return to the operating room for wound closure within 3 to 5 days.

Graft Selection

Skin graft harvest occurs with the standard technique using an electric or air-powered dermatome. Selecting donor sites should be done carefully with prioritization to limiting donor site morbidity. Prior to surgery, a discussion should occur with the patient to help select optimal donor site, especially in smaller burns where a donor site could be selected so that it is hidden under clothes and without visible scarring.[24] Generally skin grafts are harvested at an intermediate depth most commonly 10 to 12 thousandths of an inch. Pediatric and geriatric patients have thinner reticular dermis than healthy adults, and skin grafts should generally be harvested at a thinner thickness.

Unmeshed, sheet grafts are the best replacement for the debrided areas of injury. In general, they should be considered when best long-term functional and aesthetic outcomes are the priority. They are particularly useful for primary grafting of the face, hands and feet and should be standard care for most burns in children. Thicker skin grafts have the advantage of less contracture after graft take; however, the donor sites take longer to heal and have more scarring. Thinner grafts have less metabolic demand and can take more readily on suboptimal wound bed but contract more. The donor site for thinner grafts heals faster.

If necessary, the grafts can then be meshed to expand their surface area and limit donor site harvest. Meshed grafts can cover a larger wound area but have a reticulated appearance after graft takes, as the interstices in the mesh must heal by contraction. The interstices of the mesh graft allow serum or small amounts of bleeding to escape which may improve mesh graft take rates when compared to sheet grafts.

Although sheet grafts have a better overall appearance and less contracture than mesh grafts, they do require meticulous wound care postoperatively and should be checked frequently to ensure seroma or hematoma formation under the sheet graft is not occurring. If this happens, the fluid collection may be drained and evacuated with an 18-gauge needle.

Full-thickness grafts have little role in acute burn surgical management. Given the limited amount of full-thickness skin available, they are best reserved for subsequent reconstruction of areas such as the eyelids or the palmar surface of the hand.

Skin Substitutes

There are multiple alternatives to autologous skin grafts. Most commonly used is frozen cadaveric allograft, which can be used in a staged fashion to aid in wound bed preparation and temporary wound closure. It encourages angiogenesis within the wound bed and can limit evaporative losses for larger burns that must be closed in a staged fashion. Allografts are relatively expensive, however, and must be maintained frozen in an approved skin bank. As the patient regains immunocompetence, the allogenic skin will reject, which can occur from 10 to 30 days after placement. After temporizing the wound bed with allografts, autografts must ultimately be placed for durable wound coverage.

When sufficient donor site skin is not available, biosynthetic matrices such as Integra® can be used to graft wounds. These products create a neodermis after ingrowth of autologous wound cells. The silicone sheet on the Integra prevents evaporative losses and the underlying vascularized neodermis supports thinner grafts to be placed to restore epidermal coverage. Integra can also be used to bridge across and cover areas of questionable vascularity such as bone lacking periosteum or tendons denuded of paratenon. Drawbacks of such products are that they easily become infected if the burn wound was inadequate debrided and take a prolonged time, usually around 3 weeks, to become revascularized. They are all expensive.

Cultured epidermal autografts and spray on keratinocytes have also been described and have found use in coverage of massive burn areas with limited donor sites. However, they are very expensive, and outcomes are practitioner dependent.

Graft Placement

The skin graft should then be precisely adapted to the wound bed with minimal overlap of the graft with the wound edge. Grafts should not be too small as the seam between the graft and the wound margin will leave an unsightly and often hypertrophic scar.

The skin graft is then secured to the wound bed with conventional techniques such as sutures or staples. Fibrin glue has been advocated by some practitioners, in particular for shear-prone areas.

Dressings

After the skin grafts or substitutes are placed, they should be dressed in compressive dressings. Joints should be immobilized both one joint above and below the area of grafting. It is critical to be conscientious about dressing placement, because inadequate dressings may lead to shearing during the graft healing phase and partial or complete graft loss. Methods of dressings include foam bolsters, tie-over bolsters, negative pressure wound therapy dressings, and compressive therapy for extremities. There is no demonstrated superior technique from one to the other. The principle behind the dressing is such that it maintains adequate pressure downward on the skin graft and immobilizes the area to prevent sheer. In our Unit, all grafts are treated by some kind of antimicrobial dressing.

Physical Therapy and Occupational Therapy

There are no more important members of the burn team than physical and occupational therapists. Early therapeutic intervention is critical to preventing the functional deformities that can develop after burn injuries. Contractures across joints can require release but can often be entirely avoided with excellent therapeutic care from the time of injury and dedicated patient compliance. Range of motion and strengthening exercises should be initiated as soon as possible after the injury and should continue until the timing of grafting. There are inevitable lapses in therapy after grafting procedures to allow the grafts time to adhere, mature, and become shear resistant.

The timing of postoperative mobilization is controversial, and different institutions have protocols that vary widely. There is a balance between early mobilization to fully achieve normal range of motion and strength versus allowing time for graft healing and maturation to occur. Best outcomes occur when the therapists are an essential part of the decision team and are crucial for preventing scar contractures from burn injuries that could lead to worse functional outcomes.

OTHER BURN INJURIES

Chemical Burns

Chemical burn injuries are the result of chemical rather than thermal trauma. These are very often work related or industrial accidents. The acid or base denatures cutaneous proteins with acids forming coagulation necrosis and bases with liquefactive necrosis. Other chemicals can denature tissue through other mechanisms. Whatever the specifics of the chemical agent is treated by dilution, specifically the treatment is to irrigate the contact area with regular tap water for a minimum of 15 minutes. Acids and bases should not be neutralized with an opposing reagent because this could create an exothermic reaction that could add thermal damage to the already existing chemical damage. One exception to this rule is hydrofluoric acid, which should be neutralized with calcium gluconate or calcium chloride. Bases tend to create more significant injury than acids because of deeper penetration from ongoing liquefactive injury. The depth of chemical injuries may not be readily apparent on the initial evaluation and may require several days of observation before accurate diagnosis of burn depth can be made. For these reasons, treatment decisions are usually delayed for 5 to 7 days.

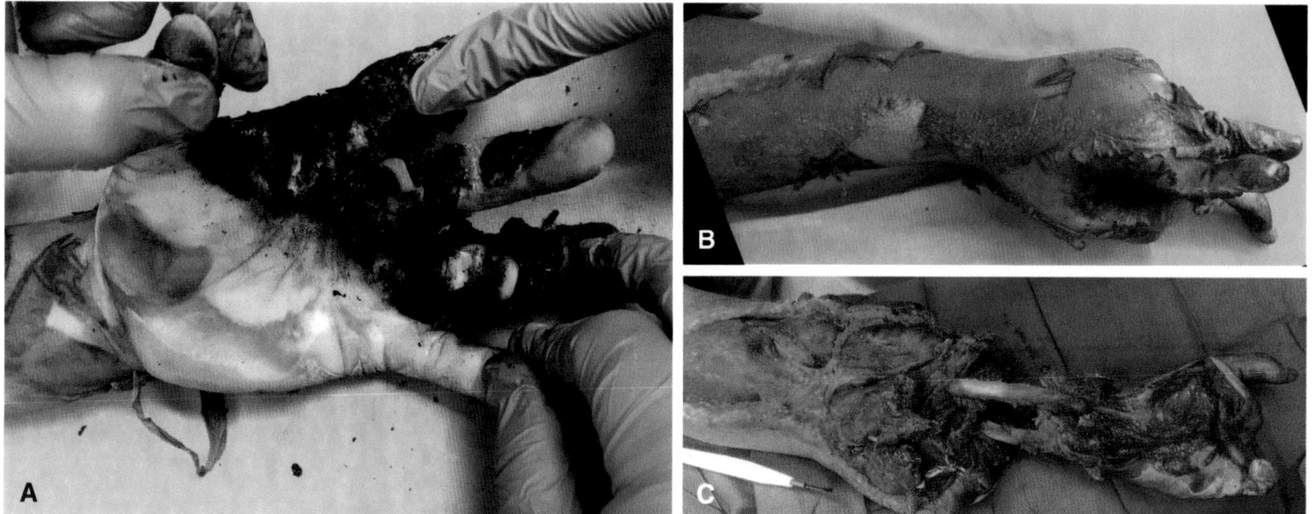

FIGURE 21.4. High-voltage electrical burns of the left arm and hand. **A and B.** Day of the burn injury, before debridement. **C.** After multiple staged debridements of nonviable tissues. This patient ultimately required a forearm amputation.

Electrical Burns

Electrical burns can be the most devastating type of burn injury (Figure 21.4). Although other etiologies of burn injury can be quantified by a careful evaluation of the skin, electrical burns can be difficult to diagnose the exact extent of the injury. These types of burns are also often associated with other traumatic injuries or secondary flash or blast injuries from the superheated air surrounding the electrical current.

In an electrical burn, electricity travels along the path of least resistance which in human tissue corresponds directly with the water content of that tissue. Heat is generated according to the resistance of various body tissues with the amount of heat generated directly proportional to the resistance encountered. Bone has the highest resistance, followed by fat, tendon, skin, muscle, blood vessels, and nerve. Injuries to deeper structures may occur at any location within the course of where the electricity traveled; thus, it is important to locate the contact points on the body and map the course of the electricity. Areas with low cross-section and high bony content, such as the wrist and ankles, are particularly susceptible to severe injury.

In the event of deeper compartment or muscular electrical injury, fasciotomies must be performed for adequate compartment release and perfusion of damage tissues. Additionally, there may be damage to myocardium or any associated organ that lies within the path of the electricity. If there is concern for cardiac damage, EKG should be obtained at the initial evaluation. Creatine kinases are drawn for quantification of muscle damage. Because of the propensity for muscular injury, rhabdomyolysis may result which can cause secondary acute kidney injuries. Peripheral nerve releases including carpal tunnel and Guyon canal should be included in surgical management if contact points involve the hand or extremity.

Cold Injuries

Frostbite injury can be insidious in presentation and preferentially affects the distal or exposed areas of the body. Ice crystal formation in the intracellular and extracellular spaces kills cells but does not alter matrix organization. Secondary inflammatory damage occurs after rewarming and can be variable. As a result, the full extent of tissue damage and subsequent healing potential can be difficult to assess on first presentation. The initial management of frostbite injuries should be to restore normothermia. Systemic hypothermia should be addressed first followed by rapid rewarming in a water bath with temperature between 40 and 42°C for 30 minutes to the affected areas. After rewarming, the damaged areas should be gently cleaned, blisters debrided, and treated with local wound care. Some evidence suggests that topical aloe vera may be a valuable adjunct. Systemic administration of nonsteroidal anti-inflammatory drugs such as ibuprofen can help prevent ongoing inflammatory damage. If the injury is less than 24 hours old, angiography with either catheter directed or systemic thrombolytic administration may decrease need for digital amputation.[25] Surgery should be delayed until full tissue demarcation has occurred, which can take anywhere from 3 weeks to 3 months.

SPECIAL ANATOMIC CONSIDERATIONS

Face

Facial burn injury should be managed nonoperatively initially even if they appear to be full-thickness injuries. The excellent perfusion of facial skin may allow deep-appearing burns to heal, thus circumventing the need for excision and grafting. After meticulous local wound care, facial burns should be reevaluated at approximately 10 to 14 days and any nonhealing areas excised and grafted. All facial burns should be sheet grafted, as mesh grafts on the face are aesthetically and functionally unacceptable. Sheet grafts should be applied with seams adhering to facial aesthetic subunits, but intact skin should *not* be removed (Figure 21.5). Scalp grafts provide optimal color match

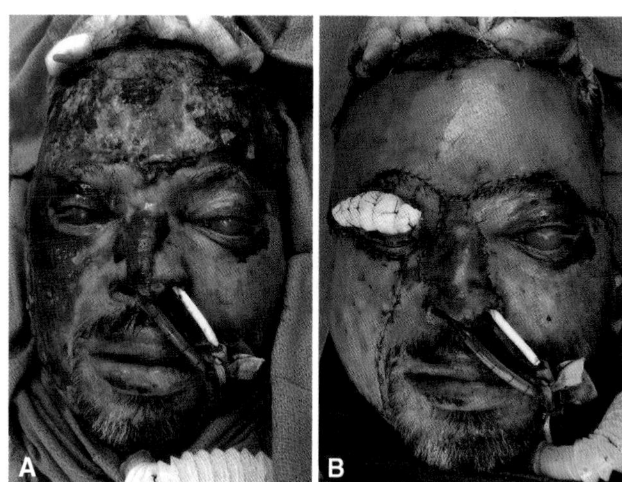

FIGURE 21.5. Deep facial burn injury. **A.** Preoperative appearance of nonhealing deep facial burns, 18 days after initial injury. **B.** Postoperative appearance after excision of burns and placement of sheet grafts to the forehead, right cheek, and right upper eyelid.

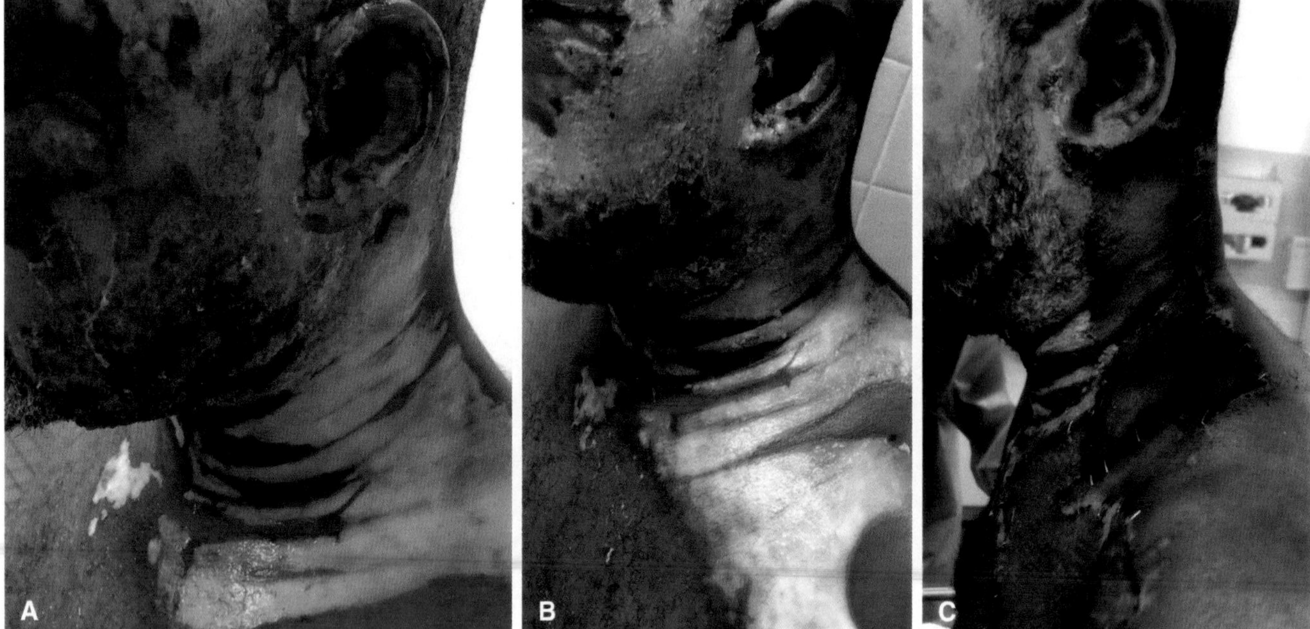

FIGURE 21.6. Deep partial-thickness facial, neck, and chest flame burns. **A.** Day of the burn injury. **B.** Seven days after burn injury. **C.** Appearance of sheet-grafted neck burn and meshed grafted of chest burn 5 days after grafting, 14 days after injury.

but are seldom wide enough to fully graft any aesthetic unit except eyelids. First-pass donor site grafts are preferred to reharvested donor sites. Sheet grafts should be maintained and dressed as indicated earlier in this chapter. A tracheostomy provides best care of facial burn wound care and postoperative graft management. Ophthalmology consultation should be obtained if there is concern for ocular involvement. If severe lid burns exist, eyelid releases or temporary tarsorrhaphies may be indicated to protect the cornea from further damage from exposure.

Neck

Isolated burns of the neck are best managed, like other isolated injuries, by early excision and sheet grafting. Early therapy will help limit neck flexion contractures. In contrast, in patients with a very large TBSA burn, facial burns, and inhalation injury, the neck should be grafted early with a meshed graft to allow early tracheostomy (Figure 21.6). A tracheostomy should not be placed through ungrafted burned areas because of the unacceptably high risk of mediastinitis. The face can be grafted with a stable airway. Although this strategy predictably results in neck contractures, it improves the ability to get superior outcomes with face grafting. A cervical immobilizing collar may be useful in postoperative graft management.

Hands

The reflex response, to flex into a fist, combined with thicker palmar skin means that most hand burns are dorsal. In general, most palmar hand burns heal reasonably well. Dorsal hand burns have best outcomes with early excision and grafting, allowing for early functional mobilization. In a seminal work from 1979, Hunt et al. described their experience with early excision and mesh grafting of 60 patients with deep dermal hand burns.[26] These authors excised and grafted all patients between 3 and 10 days after burn and reported excellent functional results with full range of motion by 10 days postoperatively. They did note the appearance of the mesh graft as a drawback to their technique. Since that time, common practice is to sheet graft dorsal hand burns because of unacceptably high rates of contracture with mesh grafts and poor appearance. Early initiation of hand therapy prevents long-term stiffness and limits contractures.

Severe hand burns with exposure of tendons or bone may require staging with coverage by skin substitutes such as Integra or vascularized soft tissue flaps. In cases for which early hand therapy is not possible and the hand will be immobilized for a prolonged period, Kirschner wires may be placed to immobilize the interphalangeal and metacarpophalangeal joints with the hand in a position of safety to prevent tightening of the collateral ligaments.

REFERENCES

1. American Burn Association. Burn Incidence Fact Sheet. https://ameriburn.org/who-we-are/media/burn-incidence-fact-sheet/. Accessed August 31, 2018.
2. Hop MJ, Polinder S, van der Vlies CH, et al. Costs of burn care: a systematic review. *Wound Repair Regen*. 2014;22(4):436-450.
3. Tricklebank S. Modern trends in fluid therapy for burns. *Burns*. 2009;35(6):757-767.
4. Hilton JG, Marullo DS. Effects of thermal trauma on cardiac force of contraction. *Burns Incl Therm Inj*. 1986;12(3):167-171.
5. Horton JW, Maass DL, White DJ, Sanders B, Murphy J. Effects of burn serum on myocardial inflammation and function. *Shock*. 2004;22(5):438-445.
6. Holm C, Hörbrand F, von Donnersmarck GH, Mühlbauer W. Acute renal failure in severely burned patients. *Burns*. 1999;25(2):171-178.
7. Chrysopoulo MT, Jeschke MG, Dziewulski P, et al. Acute renal dysfunction in severely burned adults. *J Trauma*. 1999;46(1):141-144.
8. ISBI Practice Guidelines Committee, Steering Subcommittee, Advisory Subcommittee. ISBI practice guidelines for burn care. *Burns*. 2016;42(5):953-1021.
9. CMS.gov. ICD-10. cms.gov. https://www.cms.gov/Medicare/Coding/ICD10/index.html. Accessed May 5, 2018.
10. Sen CK, Ghatak S, Gnyawali SC, et al. Cutaneous imaging technologies in acute burn and chronic wound care. *Plast Reconstre Surg*. 2016;138(suppl 3):119S-128S.
11. American Burn Association. Burn Center Referral Criteria. http://ameriburn.org/wp-content/uploads/2017/05/burncenterreferralcriteria.pdf. Accessed August 31, 2018.
12. Williams DJ, Walker JD. A nomogram for calculation of the revised Baux score. *Burns*. 2015;41(1):85-90.
13. Gibran NS, Wiechman S, Meyer W, et al. American Burn Association consensus statements. *J Burn Care Res*. 2013;34:361-385.
14. Tanaka H, Matsuda T, Miyagantani Y, Yukioka T, Matsuda H, Shimazaki S. Reduction of resuscitation fluid volumes in severely burned patients using ascorbic acid administration: a randomized, prospective study. *Arch Surg*. 2000;135(3):326-331.
In a randomized controlled trial comparing ascorbic acid (vitamin C) to lactated Ringer solution alone, these researchers found ascorbic acid at a dose of 66 mg/kg/h for 24 hours decreased overall volume requirements for resuscitation.
15. Demling RH, Orgill DP. The anticatabolic and wound healing effects of the testosterone analog oxandrolone after severe burn injury. *J Crit Care*. 2000;15(1):12-17.
In a randomized, placebo controlled trial, these researchers studied the effects of oxandrolone, a testosterone analogue, in 20 patients with between 40% to 70% TBSA. They found patients receiving the medication demonstrated decreased muscle loss and improved donor site wound healing compared with controls.

16. Herndon DN, Barrow RE, Rutan TC, et al. Effect of propranolol administration on hemodynamic and metabolic responses of burned pediatric patients. *Ann Surg.* 1988;208(4):484-492.
In a prospective case-control trial of 47 burned children in 1988, these researchers demonstrated that propranolol decreased myocardial work (heart rate, left ventricular work, and rate pressure product) while maintaining adequate oxygen delivery and cardiac output in pediatric patients.
17. Breitenstein E, Chioléro RL, Jéquier E, et al. Effects of beta-blockade on energy metabolism following burns. *Burns.* 1990;16(4):259-264.
18. Yenikomshian H, Reiss M, Nabavian R, Garner WL. Gastric feedings effectively prophylax against upper gastrointestinal hemorrhage in burn patients. *J Burn Care Res.* 2011;32(2):263-268.
19. Grunwald TB, Garner WL. Acute burns. *Plast Reconstr Surg.* 2008;121(5):311e-319e.
20. Pace N, Strajman E, Walker EL. Acceleration of carbon monoxide elimination in man by high pressure oxygen. *Science.* 1950;111(2894):652-654.
21. Burke JF, Bondoc CC, Quinby WC. Primary burn excision and immediate grafting: a method shortening illness. *J Trauma.* 1974;14(5):389-395.
These researchers were the first to promote early excision and grafting in a series of 200 patients treated between 1969 and 1973. They found that patients with early (<14 days) burn excision and immediate autografting had improvements in mortality (4% versus 11%) and faster wound closure.
22. Saaiq M, Zaib S, Ahmad S. Early excision and grafting versus delayed excision and grafting of deep thermal burns up to 40% total body surface area: a comparison of outcome. *Ann Burns Fire Disasters.* 2012;25(3):143-147.
23. Keshavarzi A, Ayaz M, Dehghankhalili M. Ultra-early versus early excision and grafting for thermal burns up to 60% total body surface area: a historical cohort study. *Bull Emerg Trauma.* 2016;4(4):197-201.
24. Garcia E, Stone E, Chan LS, Van Vliet M, Garner WL. Donor-site preferences in women during autologous skin grafting. *Plast Reconstr Surg.* 2014;133(3):378e-382e.
25. Bruen KJ, Ballard JR, Morris SE, et al. Reduction of the incidence of amputation in frostbite injury with thrombolytic therapy. *Arch Surg.* 2007;142(6):546-551.
26. Hunt JL, Sato R, Baxter CR. Early tangential excision and immediate mesh autografting of deep dermal hand burns. *Ann Surg.* 1979;189(2):147-151.
In 1979, these researchers described their experience with early excision and mesh grafting of 60 patients with deep dermal hand burns. All patients were excised and grafted between 3 to 10 days post burn and reported excellent functional results with full range of motion by 10 days postoperatively.

QUESTIONS

1. Which of the following statements regarding facial burn is correct?

a. The thin skin of the face commonly results in deeper burn injuries
b. Full-thickness facial burns should be grafted with full-thickness skin
c. Treatment of full-thickness facial burns with grafting should be delayed until all healing and contraction have completed
d. Initial treatment of face burns should not include resecting normal adjacent skin

2. A 4-year-old girl presents with 30% TBSA deep partial-thickness burn injury to her chest, back, and bilateral lower extremities. What fluid should be used to initiate resuscitation of this patient?

a. Lactated Ringer solution
b. Lactated Ringer solution with 5% dextrose
c. 0.9% (normal) saline
d. 0.9% (normal) saline with 5% dextrose
e. 0.45% (half-normal) saline

3. A 45-year-old man with 70% TBSA partial-thickness and full-thickness burns to the face, torso, and bilateral upper and lower extremities is admitted to the burn unit. He is actively undergoing resuscitation with lactated Ringer solution according to the Parkland formula. Which of the following parameters is best used to titrate his rate of intravenous fluids?

a. Heart rate less than 100 bpm
b. Arterial systolic pressure greater than 80 mm Hg
c. Urinary output of 0.5 mL/kg/h
d. Cardiac output greater than 6 L/min
e. Mean arterial pressure greater than 55 mm Hg

4. An otherwise healthy 30-year-old woman presents with 15% TBSA circumferential superficial and deep partial-thickness flame burns to her bilateral hands and arms. Her burns are cleaned in the emergency room. Her pain is controlled with oral medications. Her compartments feel soft, and she has minimal pain with passive or active range of motion of her hands. Radial pulses are palpable bilaterally. She is otherwise medically stable. What is the most appropriate next step in management?

a. Placement of silver-based dressings and close outpatient follow-up
b. Emergent escharotomy
c. Immediate surgical excision and autografting
d. Fluid resuscitation with lactated Ringer solution and the Parkland formula
e. Placement in dry dressings and referral to the closest burn center

5. A 60-year-old man has 55% TBSA deep partial-thickness burns of the face, neck, torso, and lower extremities. Which of the following is the most effective immediate method to deliver nutrition to this patient?

a. Ad lib oral intake with high-calorie protein shakes
b. Enteral nutrition through gastrostomy tube
c. Enteral nutrition through nasogastric tube
d. Parenteral nutrition through central venous catheter
e. Parenteral nutrition through peripheral intravenous injection

1. **Answer: d.** Although excision and grafting of facial burns should be done with aesthetic subunits in mind, normal skin should *not* be resected during the wound bed preparation. Face burns should be given 2 weeks for healing to occur, but grafting and wound closure should happen around 3 weeks. Grafting should not be delayed until full-thickness wounds heal. The facial skin as a whole is not particularly thin, and given the robust vascular supply, many deeper facial burns will heal without surgery.

2. **Answer: b.** Burn patients should be resuscitated with a balanced salt solution such as lactated Ringer solution, and pediatric patients require the addition of dextrose to the resuscitative fluids to prevent hypoglycemia. Normal saline should not be used for acute burn resuscitation because it perpetuates a metabolic acidosis. Lactated ringers is more physiologic. Half-normal saline is not used in acute burn resuscitation because it is hypotonic and would lead to increased volume of resuscitation.

3. **Answer: c.** Maintaining an adequate urine output between 0.5 and 1 mL/kg/h is the gold standard for resuscitation. Heart rate, systolic pressures, and cardiac output are not end points of resuscitation. Mean arterial pressure is monitored and should be maintained above 65.

4. **Answer: e.** This patient has greater than 10% TBSA involvement with partial-thickness burns and has burns to the hand—both are criteria for referral to a burn center. Failure to initiate prompt referral may lead to delays in care. Placement of silver dressings would require removal and replacement when she reaches the burn center. Although she does have circumferential burns, she does not demonstrate any evidence of compartment syndrome. She only has partial-thickness burns, which may heal without surgical intervention. Burn resuscitation with the Parkland formula is reserved for patients with 20% TBSA or greater.

5. **Answer: c.** Establishing early enteral nutrition is critical in the management of larger burns, and given the extent of this burn and the resulting increased caloric needs, this patient should have a nasogastric tube placed and tube feeds initiated as part of his initial management. Oral nutrition is reasonable in the right patient but should be regimented and calories counted. Placement of a gastrostomy tube is not indicated as the first step. Parenteral nutrition should be avoided unless enteral nutrition fails.

CHAPTER 22 Principles of Burn Reconstruction

Benjamin Levi and Rodney Chan

KEY POINTS

- Burn scars are common sequelae following acute burn care.
- Hypertrophic burn scars affect appearance and function.
- Tension is a key contributing factor for hypertrophic scarring; tension relief with tissue rearrangement (Z-plasty) or releasing and adding additional tissue (graft or flap) offers the best way to reconstruct the scar.
- Treatment of burn scars requires multimodality treatments from nonsurgical to laser to surgical procedures.
- The location of functional burn scar contractures is most common in areas of mobility including the periorbita, perioral region, neck, and upper and lower extremities.
- Minor burn contractures can be treated with local tissue and Z-plasties alone, but larger contractures require the addition of new tissue either with a graft or flap.
- Laser rehabilitation of burn scars has changed the treatment algorithm of burn scars and primarily depends on the use of CO_2 and pulsed dye lasers.

As survival of patients from large surface area burns has increased because of improved critical care and acute burn care, surgeons are presented with an increased number of patients with secondary burn deformities. Burn reconstruction represents one of the earliest types of reconstructive surgery and defined plastic surgery in World War I when it became clear that standard surgical techniques and the care of wounded soldiers require more thoughtful approach to restoring function and appearance. Whereas patients with large surface area burns and deep burn injuries would often succumb to their burns, patients are now surviving with over 80% and 90% burn injuries. This increased survival has thus led to more patients living with the social, functional, and physical challenges of burn injury. Concurrent with this improved overall survival is improved acute care burn principles of early debridement and grafting and attention to detail of functional and aesthetic subunits. Burn reconstruction spans all areas of plastic surgery from craniofacial surgery to hand surgery to microsurgery and transplant surgery. Although some reconstruction procedures can be as simple as a release and grafting, many operations and reconstructive challenges are more complex and require a multimodal approach. Advances in microsurgical techniques as well as composite tissue allotransplantation have opened up new avenues for patients with burn reconstruction. Finally, the recent improvement in fractional laser technologies has dramatically changed the approach of reconstructive burn surgery and has changed some of the paradigm for when and how to intervene for severe hypertrophic scars.

EVALUATING THE BURN SCAR AND TIMING OF RECONSTRUCTION

Thermal burn injures can cause tremendous morbidity, leaving the patient with not only cosmetic but also functional impairments. Hypertrophic scarring is a major complication after burn injury with a prevalence of 32% to 72%. Several risk factors have been identified that contribute to its development including the localization of the burn injury, burn depth, time to heal, and skin color.[1,2] Although the precise mechanism by which hypertrophic scarring occurs remains unclear, strong and persistent expression of transforming growth factor beta and its receptors have been associated with postburn hypertrophic scarring. Furthermore, a critical step in the healing process that is altered is the transition from granulation tissue into normal scarring. During this remodeling process, wound epithelization and scar collagen formation occur but are accompanied by a gradual decrease in cellularity due to apoptosis. However, early immature hypertrophic scars caused by burns are hypercellular. During the process of remodeling and maturing, fibroblast density does not resemble that of normal healing. More specifically, apoptosis of myofibroblasts occurs 12 days after injury in normal wound healing, but in hypertrophic scar tissue, the maximum apoptosis occurs much later at 19 to 30 months. These events result in a significantly higher percentage of myofibroblasts and the hypertrophy of the scar tissue following severe burn injuries. Although oftentimes hypertrophic scars cannot be avoided, there are several steps that can optimize a burn scar: (1) Wound closure of a burn that is likely not to heal on its own in 3 weeks. (2) Avoidance of sun contact of the scar during the first 6 months. (3) Compression garments for those who can tolerate treatment for up to 1 year. (4) Keeping the scar moist.

One of the key pathologic factors that needs to be addressed in any hypertrophic scar is tension. A new concept of *scar rejuvenation* has emerged with the idea being to improve the environment of the scar without actual excision of the scar. Despite not removing any tissue, a large defect is often created once the tension is released. This defect can then be treated by adding new tissue such as a full-thickness skin graft (FTSG) or a thick split-thickness skin graft (STSG). Additional way to relieve tension uses tissue rearrangements such as a Z-plasty. Alternative V-Y advancements are useful if there is healthy surrounding tissue.

Current treatment strategies for hypertrophic scars include surgical manipulation, intralesional corticosteroid injections, cryotherapy, and laser therapy. Surgical manipulation to relieve skin tension remains the traditional treatment for a hypertrophic scar. Additionally, intralesional corticosteroids suppress the inflammatory process in wounds, diminish collagen synthesis, and enhance collagen degradation.[3] Lastly, since the introduction\ of laser treatment in the mid-1980s, additional lasers with different wavelengths have been used therapeutically. The most encouraging results have been obtained with the 585 nm wavelength pulsed dye laser (PDL), which has been recognized as an excellent therapeutic option for the treatment of younger hypertrophic scars. PDL induces the dissociation of disulfide bonds in collagen fibers and leads to collagen fiber realignment, decreased fibroblast proliferation, and neocollagenesis. However, it is necessary to treat two to six times, for the optimal resolution.

Recently, an exciting research demonstrated the benefit of fractional photothermolysis in the treatment of hypertrophic scarring. Although the exact mechanism is unknown, this concept uses a CO_2 laser, which is an ablative laser that targets water in the underlying tissues (10,600 nm). The laser creates columns of tissue destruction, which stimulates collagen production in adjacent uninjured columns of tissue. The adjacent uninjured tissue regenerates tissue rapidly from their follicles and sweat glands. Overall, this creates a more smooth appearance and for meshed grafts to appear less obvious.[4] Patients described less tightness as well as decreased pruritus. An important aspect of this treatment modality is the fractionated nature of the laser for remodeling of the disorganized collagen without undue thermal injury to the surface. Different strategies are used for fractional CO_2 lasers with some clinicians preferring high density and low energy and others preferring low density and high energy. Caution must be used to avoid high energy and high density, which can cause an iatrogenic burn injury. If scars are erythematous and hypertrophic, then a combination of PDL and CO_2 laser can be used (Figure 22.1).

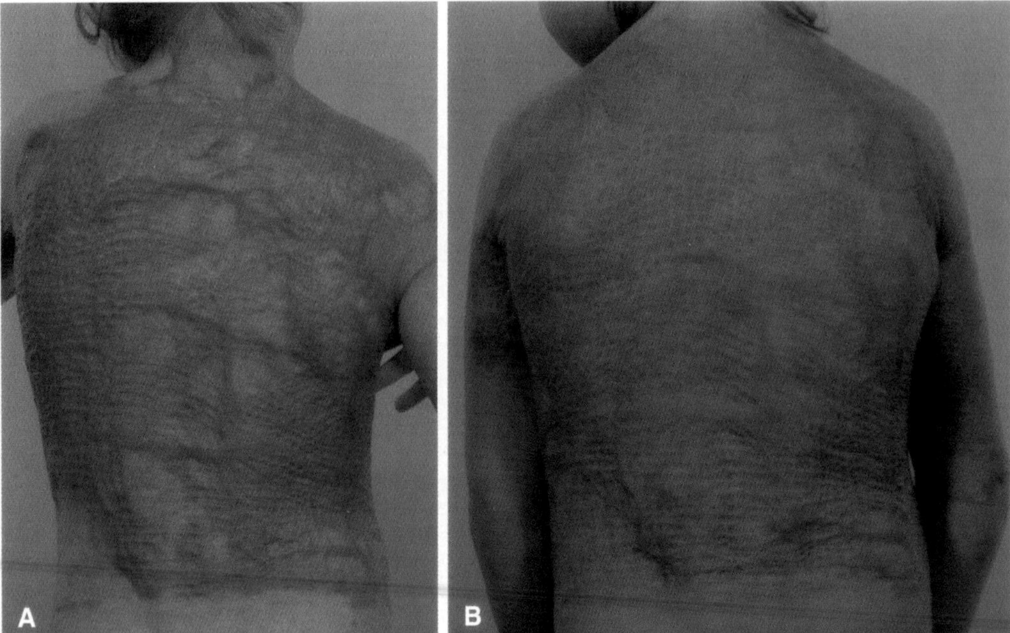

FIGURE 22.1. This patient had undergone Meek reconstruction for full-thickness burn of the back. **A.** Before laser treatment. **B.** After two treatments of pulsed dye laser and CO_2 laser.

GENERAL PRINCIPLES OF BURN SCAR REHABILITATION

Release With Local Tissue Rearrangement

Z-plasty is a commonly used form of local tissue rearrangement to release linear burn scar contractures.[5,6] In addition to lengthening a scar, it is also useful in redirecting a scar, flattening a raised or depressed scar, and recreating a webspace.[7-9] The classic Z-plasty design incorporates angles of 60° with three equal limbs to achieve a theoretical 75% lengthening. This configuration balances the desired increase in length of the contracture by taking advantage of available lateral skin laxity. Other angles and theoretical increases in lengths are detailed in **Table 22.1**. Positioning of this classic Z-plasty in series or in opposition are both reliable methods to improve burn scar contractures. The double-opposing or *jumping man* Z-plasty combines two Z-plasties oriented along a common central limb axis, with advancement of a triangular flap into a releasing incision made perpendicular to the central axis. This technique is particularly useful for releasing webspace contractures in which there is significant transverse skin laxity. Clever variations, including W-plasty and trapeze-plasty, all have their staunch supporters.[1,10-12] The advantage of a Z-plasty, when it is indicated, is that no additional donor site is incurred and recovery is short. However, not all burn scars are ideal candidates for this procedure. Use of this procedure in broad contractures often results in less than satisfactory release. Surgeons need to weigh these benefits against the risks of inadequate correction and the need for additional operations. Preserving the subdermal blood supply by maximizing thickness and meticulous handling are paramount to a successful outcome and minimizes flap-tip necrosis.

TABLE 22.1. Z PLASTY GAIN BASED ON LIMB ANGLE

Angle of Each Lateral Limb of Z-Plasty	Gain in Length of Central Limb
30°	25%
45°	50%
60°	75%
75°	100%
90°	120%

Incisional Release with Skin Graft

Broad burn scar contractures will require a generous transverse release to restore structures to their normal anatomic positions for a proper correction. Sound clinical judgment is needed to determine the adequacy of a surgical release. As a rule, most burn scar contractures that cross a mobile structure, such as an eyelid or a joint, will require an incision designed across the entire axis of rotation. For instance, an adequate eyelid release requires an incision from just medial to the medial canthus to the lateral orbital rim. An antecubital fossa release traverses the medial epicondyle to the lateral epicondyle.

A question sometimes arises whether a broad scar contracture should be excised, either in lieu of or concurrent with a release. As previously mentioned, scar excision should rarely be contemplated. A contracture implies a lack of skin. Scar excision only increases the amount of skin replacement needed. Scar excision may be considered for hypertrophic scarring of the face when the subunit concept is indicated. Even then, the use of CO_2 laser scar resurfacing as an alternative to scar excision should be considered.[13,14]

Many options exist for skin coverage of the resulting defect after a transverse release. Color-matched full-thickness skin in the form of a graft is ideal but not always available. Thick STSG is a good second choice, if available. Dermal substitutes have been touted to augment the performance of a thin STSG with reasonable successes. The superiority of a thicker graft is dependent on the greater quantity of transferred dermis. Thin grafts, on the other hand, *take* more easily but with a corollary increase in secondary graft contraction. Although STSGs can be meshed and expanded, this can result in mesh pattern scars and should be avoided, if possible, during late reconstructions.[15]

Pedicled Flaps, Tissue Expansion, and the Use of Previously Burned or Grafted Skin as Flaps

Just as thicker skin grafts provide greater amount of biology for higher quality results, proponents of flap coverage of burn releases argue that flaps contain the most biological advantage and have the added advantage of not having to rely on the blood supply of the recipient bed to survive. Should a scar release result in the exposure of nongraftable structures, pedicled flaps maybe the only option. However, before using a flap for the coverage of a graftable wound bed, one must balance donor site morbidity. Furthermore, flap debulking is almost guaranteed. Therefore, although pedicled flaps have been described for just about any type of burn reconstruction, fasciocutaneous flaps predominate, and the use of preoperative tissue expansion as a delay strategy has gained popularity to decrease the thickness and bulk while maximizing vascularity.

Tissue expansion is a valuable tool for the burn reconstructive surgeon when a large contiguous piece of skin is needed either as a full-thickness graft or a flap. The basis for tissue expansion is placement of mechanical stress to skin over time, resulting in both mechanical and biologic *creep*. Mechanical creep refers to the immediate increase in tissue surface area upon placement of mechanical forces. Biologic creep involves a series of cellular-level changes induced over time by this stress, including thickening of the epidermis, thinning of the dermis, cellular hypertrophy, and realignment of collagen fibrils. In addition, expanded skin exhibits greater vascularity than nonexpanded skin owing to the delay phenomenon and increases reliability of local flaps.

Prior to placing a tissue expander, the surgeon should understand the amount of expanded skin has to be enough to cover the width of the tissue expander as well as the width of eventual defect. The incision used for placement of the tissue expander should be carefully planned so as not to compromise the blood flow to any future flaps. Furthermore, the surgeon should have a plan for how the expanded skin will be advanced prior to the placement of the expander. Several authors have described techniques for maximizing advancements from rectangular tissue expanders. Complications of tissue expansion include infection, implant exposure, and flap ischemia.

Use of pedicled flaps to reconstruct defects in areas of functional importance or those with exposed critical structures is often "*limited*" by the presence of previously burned skin in the surrounding tissues. Many surgeons are reluctant to include this previously burned or previously grafted skin as part of a local or regional flap because of concerns about damage to its vascularity. However, these concerns are often unfounded, as the initial thermal injury is generally limited to the skin and subcutaneous fat, and the underlying fascia and its axial blood supply are often spared. Many documented cases have been performed incorporating previously burned[16] or grafted skin[17,18] into fasciocutaneous flaps for the trunk, hand, and upper extremity reconstruction without significant differences in flap necrosis.[19]

SITE-SPECIFIC SURGICAL INTERVENTIONS FOR BURN SCARS AND CONTRACTURES

General Face

The face is a complex, three-dimensional structure comprised of myriad tissue components of differing dermal thicknesses, subcutaneous fat, and underlying muscle. The simplest method of reconstruction may not be the preferred or optimal approach in burn reconstruction, and thoughtful deviation from the traditional *reconstructive ladder* is often appropriate.[20] Burned faces have readily noticeable features: contractures; decreased pliability; alopecia; variations in surface, color, and texture; and fragility of tissues.[20] Additionally, these scars frequently cause functional deficits as in ectropion, nasal stenosis, microstomia, neck contracture, and lip retraction leading to periodontal disease. The eyes, cheeks, nose, ears, scalp, and lips have different underlying dermal thicknesses, muscles, and functions and must be approached differently.

The nose and lips are central facial units; they are of critical importance to the appearance of the face.[21] The cheek is a peripheral unit of the face and is of near-critical importance.[21] In his 1995 paper, Rose describes the following goals: a *normal* appearance at conversational distance, a face that is balanced and symmetric, distinct aesthetic units connected by inconspicuous scars, a soft skin texture that will bear corrective makeup, and the ability for dynamic and natural facial expression.[22] Below, we describe typical reconstructions for each anatomic site. In addition, with increasing evidence supporting laser treatment modalities, gradual release of tension and serial laser treatments can dramatically improve patient outcomes.[13,23,24]

Periorbital Reconstruction

Periorbital reconstruction represents the most complex and functionally important regions of reconstruction. As in other regions, a good reconstructive outcome depends on appropriate acute treatment. Burns of the periorbita that are not thought to heal within the first 10 to 14 days should receive early debridement and grafting. For the actual lid tissue, we recommend thin split-thickness grafts. For the region below the lower lid, thicker split- or full-thickness grafts can be used. Immediate intervention should be instated to avoid damage to the globe if ectropion of the upper or lower lid is noted. In addition to early debridement and grafting, sometimes early release is needed. For periorbital reconstruction, it is important to address all regions including the medial canthus, lateral canthus, and upper and lower lids. Additionally, one must assess which lamellae have been damaged. Given that periorbital burns are often concurrent with cheek burns that pull on the lower lid, it is important to provide additional support to the lower lid to prevent recurrent contracture and ectropion.

Upper Lid

The skin distal to the confluence of the orbital septum and the levator is some of the thinnest skin in the body. When debriding this tissue, extreme caution must be taken to avoid debriding too deeply. Similarly, for reconstruction, scar release should ensure not to violate the orbicularis oculi. The release should be performed in the upper eyelid crease along the entire length of the eyelid just beyond the medial and lateral canthus. Traction sutures make it easer to perform a more exact release. Once release is performed, a thin STSG should be used. There should be two separate grafts with one over the palpebral lid and one proximal to the confluence of the septum and levator. This proximal graft can be slightly thicker. Donor sites should obtain color match by using a supraclavicular region or the inner proximal arm. Grafts should be bolstered for up to 7 to 10 days, and concurrent temporary tarsorrhaphy sutures should be placed to prevent recontracture. These tarsorrhaphy sutures can remain for up to 3 weeks, or permanent tarsorrhaphy sutures can remain for several months (Figure 22.2).

Lower Lid

Similar to the upper lid, depth of debridement and release must not go too deep. For the lower lid, the release should be performed using a subciliary incision extending the full length of the eyelid.[25] For the lower lid, a thicker split- or full-thickness graft can be used. Again, postoperative splinting with tarsorrhaphy or Frost sutures should be used. If the contracture on the lower lid extends onto the cheek, often additional support is needed to prevent the lower lid from retracting. If this is the case, we usually perform a graded approach. If the medial and lateral canthi are still retracted after the release, we recommend a medial and lateral canthoplasty. Additionally, through the incision made for the release, the suborbicularis oculi fat can be mobilized and suspended from the inferior orbital rim. Finally, if the inner or middle lamellae are affected, a release of the conjunctiva and placement of a palatal graft provides tissue and support.

Canthi

Webbing of the medial canthus is a common sequela of burns to the periorbita. This webbing, similar to webbing between fingers, is often best addressed with a five-flap jumping man flap (Figure 22.3). If this is concurrent with medial canthal ectropion, a concurrent medial

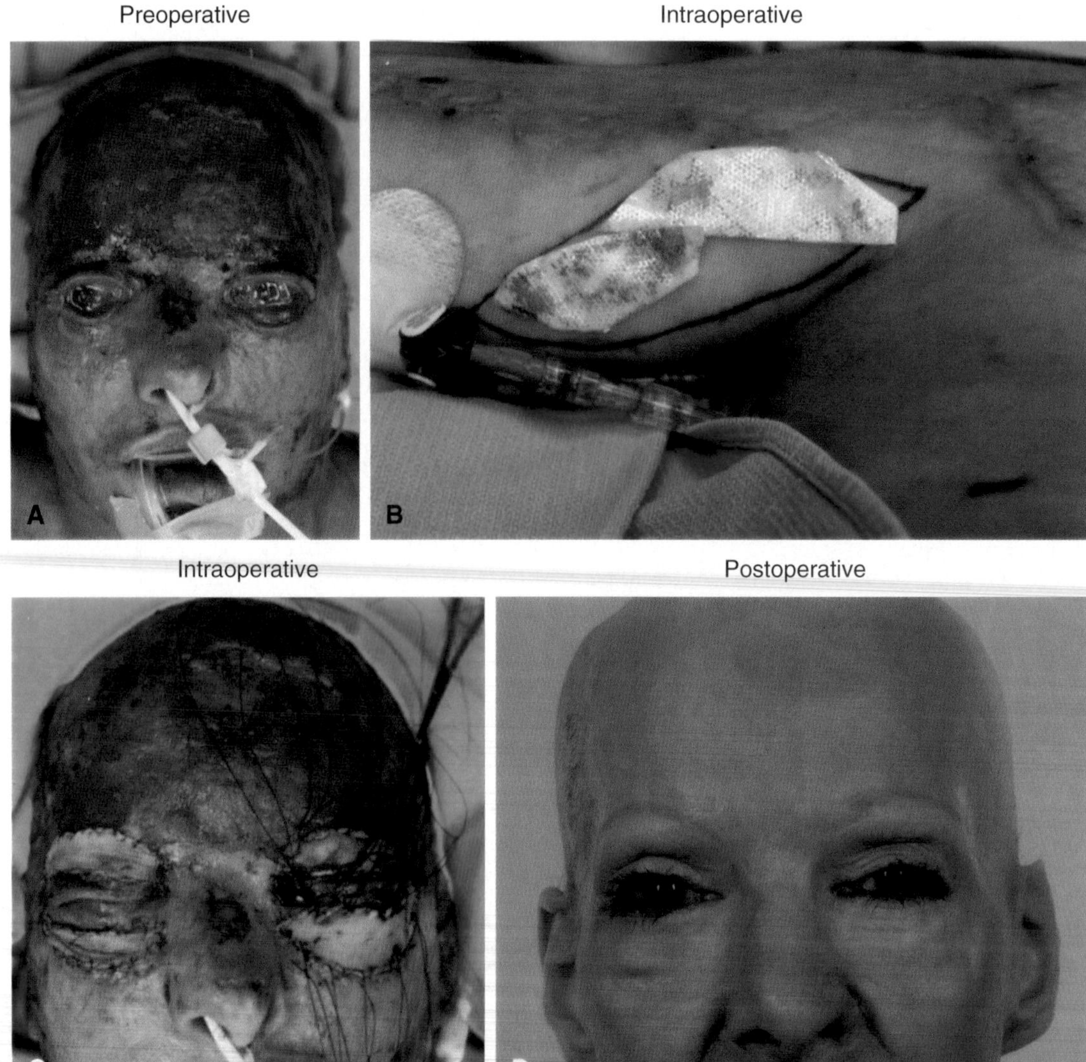

FIGURE 22.2. Burn ectropion. **A.** Burn ectropion after nontreated burn 3 weeks after injury. **B,C.** Intraoperative full-thickness skin graft and medial and lateral tarsorrhaphy. **D.** One year postoperatively.

canthoplasty should be performed. The lateral canthus usually does not form a similar web, and a canthoplasty best restores position of the lateral canthus and prevents ectropion.

Perioral Reconstruction

Acute burn care for the perioral region differs somewhat from elsewhere on the face, given their robust vascularity. Burns to the lips often heal by secondary intention, so excision and grafting of perioral burns is not typically performed.[26] Two common sequelae of burns to the lips and perioral region are microstomia and lower lip eversion, which can cause periodontal complications. Similar to periocular and neck skin, perioral muscles lie close to the surface and often contract strongly with burns in this region. Microstomia forms after burns to the lips or perioral region either from intrinsic contractures of the lip itself or from extrinsic contractures caused by burns to the surrounding tissue or even contracture of skin grafts to surrounding areas.[26] Early occupational therapy and splinting are crucial in the acute burn phase. Although splinting can prevent or manage mild perioral contractures, the durable, successful management of microstomia is typically surgical.[26] Contractures at the oral commissure can be incised, and the mucosa (along with underlying orbicularis oris) can be advanced in a Y-to-V fashion and inset into the incision to deepen the oral commissure and reconstruct the vermillion.[26]

Lip contractures and lip eversion occur when the lower lip is pulled downward and the upper lip is pulled upward, leading to excessive exposure of the vermillion causing difficulty with oral competence and drooling. Small amounts of eversion can be corrected by horizontal elliptical excision of the red lip posterior to the wet-dry border.[20] For more severe contractures and eversion, the surgeon should release along the entirety of the lip just below the white line and extend beyond the lip slightly. Placing stay sutures in the vermillion to give counter traction helps. The release should carry down to the orbicularis oris but not disturb this muscle layer. Then, the entire lip subunit should be replaced with a full- or thick split-thickness skin graft. For the upper lip, this subunit should extend up laterally to the nasal ala. For the upper and lower lips, the release should continue lateral to the modiolus.

Persistent incompetence of the lower lip, resulting from burn scarring itself or from scarring and loss of contour after reconstruction, can be addressed using strips of temporalis muscle and fascia, tunneled in a subcutaneous plane but over the zygomatic arch, and augmented with fascia lata graft to create a sling through the reconstructed lower lip. This procedure results in a durable and dynamic restoration of lower lip competence.[4]

More severe burns to the perioral region require more extensive reconstruction. Larger flaps and free flaps from the scalp,

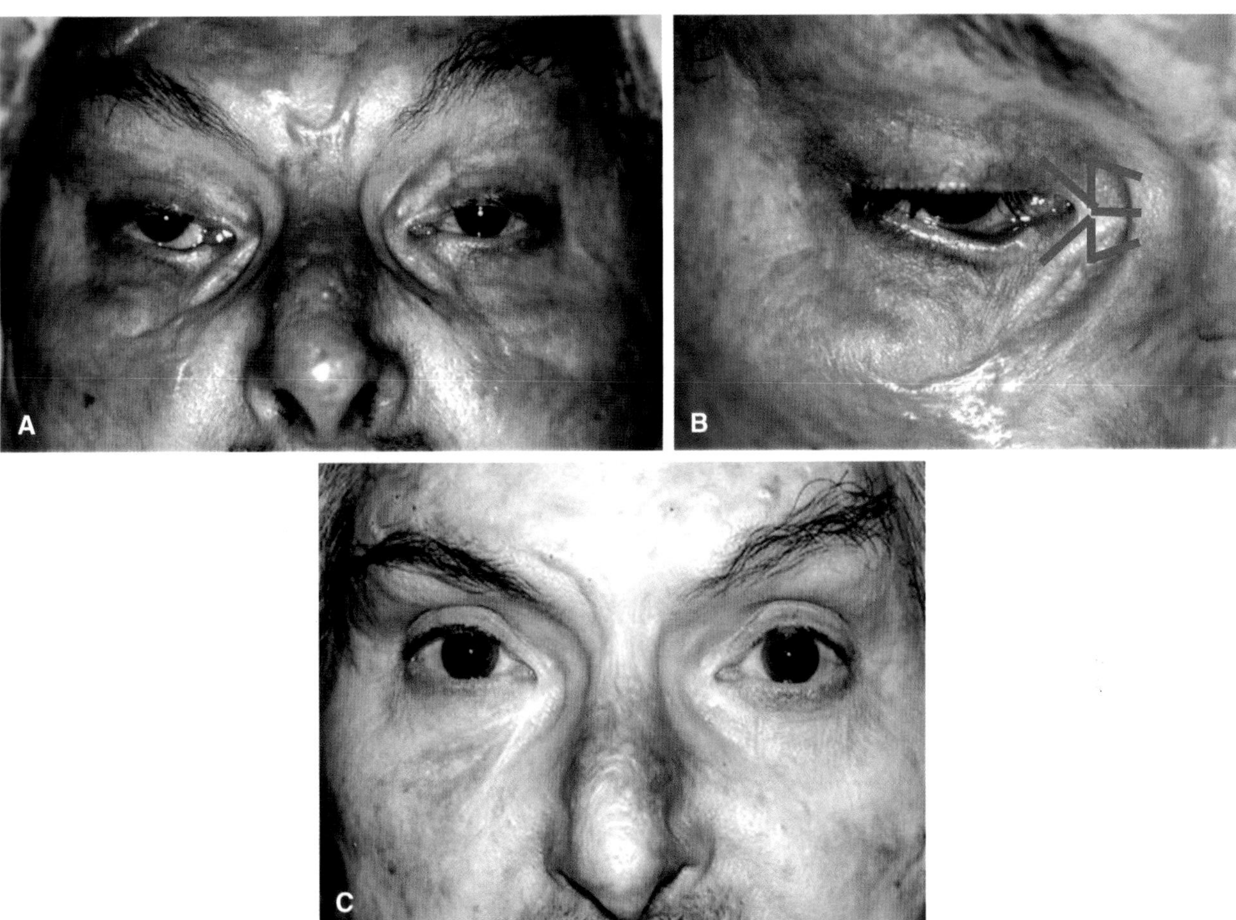

FIGURE 22.3. Preoperative **(A,B)** and postoperative **(C)** photos of five-flap jumping man rearrangement to improve medial canthal webbing. (Courtesy of Paul Cederna, MD, University of Michigan.)

temporoparietal fascia, supraclavicular region, and radial forearm have been described, in conjunction with other procedures such as fascial slings, to resurface more extensive burn injuries to the lips and perioral region.[22]

Scalp Reconstruction

The scalp is composed of five layers—skin, subcutaneous tissue, galea aponeurotica, loose areolar tissue, and periosteum or pericranium. Whereas tension release and laser have avoided tissue expansion in many regions, this often is insufficient in the scalp where hair-bearing skin needs to be brought in. Thus, tissue expansion is a useful tool in the scalp to expand and advance local hair-bearing skin. Up to 50% of the scalp can be reconstructed with tissue expansion.[27] Care should be taken to maintain the normal hair directional pattern. When choosing an expander size, we usually choose the largest possible size that a pocket can fit. Using multiple expanders is needed because the scalp will never stretch and advance as much as one would hope. The expander should be placed in the subgaleal plane above the periosteum. The region of the scar should not be dissected to prevent the expander migrating in the wrong direction. If using remote ports, a small pocket should be dissected and the port should be placed over the mastoid process if possible, as this makes it easy to find and has thin skin over the top of the port. Given the thickness of the scalp, placing a port elsewhere can at times make it hard to find. When advancing the flaps, galeal scoring can be performed perpendicular to the desired tissue gain for slightly improved reach. Standing cutaneous deformities should not be excised as in other regions of the face because they will usually flatten on their own.[28] If calvarial bone is exposed, a more complex reconstruction might be required. Small scars can be addressed with a V-Y advancement flap. Larger defect requires large rotational flaps that incorporate multiple vessels to supply the scalp. These should be bipedicled and include at least one major artery.[28] The most well described is the Orticochea flap which is most useful for defects in the occipitoparietal region. If the calvarial bone is viable, then sometimes burring the outer cortex followed by Integra placement and subsequently skin grafting might be sufficient. If this conservative approach fails, a free tissue transfer of a flap that will curve over a contoured region such as a latissimus dorsi flap can provide the most durable coverage. These flaps are plugged into the superficial temporal artery. If underlying bone is nonviable, then a more complex reconstruction with bone grafts from a split calvarial or split rib graft and free tissue transfer is required.

Nasal Reconstruction

The nose poses a unique challenge among facial structures because of its complex three-dimensional structure and underlying bony and cartilaginous skeleton. The structure is of course divided into the subunits of radix, dorsum, tip, columella, two sidewalls, two ala, and two soft triangles. These subunits, as in Mohs reconstruction, should be taken into account during reconstruction. Unlike Mohs reconstruction, however, the surrounding tissues are also often scarred or previously grafted, making large local tissue rearrangements less reliable. Thus, surgical delay should be considered when performing local tissue rearrangements. Functionally, the goal is a functional nose for normal breathing and speech. As such, the prevention and correction of nasal stenosis is crucial.[3] A common sequela of patients who are smoking while using home O_2 is intranasal burns. These should be treated with immediate nasal stenting for up to a month to prevent nasal stenosis. If stenosis does develop, it should be approached by addressing the nasal lining and the nasal aperture. For the nasal lining, depending on the severity, groups have described a simple approach of release and stenting or release and grafting. For more dramatic stenosis, additional tissue must be added either from the septal mucosa, nasolabial flaps, or gingivobuccal mucosal flaps with or without additional cartilage graft support.[29-32] If the nasal vestibule is patent but the nasal ala is missing, a different approach can be used. Inferiorly based turndown flap using the dorsum of the nose can be used to reconstruct even severely burned nose and maintain tip projection and alar contour when the forehead is not an available donor site.[33] This approach takes the skin, including scar and skin graft, of the nose, incised broadly from the lateral ala, along the nasofacial sulcus up to the radix bilaterally, and folded down 180° over itself. The resultant defect is then skin grafted, so that the skin graft makes up the exterior skin of the nose. The turnover eventually contracts down, taking advantage of the stiff, scarred tissue to recreate a projecting tip and the appearance of alar lobules even in the absence of cartilage.

If a small nasal alar defect is present, a helical composite graft offers skin and cartilage. These composite grafts, however, are limited by size and often fail if larger than 1 cm. For a larger alar defect when local options are not available, a free helical root flap can be performed based on the anterograde or retrograde branch of the superficial temporal artery (Figure 22.4). This can be plugged into the angular artery if it is available and size appropriate or to the facial artery using an A-V loop.[34]

If burn injury to the nose is superficial with adequate subcutaneous tissue remaining and bony/cartilaginous structures covered and preserved, burn scars of the external nose can be accomplished via excision and FTSG.[20] Preferred donor sites are elsewhere on the head and neck above the clavicle or on the inside of the proximal arm for non–hair-bearing color match.[1] For injuries that involve deeper structures, resection of larger portions of the nose may be necessary to control the injury and give a wound bed for reconstruction. The forehead flap is a commonly preferred method of reconstruction; it can be accomplished even with scarred skin as long as the frontalis muscle is intact.[20]

Nasolabial or melolabial flaps can be used for reconstruction of the nasal sidewall, dorsum, tip, and ala (even if retracted or notched). In the case of inferiorly based melolabial flaps, the lips and columella can also be resurfaced. These flaps come in three different geometries, all of which take advantage of the blood supply of facial artery and its anastomoses. Inferiorly and superiorly based flaps are designed with the medial incision in the melolabial sulcus and the lateral incision on the cheek; after the flaps are elevated, they are rotated into the defect, and the donor site is closed in the site of the melolabial fold, camouflaging it.

Ear Reconstruction

Early treatment of ear burns should follow similar principles of facial reconstruction with early debridement if the tissue is not expected to heal within 2 to 3 weeks. We often stage the subacute burns with Integra to cover any exposed cartilage and to support subsequent skin grafts. We typically recommend STSGs for visualization of the underlying cartilage. During the reconstruction phase, a common reconstructive challenge is a tethered lobule. This can usually be corrected with a series of Z-plasties if there is a scar band. Alternatively, a release is made with a V around the lobule and Y advancement of the tissue inferiorly. The remainder of burned ear reconstruction follows general principles of ear reconstruction discussed elsewhere in this text. The main challenge in burned ear reconstruction is that often there is no unburned surrounding tissue, making local flaps difficult. For complete ear reconstruction, we recommend autologous cartilage grafts from the costochondral cartilages or a conchal transposition covered by a temporoparietal fascial flap and a STSG (Figure 22.5). The contralateral ear should serve as a template if available. Despite increased use of porous polyethylene implants, the surgeon must ensure coverage is adequate. The patient and surgeon should expect a higher complication rate than autologous tissue.

Cheek Reconstruction

When evaluating cheek burn scars, it is important to assess if the redness or part of the deformities are caused from more proximal tension from neck scars. If the neck scars are released, often the redness of the cheeks will improve. In the cheek, it is typically unnecessary to excise all adjacent normal tissue in the unit just to resurface a segment of it. In the cheek region, muscle tissues are deeper than in the periorbital and perioral regions.

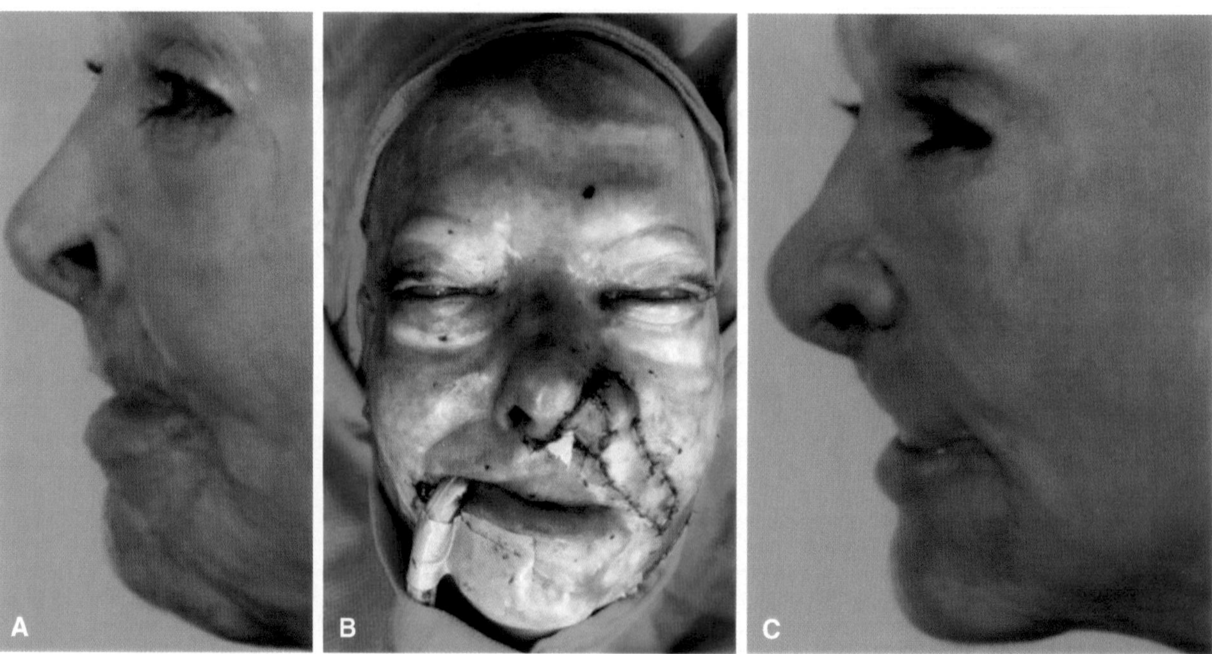

FIGURE 22.4. Preoperative **(A)**, intraoperative **(B)**, and postoperative **(C)** photos of free helical root flap reconstruction of nasal ala. (Procedure done in collaboration with Adeyiza Momoh, MD, University of Michigan.)

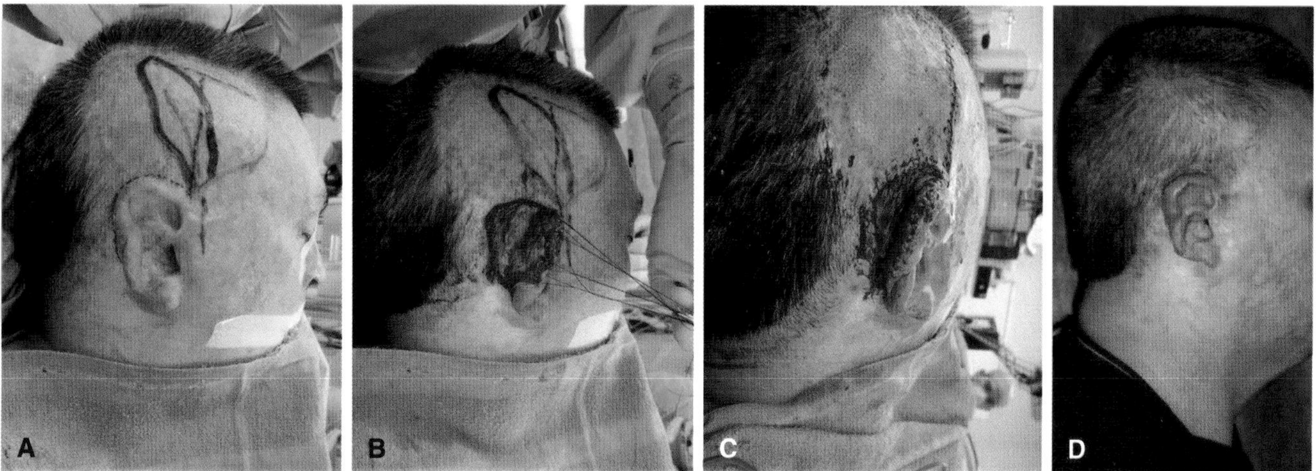

FIGURE 22.5. Preoperative **(A)**, intraoperative **(B,C)**, and postoperative **(D)** photos of ear reconstruction with conchal transposition and temporoparietal fascia flap.

Functionally, management of cheek scars is important to preserve the function of adjacent structures including the lower lid and the upper and lower lips. Thick STSGs or FTSGs can be used to resurface regions of the cheek owing to their technical simplicity, but they are almost by requirement different in color and texture from their recipient site and can cause a patchy appearance.[21] If they are to be used, care must be taken to use skin that is most like that of the recipient region, such as supraclavicular skin or skin from the inner proximal arm. Deep wounds to the cheek can be challenging because of the risk of facial nerve involvement or scarring around the facial nerve as well as the need for thick soft tissues and a functional oral lining.[30] When there are deficits of the latter two, fat grafting and de-epithelialized pedicled or free flaps can provide thickness to the buccal region and oral lining if needed.[26] As in other regions, the most important step is to relieve tension. For panfacial burns, the contractures often run along the nasolabial folds and marionette lines. These should be broken up with small Z-plasties to relieve tension but to avoid altering the normal aesthetic lines. Tissue should be handled gently with skin hooks rather than forceps. If local flaps are used, they should be made thick enough to ensure vascularized tissue is included, incorporating the fascia when possible.[1] The tips of small flaps can be blunted to decrease tip necrosis.[1] In our experience, truncating the tips of Z-plasty flaps appears to improve the viability of flap tips.

One of the primary challenges in cheek reconstruction after burn injury arises when there is a paucity of local tissue with which to reconstruct the region, and when adjacent tissues are often damaged by the precipitating injury as well. Tissue expansion improves options for local reconstruction with similar tissues including local tissue rearrangement and skin grafting. Tissue expansion is useful in postburn scars of the face and neck. In two recent series, mostly rectangular expanders were placed in a subcutaneous plane, filled until the expanded skin was 10%-20% greater in width than the scar to be excised, and the expander was then removed and the expanded skin used to reconstruct the scarred region.[35] Tissue expansion is an excellent option in the face and especially the cheek for a number of reasons (Figure 22.6). It is possible to replace part or all of the aesthetic subunit with skin of similar qualities to avoid distal donor sites and to provide sensate and hair-bearing tissue. The cheek also serves as

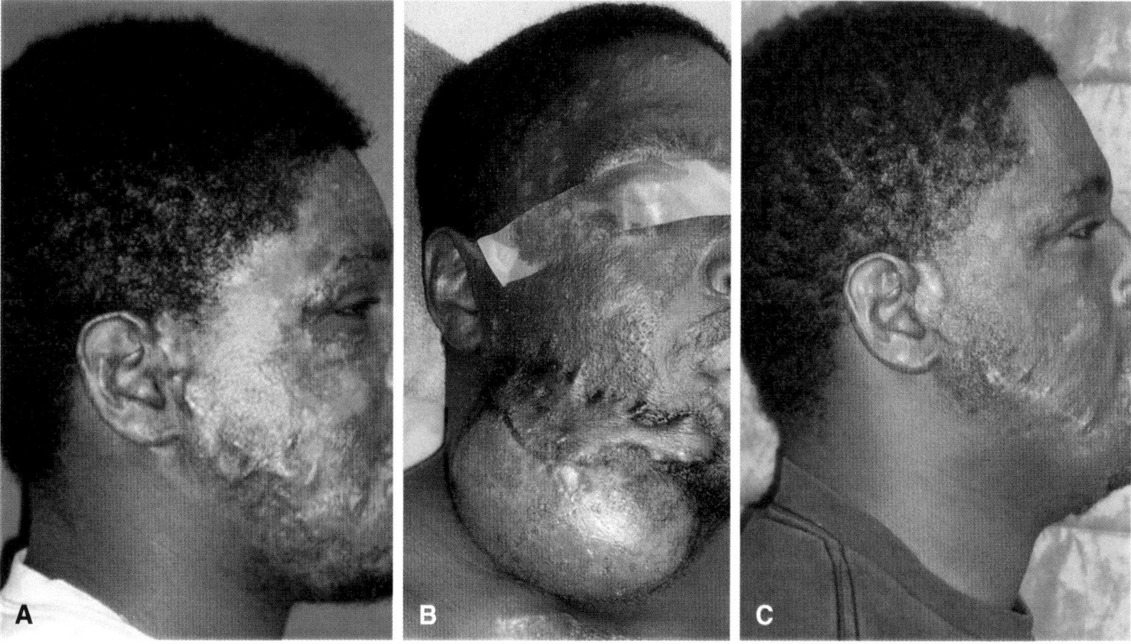

FIGURE 22.6. Preoperative **(A)**, intraoperative **(B)**, and postoperative **(C)** photos of cheek reconstruction with tissue expander reconstruction.

TABLE 22.2. ALGORITHM FOR NECK CONTRACTURE REPAIR

Neck Contracture	Reconstruction
Scar band	Z-plasty
Moderate contracture	Release plus thick STSG or FTSG
Severe contracture	Release and supraclavicular flap or free fasciocutaneous flap

STSG, split-thickness skin graft; *FTSG*, full-thickness skin graft.

an important subunit when repairing lower lid ectropion because the cheek can often pull down on the lower lid. Resuspending the superficial muscular aponeurotic system off the midface using a lower lid transconjunctival approach helps take tension off the lower lid. This is performed by creating a transconjunctival incision inferior to the lower tarsal border. Dissection is performed to reach the inferior orbital rim and then to undermine a midface flap in the subperiosteal plane. This flap is then advanced superiorly and sutured in its new, lifted position to the inferior orbital rim.[36]

Neck Reconstruction

As mentioned earlier, the neck is one of the most common locations for a functional burn contracture to form. Early debridement and grafting and aggressive splinting are crucial to prevent neck contractures. The neck is also the first region of the face that should be addressed when beginning reconstruction because tension in this region can cause disfigurement and discoloration of the entire face. For limited scar bands, series of Z-plasties can be used. Large Z-plasties (unlike in the hand) can be used owing to the robust blood supply.

Larger, more diffuse neck contractures represent a more complex challenge with several options including grafts, local flaps, regional flaps, and free tissue transfer (**Table 22.2**). Regardless of the tissue used to fill in the defect after the release, the release itself of the neck should be aggressive expanding along the entirety of the neck and should have fish tails at the end for the scar to fully open up without having to chase the scar indefinitely. In general, we do not support excising scars leading to a large defect. The release should and can include release of the underlying platysma. The placement of the release should be considered preoperatively. Some surgeons advocate releasing at the base of the chin subunit. The downside of this placement is that the tissue covering the defect can creep onto the chin by creating an aesthetically unappealing result. Others recommend releasing in the middle of the neck. If this approach is taken, attention to the patient's previous hospital course and the tracheostomy site should be assessed because an unhealed tracheal fistula can lead to a surgical emergency. We recommend intraoperative laryngoscopy to evaluate the previous tracheostomy site. The base of the neck is another location where the release can be performed (**Figure 22.7**). Benefit of this site is that it provides a flat surface to bolster a graft. The downside of this placement is that this often leads to the least amount of release. Once the scar is released, several tissue options exist. A thick split-thickness graft can be used or a large full-thickness graft from the abdomen using an abdominoplasty technique if this tissue was spared. The limitation of skin grafting is a high rate of recurrence unless a prolonged course of splinting is followed.

If the supraclavicular region is spared, these flaps serve as outstanding regional flaps with a nice thick tissue. This donor site can also be expanded preoperatively for a larger neck coverage.[37] Finally, free tissue transfer offers a good option with likely the least amount of recurrent contracture. Anterolateral thigh[38] and abdominal-based perforator flaps provide the most tissue. The main challenge with free tissue transfer is that the anterolateral thigh and abdomen in many Western countries have a significant amount of adipose tissue. This excess tissue takes away the contour of the neck making it hard to identify where the chin subunit ends and where the neck subunit begins. A groin flap free tissue transfer based on the superficial branch of the superficial circumflex iliac artery and superficial epigastric artery provides a thin flap for reconstruction.[39] The scapular or parascapular fasciocutaneous flaps also contribute to large, thin skin coverage.[40,41]

Breast and Chest

As in general breast reconstruction, reconstruction of the burned breast should focus on the breast mound as well as the nipple-areolar complex (NAC). Traditional reconstructive options, as in other regions, have often included release and grafting.[42-45] This approach is useful during development if the breast is being restricted. Although useful, at times this approach fails to address the tight skin envelope, parenchyma asymmetry, and NAC malformations, leaving the patient with suboptimal aesthetic results. Autologous tissue reconstruction, including local and regional cutaneous, fasciocutaneous, and myocutaneous flaps, has been used successfully but may not be available depending on the extent of the burn. Alternatives are placement of tissue expanders through an open or endoscopic method into the breast as well as surrounding unburned tissue.[46] In the developing breast, the expander can be placed and expanded to match the contralateral breast. When development is complete, the expander can

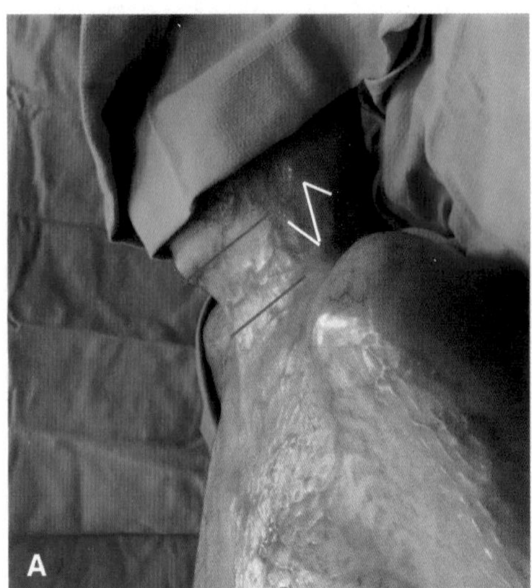

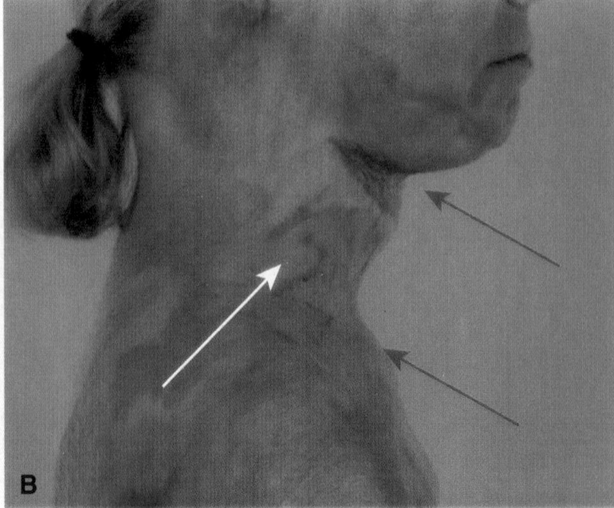

FIGURE 22.7. Preoperative **(A)** and postoperative **(B)** photos of neck reconstruction with release and graft and Z-plasty. Red lines and arrows mark area of release for graft, and white lines and arrows demonstrate Z-plasty.

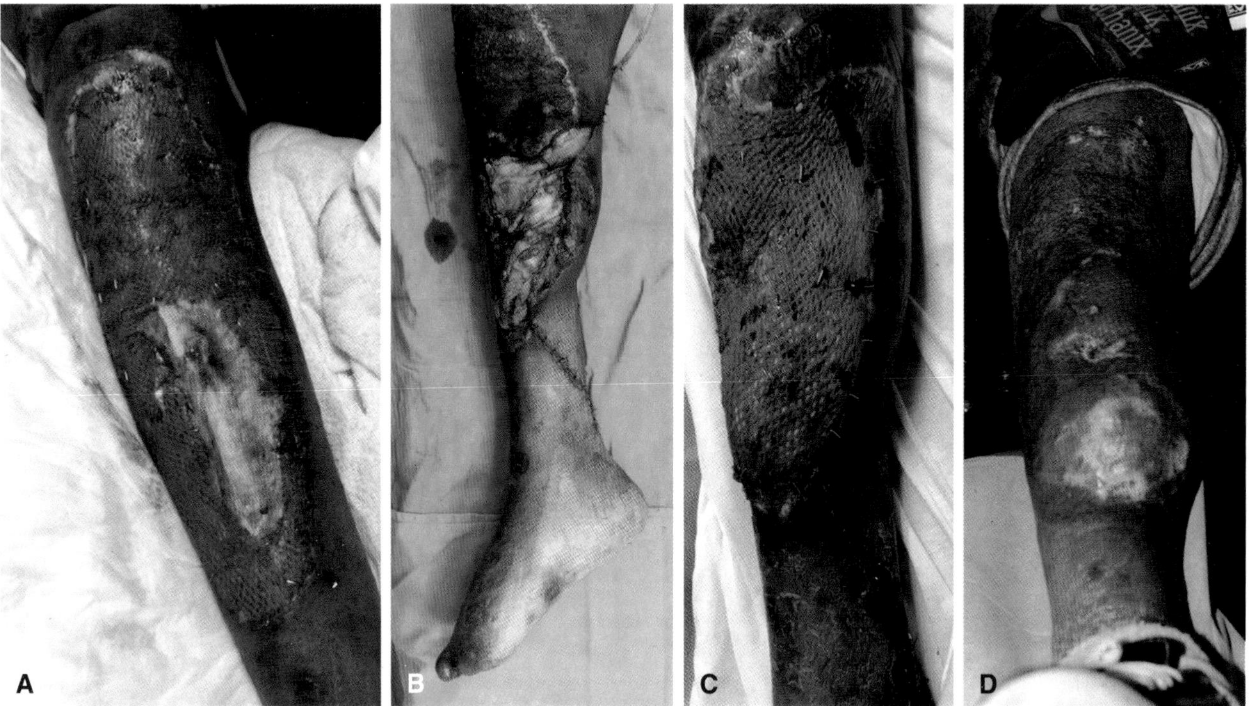

FIGURE 22.8. Preoperative **(A)**, intraoperative **(B)**, and postoperative **(C,D)** photos of gastrocnemius/soleus flap coverage of exposed bone.

be exchanged for a permanent implant alone or an implant plus a latissimus dorsi flap if a scar release is needed at the time of exchange. As the burned breast often lacks ptosis, a contralateral mastopexy can be performed to improve symmetry in the developed adult. The NAC can be reconstructed 9 to 12 months after the final breast reconstruction. Despite the burned tissue, a skate flap[47] can be used with an FTSG to redefine the areola which can also be tattooed later.

Lower Extremity and Foot

Lower extremity reconstruction in burn patients follows the same principles of lower extremity reconstruction after trauma or wound formation. For contour and aberrant scarring secondary to meshed grafts, laser treatments often suffice. If more severe wounds exist with exposed tendon or bone, principles should follow rule of thirds. For proximal third wounds, local gastrocnemius flaps can be used. For middle third wounds, a soleus or gastrocnemius and soleus flap can be used (Figure 22.8). For distal third wounds, free tissue transfer with a thin fasciocutaneous flap is indicated (Figure 22.9). If the surrounding skin is viable, sometimes a biologic reconstruction can mitigate the need for free tissue transfer.

As in the hand, reconstruction of the foot must take into place the soft tissue, tendon, joint, and bony abnormalities. Severe toe contractures cause considerable functional morbidity and often involve deeper structures, such as shortening of the tendons and fibrosis of the interphalangeal or metatarsophalangeal joint capsules; thus,

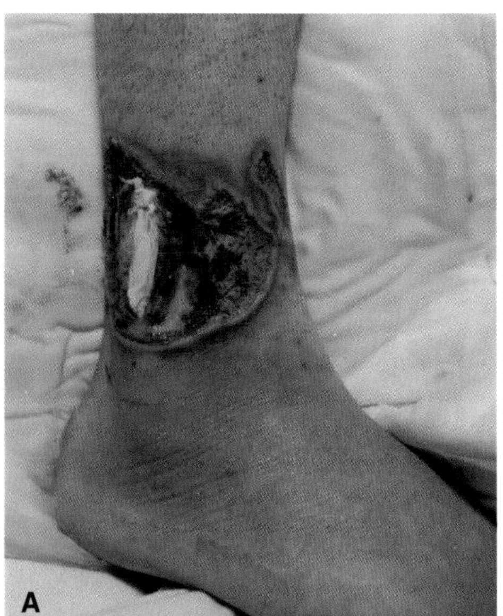

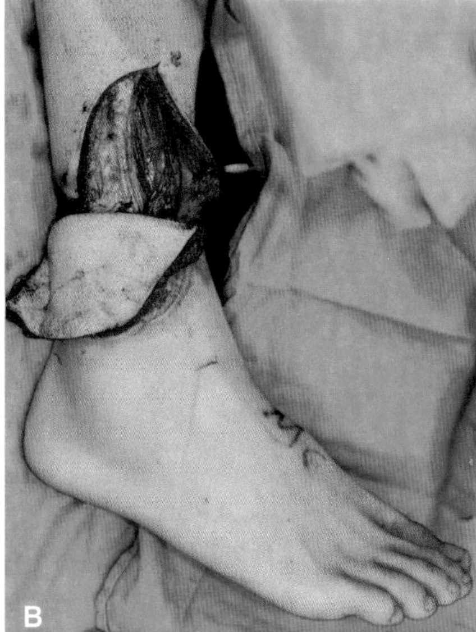

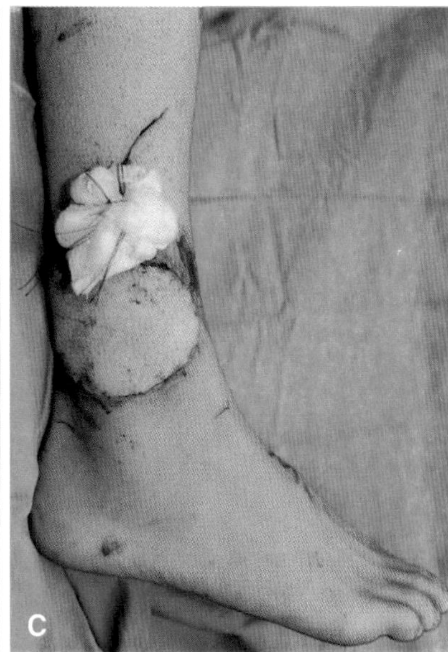

FIGURE 22.9. Preoperative **(A)**, intraoperative **(B)**, and postoperative **(C)** photos of anterolateral thigh flap to exposed lateral compartment tendon.

preoperative X-rays should be obtained. Similar to hand, burns on the dorsal skin cause tissue shortening, hyperextension of the toes, and subluxation and dislocation of the metatarsophalangeal joints. These contractures should be released aggressively. Depending on the involvement of the deeper structures, we recommend the following additional steps: a thick STSG or an FTSG for the skin, tendon lengthening, open capsulotomy, and pin fixation for several weeks to maintain the integrity of the reconstruction. If exposed white structures exist, a thick fasciocutaneous flap should be used. Webspaces are handled like the hand with five-flap jumping man Z-plasties.

TABLE 22.3. ALGORITHM FOR HAND CONTRACTURE REPAIR

Region	Reconstruction
Webspace	Five-flap jumping man
MCP and PIP	Z-plasty
Nail bed and DIP	Release and FTSG

DIP, distal interphalangeal joint; *FTSG*, full-thickness skin graft; *MCP*, metacarpophalangeal joint; *PIP*, proximal interphalangeal joint.

Hand Reconstruction

The complex anatomy of the hand must be analyzed when preparing for reconstruction of the burned hand. Even small scar bands can result in significant functional impairment. Immediate splinting is important to prevent debilitating contractures. The shoulder should be abducted at 90°, the elbow should be extended at 180°, the wrist slightly extended, and the hand in intrinsic plus position. Early aggressive debridement and grafting for the dorsum of the hand is recommended, whereas more conservative treatment and possible staging with Integra is recommended for the palm. The dorsum of the hand is especially susceptible to hypertrophic scar formation owing to the thin and pliable nature of the skin in this area, which requires less thermal force to induce burn to the deeper dermal tissues and hypertrophic scarring. Dorsal scarring may not only inhibit passive flexion but severe burns can result in hyperextension and subluxation of the joints in severe cases.[48] On the volar surface, hypertrophic scar formation of the palm can result in a cupping deformity, which is characterized by convex warping of the longitudinal and horizontal palmar arches.[49] Acute burns to the palm should give more time to heal secondarily because grafts to the palm will impair sensation for the remainder of the patient's life. Additionally, the palmar skin is more durable than any skin graft. If a graft is needed, a thick split- or full-thickness graft

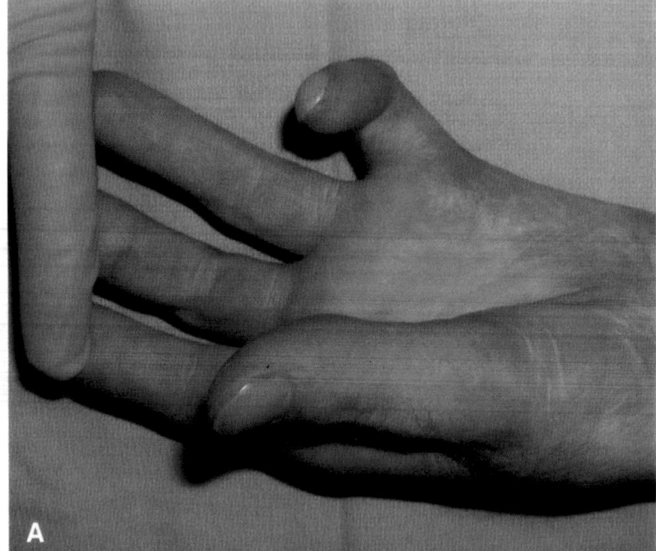

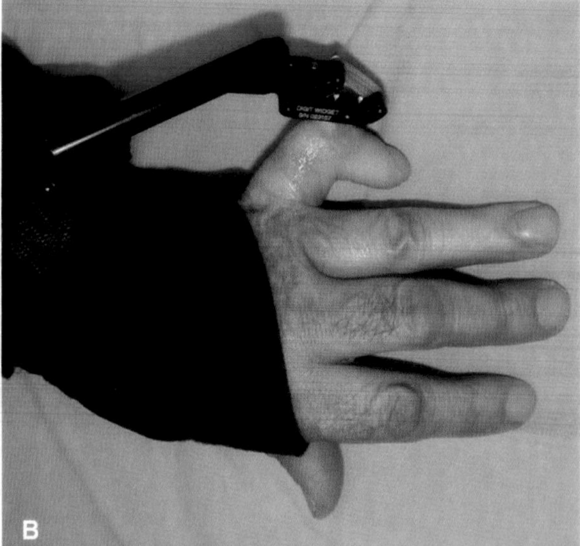

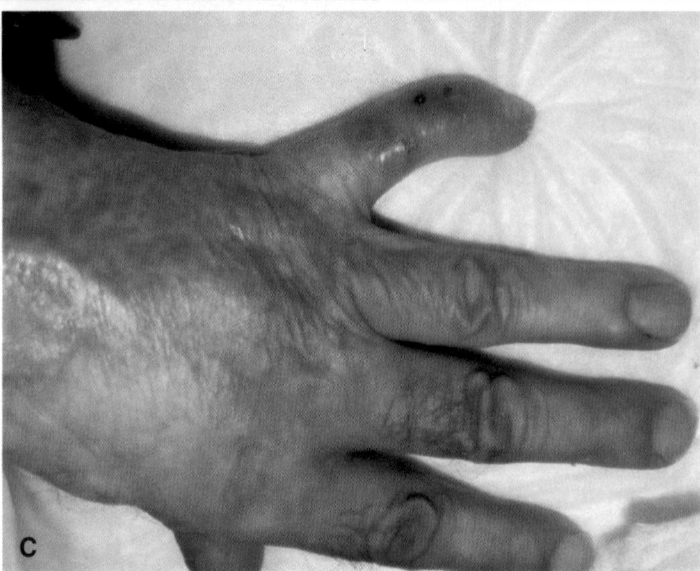

FIGURE 22.10. Digit Widget reconstruction of small finger proximal interphalangeal joint contracture. Preoperative **(A)**, postoperative digit widget placement **(B)**, and postoperative digit widget removal **(C)**. (Courtesy of Steve Haase, MD, University of Michigan)

is best used. Palmar burn scars commonly involve a large surface and can therefore result in tight contractures. Mild forms can be addressed with a sequence of Z-plasties. If the contracture is severe, release of the scar may be required which leaves a large defect. This defect can be filled with an FTSG if no crucial structures are exposed.[50] FTSGs are preferred over split-thickness graft to decrease secondary contraction and to minimize scarring. If the contracture release leads to exposed tendon or bone, local or distant flaps may be required.[51] The extensor tendons dorsally often benefit from a fascia-only reverse radial forearm flap with a skin graft for coverage or a reverse dorsal interosseous flap. Alternatives include free fascia-only or fasciocutaneous flaps, although bulky flaps should be avoided if possible.[52] Severe burns on the dorsal and volar surfaces of the hand often benefit from K-wire placement to keep the digits in an intrinsic plus position to prevent deforming contractures. Thermal injury involving opposing surfaces of border digits can result in a scar band reducing the interdigital space and limiting abduction. Furthermore, if the first webspace is involved, thumb abduction is affected causing adduction contractures, reducing grip strength and function (**Table 22.3**).

Flexion contracture of the small finger is one of the most difficult reconstructive challenges for surgeons because contracture of the collateral ligaments, flexor tendons, and skin results in shortening of the vessels and nerves. For these patients, preoperative X-rays and analysis of the level of contracture of the joint are crucial to a successful outcome. If severe joint contracture is present or the patient has a boutonnière deformity from previous debridement or injury to the extensor tendon, the finger will not be improved by an operation addressing the skin contracture alone. The surgeon should also avoid the urge to straighten the small finger in one operation, as this will often lead to venous congestion or ischemia due to the shortening of the vessels from the contracture. If the skin is the only area causing the contracture then a Z-plasty or series of Z-plasties can be used. In more severe contractures, a release and full-thickness hypothenar flap can be used. Finally, in cases with joint and skin contracture, a Digit Widget can be used for slow distraction and stretching of the contracture. This device places two K-wires in the middle phalanx and has a series of bands that connect to the wrist slowly stretching the contracture (**Figure 22.10**).[53]

Another common and stigmatic deformity of the burned hand is the finger nail. Burn injury to the dorsum of the digit can result in retraction of the soft tissue proximal to the nail fold leading to exposure of the germinal matrix and alterations in nail growth.[54] This is caused by excess vertical tension across the dorsal digit, which often restricts distal interphalangeal joint (DIP) flexion. To treat the contracture and eponychial fold deformity, we use a technique of release and full-thickness graft proximal to the DIP. This involves a distally based bipedicled flap, which is designed to release the proximal nail fold contracture. This is accompanied by an extensive release of the dorsal soft tissues and resurfacing of the resulting defect with an FTSG. Restoration of normal anatomy can thus be achieved and results in normalized nail growth and improved DIP flexion[54] (**Figure 22.11**).

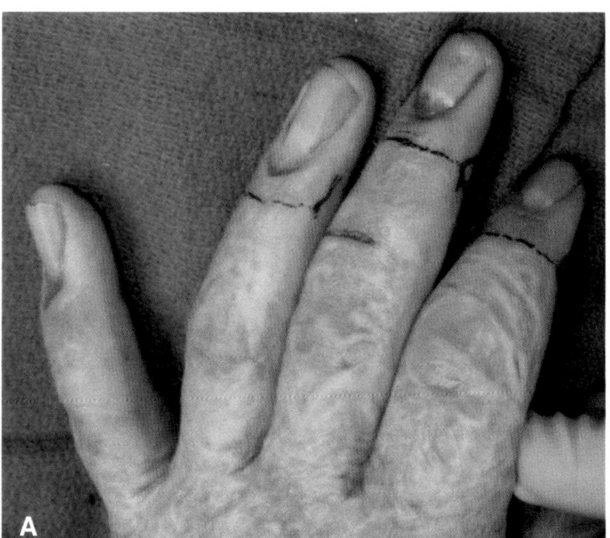

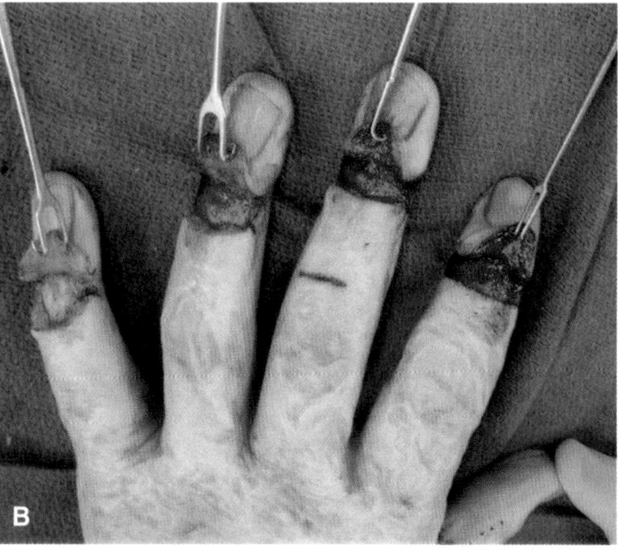

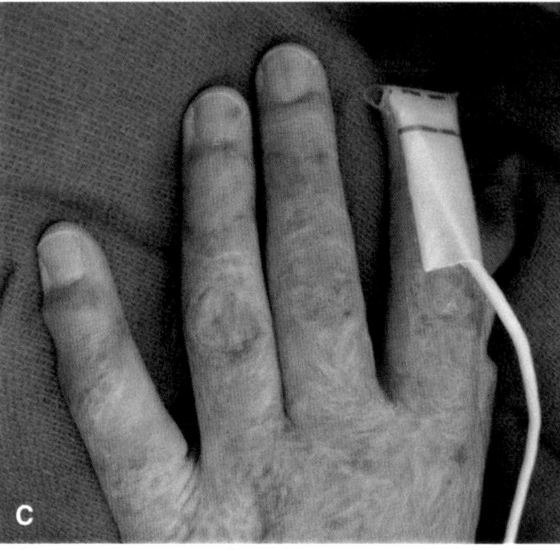

FIGURE 22.11. Preoperative **(A)**, intraoperative **(B)**, and postoperative **(C)** photos of nail bed reconstruction with release and full-thickness skin graft to restore eponychial fold and distal interphalangeal joint tightness.

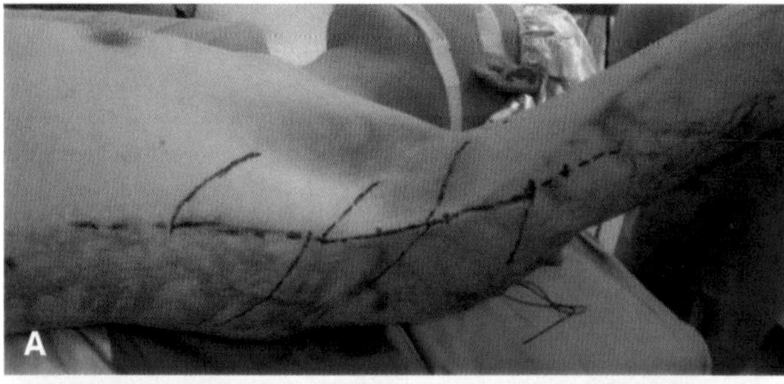

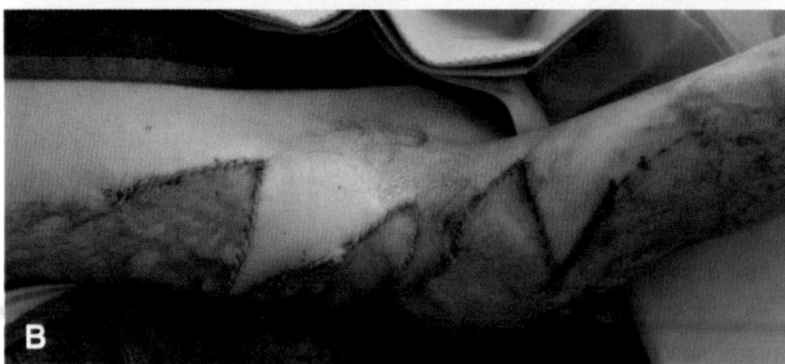

FIGURE 22.12. Preoperative **(A)** and postoperative **(B)** photos of Z-plasty reconstruction of the axilla.

Webspace contractures should be treated with modifications of Z-plasties.[55,56] The five-flap jumping man Z-plasty (two Z-plasties with an intervening Y-to-V) is frequently used and is effective in creating a concavity and lengthening within the webspace because of its geometric design. The Y-to-V region of this flap should be placed in the region of desired deepening. Other options include V-Y advancement flaps, which apply the supple dorsal tissue that is advanced into the web space. These flaps can be combined with forms of Z-plasties.[2]

Axillary scar contractures are the second most common contractures behind neck contractures and are difficult to improve. Small linear bands can be released with Z-plasties (**Figure 22.12**). Z-plasties in this region should be designed large, and flaps should be kept thick with subcutaneous fat. A five-flap jumping man offers a useful reconstruction as in the webspace because it deepens the axilla. Care must be taken during these tissue rearrangements not to move too much hair-bearing skin onto non–hair-bearing skin. Larger more restrictive contractures can be treated with release and apply thick STSG or FTSG. Others have described treatment of severe contractures with pedicled flaps or with regional and free tissue transfer.[57] As in the neck, a thin fasciocutaneous flap will provide the optimal result.

REFERENCES

1. Grishkevich VM. Flexion contractures of fingers: contracture elimination with trapeze-flap plasty. *Burns*. 2011;37(1):126-133.
2. Peker F, Celebiler O. Y-V advancement with Z-plasty: an effective combined model for the release of post-burn flexion contractures of the fingers. *Burns*. 2003;29(5):479-482.
3. Reish RG, Eriksson E. Scar treatments: preclinical and clinical studies. *J Am Coll Surg*. 2008;206:719-730.
4. Chan RK, Bojovic B, Talbot SG, et al. Lower lip suspension using bilateral temporalis muscle flaps and fascia lata grafts. *Plast Reconstr Surg*. 2012;129(1):119-122.
5. Hove CR, Williams EF, Rodgers BJ. Z-plasty: a concise review. *Facial Plast Surg*. 2001;17(4):289-294.
6. Furnas DW, Fischer GW. The Z-plasty: biomechanics and mathematics. *Br J Plast Surg*. 1971;24:144.
   This classic article discusses the power of the Z-plasty to gain scar length by increasing scar width.
7. McGregor IA. The Z-plasty. *Br J Plast Surg*. 1966;19(1):82-87.
8. Fraulin FO, Thomson HG. First webspace deepening: comparing the four-flap an five-flap Z-plasty: which gives the most gain? *Plast Reconstr Surg*. 1999;104(1):120-128.
9. Chen B, Song H. The modification of five-flap Z-plasty for web contracture. *Aesthet Plast Surg*. 2015;39(6):922-926.
10. Shockley WW. Scar revision techniques: Z-plasty, W-plasty, and geometric broken line closure. *Facial Plast Surg*. 2011;19(3):455-463.
11. Sokolowich D, Zimman O. W-plasty: make it easy. *Plast Reconstr Surg*. 1989;83(5):928-929.
12. Grishkevich VM. Trapeze-flap plasty: effective method for postburn neck contracture elimination. *Burns*. 2010;36(3):383-388.
13. Hultman CS, Friedstat JS, Edkins RE, et al. Laser resurfacing and remodeling of hypertrophic burn scars: the results of a large, prospective, before-after cohort study, with long-term follow-up. *Ann Surg*. 2014;260(3):519-529.
    This article demonstrates the benefit of laser treatment to improve scar outcomes in burn patients.
14. Cho SB, Lee SJ, Chung WS, et al. Treatment of burn scar using a carbon dioxide fractional laser. *J Drugs Dermatol*. 2010;9:173-175.
15. Klein M. *Skin grafting*. In: *Color Atlas of Burn Reconstructive Surgery*. New York, NY: Springer-Verlag; 2010:132-138.
16. Pribaz JJ, Pelham FR. Use of previously burned skin in local fasciocutaneous flaps for upper extremity reconstruction. *Ann Plast Surg*. 1994;33:272-280.
17. Tolhurst D, Haeseker B, Zeeman R. The development of the fasciocutaneous flap. *Plast Reconstr Surg*. 1983;71:597-605.
18. Cherup LL, Zachary LS, Gottlieb LJ, Petti C. The radial forearm skin graft-fascial flap. *Plast Reconstr Surg*. 1990;85:898-902.
19. Barret J HD, McCauley R. Use of previously burned skin as random cutaneous local flaps in pediatric burn reconstruction. *Burns*. 2002;28:500-502.
20. Wainwright DJ. Burn reconstruction: the problems, the techniques, and the applications. *Clin Plast Surg*. 2009;36(4):687-700.
21. Menick FJ. Reconstruction of the cheek. *Plast Reconstr Surg*. 2001;108(2):496-505.
22. Rose EH. Aesthetic restoration of the severely disfigured face in burn victims: a comprehensive strategy. *Plast Reconstr Surg*. 1995;96(7):1573-1585.
23. Levi B, Ibrahim A, Mathews K, et al. The use of CO_2 fractional photothermolysis for the treatment of burn scars. *J Burn Care Res*. 2016;37(2):106-114.
24. Anderson RR, Donelan MB, Hivnor C, et al. Laser treatment of traumatic scars with an emphasis on ablative fractional laser resurfacing: consensus report. *JAMA Dermatol*. 2014;150(2):187-193.
    This is the first article to provide a pathway for laser treatment of burn patients who would benefit from fractional CO_2 *laser.*
25. Wong S, Melin A, Reilly D. Head and neck reconstruction. *Clin Plast Surg*. 2017;44(4):845-856.
26. Egeland B, More S, Buchman SR, Cederna PS. Management of difficult pediatric facial burns: reconstruction of burn-related lower eyelid ectropion and perioral contractures. *J Craniofac Surg*. 2008;19(4):960-969.
27. Manders EK, Graham WP, Schenden MJ, Davis TS. Skin expansion to eliminate large scalp defects. *Ann Plast Surg*. 1984;12(4):305-312.
28. Leedy JE, Janis JE, Rohrich RJ. Reconstruction of acquired scalp defects: an algorithmic approach. *Plast Reconstr Surg*. 2005;116(4):54e-72e.
29. Daya M. Nostril stenosis corrected by release and serial stenting. *J Plast Reconstr Aesthet Surg*. 2009;62(8):1012-1019.
30. Daines SM, Hamilton GS, Mobley SR. A graded approach to repairing the stenotic nasal vestibule. *Arch Facial Plast Surg*. 2010;12(5):332-338.
31. Salvado AR, Wang MB. Treatment of complete nasal vestibule stenosis with vestibular stents and mitomycin C. *Otolaryngol Head Neck Surg*. 2008;138(6):795-796.
32. Copcu E. Reconstruction of total and near-total nostril stenosis in the burned nose with gingivo-mucosal flap. *Burns*. 2005;31(6):802-803.
33. Taylor HO, Carty M, Driscoll D, et al. Nasal reconstruction after severe facial burns using a local turndown flap. *Ann Plast Surg*. 2009;62(2):175-179.
34. Pribaz JJ, Falco N. Nasal reconstruction with auricular microvascular transplant. *Ann Plast Surg*. 1993;31(4):289-297.
35. Ashab Yamin MR, Mozafari N, Razi Z. Reconstructive surgery of extensive face and neck burn scars using tissue expanders. *World J Plast Surg*. 2015;4(1):40-49.
36. Chung JE, Yen MT. Midface lifting as an adjunct procedure in ectropion repair. *Ann Plast Surg*. 2007;59(6):635-640.
37. Karacaoglan N, Uysal A. Reconstruction of postburn scar contracture of the neck by expanded skin flaps. *Burns*. 1994;20(6):547-550.
38. Yang JY, Tsai FC, Chana JS, et al. Use of free thin anterolateral thigh flaps combined with cervicoplasty for reconstruction of postburn anterior cervical contractures. *Plast Reconstr Surg*. 2002;110(1):39-46.
39. Akita S, Hayashida K, Takaki S, et al. The neck burn scar contracture: a concept of effective treatment. *Burns Trauma*. 2017;5:22.
40. Inigo F, Jimenez-Murat Y, Arroyo O, et al. Free flaps for head and neck reconstruction in non-oncological patients: experience of 200 cases. *Microsurgery*. 2000;20(4):186-192.
41. Xu J, Li SK, Li YQ, et al. Superior extension of the parascapular free flap for cervical burn scar contracture. *Plast Reconstr Surg*. 1995;96(1):58-62.
42. Kunert P, Schneider W, Flory J. Principles and procedures in female breast reconstruction in the young child's burn injury. *Aesthet Plast Surg*. 1988;12(2):101-106.
43. MacLennan SE, Wells MD, Neale HW. Reconstruction of the burned breast. *Clin Plast Surg*. 2000;27(1):113-119.
44. Neale HW, Smith GL, Gregory RO, MacMillan BG. Breast reconstruction in the burned adolescent female (an 11-year, 157 patient experience). *Plast Reconstr Surg*. 1982;70(6):718-724.
45. Guan WX, Jin YT, Cao HP. Reconstruction of postburn female breast deformity. *Ann Plast Surg*. 1988;21(1):65-69.
46. Levi B, Brown DL, Cederna PS. A comparative analysis of tissue expander reconstruction of burned and unburned chest and breasts using endoscopic and open techniques. *Plast Reconstr Surg*. 2010;125(2):547-556.
47. Little JW. Nipple-areola reconstruction. *Clin Plast Surg*. 1984;11(2):351-364.

48. Graham TJ, Stern PJ, True MS. Classification and treatment of postburn metacarpophalangeal joint extension contractures in children. *J Hand Surg Am.* 1990;15(3):450-456.
49. Cartotto R, Cicuto BJ, Kiwanuka HN, et al. Common postburn deformities and their management. *Surg Clin North Am.* 2014;94(4):817-837.
50. Yotsuyanagi T, Yamashita K, Gonda A, et al. Double combined Z-plasty for wide-scar contracture release. *J Plast Reconstr Aesthet Surg.* 2013;66(5):629-633.
51. Karanas YL, Buntic RF. Microsurgical reconstruction of the burned hand. *Hand Clin.* 2009;25(4):551-556.
52. Jones NF, Jarrahy R, Kaufman MR. Pedicled and free radial forearm flaps for reconstruction of the elbow, wrist, and hand. *Plast Reconstr Surg.* 2008;121(3):887-898.
53. Houshian S, Gynning B, Schroder HA. Chronic flexion contracture of proximal interphalangeal joint treated with the compass hinge external fixator: a consecutive series of 27 cases. *J Hand Surg Br.* 2002;27(4):356-358.
54. Donelan MB, Garcia JA. Nailfold reconstruction for correction of burn fingernail deformity. *Plast Reconstr Surg.* 2006;117(7):2303-2308.
55. Sari E, Tellioglu AT, Altuntas N, et al. Combination of rhomboid flap and double Z-plasty technique for reconstruction of palmar and dorsal web space burn contractures. *Burns.* 2015;41(2):408-412.
56. Grishkevich VM. First web space post-burn contracture types: contracture elimination methods. *Burns.* 2011;37(2):338-347.
57. Ogawa R, Hyakusoku H, Murakami M, Koike S. Reconstruction of axillary scar contractures: retrospective study of 124 cases over 25 years. *Br J Plast Surg.* 2003;56(2):100-105.

QUESTIONS

1. **What flap is ideal to improve a webspace contracture between the ring and middle fingers?**
   a. Z-plasty
   b. Five-flap jumping man flap
   c. Kite flap
   d. Littler flap

2. **What laser modality would best treat an erythematous burn scar that is not hypertrophic?**
   a. Pulse dye
   b. Alexandrite
   c. CO_2 laser
   d. Erbium-yttrium aluminum garnet

3. **What is the proper degree to splint the shoulder, elbow, and hand after a burned upper extremity injury?**
   a. 120°; 120°; extrinsic plus
   b. 90°; 180°; intrinsic plus
   c. 45°; 90°; intrinsic plus
   d. 90°; 90°; intrinsic plus

4. **How can recurrent postoperative ectropion be avoided?**
   a. Bolster
   b. Tarsorrhaphy
   c. Meshed skin grafting
   d. Laser

5. **What percentage gain is provided by a Z-plasty that is 60°?**
   a. 50%
   b. 75%
   c. 100%
   d. 125%

1. **Answer: b.** Many different local flaps can be used to fix webspace contractures. A five-flap jumping man allows for both release of the contracture as well as webspace deepening. This webspace deepening comes from the Y-to-V advancement flap. Z-plasties are useful for linear contractures along fingers.

2. **Answer: a.** PDL targets chromophores at a wavelength that will heat up red tissues. Thus, the PDL is the optimal laser to treat a burn scar that is only erythematous. For scars that are erythematous and hypertrophic, the CO_2 laser with or without the PDL is often the appropriate modality. The Alexandrite laser is best used for hair removal.

3. **Answer: b.** Postoperative splinting is crucial to maintaining any releases that are performed for burn patients. For the upper extremity, the shoulder should be maintained at 90°, the elbow should be maintained at 180°, and the hand should be placed in intrinsic plus.

4. **Answer: b.** Acute burn ectropion and recurrent postoperative ectropion can be avoided with tarsorrhaphy. These can be temporary or permanent depending on the extent of the ectropion and the release. These can be placed medially, laterally, or both also depending on the location and extent of the ectropion. Once ectropion forms, a release and FTSG is often necessary. Sometimes concurrent midface lift, canthoplasty, and palatal grafts (to inner lamellae) are necessary. Meshed grafts should never be used on the face.

5. **Answer: b.**

CHAPTER 23 Radiation and Radiation Injury

Natalia Fullerton and Christine Hsu Rohde

KEY POINTS

- Radiation therapy uses ionizing radiation for the treatment of various conditions, primarily as a cancer therapy.
- Improvements in radiation therapy are aimed at increasing the radiation to the site of therapy and decreasing the radiation to surrounding tissue to reduce the injury to normal tissue through improved therapy planning and more precise therapy delivery.
- Radiation injury can be classified as acute toxicity or late toxicity.
- Acute toxicity is reversible, beginning a few weeks after the start of therapy and resolving a few weeks after the end of the therapy.
- Late toxicity is permanent, occurring 6 months after the completion of therapy, and is characterized by fibrosis.
- Primary treatment for complications of late toxicity radiation therapy is reconstruction with well-vascularized nonirradiated tissue.

The antecedent of the medical field of radiology was born in 1895, with Wilhelm Conrad von Roentgen's discovery of a new type of ray emitted from electrons in a Hittorf-Crookes tube. These rays could penetrate tissues differentially, creating an image of the structures inside the body. Given the mysterious nature of the rays, it was termed the X-ray. Following his discovery, the X-ray was developed for diagnostic application, and by World War I, radiology became an established discipline. Soon after Roentgen's discovery, Pierre and Marie Sklodowska Curie isolated and reported on the radioactivity of the radioactive element radium in 1889. A year later, the application of radiation to cure cancer was reported in Sweden. Brachytherapy, utilizing radium, expanded in the 1900s and had become the standard of care in oncology.[1,2]

Externally administered radiation therapy (RT) was also successfully developed in the 1920s, after the formulation of fractionated dosages, understanding of the relative sensitivity of different tissue to radiation, and the development of normal and neoplastic tissue response to radiation as a response to dose. Treatment was employed with peak voltage of 250 kV or less, limiting practice to superficial uses. The next great development in external beam radiation came with the advent of the megavoltage (MV) unit. In 1951, the cobalt-60 unit was developed in Canada, allowing for greater penetration of tissue, skin-sparing capability, and improved homogeneity of dosage. This technology was followed by the MV linear accelerators, or Linac systems, developed simultaneously at Stanford and Great Malvern, England. This technology has supplanted the cobalt units in more affluent countries, although the cobalt-60 units continue to be the mainstay of second and third world countries owing to ease of availability.[1,3]

Presently, RT innovations are aimed at increasing radiation dose to the site of therapy, while decreasing the radiation dose to surrounding normal tissue. This is being accomplished with improved treatment planning utilizing simulation, computed tomography, and magnetic resonance imaging; enhanced delivery of radiation to the target tissue with the use of multileaf collimators (MLC), allowing for blocking or shielding of radiation from critical structures; and the use of intensity-modulated radiation therapy (IMRT) and image-guided radiation therapy (IGRT) to more precisely deliver radiation to desired locations.[1]

BASICS OF RADIATION THERAPY

Radiation therapy (RT) utilizes ionizing radiation for the treatment of various lesions. Radiation oncology is the discipline in medicine that specializes in the treatment of cancer and other benign processes with the use of ionizing radiation. In 2016, it was reported that a significant number of cancers were being treated with some form of RT, either as a single modality or in combination with surgery and/or chemotherapy. To demonstrate a few concrete examples, in stage I and II breast cancer treatment, 59% of patients underwent some form of radiation schedule, with this number increasing to 73% of patients with stage III breast cancer; 50% of patients with stage III and IV non–small cell lung cancer undergo RT; and 32% of patients with muscle invasive bladder cancer undergo RT.[4] Given the plastic surgeon's close relationship with surgical oncologists and their role in reconstruction after tumor extirpation, it is important to be more cognizant of the management of certain cancers with RT, as well as the risks and toxicities that may result from this particular treatment.

Ionizing radiation is the propagation of energy necessary to displace one or more orbital electrons. This can result in direct ionization, wherein the charged particle of sufficient energy can directly disrupt the atomic structure of the absorbing material, such as DNA. The energy can also produce indirect ionization, in which there is ionization of an intermediary, commonly water (H_2O), producing free radicals, such as a hydroxyl radical (OH^-), which can then interact and damage DNA, cell membranes, or other critical structures, resulting in cell injury or death.

$$H_2O + e^- \rightarrow H_2O^+$$

$$H_2O^+ + H_2O \rightarrow H_3O^+ + OH^-$$

It is estimated that two-thirds of radiation from X-rays and gamma photons produce DNA damage through indirect ionization and free radicals. The exact mechanism of radiation-induced cell death is not well characterized, although it is believed to be due to damage to DNA causing apoptosis or reproductive death, in which the cell is unable to divide in an unlimited fashion.[5]

As radiation can affect both tumor and normal tissue, it is important to find ways to increase the tumor control and decrease the normal tissue complication. This dose-response relationship between tumor control and normal tissue complication is known as the therapeutic ratio (Figure 23.1). In an ideal situation, there would be no overlap between the tumor control and normal tissue complication curves. However, more frequently, there is a degree of overlap. Traditionally, it is accepted that normal tissue will have a 5% risk of complication, represented by a 5% overlap of the two curves.[5-7] A significant portion of technological advances in RT are focused at increasing the tumor control and decreasing the normal tissue complication probability, improving the therapeutic ratio.

The energy required for radiation to be ionizing is quantified in electron volts (eV). The energy used in therapeutic X-rays begins at the kilovoltage (kV) unit. This energy was the first available modality for cancer therapy. Today, therapy with these units can be subdivided into superficial therapy using 50 to 150 kV, which is suitable for lesions up to 5 mm in depth, with the delivery of 90% of the dose to the surface of the skin. These units are particularly useful for skin cancers, as the majority of the radiation does not penetrate deep and the radiation is tightly focused to the treatment zone.[8] Deep therapy, also known as orthovoltage therapy, is categorized by energies of 150 to 500 kV. The therapy has a penetration depth of 4 to 6 cm, a steep drop-off of dose with depth of penetration, and a tight penumbra of

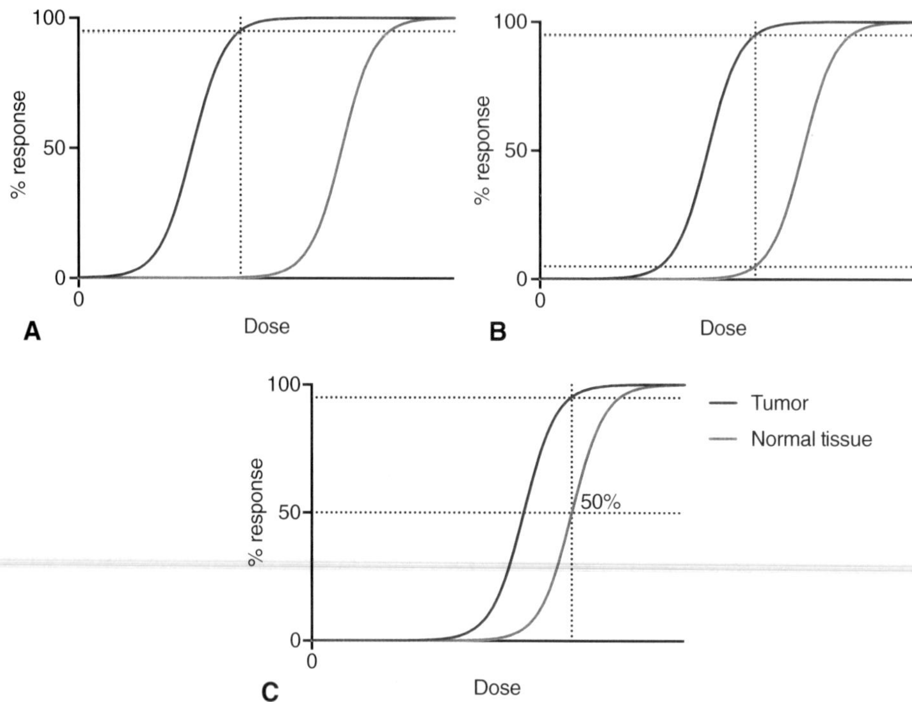

FIGURE 23.1. Therapeutic ratio. **A.** Ideal situation—no overlap between the tumor control and normal tissue complication curves. **B.** Accepted 5% risk of complication to normal tissue, represented by a 5% overlap of the two curves. **C.** Significant overlap between the tumor control curve and normal tissue complication, resulting in a significant level of normal tissue toxicity.

dose dispersion.[8,9] For increased penetration, MV therapy is used for improved skin sparing and dose homogeneity. The two main modalities that operate at the MV energy level are the cobalt-60 units, which generate gamma rays with an average energy of 1.3 MV and the linear accelerator units (Linac), with photon energies of 4 to 18 MV. As elucidated earlier, cobalt-60 units are the most widely used therapy modality in the world. However, Linac units are replacing this older technology owing to its deeper penetration, tighter penumbra, and more a uniform dose. The Linac functions by producing high-frequency electromagnetic waves that accelerate electrons, which then pass through a beamline, eventually colliding with a high-density target, emitting an MV X-ray beam. The Linac system can also emit electrons to treat superficial lesions.[3,5]

A newer system of external beam radiation utilizes particle therapy, rather than X-ray and gamma photon radiation. This group of particles is usually grouped as heavy particle therapy, as it encompasses protons, neutrons, or other positive ions such as carbon. Electron therapy is generally not classified in this subgroup, as they have a shallow depth of penetration. The slow implementation of proton therapy in the realm of RT is associated with the high start-up cost in building a large infrastructure dedicated for its use. The benefit of heavy particle therapy is the maximal deposition of energy at the end of their intended path, with minimal dose deposition along the path. This phenomenon is called the Bragg peak. After the Bragg peak, the dose falls off considerably. This advantage allows for less toxicity to surrounding normal tissue with greater effect on the target tissue. This also allows for a sharp penumbra within shallow or moderately deep tissue.[10,11] There is concern for some effect on the particle by the heterogeneity of tissue, resulting in an unknown change in effect on the target tissue.[12] This concern for variability in effect is especially prominent in tissue fields where the particle must traverse multiple organ types, such as the lung, head and neck, prostate, etc.[10,11] However, the advantage of this treatment modality is especially prominent in the pediatric population, particularly craniospinal tumors, rhabdomyosarcoma, and retinoblastoma, where salvage of radiation toxicity to normal tissue has shown to decrease secondary malignancies and decrease effects on organ growth and function.[10,13]

Similar to proton therapy, carbon therapy also portrays a Bragg peak effect, sparing radiation toxicity to normal surrounding tissue. The heavier charged carbon particle produces radiation damage within the cell nuclei, leading to increased relative biologic effectiveness compared with proton therapy. However, this technology is still in its infancy, and studies on superiority are in progress.[11]

Brachytherapy offers an additional source of RT to local tissue. As the name implies, brachy, the Greek root for *short*, is the use of a radioactive source placed in close proximity to the target tissue.[1] The close proximity of the radiation source to the target tissue imparts a high radiation dose to the target tissue with a rapid dose falloff to the surrounding tissue.[14] The main methods of brachytherapy delivery include interstitial, when the source is directly implanted into the target tissue, intracavitary, when a sealed source is inserted into the cavity of an organ (e.g., a cylindrical rod inserted into the cervix), or surface application, in which an applicator can be used to directly deliver a radiation dose to the surface of a tumor (e.g., eye plaque for uveal melanoma).[14,15] Major advances in the realm of brachytherapy include the use of newer imaging modalities to aid in the planning and positioning of brachytherapy treatments, planning algorithms to more precisely deliver appropriate doses to the tumor and avoid surrounding normal tissue, and newer delivery techniques such as high and pulsed dose rate therapies, which deliver higher dose rates through a previously placed catheter.[16-18]

Another modality of radiotherapy is intraoperative RT, whereby radiation is delivered to the tumor bed during surgical resection. This technique is typically used in combination with other modalities in a multidisciplinary approach to cancer therapy and has been shown to have efficacy in locally advanced and recurrent rectal cancer, retroperitoneal sarcomas, pancreatic cancers, early breast cancers, and some gynecological and genitourinary cancers. The advantage of this technology is that it gives precise and high-dose radiation delivery to the tumor bed while sparing local normal tissue, improving the therapeutic ratio of radiation delivery. It also delivers dose escalation or reirradiation of patients who would otherwise not be candidates with the conventional external beam radiation.[19]

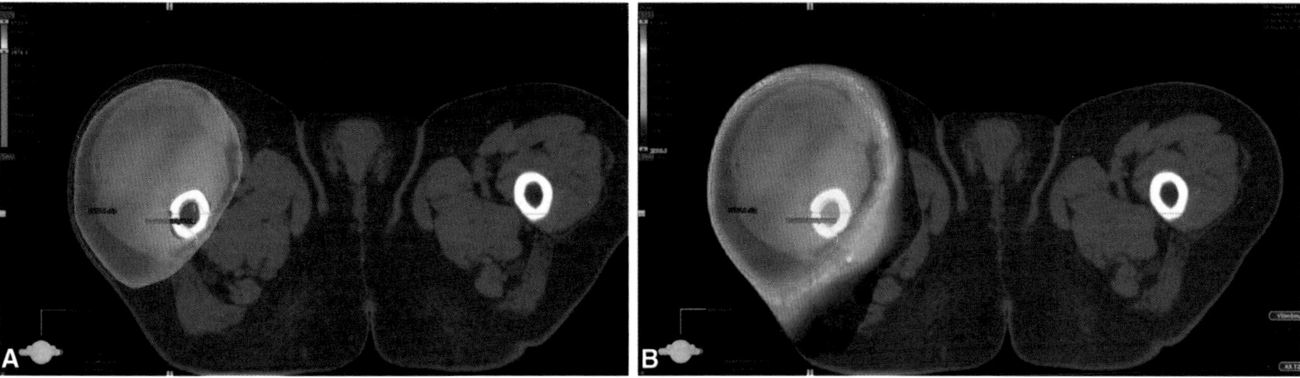

FIGURE 23.2. Intensity-modulated radiotherapy. Preoperative radiation plan for a patient with a right thigh sarcoma. **A.** Color wash of low-dose radiation, sparing a skin strip and vital midline structures. **B.** Color wash of high-dose radiation, sparing the adjacent femur.

Advances in RT are now aimed at improving RT delivery accuracy and the planning and verification of radiation, all to improve the accuracy of radiation dose to the affected tissue while decreasing the dose received by normal tissue. Conventionally, RT is delivered in a uniform field. With the use of special shields, wedges, compensators, or blocks, the beam can be modified to deliver differential doses to different tissues. Current technology makes use of a MLC, which utilizes narrow strips of metal mounted on the head of Linac machine. The MLC can be programmed to statically or dynamically conform the aperture of the radiation to adjust to differentially delivery of radiation to the various tissues, with the goal of excluding a significant amount of radiation to normal tissue. This technology is supplemented with the implementation of IMRT, a three-dimensional treatment planning, and computer-controlled RT delivery system. The system utilizes computed tomography images to specify the dose-based or dose volume–based parameters of radiation to the target tissue (tumor and margin for uncertainty) as well as the surrounding normal tissue to plan an optimized nonuniform radiation beam intensity to different tissue (Figure 23.2) This is then calculated into an algorithm for controlling the MLC to deliver the appropriate dose to the target tissue.[20] Different structures will receive varying doses of radiation during the therapy treatment. With the advent of IGRT, the therapy sessions are further tailored to the changing evolution of the tumor by evaluating alterations to the initial plan with serial imaging throughout the treatment processes. The changes in tumor size or anatomical changes facilitate adapting the treatment plan. This can further reduce the radiation exposure to surrounding structures by decreasing the margin of uncertainty that is generally applied when making the dose-based parameters in the initial planning of the therapy.[21]

RADIATION TOXICITY

As described earlier, RT affects cells through molecular injury either by direct disruption of the DNA structure or through ionization of an intermediary, producing free radicals to interact and damage DNA.[5] This damage affects both the target tissue and the normal surrounding tissue, resulting in radiation toxicity of the normal tissue. Radiation toxicity can be classified as either acute, delayed acute, or late toxicities to tissue.

DNA damage preferentially affects cells during the proliferative phase of the cell cycle, therefore primarily affecting cells with rapid turnover such as oral mucosa and epithelium. Injury to these cells causes an acute toxicity. The pathophysiology of the acute toxicity is from free radicals and irreversible breaks in DNA leading to a local inflammatory cascade of cytokines (IL-1, IL-3, IL-5, IL-6, TNF-α), chemokines (IL-8, eotaxin, CCR receptor), receptor tyrosine kinase, and adhesion molecules (ICAM-1, VCAM, E-selectin), which recruit an eosinophil and neutrophil response, driving a self-perpetuating tissue damage. In the skin, injury can also affect the epidermal permeability barrier, facilitating increased entrance of toxins and antigens to aggravate dermal inflammation, and can predispose the epidermis to infections.[22] This form of injury presents 2 to 4 weeks after the initiation of therapy, is dependent on the dose of radiation, volume of tissue irradiated, or concurrent chemotherapeutic drug use, and is generally reversible with healing beginning at about 2 weeks after the completion of therapy owing to the slow turnover of progenitor stem cells. Acute toxicity typically presents with skin erythema, edema, pigmentary changes, depilation, wet and dry desquamation, mucositis, and esophagitis (Figure 23.3). The exception to the reversibility

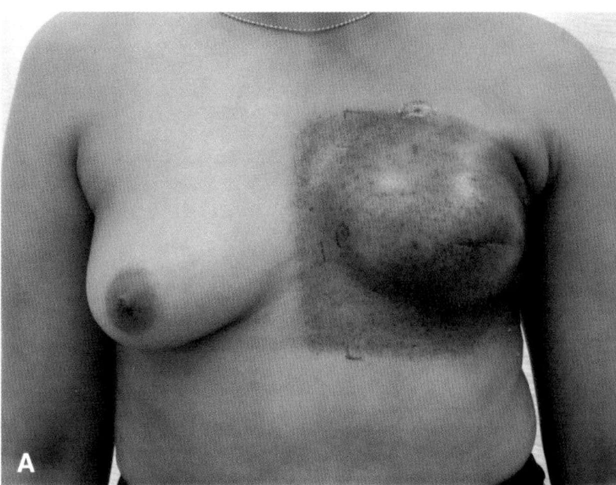

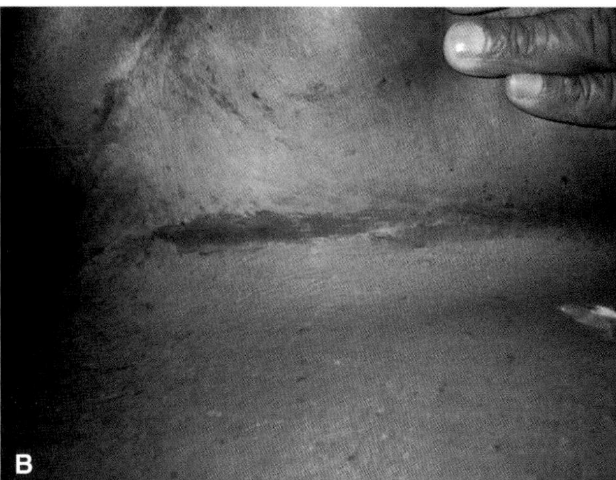

FIGURE 23.3. Acute radiation toxicity. **A.** Hyperpigmentation of left chest 1 week following completion of radiation therapy. **B.** Dry desquamation and hyperpigmentation of inframammary fold following radiation therapy.

of this injury is a result from injury to the progenitor stem cells that can occur with high doses of radiation. This is termed consequential damage and can present as ulceration or necrosis to the site of radiation toxicity.[5,23]

Similar to acute toxicity, there can be a delayed acute toxicity in certain tissues. Examples include acute radiation pneumonitis, which occurs 8 to 16 weeks following the initiation of radiation to the lung and is due to endothelial and epithelial cells death, microvascular thrombosis, and type II pneumocyte desquamation.[5] Lhermitte syndrome is a temporary demyelination of the posterior columns during spinal irradiation, presenting 2 to 6 months following RT.[5]

Late or chronic toxicity can be seen about 6 months to years following the completion of RT and is generally not reversible. The main characteristic is stromal tissue fibrosis but can also present as parenchymal tissue atrophy, as a result of cell apoptosis, necrosis, or senescence.[5] Damage can be predominantly seen in vessel endothelium, particularly capillaries, resulting in telangiectasia and tissue ischemia. Owing to poor vascularity, the tissue becomes fragile and susceptible to breakdown and poor wound healing with minor trauma. Injury can also be caused by damage to parenchymal cells with slow cell regeneration and poor repopulation from a stem cell population (Figure 23.4).

The pathophysiology behind the fibrosis response to RT is thought to be activated by cyclin-dependent kinase inhibitors p21, p27, and p16 which coordinate cell cycle arrest, ensuing in a predominantly TGF-β1 self-perpetuating expression, mediating terminal differentiation of progenitor fibroblasts into postmitotic fibroblasts, leading to an upregulation of collagen production with resultant fibrosis.[24,25]

The effect of radiation toxicity is dependent on the dose of radiation given, with more severe injury occurring with higher doses of radiation, the volume of tissue being irradiated, and the time frame at which the dose is given or the fractions.[5,23] Fractions of radiation doses are aimed at delivering lower daily doses of radiation over a prolonged period of time, so that the tumor is given high doses, while allowing normal tissue to heal, therefore decreasing the toxicity to this tissue. The biologic effects depending on the four R's of radiation biology: repopulation, redistribution, repair, and reoxygenation.[25]

Various factors can additionally exacerbate the radiation effects. These include patient related factors, including smoking, obesity, overlapping skin folds (in skin toxicity), poor nutrition, and preexisting trauma to the tissue; genetic disorders including ataxia telangiectasia, Gorlin syndrome, Fanconi anemia, Bloom syndrome, xeroderma pigmentosum, familial polyposis, Gardner syndrome, hereditary malignant melanoma, and dysplastic nevus syndrome; systemic diseases such as scleroderma, systemic lupus erythematosus, rheumatoid arthritis, hyperthyroidism, and diabetes mellitus; and certain therapeutic agents, particularly chemotherapeutic agents including doxorubicin, tamoxifen, methotrexate, bleomycin, 5-fluorouracil, and actinomycin D.[22,23,26]

Given the complexity of timing of radiation injury, it has been proposed to delay RT at least seven or more days after surgery to allow adequate time for healing. Similarly, surgery should be delayed 3 to 10 weeks after completion of RT for optimal wound healing after the effects of acute radiation toxicity has resolved but before the onset of the deleterious effects of delayed tissue toxicity. Additionally, given

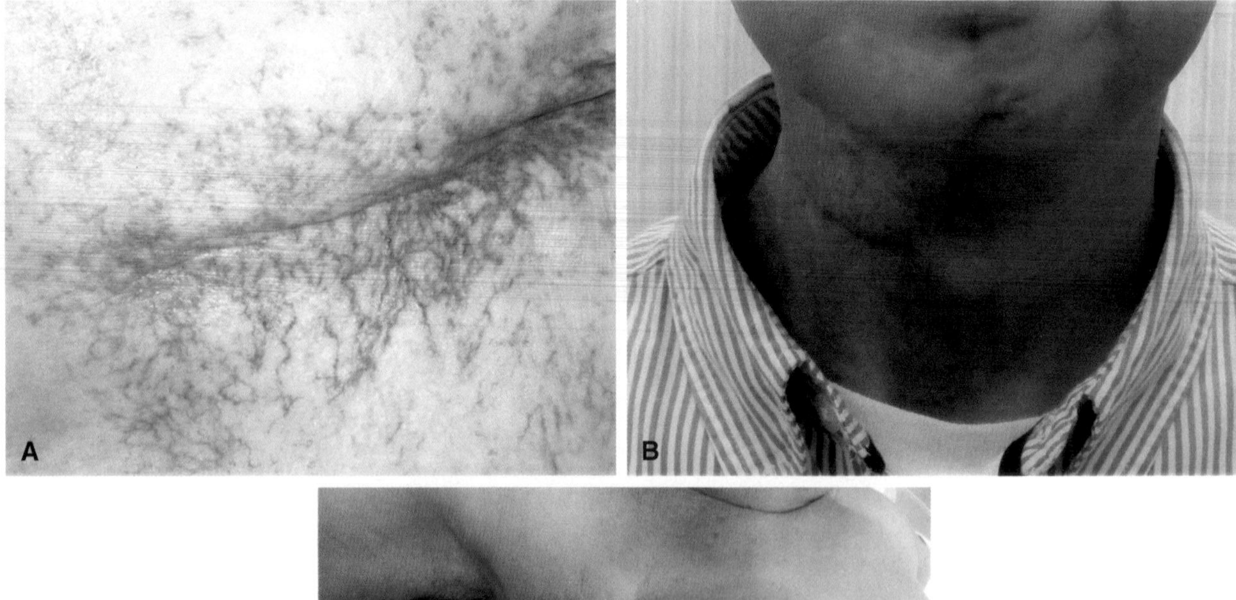

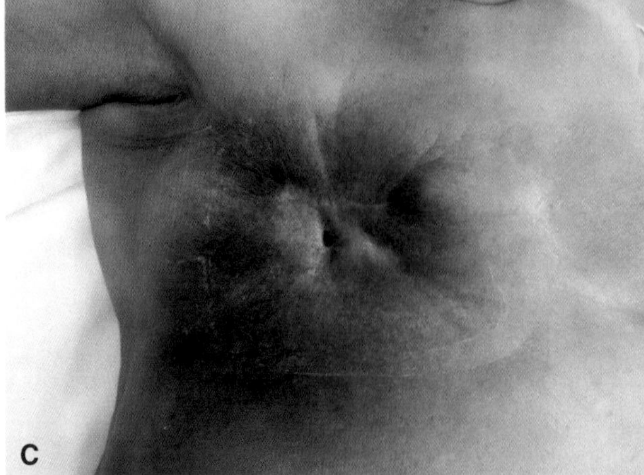

FIGURE 23.4. Chronic radiation toxicity. **A.** Telangiectasia of left chest mastectomy scar. **B.** Fibrosis of right neck. **C.** Chronic nonhealing wound for 8 months, 7 years after completion of radiation therapy.

the relative hypoxia and hypovascularity of radiated tissue, improving blood supply through the recruitment of healthy, nonirradiated tissue to the site of radiation has been shown to decrease wound complication and breakdown.[25]

SPECIFIC THERAPIES AND TOXICITIES

Breast Cancer

RT in breast cancer serves as an adjunct in eradicating microscopic disease after surgical excision of gross tumor, leading to a reduction in local recurrence and increasing breast cancer–specific survival. Guidelines for its use have been set in breast conservation therapy (BCT) and in certain postmastectomy patients.

Several randomized control trials (RCTs) have demonstrated the benefit of RT in decreasing local recurrence rates in BCT for early-stage invasive breast cancer and ductal carcinoma in situ. NSABP B-06, the largest trial, which included 1851 patients with tumors of 4 cm or less, demonstrated a local recurrence rate of 14.8% in the mastectomy group, 17.5% in the lumpectomy group compared with 8.1% in the lumpectomy and RT group at 20 years. There was no significant difference in disease-free or overall survival among the three groups. This study was substantiated by additional RCTs and a meta-analysis by the EBCTCG group that demonstrated similar results.

Absolute contraindications to RT in BCT include pregnancy, positive margins, multicentric cancer, or diffuse malignant-appearing calcifications. Relative contraindications to RT include a history of prior RT to the chest and patients with collagen vascular disease, most prominently in patients with scleroderma.

In patients over the age of 70 years who are undergoing BCT for small, node-negative, estrogen receptor–positive breast cancer, who plan on receiving hormonal therapy, local recurrence rates have been demonstrated to be sufficiently low that RT may be omitted in their cancer therapy plan.

Although specific regimens for breast RT vary among institutions, the standard course of RT for whole breast radiation consists of 50 to 50.4 grays (Gy), delivered in 25 to 26 fractions, followed by a 10 to 16 Gy boost, which is additional radiation aimed specifically at the tumor bed. Various alternative methods of treatment have been developed to improve breast RT. Hypofractionation, in which larger than standard doses of radiation over fewer fraction doses, has been devised to decrease treatment length of time. This treatment has been found to have compatible aesthetic outcome and recurrence rates compared with standard RT regimens. Currently, hypofractionation is considered appropriate in all patients, with any stage disease, provided that the intent is to treat the whole breast without an additional field to cover regional lymph nodes, with any chemotherapy, and a radiation plan with any volume of the breast receiving >105% of the prescription dose should be minimized regardless of the dose fractionation.[27] Additional alternatives include prone breast irradiation and accelerated partial breast irradiation, wherein larger doses are delivered to the postsurgical cavity with a specified surrounding margin, over 1 to 2 weeks, in order to decrease the RT dose to the normal tissue. Methods of RT delivery include multicatheter brachytherapy, intracavitary balloon brachytherapy, intraoperative RT, and external beam conformal therapy. The use of accelerated partial breast irradiation is still in clinical trials but may be acceptable in patients over the age of 50 years with negative margins by ≥2 mm, Tis or T1 stage, and ductal carcinoma in situ.

RT for postmastectomy patients is recommended in patients with four or more positive axillary lymph nodes, primary tumors greater than 5 cm with any number of positive nodes, or any T4 tumors. Postmastectomy radiation therapy (PMRT) is controversial for patients with one to three positive lymph nodes, with research still in progress to determine its efficacy.[28-30]

In plastic surgery, we are asked to perform breast reconstruction after the patient has undergone RT, either after failed BCT or as a delayed reconstruction after PMRT, or prior to radiation as in immediate breast reconstruction after mastectomy in patients who have a high likelihood of requiring PMRT. In patients with previous breast RT, studies have shown an increased incidence of implant-based reconstructive failure (14% pooled analysis) and complication rate, including capsular contracture risk, infection, mastectomy flap necrosis, and seroma.[31,32] Traditionally, it is recommended that patients with previous RT undergo autologous tissue reconstruction with either a latissimus dorsi myocutaneous flap with or without implant reconstruction, decreasing the incidence of reconstructive failure by 72%, or by means of other autologous reconstruction.[31] However, in patients who have undergone RT, the dissection for free flap reconstruction can have increased fibrosis. These patients have shown to have an in increase in intraoperative microvascular complications as well as postoperative minor complications, without an increased risk of flap loss.[33,34] In patients who are to undergo PMRT, institutional protocols differ with regard to radiation after tissue expansion or after the final implant reconstruction, depending on surgeon's or radiation oncologist's preference for improved RT to the internal mammary lymph nodes. Various systemic reviews have been conducted on the subject without clear consensus as to which, RT to tissue expander (TE) or to the permanent implant, has superior results in reconstruction. Many meta-analyses show an increased rate of reconstructive failure when RT is applied to the TE with an increased rate of capsular contracture when RT is applied to the final implant; however, there are systemic reviews that show contradictory results.[34-36] When considering autologous breast reconstruction in the setting of PMRT, there has been a move toward delayed immediate reconstruction to avoid direct radiation of the free flap, which can result in increased flap fat necrosis. The idea behind this technique is to place a TE at the time of mastectomy to act as a placeholder if RT were to be necessary to preserve the breast pocket. If radiation is not required or following radiation, the expander is removed and autologous reconstruction can proceed.[34,37]

Head and Neck Cancer

Head and neck cancers (HNC) are a group of cancers primarily involving the hypopharynx, oropharynx, lip, oral cavity, nasopharynx, or larynx, with the majority of the cancers being squamous cell carcinomas. RT plays an integral role as the primary modality in many early-stage diseases, as well as part of a multimodality treatment for the more common presentation of locally advanced HNC, which may include chemoradiation therapy, induction chemotherapy followed by cetuximab and RT or chemoradiation therapy with surgery.

The standard of RT care in HNC is the use of IMRT or other three-dimensional conformal techniques, including IGRT and proton beam therapy, to reduce the radiation dose to closely located organs, including the parotid and other salivary glands, temporal lobes, and auditory optic or intracranial structures. Additionally, various fractionation treatments exist in HNC RT. The commonly used simultaneous integrated boost technique uses differential *dose painting* of 66 to 74 Gy to gross disease and 50 to 60 Gy to subclinical disease, administered in various fractionation/hyperfractionation schedules. Given the complex interplay between various radiation technologies, fractionation regimens, and chemotherapy options, there is a large combination of therapies available that can affect local toxicity as well as tumor control.[38]

Acute radiation toxicities in HNC include mucositis, xerostomia, mucosal infection including candidiasis, pain, and sensory disturbances. Mucositis affects the majority of HNC patients undergoing RT and presents with significant pain that can result in decreased nutritional status requiring gastric tubes or other forms of nutritional supplementation. Presentation includes erythema beginning at 2 to 3 weeks after the start of RT followed by progression to ulceration and pseudomembranes, peaking at the end of RT, and continuing for 2 to 4 weeks after the end of RT. Concurrent chemotherapy or targeted therapies can prolong or amplify mucositis. Treatment is aimed at alleviating symptoms and includes oral care, pain control with morphine and doxepin mouthwashes and oral analgesics, wound healing promotion with the use of zinc, and photomodulation therapy.[39]

Xerostomia results from damage to the acinar cells of salivary glands. The damage can be transient, beginning after the first week of RT and terminating 3 months after completion of treatment. However, when the dose exceeds 52 Gy, the damage can become permanent. Changes in salivary production can have an effect on oral lubrication, oral pH (resulting in a more acidic environment), demineralization/remineralization of tooth surfaces, and oral flora equilibrium, which can cause difficulty in chewing and swallowing, periodontal disease, halitosis, pain, and contribute to changes in taste. Treatment includes saliva substitutes, saliva-stimulating medications, including parasympathomimetic medications that stimulate cholinergic receptors, including pilocarpine or cevimeline, as well as good oral hygiene.[40]

Chronic radiation toxicities include tissue fibrosis, permanent salivary gland dysfunction as previously discussed, and osteoradionecrosis (ORN) which will be discussed separately. Fibrosis can affect any number of tissues in the radiated field. Radiation can affect muscular function as with the muscles of mastication, muscles of the pharynx, and lingual muscles, which can result in trismus, dysphagia, and poor tongue function, respectively. Of note, radiation to the neck can result in fibrosis of the nerves and vessels in the neck, making microvascular anastomoses more challenging.[39]

Nonmelanoma Skin Cancers

Nonmelanoma skin cancers are the most common malignancies in the world, with basal cell cancer (BCC) and squamous cell cancer (SCC) accounting for 99% of these cancers. Other nonmelanoma skin cancers include Merkel cell carcinoma (MCC), dermatofibrosarcoma, primary cutaneous B cell lymphoma, Kaposi sarcoma, and carcinosarcoma.

RT has had a long history in the treatment of many of these malignancies. Given better-quality evidence on treatment efficacy and changing radiation technologies, the role of RT for these cancers continues to evolve. Current guidelines for RT use are delineated at the National Comprehensive Cancer Network and the American Joint Committee on Cancer. For BCC and SCC, the primary treatment remains Mohs micrographic surgery or surgical excision. However, if the patient is not a surgical candidate or has a preference for RT, then RT may be the primary therapy for low- or high-grade BCC and SCC. RT should not be chosen as a first-line agent owing to the higher recurrence rate compared with surgical excision, 7.5% versus 0.7% for BCC and between 4% and 7% for SCC. Additionally, this therapy is generally reserved for patients older than 60 years owing to concerns over long-term sequela, has been found to have poorer appearance, and has more posttreatment complications. RT is advocated as adjuvant RT for BCC with perineural involvement or positive tissue margins. It is also useful in SCC with perineural involvement, positive margins that are not candidates for re-excision, or for regional therapy after lymph node dissection.

Therapy modality varies depending on institutional preferences. Given the superficial nature of the malignancy, therapy options that deliver the majority of their energy at the surface of the skin, including kilovoltage and electron therapy, are the mainstay of treatment. Although not sanctioned by the National Comprehensive Cancer Network due to insufficient data on long-term efficacy, brachytherapy may have a role owing to its shorter treatment course, shallow dose deposition, and ability to conform to irregular surfaces.[41-43]

Unlike SCC and BCC, MCC is a neuroendocrine tumor of the skin with a highly aggressive nature and rate of local recurrence, regional, and distant metastatic rates (25%–30%, 52%–59%, and 34%–36%, respectively). RT is advocated as a primary therapy in patients who are not candidates for surgical excision and as an adjuvant therapy to surgical excision in all instances of MCC except when the tumor is less than 1 cm after undergoing wide local excision and is without lymphovascular invasion or immunosuppression of the patient. RT is also recommended for the draining nodal basin when there is a positive sentinel lymph node with or without lymph node dissection.

RT toxicities for the treatment of skin cancers have been listed previously and include erythema, hyperpigmentation, dry and moist desquamation, acute ulceration, chronic wounds and skin necrosis as consequential damage, and fibrosis, atrophy, hypo-/hyperpigmentation, and telangiectasias.[23]

Sarcoma

Malignancies of mesenchymal cell origin are classified as sarcomas. This category of cancers is a heterogeneous group of rare solid tumors that account for approximately 1% of all adult malignancies and about 15% of all pediatric malignancies. Sarcomas are subclassified into two distinct groups, including soft tissue sarcomas, which include malignancy of fat, muscle, nerve, nerve sheath, blood vessels, and other connective tissues, and malignancy of bone. The most common subtype of soft tissue sarcoma in adults is undifferentiated pleomorphic sarcoma, while the most common subtype in children is rhabdomyosarcoma. The most common location of disease is the extremity (43%) with the most common location of metastasis being the lung. One of the main risk factors for developing sarcomas includes prior RT.

Treatment of sarcoma with adjuvant RT should be considered for all adult patients, unless they present with stage I disease with negative margins after resection. There continues to be a debate of whether RT should be administered prior to surgical excision or after surgical excision. The advantages of preoperative RT include possible regression of the tumor size prior to excision, formation of a pseudocapsule to ease excision of tumor, decrease seeding of cancer during the tumor manipulation during surgery, and reduction of late toxicities when treated with IGRT. However, preoperative RT has been shown to decrease wound healing after surgery and requires the surgical team to wait 3 to 6 weeks until they can excise the tumor. For this reason, plastic surgeons are often called to aid with closure and reconstruction to improve soft tissue wound healing.

Postoperative RT facilitates excision of the tumor without delaying therapy. It has also been shown to improve local tumor control when positive surgical margins are present. The disadvantage of using this regimen, however, is its association with higher rates of long-term treatment related side effects. Despite the differences in timing, there has been no evidence to suggest differences in disease outcomes between the two regimens.[44,45]

Additional Toxicities

Osteoradionecrosis

Late radiation toxicity to bone may manifest as ORN. It is defined as chronically exposed devitalized irradiated bone for 3 to 6 months without the recurrence of tumor. About 70% to 94% of cases are seen in the first 3 years following RT but can occur at any point after RT. ORN can occur at multiple sites, including the maxilla, sternum, pelvis, temporal bone, and vertebrae, but is generally seen in the mandible after irradiation of HNC. The pathophysiology of ORN suggests that the mechanism for its development may be due to microvascular thrombosis and decreased vascularity, abnormal fibroblastic activity, and fibroblastic remodeling leading to bone fibrosis and loss of osteocytes in the bone.[39,46]

Risk factors for developing ORN include hyperfractionated irradiation regimens, with a higher total dose to the bone exceeding 6000 cGy, concomitant chemotherapy, pre- or postirradiation dental extraction or trauma to the irradiated bone (preirradiation extraction with irradiation occurring before the bone has been given time to heal), poor oral hygiene and periodontal disease contributing to local infection, and alcohol and tobacco use.[46]

Treatment of ORN includes prevention with dental care before the initiation of RT. Early-stage disease is treated with conservative management with improved oral hygiene, saline irrigation, antibiotic therapy, hyperbaric oxygen therapy, and newer medical modalities including pentoxifylline and tocopherol, with resolution in about 8%–33% of patients after 1 year. It should be noted that therapy with hyperbaric oxygen therapy is controversial with some data reporting a lack of efficacy. Later-stage ORN can be treated with wound debridement, sequestrectomy, decortication and resection of necrotic bone, and free flap reconstruction.[39,46]

Lymphedema

In the United States, the leading cause of lymphedema comes from lymph node dissection for cancer therapy. Given the prevalence of breast cancer with the primary source of metastasis to axillary lymph nodes resulting in lymph node dissection, it has become the most common cause of lymphedema in the Western countries. RT has been identified as a major risk factor for lymphedema after lymph node dissection for breast cancer as well as other malignancies.[29,47,48] In a study by Chandra et al., the 2-year incidence of lymphedema in breast cancer patients treated with RT who had undergone regional lymph node dissection ranged between 20% and 22% depending on the type of RT administered to the axilla. Risk factors for the development of lymphedema in the setting of axillary RT included axillary node dissection compared with sentinel lymph node dissection and increased body mass index.[48] The mechanism by which radiation results in lymphedema can be attributed to depletion of lymphatic vessels and endothelial cells as well as increased fibrosis.[47]

Radiation-Induced Malignancies

Radiation may cause mutations in normal tissue resulting in various other malignancies. Cahan criteria to define radiation-induced malignancies (RIMs) include: a malignancy arising in an irradiated field, sufficient latency between the initial RT and new malignancy (generally longer than 4 years), a new malignancy of different histology to the primary cancer, and tissue of the new malignancy that is genetically and metabolically normal prior to the radiation exposure. For this reason, RIM is a complication that affects cancer survivors. Histologically, sarcomas are most common RIM in tissues receiving high-dose RT. Patients who undergo RT for HNC are at increased risk of developing SCC followed by sarcoma RIM. Patients who undergo RT for breast cancer are at increased risk for developing carcinoma of the lung, contralateral breast, esophagus, and sarcoma RIM. Those patients who underwent mantle field RT for Hodgkin disease are at increased risk of developing breast, lung, and thyroid RIM. Patients who undergo craniospinal RT and total body irradiation are at increased risk of meningioma, glioma, leukemia, and lymphomas. Risk factors for developing a RIM include higher radiation doses, chemotherapy, environmental exposures such as smoking, hereditary predisposition (familial retinoblastoma, Li-Fraumeni syndrome, tuberous sclerosis, and neurofibromatosis I), and age of RT, with a significant increase in RIM in pediatric patients undergoing RT. The increased risk of RIM with age is thought to be multifactorial with genotoxic injury to stem cells and longer survival of childhood malignancies both contributing to RIM.[49]

GENERAL CONSIDERATIONS IN TREATMENT OF CUTANEOUS RADIATION TOXICITIES

Acute Toxicities

Management of acute cutaneous toxicities (ACT) can be divided into preventive and treatment therapies. Currently, there are no standardized guidelines in the management of ACT. It is up to the discretion of the treating institution to decide on best practices. A recent meta-analysis of RCTs may be able to better direct treating physicians on best practices, although further research is still warranted (**Table 23.1**).

For preventive management of ACT, oral Wobe-Mugos® (proteolytic enzyme containing 100 mg papain, 40 mg trypsin, 40 mg chymotrypsin) was found to decrease the risk of developing an ACT by 87%. It is generally recommended that patients practice good hygiene with mild soaps and water, followed by water-based lanolin-free moisturizers, and avoiding metallic-based deodorants. However, no RCT validated these practices. Additional common recommendations, not covered by the meta-analysis, include wearing loose fitting clothing and avoiding sun exposure to areas of RT.

For treatment of ACT, oral Wobe-Mugos® as well as 25 mg of zinc supplementation was found to be effective at reducing the severity of ACT. Small studies have shown that 0.1% betamethasone cream and 0.1% methylprednisolone were effective at reducing the severity of ACT. There are conflicting results on whether the use of topical hyaluronic acid is effective at reducing ACT severity. When dressings are required for treatment of moist desquamation, hydrogel, silver nylon, and Mepilex Lite® dressings may be more effective at decreasing time to healing compared with other dressings. Finally, washing with soap compared with no washing or washing with only water was found to be more effective at decreasing desquamation and severity of erythema. Of note, in severe ACT when full-thickness skin necrosis and ulceration occur, the treatment should include discontinuation of RT, debridement, and advanced wound care management.[23,50]

Late Toxicities

Unlike ACT, late cutaneous toxicities are not transient and may require intervention for resolution. For the treatment of telangiectasias associated with late cutaneous toxicities, pulsed dye laser therapy has been shown to have satisfactory results on physical appearance of the skin. Patients who present with chronic ulcerations and necrosis may be treated with local wound care with hydrophilic or lipophilic barrier creams and hydrogel or hydrocolloid dressings depending on amount of wound exudate. Infected wounds benefit from antibacterial agents with or without silver-based dressings. Finally, severe ulcerations may require surgical management with flap reconstruction. It is important to rule out secondary skin malignancies in refractory ulcers, as they can have a similar presentation.[23]

RT-induced fibrosis may be more difficult to manage with therapies consisting of rehabilitative care including several massage techniques as well as physical therapy to reduce contraction and improve movement. Pharmacotherapy with pentoxifylline, a methylated xanthine derivative, with concurrent tocopherol (vitamin E), shows promise at reducing superficial fibrosis with long-term therapy. Small trials with superoxide dismutase, an antioxidant enzyme may also be useful at decreasing fibrosis, but larger studies are required before asserting its efficacy. In severe cases of fibrosis, where there is poor quality of life, very limited mobility, and pain, surgery to remove the area of fibrosis with interposition of healthy vascularized tissue may be considered. Clinical suspicion should be heightened in these patients, as they may be at risk for tumor recurrence or an RIM. It is important to weigh the risk and benefits of such intervention, as there can exacerbate fibrosis and patients are at increased risk for wound healing.[23]

TABLE 23.1. RADIATION TOXICITY TREATMENTS

Acute Cutaneous Toxicities		
Preventive Treatment		
	Pharmacotherapy	Wobe-Mugos®
	Lifestyle modification	Hygiene with mild soap and water
		Water-based lanolin-free moisturizer
		Avoidance of metallic-based deodorants
		Wearing loose fitting clothing
		Avoidance of sun exposure
Active Treatment		
	Lifestyle modification	Hygiene with soap and water
	Pharmacotherapy	Wobe-Mugos®
		Zinc supplementation
Erythema and dry desquamation	Pharmacotherapy	0.1% betamethasone cream or 0.1% methylprednisolone cream
		Conflicting data exist on efficacy of hyaluronic acid
Moist desquamation	Dressings	Treatment with hydrogel, silver nylon, or Mepilex Lite® dressing
Full-thickness necrosis/ulceration		Treatment with discontinuation of radiation therapy, debridement, and wound care
Late Cutaneous Toxicities		
Telangiectasia		Pulsed dye laser therapy
Ulceration and necrosis	Lifestyle modification	Local wound care
	Pharmacotherapy	Hydrophilic or lipophilic barrier cream
	Dressings	Hydrogel dressing to increase moisture to wound
		Hydrocolloid dressing to decrease moisture to exudative wounds
Infected wounds	Dressings	Antibacterial agents with or without silver-based dressings
Severe ulceration		Surgical management with flap reconstruction
		Rule out radiation-induced malignancies
Fibrosis	Rehabilitative therapy	Physical therapy or massage therapy
	Pharmacotherapy	Pentoxifylline and tocopherol with long-term therapy
		Superoxide dismutase may be useful, but larger trials are warranted to determine efficacy
Severe fibrosis		Excision of fibrosis with healthy tissue interposition

CONCLUSION

There have been great advancements in the management of malignancies with the use of RT as a primary or multidisciplinary mode of therapy. With the advent of IMRT and IGRT in radiation planning and delivery to the site of interest, ionizing radiation can more accurately be directed at the tumor while minimizing the toxicity to the surrounding normal tissue, improving the therapeutic ratio.

Despite these improvements, radiation is still responsible for local tissue injury, both acute and late toxicities. Although acute local tissue toxicities are reversible and can be managed with proper wound care, late toxicities may require further and more drastic interventions for resolution. Key plastic surgery concepts can be employed to improve the detrimental effects of fibrosis, including decreased mobility, pain, or chronic wounds. For areas with contracture bands, Z-plasties can be used to improve joint range of motion or tissue pliability. Healthy, nonradiated tissue should be brought into the areas of radiation injury, as they can provide vascularized tissue to areas with contracture and poor tissue perfusion. These can include pedicled muscle flaps like a latissimus dorsi, vertical rectus myocutaneous flap or transverse myocutaneous flap, or fasciocutaneous flaps. If no local, unirradiated tissue is available, free flaps should be used for reconstruction.

Given the tremendous improvement in cancer survival with the use of RT, more patients will be requiring reconstruction of difficult-to-manage resection defects and late local toxicity injuries. It is important for the plastic surgeon to understand the pathophysiology behind radiation injury to more properly treat this patient population.

REFERENCES

1. Laughlin JS. Development of the technology of radiation therapy. *Radiographics*. 1989;9(6):1245-1266.
2. Timins JK. Communication of benefits and risks of medical radiation: a historical perspective. *Health Phys*. 2011;101(5):562-565.
3. Kaplan HS. Basic principles in radiation oncology. *Cancer*. 1977;39(2 suppl):689-693.
4. Miller KD, Siegel RL, Lin CC, et al. Cancer treatment and survivorship statistics, 2016. *CA Cancer J Clin*. 2016;66(4):271-289.
   A collaborative effort between the American Cancer Society and the National Cancer Institute estimating cancer survivorship as well as treatment patterns and treatment-related side effects in an attempt to raise awareness of survivorship issues.
5. Fajardo LF, Berthrong M, Anderson RE, Meyer JL. *Radiation Pathology*. Oxford University Press; 2001.
6. Chargari C, Magne N, Guy JB, et al. Optimize and refine therapeutic index in radiation therapy: overview of a century. *Cancer Treat Rev*. 2016;45:58-67.

7. Bloomer WD, Hellman S. Normal tissue responses to radiation therapy. *N Engl J Med*. 1975;293(2):80-83.
A description of the normal tissue response curve to radiation therapy in comparison to the tumor response curve, resulting in the understanding of the therapeutic index.
8. Wolstenholme V, Glees JP. The role of kilovoltage X-rays in the treatment of skin cancers. *Eur Oncol Haematol*. 2006;1(1):32.
9. Hill R, Healy B, Holloway L, et al. Advances in kilovoltage x-ray beam dosimetry. *Phys Med Biol*. 2014;59(6): R183-R231.
10. Mitin T, Zietman AL. Promise and pitfalls of heavy-particles therapy. *J Clin Oncol*. 2014;32(26):2855-2863.
11. Combs SE, Debus J. Treatment with heavy charged particles: systematic review of clinical data and current clinical (comparative) trials. *Acta Oncol*. 2013;52(7):1272-1286.
12. Urie MM, Sisterson JM, Koehler AM, Goitein M, Zoesman J. Proton beam penumbra: effects of separation between patient and beam modifying devices. *Med Phys*. 1986;13(5):734-741.
13. Bassal M, Mertens AC, Taylor L, et al. Risk of selected subsequent carcinomas in survivors of childhood cancer: a report from the Childhood Cancer Survivor Study. *J Clin Oncol*. 2006;24(3):476-483.
14. Sadeghi M, Enferadi M, Shirazi A. External and internal radiation therapy: past and future directions. *J Cancer Res Ther*. 2010;6(3):239.
15. Jang B-S, Chang JH, Oh S, Lim YJ, Kim IH. Surgery vs. radiotherapy in patients with uveal melanoma. *Strahlenther Onkol*. 2017;193(11):931-942.
16. Lee CD. Recent developments and best practice in brachytherapy treatment planning. *Br J Radiol*. 2014;87(1041):20140146.
17. Nicholas Lukens J, Gamez M, Hu K, Harrison LB. Modern brachytherapy. *Semin Oncol*. 2014;41(6):831-847.
18. Thomadsen BR, Erickson BA, Eifel PJ, et al. A review of safety, quality management, and practice guidelines for high-dose-rate brachytherapy: executive summary. *Pract Radiat Oncol*. 2014;4(2):65-70.
19. Pilar A, Gupta M, Laskar SG, Laskar S. Intraoperative radiotherapy: review of techniques and results. *Ecancermedicalscience*. 2017;11:1-33.
20. Boyer A, Butler B, DiPetrillo T, et al. Intensity modulated radiotherapy: current status and issues of interest. Intensity modulated radiation therapy collaborative working group. *Int J Radiat Oncol Biol Phys*. 2001;51(4):880-914.
An overview, description, guidelines, and recommendations for implementation of intensity-modulated radiation therapy by a Collaberative Working Group of experts in IMRT, formed by the National Cancer Institute.
21. Goyal S, Kataria T. Image guidance in radiation therapy: techniques and applications. *Radiol Res Pract*. 2014;2014:1-10.
22. Jaschke W, Schmuth M, Trianni A, Bartal G. Radiation-induced skin injuries to patients: what the interventional radiologist needs to know. *Cardiovasc Intervent Radiol*. 2017;40(8):1131-1140.
23. Bray FN, Simmons BJ, Wolfson AH, Nouri K. Acute and chronic cutaneous reactions to ionizing radiation therapy. *Dermatol Ther*. 2016;6(2):185-206.
A review of the clinical manifestations, pathophysiology, epidemiology, risk factors, prevention, and treatment of both acute and chronic cutaneous radiation toxicities.
24. Hill RP, Rodemann HP, Hendry JH, et al. Normal tissue radiobiology: from the laboratory to the clinic. *Int J Radiat Oncol Biol Phys*. 2001;49(2):353-365.
25. Devalia HL, Mansfield L. Radiotherapy and wound healing. *Int Wound J*. 2008;5(1):40-44.
26. Wunderle K, Gill AS. Radiation-related injuries and their management: an update. *Semin Intervent Radiol*. 2015;32(2):156-162.
27. Smith BD, Bellon JR, Blitzblau R, et al. Radiation therapy for the whole breast: executive summary of an American Society for Radiation Oncology (ASTRO) evidence-based guideline. *Pract Radiat Oncol*. 2018;8(3):145-152.
28. Jonathan Yang T, Ho AY. Radiation therapy in the management of breast cancer. *Surg Clin North Am*. 2013;93(2):455-471.
29. Castaneda SA, Strasser J. Updates in the treatment of breast cancer with radiotherapy. *Surg Oncol Clin North Am*. 2017;26(3):371-382.
30. Recht A, Comen EA, Fine RE, et al. Postmastectomy radiotherapy: an American Society of Clinical Oncology, American Society for Radiation Oncology, and Society of Surgical Oncology focused guideline update. *Pract Radiat Oncol*. 2016;6(6):e219-e234.
31. Lee KT, Mun GH. Prosthetic breast reconstruction in previously irradiated breasts: a meta-analysis. *J Surg Oncol*. 2015;112(5):468-475.
32. Ascherman JA, Hanasono MM, Newman MI, Hughes DB. Implant reconstruction in breast cancer patients treated with radiation therapy. *Plast Reconstr Surg*. 2006;117(2):359-365.
33. Fracol ME, Basta MN, Nelson JA, et al. Bilateral free flap breast reconstruction after unilateral radiation: comparing intraoperative vascular complications and postoperative outcomes in radiated versus nonradiated breasts. *Ann Plast Surg*. 2016;76(3):311-314.
34. Nelson JA, Disa JJ. Breast reconstruction and radiation therapy: an update. *Plast Reconstr Surg*. 2017;140(5):60S-68S.
A review of the current understanding and treatment options for the management of surgical reconstruction of breast cancer patients who have undergone or are to undergo radiation therapy.
35. El-Sabawi B, Carey JN, Hagopian TM, et al. Radiation and breast reconstruction: algorithmic approach and evidence-based outcomes. *J Surg Oncol*. 2016;113(8):906-912.
36. Cordeiro PG, Albornoz CR, McCormick B, et al. What is the optimum timing of postmastectomy radiotherapy in two-stage prosthetic reconstruction: radiation to the tissue expander or permanent implant? *Plast Reconstr Surg*. 2015;135(6):1509-1517.
37. Kronowitz SJ, Hunt KK, Kuerer HM, et al. Delayed-immediate breast reconstruction. *Plast Reconstr Surg*. 2004;113(6):1617-1628.
38. Head and neck cancers. National Cancer Institute Website. http://www.cancer.gov/types/head-and-neck/head-neck-fact-sheet. Reviewed Mar 29, 2017.
39. Sroussi HY, Epstein JB, Bensadoun RJ, et al. Common oral complications of head and neck cancer radiation therapy: mucositis, infections, saliva change, fibrosis, sensory dysfunctions, dental caries, periodontal disease, and osteoradionecrosis. *Cancer Med*. 2017;6(12):2918-2931.
A description of the common complications of radiation therapy in head and neck cancer, including complication grading scales, clinical manifestations, and treatment recommendations.
40. Pinna R, Campus G, Cumbo E, et al. Xerostomia induced by radiotherapy: an overview of the physiopathology, clinical evidence, and management of the oral damage. *Ther Clin Risk Manag*. 2015;11:171-188.
41. Fahradyan A, Howell A, Wolfswinkel E, et al. Updates on the management of non-melanoma skin cancer (NMSC). *Healthcare*. 2017;5(4):82.
42. Squamous cell skin cancer. Medline Plus. https://www.nlm.nih.gov/medlineplus/ency/article/000829.htm. Updated August 14, 2018.
43. Bichakjian CK, Olencki T, Aasi SZ, et al. Basal Cell Skin Cancer, Version 1.2016, NCCN Clinical Practice Guidelines in Oncology. *J Natl Compr Canc Netw*. 2016;14(5):574-597.
44. Eastley N, Green PN, Ashford RU. Soft tissue sarcoma. *BMJ*. 2016;352:i436.
45. Wang D, Zhang Q, Eisenberg BL, et al. Significant reduction of late toxicities in patients with extremity sarcoma treated with image-guided radiation therapy to a reduced target volume: results of radiation therapy oncology group RTOG-0630 trial. *J Clin Oncol*. 2015;33(20):2231-2238.
46. Rivero JA, Shamji O, Kolokythas A. Osteoradionecrosis: a review of pathophysiology, prevention and pharmacologic management using pentoxifylline, α-tocopherol, and clodronate. *Oral Surg Oral Med Oral Pathol Oral Radiol*. 2017;124(5):464-471.
47. Avraham T, Yan A, Zampell JC, et al. Radiation therapy causes loss of dermal lymphatic vessels and interferes with lymphatic function by TGF- 1-mediated tissue fibrosis. *AJP Cell Physiol*. 2010;299(3):C589-C605.
48. Chandra RA, Miller CL, Skolny MN, et al. Radiation therapy risk factors for development of lymphedema in patients treated with regional lymph node irradiation for breast cancer. *Int J Radiat Oncol Biol Phys*. 2015;91(4):760-764.
49. Kumar G, Yadav V, Singh P, Bhowmik KT. Radiation-induced malignancies making radiotherapy a " two-edged sword ": a review literature. *World J Oncol*. 2017;8(1):1-6.
50. Chan RJ, Webster J, Chung B, et al. Prevention and treatment of acute radiation-induced skin reactions: a systematic review and meta-analysis of randomized controlled trials. *BMC Cancer*. 2014;14:53.
A meta-analysis looking at the efficacy of various interventions directed at preventing and treating both acute and late radiation induced skin toxicities.

QUESTIONS

1. A 55-year-old woman with a history of a 6 cm mass of the left breast, found to be invasive ductal carcinoma with positive regional lymph node, who underwent left mastectomy and RT to the breast 15 years prior, now presents with a 1 cm nonhealing wound on the superior medial border of the chest wall. What should the next step be?

a. Local wound care and antibiotic therapy
b. Local tissue rearrangement for reconstruction
c. Pectoralis major turnover flap
d. Free transverse rectus abdominis myocutaneous flap with microvascular anastomosis to the thoracodorsal vessels for coverage of the sinus as well as breast reconstruction
e. Biopsy and culture of wound

2. When performing autologous breast reconstruction of a previously irradiated breast, there is an increased risk of

a. Mastectomy flap loss compared with implant-based reconstruction
b. Implant loss with latissimus dorsi reconstruction
c. Free flap necrosis compared with nonirradiated tissue
d. Microvascular complication compared with nonirradiated tissue
e. None of the above; there is no increased complication risk when using autologous reconstruction in an irradiated field

3. Risk factors for developing ORN of the mandible include all of the following except

a. Radiation at doses higher than 30 Gy
b. Extraction of tooth to the area of radiated bone after RT
c. Tobacco use
d. Poor oral hygiene
e. Alcohol use

4. A 40-year-old man with an undifferentiated pleomorphic sarcoma of the right lower extremity, who underwent preoperative RT 3 weeks prior to tumor excision. The sarcoma now measures 5 × 5 cm and is located on the medial lower extremity 2 cm below the knee. What is the optimal reconstructive option?

a. Lateral gastrocnemius flap
b. Medial gastrocnemius flap
c. Local random rotational flap
d. Right anterior lateral thigh flap
e. Deep inferior epigastric perforator flap

5. Fibrosis following RT is associated with all of the following except

a. Differentiation of fibroblasts to postmitotic fibroblasts resulting in the upregulation of collagen
b. Upregulation of TGF-β1 expression
c. Dose dependent
d. Usually presents 2 to 3 weeks after the completion of RT
e. Potentiated by concurrent chemotherapeutic agents including doxorubicin, tamoxifen, methotrexate, bleomycin, 5-fluorouracil, and actinomycin D

1. **Answer: e.** A patient with a history of cancer and RT 15 years prior with a new wound should be worked up for an RIM. Radiation-induced, nonbreast cancer malignancies have a 23% higher incidence in irradiated breast cancer patients compared with the general female population. This population has a higher risk of second cancer of the lung, esophagus, thyroid, and sarcoma that increases over time, peaking at 10 to 15 years after initial cancer diagnosis. The standardized incidence ratio of sarcoma is 6.54 in irradiated patients compared with 1.42 in nonirradiated patients.

2. **Answer: d.** Microvascular arterial complications are significantly more common in a radiated field compared with a nonirradiated field. Radiation, however, did not have an impact on outcomes, including fat necrosis or flap loss. There is no difference in breast-related complications when comparing implant-based or autologous reconstruction in a radiated breast. Furthermore, there is a decrease in implant loss when reconstructed with a latissimus dorsi flap compared with no autologous reconstruction.

3. **Answer: a.** Risk factors for developing ORN of the mandible include radiation at doses higher than 60 Gy, trauma or surgery to the radiated field including tooth extraction, social habits including tobacco and alcohol use, and poor oral hygiene leading to periodontal disease and caries.

4. **Answer: d.** After RT, tissue to the irradiated field has poor wound healing capabilities due to the slow turnover of progenitor cells. Chronically, there is damage to vessel endothelium, predisposing radiated tissue to poor wound healing with minor trauma. For this reason, reconstruction should recruit nonradiated tissue to improve wound healing after tumor excision. A right anterior lateral thigh flap would offer nonradiated tissue with less donor site morbidity compared with a deep inferior epigastric perforator flap.

5. **Answer: d.** Fibrosis following RT is associated with the upregulation of TGF-β1 expression, resulting in the differentiation of postmitotic fibroblasts and subsequent upregulation of collagen formation. It is dose dependent, with increased risk of fibrosis with higher doses of radiation. Many factors can exacerbate fibrosis, including smoking, obesity, overlapping skin folds, poor nutrition, preexisting trauma to the tissue, genetic disorders, systemic diseases, and chemotherapeutic agents including doxorubicin, tamoxifen, methotrexate, bleomycin, 5-fluorouracil, and actinomycin D. Fibrosis is a manifestation of late radiation toxicity, appearing about 6 months to years following the completion of RT.

CHAPTER 24 Lasers in Plastic Surgery

Nathanial R. Miletta, R. Rox Anderson, and Matthias B. Donelan

KEY POINTS

- Modern advances in laser surgery have contributed to a paradigm shift in reconstructive and aesthetic medicine, necessitating a familiarity with this valuable modality.
- Lasers generate spatially and temporally coherent electromagnetic radiation allowing the generation of very bright and focused laser beams with medium-specific, fixed wavelengths.
- Chromophores within the skin absorb specific wavelengths of light and subsequently respond with thermal, mechanical, or chemical reactions.
- The unique characteristics of lasers can be leveraged to create tools of remarkable therapeutic and diagnostic precision in order to better optimize patient outcomes.
- A conceptual overview will be presented along with representative clinical cases to better develop the physician's comfort level in utilizing laser surgery.

Modern advances in laser surgery have contributed to a paradigm shift in reconstructive and cosmetic surgery that favors minimally invasive procedures, necessitating a familiarity with this valuable modality. Laser surgery is utilized in a number of conditions germane to the plastic surgeon and may serve as a definitive treatment of choice or as an adjuvant therapy to best optimize patient outcomes. In the reconstructive realm, laser therapy for hypertrophic burn and trauma scars has led to significant improvements in scar aesthetics, functioning, and symptoms often obviating the need for more extensive surgical procedures.[1-4] Aggregated laser surgery ranks only behind botulinum toxin injections and soft tissue fillers in cosmetic procedures performed annually and has contributed to the trend of patients seeking aesthetic treatments earlier in life and with a more equal gender distribution.[5]

Most laser platforms are now equipped with manufacturer-recommended starting settings that are target and Fitzpatrick skin type (FST) specific. Although generally considered safe, the surgeon will find that a better understanding of laser surgery will allow therapeutic customization resulting in better patient outcomes. This chapter will highlight key concepts in laser surgery complete with representative case examples in order to better inform the clinical decision making of the laser surgeon.

BASIC SCIENCE

Laser Light

Laser is an acronym for light-amplified stimulated emission of radiation. Lasers generate spatially and temporally coherent electromagnetic radiation of a fixed wavelength focused into a precise beam of energy (Figure 24.1). Lasers consist of an energy source and a medium housed within an optical cavity (Figure 24.2). The electrons of the atoms within the medium are excited upon exposure to the energy source, commonly a flash lamp. The medium may be a solid, liquid, or gas. As the electrons spontaneously fall from the excited to resting state, photons with medium-specific wavelengths are emitted.[6] Using a system of reflective and semireflective mirrors, the emitted photons are redirected back into the medium allowing for (1) excitement of additional electrons within the medium (amplification) and (2) coherence and collimation due to constructive and destructive interference.[7,8] Once a sufficient amount of energy is generated, the laser beam will be allowed to exit the optical cavity. The laser light may be delivered to the tissue by a series of mirrors within an articulating arm or transported along a fiber optic cable.

Laser-Tissue Interactions

Laser light may be reflected, transmitted, scattered, or absorbed by tissue. The molecules that absorb light are known as chromophores and include hemoglobin, melanin, tattoo pigment, and water. After absorption, chromophores may reemit photons or undergo photothermal, photomechanical, or photochemical reactions.[9] Photothermal events represent the majority of medical laser reactions and result from an increase of local kinetic energy and the generation

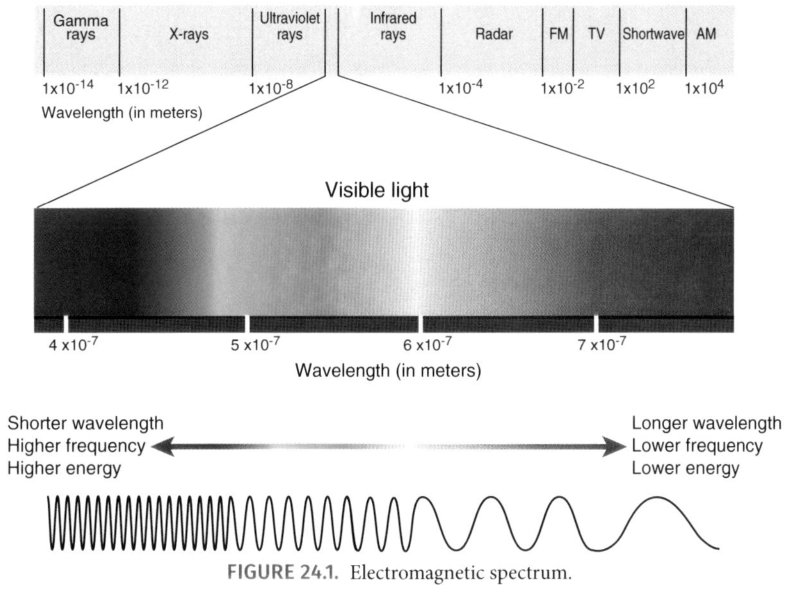

FIGURE 24.1. Electromagnetic spectrum.

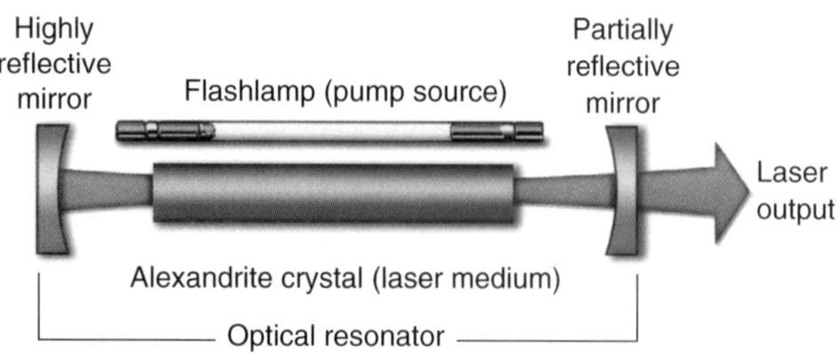

FIGURE 24.2. Basic components of a laser.

of localized heat.[7] Photomechanical reactions result in structural degradation of the chromophore through vibrations following photoexcitation of the chromophore.[9] Photochemical reactions occur when the excited state of the chromophore has markedly different physical or chemical properties than the resting state.[9]

Laser Variables

When choosing a laser, it is critical to consider the absorption spectrum of the chromophore and its location within the skin. These two factors will determine the wavelength of the laser medium chosen, both for absorption and depth of laser penetration (**Table 24.1** and Figure 24.3). Laser wavelength and depth are directly proportional until water begins to serve as the primary chromophore, at which point, laser penetration decreases owing to the ubiquity and highly absorptive nature of water. The amount of physiologic melanin present must be considered, and the wavelength selected should minimize collateral injury that could result in dyspigmentation. The pulse width of the laser may vary by several orders of magnitude and should be carefully titrated based upon the thermal relaxation time (TRT) of the target, which corresponds to its size (**Table 24.2**).[7] The pulse width should not exceed the TRT, as this can lead to collateral injury within the skin and a loss of selectivity.[7]

Once an appropriate wavelength and pulse width have been selected, the laser surgeon must choose a starting fluence, which is measured in energy/treatment area. Most laser platforms recommend starting settings from which the laser surgeon may titrate upward to the desired therapeutic end point, which is specific to each target. Increasing the laser spot size allows for more rapid treatment sessions and a decrease in the relative scatter of light. Of note, if the spot size is increased, the fluence will likely need to be decreased to prevent excessive energy delivery. Epidermal cooling mechanisms must be also considered in order to prevent damage to the superficial layer of the skin and can be achieved by contact or noncontact (spray) cooling. Hertz (Hz), or the rate in which pulses are delivered, is also important to consider in order to avoid excessive bulk heating.

As we discuss the conditions that can be treated with lasers, we will review approaches and tips for selecting appropriate settings, as well as, the desired therapeutic end points of the common targets within the skin.

Chromophores

The chromophores in the skin include oxyhemoglobin, deoxyhemoglobin, melanin, water, and tattoo pigment (**Figure 24.4**). Chromophore-wavelength selectivity allows the laser surgeon to generate photothermal, photomechanical, or photochemistry reactions limited to discrete structures or in a spatially selective manner within the skin optimizing clinical outcomes.[7]

SKIN COMPONENT-SELECTIVE PHOTOREACTIONS

Hemoglobin

The treatment of cutaneous vasculature relies upon the selective absorption of laser light by oxyhemoglobin and deoxyhemoglobin and the photothermal reaction that ensues.[7] The focal heating of intravascular hemoglobin damages vessel endothelium resulting in coagulation and vessel elimination while sparing local tissue.[7] Oxyhemoglobin displays an absorption band from 400 to 1200 nm, with major peaks at 418, 542, and 577 nm and a minor peak that encompasses 1064 nm (see Figure 24.4).[7] Deoxyhemoglobin demonstrates an absorption peak that includes the 755 and 800 nm wavelengths. When treating vasculature, it is important to remember physiologic melanin absorbs laser light particularly well at lower wavelengths. For patients with higher FSTs, longer wavelength lasers should be utilized. When selecting a pulse width, titrate to the target (blood vessel) and not the chromophore (hemoglobin). Epidermal cooling is important to prevent damage to the epidermis. Devices commonly used to treat vasculature include the 532 nm potassium titanyl phosphate (KTP), 560 nm intense pulsed light (IPL), 595 nm pulsed dye laser (PDL), 755 nm alexandrite, 810 nm diode, and

TABLE 24.1. MEDICAL LASERS

Medium	Spectrum	λ (nm)	Chromophore
Argon	Visible light	488, 514	Oxyhemoglobin, melanin
Intense pulsed light[a]		515, 560, 650	Oxyhemoglobin, melanin
Potassium titanyl phosphate (KTP)		532	Oxyhemoglobin, melanin, tattoo pigment
Yellow dye		595	Oxyhemoglobin
Ruby		694	Melanin, tattoo pigment
Alexandrite	Near infrared	755	Melanin, tattoo pigment, deoxyhemoglobin
Titanium sapphire		785	Tattoo pigment
Diode		800	Melanin, deoxyhemoglobin
Neodymium:yttrium aluminum garnet (Nd:YAG)		1064	Melanin, tattoo pigment, deoxyhemoglobin
Erbium-doped glass (Er:glass)	Mid infrared	1550	Water
Thulium-doped glass (Th:Glass)		1927	Water
Erbium:yttrium aluminum garnet (Er:YAG)	Far infrared	2940	Water
Carbon dioxide (CO_2)		10,600	Water

[a]Intense pulsed light (IPL) is filtered light.

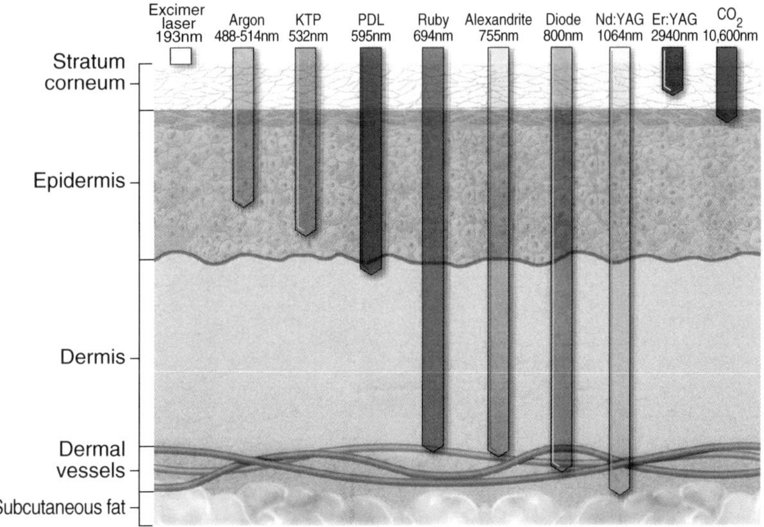

FIGURE 24.3. Penetration depth of common laser mediums.

1064 nm neodymium-doped:yttrium aluminum garnet (Nd:YAG) (Table 24.1). All of the lasers above fall in the long-pulsed domain (Table 24.2). Fully ablative lasers targeting water as a chromophore may also be used to nonselectively destroy vasculature in the treatment area. Many vascular conditions can be treated by targeting hemoglobin to include capillary vascular malformations; telangiectasias; erythema; angiomas; infantile hemangiomas; postprocedural purpura; spider veins; reticular veins; and erythematous scars.

Capillary Vascular Malformations (Port Wine Stains)

The treatment of capillary vascular malformations, or port wine stains (PWSs), illustrates the therapeutic rationale for treating vascular conditions. With one million patients in the United States and 22 million affected globally, PWSs represent a common cause of presentation to the laser surgeon.[10] Without treatment, 65% of PWSs become hypertrophic, often leading to bleeding, aesthetic deformation, and psychological stress.[11-17] Although the etiology is unclear, the clinical phenotype results from ectatic capillaries and postcapillary venules with varying degrees of oxygenation and dilatation within the superficial and deep dermis.[18,19] In infants and young children, PWSs are erythematous with increased oxyhemoglobin and respond well to shorter wavelength lasers. PWSs in adult patients are often more violaceous owing to deoxyhemoglobin and demonstrate increased thickness necessitating use of the longer wavelength lasers. Initiating treatment as early as possible is critical for minimizing laser light scatter due to dermal collagen and acquired tanning melanin (Figure 24.5).[20-25]

Infantile Hemangiomas

The serendipitous discovery of propranolol as a safe, effective treatment of infantile hemangiomas drastically changed the management of superficial, deep, and mixed infantile hemangiomas.[26] However, selective photothermolysis of the vasculature continues to play a role in the treatment of superficial or ulcerated infantile hemangiomas, as well as resolved hemangiomas with residual vasculature.[27-29] Adjuvant treatment with topical timolol 0.5% solution may help expedite resolution, but early studies have not demonstrated a cumulative benefit.[30]

TABLE 24.2. PULSE WIDTH DOMAINS

Domain	Range
Continuous wave	Seconds (s)
Long pulsed	Milliseconds (ms)
Short pulsed	Nanoseconds (ns)
Ultrashort pulsed	Picoseconds (ps) Femtoseconds (fs)

Varicose Veins and Spider Veins

Endovenous laser ablation represents the gold standard in the management of larger varicosities achieving a 90% to 100% success rate in improving cosmesis and symptoms.[31] Access to the vascular lumen is achieved with a fiber optic laser percutaneously under ultrasound guidance. Superficial spider veins are common in patients with underlying venous insufficiency. After successful endovenous laser ablation, spider veins may be treated with sclerotherapy or vascular laser treatment.[32]

Telangiectasias and Erythema

Telangiectasias (broken blood vessels) result from photodamage, inflammatory skin disease, radiation, or underlying systemic disease.[33] Optimal treatment includes longer pulse widths and the end point of durable purpura; however, patients are often willing to sacrifice clinical efficacy to minimize downtime achieved with subpurpuric settings.[34] Facial erythema represents a similar process to telangiectasia but is composed of fine dilated vessels that require magnification to be appreciated. Shorter pulse widths and subpurpuric fluences have been shown to achieve ideal outcomes in generalized erythema.[34]

Angiomas (Cherry and Spider)

Cherry angiomas represent capillary proliferations that commonly arise on the trunk of middle-aged patients. These growths can easily be treated with lasers that target hemoglobin. As they arise from capillaries, short millisecond pulse widths may be used with purpuric fluences. Spider angiomas represent a similar process and are treated in a similar fashion.

Verruca Vulgaris

Treatment of warts using laser therapy has demonstrated equivocal outcomes to cryotherapy or electrodessication.[35] Paring must be performed to eliminate keratinization, but once complete, vascular lasers are capable of destroying wart vasculature.[35] Purpuric settings should be used without epidermal cooling.

Postprocedural Purpura

Selective photothermolysis of the vasculature has been shown to significantly reduce postprocedural purpura in a small case series of patients.[36] Treatment is particularly helpful for cosmetic surgery patients that would prefer discretion after elective procedures.

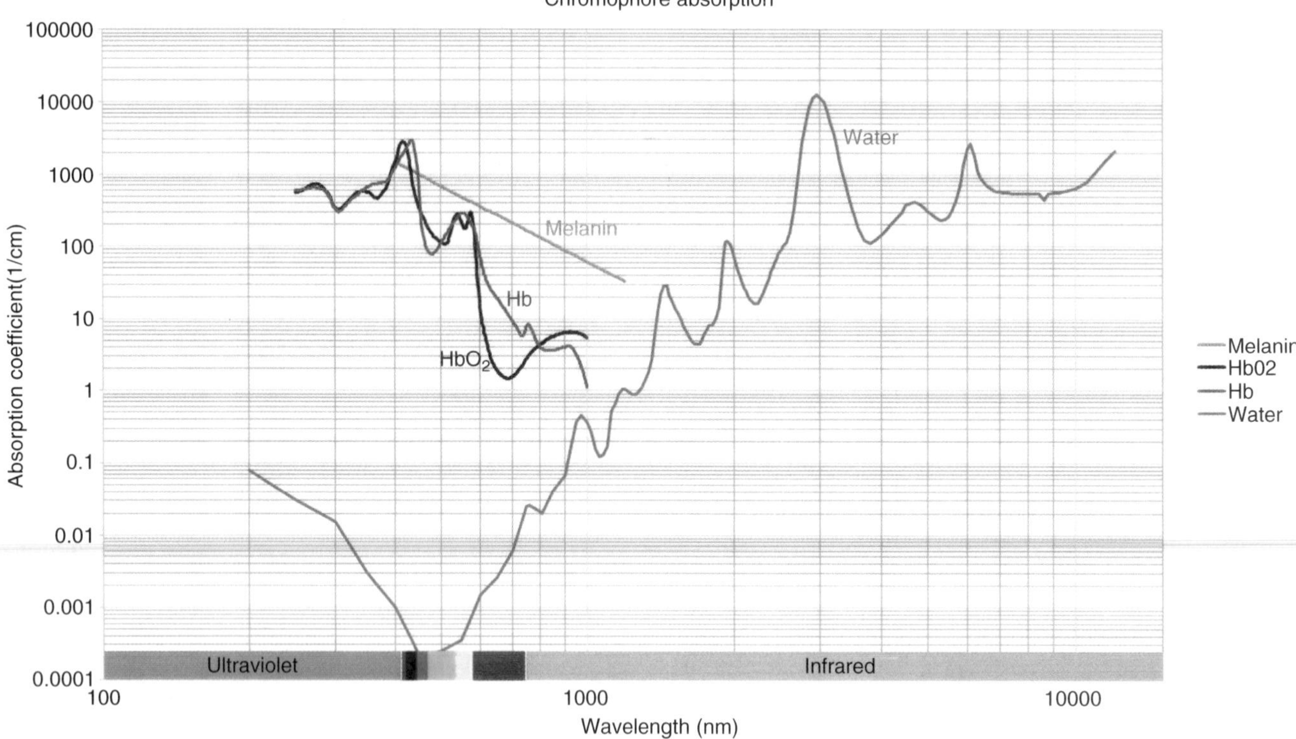

FIGURE 24.4. Chromophore absorption spectrum with common laser mediums noted. (Courtesy of Lumenis Ltd.)

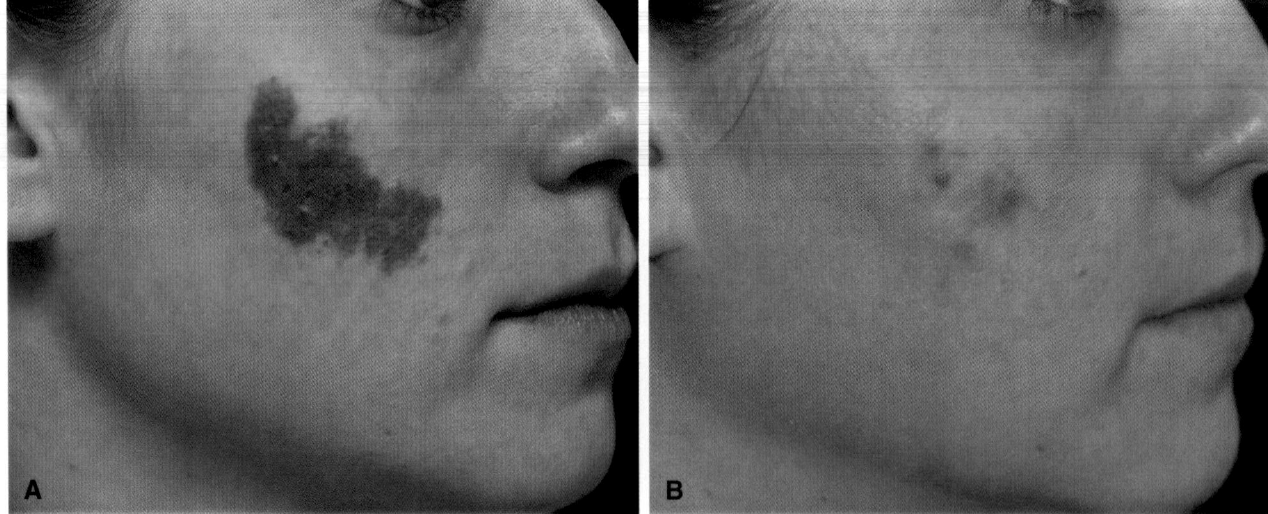

FIGURE 24.5. A. A 26-year-old, Fitzpatrick skin type (FST) II patient with an isolated facial port wine stain (PWS) presented with concern for its color and thickness. Anesthesia was achieved with topical anesthetic. The erythematous and violaceous nature of the PWS demonstrated the presence of both oxyhemoglobin and deoxyhemoglobin. Given the relative paucity of melanin in FST II patients, a shorter wavelength is appropriate to target the oxyhemoglobin. The most extensively studied device in this range for PWS and treatment of choice is the pulsed dye laser (PDL).[20,21] The long-pulsed potassium titanyl phosphate (KTP) laser, intense pulsed light (IPL), and alexandrite laser have also demonstrated efficacy in the treatment of PWS.[20,21] Given the various sizes of the vessels within the PWS, PDL was chosen with a short pulse width of 0.45 ms, fluence of 8 J/cm^2, spot size of 7 mm, and dynamic cooling device (DCD) engaged to achieve the treatment end point of durable purpura.[22] The pulse width was chosen to eliminate very fine vessels. A longer pulse width would have exceeded the TRT of the narrow diameter vessels, which could have resulted in sclerotic white patches within the PWS. At subsequent treatment sessions, the pulse width was increased to 1.5 and 3 ms with the fluence titrated to the same end point to target the larger vessels. Future visits were scheduled every 3 weeks.[23] At the fourth visit, the alexandrite laser was used prior to the PDL to better target deoxyhemoglobin in the postcapillary venules. Using a pulse width of 3 ms, an 8 mm spot size, and the DCD engaged, a fluence of 35 J/cm^2 was selected and titrated upward to 85 J/cm^2 to the end point of transient, bluish purpura.[22] Caution was used, as the risk of scarring is much greater with the infrared lasers in PWS.[24,25] An additional five treatments were performed using the principles above to achieve a desired outcome. Additional treatments could have been performed but the patient became pregnant and opted to halt therapy until after the delivery of the baby. **B.** Final result.

Erythematous Scars

Through the induction of controlled damage to the dermal microvasculature, selective photothermolysis has proven to be a cornerstone in the treatment of erythematous and symptomatic scars since its introduction.[37] Employing a PDL with the following settings is helpful: pulse width between 0.45 and 1.5 ms, 7 mm spot size, and fluence titrated upward from 5.0 J/cm^2 to the clinical end point of transient purpura. PDL excels at decreasing erythema and pruritus.[38] Improvements in scar volume, pliability, and skin elasticity have also been reported.[39]

Melanin

In the absence of external injury, melanin is the primary chromophore responsible for cutaneous pigmentation. Excess melanin may be located in the epidermis, dermis, or both. It is critical to understand the depth of the melanin when choosing a laser wavelength. A 365 nm Wood's lamp light source may be used to help determine the level. Upon exposure to Wood's lamp, epidermal melanin will strongly absorb the light, creating a stronger contrast, while dermal melanin will have less contrast.[40] The absorption spectrum of melanin is inversely proportional to laser light wavelength (see Figure 24.4). However, shorter wavelengths face increased competition from hemoglobin and have difficulty reaching dermal melanin.[7] In patient populations with increased physiologic melanin, longer wavelengths should be selected in order to avoid dyspigmentation.

Epidermal disorders of pigmentation include lentigines, ephelides (freckles), seborrheic keratoses, café-au-lait macules, and Becker nevi. Dermal disorders of pigmentation include dermal melanocytosis (nevus of Ota, nevus of Ito, and Mongolian spots), and drug-induced hyperpigmentation. Postinflammatory hyperpigmentation (PIH) and melasma often demonstrate both epidermal and dermal components. Melanin within the hair shaft can also be targeted in order to perform laser hair reduction (LHR). Devices commonly used to target melanin include the KTP, IPL, alexandrite, and Nd:YAG in the long-pulsed, short-pulsed, and ultrashort-pulsed domains (Table 24.2). Fractional and fully ablative lasers targeting water as a chromophore may also be used to nonselectively destroy pigment.

Epidermal Melanin

Lentigines

Lentigines commonly present on the face, chest, and dorsal hands as well-demarcated hyperpigmented macules. The chromophore in lentigines is epidermal melanin and can be targeted using a variety of wavelengths (Table 24.1). Effective removal can be accomplished with long-pulsed, short-pulsed, and ultrashort-pulsed lasers and lights.[41] Once melanin absorbs laser light, the ensuing photoreaction may be photothermal or photomechanical depending upon the pulse width selected. The desired treatment end point is epidermal whitening.[22] Of note, labial melanotic macules represent a subtype of lentigines and may be treated similarly (Figure 24.6).

Café-au-lait Macules

Although studies have shown less than favorable clearance of café-au-lait macules treated with laser therapy, shorter wavelength lasers may demonstrate efficacy as the pigment resides in the epidermis.[41,42] If sufficiently small, excision may represent a better treatment option.

Ephelides (Freckles)

Ephelides also demonstrate increased melanin in the epidermis but do not show an increased presence of melanocytes. Treatment approach is similar to that of lentigines and improvement often requires one to two treatments for patient satisfaction.

Dermal Melanin

Laser Hair Removal

Selective heating of hair shaft melanin can be utilized to target and destroy stem cells within the bulge of the hair follicle. Although the melanin chromophore is very small, the TRT of the entire hair follicle must be considered to achieve sustained LHR. Given the depth and size of the hair follicle, long-pulsed, longer wavelength lasers and lights (650–1064 nm) are preferred for treatment (Table 24.1). In FST I to III patients, the long-pulsed alexandrite is the laser of choice given the relative paucity of competing physiologic melanin. In FST IV to VI patients, the long-pulsed Nd:YAG laser

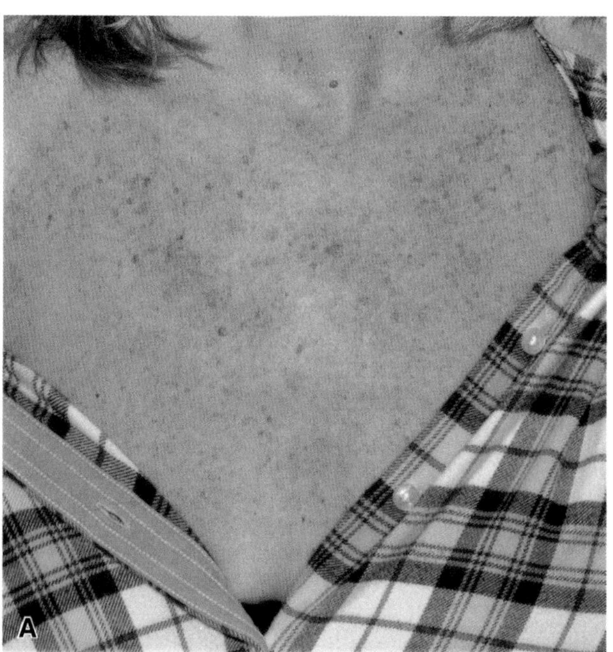

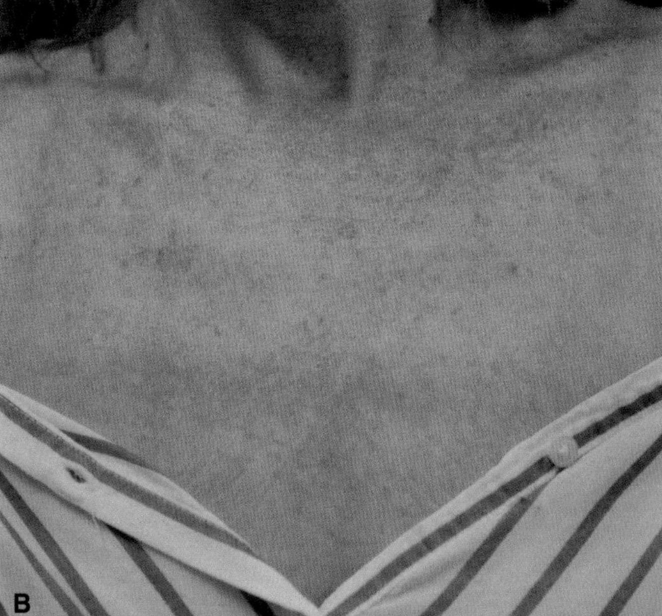

FIGURE 24.6. **A.** A 57-year-old Fitzpatrick skin type (FST) II female patient with an active tan presented for the elective removal of 2 to 6 mm hyperpigmented macules on the central chest. Owing to the surface area, an intense pulsed light (IPL) with a 515 nm filter was chosen with the following settings: fluence of 12 J/cm^2, 10 ms pulse width, and the contact cooling set to 18°C. One treatment was performed with a significant reduction in pigmentation noted at 4 weeks. **B.** Of particular interest, areas that were not treated with the IPL demonstrated a sharp pigmentary border. An additional treatment with the same settings was performed to create a more even appearance of the pigment to the patient's satisfaction.

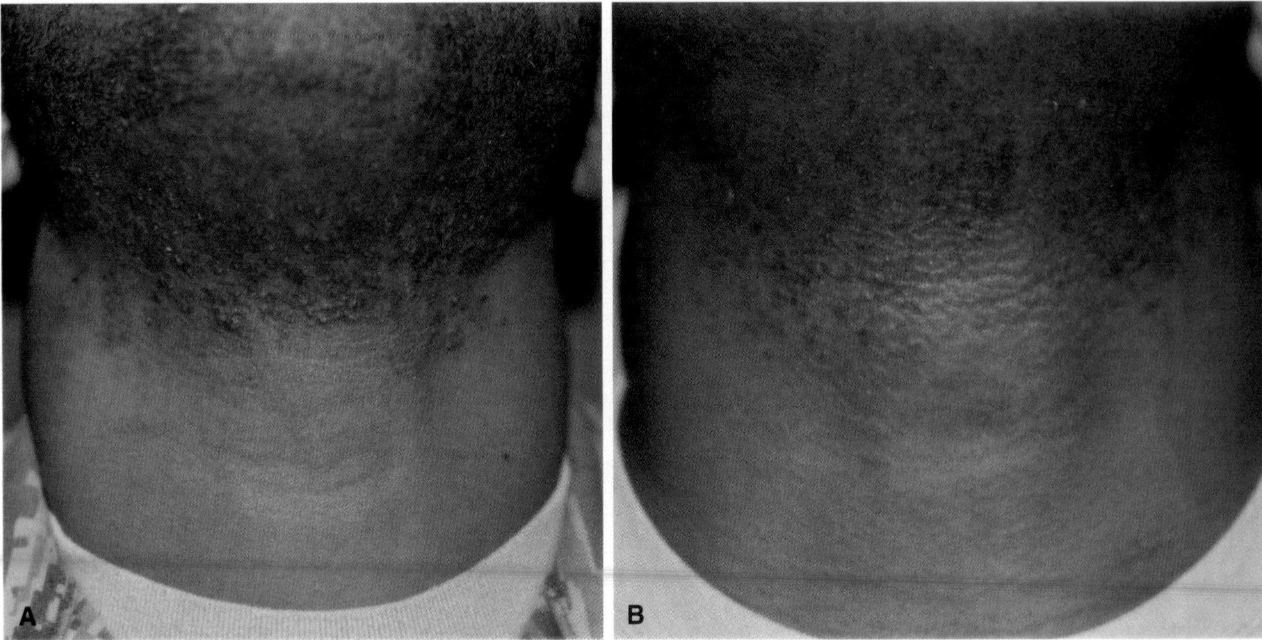

FIGURE 24.7. **A.** A 33-year-old Fitzpatrick skin type (FST) V male, active-duty military patient with pseudofolliculitis barbae (PFB) secondary to military grooming standards presented for laser hair reduction to the beard area. At the time of presentation, he demonstrated hyperpigmentation and inflammatory papules secondary to his PFB. Given the depth of the hair follicle and physiologic melanin present, the long-pulsed 1064 nm neodymium-doped:yttrium aluminum garnet (Nd:YAG) laser was selected. The patient shaved the morning of the procedure to minimize superficial absorption of energy. Superficial absorption would prevent the laser light from reaching the bulge of the hair follicle and, in extreme cases, may cause flash burns of the epidermis. Anesthesia was achieved using topical anesthetic. For the first treatment, a pulse width of 10 ms was chosen with an 18 mm spot size. The starting fluence was 16 J/cm^2 and was titrated to 18 J/cm^2 achieving the end point of perifollicular edema.[22] Four additional treatments were performed during which time the pulse width was incrementally increased to 30 ms and the fluence also increased accordingly to achieve the desired end point. **B.** After his five treatments, the patient had a significant reduction in hair and the resulting complications of hyperpigmentation and inflammatory papules. The patient was satisfied with his treatment, and a hydroquinone bleaching cream was provided to expedite resolution of his postinflammatory hyperpigmentation.

is preferred for the effective removal of hair while sparing melanin within the skin. To minimize damage to superficial structures, epidermal cooling should be used during LHR treatments (**Figure 24.7**).

Dermal Melanocytosis (Nevus of Ito, Nevus of Ota, Mongolian Spots)

Excess melanocytes are present in the dermis; therefore, longer wavelengths are often utilized. A recent study indicated that the 1064 nm Nd:YAG laser in the nanosecond domain was more efficacious and better tolerated than the nanosecond 755 nm alexandrite laser.[43,44] Of note, a small case series has demonstrated the use of the picosecond 532 nm KTP laser to adequately treat dermal melanocytosis.[45]

Mixed Epidermal and Dermal Melanin

Melasma (Chloasma)

Melasma typically presents in female patients as hyperpigmented, mottled patches on the forehead, malar cheeks, and perioral areas. It appears to have both a genetic predisposition and environmental influences from ultraviolet light and patient hormone status.[46] Laser therapy may temporarily lighten melasma, but it is often recurrent and may be exacerbated by light therapy. A growing cohort of physicians advocate for the use of low-fluence laser toning with nanosecond and picosecond lasers, but efficacy remains unclear.[46] Sun avoidance and serial superficial chemical peels can often achieve patient satisfaction with less risk for rebound hyperpigmentation.

Drug-Induced Pigmentation

Drug-induced pigmentation may result from the deposition of melanin, heavy metals (iron/silver), or drug-pigment complexes or ochronosis. Short-pulsed and ultrashort-pulsed lasers in the 700 to 1064 nm range have shown some efficacy in improving these conditions.[47,48]

Postinflammatory Hyperpigmentation

Laser treatment of PIH is rarely pursued, as it often exacerbates the condition. Sun avoidance and topical bleaching agents can improve PIH significantly.

Tattoo Pigment

It is estimated that 17% of patients with tattoos have considered elective removal.[49] Historically, options were limited to modalities that often resulted in unsightly scars, such as surgical excision and dermabrasion. Advances in laser technology have afforded patients a new option for significant pigment reduction with a decreased risk of complications. Laser tattoo removal relies upon selecting a laser wavelength that will be absorbed by the tattoo pigment (**Table 24.3**). Given the minute size of the tattoo particles, short-pulsed and ultrashort-pulsed lasers are the pulse widths of choice for removal (Table 24.2). Ensuing photothermal and photomechanical reactions cause the tattoo particles to be broken down into smaller fragments that are cleared lymphatically or become fine enough that they are difficult to appreciate visually.

In the case of multicolor tattoos, treatment should be performed with the most superficial (shortest) wavelength first. As the cutaneous edema from treatment develops, the longer laser wavelengths with increased penetration will still allow the laser surgeon to reach dermal tattoo pigment. Alternatively, a 20-minute rest period with topical cooling will also reduce edema for successive treatments. Patients with higher FSTs should be treated with caution, as shorter wavelengths of light are highly absorbed by melanin. The fluence of the tattoo laser should be titrated upward to the treatment end point of dermal whitening.[22] A growing number of laser surgeons advocate for treating over the tattoo with ablative fractional laser (AFL) to allow the release of cutaneous edema and to provide a potential path for the extravasation of tattoo remnants. Treatment intervals should be at least 6 weeks in length to allow for mobilization of tattoo pigment. It is important to

TABLE 24.3. TATTOO PIGMENTS

Color	Medium (Wavelength)
Purple	Nd:YAG (1064 nm)
Blue	Nd:YAG (1064 nm) Titanium sapphire (785 nm) Alexandrite (755 nm) Ruby (694 nm)
Green	Titanium sapphire (785 nm) Alexandrite (755 nm) Ruby (694 nm)
Yellow	KTP (532 nm)
Red	KTP (532 nm)
White	Nd:YAG (1064 nm)
Black	Nd:YAG (1064 nm) Alexandrite (755 nm) Ruby (694 nm)
Brown	Nd:YAG (1064 nm)

KTP, potassium titanyl phosphate; *Nd:YAG*, neodymium:yttrium aluminum garnet.

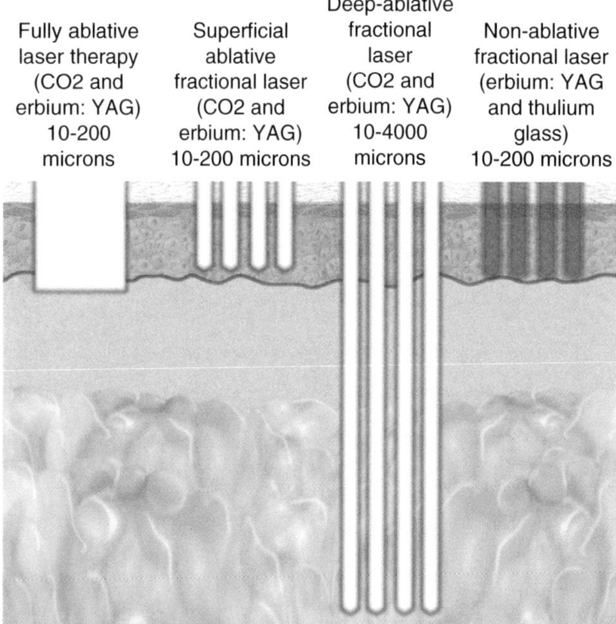

FIGURE 24.8. Overview of ablative and nonablative laser therapies.

mitigate patient expectations, as studies have shown that 15 treatments with short-pulsed (nanosecond) lasers result in only 75% of patients experiencing successful tattoo removal.[50] The newer ultrashort-pulsed (picosecond) lasers have anecdotally cleared tattoos faster and with fewer treatments, but well-powered studies have yet to be conducted.

SPATIALLY-SELECTIVE PHOTOTHERMOLYSIS

Water

As laser light wavelength increases, absorption of electromagnetic radiation by hemoglobin and melanin diminish while the absorption by water increases. Although water is a chromophore, its ubiquity in the skin and efficiency in absorbing laser light effectively eliminates structure selectivity. As such, modification of the laser beam using central pattern generators and scanners allow these lasers to be spatially selective, creating unique patterns of microinjury and preselected determination of penetration depth. Depending upon the wavelength of light, the ensuing tissue interaction may be thermal (nonablative) or ablative. Further manipulation of the beam profile allows the treatment to be either fractional or nonfractional (Figure 24.8). Lasers used to target water include the following: 1550 nm erbium-doped glass (Er:glass), 1927 nm thulium-doped glass (Th:glass), 2940 nm erbium-doped:yttrium aluminum garnet (Er:YAG), and 10,600 nm carbon dioxide (CO_2).

Fully Ablative Laser Therapy

Cosmetic Laser Resurfacing

The use of fully ablative laser therapy (nonfractional) first gained popularity in the 1980s for skin resurfacing as an alternative to mechanical and chemical resurfacing procedures.[51] The continuous wave CO_2 laser was the first to ablate successive layers of tissue in order to treat rhytidosis, dyschromia, and rhinophyma and to remove focal skin growths. Although clinically effective, the continuous wave pulse width demonstrated significant risk of scarring, hyperpigmentation, hypopigmentation, prolonged erythema, and secondary infections.[51] As technology and the understanding of laser-tissue interactions evolved, risk was mitigated by using pulse widths less than the TRT of the skin and laser scanners that helped decrease bulk heating.[51,52] These changes helped usher in the peak popularity of fully ablative resurfacing in the 1990s and early 2000s.[52]

The development of the Er:YAG in the 1990s provided laser surgeons with an additional option for fully ablative resurfacing with decreased thermal injury. Although both CO_2 and Er:YAG lasers are used for resurfacing, studies have shown the thermal injury from the CO_2 laser results in greater long-term skin contraction and fibroplasia.[52] Important considerations in fully ablative laser therapy include the depth of ablation (determined by the fluence), the rate in which the ablation is performed (hertz), and the scanner utilized. Scanners can be used to place individual pulses at small distances from one another within a treatment area to minimize bulk heating and potential injury. It is also important to consider the thickness of the skin in the treatment area and the density of adnexal structures containing stem cells necessary for recapitulating the epidermis (Figure 24.9).

Skin Growths

Fully ablative resurfacing may be used for the destruction of localized skin growths. To selectively remove these growths, the spot size of a fully ablative laser is titrated to the size of the lesion. Repeated passes are performed until the goal end point is achieved, which is visualization of the pink papillary dermis. Examples of epidermal growths include adenoma sebaceum, neurofibromas, syringomas, cylindromas, actinic keratoses, actinic cheilitis, verruca vulgaris, nevus sebaceus, epidermal nevi, and lymphatic malformations.

Fractional Photothermolysis

In 2004, the concept of fractional photothermolysis was introduced as a less aggressive alternative to fully ablative laser therapy.[53] Fractional lasers generate discrete columns of thermal injury within the epidermis and dermis referred to as microscopic treatment zones.[53] These columns vary from a few to several hundred micrometers (microns) in diameter and allow increased penetration up to 4 mm in depth.[53] By placing these columns in a gridlike pattern set distances from one another, intervening untreated skin acts as a reservoir of epidermal stem cells. This approach induces controlled remodeling and regeneration of collagen with shorter healing times.[54] A reduced risk of side effects comes at the cost of clinical benefit, often requiring serial treatments to achieve the same outcome as fully ablative laser. The increased depth of penetration afforded by fractional photothermolysis has demonstrated unique benefit when treating hypertrophic and keloid scars.[2-5]

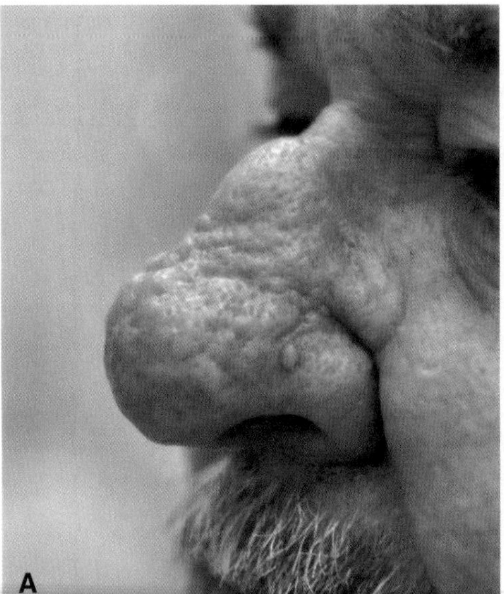

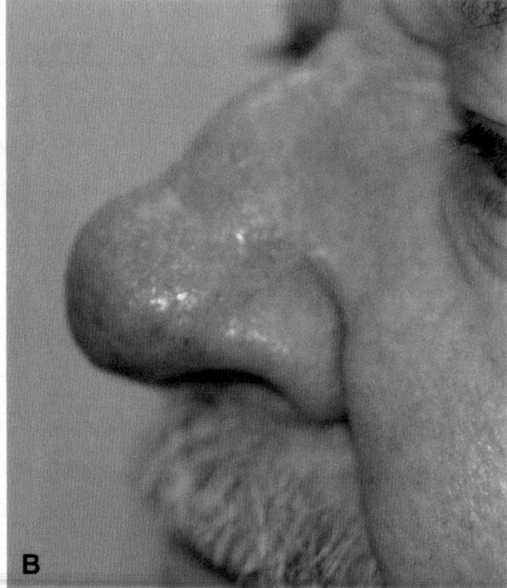

FIGURE 24.9. A. A 61-year-old Fitzpatrick skin type (FST) II male presented with a moderate case of rhinophyma. Prior to treatment, the patient was placed on viral prophylaxis with valacyclovir 1000 mg daily for 10 days beginning the day before the procedure. Preprocedural anxiolytic was given, and local anesthesia was achieved with 9 mL of 1% lidocaine with epinephrine 1:100,000. Once anesthesia was achieved, the patient was treated with several passes of fully ablative CO_2 laser with the goal of eliminating sebaceous glands and optimizing contouring of the nose using a stamping technique. A 4 × 4 gauze wetted with sterile water was used to cleanse the nose between passes. Once the shape and contour of the nose was returned to a more aesthetically optimal level, a thick layer of white petrolatum was applied. Over the next 14 days, the patient cleaned his face with diluted vinegar soaks three or four times daily and ensured continued application of white petrolatum. Occlusive bandages were not employed. **B.** A full recovery with near-optimal clinical outcome was achieved in 21 days.

Ablative Fractional Laser

Burn and Trauma Scars

Ablative fractional laser (AFL) was found to be beneficial in the treatment of burn and trauma scars in the mid-2000s. Areas, up to 4 mm deep, treated with AFL were shown to repopulate with collagen demonstrating a profile consistent with nonwounded skin.[55] AFL, in conjugation with PDL, has been shown to significantly reduce thickness and tension of the scars and improve cosmesis[2-5] (**Figure 24.10**).

Nonablative Fractional Laser

Nonablative fractional lasers (NAFLs) operate by creating pixilated patterns of injury similar to AFL but with thermal coagulation injury rather than tissue ablation. Selective heating and coagulation of tissue columns stimulates collagen remodeling, improving skin texture and tone without the potential complications or downtime associated with ablative lasers.[56] NAFL therapy typically requires a more extensive series of treatment sessions to achieve the desired clinical outcomes.

Acne Scars

Acne scars can be managed by a variety of therapeutic modalities to include NAFL. Other options include dermabrasion, subcision, surgical excision, chemical peels, and AFL. Although both AFL and NAFL can be used to treat acne scars, many patients prefer the decreased downtime of 3 or 4 days with NAFL. With four or five treatments performed every 4 to 6 weeks, patients can see significant improvement in acne scars (**Figure 24.11**).

LASER SAFETY

A protocol promoting the safety and well-being of the laser surgeon and the patient should be established in every practice. Cases have been reported of fire caused by PDLs, severe eye injury from misguided laser light, and a risk of the laryngeal papillomatosis caused by aerosolized viral particles in laser-generated smoke.[57] The Occupational Safety and Health Administration provides specific information regarding workplace hazards and appropriate

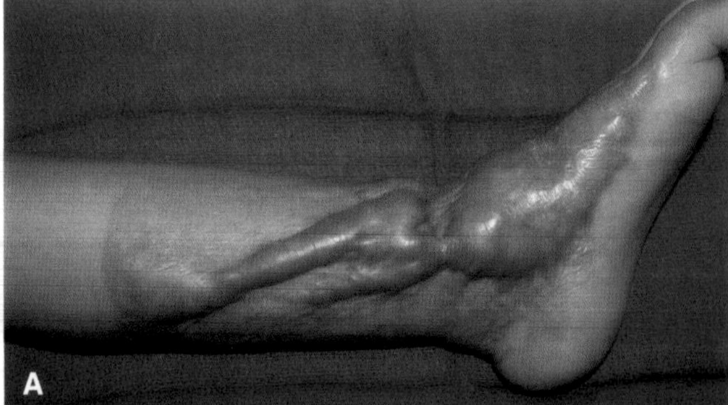

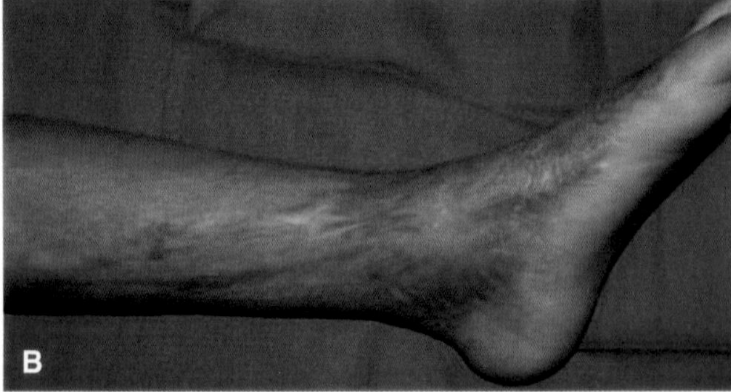

FIGURE 24.10. A. A 10-year-old Fitzpatrick skin type (FST) III male patient presented with hypertrophic burn scarring of the left lower leg and foot due to second- and third-degree scald burns incurred 2 years prior. Marked reduction of cutaneous extensibility and elasticity were noted upon physical examination. Initially, the patient was treated with the pulsed dye laser (PDL) every 4 weeks with the following settings: 0.45 ms pulse width, 5.5 J/cm^2, 7 mm spot size, and dynamic cooling device (DCD) engaged to the end point of transient purpura.[22] Adjuvant Z-plasties were performed in areas of high tension. At the initial treatment session, the patient was also treated with CO_2 ablative fractional laser (AFL), which was repeated every 3 months with the following settings: 15 to 40 mJ, 5% to 10% density, and 150 to 200 Hz. Triamcinolone solution with a concentration of 10 mg/mL was applied topically following CO_2 treatment. Intralesional triamcinolone with a concentration of 20 mg/mL was injected into the area, as well. **B.** Marked clinical improvement was observed aesthetically, and improvement in elasticity and extensibility resulted in improved function for the patient.

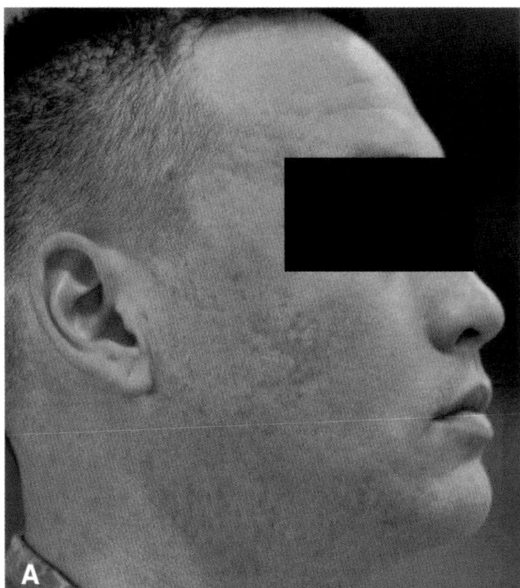

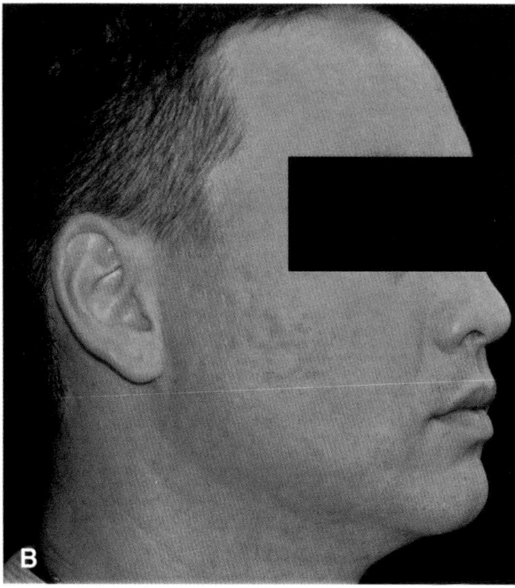

FIGURE 24.11. **A.** A 29-year-old Fitzpatrick skin type (FST) III male patient presented to the clinic with concern for acne scars on the temples, malar cheeks, jawline, and neck. Anesthesia was achieved using topical anesthetic. Using a long-pulsed 1550 nm erbium:glass laser, the patient was treated with the following settings: 70 mJ, density 14%, and a total dose of 2.5 kJ, delivered over eight passes. Complications were minimal to include swelling and erythema. Treatment was repeated for four additional sessions. **B.** Clinical outcome 3 months after the final treatment. The patient was satisfied with this 50% to 60% reduction in his acne scarring but could have chosen to seek additional treatments for greater benefit, if desired.

countermeasures related to medical laser use.[58] Categories of safety concern include severe eye injuries from direct or reflected laser light, skin burns from misdirected beams of surgical lasers, and respiratory hazards from laser-generated airborne contaminants.

The American National Standard Institute Z136 series of laser safety standards provides guidance for the safe use of lasers in diagnostic, cosmetic, preventative, and therapeutic applications in health care facilities.[59] These guidelines are considered to be the gold standard for safe practice and are recommended for review and implementation. These standards can be incorporated into a laser safety program that may also include standardized laser safety training for all health professionals working with laser equipment, annual training reviews, quarterly self-inspections, and incorporation of preprocedure laser safety checklists.

CONCLUSION

Laser surgery offers an effective and value-added modality to treat conditions that commonly present to the plastic surgeon. Optimal patient outcomes depend upon a thorough understanding of laser technology and customization to the individual patient. Laser surgery, alone or as an adjuvant therapy, offers patients the best chance to achieve their goals with minimal downtime and maximum efficacy.

REFERENCES

1. Donelan MB, Parrett BM, Sheridan RL. Pulsed dye laser therapy and z-plasty for facial burn scars: the alternative to excision. *Ann Plast Surg*. 2008;60:480-486.
   The first study to demonstrate that laser therapy can decrease the indications for burn scar excision in reconstructive surgery.
2. Levi B, Ibrahim A, Mathews K, et al. The use of CO_2 fractional photothermolysis for the treatment of burn scars. *J Burn Care Res*. 2016;37(2):106-114.
3. Miletta N, Lee K, Siwy K, et al. Objective improvement in burn scars after treatment with fractionated CO_2 laser. In: Presented at American Society for Laser Medicine and Surgery, Cutaneous Applications, April 2016, Boston, MA.
4. Issler-Fisher AC, Fischer OM, Smialkowski AO, et al. Ablative fractional CO2 laser for burn scar reconstruction: an extensive subjective and objective short-term outcome analysis of a prospective treatment cohort. *Burns*. 2017;43(3):573-582.
5. *2017 Cosmetic Plastic Surgery Statistics. American Society of Plastic Surgery, Plastic Surgery Statistics Report*. 2017. https://www.plasticsurgery.org/documents/News/Statistics/2017/plastic-surgery-statistics-report-2017.pdf. Accessed March 14, 2018.
6. Einstein A. On the quantum theory of radiation. *Physikal Zeitschr*. 1917;18:121.
   Einstein's paper on the quantum theory of radiation is the seminal work in the field of laser surgery and the foundation that allowed for the invention of lasers as we know them today.
7. Anderson RR, Parrish JA. Selective photothermolysis: precise microsurgery by selective absorption of pulsed radiation. *Science*. 1983;220:524-527.
   The concept of selective photothermolysis for skin conditions described for the first time. This approach allows the precise elimination of targets within the skin without damaging surrounding tissue. Nearly all medical lasers we use today are founded upon the principle of selective photothermolysis.
8. Nelson JS, Berns MW. Basic laser physics and tissue interactions. *Contemp Dermatol*. 1988;2:1.
9. Jacques SL. Laser–tissue interactions: photochemical, photothermal, and photomechanical. *Surg Clin North Am*. 1992;72:531-558.
10. Renfro L, Geronemus RG. Anatomical differences of port wine stains in response top treatment with pulsed dye laser. *Arch Dermatol*. 1993;129:182-188.
11. Klapman MH, Yao JF. Thickening and nodules in port-wine stains. *J Am Acad Dermatol*. 2001;449(2):300-302.
12. Lanigan SW, Cotterill JA. Psychological disabilities amongst patients with port-wine stains. *Br J Dermatol*. 1989;121:209-215.
13. McClean K, Hanke CW. The medical necessity for treatment of port-wine stains. *Dermatol Surg*. 1997;23(8):663-667.
14. Wagner KD, Wagner RF Jr. The necessity for treatment of childhood port-wine stains. *Cutis*. 1990;45(5):317-318.
15. Strauss RP, Resnick SD. Pulsed dye laser therapy for port-wine stains in children: psychosocial and ethical issues. *J Pediatr*. 1993;122(4):505-510.
16. Hansen K, Kreiter CD, Rosenbaum M, et al. Long-term psychological impact and perceived efficacy of pulsed dye laser therapy for patients with port-wine stains. *Dermatol Surg*. 2003;29(1):49-55.
17. Hagen SL, Grey KR, Korta DZ, et al. Quality of life in adults with facial port-wine stains. *J Am Acad Dermatol*. 2017;76(4):695-702.
18. Smoller BR, Rosen S. Port-wine stains: a disease of altered neural modulation of blood vessels? *Arch Dermatol*. 1986;122(2): 177-179.
19. Chang CJ, Yu JS, Nelson JS. Confocal microscopy study of neurovascular distribution in facial port wine stains (capillary malformation). *J Formos Med Assoc*. 2008;107:559.
20. Faurschou A, Olesen AB, Leonardi-Bee J, et al. Lasers or light sources for treating port-wine stains. *Cochrane Database Syst Rev*. 2011;(11):CD007152.
21. Reddy KK, Brauer JA, Idriss MH, et al. Treatment of port-wine stains with a short pulse width 532 nm Nd:YAG laser. *J Drug Dermatol*. 2013;12(1):66-71.
22. Wanner M, Sakamoto FH, Avram MM, et al. Immediate skin responses to laser and light treatments. Therapeutic endpoints: how to obtain efficacy. *J Am Acad Dermatol*. 2016;74(5):821-833.
    Clear and succinct outline of the therapeutic end points for the most common conditions presenting for laser surgery. This concept is critical in order to optimize patient outcomes and prevent adverse events.
23. Anolik R, Newlove T, Weiss ET, et al. Investigation into optimal treatment intervals of facial port-wine stains using the pulsed dye laser. *J Am Acad Dermatol*. 2012;67(5):985-990.
24. Izikson L, Nelson JS, Anderson RR. Treatment of hypertrophic and resistant port wine stains with a 755 nm laser: a case series of 20 patients. *Lasers Surg Med*. 2009;41(6):427-432.

25. Carlsen BC, Wenande E, Erlendsson AM, et al. A randomized side-by-side study comparing alexandrite laser at different pulse durations for port-wine stains. *Lasers Surg Med.* 2017;49(1):97-103.
26. Léauté-Labrèze C, Dumas de la Roque E, Hubiche T, et al. Propranolol for severe hemangiomas of infancy. *N Engl J Med.* 2008;358(24):2649-2651. doi:10.1056/NEJMc0708819.
27. Rizzo C, Brightman L, Chapas AM, et al. Outcomes of childhood hemangiomas treated with the pulsed dye laser with dynamic cooling: a retrospective chart analysis. *Dermatol Surg.* 2009;35(12):1947-1954.
28. Hohenleutner S, Badur-Ganter E, Landthaler M, et al. Long-term results in the treatment of childhood hemangioma with the flashlamp-pumped pulsed dye laser: an evaluation of 617 cases. *Lasers Surg Med.* 2001;28(3):273-277.
29. Darrow DH, Greene AK, Mancini AJ, et al. Diagnosis and management of infantile hemangioma. *Pediatrics.* 2015;136(4):e1060-e1104.
30. Passeron T, Maza A, Fontas E, et al. Treatment of port wine stains with pulsed dye laser and topical timolol: a multicenter randomized controlled trial. *Br J Dermatol.* 2014;170(6):1350-1353.
31. Van den Bos R, Arends L, Kockaert M, et al. Endovenous therapies of the lower extremity varicosities: a meta-analysis. *J Vasc Surg.* 2009;49(1):230-239.
32. Bernstein EF, Lee J, Lowery J, et al. Treatment of spider veins with the 595 nm pulsed dye laser. *J Am Acad Dermatol.* 1998;39(5 Pt 1):746-750.
33. Hare McCoppin HH, Goldberg DJ. Laser treatment of facial telangiectasias: an update. *Dermatol Surg.* 2010;36(8):1221-1230.
34. Iyer S, Fitzpatrick RE. Long-pulsed dye laser treatment for facial telangiectasias and erythema: evolution of a single purpuric pass versus multiple subpurpuric passes. *Dermatol Surg.* 2005;31(8 Pt 1):898-903.
35. Robson KJ, Cunningham NM, Kruzan KL, et al. Pulsed dye laser versus conventional therapy in the treatment of warts: a prospective randomized trial. *J Am Acad Dermatol.* 2000;43(2 Pt 1):275-280.
36. Karen JK, Hale EK, Geronemus RG. A simple solution to the common problem of ecchymosis. *Arch Dermatol.* 2010;146(1):94-95.
37. Alster TS. Improvement of erythematous and hypertrophic scars by the 585-nm flashlamp-pumped pulsed dye laser. *Ann Plast Surg.* 1994;32(2):186-190.
38. Nast A, Eming S, Fluhr J, et al. German S2k guidelines for the therapy of pathological scars (hypertrophic scars and keloids). *J Dtsch Dermatol Ges.* 2012;10(10):747-762.
39. Jin R, Huang X, Li H, et al. Laser therapy for prevention and treatment of pathologic excessive scars. *Plast Reconstr Surg.* 2013;132(6):1747-1758.
40. Gilchrest BA, Fitzpatrick TB, Anderson RR, et al. Localization of melanin pigmentation in the skin with Wood's lamp. *Br J Dermatol.* 1977;96(3):245-248.
41. Shimbashi T, Kamide R, Hashimoto T. Long-term follow-up in treatment of solar lentigo and café-au-lait macules with Q-switched ruby laser. *Aesthet Plast Surg.* 1997;21(6):445-448.
42. Kim HR, Ha JM, Park MS, et al. A low-fluence 1064-nm Q-switched neodymium-doped yttrium aluminium garnet laser for the treatment of café-au-lait macules. *J Am Acad Dermatol.* 2015;73(3):477-483.
43. Chan HH, Ying SY, Ho WS, et al. An in vivo trial comparing the clinical efficacy and complications of Q-switched 755 nm alexandrite and Q-switched 1064 nm Nd:YAG lasers in the treatment of nevus of Ota. *Dermatol Surg.* 2000;26(10):919-922.
44. Chan HH, King WW, Chan ES, et al. In vivo trial comparing patients' tolerance of Q-switched Alexandrite (QS Alex) and Q-switched neodymium:yttrium-aluminum-garnet (QS Nd:YAG) lasers in the treatment of nevus of Ota. *Lasers Surg Med.* 1999;24(1):24-28.
45. Jerdan K, Hsu JT, Schnurstein E. Successful treatment of Ota nevus with the 532-nm solid-state picosecond laser. *Cutis.* 2017;99(3):E29-E31.
46. Jeong SY, Shin JB, Yeo UC, et al. Low-fluence Q-switched neodymium-doped yttrium aluminum garnet laser for melasma with pre- or post-treatment triple combination cream. *Dermatol Surg.* 2011;37(1):126-127.
47. Tsao H, Busam K, Barnhill RL, et al. Treatment of minocycline-induced hyperpigmentation with the Q-switched ruby laser. *Arch Dermatol.* 1996;132(10):1250-1251.
48. Bellew SG, Alster TS. Treatment of exogenous ochronosis with a Q-switched alexandrite (755 nm) laser. *Dermatol Surg.* 2004;30(4 Pt 1):555-558.
49. Laumann AE, Derick AJ. Tattoos and body piercings in the United States: a national data set. *J Am Acad Dermatol.* 2006;55(3): 413-421.
50. Bencini PL, Cazzaniga S, Tourlake A, et al. Removal of tattoos by Q-switched laser: variables influencing outcome and sequelae in a large cohort of treated patients. *Arch Dermatol.* 2012;148(12):1364-1369.
51. Nanni CA, Alster TS. Complications of carbon dioxide laser resurfacing: an evaluation of 500 patients. *Dermatol Surg.* 1998;24(3):315-320.
52. Ross EV, McKinlay JR, Anderson RR. Why does carbon dioxide resurfacing work? A review. *Arch Dermatol.* 1999;35(4):444-454.
53. Manstein D, Herron GS, Sink RK, et al. Fractional photothermolysis: a new concept for cutaneous remodeling using microscopic patterns of thermal injury. *Lasers Surg Med.* 2004;34(5):426-438.
The seminal work on the concept of fractional photothermolysis. This concept has been developed and allows improved patient outcomes while minimizing side effects. This concept of fractional photothermolysis has been instrumental in both the reconstructive and aesthetic laser surgery domains.
54. Laubach HJ, Tannous Z, Anderson RR, et al. Skin responses to fractional photothermolysis. *Lasers Surg Med.* 2006;38(2):142-149.
55. Ozog DM, Liu A, Chaffins ML, et al. Evaluation of clinical results, histological architecture, and collagen expression following treatment of mature burn scars with a fraction carbon dioxide laser. *JAMA Dermatol.* 2013;149(1):50-57.
The most extensive review of burn scars to date. A thorough discussion of the clinical, histologic, and chemical reactions to treatment with a fractional carbon dioxide laser is provided further advancing the understanding of burn scars.
56. Kim KH, Geronemus RG. Nonablative laser and light therapies for skin rejuvenation. *Arch Facial Plast Surg.* 2004;6(6):398-409.
57. Bargman H. Laser safety guidelines. *J Clin Aesthet Dermatol.* 2010;3(5):18-19.
58. Occupational Safety and Health Administration. Surgical Suite: Laser Hazards. https://www.osha.gov/SLTC/etools/hospital/surgical.html#Lasers. Accessed March 12, 2018.
59. American National Standards Institute. *ANSI Z136: American National Standard for Safe Use of Lasers.* 2014. http://webstore.ansi.org/RecordDetail.aspx?sku=ANSI+Z136.1-2014&source=blog. Accessed March 15, 2018.

QUESTIONS

1. **A 36-year-old FST I patient presents with a 3 cm erythematous hypertrophic scar on the chest that is pruritic. What would be the optimal laser treatment mediums to improve the function and cosmesis of the scar?**
   a. 1064 nm Nd:YAG and fractional 10,600 nm CO_2 laser
   b. 595 nm PDL and fractional 10,600 nm CO_2 laser
   c. 694 nm ruby and 2940 nm erbium:YAG
   d. 1064 nm Nd:YAG and 595 nm PDL

2. **A 60-year-old FST II patient presents with diffuse photodamage and deep, static rhytides presents for consultation. What laser treatment modality would you recommend for this patient?**
   a. 755 nm alexandrite
   b. 595 nm pulsed dye
   c. 1064 nm Nd:YAG
   d. 10,600 nm carbon dioxide

3. **What is the chromophore for PDL?**
   a. Hemoglobin
   b. Melanin
   c. Water
   d. Bilirubin

4. **Which of the following lasers penetrates the skin the deepest?**
   a. 595 nm PDL
   b. 694 nm ruby laser
   c. 755 nm alexandrite laser
   d. 1064 Nd:YAG laser

5. **What is the treatment of choice for a facial capillary vascular malformation (PWS)?**
   a. 595 nm PDL
   b. 10,600 nm CO_2 laser
   c. 2940 nm erbium:YAG laser
   d. 1550 nm erbium-doped glass laser

1. **Answer: b.** The use of the 595 nm and 10,600 nm fractional CO_2 lasers serve as the cornerstones of laser treatment for hypertrophic scars. Through controlled damage to the dermal microvasculature, the 595 nm PDL generates a hypoxic environment that results in collagen fiber heating, realignment, and decreased collagen type III deposition; decreased fibroblast proliferation; and histamine release that decreases fibroblast activity. The 10,600 nm fractional CO_2 laser has been shown to increase elasticity and extensibility of hypertrophic scars through the ablation of scar tissue, upregulation of matrix metalloproteinases facilitating the degradation of fibrotic collagen and clearing the way for neocollagenesis. This benefit has been shown to extend beyond the area of treatment and create a collagen subtype profile similar to that of nonwounded skin.

2. **Answer: d.** Of the laser treatment modalities listed, the fully ablative 10,600 nm fractional carbon dioxide laser is the best treatment option to perform cosmetic laser resurfacing. Through the ablation and coagulation of the epidermis and superficial papillary dermis, the patient will experience significant improvements in photodamage and rhytidosis.

3. **Answer: a.** Hemoglobin, particularly the oxyhemoglobin subtype, is the chromophore for the 595 nm PDL (see Figure 24.4).

4. **Answer: d.** Laser wavelength and depth are directly proportional until water transitions to the primary chromophore (>1100 nm), at which point laser penetration decreases owing to the ubiquity and highly absorptive nature of water (see Figure 24.3).

5. **Answer: a.** Capillary vascular malformations (PWSs) are heterogeneous and are composed of blood vessels of varying sizes and oxygenation located within the superficial and deep dermis. The 595 nm PDL has represented the gold standard of treatment for PWSs over the past 30 years. Early initialization of treatment may result in virtual elimination of the PWS.

PART III

■ CONGENITAL ANOMALIES AND PEDIATRIC PLASTIC SURGERY

CHAPTER 25 Cleft Lip and Palate: Embryology, Principles, and Treatment

Russell E. Ettinger and Steven R. Buchman

KEY POINTS

- Cleft lip and palate exist along a morphologic continuum, whereas isolated cleft palate is a distinct entity with a unique etiopathogenesis.
- The critical period for cleft lip and palate embryologic development is 4 to 7 weeks. Cleft lip results from failure of fusion of the medial nasal process and the maxillary prominence. Cleft palate results from failure of fusion of the palatal shelves.
- A key tenant of unilateral cleft lip repair is to restore vertical lip height which is done through the application of well-known plastic surgery principles including curvilinear incisions, Z-plasties, geometric flaps, and by borrowing from adjacent tissues.
- Timing of cleft palate repair should occur before 1 year of age when critical language develops. Failure to repair the palate leads to maladaptive compensatory misarticulations.
- The hard palate and soft palate clefts should be considered as individual entities with the repair technique dictated by the underlying cleft morphology.
- Optimal management of patients with cleft lip and palate is provided by a coordinated multidisciplinary team of professionals including plastic surgeons, pediatricians, pediatric otolaryngologists, speech pathologists, pediatric dentists, orthodontists, oral surgeons, audiologists, neuropsychologists, social workers, geneticists, and clinic coordinators.
- Secondary surgical correction of hypernasal speech–associated velopharyngeal insufficiency must be balanced with the risk of the emergence of obstructive sleep apnea secondary to narrowing of the nasopharyngeal airway.
- Many cleft lip and palate patients will require secondary orthognathic surgery to correct persistent dentofacial deformity and midface hypoplasia with either conventional orthognathic osteotomies or via distraction osteogenesis for larger advancements.

Cleft lip and cleft palate are the most common congenital craniofacial anomalies treated by plastic surgeons. The degree of phenotypic variation within cleft lip and palate (CL/P) remains one of the most challenging aspects of cleft care and necessitates a broad understanding of the embryologic development, normative and anomalous anatomy, functional impairments, and the social impact of cleft deformities. Although plastic surgeons maintain a central role in treating cleft pathology, a multidisciplinary team of pediatricians, otolaryngologists, oral surgeons, sleep medicine specialists, orthodontists, dentists, nurses, speech pathologists, audiologists, social workers, geneticists, and cleft team coordinators are all required to provide the highest level of longitudinal care for patients.

EMBRYOLOGY

During the third week of gestation, proliferation of neural crest–derived mesenchyme from the first and second pharyngeal arches form the frontonasal prominence, paired maxillary, and mandibular prominences. The neural crest cells within these primordial structures ultimately differentiate into skeletal muscle, connective tissue, bone, and cartilage that comprise the face. At the end of the fourth week of gestation, nasal placodes develop within the frontonasal prominence and invaginate to form nasal pits. The ridges of tissue along the medial and lateral aspects of these pits form into the medial and lateral nasal prominences (**Figure 25.1**). The medial nasal prominence serves as the precursor to the nasal tip, columella, philtrum, and premaxilla. The lateral nasal prominence is the precursor to the nasal ala. During the subsequent 2 weeks the paired maxillary prominences grow and push the medial nasal prominences toward the midline and eventually obliterate the cleft between the medial nasal prominences and the maxillary prominences. Failure of the medial nasal prominence and maxillary prominence to fuse gives rise to the various forms of cleft lip. The upper lip is therefore a composite structure composed of the philtrum from the fused medial nasal prominences and the lateral lip elements from the maxillary prominences (see Figure 25.1). The lower lip and jaw derive from the bilateral mandibular prominences, which fuse across the midline.

Palatogenesis initiates during the sixth week of development and coincides with the medial growth of the maxillary prominences. As the medial nasal prominences are pushed toward the midline, they fuse to form the intermaxillary segment. The intermaxillary segment is made up of an outer labial component which gives rise to the philtrum and an inner bony palatal component that includes the four maxillary incisors and the primary palate to lie anterior to the incisive foramen. The portion of the palate posterior to the incisive foramen is derived from two outgrowths from the paired maxillary prominences called the lateral palatine shelves. The initial growth of the palatine shelves is obliquely downward on either side of the embryologic tongue. In the seventh week of development, the palatine shelves assume a horizontal orientation, right before left, and fuse in the midline with each other and the nasal septum. As such the palatal midline fuses in an anterior to posterior direction with fusion of the hard palate complete by the 10th week and soft palate fusion achieved by the 12th week. Failure of fusion along the axis of the primary to secondary palate results in the development of cleft palate and explains varying degrees of cleft palate phenotypes. Direct obstruction of palatine shelf fusion is also implicated in Pierre Robin sequence, whereby a small mandible results in a retropositioned tongue (glossoptosis) and a cleft palate originating from mechanical obstruction rather than from a failure of embryologic fusion.

EPIDEMIOLOGY

The incidence of CL/P varies depending on ethnicity, geographic location, and socioeconomic factors. Reported rates for CL/P are highest among Native Americans, 3.6/1000 newborns; followed by

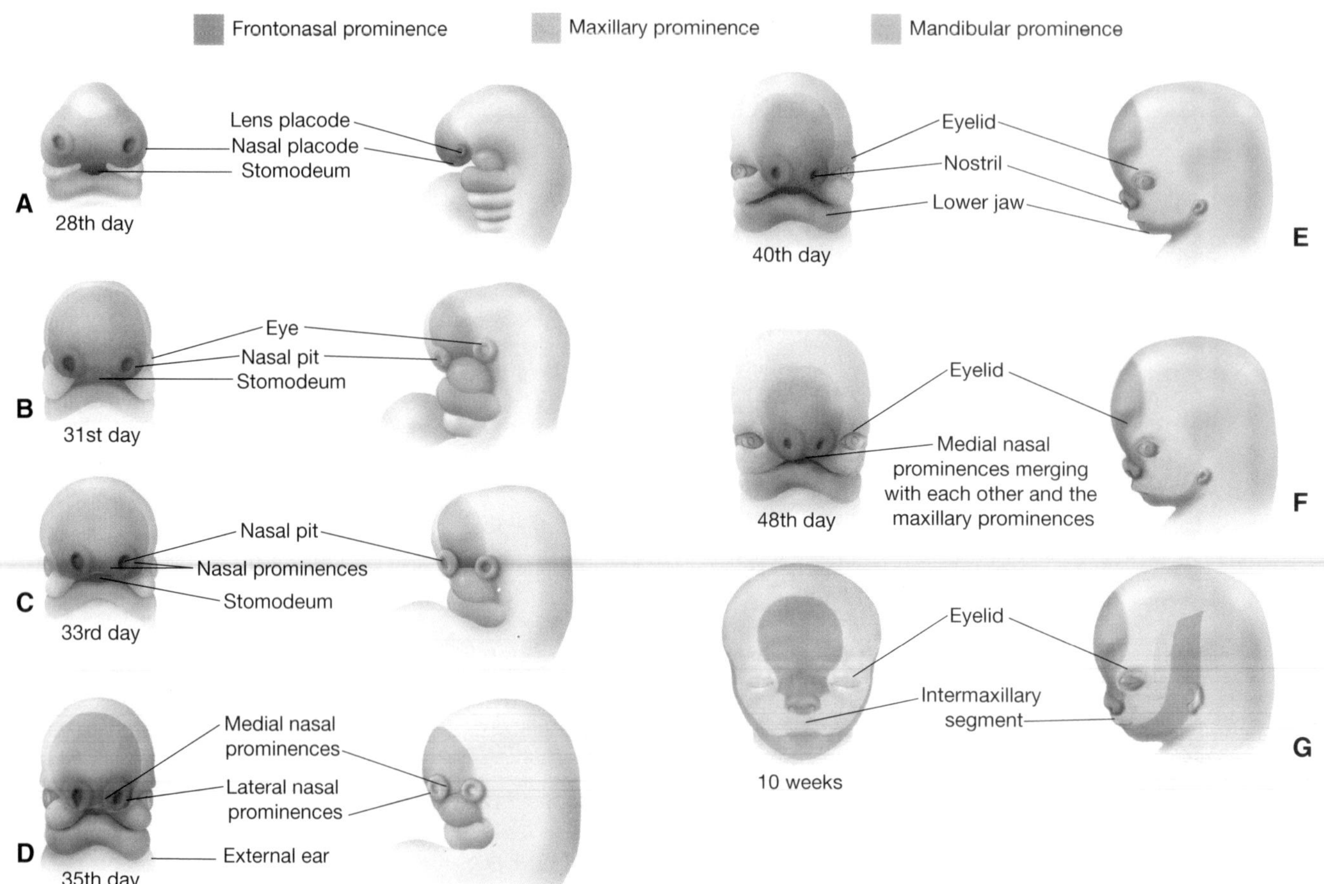

FIGURE 25.1. Embryologic development of the human face from the gestational age of 28 days through 10 weeks. **F.** Fusion of maxillary prominences with the medial nasal prominence during the seventh to eighth week of development.

Japanese, 2.1/1000 newborns; Chinese, 1.7/1000 newborns; and Caucasians, 1.0/1000 newborns. Rates remain the lowest among African Americans, 0.3/1000 newborns.[1,2] Geographic variation is also seen as children of Asian descent born in the United States demonstrate a lower incidence of CL/P relative to Asian children born in their ethnic country of origin. Epidemiologic studies also reveal a higher incidence of CL/P at lower socioeconomic levels.[3] Gender variation is also observed with 2:1 male-to-female gender predominance for CL/P versus a 1:2 male-to-female gender predominance for isolated cleft palate.[4] Delayed fusion of the palatal shelves in females has been proposed as a contributing factor for the higher incidence of isolated cleft palate in females. Morphologically, left unilateral clefts are the most common followed by right unilateral clefts and bilateral clefts with a 6:3:1 ratio. This phenomenon may have its origin in embryogenesis as the left palatine process attains a horizontal position after the right palatine process, giving rise to a higher incidence of left unilateral cleft palates. Isolated CL/P remains more common than isolated cleft palate which is more common than isolated cleft lip with a 5:3:2 ratio. The inheritance of CL/P has a multifactorial etiology, comprising both environmental and genetic factors. For families with a history of CL/P, the risk to subsequent children is dependent on familial involvement. If one child or one parent has CL/P, then there is a 4% risk to subsequent children. If two children have CL/P, the risk increases to 9%. If one child and a parent have CL/P, then the risk increases to 17%. For patients with syndromic etiologies for CL/P, such as van der Woude syndrome, the risk to subsequent children follows Mendelian inheritance patterns. Therefore, if one parent has van der Woude syndrome (autosomal dominant inheritance), the risk to subsequent children being born with CL/P is 50%.

CLASSIFICATION AND SPECTRUM OF CLEFT PATHOLOGY

Although CL/P exist on a morphologic continuum, isolated cleft palate (CP) is a separate entity with its own unique etiopathogenesis. Orofacial clefts limited to the lip and palate are distinct from craniofacial clefts as classified by Tessier, which can involve the mouth, cheeks, eyes, ears, nose, forehead, and hairline.[5] Orofacial clefts are broadly categorized as nonsyndromic CL/P, nonsyndromic CP, syndromic CL/P, and syndromic CP. Syndromic clefts occur as a component of a multiple congenital anomaly syndrome, follow Mendelian genetic inheritance patterns, or arise in the setting of a known teratogenic exposure.[6] Nonsyndromic clefts are isolated anomalies without concurrent physical or developmental defects. When clefts are classified anatomically based on the extent of tissue involvement, they are noted to be unilateral or bilateral and incomplete or complete. Unilateral CL/P involves a cleft of the lip and/or premaxilla on a single side of the face versus a bilateral CL/P which demonstrates clefts of both the right and left lip and premaxilla. Incomplete cleft lip is defined as a partial cleft of the lip without extension across the nasal sill. Complete cleft lips are defined as a confluent cleft of the lip extending into the nasal floor. Incomplete cleft palate is a partial cleft of the soft palate (velum) and/or secondary hard palate but does not involve the primary palate (alveolus). A complete cleft palate is defined as a cleft extending the entire length of the primary and secondary palate (**Figure 25.2**).

Numerous classification systems for CL/P have previously been described. No system is ubiquitous; knowledge of the common classification schemes helps solidify an understanding of the different cleft

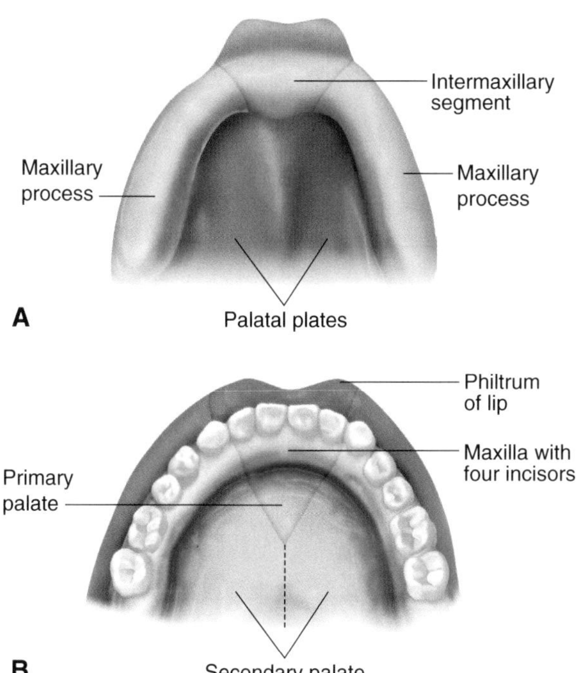

FIGURE 25.2. A. Intermaxillary segment and the maxillary processes. **B.** Intermaxillary segment giving rise to the philtrum of the upper lip, four incisor teeth, and primary palate. Bilateral maxillary processes form palatal plates which fuse in the midline to form the secondary palate.

subtypes. Veau classification delineates clefts into four categories[7] (**Figure 25.3**).

Class I: cleft of the soft palate
Class II: cleft of the hard and soft palate up to the incisive foramen
Class III: clefts of the soft and hard palate extending unilaterally through the alveolus
Class IV: clefts of the soft and hard palate extending bilaterally through the alveolus

The critique of the Veau classification system is that it lacks terminology to describe isolated clefts of the lip. Kernahan and Stark challenged the use of morphology alone for the basis of cleft classification and suggested that characterization should be based on the embryologic origins of the primary and secondary palate. Kernahan and Stark therefore classified clefts into three groups[8]:

1. Clefts of structures anterior to the incisive foramen
2. Clefts of structures posterior to the incisive foramen
3. Clefts affecting structures anterior and posterior to the incisive foramen

This mostly descriptive classification was later refined into a pictorial form of the Kernahan striped-Y diagram (**Figure 25.4A**).[9] The striped-Y simplified record keeping and allowed classification of clefts to become a visual rather than cognitive exercise. An extension of Kernahan striped-Y was Kriens LAHSHAL classification involving a right-to-left palindromic/pictorial system to characterize cleft patterns. The LAHSHAL system used periods (.) to denote normal anatomy, asterisks (*) for microform or submucous clefts, lowercase letters (l, a, h, s) for incomplete clefts of a region, and uppercase letters (L, A, H, S) to denote complete clefts of a region (**Figure 25.4B**).

Each of these classification systems has its merits and shortcomings, and they are currently implemented to varying degrees in cleft centers across the country. Agreement on the best classification system for CL/P remains elusive with ongoing research directed toward new acronymic shorthand forms. Until consensus is achieved, the clinician should be well versed at providing an accurate description of the cleft phenotype in longhand form to include a description of the side (right versus left), laterality (unilateral or bilateral), severity of the cleft (complete or incomplete), and anatomic location structures involved (lip, alveolus, hard palate, and soft palate).[10]

Microform Cleft Lip

The microform cleft lip is characterized by mild notching at the vermillion cutaneous junction, deficiency of vermillion, indented mucosa, and an elevation of the involved cupid's bow relative to the uninvolved side (**Figure 25.5A**). Although the external deformity appears mild, there is typically aberrant insertion of the underlying orbicularis oris muscle into the philtral ridge on the involved side resulting in muscular depression along the philtral line with prominence of the medial component of the philtral ridge. The nasal deformity associated with microform cleft lip is variable but typically demonstrates some degree of lower lateral alar slumping, horizontal orientation of the nostril, depression of the nostril sill, and cephalo-retrodisplacement of the alar base. Surgical repair of the microform cleft can be tailored to the degree of the labial and nasal deformity with lenticular excision (straight-line), modified Z-plasty, or full cheiloplasty repairs all being reported.[11,12]

Unilateral Cleft Lip

Incomplete unilateral cleft lip is the morphologic continuation from a microform cleft with varying degrees of separation of the central and lateral lip elements. Separation that is greater than 3 mm in height compared with the Cupid's bow on the uninvolved side defines a true incomplete cleft lip from a microform cleft. Complete orbicularis oris muscle disruption is the hallmark of a true cleft lip; however, if the cleft extends to less than two-thirds the height of the lip, there may be intact orbicularis oris muscle fibers traversing the superior aspect of an incomplete cleft. A cleft maintaining only a small skin bridge at the nasal sill is known as a Simonart band and intrinsically lacks underlying orbicularis fibers. A complete cleft with a Simonart band can be differentiated from an incomplete cleft by the presence of an underlying complete alveolar cleft. In complete unilateral cleft lip, there is pathologic insertion of the orbicularis oris muscle onto the alar base on the cleft side and the base of the columella on the noncleft side. The pars marginalis (the orbicularis oris below the vermillion lip) is attenuated with loss of the white roll as it continues into the cleft margin. Noordhoff point is a critical landmark for cleft lip repair and

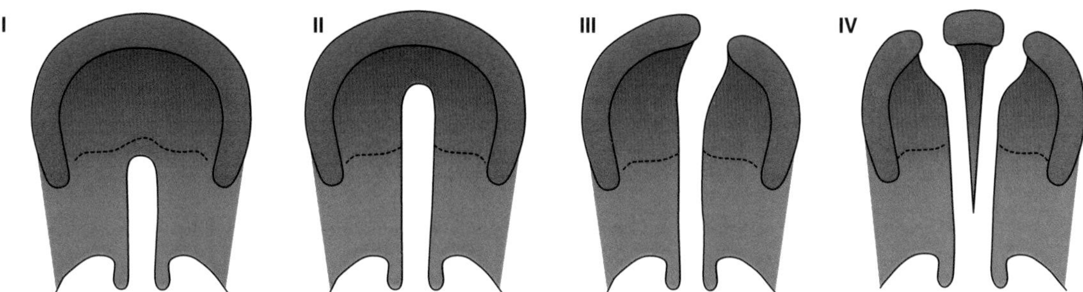

FIGURE 25.3. Veau classification of cleft palate. Class I: Soft palate cleft. Class II: Incomplete cleft of hard and soft palate. Class III: Unilateral complete cleft. Class IV: Bilateral complete cleft.

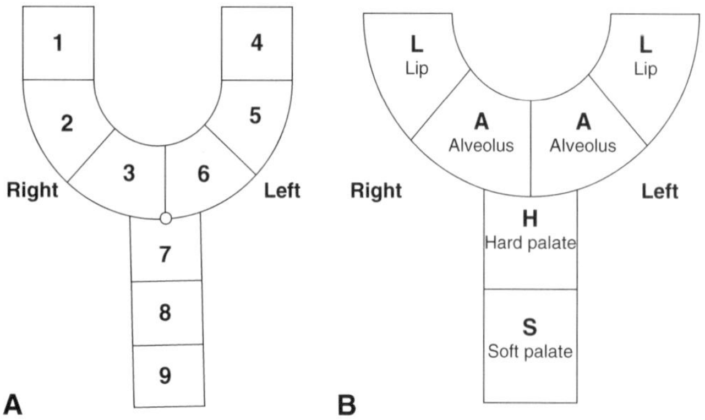

1 4 2 5 3 6 Right Left 7 8 9

A

L Lip L Lip A Alveolus A Alveolus Right Left H Hard palate S Soft palate

B

FIGURE 25.4. **A.** Kernahan striped-Y. **B.** LAHSHAL nomenclature system. Periods (.) denote normal anatomy, asterisks (*) signify microform or submucous clefts, lowercase letters (l, a, h, s) denote for incomplete clefts, and uppercase letters (L, A, H, S) signify complete clefts. For example LAHS… signifies a complete right unilateral cleft lip, alveolus, hard palate, and soft palate.

is determined where the cleft side vermillion height is at its greatest and typically coincides with the last point at which the white is fully defined.[13] Vertical lip height is diminished on the noncleft side with an increasing paucity of vermillion as it tracks into the cleft margin. The cleft nasal deformity associated with unilateral cleft lip is well characterized and includes lower lateral cartilage hypoplasia, flattening of the cleft side alar dome, lack of upper lateral and lower lateral cartilage overlap, subluxation of the lower lateral cartilage, a horizontal orientation of the nostril, and alar base displacement posteriorly and superiorly due to the underlying maxillary hypoplasia. The caudal septum and anterior nasal spine are typically deviated toward the noncleft side, resulting in deflection of the nasal tip to the noncleft side.

Bilateral Cleft Lip

Bilateral cleft lip exists on a morphologic spectrum analogous to unilateral cleft lip with varying degrees of cleft severity. Although the most common presentation is symmetrical bilateral complete clefts, incomplete forms and microform clefts can be seen with asymmetry in cleft severity from side to side. The hallmark of bilateral cleft lip includes two lateral labial-alveolus-palatine elements (lateral segments) and an intervening central prolabial and premaxillary segment. In complete clefts, the lack of connection of the premaxillary segment to the lateral segments results in varying degrees of premaxillary protrusion with concurrent posterior and medial collapse of the lateral segments. The ultimate extension of this process can result in a *locked out* premaxilla whereby the premaxilla sits entirely outside the arch of the collapsed lateral segments making correction exceedingly challenging without adjunctive interventions.

The bilateral cleft nasal deformity includes widening of the alar bases and fattening of the alar domes secondary to subluxation of the lower lateral cartilages from their normal anatomic position overlying the upper lateral cartilages.[14,15] Underdevelopment or absence of the anterior nasal spine causes posterolateral displacement of the medial crural footplates and contributes to a lack of nasal projection, a broad nasal tip, and significant foreshortening of the columella. There is an absence of a normal gingival labial sulcus within the premaxillary/prolabial segment which is devoid of orbicularis muscle. The lack of orbicularis fibers within the prolabium results in the absence of philtral columns, midline philtral depression, and central vermillion tubercle, all of which are established by the intricate decussation of orbicularis oris fibers in the normal lip. Invariably, the foreshortened columella and paucity of prolabial skin makes primary reconstruction of both the cutaneous lip and columella difficult without causing secondary tethering and further deprojection of the nasal tip. This challenge has been lessened with the advent of presurgical molding

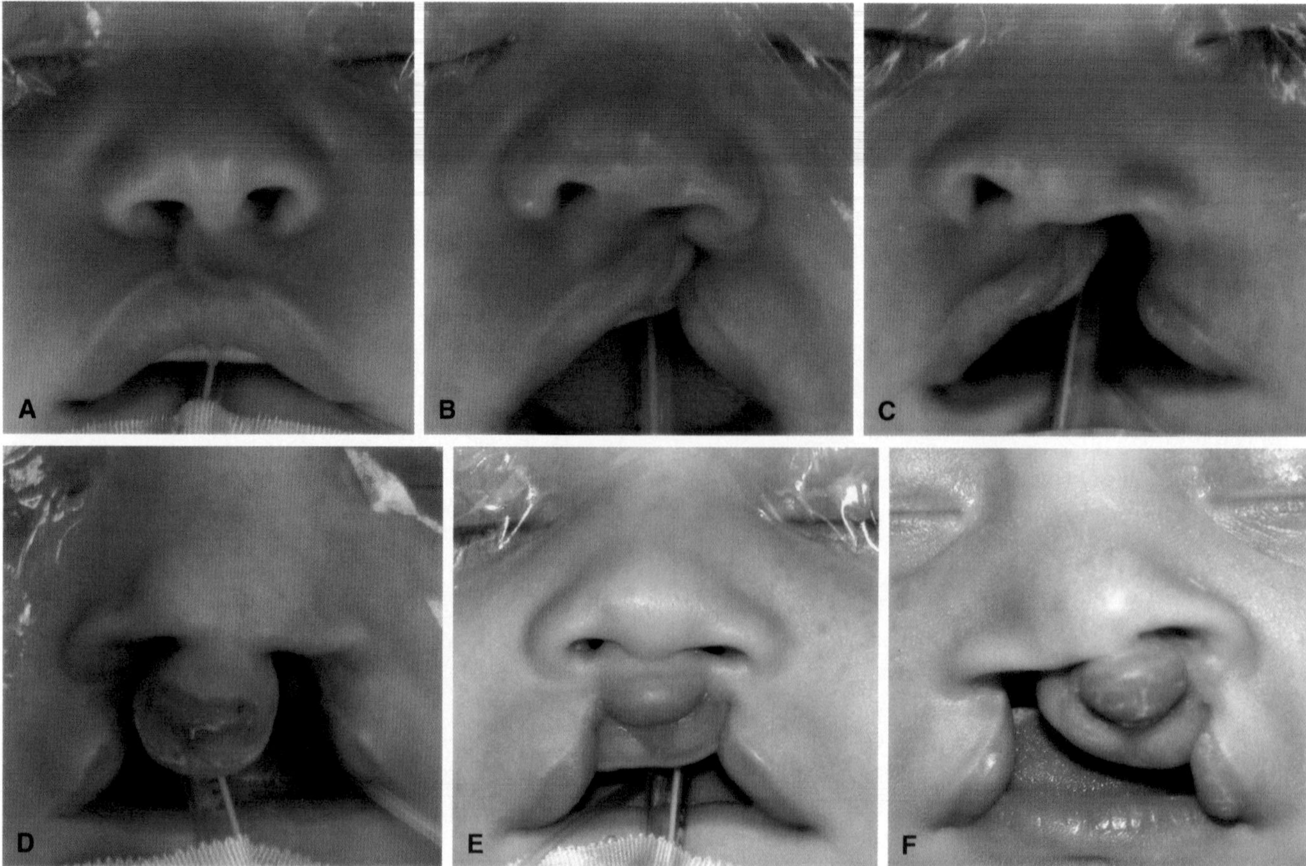

FIGURE 25.5. The spectrum of cleft lip types. **A.** Microform unilateral cleft lip. **B.** Incomplete unilateral cleft lip. **C.** Complete unilateral cleft lip. **D.** Complete bilateral cleft lip. **E.** Incomplete bilateral cleft lip. **F.** Right unilateral complete cleft lip and left unilateral incomplete cleft lip.

techniques to aid in restoring the arch form, narrowing the nasal base, and elongating the columella.

Cleft Lip and Palate

The presence of a cleft palate in addition to a cleft lip introduces additional functional concerns beyond the appearance of the patient. Combined clefts of the lip and palate can affect the nasal floor, alveolus, secondary hard palate, or soft palate. Infants with cleft palate have open communication between the oral cavity and nasal cavity often preventing them from generating the prerequisite negative intraoral pressure for nursing. Therefore, infants with cleft palate may require specialty bottles and nipples for free flow of breast milk or formula without the reliance on negative pressure for delivery. Soft palate clefts result in disruption of the underlying muscles which are responsible for palatal elevation and velopharyngeal closure, as well as inner ear drainage via the Eustachian tube. Specifically, the levator veli palatini (primary palatal elevator) and the tensor veli palatini (secondary palatal elevator and modulator of the Eustachian tube) demonstrate anomalous insertion into the posterior hard palate instead of the midline palatal aponeurosis. The inability to close the velopharyngeal port results in pathologic speech development and compensatory misarticulations due to the inability to separate the nasopharynx and oropharynx with phonation. Impaired Eustachian tube function increases the risk of middle ear infections in patients with cleft palate, leading to hearing loss if not properly treated.[16] The presence of a cleft palate in addition to a cleft lip requires additional surgery for palatal closure around 12 months of age prior to the emergence of early speech development. Tympanostomy and placement of pressure equalization tubes are typically performed at the time of primary palatoplasty.

Isolated Cleft Palate

The presence of an isolated cleft palate should warrant additional genetic evaluation because nearly half of all isolated clefts occur in the setting of an associated syndrome or anomaly. Isolated cleft patients should also be evaluated for the findings associated with Pierre Robin sequence including micrognathia, glossoptosis, cleft palate, airway obstruction, and feeding difficulties. Pierre Robin is not a syndrome but rather a sequence whereby a single event leads to a sequential chain of anomalies. By contrast, a syndrome represents a group of anomalies that occur together due to a single underlying abnormality such as a gene mutation. In the case of Pierre Robin sequence, micrognathia results in decreased oral cavity volume and glossoptosis or an abnormal posterior and superior positioning of the tongue. The retroposition of the tongue during embryogenesis physically impedes of the descent and fusion of the lateral palatal shelves resulting in a characteristic wide U-shaped cleft palate. Although feeding difficulties are commonly seen in Pierre Robin sequence as with any cleft palate, management of airway obstruction secondary to micrognathia and glossoptosis dominate the early treatment. Supplemental oxygen and prone positioning may be adequate to stabilize the airway, but temporary intubation, tongue lip adhesions, and mandibular distraction may be required in severe cases.[17]

Submucous Cleft Palate

Submucous cleft palate is defined by a classic triad of findings including a bifid uvula, notching of the posterior hard palate, and midline mucosal attenuation known as the zona pellucida. Anatomically, there is anterior displacement of the levator veli palatini muscles onto the notched hard palate leading to variable degrees of velopharyngeal dysfunction (VPD) despite the lack of an overt cleft. The subtle physical examination findings in submucous cleft palate can result in delayed diagnosis, although evidence suggests that late-presenting patients may still benefit from palatoplasty beyond the age of critical language development.[18-20]

PRESURGICAL ORTHOPEDICS AND SURGICAL MOLDING

There are several different modalities that harness the plasticity of developing facial tissue and aid in the correction of the cleft deformity prior to definitive surgical repair. Methods include both active and passive forms of presurgical molding. Passive methods include lip taping, nasoalveolar molding, and lip adhesion which rely on applying a static tension or compressive force to enact change in the facial form. Active methods such as the Latham device exert a progressive and tunable force across tissues to create the desired effect.

Lip taping applies surgical tape across the lip elements and is initiated as early as the first week of life. Taping provides a preliminary approximation of the greater and lesser lip elements with medialization of the cleft side alar base. The restraining force provided by taping has been shown to significantly reduce alveolar gaps.[21] Lip taping is simple and cost-effective but requires a substantial degree of diligence on behalf of the parents or caregivers. Lip adhesion is an operative procedure to reapproximate lip elements surgically without disruption of the key landmarks required for definitive lip repair. Lip adhesions have been demonstrated to significantly reduce alveolar gaps and normalize preoperative cleft severity but at the cost of an additional operation prior to definitive repair.[22]

Nonalveolar molding (NAM) uses the serial application of a custom intraoral appliance with nasal extensions with the goal of aligning the alveolar segments and helping to correct the preoperative cleft nasal deformity by supporting the alar domes, lengthening the columella, and improving nasal tip projection and symmetry.[23] Although many studies have demonstrated initial improvement in preoperative nasal and alveolar arch forms, the longevity of these changes on longitudinal follow-up remain uncertain.[24-26] Frequent visits and expertise in the fabrication and modification of NAM appliances limits the generalizability of this technique despite its clear presurgical benefits.

Active presurgical molding, as advocated by Latham, uses a pin-retained device that is surgically implanted into the alveolar segments.[27] Following placement, the device is activated by turning an orthodontic screw to bring the alveolar segments into approximation. In bilateral cases the device was used to rein in the premaxilla while simultaneously expanding the palatal arch. However, active methods of presurgical molding are less ubiquitous owing to concerns over secondary growth disturbance.[28]

Ultimately, presurgical orthopedics and molding is a beneficial adjunct to definitive cleft repair and aids the surgeon by reducing tension, aligning the alveolar arch form, restricting unwanted growth, and mitigating secondary deformities. The choice of modality should be determined based on cleft morphology, patient and family factors, hospital resources, and surgeon preference, as each technique has its own merits and drawbacks.

SURGICAL CORRECTION

Timing

Cleft care is truly a longitudinal and multidisciplinary endeavor requiring numerous interventions. The operations start in the postnatal period and extending into early adulthood. A timeline for interventions and operations in CL/P care is summarized in Table 25.1.

Unilateral Cleft Lip

The primary hallmark of the unilateral cleft lip deformity is a lack of vertical lip height caused by attenuation of the lip tissues as they enter the cleft margin. Recognition of this soft tissue deficiency by plastic surgeons throughout history has been the primary driving force behind the development of nearly all forms of unilateral cleft lip repair. Despite increasing complexity and nuance, all cleft lip repair techniques function to increase vertical lip height through the

TABLE 25.1. TIMING OF CLEFT LIP AND PALATE TREATMENT

Age	Treatment/Intervention	Cleft Team Member
Prenatal	In utero diagnostic ultrasound of lip and palate and referral to cleft team if cleft identified	Multidisciplinary
Newborn	Feeding assessment, medical evaluation, newborn hearing screening, parent/caregiver counseling, genetic referral	Multidisciplinary
0–3 months	Presurgical versus surgical molding. Additional audiologic assessment if newborn screening abnormal	Orthodontist, plastic surgeon, audiologist
3 months (or following completion of molding)	Primary cleft lip repair, +/– primary tip rhinoplasty, gingivoperiosteoplasty	Plastic surgeon
9–12 months	Primary cleft palate repair and placement of myringotomy tubes	Plastic surgeon, otolaryngologist
12–36 months	Prelinguistic speech screening (<2 years) versus formal speech evaluation (>2 years) for diagnosis of velopharyngeal insufficiency (VPI)	Speech pathologist
3–5 years	Secondary speech surgery (palatal lengthening, dynamic sphincter pharyngoplasty, or posterior pharyngeal flap)	Plastic surgeon
School-aged years	Treatment or revision of secondary cleft lip and nasal deformities	Plastic surgeon
7–9 years (mixed dentition prior to eruption of permanent canine)	Alveolar cleft bone grafting	Plastic surgeon, oral surgeon
Adolescent years 10–19 years	First-stage orthodontics, definitive versus revision open tip rhinoplasty, second-stage decompensating presurgical orthodontics	Orthodontist, plastic surgeon, oral surgeon
Early adulthood/skeletal maturity (around 16 years for female, 18 years or later for males)	Orthognathic surgery (LeFort I advancement +/– mandibular osteotomy)	Plastic surgeon, oral surgeon

application of well-known plastic surgery principles. These principles include the use of curvilinear incisions, Z-plasty, and geometric flaps to borrow from adjacent tissue to augment the deficient central elements. When one approaches cleft lip repair from this mindset, the rationale and complexities of the varying techniques becomes more evident.

Vertical lip height deficiency was first addressed in the modern era by Rose and Thompson who utilized curvilinear or *paring* incisions around the cleft margin to functionally increase the length of the incision line during subsequent straight-line closure (**Figure 25.6A**).[29] The lengthening of the incision line via curvilinear incisions, now known as the *Rose-Thompson effect*, was a significant improvement over earlier straight-line techniques which simply approximated the lip elements with preservation of the vertical height discrepancy to the noncleft side. Introduction of the Z-plasty to cleft lip repair to further correct vertical lip height deficiency is credited to LeMesurier (**Figure 25.6B**).[30] The application of a Z-plasty was an elegant solution to cleft lip repair in that it gained lip height at the expense of width to simultaneously correct the rotational component of the medial lip element. The main critique of LeMesurier technique is the low placement of the Z-plasty limbs, which inevitably cross both the cleft side philtral column and central philtrum.

Tennison modified the LeMesurier repair and reoriented the Z-plasty so that one limb would coincide with the peak of the cleft side Cupid's bow, thereby preserving the natural curvature of the central Cupid's bow nadir (Figure 25.6B).[31] Tennison's use of a malleable wire to mark the Z-plasty limbs was refined by Randall, who introduced standardized measurements of the cleft and noncleft side philtral heights.[32] The difference between the normal and cleft side philtral columns was used to determine the base width of the triangular flap used to augment the vertical lip height on the cleft side (**Figure 25.6C**). The formulaic and numerically driven Randall-Tennison repair is highly reproducible and can be used for wide clefts but has the drawback of creating a long lip with the laterally based triangular flap which also results in a visible scar on the lower philtrum.

Attempts to preserve anatomic boundaries and move incision lines to less conspicuous locations gave rise to the rotation advancement flap repair popularized by Millard.[33] This technique elevates the Z-plasty to just below the nasal sill while simultaneously rotating the central lip element to its normal anatomic position (**Figure 25.6D**). The ability of the rotation flap to reconstitute the deficiency in vertical lip height is contingent upon the back-cut which is made across the midline of the columellar labial junction back toward, but not violating, the noncleft side philtral column. The length of the back-cut is determined in a *cut as you go* fashion relying on the experience of the surgeon to determine the appropriate degree of downward rotation required. The resultant defect created by the back-cut is filled by the leading edge of the advancement flap from the lateral lip correcting the deficiency in vertical lip height. Mobilization of the advancement flap into the defect of the rotation flap simultaneously corrects alar flare and reconstitutes the cleft side nasal sill. The superiorly based triangular *C-flap* then can be rotated medially to lengthen the columella or rotated laterally into the nose to assist with nasal floor closure if there is adequate columellar length. The benefits of the rotation advancement technique include its maximal tissue preservation, versatility, and well-hidden scar within the line of the new philtral column. Numerous modifications have been made to the rotation advancement flap technique including the use of a vertical back-cut onto the columella by Mohler (**Figure 25.6E**) to obviate the need for a horizontal scar across the philtrum and leverage the columellar skin to lengthen the lip.[34] The resultant columellar defect is reconstituted by the C-flap which also contributes to the closure of the nasal floor. Further modification of the Mohler technique by Cutting introduced a laterally based triangular flap within the vermillion at the wet-dry border to further augment the vertical lip height.[35] In total, the Millard rotation advancement flap and its subsequent refinements have made it the most common technique of unilateral left lip repair among plastic surgeons today.[36]

In contrast to the Z-plasty principle used in the rotation advancement flap, the Fisher technique applies several principles from earlier forms of cleft repair to correct the vertical lip height deficiency while creating a scar that fully preserves the anatomic subunits of the lip. The Fisher repair employs a geometric design with triangular flaps akin to the Randall-Tennison technique that further increases vertical lip height by creating *paring* incisions that result in a *Rose-Thompson effect* with the final straight-line closure (**Figure 25.6F**). Although the

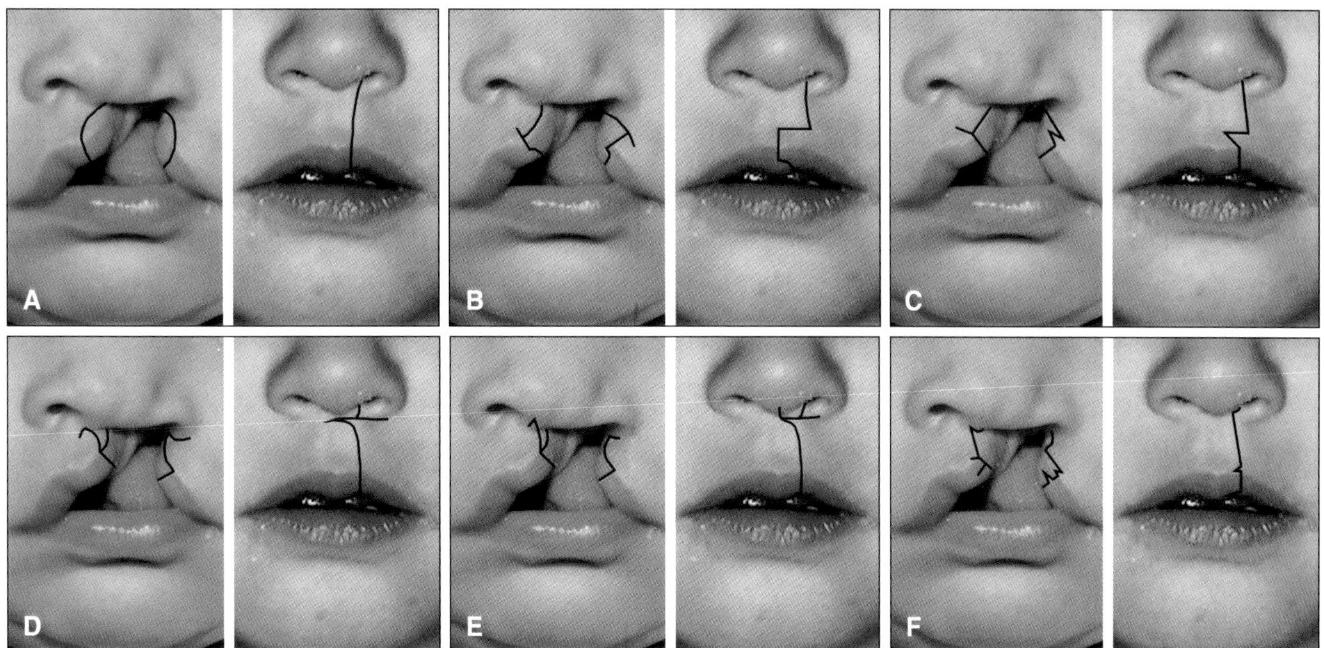

FIGURE 25.6. Cleft lip repairs. **A.** Rose-Thompson. **B.** LeMesurier. **C.** Randall-Tennison. **D.** Millard. **E.** Mohler. **F.** Fisher

Millard repair relies on experience and *cut as you go* methodology, the Fisher repair is highly systematic by relying on 25 landmarks and is much more exacting in its preincision planning. The critique of the Fisher method is that it can be more time-consuming, but its grounding in geometric planning, preservation of anatomic landmarks, and favorable scar positioning has led to its adoption by a subset of plastic surgeons.

Irrespective of the skin incision utilized for cleft lip repair, the appropriate mobilization of the underlying orbicularis oris muscle from its abnormal insertion to the maxilla and its meticulous reapproximation is paramount to the success of the operation. Repair of the muscle reduces tension on the skin closure in addition to reconstituting the oral sphincter. Care should be taken at the inferior border of the muscle to recreate the J shape of the caudal orbicularis or pars marginalis which contributes to the natural pout of the lip. The use of primary rhinoplasty at the time of initial cleft lip repair remains controversial and depends on the severity of the associated cleft nasal deformity. Although some surgeons advocate for formal open rhinoplasty techniques during lip repair, most others have adopted a more conservative approach with judicious undermining of nasal cartilages and percutaneous suturing and/or placements of intranasal stents to achieve significant restoration and reconstruction of the nasal tip at the time of lip repair.

Bilateral Cleft Lip

Historically, bilateral cleft lip repair presented one of the greatest challenges for plastic surgeons. The early difficulties of bilateral cleft lip repair revolved around management of the protruded premaxilla, hypoplastic prolabium, and foreshortened columella. The recognition of significant soft tissue deficiency within the central lip elements gave rise to staged procedures whereby the lateral lip elements were brought into continuity with the prolabium resulting in a widening of the prolabial skin. The additional prolabial skin was then used in a second stage to lengthen the columella via fork flaps or V-Y advancement flaps functioning to bring labial tissue into the foreshortened columella. Unfortunately, early techniques that relied on approximation of the lateral lip segments directly to the prolabium and secondary operations for lengthening the columella led to suboptimal outcomes for several reasons. Relying on the prolabium to reconstitute the entirety of central lip is ill advised given its lack of orbicularis muscle, inadequate vermillion and cutaneous height, and lack of a well-defined white roll. These factors lead to unnatural lip animation, lateral lip bulging from discontinuity of the orbicularis, and a static *whistle deformity* due to an intrinsic lack of vertical lip height of the prolabial segment. Labial and columellar scarring and resultant asymmetry were also a concern given the multiple operations and the use of local flaps for secondary columellar elongation.

A relatively recent paradigm shift in bilateral cleft lip repair occurred with the realization that primary correction of the nasal deformity with alar repositioning could create columellar length rather than relying on cutaneous augmentation from the lip. Early proponents of this technique included McComb and Mulliken, who used rhinoplasty techniques to medialize the domal segments of the lower lateral cartilages, thereby enhancing nasal projection and increasing columellar length.[37,38] The introduction of this concept eliminated the reliance on the hypoplastic prolabium to recreate both the columella and the central lip element. Instead, recruitment of nasal skin allowed the prolabium to be utilized for philtral reconstruction, thereby ushering in the development of the modern bilateral cleft lip repair. Much of the subsequent refinement of the modern bilateral cleft lip repair is attributed to Mulliken, who described several key principles[39]:

- A single-stage repair of both sides of the cleft controls lip symmetry in comparison to staged approaches
- Continuity of the muscular oral sphincter should be achieved via complete mobilization of the orbicularis oris from the lateral lip elements with midline approximation throughout the vertical extent of the lip
- The size and shape of the philtrum should account for subsequent growth of the child to prevent lateral bowing and excessive elongation commonly seen with previous repair techniques
- The tubercle should be constructed from the vermillion of the lateral lip elements and not from the prolabial vermillion
- Deficient nasal tip projection and columellar length can be corrected by repositioning and supporting the lower lateral cartilages at the time of primary lip repair

Today, adherence to these principles as well as the advent of presurgical molding has revolutionized bilateral cleft lip repair (**Figure 25.7**) to the point that the aesthetic results for bilateral lip repairs are on par with or even exceed that of unilateral cleft lips.

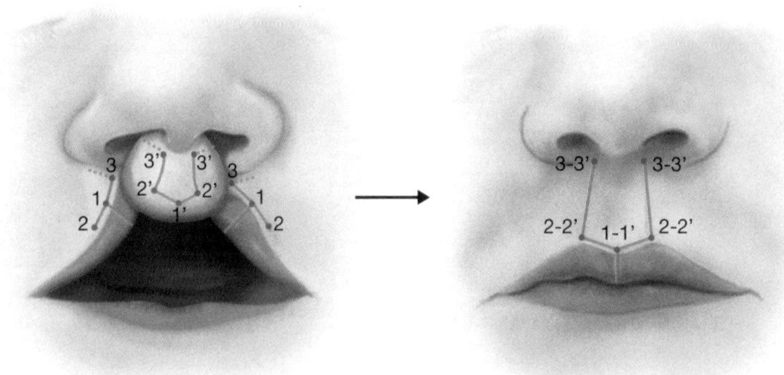

FIGURE 25.7. Preoperative markings (left) and final closure of bilateral cleft lip repair (right). Note the use of the lateral lip elements to recreate the midline vermillion tubercle and the substitution of incision lines for the prolabial white roll. (From Chetta MD, Oppenheimer AJ. Cleft lip. In: Brown DL, Borschel GH, Levi B, eds. *Michigan Manual of Plastic Surgery*. 2nd ed. Philadelphia, PA: Lippincott Williams & Wilkins; 2014:241-252.)

Cleft Palate

In comparison to cleft lip repair which exemplifies the fine balance between aesthetics and function, the objectives of palatoplasty are largely functional in nature. Clefts of the hard palate lead to feeding difficulties due to the inability to generate negative intraoral pressure and allow reflux of food between the nose and mouth. Clefts of the soft palate result in disruption of the velopharyngeal port and subsequent speech dysfunction. Therefore, the primary goals of palatoplasty are to separate the oral and nasal cavities and create a competent velopharyngeal port. Secondary goals include the avoidance of a palatal fistula and the prevention of maxillary growth disturbance.

When attempting to understand the various techniques of palatoplasty, it is beneficial to visualize the hard and soft palate as separate entities. In classic descriptions and illustrations of cleft palate repairs, the hard and soft palate closures were often amalgamated together to encompass a single repair technique. Although this is accurate to the technique of the individual surgeon, it may be confusing to the novice learner. A better approach is to realize that the various hard and soft palate repair techniques can be used interchangeably. The decision of which techniques to employ should be dictated by the underlying cleft morphology (**Table 25.2**).

Hard Palate Closure Techniques

The techniques for hard palate repair are all variations around the design of axially based mucoperiosteal flaps supplied primarily by the greater palatine vessels. Flap elevation in the hard palate universally requires separation of the oral and nasal mucosa which are then mobilized to the midline and reapproximated separately to provide two-layer closure of the hard palate cleft. One of the earliest forms of hard palate repair was the von Langenbeck technique introduced in 1849, which is still used today. The von Langenbeck employs two lateral releasing incisions just medial to the alveolar ridge ending just posterior to the maxillary tuberosity. The midline incision follows the cleft margin at the junction of the oral and nasal mucosa which is then separated to form two leaflets. The bilateral mucoperiosteal flaps are undermined and elevated off the intervening palatal bone between the two incisions by creating two bipedicled flaps based off the greater palatine vessels posteriorly and the sphenopalatine arteries emanating from the incisive foramen anteriorly (**Figure 25.8A**). Nasal closure is achieved first, followed by medialization of the bipedicled flaps to close the oral side in the midline. In the original description, the lateral relaxing incisions are left to heal by secondary intention.

A variation of the von Langenbeck repair is the Veau-Willard-Kilner technique, also known as a V-Y pushback. A similar lateral releasing incision is performed just within the alveolar ridge but is then angled back toward the anterior aspect of the cleft margin to create two posteriorly based mucoperiosteal flaps that can then be *pushed back* in V-Y fashion (**Figure 25.8B**). The Veau-Willard-Kilner repair offers the added benefit of increasing palatal length through the retropositioning of the mucoperiosteal flaps to assist with velopharyngeal competency. The primary critique of this repair is that it results in a large area of denude palate centrally leading to potential maxillary growth disturbance and secondary scar contracture with foreshortening of the initial palatal pushback.[40,41]

The Bardach two-flap palatoplasty was originally described in 1967 and involves extending the lateral releasing incisions around alveolar margin in continuous fashion into the cleft margin. The posteriorly based mucoperichondrial flaps are then extensively undermined to the level of the posterior hard palate. The greater palatine neurovascular bundles are identified and circumferentially dissected for additional mobilization of the mucoperiosteal flaps. The flaps can then be mobilized to the midline following nasal mucosal closure to provide a robust oral closure to the cleft **Figure 25.8C**. In the case of a complete cleft palate, the apices of the Bardach flaps can be transposed across the cleft anteriorly and closed directly behind the

TABLE 25.2. SELECTION OF PALATE REPAIR TECHNIQUE BASED ON CLEFT MORPHOLOGY

Cleft Type	Hard Palate Repair	Soft Palate Repair
Isolated cleft of soft palate (Veau 1)	None, or small midline extension onto hard palate	Intravelar veloplasty or Furlow
Incomplete cleft of hard and soft palate (Veau II)	von Langenbeck, V-Y pushback, or Bardach 2-flap	Intravelar veloplasty or Furlow
Unilateral complete cleft palate (Veau III)	Bardach 2-flap	Intravelar veloplasty or Furlow
Bilateral complete cleft palate (Veau IV)	Bardach 2-flap + vomer flaps	Intravelar veloplasty or Furlow
Submucous cleft palate	None	Intravelar veloplasty or Furlow

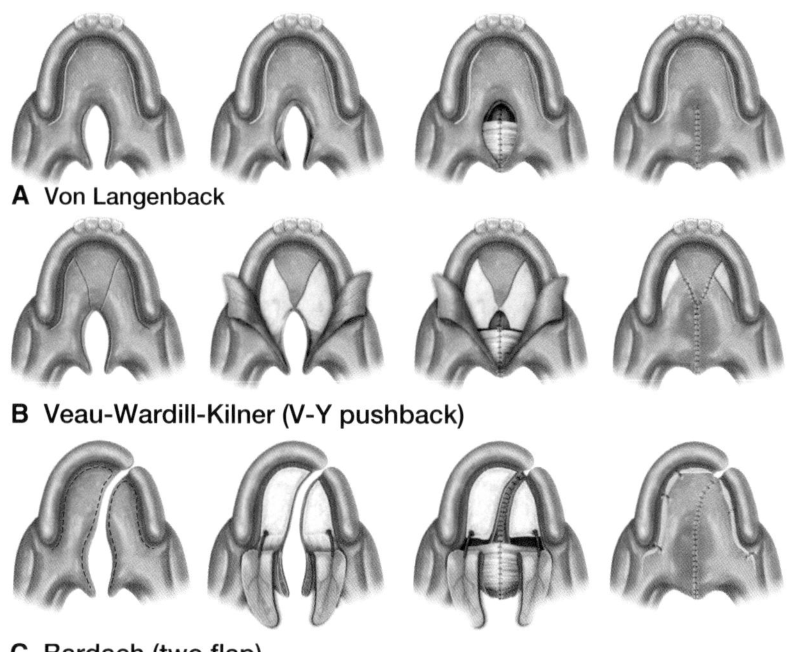

FIGURE 25.8. Hard palate closure techniques. Note that each closure is paired with a soft palate intravelar veloplasty repair in these example images.

alveolar margin, thereby providing an oral closure over the alveolar fistula from the palatal side. The lateral relaxing incision lines can usually be closed loosely. Despite the versatility of the Bardach technique, it does not increase palatal length following flap elevation and inset and therefore is usually paired with a lengthening soft palate repair technique.

For bilateral complete cleft palates, additional flap elevation is required to achieve a durable two-layer hard palate closure. In these instances, mucoperiosteal flaps elevated from the vomer provide additional tissue that can be recruited into the nasal side closure. The original vomer flaps were inferiorly based with incisions high up on the nasal septum with subsequent downward reflection of the mucoperichondrium. Unfortunately, these inferiorly based vomer flaps resulted in a high incidence of maxillary growth disturbance and fistula, leading to their abandonment. The technique was modified with a midline incision on the caudal margin of the vomer with superior reflection of the two septal mucosa flaps in opposite directions. These superiorly based vomer flaps can then be inset to the lateral nasal mucosa to reconstitute the nasal side closure in bilateral clefts. The oral side closure can then be achieved as previously described with the Bardach technique by providing durable two-layer hard palate closure.

Soft Palate Closure Techniques

The soft palate consists of three distinct layers: oral mucosa, muscle layer, and nasal mucosa. Early forms of palate repair consisted of simple midline reapproximation of these structures but failed to correct the aberrant levator muscle insertion to the posterior hard palate. The intravelar veloplasty was the first technique to address the underlying muscle abnormality. This technique requires delamination of all three soft palate layers with complete release of the anterior insertion of the levator muscles from the posterior aspect of the hard palate and midline cleft margin. The levator muscles are then transposed across the midline and reapproximated at the posterior aspect of the soft palate. This technique reconstitutes the velopharyngeal sling resulting in dynamic palatal elevation to separate the oropharynx and nasal pharynx during swallowing and phonation. Additional modifications of this technique including transection of the tensor veli palatini tendon and extensive dissection of the levator muscle from the oral and nasal mucosa for greater mobility of the levator muscles. Despite effectively recreating the normal orientation of the velopharyngeal musculature, the primary critique of the intravelar veloplasty is that it does not significantly increase palatal length.

One of the greatest contributions to cleft palate repair was the introduction of the double opposing Z-plasty technique by Furlow.[42] This elegant repair uses reversed Z-plasties based on the cleft midline to attain simultaneous levator muscle repositioning as well as palatal lengthening through the transposition of the Z-plasty limbs. The first step in the Furlow palatoplasty is to design the oral side Z-plasty. In the Furlow repair, each Z-plasty consists of a combined musculomucosal flap and a contralateral mucosal flap. The musculomucosal flaps are always posteriorly based, and the mucosal flaps are anteriorly based. The most challenging aspect of elevating the Z-plasty flaps is separating the delicate nasal mucosa from the overlying levator muscle. Therefore, for the right-handed surgeon, the left-sided oral Z-plasty is oriented from anterior to posterior and a posteriorly based musculomucosal flap elevated away from the nasal mucosa (**Figure 25.9A**) in forehand fashion. The contralateral right-sided oral Z-plasty incision is oriented posterior to anterior, and an anteriorly based oral mucosa flap is elevated. The subsequent nasal-side Z-plasty is designed as the inverse of oral side with the same principle of the musculomucosal flap being posteriorly based and the mucosal flap being anteriorly based. The nasal-side Z-plasty is transposed moving musculomucosal flap posteriorly and bringing the levator muscle to its normal transverse orientation across the posterior soft palate (**Figure 25.9B**). The oral-size Z-plasty limbs are then transposed and the levator muscles secured to one another under appropriate tension followed by completion of the oral-side closure (**Figure 25.9C**). The primary drawback to the Furlow technique is the sacrifice of width to achieve length resulting in tension transversely across the palatal closure. This makes application of the Furlow technique to wide clefts more challenging. This shortcoming can be remedied through additional hard palate mucoperiosteal undermining, infracturing of the hamulus, or dissection of the greater palatine neurovascular bundle. In addition, moving the cuts of the Z-plasties more posteriorly will result in greater mobility in the flaps, as they are less anchored to the bony tethers of the hard palate and gain distensibility from the looser attachments of the lateral pharyngeal mucosa. The palatal lengthening achieved with the Furlow repair makes it versatile as both a primary repair and a secondary revision procedure for

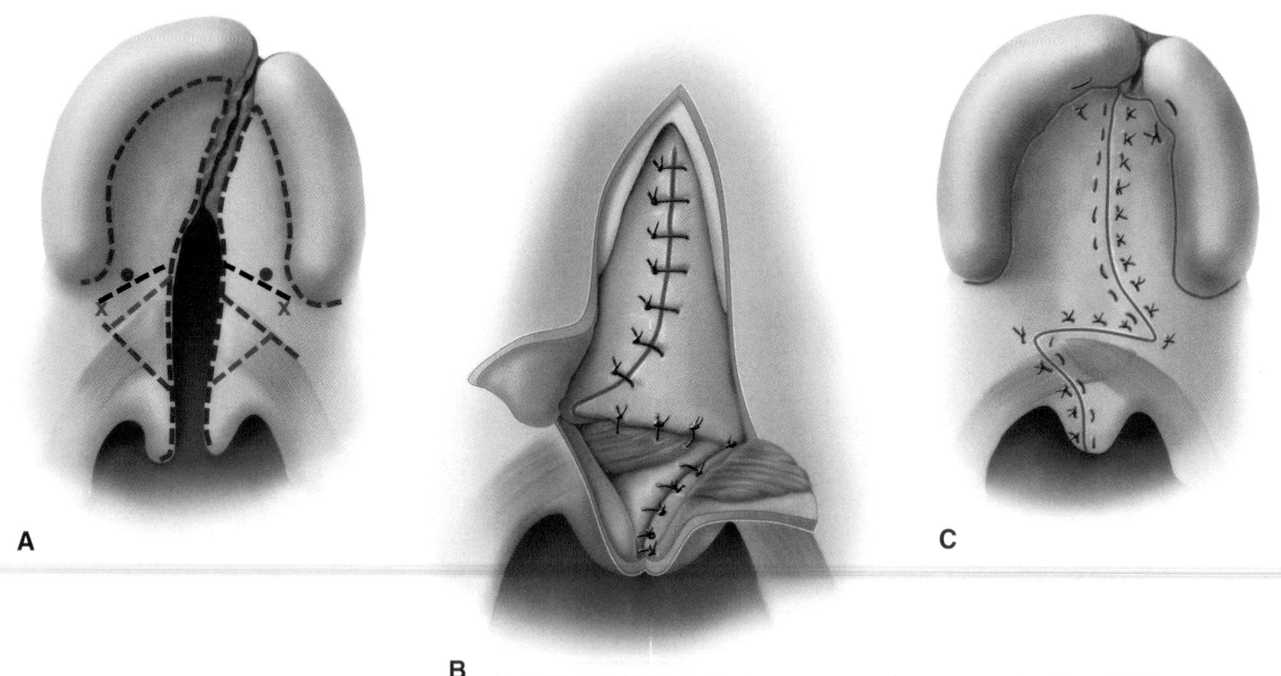

FIGURE 25.9. Furlow double opposing Z-plasty technique. **A.** Design of the incisions: Dotted blue lines mark the oral side Z-plasty with the central limb as the cleft margin. Dotted red lines on the soft palate mark the nasal side Z-plasty. Black dotted lines denote the junction of the hard and soft palate. The X marks the point where the tensor tendon traverses the hamulus and fuses with the levator aponeurosis. Red circles delineate the location of the greater palatine pedicle. **B.** Transposition and inset of the nasal side Z-plasty with reorientation of the right levator muscle to its normal transverse orientation. **C.** Final closure after transposition of the oral side Z-plasty with overlap of the levator muscles in the midline and restoration of the levator sling.

patients with persistent velopharyngeal insufficiency (VPI). Recent retrospective studies have demonstrated that patients undergoing Furlow palatoplasty have improved speech outcomes in comparison with other techniques.[43]

Buccal Fat Pad Flaps

Recent publications have described the significant utility of the buccal fat pads as flaps that can be employed in primary cleft closure.[44] The buccal fat pad can be harvested and delivered into the oral cavity via a simple incision in the buccal sulcus. Once located the fat pad can be mobilized and used to line the open lateral relaxing incision defects in hard palate repairs to protect the exposed palatine vessels as well as prevent secondary scarring and contracture thought to lead to restriction of transverse growth over time. In addition, the buccal fat pad flaps can be used as a middle lamella in the space just behind the posteriorly transposed muscles of an intravelar veloplasty and a Furlow repair. Filling the void with the buccal fat pad flap has the potential to decrease the incidence of fistula formation as well as prevent secondary contracture and retropositioning of the transposed muscles of the soft palate after primary repair.[44]

Secondary Speech Surgery

VPD refers to the inability of the soft palate to close consistently and completely against the posterior pharynx during phonation causing nasal air escape and hypernasal resonance. If allowed to persist, cleft patients with VPD can develop compensatory misarticulations such as glottal stops, pharyngeal fricatives, nasal fricatives, and pharyngeal plosives due to the inability to produce sounds normally with a functional velopharyngeal port. VPD is further subdivided into VPI, velopharyngeal incompetence, and velopharyngeal mislearning depending on the underlying abnormality. VPI is caused by insufficient palatal length to achieve velopharyngeal port closure despite normal palatal elevation with phonation. In contrast, velopharyngeal incompetence refers to aberrant palatal elevation or motion resulting in lack of velopharyngeal port closure despite adequate palatal length. Velopharyngeal mislearning results when a patient continues to use abnormal speech patterns despite a normally functioning palate with adequate length and closure. Differentiation of the subtype of VPD is critical, as it dictates the subsequent treatment. VPI is an anatomic problem and will not improve with speech therapy and therefore requires surgical intervention. Velopharyngeal incompetence can be improved with speech therapy if normal palatal motion can be learned by the patient. In rare circumstances this is not possible and surgical intervention may be required. Velopharyngeal mislearning is treated with speech therapy alone.

The determination of VPD subtype is contingent upon perceptual speech evaluation by a qualified speech pathologist who has specialized training in cleft pathology and speech patterns. Additional modalities such as pressure-flow testing and video nasendoscopy are important adjuncts that can assist with classification of the VPD. Video nasendoscopy is essential for surgical candidates with velopharyngeal incompetence to characterize the closure pattern of the velopharyngeal port. The surgical options for persistent VPI after palate repair include Furlow conversion, posterior pharyngeal fat grafting (PPFG), posterior pharyngeal flap (PPF), and dynamic sphincter pharyngoplasty (DSP).

A Furlow conversion can be performed for patients who underwent a straight-line closure or intravelar veloplasty during their primary cleft palate operation. Converting to a Furlow palatoplasty will provide additional palatal length at the expense of palatal width and can be applied to mild to moderate velopharyngeal gaps. PPFG can also be utilized as an adjunctive procedure for modest (<2 cm^2) gaps. The volume of autologous fat required and regions for augmentation are determined from preoperative nasendoscopy. Results with PPFG have demonstrated favorable outcomes with reduction in hypernasal speech and improved velopharyngeal closure without significant increases in postoperative obstructive sleep apnea.[45]

The PPF is utilized in cases with large velopharyngeal gaps and often preferred if the lateral pharyngeal wall motion is preserved. The technique makes two longitudinal incisions through the mucosa and muscle of the posterior pharyngeal wall to the level of the prevertebral fascia. Elevation of PPF flaps has been described with both superiorly and inferiorly based designs although the superiorly based flap is most commonly practiced today. Following elevation, the flap apex is inserted into the posterior aspect of the soft palate creating a midline subtotal obstruction of air flow with two lateral nasopharyngeal ports. The elevated raw surface of the PPF can be relined with reflected nasal mucosal flaps off the posterior palate to limit the degree of secondary flap contracture. The resultant posterior pharyngeal wall donor site is closed primarily.

Patients exhibiting large velopharyngeal gaps are also candidates for DSP. The DSP technique elevates superiorly based musculomucosal flaps from the posterior tonsillar pillars and include the underlying palatopharyngeus muscle. Prior to flap elevation, a red rubber catheter is passed through the nose, secured to the uvula, and then placed on tension to retract the soft palate and facilitate visualization. The flaps are then raised to the height of the anticipated level of the velopharyngeal port just inferior to the adenoid pad. The medial incisions for each flap are extended transversely to meet in the midline along the posterior pharyngeal wall. Each flap is transposed 90 degrees and inset sequentially into the transverse pharyngeal wall incision. The result is a circular DSP port with a central opening. The diameter of the DSP port is modulated by the degree of overlap and tension on the flaps during inset.

The use of PPF and DSP is largely center and surgeon dependent, with conflicting reports regarding the effectiveness and safety profiles of each procedure.[46,47] However, a recent randomized multicenter trial comparing PPF to DSP through standardization of technique demonstrated equivalent results between PPF and DSP for speech resonance, nasalance, endoscopic outcomes, and surgical complications at 1-year follow-up.[48] Postoperative obstructive sleep apnea was observed in both groups; therefore, pre- and postoperative polysomnographic evaluation is warranted for patients requiring either procedure.

Alveolar Cleft Closure

Methods for addressing the alveolar cleft include early primary bone grafting, gingivoperiosteoplasty (GPP), and secondary bone grafting during mixed dentition. The rationale for early primary bone grafting (<2 years old) is that bony reconstruction of maxillary arch will prevent collapse of the greater and lesser segments, thereby diminishing the need for extensive orthodontic treatment and future orthognathic surgery. Split rib corticocancellous grafts were typically used with a segment of cortex on-laid to the labial cleft margin and morselized cortical and cancellous bone interposed into the alveolar cleft. However, concern for disruption of maxillary growth with early primary bone grafting has caused this approach to largely fall out of favor despite modifications to the technique.

Early intervention on the alveolar cleft can also be achieved with the use of GPP. Centers advocating the use of GPP typically use it in conjunction with nasoalveolar molding to closely approximate the greater and lesser alveolar segments. This allows for limited gingivoperiosteal flaps to be elevated off the cleft margins and approximated to each other thereby forming a periosteum-lined tunnel through which nascent bone formation can occur. GPP is typically performed at the time of the primary lip repair and theoretically obviates the need for a secondary surgery and additional donor site morbidity. However, GPP remains limited in implementation owing to the resource-intensive nature of NAM and questions regarding the quantity and quality of bone formed through periosteal induction. Studies have demonstrated that up to 40% of patients treated with GPP still require secondary bone grafting and significantly higher failure rates of both primary and secondary GPP compared with secondary bone grafting alone.[49,50]

Secondary bone grafting is typically performed just prior to eruption of the permanent maxillary canine into the cleft margin (8–9 years of age). Cancellous bone is harvested from the iliac crest and utilized to definitively close the anterior oral-nasal fistula remaining after definitive lip and palate repair, augment the cleft-side piriform rim, and restore continuity to the maxillary dental arch. Reported success rates for secondary alveolar cleft bone grafting in the literature approach 80% to 90%.[50-52] However, the potential for donor site morbidity, including remote scarring, infection, hematoma, meralgia paresthetica, and iatrogenic fracture, has stimulated the investigation of allograft bone substitutes and osteogenic growth factors in lieu of autologous bone. Preliminary reports of supplementing autologous iliac crest bone graft with demineralized bone matrix and cancellous autograft[53] as well as the use of recombinant human bone morphogenic protein-2 with demineralized bone matrix alone without autogenous bone have shown favorable results. However, additional studies evaluating the long-term outcomes, complications, cost-effectiveness, and safety of these novel therapies are required prior to widespread adoption.

Orthognathic Surgery

Patients with CL/P require longitudinal care spanning infancy through early adulthood. Throughout this time, they require multiple operations which carry additive potential for maxillary growth inhibition through disruption of facial growth centers and postoperative scarring of the soft tissue envelope. When combined with the congenital limitations in growth potential, CL/P patients often develop maxillary hypoplasia and resultant Angle Class III malocclusion. Cleft patients can also exhibit transverse maxillary hypoplasia with unilateral or bilateral collapse of the alveolar segments with resultant narrowing of the maxillary arch. The mandibles in individuals with CL/P tend to have preserved growth potential further compounding the Class III dentofacial relationship. This results in the mandible overriding of the hypoplastic maxilla and autorotating into a pseudoprognathic position with loss of vertical facial height and an undesirable *edentulous* appearance. Therefore, the typical orthognathic correction for cleft patients is a LeFort I maxillary advancement with variable need for palatal osteotomies depending on the degree of transverse maxillary deficiency.

The reported incidence of cleft patients requiring orthognathic surgery varies but has recently been reported at 48% for unilateral clefts and 65% for bilateral clefts after a 30-year review at a single institution.[54] In the noncleft population, the standard prerequisites for undertaking orthognathic surgery include full eruption of the permanent dentition, completion of presurgical orthodontia to level and align the dental arches, and completion of maxillomandibular growth. Serial cephalograms to evaluate vertebral body morphology or wrist films documenting epiphyseal plate closure can aid in the determination of a patient's skeletal maturity. In the cleft population, the degree of dentofacial deformity can be severe, leading to significant psychosocial or functional concerns that necessitate orthognathic correction prior to achieving skeletal maturity. In these instances, distraction osteogenesis (DO) or a finalizing osteotomy after completion of facial growth may be required. The indications for DO versus conventional orthognathic surgery are also predicated on the degree of maxillary movement required to reestablish normal maxillomandibular occlusion. The literature reports that DO is indicated for correction of a negative overjet of greater than 6 mm in cleft patients and greater than 10 mm in noncleft patients.[55] The decision to proceed with DO versus conventional orthognathic surgery techniques remains at the discretion of the treating cleft surgeon, as both methods have yielded reliable and stable postoperative results.[56-58] Severe maxillary hypoplasia that presents early can often be rectified with early DO, with overcorrection. Strategic distraction at a younger age in severe patients will often preclude any *compromises* in the plan for orthognathic surgery at maturity resulting in the best aesthetic and functional result. Cleft-specific considerations for orthognathic surgery include counseling patients on the development of postoperative VPI following midface advancement. Patients with borderline preoperative velopharyngeal function or who require large advancements (>10 mm) are at higher risk for this complication, although patients may note improvements in articulation and speech intelligibility secondary to improved maxillomandibular occlusion. Finally, the surgical plan for cleft orthognathic cases should factor in a modest degree of overcorrection to account for surgical relapse owing to the larger osteotomy gaps frequently necessitated for cleft cases and remodeling relapse due to the tension from a restricted and scared soft tissue envelope.

REFERENCES

1. Tolarova MM, Cervenka J. Classification and birth prevalence of orofacial clefts. *Am J Med Genet*. 1998;75:126-137.
2. Croen LA, Shaw GM, Wasserman CR, Tolarova MM. Racial and ethnic variations in the prevalence of orofacial clefts in California, 1983-1992. *Am J Med Genet*. 1998;79:42-47.
3. Cembrano JRJ, Joaquino JB, Ng EF, et al. Familial risk of recurrence of cleft lip and palate. *Philipp J Surg Surg Spec*. 1995;50:37-40.
4. Meng T, Shi B, Zheng Q, et al. Clinical and epidemiologic studies of nonsyndromic cleft lip and palate in China: analysis of 4268 cases. *Ann Plast Surg*. 2006;57:264-269.
5. Tessier P. Anatomical classification of facial, cranio-facial and latero-facial clefts. *J Maxillofac Surg*. 1976;4:69-92.
6. Schutte BC, Murray JC. The many faces and factors of orofacial clefts. *Hum Mol Genet*. 1999;8:1853-1859.
7. Veau V, Borel S. *Division Palatine: Anatomie, Chirurgie Phonétique*: Paris: Masson; 1931.
8. Kernahan DA, Stark RB. A new classification for cleft lip and cleft palate. *Plast Reconstr Surg Transpl Bull*. 1958;22:435-441.
9. Kernahan DA. The striped Y: a symbolic classification for cleft lip and palate. *Plast Reconstr Surg*. 1971;47:469-470.
10. Allori AC, Mulliken JB, Meara JG, et al. Classification of cleft lip/palate: then and now. *Cleft Palate Craniofac J*. 2017;54:175-188.
11. Yuzuriha S, Mulliken JB. Minor-form, microform, and mini-microform cleft lip: anatomical features, operative techniques, and revisions. *Plast Reconstr Surg*. 2008;122:1485-1493.
This manuscript provides a comprehensive review of the nomenclature, anatomic features, and repair techniques for the spectrum of incomplete cleft lip phenotypes. The manuscript illustrations of the repair techniques serve as an excellent reference for resident education and surgical planning.
12. Mulliken JB. Double unilimb Z-plastic repair of microform cleft lip. *Plast Reconstr Surg*. 2005;116:1623-1632.
13. Noordhoff MS. Reconstruction of vermilion in unilateral and bilateral cleft lips. *Plast Reconstr Surg*. 1984;73:52-61.
14. Mulliken JB. Principles and techniques of bilateral complete cleft lip repair. *Plast Reconstr Surg*. 1985;75:477-487.
15. McComb H. Primary repair of the bilateral cleft lip nose: a 10-year review. *Plast Reconstr Surg*. 1986;77:701-716.
16. Sheahan P, Miller I, Sheahan JN, et al. Incidence and outcome of middle ear disease in cleft lip and/or cleft palate. *Int J Pediatr Otorhinolaryngol*. 2003;67:785-793.
17. Flores RL, Tholpady SS, Sati S, et al. The surgical correction of Pierre Robin sequence: mandibular distraction osteogenesis versus tongue-lip adhesion. *Plast Reconstr Surg*. 2014;133:1433-1439.
18. Ettinger RE, Kung TA, Wombacher N, et al. Timing of Furlow palatoplasty for patients with submucous cleft palate. *Cleft Palate Craniofac J*. 2018;55:430-436.
19. McWilliams BJ. Submucous clefts of the palate: how likely are they to be symptomatic? *Cleft Palate Craniofac J*. 1991;28:247-249.
20. Sullivan SR, Vasudavan S, Marrinan EM, Mulliken JB. Submucous cleft palate and velopharyngeal insufficiency: comparison of speech outcomes using three operative techniques by one surgeon. *Cleft Palate Craniofac J*. 2011;48:561-570.
21. Pool R, Farnworth TK. Preoperative lip taping in the cleft lip. *Ann Plast Surg*. 1994;32:243-249.
22. Vander Woude DL, Mulliken JB. Effect of lip adhesion on labial height in two-stage repair of unilateral complete cleft lip. *Plast Reconstr Surg*. 1997;100:567-572.
23. Grayson BH, Cutting CB. Presurgical nasoalveolar orthopedic molding in primary correction of the nose, lip, and alveolus of infants born with unilateral and bilateral clefts. *Cleft Palate Craniofac J*. 2001;38:193-198.
The development of presurgical nasoalveolar molding (NAM) by the group at NYU has greatly faciltated the cleft surgeon's ability to manage difficult clefts and optimize the definitive repair result. Although NAM is not universally practiced at all cleft centers, an understanding of its principles and merits are critical for every cleft surgeon.
24. Liou EJ, Subramanian M, Chen PK, Huang CS. The progressive changes of nasal symmetry and growth after nasoalveolar molding: a three-year follow-up study. *Plast Reconstr Surg*. 2004;114:858-864.
25. Clark SL, Teichgraeber JF, Fleshman RG, et al. Long-term treatment outcome of presurgical nasoalveolar molding in patients with unilateral cleft lip and palate. *J Craniofac Surg*. 2011;22:333-336.
26. Uzel A, Alparslan ZN. Long-term effects of presurgical infant orthopedics in patients with cleft lip and palate: a systematic review. *Cleft Palate Craniofac J*. 2011;48:587-595.
27. Latham RA. Orthopedic advancement of the cleft maxillary segment: a preliminary report. *Cleft Palate J*. 1980;17:227-233.
28. Berkowitz S, Mejia M, Bystrik A. A comparison of the effects of the Latham-Millard procedure with those of a conservative treatment approach for dental occlusion and facial aesthetics in unilateral and bilateral complete cleft lip and palate: part I. Dental occlusion. *Plast Reconstr Surg*. 2004;113:1-18.
29. Thompson JE. An artistic and mathematically accurate method of repairing the defect in cases of harelip. *Surg Gynecol Obstet*. 1912;14:498-505.
30. LeMesurier A. A method of cutting and suturing the lip in the treatment of complete unilateral clefts. *Plast Reconstr Surg*. 1949;4:1-12.
31. Tennison CW. The repair of the unilateral cleft lip by the stencil method. *Plast Reconstr Surg*. 1952;9:115 120.
32. Randall P. A triangular flap operation for the primary repair of unilateral clefts of the lip. *Plast Reconstr Surg Transpl Bull*. 1959;23:331-347.
33. Millard DR Jr. A radical rotation in single harelip. *Am J Surg*. 1958;95:318-322.
34. Mohler LR. Unilateral cleft lip repair. *Plast Reconstr Surg*. 1987;80:511-517.
35. Cutting CB, Dayan JH. Lip height and lip width after extended Mohler unilateral cleft lip repair. *Plast Reconstr Surg*. 2003;111:17-23.
36. Sitzman TJ, Girotto JA, Marcus JR. Current surgical practices in cleft care: unilateral cleft lip repair. *Plast Reconstr Surg*. 2008;121:261e-270e.
37. McComb H. Primary repair of the bilateral cleft lip nose: a 15-year review and a new treatment plan. *Plast Reconstr Surg*. 1990;86:882-889.
38. Mulliken JB. Correction of the bilateral cleft lip nasal deformity: evolution of a surgical concept. *Cleft Palate Craniofac J*. 1992;29:540-545.
39. Mulliken JB. Primary repair of bilateral cleft lip and nasal deformity. *Plast Reconstr Surg*. 2001;108:181-194.
The contributions to bilateral cleft lip repair by Dr. Mulliken cannot be understated. His multiple manuscripts and technique descriptions have become the foundation of the modern bilateral cleft lip repair. His entire series of manuscripts describing the creation and evolution of his technique are essential reading for any plastic surgeon.
40. LaRossa D. The state of the art in cleft palate surgery. *Cleft Palate Craniofac J*. 2000;37:225-228.
41. Pigott RW, Albery EH, Hathorn IS, et al. A comparison of three methods of repairing the hard palate. *Cleft Palate Craniofac J*. 2002;39:383-391.
42. Furlow L Jr. Cleft palate repair by double opposing Z-plasty. *Plast Reconstr Surg*. 1986;78:724-738.
Dr. Furlow's description of the double opposing Z-plasty for soft palate repair is one of the seminal contributions to cleft care. His technique provided a novel and elegant technique to provide soft palate closure with levator muscle repositioning with simultaneous lengthening of the palate.
43. McWilliams BJ, Randall P, LaRossa D, et al. Speech characteristics associated with the Furlow palatoplasty as compared with other surgical techniques. *Plast Reconstr Surg*. 1996;98:610-619.
44. Levi B, Kasten SJ, Buchman SR. Utilization of the buccal fat pad flap for congenital cleft palate repair. *Plast Reconstr Surg*. 2009;123:1018-1021.
45. Lau D, Oppenheimer AJ, Buchman SR, et al. Posterior pharyngeal fat grafting for velopharyngeal insufficiency. *Cleft Palate Craniofac J*. 2013;50:51-58.
46. Sloan GM. Posterior pharyngeal flap and sphincter pharyngoplasty: the state of the art. *Cleft Palate Craniofac J*. 2000;37:112-122.
47. de Serres LM, Deleyiannis FW, Eblen LE, et al. Results with sphincter pharyngoplasty and pharyngeal flap. *Int J Pediatr Otorhinolaryngol*. 1999;48:17-25.
48. Abyholm F, D'Antonio L, Davidson Ward SL, et al. Pharyngeal flap and sphincterplasty for velopharyngeal insufficiency have equal outcome at 1 year postoperatively: results of a randomized trial. *Cleft Palate Craniofac J*. 2005;42:501-511.
49. Santiago PE, Grayson BH, Cutting CB, et al. Reduced need for alveolar bone grafting by presurgical orthopedics and primary gingivoperiosteoplasty. *Cleft Palate Craniofac J*. 1998;35:77-80.
50. Matic DB, Power SM. Evaluating the success of gingivoperiosteoplasty versus secondary bone grafting in patients with unilateral clefts. *Plast Reconstr Surg*. 2008;121:1343-1353.
51. Dempf R, Teltzrow T, Kramer FJ, Hausamen JE. Alveolar bone grafting in patients with complete clefts: a comparative study between secondary and tertiary bone grafting. *Cleft Palate Craniofac J*. 2002;39:18-25.
52. Kortebein MJ, Nelson CL, Sadove AM. Retrospective analysis of 135 secondary alveolar cleft grafts using iliac or calvarial bone. *J Oral Maxillofac Surg*. 1991;49:493-498.
53. Macisaac ZM, Rottgers SA, Davit AJ III, et al. Alveolar reconstruction in cleft patients: decreased morbidity and improved outcomes with supplemental demineralized bone matrix and cancellous allograft. *Plast Reconstr Surg*. 2012;130:625-632.
54. Daskalogiannakis J, Mehta M. The need for orthognathic surgery in patients with repaired complete unilateral and complete bilateral cleft lip and palate. *Cleft Palate Craniofac J*. 2009;46:498-502.
55. Cheung LK, Chua HD, Hagg MB. Cleft maxillary distraction versus orthognathic surgery: clinical morbidities and surgical relapse. *Plast Reconstr Surg*. 2006;118:996-1008.
56. Posnick JC, Tompson B. Cleft-orthognathic surgery: complications and long-term results. *Plast Reconstr Surg*. 1995;96:255-266.
Adjunctive cleft operations including orthognathic surgery are required for a subset of cleft lip and palate patients once they reach skeletal maturity. Dr. Posnick's manuscript reports on his a longitudinal experience treating the secondary dentofacial deformity associated with cleft lip and palate with LeFort I with or without mandibular osteotomies. His series demonstrates favorable outcomes with low rates of relapse on long-term follow-up and low rate of perioperative and postoperative complications.
57. Scolozzi P. Distraction osteogenesis in the management of severe maxillary hypoplasia in cleft lip and palate patients. *J Craniofac Surg*. 2008;19:1199-1214.
58. Gursoy S, Hukki J, Hurmerinta K. Five-year follow-up of maxillary distraction osteogenesis on the dentofacial structures of children with cleft lip and palate. *J Oral Maxillofac Surg*. 2010;68:744-750.

QUESTIONS

1. **Failure of fusion of which of the following structures gives rise to a cleft lip?**
   a. Frontonasal prominence and lateral nasal prominence
   b. Medial nasal prominence and maxillary prominence
   c. Medial nasal prominence and lateral nasal prominence
   d. Maxillary prominence and mandibular prominence
   e. Lateral nasal prominence and frontonasal prominence

2. **The parents of a 2-month-old infant with CL/P come to your office for consultation. This is the parents' second child; their first was also born with CL/P. They want to know what are the chances that their next child will have CL/P.**
   a. 2%
   b. 4%
   c. 9%
   d. 17%
   e. 50%

3. **A 5-year-old girl with a history of repaired unilateral complete CL/P presents to clinic for evaluation. She has a persistent alveolar fistula but good alignment of her maxillary arch segments. Alveolar cleft bone grafting is planned. Which of the following dictates timing for this intervention?**
   a. Patient age
   b. Patient and family preference
   c. Permanent canine eruption on periapical radiographs
   d. Degree of compensatory misarticulations
   e. Completion of maxillary growth

4. **A 28-month-old female child is brought to clinic for evaluation of CL/P. She was adopted from China where her lip was previously repaired. No additional operations have been performed. Examination demonstrates a vermillion cutaneous step-off of 3 mm, inadequate vertical lip height, and unfavorable scaring. Intraoral examination demonstrates complete unilateral cleft palate. Nasal examination demonstrates persistent alar slumping and tip deviation to noncleft side. Which of the following is the most appropriate next step in management?**
   a. Cleft palate repair
   b. Minor lip revision with realignment of the white roll
   c. Complete lip revision with reapproximation of orbicularis muscle and cutaneous lip elements
   d. Complete cleft lip revision with concurrent cleft rhinoplasty
   e. Observation

5. **Which of the following muscles is utilized to construct the sphincter during DSP for treatment of refractory velopharyngeal dysfunction?**
   a. Tensor veli palatini
   b. Palatoglossus
   c. Levator veli palatini
   d. Palatopharyngeus
   e. Superior pharyngeal constrictor

1. **Answer: b.** During the sixth to eighth weeks of gestation, the medial nasal prominence fuses with the maxillary prominence to form the upper lip. The medial nasal prominence gives rise to the philtrum, and the maxillary prominences become the lateral lip element with the philtral column delineating the fusion plane. The frontonasal prominence is the precursor to the medial and lateral nasal prominences. The mandibular prominence does not contribute to the formation of the upper lip.

2. **Answer: c.** The risks for having a child with CL/P are multifactorial. Familial cases have a risk that is dependent on family history, parental involvement, and genetics. The risk of clefting in subsequent children is as follows. If one child or one parent has CLP then there is a 4% chance of a subsequent child being born with a cleft. If two children have CLP then there is a 9% chance of a subsequent child being born with a cleft. If one child and one parent both have CLP then there is a 17% chance a subsequent child being born with a cleft. For an affected parent with CL/P and lip pits who has van der Woude syndrome, the risk for the affected child would be 50%, as van der Woude follows an autosomal dominant inheritance pattern.

3. **Answer: c.** Timing of alveolar cleft bone grafting should precede eruption of the cleft side permanent canine. This is best judged from periapical radiographs. Performing bone grafting at this time will unite the maxillary arches and provide bone stock to support the erupting canine. Although alveolar cleft bone grafting is typically performed around 8 or 9 years of age, the timing is dictated by canine eruption, and therefore age cannot be utilized as a strict criterion. Persistent alveolar clefts can contribute to hypernasal speech, but speech disturbance is not a primary indication for bone grafting. Family and patient preference do not typically dictate the timing for alveolar cleft bone grafting.

4. **Answer: a.** The patient described is already reaching the age of critical language development and has an unrepaired cleft palate. An unrepaired cleft during this phase of development can lead to severe speech dysfunction; therefore, performing cleft palate repair is the first objective. Despite an unfavorable appearance to the previous cleft lip repair, revisionary surgery should be deferred until after palatoplasty is performed. Observation is not indicated, as the child has already surpassed the ideal age for performing palatoplasty.

5. **Answer: d.** In cleft patients, VPI can persist despite initial palatoplasty. Secondary interventions for VPI include Furlow palatoplasty conversion, posterior PPFG, PPF, and DSP. To perform a DSP, superiorly based musculomucosal flaps are elevated from the posterior tonsillar pillars including the underlying palatopharyngeus muscle. These flaps are then transposed and overlapped in the midline to create a circular velopharyngeal port.

CHAPTER 26 Congenital Melanocytic Nevi and Other Common Skin Lesions

David W. Low and Oksana A. Jackson

KEY POINTS

- Congenital nevi may be classified by depth of involvement (epidermal, junctional, dermal, compound), predominant type of cells (melanocytic, sebaceous), cellular atypia (mild, moderate, severe, dysplastic, Spitz), size (small, medium, giant), and in certain cases, location (nevus of Ota on the face, nevus of Ito on the shoulder, Mongolian spots on the buttocks).
- The malignant potential of melanocytic nevi depends largely upon size, but a family history of dysplastic nevi and melanoma significantly increases the potential for malignant melanoma.
- Although the ABCDs of pigmented lesions may be useful indicators of suspicious moles (asymmetry, border irregularity, color variegation, diameter >6 mm), the most important feature is E (evolving)—a nevus that is changing.
- Small and medium-sized melanocytic nevi have a lifetime risk of melanoma of less than 1%. Giant congenital nevi may have a lifetime risk of 5% to 10%.
- The surgical management of congenital melanocytic nevi may include incisional biopsy, excisional biopsy, serial excision, excision and skin grafting, and tissue expansion prior to excision of large or giant nevi. The role of lasers may be useful for epidermal nevi, but it remains controversial for melanocytic nevi.
- Sebaceous nevi often become oily and crusty during puberty, and they have a 10% to 15% risk of basal cell carcinoma in adulthood. Surgical excision is usually straightforward on the scalp, but on the face, significant scars can result.
- Other common pediatric skin lesions include epidermal cysts, pilomatrixomas, and dermoid cysts. Surgical excision is recommended and is usually curative.

LAYERS OF THE SKIN

The skin is divided into the epidermis and the dermis, and in most areas of the body, the next deepest layer is subcutaneous tissue. (Eyelid skin is directly attached to the orbicularis muscle.) The epidermis can be microscopically subdivided into five layers (from superficial to deep: corneum, lucidum, granulosum, spinosum, and germinativum), but what is important to plastic surgeons is that malignant tumors confined to the epidermis are regarded as premalignant *in situ* carcinomas, rather than invasive skin cancers. The dermis is divided into two clinically important layers, the papillary and reticular dermis. The papillary dermis interdigitates with the epidermis and lies above the reticular dermis. This distinction is clinically important in classifying the depth of invasion of melanomas, but it is also important in skin resurfacing as ablative techniques that penetrate into the reticular dermis can cause undesirable scar formation.

NEVI

Congenital Melanocytic

Classification

Congenital nevi are classified by a variety of features, including layer(s) of skin involvement, size, and location on the body. Epidermal nevi have no malignant potential but become increasingly verrucous over time, posing significant cosmetic concerns. Similarly, dermal nevi have low malignant potential but typically protrude above the surface of the skin as flesh-colored papules. Acquired nevi are often located at the junction of the epidermis and dermis, so they are called junctional nevi. Nevi that are located in both layers are compound nevi. Nevi that are characterized as having congenital features follow hair follicles through the dermis and into the superficial subcutaneous tissues (**Figure 26.1**).

Congenital nevi are also classified by their size as small, medium, and giant. This rather imprecise method groups them into nevi that are less than 1.5 cm, 1.5 to 20 cm, and greater than 20 cm. Small nevi are the most common, occurring in 1:100 births. Medium nevi occur in 1:1000 births. Giant nevi are the least frequent at 1:20,000 births and often have associated satellite nevi. Giant nevi may occupy an entire back, buttock, or thigh. A large part of the face and scalp may be classified as a giant hairy nevus, even if the exact measurement is less than 20 cm. Nevi greater than 50 cm in dimension are very rare, occurring in 1:500,000 births.

Some congenital nevi are classified by location. Nevus of Ota is a dermal melanocytic nevus located on the face (V1 and V2 distribution), which occurs more commonly in women, rarely in Caucasians, and may be associated with glaucoma (**Figure 26.2**). Similarly, nevus of Ito is characterized by dermal melanocytosis, except that its location is on the shoulder, upper chest, and back. It is also most commonly seen in Asians. Mongolian spots are found on the lumbosacral area and are characterized by dermal melanocytic pigmentation, but curiously disappear in most patients by 3 to 5 years of age and in the remainder by puberty. They are sometimes misdiagnosed as child abuse because the pigment can be mistaken for a bruise (**Figure 26.3**).

Congenital nevi are most accurately classified by their microscopic appearance, and the pathology report may include terms such as epidermal nevus, nevus with congenital features, Spitz nevus, sebaceous nevus, cellular blue nevus, halo nevus, and dysplastic nevus with varying degrees of cellular atypia. As noted earlier, epidermal nevi are confined to the most superficial skin layer, whereas *congenital* nevi have melanocytic pigment throughout all layers of the skin. Spitz nevi resemble melanomas but do not carry the same oncologic risk. Sebaceous nevi are composed of sebaceous units. Cellular blue nevi have densely packed melanocytes. Halo nevi show loss of melanin (probably an autoimmune phenomenon) and clinically have a peripheral zone of hypopigmentation. Dysplastic nevi demonstrate variable degrees of cellular atypia (mild, moderate, severe) with increased risk of neoplastic transformation.

Spitz Nevi

In 1948, an American pathologist, Sophie Spitz, described 12 pediatric patients whose nevi resembled melanoma microscopically but did not carry the same biologic risk. She coined the term *juvenile*

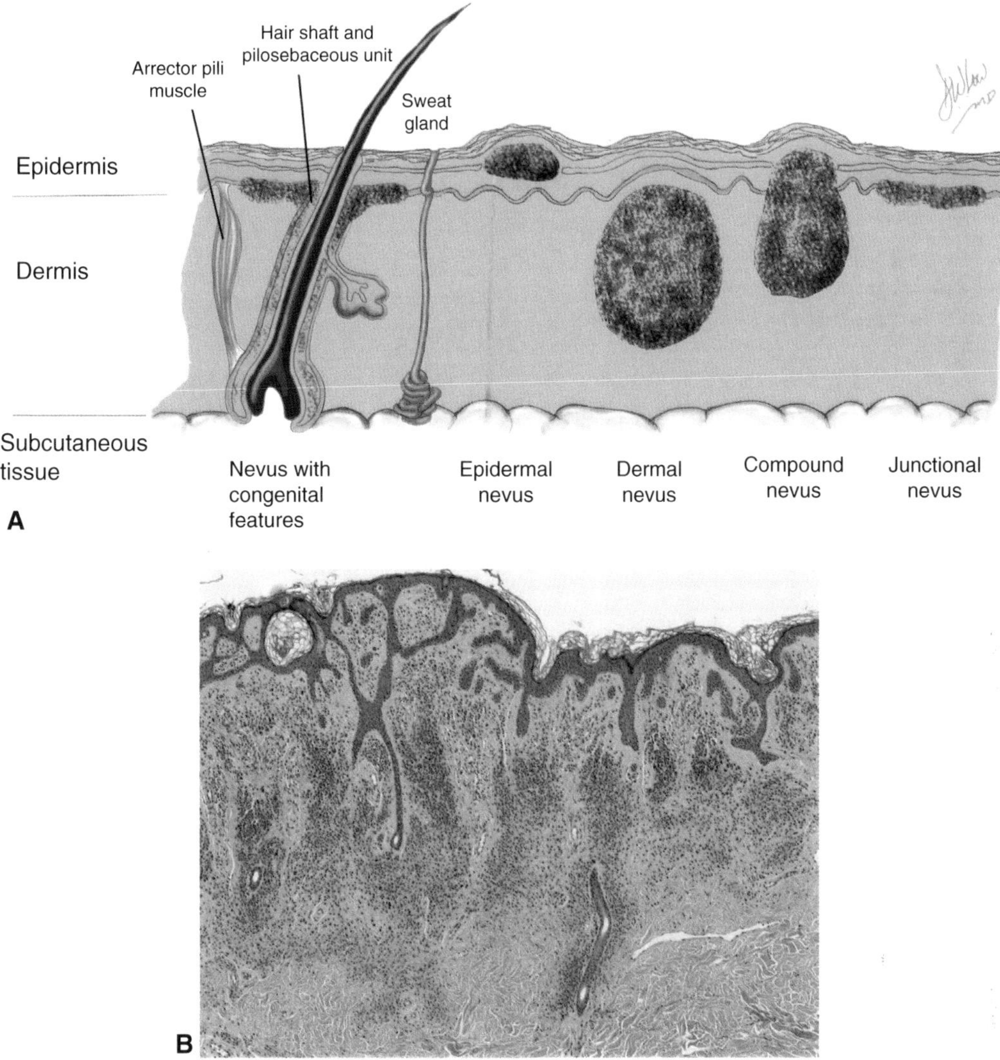

FIGURE 26.1. **A.** Classification of nevi based on location. Nevi can be located in the epidermis, the dermis, both layers (compound), at the interface (junctional), or may extend down the hair follicle into the fat (nevus with congenital features). **B.** Photomicrograph of a congenital nevus. The nevus cells extend into the mid or deep reticular dermis. The cells typically surround or extend into hair follicles, sebaceous glands, and eccrine ducts. (Courtesy of Rosalie Elenitsas, MD.)

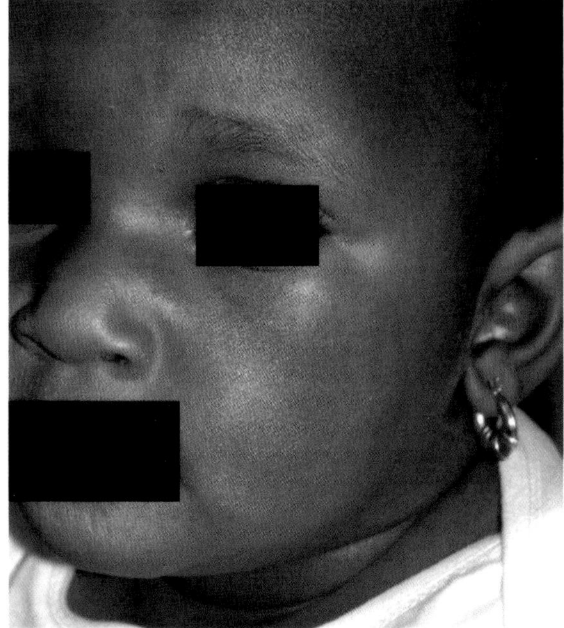

FIGURE 26.2. Nevus of Ota. This dermal melanocytic nevus is located in the V1 and V2 distribution of the face and can be associated with glaucoma. (Courtesy of Albert Yan, MD.)

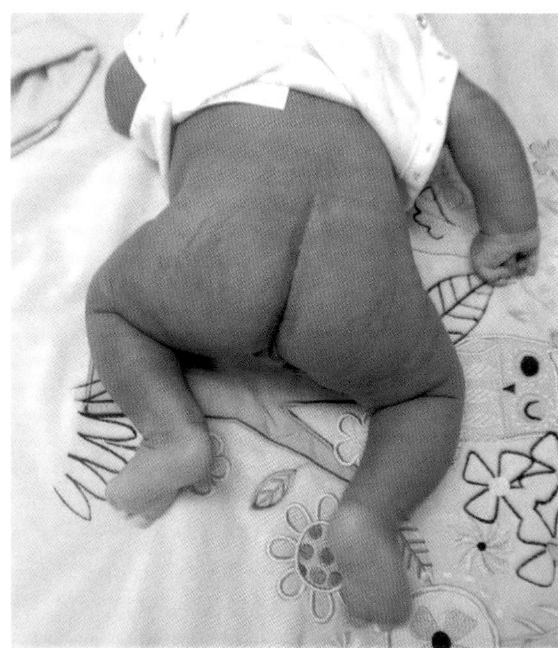

FIGURE 26.3. Mongolian spots. The dermal melanocytic pigmentation of the buttocks resolves with time but can be mistaken for bruising associated with child abuse.

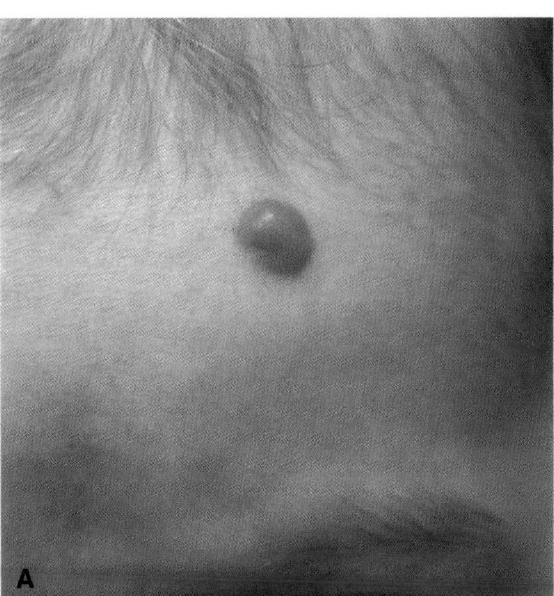

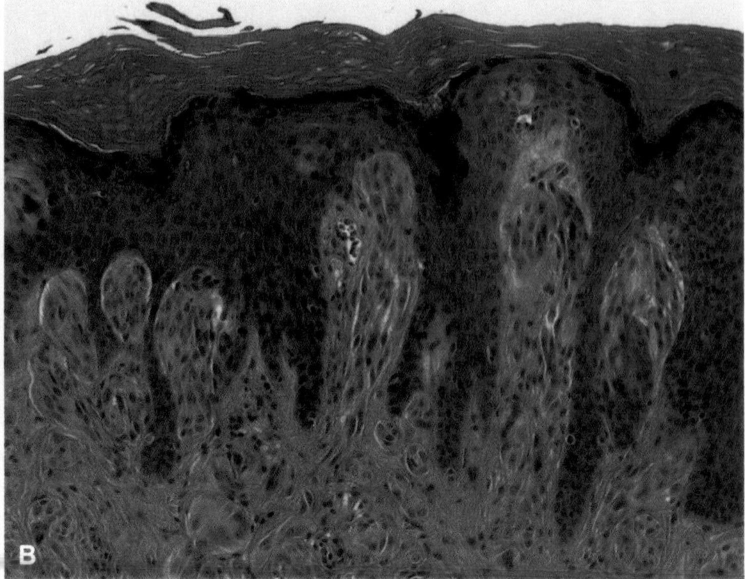

FIGURE 26.4. A. Spitz nevi can exhibit rapid growth, and their nickname juvenile melanoma is intimidating, but they are actually no more dangerous than other congenital nevi. **B.** These lesions are composed of nests of large epithelioid melanocytes that have an abundance of pink cytoplasm. The cells are often present in both the epidermis and dermis and show many overlapping features with melanoma cells. (Courtesy of Rosalie Elenitsas, MD.)

melanoma to distinguish them from malignant melanoma. They occur most commonly on the face and neck between the ages of 3 and 13, are usually less than 1 cm in diameter, and have a well-circumscribed border (**Figure 26.4**). However, because they may exhibit rapid growth, they are commonly tangentially biopsied by pediatric dermatologists and then referred to plastic surgeons for full-thickness excision. Although the potential for malignant transformation is no greater than other small melanocytic nevi, the resemblance to melanoma gives Spitz nevi an undeserved ominous reputation. Excision with a small margin of normal skin is sufficient.

Halo Nevi

A nevus with a surrounding zone of hypopigmented skin occurs most commonly in late adolescence and is believed to represent autoimmune destruction of melanocytes. The central nevus may disappear over the course of months or years, and it is not uncommon for the pigment to return. This is generally a benign process, but biopsy is indicated if the central nevus appears atypical. The most common location is on the trunk, especially the back, and patients may have more than one such lesion (**Figure 26.5**).

Dysplastic Nevi and Dysplastic Nevus Syndrome

Dysplastic nevi are clinically suspected when patients have asymmetric moles with irregular borders and variegation in pigmentation (**Figure 26.6**). Patients may have >50 dysplastic moles and a family history of dysplastic nevi. Wallace Clark first described dysplastic nevus syndrome while at Penn, and noted that patients with many dysplastic nevi and two or more first-degree relatives with melanoma have perhaps a lifetime risk of melanoma approaching 100%. Clark is best known for describing the depth of invasion of a melanoma (Clark levels I–V), the deeper the level, the worse the prognosis (**Figure 26.7**). In most patients, Clark level correlates with the tumor thickness, measured in millimeters (Breslow classification). Tumor thickness, however, is the most important prognostic indicator. A full-thickness biopsy is indicated for any suspicious lesion. Patients with large numbers of dysplastic nevi are best followed with full body photographs to help determine which nevi are truly changing and deserve biopsy.

Surgical Management of Melanocytic Nevi

The malignant potential for most melanocytic nevi is less than 1% over a lifetime; therefore guidelines have been established to alert the patient and the clinician to suspicious nevi warranting biopsy. The ABCDEs of suspicious nevi include *a*symmetry, irregular *b*order, variegation in *c*olor, *d*iameter larger than a pencil eraser (>6 mm, probably the least important feature), and most importantly a changing nevus (*e*volution). Changing features may also include crusting, bleeding, and itching.

A full-thickness biopsy rather than a shave biopsy is indicated to include all skin layers and subcutaneous tissue, and it may include a punch biopsy, an incisional biopsy, or an excisional biopsy. If a melanoma is diagnosed, a wide local excision is indicated down to the muscle fascia, and the thickness and depth of the melanoma, mitosis per square mm, presence of tumor infiltrating lymphocytes, presence or absence of regression, and other features such as tumor ulceration,

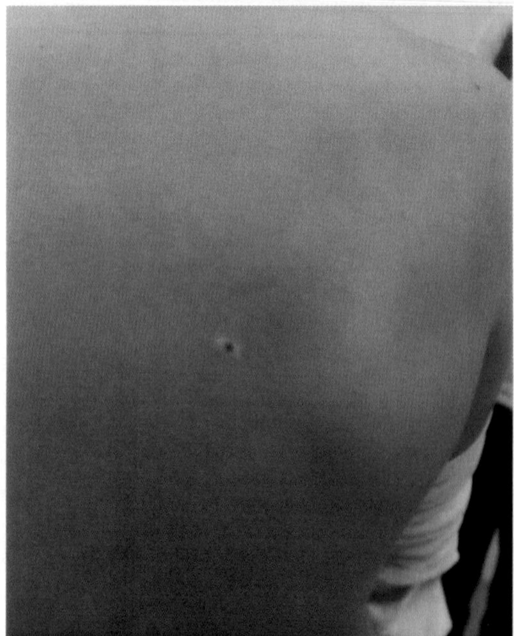

FIGURE 26.5. Halo nevi have a zone of hypopigmentation surrounding the central nevus. Although the process is thought to be a benign autoimmune phenomenon, the presence of a changing nevus usually warrants a confirmatory biopsy for parents' peace of mind.

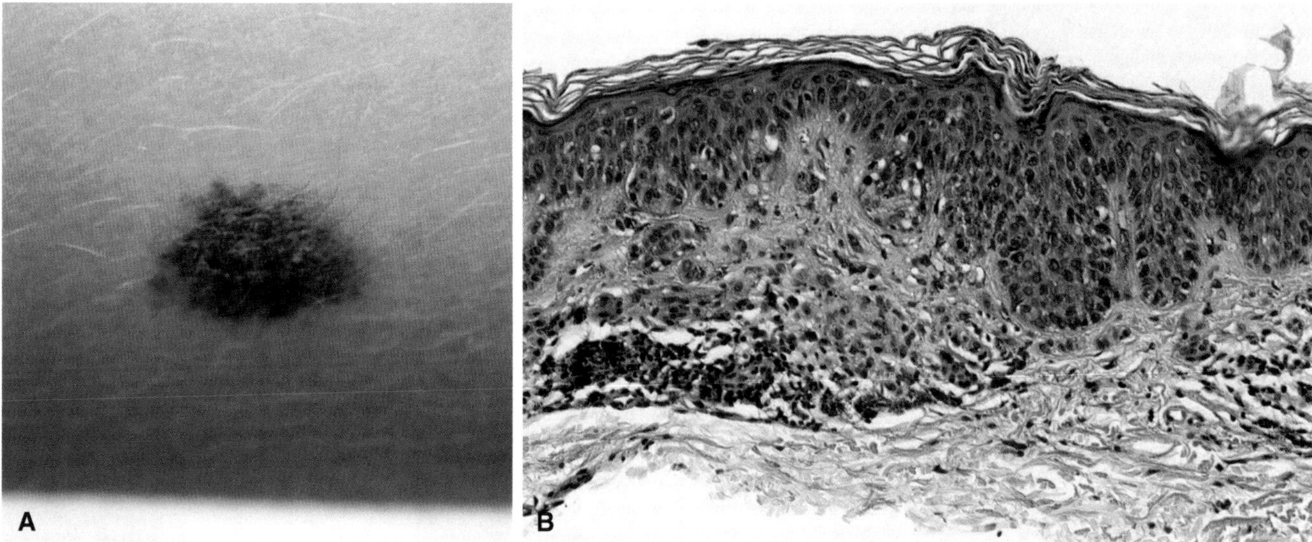

FIGURE 26.6. A. Dysplastic nevi have irregular fuzzy borders and variegation in pigmentation. A family history of melanoma and many dysplastic nevi warrants close dermatologic surveillance, usually with full body photographs to determine which nevi are changing and require biopsy. **B.** Dysplastic nevus with severe atypia. In the epidermal component of this dysplastic nevus, there is high cellularity and focal pagetoid growth of nevomelanocytes. (Courtesy of Rosalie Elenitsas, MD.)

tumor satellitosis, and neurotropism may dictate the need for sentinel lymph node staging, node dissection, metastatic screening, and periodic follow-up.

Small benign nevi can be excised in their entirety during initial biopsy. Large nevi may be managed with serial excision (**Figure 26.8**), excision and skin grafting, or tissue expansion of adjacent skin for large or giant congenital nevi (**Figure 26.9**). The role of lasers for congenital nevi has remained controversial over the past three decades. Lasers that target melanin can destroy melanocytes, but one can never guarantee complete removal of the nevus. Therefore, concerns that melanoma transformation may still occur and the lack of pigment may delay the diagnosis of melanoma that discourages most clinicians from offering laser as an option. However, in cosmetically challenging areas such as the eyelid where surgical options for nevi usually result in poor results, laser may provide a reasonable option where the cosmetic benefit outweighs the very small risk of melanoma transformation.

Neurocutaneous melanosis is a rare condition thought to arise from abnormal development of the neuroectoderm that results in melanotic tissue in both the skin and meninges. It can be associated with large (>20 cm) congenital nevi, or with multiple nevi in association with meningeal melanosis or melanoma. A screening MRI can be done at 4 to 6 months, but the prognosis is poor, even in the absence of meningeal melanoma, as patients may exhibit hydrocephalus, seizures, developmental delay, cranial nerve palsies, and a tethered spinal cord.

Epidermal Nevi

Epidermal nevi have no malignant potential, but they may carry significant psychologic burden as they typically become increasingly verrucous and unsightly over time (**Figure 26.10**). The skin lesions may resemble warts, and in some cases, there are associated ocular, neurologic, skeletal, and endocrine abnormalities. Cataracts, colobomas, seizures, developmental delay, hemiparesis, scoliosis, growth abnormalities of the extremities, and vitamin D–resistant rickets have been described. When these extracutaneous associated findings are present, the term *epidermal nevus syndrome* may be applied, but fortunately the vast majority of patients have random occurrence of epidermal nevi with no other symptoms.

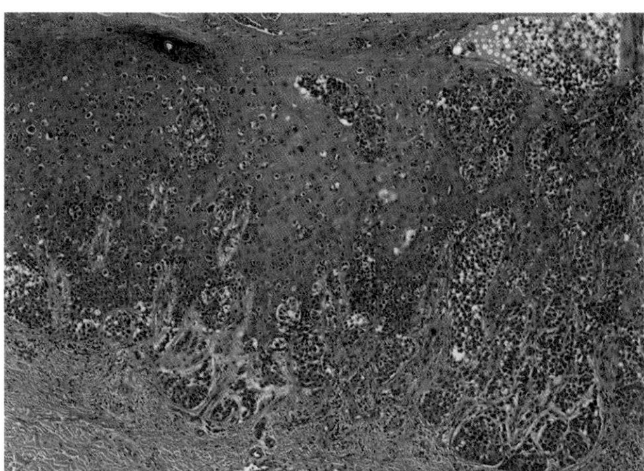

FIGURE 26.7. Malignant melanoma characteristically shows pagetoid growth of melanocytes in the epidermis. This term refers to the proliferation of these atypical melanocytic cells at all layers of the epidermis. Invasive melanoma is demonstrated by the presence of the atypical cells in the dermis (lower right-hand corner of photomicrograph). (Courtesy of Rosalie Elenitsas, MD.)

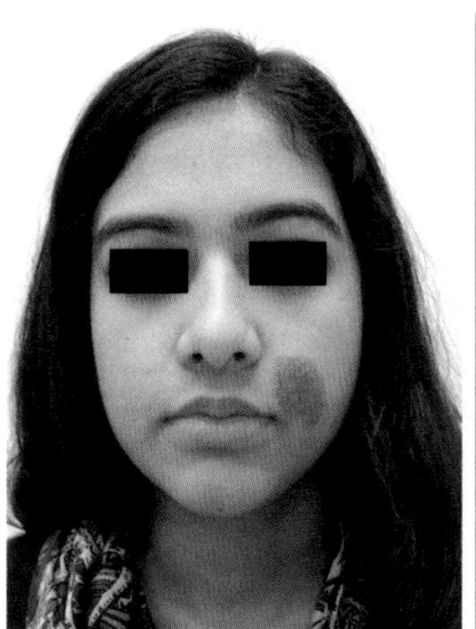

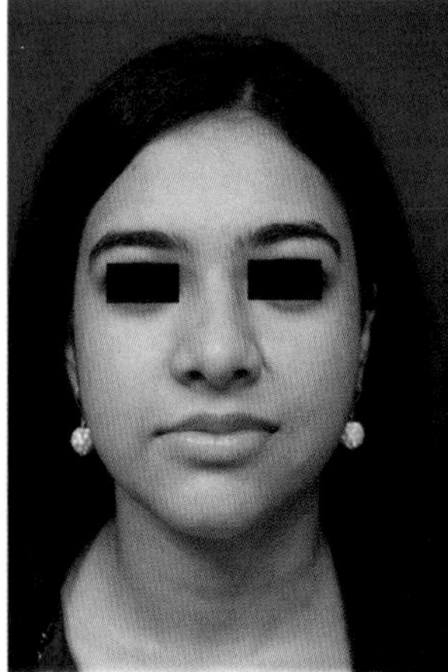

FIGURE 26.8. A. Nevi that are too large to be excised in a single stage and too small to warrant tissue expansion can be approached by serial excision. **B.** Fortunately, this nevus allowed the surgical scar to be hidden in the nasolabial crease after a series of 3 excisions.

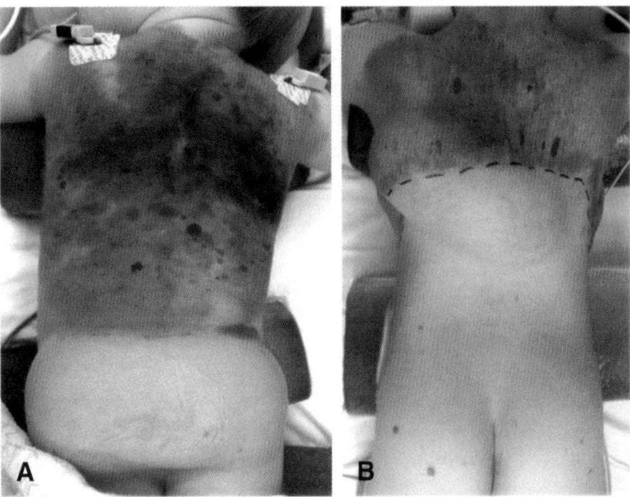

FIGURE 26.9. Giant congenital nevi can either be followed conservatively or excised with the help of tissue expansion. Parents should be advised that multiple cycles of expander insertion/removal and skin advancement may be necessary to serially excise these nevi, obligating the patient and family to endure considerable pain and morbidity. **A.** Expander placed under normal skin below the nevus. **B.** Same patient 4 years later after serial expansion and nevus excision.

Treatment includes tangential shave excision (scalpel or iris scissors), dermabrasion, CO_2 laser vaporization (**Figure 26.11**), or surgical excision. Partial-thickness removal appears to be more effective if it is performed before the nevus becomes verrucous as the cleavage plane between the epidermis and dermis appears to separate more uniformly. However, despite being in an epidermal plane, some degree of nevus recurrence is common, and repeat treatments may be indicated. In cases where the shape of the nevus lends itself to complete full-thickness excision, permanent removal is possible at the expense of a surgical scar.

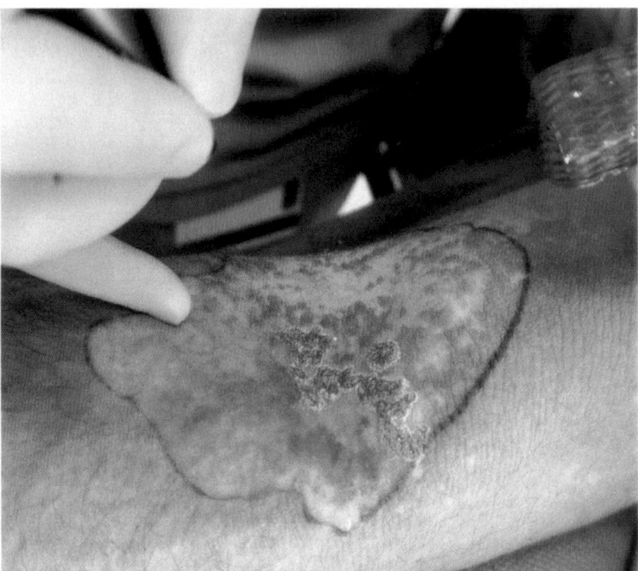

FIGURE 26.11. Epidermal nevi can be vaporized with a CO_2 laser if a large surface area is involved. Laser may be more precise, less bloody, and less likely to catch regional hairs compared with sharp dissection or dermabrasion. It works best if done while the nevus is relatively flat, as the nevus separates at a nice dermal cleavage plane.

Sebaceous Nevi (Nevus Sebaceous of Jadassohn)

Described in 1885 by German dermatologist Josef Jadassohn, these congenital nevi have a fleshy, tan, and cobblestone appearance and are often located on the scalp and face (**Figure 26.12**). Unlike congenital melanocytic nevi, they have prominent sebaceous glands, and when located on the scalp they are non–hair bearing. During puberty they commonly become oily and crusty, presenting a cosmetic nuisance. More significantly, they have a 10% to 15% risk of basal cell skin cancer in adulthood. For these reasons, the treatment of choice for scalp sebaceous nevi is surgical excision. Evaluation of the surgical margins can be difficult for pathologists, but wide excision is overly aggressive and unnecessary. When these nevi occur on the face, conservative observation, tangential shave excision, and CO_2 laser vaporization may be chosen to avoid an obvious surgical scar, as long as parents understand the risk of basal cell skin cancer will not be removed.

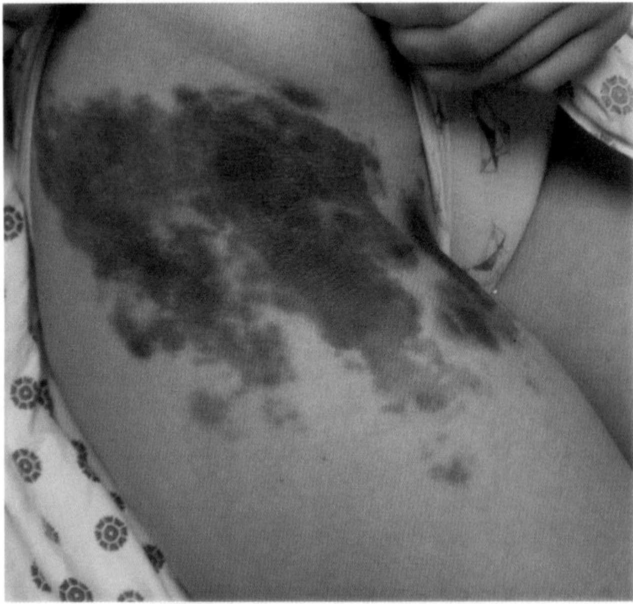

FIGURE 26.10. An epidermal nevus is benign, but the texture of the skin often becomes increasingly verrucous and unsightly. Removal by shave excision, dermabrasion, and laser vaporization may provide adequate palliation. Full-thickness excision is curative for small or linear lesions at the expense of a permanent surgical scar.

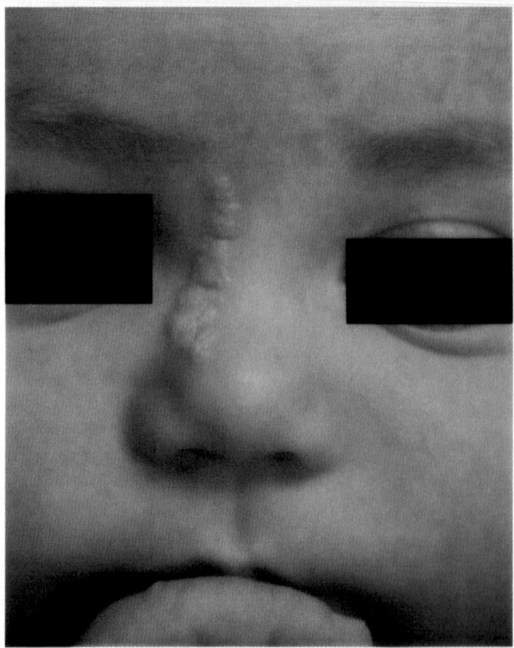

FIGURE 26.12. A sebaceous nevus has a cobblestone texture that worsens during puberty. There is a 10% to 15% risk of basal cell carcinoma in adulthood. Most parents will opt for removal and accept a surgical scar prior to the patient's teenage years.

CYSTS

Epidermal Cysts

Epidermal cysts will forever be inaccurately called sebaceous cysts, owing to the assumption that they are filled with sebum because of a blocked pore. In fact, they are actually lined by epidermis and filled with desquamated epidermal cells and fatty acids, which give them a cheesy texture and odor. Complete excision of the capsule with a small amount of adherent overlying skin is necessary to minimize the risk of recurrence. Some surgeons will intentionally evacuate the contents of a large cyst and allow the capsule to contract, resulting in a smaller scar when the residual cyst is excised at a later date. If they become secondarily infected, they become inflamed and painful, and also contain purulent drainage under pressure. In this setting, incision and drainage is usually palliative rather than curative, and patients return after the inflammation subsides for definitive excision. Unruptured and noninflamed cysts usually shell out easily from the surrounding subcutaneous tissue (**Figure 26.13**), whereas previously inflamed or recurrent cysts often have dense adhesions to the surrounding fat.

Pilomatrixomas (Calcifying Epithelioma of Malherbe)

French physician Albert Malherbe described a benign tumor of hair cell origin (*pilo = hair*) that clinically appears similar to an epidermal cyst, but with a rock-hard texture. They are usually adherent to the overlying skin, and sometimes may be mistaken for a vascular malformation as the overlying skin may contain a bluish hue and small telangiectasias, which resolve after excision. The capsule is thin and fragile, and clusters of calcified granules are easily visualized through it. Complete excision with a small amount of adherent overlying skin is curative (**Figure 26.14**).

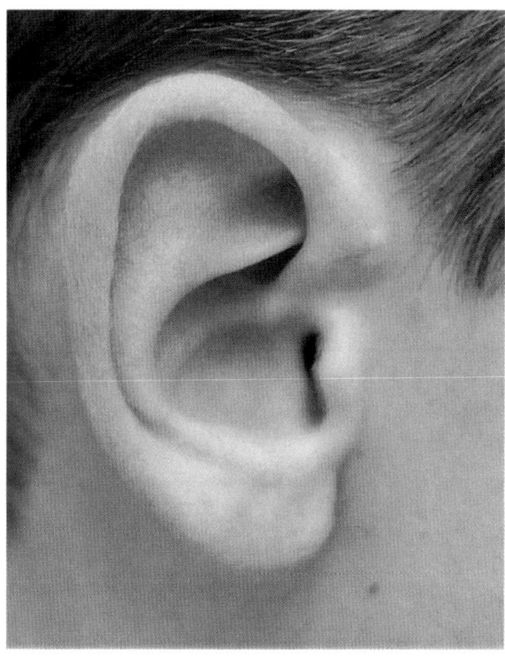

FIGURE 26.14. Pilomatrixoma (calcifying epithelioma of Malherbe). Unlike an epidermal cyst, a pilomatrixoma contains hard calcified granules. The overlying skin may have telangiectasias or a bluish pigmentation, mimicking a vascular lesion. The pigmentation resolves once the pilomatrixoma is excised.

Dermoid Cysts

Dermoid cysts can occur anywhere along sites of embryologic fusion, but in the head, they can commonly occur in the periorbital, glabellar, and nasal regions as well as the scalp and temporal region. They contain dermis, epidermis, sebaceous glands, and hair and exhibit slow growth. Intracranial extension can occur with midline nasal, glabellar, and temporal dermoids; therefore, dermoids in these locations are best worked up with MRI or CT scans. Collaboration with neurosurgery may be required for complete cyst removal in these cases. Lateral brow dermoids are best approached through lateral supratarsal fold incisions that leave an imperceptible scar rather than through the eyebrow (**Figure 26.15**). They are commonly adherent to the periosteum and may even cause bony indentations that resolve after cyst removal.

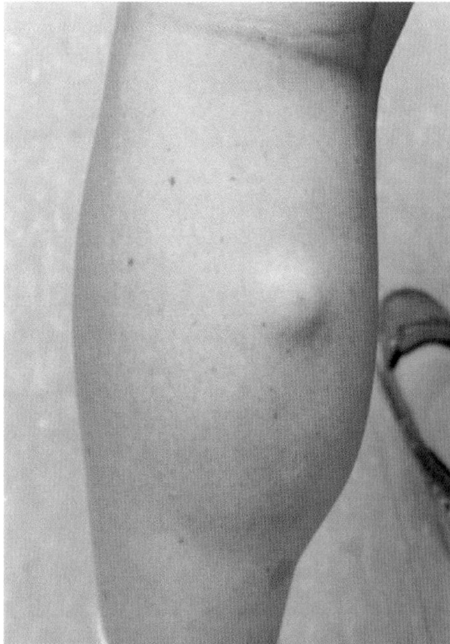

FIGURE 26.13. An epidermal inclusion cyst is adherent to the overlying dermis and can sometimes be confused with a superficial lipoma. Excision of the entire capsule is necessary to minimize the risk of recurrence.

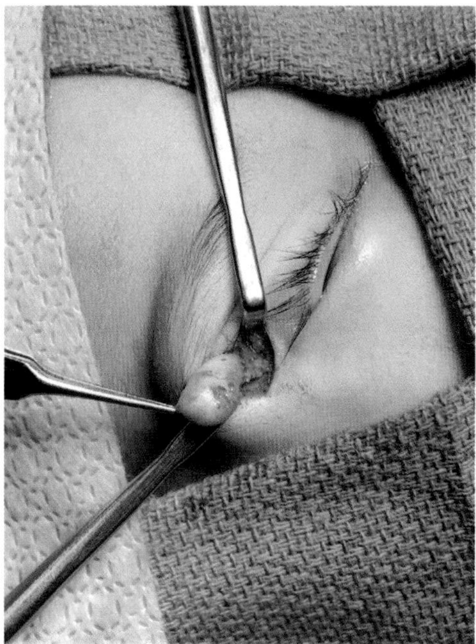

FIGURE 26.15. A dermoid cyst in the periorbital area is usually adherent to the underlying periosteum. Lateral brow dermoids are best approached through a lateral upper eyelid incision, which leaves an imperceptible scar.

ACKNOWLEDGMENTS

The authors are indebted to the contributions of Albert Yan, MD, Professor of Pediatrics and Dermatology, and Rosalie Elenitsas, MD, Herman Beerman Professor of Dermatology, Perelman School of Medicine at the University of Pennsylvania.

BIBLIOGRAPHY

1. Arad E, Zuker RM. The shifting paradigm in the management of giant congenital melanocytic nevi: review and clinical applications. *Plast Reconstr Surg.* 2014;133(2):367-376.
   An updated review is presented of controversial topics in the management of congenital melanocytic nevi, and clinical applications are demonstrated through clinical cases.
2. Chung C, Forte AJ, Narayan D, Persing J. Giant nevi: a review. *J Craniofac Surg.* 2006;17(6):1210-1215.
   A comprehensive review article describing the incidence, histology, and management of giant melanocytic nevus.
3. Ferguson RE Jr, Vasconez HC. Laser treatment of congenital nevi. *J Craniofac Surg.* 2005;16(5):908-914.
   Review of laser terminology is presented along with a review of nevus of Ota, nevus of Ito, and congenital melanocytic nevi.
4. Gosain AK, Santoro TD, Larson DL, Gingrass RP. Giant congenital nevi: a 20-year experience and an algorithm for their management. *Plast Reconstr Surg.* 2001;108(3):622-636.
   A retrospective review of 61 patients with giant congenital nevi is presented including the surgical treatments used. An algorithm for management is presented by the authors based on their experience over time.
5. Schaffer JV. Update on melanocytic nevi in children. *Clin Dermatol.* 2015;33(3):368-386.
   This review article summarizes the natural history and clinical spectrum of nevi in pediatric patients, and provides an update in their dynamic evolution over time, molecular insights into nevogenesis, and phenotypic markers for increased risk of melanoma.
6. Schaffer JV, Bolognia JL. The clinical spectrum of pigmented lesions. *Clin Plast Surg.* 2000:27(3):391-408.
   Review article presenting the clinical features of a spectrum of pigmented lesions, including congenital, Spitz, and blue nevi, as well as each subtype of cutaneous melanoma.

QUESTIONS

1. **Sebaceous nevi (nevus sebaceous of Jadassohn) may demonstrate all of the following except:**
   a. Lack of hair growth when located on the scalp
   b. Crusting and oily discharge during puberty
   c. 10% to 15% risk of basal cell carcinoma in adulthood
   d. 10% to 15% risk of squamous cell carcinoma in adulthood
   e. Difficult margins for the pathologist to interpret

2. **Appropriate treatment of congenital melanocytic nevi may include all of the following except:**
   a. Photographic documentation and periodic physical examination
   b. Punch biopsy or incisional biopsy
   c. Tangential shave biopsy
   d. Excisional biopsy
   e. Serial excision

3. **The ABCDEs of suspicious nevi include all of the following except:**
   a. Asymmetry
   b. Border irregular
   c. Color variegation
   d. Diameter >1 cm
   e. Evolution

4. **The following lesions are benign without malignant potential except:**
   a. Spitz nevus
   b. Pilomatrixoma
   c. Sebaceous nevus
   d. Nevus of Ota
   e. Nevus of Ito

5. **Which of the following statement is *not* true?**
   a. Dermoid cysts are present at birth.
   b. Dermoid cysts can contain hair in addition to dermis, epidermis, and sebaceous glands.
   c. Intracranial extension can occur with temporal dermoid cysts.
   d. Intracranial extension does not occur with lateral brow dermoid cysts.
   e. Dermoid cysts in the periorbital region may be adherent to the periosteum and cause bony indentations.

1. **Answer: d.** Parents will usually elect surgical excision when sebaceous nevi are located in their child's scalp because they are typically non–hair bearing and will develop oily crusts because of hormonal stimulation of the sebaceous glands during puberty, and because of the malignant potential (basal cell, not squamous cell carcinoma). Pathologists note that complete excision can be difficult to confirm because the margins can be challenging to interpret since normal skin contains sebaceous glands.

2. **Answer: c.** Photodocumentation of a congenital nevus allows the clinician to determine whether it is changing, and an evolving nevus warrants a biopsy. This is particularly useful when patients have many dysplastic nevi and excision of all of them is impossible or impractical. Periodic follow-up every 6 to 12 months with good-quality photographs is an appropriate way to monitor patients. A full-thickness biopsy is appropriate because it will allow one to determine tumor thickness and the level of invasion in the event of a melanoma. A shave biopsy can establish the diagnosis of melanoma, but it may make it impossible to ever know the true tumor thickness of a melanoma, and therefore removes the most import prognostic indicator (Breslow tumor thickness in millimeters). A punch or incisional biopsy of the thickest part of the nevus should include subcutaneous fat. An excisional biopsy or a serially excised nevus should also include superficial subcutaneous tissue.

3. **Answer: d.** Nevus size that should raise concern and prompt closer evaluation is >6 mm or about the size of a pencil eraser. Size, however, is probably the least important feature. The most important feature to note by history or repeated examination is changes in the appearance or evolution of the nevus over time. Other concerning symptoms may include crusting, bleeding, and itching.

4. **Answer: c.** Sebaceous nevi have a 10% to 15% risk of basal cell skin cancer in adulthood. Spitz nevi resemble melanoma histologically; however, their potential for malignant transformation is no greater than other small melanocytic nevi. Pilomatrixomas are benign tumors of hair cell origin that are adherent to the overlying skin and have a rock-hard texture due to the presence of calcified granules. Nevus of Ota is a dermal melanocytic nevus located on the face (V1 and V2 distribution). Nevus of Ito is characterized by dermal melanocytosis and location on the shoulder, upper chest, and back.

5. **Answer: d.** Dermoid cysts develop during pregnancy and can occur anywhere along sites of embryologic fusion. They contain dermis, epidermis, sebaceous glands, and hair and exhibit slow growth. Intracranial extension can occur with midline nasal, glabellar, and temporal dermoids; therefore, dermoids in these locations are best worked up with MRI or CT scans. Lateral brow dermoids are commonly adherent to the periosteum and may even cause bony indentations that resolve after cyst removal.

CHAPTER 27 Vascular Anomalies

Kavitha Ranganathan and Steven J. Kasten

KEY POINTS

- Vascular malformations fall into two broad categories: neoplastic and nonneoplastic.
- Vascular malformations are present at birth and grow concurrently with the patient, whereas hemangiomas present postnatally and commonly involute by adolescence.
- First-line pharmacologic treatments for hemangiomas include beta blockers, systemic steroids, and intralesional steroids.
- Vascular malformations are characterized based on whether they are slow or fast flow; lesions with an arterial component are fast flow, whereas all other lesions including venous, capillary, and lymphatic malformations are slow flow.
- Treatment for malformations is by multiple modalities depending on classification and anatomic location.
- Sclerotherapy is one potential intervention for venous and lymphatic malformations.
- Asymptomatic vascular malformations can be observed, but it is important to rule out other comorbid conditions and syndromes first.
- It is critical to remember that vascular anomalies can present as part of a syndrome; recognizing the associated symptoms and pathology is of utmost importance.

HISTORICAL PERSPECTIVE

In the 1800s, Virchow developed one of the first methods of characterizing vascular anomalies.[1,2] Subsequently, in 1996, the International Society for the Study of Vascular Anomalies (ISSVA) stratified these vascular anomalies into two main types: vascular malformations and vascular tumors. This work was heavily influenced by the work of Mulliken and Glowacki, whose initial research defined these types of lesions according to vessel composition, namely by whether the vessel is a capillary, venous, lymphatic, arterial, or combined malformation.[3] These guidelines were subsequently updated in 2014 and represent the most recent consensus on the definitions and clinical manifestations of vascular malformations and tumors.

Accurate diagnosis of vascular anomalies and tumors relies on obtaining a thorough history and physical examination, with timing of onset of the condition being one of the most critical considerations. Imaging is useful when determining the extent of the lesion as well as the amount of flow, particularly for vascular malformations. Slow-flow lesions include capillary, venous, and lymphatic malformations, whereas fast-flow lesions include any malformation with an arterial component. Historically, one of the most difficult aspects of caring for patients with such congenital anomalies has been the use of inconsistent terminology.[3] As the treatment and time course are quite different between vascular malformations and tumors, these variations in terminologies have affected progress within the field and have led to inconsistencies in treatment. The goal of the current chapter is to educate the reader on how to properly diagnose and differentiate vascular malformations from vascular tumors including hemangiomas, and manage these lesions based on the initial presentation of the patient as well as over time.

VASCULAR TUMORS

Infantile Hemangiomas

Epidemiology and Clinical Course

Hemangiomas are the most common tumor of infancy and occur at a rate of 11 in 10 infants. These lesions are not present at birth and are commonly visualized at approximately 2 weeks after birth. These tumors are more common in females (3:1) and Caucasians (1 in 10) with the most common location occurring in the head and neck region.[4,5] Diagnosis is largely clinical, when the diagnosis is in question based on history and physical examination. Hemangiomas are distinguished from vascular malformations by the timing of onset occurring after birth; conversely, vascular malformations are always present at birth. These benign vascular proliferations of endothelial cells go through three main phases during development: proliferation (0 to 12 months), involution (12 months to 10 years), and finally, regression (after 10 years).[4,5] Consideration for early intervention is critical for patients presenting with functional deficits associated with the presence of the anomaly. For example, early surgical or medical resection should be considered among patients presenting with hemangiomas that result in amblyopia, distortion of critical anatomic structures, ulceration and bleeding complications, or airway compromise. As infantile hemangiomas can present as part of a defined syndrome, patients may need to be evaluated for additional anomalies based on their clinical presentation (**Table 27.1**). Infantile hemangiomas are positive for glucose transporter 1 (GLUT-1) on biopsy of the lesion as well as within the urine.

Pathophysiology

Hemangiomas are thought to occur as a result of clonal mutations in hematopoietic endothelial stem cell populations that express mesenchymal stem cell markers.[6] Growth can be stimulated by hypoxic conditions within these stem cell populations and/or abnormal responses from vasculogenic endothelial growth factor receptor function.[6-12] Although the exact pathway responsible for hemangioma involution remains unclear, it is thought to occur via decreased endothelial cell proliferation and increased cell death. Hormonal alterations over time can also affect this process.

Imaging

As history and physical examination are the most important diagnostic tools for the proper diagnosis and evaluation of patients

TABLE 27.1. SYNDROMES/ANOMALIES ASSOCIATED WITH HEMANGIOMAS

Syndrome	Characteristic Features
Kasabach-Merritt syndrome	Thrombocytopenia (<10,000), hemangiomas
PHACES	Posterior fossa anomalies, hemangiomas, arterial anomalies, cardiac anomalies, eye/ear anomalies, sternal cleft, and supraumbilical raphe syndrome
Maffucci syndrome	Numerous enchondromas, hemangiomas
Von Hippel-Lindau disease	Retinal hemangiomas, cerebellar hemangioblastomas, visceral cysts and hemangiomas, developmental delay

presenting with hemangiomas, imaging is not commonly required. In fact, imaging may further complicate the diagnosis given that these are not the only lesions that demonstrate fast flow on ultrasound; any lesion with an arterial component, particularly arteriovenous malformations (AVMs), will demonstrate fast flow. Additional ultrasound findings include a shunting pattern of flow. MRI is an alternative imaging strategy; proliferating hemangiomas are isointense on T1 view and hyperintense on T2 view, with confluent enhancement and flow voids with contrast. As the hemangioma begins to involute, imaging may demonstrate an increase in fat content of the lesion. Given that most hemangiomas are treated nonoperatively, imaging is not commonly required and must be approached with caution particularly in pediatric populations.

Treatment

The most common nonsurgical treatment for hemangiomas is observation because many of these lesions completely involute over the course of the child's early life. As such, reassurance of the parents is critical during this phase of care. Observation is appropriate in the absence of functionally restricting features such as severe bleeding/ulceration, obstruction of the visual field or airway, or when the hemangioma does not involve critical structures such as the eyelid, ear, nose, or lips. As plastic surgeons see a select subset of patients presenting with hemangiomas, these patients oftentimes require treatment. Other nonsurgical treatment options include use of the pulsed dye laser to lighten the color of the hemangioma and improve skin texture while reducing bleeding from the site. This is particularly effective for superficial hemangiomas with minimal skin change in noncritical anatomic areas, but less effective for deeper lesions as the depth of penetration of the pulsed dye laser is approximately 0.75 to 1.2 mm.

For larger, deforming lesions, pharmacologic therapy represents an important mainstay of treatment, particularly for those hemangiomas that are in cosmetically sensitive areas or within anatomic structures of functional importance (**Figure 27.1**). These treatments are commonly instituted under the guidance of a multidisciplinary team, which can include dermatologists, hematologists, pediatricians, and plastic surgeons.

Systemic corticosteroids were previously considered the first-line pharmacologic treatment of choice. At doses of 2 to 3 mg/kg/d given for 4 to 6 weeks, corticosteroids (i.e., prednisone or prednisolone) are particularly effective when given during the proliferative period of hemangioma growth; this dose is subsequently tapered slowly toward the end of the treatment course. Approximately 85% to 88% of lesions stabilize after completion of treatment, and an initial response is seen within 1 or 2 weeks.[13] However, this treatment option is not without risk, causing cushingoid facies, cardiac disturbances, endocrine dysfunction, femoral head necrosis, and myopathy are potential side effects.[13-19]

Intralesional corticosteroid delivery is another method of drug administration that has lower risks of systemic side effects, but similar potential to prevent further growth and induce tumor regression.[20] During administration, clinicians must be cautious to perform the injection within the bulk of the hemangioma to prevent attenuation and atrophy of the surrounding normal tissues. Dosage is dependent on the size of the lesion. Although injectable steroid is known to be effective, topical corticosteroid application is ineffective.

Beta blockers have recently come into favor for management of hemangiomas and are utilized under similar indications as systemic corticosteroids. As it remains unclear whether beta blockers are more or less effective than steroids, the utilization of one pharmacologic agent over another may be tailored to the resources available at an individual institution. Beta blockers, most commonly propranolol, are administered at a dose of 2 mg/kg/d and are most effective when initiated during the proliferative phase of hemangioma growth. At many institutions, patients are admitted to the hospital for observation, while the first dose of the beta blocker is administered to monitor for hypoglycemia and hypotension. Patients must also pass a thorough cardiopulmonary evaluation prior to drug initiation, given the potential for serious adverse effects. Topical beta blockers such as timolol are also effective.[21-28]

Interferon alpha-2A is considered a second-line treatment for patients who are not responding to corticosteroid therapy or who are unable to tolerate beta blockade. At a subcutaneous dose of 2 to 3 mU/m^2, a response is usually seen within 6 to 10 months.[29] Although the most serious side effect to monitor is spastic diplegia, fevers, transaminitis, neutropenia, and anemia are other potential complications. This treatment is thought to be particularly effective for patients with Kasabach-Merritt syndrome.

Another second-line agent for the treatment of infantile hemangiomas is vincristine.[22,23] As this is a chemotherapeutic agent, side effects include peripheral neuropathy, infections, and hair loss. Although the response rate is thought to approach over 80%, patients are required to have a central line for administration. Thus, this agent is not commonly used in lieu of other less hazardous pharmacologic treatment strategies.[30,31]

Surgical management is required for hemangiomas that cause functionally disruptive symptoms as described (**Figure 27.2**).[32-34] Excision can be performed in a single-stage fashion for smaller lesions or in a staged fashion for larger lesions; management is dependent on the location and size of the lesion. Because there is no future neoplastic potential, it should be kept in mind that complete excision of the hemangioma in one stage is not required, and partial excision may facilitate reconstruction. Historically, circular excision with purse-string closure is one potential technique

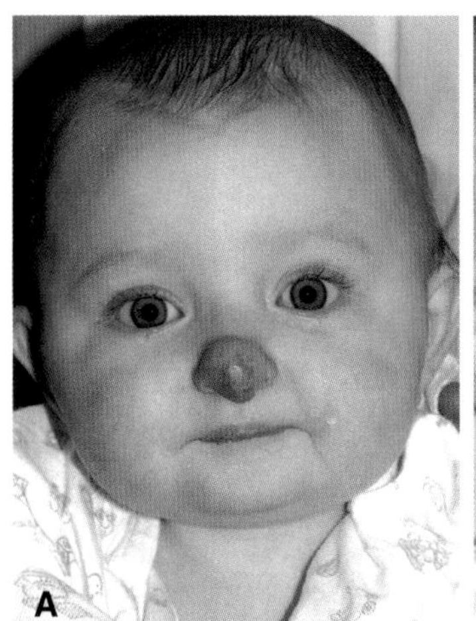

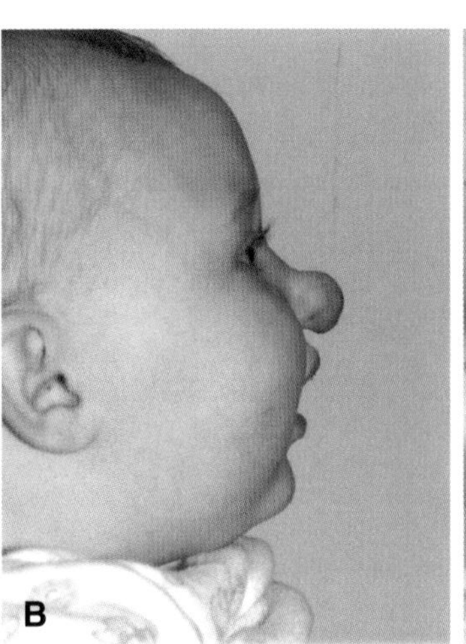

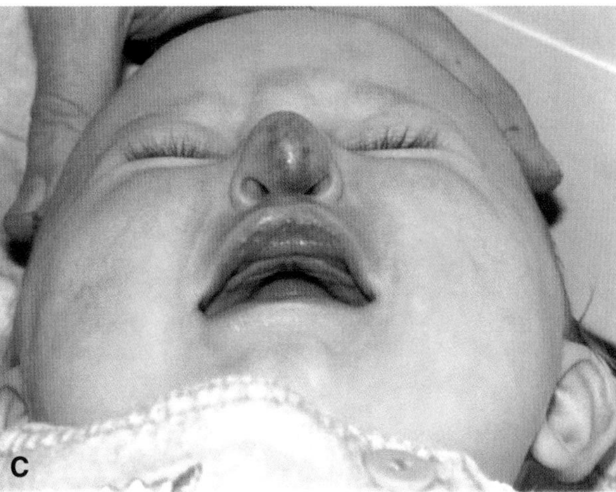

FIGURE 27.1. Nasal hemangiomas can dramatically distort the underlying anatomy and result in significant residual deformity. Prompt treatment with intralesional steroid, beta blockers, or systemic steroids is critical.

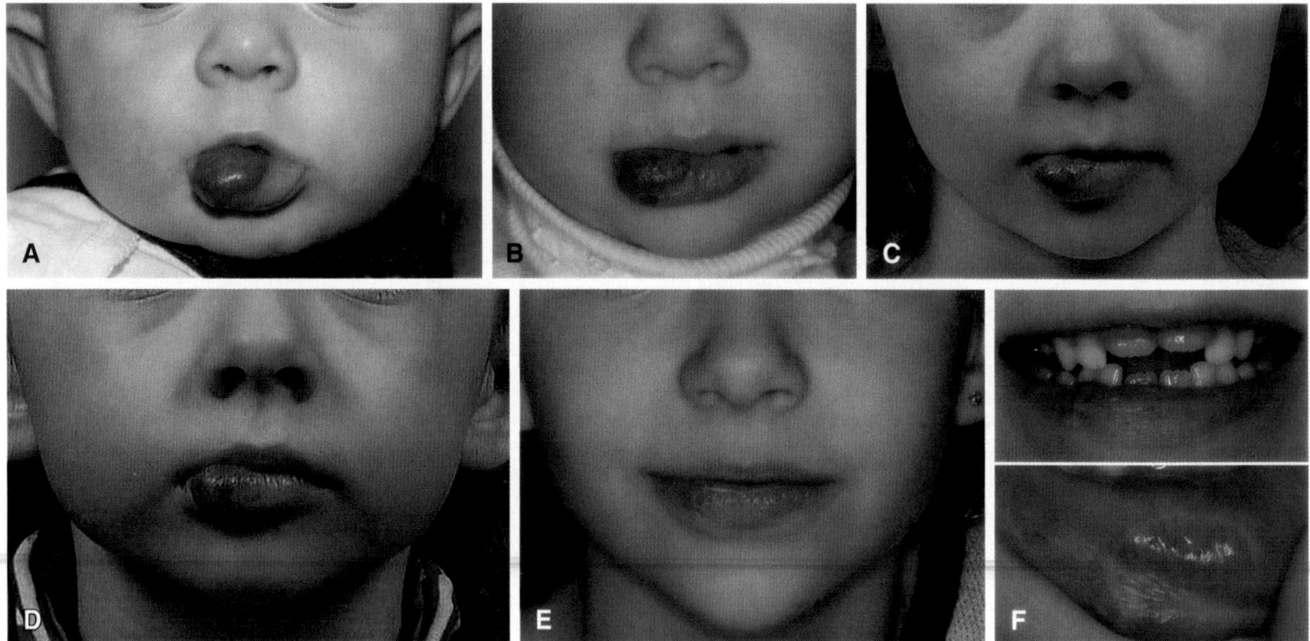

FIGURE 27.2. Hemangiomas of the lip can also cause significant deformity that even after involution results in soft-tissue laxity and discoloration. **A.** Initial presentation of lower-lip hemangioma. **B.** Two-year follow-up. **C.** Three-year follow-up. **D.** Four-year follow-up. **E,F.** Surgical excision performed six years after initial presentation resulted in significant improvement in contour and overall appearance.

for excision to decrease the dimensions of the scar. For larger lesions, concomitant tissue expansion may be required to facilitate soft-tissue coverage. Although previous reports of the use of tissue expanders in the back and extremities have high complication rates particularly due to infection and extrusion, it is our experience that tissue expansion remains an excellent option for vascular anomalies in these locations in pediatric patient populations. Regardless of the technique used, surgeons must approach excision with utmost caution, as these lesions may remain highly vascular even in the resolution phase and can result in significant blood loss intraoperatively. For this reason, preoperative embolization may be required.

Congenital Hemangiomas

Although infantile hemangiomas are typically defined by their postnatal origins and development, a subgroup of hemangiomas known as congenital hemangiomas arise within the fetus and are fully grown at birth. Congenital hemangiomas have a characteristic appearance associated with their development, which includes a surrounding whitish halo, pale central portion of the lesion, and otherwise reddish hue. There are two main types of congenital hemangiomas: noninvoluting congenital hemangiomas (NICH) and rapidly involuting congenital hemangiomas. Although both commonly present within the head and neck region, noninvoluting hemangiomas demonstrate persistent fast flow and do not regress, whereas rapidly involuting hemangiomas substantially regress within a few months of birth. Additionally, congenital hemangiomas are distinguished from infantile hemangiomas based on the expression of glucose transporter protein-1 (GLUT-1); congenital hemangiomas are negative for GLUT-1, whereas infantile hemangiomas are positive.[35-37]

Hemangioendotheliomas

Hemangioendotheliomas are lesions that can manifest at birth or postnatally. Like other types of vascular anomalies, history and physical examination is the key to proper diagnosis. Although these lesions do not metastasize, hemangioendotheliomas are locally aggressive and characteristically enlarge beyond 5 cm in diameter. They are most commonly located in the head and neck region and are equally common in males and females. When these lesions are suspected, biopsy should be considered to rule out malignancy.[38-40] Importantly, hemangioendotheliomas can present as part of Kasabach-Merritt phenomenon.[41,42] In addition to causing pain and local-tissue destruction, hemangioendotheliomas are also associated with thrombocytopenia and bleeding in this setting; platelet transfusions may exacerbate swelling so should be avoided unless indicated for uncontrolled bleeding in this circumstance. Given the aggressive, invasive nature of hemangioendotheliomas, resection is not commonly possible. Thus, symptomatic control is the mainstay of care for these patients. For those with Kasabach-Merritt phenomenon, vincristine is the first-line treatment; agents used to treat hemangiomas including beta blockers and steroids are usually ineffective for this indication.[41,42] Although some hemangioendotheliomas regress by 2 years of age, many of these lesions do not involute with time, necessitating symptomatic management as the main goal of care.

VASCULAR MALFORMATIONS

Epidemiology and Clinical Course

The key distinguishing factor between vascular malformations and hemangiomas is the timing of onset. Unlike hemangiomas, vascular malformations are always present at birth because of aberrancies in vessel formation in utero.[43-45] Although the lesion may not be clinically evident, vascular malformations are characterized by this timeline. These lesions are equally common among males and females and grow proportionately with the child over time. These lesions often enlarge to become symptomatic or clinically evident at puberty because of the impact of hormonal changes on these lesions. Vascular malformations do not involute. Many lesions are composed of a mixture of these vessel types and are therefore classified as combined lesions; biopsy should be considered for any lesion when there is uncertainty regarding the diagnosis. Similar to hemangiomas, vascular malformations can be associated with a variety of concomitant conditions including platelet trapping and coagulopathy that may require further workup.

TABLE 27.2. SYNDROMES/ANOMALIES ASSOCIATED WITH CAPILLARY MALFORMATIONS

Syndrome	Characteristic Features
Sturge-Weber syndrome	Capillary malformations in V1/V2 distribution, leptomeningeal capillary malformations (presents as seizures, hemiplegia), ocular symptoms, developmental delay
Klippel-Trenaunay syndrome	Capillary malformations, lymphatic malformations, hypertrophy of extremity (commonly lower extremity)
Parkes Weber syndrome	Capillary malformation, AVMs, hypertrophy of extremity
Cobb syndrome	Capillary malformation of trunk, spinal AVM

AVM, arteriovenous malformation.

Capillary Malformations

Composed of collections of thin-walled capillaries within the dermis, capillary malformations are slow-flow lesions. As capillary malformations often manifest within a characteristic dermatomal distribution, it is thought that these lesions are at least in part influenced by the autonomic nervous system. For example, Sturge-Weber syndrome is defined by a capillary malformation within the V1 trigeminal nerve distribution. These lesions are present at birth, do not involute, and grow concurrently with the patient.[45-47] Capillary malformations occur with greater frequency among female children and can be associated with various syndromes (**Table 27.2**).

Isolated cutaneous capillary malformations do not require imaging for further characterization unless uncertainty exists with regard to the presence of visceral lesions or to more clearly define the extent of these lesions. If imaging is required for these purposes, MRI is one potential option. Ultrasound is another option, but may simply demonstrate the presence of a high-flow lesion and is of limited value.

Three main lines of treatment are utilized in the management of capillary malformations. Observation is the first option; this strategy is suitable for asymptomatic vascular malformations. For lesions that are ulcerated and/or pigmented, pulsed dye laser represents an effective treatment when delivered in a serial fashion.[48-50] Finally, excision is another option. In the setting of capillary malformations, excision in the form of debulking is mainly indicated for patients presenting with soft-tissue/skeletal hypertrophy of the tissues underlying the malformation (**Figure 27.3**). Once again, care must be taken to address the potential for significant blood loss in these cases.

Lymphatic Malformations

Lymphatic malformations are slow-flow lesions. Similar to other vascular malformations, these lesions can also cause hypertrophy of the underlying soft tissues. The extent of these lesions is commonly characterized by MRI. Imaging findings and the extent of symptoms dictate the need for treatment in these cases. MRI findings include a soft-tissue mass with low signal on the T1 window and high signal with fluid levels on the T2 window. Symptoms can range from mild pain to severe swelling, edema, and recurrent infections. As with capillary malformations, observation is an option for asymptomatic lesions; compression garments and wraps serve as important adjuncts. Conversely, well-defined, symptomatic lesions that are not adjacent to anatomic structures of importance are amenable to intervention. Two main interventions are commonly utilized: sclerotherapy and surgical excision. Macrocystic lesions are commonly treated with sclerosing agents such as doxycycline, ethanol, and sodium tetradecyl sulfate. Microcystic lesions are less amenable to sclerotherapy and are instead treated with surgical excision.[51,52] Direct excision and liposuction are potential techniques utilized for operative intervention.[53-55] Sirolimus has recently been reported as an effective medical treatment, but convincing evidence is lacking.

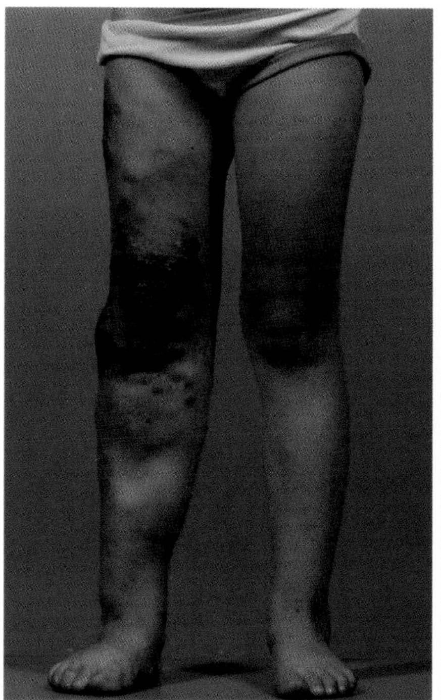
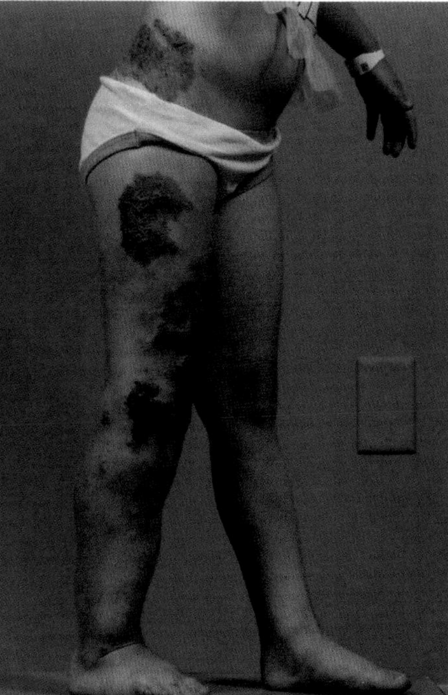
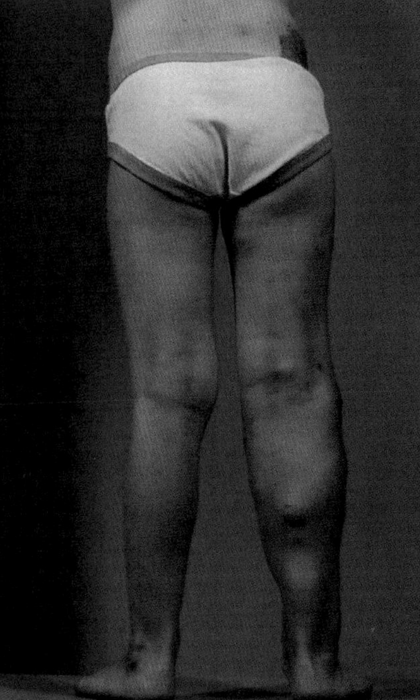

FIGURE 27.3. Klippel-Trenaunay syndrome manifests as limb hypertrophy as a result of soft-tissue and bone overgrowth in the presence of vascular malformations composed of lymphatics, venous, and/or capillaries. These lesions are very difficult to manage depending on the severity of the disease process. Observation, pulsed dye laser, and excision are potential options of treatment.

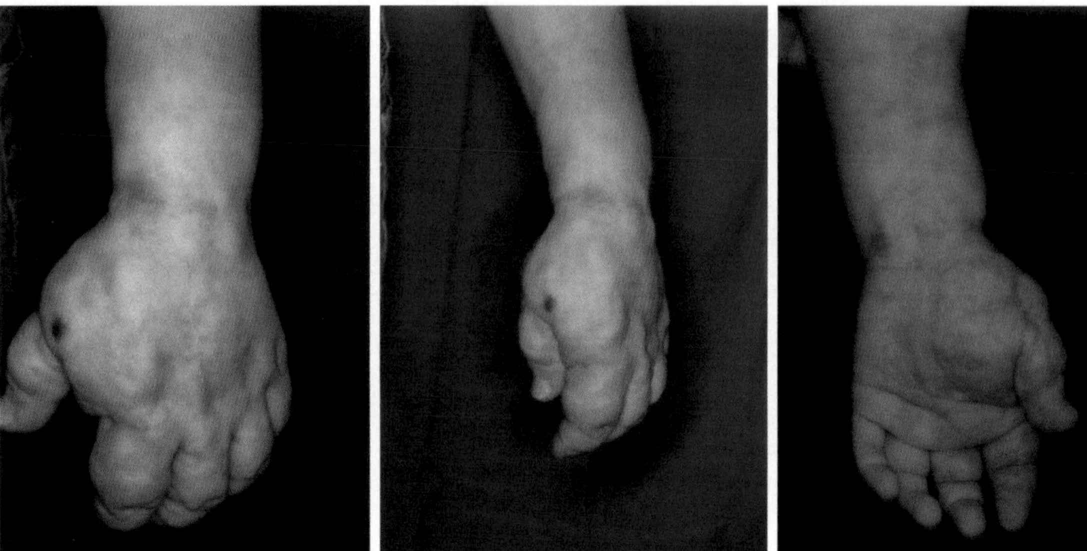

FIGURE 27.4. Venous malformations are slow-flow lesions that can be distinguished by a history of swelling when the extremity is placed in a dependent position. Such malformations can cause pain as a result of phleboliths and chronic inflammation. Compression garments, sclerotherapy, and surgical excision are potential treatment options.

Venous Malformations

Venous malformations are composed of numerous thin-walled veins, many of which lack valves and normal smooth muscle control. Consequently, these lesions are associated with swelling and edema at the site of the malformation when in a dependent position; this characteristic feature is an important component to isolate in the history and physical examination when a venous malformation is part of the differential diagnosis (**Figure 27.4**). MRI demonstrates isointense signal within the lesion on the T1 window and high signal with signal voids at sites of phleboliths on the T2 window. Treatment of venous malformations is similar to that of lymphatic malformations. Options include observation, compression wraps, sclerotherapy, and excision for debulking. Low-dose aspirin therapy is helpful for pain due to microthrombi.[56-59]

Arteriovenous Malformations

AVMs are high-flow lesions that result from an abnormal connection between an artery and vein (**Figure 27.5**).[60,61] These malformations are thought to go through four main stages of development. In the first stage, AVMs begin as quiescent lesions that may or may not be evident at birth. On imaging, however, shunting is seen within these lesions on ultrasound. MRI demonstrates soft tissue thickening with flow voids on the T1 window with a variable increase in signal and similar flow voids in the T2 window. Stage 2 consists of expansion of the AVM, which can manifest as a thrill or bruit on physical examination. As the lesion progresses to the destructive phases (stage 3), episodes of bleeding, pain, and local-tissue damage become apparent. Finally, stage 4 is associated with heart failure and continued local-tissue destruction. Given the extensive blood loss commonly associated with AVMs as a result of the shunting of blood between the arterial and venous systems, surgeons must be cautious prior to proceeding directly to surgical resection. Thus, observation is one potential option for care. Importantly, however, AVMs can progress and lead to significant sequelae including cardiac failure. Consequently, early intervention should be considered to minimize the risk of subsequent complications. Treatment may be operative or nonoperative, depending on the symptoms and anatomic location. When surgery is required, preoperative embolization or ligation of the AVM can decrease blood loss and facilitate surgical resection. These lesions may also be associated with syndromes and additional anomalies (**Table 27.3**).[62-68]

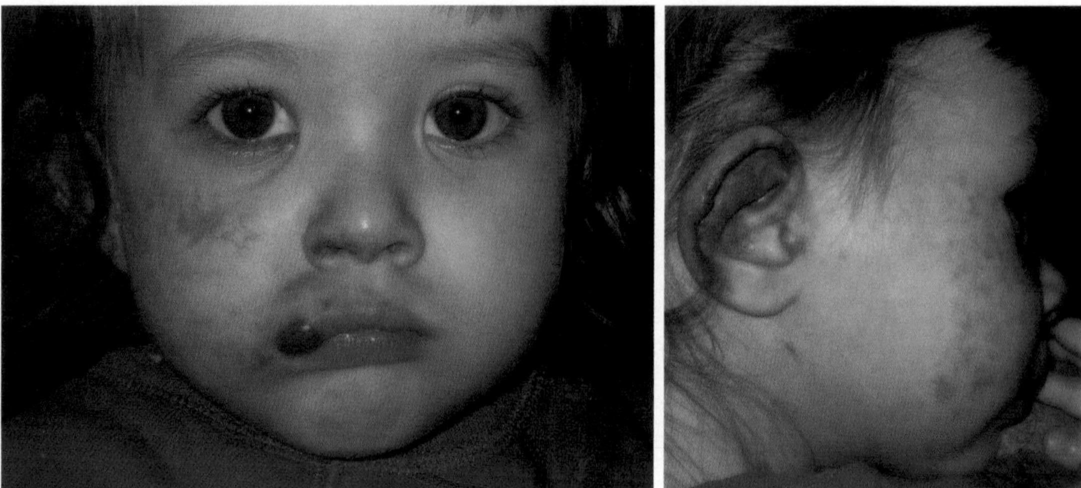

FIGURE 27.5. Arteriovenous malformations are fast-flow lesions that are commonly treated with observation given their invasive nature. Such malformations are present at birth and do not involute with time.

TABLE 27.3. SYNDROMES/ANOMALIES ASSOCIATED WITH ARTERIOVENOUS MALFORMATIONS (AVMS)

Syndrome	Characteristic Features
Bannayan-Zonana syndrome	AVMs, microcephaly, lipomas
Riley-Smith syndrome	AVMs, microcephaly, pseudopapilledema
Osler-Weber-Rendu disease	Cutaneous telangiectasias, frequent nosebleeds, AVMs of viscera

CONCLUSION

Vascular anomalies represent common conditions among pediatric plastic surgery patients. Accurate, timely diagnosis is imperative so that a proper treatment plan can be designed and implemented (**Figure 27.6**). Hemangiomas commonly regress without the need for intervention, whereas vascular malformations grow in conjunction with the patient. Although pharmacologic agents are particularly effective to prevent growth and potentially induce involution for hemangiomas, only interventions such as sclerotherapy and surgical resection are used for vascular malformations. Thus, by understanding the principles that guide the diagnosis of vascular anomalies to

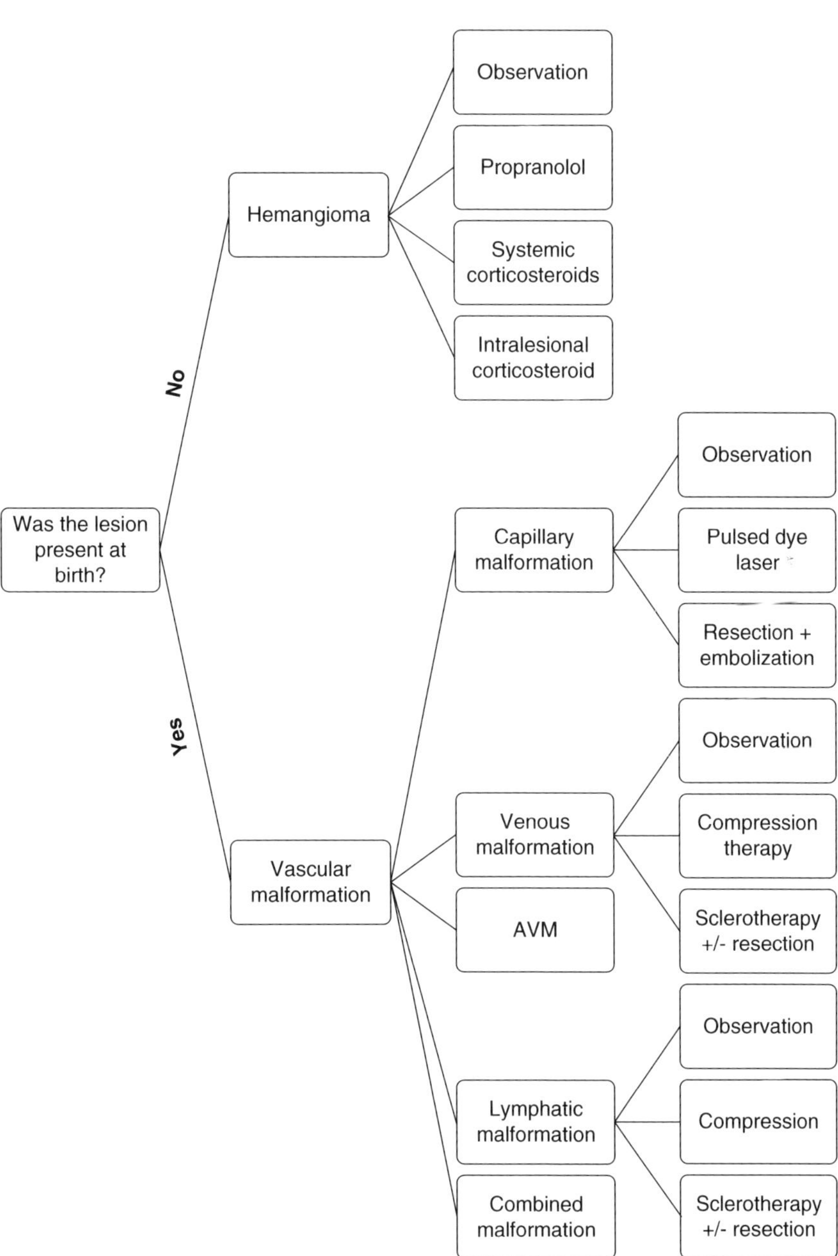

FIGURE 27.6. Algorithm for management of common vascular anomalies.

differentiate vascular tumors from malformations, and properly diagnose and differentiate vascular malformations from vascular tumors including hemangiomas, and recognizing the differences in treatment algorithms between these two conditions, clinicians can improve outcomes among patients presenting with these common anomalies.

REFERENCES

1. Mulliken JB, Young A. *Vascular Birthmarks: Hemangiomas and Malformations.* Philadelphia: WB Saunders; 1988.
2. Virchow R. *Angioma in die Krankhaften Geschwulste.* Vol. 3. Berlin: Hirschwald; 1863:306-425.
3. Mulliken JB, Glowacki J. Hemangiomas and vascular malformations in infants and children: a classification based on endothelial characteristics. *Plast Reconstr Surg.* 1982;69:412-422.
   In this landmark manuscript, Mulliken and Glowacki classify vascular anomalies into two main categories: vascular malformations and hemangiomas. Using 49 specimens from various types of vascular lesions, the authors found that hemangiomas were distinguished by endothelial hyperplasia and rapid growth during early infancy in the proliferative phase and by fibrosis and fatty infiltration in the involuting phase. Vascular malformations were noted at birth and grew proportionately with the child. This manuscript has served as the foundation for our current principles regarding the diagnosis of hemangiomas and vascular malformations.
4. Smoller BR, Apfelberg DB. Infantile (juvenile) capillary haemangioma: a tumor of heterogeneous cellular elements. *J Cutan Pathol.* 1993;20:330-336.
5. Mancini AJ, Smoller BR. Proliferation and apoptosis within juvenile capillary hemangiomas. *Am J Dermatopathol.* 1996;18:505-514.
6. Khan ZA, Boscolo E, Picard A, et al. Multipotential stem cells recapitulate human infantile hemangioma in immunodeficient mice. *J Clin Invest.* 2008;118:2592-2599.
7. Yu Y, Flint AF, Mulliken JB, et al. Endothelial progenitor cells in infantile hemangioma. *Blood.* 2004;103:1373-1375.
8. Khan ZA, Melero-Martin JM, Wu X, et al. Endothelial progenitor cells from infantile hemangioma and umbilical cord blood display unique cellular responses to endostatin. *Blood.* 2006;108:915-921.
9. Kleinman ME, Tepper OM, Capla JM, et al. Increased circulating AC133+ CD34+ endothelial progenitor cells in children with hemangioma. *Lymphat Res Biol.* 2003;1:301-307.
10. Kleinman ME, Greives MR, Churgin SS, et al. Hypoxia- induced mediators of stem/progenitor cell trafficking are increased in children with hemangioma. *Arterioscler Thromb Vasc Biol.* 2007;27:2664-2670.
11. Kilcline C, Frieden IJ. Infantile hemangiomas: how common are they? A systematic review of the medical literature. *Pediatr Dermatol.* 2008;25:168-173.
12. Finn MC, Glowacki J, Mulliken JB. Congenital vascular lesions: clinical application of a new classification. *J Pediatr Surg.* 1983;18:894-900.
13. Sloan GM, Renisch JF, Nichter LS, et al. Intralesional corticosteroid therapy for infantile hemangiomas. *Plast Reconstr Surg.* 1989;83:459-467.
   Sloan et al. administered intralesional corticosteroid injections consisting of a mixture of betamethasone and triamcinolone to 31 patients with hemangiomas; most of these lesions were located in the craniofacial region. Of these lesions, 13% almost completely resolved, 32% showed greater than 50% reduction in volume, 32% demonstrated less than 50% reduction in volume, and 23% showed no change. As none of these lesions grew and there were no complications, intralesional steroid injections were found to be a safe and potentially effective treatment for hemangiomas.
14. Barlow CF, Priebe C, Mulliken JB, et al. Spastic diplegia as a complication of interferon-alfa-2a treatment of hemangiomas of infancy. *J Pediatr.* 1998;132:527-530.
15. Haisley-Royster C, Enjolras O, Frieden IJ, et al. Kasabach-merritt phenomenon: a retrospective study of treatment with vincristine. *J Pediatr Hematol Oncol.* 2002;24:459-462.
16. Enjolras O, Breviere GM, Roger G, et al. Vincristine treatment for function- and life-threatening infantile hemangioma. *Arch Pediatr.* 2004;11:99-107.
17. Zarem HA, Edgerton MT. Induced resolution of cavernous hemangiomas following prednisolone therapy. *Plast Reconstr Surg.* 1967;39:76-83.
18. Boon LM, MacDonald DM, Mulliken JB. Complications of systemic corticosteroid therapy for problematic hemangiomas. *Plast Reconstr Surg.* 1999;104:1616-1623.
19. Bennett ML, Fleischer AB, Chamlin SL, et al. Oral corticosteroid use is effective for cutaneous hemangiomas. *Arch Dermatol.* 2001;137:1208-1213.
20. Greene AK, Rogers G, Mulliken JB. Management of parotid hemangioma in 100 children. *Plast Reconstr Surg.* 2004;113:53-60.
21. Greene AK. Corticosteroid treatment for problematic infantile hemangioma: evidence does not support an increased risk for cerebral palsy. *Pediatrics.* 2008;126:1251-1252.
22. Greene AK. Systemic Corticosteroid is effective and safe treatment for problematic infantile hemangioma. *Pediatr Dermatol.* 2010;23:322-323.
23. Greene AK, Couto RA. Oral prednisolone for infantile hemangioma: efficacy and safety using a standardized treatment protocol. *Plast Reconstr Surg.* 2011;128:743-752.
   Hemangiomas in 25 patients were treated with oral prednisolone to determine the safety and efficacy of oral corticosteroid treatment. Patients received a dose of 3 mg/kg/d for one month followed by a gradual taper. Of these hemangiomas, 88% regressed and 12% demonstrated stability in size. The most common complication was a transient cushingoid appearance.
24. Leaute-Labreze C, Dumas de la Roque E, Hubiche T, et al. Propranolol for severe hemangiomas of infancy. *N Engl J Med.* 2008;358:2649-2651.
   In this letter to the editor, Leaute-Labreze et al. use data obtained from eleven patients to demonstrate the safety and efficacy of propranolol for hemangiomas. It is thought that propranolol may exert its effect by decreasing the expression of vascular endothelial growth factors, triggering apoptosis within capillary endothelial cells, and inducing vasoconstriction.
25. Sans V, Dumas de la Roque E, Berge J, et al. Propranolol for severe infantile hemangiomas: follow-up report. *Pediatrics.* 2009;124:423-431.
26. Lawley LP, Siegfried E, Todd JL. Propranolol treatment for hemangioma of infancy: risks and recommendations. *Pediatr Dermatol.* 2009;26:610-614.
27. Frieden IL, Drolet BA. Propranolol for infantile hemangiomas: promise, peril, pathogenesis. *Pediatr Dermatol.* 2009;26:642-644.
28. Holland KE, Frieden IJ, Frommelt PC, et al. Hypoglycemia in children taking propranolol for the treatment of infantile hemangioma. *Arch Dermatol.* 2010;146:775-778.
29. Pavlakovic H, Kietz S, Lauerer P, et al. Hyperkalemia complicating propranolol treatment of an infantile hemangioma. *Pediatrics.* 2010;126:e1589-e1593.
30. Buckmiller LM, Munson PD, Dyamenahalli U, et al. Propranolol for infantile hemangiomas: early experience at a tertiary vascular anomalies center. *Laryngoscope.* 2010;120:676-681.
31. Goswamy J, Rothera MP, Bruce IA. Failure of propranolol in the treatment of childhood haemangiomas of the head and neck. *J Laryngol Otol.* 2011;125:1164-1172.
32. Scarcella JV, Dykes ER, Anderson R. Hemangiomas of the parotid gland. *Plast Reconstr Surg.* 1965;36:38-47.
33. Williams HB. Hemangiomas of the parotid gland in children. *Plast Reconstr Surg.* 1975;56:29-34.
34. Little KE, Cywes S, Davies MR, et al. Complicated giant hemangioma: excision using cardiopulmonary bypass and deep hypothermia. *J Pediatr Surg.* 1976;11:533-536.
35. Boon LM, Enjolras O, Mulliken JB. Congenital hemangioma: evidence of accelerated involution. *J Pediatr.* 1996;128:329-335.
36. Enjolras O, Mulliken JB, Boon LM, et al. Noninvoluting congenital hemangioma: a rare cutaneous vascular anomaly. *Plast Reconstr Surg.* 2001;107:1647-1654.
37. Berenguer B, Mulliken JB, Enjolras O, et al. Rapidly involuting congenital hemangioma: clinical and histopathologic features. *Pediatr Dev Pathol.* 2003;6:495-510.
38. Lyons LL, North PE, Mac-Moune Lai F, et al. Kaposiform hemangioendothelioma: a study of 33 cases emphasizing its pathologic, immunophenotypic, and biologic uniqueness from juvenile hemangioma. *Am J Surg Pathol.* 2004;28:559-568.
39. Debelenko LV, Perez-Atayde AR, Mulliken JB, et al. D2–40 immunohistochemical analysis of pediatric vascular tumors reveals positivity in kaposiform hemangioendothelioma. *Mod Pathol.* 2005;18:1454-1460.
40. Zukerberg LR, Nikoloff BJ, Weiss SW. Kaposiform hemangioendothelioma of infancy and childhood: an aggressive neoplasm associated with Kasabach–Merritt syndrome and lymphangiomatosis. *Am J Surg Pathol.* 1993;17:321-328.
41. Sarkar M, Mulliken JB, Kozakewich HP, et al. Thrombocytopenic coagulopathy (Kasabach–Merritt phenomenon) is associated with kaposiform hemangioendothelioma and not with common infantile hemangioma. *Plast Reconstr Surg.* 1997;100:1377-1386.
42. Enjolras O, Wassef M, Mazoyer E, et al. Infants with Kasabach-Merritt syndrome do not have "true" hemangiomas. *J Pediatr.* 1997;130:631-640.
43. Johnston M. Radioautographic study of the migration and fate of cranial neural crests in the chick embryo. *Anat Rec.* 1966;156:143-155.
44. Nozue T, Tsuzaki M. Further studies on distribution of neural crest cells in prenatal or postnatal development in mice. *Okajimas Folia Anat Jpn.* 1974;51:131-160.
45. Smoller BR, Rosen S. Port-wine stains. A disease of altered neural modulation of blood vessels? *Arch Dermatol.* 1986;122:177-179.
46. Cunha e Sa M , Barroso CP , Caldas MC , et al. Innervation pattern of malformative cortical vessels in Sturge–Weber disease: a histochemical, immunohistochemical, and ultrastructural study. *Neurosurgery.* 1997;41:872-876.
47. Enjolras O, Riché MC , Merland JJ . Facial port-wine stains and Sturge–Weber syndrome. *Pediatrics.* 1985;76:48-51.
48. Tan OT, Sherwood K, Gilchrest BA. Treatment of children with port-wine stains using the flashlamp- pulsed tunable dye laser. *N Engl J Med.* 1989;320:416-421.
   Tan et al. treated port wine stains in 35 children with the pulsed dye laser. The authors reported that all lesions cleared after an average of 6.5 laser treatments, and review the demographic and clinical characteristics associated with improved responsiveness in this manuscript.
49. Chapas AM, Eickhorst K, Geronemus RG. Efficacy of early treatment of facial port wine stains in newborns: a review of 49 cases. *Lasers Surg Med.* 2007;39:563-568.
50. Huikeshoven M, Koster PH, de Borgie CA, et al. Redarkening of port-wine stains 10 years after pulsed- dye-laser treatment. *N Engl J Med.* 2007;356:1235-1240.
51. Padwa BL, Hayward PG, Ferraro NF, et al. Cervicofacial lymphatic malformation: clinical course, surgical intervention, and pathogenesis of skeletal hypertrophy. *Plast Reconstr Surg.* 1995;95:951-960.
52. Smith MC, Zimmerman B, Burke DK, et al. Efficacy and safety of OK-432 immunotherapy of lymphatic malformations. *Laryngoscope.* 2009;119:107-115.
53. Choi DJ, Alomari AI, Chaudry G, et al. Neurointerventional management of low-flow vascular malformations of the head and neck. *Neuroimaging Clin N Am.* 2009;19:199-218.
54. Alomari AI, Karian VE, Lord DJ, et al. Percutaneous sclerotherapy for lymphatic malformations: a retrospective analysis of patient-evaluated improvement. *J Vasc Interv Radiol.* 2006;17:1639-1648.

55. Burrows PE, Mitri RK, Alomari A, et al. Percutaneous sclerotherapy of lymphatic malformations with doxycycline. *Lymphat Res Biol.* 2008;6:209-216.
56. Padwa BL, Hayward PG, Ferraro NF, et al. Cervicofacial lymphatic malformation: clinical course, surgical intervention, and pathogenesis of skeletal hypertrophy. *Plast Reconstr Surg.* 1995;95:951-960.
57. Edwards PD, Rahbar R, Ferraro NF, et al. Lymphatic malformation of the lingual base and oral floor. *Plast Reconstr Surg.* 2005;115:1906-1915.
58. Upton J, Coombs CJ, Mulliken JB, et al. Vascular malformations of the upper limb: a review of 270 patients. *J Hand Surg (Am).* 1999;24:1019-1035.
59. Hein KD, Mulliken JB, Kozakewich HP, et al. Venous malformations of skeletal muscle. *Plast Reconstr Surg.* 2002;110:1625-1635.
60. Enjolras O, Ciabrini D, Mazoyer E, et al. Extensive pure venous malformations in the upper or lower limb: a review of 27 cases. *J Am Acad Dermatol.* 1997;36:219-225.
61. Adams DM, Wentzel MS. The role of the hematologist/oncologist in the care of patients with vascular anomalies. *Pediatr Clin North Am.* 2008;55:339-355.
62. Halsted W. Congenital arteriovenous and lymphaticovenous fistulae: unique clinical and experimental observations. *Proc Natl Acad Sci USA.* 1919;5:76-79.
63. Holman E. The physiology of an arteriovenous fistula. *Am J Surg.* 1955;89:1101-1108.
64. Mulliken JB, Fishman SJ, Burrows PE. Vascular anomalies. *Curr Probl Surg.* 2000;37:517-584.
65. Kohout MP, Hansen M, Pribaz JJ, et al. Arteriovenous malformations of the head and neck: natural history and management. *Plast Reconstr Surg.* 1998;102:643-654. *In this retrospective review of 81 patients with arteriovenous malformations at a single institution, the authors review the natural history of these lesions. The most common site of arteriovenous malformations was in the midface. Lesions were more common in females than in males. Characteristics associated with both positive and negative outcomes after treatment are discussed in this article.*
66. Wu IC, Orbach DB. Neurointerventional management of high-flow vascular malformations of the head and neck. *Neuroimaging Clin North Am.* 2009;19:219-240.
67. Liu AS, Mulliken JB, Zurakowski D, et al. Extracranial arteriovenous malformations: natural progression and recurrence after treatment. *Plast Reconstr Surg.* 2010;125:1185-1194.
68. Burrows P, Laor T, Paltiel H, Robertson R. Diagnostic imaging in the evaluation of vascular birthmarks. *Pediatr Dermatol.* 1998;16(3):455-488.

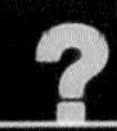

QUESTIONS

1. Which of the following syndromes is characterized by hemihypertrophy of a limb in the presence of lymphaticovenous malformations?

   a. Klippel-Trenaunay syndrome
   b. Sturge-Weber syndrome
   c. Osler-Weber-Rendu disease
   d. Parkes Weber syndrome
   e. Riley-Smith syndrome

2. A 3-week-old boy presents with a well-circumscribed but growing vascular lesion of the nasal tip, which presented immediately after birth that is deforming the underlying anatomic structures. What is the best first step in management that will decrease the extent of deformity?

   a. Observation
   b. Obtain additional imaging to confirm the diagnosis prior to treatment
   c. Biopsy the lesion
   d. Intralesional steroid injection
   e. En bloc resection with lymph node biopsy

3. Which of the following lasers is commonly used to reduce the red discoloration associated with superficial capillary malformations?

   a. Pulsed dye laser
   b. Yag laser
   c. Erbium laser
   d. Alexandrite laser
   e. None of the above

4. A 10-year-old girl presents to you with Kasabach-Merritt syndrome. Which of the following consultants should also be involved prior to surgical intervention?

   a. Neurologist
   b. Hematologist
   c. Infectious disease specialist
   d. No consultants needed

5. Which of the following congenital anomalies is defined by its presence as a fast-flow lesion present upon birth?

   a. Venous malformation
   b. Epidermoid cyst
   c. Infantile hemangioma
   d. AVM
   e. Dermoid cyst

1. **Answer: a.** Klippel-Trenaunay syndrome. This syndrome is defined by the presence of a vascular malformation commonly composed of lymphatics, venous structures, and capillaries within a limb that results in hypertrophy compared with the contralateral side (see **Figure 27.5**). Resection can be difficult, as the malformation is commonly embedded within the surrounding anatomic structures.

2. **Answer: d.** Intralesional steroid injection. This lesion is likely a hemangioma of the nasal tip based on the history and physical examination findings. During the proliferative phase, intralesional steroid injection can prevent further growth of the lesion and minimize deformity in this manner. Additional imaging and biopsy are unnecessary in these circumstances as the history and physical examination are characteristic for a hemangioma.

3. **Answer: a.** The pulsed dye laser is commonly used to treat the discoloration associated with capillary malformations and hemangiomas. This laser targets oxyhemoglobin, which is why it is useful for this indication, and delivers energy at a wavelength of 595 nm.

4. **Answer: b.** A hematologist should be consulted for patients presenting with Kasabach-Merritt syndrome. Workup and evaluation of thrombocytopenia is critical for this patient population, particularly prior to surgical intervention.

5. **Answer: d.** AVMs are fast-flow lesions. One of the key distinguishing features between hemangiomas and vascular malformations is that the latter are present at birth. Venous malformations are slow-flow lesions that are present at birth. Epidermoid cysts and dermoid cysts can originate any time after birth and are not vascular structures. Infantile hemangiomas present after birth and are one of the most common benign tumors among children.

CHAPTER 28 Nonsyndromic Craniosynostosis and Deformational Plagiocephaly

Jesse A. Taylor and Ian C. Hoppe

KEY POINTS

- The pathogenesis of nonsyndromic craniosynostosis is multifactorial, with some evidence that certain forms may be related to genetic mutations, but less so than with cases of syndromic craniosynostosis.
- The growth of the infant's cranial vault is directly related to the growing brain, and in some cases, its restriction may lead to changes in skull shape and increased intracranial pressure (ICP). The effects of elevated ICP as a result of craniosynostosis on neurodevelopment in children is controversial, but treatment of the calvarial/orbital deformity may lead to improved skull shape and neuropsychological well-being.
- Differentiation between positional posterior plagiocephaly and lambdoid craniosynostosis is made based on the shape of the head, position of the ears, the presence of a mastoid bulge, and the appearance of the forehead on the affected side.
- Although significant variability exists in type and timing of treatment, most centers intervene during the first year of life to release any restriction on the growing brain, normalize appearance differences, and minimize the risk of secondary deformities.
- Certain craniosynostotic deformities are amenable to minimally invasive treatments that can result in less perioperative morbidity and more rapid recovery. Enthusiasm for minimally invasive techniques must be tempered by the lack of long-term follow-up and some reports of high revision rates.
- Complications in craniosynostosis surgeries are fortunately rare but can be serious in nature and warrant timely intervention.

Craniosynostosis is the premature fusion of one or more cranial sutures resulting in distinctive calvarial and facial deformities, as well as the potential for neurocognitive impairment. Most interventions attempt to address both of these concerns. Most cases are idiopathic, with a small number having genetic underpinnings. Genetic forms of craniosynostosis may be associated with other noncraniofacial deformities including limb and spine anomalies.

The pathophysiology of craniosynostosis is still poorly understood. Of historical note, Virchow correlated the premature closure of cranial sutures with the development of distinctive deformities of the cranial vault and made one of the first attempts to describe the deformities of the cranial vault and cranial base seen in craniosynostosis.[1] His hypothesis was that the environment of the suture solely determined whether it would remain patent, completely independent of any external influences (intracranial contents). *Virchow* law states that closure of a cranial suture results in compensatory growth parallel to the fused suture, with arrest of growth in a perpendicular fashion to the suture.

In the mid 20th century, Moss and Salentijn described the *functional matrix theory*, which dictates that normal cranial vault development is dependent on a normal *neural mass* and its subsequent expansion.[2] Consequently, the suture itself may not be the primary source of the deformity; instead a complex interplay between the cranial base and expanding brain may be the culprit.

The modern management of craniosynostosis involves early diagnosis with interventions aimed at minimizing constricted brain growth and craniofacial deformities. A wide variety of procedures have been developed, including limited craniectomy with or without molding helmets, regional cranial vault remodeling, whole vault remodeling, and cranial distraction osteogenesis.

ANATOMY AND EMBRYOLOGY

The skull consists of the neurocranium (cranial vault and base) and the viscerocranium (facial bones). The mammalian cranial vault is predominantly comprised of five bones: the paired frontal and parietal bones and the interparietal bone, with contributions from parts of the temporal and sphenoid bones. These bones derive from neural crest cells and form via intramembranous ossification. The boundaries between these bones form sutures, specifically the paired coronal and lambdoid sutures and the sagittal and metopic sutures. All sutures, with the exception of the metopic suture, are initiated at a point where neural crest cells and mesoderm are in close approximation. Growth occurs perpendicular to the orientation of sutures and is predominantly driven by the rapidly expanding brain during the infant period. When a suture closes prematurely, this normal perpendicular growth does not occur and compensatory growth occurs parallel to the affected suture.[3] A depiction of the various forms of craniosynostosis are presented in **Figure 28.1**.

EPIDEMIOLOGY

The incidence of craniosynostosis is estimated to be between 1 in 2000 and 1 in 2500 live births,[4,5] with the most common suture fused being sagittal, followed by coronal, metopic, and lambdoid.[6] Recently it has been observed that metopic craniosynostosis is increasing in prevalence, with various hypotheses explaining the phenomenon.[4,7,8] There is a paucity of literature on the evolving incidence of craniofacial malformations, although sporadic reports have indicated a decreased incidence of live births given increased utilization of prenatal genetic testing and imaging, which may have led to an increased rate of termination of pregnancy in some parts of the world.[9,10]

PATHOGENESIS

Numerous theories and explanations have been set forth for the development of premature sutural fusion and include genetic processes and external environmental causes.

Genetics

The genetics of syndromic forms of craniosynostosis are fairly well described, but nonsyndromic single sutural forms are more diverse and generally do not demonstrate as much uniformity. A very small percentage of these are thought to be familial.[11] It is controversial to include genetic forms of craniosynostosis in the syndromic versus the nonsyndromic category, although others have reported the most common genetic mutations associated

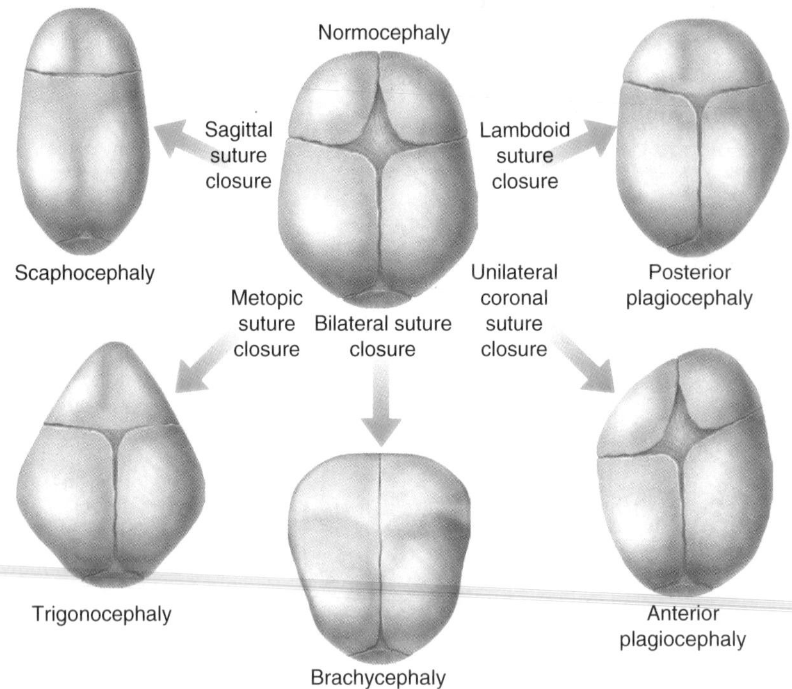

FIGURE 28.1. Clinical presentation of craniosynostosis.

with nonsyndromic craniosynostoses to be FGFR3, FGFR2, and TWIST1.[12] It is not entirely clear how these mutations cause craniosynostosis, but it is likely as a result of abnormal signaling of growth factors and stem cells at the dura mater-cranial suture interface. An examination of each suture and specific pathogenetic factors is presented in **Table 28.1**.

In general, genetic counseling is recommended in all cases of craniosynostosis but is of particular importance in the presence of coronal craniosynostosis or when multiple sutures are involved.[12] A telomeric fluorescent in situ hybridization analysis may be indicated for complex cases involving trigonocephaly.[11] This is an area of rapid clinical progress, and it is likely that genetic testing will become increasingly prevalent and useful in the coming years. As the price of whole genome sequencing and RNA sequencing drops, these more in-depth analyses will likely replace existing clinical tests.[13]

Other Potential Causes of Craniosynostosis

Intrauterine constraint has long been thought to contribute to certain presentations of craniosynostosis; however, the actual relationship remains unclear.[14] The association of some forms of craniosynostosis with plural births[15] seems to support this hypothesis, and the finding that fetal constraint can upregulate FGFR2 along fusing coronal sutures and induce changes in the cranial base in a murine model further strengthens the connection.[16,17] In addition, it has been found that lambdoid craniosynostosis is more common in male infants and in mothers experiencing preterm labor.[18] Maternal smoking and exposure to nitrosatable drugs in utero have been associated with certain forms of craniosynostosis.[19,20] The development of craniosynostosis has been associated with a paternal occupation of mechanic or repairman and in the agriculture and forestry sector.[21]

In summary, the pathogenesis of craniosynostosis is likely multifactorial, with some cases attributable to a germline genetic mutation. The exact cause of nonsyndromic craniosynostosis remains unknown and is an active area of investigation.

Deformational Plagiocephaly

The 1992 American Academy of Pediatrics *Back to Sleep* campaign began recommending a supine sleeping position for all infants to reduce the rate of sudden infant death syndrome. The unintended side effect is an increase in the number of cases of nonsynostotic positional cranial deformities.[22] These cases present with a marked flattening of one or both sides of the occiput, oftentimes with compensatory changes in the forehead and face. It is important to differentiate this condition from the similarly appearing, but extremely rare, lambdoid craniosynostosis. This distinction can almost always be based on physical examination (**Table 28.2**). The presence of a mastoid bulge on the involved side (**Figure 28.2**) is nearly pathognomonic for lambdoid craniosynostosis and is rarely found in cases of positional plagiocephaly. Correctly diagnosing positional plagiocephaly avoids unnecessary radiologic examinations and intracranial procedures

TABLE 28.1. PATHOGENETIC FACTORS OF CRANIOSYNOSTOSIS

	Sex Predominance	Familial Transmission Rate	Genetics
Sagittal	Male	2%–6%	No consistent gene mutation identified
Coronal	Female	8%–14%	Mutations in FGFR3 (Muenke syndrome) and TWIST (Saethre-Chotzen syndrome) identified
Metopic	Male	~5%	No consistent gene mutation identified. Associated with cytogenetic abnormalities (deletion of chromosome 11q24, trisomy/deletion of 9p, and deletion of 7p)
Lambdoid	Male	Several case reports of familial transmission	No consistent gene mutations identified

TABLE 28.2. DIFFERENTIATING POSITIONAL PLAGIOCEPHALY FROM LAMBDOID CRANIOSYNOSTOSIS

Characteristic	Positional Plagiocephaly	Unilateral Lambdoid Craniosynostosis
Head shape (vertex view)	Parallelogram	Trapezoid
Frontal bossing	Ipsilateral	Contralateral
Ipsilateral forehead	Anteriorly displaced	Retruded
Ipsilateral occipitomastoid bulge	Absent	Present
Ipsilateral ear position when viewed from above	Anteriorly displaced	Posteriorly displaced
Ipsilateral ear position when viewed from behind	Level	Inferiorly displaced
Ipsilateral mastoid bulge	Absent	Present
Ridging of ipsilateral lambdoid suture	Absent	Present
Onset	After birth	Present at birth
Incidence	Very common	Very rare

with their associated risks. The treatment of this condition is nonsurgical, with encouragement of head turning, treatment of any underlying torticollis, physical therapy, and in some cases helmet molding therapy.

DIAGNOSIS

Radiologic Investigation

Although the diagnosis of many forms of craniosynostosis can be made on physical examination alone,[23] a computed tomography (CT) scan is considered the standard for radiological imaging of cranial sutures, with a sensitivity and specificity for craniosynostosis close to 98%.[23] The high resolution obtained with a thin-slice CT scan provides a high-fidelity view of the bony and sutural architecture, can provide a high-level view of any underlying intracranial pathology, and may assist in treatment planning. However, the risk of subjecting an infant's brain to the effects of ionizing radiation must be weighed against the potential downsides.[23-26]

In an effort to minimize or avoid exposure to ionizing radiation, some centers have developed ultrasound and low-dose CT protocols.[27,28] Importantly, consultation with a specialist is recommended prior to performance of imaging, as this will usually avoid any unnecessary tests.

Intracranial Pressure and Neurodevelopmental Implications

When cranial sutures fuse prematurely, there can be growth restriction of the growing brain, potentially leading to increased intracranial pressure (ICP) and neurocognitive impairment. In 1982, Renier and colleagues published a landmark paper examining the incidence of ICP in patients with varying forms of craniosynostosis[29] and found that approximately 14% of patients with single suture and 47% with multisuture craniosynostosis experienced obviously elevated ICP. This was found to decrease significantly following surgery to correct the deformity. These findings have been replicated, with some studies suggesting that the number of patients with increased ICP may be underestimated.[30]

Directly measuring ICP via placement of an intraventricular or intraparenchymal device is not practically performed in every patient with craniosynostosis. Thus, there has been much effort to determine a less invasive means of measuring it indirectly. Some of these methods include lumbar puncture (although oftentimes this still requires anesthesia in the pediatric patient), visual-evoked potentials, hemodynamic response to neonatal fontanelle compression, optic nerve sheath diameter,[31] and ocular coherence tomography.[32]

The ultimate concern with increased ICP in children with craniosynostosis is the effect that this has on neuropsychological development. Most research in this area is confounded by the difficulty

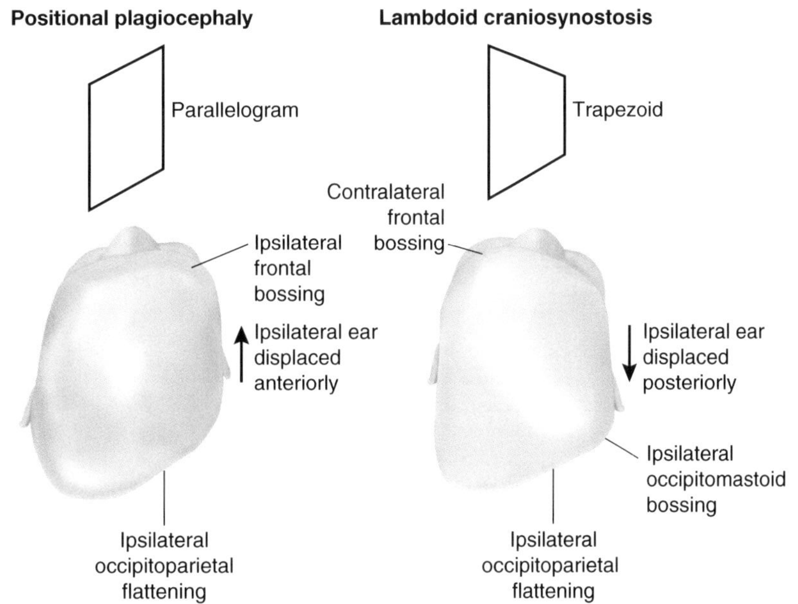

FIGURE 28.2. Clinical distinctions between posterior positional plagiocephaly and lambdoid craniosynostosis.

associated with measuring cognitive function in young children but seem to point to a mild neurocognitive deficit in this patient population.[33] A recent publication examining the difference between school-age children with craniosynostosis and unaffected controls found lower scores on measures of intelligence quotient and math in the group with craniosynostosis.[34] Another study found that timing of surgery, and specifically an earlier age at correction, may correlate with improved long-term neurological outcomes.[35] Many questions remain to be answered relating to pathophysiology of craniosynostosis, the role of ICP, and neurocognition. Based on the findings of the literature, it would seem prudent to refer patients with craniosynostosis for routine neurodevelopmental screening.

OPERATIVE MANAGEMENT OF CRANIOSYNOSTOSIS

General Considerations

Safety

Surgery for craniosynostosis is generally performed in large centers where a dedicated craniofacial team exists. A team of craniofacial anesthesiologists who understands the unique needs of these patients minimizes intraoperative complications such as under-resuscitation and other more catastrophic sequelae. In addition, the ability to establish invasive monitoring in a timely manner results in more expedient procedures. A dedicated nursing staff ensures that procedures are performed efficiently to minimize anesthetic time for patients. A pediatric intensive care unit that understands these procedures and how to care for these patients facilitates postoperative management.

Timing

The optimal timing of surgery for craniosynostosis is controversial, with most centers performing surgery within the first year of life.[36] Uncorrected restrictive deformities can be exacerbated by rapid brain growth, but brain growth may also be harnessed with surgical intervention to aid in their correction.[37–39] Generally speaking, minimally invasive procedures such as strip craniectomy ± molding helmet, spring-mediated cranial vault remodeling, and distraction-mediated cranial vault remodeling are performed earlier, with most centers targeting 3 to 6 months of age. Open cranial vault remodeling techniques are performed later, between 8 and 11 months of age.[36]

Informed Consent

Important things to include on informed consent for any cranial vault remodeling procedure include those that you would include for any surgical procedure (infection, bleeding, scars, wound healing complications, hematoma, seroma) as well as the possibility of skull contour irregularities, persistent bone gaps, cerebrospinal fluid leak, bone malunion/nonunion, hardware infection/extrusion, the need for additional procedures, and injury to the brain/eyes/nerves. It is important to stress that secondary procedures are sometimes needed later in life to correct contour irregularities, orbital deformities, or slight asymmetries or to close persistent bone gaps.

Sagittal Craniosynostosis

A scaphocephalic head shape (elongated skull with bitemporal/biparietal narrowing, frontal bossing, and occipital bulleting) and oftentimes a palpable ridge over the sagittal suture characterize this deformity (**Figure 28.3**). The deformity may predominantly affect the anterior and/or posterior skull depending upon what part of the sagittal suture is involved.

The goals of surgical intervention include reducing the anteroposterior dimension of the skull, increasing the skull height and width, and decreasing the frontal bossing/occipital bulleting. Numerous methods have been advocated to accomplish this including simple strip craniectomy, the π-procedure,[40] subtotal calvarial vault remodeling, endoscopic strip craniectomy with postoperative helmet therapy, and strip craniectomy with placement of transutural springs. Each method presents with unique advantages and challenges, with no single method being best for every patient. The more involved procedures (subtotal vault remodeling, π procedure) have the advantage of attempting to correct the deformity in one stage but carry the risks of maximally invasive surgery.[40] The minimally invasive procedures (suturectomies with either helmeting or springs) carry less operative risk of bleeding and anesthesia time but need to be performed earlier (2–4 months of age) to harness the rapid growth of the brain and skull at this age. Endoscopic suturectomy with postoperative helmet therapy requires a prolonged period (9–18 months) of intensive helmet therapy for which some families may be ill equipped.[41] Placement of springs following suturectomy requires a second anesthetic for removal of the devices. Another method of managing the deformity in sagittal craniosynostosis is to perform staged posterior and anterior vault remodeling procedures. The posterior vault is traditionally performed first, as there have been reports of an improvement in the anterior deformity following this intervention.[42] The posterior vault reconstruction is performed at 9 to 12 months of age, followed by a traditional fronto-orbital advancement (FOA) if needed at 18 to 24 months of age.

Coronal Craniosynostosis

The cranial deformity caused by premature closure of one of the coronal sutures includes ipsilateral forehead/supraorbital rim retrusion and brow elevation and contralateral forehead bossing (**Figure 28.4**). This is caused by restriction of anterior growth of the anterior cranial vault on the affected side causing compensatory growth on the unaffected side. The anterior restriction in growth is translated to the cranial base through the greater wing of the sphenoid, resulting in the *harlequin* orbital deformity that is seen on anteroposterior radiographs of patients with unicoronal craniosynostosis (**Figure 28.5**). The deformity of the cranial base results in characteristic facial features, including nasal radix deviation toward the affected side and chin point deviation toward the unaffected side.

Different treatment modalities have been proposed for this asymmetric condition including endoscopic craniectomy with helmet therapy, spring-mediated distraction, formal distraction osteogenesis, and conventional anterior cranial vault remodeling in the form of FOA. It is desirable to perform an overcorrection of the deformity to accommodate future growth of the child.[43] If the patient presents early (2–3 months of age), it may be possible to perform distraction osteogenesis for this deformity. A description of these two methods is as follows.

Fronto-Orbital Advancement Technique

The surgical procedure begins with placement of the child in the supine position, elevation of a bicoronal flap to expose the supraorbital region, and elevation of the temporalis muscle on the affected side. It is important to perform a subperiosteal dissection into the superior orbit (with care to protect the supraorbital nerve) with exposure of the entire fronto-orbital region. A neurosurgeon performs a frontal craniotomy and dissects the anterior cranial base and temporal region to facilitate access for osteotomies of the fronto-orbital bandeau. Osteotomies are performed as illustrated in **Figure 28.6**. The affected side is advanced (hinging on the unaffected side, supraorbital region); a bone graft is placed in the temporal region to maintain the advancement, and a resorbable plate is used to fixate it in place. The frontal bone is recontoured and replaced with resorbable plates and sutures. Any resultant bone gaps are filled with shavings from the frontal bone flap, and the scalp is closed over a closed suction drain.

Fronto-Orbital Distraction Technique

The positioning and exposure is the same as for a traditional FOA. The anticipated craniotomy is marked, usually extending from the contralateral mid-orbit to the ipsilateral pterion. It is important that the neurosurgeon places a bur hole at the pterion for osteotomy of the greater wing of the sphenoid. When performing distraction, it is critical to minimize dural dissection of the bone flap to preserve a *pedicle* to the segment undergoing transport. A traditional craniotomy

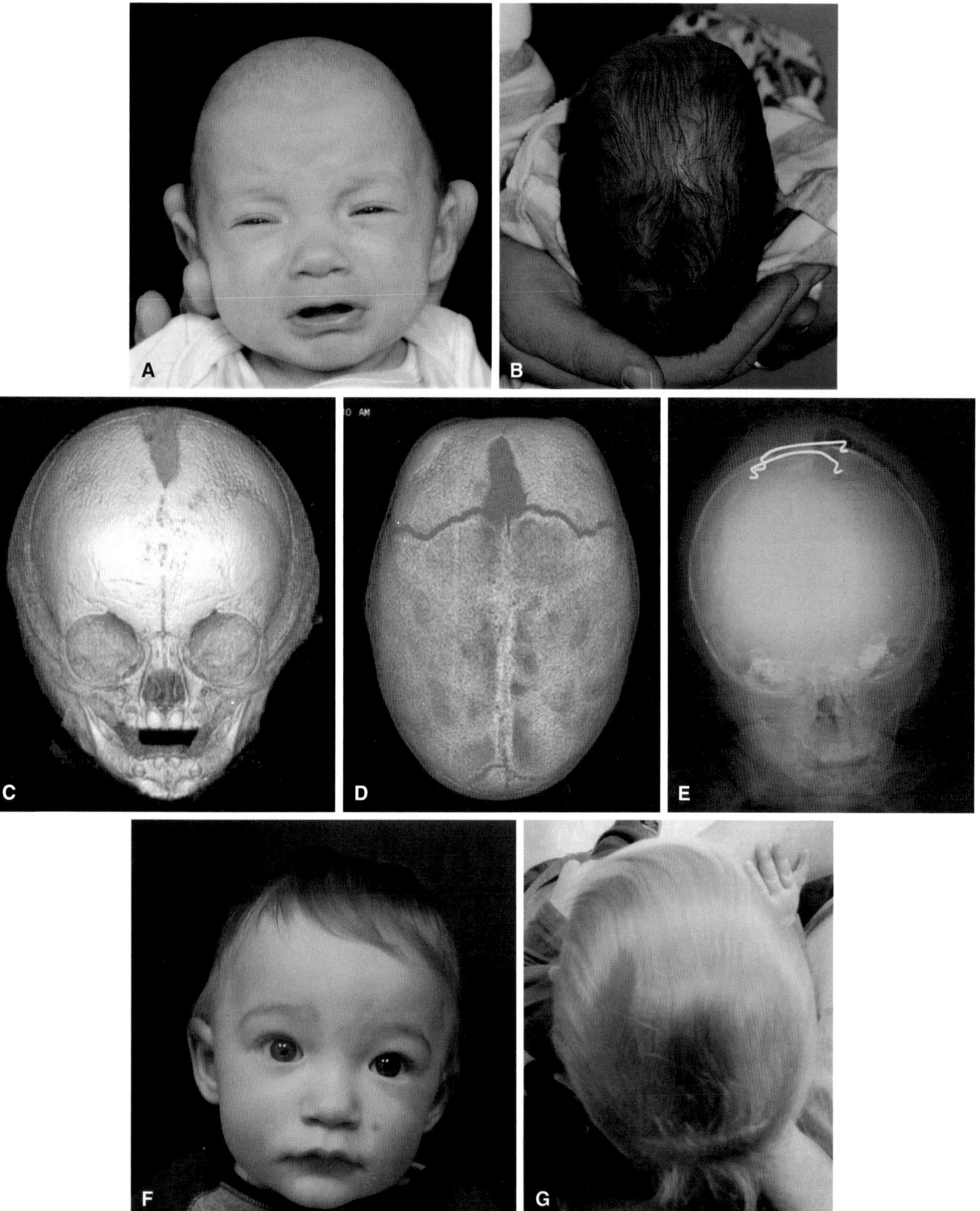

FIGURE 28.3. Sagittal craniosynostosis. Preoperative patient photos **(A,B)** and computed tomography images **(C,D)**. **E.** Postoperative radiograph demonstrating spring placement. **F,G.** Postoperative photos after removal of springs.

is performed posteriorly and carried into the lateral portion of the fronto-orbital bandeau. An osteotome is introduced through the pterional *window* and used to cut the greater wing of the sphenoid into the orbital roof. A *perforating* or interrupted osteotomy is then performed from the contralateral mid-orbit to the posterior extent of the previously made craniotomy (**Figure 28.7**). Finally, radial osteotomies of the ipsilateral orbital roof are performed to correct the horizontally short orbit. A distractor is secured to the stable skull and the now completely osteotomized bone flap with an anterior and slightly inferior vector.

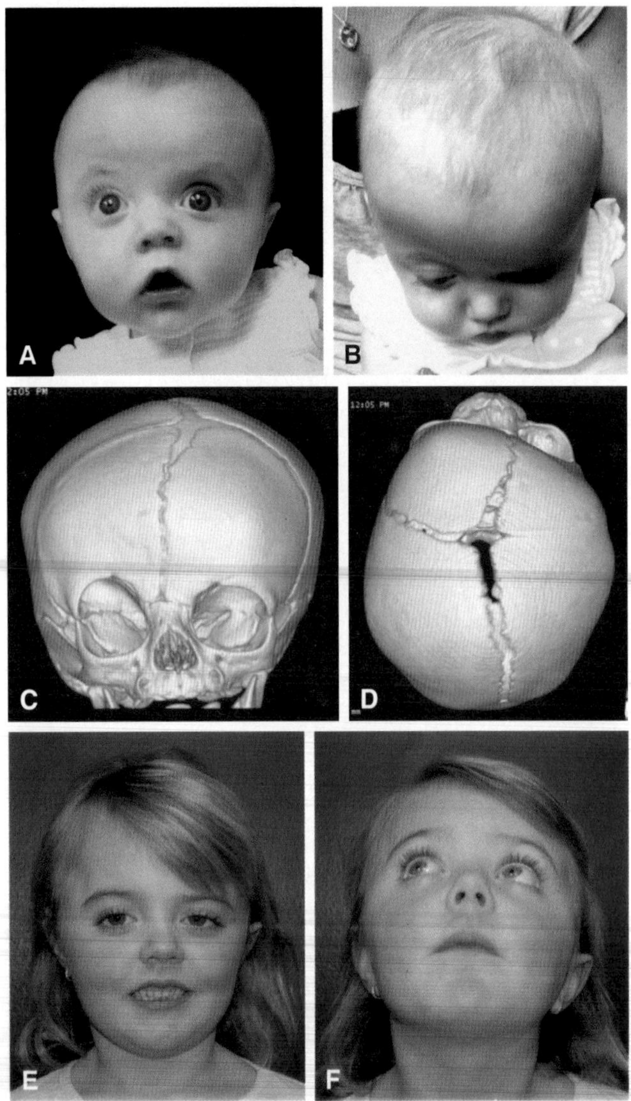

FIGURE 28.4. Right coronal craniosynostosis. Preoperative patient photos **(A,B)** and computed tomography images **(C,D)**. **E,F.** Postoperative photos after right-sided fronto-orbital advancement.

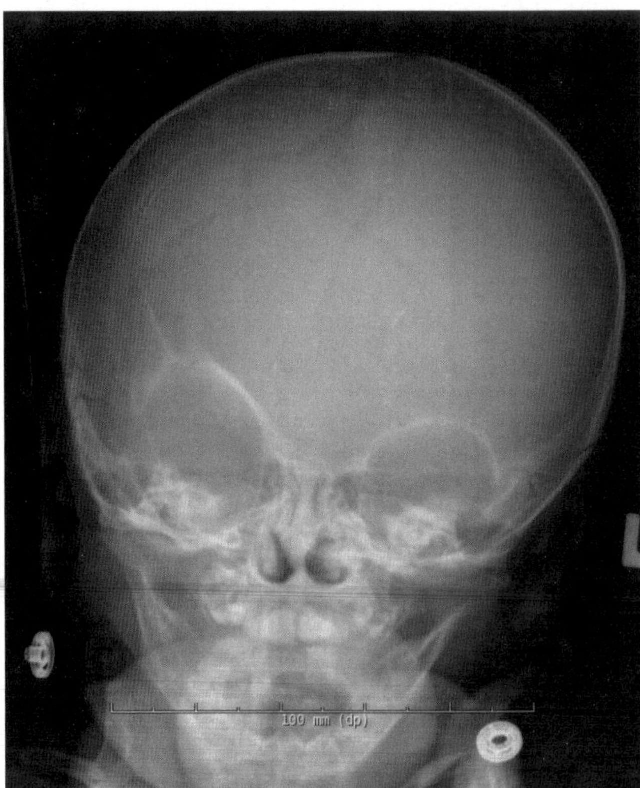

FIGURE 28.5. Anteroposterior radiograph demonstrating harlequin eye deformity seen in coronal craniosynostosis.

Metopic Craniosynostosis

The deformity associated with premature closure of the metopic suture is termed *trigonocephaly* and includes a keel-shaped forehead, hypotelorism, bitemporal narrowing, and oftentimes a palpable ridge over the fused suture (**Figure 28.8**). The deformity can be extremely variable because of the fact that the metopic suture normally closes before 8 months of age. The decision to intervene surgically is most often based on the severity of the trigonocephaly, not the fact that the suture is closed.

Although some centers advocate endoscopic suturectomy and helmet therapy or spring-mediated distraction, the most widely accepted treatment of trigonocephaly is a bilateral FOA. The osteotomies are performed bilaterally in a similar fashion to that described for unicoronal craniosynostosis. Following the removal of the bandeau, it is often split in the midline and widened with an interpositional bone graft. The lateral orbits are then bent inward to correct the bitemporal narrowing. The bandeau is then replaced, and the frontal bone is often split in the middle and barrel staved to decrease projection.

Lambdoid Craniosynostosis

Premature closure of the lambdoid suture is the least common form of craniosynostosis and results in ipsilateral occipital flatness and a mastoid bulge, posteroinferior displacement of the ipsilateral ear, and sometimes an ipsilateral frontal flattening. The most critical aspect in the diagnosis of lambdoid craniosynostosis is differentiating it from positional plagiocephaly, which is far more common and treated in a nonsurgical manner (see Figure 28.2 and Table 28.2).

The surgical treatment of lambdoid craniosynostosis is traditionally a posterior vault remodeling procedure. This is accomplished by putting the patient in the prone position and elevating the scalp over the occipital region. A posterior craniotomy is performed, and the

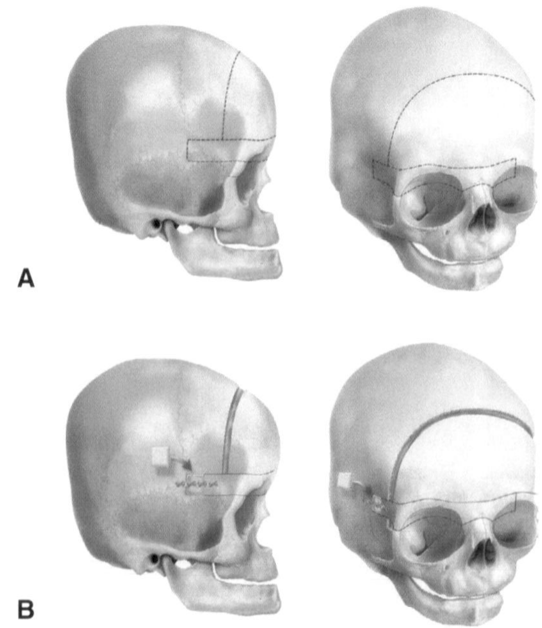

FIGURE 28.6. Technique of two-thirds fronto-orbital advancement for the treatment of unicoronal craniosynostosis. **A.** Osteotomies. **B.** Fixation.

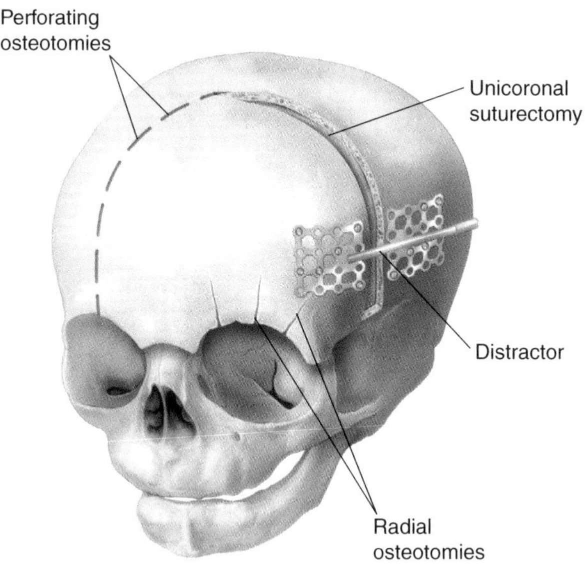

FIGURE 28.7. Technique of fronto-orbital distraction for treatment of unicoronal craniosynostosis.

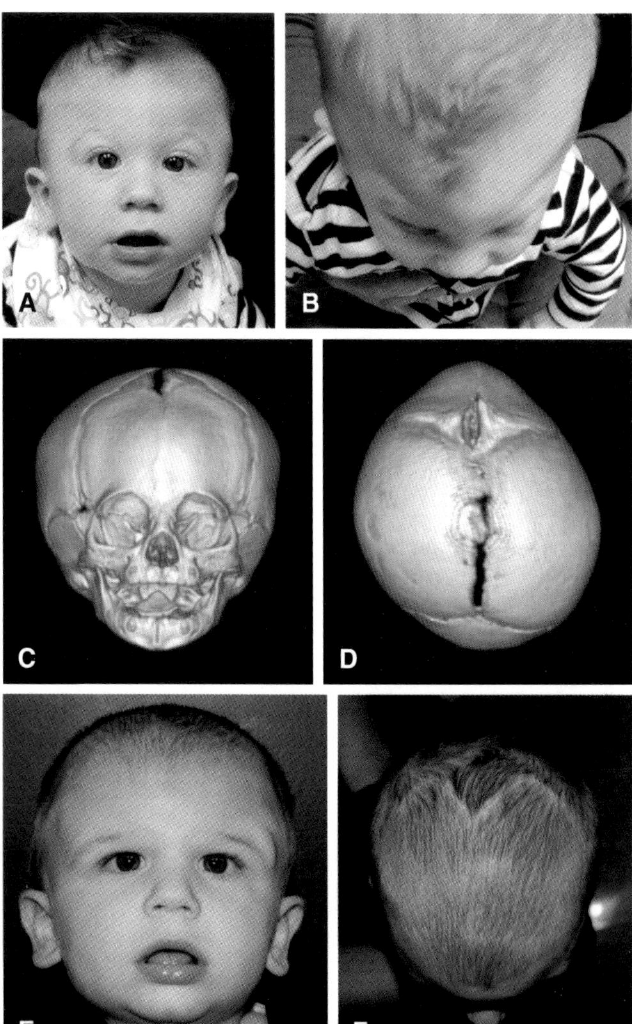

FIGURE 28.8. Metopic craniosynostosis. Preoperative patient photos **(A,B)** and computed tomography images **(C,D)**. **E,F.** Postoperative photos after bilateral fronto-orbital advancement.

misshaped occipital bones are contoured and replaced with resorbable plates and screws. If extended reshaping is needed outside of the region of the posterior craniotomy, barrel staves can be performed anteriorly and posteroinferiorly.

COMPLICATIONS

Complications following surgery for craniosynostosis are reported in 1.1% to 3.5% of cases.[44] The types of complications can be separated into acute perioperative complications (death, hemorrhage, venous air embolism, cerebrospinal fluid fistula, blindness, infection) and those occurring months to years following surgery (strabismus, sensory disturbances, contour irregularities).

Among the acute complications, perioperative death is the most feared and is estimated to be between 0.08% and 0.1% of cases, most often due to exsanguination.[45,46] Intraoperative hemorrhage is not necessarily a complication, as a certain degree of blood loss is expected. However, inadvertent injury to a sinus can result in catastrophic bleeding. Venous air embolism can occur whenever surgery is performed above the level of the heart and noncollapsible veins are exposed to air. A pressure gradient develops between atmospheric air and the bleeding vein (which can be worsened by hypotension) eventually favoring air entry into the vein as opposed to blood egress from the vein. Venous air emboli are fairly common during craniosynostosis surgery (up to 82% of patients experience an event) but few are symptomatic.[47] If an air embolus is suspected and the patient is symptomatic, the treatment is placement of a wet sponge over the operative field and putting the patient in the left lateral decubitus and Trendelenburg position to discourage continued air entry into the venous system and position the right ventricular outflow tract inferior to the right ventricular cavity. Cerebrospinal fluid leaks and pseudomeningoceles can be caused by inadvertent injury to the dura during intracranial procedures. Treatment of an asymptomatic cerebrospinal fluid leak is conservative with the removal of drains from suction and elevation of the head of bed.[48]

Ophthalmologic complications (strabismus, astigmatism, and amblyopia) following craniosynostosis surgery are seen in cases of unicoronal craniosynostosis. Prior to surgery, patients with unicoronal craniosynostosis are at higher risk for strabismus in the eye on the affected side and FOA appears to increase the risk for its development.[49] It is not infrequent for these patients to require surgical correction of the unbalanced extraocular muscles. A common concern for the craniofacial surgeon is preservation of the supraorbital nerve during dissection of the orbits from a coronal approach. One of the more frequent indications for reoperation in patients with craniosynostosis is the presence of bone gaps and contour irregularities at skeletal maturity.[50] It is unclear what causes poor ossification in some patients leading to the need for secondary cranioplasty. It is accepted practice to perform primary bone grafting from the inner table of bone at the time of the initial procedure to try to minimize the development of these sequelae. If persistent bony defects continue into the period of skeletal maturity, a secondary cranioplasty may be performed to address the gaps and at the same time provide final contouring of any irregularities.

OUTCOMES

One of the most difficult things to measure with regard to surgery for nonsyndromic craniosynostosis is an objective outcome. In the simplest of terms, there are two major outcome measures: aesthetic and neuropsychological. The most enduring measure of aesthetic outcome available in craniofacial surgery is the Whitaker classification, which rates a result from I to IV.[39] A Whitaker class I is a patient in whom no additional procedure is required. A class II indicates the need for a soft tissue or bone-contouring procedure. Class III necessitates additional major osteotomies to be performed. Finally, a class

IV result is a patient in whom an additional major craniofacial procedure is required, essentially duplicating or exceeding the original procedure.

Neuropsychological outcomes are even more difficult to quantify, as the changes that have been noted in this population are extremely subtle and may not present in a typical fashion. In addition, it is very difficult to reliably measure preoperative and postoperative metrics in this extremely young patient population. Developmental milestones are used as a surrogate to determine patients who may be at risk for untoward neuropsychological outcomes, but the use of these is far from precise and further research needs to be performed to more accurately identify these at-risk patients.

REFERENCES

1. Persing JA, Jane JA, Shaffrey M. Virchow and the pathogenesis of craniosynostosis: a translation of his original work. *Plast Reconstr Surg.* 1989;83(4):738-742.
2. Moss ML, Salentijn L. The primary role of functional matrices in facial growth. *Am J Orthod.* 1969;55(6):566-577.
3. Morriss-Kay GM, Wilkie AO. Growth of the normal skull vault and its alteration in craniosynostosis: insights from human genetics and experimental studies. *J Anat.* 2005;207(5):637-653.
4. Di Rocco F, Arnaud E, Renier D. Evolution in the frequency of nonsyndromic craniosynostosis. *J Neurosurg Pediatr.* 2009;4(1):21-25.
5. Shuper A, Merlob P, Grunebaum M, Reisner SH. The incidence of isolated craniosynostosis in the newborn infant. *Am J Dis Child.* 1985;139(1):85-86.
6. Shillito J Jr, Matson DD. Craniosynostosis: a review of 519 surgical patients. *Pediatrics.* 1968;41(4):829-853.
7. Selber J, Reid RR, Chike-Obi CJ, et al. The changing epidemiologic spectrum of single-suture synostoses. *Plast Reconstr Surg.* 2008;122(2):527-533.
8. van der Meulen J, van der Hulst R, van Adrichem L, et al. The increase of metopic synostosis: a pan-European observation. *J Craniofac Surg.* 2009;20(2):283-286.
9. Maarse W, Boonacker CW, Lapid O, et al. Professional opinion on oral cleft during pregnancy: a comparison between Israel and The Netherlands. *Prenatal Diagn.* 2015;35(6):544-548.
10. Zlotogora J, Haklai Z, Rotem N, Georgi M, Rubin L. The impact of prenatal diagnosis and termination of pregnancy on the relative incidence of malformations at birth among Jews and Muslim Arabs in Israel. *Isr Med Assoc J.* 2010;12(9):539-542.
11. Boyadjiev SA, International Craniosynostosis C. Genetic analysis of non-syndromic craniosynostosis. *Orthodont Craniofac Res.* 2007;10(3):129-137.
12. Johnson D, Wilkie AO. Craniosynostosis *Eur J Hum Genet.* 2011;19(4):369-376.
13. National Institute of Health. The Cost of Sequencing a Human Genome. https://www.genome.gov/sequencingcosts/. Updated July 6, 2016. Accessed November 2, 2017.
14. Higginbottom MC, Jones KL, James HE. Intrauterine constraint and craniosynostosis. *Neurosurgery.* 1980;6(1):39-44.
15. Alderman BW, Lammer EJ, Joshua SC, et al. An epidemiologic study of craniosynostosis: risk indicators for the occurrence of craniosynostosis in Colorado. *Am J Epidemiol.* 1988;128(2):431-438.
16. Hunenko O, Karmacharya J, Ong G, Kirschner RE. Toward an understanding of nonsyndromic craniosynostosis: altered patterns of TGF-beta receptor and FGF receptor expression induced by intrauterine head constraint. *Ann Plast Surg.* 2001;46(5):546-553.
17. Smartt JM Jr, Karmacharya J, Gannon FH, et al. Intrauterine fetal constraint induces chondrocyte apoptosis and premature ossification of the cranial base. *Plast Reconstr Surg.* 2005;116(5):1363-1369.
18. Shahinian HK, Jaekle R, Suh RH, et al Obstetrical factors governing the etiopathogenesis of lambdoid synostosis. *Am J Perinatol.* 1998;15(5):281-286.
19. Gardner JS, Guyard-Boileau B, Alderman BW, et al. Maternal exposure to prescription and non-prescription pharmaceuticals or drugs of abuse and risk of craniosynostosis. *Int J Epidemiol.* 1998;27(1):64-67.
20. Kallen K. Maternal smoking and craniosynostosis. *Teratology.* 1999;60(3):146-150.
21. Bradley CM, Alderman BW, Williams MA, et al. Parental occupations as risk factors for craniosynostosis in offspring. *Epidemiology.* 1995;6(3):306-310.
22. American Academy of Pediatrics AAP Task Force on Infant Positioning and SIDS. Positioning and SIDS. *Pediatrics.* 1992;89(6 Pt 1):1120-1126.
Prior to the release of this report positional plagiocephaly was not recognized as a disease process. The meteoric rise in the diagnosis of posterior plagiocephaly following its release resulted in the establishment of the differences between this deformity and true lambdoid craniosynostosis.
23. Fearon JA, Singh DJ, Beals SP, Yu JC. The diagnosis and treatment of single-sutural synostoses: are computed tomographic scans necessary? *Plast Reconstr Surg.* 2007;120(5):1327-1331.
24. Agrawal D, Steinbok P, Cochrane DD. Diagnosis of isolated sagittal synostosis: are radiographic studies necessary? *Child Nerv Syst.* 2006;22(4):375-378.
25. Cerovac S, Neil-Dwyer JG, Rich P, et al. Are routine preoperative CT scans necessary in the management of single suture craniosynostosis? *Br J Neurosurg.* 2002;16(4):348-354.
26. Domeshek LF, Mukundan S Jr, Yoshizumi T, Marcus JR. Increasing concern regarding computed tomography irradiation in craniofacial surgery. *Plast Reconstr Surg.* 2009;123(4):1313-1320.
27. Soboleski D, Mussari B, McCloskey D, et al. High-resolution sonography of the abnormal cranial suture. *Pediatr Radiol.* 1998;28(2):79-82.
28. Craven CM, Naik KS, Blanshard KS, et al. Multispiral three-dimensional computed tomography in the investigation of craniosynostosis: technique optimization. *Br J Radiol.* 1995;68(811):724-730.
29. Renier D, Sainte-Rose C, Marchac D, Hirsch JF. Intracranial pressure in craniostenosis. *J Neurosurg.* 1982;57(3):370-377.
This landmark article established the rate of elevated intracranial pressure in patients with craniosynostosis. In addition, it was found that patients were at an increased risk of this complication if multiple sutures were fused.
30. Wall SA, Thomas GP, Johnson D, et al. The preoperative incidence of raised intracranial pressure in nonsyndromic sagittal craniosynostosis is underestimated in the literature. *J Neurosurg Pediatr.* 2014;14(6):674-681.
31. Wiegand C, Richards P. Measurement of intracranial pressure in children: a critical review of current methods. *Dev Med Child Neurol.* 2007;49(12):935-941.
32. Swanson JW, Aleman TS, Xu W, et al. Evaluation of optical coherence tomography to detect elevated intracranial pressure in children. *JAMA Ophthalmol.* 2017;135(4):320-328.
33. Kapp-Simon KA, Speltz ML, Cunningham ML, et al. Neurodevelopment of children with single suture craniosynostosis: a review. *Child's Nervous Syst.* 2007;23(3):269-281.
34. Speltz ML, Collett BR, Wallace ER, et al. Intellectual and academic functioning of school-age children with single-suture craniosynostosis. *Pediatrics.* 2015;135(3):e615-e623.
35. Patel A, Yang JF, Hashim PW, et al. The impact of age at surgery on long-term neuropsychological outcomes in sagittal craniosynostosis. *Plast Reconstr Surg.* 2014;134(4):608e-617e.
36. Warren SM, Proctor MR, Bartlett SP, et al. Parameters of care for craniosynostosis: craniofacial and neurologic surgery perspectives. *Plast Reconstr Surg.* 2012;129(3):731-737.
37. Faber HK, Towne EB. Early craniectomy is a preventive measure in oxycephaly and allied conditions: with special reference to the prevention of blindness. *Am J Med Sci.* 1927;173(5):701-711.
This landmark article established the concept of preventative treatment of patients with craniosynostosis.
38. McCarthy JG, Glasberg SB, Cutting CB, et al. Twenty-year experience with early surgery for craniosynostosis. I. Isolated craniofacial synostosis—results and unsolved problems. *Plast Reconstr Surg.* 1995;96(2):272-283.
39. Whitaker LA, Bartlett SP, Schut L, Bruce D. Craniosynostosis: an analysis of the timing, treatment, and complications in 164 consecutive patients. *Plast Reconstr Surg.* 1987;80(2):195-212.
This landmark article established the concept of early intervention during infancy as the standard of care for the treatment of patients with craniosynostosis. This article also served to introduce the now widely used Whitaker classification of postoperative outcomes in craniosynostosis.
40. Jane JA, Edgerton MT, Futrell JW, Park TS. Immediate correction of sagittal synostosis. *J Neurosurg.* 1978;49(5):705-710.
41. Wilbrand JF, Wilbrand M, Malik CY, et al. Complications in helmet therapy. *J Craniomaxillofac Surg.* 2012;40(4):341-346.
42. Khechoyan D, Schook C, Birgfeld CB, et al. Changes in frontal morphology after single-stage open posterior-middle vault expansion for sagittal craniosynostosis. *Plast Reconstr Surg.* 2012;129(2):504-516.
43. Taylor JA, Paliga JT, Wes AM, et al. A critical evaluation of long-term aesthetic outcomes of fronto-orbital advancement and cranial vault remodeling in nonsyndromic unicoronal craniosynostosis. *Plast Reconstr Surg.* 2015;135(1):220-231.
44. Tahiri Y, Paliga JT, Wes AM, et al. Perioperative complications associated with intracranial procedures in patients with nonsyndromic single-suture craniosynostosis. *J Craniofac Surg.* 2015;26(1):118-123.
45. Allareddy V. Prevalence and impact of complications on hospitalization outcomes following surgical repair for craniosynostosis. *J Oral Maxillofac Surg.* 2014;72(12):2522-2530.
46. Czerwinski M, Hopper RA, Gruss J, Fearon JA. Major morbidity and mortality rates in craniofacial surgery: an analysis of 8101 major procedures. *Plast Reconstr Surg.* 2010;126(1):181-186.
This article discusses the safety of intracranial procedures in craniofacial surgery. In addition, an in-depth analysis of deaths associated with these procedures is performed.
47. Faberowski LW, Black S, Mickle JP. Incidence of venous air embolism during craniectomy for craniosynostosis repair. *Anesthesiology.* 2000;92(1):20-23.
48. Golinko MS, Harter DH, Rickert S, Staffenberg DA. Cerebrospinal fluid fistula for the craniofacial surgeon: a review and management paradigm. *J Craniofac Surg.* 2017. doi:10.1097/SCS.0000000000003148.
49. Gencarelli JR, Murphy A, Samargandi OA, Bezuhly M. Ophthalmologic outcomes following fronto-orbital advancement for unicoronal craniosynostosis. *J Craniofac Surg.* 2016;27(7):1629-1635.
50. Prevot M, Renier D, Marchac D. Lack of ossification after cranioplasty for craniosynostosis: a review of relevant factors in 592 consecutive patients. *J Craniofac Surg.* 1993;4(4):247-254.

QUESTIONS

1. A 5-month-old girl presents to your office with her mother who is concerned about the appearance of the back of her head. Which of the following clinical characteristics favors a diagnosis of lambdoid craniosynostosis over positional posterior plagiocephaly?

a. Ears at same level when viewed from behind
b. Forehead on affected side retruded
c. Ear on affected side displaced anteriorly when viewed from above
d. Lack of deformity at birth, with gradual worsening

2. Which of the following clinical findings favors a diagnosis of *right-sided* unicoronal craniosynostosis?

a. Left-sided brow elevation
b. Left-sided chin point deviation
c. Left-sided nasal radix deviation
d. Left-sided brow retrusion

3. Which of the following forms of craniosynostosis has most reliably been linked to testable genetic mutations?

a. Sagittal
b. Metopic
c. Coronal
d. Lambdoid

4. What is the treatment of a suspected symptomatic intraoperative venous air embolism?

a. Abort procedure, close incision, and transfer to intensive care unit
b. Cover operative field with moist sponge and placement of patient in reverse Trendelenburg position
c. Cover operative field with moist sponge and placement of patient in Trendelenburg position
d. Emergent cardiac catheterization

5. Which of the following operative strategies is most likely to result in a Whitaker I result following treatment for nonsyndromic craniosynostosis?

a. Intervention after 1 year of age
b. Overcorrection of the deformity
c. Use of minimally invasive techniques
d. Limited incisions

1. **Answer: b.** Differentiating positional posterior plagiocephaly from true lambdoid craniosynostosis is important to avoid unnecessary imaging or treatment. Table 28.2 provides a comparison of the clinical features seen in the two conditions.

2. **Answer: b.** Unicoronal craniosynostosis is characterized by ipsilateral brow elevation and retrusion, ipsilateral nasal radix deviation, and contralateral chin point deviation.

3. **Answer: c.** Mutations in FGFR3 (Muenke syndrome) and TWIST (Saethre-Chotzen syndrome) have been identified in cases of coronal craniosynostosis. The other forms of craniosynostosis have not been reliably linked to specific mutations.

4. **Answer: c.** Venous air embolism can occur whenever surgery is performed above the level of the heart and noncollapsible veins are exposed to air. A pressure gradient develops between atmospheric air and the bleeding vein (which can be worsened by hypotension) eventually favoring air entry into the vein as opposed to blood egress from the vein. If air emboli are suspected and the patient is symptomatic, the treatment is placement of a wet sponge over the operative field and putting the patient in the left lateral decubitus and Trendelenburg position to discourage continued air entry into the venous system and position the right ventricular outflow tract inferior to the right ventricular cavity.

5. **Answer: b.** A Whitaker I result is any patient in whom no additional surgical procedures would be recommended. The most important factor in obtaining a stable long-term postoperative result is overcorrection of the deformity to account for continued growth of the child. Intervention prior to 1 year of age is desirable to harness the rapid growth of the infant brain. The use of minimally invasive techniques and limited incisions has not been shown to result in less operative reinterventions (Whitaker I result).

CHAPTER 29 Syndromic Craniosynostosis

Wayne Ozaki and Thomas D. Willson

KEY POINTS

- The common syndromic craniosynostoses are primarily autosomal dominant and FGFR-related with bicoronal synostosis being the most common pattern.
- Phenotypic differences in the hands and feet can usefully distinguish among FGFR-related craniosynostoses.
- Early surgical interventions are aimed at reducing intracranial pressure and normalizing skull shape.
- Timing of cranial vault remodeling balances the need for cranial decompression with the limited advancement and weaker bone available in younger children.
- Later surgical interventions are aimed at correcting midface hypoplasia.
- Limited data are available regarding reoperation rates in syndromic craniosynostosis, but overall complication rates are low, and there is a correlation between early vault remodeling and later neuropsychological assessment scores.

Craniosynostosis is the abnormally early fusion of one or more ranial sutures. Although the metopic suture normally fuses in the first year of life, the remaining major sutures typically fuse in the second or third decade. As such, early fusion can be expected to have significant effects on not only head shape but also the ability of the brain to grow normally. When this condition occurs without other anomalies or in combination with anomalies that do not form a defined syndrome, it is referred to as *isolated* or *nonsyndromic* craniosynostosis. This chapter concerns craniosynostosis in combination with defined patterns of other anomalies: the syndromic craniosynostoses.

A review of syndromic craniosynostoses shows that there are now more than 150 described craniosynostosis syndromes. In this chapter, we will focus our attention on the syndromes most commonly encountered by practicing plastic surgeons: Apert, Crouzon, Saethre-Chotzen, Muenke, and Pfeiffer syndromes. Syndromic craniosynostoses are nearly as common as isolated forms, making up 46% of patients in one prospectively gathered database. Although a plastic surgeon in a nonpediatric practice may never treat such a patient themselves, recognizing the signs of syndromic craniosynostosis is critical for providing appropriate guidance and referral to the patient, their family, and other involved practitioners.

Team-based approaches are the cornerstone of syndromic craniosynostosis treatment. Whereas in isolated cases, cranial decompression may be the only intervention the patient requires; syndromic children often require involvement of multiple specialists including pediatricians; geneticists; cardiologists; pulmonologists; speech, behavioral, and occupational therapists; otolaryngologists; and plastic surgeons. Treatment of these patients is best accomplished in either specialized practices or at tertiary children's facilities with experienced, dedicated craniofacial teams.

CLINICAL FINDINGS

Head shape is certainly the most striking feature of many of the craniosynostosis syndromes, but as the term syndrome implies, it is far from the only feature these patients exhibit. Brachycephaly, a head shape with biparietal widening and anterior-posterior restriction, results from bilateral coronal synostosis. Turricephaly (also called oxycephaly), a steeple-shaped head with a long, high forehead resulting from synostosis of the coronal plus another major suture, is another common head shape among these patients. Cloverleaf-shaped head, known by its German term Kleeblattschädel, is uncommon, resulting from the fusion of multiple major sutures, but is encountered in severe Pfeiffer syndrome patients. Other less common head shapes in syndromic craniosynostosis include trigonocephaly, scaphocephaly, and plagiocephaly. Trigonocephaly is typically seen with fusion of the metopic suture and leads to a triangular forehead shape with temporal narrowing and, depending on severity, hypotelorism. Scaphocephaly, from Greek skaphe meaning boat, results from fusion of the sagittal suture, elongating the head in the anterior-posterior dimension and giving it a boatlike appearance. Plagiocephaly can be seen with either prolonged positioning or preferential lying on one side of the head as well as with unilateral fusions of the lambdoid or coronal sutures. In the synostotic cases, there is flattening on the affected side with compensatory bossing of the head diagonally across from the fused suture.

Many of the common syndromes have similar patterns of craniosynostosis in addition to midface hypoplasia and limb anomalies. The facial and cranial features among the syndromes are so similar in some cases that differences in the limbs may be the main clinical differentiator between one syndrome and another. Both simple and complex syndactylies are seen in syndromic craniosynostosis alongside more subtle digital differences including overly broad digits and shortened digits. Anomalies of limb length and long bone development are also described.

Advances in genetics have provided significant insight into the syndromic craniosynostoses, allowing differentiation among phenotypically similar conditions, discussion of heritability, and explaining connections among the various features of the syndromes. Autosomal recessive, autosomal dominant, and X-linked inheritance patterns have all been observed among craniosynostosis syndromes. Among those discussed in this chapter, all have autosomal dominant modes of inheritance, although in some cases sporadic mutations are more common than familial forms. With the exception of Saethre-Chotzen syndrome, which is associated with mutations in the TWIST1 gene, the other four syndromes are associated with mutations in the fibroblast growth factor receptor (FGFR) family of genes.

The following subsections discuss findings of the common craniosynostosis syndromes in detail. A summary of the information can be found in **Table 29.1**.

Crouzon Syndrome

Craniosynostosis, usually bicoronal, associated with midface hypoplasia, shallow orbits, and exophthalmos defines Crouzon syndrome, first described in 1912 by a French neurologist. When familial, it is inherited in autosomal dominant fashion via mutations of the FGFR2 gene, although there is variable expression of the characteristics, even within a single family. The prevalence of Crouzon syndrome at birth is about 1:60,000, making it responsible for about 4.8% of cases of craniosynostosis.

As mentioned, brachycephaly is the most common calvarial deformity, although trigonocephaly and scaphocephaly, from fusion of the metopic and sagittal sutures, respectively, have also been reported. Other associated features include hypertelorism, parrot-beaked nose, maxillary hypoplasia, and mandibular prognathism. Involvement of the cranial base sutures is responsible for the maxillary hypoplasia component and when combined with normal mandibular growth results in class III malocclusion and relative prognathism.

Exophthalmos in this syndrome can be particularly severe. Exposure keratoconjunctivitis is common; lagophthalmos is near universal.

TABLE 29.1. SUMMARY OF COMMON CRANIOSYNOSTOSIS SYNDROMES AND CHARACTERISTICS

Syndrome	Frequency	Common Head Shape	Facial Features	Limb Features	Other Associations	Intelligence	Gene	Inheritance
Crouzon	1:60,000	Brachycephaly	Shallow orbits Exophthalmos Midface hypoplasia Anterior open bite	Normal extremities		Normal	*FGFR2*	AD
Apert	1:64,000 to 1:80,000	Brachycephaly Turribrachycephaly	Shallow orbits Exophthalmos Negative canthal tilt *Parrot beak* nose Midface hypoplasia Anterior open bite	Symmetric syndactyly of hands and feet, usually complex (2nd, 3rd, 4th digits)	Severe acne during adolescence	Increased incidence of disability	*FGFR2*	AD possible, mostly sporadic
Saethre-Chotzen	1:25,000 to 1:50,000	Heterogenous; brachycephaly common	Low frontal hairline Eyelid ptosis Facial asymmetry Overall mild facial features	Simple syndactyly Brachydactyly Clinodactyly Radioulnar synostosis	Short stature Vertebral anomalies	Usually normal	*TWIST1* (rare *FGFR2/3*)	AD, sporadic
Muenke	1:130,000	Brachycephaly; usually mild	Eyelid ptosis Negative canthal tilt Overall mild facial features	*Thimble-like* middle phalanges Carpal fusion Calcaneal-tarsal fusion	Hearing loss	Increased incidence of disability	*FGFR3* (Pro250Arg)	AD, sporadic
Pfeiffer Type 1 (classic) Type 2 Type 3	1:100,000	 Turribrachycephaly *Kleeblattschädel* Brachycephaly or turribrachycephaly	Exophthalmos Hypertelorism Strabismus Negative canthal tilt Midface hypoplasia Shallow orbits Severe exophthalmos (types 2 and 3)	All: broad thumbs and great toes; partial soft tissue syndactyly Types 2 and 3: elbow ankylosis	Survival to adulthood Childhood demise common (types 2 and 3)	Normal (type 1) Profound disability (types 2 and 3)	*FGFR1/2*	AD (types 2 and 3 sporadic)

AD, autosomal dominant; FGFR, fibroblast growth factor receptor.

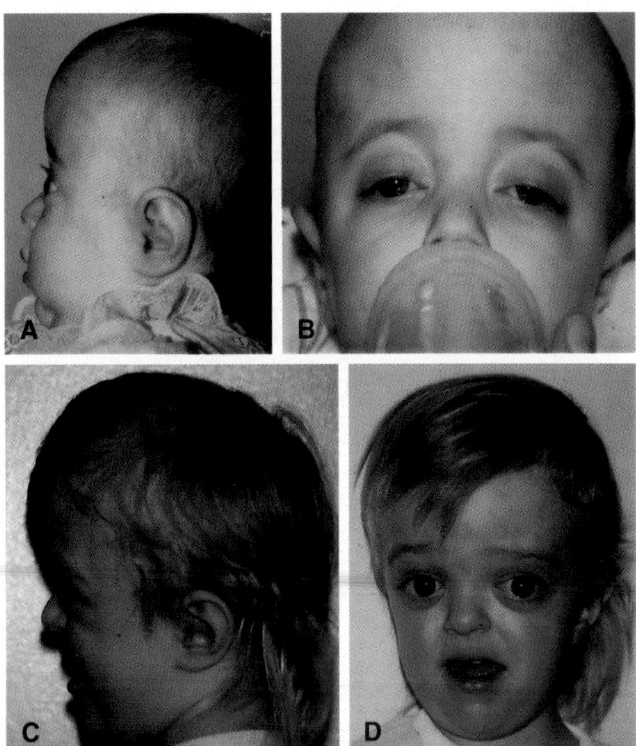

FIGURE 29.1. A, B. Preoperative lateral and anterior views of an infant with Crouzon syndrome. **C, D.** Lateral and anterior views of the same child 2 years after cranial vault remodeling and fronto-orbital advancement.

On occasion, exophthalmos can be so severe that the globes herniate through the eyelids. Immediate reduction is necessary to preserve vision, and tarsorrhaphy may be indicated. Other visual changes including strabismus have also been reported.

The hands and feet are usually normal and intelligence is normal or near-normal. **Figure 29.1** shows a child with typical findings of Crouzon syndrome.

Apert Syndrome

Apert syndrome, first described in France in 1906, shares cranial and facial features with Crouzon syndrome. The syndrome is defined by craniosynostosis, again usually resulting in a brachycephalic or turribrachycephalic head shape, in association with midface hypoplasia, shallow orbits, and syndactyly. The presence of syndactyly is a distinguishing feature between Apert and Crouzon syndromes.

Although it can be inherited in an autosomal dominant fashion, there are very few reports of patients with Apert syndrome having children. Most cases of Apert syndrome are, therefore, sporadic and result from point mutations in exon 7 of the FGFR2 gene (amino acids 252 or 253). Estimates of the birth prevalence of Apert syndrome vary significantly with early reports suggesting about 1:160,000, while more recent findings suggest a rate between 1:64,000 and 1:80,000 live births.

Symmetrical hand syndactyly, the pathognomonic finding, usually affects the index, long, and ring fingers, although the thumb and the small finger can also be involved **(Figure 29.2)**. The syndactyly is usually complex, involving the bone as well as soft tissue. Syndactyly of the foot similarly involves the second, third, and fourth toes. Early referral to an experienced hand surgeon for staged syndactyly release is essential to provide maximal function and prevent growth restriction.

Other associated findings in Apert syndrome largely mirror Crouzon syndrome. The nose has a parrot-like tip with flattening of the dorsum. The eyes display characteristic exorbitism due to shallow orbits as well as a negative canthal vector. Maxillary hypoplasia with normal mandibular growth again results in class III malocclusion. Severe acne, responsive to standard treatments, develops as children with Apert syndrome reach adolescence. Children with Apert syndrome have, on average, some degree of intellectual disability. The overall phenotype is typically more severe than in Crouzon syndrome. **Figure 29.3** shows the typical facial features of a child with Apert syndrome.

Saethre-Chotzen Syndrome

Saethre-Chotzen syndrome was first described in 1931 and is defined by craniosynostosis in association with facial dysmorphia and limb anomalies. Coronal synostosis is once again the most common form. Inheritance is autosomal dominant, and unlike the other syndromes discussed in this chapter, the majority of mutations in Saethre-Chotzen syndrome occur in the TWIST1 gene (although FGFR2 and FGFR3 mutations have been described). Despite being autosomal dominant and highly penetrant, there is a high degree of variability in the physical manifestations of Saethre-Chotzen. Mild phenotypes **(Figure 29.4)** may go undiagnosed, whereas Crouzon-like phenotypes may be misclassified without genetic testing. The estimated birth prevalence of 1:25,000 to 1:50,000 makes this the most common of the syndromic craniosynostoses.

Other facial findings in Saethre-Chotzen syndrome include facial asymmetry, hypertelorism, eyelid ptosis, lacrimal anomalies, and a low frontal hairline. Exorbitism is not typical of the syndrome. The most common limb anomalies are simple (cutaneous) syndactyly, brachydactyly, clinodactyly, broad great toes, and radioulnar synostosis. Patients are typically short in stature and vertebral anomalies are also common. Mild to moderate intellectual disability has been reported in some cases.

Muenke Syndrome

Muenke syndrome was described in 1996 and epitomizes the contributions molecular genetics have made to our understanding of craniosynostosis syndromes. Sixty-one individuals from 20 unrelated families were found to have identical point mutations (Pro250Arg) in the FGFR3 gene along with phenotypic characteristics that define the syndrome. Inheritance is autosomal dominant, but expression is variable, even within families. Incidence is estimated to be about 1:130,000.

Unicoronal or bicoronal craniosynostosis is by far the most common cranial manifestation, although some carriers do not have premature suture fusion and instead have either macrocephaly or a normal head size and shape. Facial features in Muenke syndrome patients, like Saethre-Chotzen, tend not to be strikingly abnormal

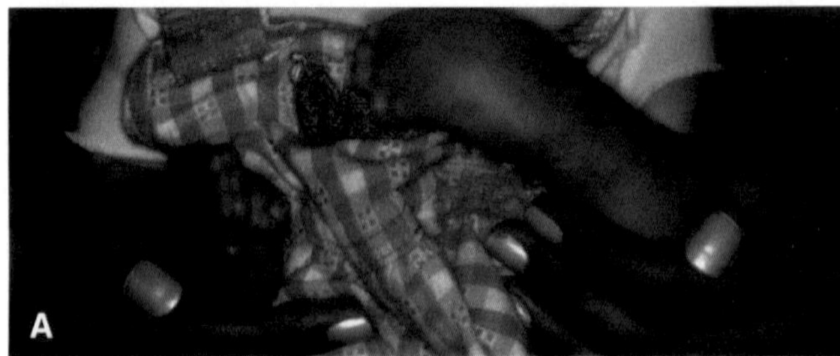

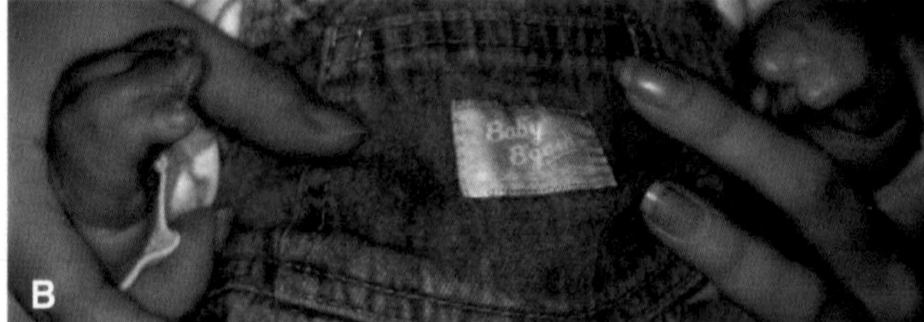

FIGURE 29.2. Syndactyly of the hands of two different children with Apert syndrome. **A.** *Mitten hand* appearance, with the four fingers fused and only the thumb free. **B.** Complex symmetric syndactyly, but not mitten hand.

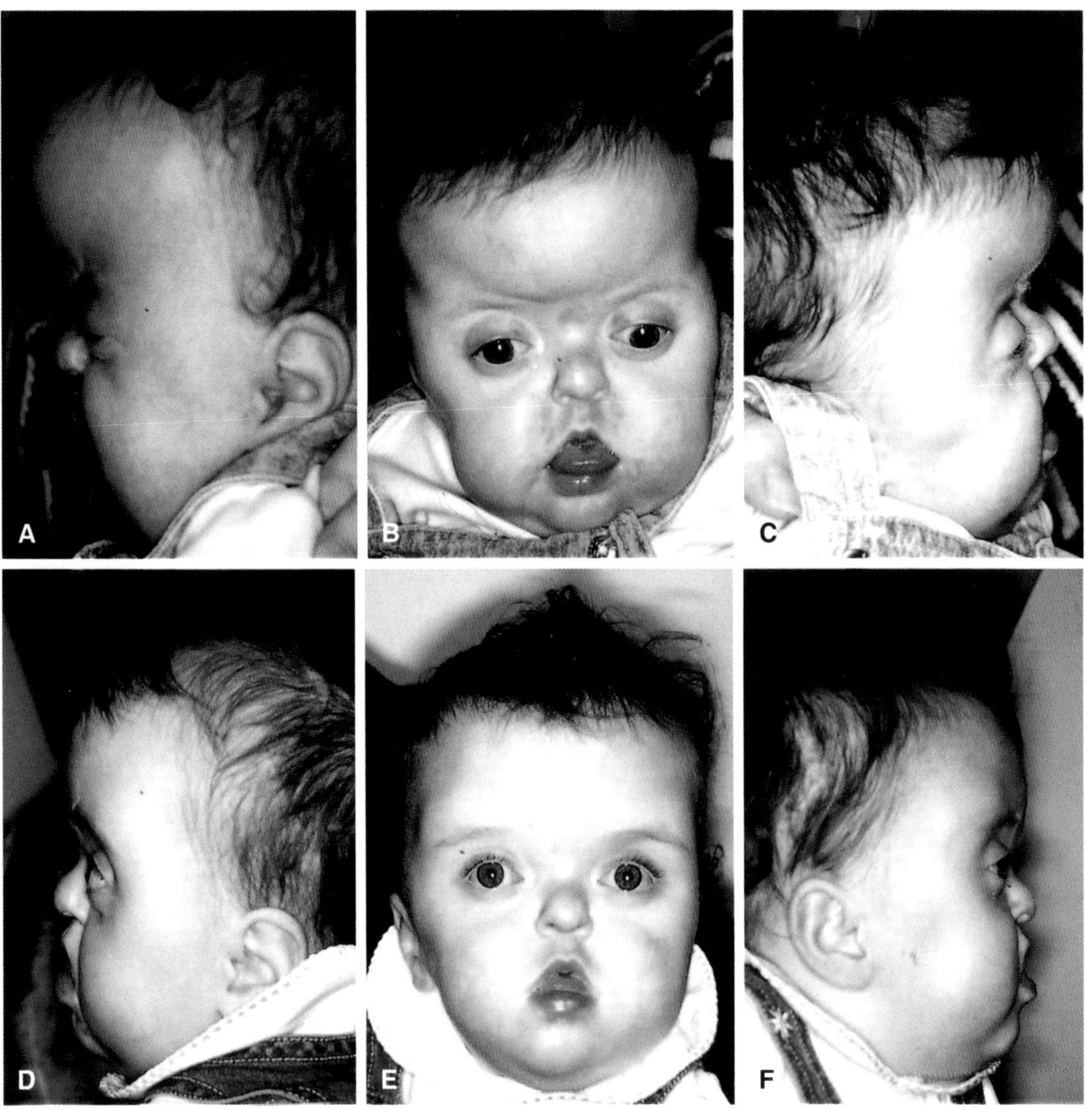

FIGURE 29.3. Preoperative **(A–C)** and postoperative **(D–F)** views of an infant with Apert syndrome.

and as such the condition may be underdiagnosed and underreported; genetic testing is advisable in cases of apparently isolated coronal synostosis. Common facial features include negative canthal vector, eyelid ptosis, and midface hypoplasia. Sensorineural hearing loss is very common and is usually bilateral. Developmental delay has been noted in about two-thirds of patients, although intellectual disability is only present in about one-third.

Limb phenotypes may be suggestive of the syndrome with brachydactyly, clinodactyly, or broad thumbs and great toes, but radiographic findings of the extremities are dispositive. *Thimble-like* middle phalanges are often seen, although there is no functional significance. Other radiographic findings include calcaneal-tarsal fusion and carpal bone fusion which, although not cardinal signs of the syndrome, are nearly pathognomonic when present.

Pfeiffer Syndrome

Pfeiffer syndrome was originally described in 1964 as an association among craniosynostosis, broad thumbs and great toes with radial deviation, and partial soft tissue syndactyly of the hands and feet. Since then, it has been subdivided into three types, of which one is autosomal dominant and the others are sporadic mutations owing to demise prior to childbearing. The heterogeneity of Pfeiffer syndrome is attributable to a heterogeneity of underlying mutations, which occur in either the FGFR1 or FGFR2 genes. The syndrome is estimated to affect about 1:100,000 individuals.

Type 1 or *classic* Pfeiffer syndrome is as described. Intelligence is typically normal, although intellectual disability has been reported. Other anomalies are uncommon. Type 2 Pfeiffer syndrome consists of a Kleeblattschädel skull shape with severe exophthalmos, broad thumbs and great toes, brachydactyly, and syndactyly. Elbow ankyloses or synostosis is found commonly in both type 2 and type 3 but rarely in type 1 Pfeiffer syndrome. Type 3 Pfeiffer syndrome has the same findings as type 2 save for the cloverleaf skull (**Figure 29.5**). Multiple visceral anomalies are also common. Both type 2 and type 3 Pfeiffer syndrome result in mortality in infancy or childhood in the vast majority of cases.

SURGICAL MANAGEMENT

Goals

First and foremost, the surgical goals in syndromic craniosynostosis are functional. Reduction of intracranial pressure (ICP), preservation of vision, and provision of functional extremities are the goals

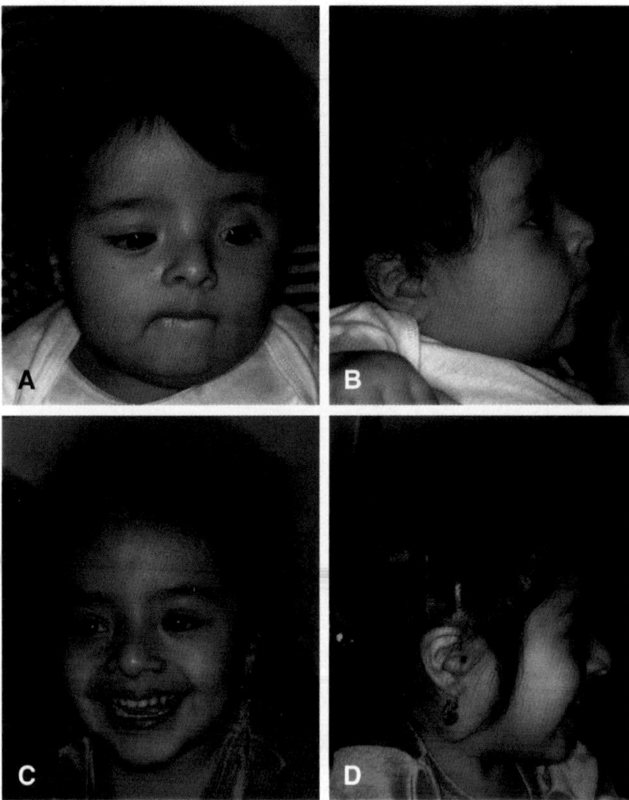

FIGURE 29.4. A, B. Preoperative anterior and lateral views of a child with Saethre-Chotzen syndrome. Despite being highly penetrant, physical manifestations can be extremely mild, as in this case, or Crouzon-like in more severe cases. **C, D.** Two years after vault remodeling.

of early interventions. Aesthetic considerations and normalization of appearance, although important, are secondary goals and require refinement as the child grows and matures.

Intracranial hypertension results from mismatch between brain size and intracranial volume. Classic situations involve space-occupying lesions such as blood or tumors, but craniosynostosis, which restricts skull growth effectively, reduces the space available for the growing brain. The brain triples in size during the first year of life and continues to grow throughout childhood. Direct recordings have demonstrated that about one-third of children with craniosynostosis have increased ICP; another third have borderline pressures, but such approaches are invasive. Indirect measures, such as papilledema on fundoscopic examination are operator dependent and may not always be present. Radiographic findings such as thumb-printing and copper-beaten appearance of the skull demonstrate increased ICP but do not appear until later in development. Because there is an association between increased ICP and intellectual achievement, and it is difficult to determine whether ICP is increased in any given case (and it is impossible to say whether increased ICP will automatically lead to intellectual disability), skull remodeling is recommended for these patients. Aesthetic improvement is a secondary benefit.

Vision represents another important surgical consideration in syndromic craniosynostoses. Bicoronal synostosis, the most common form in the syndromes discussed, results in relatively shallow orbits; globe size, however, is unchanged. This leads to a size mismatch between the orbits and their contents resulting in the characteristic exophthalmic appearance of many syndromic craniosynostosis patients. Lagophthalmos is common, and over time corneal damage can accumulate, resulting in loss of vision. In extreme cases, the globes have been seen to herniate beyond the eyelids, becoming incarcerated and requiring reduction to preserve vision. Ocular muscle problems including malposition and strabismus are also common, owing to the abnormal size and shape of the orbits. Fronto-orbital advancement (FOA) as well as the midface advancement techniques described help to deepen the orbits, providing enough room for the globes and preserving vision. Again, there is a secondary benefit in improving upper- and midface appearance.

Safety is of paramount importance in treating patients with syndromic craniosynostosis. These patients will require multiple surgeries over their lifetimes, and complications can have knock-on effects not only in terms of patient function, quality of life, and compliance outcomes but also on the need for and difficulty of revisional procedures. None of the plastic surgery procedures patients with syndromic craniosynostosis undergo is an emergency nor should they be done on an emergency basis. As with their ongoing, outpatient treatment, an experienced team operating under controlled conditions is among the most effective methods for reducing complications.

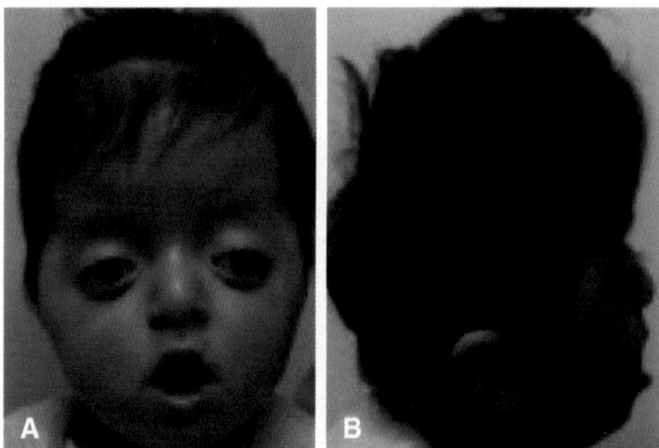

FIGURE 29.5. Pfeiffer syndrome is classified into three subtypes with type 1 representing the mildest form. **A.** Note the exophthalmos, negative canthal tilt, and mild hypertelorism. **B.** The lateral view clearly demonstrates the turribrachycephaly commonly found in type 1.

Cranial Vault Remodeling

The first plastic surgery intervention these patients will experience is a procedure to reshape the skull. Depending upon the sutures involved, this may take the form of FOA with anterior remodeling of the cranial vault or, more recently, preferential posterior fossa expansion and the use of distraction osteogenesis for both anterior and posterior cranial expansion. Suffice it to say, there are many approaches to reshaping the skull depending on the underlying synostosis, and the traditional methods are being supplemented, and in some cases supplanted, by new practices. For mild or moderate cranial vault restrictions, such as in single suture synostosis, an anterior vault correction is performed at 6 months. In more severe conditions, such as the syndromic craniosynostoses, many high-volume centers now perform posterior fossa expansion as the first intervention between 3 and 6 months of age followed by FOA at around age 1 year and midface procedures on an as-needed basis.

Posterior Fossa Distraction

Although the primary skull deformity in the syndromic craniosynostoses discussed thus far is brachycephaly, distraction of the posterior fossa has emerged as a valuable addition to the surgical armamentarium. The human brain nearly triples in size during the first year of life. This rapid growth combined with restriction by fused calvarial sutures is responsible for the abnormal head shapes seen in craniosynostosis patients. Timely intervention is, therefore, recommended. Early surgery, however, is associated with higher morbidity; is more technically challenging owing to the small size and relatively thin immature skull; and is more complicated from an anesthesia standpoint, and the volume gains from early surgery are rapidly obliterated by the growing brain.

Distraction osteogenesis is a logical solution to some of these problems. It has been described in anterior, mid-vault, and posterior forms. The procedure is less invasive, requiring only osteotomies in the desired

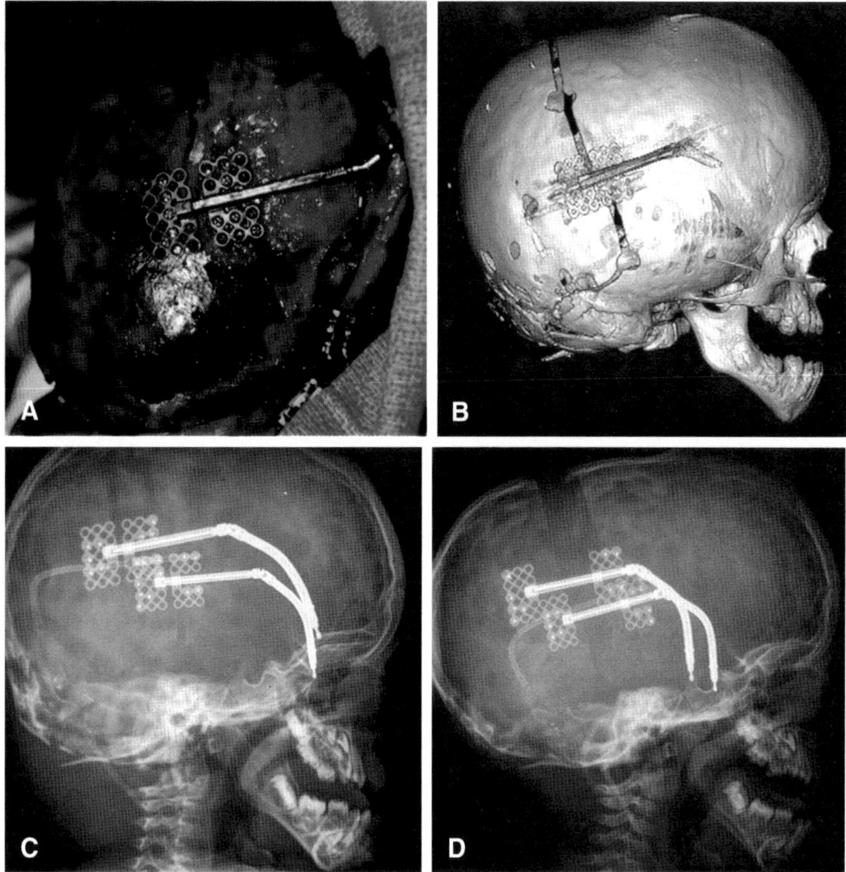

FIGURE 29.6. Posterior fossa distraction. **A.** Osteotomies are made to free the posterior calvarium, and distractors are placed parallel to the sagittal sinus. **B.** Three-dimensional computed tomography demonstrating distractor placement preexpansion. **C, D.** Preexpansion and postexpansion lateral cephalograms, respectively. This technique allows greater expansion than can be achieved with anterior remodeling and fronto-orbital advancement alone.

area and distractor placement (**Figure 29.6**). Dural dissection is minimal. This preserves growth potential of the bone and minimizes blood loss. Distraction allows the adherent dura to expand with the overlying bone, and the slow stretching of the overlying soft tissue permits more volume gain than is possible in a single-stage advancement. The posterior approach also allows greater expansion than can be achieved anteriorly.

Once the device has been placed, most reported protocols wait for a latency period of up to 5 days before beginning distraction. Patients are distracted at home at a rate of about 1 mm per day, usually divided half in the morning and half in the evening. Bony regenerate fills in the gaps left by the distraction. The distraction rate is a balance: too slow a rate will result in premature consolidation, potentially requiring additional surgery to reosteotomize the bone or breakage of the device; too fast a rate will result in low-quality regenerate or no regenerate. Once the desired distraction has been achieved, the activation period ends. A consolidation period of twice the activation period follows for the bony regenerate to solidify. The distractors can then be removed on an outpatient basis.

Fronto-Orbital Advancement

Fronto-orbital advancement (FOA) has been a mainstay of treatment for craniosynostosis for more than 40 years. Originally described by Marchac in 1978, it remains the initial treatment of choice for cranial vault expansion in bicoronal craniosynostosis and many centers. Although there is less gain in intracranial volume than with posterior procedures, FOA simultaneously provides anterior-posterior expansion and attempts to reproduce the normal forehead appearance.

The frontal bone is removed, typically in one or two pieces. Depending upon the exact nature of the deformity, the pieces can then be advanced forward and either reoriented or cut and shaped to produce the gentle backward slope of a normal forehead. Removal of the supraorbital bar as a single piece allows the surgeon to address the lower forehead. Externally, vertical osteotomies are made at the pterion followed by horizontal osteotomies up to the lateral orbital rim, oblique osteotomies through the rim itself, and a transverse osteotomy at the nasofrontal junction; the brain and globes are retracted and protected throughout this process using malleable retractors. From an intracranial position, osteotomies are made through the orbital roofs beginning at the pterion and progressing medially to the nasofrontal junction, again protecting the brain and globes. The bar can then be advanced and reshaped by greenstick fracturing. Resorbable plates and screws fix the construct in its final position. The osteotomies and final position are depicted in **Figure 29.7**.

Midface Procedures

After cranial vault expansion, the next major procedure syndromic craniosynostosis patients undergo is surgical reshaping of the midface. This is typically done in childhood, usually between the ages of 5 and 8 years, and is delayed as long as functional considerations will allow to permit the orbits to attain their adult size; there is essentially no further vertical maxillary growth following midface osteotomy. Although normalizing the facial appearance is an important outcome of midface surgery, the operations are still functional, and functional considerations ultimately dictate timing. Severe exorbitism can threaten vision; severe sleep apnea increases the risk of sudden death and reduces overall functioning and achievement; severe hypertelorism can make fitting glasses difficult: these and other problems can be addressed with the procedures described. Monobloc and Le Fort III operations move the midface in a primarily anterior-posterior plane; facial bipartition controls horizontal and vertical orbital position as well as midface width and can be combined with monobloc advancement. The choice of surgery depends upon the patient's functional needs and phenotype.

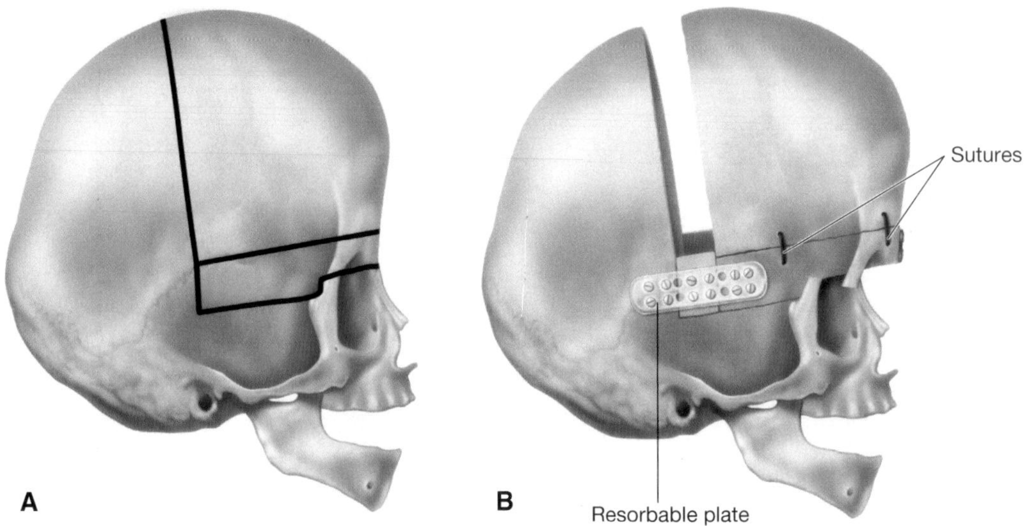

FIGURE 29.7. A. Preoperative position and osteotomies for frontal craniotomy and supraorbital bandeau for fronto-orbital advancement. **B.** Postoperative position. The position can be maintained with resorbable plates, sutures, tongue-and-groove cuts, or a combination of methods at the surgeon's discretion.

Monobloc

The monobloc procedure moves the midface and supraorbital bar as a unit. As a result, it can be used to correct exorbitism, midface retrusion, and forehead retrusion and offers a small increase in intracranial volume. It is, therefore, a good option in patients for whom the forehead and midface need to be moved the same or similar distances. Monobloc can also be combined with facial bipartition, discussed later, to address orbital position and midface width. Both acute advancement and distraction osteogenesis are possible, with the latter now preferred owing to a more favorable complication profile and greater potential for advancement. The main drawback of distraction procedures is the need for two surgeries: distractor placement and removal.

As in FOA, a frontal craniotomy allows access to the anterior cranial fossa and orbits. Orbital roof osteotomies are made in similar fashion, continuing to and then down the lateral edge of the orbit. Next, the body of the zygoma is osteotomized followed by the orbital floor. Pterygomaxillary osteotomies are performed transorally. Medial orbital wall osteotomies are performed just posterior to the posterior lacrimal crest. Finally, the orbital roofs and cranial base are osteotomized just anterior to the cribriform plate. The segment can then be mobilized and repositioned. If acute advancement is performed, bone grafts as well as plates and screws are used to help maintain the advancement (**Figure 29.8**). In the case of distraction, we adapt the distractors to the monobloc prior to the osteotomies with one or two holes predrilled to mark the planned position and alignment. Once the segment has been mobilized, the distractors are reapplied. After a latency period of about 7 days, distraction proceeds at 1 mm per day. We aim to overcorrect our patients in anticipation of further growth and inevitable relapse. The turning arms for internal distractors can then be removed, allowing a longer consolidation period with removal of the internal portion of the devices at about 3 months.

Early experience with monobloc surgery was fraught with complications including meningitis, persistent cerebrospinal fluid (CSF) leaks, and nasocranial fistulae alongside the more garden variety wound infections and relapse. Modifications to the conventional technique have significantly reduced serious complications, from 50% to 36% in one study. The same work demonstrated a reduction of serious complications to 0% (and overall complications from 67% to 8%) in the distraction osteogenesis group while achieving a much larger advancement and significantly less relapse. The primary drawback of distraction remains the need for a secondary surgery to remove the distractors.

Le Fort III

The Le Fort III procedure moves the midface separately from the frontal bar. Under appropriate circumstances, it can provide several advantages over the monobloc. Chief among those advantages is the improved complication profile of separating the intracranial (FOA) component from the extracranial component (subcranial Le Fort III). Although this obviously results in an additional surgery, a second advantage is that it allows differential advancement of the forehead and midface, which is commonly called for. Finally, the timing of indications for forehead and midface advancement rarely matches; separating the surgeries allows each to be done at the appropriate time rather than compromising the timing of one, the other, or both. Like monobloc surgery, Le Fort III can be performed either as a distraction procedure or with acute advancement. Distraction can be done either using partially buried internal devices or an external halo system **(Figure 29.9)**.

We use a coronal approach with subperiosteal dissection beginning in the supraorbital area, if an extracranial procedure is planned, and continue medially to the nasal bones, down the lateral orbital rims and zygomatic arches, and across the infraorbital area. The orbits are also dissected in the same subperiosteal plane. Osteotomies are made first at the zygomatic arch followed by the zygomaticofrontal suture to enter the orbit. The osteotomy continues across the lateral orbit to the inferior fissure then through the medial orbit taking care to remain posterior to the lacrimal apparatus. The nasal bone is cut at the frontonasal suture below the ethmoidal arteries. Intraoral pterygomaxillary and posterior maxillary osteotomies are performed. We begin the downfracture and then perform septal, perpendicular plate, and vomer osteotomies. The segment can then be mobilized and repositioned. In acute advancement, a combination of bone grafts, plates, and screws is used to stabilize the advanced segment. In the case of distraction, we preadapt the distractors to the bony framework with pilot holes predrilled to mark position and alignment. The distractors are reapplied and tested once the segment has been mobilized. After a latency period of 7 days, distraction proceeds at 1 mm per day with some overcorrection to account for growth and relapse. The distractor turning arms are removed immediately following distraction, and buried internal devices are then removed at 3 months.

Complications of subcranial Le Fort III are less common than for monobloc advancement. A completely extracranial approach reduces the risk of CSF leak and meningitis substantially, although not to zero. It is important to confirm the position of structures such as the cribriform plate and the anterior extent of the temporal lobes radiographically to avoid unplanned intracranial surgery, as these can be lower and more anterior, respectively, in syndromic patients than

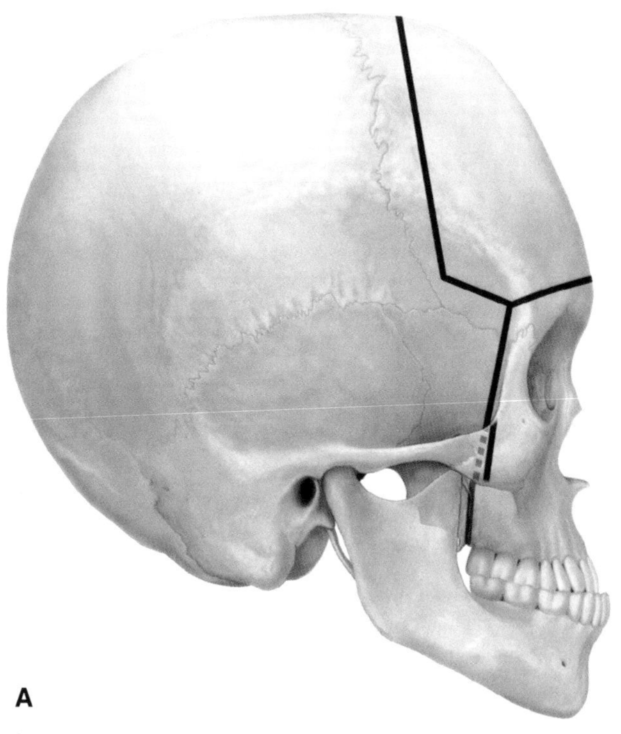

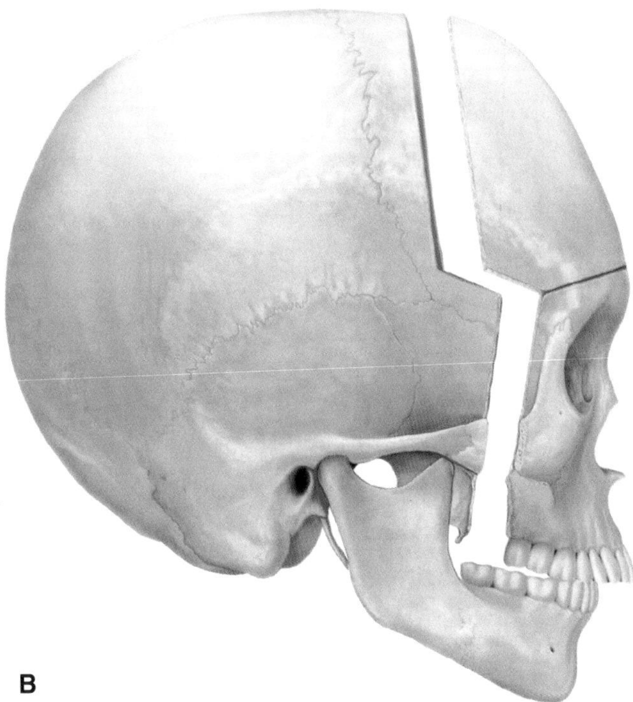

FIGURE 29.8. A. Preoperative position and osteotomies for monobloc advancement. The same osteotomies can be used for both distraction and acute advancement. **B.** Postoperative positioning. The position is maintained with plates and screws, tongue-and-groove cuts, or by the distractors as bony regenerate forms. Note the bone graft at the zygomatic arch.

might be expected. Other complications such as anosmia and visual disturbances are uncommon. Altered sensation of the forehead, palate, and midface occurs with some frequency. Wound healing and distractor-related complications make up the bulk of postoperative problems. Relapse does occur, particularly with large acute advancements. In skeletally immature patients, overcorrection of the malar eminences is critical; occlusion is addressed later, at maturity.

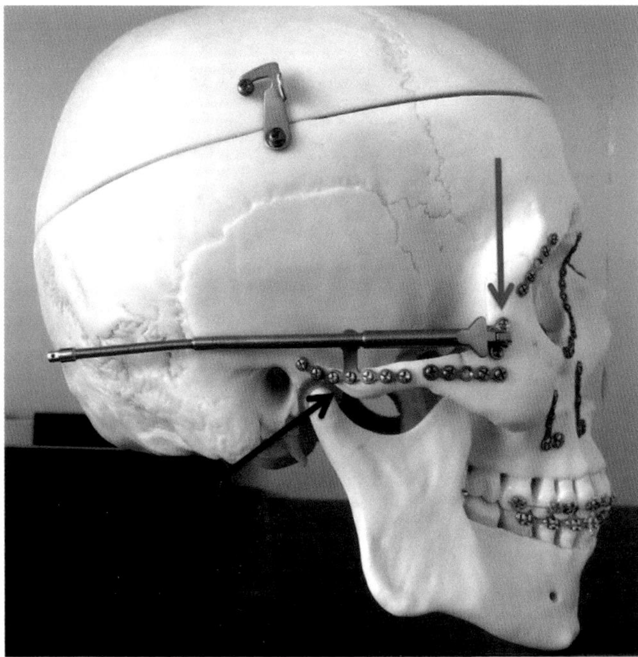

FIGURE 29.9. Placement of distractors for Le Fort III distraction. Note that the footplates rest on the zygomatic arch (black arrow) and body of the zygoma (blue arrow). The distractor arms exit posteriorly in the temporal scalp.

Facial Bipartition

Facial bipartition can be used alone or in combination with monobloc surgery to move the orbits and reshape the midface (**Figure 29.10**). Potential exists for simultaneous correction of hypertelorism as well as facial advancement and sagittal bending of the midface to correct the *dish face* deformity seen in syndromic craniosynostoses, particularly Apert syndrome.

Coronal and upper gingival-buccal sulcus approaches are used to deglove the forehead and midface. A bifrontal craniotomy is performed, and the bone is set aside. Typically, a triangular piece is removed from the midline of the frontonasal bone to permit upward and medial rotation of the orbits. This also increases the projection of the central face by increasing the curvature of the frontal bone when the two pieces are rejoined. If the orbits are asymmetric, the osteotomies may be made asymmetric to compensate. This and other contouring to account for movement of the supraorbital ridges are performed after the bipartition. First, monobloc osteotomies are performed as previously described. The bony medial intercanthal distance is measured on the table and the amount of bone to be removed is determined based on the patient's age, gender, and ethnicity, with an additional 5 mm overcorrection. The bone is removed in a wedge shape corresponding to an imaginary triangle with its base at the nasofrontal junction and tip at the midline of the maxillary alveolar ridge. The two bipartition segments are then wired together. This closure causes separation at the palate; dissecting the midline palatal mucosa before wiring the segments together reduces the risk of palatal tears. Pericranial flaps are used to separate the floor of the anterior cranial fossa from the nasal cavity and are sutured in place. At this point, after the two segments have been stabilized to each other, any planned acute advancement is performed and the construct is plated in place, or distractors are applied.

Bipartition with monobloc advancement results in differential movement of the central and lateral face, with greater advancement centrally. Patients and physicians note significant aesthetic as well as functional improvements in sleep apnea and corneal exposure. Bipartition results in malocclusion due to expansion of the maxilla,

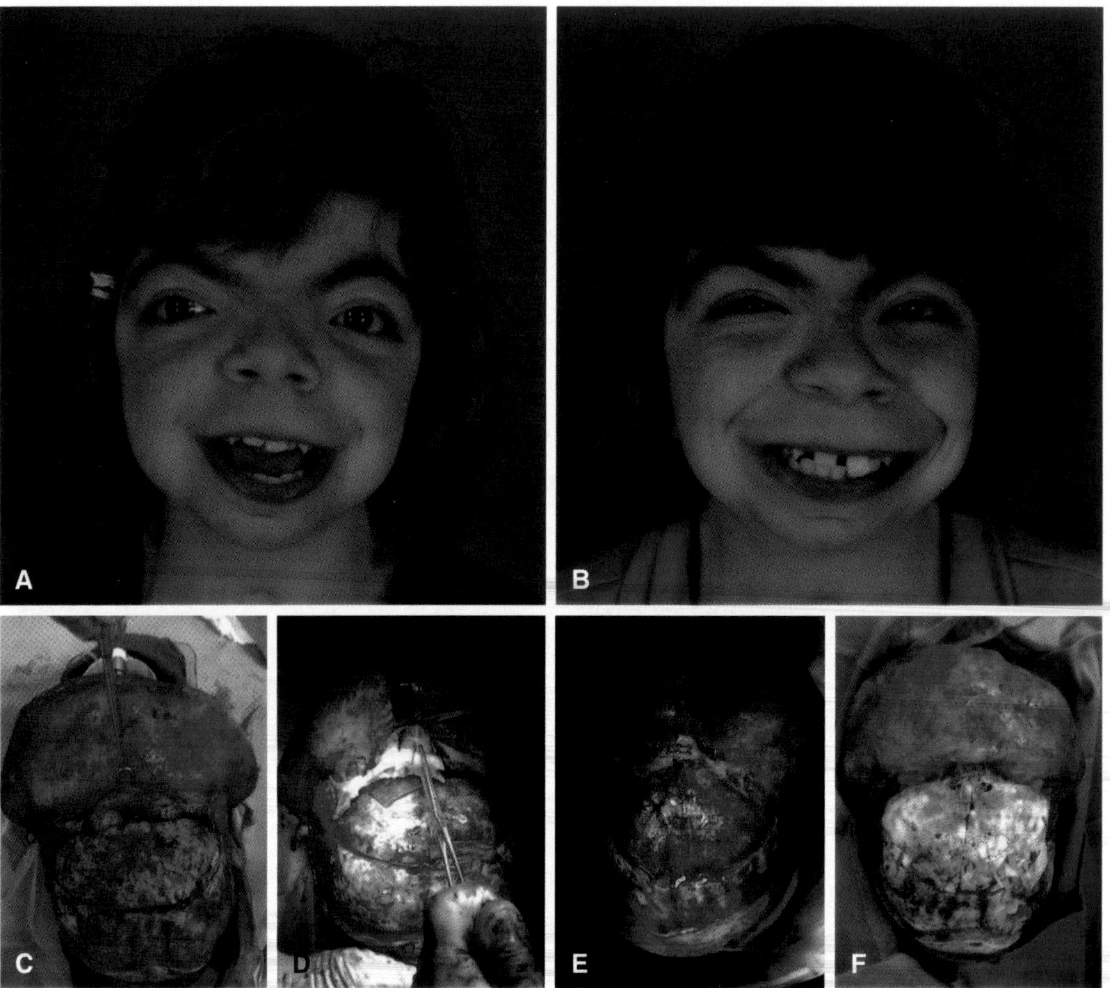

FIGURE 29.10. Preoperative **(A)** and postoperative **(B)** photographs of a patient undergoing monobloc and facial bipartition. Note the change in canthal position and the reduced intercanthal distance in the postoperative photograph. **C.** Intraoperative view with markings for frontal craniotomy (top is anterior). **D.** The triangular central midface segment has been osteotomized and is being removed. **E.** Fixation of the two hemifaces after the triangular wedge has been removed and the orbits repositioned. **F.** Final position of the construct with all fixation in place.

which is often asymmetric. Postoperative orthodontic treatment is needed after consolidation and in preparation for orthognathic surgery at maturity. In addition to wound and distractor-related complications, less common problems after bipartition include persistent CSF leak, meningitis, and visual disturbances. Relapse does occur, but can be overcome by planned overcorrection of the intercanthal distance.

OUTCOMES AND REVISIONS

Treatment outcomes in syndromic craniosynostoses are notoriously difficult to measure. Prevention of developmental delay is difficult to determine statistically given the relative rarity of syndromic craniosynostoses in any center and the association between some syndromes and impaired neuropsychosocial development. Similarly, normalization of aesthetics is by definition subjective and is strongly influenced by the starting phenotype; patients with milder differences to start with tend to have more aesthetically pleasing results.

McCarthy and colleagues reported a 20-year experience with syndromic craniosynostosis with satisfactory results in 73% of patients, although reoperation was recommended in 37%. Their outcomes are reported using Whitaker classification (**Table 29.2**), but

TABLE 29.2. WHITAKER CLASSIFICATION OF CRANIOSYNOSTOSIS SURGERY OUTCOMES

Classification	Interpretation
I	Excellent result No refinement recommended by surgeon or patient
II	Adequate result Minor soft tissue refinement or bony contouring; outpatient surgery
III	Poor result Major bony revision, bone grafting, orbital repositioning; not as extensive as the original surgery
IV	Unsatisfactory result Major craniofacial surgery recommended; essentially reproducing the extent of the original operation if not more

Adapted with permission from Whitaker LA, Bartlett SP, Schut L, et al. Craniosynostosis: an analysis of the timing, treatment, and complications in 164 consecutive patients. *Plast Reconstr Surg*. 1987;80(2):195-206.

the exact criteria for revision remain to be decided on a case-by-case basis. Mulliken and colleagues reported on reoperation rates in syndromic craniosynostoses initially treated with FOA finding high rates in Apert (100%) and Saethre-Chotzen (65%) syndromes with much lower rate in Crouzon syndrome (5%), although they note the possibility of selection bias among the Saethre-Chotzen group, as milder phenotypes may require no frontal surgery or go completely undetected.

Authors reporting on midface procedures uniformly note improvements in both exorbitism and sleep apnea, although complete resolution is not seen in all patients. Distraction patients fare better in terms of relapse than acute advancements. McCarthy and colleagues reported stable advancements after Le Fort III distraction in both the medium and long term including some minimal additional maxillary growth.

Fat grafting is an important adjunct to the surgeries described thus far. Relatively minor postoperative deformities or deficiencies such as mild temporal hollowing that used to require a second major cranial vault or midface procedure can now be camouflaged by injecting fat in an outpatient setting. The combination of minimal downtime, low morbidity, and the ability to address only the specific areas that the patient finds bothersome has made fat grafting popular among our patients and is a standard part of our armamentarium for treating syndromic craniosynostosis.

The treatment of syndromic craniosynostosis patient is more complex than in isolated cases. Rather than a single procedure, these patients undergo multiple operations to reshape the cranium, to correct midface hypoplasia, and to camouflage their differences throughout their childhood. Behavioral and social interventions starting from an early age also play an important role in maximizing quality of life. Although a plastic surgeon in general practice may never treat a syndromic craniosynostosis patient themselves, understanding the common syndromes, findings, and treatment timelines can aid other specialists in recognizing the condition and making a referral to a craniofacial team.

BIBLIOGRAPHY

1. Bradley JP, Gabbay TS, Taub PJ, et al. Monobloc advancement by distraction osteogenesis decreases morbidity and relapse. *Plast Reconstr Surg.* 2006;118(7):1585-1597.
Bradley and colleagues describe the evolution of the monobloc procedure at a single institution. Complications are somewhat decreased with their modified acute advancement technique but are substantially improved with distraction osteogenesis. Significantly less relapse is also noted in the distraction osteogenesis group compared with more conventional techniques.
2. Cohen MM. Perspectives on craniosynostosis. *West J Med.* 1980;32(6):507-513.
3. Cohen MM Jr. Craniosynostosis: phenotypic/molecular correlations. *Am J Med Genet.* 1995;56(3):334-339.
4. Cohen MM Jr. Pfeiffer syndrome update, clinical subtypes, and guidelines for differential diagnosis. *Am J Med Genet.* 1993;45(3):300-307.
5. Cohen MM Jr, Kreiborg S. Hands and feet in the Apert syndrome. *Plast Reconstr Surg.* 1995;57(1):82-96.
6. de Jong T, Bannink N, Bredero-Boelhouwer HH, et al. Long-term functional outcome in 167 patients with syndromic craniosynostosis; defining a syndrome-specific risk profile. *J Plast Reconstr Aesthet Surg.* 2010;63(10):1635-1641.
7. de Jong T, Maliepaard M, Bannink N, et al. Health-related problems and quality of life in patients with syndromic and complex craniosynostosis. *Childs Nerv Syst.* 2012;28(6):879-882.
8. Dederian C, Seaward J. Syndromic craniosynostosis. *Semin Plast Surg.* 2012;6(2):64-75.
9. Fearon JA, Rhodes J. Pfeiffer syndrome: a treatment evaluation. *Plast Reconstr Surg.* 2009;123(5):1560-1569.
10. Fearon JA, Vakarakis GM, Kolar J. A comparative study of anterior cranial vault distraction versus remodeling. *J Craniofac Surg.* 2014;25(4):1159-1163.
11. Fernandes MB, Maximino LP, Perosa GB, et al. Apert and Crouzon syndromes: cognitive development, brain anomalies, and molecular aspects. *Am J Med Genet A.* 2016;170(6):1532-1537.
12. French LR, Jackson IT, Melton LJ III. A population-based study of craniosynostosis. *J Clin Epidemiol.* 1990;43(1):69-73.
13. Gillies H, Harrison SH. Operative correction by osteotomy of recessed malar maxillary compound in a case of oxycephaly. *Br J Plast Surg.* 1950;3(2):123-127.
Although modern osteotomies are placed somewhat differently, the authors describe the first subcranial Le Fort III–type procedure for treatment of craniosynostosis-associated midface hypoplasia and malocclusion in this case report.
14. Goldstein JA, Paliga JT, Taylor JA, Bartlett SP. Complications in 54 frontofacial distraction procedures in patients with syndromic craniosynostosis. *J Craniofac Surg.* 2015;26(1):124-128.
15. Goldstein JA, Paliga JT, Wink JD, et al. A craniometric analysis of posterior vault distraction osteogenesis. *Plast Reconstr Surg.* 2013;131(6):1367-1375.
16. Greig AV, Britto JA, Abela C, et al. Correcting the typical Apert face: combining bipartition with monobloc distraction. *Plast Reconstr Surg.* 2013;131(2):219e-230e.
17. Kruszka P, Addissie YA, Yarnell CM, et al. Muenke syndrome: an international multicenter natural history study. *Am J Med Genet A.* 2016;170A(4):918-929.
18. Maliepaard M, Mathijssen IM, Oosterlaan J, Okkerse JM. Intellectual, behavioral, and emotional functioning in children with syndromic craniosynostosis. *Pediatrics.* 2014;133(6):1608-1615.
19. Marchac D. Radical forehead remodeling for craniostenosis. *Plast Reconstr Surg.* 1978;61(6):823-835.
Marchac describes his technique for remodeling of the cranial vault in the treatment of craniosynostosis. This article marks a departure from strip craniectomy, which was the standard procedure at the time. The article also describes normal forehead anatomy and the addition of a supraorbital bar to separately correct changes in the brow and forehead.
20. McCarthy JG, Glasberg SB, Cutting CB, et al. Twenty-year experience with early surgery for craniosynostosis: I. isolated craniofacial synostosis—results and unsolved problems. *Plast Reconstr Surg.* 1995;96(2):272-283.
21. McCarthy JG, Glasberg SB, Cutting CB, et al. Twenty-year experience with early surgery for craniosynostosis: II. the craniofacial synostosis syndromes and pansynostosis—results and unsolved problems. *Plast Reconstr Surg.* 1995;96(2):284-295.
The authors present a treatment algorithm for syndromic craniosynostosis patients developed over their 20-year experience. Surgical outcomes, ICP outcomes, complications, and pearls for each syndromic group are discussed.
22. Morriss-Kay GM, Wilkie AO. Growth of the normal skull vault and its alteration in craniosynostosis: insights from human genetics and experimental studies. *J Anat.* 2005;207(5):637-653.
23. Muenke M, Gripp KW, McDonald-McGinn DM, et al. A unique point mutation in the fibroblast growth factor receptor 3 gene (FGFR3) defines a new craniosynostosis syndrome. *Am J Hum Genet.* 1997;60(3):555-564.
24. Ortiz-Monasterio F, del Campo AF, Carrillo A. Advancement of the orbits and the midface in one piece, combined with frontal repositioning, for the correction of Crouzon's deformities. *Plast Reconstr Surg.* 1978;61(4):507-516.
Ortiz-Monasterio orbitofacial advancement laid the groundwork for what would eventually become the monobloc procedure. This article discusses the original surgical technique, results, and follow-up of a seven-patient cohort.
25. Patel PA, Shetye PR, Warren SM, et al. Five-year follow-up of midface distraction in growing children with syndromic craniosynostosis. *Plast Reconstr Surg.* 2017;140(6):794e-803e.
26. Paznekas WA, Cunningham ML, Howard TD, et al. Genetic heterogeneity of Saethre-Chotzen syndrome, due to TWIST and FGFR mutations. *Am J Hum Genet.* 1998;62(6):1370-1380.
27. Renier D, Sainte-Rose C, Marchac D, Hirsch JF. Intracranial pressure in craniostenosis. *J Neurosurg.* 1982;57(3):370-377.
28. Sabatino G, Di Rocco F, Zampino G, et al. Muenke syndrome. *Childs Nerv Syst.* 2004;20(5):297-301.
29. Shetye PR, Boutros S, Grayson BH, McCarthy JG. Midterm follow-up of midface distraction for syndromic craniosynostosis: a clinical and cephalometric study. *Plast Reconstr Surg.* 2007;120(6):1621-1632.
30. Spruijt B, Joosten KF, Driessen C, et al. Algorithm for the management of intracranial hypertension in children with syndromic craniosynostosis. *Plast Reconstr Surg.* 2015;136(2):331-340.
31. Swanson JW, Samra F, Bauder A, et al. An algorithm for managing syndromic craniosynostosis using posterior vault distraction osteogenesis. *Plast Reconstr Surg.* 2016;137(5):829e-841e.
32. Taylor JA, Bartlett SP. What's new in syndromic craniosynostosis surgery? *Plast Reconstr Surg.* 2017;140(1):82e-93e.
33. Tessier P. Relationship of craniostenosis to craniofacial dysostoses, and to faciostenoses: a study with therapeutic implications. *Plast Reconstr Surg.* 1971;48(3):224-237.
34. Tessier P. The definitive plastic surgical treatment of the severe facial deformities of craniofacial dysostosis, Crouzon's and Apert's diseases. *Plast Reconstr Surg.* 1971;48(5):419-442.
Tessier describes his early techniques for treating the facial deformities associated with Crouzon and Apert syndromes. Morphologic and functional considerations for each syndrome are described in detail in addition to step-by-step approach to subcranial Le Fort III. Complications and subsequent complementary surgeries are also discussed.
35. Tiwana PS, Turvey TA. Subcranial procedures in craniofacial surgery: the Le Fort III osteotomy. *Oral Maxillofac Surg Clin North Am.* 2004;16(4):493-501.
36. Tolarova MM, Harris JA, Ordway DE, Vargervik K. Birth prevalence, mutation rate, sex ratio, parents' age, and ethnicity in Apert syndrome. *Am J Med Genet.* 1997;72(4):394-398.
37. Utria AF, Mundinger GS, Bellamy JL, et al. The importance of timing in optimizing cranial vault remodeling in syndromic craniosynostosis. *Plast Reconstr Surg.* 2015;135(4):1077-1084.
38. Van der Meulen JC. Medial fasciotomy. *Br J Plast Surg.* 1979;32(4):339-342.
Van der Meulen medial faciotomy is an early approach to the facial bipartition for simultaneous correction of hypertelorism and maxillary malposition.
39. Vogels A, Fryns JP. Pfeiffer syndrome. *Orphanet J Rare Dis.* 2006;1:19.

40. Whitaker LA, Bartlett SP, Schut L, Bruce D. Craniosynostosis: an analysis of the timing, treatment, and complications in 164 consecutive patients. *Plast Reconstr Surg*. 1987;80(2):195-212.
41. Whitaker LA, Munro IR, Salyer KE, et al. Combined report of problems and complications in 793 craniofacial operations. *Plast Reconstr Surg*. 1979;64(2):198-203.
42. Wilkie AO, Byren JC, Hurst JA, et al. Prevalence and complications of single-gene and chromosomal disorders in craniosynostosis. *Pediatrics*. 2010;126(2):e391-e400.
43. Wong GB, Kakulis EG, Mulliken JB. Analysis of fronto-orbital advancement for Apert, Crouzon, Pfeiffer, and Saethre-Chotzen syndromes. *Plast Reconstr Surg*. 2000;105(7):2314-2323.

QUESTIONS

1. You are asked to evaluate a 12-month-old infant with bicoronal craniosynostosis, complete syndactylies of the hands and feet, and midface hypoplasia. Genetic testing is most likely to reveal a mutation in

a. TWIST
b. FGFR
c. Chromodomain-helicase-DNA-binding protein 7
d. Treacle ribosome biogenesis factor 1
e. Collagen type II alpha 1 chain

2. Which of the following is an advantage of posterior fossa distraction compared with FOA for the initial treatment of craniosynostosis?

a. More immediate correction of frontal aesthetics with posterior fossa distraction
b. Need for only one surgery in infancy with posterior fossa distraction
c. More increase in intracranial volume with posterior fossa distraction
d. Shorter operative time with FOA
e. Less need for blood transfusion with FOA

3. Which of the following is an advantage of Le Fort III compared with monobloc surgery for correction of midface hypoplasia in syndromic craniosynostosis?

a. Monobloc allows differential correction of frontal and midface deficiencies
b. Le Fort III can be performed as a distraction procedure whereas monobloc cannot
c. Le Fort III has a favorable complication profile compared with monobloc
d. Le Fort III can be combined with facial bipartition to simultaneously correct orbital position and facial width
e. There is no risk of meningitis or CSF leak with Le Fort III

4. A 10-year-old child who underwent surgery for craniosynostosis as an infant presents to your office with concerns about her appearance. On examination, she is short for her age and has a low frontal hairline as well as subtle eyelid ptosis. She has met all of her developmental milestones and is an average student. Which is the most likely underlying craniosynostosis syndrome?

a. Muenke
b. Crouzon
c. Pfeiffer
d. Saethre-Chotzen
e. Apert

5. Which craniosynostosis syndrome is least associated with limb anomalies?

a. Apert
b. Crouzon
c. Muenke
d. Pfeiffer
e. Saethre-Chotzen

1. **Answer: b.** This child has the characteristics of Apert syndrome (craniosynostosis, polysyndactyly, midface hypoplasia), one of the FGFR-associated craniosynostosis syndromes. Apert syndrome is associated with a mutation in the FGFR2 gene, which is usually autosomal dominant. Mutations of the TWIST gene are associated with Saethre-Chotzen syndrome. Although patients with Saethre-Chotzen syndrome often have syndactyly of the second and third digits, involvement of the fourth digit and complete syndactyly are less common. Anomalies in chromodomain-helicase-DNA-binding protein 7 are associated with CHARGE syndrome, a craniofacial syndrome that is not typically associated with craniosynostosis. Findings in CHARGE syndrome include coloboma, heart defects, choanal atresia, growth retardation, genital anomalies, and ear anomalies. Treacle ribosome biogenesis factor 1 mutations are responsible for Treacher Collins syndrome. Findings include bilateral Tessier 6, 7, and 8 clefts. There is no association with craniosynostosis, but like the FGFR-associated craniosynostosis syndromes, it is inherited in an autosomal dominant pattern. Collagen type II alpha 1 chain mutations are associated with Stickler syndrome. In addition to hypoplasia of the midface and Pierre Robin sequence, Stickler syndrome is associated with hearing loss, joint problems, and eye abnormalities.

2. **Answer: c.** Posterior fossa distraction offers a greater increase in intracranial volume than fronto-orbital distraction. FOA offers the opportunity to immediately correct frontal aesthetics while expanding the intracranial volume. Some authors do report that FOA is not always required after posterior fossa distraction owing to spontaneous correction. Posterior fossa distraction requires two operations in infancy: one to place the distractors and one to remove them; this is frequently cited as a disadvantage of posterior fossa distraction. FOA is a more invasive surgery than posterior fossa distraction with both longer operative times and higher rates of blood transfusion.

3. **Answer: c.** Le Fort III generally has fewer and less serious complications than monobloc surgery. Although the risk of meningitis and CSF leak with Le Fort III is much lower than monobloc because the procedure is intended to be extracranial, the risk is not zero. Facial bipartition can be combined with monobloc surgery but not with Le Fort III; intracranial access and movement of the frontal bones are necessary to accommodate the orbital movements associated with facial bipartition. As suggested by the name, monobloc involves movement of the upper and midface as one unit, so it does not permit differential correction of frontal and midface deficiencies. Both procedures can be performed as either acute advancement or distraction.

4. **Answer: d.** Saethre-Chotzen is an autosomal dominant craniosynostosis syndrome that is characterized by low frontal hairline, eyelid ptosis, and short stature with normal intelligence. Limb anomalies are sometimes seen. The overall phenotype is typically mild. Crouzon syndrome is characterized by midface hypoplasia and exorbitism with normal intelligence. Apert syndrome is characterized by midface hypoplasia and exorbitism associated with complex syndactyly, severe acne in adolescence, and frequently developmental delay. In Pfeiffer syndrome, findings include midface hypoplasia, exophthalmos, and negative canthal tilt with broad thumbs and toes and simple syndactyly; childhood mortality is common in types 2 and 3. Muenke syndrome is characterized by ptosis, negative canthal tilt, and mild overall facial findings; thimble-like middle phalanges are pathognomonic.

5. **Answer: b.** Crouzon syndrome is associated with facial and skull findings including craniosynostosis, midface hypoplasia, and exophthalmos, but limb findings are typically absent. Apert syndrome limb findings include complex, symmetric syndactyly of the fingers and toes. Limb findings in Muenke syndrome include thimble-like middle phalanges on radiography as well as carpal bone fusions. Pfeiffer syndrome limb findings include broad thumbs and toes, soft tissue syndactyly, and, in types 2 and 3, elbow ankyloses. Saethre-Chotzen patients may have simple syndactyly, brachydactyly, clinodactyly, and radioulnar synostosis.

CHAPTER 30 Craniofacial Microsomia and Principles of Craniofacial Distraction

Sergey Y. Turin and Arun K. Gosain

KEY POINTS

- Craniofacial microsomia
  - This is the second most common congenital craniofacial anomaly after cleft lip or palate.
  - Abnormality of structures arises from the first and second branchial arches, with multiple tissue types affected (skeletal structures, ear, nerve, and muscle).
  - May be bilateral or unilateral—thus craniofacial is the preferred term.
  - Comprehensive treatment of the patient's unique constellation of symptoms is the cornerstone of management.
  - Controversy is in timing of surgery and osteotomies required—early distraction of mandible and orthodontic control of growing maxilla (as per McCarthy's group) versus waiting for skeletal maturity to perform orthognathic surgery for correction of both jaws (Obwegeser method).
- Craniofacial distraction
  - Only process to create new bone and avoid grafts/flaps; bone formation takes places without cartilaginous intermediate.
  - This is the only process to also provide gradual expansion of soft-tissue envelope.
  - There are three phases—latency (4–5 days), distraction (4–6 weeks, or until desired amount of advancement is obtained), and consolidation (6–8 weeks).
  - Distraction rate standard is 1 mm per day, but may be higher if mandibular distraction is done in infancy.
  - Early distraction of midface (Le Fort I or III osteotomies) can be considered if maxillary and malar asymmetry is significant before skeletal maturity.

CRANIOFACIAL MICROSOMIA

Craniofacial microsomia (CFM) is one of a large set of craniofacial disorders characterized by failure or inadequacy of facial skeleton and soft-tissue development. Although initially termed *hemifacial microsomia*, the term *craniofacial microsomia* is more accurate as a number of patients present with bilateral findings, as well as findings beyond the face per se (i.e., the ear). This same entity has also been previously referred to as first and second branchial arch syndrome, otomandibular dysostosis, lateral facial dysplasia, and oculoauriculovertebral (OAV) sequence or equivalent. In 1963, Gorlin[1] proposed the term oculoauriculovertebral dysplasia spectrum to represent a more inclusive set of disorders. The OAV spectrum includes a variable phenotype and affects a greater range of structures, including the skeletal and soft-tissue components of the face, orbits, and cranium, as well as the axial skeleton and visceral structures.

It is likely more accurate to consider CFM as a subset of OAV dysplasia, with a presentation limited to disorders of tissues stemming from the first and second branchial arches, most commonly thought of as involving the ear and the mandible. In turn, Goldenhar syndrome may be considered as a subset of both OAV spectrum and CFM, defined by *ocular* anomalies (most commonly epibulbar dermoids or lipodermoids), *auricular* anomalies (ranging from microtia to accessory tragal remnants), and *vertebral* anomalies.

Epidemiology

CFM is regarded as the second most common craniofacial anomaly after cleft lip/palate. Grabb's seminal 1965 article on the topic estimated the prevalence to be approximately 1 in 5600 based on the local hospitals' data,[1] but incidence as frequent as 1 in 3000 has been cited.[2] Owing to the variable presentation and relatively low incidence, it is difficult to obtain a more accurate estimate of the true incidence of CFM.

Pathophysiology

The exact pathogenesis of CFM is yet to be determined, but two hypotheses are currently dominant: tissue insult due to hemorrhage/ischemia caused by stapedial artery malformation, or disruption of neural crest cell migration. Thalidomide, retinoic acid, and maternal diabetes have also been linked to this disorder,[3] but the exact mechanism of their effect is also still under investigation.

The vascular insult hypothesis describes a defect in the stapedial artery, which is a temporary hyoid artery collateral, causing a hematoma or hemorrhage. This hemorrhage, in turn, compromises the developing first and second branchial arches. A variation of this hypothesis was first advanced by Braithwaite in 1949, supposing a deficiency of the stapedial artery in irrigating the affected tissues in the period prior to formation of the external carotid artery. This hypothesis was further supported experimentally by Poswillo, who showed that triazene and thalidomide led to development of a focal area of hemorrhage and disruption of the forming stapedial artery in the developing faces of mice and monkeys. The animals then went on to exhibit the microtia and mandible hypoplasia consistent with a CFM phenotype.[4] However, later reexamination of these experiments cast doubt on the vascular insult hypothesis because of the timing of hemorrhage inconsistent with drug administration and lack of explanation for associated anomalies present in OAV dysplasia, such as renal or vertebral defects.[5]

More recently, Johnston and Bronsky proposed that a disruption in neural crest cell migration may be responsible for the findings seen in OAV dysplasia and CFM.[6] The widely varied roles of neural crest cells in the development of the craniofacial skeleton and soft tissues provide a possible explanation for the rather heterogeneous OAV dysplasia phenotypes due to different populations of neural crest cells affected. There are also data correlating retinoic acid and diabetes (i.e., hyperglycemia) with neural crest cell apoptosis in embryogenesis, lending further credence to this hypothesis.[7]

It has been believed traditionally that most cases are sporadic: a relatively large cohort study in 1983 showed 45% of patients with OAV dysplasia/Goldenhar syndrome/CFM had some family history of similar findings, but only 6% to 8% of first-degree relatives were affected.[8] Since then, a number of chromosomal anomalies have been loosely tied to CFM[9] and the related disorders falling under the OAV dysplasia umbrella, including trisomies of chromosomes 7, 9, 18, and 22, among a number of other rearrangements and deletions. Some recent studies suggest that CFM may, in fact, exhibit an autosomal dominant pattern of inheritance with variable penetrance.[10] Nevertheless, identification of a responsible genetic locus remains elusive, supporting multifactorial inheritance.

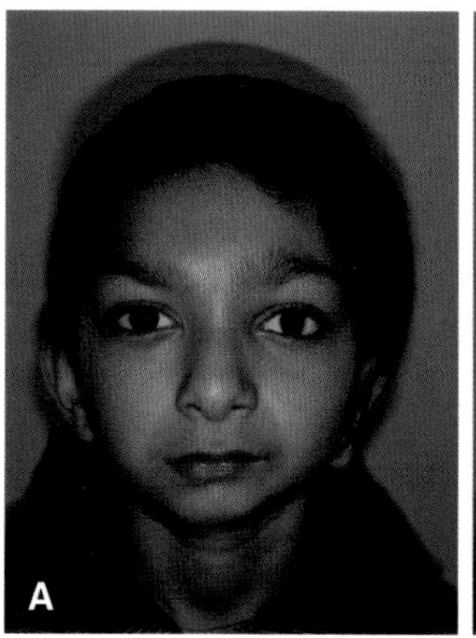

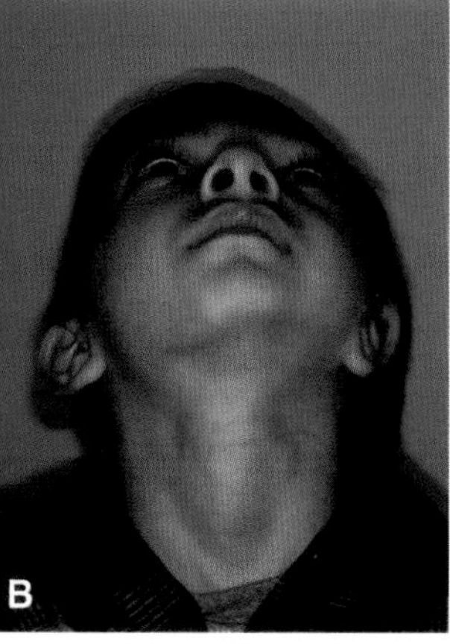

FIGURE 30.1. This patient first presented for facial asymmetry evaluation at 7 years of age. **A.** The typical asymmetry of the mandible, chin, and ear position is typical of the natural progression of a patient with CFM. **B.** Note also the decreased cheek projection and midface volume on the affected left side as seen in the basilar view.

Presentation

Interestingly, CFM more commonly tends to affect the right side (~60%) and is more frequent in males (up to 65% males).[11] The true rate for bilateral versus unilateral presentation is difficult to determine often because of unclear diagnostic criteria used (e.g., including a preauricular tag or not as an affected hemiface), but the literature supports a rate of bilateral presentation ranging from as low as 5% to over 30% of cases.[12]

CFM can affect many structures with variable degrees of severity, producing a wide spectrum of clinical presentations (**Figures 30.1** and **30.2**). The mandible, soft tissue, facial skeleton, facial muscles, ears, and related nervous system structures can all be affected. The frequency of involvement of any particular structure has not been definitively determined, and the current best data as noted in the following sections are compiled from existing case series.[9,13-15]

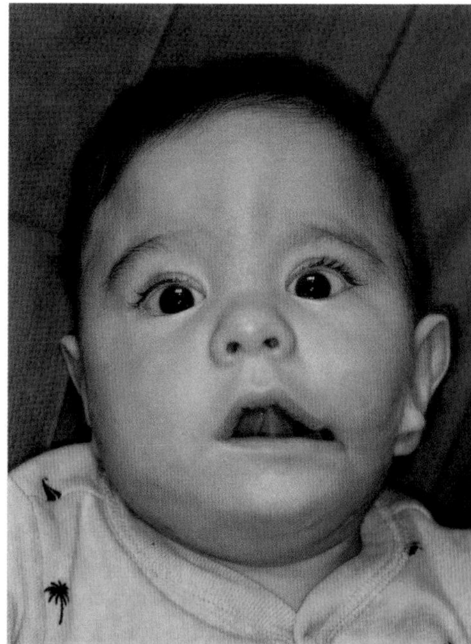

FIGURE 30.2. This 7-month-old infant with Goldenhar syndrome was found to exhibit a complex accessory tragus and cervical spine vertebral anomalies, but not the commonly found epibulbar dermoids. His macrostomia (Tessier cleft #7) is also a common secondary finding in CFM.

Mandible

Mandibular hypoplasia is usually the most obvious finding, as well as the most common, present in over 90% of patients. The ramus and condyle are usually affected much more than the body or ipsilateral parasymphysis, with some authors maintaining that the condyle is affected to some degree in every patient with CFM. The degree of hypoplasia can vary from a mandible that is morphologically normal but overall small in size to a mandible with absent condyle, ramus, and angle. With progressing degrees of severity, the body of the mandible becomes short and hypoplastic, curving superiorly in the direction of the malformed temporomandibular joint (TMJ). The degree of condyle and ramus malformation corresponds to changes in the glenoid fossa. The glenoid fossa loses concavity and flattens and can be malformed frankly in approximately 27% of patients. The *pivot point* for the hypoplastic ramus or condyle is translated anteriorly when compared with the contralateral TMJ. The double joint function of a normal TMJ may be lost, resulting in a simple hinge joint, limiting mandible depression and mouth opening. In unilateral cases, the chin will deviate to the affected side, and there will be corresponding loss of facial contour over the hypoplastic angle. Loss of mandibular height at the angle will produce loss of facial height posteriorly and creates an occlusal cant. Up to 27% of patients also present with hypodontia, which correlates in severity to the degree of mandibular hypoplasia.

Maxilla and Zygoma

Both of these arise from maxillary process of the first branchial arch and are frequently hypoplastic as well. The maxilla and zygoma may be deficient in the axial, sagittal, or coronal planes, with some severe cases showing an absence of the zygomatic arch. These changes correlate to the less projecting, flattened cheek and deficient lateral facial contour seen in these patients. Moreover, the smaller maxilla is associated with a superior displacement of the maxillary sinus and nasal base, in line with the general elevation of the occlusal plane on the affected side.

Cranial Base and Other Skeletal Involvement

Skeletal changes in CFM extend beyond the facial skeleton and glenoid fossa, involving the temporal and sometimes frontal bones, where flattening akin to plagiocephaly may be seen in up to 12% of patients. The cranial base itself may be affected as well, as shown in recent imaging-based studies noting asymmetry of cranial base landmarks in CFM patients.[16,17]

Importantly, the most common site of extracranial bony involvement is the axial skeleton, with vertebral or rib anomalies in 8% to 79% of patients. The manifestations of vertebral anomalies are varied and include hemivertebrae, block vertebrae, scoliosis/kyphoscoliosis, and spina bifida.

Nervous System, Eye, and Orbit

The nervous system may be involved in CFM in 2% to 69% of patients, as manifested by abnormalities of the cranial nerves and the eye as an extension of the central nervous system. Facial nerve paresis and palsies have been reported, as well as involvement of the vestibulocochlear nerve (CN VIII), but any cranial nerve may be involved. Eye anomalies may range from microphthalmia, vertical dystopia, impairment of extraocular movements to frank anophthalmia.[3] Epibulbar dermoids are more frequently associated with Goldenhar syndrome but may also be seen in CFM.

The central nervous system defects commonly include neural tube defects, corpus callosum agenesis or hypoplasia, intracranial lipoma, Arnold-Chiari malformations, hydrocephaly, ventriculomegaly, and cerebral hypoplasia. Developmental disorders including intellectual disability, language or speech developmental delay, and neuropsychomotor delay have been seen in 8% to 73% of patients. The presence of brain anomalies is well correlated with ocular findings, and epibulbar dermoids specifically.[18]

The cranial nerve most commonly involved is the facial nerve (CN VII), which can be due to hypoplasia or agenesis of the nerve trunk peripherally or of the facial nerve nucleus in the brainstem, so facial animation should be thoroughly documented for these patients.

Skin and Soft Tissue

Aside from the auricular appendage, macrostomia, muscles of mastication, and salivary glands are probably the soft-tissue structures that are significantly involved.

Macrostomia can be seen in up to 35% of patients, with wide variations in severity. This can be manifested as lateral displacement of the oral commissure due to hypoplasia of the mandible and cheek soft tissues or as a frank full-thickness defect, essentially constituting a facial cleft. Clefting of the lip and palate has also been reported and has been raised as an argument against the hematoma pathogenesis hypothesis because it would be less likely that an insult primarily affecting the mandible and lateral face would also be responsible for fusion of the palatal shelves or maxillary prominences anteriorly.

Hypoplasia of the muscle tissues is seen in muscles derived from the first and second branchial arches, thereby encompassing the muscles of mastication as well as the muscles of facial expression. The weakness and loss of bulk exacerbate the facial contour changes on the affected side as well as animation asymmetry. The severity of muscle hypoplasia appears to be correlated to the overall severity of the disorder.[19] Interestingly, one study of patients with Pruzansky grade I and II mandibular hypoplasia found this relationship to hold in regard to the masseter, but not the temporalis muscle, perhaps suggesting a differential effect on these two structures, although more data would be needed from more severe cases before drawing a conclusion.[20]

Salivary gland involvement tends to be predominantly confined to hypoplasia or agenesis of the parotid duct or the gland itself.

Systemic

Less commonly, systemic anomalies are encountered as well. There are cardiovascular findings in up to 33% of patients, including tetralogy of Fallot, ventricular septal defects, transposition of the great vessels, and aortic arch anomalies. Genitourinary defects are seen in up to 18% of patients, including absent kidney, double ureter, crossed renal ectopia, hydronephrosis, and hydroureter. More rarely, pulmonary and gastrointestinal anomalies may be encountered in up to 15% and 12% of patients, respectively. Notably, the presence of a single extracraniofacial anomaly is associated with an increased chance of others being present, so any findings in one of the cardiac/renal/vertebral systems should prompt a thorough workup of the rest.[11,15]

Ears

Malformation or hypoplasia of the auricular structures is a sine qua non for CFM, with all patients presenting with some abnormality. This may be a mild manifestation, such as a preauricular tag, which is usually an accessory cartilaginous appendage representing an accessory tragus or tragal remnants and not simple skin tags or acrochordons, for which these may be commonly confused. More severe presentations include all degrees of microtia, anotia, and aural atresia. There is some thought that an isolated accessory tragal remnant may be the only clinical manifestation in a number of patients with milder forms of OAV dysplasia or CFM. Without other, more severe, anomalies, these patients may avoid diagnosis of OAV dysplasia or CFM, suggesting that the incidence for these disorders may be higher than otherwise reported. Isolated microtia or aural atresia likely does not warrant imaging of the spine or kidneys as the prevalence of abnormalities does not appear increased in this population.[21] However, isolated microtia may serve as a useful marker to trigger screening in patients for other manifestations of OAV dysplasia, as it has been shown to predict later facial growth asymmetry in up to 40% of screened patients.[22]

The middle ear is also often frequently affected, with moderate hypoplasia or atresia seen in up to 90% of patients.[23] If present, hearing loss is conductive in the vast majority of cases (73%–86%) and may be present on the contralateral side in unilateral CFM cases. Notably, the severity of craniofacial features does not appear to correlate with the degree of hearing loss, so all patients suspected to be at risk should undergo formal audiologic evaluation.[23]

Classification Schemes

Classification schemes for the overall total presentation have been proposed by Harvold, Vargevik, and Chierici in 1983, and then by Munro and Lauritzen in 1985, among others. The classification most widely adopted at this time is the OMENS+ classification. Vento, LaBrie, and Mulliken originally proposed the OMENS scheme in 1991, describing the components most frequently affected: orbit, mandible, ear, nerve, and soft tissue (**Figure 30.3**).[13] Each component is rated 0 to 3, with 0 indicating normal phenotype and 3 indicating maximal abnormality, for a total score ranging from 0 to 15. This was revised to OMENS+ in 1995 by Horgan et al. to include extracraniofacial abnormalities, as their study showed a correlation between a higher OMENS score and likelihood of other, noncraniofacial anomalies.[24]

Classification schemes for the individual features affected have also been proposed. The auricular deformity has been classified by Meurman,[25] although Nagata's microtia classification remains the more clinically relevant one as its stages better correlate to conditions guiding surgical reconstruction. The commonly recognized *Pruzansky* classification for mandible hypoplasia was first proposed by Pruzansky in 1969[26] but was modified to the currently used schema by Kaban, Moses, and Mulliken in 1988 by subdividing the type II hypoplastic mandible into type IIa and IIb based on the status of the TMJ.[27] This alteration aligned the classification scheme with the surgical treatment algorithm and thus greatly improved its usefulness. **Figure 30.4** illustrates the modified Pruzansky classification for mandibular hypoplasia, which will be the basis of the following discussion regarding treatment.

Workup

Initiating care for a child with CFM begins with a thorough history:

- Family history should focus on craniofacial disorders, facial asymmetry, auricular and periauricular anomalies, hearing loss, ophthalmologic anomalies (epibulbar dermoids, colobomas), and mandible asymmetry or malformation.
- Maternal and pregnancy history should focus on use of any known teratogens (specifically retinoic acid) and maternal diabetes mellitus.

Physical examination should include the following:

- Following the OMENS+ classification template is useful to ensure completeness and relevant documentation. Ophthalmologic examination should include assessment for epibulbar dermoids and colobomas; there should be a low threshold for ophthalmologic consultation to perform a funduscopic examination, especially if there is a suspicion of Goldenhar syndrome. The mandible, auricle, soft tissues, and facial nerve function are all documented and assigned a grade.
- Pictorial tools are available to aid in documentation of the present deformities.[28]
- Evaluation of the mandible should document interincisal opening and TMJ function. Together with the cephalogram or CT/MRI imaging (if obtained), a modified Pruzansky grade should be assigned for any child with mandibular hypoplasia.

At this time, there is no indication for routine genetic testing of patients with CFM, but engaging a genetic counselor may improve the parents' and patients' understanding of the condition and can be an important part of provided comprehensive care. Genetic testing and referral should be considered for any patients whose presentation might suggest the presence of another syndrome (e.g., CHARGE or Treacher Collins syndrome).

Modified O.M.E.N.S. (+) Classification of Hemifacial Microsomia'
(check all that apply)

Side (Each side evaluated separately in cases of bifacial microsomia)
_R_L

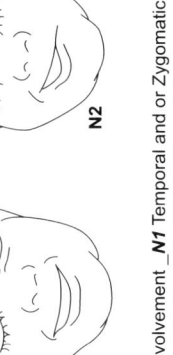

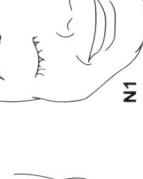

Orbit[2]

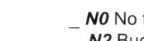

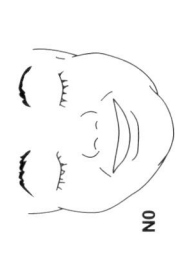

00 01 02↓ 02↑ 03

***00*** Normal orbital size and position***O1*** Abnormal orbital size_***O2***↓ Inferior orbital displacement_***O2***↑ Superior orbital displacement_***O3*** Abnormal orbital size and position

Mandible

M0 M1 M2A M2B M3

_ ***M0*** Normal mandible _ ***M1*** Small mandible and glenoid fossa with short ramus _ ***M2A*** Abnormally shaped and short ramus[3] (Glenoid fossa in acceptable position with reference to contralateral TMJ) _ ***M2B*** Abnormally shaped and short ramus (Glenoid fossa is inferiorly, medially and anteriorly displaced with hypoplastic condyle) _ ***M3*** Absence of ramus and glenoid fossa (no TMJ)

Ear

E0 E1 E2 E3

_ ***E0*** Normal auricle _ ***EI*** Mild hypoplasia and cupping with presence of all structures _ ***E2*** Absence of external canal with variable hypoplasia of concha _ ***E3*** Malpositioned lobule with absent auricle; lobular remnant typically inferiorly and anteriorly displaced

Nerve

N0 N1 N2 N3

_ ***N0*** No facial nerve involvement _***N1*** Temporal and or Zygomatic branch involvement _***N2*** Buccal and/or Mandibular and/or Cervical branch involvement _***N3*** All branches affected

Soft Tissue

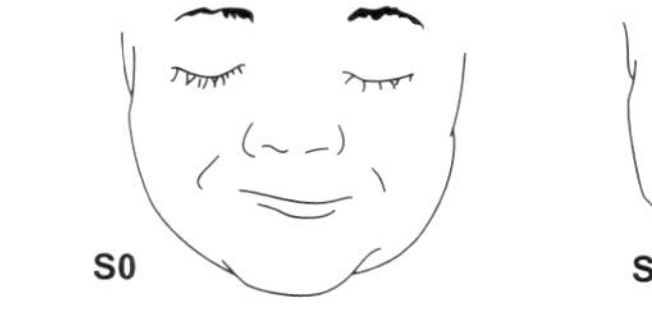
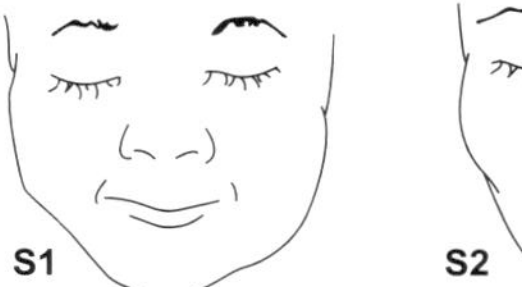
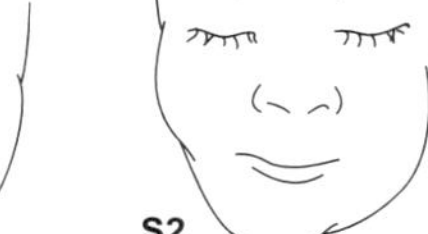
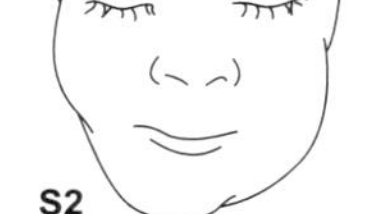
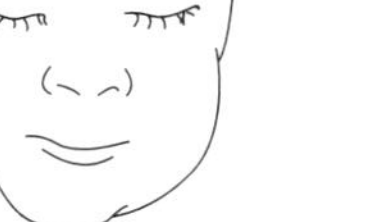
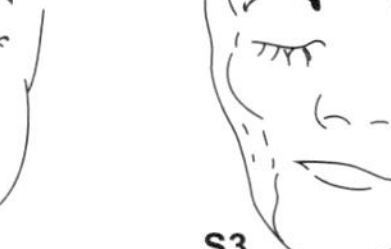

S0 S1 S2 S3

_***S0*** No soft tissue deficiency _ ***S1*** Minimal soft tissue deficiency _***S2*** Moderate soft tissue deficiency (between SI and S3) _ ***S3*** Severe soft tissue deficiency

Macrostomia (Tessier # 7 Cleft)

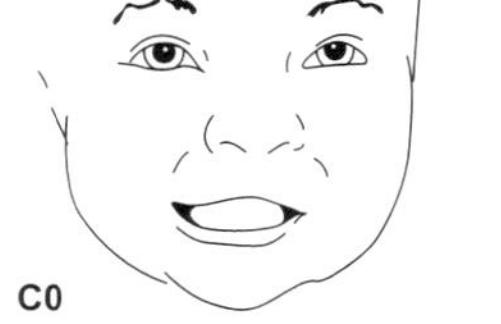
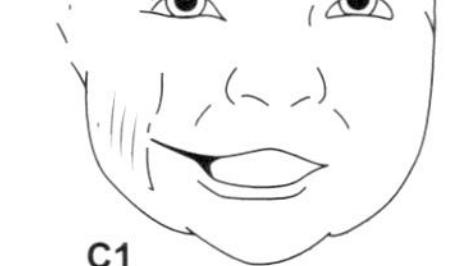
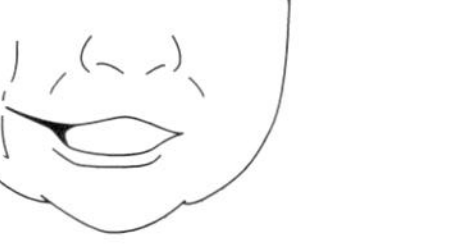
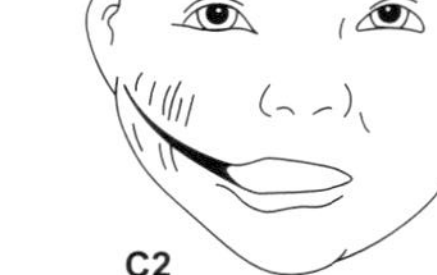

C0 C1 C2

_ ***C0*** No cleft _ ***C1*** Cleft terminates medial to anterior border of masseter _***C2*** Cleft terminates lateral to anterior border of masseter

Miscellaneous

O.M.E.N.S. (+)[4] { _ *Yes* / _ *No*

_ ***Goldenhars*** (Hemifacial Microsomia with epibulbar lipodermoids and fused/hemivertebrae)

FIGURE 30.3. These pictographs developed by Gougoutas and colleagues are useful visual aids in applying the OMENS+ classification system. (From Gougoutas AJ, Singh DJ, Low DW, Bartlett SP. Hemifacial microsomia: clinical features and pictographic representations of the OMENS classification system. *Plast Reconstr Surg.* 2007;120(7):112e-120e.)

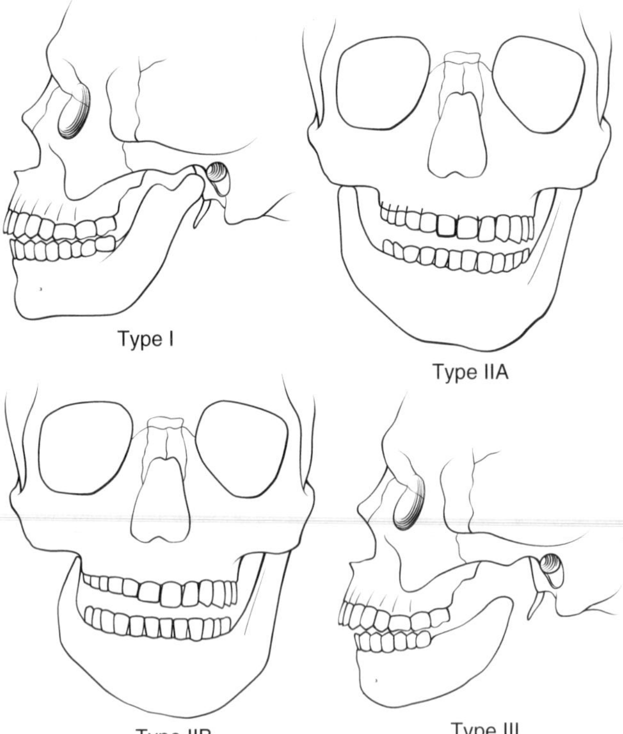

FIGURE 30.4. Kaban and colleagues' modification[27] of the original CFM classification system proposed by Pruzansky.[26] **A.** Type I: The condyle and ramus are reduced in size, but the overall morphology is maintained. **B.** Type IIA: The ramus and condyle demonstrate abnormal morphology, but the glenoid fossa has maintained a position in the temporal bone similar to that of the contralateral side. **C.** Type IIB: The ramus/condyle is hypoplastic, malformed, and displaced toward the midline. **D.** Type III: The ramus is essentially absent without any evidence of temporomandibular joint.

Imaging and Testing

- Auditory testing should be routinely performed for all patients with auricle malformations to assess for hearing loss.
- Swallow evaluation for dysphagia should be considered for all patients with CFM. Up to 13.5% of patients may have swallowing difficulties, with the degree of dysphagia correlating to the severity of the presentation. Video fluoroscopic swallow studies should be strongly considered for patients with Pruzansky grade III mandible hypoplasia.
- Children with findings on physical examination or history concerning for upper airway obstruction (tachypnea, increased work of breathing, apnea, or snoring) should be evaluated with a sleep study and/or airway endoscopy.
- Standardized photography is crucial to document the patient's appearance at presentation and through his or her growth and treatment.
- Cephalograms are routinely obtained to evaluate the shape and size of the mandible and maxilla. These may be supplemented or replaced with CT imaging, particularly if virtual surgical planning is anticipated to be used in future treatment.
- It is important to diagnose any vertebral anomalies at an early stage because these can result in cervical spine instability and risk neurologic compromise. Routine plain film X-ray evaluation of the cervical spine is recommended for all patients with CFM; a spine specialist should be consulted should any such anomalies be identified.
- In cases with hearing loss, CT or MRI should be considered to image the middle and inner ear to evaluate the degree of anatomic constriction or ossicle malformation.
- Echocardiogram and renal ultrasound studies are recommended given the relatively high prevalence and high impact of these anomalies in children with CFM.

Management and Treatment

Treatment for CFM is complex because no single approach or algorithm can address the wide variety of CFM presentation, and there is still debate regarding the timing of surgical intervention. Patients with CFM should be treated in a multidisciplinary fashion, to ensure that all aspects of the affected systems are correctly diagnosed and treated in a coordinated fashion. The already high likelihood of multiple surgeries (microtia reconstruction, primary and/or secondary orthognathic surgery, soft-tissue or macrostomia reconstruction, etc.) underscores the importance of coordinating care. Moreover, the reconstructive surgeon should be familiar with the spectrum of procedures needed for a patient with CFM to thoughtfully plan the earlier surgeries. This is well illustrated in patients with severe microtia, in whom periauricular and temporal tissues are highly likely to be used in subsequent procedures, and thus external incision planning for mandibular surgery must be undertaken with great care.

The treatment of orbital dystopia, microtia, and cranial vault deformities is addressed elsewhere in this text so that the present discussion will focus on correction of the maxilla and mandible that is specific to CFM.

As one of the focal points of CFM, treatment of the mandible forms the centerpiece of the overall surgical plan, together with complementary intervention for the maxilla. The goal is to create functional occlusion, construct a functional TMJ, and improve the facial skeletal bulk and contour to create facial symmetry. The basic intervention layout has changed little since Kaban's modification of the Pruzansky classification, which hinges the operative decision-making on the functional status of the temporomandibular articulation (**Table 30.1**).

An important variable to consider is the status of the patient's airway. In the newborn or infant with CFM, the mandibular hypoplasia may lead to tongue retropositioning and tongue-based airway obstruction, particularly in bilateral cases. If sleep study evaluation suggests significant apnea or hypopnea and nasoendoscopy demonstrates airway obstruction limited to the tongue-base, early mandibular advancement can improve the airway and facilitate decannulation if a tracheostomy has been previously placed, accompanied by improvement in feeding/swallowing. Distraction is currently the favored method of advancing the mandible in children, providing low relapse rates and expansion of the soft-tissue envelope.

The techniques and outcomes of sagittal split osteotomy have been extensively researched since Obwegeser's initial description of the procedure.[29] One of the more common complications in SSO (surgical site occurrence) is injury to the inferior alveolar nerve. It should be noted that in CFM patients, the mandibular foramen is shifted superiorly, where it is found one-third of the way down as measured

TABLE 30.1. MODIFIED PRUZANSKY CLASSIFICATION

Type	Description	Surgical Treatment Goals and Techniques
I or IIa	Varied degree of hypoplasia and condyle/ramus deformity TMJ is functional	Expand existing bone stock to increase ramus height and facial contour, accomplished via sagittal split osteotomy with or without a bone graft, or via distraction osteogenesis
IIb or III	Severe hypoplasia or absence of the ramus/condyle and deformity of the body TMJ is nonfunctional or absent Zygomatic arch may be absent	Some type IIb with adequate bone stock may be distracted. Otherwise, as for all type III patients, new bone stock must be brought in, accomplished via costochondral and osseous grafts to reconstruct the ramus and TMJ/zygomatic arch

from the sigmoid notch to the angle of the mandible, as opposed to halfway between these landmarks in control patients. In addition, the nerve is located closer to the buccal cortex in patients with CFM.[30]

Treatment of the type IIb mandible with adequate bone stock can be similar to the type I/IIa in that distraction may suffice to expand the existing structure as long as the condyle is adequately developed and properly directed toward the glenoid fossa to create a vertical stop and allow elongation of the ramus with distraction (**Figures 30.5** and **30.6**). By carrying out expansion in a vertical vector posteriorly, the distracted segment can be brought up to about the glenoid fossa where it can form a pseudoarthrosis. If successful, expansion of even a hypoplastic condyle avoids the need to formally reconstruct the TMJ as long as the condyle creates a vertical stop to facilitate distraction. Type IIb mandibles are too hypoplastic to carry out distraction, or type III mandibles are treated with graft reconstruction of the ramus, zygoma, and TMJ. Commonly, a costochondral graft is affixed to the mandible with lag screws and placed in opposition to a cartilaginous graft or fascial inlay at the base of the temporal bone to recreate a glenoid fossa. This construct is most stable if the zygomatic arch is present and can prevent lateral displacement of the neocondyle. In the absence of a zygomatic arch, reconstruction of the arch with a rib graft should be considered to provide lateral stability to the reconstructed TMJ (**Figure 30.7**).

Timeline

The controversy regarding surgical treatment of the mandible and maxilla in CFM centers around the questions of intervening in early childhood or waiting until skeletal maturity, with the choice of distraction osteogenesis or one-stage surgery as a secondary debate. The argument for early intervention is in part that correcting the mandible in childhood will normalize the patient's appearance throughout their childhood, correct some of the soft-tissue contours, and facilitate downward growth of the maxilla, potentially sparing the child a subsequent surgical procedure to correct the maxilla. These benefits come at the cost of the increased difficulty of working with the immature mandible bone stock and the increased likelihood of needing repeat surgery at skeletal maturity to correct for any occlusion changes that will happen with growth. The alternative is waiting until skeletal maturity and then performing orthognathic surgery on the developed bony stock, usually comprised of a *three-jaw* surgery: Le Fort I osteotomy of the maxilla, BSSO (bilateral sagittal split osteotomy), and asymmetric osseous genioplasty. Although this is likely to provide a one-stage orthognathic correction, it does not address the soft-tissue paucity nor the psychological cost to the child in growing up with an uncorrected deformity. **Table 30.2** summarizes the basic arguments for earlier or later intervention.

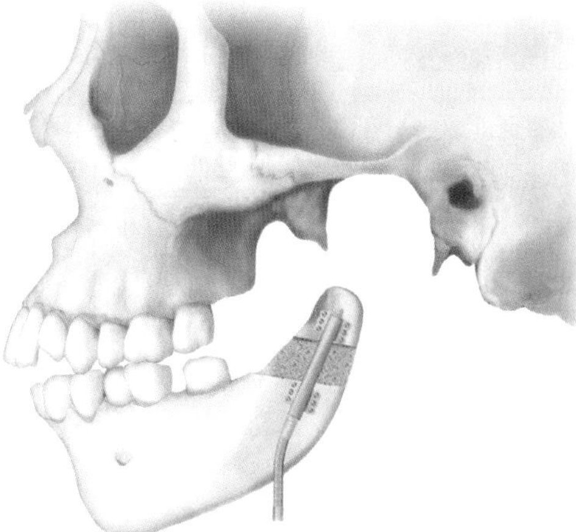

FIGURE 30.5. Distraction of the hypoplastic mandible with an internal (buried) distractor. Note the need for adequate bony stock on either side of the osteotomy to affix the hardware.

In a study of children with craniofacial anomalies, self-awareness of facial differences began at a mean age of 3 years and teasing at a mean age of 6, with 43% of individuals 4 years or older reporting teasing.[31] There is also evidence of worse psychological outcomes in children with CFM,[32] lending credence to the idea of earlier surgery to improve children's psychosocial development.

Earlier surgery on the mandible also affects the growth of the maxilla, as Kaban et al. showed that correction of the mandible at an early age and creation of an open bite on the affected side can lead to responsive downward growth of the maxilla, resulting in an overall level occlusal plane and sparing patients from the need for Le Fort maxillary osteotomies to level the maxillary occlusal plane in the future.[27]

Choosing distraction versus osteotomy and advancement (with bone grafting, if needed) in a single step depends on the patient's age, bone stock, soft tissue, and surgeon preference. It has been thought that by the virtue of gradually stretching soft tissue with distraction, these forces would be lessened at the end of the distraction course and thus lead to lower relapse rates. However, a prospective randomized controlled trial in adults >35 years of age did not show any significant difference in relapse rates for advancements <10 mm.[33] Whereas 10 mm advancement is a modest distraction distance, differences between the stability of distraction and orthognathic advancement of the mandible may become apparent in advancements >10 mm.

One of the other controversial topics in this discussion is the natural growth of the affected mandible, maxilla, and soft tissues. Although it is clear that the affected tissues do not catch up in growth when compared with the contralateral side, it is less clear whether it is the relative or absolute size discrepancy of the affected side that worsens over time. The mandible that has been distracted or reconstructed with a graft can exhibit growth, albeit at a slower rate than the contralateral side, thus sometimes necessitating a revision surgery at maturity if the initial correction was done at a young age.

The overall timeline is as follows:

- Infancy (up to 2 years of age)
  - Correction of macrostomia, clefts, and minor auricular anomalies (pits, accessory appendages) should be performed early on to improve function and make a dramatic improvement in appearance.
  - Distraction of the affected mandible is considered at this early stage for patients with airway compromise.
- Early childhood (to 6 years of age)
  - **Type I:** If the deformity is mild, treatment is delayed until skeletal maturity.
  - **Type IIa/IIb:** If the aesthetic deformity is severe or airway problems exist, which were not addressed in infancy, distraction osteogenesis is considered for type IIa and type IIb mandibles with adequate bone stock.
  - **Type III:** The ramus, zygomatic arch, and the temporomandibular articulation is reconstructed using costochondral grafts at approximately 4 years of age or older, with secondary distraction if needed to expand the construct once healed.
- Late childhood/adolescence (6–16 years of age)
  - Orthodontic treatment is applied during this period. If the mandible has already been corrected, orthodontia can help bring the maxilla into occlusion. The goal is to correct the maxilla enough to avoid a Le Fort I osteotomy in the future.
- Adolescence and later (after age 16)
  - If the mandible has already been operated on:
    - Once the patient is deemed to be at skeletal maturity, the occlusion and results of orthodontic treatment are assessed. There is a high likelihood that secondary surgery will be needed to correct the maxilla, to revise the mandible to account for the unaffected side's growth, or to perform an asymmetric genioplasty to restore the chin to the midline.
  - If the patient has not yet had mandibular surgery (typically type I mandibles or if the decision was made to delay treatment):
    - The surgical plan must be customized to each patient, but will usually include:

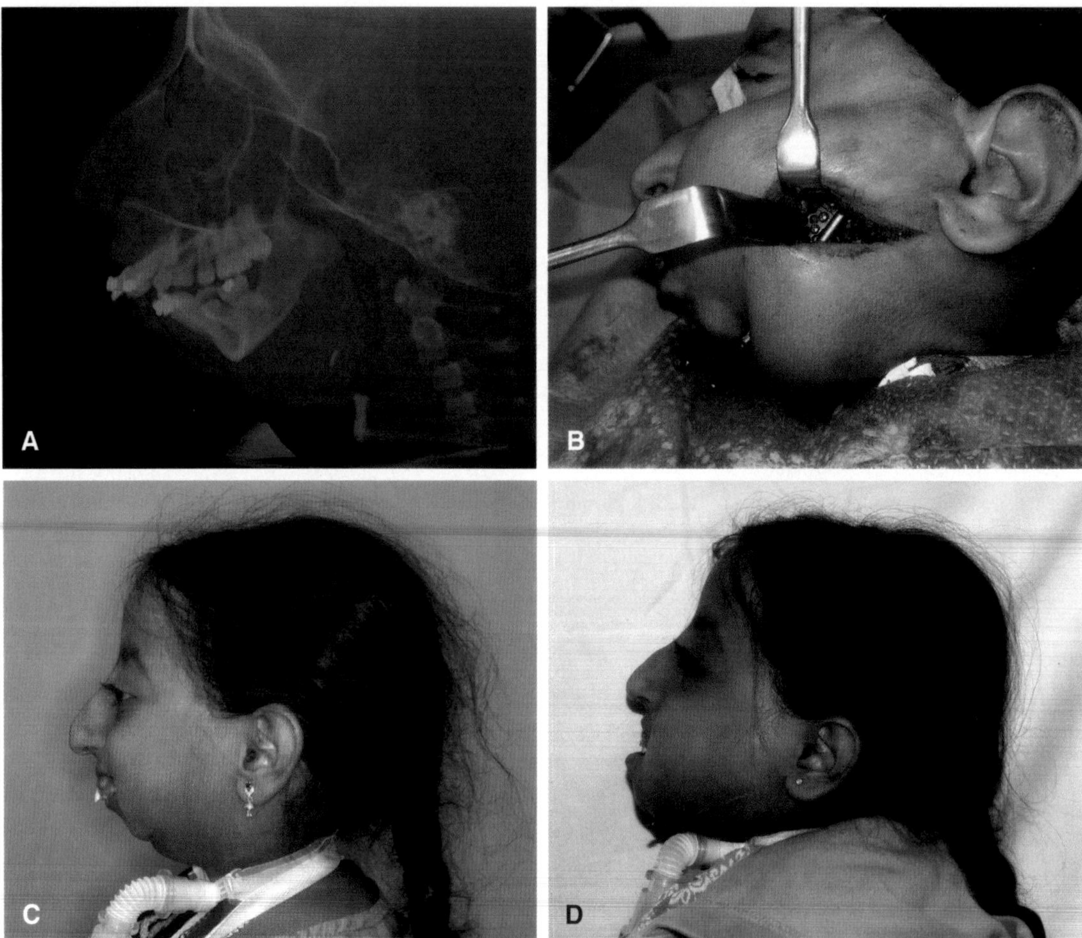

FIGURE 30.6. This patient presented for treatment at 7 years of age. The etiology of her craniofacial anomalies has not been described. A large part of the problem was the hypoplastic mandible—Pruzansky type IIa. Because adequate bony stock was present and there was a rudimentary TMJ, internal distractors were placed as diagrammed in Figure 30.5, yielding a total of 31 mm of advancement. **A.** Mandible contour on lateral X-ray. **B.** Orientation of the distractor application. **C,D.** Patient's predistraction and postdistraction appearances, respectively, reflecting the significant advancement achieved.

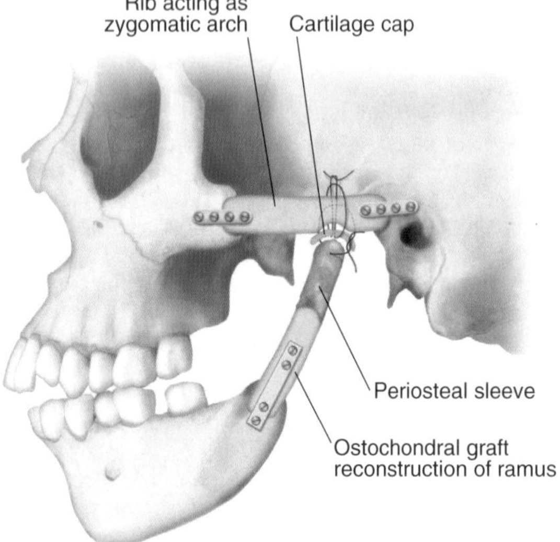

FIGURE 30.7. Pruzansky grade IIb and above mandibles can be reconstructed using a rib graft to recreate the zygomatic arch if absent; costochondral rib grafts to recreate the ramus of the mandible, and careful positioning of a cartilaginous cap of the costochondral graft to serve as a neocondyle within the reconstructed glenoid fossa.

- Sagittal split osteotomy with or without bone graft to address the mandibular vertical deficiency.
- Le Fort I osteotomy, often with impaction on the affected side, to level the occlusal plane.
- Asymmetric osseous genioplasty, to correct the facial asymmetry.

□ Advanced soft-tissue correction can also be undertaken at this time. Severe soft-tissue deficit is best addressed by choosing distraction for the mandible: as the bone is expanded, so is the overlying soft-tissue envelope. For residual defects, an adipofascial free flap or serial fat injection may be used to correct volume deficiency, depending on the defect size.

□ Adipofascial free flaps have been associated with ptosis and less predictable volume over time with patient weight loss or gain. There is currently an increasing trend for serial fat injection to treat facial soft-tissue deficit because this is less likely to undergo ptosis and patients can be regrafted with much less morbidity.

CRANIOFACIAL DISTRACTION

The problem of deficient bone stock has long been present in both the pediatric population (e.g., hypoplastic mandible in children with CFM or Pierre Robin sequence) and in adults (e.g., bone loss

TABLE 30.2. ARGUMENTS FOR EARLIER OR LATER INTERVENTION

Factor	Early Childhood Intervention	Surgery at Skeletal Maturity
Need for revision orthognathic surgery	High	Low
Soft tissue	Partially addressed during distraction	Must be addressed separately
Psychosocial factors	Provides early improvement prior to school age	Patient bears burden of deformity until adolescence
Need for maxillary surgery	Variable based on orthodontic Rx	Almost always

due to trauma or need of orthognathic surgery with large [>1 cm] advancements). Solutions such as vascularized bone transfer are often impractical and carry a large donor site burden, and an avascular graft carries the risks of infection, nonunion, and resorption. Distraction osteogenesis solves this problem by expanding the existing bone stock along the vector specified by the surgeon, essentially replicating for bone what tissue expansion has done for the skin. Although it was described earlier, Ilizarov is credited with proving the concept and establishing its efficacy in long bones.[34] McCarthy and colleagues later applied these principles to craniofacial scenarios, supporting the clinical efficacy of this technique.[35]

The basic principle of distraction osteogenesis consists of an osteotomy across the bone to be distracted and then carefully controlled separation of the two segments at a rate that promotes bony regeneration to close the gap. Although details may differ based on surgeon preference and patient age, the basic timeline is as follows:

- Osteotomy and hardware placement
  - The bone to be distracted is divided into segments with an osteotomy or corticotomy, creating the *distraction zone.* The surgeon must ensure that the segments are mobile so that distraction can take place—an incomplete osteotomy/corticotomy will skew the vector of distraction or cause hardware failure.
  - The distractor hardware is placed across the distraction zone aligned with the desired vector of movement to promote new bone deposition. No distraction takes place at this time, and the bony segments remain in opposition.
- Latency period
  - Approximately 1 week (5–7 days) is allowed for healing and initial callus formation in the distraction zone prior to initiation of distraction.
- Activation period
  - The distraction hardware is used to separate the bony segments at some predetermined rate (usually 0.5 mm twice per day). Faster rates are commonly seen in infants because of their ability to quickly deposit bone regenerate—the guiding principle here is to set such a rate that separation of the bony segments will not outpace the deposition of new callus, yet will also not be so slow so that ossification leading to bony union causes premature end of distraction.
  - The device is periodically checked for alignment and solid fixation to ensure the desired vector of distraction is maintained.
- Consolidation period
  - Once the desired amount of travel is achieved, distraction is stopped and the callus formed in the distraction space ossifies. This period is usually 8 weeks in length, after which time the new bony construct should be stable and hardware can be removed. However, in infants, the consolidation period is often shortened to 6 weeks because of rapid bone consolidation.

McCarthy and colleagues examined the histology of the bony generate[36] in the distraction zone, with later studies providing further detail (**Figure 30.8**).[37] The healing response is initiated similar to any other fracture with hematoma formation and inflammatory cell influx during the latency period, producing the initial callus. Infiltration of fibroblast-like cells and neovascularization are noted after beginning of activation. Osteogenesis is noted at 2 weeks after activation is started with osteoid deposition and mineralization, and osteoblasts seen another week later. The basic histologic structure shown in Figure 30.8 reflects the findings of McCarthy et al., although later studies revealed a more stratified organization to the generate. The key findings agree in that bony trabeculae start forming along the axis of distraction with concomitant neovascularization and then continue this process after distraction is stopped until mature lamellar bone is produced. In an in vitro model, Slack et al.[38] found that skipping the latency period and starting distraction immediately appears to lead to marked delays in cell proliferation, alkaline phosphatase activity, osteogenic gene expression, and higher apoptosis at the osteotomy site; however, the bone volume and quality at the clinical endpoints were unaffected. Of note is that latency periods are often shortened to 1 day or completely eliminated in infants. Future studies are required to further investigate the importance, duration, and age-dependence of the latency period.

The cellular-level processes underlying osteogenesis in this scenario are understandably complex, but one of the key factors is TGF-B1 (transforming growth factor B1), which peaks during the activation period, ostensibly inducing deposition of collagen and extracellular matrix necessary for further ossification.[39] TGF-B1 subsequently induced VEGF and FGF, which in turn are key to neovascularization of the bony generate and fibroblast activity necessary for the process.[40] Bone morphogenic protein, insulin-like growth factor, and osteonectin/osteopontin also appear to play key roles.[37]

Hardware

A major decision for each distraction case is whether to use internal or external hardware. Applications in the mandible can use either type with no significant difference in efficacy, whereas others, such as posterior vault distraction, appear to be better suited for buried (internal)

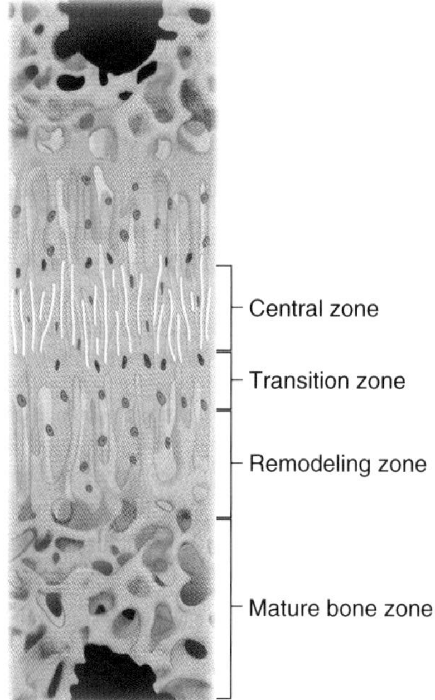

FIGURE 30.8. Diagram of the bony generate in the setting of distraction.[36] Central zone is area of mesenchymal proliferation and collagen deposition. Transition zone has osteoid formation on the scaffold of collagen bundles. Remodeling zone is area of osteoclast activity and new bone remodeling, leading up to mature bone zone.

TABLE 30.3. KEY DIFFERENCES BETWEEN INTERNAL AND EXTERNAL DISTRACTION HARDWARE

	Internal	External
Profile	Lower profile, only the activator arm needs to be externalized	Bulkier profile, multiple pin sites require more hygienic care
Incisions	Requires a larger incision for the bulky hardware and wide exposure of the bony for footplate fixation	Smaller stab incisions for pins may reduce external incision burden if other approach (intraoral) can be used to complete osteotomy
Monitoring	Difficult to assess distraction and hardware position/security because only the activator arm is visible	Position and movement of hardware is easily examined; however, correlation with bone movement is speculative
Adjustments	No adjustments can be made once the hardware is in place	Vector can be manipulated and multivector distraction can be carried out

hardware. In general, the external distractors act similarly to an external fixator with a mechanism for applying a distracting force between two sets of pins. Each center has its own preference for internal versus external hardware for mandibular distraction. There are some data that buried devices lead to higher satisfaction with quality of life and the decision to undergo the procedure in the face of equivalent functional and aesthetic outcomes.[41] However, internal distraction devices have the disadvantage of requiring a second surgical procedure for device removal. This is a significant consideration given that injury to the marginal mandibular nerve with long-term weakness of depressor function of the oral commissure has been reported in 15% of cases following internal mandibular distraction in patients with Pierre Robin sequence.[42] One must consider the increased risk of nerve injury following internal distractor placement, given the need for reentry into the incision for distractor removal when the nerve may be obscured by scar following the initial procedure. In summary, the guiding principle for hardware choice is to ensure that fixation will be secure, and the desired vector of distraction will be maintained, with remaining factors determined by surgeon preference and experience. **Table 30.3** shows the general pros and cons of each design.

With the establishment of distraction osteogenesis as a clinically effective and safe technique, its indications have widened. Large early analyses reported pooled complication rates approximating 1 in 3 patients, with markedly lower rates reported by surgeons experienced in the technique.[43] As the specialty's collective experience has grown, so has the safety profile, as shown below for the specific applications.

Figure 30.6 shows the application of internal distraction hardware for mandible distraction. In the same setting of mandibular distraction, it is easy to appreciate the differences when compared with external distraction, as shown in **Figure 30.9**.

Mandibular Distraction

The mandible was the first bone where craniofacial distraction was successfully implemented—it is accessible, the progress of distraction is easy to assess, and it addresses a significant clinical need. Mandibular distraction has enabled craniofacial surgeons to address mandibular hypoplasia at a younger age with less morbidity than traditional methods. It has shown to be effective in infants with Pierre Robin sequence, Treacher Collins syndrome, and CFM. Patients with these conditions suffering from airway compromise often find significant improvement after distraction and can be successfully decannulated.

One of the key decisions in mandibular distraction is the choice of vector. This hinges on the morphology of the patient's mandible: adequate bony stock in the body with a deficient or absent ramus dictates a vertical vector (perpendicular to the occlusal plane), whereas the converse (short body but adequate ramus) dictates a horizontal vector. If both the body and ramus are deficient, an oblique vector can be chosen. It is important to account for autorotation when distracting with a vertical or oblique vector, as the extraposterior height will result in anterior movement of the body and increase chin projection. In unilateral cases, there will also be some correction of the chin point deviation. When performing this in infants or children who have not yet reached skeletal maturity, the goal should be to achieve overcorrection as the distracted mandible exhibits slower growth than age-matched controls.[44] One must also determine whether unilateral or bilateral mandibular distraction is indicated based on the relative asymmetry of mandibular position relative to the maxilla.

Monobloc and Le Fort III Distraction

Despite over two decades of experience with monobloc and Le Fort III distraction,[45] in a review of Monobloc and Le Fort III advancement, it appears there are mixed data regarding the complication profiles for distraction versus traditional advancement. Monobloc advancements incurred higher complication rates with distraction, and the opposite was seen in Le Fort III advancements, indicating that further refinement of these techniques is needed.[46] Nevertheless, for younger children in need of significant midface advancement, distraction has been[47] and continues to be the preferred method of midfacial advancement. Both rigid external devices and buried distraction hardware have been successfully used in this setting.

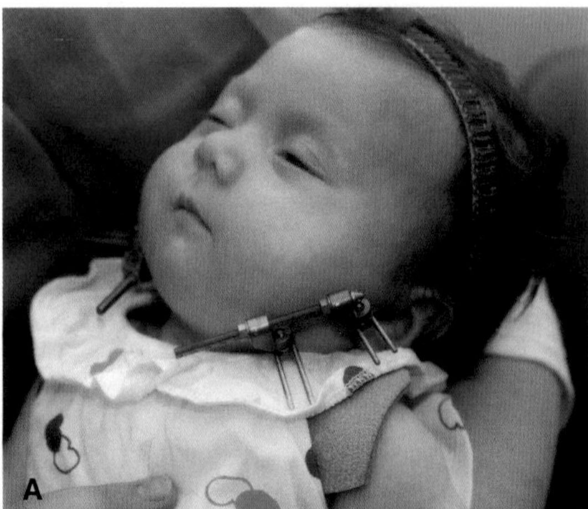

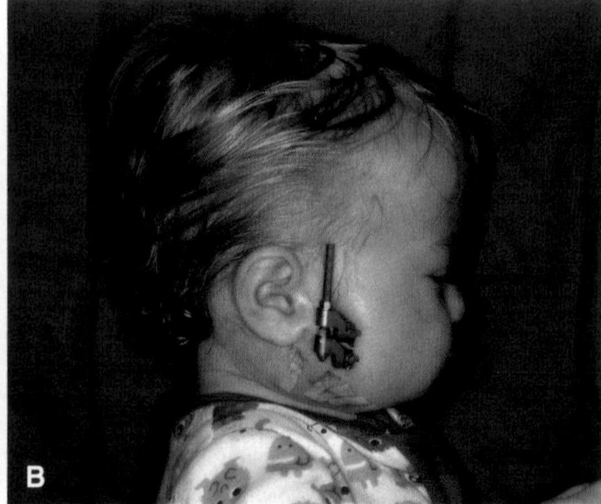

FIGURE 30.9. Mandible distraction using external hardware. An oblique vector addressing the mandibular body is shown in (**A**) and a vertical vector addressing a ramus height deficiency is shown in (**B**).

Cranial Vault Distraction

Distraction of the cranial vault, and the posterior vault specifically, is a relatively new application of distraction osteogenesis. The intracranial volume gained by posterior vault distraction is markedly higher when compared with fronto-orbital advancement,[48] and compared with traditional methods of posterior vault cranioplasty, the complication rate appears to be comparable.[49] Notably, great care must be paid to avoid inadvertently injuring the dura with the screws, as the multiple footplates will likely span areas of variable bone thickness (**Figure 30.10**). Although the argument exists for distraction to obtain the maximal possible gain in intracranial volumes, there are not yet enough data to show clear superiority of distraction to traditional cranioplasty for posterior vault expansion.[33]

Complications of Distraction Osteogenesis

The complex nature of the deformity and surgical course is associated with complications at any point. Complications more specific to distraction include hardware problems, soft-tissue ulceration and breakdown, incorrect distraction vectors, and postdistraction sequelae. The practice of distraction osteogenesis is heterogeneous because of the varied indications, patient scenarios, hardware types,

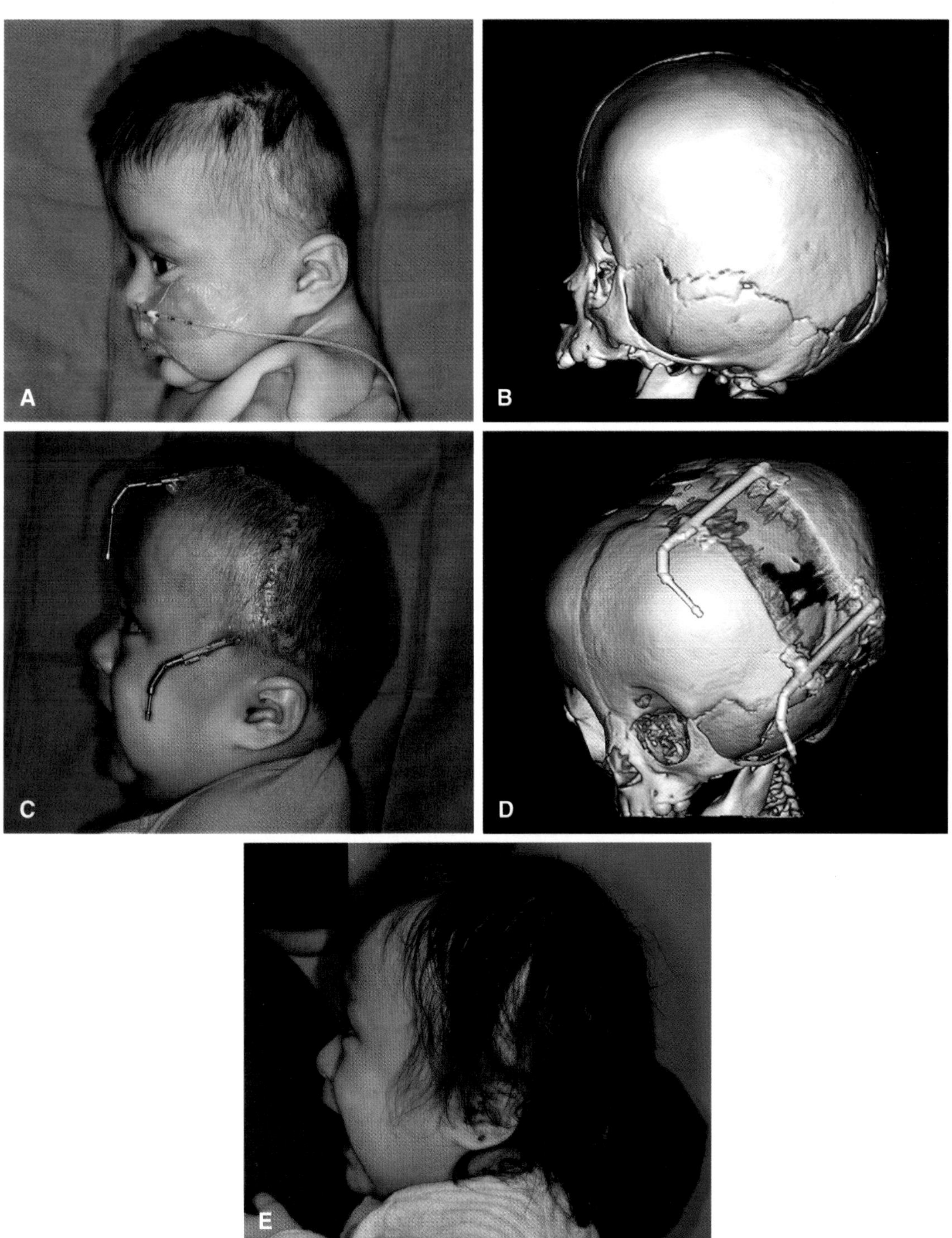

FIGURE 30.10. This patient demonstrates the application of posterior cranial vault distraction for correction of brachycephaly because of bilateral coronal synostosis. Note that internal hardware was used, as is the norm for these cases, with three distractors placed to stabilize the distracted segment against rotation. **A, B.** Pre-operative clinical and radiographic appearance prior to distractor placement. **C.** Patient appearance at 10 days of distraction at 1 mm per day. **D.** Radiographic results of distraction after 40 mm of distraction. **E.** Patient appearance at 6 months follow up after distractor hardware removal.

and surgeon experience. Accordingly, although there is evidence that surgeon experience is associated with lower complication rates, complication rates vary widely.

Infectious complications include infection of the hardware, but the more common finding is localized cellulitis at the pin or activator arm sites, which may be due to poor hygiene. This can often be treated medically and with improved pin site care. With internal hardware, breakage can occur, leading to premature distraction termination or repeat surgery for distractor replacement. With external hardware, distractors can be replaced without requiring repeat surgical procedures. Inappropriate distraction vectors will lead to poor occlusal outcomes and asymmetry. Cranial distraction has its own unique complications with dural injury or CSF leaks.

Some of the complications of distractions are less avoidable, such as decreased growth of the distracted bones or loss of dentition at the site of the osteotomy in cases of mandible distraction. These, as well as some mild relapse in the year after distraction is complete, appear to be sequelae of the techniques themselves.

REFERENCES

1. Grabb WC. The first and second branchial arch syndrome. *Plast Reconstr Surg.* 1965;36(5):485.
2. Poswillo D. The aetiology and pathogenesis of craniofacial deformity. *Development.* 1988;103(suppl):207.
3. Cohen MM, Rollnick BR, Kaye CI. Oculoauriculovertebral spectrum: an updated critique. *Cleft Palate J.* 1989;26(4):276.
4. Poswillo D. The pathogenesis of the first and second branchial arch syndrome. *Oral Surg Oral Med Oral Pathol.* 1973;35(3):302.
5. Sadler TW, Rasmussen SA. Examining the evidence for vascular pathogenesis of selected birth defects. *Am J Med Genet A.* 2010;152A(10):2426-2436.
6. Johnston MC, Bronsky PT. Prenatal craniofacial development: new insights on normal and abnormal mechanisms. *Crit Rev Oral Biol Med.* 1995;6(4):368-422.
7. Luquetti DV, Heike CL, Hing AV, et al. Microtia: epidemiology and genetics. *Am J Med Genet A.* 2012;158A(1):124-139.
8. Rollnick BR, Kaye CI. Hemifacial microsomia and variants: pedigree data. *Am J Med Genet.* 1983;15(2):233-253.
9. Heike C, Luquetti D, Hing A. Craniofacial microsomia overview. In: Adam MP, Ardinger HH, Pagon RA, et al, eds. *GeneReviews® [Internet].* Seattle, WA: University of Washington. March 19, 2009; Updated October 9, 2014.
10. Kaye CI, Martin AO, Rollnick BR, et al. Oculoauriculovertebral anomaly: segregation analysis. *Am J Med Genet.* 1992;43(6):913-917.
11. Rollnick BR, Kaye CI, Nagatoshi K, et al. Oculoauriculovertebral dysplasia and variants: phenotypic characteristics of 294 patients. *Am J Med Genet.* 1987;26(2):361.
12. Converse JM, Wood-Smith D, McCarthy JG, et al. Bilateral facial microsomia. Diagnosis, classification, treatment. *Plast Reconstr Surg.* 1974;54(4):413.
13. Vento AR, Labrie RA, Mulliken JB. The O.M.E.N.S. classification of hemifacial microsomia. *Cleft Palate Craniofac J.* 1991;28(1):68.
14. Tuin AJ, Tahiri Y, Paine KM, et al. Clarifying the relationships among the different features of the OMENS+ classification in craniofacial microsomia. *Plast Reconstr Surg.* 2015;135(1):149e.
This article delineated the development and criteria for the most widely used classification system at this time.
15. Caron CJJM, Pluijmers BI, Wolvius EB, et al. Craniofacial and extracraniofacial anomalies in craniofacial microsomia: a multicenter study of 755 patients. *J Craniomaxillofac Surg.* 2017;45(8):1302.
16. Chen X, Zin AM, Lin L, et al. Three-dimensional analysis of cranial base morphology in patients with hemifacial microsomia. *J Craniomaxillofac Surg.* 2018;46(2):362.
17. Schaal SC, Ruff C, Pluijmers BI, et al. Characterizing the skull base in craniofacial microsomia using principal component analysis. *Int J Oral Maxillofac Surg.* 2017;46(12):1656.
18. Renkema RW, Caron CJJM, Wolvius EB, et al. Central nervous system anomalies in craniofacial microsomia: a systematic review. *Int J Oral Maxillofac Surg.* 2018;47(1):27.
19. Marsh JL, Baca D, Vannier MW. Facial musculoskeletal asymmetry in hemifacial microsomia. *Cleft Palate J.* 1989;26(4):292.
20. Suzuki N, Miyazaki A, Igarashi T, et al. Relationship between mandibular ramus height and masticatory muscle function in patients with unilateral hemifacial microsomia. *Cleft Palate Craniofac J.* 2017;54(1):43.
21. Zim DS, Lee DJ, Rubinstein DB, Senders DC. Prevalence of renal and cervical vertebral anomalies in patients with isolated microtia and/or aural atresia. *Cleft Palate Craniofac J.* 2017;54(6):664-667.
22. Keogh IJ, Troulis MJ, Monroy AA, et al. Isolated microtia as a marker for unsuspected hemifacial microsomia. *Arch Otolaryngol Head Neck Surg.* 2007;133(10):997-1001.
23. Rahbar R, Robson CD, Mulliken JB, et al. Craniofacial, temporal bone, and audiologic abnormalities in the spectrum of hemifacial microsomia. *Arch Otolaryngol Head Neck Surg.* 2001;127(3):265.
24. Horgan JE, Padwa BL, Labrie RA, Mulliken JB. OMENS-Plus: analysis of craniofacial and extracraniofacial anomalies in hemifacial microsomia. *Cleft Palate Craniofac J.* 1995;32(5):405.
Horgan et al. studied the relationships between varied manifestations of CFM that may be treated by the craniofacial surgeon and the multiple other developmental anomalies that may be found in these patients.
25. Meurman Y. Congenital microtia and meatal atresia; observations and aspects of treatment. *AMA Arch Otolaryngol.* 1957;66(4):443-463.
26. Pruzansky S. Not all dwarfed mandibles are alike. *Birth Defects.* 1969;4:120.
27. Kaban LB, Moses MH, Mulliken JB. Surgical correction of hemifacial microsomia in the growing child. *Plast Reconstr Surg.* 1988;82(1):9.
Landmark article modifying the original Pruzansky classification to produce what is currently used to stratify hypoplastic mandibles.
28. Birgfeld CB, Luquetti DV, Gougoutas AJ, et al. A phenotypic assessment tool for craniofacial microsomia. *Plast Reconstr Surg.* 2011;127(1):313.
29. Patel PK, Novia MV. The surgical tools: the LeFort I, bilateral sagittal split osteotomy of the mandible, and the osseous genioplasty. *Clin Plast Surg.* 2007;34(3):447.
This excellent publication lays out the fundamentals of the surgical techniques that are the foundation of correcting the findings in CFM.
30. Tiwari P, Chin DHL, Cutting CB, et al. The course of the inferior alveolar nerve in craniofacial microsomia: virtual dissection using three-dimensional computed tomography image analysis. *Plast Reconstr Surg.* 2002;109(5):1513.
31. Luquetti DV, Brajcich MR, Stock NM, et al. Healthcare and psychosocial experiences of individuals with craniofacial microsomia: patient and caregivers perspectives. *Int J Pediatr Otorhinolaryngol.* 2018;107:164.
32. Dufton LM, Speltz ML, Kelly JP, et al. Psychosocial outcomes in children with hemifacial microsomia. *J Pediatr Psychol.* 2011;36(7):794.
33. Fearon JA. Discussion: an algorithm for managing syndromic craniosynostosis using posterior vault distraction osteogenesis. *Plast Reconstr Surg.* 2016;137(5):842e.
34. Ilizarov GA. The tension-stress effect on the genesis and growth of tissues. Part I. The influence of stability of fixation and soft-tissue preservation. *Clin Orthop Relat Res.* 1989(238):249.
35. Karp NS, Thorne CH, McCarthy JG, Sissons HA. Bone lengthening in the craniofacial skeleton. *Ann Plast Surg.* 1990;24(3):231.
This is one of multiple publications from this very productive group describing their development of the tools and techniques of craniofacial distraction.
36. Karp NS, McCarthy JG, Schreiber JS, et al. Membranous bone lengthening: a serial histological study. *Ann Plast Surg.* 1992;29(1):2.
37. Rachmiel A, Rozen N, Peled M, Lewinson D. Characterization of midface maxillary membranous bone formation during distraction osteogenesis. *Plast Reconstr Surg.* 2002;109(5):1611-1620.
38. Slack GC, Fan KL, Tabit C, et al. Necessity of latency period in craniofacial distraction: investigations with in vitro microdistractor and clinical outcomes. *J Plast Reconstr Aesthet Surg.* 2015;68(9):1206.
39. Mehrara B, Rowe N, Steinbrech D, et al. Rat mandibular distraction osteogenesis: II. Molecular analysis of transforming growth factor beta-1 and osteocalcin gene expression. *Plast Reconstr Surg.* 1999;103(2):536.
40. Davidson EH, Sultan SM, Butala P, et al. Augmenting neovascularization accelerates distraction osteogenesis. *Plast Reconstr Surg.* 2011;128(2):406.
41. Hindin DI, Muetterties CE, Lee JC, et al. Internal distraction resulted in improved patient-reported outcomes for midface hypoplasia. *J Craniofac Surg.* 2018;29(1):139.
42. Steinberg JP, Brady CM, Waters BR, et al. Mid-term dental and nerve-related complications of infant distraction for robin sequence. *Plast Reconstr Surg.* 2016;138(1):82e-90e.
43. Mofid MM, Manson PN, Robertson BC, et al. Craniofacial distraction osteogenesis: a review of 3278 cases. *Plast Reconstr Surg.* 2001;108(5):1103.
44. Peacock ZS, Salcines A, Troulis MJ, Kaban LB. Long-term effects of distraction osteogenesis of the mandible. *J Oral Maxillofac Surg.* 2018;76(7):1512-1523.
45. Polley JW, Figueroa AA, Charbel FT, et al. Monobloc craniomaxillofacial distraction osteogenesis in a newborn with severe craniofacial synostosis: a preliminary report. *J Craniofac Surg.* 1995;6(5):421.
The authors describe their novel application of distraction principles to the complex monobloc advancement scenario and demonstrate the feasibility of the distraction techniques in these settings.
46. Knackstedt R, Bassiri Gharb B, Papay F, Rampazzo A. Comparison of complication rate between LeFort III and monobloc advancement with or without distraction osteogenesis. *J Craniofac Surg.* 2018;29(1):144.
47. Fearon JA. The Le Fort III osteotomy: to distract or not to distract? *Plast Reconstr Surg.* 2001;107(5):1091.
48. Derderian CA, Wink JD, McGrath JL, et al. Volumetric changes in cranial vault expansion: comparison of fronto-orbital advancement and posterior cranial vault distraction osteogenesis. *Plast Reconstr Surg.* 2015;135(6):1665.
This important study showed that posterior cranial vault distraction resulted in greater intracranial volume gain compared with front-orbital advancement, supporting the growing use of distraction techniques for cranial vault remodeling.
49. Taylor JA, Derderian CA, Bartlett SP, et al. Perioperative morbidity in posterior cranial vault expansion: distraction osteogenesis versus conventional osteotomy. *Plast Reconstr Surg.* 2012;129(4):674e.

QUESTIONS

1. **A new patient shown in the photograph is referred to your clinic by the pediatrician for facial asymmetry. You tentatively diagnose the patient with CFM and assign which of the following grades?**
   a. 1
   b. 2a
   c. 2b
   d. 3
   e. 4
   f. None of the above

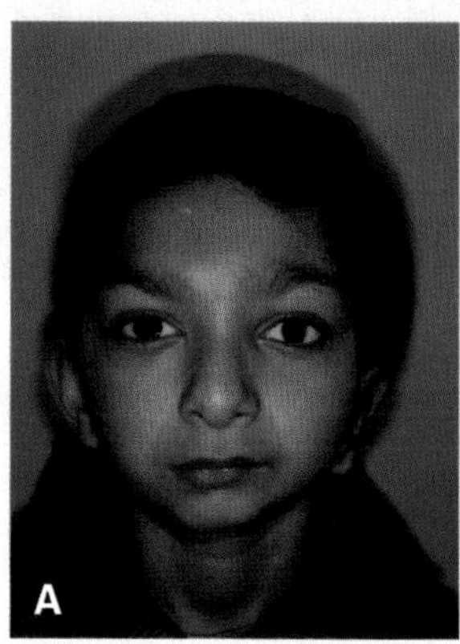

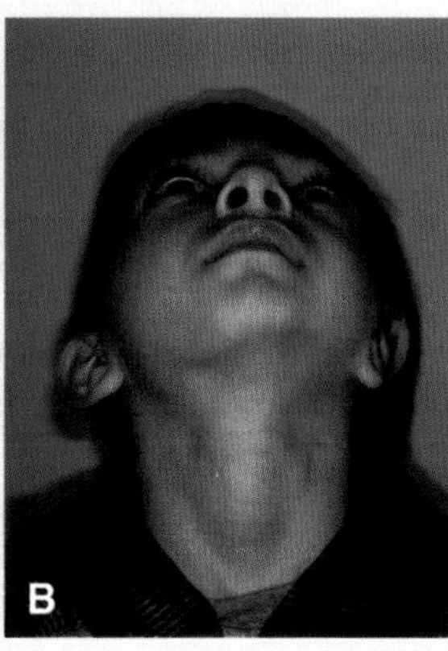

2. **During the initial evaluation of a new patient suspected of having CFM, which of the following testing or imaging modalities are recommended?**

   I. Echocardiogram
   II. Renal ultrasound
   III. Cervical spine X-rays
   IV. Skeletal survey

   a. I only
   b. I and II
   c. I, II, and III
   d. All four are recommended

3. **Which of these answers correctly associates a category of mandible hypoplasia seen in the setting of a patient with CFM, with the correct treatment strategy?**
   a. Type III, treat at 2 years of age with a costochondral graft to definitively reconstruct the TMJ
   b. Type I, treat at 5 to 7 years of age with unilateral sagittal split osteotomy to improve facial symmetry and contour
   c. Type IIb, treat at 5 to 7 years of age with distraction osteogenesis to create a pseudo-TMJ
   d. Type III, treat at 2 to 3 years of age with a costochondral graft to reconstruct TMJ and free soft-tissue transfer to improve facial contour

4. **Which of the following is true regarding distraction osteogenesis?**
   a. Exposure of the bone that is to be distracted is similar for both internal and external hardware placement, despite different external incision patterns.
   b. A latency period is necessary to prevent overly fast distraction.
   c. Distraction of a hypoplastic mandibular ramus should not affect chin projection or asymmetry; an asymmetric genioplasty is always necessary to correct these.
   d. The optimal rate of distraction is 0.25 mm twice per day or slower in adults.
   e. Distraction osteogenesis has proven efficacy in both long bones of the extremities as well as the flat bones of the skull.

5. **Which of the following is true regarding the treatment of CFM?**
   a. Distraction of the hypoplastic mandible in early childhood mandates maxillary surgery at maturity.
   b. Distraction of the hypoplastic mandible in early childhood resolves any appearance concerns until secondary correction is necessary.
   c. Correctly executed distraction of the hypoplastic mandible will obviate any need for osseous genioplasty at maturity.
   d. Aside from difference in size, the anatomy of the hypoplastic mandible in CFM is otherwise the same.
   e. When a costochondral graft is used for ramus reconstruction, a TMJ prosthesis is not necessary to obtain a functional outcome.

1. **Answer: f.** The morphology and functional status of the TMJ are key to grading and treatment planning in a patient with CFM. Without clear information regarding the status of the TMJ, no definitive grade can be assigned.

2. **Answer: c.** Cardiac, renal, and cervical spine evaluation is recommended for all CFM patients because of the high prevalence of associated anomalies in these systems. There is no evidence that shows any benefit to evaluating the rest of the skeleton aside from the cervical spine.

3. **Answer: c.** Although there are multiple points of view regarding the specific timing of surgical intervention for craniofacial macrosomia, certain guidelines are agreed upon. For type III mandibular hypoplasia, treatment should be considered at 4 years of age and they will likely need revision procedures after they reach skeletal maturity. Type I mandible hypoplasia is better addressed with distraction to produce a lower relapse rate and may also require revision in adulthood. Type IIb may be treated with either distraction and creating of a pseudo-TMJ or a costochondral graft to create a neo-TMJ. However, type III hypoplasia is not amenable to treatments solely with distraction and requires bone graft to fabricate an acceptable neomandible and TMJ. Moreover, free soft-tissue transfer for facial contour would likely be more appropriately performed in a delayed fashion, 6 to 8 months after the bony skeleton reconstruction is in place.

4. **Answer: e.** Internal and external hardware requires the same osteotomy, but internal hardware requires much greater periosteal stripping and bony dissection to gain access for securing the hardware footplates. A latency period is often skipped in very young patients and has been shown to not significantly alter the final bony generate. Distraction of a mandibular ramus will lead to autorotation of the mandible on that side, moving the chin toward the contralateral side and increasing its projection. The most widely used rate of distraction is 0.5 mm twice per day in adults, with higher rates possible in infants. Distraction osteogenesis has been shown to be an effective technique in both the extremities (as originally described by Ilizarov) as well as in the bones of the craniofacial skeleton.

5. **Answer: e.** Distraction of the hypoplastic mandible in early childhood, coupled with orthodontia, may often obviate the need for maxillary surgery maturity. Hypothetically, this is due to allowing the maxilla to resume its normal downward growth on the affected side once the obstruction presented by the mandible is addressed. Although addressing the mandible in early childhood improved patients' appearance as they grow, there is no guarantee the correction will be complete. Moreover, other associated anomalies (macrostomia, microtia) may continue to cause psychosocial distress until they are addressed as well. If the size of the affected hemimandible is corrected, the shape will likely still be asymmetric, with some deviation of the chin, and thus an osseous genioplasty is often needed at maturity to obtain the best possible result. The anatomy of the hypoplastic mandible in CFM is different both in terms of altered shape, hypoplasia or lack of condylar or coronoid processes, as well as displacement of the inferior alveolar foramen superiorly and the canal buccally.

CHAPTER 31 Orthognathic Surgery

Reza Jarrahy and Thomas D. Willson

KEY POINTS

- Orthognathic surgery repositions the maxilla, mandible, or both to correct improper occlusal relationships and improve facial aesthetics. Patients with clefts and syndromic dentofacial deformities frequently require orthognathic surgery. Members of the general population without clefts or congenital facial syndromes, however, may also require orthognathic correction.
- Virtual surgical planning (VSP) has largely supplanted traditional dental impression/cast stone model surgery in developing and executing a treatment plan for orthognathic surgery. Close collaboration between the orthodontist and surgeon remains critical to successful outcomes.
- Skeletal movements significantly impact the position of overlying soft tissues and the overall appearance of the patient. Movements that expand the face can smooth rhytids and provide support to otherwise ptotic tissues, resulting in a rejuvenated appearance. In contrast, contraction of the facial skeleton may decrease soft tissue support and contribute to undesirable aesthetic results.
- Following the completion of skeletal movements and rigid fixation of the mobilized jaw segments, the surgeon must meticulously confirm the final occlusion to ensure it specifically corresponds to the preoperative plan. Minor misalignments can usually be corrected with postsurgical orthodontics, but lack of attention to detail can result in persistent malocclusion that may require secondary surgical correction.

Orthognathic surgery is a discipline that focuses on surgical manipulation of the maxilla and mandible to optimize the occlusal relationship between the upper and lower jaws. The primary goal of most orthognathic procedures is to restore function. Malocclusion can result in a variety of functional deficits of varying severity. These include the development of dental pathology, temporomandibular joint (TMJ) dysfunction, speech abnormalities, airway obstruction, and problems with deglutition. Surgical restoration of normal maxillomandibular relationships can successfully correct aberrancies in all of these areas.

Although the functional impact of jaw surgery is usually the driving force behind orthognathic procedures, we cannot underestimate the profound effect that surgical movements of the jaws have on facial aesthetics. Normal dentofacial skeletal relationships help define human standards of beauty and balance. All surgical planning for orthognathic procedures must therefore consider the aesthetic implications of specific maneuvers. Similarly, the aesthetic changes that are predictably associated with certain techniques must be considered when developing the surgical plan.

The most common indication for orthognathic surgery is malocclusion associated with a history of cleft lip and palate. Up to 25% of cleft lip and palate patients will require orthognathic surgery by the time they complete adolescence. Similarly, patients with syndromic craniofacial differences, including the various craniofacial dysostoses, represent another group of patients where the need for orthognathic surgery is predictably higher than that seen in the general population, where the incidence of jaw surgery rests at around 2.5%.

Orthognathic surgery is a truly multidisciplinary endeavor. Our best and most stable surgical outcomes are achieved when surgeon and orthodontist work closely with their patients to develop a unique plan that is best suited to each individual.

DENTAL ANATOMY AND JAW DEVELOPMENT

A comprehensive review of dental anatomy and physiology is beyond the scope of this chapter, but a working knowledge of dental development is important for all surgeons who engage in orthognathic procedures.

Dental development begins in utero. The primary, or deciduous, teeth form during the sixth to eighth weeks of gestation, and permanent teeth begin development around the 20th week. In an individual with no dental anomalies, there are a total of twenty deciduous teeth: two central and two lateral incisors, two canines (or cuspids), and four molars in each of the maxillary and mandibular dental arches. Each quadrant contains one central incisor, one lateral incisor, one cuspid, and two molars. By comparison, an adult with complete dentition has thirty-two teeth. The most mesial (anterior) teeth are the central incisors. These are flanked by the lateral incisors. Distal (posterior) to the lateral incisors are the canine teeth. They have a single cusp and typically contain a single root. Distal to the canine teeth are the two bicuspids, or premolars, each with two cusps and a single root (except the first maxillary premolar, which has two roots). Distal to the premolars are three molars, which have four or five cusps and two or three roots each.

Shedding of the deciduous teeth begins at around age six with the appearance of the first mandibular molar. The period when an individual has both deciduous and permanent dentition in place is called the period of *mixed dentition*. This period usually lasts until age 12 years, at which time the deciduous teeth have all typically been lost. The third molars are the last teeth to erupt, late in the second decade of life.

Jaw growth generally proceeds in a cranial to caudal pattern and is mediated by multiple factors, including dental eruption and movement. The maxilla typically reaches its adult size in the mid-teenage years. Growth of the mandible typically continues for several years after the maxillary growth has ceased, as the mandible is usually the last of the bones of the craniofacial skeleton to cease its growth.

TERMINOLOGY

In the care of patients requiring orthognathic surgery, clear communication between treating specialists, including pediatric and adult dentists, orthodontists, prosthodontists, and orthognathic surgeons, is critical to making an accurate diagnosis and creating an effective treatment plan. Common knowledge of relevant terminology is a requisite to effective communication between treating specialists. Some of the more common terms used to discuss dental and oral anatomy are discussed below.

Because the dental arches are U-shaped, terms such as anterior and posterior are not always applicable in describing the position of dental structures, nor to their movements in orthodontic or orthognathic interventions. Instead, the terms *mesial*, meaning toward the midline sagittal plane along the dental arch, and *distal*, meaning away from the midline along the dental arch, are used to describe dental positions.

Occlusion is most commonly described using a classification proposed by Edward Angle in the late 19th century. The nomenclature is based on the relationship between the mesiobuccal cusp of the maxillary first molar and the buccal groove of the mandibular first molar. In an Angle class I malocclusion, the mesiobuccal cusp of first maxillary molar aligns with the buccal groove of the mandibular first molar. In an Angle class II malocclusion, the mesiobuccal cusp of the maxillary first molar is located *mesial* to the buccal groove of the mandibular first molar. Patients with class II malocclusion have a *retrognathic* appearance, where the mandible appears posteriorly positioned relative to the maxilla. By comparison, in an Angle class III malocclusion, the mesiobuccal cusp of the maxillary first molar is located *distal* to the buccal groove of the mandibular first molar, giving the patient a relatively *prognathic* appearance.

Overbite, in dental terms, refers to the vertical overlap between the maxillary and mandibular incisors. It is usually reported either as a percentage of the tooth covered or in millimeters. By comparison, *overjet* refers to the space in millimeters between the labial surfaces of the most distal incisor in each arch. A normal overjet is 2 to 4 mm. When the mandibular incisor is more prominent (e.g., in a prognathic patient with Angle class III malocclusion), the overjet is referred to as negative.

Retrognathia and *prognathia* can refer to the position of either jaw, but in common usage, these terms refer to the position of the mandible relative to the maxilla and help describe the appearance of an individual's facial profile. In *retrognathia*, the mandible appears to be posterior relative to the maxilla. In the *prognathic patient*, the mandible appears to be positioned anterior to the maxilla. Note that with either a retrognathic or prognathic appearance, both of the jaws may actually be malpositioned; the anatomically correct position of the maxilla and mandible can be specifically determined by cephalometric analysis.

CEPHALOMETRICS

Cephalometry refers to the study and measurement of the bones of the head and the face. In the setting of orthognathic surgery, cephalometry specifically focuses on measuring the spatial relationships of the maxilla and mandible to each other, to the upper face, and to the cranial base. Cephalometric analysis has, and continues to be, foundational in making accurate diagnoses and generating appropriate surgical plans for patients presenting with malocclusion.[1,2]

Historically, cephalometric analysis has been performed manually, using overlay acetate tracings of lateral cephalograms upon which markings of skeletal and soft tissue landmarks are placed. Once these landmarks are identified, numerous types of formal analyses can be performed that quantify a myriad of facial planes and angles to determine the contribution of each jaw to the patient's deformity. The orthodontist and surgeon can move the tracings to position the maxilla, mandible, and genioplasty segment into optimal positions. The sella-nasion-subspinale (SNA) and sella-nasion-supramentale (SNB) angles are the two most critical measurements in determining the relative positions of the maxilla and mandible and their relationships to the cranial base. SNA and SNB angles that are less than normal indicate that the maxilla or mandible, respectively, is positioned more posteriorly than normal relative to the cranial base; angles that are greater than the norm indicate relative anterior positions.

The cephalometric measurements and movements are then used to guide *model surgery*, or manipulation of dental models that are based on impressions taken from the patient's upper and lower dental arches, as further described below. The model surgery process yields acrylic splints that capture the new spatial relationship between the jaws. These splints are used in the operating room, where the surgeon replicates the same movements made in the dental laboratory to achieve the same occlusion obtained in the model surgery planning process.

In recent years, however, this manual process has been supplanted by computer-based software systems that can rapidly and accurately perform an endless number of cephalometric analyses using the same anatomic landmarks (**Figure 31.1**). Surgeons are increasingly turning to these digital platforms to render accurate diagnoses and plan optimal surgical movements via VSP, which is discussed in greater detail below.

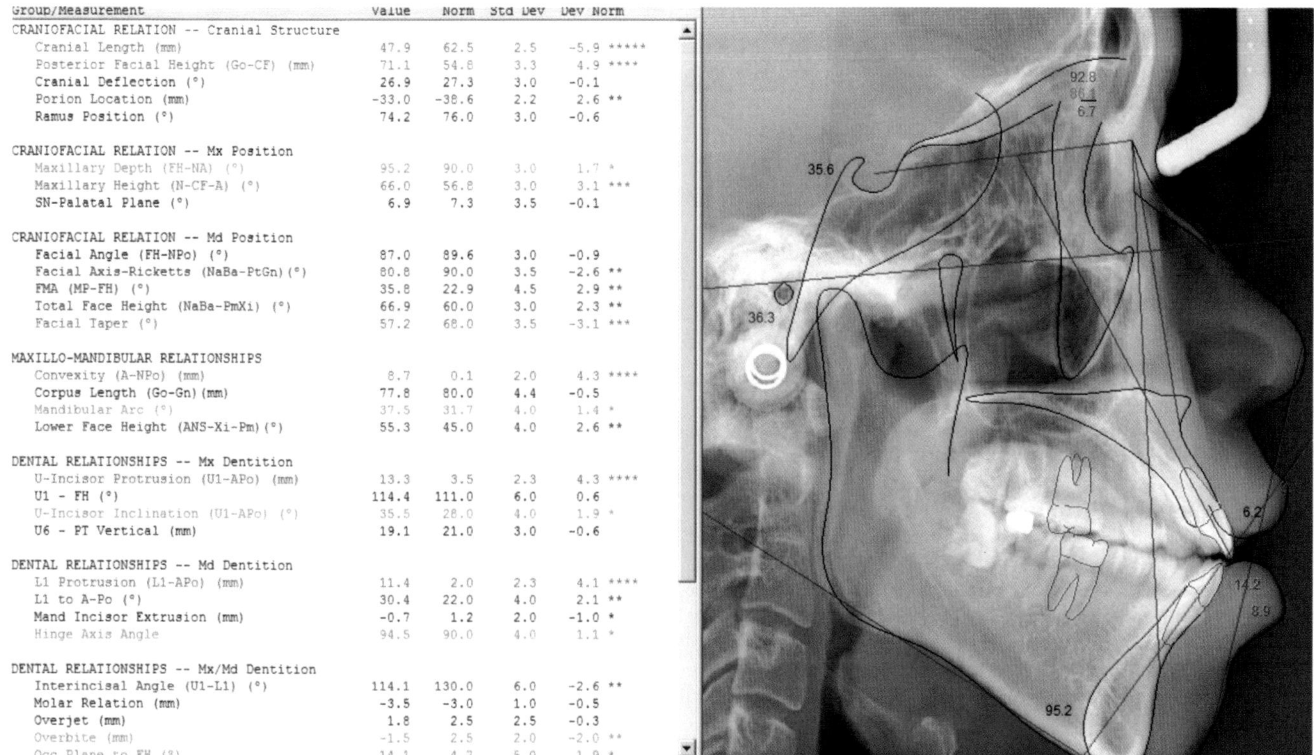

Group/Measurement	Value	Norm	Std Dev	Dev Norm
CRANIOFACIAL RELATION -- Cranial Structure				
Cranial Length (mm)	47.9	62.5	2.5	-5.9 *****
Posterior Facial Height (Go-CF) (mm)	71.1	54.8	3.3	4.9 ****
Cranial Deflection (°)	26.9	27.3	3.0	-0.1
Porion Location (mm)	-33.0	-38.6	2.2	2.6 **
Ramus Position (°)	74.2	76.0	3.0	-0.6
CRANIOFACIAL RELATION -- Mx Position				
Maxillary Depth (FH-NA) (°)	95.2	90.0	3.0	1.7 *
Maxillary Height (N-CF-A) (°)	66.0	56.8	3.0	3.1 ***
SN-Palatal Plane (°)	6.9	7.3	3.5	-0.1
CRANIOFACIAL RELATION -- Md Position				
Facial Angle (FH-NPo) (°)	87.0	89.6	3.0	-0.9
Facial Axis-Ricketts (NaBa-PtGn) (°)	80.8	90.0	3.5	-2.6 **
FMA (MP-FH) (°)	35.8	22.9	4.5	2.9 **
Total Face Height (NaBa-PmXi) (°)	66.9	60.0	3.0	2.3 **
Facial Taper (°)	57.2	68.0	3.5	-3.1 ***
MAXILLO-MANDIBULAR RELATIONSHIPS				
Convexity (A-NPo) (mm)	8.7	0.1	2.0	4.3 ****
Corpus Length (Go-Gn) (mm)	77.8	80.0	4.4	-0.5
Mandibular Arc (°)	37.5	31.7	4.0	1.4 *
Lower Face Height (ANS-Xi-Pm) (°)	55.3	45.0	4.0	2.6 **
DENTAL RELATIONSHIPS -- Mx Dentition				
U-Incisor Protrusion (U1-APo) (mm)	13.3	3.5	2.3	4.3 ****
U1 - FH (°)	114.4	111.0	6.0	0.6
U-Incisor Inclination (U1-APo) (°)	35.5	28.0	4.0	1.9 *
U6 - PT Vertical (mm)	19.1	21.0	3.0	-0.6
DENTAL RELATIONSHIPS -- Md Dentition				
L1 Protrusion (L1-APo) (mm)	11.4	2.0	2.3	4.1 ****
L1 to A-Po (°)	30.4	22.0	4.0	2.1 **
Mand Incisor Extrusion (mm)	-0.7	1.2	2.0	-1.0 *
Hinge Axis Angle	94.5	90.0	4.0	1.1 *
DENTAL RELATIONSHIPS -- Mx/Md Dentition				
Interincisal Angle (U1-L1) (°)	114.1	130.0	6.0	-2.6 **
Molar Relation (mm)	-3.5	-3.0	1.0	-0.5
Overjet (mm)	1.8	2.5	2.5	-0.3
Overbite (mm)	-1.5	2.5	2.0	-2.0 **
Occ Plane to FH (°)	14.1	4.7	5.0	1.9 *

FIGURE 31.1. Digital cephalometric analysis. Cephalometric landmarks can be labeled on a digital lateral cephalogram. Multiple detailed analyses of the positions of the upper and lower jaws and the teeth can be instantaneously calculated for use in surgical planning.

PATIENT EVALUATION

Cephalometric analysis is critical to making an accurate diagnosis, counseling the patient, and planning for the most appropriate surgical intervention. However, a thorough history and detailed physical examination are prerequisites to successful surgical outcomes.

History

A thorough medical history is important in any surgical patient. General questions should include inquiry into any underlying medical conditions that may have a negative impact upon surgery, such as diabetes, connective tissue disease, or autoimmune problems. Medications including steroids and anticoagulants that may affect wound healing or bleeding and clotting should be noted and managed perioperatively as appropriate. Any history of adverse reaction to anesthesia should be thoroughly investigated, as should any prior or current manifestation of cardiac disease, venous thromboembolic disease, or other disease process that might contribute to the development of potentially life-threatening complications.

A specific history related to dental and jaw surgery should also be elicited. Previous surgical interventions, such as mandibular or maxillary distraction, surgically assisted rapid palatal expansion (SARPE), or fracture repair, can significantly impact treatment planning. Patients should be questioned about a history of (TMJ) symptoms such as pain, clicking, popping, and trismus. When jaw asymmetries are noted on physical examination, potential etiologies should be investigated, including syndromic, neoplastic, or traumatic causes of unilateral mandibular hypoplasia or hyperplasia.

The surgeon should have an open discussion with the patient regarding his or her expectations for surgical outcomes. Orthognathic surgery is a major undertaking, frequently preceded by months of orthodontic preparation followed by additional postoperative treatment. The surgery itself results in weeks of swelling and can dramatically alter a patient's appearance. The surgeon should describe the perioperative process in detail, including specific goals of surgery and the potential risks that are inherent to a surgical procedure of such magnitude.

Physical Examination

A general physical examination should be performed on every patient before surgery. Specific evaluation for patients scheduled to undergo orthognathic surgery begins with an objective evaluation of the face, including analysis of the standard horizontal thirds and vertical fifths of the face. This assessment can help identify clinical entities such as vertical maxillary excess (VME) or deficiency or transverse deficiencies because of a narrow or constricted palate. The width of the alar bases should be evaluated, as maxillary advancement may widen the base of the nose, potentially resulting in an unexpected and unappreciated alteration in the nasal appearance if this is not addressed during the surgical procedure. The malar eminence, inferior orbital rim, and pyriform aperture projections are evaluated. Deficiencies in these areas are a relative indication for maxillary advancement. Soft tissue coverage and contours of the midface, lower face, and neck are noted. Mentalis strain and lip incompetence should be noted if present, as these are additional signs of vertical maxillary excess, as is excessive gingival show when smiling (a *gummy smile*). The dental midlines of the maxilla and mandible should be noted and any deviation from the facial midline documented. Any other asymmetries of the maxilla or mandible, particularly those associated with facial clefting or occlusal cant, should be documented.

Oral evaluation should focus on hygiene and periodontal health. Patients must demonstrate good hygiene before and during orthodontic preparation to proceed with surgery. Damaged, loose, or missing teeth should be noted, as should any retained deciduous teeth. If present, the third molars should be extracted several months before surgery to facilitate safe osteotomies at the time of surgery.

Evaluation of the patient's profile should note the projection of the forehead, malar eminences, nose, maxilla, mandible, and chin. An experienced orthognathic surgeon can frequently determine which jaw or jaws are responsible for the patient's dentofacial deformity on profile view before confirming the diagnosis with cephalometric analysis. Careful evaluation of the nose and its spatial relation to the maxilla is critical, as maxillary movements can potentially change the position of the nose and the nasolabial angle. Similarly, the predicted postoperative position of the chin should factor into the presurgical discussion and guide any discussion of the potential need for genioplasty.

Common Diagnoses

Prognathism

Prognathism technically refers to prominence of either jaw but is generally used to indicate prominence of the mandible relative to the maxilla. Mandibular prognathism is most often associated with class III malocclusion. On profile, the patient often demonstrates a *strong* chin and a long jaw line. Cephalometric analysis will typically reveal posterior positioning of the maxilla relative to the cranial base (small SNA), anterior positioning of the mandible compared with the cranial base (large SNB), or both. Treatments may include maxillary advancement, mandibular setback, or a combination of both procedures (**Figure 31.2A–C**).

Retrognathism

Retrognathism refers to a relative prominence of the maxilla compared with the mandible. Cephalometry usually shows anterior positioning of the maxilla relative to the cranial base (large SNA), posterior positioning of the mandible relative to the cranial base (small SNB), or a combination of both. Most commonly, the retrognathic patient presents with a class II malocclusion because of a small mandible; in these cases, mandibular advancement is the procedure of choice to correct the condition (**Figure 31.2D–F**).

Vertical Maxillary Excess

VME is also known as long face syndrome. Patients with VME have facies that appear long with excessive gingival show in repose and with smiling. Mentalis strain and lip incompetence are also frequently seen. Surgical correction involves maxillary impaction with cephalad repositioning of the maxilla to shorten the midface. The mandible rotates counterclockwise in a compensatory movement. Resultant changes in chin position should be noted in the preoperative planning phase to determine whether simultaneous genioplasty is indicated.[3]

Vertical Maxillary Deficiency

In vertical maxillary deficiency, the patient's lower face appears short, with little or no incisor show on repose and minimal show with smiling. Appropriate surgical treatment includes downfracture and caudal repositioning of the maxilla to lengthen the face.[4] Bone grafting to the resultant maxillary gap ensures a stable result.[5] The mandible compensates with a clockwise rotation, and the chin moves inferiorly and posteriorly. Again, preoperative planning should include an assessment of the potential need for genioplasty.

Maxillary Constriction

Maxillary constriction refers to a deficiency in the transverse dimension of the maxilla. It is commonly seen in patients with cleft palate. This results in a posterior crossbite on one or both sides of the maxilla. The condition can be treated, at least in part, with orthodontic palatal expansion. If orthodontic expansion fails, the palate can be transversely expanded surgically.

PRESURGICAL PLANNING

In addition to taking a history, performing a physical examination, and completing a cephalometric analysis, several additional steps must be taken before performing orthognathic surgery. Initial

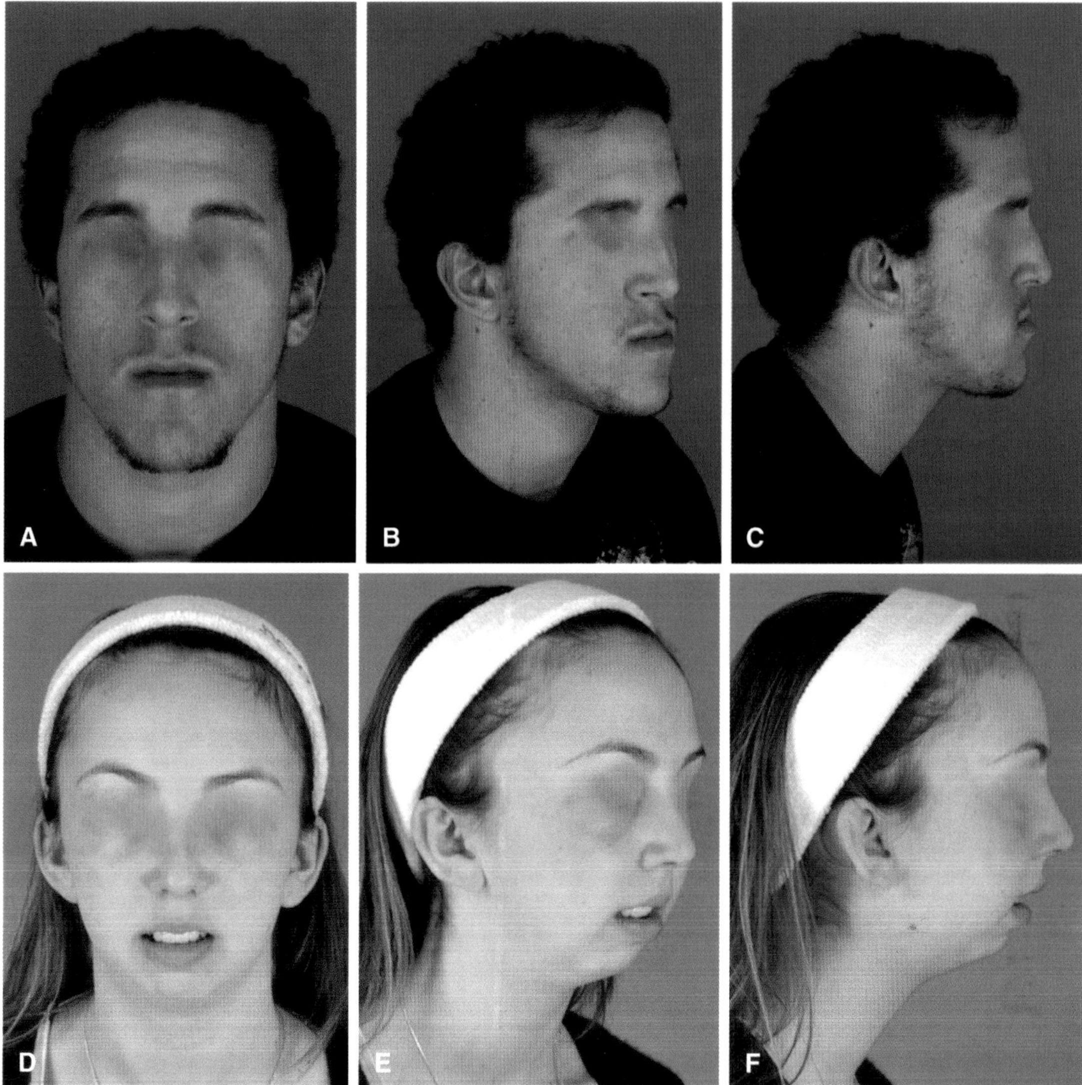

FIGURE 31.2. Relative contributions of maxilla and mandible to retrognathism and prognathism. **A–C.** Frontal, oblique, and lateral views, respectively, of a patient with mandibular prognathism and a class III malocclusion with decreased sella-nasion-subspinale and increased sella-nasion-supramentale. Both jaws are malpositioned. A maxillary advancement and mandibular setback are both indicated to achieve a normal jaw relationship. **D–F.** Frontal, oblique, and lateral views, respectively, of a patient with mandibular retrognathism and a class II malocclusion with decreased sella-nasion-supramentale. A mandibular advancement is an appropriate correction.

preparation for surgery is carried out by an orthodontist, including obtaining dental models, radiographic records, and composite facial and occlusal photos. Based on the cephalometric analysis, the planned surgical movements are then executed on traditional models of the teeth or on three-dimensional (3D) digital renderings. Regardless of the technique used, the process yields splints that index the desired final positions of the jaws following the orthognathic correction. These splints are used in the operating room to confirm that the planned movements are precisely replicated in the surgical procedure.

Planning should not only focus exclusively on correction of abnormal values identified in the cephalometric analysis but also account for the effect of skeletal movements on the overlying soft tissues to optimize the aesthetic outcomes.[6] Movements that reduce the size of the skeleton, such as maxillary impactions and maxillary or mandibular setbacks, can have aging effects on the face. When the soft tissue envelope covers a relatively contracted skeletal framework, deeper creases, more jowling, and an overall aged appearance may result. By contrast, movements that expand the skeleton tend to flatten creases and provide greater support to the soft tissues, contributing to a more youthful appearance[7] (**Figure 31.3**).

As noted above, clockwise or counterclockwise autorotation of the mandible secondary to maxillary movements—and the impact of these movements on chin position—must be considered in the presurgical plan to achieve balanced facial aesthetics along with a functional postoperative occlusion.

Orthodontic Preparation

The goal of preoperative orthodontia is to position the teeth, so that at the end of the surgical procedure, the patient is in a class I malocclusion with optimal dental intercuspation. This requires a considerable degree of skill on the part of the orthodontist, but also clear communication between the orthodontist and the surgeon regarding the planned operation. Orthodontic preparation for a single-jaw movement differs from that for two-jaw surgery; the surgical plan should therefore be clear to all caregivers and the patient from the outset.

In addition to straightening and appropriately spacing the teeth, the orthodontist is charged with reversing any natural dental compensations that the patient develops in association with his or her malocclusion. This includes correcting the aberrant orientation of

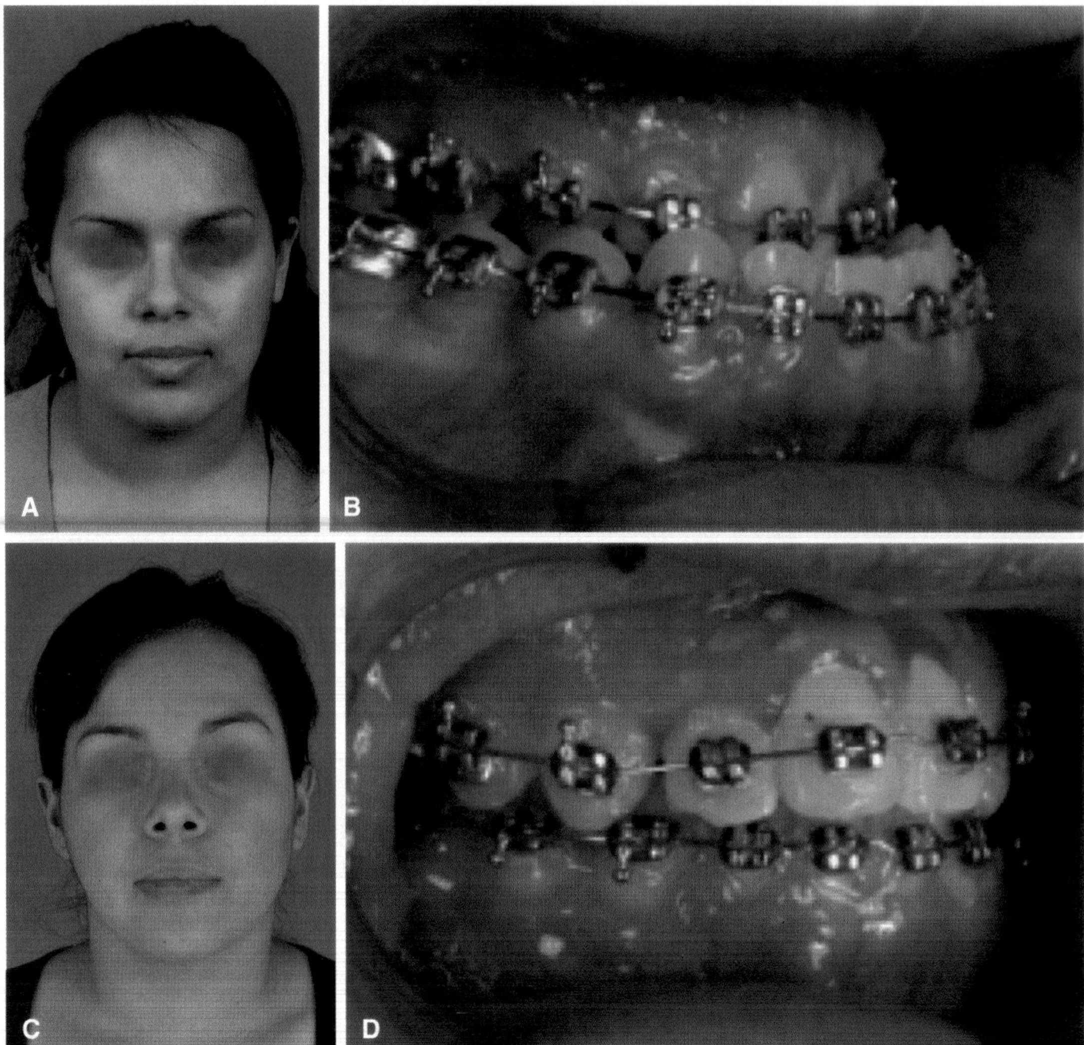

FIGURE 31.3. Impact of skeletal movements on soft tissue support and aesthetics. **A,B.** The impact of a high Le Fort I osteotomy and advancement on soft tissue support and facial aesthetics is demonstrated in this 18-year-old patient who presented with class III malocclusion and prematurely aged appearance characterized by ptotic malar soft tissues, deep nasolabial folds, marionette lines, and upper lip ptosis. **C,D.** Her malocclusion is corrected with maxillary advancement, which also results in a more youthful appearance with improved malar soft tissue support, softening of the perioral skin creases, and improved upper lip projection.

any proclined or retroclined teeth that have become malpositioned in the absence of normal anatomic relationships between the upper and lower dental arches.

Dental Models and Model Surgery

As practitioners of orthognathic surgery increasingly adapt VSP to their perioperative practices, a thorough understanding of the fundamentals of traditional model surgery remains requisite to a true appreciation of the intricacies of jaw surgery and how best to implement VSP platforms in its execution.

Before surgery, the surgeon or the orthodontist will obtain wax-bite registrations and plaster models of the patient's presurgical occlusion. These models can be mounted on an articulator, which mimics the relationship of the maxilla to the cranial base and the relationship of the mandible to the maxilla as it hinges on the articulator's joints. In a planned single-jaw surgery, the jaw that is to be cut and moved during surgery is repositioned on the articulator based on the cephalometric analysis and intended surgical movement. An acrylic splint that captures the new relationship between the maxillary and mandibular models is fabricated and brought to the operating room for use in surgery **(Figure 31.4)**.

In two-jaw surgery, the model of the jaw that is to receive the first movement is repositioned on the articulator, again according to the cephalometric analysis and surgical plan. This temporary relationship between upper and lower jaws is indexed with an *intermediate* splint that is used to guide the position of the first jaw undergoing osteotomy. Once this splint is fabricated, the second jaw to be moved in surgery is repositioned on the articulator to arrive at the appropriate occlusal relationship. A *final* splint is then created based on this occlusion and used to guide the upper and lower jaws into their final desired positions in the operating room while rigid fixation is obtained.

Virtual Surgical Planning

Although traditional model surgery has historically allowed surgeons to achieve excellent results, it is a laborious and time-consuming process. By comparison, the combination of high-resolution maxillofacial CT scanning, 3D printing, and sophisticated software platforms now allows surgeons to engage in a more streamlined but equally accurate approach to cephalometric analysis and presurgical planning that obviates many of the manual components described earlier. As a result, VSP protocols are rapidly replacing more traditional approaches to orthognathic surgery.

VSP begins with the acquisition of a high-resolution CT scan of the face. These radiographic images are imported into specialized

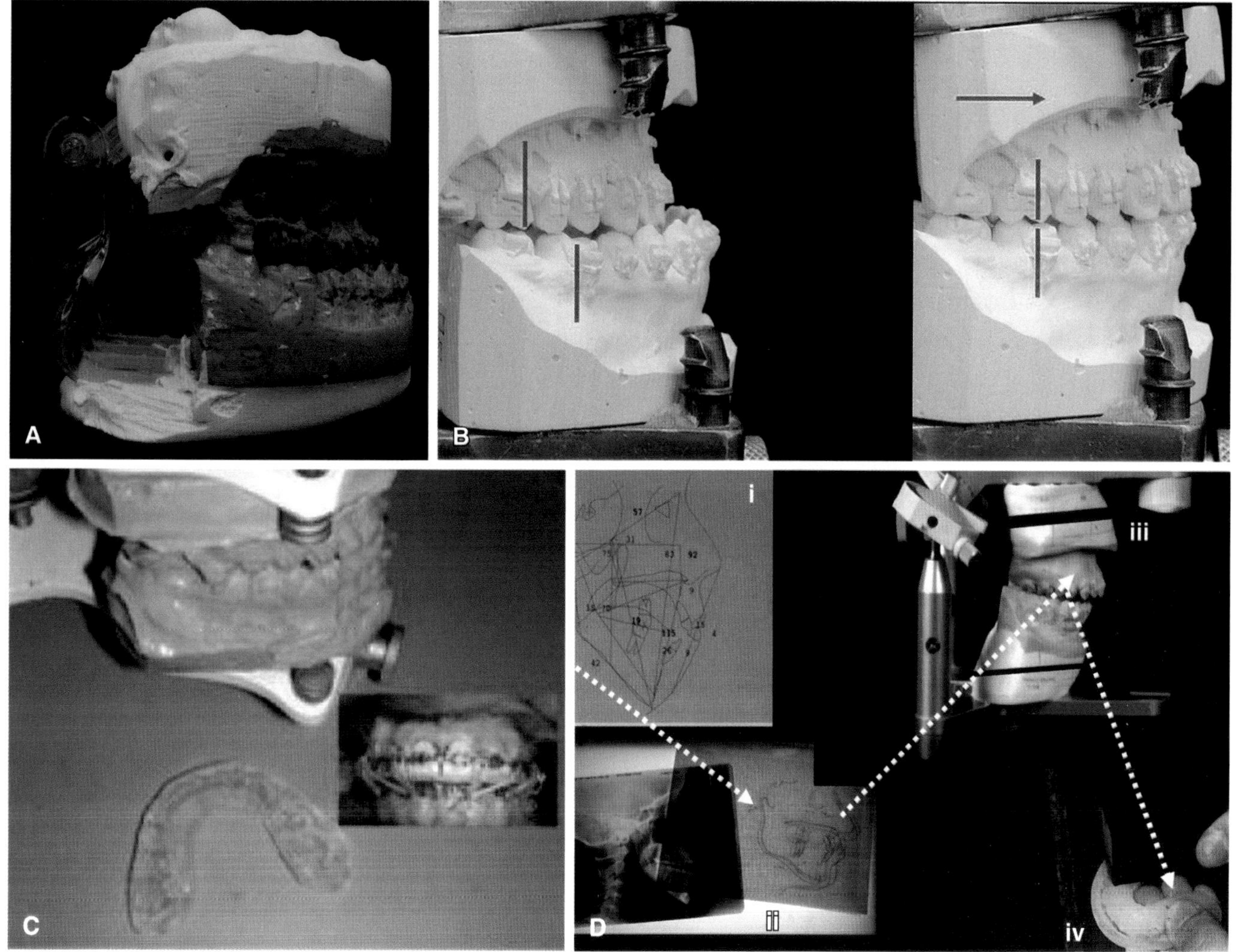

FIGURE 31.4. Model surgery. **A.** An articulator is used to mount maxillary and mandibular dental models in their baseline occlusal relationship (in this case, a class III malocclusion). **B.** The maxillary model is repositioned to achieve a class I relationship. The red arrow indicates the vector of movement, simulating a Le Fort I osteotomy and advancement. **C.** An acrylic splint is fabricated to capture this new occlusal relationship and will be used in the operating room. **D.** These images demonstrate typical steps taken to plan an orthognathic surgery procedure. Preparation begins with cephalometric analysis (i). The arrow indicates the next step in the process: tracings and planned jaw movements (ii). After the jaw movements are planned on paper, they are replicated on the mounted dental models (iii). Model surgery results in splint fabrication to facilitate the actual surgery (iv).

computer-assisted design software, which generates 3D renderings of the craniofacial skeleton. Incorporating digital scans of the patient's dental models into the renderings can increase the level of detail of the 3D images. The surgeon can perform digital osteotomies on these renderings, and the positions of the jaws can be subsequently altered to achieve a desired occlusion (**Figure 31.5**). A 3D printer can then fabricate splints that capture the new occlusal relationship for use in the operating room. VSP software can also generate 3D renderings of how the soft tissues of the face may change as the underlying skeletal components are repositioned, although these renderings are digital projections only; they should not be used to guide specific patient expectations.

Although VSP represents a resource that has transformed the process of planning for orthognathic surgery without any compromise of surgical results, users of this technology must be aware that like any computer program, VSP outputs are only as good as their inputs. Computer-assisted design software allows one to make unrestricted movements on a screen, regardless of whether those movements might be stable or desirable in an actual clinical setting. The surgeon must therefore always rely on his or her experience and fundamental cephalometric and surgical principles to determine the optimal technique for each individual patient.

SURGICAL TECHNIQUES

General Principles

Orthognathic surgery is a true *team sport*. Active and effective communication between the surgeon and multiple other specialists is necessary for a successful surgical outcome. Before surgery, the surgeon must confer with the patient's orthodontist to confirm that the patient has been adequately prepared for surgery. On the day of surgery, the surgeon must confirm with the operating room nursing staff that all necessary equipment is available and in good working order, including powered and manually driven bone-cutting tools, procedure-specific instruments, and rigid fixation hardware. Ongoing communication with the anesthesiologist throughout the surgery is of paramount importance. Elective jaw surgery patients are nasotracheally intubated, preferably with a Ring-Adair-Elwyn (RAE) tube that is secured to prevent unintentional extubation during surgical manipulation of the jaws. Preoperative antibiotics covering oral flora are administered intravenously. Hypotensive anesthesia during osteotomies and maxillary downfracture can help to reduce blood loss.

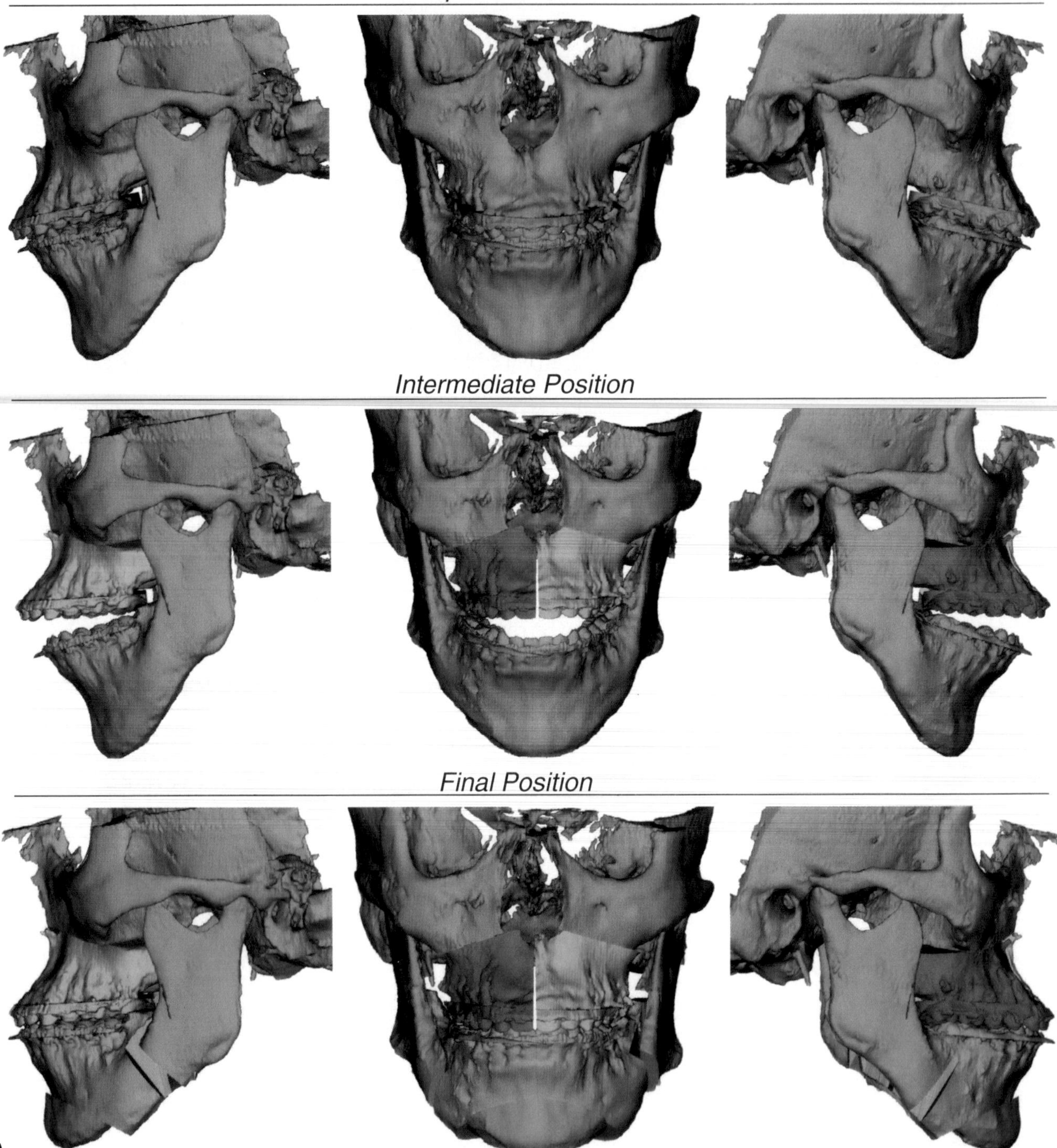

FIGURE 31.5. Virtual surgical planning for orthognathic surgery. **A.** The virtual surgical planning summary for this maxilla-first two-jaw surgery demonstrates the preoperative condition (top), the intermediate position of the jaws (center), and the final occlusion (bottom). In this case, the maxilla was split and expanded transversely to correct a posterior crossbite, impacted to correct for vertical maxillary excess, and advanced. Next a bilateral sagittal split osteotomy was used to rotate the mandible in a counterclockwise direction. A reduction and advancement genioplasty was added to the surgical plan to provide facial balance and optimize aesthetic results. Cephalometric measurements such as sella-nasion-subspinale and sella-nasion-supramentale can easily be incorporated into the planning process **(B)**, as can other data such as facial height measurements before and following planned jaw movements **(C)**.

Preoperative Position

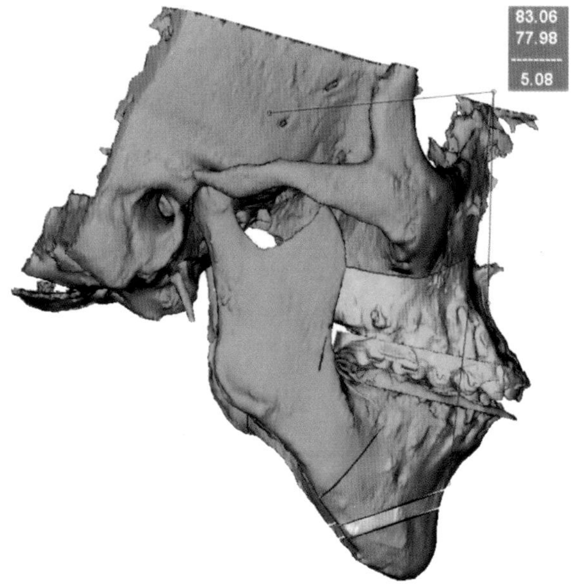

Preoperative Position

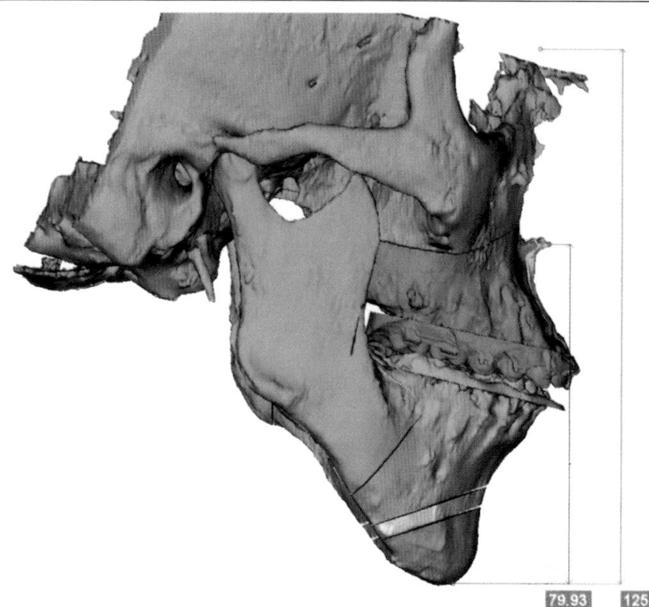

Postoperative Position

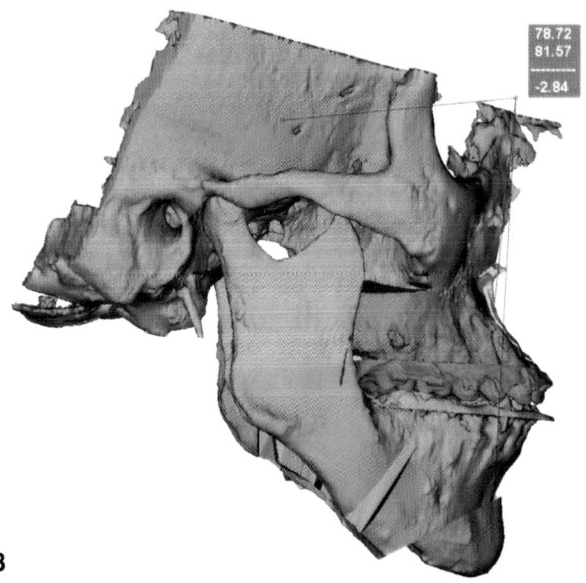

B

Postoperative Position

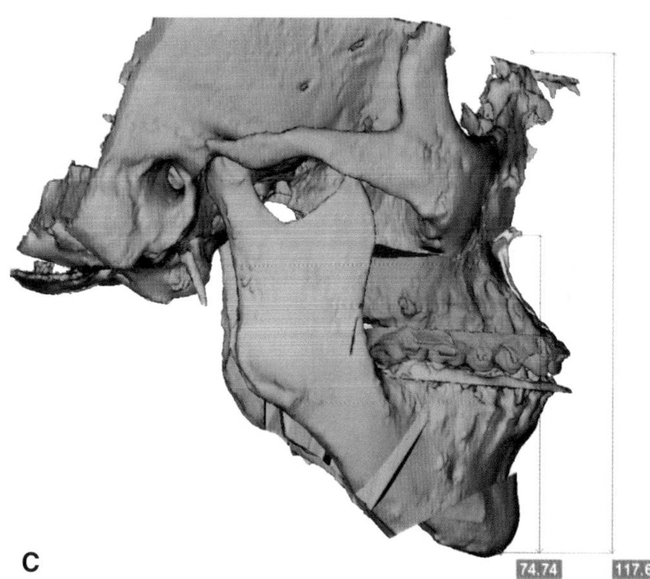

C

FIGURE 31.5. *Continued*

Maxillary Osteotomies

Le Fort I

The Le Fort I osteotomy allows for multivector movement of the maxilla. Anterior-posterior, cranial-caudal, and rotational movements in axial, coronal, and sagittal planes are all possible. This flexibility permits correction of occlusal cants, midline shifts, and overjet.[8]

The medial canthi are marked with ink, and the vertical height of the maxilla between the canthi and the maxillary dental arch is measured with a caliper. These measurements are important when correcting occlusal cants or altering the maxillary height (e.g., in cases of maxillary impaction or lengthening). An upper gingivobuccal sulcus incision is made. The anterior wall of the maxilla is dissected in the subperiosteal plane with careful preservation of the infraorbital nerve. Lateral dissection continues around the lateral maxillary walls to the pterygomaxillary buttresses. Subperiosteal dissection of the floor of the nasal cavity is performed through the pyriform aperture.

When designing the Le Fort osteotomy, the surgeon must note the vertical height of the dental roots to avoid injury to the teeth. In addition, higher osteotomies that incorporate the upper maxilla and even the caudal portion of the zygoma into the Le Fort segment can be designed when more soft tissue support is indicated.

The osteotomies through the medial and lateral buttresses and the anterior maxillary wall are performed with a reciprocating saw or an ultrasonic bone cutter. The nasal septum is released from the vomer with either a double-guarded osteotome or the saw blade. Finally, pterygomaxillary osteotomes are used to create controlled vertical fractures of pterygoid plates and release the Le Fort segment from the skull base. Downfracture can then be performed (**Figure 31.6A**).

The Le Fort segment is completely mobilized to allow for easy positioning into the splint. Maxillomandibular fixation (MMF) is obtained using wires or elastics (**Figure 31.6B**). L-shaped plates fixed to the medial and lateral buttresses are used to secure the position of

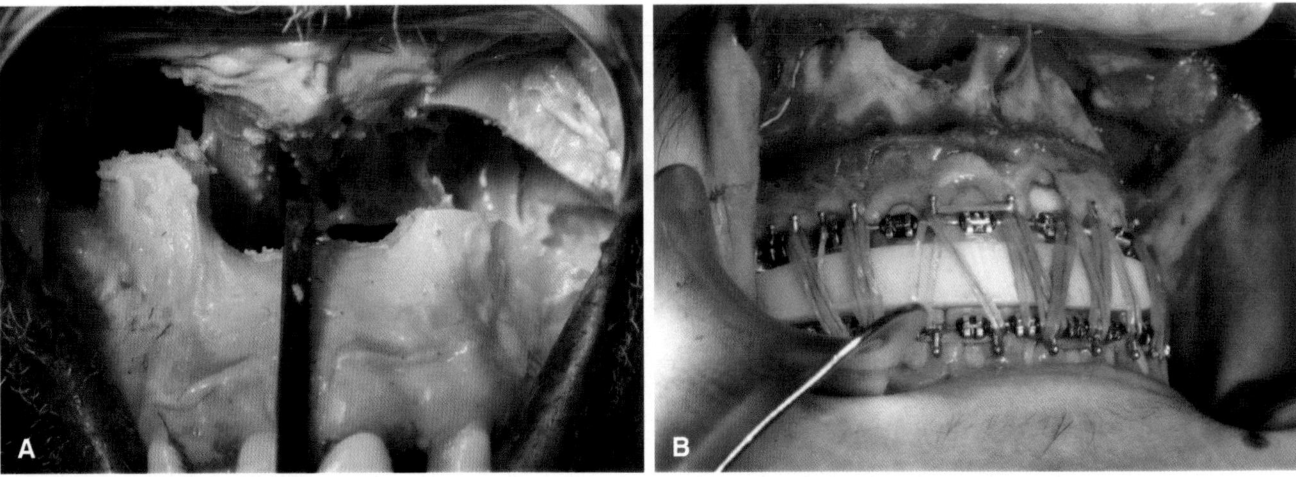

FIGURE 31.6. Maxillary osteotomies. **A.** In this cadaver, differential Le Fort I osteotomy levels have been performed for demonstration purposes. The high osteotomy on the patient's right will provide increased soft tissue support in the upper midface if the maxilla is advanced. Regardless of the vertical level, osteotomies are made above the levels of the dental roots to avoid injury to the teeth. The nasal septum and maxillary sinuses are clearly visible following downfracture. **B.** In maxilla-first two-jaw surgery, a bulky intermediate splint is used to index the temporary relationship between the jaws following the Le Fort I manipulation and before the mandibular movement.

the Le Fort segment. During fixation, the surgeon must ensure that the condyles are properly seated to avoid a postoperative malocclusion.

Once rigid fixation is achieved, the splint is removed and the new occlusion is evaluated. If the surgery was planned as a maxilla-only procedure and the position of the maxilla is consistent with the presurgical plan, the incision is closed and guiding elastics are placed. The patient is followed closely during the first few weeks after surgery to monitor stability of the maxillary movement. If the surgery was designed as a maxilla-first two-jaw manipulation, MMF is reestablished after the appropriate intermediate position of the maxilla in confirmed and the surgeon proceeds with the mandibular osteotomies.

Surgically Assisted Rapid Palatal Expansion

In adolescence, transverse maxillary deficiency can usually be corrected orthodontically with palatal expansion devices. Once the midline palatine suture fuses, however, surgical assistance may be required to effectively expand the maxilla if correction of posterior crossbite is needed. In these cases, a Le Fort I osteotomy is then performed as described earlier. The maxilla is then bisected between the roots of the central incisors and through the hard palate in the midline. Great care must be taken to preserve the palate mucosa to avoid development of an iatrogenic oronasal fistula. The Le Fort I segment is not rigidly fixed as in a traditional Le Fort I procedure. Following surgery, a palatal expander is placed and activated by the orthodontist to correct the transverse deficiency. This approach offers the best correction of transverse maxillary deficiency with the lowest rate of relapse in skeletally mature patients or in patients for whom traditional expansion techniques fail.

Mandibular Osteotomies

Numerous types of mandibular osteotomies have been described for implementation in orthognathic surgery. The sagittal split osteotomy (SSO) and the vertical ramus osteotomy (VRO) are by far the most commonly used and are discussed in further detail below. These techniques provide great versatility to surgeons and consistent, stable results for patients.

Sagittal Split Osteotomy

SSO is the most common technique used in orthognathic procedures involving the mandible. It is technically straightforward, can be performed intraorally, and allows for advancement, setback, rotation, and closure of anterior open bites. Bony overlap between the proximal and distal segments facilitates stable healing, but the proximity of the inferior alveolar nerve to the osteotomy line contributes to the risk of permanent sensory changes associated with this approach.[9,10]

Surgery begins with an incision in the gingivobuccal sulcus at the level of the first molar that is extended along the anterior border of the ascending mandibular ramus. Subperiosteal dissection is used to elevate the soft tissues from the buccal surfaces of the body and ramus, as well as the anterior and lingual surfaces of the ramus.

The osteotomy begins on the lingual surface of the ramus, above the occlusal plane, to avoid injury to the inferior alveolar nerve at the level of the lingula. A reciprocating saw or ultrasonic bone cutter is used to cut the medial ramus. The osteotomy continues across the anterior border of the ramus and along the external oblique line of the mandible to the first molar, where a vertical cut is made from the oblique line to the inferior border (**Figure 31.7**).

These bone cuts are corticotomies; once they are made, the sagittal split is completed using osteotomes and a mallet. A successful split results in a mandibular segment that contains the buccal plate, ascending ramus, condyle, and coronoid process (the *proximal segment*) and a distinct segment that contains the tooth-bearing portion of the body and symphysis (the *distal segment*).

Once the proximal and distal segments are mobilized, the mandible is advanced or set back as dictated by the surgical plan and brought into the prefabricated occlusal splint.[11,12] Rigid fixation is achieved with either bicortical positional screws or monocortical plates and screws (**Figure 31.7D**). Again, during fixation, the surgeon must ensure that the condyles are properly seated in the glenoid fossae. MMF is released, the occlusion is checked, and guiding elastics are placed as indicated. The incisions are closed in the surgeon's preferred fashion.

Vertical Ramus Osteotomy

In contrast to the SSO, the VRO creates a distal segment that includes the tooth-bearing portion of the mandible, coronoid process, inferior alveolar nerve, and anterior ramus, and a proximal segment that includes the mandibular condyle and the posterior ramus. The procedure can be performed via an external or internal approach, and subperiosteal exposure of the mandible is similar to that of the SSO. The osteotomy is placed 7 to 8 mm in front of the posterior border of the ramus between the sigmoid notch and the inferior border of the mandible. Adequate bone stock must be preserved on the posterior segment to accommodate fixation hardware.

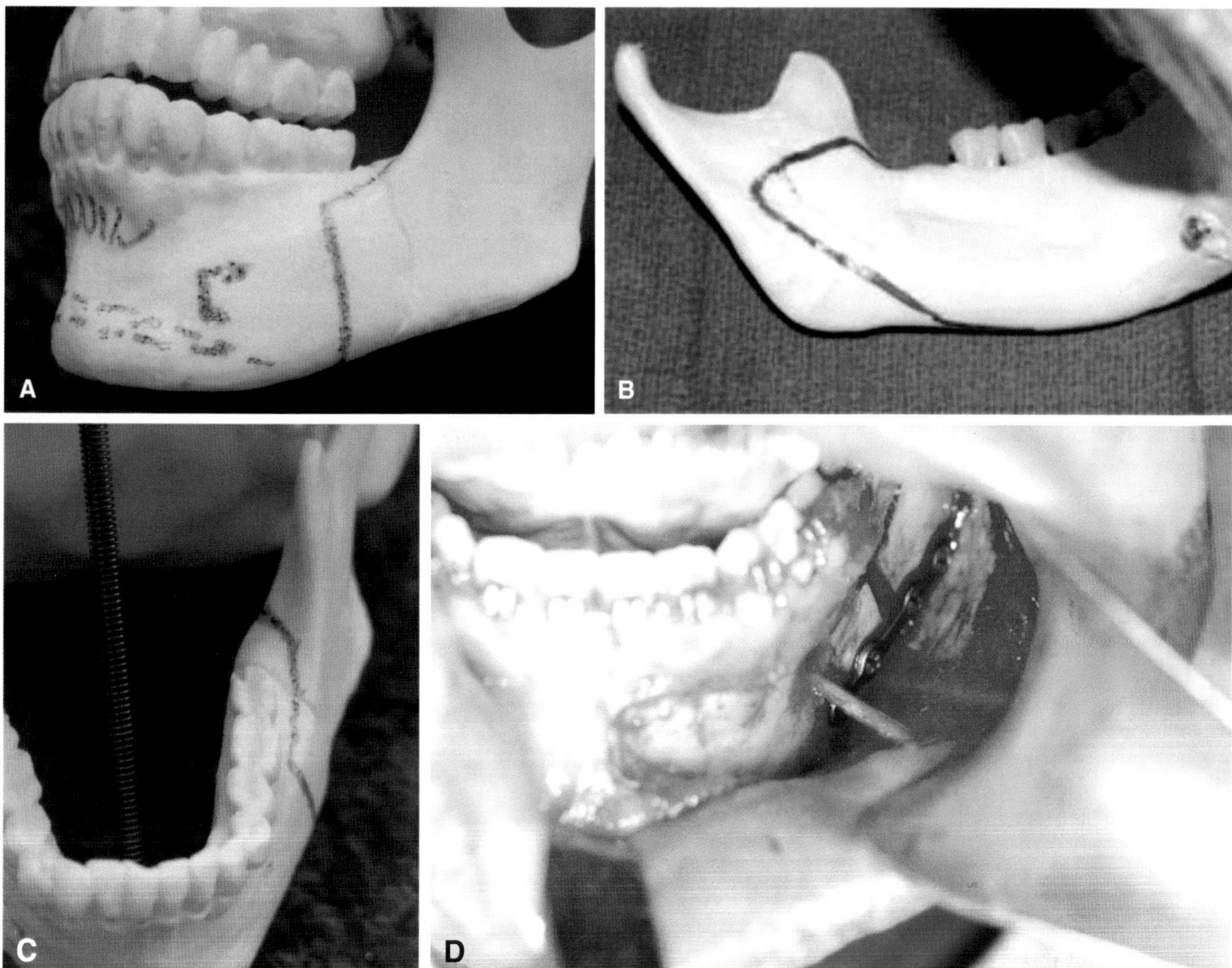

FIGURE 31.7. Mandibular osteotomies. **A–C.** A typical line of corticotomy for the SSO is demonstrated on this skull model from buccal, lingual, and frontal perspectives. **D.** This intraoperative photo demonstrates the proximity of the mental nerve exiting its foramen in a patient undergoing SSO with mandibular advancement. Rigid fixation is achieved with locking titanium alloy plates and screws.

The procedure is of limited utility when mandibular advancement is indicated: significant advancement creates a long vertical gap between the two segments, increasing the risk of nonunion and relapse. However, VRO is particularly suited to address horizontal mandibular excess and asymmetries requiring setback.[13]

As with the SSO, occlusion is established intraoperatively using a splint and MMF. Once rigid fixation is obtained, the patient is taken out of interdental fixation to confirm the position of the jaws. If all is satisfactory, the incision is closed and guiding elastics are placed.

Osseous Genioplasty (Horizontal Osteotomy of the Mandible)

Genioplasty, or horizontal osteotomy of the mandible, can significantly complement the orthognathic surgery plan and optimize the aesthetic surgical result. Osseous genioplasty is an extremely powerful tool, allowing for advancement, setback, reduction, lengthening, widening, narrowing, and rotation of the chin.[14-16]

The procedure is performed via a central gingivobuccal sulcus incision, with subperiosteal dissection to the inferior border of the mandible and lateral dissection to the mental foramina. Surgeons should carefully consider the anatomy of the inferior alveolar nerve, which drops 5 to 6 mm bselow the mental foramen before exiting the bone, when planning their osteotomies (**Figure 31.8A**). A cuff of mentalis at the incision line and muscle attachments to the caudal symphysis are preserved to allow resuspension of the muscle at the end of the procedure and prevent development of a witch's chin deformity (**Figure 31.8B**). Once the genioplasty segment is freed, it is manipulated to correct the identified deformity and rigidly fixed in place with titanium plates and screws. The mentalis muscle is resuspended, and the gingivobuccal sulcus incision is closed with absorbable sutures.

Two-Jaw Surgery

Moving the maxilla and the mandible in a single surgery is more involved than simply combining individual Le Fort and SSO techniques. Two-jaw surgery requires precision at every step, from orthodontic preparation to presurgical planning to performing the osteotomies to rigid fixation to the use of postoperative guiding elastics.[17-20]

The maxillary and mandibular movements are performed in series. Traditionally, the Le Fort I osteotomy is performed first, followed by the mandibular movement. More recently, mandible-first surgery has been widely adopted with results that are equal to the more time-honored maxilla-first approach. Currently, the choice of technique is often an arbitrary one based on surgeon preference.[21]

Regardless of the order of osteotomy, as described earlier, an intermediate splint is generated during the presurgical planning process that indexes the position of the jaws following the first movement. Interdental fixation is obtained and the intermediate splint holds the jaws in the desired position while rigid fixation is achieved. MMF is then released, bone cuts for the second jaw movement are made, and the final splint is used to stabilize the mandible and maxilla in the final desired occlusion while rigid fixation is obtained.

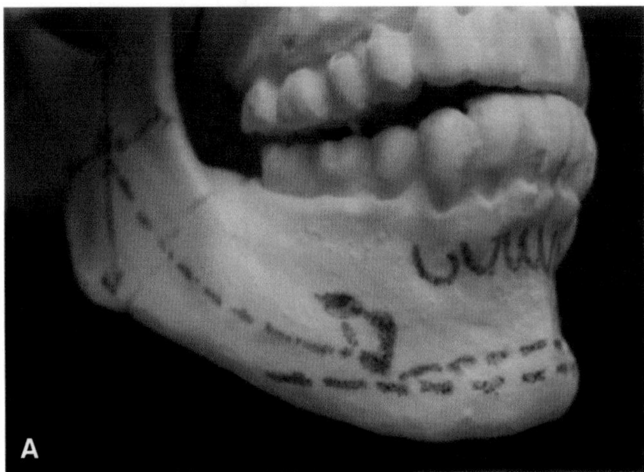

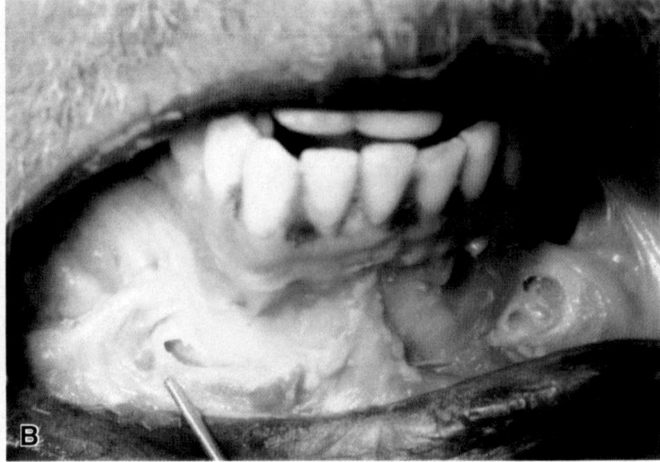

FIGURE 31.8. Osseous genioplasty. **A.** The anatomy of the mental nerve should be appreciated before performing a genioplasty. Specifically, the surgeon should be aware that the intraosseous excursion of the nerve carries it 5 to 6 mm below the mental foramen before it curves cephalad and exits the bone. **B.** This cadaver dissection demonstrates exposure of the nerves bilaterally with preservation of caudal central muscle attachments. A reciprocating saw or other bone-cutting instrument can make the osteotomy with preservation of the soft tissue attachments.

PERIOPERATIVE CARE AND MANAGEMENT OF COMPLICATIONS

Postoperative management focuses on patient comfort and the prevention of complications. Cold packs or compresses and head elevation can significantly decrease edema. In addition, a short course of oral steroid therapy may help minimize swelling, as well as the risk of postanesthesia nausea and vomiting. Antiemetics are routinely provided to the patient. Chlorhexidine oral rinses after and between meals help maintain an antiseptic environment in the mouth and mitigate against oral wound infection. Oral antibiotic administration following surgery has been shown to reduce the risk of infection.

A liquid diet is instituted immediately after surgery, progressing to a mechanical soft diet at postoperative follow-up. Patients should be counseled that they may experience significant weight loss because of limited caloric intake in the immediate postoperative period, and the importance of adequate nutritional intake should be emphasized. Guiding elastics are used to help maintain the stability of the new occlusion and begin musculoskeletal training, so patients may get accustomed to their new jaw and dental relationships.

Every orthognathic surgery patient will require some degree of postsurgical orthodontic therapy to complete their rehabilitation. The length of orthodontic care following orthognathic surgery varies greatly and is largely dependent upon the presurgical plan, the extent of presurgical orthodontic preparation, and the specific endpoints set forth by the orthodontist.

Postoperative bleeding is rare, as most bleeding is encountered and controlled during surgery. In unusual circumstances, injury to the internal maxillary artery or the plexus of vessels at the skull base behind the maxilla may manifest following completion of the procedure. In these cases, evaluation and intervention must be immediate and aggressive, potentially involving interventional radiology services or surgical exploration.[22]

After mandibular and two-jaw surgery, most patients will experience transient decrease in sensation in the distribution of the inferior alveolar nerve. It is important during the SSO to identify and preserve the nerve as it enters the mandible proximally, throughout its course within its bony canal, and as it exits the mental foramen. If a transection is identified, neurorrhaphy should be performed immediately.

Postoperative malocclusion is a rare but serious complication of orthognathic surgery. Technical errors during surgery may predispose a patient to this adverse outcome. The final occlusion should be thoroughly checked with the condyles seated in the glenoid fossae after rigid fixation is achieved. If the occlusion does not exactly correlate with the presurgical plan, rigid fixation should be removed, and the position of one or both jaws must be adjusted. Bony nonunion and malunion are also rare outcomes following orthognathic surgery. Both require reoperation. Repeat osteotomy and bone grafting may be necessary in these situations.

SUMMARY

With appropriate planning and preparation, orthognathic surgery is associated with excellent outcomes, low-risk profiles, and very satisfied patients. A wide range of versatile techniques exist that can be implemented in the treatment of malocclusion, and new technologies allow for detailed VSP and other streamlined perioperative processes that contribute to surgical success. Careful consideration of the impact of planned jaw movements on the position of both skeletal and soft tissue components of the face allows surgeons to achieve desired functional outcomes, optimize facial aesthetics, and meet patient expectations.

REFERENCES

1. Reyneke JP. Surgical cephalometric prediction tracing for the alteration of the occlusal plane by means of rotation of the maxillomandibular complex. *Int J Adult Orthodon Orthognath Surg.* 1999;14(1): 55-64.
2. Ricketts RM. Cephalometric analysis and synthesis. *Angle Orthod.* 1961;31(3):141-156.
   This article describes the cephalometric tracings and analysis that have come to be known as a Ricketts analysis for the diagnosis of dentofacial deformities. Ricketts also describes how cephalometric analysis relates to, and is distinct from, treatment planning for orthognathic surgery.
3. Schendel SA, Eisenfeld J, Bell WH, et al. The long face syndrome: vertical maxillary excess. *Am J Orthod.* 1976;70(4):398-408.
4. Reyneke JP, Masureik CJ. Treatment of maxillary deficiency by Le Fort I downsliding technique. *J Oral Maxillofac Surg.* 1985;43(11):914-916.
5. Wagner S, Reyneke JP. The Le Fort I downsliding osteotomy: a study of long-term hard tissue stability. *Int J Adult Orthodon Orthognath Surg.* 2000;15(1):37-49.
6. Selber JC, Rosen HM. Aesthetics of facial skeletal surgery. *Clin Plast Surg.* 2007;34(3):437-445.
7. Rosen HM. Facial skeletal expansion: treatment strategies and rationale. *Plast Reconstr Surg.* 1992;89(5):798-808.
   This article describes Rosen's philosophical and clinical preference for skeletal expansion rather than contraction in orthognathic surgery. It emphasizes the paramount importance of aesthetics over orthognathic perfection and illustrates this approach using case examples in which facial disproportion was created or maintained to optimize the aesthetic outcome.
8. Bell WH. Le Forte I osteotomy for correction of maxillary deformities. *J Oral Surg.* 1975;33(6):412-426.
9. Trauner R, Obwegeser H. The surgical correction of mandibular prognathism and retrognathia with consideration of genioplasty. Part I. Surgical procedures to correct mandibular prognathism and reshaping of the chin. *Oral Surg Oral Med Oral Pathol.* 1957;10(7):677-689.

In the first of a series of classic articles, the authors describe various mandibular osteotomies that are still in use today, including the sagittal split and inverted L sliding genioplasty technique that are also described.

10. Bell WH. Surgical correction of mandibular retrognathism. *Am J Orthod.* 1966;52(7):518-528.
11. Bell WH. Correction of mandibular prognathism by mandibular setback and advancement genioplasty. *Int J Oral Surg.* 1981;10(4):221-229.
12. Bell WH, Jacobs JD, Legan HL. Treatment of the class II deep bite by orthodontic and surgical means. *Am J Orthod.* 1984;85(1):1-20.
13. Al-Moraissi EA, Ellis E III. Is there a difference in stability or neurosensory function between bilateral sagittal split osteotomy and intraoral vertical ramus osteotomy for mandibular setback? *J Oral Maxillofac Surg.* 2015;73(7):1360-1371.
14. Converse JM, Wood-Smith D. Horizontal osteotomy of the mandible. *Plast Reconstr Surg.* 1964;34(5):464-471.
15. Posnick JC, Choi E, Chang RP. Osseous genioplasty in conjunction with bimaxillary orthognathic surgery: a review of 262 consecutive cases. *Int J Oral Maxillofac Surg.* 2016;45(7):904-913.
16. Trauner R, Obwegeser H. The surgical correction of mandibular prognathism and retrognathia with consideration of genioplasty. Part II. Operating methods for microgenia and distoclusion. *Oral Surg Oral Med Oral Pathol.* 1957;10(8):787-792.
17. Bell WH, Jacobs JD, Quejada JG. Simultaneous repositioning of the maxilla, mandible, and chin. Treatment planning and analysis of soft tissues. *Am J Orthod.* 1986;89(1):28-50.
 Cephalometric and aesthetic analysis as well as indications for two-jaw orthognathic surgery are described. Case examples illustrate the diagnostic, analytic, and orthodontic and surgical treatment processes.
18. Bell WH, Sinn DP, Finn RA. Cephalometric treatment planning for superior repositioning of the maxilla and concomitant mandibular advancement. *J Maxillofac Surg.* 1982;10(1):42-49.
19. Brammer J, Finn R, Bell WH, et al. Stability after bimaxillary surgery to correct vertical maxillary excess and mandibular deficiency. *J Oral Surg.* 1980;38(9):664-670.
20. Park N, Posnick JC. Accuracy of analytic model planning in bimaxillary surgery. *Int J Oral Maxillofac Surg.* 2013;42(7):807-813.
21. Perez D, Ellis E III. Sequencing bimaxillary surgery: mandible first. *J Oral Maxillofac Surg.* 2011;69(8):2217-2224.
 The article is a commentary on mandible-first two-jaw orthognathic surgery and its advantages over more traditional maxilla-first approaches. Requirements for a mandible-first approach as well as circumstances favoring mandible-first, unique aspects of planning, and disadvantages are also described.
22. Bradley JP, Elahi M, Kawamoto HK. Delayed presentation of pseudoaneurysm after Le Fort I osteotomy. *J Craniofac Surg.* 2002;13(6):746-750.

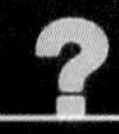

QUESTIONS

1. A 30-year-old man presents to your office because he is bothered by his prominent chin. On physical examination, he has class III malocclusion. Cephalometric evaluation shows an SNA of 81° (normal 80–84) and an SNB angle of 83° (normal 78–80). There are no other abnormalities. Which of the following procedures is most appropriate in this patient?
   a. Setback genioplasty
   b. SSO and setback
   c. Le Fort I maxillary advancement
   d. Two-jaw surgery

2. A skeletally mature patient presents to your office after referral from her orthodontist. She has transverse maxillary deficiency with bilateral posterior crossbite. What is the most appropriate intervention?
   a. Orthodontic palatal expansion
   b. SARPE
   c. Le Fort I advancement
   d. Bilateral SSO mandibular setback

3. Which of the following orthognathic movements is likely to cause the appearance of facial aging?
   a. Le Fort I advancement
   b. Le Fort I with downward repositioning
   c. Le Fort I with upward repositioning
   d. Bilateral sagittal split and advancement
   e. Advancement genioplasty

4. A 22-year-old woman comes to your office with concerns about her lower-third facial appearance, specifically her weak chin. She has no concerns about her midfacial appearance. She has had previous orthodontia and is in class I malocclusion. Her overall facial height is proportional in all views, but on profile, her chin appears weak in an anterior-posterior direction. Cephalometric analysis demonstrates that her SNA angle is 82° (normal 78–82) and her SNB angle is 80° (normal 78–80). What is the most appropriate surgical management?
   a. Bilateral sagittal split and advancement
   b. Two-jaw surgery with maxillary and mandibular advancement
   c. Vertical lengthening genioplasty and bone grafting
   d. Horizontal sliding genioplasty and advancement
   e. Le Fort I setback

5. A 25-year-old man is referred to your office for concerns about lower facial asymmetry. On examination, his maxillary dental midline is in line with his overall facial midline, but his mandibular dental midline is shifted 5 mm to the right. His chin point is in line with his mandibular dental midline. With appropriate orthodontics, which orthognathic procedure would best treat this patient's lower facial asymmetry?
   a. SSO with leftward shift alone
   b. SSO with rightward shift alone
   c. SSO with leftward shift and sliding genioplasty to the right
   d. SSO with rightward shift and sliding genioplasty to the left
   e. Le Fort I osteotomy with rightward shift

1. **Answer: b.** The patient has prognathism with an abnormal SNB angle. Mandibular osteotomies and setback will address both the patient's prominent chin and his malocclusion. Given that his SNA angle is within the normal range, Le Fort I maxillary advancement is not the ideal choice in this scenario. Likewise, two-jaw surgery is unnecessary with a normal SNA angle and a relatively small overall movement. Setback genioplasty may address the patient's concerns about his prominent chin, but will not address his malocclusion.

2. **Answer: b.** The key to this question is that the patient is skeletally mature. This means that the palatal suture is likely to be fused and orthodontic palatal expansion alone is unlikely to correct her transverse maxillary deficiency. Both Le Fort I and bilateral SSOs are incorrect because both primarily address anterior-posterior discrepancies. SARPE involves surgically splitting the palatal suture followed by orthodontic expansion. This will allow transverse expansion of the maxilla without changes in the anterior-posterior direction.

3. **Answer: c.** All of the movements described expand the facial skeleton except for Le Fort I with upward repositioning (impaction). Le Fort I impaction reduces facial height, but because the existing soft tissue envelope is draped over a smaller skeletal frame, this may result in deeper rhytids and the appearance of facial aging. In contrast, movements that expand the facial skeleton cause the existing soft tissue envelope to be draped over a larger frame, softening and flattening rhytids.

4. **Answer: d.** The patient described has microgenia, but normal facial height and would benefit from augmenting her chin by advancing it horizontally (a chin implant, although not one of the answer choices, would also be a reasonable option). This patient has normal SNA and SNB angles on cephalometric analysis and is in class I malocclusion; she also has no concerns about her midfacial appearance. These factors all argue against two-jaw surgery with advancements; additionally, this would not change her relative microgenia. Vertical lengthening genioplasty and bone grafting is not indicated because her overall facial height is proportionate (vertical thirds are similar). Le Fort I setback and bilateral sagittal split with advancement would both create malocclusion and neither would address the patient's weak chin.

5. **Answer: a.** This patient's maxillary midline is coincident with his overall facial midline; only the mandibular midline is malpositioned. Although Le Fort I osteotomy and rightward shift could align the dental midlines, this would actually make the patient appear more asymmetric and is, therefore, incorrect. Additionally, the patient's chin point is coincident with his mandibular dental midline, meaning that moving the mandibular dental midline into the correct position will move the chin point at the same time, rendering genioplasty unnecessary. If the chin point was coincident with the facial midline rather than the mandibular dental midline, a compensatory genioplasty in the opposite direction of the mandibular movement would be needed. This leaves sagittal split alone as the only option, and in this case the patient is already off to the right, so his midline needs to be shifted to the left.

CHAPTER 32 Craniofacial Clefts and Orbital Hypertelorism

Jesse A. Goldstein and Joseph E. Losee

KEY POINTS

- Treat each with a craniofacial cleft and/or hypertelorism individually
- Soft tissue contours follow the underlying bony abnormality
- Establishing the brain/nose barrier is critical early in life
- Definitive surgical intervention for orbital hypertelorism should wait until the orbit has reached maturity (at least 5 to 7 years of age)
- Maintain medial canthal attachments if possible; if not, resuspend with transnasal wiring
- No. 7 craniofacial clefts are the most prevalent
- Orbital hypertelorism is a physical finding, not a syndrome

Craniofacial clefts and orbital hypertelorism (OHT) represent two distinct entities that have in common an extreme variation in presentation. They span severity from subtle anomalies of little clinical consequence to the most profound forms of craniofacial disfigurement encountered in plastic surgery. With few exceptions, these entities are rare and result from uncharacterized disruptions during embryogenesis; however, several well-defined syndromes and diagnoses exist whose primary manifestation is hypertelorism or craniofacial clefting. As a whole, these entities should be thought of as part of a phenotypical spectrum and not as those that share a clearly delineated etiopathogenesis. Even so, developing a comprehensive framework for understanding, evaluating, and treating patients with these complex anomalies is crucial to success. This chapter is meant to provide the framework for assessing and categorizing these complex anomalies as well as provide some basic principles of treatment that may be broadly applied.

TESSIER CLASSIFICATION

Craniofacial clefts are often referred to as *Tessier clefts*, a reference to Paul Tessier (1917–2008) who founded the field of craniofacial surgery and developed a system for understanding these diverse entities.[1] The Tessier classification[2] is the most complete and commonly utilized framework today, describing both the soft tissue anomalies and the underlying bony abnormalities. Tessier's classification was a synthesis of anatomic and clinical study of patients and was developed before the advent of computed tomography (CT).[3] It has withstood the transition into the modern era of imaging including 3D CT and magnetic resonance imaging technologies.

The Tessier classification of rare craniofacial clefts centers around the orbits and eyelids, which represent the region of interface between the cranium and the facial structures (**Figure 32.1**). Therefore, the clefts that occur cephalad to the orbits are defined as cranial clefts, and those occurring caudal to the orbit represent the facial clefts. Tessier's numbering system helps reinforce this point: facial clefts are numbered 0 to 7, whereas cranial clefts are numbered 8 to 14. Furthermore, cranial and facial clefts often occur in distinct patterns. When Tessier clefts occur in combination, they often include a facial cleft and a cranial cleft such that the sum of the cleft numbers is 14. For example, a midline cleft may begin at the lip and nose (no. 0 cleft) but extend up through the forehead (no. 14 cleft). Other common combinations of craniofacial clefts include 1 and 13, 2 and 12, 3 and 11, etc. (**Table 32.1**) Craniofacial clefts rarely exhibit the same extent of soft tissue and skeletal involvement. A diagnosis of a craniofacial cleft can be made more reliably based on the skeletal manifestations which are more consistent than the soft tissue manifestations.

FEATURES OF CRANIOFACIAL CLEFTS

Median Clefts: No. 0 and No. 14 Clefts

Median craniofacial clefts represent a unique form of facial clefting which can be associated with both hypoplasia of midline structures and tissue hyperplasia. The no. 0 clefts define the facial component of the spectrum of median clefts, whereas the no. 14 clefts define the cranial, or frontoethmoidal, component of median clefts. Median clefts can be further divided into hypoplasia or agenesis, dysraphia, and hyperplasia.[4]

Median Craniofacial Hypoplasia

Hypoplasia associated with no. 0 clefts can range from small but normal to complete agenesis of the midline facial structures, whereas their extension into a no. 14 cleft can present with mild or severe hypotelorism and central nervous system (CNS) anomalies. Severe forms of median craniofacial hypoplasia fall under the diagnosis of holoprosencephaly and include cyclopia, ethmocephaly with midline proboscis, and cebocephaly, and there is a positive correlation between the severity of the facial findings and degree of CNS anomalies resulting in significantly limited life expectancy or intrauterine demise. In patients with milder forms, assessing CNS anatomy

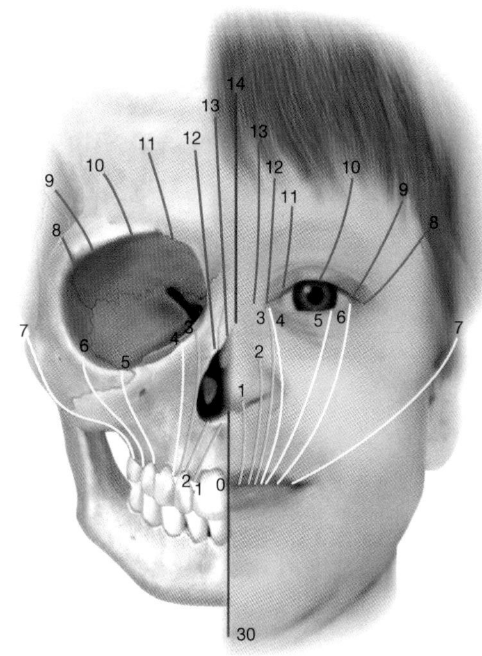

FIGURE 32.1. Tessier classification of craniofacial clefts. Soft tissue clefts are demonstrated on the left. The skeletal clefts are depicted on the right. The facial clefts are numbered 0 through 7 and the cranial clefts are numbered 8 to 14.

TABLE 32.1. COMPREHENSIVE LIST OF CRANIOFACIAL (TESSIER) CLEFTS WITH ASSOCIATED BONY AND SOFT TISSUE LANDMARKS

	Cleft Number	Soft Tissue	Skeletal	
Medial → Lateral	0	Mouth: True or False Median cleft lip Nose: Absent columella to bifid nose with disorganized nasal cartilage	Midline Hypoplasia: absence of premaxilla/primary palate, hypotelorism Midline Hyperplasia: Duplicated nasal spline, anterior open bite, broad nose, hypertelorism	Facial Clefts
	1	Mouth: Cupids bow Nose: soft triangle/alar dome Eye: medial to the medial canthus	Maxilla: Keel shaped, anterior op en bite, lateral to nasal spine Nose: Between nasal bone and frontal process of maxilla Orbits: Hypertelorism	
	2	Mouth: Cupids bow peak Nose: middle third of the ala Eye: medial to the palpebral fissure	Maxilla: Piriform/nasal sill/primary and secondary palate. Nose: Between nasal bone and frontal process of maxilla Orbits: Hypertelorism	
	3	Mouth: Philtral column Nose: lateral ala Eye: between medial canthus and inferior lacrimal punctum	Maxilla: Alveolus between lateral incisor and canine to lateral piriform. Nose: Absent lateral nasal wall which is confluent with Orbit: Inferio-medial orbit including lacrimal crest	
	4	Mouth: Lateral to cupids bow peak but medial to the oral commissure Nose: lateral to the lateral ala Orbit: medial lower lid, lateral to inferior punctum	Maxilla: Alveolus between lateral incisor and canine Nose: Lateral to piriform aperture Orbit: Inferior orbit between infraorbital foramen and frontal process of maxilla	
	5	Mouth: Medial to oral commissure Nose: lateral to the lateral ala Orbit: lateral lower lid	Maxilla: Alveolus between canine and first pre -molar Nose: Lateral to piriform aperture Orbit: Inferior orbit lateral to infraorbital foramen	
	6	Mouth: Oral commissure Nose: lateral to the lateral ala Orbit: lateral to the lateral canthus	Maxilla: Zygomatico-maxillary suture to pterygomaxillary buttress Orbit: Infero-lateral orbit including the inferior orbital fissure	
	7	Mouth: Oral commissure Ear: Pre-auricular area, +/- skin tag	Maxilla: Pterygomaxillary junction cleft Zygoma: Dysplastic zygomatic body and absent arch Mandible: Vertically shortened ramus	
Lateral → Medial	8	Orbit: Lateral canthus to temporal region	Orbit: Lateral orbital wall	Cranial Clefts
	9	Orbit: lateral third of the upper lid, lateral third of the brow Scalp: Temporoparietal hairline anteriorly displaced	Orbit: Supero-lateral orbit with posterior rotation of lateral wall Neurocranium: Lateral temporal and parietal bone abnormalities	
	10	Orbit: middle third of the upper lid, middle third of the brow Scalp: Fronto-temporoparietal hairline anteriorly displaced	Orbit: Mid superior orbital rim, lateral to the supraorbital foramen. Encephalocele may be present with infero-lateral orbital displacement and hypertelorism Forehead: Variable lateral frontal bone cleft	
	11	Orbit: medial third of the upper lid, medial third of the brow Scalp: Frontal hairline anteriorly displaced	Orbit: Medial third of the supra -orbital rim, variable hypertelorism Forehead: Variable medial frontal bone cleft	
	12	Orbit: medial to the medial canthus with lateral displacement, medial third of the brow Scalp: Paramedian frontal hairline anteriorly displaced	Orbit: Associated with the frontal process of the maxilla, extending into the ethmoid sinus with resulting hypertelorism and telocant hus. Forehead: Variable medial frontal bone cleft without encephalocele.	
	13	Orbit: Eyelid and eyebrow are unaffected Scalp: V-shaped frontal hair projection	Orbit: Associated with the frontal process of the maxilla, extending into the ethmoid sinus with resulting hypertelorism, and variable encephalocele. Cranium Cribiform widening and depression.	
	14	Orbit: Hypotelorism or hypertelorism, with or without nasofrontal encephalocele Scalp: Microcephaly or wide forehead with soft tissue atrophy, widow's peak	Midline Hypoplasia: Hypotelorism, microcephaly Midline Hyperplasia: Hyperplasia, inferiorly displaced cribiformplate, wide, persistent anterior fontanelle	

■ Midline clefts
■ Clefts that involve the mouth, nose and eye
■ Clefts that involve the mouth and eye, but are lateral to the nose
■ Clefts at the level of the orbit and above

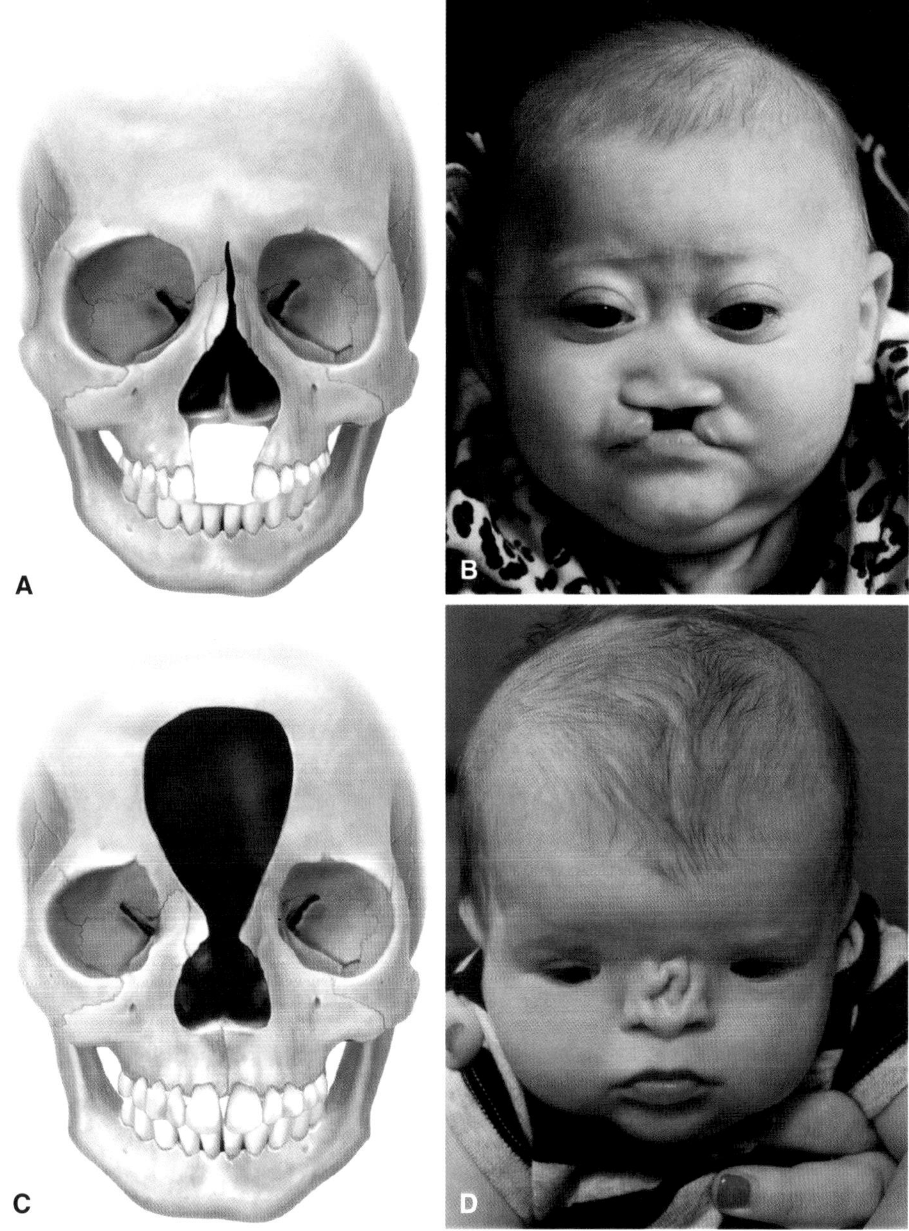

FIGURE 32.2. No. 0–14 cleft. **A.** Skeletal involvement demonstrating midline palatal hypoplasia and hypotelorism. **B.** Patient with midline craniofacial hypoplasia associated with a false medial cleft lip, absent columella, flat nasal bridge, and hypotelorism. **C.** Skeletal involvement demonstrating midline craniofacial hypertrophy and hypertelorism. **D.** Patient with midline craniofacial hyperplasia associated with hypertelorism and excess and disorganized nasal cartilage.

is crucial with CT or magnetic resonance imaging to differentiate between lobar and alobar holoprosencephaly and to determine the integrity of the hypothalamic-pituitary axis.

Soft Tissue Deficiencies

No. 0 clefts can affect the soft tissues of the upper lip and nose and can range from agenesis to subtle hypoplasia. A false median cleft lip may be present with absence of the philtrum and central tubercle. The columella may be narrowed, shortened, or absent, and the nasal tip may lack projection because of a hypoplastic or absent caudal septum. Hypotelorism and midline fusion of the eyebrows can occur in no. 14 clefts.

Skeletal Deficiencies

As with all aspects of craniofacial clefts, the skeletal involvement in no. 0/14 clefts can range from subtle separation between the maxillary central incisors to complete absence of the premaxilla and primary palate resulting in a large central palatal cleft. Hypoplastic nasal structures can also be present including septal, ethmoidal, and nasal bone deficiencies resulting in a flat nasal bridge, hypotelorism, and microcephaly (**Figure 32.2**). Additionally, intrinsic dental anomalies may also be present including absent or hypoplastic maxillary central incisors or a midline central incisor.

Midline Craniofacial Dysraphia

Dysraphia represents a failure of fusion, or cleft, of midline structures without deficiency or excess. The two diagnoses associated with a no. 0/14 cleft are a median cleft lip and an encephalocele.

Soft Tissue Involvement

This includes a true median cleft lip where all central structures are present. These clefts represent an embryological failure of fusion of the paired medial nasal processes and results in a narrow median

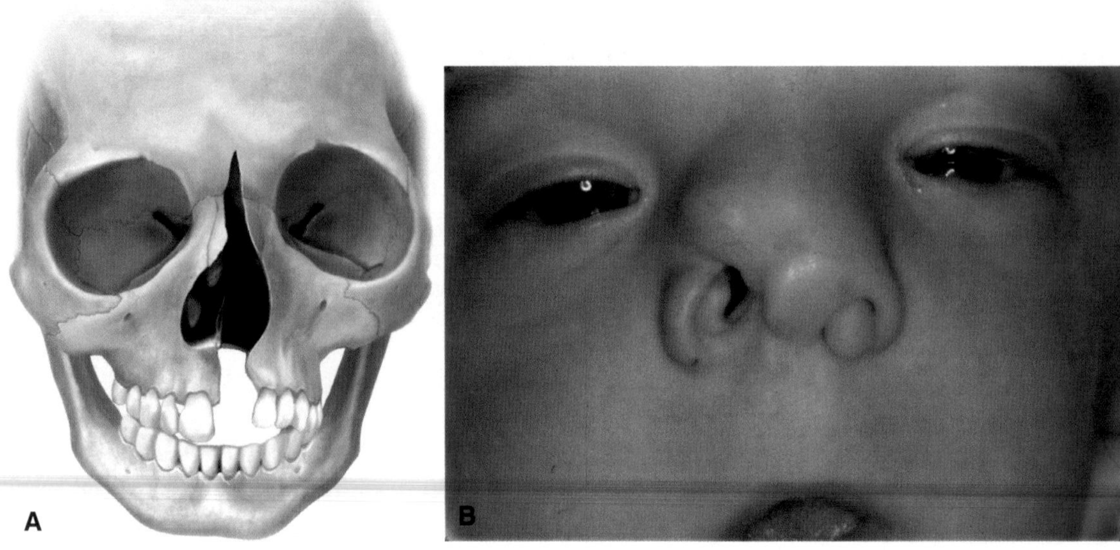

FIGURE 32.3. No. 1 cleft. A. Skeletal involvement is through the piriform aperture just lateral to the nasal spine and septum. The orbit is displaced laterally. B. Patient with a notched alar dome and mild orbital dystopia. (Reproduced from Losee JE, Kirschner RE. *Rare craniofacial defects.* In: *Comprehensive Cleft Care.* Vol 2. 2nd ed. New York, NY: Thieme Medical Publishing; 2016.)

cleft with present philtral columns. An encephalocele is a herniation of CNS structures including brain and cerebrospinal fluid through a weakened midline space and can result in a mass effect and further separation of normal facial structures.

Skeletal Involvement

True median clefts can result in a midline alveolar cleft and a midline primary palatal cleft, as well as hypertelorism if the cleft extends cephalad toward the orbits. Anterior encephaloceles can be divided into basal encephaloceles, where the CNS herniates through a defect in the cribriform plate or sphenoid bone into the ethmoidal space and frontoethmoidal encephaloceles, where the herniation occurs anterior to the crista galli at the junction of the frontal and ethmoidal bones.

Midline Craniofacial Hyperplasia

The spectrum of midline craniofacial hyperplasia ranges from clinically minor duplication of the nasal septum and subclinical hypertelorism to severe forms of frontonasal dysplasia together with severe hypertelorism and nasal duplication.[5-7]

Soft Tissue Involvement

Soft tissue excess may manifest as a widened philtrum, a bifid nasal tip or duplication, and abnormal nasal cartilage as well as widely spaced nasal soft tissue structures (Figure 32.2).

Skeletal Involvement

Skeletal excess in a hyperplastic no. 0/14 cleft can range from a widening of the maxillary alveolar process resulting in a central incisor diastema to a widened and shortened central dental arch resulting in an anterior open bite. A duplicated nasal spine may be present, and the nasal bones and maxillary processes of the maxilla may be flat, broad, and laterally displaced. Hypertelorism and frontal bossing/diastasis may be present because of varying degrees due to widening of the ethmoid sinuses and anterior cranial fossa, while the cribiform plate is low.

No. 1 Cleft

Soft Tissue Involvement

No. 1 Tessier clefts can often be confused with common cleft lips, as the cleft passes through Cupid's bow to the nasal base. The distinguishing feature of a no. 1 cleft, however, is the involvement of the medial nose including notched soft triangle and alar dome. This cleft can extend up the nose, lateral to midline, and be associated with soft tissue furrows and medial canthal displacement resulting in telecanthus (**Figure 32.3**). The eyelids are unaffected. No. 1 clefts can continue cephalad as no. 13 clefts, which can result in orbital dystopia.

Skeletal Involvement

An anterior open bite and keel-shaped maxilla are present, whereas a paramedian cleft may extend from between the central and lateral incisor to the nasal floor lateral to the nasal spine. A primary and secondary palatal cleft may be present. The cephalic extension of the cleft occurs between the nasal bone and the frontal process of the maxilla and can result in flattening and widening of the nasal dorsum. Widened ethmoids can result in hypertelorism.

No. 2 Cleft

Soft Tissue Involvement

Similar to no. 1 clefts, no. 2 Tessier clefts can also mimic common cleft lips. They are also paramedian, originating at the peak of Cupid's bow before extending up to the nasal sill. Unlike no. 1 clefts, however, no. 2 clefts pass through the middle third of the ala, lateral to the soft triangle, resulting in a hypoplastic ala rather than a notch. The nose can be broad and flat, and the medial canthus can be displaced. The lacrimal system and eyelids are unaffected (**Figure 32.4**). No. 2 clefts can continue cephalad as no. 12 clefts, which can lead to orbital dystopia and medial brow distortion.

Skeletal Involvement

This cleft originates lateral to the lateral maxillary incisor and extends up to the piriform aperture and primary/secondary palate similar to a common cleft lip/palate. Similar to a no. 1 cleft, the cephalic extension of the no. 2 cleft occurs between the nasal bone and the frontal process of the maxilla and can result in flattening and widening of the nasal dorsum as well as ethmoidal involvement and hypertelorism.

No. 3 Cleft

The no. 3 cleft is a common Tessier cleft and is often referred to as a Tessier oro-naso-ocular cleft (**Figure 32.5**).

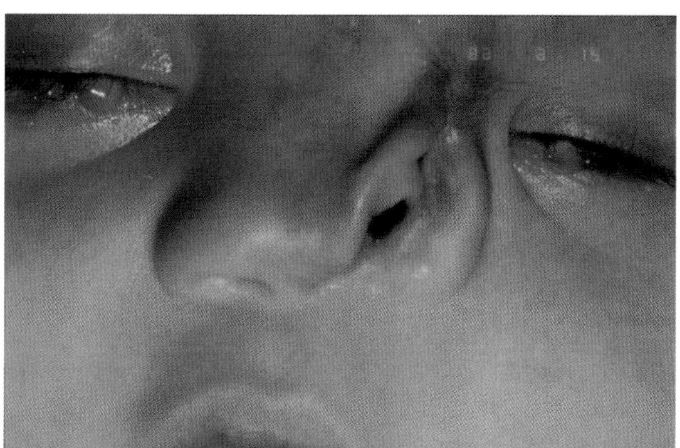

FIGURE 32.4. No. 2 cleft. Patient with a lateral alar deficiency and mild orbital dystopia. (Reproduced from Losee JE, Kirschner RE. *Rare craniofacial defects*. In: *Comprehensive Cleft Care*. Vol 2. 2nd ed. New York, NY: Thieme Medical Publishing; 2016.)

Soft Tissue Involvement

When isolated to the lip, no. 3 clefts manifest as a common cleft lip, starting at Cupid's bow peak and extending to the lateral nasal sill. The cleft extends through the lateral ala, which can be notched or clefted, to the lower eyelid between the medial canthus and the inferior punctum. There can be a significant soft tissue deficit in the midface with inferior displacement of the lower lid and globe, leading to a risk of exposure keratopathy. The globe may also be microphthalmic in some cases.

Skeletal Involvement

Skeletal involvement of the no. 3 cleft begins at the alveolar process, between the lateral incisor and canine, extending up to the lateral piriform aperture and into the medial orbit. The medial wall of the maxillary sinus is absent. The frontal process of the maxilla is disrupted as the bony component of the cleft terminates in the lacrimal groove in the inferior-medial orbit.

No. 4 Cleft

Soft Tissue Involvement

As with other craniofacial clefts, soft tissue involvement in no. 4 clefts presents as a wide spectrum of deformities.[8] The cleft begins lateral to the peak of Cupid's bow, midway between the commissure and the philtrum. This is the first of the clefts to travel lateral to the nose, although nasal anatomy can still be indirectly displaced superiorly. The cleft extends to the lower lid lateral to the medial canthus, which is displaced inferior-laterally, and can involve the lacrimal system at the level of the punctum and the lacrimal sac. The distance between the lower eyelid and the upper lip is foreshortened and can result in significant corneal exposure (Figure 32.5).

Skeletal Involvement

The skeletal involvement affects the inferior maxilla similarly to a no. 3 cleft; however, the no. 4 cleft courses lateral to the piriform region through the maxillary sinus, including the palate and choanae, superiorly to the infraorbital rim between the frontal process of the maxilla and the infraorbital foramen. The lacrimal system is usually spared. Variable orbital floor defects can be present.

No. 5 Cleft

No. 5 clefts are the least common of the oblique facial clefts.

Soft Tissue Involvement

Soft tissue involvement begins medial to the lateral oral commissure and proceeds cephalad toward the lower eyelid in the middle third. Similar to no. 4 clefts, there is often a soft tissue deficiency between the mouth and the lower lid, resulting in higher risk of corneal exposure (**Figure 32.6**).

Skeletal Involvement

The no. 5 cleft affects the alveolus lateral to the canine and extends through the maxillary sinus by encountering the inferolateral orbit lateral to the infraorbital foramen.

No. 6 Cleft

The no. 6 cleft is associated with mild forms of Treacher Collins syndrome and Nager syndrome, both of which present with zygomaticomaxillary dysplasia.

Soft Tissue Involvement

The soft tissue involvement often presents as a vertical cleft or furrow originating in the oral commissure and extending cephalad to the lateral lower eyelid. This can result in inferior displacement of the lateral

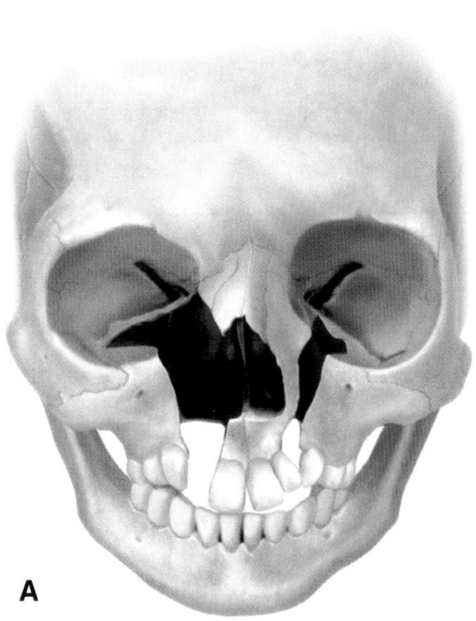

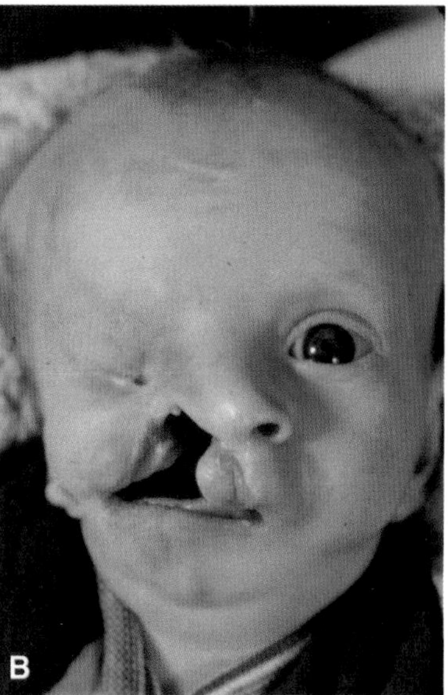

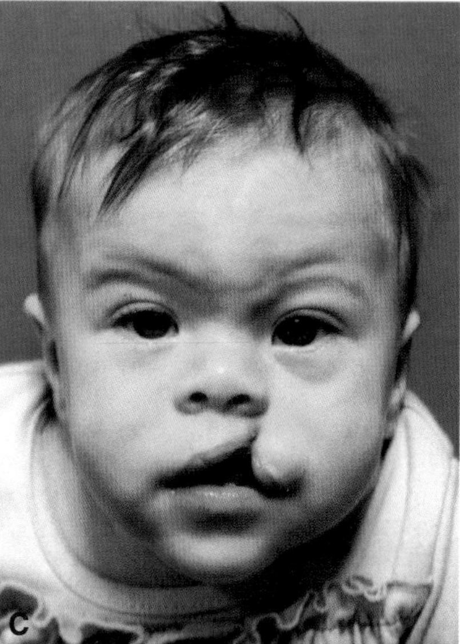

FIGURE 32.5. Right no. 3 cleft; left no. 4 cleft. **A.** Skeletal involvement demonstrates deformity of right medial maxilla and inferior orbital rim/floor with orbital dystopia and left-sided involvement lateral to the piriform extending to the inferior orbital rim/floor with orbital dystopia. **B.** Patient with deficiency extending from the alveolus into the piriform with microphthalmia and orbital dystopia. **C.** Patient with mild no. 4 cleft demonstrating cleft lip lateral to the nasal sill and subtle inferior displacement of the medial canthus.

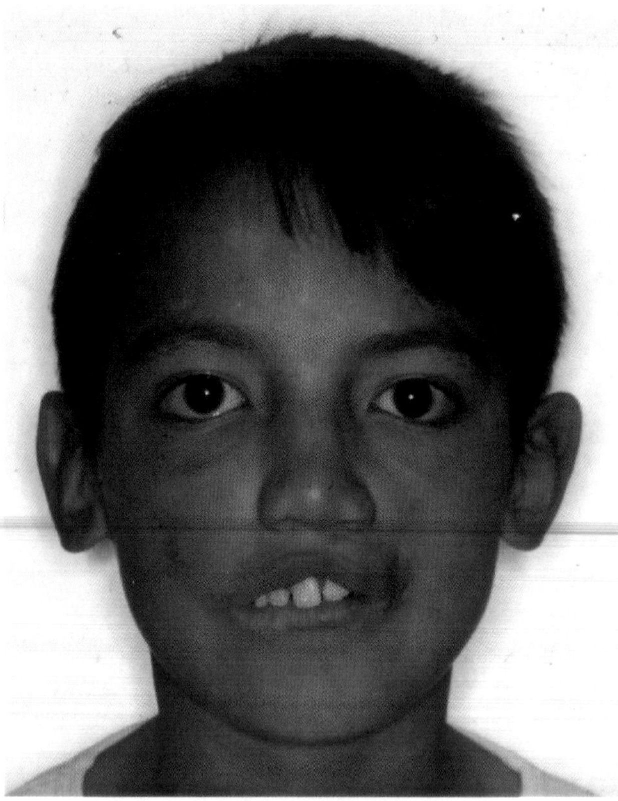

FIGURE 32.6. Right no. 5 cleft; left no. 6 cleft. The right no. 5 cleft is demonstrated by a subtle soft tissue furrow that begins medial to the oral commissure and extends toward the middle lower lid. The no. 6 cleft begins at the commissure and extends toward the lateral lower lid. (Reproduced from Losee JE, Kirschner RE. *Rare craniofacial defects*. In: *Comprehensive Cleft Care*. Vol 2. 2nd ed. New York, NY: Thieme Medical Publishing; 2016.)

canthus, ectropion, and an oblique orientation of the palpebral axis, oftentimes referred to as an antimongoloid slant. Colobomas can be present at the inferior lateral eyelid (Figure 32.6).

Skeletal Involvement

Skeletal involvement tracks along the zygomaticomaxillary suture and excludes the alveolar process. The posterior maxillary buttress (pterygomaxillary buttress) can be foreshortened resulting in a steep maxillary occlusal plane and choanal atresia. The cephalad extend of the no. 6 cleft is the lateral orbital floor with a communication with the inferior orbital fissure.

No. 7 Cleft

No. 7 clefts are by far the most common of the craniofacial clefts. When they occur in isolation, they result in isolated macrostomia (**Figure 32.7**) often associated with a preauricular remnant. Conversely, they can occur as part of a known syndrome such as hemifacial macrosomia or Goldenhar syndrome which are associated with isolated no. 7 clefts,[9-12] or Treacher Collins and Nager syndromes which are associated with no. 6 to 8 craniofacial clefts.

Soft Tissue Involvement

The no. 7 cleft begins at the lateral commissure and extends to a variable extent posteriorly to the preauricular region. Most commonly, the cleft terminates medial to the masseter. A preauricular remnant may be present as well as varying degrees of microtia. Cranial nerve V may be involved as can the tongue and palate on the affected side.

Skeletal Involvement

The skeletal cleft passes through the pterygomaxillary junction and may affect the ipsilateral posterior maxillary and mandibular ramus, which can be vertically foreshortened contributing to a steel occlusal plane. The zygomatic body is variably dysplastic with an incomplete or absent arch. The cranial base can also be affected leading to asymmetry of the glenoid fossa and sphenoid bone.

No. 8 Cleft

The no. 8 cleft divides the facial clefts from the cranial clefts and is centered around the frontozygomatic suture. It is the lateral most of the cranial clefts. It is associated with several syndromes including Treacher Collins and Goldenhar syndromes.

Soft Tissue Involvement

The no. 8 cleft extends from the lateral canthus laterally to the temporalis region and can be associated with a coloboma of the iris or lateral canthal region.[13] In Goldenhar syndrome, an epibulbar dermoid cyst is present on the globe (Figure 32.7).

Skeletal Involvement

The no. 8 cleft is a cleft in the frontozygomatic suture.

Treacher Collins and Nager Syndromes

Treacher Collins and Nager syndromes are discussed elsewhere in this text. However, it is important to present these anomalies here to demonstrate how this specific syndrome relates to the Tessier classification of craniofacial clefts. It was Tessier who first attributed the no. 6, 7, and 8 cleft to Treacher Collins syndrome.[14,15] The classic findings of Treacher Collins syndrome include zygomatic hypoplasia (no. 6 cleft), vertical pterygomaxillary deficiency with a steep occlusal plane (no. 7 cleft), inferior-lateral decent of the lateral canthus (no. 7 cleft), and absence of the inferior and lateral orbit as zygomatic arch (no. 7 and 8 clefts). Nager syndrome has a similar phenotype to Treacher Collins syndrome but also includes limb anomalies.[16]

No. 9 Cleft

The no. 9 cleft is the rarest of the isolated cranial clefts and begins the medial movement of the cranial clefts. This cleft has been termed fronto-sphenoid dysplasia and is the cranial extension of the no. 5 cleft.

Soft Tissue Involvement

Soft tissue involvement includes abnormalities in the lateral third of the upper eyelid and brow. It extends up to the temporoparietal hairline which can be anteriorly displaced with a projection of hair in the temporal region. The orbit may be displaced laterally and microphthalmia may also be present. The frontotemporal branch of the facial nerve can be affected (**Figure 32.8**).

Skeletal Involvement

The no. 9 cleft extends superiorly through the superior-lateral orbit displacing the greater wing of the sphenoid and the squamosal temporal bone. This can lead to posterior rotation of the lateral orbital wall.

No. 10 Cleft

The no. 10 cleft is centered on the middle orbit and cephalic extensions and is a continuation of a no. 4 cleft.

Soft Tissue Involvement

Soft tissue involvement includes the middle third of the upper eyelid and central eyebrow. Eyelid deficiencies are common, ranging from colobomas to complete ablepharon. A paramedian forehead soft tissue furrow may extend to a frontal hair projection in the temporoparietal scalp (see Figure 32.8).

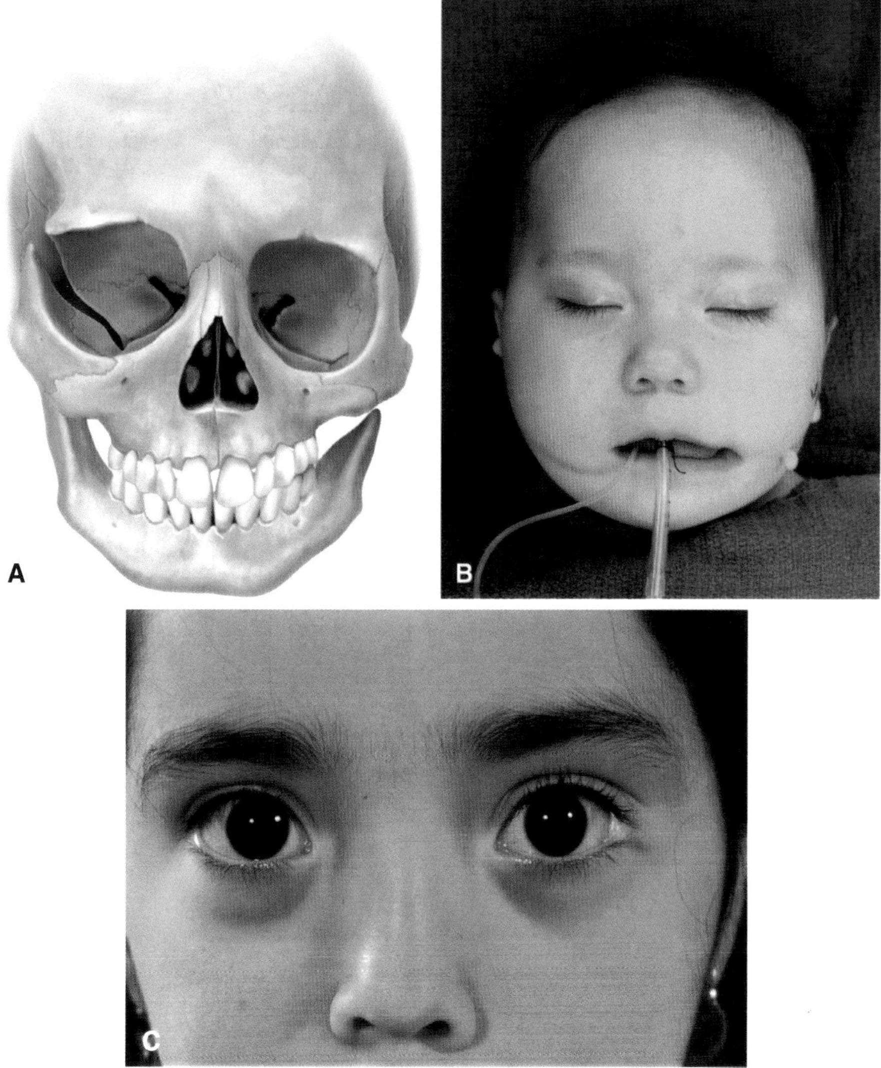

FIGURE 32.7. Left no. 7; right no. 8 cleft. **A.** Skeletal involvement demonstrates deformity of the lateral alveolus, extending through the pterygomaxillary junction to the zygomatic arch and involvement of the lateral orbital rim centered around the zygomaticofrontal suture. **B.** The right soft tissue no. 7 cleft is shown with obliteration of the lateral commissure and a preauricular skin tag. **C.** Left no. 8 cleft is shown with subtle changes at the lateral canthal region including brow malposition. (**B,C.** Reproduced from Losee JE, Kirschner RE. *Rare craniofacial defects*. In: *Comprehensive Cleft Care*. Vol 2. 2nd ed. New York, NY: Thieme Medical Publishing; 2016.)

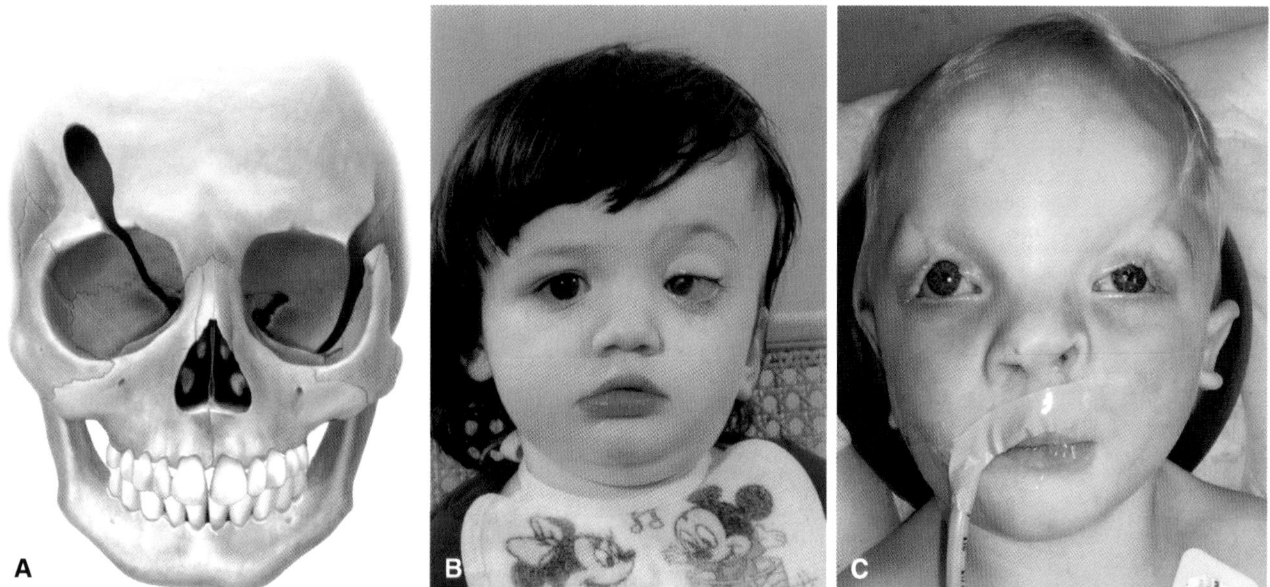

FIGURE 32.8. Left no. 9; right no. 10 cleft. **A.** Skeletal involvement of the no. 9 cleft demonstrates disruption of the superolateral orbit and frontotemporal region. Skeletal involvement of the no. 10 cleft originates with the superior orbital fissure and extends through the central supraorbital rim into the frontal bone. **B.** Patient with no. 9 cleft demonstrating orbital rim, brow, and forehead irregularities. **C.** Patient with bilateral no. 10 clefts demonstrating soft tissue colobomas of the medial third of the upper eyelid and brown and forehead involvement. (**B.** Reproduced from Losee JE, Kirschner RE. *Rare craniofacial defects*. In: *Comprehensive Cleft Care*. Vol 2. 2nd ed. New York, NY: Thieme Medical Publishing; 2016.)

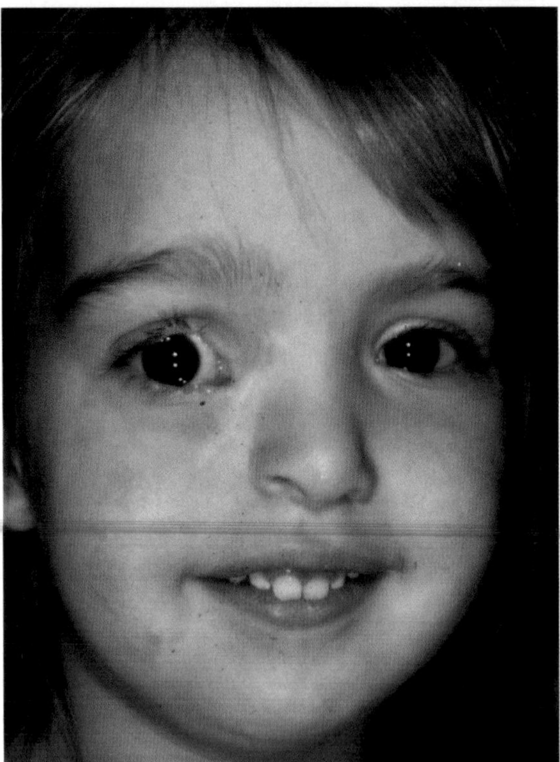

FIGURE 32.9. No. 11 cleft. Patient with right-sided no. 11 cleft demonstrating involvement of the medial third of the upper lid, canthal involvement, and orbital malposition. (Reproduced from Losee JE, Kirschner RE. *Rare craniofacial defects*. In: *Comprehensive Cleft Care*. Vol 2. 2nd ed. New York, NY: Thieme Medical Publishing; 2016.)

Skeletal Involvement

Skeletal involvement begins at the superior orbit, lateral to the supraorbital foramen, and extends cephalad. An encephalocele may develop through the anterior cranial fossa resulting in inferior-lateral displacement of the orbit and hypertelorism.

No. 11 Cleft

The no. 11 cleft is the cranial extension of the no. 3 facial cleft.[17]

Soft Tissue Involvement

This cleft originates in the medial orbit, and as such, the medial upper lid is often involved. Similar to a no. 10 cleft, eyelid involvement may range from a coloboma to ablepharon. The cleft may extend into the eyebrow and up to the frontal hairline with a fingerlike projection of hair extending into the medial third of the forehead (**Figure 32.9**).

Skeletal Involvement

The bony involvement of the no. 11 cleft involves the medial third of the orbital rim and may extend cephalad similarly to a no. 10 cleft. If the ethmoid sinus is involved, significant hypertelorism can be seen. The cranial base and anterior cranial fossa are uninvolved.

No. 12 Cleft

The no. 12 cleft is the cranial extension of the no. 2 facial cleft.[18]

Soft Tissue Involvement

The soft tissue cleft lies medial to the medial canthus, which is laterally displaced and extends cephalad to the medial eyebrow with effacement of the eyebrow root. A short anterior projection of the hairline occurs just lateral to midline.

Skeletal Involvement

The bony component of the no. 12 cleft originates from the frontal process of the maxilla and extends superiorly. The ethmoid sinuses are widened which contributes to hypertelorism and telecanthus. The anterior and middle cranial fossa may be widened but encephaloceles are uncommon. The cribriform plate and olfactory groove are unaffected.

No. 13 Cleft

The no. 13 cleft represents the paramedian cranial extension of the no. 1 facial cleft.

Soft Tissue Involvement

The eyelid and eyebrow are intact in this cleft; however, the medial brow may be inferiorly displaced. A frontal encephalocele may be present, along with a paramedian V-shaped frontal hair projection (**Figure 32.10**).

Skeletal Involvement

This cleft originates from between the nasal bone and frontal process of the maxilla where an encephalocele may be present leading to cribriform displacement and vertical ocular dystopia. A classic finding of the no. 13 cleft is the involvement of the cribriform plate, leading to widening of the olfactory groove, cribriform plate, and ethmoid sinuses. Especially when bilateral, this involvement can produce some of the most severe forms of hypertelorism encountered.

No. 30 Cleft

The no. 30 cleft is exceedingly rare with few cases reported.[19] It presents as an extension of the no. 0 cleft inferiorly into the mandible and cervical structures (**Figure 32.11**) and can range in presentation.

Soft Tissue Involvement

In microforms/mild forms, a lower lip notch may be the only sign of a no. 30 cleft. In more severe cases, the lip and chin may be completely cleft, with the addition of a bifid tongue, ankyloglossia, or tongue agenesis. There may be diastatic or atrophic cervical strap muscles with scarring and neck contracture.

Skeletal Involvement

Skeletal involvement includes an alveolar cleft between the mandibular central incisors that extends into the symphysis. The hyoid bone may be clefted, or absent, as well as the thyroid cartilage and rarely the sternum.

ORBITAL HYPERTELORISM

OHT is an uncommon malformation which results in an abnormally wide spacing of the orbits, eyes, and periorbita.[20] It may be isolated, associated with a craniofacial cleft or encephalocele as detailed above, or one of a variety of findings in any of several craniofacial syndromes. It is important to distinguish hypertelorism from telecanthus (or pseudohypertelorism). Telecanthus is the widening of the intercanthal distance often a result of medial canthal tendon avulsion or nasoorbitalethmoid fracture. In telecanthus, the bony orbits are in a normal position. In contrast, the hyperteloric orbit is entirely displaced and the bony distance between the orbits (interdacryon distance) is increased. In addition to the horizontal vector, orbits can be displaced vertically (orbital dystopia), anteriorly or posteriorly, and rotationally. It is crucial to identify the complete extent of orbital malposition to assist in the diagnosis and correctly identify the most appropriate treatment modality.

The classification of hypertelorism is based on the interdacryon distance, sometimes referred to the interorbital distance, which is defined as the distance between the junction points of the contralateral

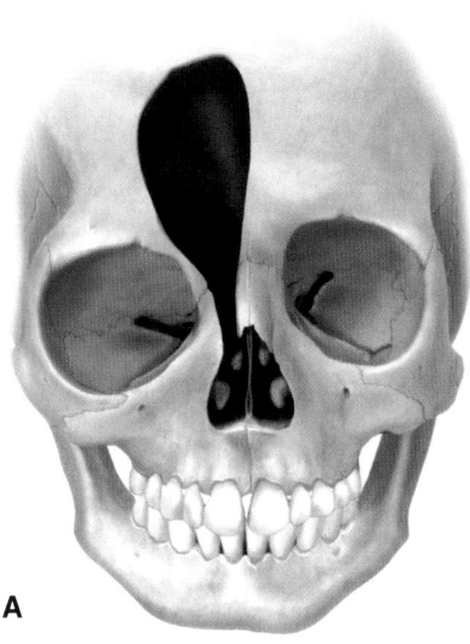

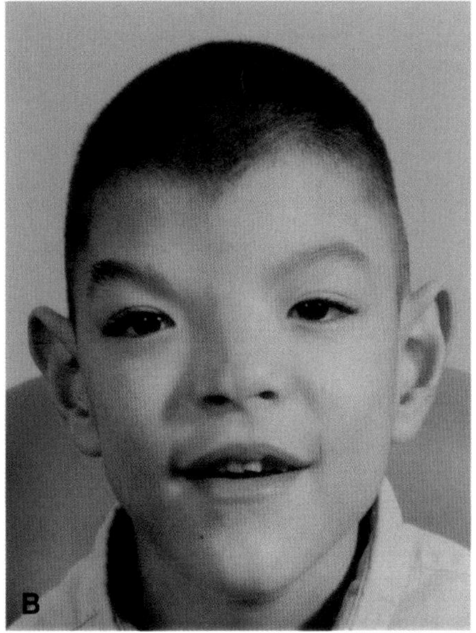

FIGURE 32.10. No. 13 cleft. **A.** Skeletal involvement occurs between the nasal bone and frontal process of the maxilla and is associated with widened ethmoids and hypertelorism. **B.** Patient demonstrating right-sided no. 13 cleft with preservation of the lid and canthal structures, orbital dystopia, and frontal soft tissue and bony abnormalities. (**B.** Reproduced from Losee JE, Kirschner RE. *Rare craniofacial defects*. In: *Comprehensive Cleft Care*. Vol 2. 2nd ed. New York, NY: Thieme Medical Publishing; 2016.)

lacrimal bones, frontal processes of the maxilla, and frontal bones.[21] This measurement is best made radiographically or intraoperatively; however, a rough approximation can be made clinically by subtracting 4 to 6 mm from the caliper measurement to account for the soft tissue. In an adult, the average interdacryon distance is 25 mm in a female and 28 mm in a male. *First-degree hypertelorism* is defined as an interdacryon distance of 30 to 34 mm, *second degree* is defined as 34 to 40 mm, and *third degree* is defined as an interdacryon distance of greater than 40 mm.[22,23] In contrast, in a growing child, the distance between the orbits changes over time. Table 32.2 demonstrates the normal interdacryon distance at varying times during development. In children, *first-degree hypertelorism* is defined as an interdacryon distance 2 to 4 mm greater than normal, *second degree* is 4 to 8 mm greater than normal, and *third degree* is more than 8 mm greater than normal (**Table 32.2**).

Craniofrontonasal dysplasia is a unique inherited form of hypertelorism associated with the X-linked EFNB1 gene.[24] It occurs in both inherited and sporadic forms; the typical manifestations include unicoronal or bicoronal craniosynostosis, hypertelorism, bifid or absent nasal tip, widow's peak, and wiry hair. Additionally, patients may have cleft lip and/or palate and limb anomalies including syndactyly.

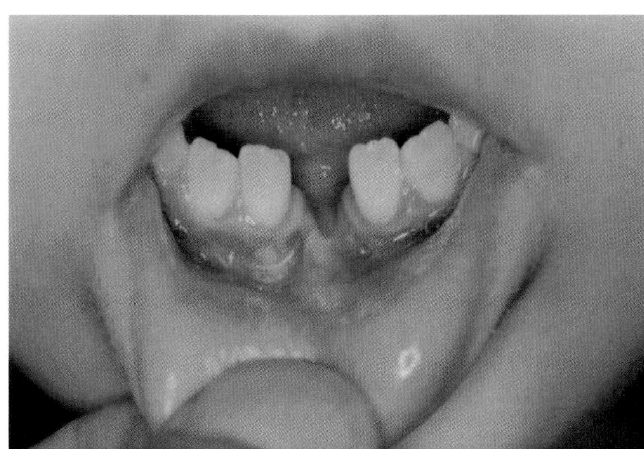

FIGURE 32.11. No. 30 cleft. Patient demonstrating a no. 30 cleft with bony and soft tissue deficiency. (Reproduced from Losee JE, Kirschner RE. *Rare craniofacial defects*. In: *Comprehensive Cleft Care*. Vol 2. 2nd ed. New York, NY: Thieme Medical Publishing; 2016.)

PRINCIPLES OF TREATMENT

Craniofacial Clefts

Each patient with a craniofacial cleft is unique and should be treated with an individualized plan based on the specific anomalies, functional issues, and social situation. It is helpful to break down various treatment modalities based on the ideal age at which they are performed. For patients with frontonasal dysplasia, frontoethmoidal encephaloceles, or any of the medial cranial clefts (nos. 11–14), early intervention may be warranted to reduce and separate the intracranial compartment from the paranasal sinuses. To avoid the dangerous sequelae of an ascending CNS infection such as meningitis, surgery should be performed as soon as the patient is old enough to tolerate the procedure (>3 months). Additionally, patients with significant ocular involvement including eyelid deficiency or displacement may require earlier intervention if eye lubrication is insufficient to prevent corneal damage.

Soft tissue reconstruction of isolated perioral clefts (nos. 0–7) can be performed at 3 to 6 months of age, similar to repairing a common cleft lip deformity. Similarly, palatal involvement should be considered around 9 to 12 months of age to maximize potential for speech

TABLE 32.2. NORMATIVE INTERDACRYON (INTERORBITAL) DISTANCE BY AGE

Age (years)	Interdacryon Distance (mm)
1	18.5
2	20.5
3	21
5	22
7	23 ± 4
10	25 ± 2
12	26 ± 1

development. Nasal anomalies can be treated at the time of perioral cleft repair; however, patients with frontonasal dysplasia and disorganized accessory nasal cartilage may benefit from surgery at an older age to minimize growth restriction. Medial orbital (nos. 3/11 and 4/10) clefts may require dacryocystorhinostomy if symptomatic.

Bony anomalies should be reconstructed in a delayed manner unless causing functional impairment. In general, cranial bone grafts are necessary to reconstruct the orbits, facial buttresses, and nose, whereas cancellous iliac crest bone grafts can be used to treat persistent alveolar clefts. Repair of orbital dystopia and hypertelorism should be avoided before school age and preferably performed at orbital maturity (6–9 years of age).

Hypertelorism

Hypertelorism is not a diagnosis. Rather, it is a physical finding which can occur in a range of abnormalities. When determining the correct treatment, it is crucial to consider patient's overall diagnosis as well as other pertinent physical findings. For example, hypertelorism secondary to Apert syndrome should be treated in a completely different manner than that caused by a no. 0/14 cleft.

When hypertelorism occurs, treatment should focus on safely decreasing the interorbital distance to less than 17 mm by performing a box osteotomy or a facial bipartition. Although these two operations both reduce the interdacryon distance, they differ significantly in the degree of other facial changes they produce.[25-28] A box osteotomy is limited to repositioning the orbits and the zygomas and can effectively narrow the interorbital distance while preserving midfacial and occlusal relationships. It is performed by mobilizing the orbits via a coronal incision, intracranial exposure, and orbital osteotomies in all four walls. Conversely, a facial bipartition procedure is ideal for patients who, in addition to OHT, also have maxillary hypoplasia, a narrow maxillary arch, and malocclusion. The bipartition requires mobilizing the orbits laterally and superiorly and by removing a central wedge of bone from the crista galli extending inferiorly to include the central frontal bone, ethmoids, nasal bones, and nasal septum. A central maxillary osteotomy/ostectomy is made inferior to the piriform and extending to the alveolus to complete the separation of the facial skeleton into two pieces. As the interorbital distance is narrowed, the lower facial skeleton is widened. In both procedures, rigid fixation with titanium miniplates are used to secure the bone segments, medial canthopexies are required to resuspend the soft tissue, and cantilevered bone grafts are used to maintain nasal projection.[29]

REFERENCES

1. Wolf SA. *A Man from Héric: The Life and Work of Paul Tessier, MD, Father of Craniofacial Surgery*. Lulu Enterprises; 2012.
2. Tessier P. Anatomical classification of facial, craniofacial, and latero-facial clefts. *J Maxillofac Surg*. 1976;4:69.
3. Kawamoto HK Jr. The kaleidoscopic world of rare craniofacial clefts: order out of chaos (Tessier classification). *Clin Plast Surg*. 1976;3(4):529-572.
4. Allam KA, Wan DC, Kawamoto HK, et al. The spectrum of median craniofacial dysplasia. *Plast Reconstr Surg*. 2011;127(2):812-821.
5. Gaball CW, Yencha MW, Kosnik S. Frontonasal dysplasia. *Otolaryngol Head Neck Surg*. 2005;133(4):637-638.
6. Guion-Almeida ML, Richieri-Costa A, Saavedra D, Cohen MM. Frontonasal dysplasia: analysis of 21 cases and literature review. *Int J Oral Maxillofac Surg*. 1996;25(2):91-97.
7. Jones MC. Etiology of facial clefts: prospective evaluation of 428 patients. *Cleft Palate J*. 1988;25(1):16-20.
8. Resnick JI, Kawamoto HK. Rare craniofacial clefts: Tessier no. 4 clefts. *Plast Reconstr Surg*. 1990;85(6):843-849.
9. Stark RB, Saunders DE. The first branchial syndrome. The oral-mandibular-auricular syndrome. *Plast Reconstr Surg Transpl Bull*. 1962;29:229-239.
10. Longacre JJ. The surgical management of the first and second branchial arch syndrome. *Br J Plast Surg*. 1965;18:243-253.
11. Converse JM, Coccaro PJ, Becker M, Wood-Smith D. On hemifacial microsomia: the first and second branchial arch syndrome. *Plast Reconstr Surg*. 1973;51(3):268-279.
12. Grabb WC. The first and second branchial arch syndrome. *Plast Reconstr Surg*. 1965;36(5):485-508.
13. Limaye SR. Coloboma of the iris and choroid and retinal detachment in oculo-auricular dysplasia (Goldenhar syndrome). *Eye Ear Nose Throat Mon*. 1972;51(10):384-386.
14. Raulo Y, Tessier P. Mandibulo-facial dysostosis: analysis; principles of surgery. *Scand J Plast Reconstr Surg*. 1981;15(3):251-256.
15. Roddi R, Vaandrager JM, van der Meulen JC. Treacher Collins syndrome: early surgical treatment of orbitomalar malformations. *J Craniofac Surg*. 1995;6(3):211-217.
16. Halal F, Herrmann J, Pallister PD, et al. Differential diagnosis of Nager acrofacial dysostosis syndrome: report of four patients with Nager syndrome and discussion of other related syndromes. *Am J Med Genet*. 1983;14(2):209-224.
17. Bodin F, Salazard B, Bardot J, Magalon G. Craniofacial cleft: a case of Tessier no. 3, 7 and 11 cleft. *J Plast Reconstr Aesthet Surg*. 2006;59(12):1388-1390.
18. Ozek C, Gundogan H, Bilkay U, et al. Rare craniofacial anomaly: Tessier no. 2 cleft. *J Craniofac Surg*. 2001;12(4):355-361.
19. Ladani P, Sailer HF, Sabnis R. Tessier 30 symphyseal mandibular cleft: early simultaneous soft and hard tissue correction: a case report. *J Craniomaxillofac Surg*. 2013;41(8):735-739.
20. Tan ST, Mulliken JB. Hypertelorism: nosologic analysis of 90 patients. *Plast Reconstr Surg*. 1997;99(2):317-327.
21. Tessier P. Orbital hypertelorism. I. Successive surgical attempts. Material and methods: causes and mechanisms. *Scand J Plast Reconstr Surg*. 1972;6(2):135-155.
22. Costaras M, Pruzansky S, Broadbent BH. Bony interorbital distance (BIOD), head size, and level of the cribriform plate relative to orbital height: I. Normal standards for age and sex. *J Craniofac Genet Dev Biol*. 1982;2(1):5-18.
23. Costaras M, Pruzansky S. Bony interorbital distance (BIOD), head size, and level of the cribriform plate relative to orbital height: II. Possible pathogenesis of orbital hypertelorism. *J Craniofac Genet Dev Biol*. 1982;2(1):19-34.
24. Wolfswinkel EM, Weathers WM, Correa B, et al. Craniofrontonasal dysplasia: variability of the frontonasal suture and implications for treatment. *J Craniofac Surg*. 2013;24(4):1303-1306.
25. Marchac D, Sati S, Renier D, Deschamps-Braly J, Marchac A. Hypertelorism correction: what happens with growth? Evaluation of a series of 95 surgical cases. *Plast Reconstr Surg*. 2012;129(3):713-727.
26. Kawamoto HK, Heller JB, Heller MM, et al. Craniofrontonasal dysplasia: a surgical treatment algorithm. *Plast Reconstr Surg*. 2007;120(7):1943-1956.
27. McCarthy JG, La Trenta GS, Breitbart AS, et al. Hypertelorism correction in the young child. *Plast Reconstr Surg*. 1990;86(2):214-225.
28. Tessier P, Guiot G, Derome P. Orbital hypertelorism. II. Definite treatment of orbital hypertelorism (OR.H.) by craniofacial or by extracranial osteotomies. *Scand J Plast Reconstr Surg*. 1973;7(1):39-58.
29. Wan DC, Levi B, Kawamoto H, et al. Correction of hypertelorbitism: evaluation of relapse on long-term follow-up. *J Craniofac Surg*. 2012;23(1):113-117.

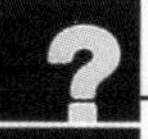

QUESTIONS

1. **The proper assessment of hypertelorism most appropriately includes measurement of which of the following?**
   a. Distance between lacrimal crests
   b. Distance between medial canthi
   c. Distance between pupils
   d. Distance between lateral canthi
   e. Distance between zygomaticofrontal sutures

2. **A one-year-old presents with brachycephaly, bilateral superior orbital rim retrusion with an interorbital distance of 28 mm, and a wide nasal root. Mutation in which of the following genes is associated with these findings:**
   a. FGFR2
   b. EFNB1
   c. IRF6
   d. TWIST
   e. TCOF1

3. **After cleft lip, the most common craniofacial cleft is:**
   a. no. 2 cleft
   b. no. 15 cleft
   c. no. 7 cleft
   d. no. 11 cleft

4. **Which of the following disorders is not associated with a craniofacial cleft?**
   a. Hemifacial microsomia
   b. Treacher Collins syndrome
   c. Cleft lip/palate
   d. Ethmocephaly
   e. Nasofrontal encephalocele

1. **Answer: a.** OHT is a lateral displacement of the orbits with an increase in the interorbital distance. In patients with OHT, all of the distances in the answer choices are increased; however, OHT is defined by the bony widening between the eyes best measured by the interdacryon distance, or the distance between the anterior lacrimal crests. Pseudohypertelorism, or telecanthus, can be seen after nasoorbitalethmoid fractures and results in an isolated widening of the medial canthi without lateral displacement of the globes. In skeletally mature patients, first-degree hypertelorism is defined as an interdacryon distance greater than 30 mm.

2. **Answer: b.** The patient described has bicoronal craniosynostosis and hypertelorism (defined as an interorbital difference of greater than a standard deviation over the age-corrected mean; 18.5 mm in a 1 year-old) and nasal anomalies. These findings are typical of patients with craniofrontonasal dysplasia, an X-linked disorder associated with mutations in the EFNB1 gene. Additionally, patients may have cleft lip/cleft palate, curly hair, and syndactyly. FGFR2 is associated with Crouzon, Apert, and Pfeiffer syndromes. IRF6 is the mutation associated with van der Woude syndrome, TCOF1 is associated with Treacher Collins syndrome, and TWIST is associated with Saethre-Chotzen syndrome. None of these syndromes is associated with the constellation of symptoms described earlier.

3. **Answer: c.** The Tessier rare craniofacial cleft classification describes both bony and soft tissue clefts. The Tessier no. 7 cleft describes a soft tissue cleft which starts at the lateral oral commissure and extends to varying extents toward the tragus. It is the most common of the Tessier clefts and is associated with multiple craniofacial syndromes including Treacher Collins syndrome and hemifacial microsomia.

4. **Answer: c.** Hemifacial microsomia is often associated with a no. 7 (lateral commissure) cleft. Treacher Collins syndrome is associated with no. 6, 7, and 8 clefts. Ethmocephaly is associated with midline craniofacial hypoplasia and no. 14 cleft. Craniofrontonasal dysplasia and nasofrontal encephaloceles are associated with no. 14 or 0/14 clefts. The Tessier (rare craniofacial) cleft classification is not used to describe common facial clefts such as those that occur in unilateral or bilateral cleft lip and/or palate.

CHAPTER 33 Ear Reconstruction

Akira Yamada and Arun K. Gosain

KEY POINTS

- The understanding of precise location, dimension, and proportion of the normal auricle is the foundation for optimal ear reconstruction.
- There are four principles in ear reconstruction: proper ear location, well-vascularized thin skin envelope, anatomical 3D framework, and beautiful curves.
- Team approach to address both hearing and external ear shape from infancy to adulthood will give patients optimal integration to the society.
- Timely ear molding less than 3 months of age, ideally less than 1 month of age, is a powerful option for miscellaneous ear anomalies to obviate the need for surgery.
- Current three major options for microtia reconstruction are autogenous rib reconstruction, Medpor reconstruction, and prosthesis. Surgeons should explain to patients the pros and cons of each option.
- Precise 3D framework is the essential foundation for total auricular construction.
- Secondary ear reconstruction may require total replacement of 3D framework, new skin flap/fascial flap coverage, and correction of the ear location.

THE NORMAL AURICLE

Anatomy

The auricle is difficult to reproduce surgically because it is made up of a complexly convoluted frame of delicate elastic cartilage surrounded by a thin skin envelope. Like spiral architecture in the inner ear, the external ear also has a spiral architecture, connecting the basal layer to the top layer. The auricle's rich vascular supply comes from the superficial temporal anteriorly and posterior auricular vessels posteriorly. The sensory supply to the auricle is mainly derived from the inferiorly coursing greater auricular nerve (C_2-C_3). Upper portions of the auricle are supplied by lesser occipital (C_2-C_3) and auriculotemporal nerves (V_3) (tragus and crus helicis), whereas the concha region is supplied by a branch of vagal nerve. Arnold nerve (CN 7,9,10) is an auricular branch of vagus nerve that receives contributions from facial nerve and glossopharyngeal nerve. Arnold nerve supplies posterior inferior external auditory canal and meatus, and inferior conchal bowl. This nerve mediates clinical phenomena, such as otalgia. Lymphatic drainage correlates with six embryonic hillocks. The tragus, root of the helix, and superior helix arise from first branchial arch (anterior hillocks 1–3) and drain into parotid nodes. The antihelix, antitragus, and lobule arise from second branchial arch (posterior hillocks 4–6) and drain into cervical nodes.

Embryology

The auricle begins to protrude from the developing face at approximately 3 to 4 months of gestation (**Figure 33.1**). The auricle arises from two branchial arches: mandibular branchial arch (first) and hyoid branchial arch (second). First branchial arch (anterior hillocks 1–3) contributes the tragus, root of helix, and superior helix (upper third of auricle). Second branchial arch (posterior hillocks 4–6) contributes the rest (antihelix, antitragus, lobule) (lower two-thirds of auricle).

Location and Dimensions

The auricle is located one ear length posterior to the lateral orbital rim, with superior pole level with brow and inferior pole level with alar base. Vertical height of an adult auricle is approximately 55 to 65 mm. Width is approximately 50% to 55% of its length[1] (**Figure 33.2**). Lateral protrusion of the helix is 1 to 2 cm from the scalp. The long axis tilts posteriorly 15° to 20°. Projection from mastoid to helix: superior 10 to 12 mm; middle 16 to 18 mm; and inferior 20 to 22 mm. The normal auricle is located immediately behind the face mask. Surgeons should avoid placing the new auricle inside the face mask: This is especially important in hemifacial microsomia because the vestige lobule tends to be located anteriorly and inferiorly and may be located inside the face mask. An anthropological study shows that the auricle is normally located approximately 20 mm behind the sideburn.[2] There is a trapezium-shape nonhair-bearing skin space, between the sideburn and the auricle in normal anatomy (**Figure 33.3**). Avoiding placing ear framework in this preauricular trapezium is important to prevent anterior inclination of the auricle.

MISCELLANEOUS EAR ANOMALIES

Cryptotia

Cryptotia is a congenital ear deformity in which upper pole of ear cartilage is buried underneath the scalp. The superior auriculocephalic sulcus is absent but can be demonstrated when you pull up the helical pole. Various surgical corrections are reported from Japan, due to the high prevalence of cryptotia, as frequently as 1:400. Nonsurgical ear-molding treatment may be applied if the child is in early neonate stage. The goal of surgical treatment is to create the retroauricular sulcus by skin grafts, Z-plasty, V-Y advancement, or

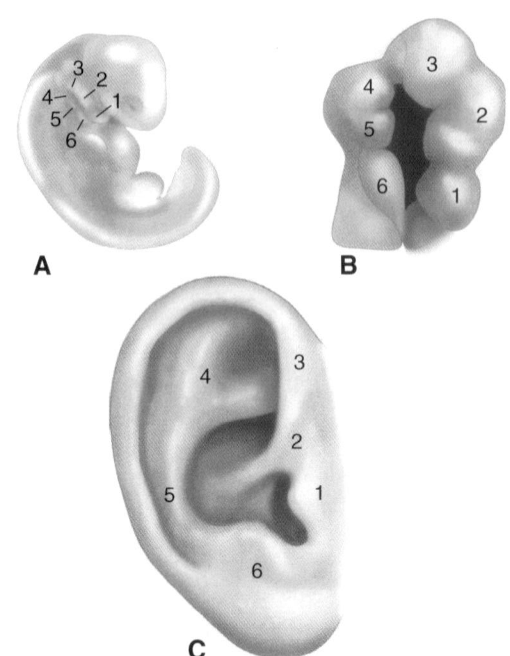

FIGURE 33.1. Embryology of the external ear. **A.** Hillock formation in an 11-mm human embryo. **B.** Hillock configuration in a 15-mm embryo at 6 weeks of gestation. **C.** Adult auricle depicting hillock derivations.

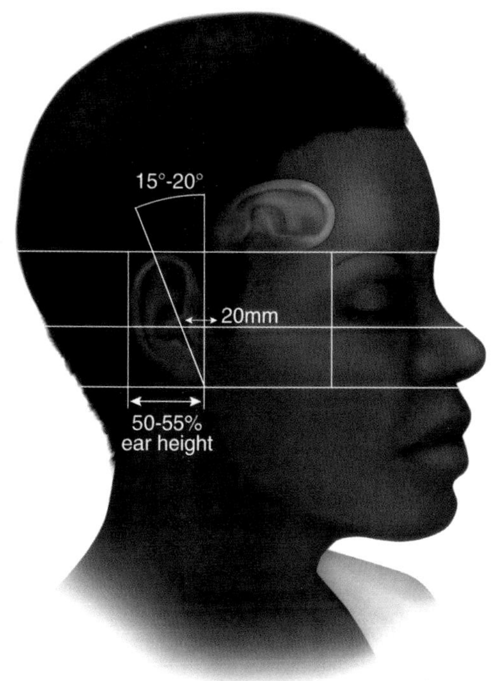

FIGURE 33.2. The normal location and dimensions of the auricle, in relation to the surrounding facial anatomy. FH, Frankfurt horizontal line.

rotation flap.[3] Common cartilage deformity associated with cryptotia is helix-scapha adhesion, which may be addressed by cartilage remodeling techniques.

Stahl Ear

Stahl ear, a rare congenital auricular deformity, is characterized by the third crus extending toward the helical rim. Stahl ear is classified into three types:

Type 1: Obtuse-angled bifurcation of antihelix; looks as though superior crus is missing
Type 2: Trifurcation of antihelix
Type 3: Broad superior crus and broad third crus (protruded scaphoid fossa)

Ear molding may work well if ear molding is started in early infancy. Surgical treatment is broadly categorized into two types: cartilage/skin excision and cartilage alteration. Type 1 Stahl ear needs special attention, to reconstruct missing superior crus, by using excised third crus or rib cartilage graft or creating superior crus by sutures or cartilage cutting.

Constricted Ear

Constricted ear is a concept proposed by Tanzer in 1975,[4] and his classification is shown in **Table 33.1**. In constricted ear, helix and scapha fossa are hooded, and crura of antihelix is flattened in various degrees. One gains an impression that the rim of helix has been

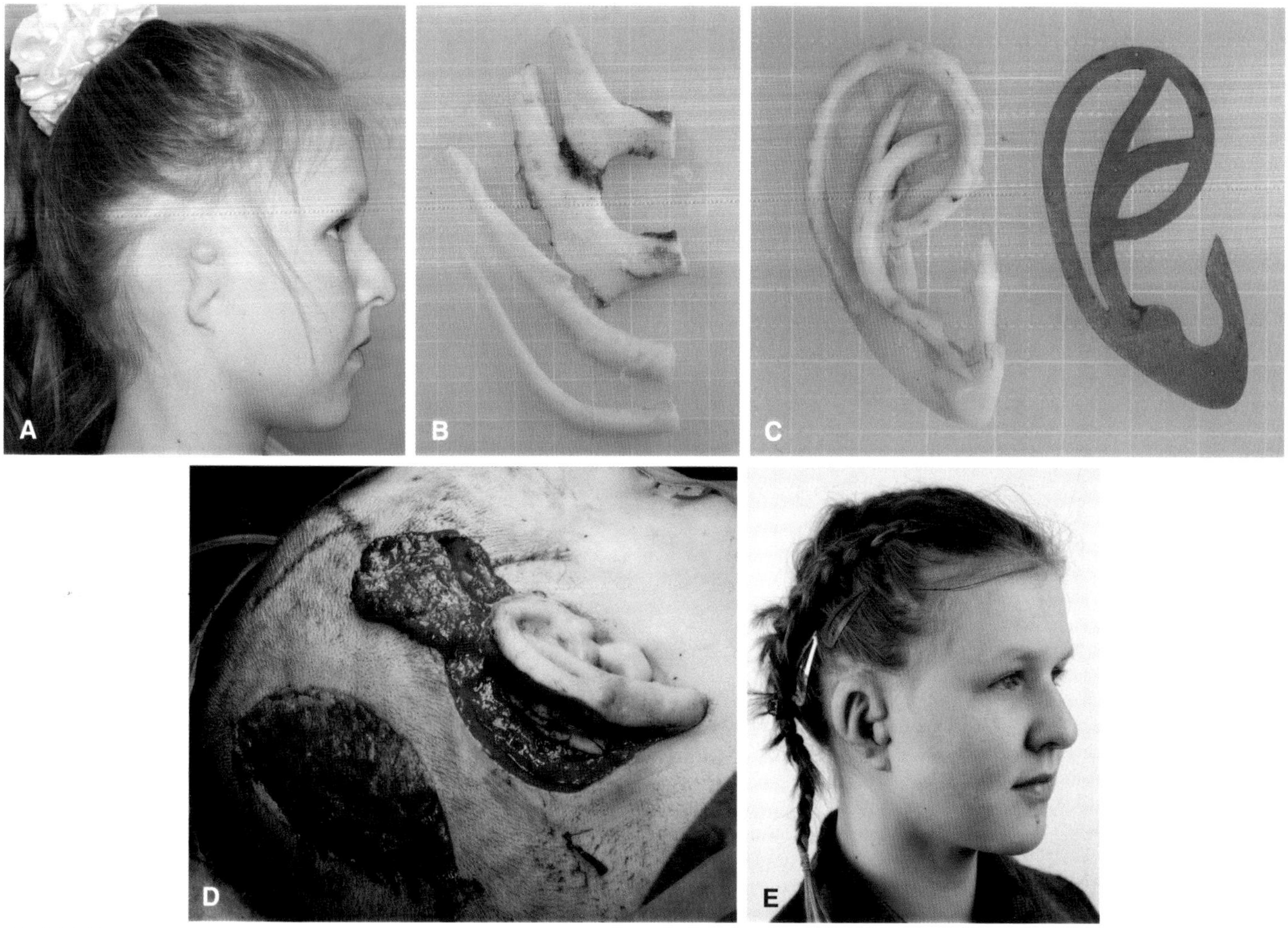

FIGURE 33.3. Nagata-type microtia construction: **A.** Preoperative view of an 11-year-old girl with lobule-type microtia. **B.** Harvested ipsilateral six to nine rib cartilage. Note the color of cartilage is white, meaning the perichondrium is completely left intact at the donor site for regeneration. **C.** 3D Framework with 52 mm type A2 template. **D.** Appearance at second-stage surgery. Temporoparietal fascia flap is raised, and the cartilage block is fabricated according to thermos-elastic template. **E.** The final view of the patient 1 year after surgery.

TABLE 33.1. TANZER CLASSIFICATION OF CONSTRICTED EAR

Group	Description
I	Involvement of helix only
II	Involvement of helix and scapha
IIA	No supplemental skin needed at margin of auricle
IIB	Supplemental skin needed at margin of auricle
III	Extreme cupping deformity; often associated with incomplete migration, forward title, stenosis of external auditory canal, and deafness

(From Tanzer RC. The constricted ear (cup and lop) ear. *Plast Reconstr Surg*. 1975;55:406.)

tightened. Constricted ear is often referred as cup or lop ear. Tanzer classified constricted ear into three groups based on the severity of defect/deformities.

Tanzer group 1: Mild deformities of helix, often called lop ear. Defect involves helical cartilage with minimum skin defect. Musgrave technique is a useful method to expand the helix. Through either anterior or posterior skin incision, multiple cuts were made to the curled cartilage, fan upward and backward, fixed to the curved strut made of concha cartilage graft. The skin is then redraped across the reconstructed framework. For milder constricted ear (group 1,2A), focusing surgical correction to construct helical curve is the reasonable option while keeping the original elastic cartilage framework, avoiding hard rib cartilage framework. When superior crus is deficient, partial helix plus superior crus frame from rib cartilage[5] can normalize the deformity.

Tanzer group 2B: Has both skin and cartilage defect in the upper one-third of the auricle. The loss of folding may involve antihelical crura, and hooding is more pronounced. The height of the ear is sharply reduced. Park[6] proposed versatile solution for group 2B constricted ear. For helical skin defect, Park modified the Grotting flap (postauricular flap), creating both skin flap and fascia flap with the same pedicle. For helical cartilage defect, eight rib cartilage is harvested, the helix is fabricated, and the entire length of helix is constructed.

Tanzer group 3: Most severe cupping and failure of migration. Brent recommends to treat severe constricted ear as if it is a form of microtia, when the construction is severe enough to produce a height difference of 1.5 cm. Nagata recommends treating severe constricted ear as a concha-type microtia, to replace the defective framework with a full rib cartilage framework.[7]

Based on the degree of defects, for both skin defects and cartilage defects, the authors' recommendations for treatment are summarized in **Figure 33.4**.

Ear Molding in Miscellaneous Ear Anomalies

Matsuo, who first reported ear molding treatment for congenital ear deformities, states that when the ear deformities are not hypoplastic, nonsurgical correction is easy and reliable.[8] Stahl ear responds well to the nonsurgical correction only during the neonatal period, whereas protruding ears and cryptotia respond until approximately 6 months of age (Matsuo). It is widely believed that the early initiation of molding is more effective because maternal estrogen in the neonate keeps ear cartilage soft and elastic. Most agree that if ear molding is started after 3 months of age, the response tends to be poor. Helix-antihelix adhesion responds poorly to the ear molding treatment and may not be the indication of the ear molding. Skin irritation is probably the most frequent complication, possibly due to tape or adhesive.

MICROTIA

Epidemiology and Pathophysiology

Microtia (small ear) is a congenital condition with unknown cause. Prevalence of microtia varies significantly among ethnic groups (0.83–17.4 per 10,000 births) and is higher in Asian countries for unknown reason. 80% to 90% of microtia is unilateral, and 10% to 20% is bilateral. There are more than 18 different microtia-associated syndromes with single-gene or chromosomal aberrations; however, there is no causal genetic mutation confirmed to date. A relatively common syndrome associated with microtia is hemifacial microsomia and Treacher-Collins syndrome. Isolated microtia rarely run in families. Treacher-Collins syndrome, inherited in an autosomal dominant fashion, often presents with bilateral microtia.

Classification

Many attempts have been made to classify microtia based on embryogenic development and severity of the deformities. Nagata's classification is based on surgical correction of the deformity[9–11]:

Anotia: Absence of auricular tissue

Lobule type: Vestige ear with lobule, without concha, acoustic meatus, and tragus

Concha type: Vestige ear with lobule, concha, acoustic meatus, and tragus

Small concha type: Vestige lobule with small indentation of concha (need lobule-type construction)

Atypical microtia: Cases do not fall into previous categories

Patient Assessment and Workup

About 20% to 60% of children with microtia have associated anomalies or an identifiable syndrome; therefore, individuals with microtia should be examined for other dysmorphic features. Microtia is a common feature of craniofacial microsomia, mandibular dysostoses (eg, Treacher-Collins and Nager syndromes), and Townes-Brocks syndrome, and these conditions should be considered among the differential diagnosis when evaluating an individual with microtia. If there is family history of syndrome, genetic counseling may be necessary.

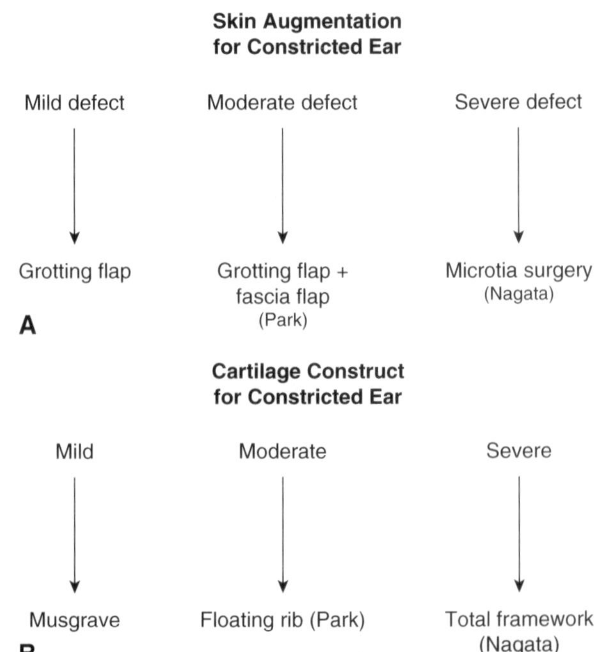

FIGURE 33.4. Recommended strategy for constricted ear. **A.** Skin augmentation strategy based of the tissue defect severity. **B.** Cartilage modification strategy based on the severity of defect.

Physical Examination

Identify the type of microtia, size, dimension, and type of normal auricle, if unilateral. Normal side may not be normal and may have subtle ear deformity such as helix-antihelix adhesion. Evaluate the symmetry of face, facial animation (partial facial paralysis is frequent finding), and dental occlusion. Hemifacial microsomia is often associated with difficult airway for intubation.

Diagnostic Studies

- Audiologic testing to determine conductive versus sensorineural defect
- Temporal bone imaging
  - High-resolution CT scan for evaluating middle ear ossicles to assess the possibilities of future otologic surgery
  - MRI to determine the course of facial nerve, often displaced, especially in the absence of pneumatized mastoid
- Rule out the presence of cholesteatoma (squamous epithelium trapped in the middle ear), present in 4% to 7% of atresia

Atresia and Middle Ear Anomalies

In bilateral microtia, early and conscientious use of bone-conductive hearing aid is imperative for hearing and speech development. Most of hearing deficits in children with bilateral microtia are managed with hearing aids. Treatments of microtia ideally involve reconstruction of the external ear and the restoration of normal hearing.[12] Hearing impairment in microtia is related to abnormal auditory canal, tympanic membrane, and middle ear. The problem is conduction. Typically, microtia patients have a hearing threshold of 40 to 60 dB on the affected side. By comparison, normal function allows us to hear sounds between 0 and 20 dB. Regarding middle ear surgery for hearing restoration, most surgeons presently feel that potential gains from middle ear surgery in unilateral microtia are outweighed by the potential risks and complications for the surgery, and this surgery should be reserved for bilateral cases. Careful selection of the atresia surgery candidate is important to achieve optimal outcome and more importantly to avoid unnecessary surgery and its complications. Jahrsdoerfer criteria are a widely accepted guideline to select atresia surgery candidates.[13] The bone-anchored hearing aid (BAHA; Cochlear, Mölnlycke, Sweden; and Ponto; Oticon, Kongeballen, Denmark) has been used since 1977, which does not need functioning middle ear or patent canal. In microtia patients, BAHA was initially started to use for bilateral microtia with bilateral conducting hearing loss: Unilateral BAHA is usually placed because a single aid will stimulate both cochlea simultaneously. The drawback of BAHA is the interface between titanium and skin: It may cause skin irritation or infection. BAHA has a retention rate of over 95% on long-term follow-up, with a soft-tissue reaction rate of 30%.[14]

Syndromes Associated With Microtia

Craniofacial Microsomia

Microtia associated with craniofacial microsomia needs attention for specific characteristics.[15]

Dystopic vestige: To achieve symmetry of the vertical dimension of the auricles, dystopic vestige must be transposed backward, and upward, either as a surgery before 3D framework placement, or simultaneous transposition[16] with 3D framework placement. Mistakes are often made to use vestige lobule in the face mask, without transposing it.

Low hairline: Low hairline is a part of abnormal hairline most often seen in hemifacial microsomia and Treacher-Collins syndrome. Abnormally low hairline is often associated with missing sideburns, which can confuse surgeons on where to place the new auricle. Avoiding hairline may cause abnormal location of the new auricle too inferiorly.

Soft-tissue defect: As a part of manifestation of hemifacial microsomia, microtia is often associated with relatively large depression of soft tissue around the auricular site. Fat grafting may help to improve it.

Vascular anomalies: The course of STA is often abnormal. To avoid injury to STA, preoperative Doppler ultrasound tracing of the STA course is advisable.

Treacher-Collins Syndrome

Because a patient with Treacher-Collins syndrome has a relatively smaller face, the size of a new ear has to balance with the smaller face. When you assess microtia in Treacher-Collins syndrome, two specific findings are important not to miss:

Low hairline: To eliminate hair on the new auricle, either temporoparietal fascia (TPF) flap or random-pattern fascia flap[17] is necessary to eliminate hair over the framework.

Coronal scar: When the patient already has a coronal scar, surgeons should be aware that STA is severed. That means TPF is not available for either low hairline case to cover the anterior surface or for Nagata-type ear elevation to cover the posterior surface. Occipital fascia flap may be indicated.

Surgical Management

History of Microtia Reconstruction

Sushuruta (6 BC) was probably the earliest surgeon who performed auricular construction, repairing the earlobe with cheek flap. Tagliacozzi described repair of ear deformities with retroauricular flaps. In 1845, Dieffenbach reported the repair of the middle third of the ear with an advancement flap. This technique may have application today. Early surgical attention focused mainly on traumatic deformities. However, by the end of the 19th century, surgeons began to address congenital defects, in particular prominent ears. The concept of microtia repair began in 1920, when Gillies buried carved costal cartilage under masts skin and elevated it with cervical flap. In 1937, Gillies also used maternal ear cartilage for more than 30 microtic ears; these were found to have progressively resorbed. Peer diced autogenous rib cartilage and placed it in a vitallium ear mold beneath the abdomen in 1948. After 5 months, he retrieved the banked mold, opened it, and harvested the ear framework for microtia repair. Steffensen's 1955 attempt to use preserved cartilage resulted in progressive resorption of the grafted cartilage. Tanzer, whose excellent results established autogenous construction with rib cartilage,[18] is considered to be the father of modern auricular construction. Surgeons from around the world visited Dartmouth-Hitchcock Medical Center, and autogenous construction spread across the globe. In the United States, Brent succeeded Tanzer in early 1970s, and Brent's artistry has influenced reconstructive surgeons for more than 40 years until today. Nagata's two-stage method emerged in the 1990s and has gradually gained popularity, becoming the strongest alternative to Brent's four-stage method. Autogenous cartilage remains the most reliable material that produces results with the least complications.

Timing of Surgery

The timing of auricular construction is governed by both psychological and physical considerations. From a psychological perspective, it would be ideal to begin construction before the child enters school, but autogenous construction should be postponed until rib growth provides substantial cartilage to permit a quality framework fabrication. Brent begins ear construction at age 6 years, when normal ear has grown to within 6 to 7 mm of its full vertical height and the amount of cartilage is enough for Brent-type framework. Nagata begins auricular construction at the age of 10 years, and chest circumference grows over 60 cm, at the xiphoid level. These two different timings could be explained by the difference of the amount of cartilage required: Nagata-type 3D framework needs larger amount of cartilage from ribs six to nine. In other words, surgeons are less likely to able to fabricate Nagata-type framework at the age 6 years.

Autogenous Construction

The two main techniques described for autogenous auricular construction using a rib cartilage are the Brent and Nagata techniques (see Figure 33.3).

- **Brent technique:** Four-stage reconstruction beginning at 6 years of age[19]:
  - Creation and placement of a rib cartilage auricular framework
  - Rotation of the malpositioned ear lobule into the correct position
  - Elevation of the reconstructed auricle and creation of a retroauricular sulcus
  - Deepening of the concha and creation of the tragus
- **Autogenous rib cartilage framework:** Rib cartilage framework has evolved from Tanzer-type in the 1950s to anatomically most complete Nagata-type 3D framework architecture (**Figure 33.5**).[20]
- **Harvesting rib cartilage method:** Brent harvested rib cartilage with perichondrium attached to it. Because the perichondrium is the scaffold of cartilage matrix regeneration, after harvesting rib cartilage, chest depression deformities are the usual consequences. Nagata harvests rib cartilage without perichondrium.[32] By leaving 100% perichondrium to the donor site, and bringing back diced leftover cartilage to the donor site, by creating a perichondrium pocket, Nagata stated that chest deformities are less likely to occur.[22,23]

Synthetic Framework

Although silicone breast implants are used, silicone ear framework is discontinued today. Silicone framework, introduced by Cronin in 1966, extrudes, causes infection, and loses definition in the long term. Porous polyethylene implant framework, newer synthetic material, was first introduced by Reinisch in 1991.[24] The advantage of porous polyethylene implant over autogenous construction is that it can be applied to younger children whose costal cartilage are less mature and not ready for autogenous reconstruction. The disadvantage of porous polyethylene framework includes use of TPF flap, long-term risk of alloplastic implant exposure or loss, and compromise of any future autogenous options. Early attempts were associated with a 42% incidence of framework extrusion leading to modifications of the original technique and coverage of the framework using a TPF flap. This drastically reduced the complication rate and is the technique of choice in his opinion. Long-term data to prove sustainability of porous polyethylene implant are not available.

Prosthesis

Osseointegrated auricular prosthetic reconstruction is complementary to other approaches and provides a reasonable alternative to poor autogenous options and poor synthetic framework outcomes. The disadvantages of prosthesis include intermittent soft-tissue problems, long-term maintenance, prosthetic remakes every 2 to 5 years, ongoing cost, compromise of future autogenous options, and need for a compliant patient.[9]

Secondary Total Auricular Reconstruction

The cause of unsatisfactory ear reconstruction can be divided into three main categories: inappropriate skin envelope, inappropriate ear framework, and inappropriate ear location. Most unsatisfactory cases have all three components. Therefore, radical total redo of everything (skin envelope, 3D framework, and ear location) may be the solution for the patients/family who are willing to go through the long and challenging surgery. Assessment of the patients is important to know what kind of surgical option would be optimal for the patients. TPF flap is the workhorse for secondary ear reconstruction.[25] The surgeon must assess the presence of STA from the base (near the caudal end of the auricle location) up to the parietal area (10 cm above the upper helix portion), by Doppler ultrasound. If TPF is not available, pedicle-occipital facial flap, or free vascularized fascia flap transfer are the option for the new skin envelope.[26]

Complications of Microtia Construction

Complication of both Brent technique and Nagata technique is rare in experienced hands. Most common complication from surgery is that the construct does not look like a normal auricle.

Framework problem: Surgeons must understand the basic aesthetic and proportion of the normal auricle to create appropriate 3D framework. Surgeons should receive intense hands-on laboratory training before starting clinical cases.

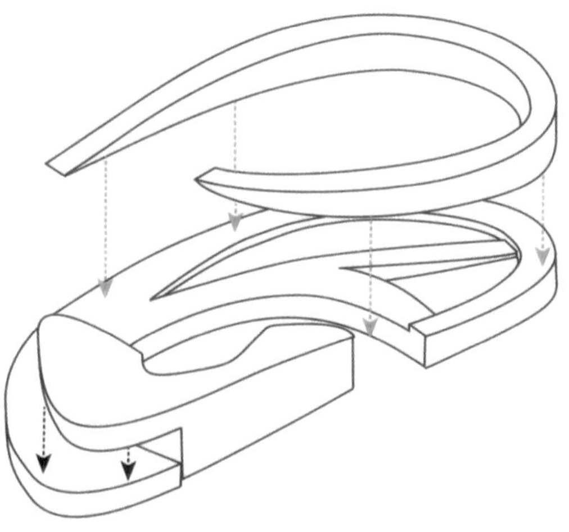

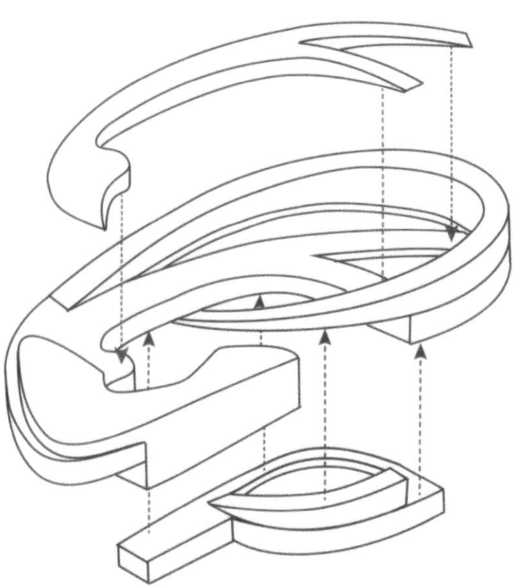

FIGURE 33.5. Architecture of 3D framework.

Skin envelope problem: There has been scarce discussion on what is the optimal thickness of the skin flap for ear reconstruction. Too thick skin flap will make ear definition poor; on the other hand, too thin skin flap may die: Surgeons have to walk on a fine line between the two. Nagata stated that proper skin thickness for ear reconstruction is 2 mm.

Ear position problem: Various types of ear malposition are possible. Surrounding pathological anatomy influences surgeon's judgment. To avoid misjudgment of ear positioning, careful assessment of anatomy around the microtia site is important: overall facial symmetry, distance between lateral canthus to the vestige, location of vestige lobule, presence of low hairline. Low hairline is easy to miss and that may cause low-set ear. To avoid hair in the reconstructed ear, ear position may be compromised by some surgeons: Ear may be located too low or inclined forward. Ear positioning in secondary reconstruction is challenging because of inherent and acquired abnormal anatomy around the ear site.

Poor definition: Poor definition is one of the most frequent unfavorable outcomes of total ear reconstruction. To create ear definition, skin flaps have to be balanced perfectly with 3D framework, have to have adequate thickness of skin flap—not too thick, not too thin—and must have enough space between cartilage to set in the skin flap. For example, if both helix and antihelix are too wide, there is minimum space between two structures, thus skin flap will not go into that space.

Atelectasis: Postoperative pain from rib cartilage harvest may aggravate atelectasis. This can be improved with infusion pumps of local anesthetics.

Skin flap necrosis: In the Nagata technique, lobule split technique requires a delicate, meticulous split of the lobule right in the middle. If the lobule was not split in the middle, uneven split may cause partial skin necrosis. To make split lobule more mobile, the split must be performed down to the fascia level. Incomplete, shallow split may cause insufficient rotation and may cause tension to the skin flap that may lead to skin flap necrosis. Relatively large subcutaneous pedicle for posterior skin flap must be preserved to prevent skin flap necrosis.[27]

Infection: Immediate postoperative infection after total ear reconstruction is rare (<0.5%). Brent stated that if the patient is free of infection at 10 days after surgery, infection is less likely to happen afterward. If you see any sign of infection, such as redness, pain, fever, and fluctuation or discharge from the wound, careful monitoring is mandatory, and incision and drainage may be necessary. If wires are used for framework, the wires should be removed, otherwise infection may persist. Prevention: For concha-type microtia, it is important to understand and recognize the middle ear pathology (otitis media/cholesteatoma) preoperatively.

Hematoma: Condition is rare (0.3%), but devastating. Early recognition is vital. Treatment is immediate draining.

Cartilage resorption: Cartilage gets nutritional supply from the surrounding environment not via vessels but through diffusion. Therefore, cartilage resorption is believed to be caused by insufficient blood supply to the tissue surrounding the cartilage. Traditional ear elevation is performed by cutting posterior vascular supply and simply placing the skin graft behind the auricle. Nagata believes that placing TPF flap, covering the entire posterior surface of the auricle, will augment vascular supply to the cartilage framework and prevent the cartilage resorption.

Hypertrophic scar: Oblique donor site skin incision is more likely to cause hypertrophic scar. Transverse skin incision parallel to skin wrinkle is better to prevent hypertrophic scar.

Framework extrusion: Exposure of framework is more common in synthetic framework than autogenous rib cartilage framework. Conservative treatment with frequent dressing change may heal the wound for autogenous framework, but less likely to heal for synthetic framework. Because of scar tissue surrounding the exposure, attempting primary closure is difficult, and well-perfused flap coverage may be the only solution. If the local skin flap is not available, fascial flap such as TPF, deep temporal fascia flap, or occipital flap may be necessary.

Wire extrusion: Brent uses nylon sutures for framework fixation to avoid wire extrusion. Nagata and Firmin use fine wires (38G) for fixation. Nagata believes that rigid fixation is optimal for cartilage framework fixation because cartilage pieces, unlike bone pieces, are less likely to fuse together, simply getting fibrous union. Once the patient/family notice the wire exposure, it is important to remove it immediately, otherwise it may cause resorption of cartilage or infection.

Thinning of temporal hair from fascia flap harvest: The Nagata technique routinely uses TPF flap for ear elevation to cover the entire posterior aspect of the new auricle.[28] TPF may also be used in low hairline cases or Medpor framework to cover anterior surface of the framework. TPF is located immediately below the hair follicles. Therefore, aggressive dissection or too much heat from coagulation hemostasis may knock out hair follicles located just above the TPF layer sharp flap dissection with scalpel usually does not cause alopecia.

PARTIAL AURICULAR DEFECT

The key of partial ear reconstruction is how you connect the new parts blending smoothly with existing anatomical architecture. Defects involves helical rim especially need careful planning how the smooth curve transition between old and new helix will be made. Pure helical rim defects are best closed by advancing the helix in both directions, as described by Antia and Buch.[29] This technique also may be applied to correct the asymmetry of ear size (make larger auricle small) for otoplasty. Major middle-third auricular defects are classically repaired with a cartilage graft that is either covered by an adjacent skin flap, rotated postauricular island flap (flip-flop flap),[30] or inserted via Converse tunnel procedure. Pearl[31] applied two-stage total ear reconstruction principle to the partial amputation of the auricle. He created partial ear framework made of rib cartilage, then attached to the remaining framework, covered it with posterior-based skin flap. Partial auricular defect can be repaired by one-stage auricular reconstruction with rib cartilage framework covered with TPF flap and scalp skin graft. Techniques for managing specific regional defects follow.

- **Upper-third defects** (in increasing order of size and complexity):
  - □ Local skin flaps
  - □ Helical advancement
  - □ Contralateral conchal cartilage graft covered with a retroauricular flap
  - □ Chondrocutaneous composite flap
  - □ Rib cartilage graft covered with retroauricular skin or temporoparietal flap/skin graft
- **Middle-third defects:**
  - □ Primary closure with excision of accessory triangles
  - □ Helical advancement
  - □ Conchal cartilage graft and retroauricular flap
  - □ Rib cartilage graft and retroauricular flap and/or temporoparietal flap
- **Lower-third auricular defects:** Most of the available method use two-stage retroauricular flap to create the lobule.[32] Earlobe does not contain cartilage. A reconstructed earlobe, however, will maintain its contour only if cartilage is included, analogous to nonanatomic alar rim grafts. The cartilage is placed beneath the cheek/retroauricular skin in the first stage. In the second stage, an incision is made around the cartilage graft, and the flap is advanced beneath the earlobe as in a facelift.[33].
- **External auditory canal:** Stenosis can be treated by a full-thickness graft applied over an acrylic mold, provided a reasonable recipient vascular bed can be prepared. Occasionally, multiple Z-plasties are used to relieve webbing of the orifice, or a local

flap is employed to line the canal and break up the contracture. Restenosis after skin grafting is common. As a preventive measure, an acrylic stent is recommended for several months to prevent restenosis.

AMPUTATED EAR

Replantation

Replantation of amputated ears has been reported, and some excellent results have been obtained. If the replantation is successful, it yields superior aesthetic result compared with secondary reconstruction. However, the vessels are small and failure is common. Reattaching large pieces of auricular tissue as composite grafts is doomed to failure. The superficial temporal artery or posterior auricular artery must be available for microvascular anastomosis to consider replantation.

Banking of Ear Cartilage

Amputated cartilage can be banked under postauricular skin, TPF, or volar forearm. The success of banking is inconsistent.

Mladick's pocket principle[34]**:** Dermabrased amputated cartilage is reattached to the remaining auricle, then buried underneath the retroauricular skin pocket. The graft is left in place for 3 weeks, then at the second-stage surgery, cartilage is exposed with soft tissue attached on the cartilage, and the skin is grafted to complete the reconstruction.

Baudet's fenestration techniques[35]**:** Posterior skin of the amputated part is removed. Fenestration is made in avulsed auricular cartilage to increase the vascular recipient area.

CAULIFLOWER EAR

A hematoma may result from trauma and frequently occurs in aggressive contact sports such as wrestlers. Unless evacuated, the blood tends to become cartilaginous, resulting in the so-called cauliflower ear. Once fully developed, the cauliflower ear requires surgical correction. Hematomas may require repeated aspirations or an incision to fully evacuate. Bolster sutures to the auricle to eliminate the space between the skin against the cartilage usually prevent reoccurrence.

REFERENCES

1. Tolleth H. Artistic anatomy, dimensions, and proportions of the external ear. *Clin Plast Surg.* 1978;5(3):337-345.
   A must-read to understand the aesthetics of the auricle for both cosmetic and reconstructive surgery.
2. Yamada A. Anthropometric study of ear position and its clinical application to the total external ear reconstruction. *Bull Osaka Med Coll.* 2009;55(2):81-89.
3. Yanai A, Tange I, Bandoh Y, et al. Our method of correcting cryptotia. *Plast Reconstr Surg.* 1988;82(6):965-972.
4. Tanzer RC. The constricted ear (cup and lop) ear. *Plast Reconstr Surg.* 1975;55:406.
   The concept of constricted ear is described in detail.
5. Kon M, van Wijk MP. T-bar reconstruction of constricted ears and a new classification. *J Plast Reconstr Aesthet Surg.* 2014;67(3):358-361.
6. Park C. A new corrective method for the Tanzer's group IIB constricted ear: helical expansion using a free-floating costal cartilage. *Plast Reconstr Surg.* 2009;123(4):1209-1219.
7. Nagata S. Alternative surgical methods of treatment for the constricted ear. *Clin Plast Surg.* 2002;29(2):301-315.
8. Matsuo K, Hirose T, Tomono T, et al. Nonsurgical correction of congenital auricular deformities in the early neonate: a preliminary report. *Plast Reconstr Surg.* 1984;73(1):38-51.
9. Nagata S. The modification stages involved in the total reconstruction of the auricle: part I. The modification in the grafting of the three-dimensional costal cartilage framework (3-D frame) for the lobule type microtia. *Plast Reconstr Surg* 1994;93:221-230.
10. Nagata S. The modification stages involved in the total reconstruction of the auricle: part II. The modification in the grafting of the three-dimensional costal cartilage framework (3-D frame) for the concha type microtia. *Plast Reconstr Surg.* 1994;93:231-242.
11. Nagata S. The modification stages involved in the total reconstruction of the auricle: part III. The modification in the grafting of the three-dimensional costal cartilage framework (3-D frame) for the small concha type microtia. *Plast Reconstr Surg.* 1994;93:243-253.
    References 9 to 11 cover the original Nagata techniques in detail.
12. Wilkes GH, Wong JW, Guilfoyle R. Microtia reconstruction. *Plast Reconstr Surg.* 2014;134(3):464e-479e.
13. Jahrsdoerfer RA, Yeakley JW, Aguilar EA, et al. Grading system for the selection of patients with congenital aural atresia. *Am J Otol.* 1992;13(1):6-12.
14. Roman S, Nicollas R, Triglia JM. Practice guidelines for bone anchored hearing aids in children. *Eur Ann Otorhinolaryngol Head Neck Dis.* 2011;128:253-258.
15. Yamada A, Ueda K, Yorozuya-Shibasaki R. External ear reconstruction in hemifacial microsomia. *J Craniofac Surg.* 2009;20(suppl):1787-1793.
16. Park C. Balanced auricular reconstruction in dystopic microtia with the presence of the external auditory canal. *Plast Reconstr Surg.* 2002;109(5):1489-1500.
17. Oyama A, Sasaki S, William M, et al. Salvage of cartilage framework exposure in microtia reconstruction using a mastoid fascial flap. *J Plast Reconstr Aesthet Surg.* 2008;61(suppl 1):S110-S113.
18. Tanzer RC. Total reconstruction of the external ear. *Plast Reconstr Surg.* 1959;23:1.
    Landmark article of the start of modern autogenous ear reconstruction.
19. Brent B. Technical advances in ear reconstruction with autogenous rib cartilage grafts: personal experience with 1200 cases. *Plast Reconstr Surg.* 1999;104(2):319-334.
    The artistry of Dr. Brent is well described in this article.
20. Yamada A. Autologous rib microtia construction: Nagata technique. *Facial Plast Surg Clin North Am.* 2018;26(1):41-55.
21. Kawanabe Y, Nagata S. A new method of costal cartilage harvest for total auricular reconstruction: part I. Avoidance and prevention of intraoperative and postoperative complications and problems. *Plast Reconstr Surg.* 2006;117(6):2011-2018.
22. Kawanabe, Nagata S. A new method of costal cartilage harvest for total auricular reconstruction: part II. Evaluation and analysis of the regenerated costal cartilage. *Plast Reconstr Surg.* 2007;119(1):308-315.
23. Yamada A, Imai K, Fujimoto T, et al. New training method of creating ear framework by using precise copy of costal cartilage. *J Craniofac Surg.* 2009;20(3):899-902.
24. Reinisch JF, Lewin S. Ear reconstruction using a porous polyethylene framework and temporoparietal fascia flap. *Facial Plast Surg.* 2009;25:181-189.
25. Brent B, Byrd HS. Secondary ear reconstruction with cartilage graft covered by axial, random, and free flaps of temporoparietal fascia. *Plast Reconstr Surg.* 1983;72:141.
    Decent secondary ear reconstruction was started from here.
26. Nuri T, Ueda K, Yamada A. Application of free serratus anterior fascial flap for reconstruction of ear deformity due to hemifacial microsomia: a report of two cases. *Microsurgery.* 2017;37(5):436-441.
27. Firmin F. Ear reconstruction in cases of typical microtia: personal experience based on 352 microtic ear corrections. *Scand J Plast Reconstr Surg Hand Surg.* 1998;32(1):35-47.
28. Nagata S. Modification of the stages in total reconstruction of the auricle: part IV. Ear elevation for the constructed auricle. *Plast Reconstr Surg.* 1995;93(2):254-266.
    Nagata-type ear elevation technique is described.
29. Antia NH, Buch VI. Chondrocutaneous advancement flap for the marginal defect of the ear. *Plast Reconstr Surg.* 1967;39(5):472-477.
30. Talmi YP, Wolf M, Horowitz Z, et al. "Second look" at auricular reconstruction with a postauricular island flap: "flip-flop flap". *Plast Reconstr Surg.* 2002;109(2):713-715.
31. Pearl RA, Sabbagh W. Reconstruction following traumatic partial amputation of the ear. *Plast Reconstr Surg.* 2011;127(2):621-629.
32. Brent B. Earlobe construction with an auriculo-mastoid flap. *Plast Reconstr Surg.* 1976;57(3):389-391.
33. Bastidas N, Jacobs JM, Thorne CH. Ear lobule reconstruction using nasal septal cartilage. *Plast Reconstr Surg.* 2013;131(4):760-762.
34. Mladick RA, Horton CE, Adamson JE, Cohen BI. The pocket principle: a new technique for the reattachment of a severed ear part. *Plast Reconstr Surg.* 1971;48(3):219-223.
35. Baudet J, Tramond P, Goumain A. A new technic for the reimplantation of a completely severed auricle. *Ann Chir Plast.* 1972;17(1):67-72.

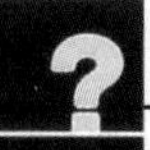

QUESTIONS

1. A 5-year-old boy is brought to your office by his parents regarding their concern for the appearance of his right ear. He is an otherwise healthy boy. On examination, the superior helix of the right ear is abnormally adherent to the temporal skin. Gentle retraction on the helix allows it to be pulled out to a normal position. What is the most likely diagnosis?

a. Stahl ear
b. Cup ear
c. Lop ear
d. Cryptotia
e. Helix-antihelix cartilage adhesion

2. Which of the following statements is correct regarding the normal size, dimension, and size of the auricle?

a. The long axis tilt is consistently within 1° to 5° in most individuals.
b. Ear height varies between 5.5 and 6.6 cm in adults.
c. The auricle is located approximately one ear width posterior to the lateral orbital rim.
d. Maximum projection from the mastoid to the helix occurs superiorly.
e. Ear width is usually less than one-third the height.

3. A child presents with vestige lobule with conchal bowl, acoustic meatus, and tragus. Based on current classification of microtia, what type of microtia does the child have?

a. Anotia type
b. Lobule type
c. Small concha type
d. Concha type
e. Atypical type

4. The lobule of the auricle arises from the:

a. first branchial arch
b. first branchial cleft
c. second branchial arch
d. second branchial cleft
e. third branchial arch

5. Which one of the following statements is correct regarding complications from autogenous microtia reconstruction?

a. The risk of chest wall deformities can be reduced by harvesting rib cartilage without perichondrium.
b. The procedure carries a relatively high risk of postoperative infection.
c. Hematoma formation is rare and is usually self-limiting.
d. The constructed auricle will remain a static size as the child continues to grow.
e. If the skin loss develops over the construct, a further surgical procedure will be almost always required.

1. **Answer: d.** Cryptotia is characterized by an abnormal adherence of the superior helix to the temporal skin, with varying degree of severity. Gentle retraction on the helix allows it to be pulled out to a normal position. If the child is less than 6 months of age, ear molding may correct the deformity according to Matsuo. Over 6 month of age, surgery is currently the only option for treatment. Cryptotia may be associated with helix-antihelix adhesion, which causes helix deformity.

2. **Answer: b.** The auricle is posteriorly tilted 15° to 20° (Farkas). The study shows that too upright or anteriorly inclined auricle to be aesthetically less pleasing. The vertical height of the auricle varies between 5.5 and 6.6 cm, and the width is usually 0.5 to 0.55 of the height (Tolleth). Projection is greatest inferiorly (~2 cm) and smallest superiorly.

3. **Answer: d.** The currently favored classification system for microtia is based on the surgical correction of the deformity, proposed by Nagata. Anotia: absence of auricular tissue. Lobule type: Vestige ear with lobule, without concha, acoustic meatus, and tragus. Concha type: Vestige ear with lobule, concha, acoustic meatus, and tragus. Small concha type: Vestige lobule with small indentation of concha (need lobule-type construction). Atypical microtia: Cases do not fall into previous categories. In concha-type microtia, 3D framework or may not accompany tragus portion.

4. **Answer: c.** The auricle develops from six auricular hillocks that form around the first branchial groove or cleft. Hillocks one to three (anteriorly) are formed from the first branchial arch (mandibular arch) and form the tragus, root of helix, and superior helix. Hillocks four to six (posterior) are formed from the second arch (hyoid arch) and form the posterior helix, antihelix, and lobule. The lobule is the last part of the auricle to develop. The external acoustic meatus develops from the first branchial groove, and the middle ear and eustachian tube develop from the first pharyngeal pouch. Part of the first arch cartilage (Meckel cartilage) ossifies and forms the malleus and incus of the middle ear. The ventral portion of Meckel cartilage disappears, and the mandible develops around it. Part of the second arch cartilage (Reichert cartilage) ossifies to form the stapes of the middle ear and styloid process. The portion between the styloid process and the hyoid bone forms the stylohyoid ligament. The third branchial arch forms the greater cornu and the lower part of the hyoid bones. The fourth to sixth arch cartilages fuse to become the laryngeal cartilages.

5. **Answer: a.** The most common late complication in auricular reconstruction is chest wall deformity, which occurs in approximately two-thirds of cases. Earlier surgery can cause more frequent chest wall deformity. Because the perichondrium is the scaffold of cartilage regeneration, harvesting rib cartilage without perichondrium will reduce the degree and frequency of chest wall deformity, although even with this method, the chest deformity may occur. The most significant early complications are skin loss, infection, and hematoma, all of which are rare; however, each must be identified early and managed accordingly to prevent extrusion of cartilage framework. The area of skin loss should be debrided and only reconstructed if the area is greater than 1 cm. Smaller defects can be managed by dressing. This is the advantage of autogenous rib cartilage framework over Medpor framework. Even a small defect in Medpor framework may be difficult to close spontaneously. Hematomas are not self-limiting and must be drained immediately to minimize the risk of skin loss. New constructed auricle commonly remains the same size over time (48%) but may increase in size as the child grows, (42%) in Brent's series.

CHAPTER 34 Management of Velopharyngeal Dysfunction

Asra Hashmi and Amanda A. Gosman

KEY POINTS

- In the normal palate, the levator veli palatini muscle rests horizontally within the middle third of the soft palate and functions to elevate and lengthen the velum posteriorly, against the posterior pharyngeal wall.
- Velopharyngeal dysfunction may be from velopharyngeal insufficiency, mislearning, and/or incompetence.
- Velopharyngeal competence results from apposition of the velum against the posterior pharyngeal wall and from motion of the lateral pharyngeal wall that causes closure of the velopharyngeal port.
- Sphincter pharyngoplasty entails 90° transposition of the palatopharyngeal muscles from the posterior tonsillar pillar to effectively obliterate the lateral ports of the velopharyngeal mechanism and decrease the diameter of the central port while still maintaining the centric opening.
- A sagittal or circular velopharyngeal closure pattern with good lateral wall motion is treated with a pharyngeal flap, which elevates the flap from the posterior pharyngeal wall after inset into the soft palate.

VELOPHARYNGEAL FUNCTION

Normal Function

Velopharyngeal competence results from apposition of the velum against the posterior pharyngeal wall and from motion of the lateral pharyngeal wall that causes closure of the velopharyngeal port. Inadequate closure of the velopharyngeal port, broadly termed velopharyngeal dysfunction (VPD), results in hypernasality and nasal air emission, which can be due to a variety of causes. In patients with a history of cleft palate surgery, the incidence of VPD is approximately 20% to 30 %.[1,2] It is important to accurately identify the etiology of VPD so that a customized treatment plan may be generated specific to patient's needs. A multidisciplinary team approach is essential in formulation of a plan. There are several radiologic, invasive, and noninvasive diagnostic options that can be utilized to correctly identify the problem. These include perceptual speech evaluation, nasal endoscopy, videofluoroscopy (VFS), magnetic resonance imaging (MRI), and nasometry. Once the cause is identified, surgical and nonsurgical treatment options can be employed to ensure best outcome for the patient.

Velopharyngeal Dysfunction

VPD is typically classified into three main subtypes based on its cause.

Velopharyngeal Incompetence

Velopharyngeal incompetence is physiologic VPD that results from neurologic or neuromuscular dysfunction, for example, myotonic dystrophy or amyotrophic lateral sclerosis. Acquired causes of velopharyngeal incompetence include head injury or stroke. It is important to note that even though most patients with velocardiofacial syndrome (also known as 22q11.2 deletion syndrome, caused by a microdeletion from chromosome 22 at the q11.2 band) present with cleft palate (overt or submucous cleft), a subset of patients with this syndrome may have velopharyngeal incompetence resulting from neuromuscular dysfunction, highlighting the necessity of correctly identifying the underlying problem.[3,4]

Velopharyngeal Mislearning

Mislearning results from inadequate closure of the velopharyngeal port, due to learned disarticulation. Hearing loss or deafness can also contribute to velopharyngeal mislearning. Speech therapy is indicated as there is no anatomic or physiologic cause associated with this type of VPD.[5]

Velopharyngeal Insufficiency

Velopharyngeal insufficiency (VPI) results from structural defect causing inadequate closure of velopharyngeal port. Patients with history of cleft palate surgery may have a short velum resulting in anatomic defect associated with VPD. Patients with submucous cleft (triad of bifid uvula, notch in the hard palate, and zona pellucida) may also present with VPI. Other anatomic causes include deep pharynx resulting from cervical spine or cranial base abnormalities, for example, in patients with Klippel-Feil syndrome.[5]

ANATOMY AND PHYSIOLOGY

Muscles of the Velopharynx

There are six muscles that play an important role in the velopharyngeal closure and speech production.

Levator Veli Palatini

This is the most important muscle in the soft palate, comprising middle 40% of the velum. Normally, the levator veli palatini (LVP) takes origin from the petrous part of the temporal bone and the Eustachian tube and decussates with the contralateral levator muscle forming a horizontally oriented sling in the soft palate. It is innervated by the pharyngeal plexus from glossopharyngeal nerve (CN IX) and vagus nerve (CN X) and functions to lengthen the velum and elevates it in the posterior direction. In patients with cleft palate, this muscle is oriented in an anterior-posterior direction (instead of normal horizontal orientation) and patients with submucous cleft tend to have diastasis of the LVP muscle (also known as zona pellucida) resulting in VPI in 15% of the cases.

Superior Pharyngeal Constrictor

This is a broad paired muscle that takes origin from the medial pterygoid and pterygomandibular raphe and inserts onto the median pharyngeal raphe. Contraction of this muscle results in anterior and medial movement of the posterior pharyngeal wall resulting in closure of the velopharyngeal port.

Palatoglossus and Palatopharyngeus Muscles

These muscles lie in the anterior and posterior tonsillar pillars, respectively, and serve to depress the soft palate. Some studies suggest that these muscles provide fine motor control of velar position during speech, by acting as an antagonist to LVP muscle.[6]

Tensor Veli Palatini

Tensor veli palatini (TVP) originates from the Eustachian tube and from the scaphoid fossa of the sphenoid bone, at the base of the medial pterygoid plate. Its tendon winds around the pterygoid hamulus and then inserts into the palatal aponeurosis by joining the muscle of the opposite side in the anterior 25% of the soft palate. As the name suggests, its action is to tense the soft palate, in addition to opening the Eustachian tube.

Musculus Uvulae

Musculus uvulae is the only intrinsic muscle of the soft palate and takes origin from the palatal aponeurosis. It likely contributes to the VP closure by providing bulk to it, by acting as a space occupying structure and a velar extensor. Studies suggest that anatomic reconstruction of musculus uvulae muscle may improve VP port closure and assists in the production of plosive sounds.[7]

All velopharyngeal muscles are innervated by the pharyngeal plexus, which receives contributions from CN IX, CN X), and accessory nerve (CN XI). The only exception is the TVP muscle, which is innervated by the mandibular branch of trigeminal nerve (CN V).

Physiology

Velopharyngeal mechanism separates oral cavity from nasal cavity for the purpose of speech and swallowing. During closure of velopharyngeal port, soft palate moves in a superior-posterior direction, the posterior pharyngeal wall moves anteriorly, and the lateral pharyngeal wall moves medially to achieve closure of the port. In some patients, the anterior motion of posterior pharyngeal wall forms a distinct bulge called the Passavant ridge. Velopharyngeal valve is typically closed for oral sounds (most consonants and vowels) and is open for nasal sounds (m, n, ng).

Closure Patterns

Croft et al. examined the velopharyngeal closure pattern on VFS and endoscopy and identified five closure patterns in normal and abnormal subjects[8] (**Figure 34.1**). Most common closure patterns in normal subjects are coronal patterns, which are caused by posterior movement of velum with less contribution from the lateral pharyngeal wall. Sagittal closure is predominantly attributed to medial movement of the lateral pharyngeal wall. Circular closure is seen when there is good motion of velum as well as lateral pharyngeal wall. Sometimes a Passavant ridge is also seen to contribute to this closure pattern, resulting in circular Passavant ridge closure pattern. Bowtie closure is seen primarily with movement of velum and posterior pharyngeal wall causing poor or minimal motion of the lateral pharyngeal wall. Jordan et al. used three-dimensional MRI to examine the closure pattern of patients with VPI and concluded that closure pattern also varied by sex with females demonstrating more circular closure patterns and males demonstrating more coronal closure patterns. Their study also suggested that length of the velum and thickness of adenoids may have the greatest impact on closure patterns.[9]

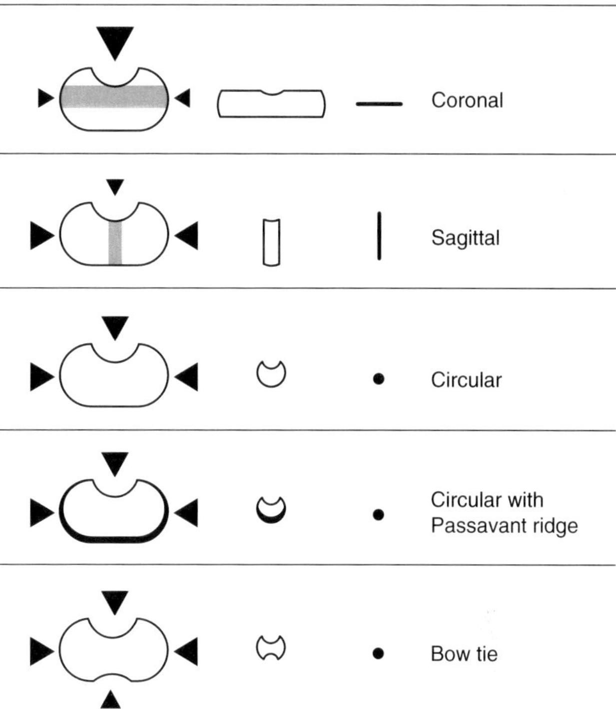

FIGURE 34.1. Velopharyngeal closure patterns. (Adapted with permission from Croft CB, Schprintzen RJ, Rakoff SJ. Patterns of velopharyngeal valving in normal and cleft palate subjects: a multi-view videofluoroscopic and nasoendoscopic study. *Laryngoscope*. 1981;91:265-271.)

DIAGNOSIS

History and Physical Examination

Obtaining a detailed history in multidisciplinary setting is important. Information should be obtained regarding feeding, swallowing difficulties, nasal regurgitation, hearing difficulties, and previous surgical procedures including surgery for cleft lip and palate repair, tonsillectomy, and adenoidectomy. History should also be obtained regarding any genetic testing for possible 22q11.2 deletion syndrome. If there is any concern for sleep apnea, then polysomnography may be obtained to evaluate the severity of sleep apnea and to identify whether it is central or obstructive in nature. Physical examination should assess dentition, occlusion, soft palate length, movement during phonation, and presence of fistula. Patients with clefts of only primary palate (especially those involving the alveolus) may have dental abnormalities, which can also cause speech disturbances because of interference with tongue movement. Jaw malocclusion may also be a major contributor to speech problems. Patients with history of cleft palate repair often present with class III malocclusion, where tongue tip is positioned anterior to the maxillary alveolar ridge. This can affect production of lingual-alveolar sounds (t,d,n,s,z) and even bilabial sounds (p,b,m).[10] The information obtained from history and physical examination should be appraised with speech evaluation to make a decision regarding the need for surgical intervention versus further diagnostic testing. For example, if a patient with a history of submucous cleft presents with absence of speech disturbances, then surgical intervention may not be necessary. On the other hand, if oral examination reveals normal anatomy despite speech abnormality, then diagnostic tests should be obtained to further investigate the cause of VPD.

Perceptual Speech Evaluation

A formal perceptual speech evaluation by a speech and language pathologist (SLP) is perhaps the most important modality in the evaluation of a patient with VPD. During speech evaluation, a skilled SLP examines the speech sample of a patient during normal conversation and with provocative sentences, by having the patient repeat some sentences with pressure-sensitive consonants (e.g., *Buy bobby a puppy*). The main components of speech assessed include language (receptive and expressive), nasal air emission, resonance (hyponasality or hypernasality), articulation, voice (hoarseness, high or low pitch), and intelligibility. It is important to familiarize oneself with the terminology commonly used while assessing a patient with VPD (**Table 34.1**). Some commonly used speech evaluation assessment tools are McWilliam Scale and the Pittsburgh Weighted Speech Scale. The Pittsburgh scale rates five aspects of speech including nasality, phonation, articulation, nasal air emission, and facial grimace. By assigning points to each component, an overall score is reached which can be used as an objective assessment of speech. CAPS-A (cleft audit protocol for speech—augmented) and UPS (universal parameters for reporting speech outcomes) are some other protocols that are utilized in speech assessment. Even though several protocols and speech assessment tools are available, the ear of the listener is considered to be the standard, and use of a set of standard sentences that isolates each pressure consonant is recommended.[11] The typical

TABLE 34.1. COMMONLY USED TERMINOLOGIES FOR PERCEPTUAL SPEECH EVALUATION

Intelligibility: Measure of comprehensibility of speech

Nasal emission: Escape of air through the nose during consonant production

Resonance: Relationship between sound reverberating in the oral versus nasal cavities, most perceptible during vowel production. In hypernasality, too much sound resonates in the nasal cavity usually seen with velopharyngeal insufficiency or fistula. In hyponasality, not enough sound resonates through nasal cavity, such as with the common cold.

Consonant: A speech sound produced by complete or partial closure of vocal cords (as apposed to vowels)

Fricatives: Consonants produced by forcing air through a narrow channel, such as (f) and (s)

Sibilant: A subset of fricatives where one still is forcing air through a narrow channel but, in addition, the tongue is curled lengthwise to direct the air over the edge of the teeth. English (s), (z), and (ʃ) are examples of sibilants

Plosives (or stop consonants): Consonant sounds that are formed by completely stopping airflow, such as (p) (lips), (t) (teeth), and (k) (back of the tongue)

Compensatory articulation: Articulation errors seen in velopharyngeal dysfunction patients resulting from an effort to compensate for increased pressure and airflow during speech

Nasal substitution: Replacement of oral sounds (p), (b), (t), and (d) for nasal sounds (m) and (n)

Sibilant distortion: Incorrect production of (s) and (z) sounds resulting from incorrect tongue placement

speech sample of a patient with VPD often reveals poor intelligibility, hypernasality, nasal substitution and glottal compensations, and weak pressure consonants.

Speech Videofluoroscopy

A static lateral radiographic view obtained during quiet breathing and production of sound can give information regarding palatal length, tonsil, and adenoids, as well as cranial base angle. Earliest reports of radiographic assessment of velopharyngeal mechanism appeared in 1909.[12] The concept of speech VFS was introduced nearly five decades ago by Skolnick,[13] which is a collaborative test between speech therapist and radiologist that provides information regarding lateral and posterior wall of the pharynx as well as length and movement of the soft palate based on sagittal and lateral radiographic views. Usually barium is instilled through the nose to coat the posterior pharyngeal wall and nasal surface of the velum. This highlights the velopharyngeal sphincter mechanism during its assessment. Subsequently speech sample is obtained by an SLP as the patient repeats some standardized words and sentences. Information can be obtained regarding velopharyngeal gap size, palatal length and stretch, pharyngeal depth, as well as the size of tonsil and adenoids. Depending upon patients' level of cooperation, this test can be performed as early as 2 or 3 years of age. VFS seems to be better tolerated by patients compared with nasopharyngoscopy (NPS), as it requires less level of cooperation from patients. Another advantage is that some objective assessment of the velopharyngeal gap can also be obtained with this test, as opposed to an NPS which does not allow any objective measurement. VFS does expose the patient to radiation, which is a downside of this test.

Nasopharyngoscopy

NPS directly visualizes the location of the defect and movement of velum during phonation. The test begins by instillation of local anesthetic and decongestant into the nose to increase patient comfort. A well-lubricated scope is then passed into the nose and views of velum, posterior and lateral pharynx, and velopharyngeal gap can be obtained while the scope sits in the middle meatus. This test is usually performed by the surgeon, and/or otorhinolaryngologist in collaboration with a trained SLP. An assessment of velopharyngeal closure pattern is obtained while the patient is asked to repeat standardized speech sample consisting of oral and nasal consonants and vowels. NPS is especially useful for small and asymmetric gaps, submucous cleft, and VPD persisting post pharyngeal flap. The patient ideally should be at least 4 to 5 years of age for this test, although it may be possible to successfully perform NPS on a very mature three-year-old patient.[12]

Magnetic Resonance Imaging

There has been a recent surge of interest in the utility of MRI in the assessment of patients with VPD.[14,15] MRI allows morphologic assessment of velopharyngeal anatomy, especially the levator muscle. It also provides information regarding the vascular anatomy of the neck which is especially important in patients with 22q11.2 deletion syndrome who may have medialized internal carotid arteries.[16] The advantage of MRI over NPS and VFS is that it is noninvasive and avoids the exposure to ionizing radiation. A major hurdle is the poor image quality, when images are obtained during active phonation, as children are usually only able to sustain phonation for 15 to 20 seconds, which limits the image acquisition time.[15] A three-dimensional dynamic, fast MRI obtained in oblique coronal plane has been proposed to provide better assessment and more precise measurements for patients with VPD.[14]

Nasometry

Warren and colleagues popularized the concept of nasometry, which allows measurement of oral and nasal air pressure and flow and calculation of velopharyngeal port size.[17] In the original design, a pressure transducer was placed in one of the nares and mouth and air flow meter was placed in the other nares. Quantitative measurement of oral and nasal pressure and airflow was made which was subsequently used to estimate velopharyngeal port size.[18] Warren in his study in 1985 suggested the use of the word *hamper* for assessment of speech because this word has a nasal-plosive blend/mp/. An orifice of >10 mm^2 has been shown to correlate with hypernasality.[19]

Nasalance (defined as the ratio of nasal sound energy divided by sum of oral and nasal sound) is the acoustic index of nasality that is primarily measured during this assessment. As the patient reads (or repeats) a standardized speech passage, computer-based analysis is done and a nasalance score is calculated (range 0%–100%). Even though a variety of cut-off values for normal versus abnormal are used (depending upon the speech stimulus), in general a higher score suggests more nasality. Nasometry is one of the few tools that indirectly provide objective assessment of velopharyngeal mechanism but the criticism to its use is its oversimplification of the VPD mechanism and its inability to predict the location of gap size.[20]

SURGICAL MANAGEMENT

If a patient is deemed a surgical candidate, then the choice of surgical procedure should be individualized and based on a host of factors. The goal of all surgical procedures is to decrease the area of velopharyngeal port and reduce nasal air escape during phonation. Size of the defect, closure pattern, and lateral wall motion are the three most

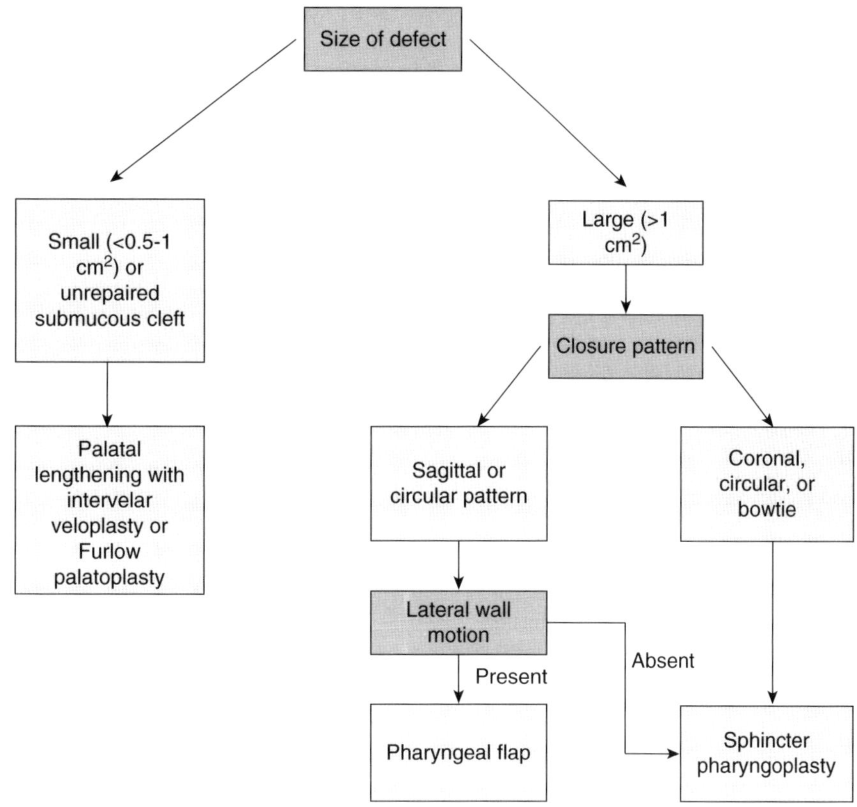

FIGURE 34.2. An algorithm for choosing the optimal surgical procedure for the treatment of velopharyngeal insufficiency.

important anatomic factors that should be considered in selecting an optimal surgical procedure for the treatment of VPI. **Figure 34.2** shows an algorithm for choosing the suitable surgical procedure for the treatment of VPI. It is important to keep in mind that functional repairs (see description later) yield a more anatomic local tissue rearrangement of structures in the soft palate, without adding tissue from neighboring areas (e.g., in pharyngeal flap, sphincter pharyngoplasty, or posterior wall augmentation procedures). Hence, functional repairs inherently have less risk of obstructive sleep apnea (OSA) and should be attempted whenever possible to reduce the risk of long-term airway complications as the patient ages.

Functional Palatal Lengthening

Functional palatal lengthening can be achieved by Furlow palatoplasty, or intervelar veloplasty. The main anatomic objective of these procedures is to achieve lengthening of the soft palate with retropositioning of levator muscle in the velum and closure of a small gap in the VP port. Sommerlad popularized the concept of radical intervelar veloplasty, described as complete dissection of the velar muscle complex off the nasal and oral mucosal layer in the soft palate as far laterally as the hamulus, where tensor tendon is visualized and divided medial to the hamulus. The muscle is then divided from the posterior border of the hard palate and then retropositioned and repaired in at least middle third of the velum (or more posterior to it).[21] Sommerlad prospectively studied pre- and postoperative speech outcomes in 129 patients with previous cleft palate repair, anterior insertion of levator muscle, and symptoms of VPI, who underwent palatal repairs by radical intervelar veloplasty technique and noted significant improvement in hypernasality, nasal air emission, and velopharyngeal gap closure.[22] Sommerlad et al. advocated that radical intervelar veloplasty should be considered as the first-line option in patients with VPI (especially those with levator knee or point of maximum velar excursion on lateral VFS more anteriorly located). However, if the palate is scarred and immobile, then rerepair is unlikely to improve symptoms of VPI and should not be attempted.

The more commonly performed palatal lengthening procedure was introduced by Leonard Furlow in 1986.[23] This procedure entails creation of two double opposing Z-plasties of oral and nasal mucosa with attached levator muscle. Lengthening is achieved by the concept of Z-plasty and reorientation of the levator muscle to a more anatomic posterior position, which is achieved by its double opposition technique. A recent study retrospectively analyzed the anatomic and speech changes of 29 patients with VPI in the setting of previous cleft palate repair or submucous cleft and confirmed that Furlow resulted in significant velar elongation, increased acuity of the genu angle, and retropositioning of the levator sling. In their study, Furlow resulted in improvement of the resting genu angle which was noted to be 10° more acute than preoperative assessment. Additionally, speech improvement and the absence of need for reoperation were most consistently associated with tightening of the genu angle.[24]

The advantage of functional repair (over more obstructive or nonanatomic surgical procedures for VPI) is that it reduces the long-term distortion of the airway which places patients at a lower risk for OSA, as they grow older and/or gain weight. This reduced risk of OSA is at the cost of up to 30% risk of failure (or incomplete resolution of VPI), which may be a risk worth taking to avoid long-term morbidity of OSA.[21,22,25] However, it is important to counsel patients about the possibility of failure and need for a more obstructive procedure in future if functional repair is selected for the management of VPI. Other methods of palatal lengthening include interpositional buccal flap and V-Y pushback palatoplasty.

Next category of surgical procedures aims to physically decrease the area of velopharyngeal port and resulting nasal air escape and hypernasality. These procedures include pharyngeal flap, sphincter pharyngoplasty, or posterior wall augmentation.

Posterior Pharyngeal Flap

Pharyngeal flap was first described by Schoenborn in 1876. This is a rectangular-shaped myomucosal flap, raised from the posterior pharyngeal wall and insetted into the velum.[26] This flap converts a

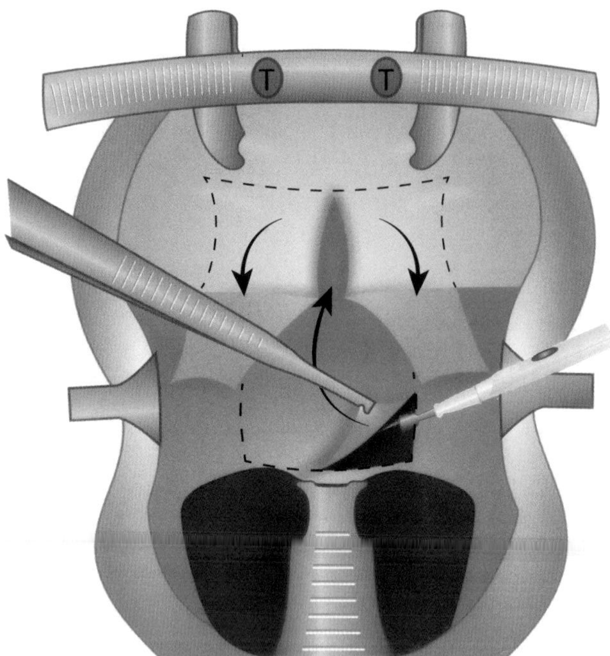

FIGURE 34.3. Pharyngeal flap.

large velopharyngeal port into two small lateral ports by creating a midline obstruction between oral and nasal cavities (**Figure 34.3**). Even though Schoenborn's original design for pharyngeal flap was inferiorly based, various modifications of posterior pharyngeal flap have been described in the literature. In general, inferiorly based flaps are considered easier to attach, and superiorly based flap have the advantage of giving a larger flap; however, data are not conclusive on superiority of one flap design over another.[27] Some of the demerits of inferiorly based flap include limitation of its length and possible inferiorly directed pull onto the velum, which is in contradiction to the goals of effective velopharyngeal closure mechanism. Even though theoretically decreasing the port size by virtue of flap attachment into the velum should decrease the symptoms of VPI secondary to all types of ports, pharyngeal flap is best suited for patients with a sagittal or circularly oriented closure patterns. Additionally, adequate lateral wall motion is also important for the success of the flap.[28] Other factors that may play a role in the success of pharyngeal flap are flap width and level of attachment. Flaps that are too wide may be counterproductive by causing symptoms of hyponasality and sleep apnea; on the other hand, flaps that are not wide enough may be ineffective. Width of the flap is generally driven by surgeon experience and supplemented by preoperative diagnostic workup and information gained by videoflouroscopy and/or nasal endoscopy regarding port size, orientation, and lateral pharyngeal wall motion.[29] Pharyngeal flap is ideally inserted at the level of C1 to allow adequate elevation of the velum.

Sphincter Pharyngoplasty

Sphincter pharyngoplasty procedure was introduced by Hynes in 1950, who described the use of bilateral salpingopharyngeus muscles for decreasing the dimension of velopharyngeal port.[30] Since the first description, several modifications of this procedure have been reported in literature.[31,32] Currently, the most commonly used design of this procedure entails 90° transposition of the superiorly based palatopharyngeal muscles from the posterior tonsillar pillars to the posterior pharyngeal wall (**Figure 34.4**). It is best suited for a large posterior gap with coronal, circular, or bowtie closure pattern and/or poor lateral wall motion. An advantage of sphincter pharyngoplasty procedure is the ability to adjust the port size postoperatively, if needed by tightening or loosening the muscles.

There is not enough evidence to suggest the superiority of sphincter pharyngoplasty or pharyngeal flap for the treatment of VPI.[33,34] Large multicenter, randomized, blinded, and prospective studies are required to determine the optimal procedure for VPI secondary to each type, size, and port orientation.

Posterior Pharyngeal Wall Augmentation

Various autologous and alloplastic materials have been reported in the literature with a goal to reduce the size of velopharyngeal port. Some of the synthetic materials used for posterior wall augmentation include silicone, Teflon, proplast, etc.[35] Fat, fascia, cartilage, dermis, and rolled posterior pharyngeal flap are some of the autologous materials that have been used for posterior wall augmentation.[36,37] Infection, resorption, extrusion, migration, and unreliability of the results are some of the reported complications and criticisms of posterior wall augmentation procedures. Another risk associated with posterior wall augmentation with fat is its enlargement with weight gain and the consequent risk of OSA, at which point the grafted fat may be difficult to remove.[36,37]

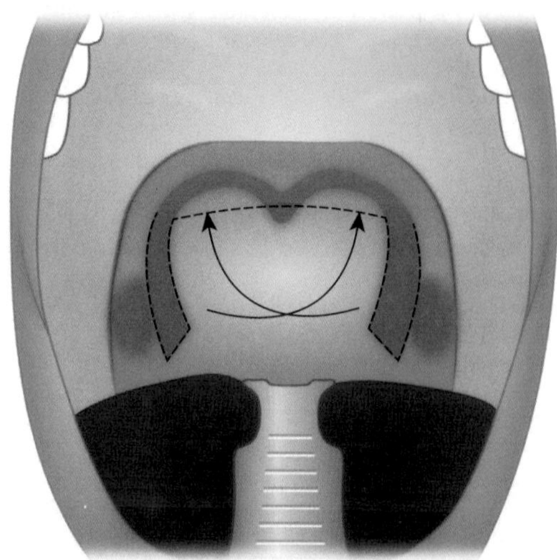

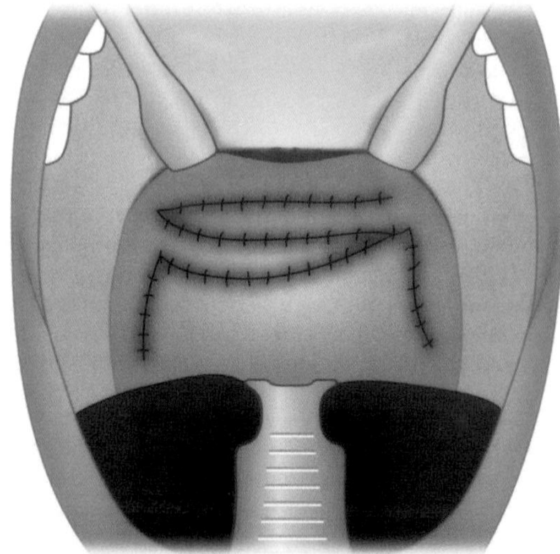

FIGURE 34.4. Sphincter pharyngoplasty.

Complications

Complications after surgery for VPI include OSA, bleeding, dehiscence, airway obstruction, injury to anomalous internal carotid artery, and persistent hypernasality, hyponasality, or reoperation. In a 10-year review of perioperative complications following pharyngeal flap surgery, overall complication rate was reported to be 6%.[38] Another series reported a 38% incidence of symptoms of upper airway obstruction acutely after pharyngeal flap surgery, but persistent symptoms beyond five months was only seen in 6% of the patients.[39] Witt et al. reported a 13% incidence of OSA following sphincter pharyngoplasty.[40] Symptoms of OSA can vary from snoring without any airway obstruction to obstruction with desaturation, hence randomized controlled studies comparing complications secondary to various surgical interventions utilized in the management of VPI patients are needed.

Another study on salvage of failed pharyngoplasties reported equivalent rates of failure with pharyngeal flap (20%) and sphincter pharyngoplasty (16%) and successful denasalization of speech following revision surgery.[41]

Special Considerations

Velopharyngeal Dysfunction and Chromosomal Syndromes

Many chromosomal syndromes are associated with VPD. Among the syndromic presentations, 22q11.2 deletion syndrome (sometimes referred to as velocardiofacial or Shprintzen syndrome) is known to be the most common syndrome associated with cleft palate and VPI. These patients commonly have submucous cleft; however, they may have a higher risk of associated VPD compared with patients with submucous cleft in the absence of 22q11.2 deletion syndrome. This higher risk is thought to be multifactorial, and the most commonly reported factor is neuromuscular dysfunction of the muscles of velopharyngeal mechanism. Other contributing factors include increase in the width of space between velum and posterior pharyngeal wall, asymmetric displacement of lateral pharyngeal wall, reduced adenoid size, and intellectual disabilities. Hence, vigilance during interpretation of diagnostic tests such as VFS and nasal endoscopy becomes even more important in the setting of syndromic presentation, so that the accurate diagnosis can be made and precise prognosis of improvement with surgical intervention can be established. During nasal endoscopy, attention should also be paid to the presence of pulsations in the posterior or lateral pharyngeal wall which may suggest medialization of internal carotid arteries. Medial displacement of internal carotid arteries can be frequently seen in patients with 22q11.2 deletion or Kabuki syndrome.[42] Shprintzen and colleagues in their study of magnetic resonance angiography for patients with 22q11.2 deletion syndrome noted anomalies in vertebral, carotid arteries or both, in all patients with 22q11.2 deletion syndrome, highlighting the importance of obtaining imaging prior to the performance of pharyngeal flap surgery in this patient population.[43] Ross and colleagues also studied the risk of medially displaced carotid arteries in this patient population and concluded that a routine superiorly based pharyngoplasty may be safe in 52%, whereas in others it should be custom designed based on the individual anatomy of the patient.[44] Another concern for 22q11.2 deletion and other syndromes with a developmental delay is that these patients may have intellectual disability, making it more challenging for them to relearn and correct some of the articulation errors with speech therapy after surgery. For this reason, in this patient population, physical management of VPI by utilizing pharyngeal flap or sphincter pharyngoplasty may be warranted so that less reliance is placed on patient's ability to relearn, to control airflow, and to use their tongue, lips, and jaw correctly to make sounds, after surgery.

Other syndromes that may present with VPD include Opitz G/BBB syndrome, Kabuki syndrome, and Jacobsen syndrome.

Submucous Cleft

Controversy exists regarding the timing and optimal surgical intervention for submucous cleft (defined as having varying degrees of phenotypic expressions of zona pellucida, notched hard palate, and bifid uvula). In a study of 353 patients with submucous cleft, only 49.8 % were noted to have VPD, with the rest of the patients demonstrating complete or marginal VPD.[45] Hence, it is reasonable to wait on the surgical intervention till the patient is old enough to provide an adequate speech sample for perceptual speech evaluation. If the patient is deemed a surgical candidate, then depending on the size of the defect, it maybe reasonable to start with palatoplasty (either intervelar veloplasty or Furlow repair). Sommerlad and colleagues performed a systemic review of 26 studies analyzing surgical management of VPI in patients with submucous cleft. Speech outcomes were compared following sphincter pharyngoplasty, pharyngeal flap, and palatal reconstruction (Furlow palatoplasty, intravelar veloplasty, and palatal *pushback*), and little evidence was found to support one intervention over another.[46]

Tonsillectomy and Velopharyngeal Insufficiency

The effect of tonsils on VPI is complex. VPI can be associated with superior pole tonsillar hypertrophy, especially when the upper pole extends above the level of the velum, into the lateral port and displaces the palatopharyngeus muscle anteriorly. On the contrary and more importantly, VPI can worsen after tonsillectomy, and hence these cases should be carefully evaluated with NPS prior to any surgical intervention. If tonsillectomy is indicated, then it may be best to perform it prior to the performance of surgical intervention for VPI, and after tonsillectomy, velopharyngeal closure should be carefully reevaluated. Additionally, during tonsillectomy procedure, the posterior tonsillar pillar should be protected, in case sphincter pharyngoplasty is indicated (which uses palatopharyngeus muscle from the posterior tonsillar pillar).[47]

NONSURGICAL MANAGEMENT

Palatal prosthesis is indicated for patients who have contraindications to surgery or for patients with poor prognosis of improvement with surgery.[48,49] These devices are typically made in coordination with a prosthodontist and a speech pathologist. The device fits along the hard palate and has a posterior extension that pushes the soft palate upwards in a patient with hypomobile velopharyngeal mechanism for closure of the port.

PROGNOSIS AND OUTCOMES

Based on a systemic review with a goal to reach consensus in the literature regarding surgical management of VPD, 71% of patients attained normal resonance and 65% attained normal nasal emission. Additionally, no difference was noted in terms of speech outcomes, sleep apnea, or need for further surgery, for patients treated with pharyngeal flap, sphincter pharyngoplasty, palatoplasty, and posterior pharyngeal wall augmentation.[50] Once the patient undergoes surgery, speech therapy becomes important in the postoperative period again so that the child can relearn and correct the articulation errors with biofeedback and speech therapy.

REFERENCES

1. Drissi C, Mitrofanoff M, Talandier C, et al. Feasibility of dynamic MRI for evaluating velopharyngeal insufficiency in children. *Eur Radiol.* 2011;21(7):1462-1469.
2. Vadodaria S, Goodacre TEE, Anslow P. Does MRI contribute to the investigation of palatal function? *Br J Plast Surg.* 2000;53(3):191-199.
3. Mehendale FV, Birch MJ, Birkett L, et al. Surgical management of velopharyngeal incompetence in velocardiofacial syndrome. *Cleft Palate Craniofac J.* 2004;41(2):124-135.

4. Shprintzen RJ. Velo-cardio-facial syndrome: 30 years of study. *Dev Disabil Res Rev*. 2008;14(1):3-10.
5. Kummer AW. Disorders of resonance and airflow secondary to cleft palate and/or velopharyngeal dysfunction. *Semin Speech Lang*. 2011;32:141-149.
6. Moon JB, Smith AE, Folkins JW, et al. Coordination of velopharyngeal muscle activity during positioning of the soft palate. *Cleft Palate Craniofac J*. 1994;31(1):45-55.
7. Inouye JM, Lin KY, Perry JL, Blemker SS. Contributions of the musculus uvulae to velopharyngeal closure quantified with a 3-dimensional multimuscle computational model. *Ann Plast Surg*. 2016;77(suppl 1):S70-S75.
8. Croft CB, Schprintzen RJ, Rakoff SJ. Patterns of velopharyngeal valving in normal and cleft palate subjects: a multi-view videofluoroscopic and nasoendoscopic study. *Laryngoscope*. 1981;91:265-271.
The authors examined the velopharyngeal closure pattern on videofluoroscopy and endoscopy and identified five closure patterns in normal and abnormal subjects. These closure patterns are typically reported when describing the orientation of nasopharyngeal gap on nasal endoscopy.
9. Jordan HN, Schenck GC, Ellis C, et al. Examining velopharyngeal closure patterns based on anatomic variables. *J Craniofac Surg*. 2017;28(1):270-274.
10. Kummer AW. Evaluation of speech and resonance for children with craniofacial anomalies. *Facial Plast Surg Clin North Am*. 2016;24(4):445-451.
11. Chapman KL, Baylis A, Trost-Cardamone J, et al. The Americleft Speech Project: a training and reliability study. *Cleft Palate Craniofac J*. 2016;53(1):93-108.
12. Ysunza PA, Repetto GM, Pamplona MC, et al. Current controversies in diagnosis and management of cleft palate and velopharyngeal insufficiency. *Biomed Res Int*. 2015;2015:196240.
13. Skolnick ML. Videofluoroscopic examination of the velopharyngeal portal during phonation in lateral and base projections: a new technique for studying the mechanics of closure. *Cleft Palate J*. 1970;7:803-816.
14. Perry JL, Sutton BP, Kuehn DP, Gamage JK. Using MRI for assessing velopharyngeal structures and function. *Cleft Palate Craniofac J*. 2014;51:476-485.
15. Kao DS, Soltysik DA, Hyde JS, et al. Magnetic resonance imaging as an aid in the dynamic assessment of the velopharyngeal mechanism in children. *Plast Reconstr Surg*. 2008;122:572-577.
16. Tatum SA III, Chang J, Havkin N, Shprintzen RJ. Pharyngeal flap and the internal carotid in velocardiofacial syndrome. *Arch Facial Plast Surg*. 2002;4(2):73-80.
17. Warren DW, Dubois AB. A pressure-flow technique for measuring velopharyngeal orifice area during continuous speech. *Cleft Palate J*. 1964;16:52-71.
The authors popularized the concept of nasometry, which allows measurement of oral and nasal air pressure and flow and calculation of velopharyngeal port size.
18. D'Antonio LL. Evaluation and management of velopharyngeal dysfunction: a speech pathologist's viewpoint. *Probl Plast Reconstr Surg*. 1992;2:86-111.
19. Warren DW, Dalston RM, Trier WC, Holder MB. A pressure-flow technique for quantifying temporal patterns of palatopharyngeal closure. *Cleft Palate J*. 1985;22(1):11-19.
20. Naran S, Ford M, Losee JE. What's new in cleft palate and velopharyngeal dysfunction management? *Plast Reconstr Surg*. 2017;139(6):1343e-1355e.
21. Sommerlad BC, Henley M, Birch M, et al. Cleft palate re-repair—a clinical and radiographic study of 32 consecutive cases. *Br J Plast Surg*. 1994;47(6):406-410.
22. Sommerlad BC, Mehendale FV, Birch MJ, et al. Palate re-repair revisited. *Cleft Palate Craniofac J*. 2002;39(3):295-307.
23. Furlow LT. Cleft palate repair by double opposing Z-plasty. *Plast Reconstr Surg*. 1986;78:724-736.
In 1986, Leonard Furlow introduced the Furlow palatoplasty procedure. This procedure entails creation of two double opposing Z-plasties of oral and nasal mucosa with attached levator muscle.
24. Pet MA, Marty-Grames L, Blount-Stahl, et al. The Furlow palatoplasty for velopharyngeal dysfunction: velopharyngeal changes, speech improvements, and where they intersect. *Cleft Palate Craniofac J*. 2015;52(1):12-22.
25. Perkins JA, Lewis CW, Gruss JS, et al. Furlow palatoplasty for management of velopharyngeal insufficiency: a prospective study of 148 consecutive patients. *Plast Reconstr Surg*. 2005;116:72-80.
26. Schoenborn D. Uber eine neue methode der staphylorraphies. *Arch F Klin Chir*. 1876;19:528-531.
Pharyngeal flap was first described by Schoenborn in 1876. This is a rectangular-shaped myomucosal flap, raised from the posterior pharyngeal wall and insetted into the velum.
27. Whitaker LA, Randall P, Graham WP III, et al. A prospective and randomized series comparing superiorly and inferiorly based posterior pharyngeal flaps. *Cleft Palate J*. 1972;9:304-311.
28. Argamaso RV, Shprintzen RJ, Strauch B, et al. The role of lateral pharyngeal wall movement in pharyngeal flap surgery. *Plast Reconstr Surg*. 1980;66:214-219.
29. Boutros S, Cutting C. The lateral port control pharyngeal flap: a thirty-year evolution and followup. *Plast Surg Int*. 2013;2013:237308.
30. Hynes W. Pharyngoplasty by muscle transplantation. *Br J Plast Surg*. 1950;3:128-135.
The Sphincter pharyngoplasty procedure was introduced by Hynes in 1950, where he described the use of bilateral salpingopharyngeus muscles for decreasing the dimension of velopharyngeal port.
31. Orticochea M. Construction of a dynamic muscle sphincter in cleft palates. *Plast Reconstr Surg*. 1968;41:323-327.
32. Jackson IT, Silverton JS. The sphincter pharyngoplasty as a secondary procedure in cleft palates. *Plast Reconstr Surg*. 1977;59:518-554.
33. Abyholm F, D'Antonio L, Davidson Ward SL, et al. Pharyngeal flap and sphincterplasty for velopharyngeal insufficiency have equal outcome at 1 year postoperatively: results of a randomized trial. *Cleft Palate Craniofac J*. 2005;42:501-511.
34. Ysunza A, Pamplona C, Ramírez E, et al. Velopharyngeal surgery: a prospective randomized study of pharyngeal flaps and sphincter pharyngoplasties. *Plast Reconstr Surg*. 2002;110:1401-1407.
35. Lewy R, Cole R, Wepman J. Teflon injection in the correction of velopharyngeal insufficiency. *Ann Otol Rhinol Laryngol*. 1965;74(3):874-879.
36. Lau D, Oppenheimer AJ, Buchman SR, et al. Posterior pharyngeal fat grafting for velopharyngeal insufficiency. *Cleft Palate Craniofac J*. 2013;50(1):51-58.
37. Lypka M, Bidros R, Rizvi M, et al. Posterior pharyngeal augmentation in the treatment of velopharyngeal insufficiency: a 40-year experience. *Ann Plast Surg*. 2010;65(1):48-51.
38. Hofer SO, Dhar BK, Robinson PH, et al. A 10-year review of perioperative complications in pharyngeal flap surgery. *Plast Reconstr Surg*. 2002;110(6):1393-1397.
In a 10-year review of perioperative complications following pharyngeal flap surgery, the overall complication rate was reported to be 6%.
39. Lesavoy MA1, Borud LJ, Thorson T, et al. Upper airway obstruction after pharyngeal flap surgery. *Ann Plast Surg*. 1996;36(1):26-30.
40. Witt PD, Marsh JL, Muntz HR, et al. Acute obstructive sleep apnea as a complication of sphincter pharyngoplasty. *Cleft Palate Craniofac J*. 1996;33(3):183-189.
41. Witt PD, Myckatyn T, Marsh JL. Salvaging the failed pharyngoplasty: intervention outcome. *Cleft Palate Craniofac J*. 1998;35(5):447-453.
A study on salvage of failed pharyngoplasties reported equivalent rates of failure with pharyngeal flap (20%) and sphincter pharyngoplasty (16%) and successful denasalization of speech following revision surgery.
42. Ysunza A, Pamplona MC, Molina F, Hernández A. Surgical planning for restoring velopharyngeal function in velocardiofacial syndrome. *Int J Pediatr Otorhinolaryngol*. 2009;73(11):1572-1575.
43. Mitnick RJ, Bello JA, Golding-Kushner KJ, et al. The use of magnetic resonance angiography prior to pharyngeal flap surgery in patients with velocardiofacial syndrome. *Plast Reconstr Surg*. 1996;97:908-919.
44. Ross DA, Witzel MA, Armstrong DC, Thompson HG. Is pharyngoplasty a risk in velocardiofacial syndrome? An assessment of medially displaced carotid arteries. *Plast Reconstr Surg*. 1996;98:1182-1190.
45. Heng Y, Chunli G, Bing S, et al. Velopharyngeal closure pattern and speech performance among submucous cleft palate patients. *Hua Xi Kou Qiang Yi Xue Za Zhi*. 2017;35(3):296-300.
In a study of 353 patients with submucous cleft, only 49.8% were noted to have velopharyngeal dysfunction, with the rest of the patients demonstrating complete or marginal VPD.
46. Gilleard O, Sell D, Ghanem A, et al. Submucous cleft palate: a systematic review of surgical management based on perceptual and instrumental analysis. *Cleft Palate Craniofac J*. 2014;51(6):686-695.
The authors performed a systemic review of 26 studies analyzing surgical management of velopharyngeal insufficiency in patients with submucous cleft. Speech outcomes were compared following sphincter pharyngoplasty, pharyngeal flap, and palatal reconstruction (Furlow palatoplasty, intravelar veloplasty, and palatal 'push-back') and little evidence was found to support one intervention over another.
47. Paulson LM, Macarthur CJ, Beaulieu KB, et al. Speech outcomes after tonsillectomy in patients with known velopharyngeal insufficiency. *Int J Otolaryngol*. 2012;2012:912767.
48. Raj N, Raj V, Aeran H. Interim palatal lift prosthesis as a constituent of multidisciplinary approach in the treatment of velopharyngeal incompetence. *J Adv Prosthodont*. 2012;4:243-247.
49. Aboloyoun A, Ghorab S, Farooq MU. Palatal lifting prosthesis and velopharyngeal insufficiency: preliminary report. *Acta Med Acad*. 2013;42:55-60.
50. de Blacam C, Smith S, Orr D. Surgery for velopharyngeal dysfunction: a systematic review of interventions and outcomes. *Cleft Palate Craniofac J*. 2018;55(3):405-422.
In a systemic review regarding surgical management of velopharyngeal dysfunction, 70.7% of patients attained normal resonance and 65.3% attained normal nasal emission. Additionally, no difference was noted in terms of speech outcomes, sleep apnea, or need for further surgery for patients treated with pharyngeal flap, sphincter pharyngoplasty, palatoplasty, and posterior pharyngeal wall augmentation.

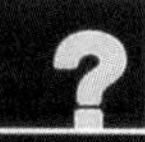

QUESTIONS

1. 1. A six-year-old boy is brought to the cleft clinic for a follow-up visit. The patient had intravelar veloplasty at 10 months of age. On perceptual speech evaluation, he was noted to have hypernasality and nasal emission. On physical examination, no fistula was noted. Nasal endoscopy showed a large coronal gap with poor lateral wall motion. Which of the following is the most appropriate management?

   a. Continued speech therapy
   b. Furlow palatoplasty
   c. Sphincter pharyngoplasty
   d. Posterior pharyngeal flap
   e. Palatal lift prosthesis

2. A six-year-old patient with a history of bilateral complete cleft palate repair in infancy undergoes sphincter pharyngoplasty for her VPI. Which of the following muscles was primarily incorporated during pharyngoplasty for this patient?

   a. Tensor veli palatini
   b. LVP
   c. Palatopharyngeus muscle
   d. Palatoglossus muscle
   e. Musculus uvulae

3. A four-year-old patient, adopted from China, is diagnosed with submucous cleft palate. He is noted to have a notch of the posterior hard palate and a bifid uvula. Which of the following is an additional feature that he is likely to have?

   a. Incomplete cleft lip
   b. Cleft of the anterior alveolus
   c. Medialized internal carotid arteries
   d. Zona pellucida
   e. Syndactyly

4. A six-year-old boy presented to the multidisciplinary craniofacial team for evaluation of his VPI. He is noted to have Tetralogy of Fallot, submucous cleft palate, learning disabilities, and hypocalcemia. On perceptual speech evaluation, he is noted to have hypernasal speech with nasal air escape. The most likely diagnosis is

   a. Apert syndrome
   b. Van der Woude syndrome (VWS)
   c. 22q11.2 deletion syndrome
   d. Nager syndrome
   e. Stickler syndrome

5. A 5-year-old patient with a history of repaired cleft palate at 12 months of age presents to the clinic for evaluation of her VPD. She is noted to have poor intelligibility, hypernasality, and weak pressure consonants on perceptual speech evaluation. She undergoes nasal endoscopy which reveals a moderate to large sized, sagittally oriented gap with good lateral wall motion and limited palatal motion because of scarring. The patient has no contraindications for surgery. Which of the following is the most appropriate treatment for this patient?

   a. Intervelar veloplasty
   b. Superiorly based pharyngeal flap
   c. Posterior wall augmentation with fat
   d. Palatal obturator
   e. Sphincter pharyngoplasty with transposition of salpingopharyngeus muscle

1. **Answer: c.** The patient described has VPI because of inadequate closure of the velopharyngeal port. The first step in the evaluation of VPD is perceptual speech assessment, which is usually performed around 3 or 4 years of age. Any nasal emission and/or hypernasality with speech are indicative of inadequate approximation of velum against the posterior pharyngeal wall. Nasoendoscopy provides qualitative assessment of the closure pattern and port size and can be performed at 4 to 5 years of age. Surgical treatment is based on the severity of speech discrepancy and the location and size of port closure defect. A large posterior gap with coronal, circular, or bowtie closure pattern and poor lateral wall motion should be treated with a sphincter pharyngoplasty, where palatopharyngeal muscles in bilateral posterior tonsillar pillars are elevated and rotated through 90°. The flaps are overlapped and sutured to each other and to the posterior pharyngeal wall.

Continued speech therapy will not correct hypernasality associated with a large coronal defect. Furlow palatoplasty with its Z-plasty design provides palatal lengthening and is well suited for the management of VPD in patients with unrepaired submucous cleft and with repaired overt clefts. Although it can be done, it is not the best technique for patients in whom the levator muscles are not sagittally oriented, as transposition would disrupt anatomically normal previously reconstructed levator sling. Posterior pharyngeal flap requires raising a myomucosal rectangular flap from the posterior pharyngeal wall and insetting it in the velum. It can be superiorly or posteriorly based and is best suited for sagittal or circular closure patterns. Palatal prosthesis is indicated in cases of failed speech therapy, when surgery is contraindicated.

2. **Answer: c.** Sphincter pharyngoplasty involves 90° transposition of the palatopharyngeus muscle from the posterior tonsillar pillar and is best suited for a moderate to large coronally oriented gap. TVP originates from the Eustachian tube and the scaphoid fossa of the sphenoid bone, and inserts into the palatal aponeurosis by joining the muscle of the opposite side in the anterior 25% of the soft palate. Its action is to tense the soft palate, in addition to opening the Eustachian tube. LVP takes origin from the petrous part of the temporal bone and decussates with the contralateral levator muscle forming a horizontally oriented sling in the soft palate. It functions to lengthen the velum and elevates it in the posterior direction. Palatoglossus muscles lie in the anterior tonsillar pillars, where the palatopharyngeus muscle is found in the posterior tonsillar pillar. They both serve to depress the soft palate. Musculus uvulae is the only intrinsic muscle of the soft palate and takes origin from the palatal aponeurosis. It likely contributes to the VP closure by providing bulk to it, by acting as a space-occupying structure and a velar extensor. Among the muscles listed, palatopharyngeus muscle is the only muscle that is used in sphincter pharyngoplasty procedure.

3. **Answer: d.** Patients with submucous cleft tend of have varying degrees of notched hard palate, bifid uvula, and diastasis of the LVP muscle (also known as zona pellucida). This results in VPI in 15% of the cases. Incomplete cleft lip, cleft of the anterior alveolus, medialized internal carotid arteries, and syndactyly are not standard features of a submucous cleft.

4. **Answer: c.** 22q11.2 deletion syndrome (commonly known as, DiGeorge syndrome, Shprintzen syndrome, velocardiofacial syndrome) is a disorder caused by the deletion mutation

on chromosome 22. The typical features of this syndrome include cleft palate, heart defects, recurrent infections, unique facial characteristics, feeding problems, kidney abnormalities, hypoparathyroidism (resulting in hypocalcemia), hearing loss, developmental delay, and learning disabilities. Apert syndrome is an autosomal dominant syndrome characterized by bicoronal synostosis with complex syndactyly, midfacial hypoplasia, exorbitism, etc. Patients with Apert syndrome can have cleft palate and 70% have decreased IQ but they typically do not have hypocalcemia and cardiac abnormalities. VWS is an autosomal dominant syndrome characterized by lower lip pits, cleft lip with or without cleft palate, or cleft palate alone. Patients with VWS can have congenital heart problems but do not tend to have hypocalcemia. Patients with Nager acrofacial dysostosis are distinguished by radial-sided limb abnormalities, malar hypoplasia, micrognathia, cleft palate, coloboma, and ear abnormalities. These patients have many other anomalies including renal and cardiac anomalies but do not typically have hypocalcemia. Stickler syndrome is another autosomal dominant syndrome with features of cleft palate, Pierre Robin sequence, ocular malformations, hearing loss, and arthropathies. Patients with Stickler syndrome can have mitral valve prolapse but hypocalcemia is not a typical feature of this syndrome.

5. Answer: b. In a superiorly based pharyngeal flap, a rectangular-shaped myomucosal flap, based superiorly, is raised from the posterior pharyngeal wall and insetted into the velum. This flap converts a large velopharyngeal port into two small lateral ports by creating a midline obstruction between oral and nasal cavities, and it is best suited for moderate to large sized gap that is a sagittally oriented gap with good lateral wall. This patient has a surgical history of cleft palate repair and now has limited palatal motion with scarring, so palatal rerepair with intervelar veloplasty is not likely to help his VPI in the presence of a moderate to large sized gap. Posterior wall augmentation with fat grafting will likely not resolve the VPI secondary to a moderate to large sized gap. Additionally, fat grafting to posterior pharynx carries the risk of increase in size (and resulting obstructive sleep apnea) if the patient gains weight. This patient has no contraindications to surgery so palatal obturator is not the best long-term solution for his VPI. Sphincter pharyngoplasty uses palatopharyngeus muscles and is best suited for a coronally oriented moderate to large sized gap.

CHAPTER 35 Craniofacial Tumors and Conditions

James P. Bradley and Justine C. Lee

KEY POINTS

- Fibrous dysplasia, a benign, spongy bone disorder, may be monostotic (single area of bone involvement) or polyostotic (multiple involved bony areas) and treated with operative recontour burring or with partial resection and bone graft reconstruction.
- Parry-Romberg syndrome, a progressive, acquired atrophy of the soft (skin/fat) and hard tissues (cartilage/bone) of the face requires, depending on severity of the case, fat grafting, free adipofascial flap, or even bony reconstruction.
- Treacher Collins syndrome, a congenital bilateral deficiency of orbitozygomatic, mandibular, and ear regions (Tessier no. 6, 7, and 8 clefts), may require staged reconstruction with bone grafts/eyelid switch flaps for orbital reconstruction, total ear reconstruction for microtia, and mandibular ramus distraction or orthognathic surgery for mandibular abnormalities.
- Neurofibromatosis of the periphery (NF-1) or centrally (NF-2) is an autosomal dominant disorder that causes (usually) benign growths within nerves and may require resection and the sacrificing of involved nerves.
- Pierre Robin sequence, a congenital anomaly with a triad of manifestations: micrognathia, glossoptosis, and upper airway obstruction, may require early operative intervention in severe cases with glossopexy or mandibular distraction to avoid a tracheostomy.
- Moebius syndrome is characterized by bilateral absence of cranial nerves VI and VII resulting in mask facies and inability to lateral deviate the eye and may be treated with functional muscle transfers to give oral commissure animation.
- Dermoid cysts are benign inclusion cysts typically located in the lateral supraorbital rim; but central lesions require imaging to rule out intracranial extension that would require an intra- and extracranial approach for resection.

FIBROUS DYSPLASIA

Definition and Clinical Findings

Fibrous dysplasia is a benign anomaly of the bone characterized by replacement of normal bone with fibro-osseous tissue. It is the most common craniofacial tumor encountered by plastic surgeons.[1] Fibrous dysplasia ranges from mild to severe and presents with monostotic or polyostotic distribution.[2,3] Skull involvement occurs in 27% of monostotic patients and up to 50% of polyostotic patients. Clinical manifestations of fibrous dysplasia depend on the location, duration, and the extent of disease. Craniofacial fibrous dysplasia most commonly begins in childhood then progresses through adolescence. It was previously thought that the disease progression halted after childhood, but this is not universally true; the disease frequently continues well into adulthood.[2] Anatomic location of the monostotic disease in the craniofacial skeleton most often affects the frontal and sphenoid bones and the maxilla[3,4] (**Figure 35.1**). Signs and symptoms of craniofacial disease are diverse and may include swelling of the affected side (most commonly), facial pain, headaches, cranial nerve (CN) palsies, anosmia, deafness, blindness, malocclusion with tooth displacement, diplopia, proptosis, and orbital dystopia.[3,5]

Etiology and Pathogenesis

Fibrous dysplasia occurs as a result of abnormal activity of the bone forming mesenchyme with an arrest of bone maturation in the woven bone stage.[3] Normal bone matrix is replaced by fibroblastic proliferation and there are resultant irregular trabeculae of partially calcified osteoid.[2] Fibrous dysplasia is caused by somatic activating mutations in the alpha subunit of the stimulatory G protein encoded by the GNAS gene.[2] A subset of patients have an associated endocrinopathy called McCune-Albright syndrome.[6,7] This condition includes precocious puberty, café au lait spots, and other endocrinopathies due to the hyperactivity of various endocrine glands.[6,7] Cherubism or familial fibrous dysplasia is a self-limited disease of the maxilla and mandible in children. This genetic giant cell disorder differs from

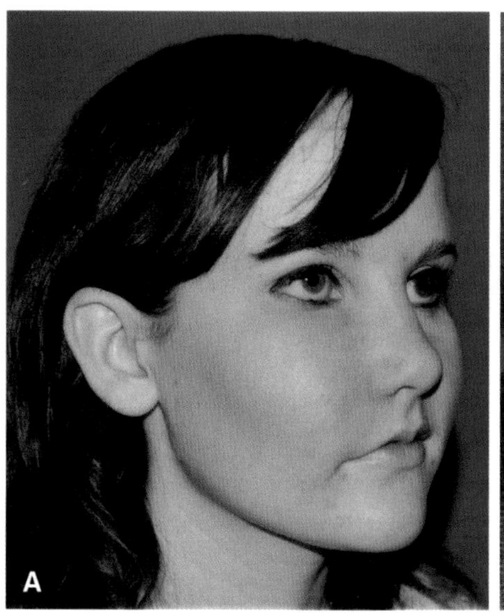

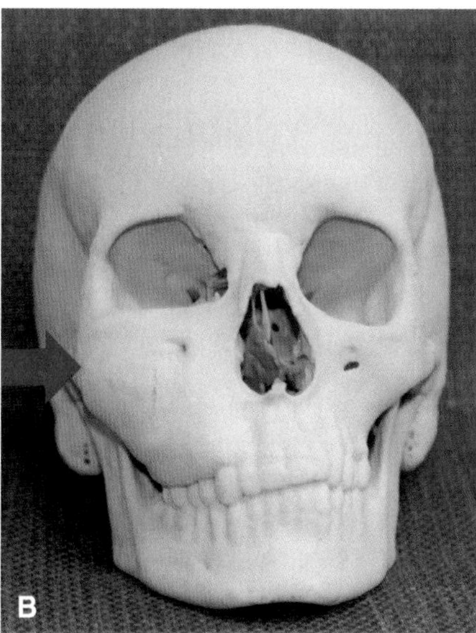

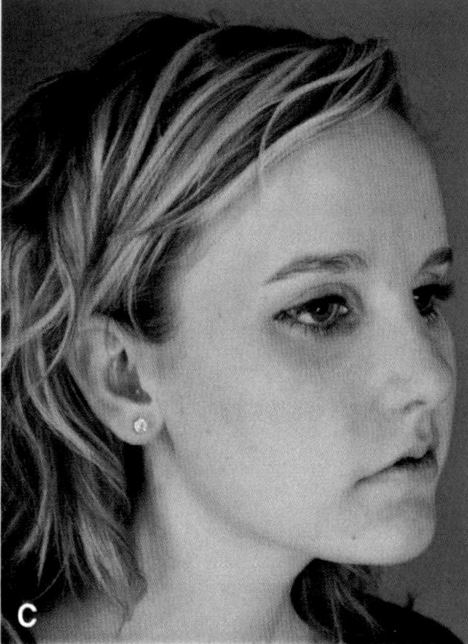

FIGURE 35.1. Fibrous dysplasia limited to zygomatic maxillary complex (monostotic). **A.** Preoperative right oblique image. **B.** 3D model depicting fibrous dysplasia mass (arrow). **C.** Postoperative right oblique image after limited resection, cranial bone graft to orbital rim/arch, and alveolar recontouring. (Courtesy of J.P. Bradley.)

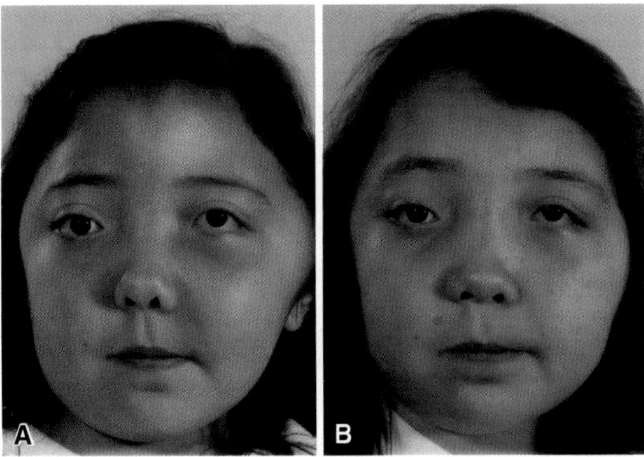

FIGURE 35.2. Fibrous dysplasia involving the left orbit, temporal, and zygomatic, regions (polyostotic). **A.** Preoperative frontal image demonstrating vertical dystopia and temporal fullness. **B.** Postoperative frontal image improvement after orbital box repositioning and recontouring of temporal bone. (Courtesy of H.K. Kawamoto.)

other forms of fibrous dysplasia; in that, it typically regresses without operation and leaves no deformity.[3] A histologic biopsy should be sent at the time of surgical exploration of fibrous dysplasia (especially for polyostotic cases) because malignant transformation may be seen in 3.2% of patients. When regions of fibrous dysplasia undergo cystic or malignant degeneration, rapid enlargement and mass effect are typically seen.[2,8] In cases of malignant degeneration, fibrous dysplasia most commonly transforms to osteosarcoma, and occasionally to chondrosarcoma or fibrosarcoma.[3,8]

Diagnosis of fibrous dysplasia depends on a combination of clinical, radiographic, and histological criteria, as diagnosis based on any individual factor alone can be difficult (exclusive of McCune-Albright syndrome).[2] The typical plain radiographic appearance is of radiolucent lytic lesions with a homogenous ground-glass appearance and ill-defined borders. However, this nonspecific appearance makes it difficult to differentiate from other conditions such as ossifying fibroma and Paget disease. Computerized tomography (CT) provides substantially better radiographic information. Fibrous dysplasia has a ground-glass pattern (56%), homogeneously dense pattern (23%), or a cystic variety (21%). In addition to improved diagnostic information, CT also improves operative planning by evaluating the extent of disease, particularly in evaluating the extent of optic nerve canal involvement.

Treatment and Complications

Management protocols for the surgical treatment of craniofacial fibrous dysplasia differ. On the radical end, complete excision of all diseased bone with reconstruction is advocated, whereas on the more conservative end, skeletal reshaping with burring to restore normal skeletal morphology is performed.[2,9] Between these two surgical protocol extremes, limited resection (without sacrificing or injuring vital structures) with osseous reconstruction is offered **(Figure 35.2)**. Chen and Nordhoff based their treatment approach to the occurrence in four designated zones in the craniofacial skeleton[2]:

- Total excision for zone 1 (fronto-orbital, zygomatic, and upper maxillary regions)
- Conservative excision (contouring) for
  - Zone 2 (hair-bearing cranium),
  - Zone 3 (the central cranial base), and
  - Zone 4 (the tooth-bearing regions of the maxillary alveolus and mandible).

When comparing limited resection with reconstruction to bone contouring, patients undergoing resection had a lower recurrence rate and required fewer total operations but had a slightly increased postoperative complication rate.[9] Medical adjuncts for fibrous dysplasia hold an adjunctive role only and include bisphosphonates, steroids, and tamoxifen.[2] Radiotherapy has no role in treatment of fibrous dysplasia and should be avoided.

Optic nerve decompression for optic canal involvement is controversial. Optic canal decompression without any vision loss is generally deemed too risky even with radiographic evidence of involvement.[2,10] However, when vision loss is first noted, optic canal decompression is advised. The outcome of optic nerve decompression ranges from (1) halting vision loss, (2) improvement in vision, to (3) worsening in vision.[2,9]

PARRY-ROMBERG SYNDROME

Definition and Clinical Findings

Parry-Romberg syndrome is characterized as a progressive hemifacial hypoplasia with regional fat atrophy, medial canthal malpositioning, enophthalmos, dystopia, and skin hyperpigmentation.[11] It manifests as unilateral atrophy of the subcutaneous facial fat in the paramedial area with equal frequency on both sides of the face. Atrophy of the skin, muscle, fascia, cartilage, and bone may follow **(Figure 35.3)**. The most evident sign is loss of fullness in 3-D parameters (atrophy of orbital, palpebral, zygomatic, and masseter muscles). The classic linear vertical deficiency is called *coup de sabre* sign (or *mark of the sword*).[12]

Etiology and Pathogenesis

Parry-Romberg syndrome results in progressive hemifacial atrophy and may be highly variable. Although primarily characterized by soft tissue involvement including fat, skin, muscle, and connective tissue, in more severe cases, bony, ophthalmological, and/or neurological involvement occurs **(Figure 35.4)**. Onset can vary from infancy, to early or mid-childhood, to adolescence, or even adulthood. Rate of progression of disease is also unpredictable and may vary. Some (but not all) cases are believed to undergo remission or *burnout* after puberty.[13]

Treatment and Complications

Current treatment options to fill deficient tissues include fat or dermal grafts, dermal fillers (hyaluronic acid or calcium hydroxyapatite), bone and/or cartilage grafts, and/or free tissue transplantation.[11] Many authors advocate waiting for the disease to reach a stable phase

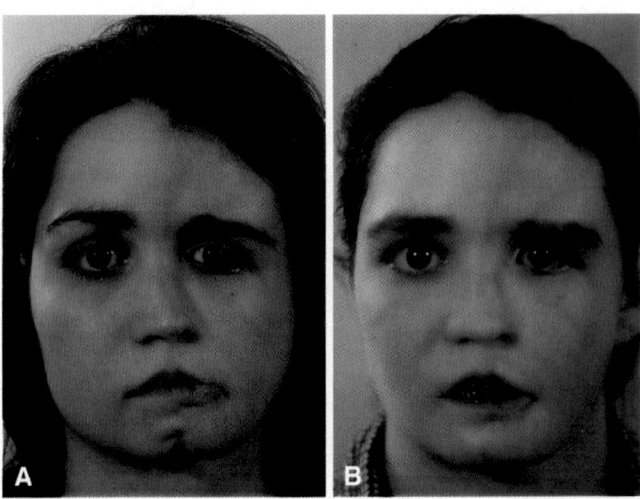

FIGURE 35.3. Romberg syndrome with left side involvement. **A.** Preoperative image shows C-shaped linear coup de sabre deficiency. **B.** Postoperative image shows correction after serial fat grafting, septorhinoplasty, and lateral canthoplasty. (Courtesy of H.K. Kawamoto.)

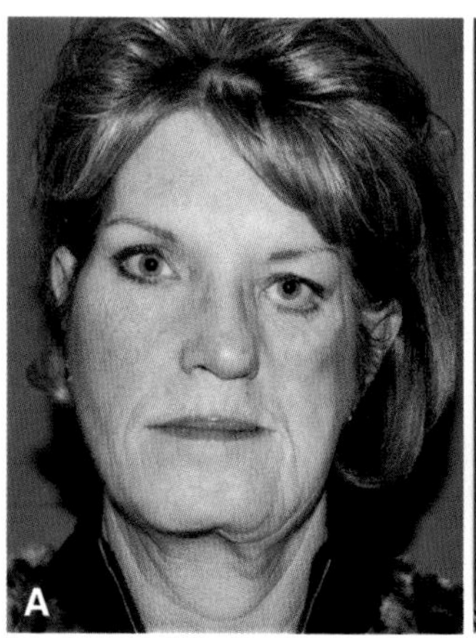
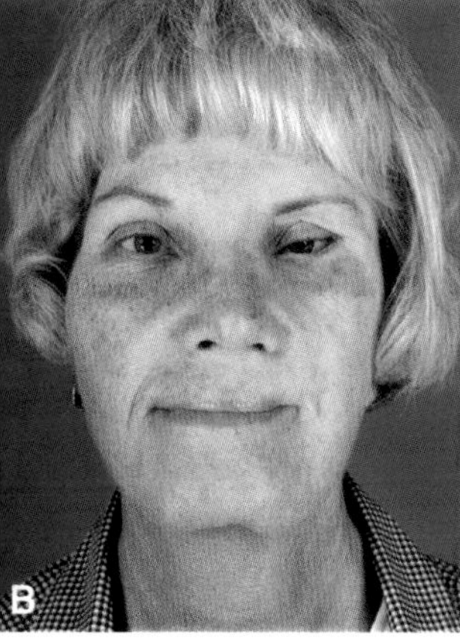

FIGURE 35.4. Romberg syndrome with left side involvement. **A.** Preoperative image shows both hard and soft tissue disruption with left vertical orbital dystopia, nasal deviation, and skin changes. **B.** Postoperative image shows correction after left orbital box elevation, lateral canthoplasty, septorhinoplasty, fat grafting, and face-lift. (Courtesy of J.P. Bradley.)

after facial growth completion in late adolescence before beginning surgical procedures.[11] *Burnout* of disease may not occur for 10 years or more. By contrast, children living with the deformity, while waiting for surgical correction, may have psychosocial difficulties at home and school.

Patients with mild to moderate deformity are typically treated with serial fat grafting procedures because of the effectiveness and low risk. Fat grafting is preferred to injection of silicone and other synthetic injectables because of higher rates of infection, seroma, capsule formation, exposure, migration, and long-term scar formation. The *take* of fat grafting in the diseased Romberg region is less than fat graft *take* in *normal* regions.[11] Interestingly, the fat graft take improves in subsequent fat grafting procedures for Romberg patients. This improved take is thought to be due to improved vascular milieu of the grafted bed. For skeletally mature patients with severe deformity, dermal fat grafts or adipofascial free flaps (such as a parascapular or inframammary extended circumflex scapular [IMECS] flaps) are accepted alternatives[14] (**Figure 35.5**). The back region provides better adipose-fascial fill for facial contouring than that of other free flaps. Although excellent results may be obtained with an IMECS flap, this is a major procedure compared with fat grafting, and subsequent revisions or debulking procedures are typically necessary. In more severe manifestations of the disease, skeletal reconstruction and soft tissue rearrangement are required to restore anatomic landmarks and facial symmetry.

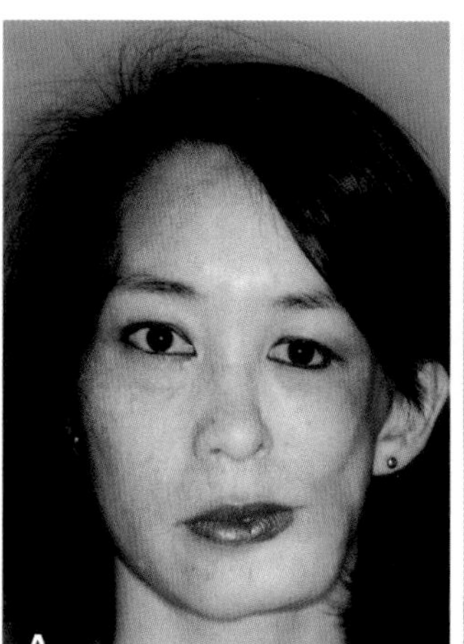
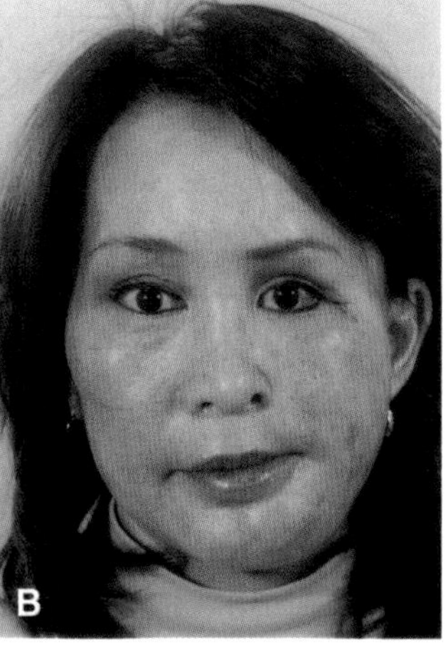

FIGURE 35.5. Romberg syndrome with left side involvement. **A.** Preoperative image shows significant soft tissue atrophy, nasal deviation, and skin changes. **B.** Postoperative image shows correction after IMECS flap, lateral canthoplasty, and composite graft to nose. (Courtesy of H.K. Kawamoto and S.W. Seibert.)

In summary, Romberg patients required multiple corrective surgeries but showed improvements even when beginning before puberty. Fat graft take is poorer in diseased regions compared with normal regions, but the procedure is still beneficial. For severe Romberg deformities, soft and hard tissue reconstruction is necessary to improve symmetry.

TREACHER COLLINS SYNDROME

Definition and Clinical Findings

Treacher Collins syndrome (TCS) is generally characterized by bilaterally symmetrical dysostosis of craniofacial structures derived from the first and second branchial arches.[15] Although there is a wide variation in phenotypic expression, common clinical features include hypoplasia of the zygomatic complex and the mandible, antimongoloid slanting of palpebral fissures, coloboma of the lower eyelids, complete or partial cleft palate, and atresia of external ear canals with abnormalities of the external ears accompanied by conductive hearing loss[15-17] (**Figure 35.6**).

Etiology and Pathogenesis

Genetic, physical, and transcript mapping techniques have demonstrated that approximately 93% of TCS is caused by loss-of-function mutations in the *TCOF1* gene (for Treacle) located on chromosome 5 (5q32-33.1).[18,19] TCS resulting from mutations in the *TCOF1* gene is inherited in an autosomal dominant fashion, with only 40% of patients inheriting a mutated copy of the gene and 60% of cases arising from de novo mutagenesis.[19,20] On a cellular basis, *TCOF1* knockout mice have a diminished number of migrating neural crest cells from extensive apoptosis and decreased proliferation.

Treatment and Complications

The treatment of TCS usually begins during infancy (when airway management at birth may be required), continues during mid-childhood (with bilateral total ear reconstruction and malar/orbital bony and soft tissue reconstruction), and is completed at facial maturity (with orthognathic procedures and a septorhinoplasty) (**Figure 35.7**).[16,17] In the newborn, severe airway obstruction may require a tracheostomy (the standard). If obstruction is limited to the tongue base and epiglottis, mandibular distraction can be effective in the newborn age or at a later age if sleep apnea develops. Choanal atresia, obstructing the posterior nasopharyngeal airway, may also need to be treated with dilatation or bony removal. Before 2 years of age, other

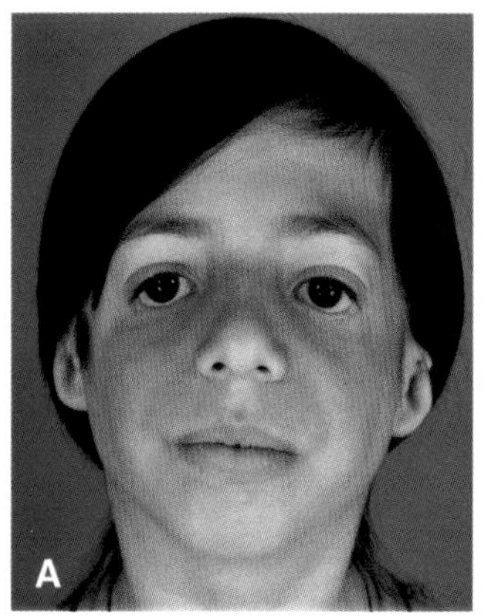
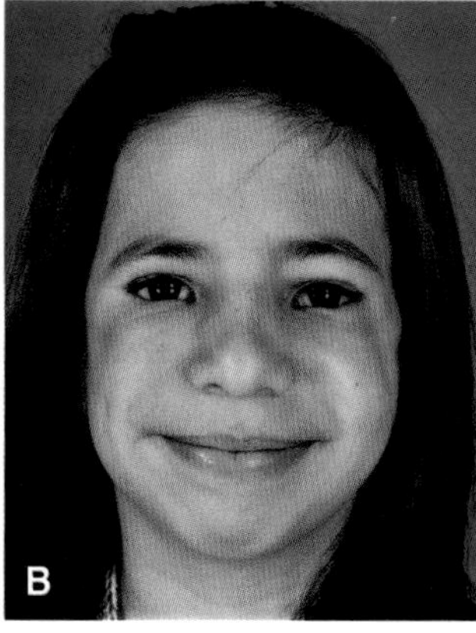

FIGURE 35.6. Treacher Collins syndrome. **A.** Preoperative image shows bilateral symmetric malar deficiency, down-slanting lateral canthus. **B.** Postoperative image shows correction after cranial bone grafting to zygomatic arches, lateral orbital wall, and upper to lower eyelid switch flaps. (Courtesy of J.P. Bradley.)

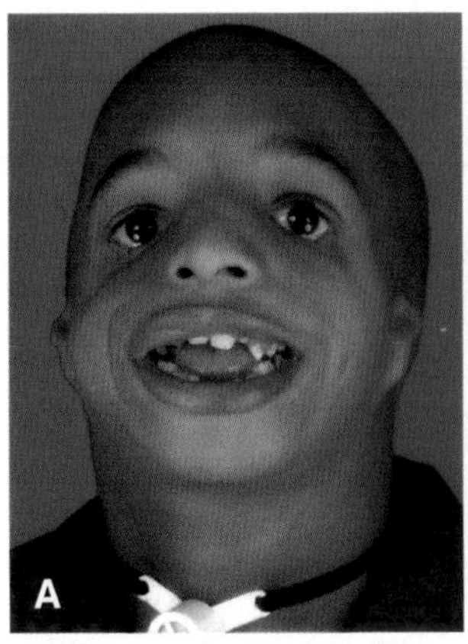

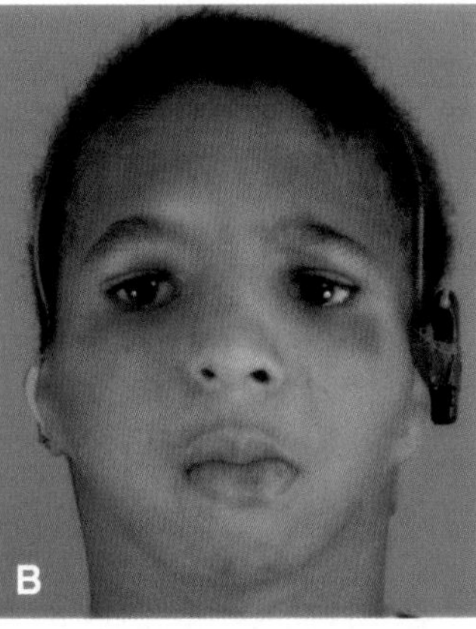

FIGURE 35.7. Treacher Collins syndrome. **A.** Preoperative image shows bilateral anterior open-bite malocclusion and symmetric malar deficiency. **B.** Postoperative image shows correction after bilateral mandibular distraction (for tracheostomy removal), cranial bone grafting to zygomatic arches, lateral orbital wall, and upper to lower eyelid switch flaps. (Courtesy of J.P. Bradley.)

procedures may be required, including cleft lip repair, cleft palate repair, macrostomia (Tessier no. 7 cleft), or removal of preauricular skin tags. In addition, optimizing hearing with BAHA (bone-anchored hearing apparatus) is beneficial in early childhood.

In mid-childhood (ages 6–9 years of age), corrective procedures may include[16]:

- mandibular distraction lengthening
- malar, zygomatic, and eyelid reconstruction
- total external ear reconstruction

Both distraction and total ear reconstruction require staged procedures in which fat grafting may be added at each stage.[21] This addition of soft tissue to the malar region helps while waiting on malar reconstruction, especially when adverse psychosocial peer experiences are occurring.

For mandibular distraction, a vertical vector is recommended to correct the short ramus; strong guiding elastics are used to close the open bite and improve the obtuse gonial angle. Relapse of this abnormal mandibular morphologic shape has been noted in long-term follow-up from the strong genioglossal muscle pull. Relapse and malocclusion may be addressed later during an orthognathic procedure.

For total ear reconstruction, the two-stage Firmin technique is preferred unless there is paucity of skin as in a very low lobule or anotia.[16] For these patients, the four-stage Brent technique may be used. Laser hair removal is performed for low-set hairlines and preauricular sideburns before first-stage ear reconstruction.

Malar/orbital reconstruction should not be attempted too early to avoid premature resorption of bone grafts. At age 8 to 12 years, malar/orbital reconstruction may be undertaken with full-thickness parietal skull bone grafts for the zygomatic arch and lateral orbit, with split thickness grafts for the orbital floor, and with simultaneous upper to lower eyelid switch flaps with lateral canthopexies.[22]

After facial skeletal maturity (16–18 years), correction of residual jaw abnormalities using orthognathic techniques and a septorhinoplasty are performed. Although a common procedure to close an open bite is Le Fort I posterior impaction, for the Treacher Collins patient, this will likely worsen the airway and aesthetics because of the short cranial base and abnormal mandible. Tessier described l'integrale procedure combining a Le Fort II osteotomy, bilateral mandibular advancement, orbital bone grafting, and genioplasty for the severe, uncorrected form of TCS with airway compromise. With distraction osteogenesis, similar osseous movements may be performed while reducing the relapse.[23] Genioplasty distraction with hyoid advancement has also been used for airway improvement and reduces relapse from genioglossal downward pull.[24] In summary, TCS remains a difficult entity to treat, often requiring multiple-staged procedures throughout childhood for functional and aesthetic improvements.

NEUROFIBROMATOSIS

Definition and Clinical Findings

Neurofibromatoses are a common group of conditions separated into five types, of which type I and type II are the most relevant for plastic surgery. Neurofibromas are benign peripheral nerve sheath tumors and may appear as discreet masses or as diffuse, plexiform masses without distinct borders.

Clinical manifestations of neurofibromatosis are detected at birth in about 40% of patients, and over 60% have manifestations by the second year of life starting with café au lait spots. Café au lait spots are pigmented macules present in over 99% of patients with neurofibromatosis. They are frequently present at birth and increase in size in childhood. Cutaneous neurofibromas appear around puberty and increase throughout life. Approximately one-third of patients develop plexiform neurofibromas and about 6% may develop malignancy. Neurologic problems occur in 10%, scoliosis in 5%, learning disabilities in 25%, and intellectual developmental delay in 8% to 9%. In young children, macrocephaly without hydrocephalus, short stature, hypertelorism, and thoracic abnormalities are frequently found.

Malignant peripheral nerve sheath tumors, also called neurosarcoma or neurofibrosarcoma, may develop in patients, particularly those with plexiform neurofibromas. The lifetime risk of development is 5% to 10% with the mean age of diagnosis at 41 years of age. Pain is the most reliable sign of malignant transformation.

- **Neurofibromatosis, type I (NF1):** NF1 accounts for 90% of all cases. Clinical diagnosis is suspected when six or more café au lait spots, cutaneous neurofibromas, and melanocytic hamartomas projecting from the surface of the iris (Lisch nodules) are found.[25]
- **Neurofibromatosis, type II (NF2):** NF2 is characterized by bilateral acoustic neuromas with hearing loss usually present as a teenager or young adult. Café au lait spots and cutaneous neurofibromas are present but usually less common than NF1. Plexiform neurofibromas and central nervous system tumors may also be present occasionally.
- **Craniofacial plexiform neurofibromas:** Craniofacial involvement in neurofibromatosis is a significant reconstructive challenge, as it is likely to be plexiform in nature with widespread destruction of facial structures and potential intracranial extension. Two types of craniofacial neurofibromas are generally considered separately:
  - Orbitotemporal neurofibromas
  - Plexiform neurofibromas resulting in hemifacial hypertrophy

The specific variety of neurofibromas localized to the orbitotemporal region involves the orbit, the eyelids, and the temporal area (**Figure 35.8**). It may have an intracranial component associated with headaches and seizures.[26] Manifested during childhood with lid swelling, it becomes worse over time with severe involvement of the subcutaneous tissues of the eyelids and variable degrees of ptosis and proptosis of the globe (see Figure 35.8). In the most severe of cases, involvement of the globe leads to blindness. The skeletal changes in orbitotemporal neurofibromas consist of an absence of the greater wing of the sphenoid and a defect of the posterolateral wall of the orbit or an enlargement of the superior orbital fissure. The orbit is enlarged and hypoplasia of the supraorbital and infraorbital rims is present. The zygoma is hypoplastic and the orbital floor is inferiorly positioned.

A second type of craniofacial involvement by plexiform neurofibromas results in a unilateral overgrowth of face because of diffuse proliferation of Schwann cells and axons associated with bony hypertrophy. This type typically forms from the trigeminal, facial, or glossopharyngeal nerves.

Etiology and Pathogenesis

Neurofibromatosis occurs in 1 in 2500 to 3000 births. NF1 is caused by mutations in neurofibromin, a tumor suppressor gene on

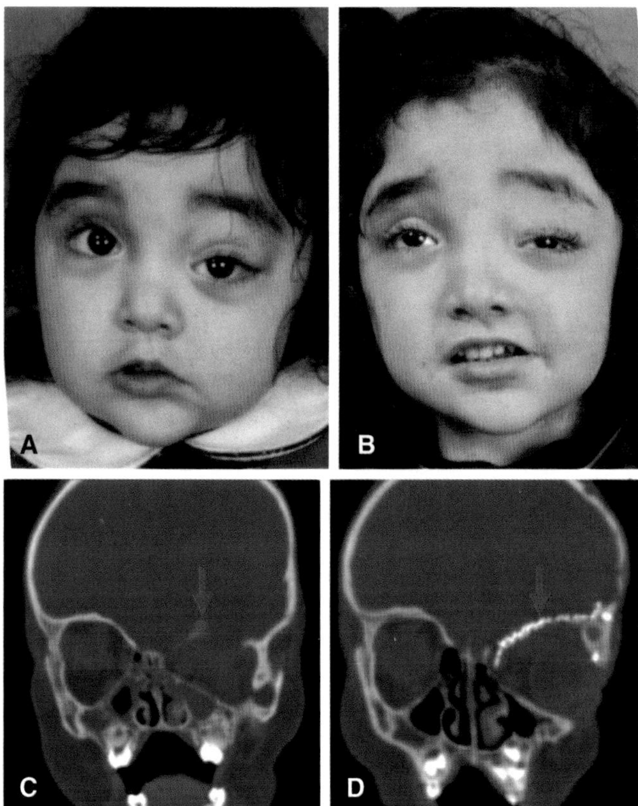

FIGURE 35.8. Neurofibromatosis type 1: left orbital involvement. **A.** Preoperative image shows vertical dystopia; patient had pulsatile globe. **B.** Postoperative image shows correction after left orbital box osteotomy with elevation and orbital roof reconstruction. **C.** Preoperative coronal CT scan depicts absent orbital roof (arrow). **D.** Postoperative coronal CT scan depicts titanium plate reconstruction of orbital roof (arrow). (Courtesy of J.P. Bradley and J.C. Lee.)

chromosome 17q, and inherited in an autosomal dominant manner. NF2 is caused by mutations in the neurofibromin-2, a tumor suppressor gene on chromosome 22q.

Treatment and Complications

Treatment of craniofacial neurofibromatosis is complex due to the variability in presentations and destructive nature of the tumors. Orbitotemporal neurofibromas associated with sphenoid wing dysplasia and plexiform neurofibromas involving the soft tissue of the face are the two main classifications of the types of neurofibromas addressed. Because surgery cannot cure the process, the goal of surgical resection is to debulk and lessen the visual impact of the deformity.

Orbitotemporal Plexiform Neurofibromas

An algorithm for the treatment of orbitotemporal neurofibromas has been described in detail by Jackson.[26] In the presence of orbital soft tissue involvement without significant bony involvement and intact vision, resection of the neurofibroma through a supratarsal incision may proceed. If the neurofibroma is found to be a discreet mass, dissection and complete resection should be undertaken. However, if there is more widespread involvement of the intraconal tissues, partial resection must be undertaken with every effort to preserve vision. A bony defect of the orbit may be found in the orbital roof which should be reconstructed at the same time to prevent enlargement of the defect due to prolapse of the intracranial contents. Although bone grafts are usually the best choice for reconstruction of most osseous defects, in the orbital roof region, resorption of the graft is common because of the pulsatile intracranial contents. Thus, in this particular location, alloplast (titanium or methylmethacrylate) should be used. Shortening of the levator aponeurosis may be necessary at the time of closure to account for the reduction of proptosis of the globe from neurofibroma resection. In addition to reconstruction of the orbital roof, vertical orbital dystopia may be present with inferior displacement of the orbit due to a mass effect from the neurofibroma. When this occurs, an orbital box repositioning may be necessary.

In the most severe of presentations, the neurofibroma is present in the temporal area and the orbit with pulsating exophthalmos because of a massive bony defect. In such cases, vision is not present. Neurosurgical involvement is necessary to reduce the temporal lobe back into the middle cranial fossa. Resection is performed with globe exenteration and reconstruction of the bony defect in preparation for prosthesis. A recent Australian study focused on visual outcomes demonstrated that vision loss and amblyopia are common in this cohort.[27]

Facial Plexiform Neurofibromas With Hemifacial Hypertrophy

Similar to the orbitotemporal neurofibromas, consideration for significant bleeding should be taken into account. In the treatment of hemifacial hypertrophy, it is necessary to sacrifice a certain amount of normal soft tissue structures, as it is not possible to separate the neurofibroma from unaffected tissues. One method of soft tissue excision was proposed based on transposition of aesthetic units from the contralateral normal side to the affected side.[28] Following transposition, the remaining tissue is excised en bloc with incisions hidden in the areas such as the nasolabial fold. Underlying bony abnormalities are also found, thus frequently requiring bone grafting for reconstruction of the mandible, maxilla, or zygoma as necessary.[29]

Pierre Robin Sequence

Definition and Clinical Findings

Pierre Robin sequence (PRS) describes a triad of manifestations in neonates that included micrognathia, glossoptosis, and upper airway obstruction; cleft palate deformity is an associated abnormality but not a requirement for the sequence.[30] Because PRS has been associated with other anomalies, it is often divided into:

- *PRS*: isolated (**Figure 35.9**)
- *PRS plus:* with comorbidities, Stickler, 22q deletion
- *Syndromic PRS:* Treacher Collins syndrome, Nager syndrome (**Figure 35.10**)

Etiology and Pathogenesis

When genetic syndromes or deformational factors disrupt prenatal growth, micrognathia ensues and causes the retropositioning of the tongue. If this process occurs before the eighth week of gestation, closure of the palatal shelves is prevented, thereby resulting in the formation of

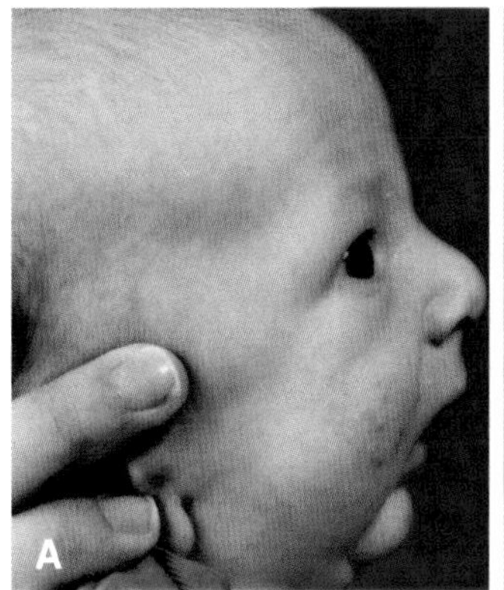

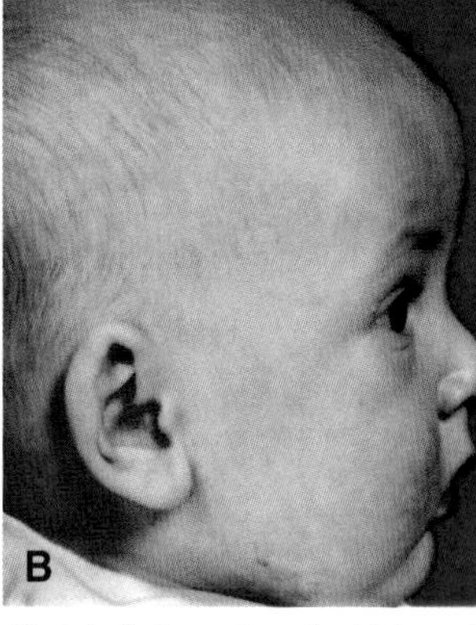

FIGURE 35.9. Pierre Robin sequence (isolated) in a 6-week-old boy. **A.** Preoperative image shows significant micrognathia (workup revealed upper airway obstruction). **B.** Postoperative image shows mandibular position improvement after bilateral mandibular distraction (and relief of airway obstruction). (Courtesy of J.P. Bradley.)

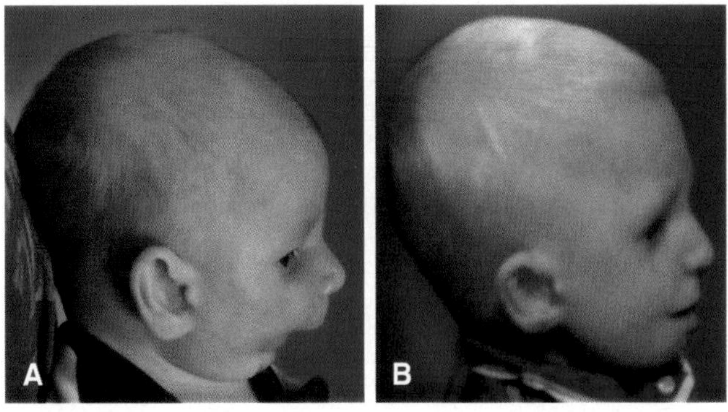

FIGURE 35.10. Syndromic Pierre Robin sequence (Nager Syndrome) in a 3-month-old boy. **A.** Preoperative image shows significant micrognathia (workup revealed upper airway obstruction). **B.** Postoperative image shows correction of chin point (and improvement in airway). (Courtesy of J.P. Bradley.)

a U-shaped cleft palate.[31] When PRS occurs in isolation, in utero deformational factors such as intrauterine growth restriction are generally considered to be important. Although neonates born with PRS may have clinically significant symptoms, a portion of children may escape surgical intervention because of postnatal mandibular *catch-up* growth. This phenomenon is generally more common to patients with isolated PRS, likely because of the release of interference by deformational intrauterine factors after delivery. However, some patients treated conservatively continued to have respiratory disturbances throughout life.[32]

Treatment and Complications

The most critical consequence of PRS is upper airway obstruction in the neonatal period. The severity of airway obstruction may not always correlate with the degree of anatomic deformity (micrognathia). An algorithmic workup is often warranted to determine the degree of tongue-based obstruction and indication for surgical treatment to maintain airway patency.[32] In the mildest of circumstances, side or prone positioning may be sufficient to prevent respiratory compromise. These mild PRS cases must still be monitored closely. When cleft palate exists, delay in the repair is recommended (at 18 months or more, as opposed to 10–12 months). In patients who cannot maintain airway patency with positioning alone, intubation using a nasopharyngeal tube or an endotracheal tube may be necessary. In neonates who require endotracheal intubation for survival, a surgical procedure is virtually universal to extubate the child.[33] The current surgical armamentarium for relief of airway obstruction includes glossopexy, subperiosteal mandibular stripping, mandibular distraction, and tracheostomy.

In PRS, retrodisplacement of the mandibular attachment of the genioglossus diminishes the ability to hold the tongue out of the pharyngeal airway. Although glossopexy has the ability to temporarily relieve obstruction with anterior movement of the tongue, this procedure depends on sufficient mandibular *catch-up* growth for long-term reversal of airway obstruction. In addition, glossopexy does not address the core anatomical disturbance.

When considering neonatal mandibular distraction for PRS patients, a decision tree model or management algorithm is recommended (**Figure 35.11**).[32] Patients who exhibit other abnormalities such as central apnea, multilevel airway obstruction, neurologic compromise, or severe airway edema from reflux are precluded from mandibular distraction. Outcome studies on neonatal mandibular distraction have shown improvements in oxygen saturation, apneic events, reflux, and feeding in neonates who received mandibular distraction.[34] In patients who are not eligible for distraction based on the management algorithm, a standard tracheostomy is performed. These tracheostomy patients will need decannulation at a later age after growth and resolve their airway abnormalities. Mandibular distraction and laryngotracheal reconstruction may be needed before tracheostomy removal. Skeletally mature, untreated PRS patients may require mandibular advancement with a sagittal split osteotomy for class II malocclusion after orthodontic preparation.

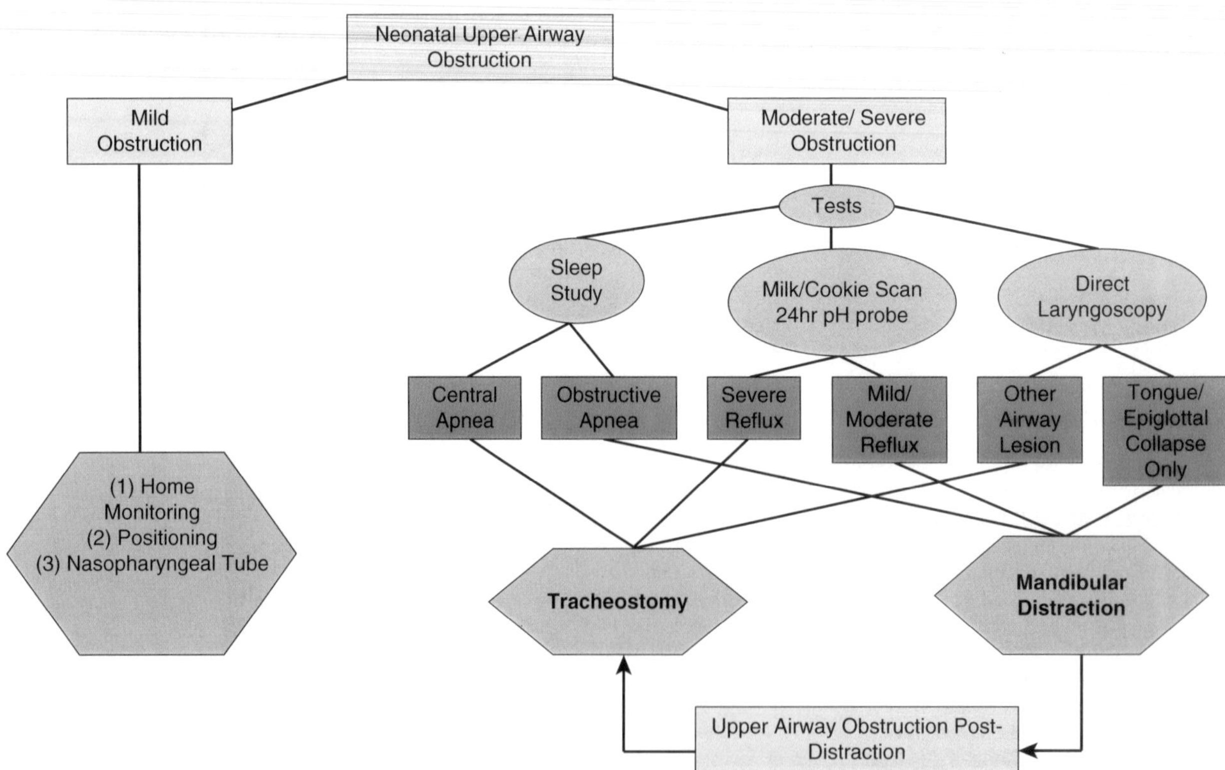

FIGURE 35.11. Pierre Robin sequence decision-tree model (algorithm) for all infants admitted to the pediatric intensive care unit (PICU) with upper airway obstruction. Mild obstruction is treated as an outpatient with monitoring. Moderate/severe obstruction undergoes multidisciplinary consultations and tests (sleep study, direct laryngoscopy, reflux study). Infants with central apnea, airway lesions (other than tongue-based obstruction), or severe reflux undergo a tracheostomy. All other infants have internal mandibular distraction.

The reported complications of mandibular distraction are respiratory failure, relapse, nerve injury, tooth injury, infection, incorrect distraction vector, and device failure.[35] These complications can be minimized with the use of proper operative indications and perioperative protocols including appropriate rate (2 mm), length (15–30 mm), and extubation times (after 7 days). In syndromic PRS patients, there is a higher rate of temporomandibular joint ankylosis after distraction.[36] Elastic condylar unloading reduces the risk of these ankylosis events.

Neonatal morbidity and mortality associated with PRS have significantly decreased with improved nonsurgical and surgical methods for airway protection. With the understanding that improved outcomes occur with mandibular distraction in a management algorithm, the majority of severely micrognathic patients are no longer destined to tracheostomies. The challenge to institutions is to implement and optimize systematic methods for evaluation and treatment for PRS neonates to achieve timely, consistent, and cost-effective outcomes.

MOEBIUS SYNDROME

Definition and Clinical Findings

In 1888 and 1892, Moebius classically described combined palsies of the abducens (CN VI) and facial (CN VII) nerves as a composite entity.[37] This description was later expanded by others to include other CNs, limb abnormalities, chest wall defects, and developmental delay.

The typical craniofacial manifestations of Moebius syndrome include mask-like facies, bilateral facial paralysis, and the inability to abduct the globes (palsy of the abducens or sixth CN) (**Figure 35.12**). Despite the classic description, there are variable presentations for Moebius syndrome including incomplete or unilateral facial palsy. Several other CNs have also been associated with Moebius syndrome, most frequently the third, fifth, ninth, and twelfth. Clinically, paralysis of the orbicularis oculi is the first sign of Moebius syndrome detected in the neonate, prompting consultation by pediatricians and neonatologists.[38] Ptosis, nystagmus, strabismus, epicanthal folds, hypertelorbitism, and lagophthalmos are all frequently manifested. The nasal root is frequently widened. The mouth opening is usually small and the commissures are downturned. Intraoral manifestations include tongue hypoplasia, oligodontia, mandibular hypoplasia, cleft palate, and poor palatal mobility associated with difficulties in feeding and speech. Feeding difficulties may resolve over time.

In addition to craniofacial manifestations, both trunk and limb differences may be found. Absence or hypoplasia of the sternal head of the pectoralis major is a common finding.[39] Moebius combined with Poland syndrome has been reported in combination in 15% to 20% of cases.[40] Scoliosis is also found in approximately 14% of cases.[40] Limb abnormalities occur in over half of all patients diagnosed with Moebius syndrome. The most common abnormality is clubfoot in 40% to 50% of patients followed by limb reduction abnormalities in approximately 20% of patients. Intellectual developmental delay occurs in 10% to 30% of patients with Moebius syndrome and ranges in severity. Autism has been associated with Moebius syndrome. Motor delay, independent of the limb abnormalities, and speech delay are frequently seen.

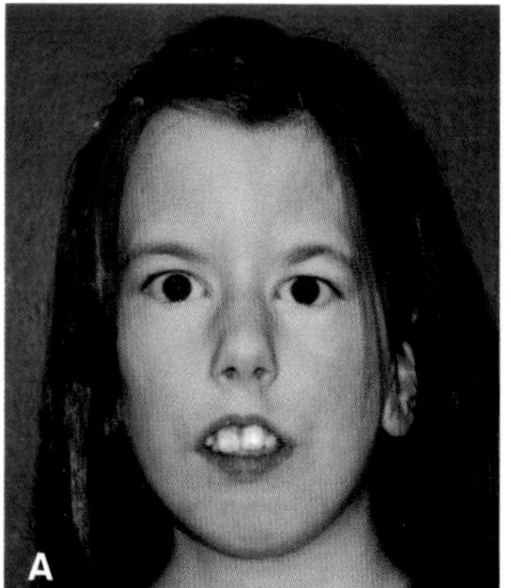

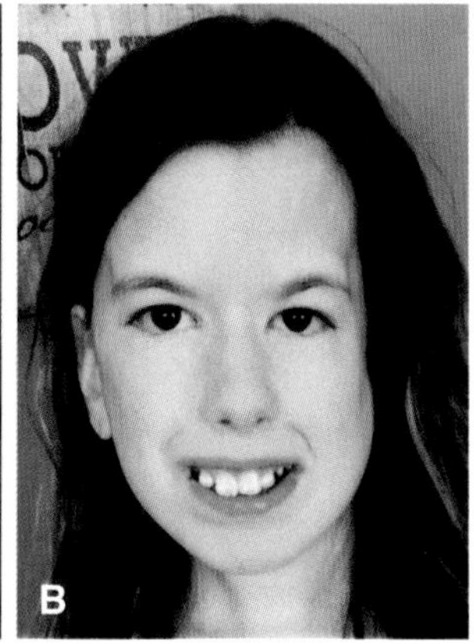

FIGURE 35.12. Moebius syndrome in a 10-year-old patient. **A.** Preoperative image (when asked to smile) shows mask faces with no expression. **B.** Postoperative image (2 years) shows correction after bilateral lengthening temporalis myoplasty. (Courtesy of P.D. Nguyen.)

Etiology and Pathogenesis

The prevalence of Moebius syndrome is estimated at 1 in 50,000 with equal distribution between male and female. Although the pathogenesis is not well understood, both environmental and genetic relationships have been described. The correlation between Moebius syndrome and misoprostol, a synthetic prostaglandin E1 analogue, was described in Brazil in the early 1990s.[41] Within 96 infants with Moebius syndrome identified in the Brazilian multicenter study, 49% of the mothers had taken misoprostol during the first trimester of pregnancy. Moebius syndrome may also be related to genetic causes inherited in an autosomal dominant, autosomal recessive, or X-linked pattern. Four genetic loci have been identified (MBS1-4) located on chromosomes 13q, 1p, 3p, and 10q, respectively.

Treatment and Complications

Reconstructive surgery in Moebius syndrome is a multidisciplinary endeavor requiring plastic surgery, ophthalmology, and orthopedic surgery. The main procedures performed by the latter two specialties are strabismus correction and clubfoot correction. For plastic surgery, the primary reconstructive procedure for the treatment of Moebius syndrome is facial reanimation for smile restoration. The ability to reconstruct facial motion using functional muscle transfers has undergone a renaissance age over the past 40 years. In the treatment of Moebius patients, the majority of patients suffer from bilateral complete paralysis. Thus, functional muscle transfers frequently require innervation by nonfacial nerves such as the masseteric nerve.

In the absence of suitable facial nerves as the donor innervator, functional muscle transfers for reanimation are typically performed in one stage.[42,43] The most commonly used one-stage procedure is the innervated, partial gracilis free muscle flap. Preoperatively, the new nasolabial fold is marked on the face and a vector connecting the modiolus and the cephaloauricular junction at the root of the helix is marked, mimicking the pull of the zygomaticus major muscle. Intraoperatively, a preauricular incision is made and a dissection is performed in a sub-SMAS plane to the new nasolabial fold and the modiolus. The masseteric nerve is then identified and dissected within an area bordered by the zygomatic arch, coronoid process of the mandible, sigmoid notch, and condyle of the mandible. Dissection is carried out through the parotid and between the superficial and middle heads of the masseter muscle, upon where the nerve is visualized and coapted with the anterior branch of the obturator nerve from the gracilis muscle flap. The harvested partial gracilis muscle is then inset to the insertion on the new nasolabial fold and modiolus and to the origin at the deep temporal fascia following the premarked vector. Microsurgical anastomoses of the vascular supply of the gracilis muscle are performed last, typically to the facial vessels.

Alternatively, if CN V is functional, lengthening temporalis myoplasty or Labbe procedure may be performed.[44] In this procedure, the nasolabial fold is marked out preoperatively. Intraoperatively, a coronal incision is made, a scalp flap is elevated, and the temporalis muscle is dissected immediately on the deep temporal fascia down to the zygomatic arch. Subperiosteal dissection is then carried over the zygomatic arch and osteotomized for access. Next, the temporalis aponeurosis is incised 1 cm below the temporal crest and the muscle is dissected away from the bone preserving the temporal nerve and vessels. To inset the muscle, the new nasolabial fold is incised and dissected down to the coronoid process. The temporalis tendon is detached from the coronoid process and sutured to the new nasolabial fold. The temporalis muscle is then stretched and resuspended to the remaining strip of aponeurosis.

Although static procedures for smile restoration are not generally considered standard of care for Moebius syndrome, auxiliary static procedures for the treatment of lagophthalmos are common and beneficial for globe protection. The mechanism of lagophthalmos in Moebius syndrome is due to the lack of opposition of the levator palpebrae muscle by the paralyzed orbicularis oculi muscle. Although a number of modalities have been described to treat lagophthalmos, the most common and widely used is the placement of a gold or platinum weight in the upper eyelid. Preoperatively, an appropriate weight is estimated by taping the weight on the patient's eyelid. Intraoperatively, an incision is made within the supratarsal fold and dissection is carried out through the orbicularis oculi muscle. Two positions have been described for the weight placement: (1) pretarsal and (2) postseptal.[45] In the pretarsal position, the weight is secured to the tarsus underneath the orbicularis oculi muscle. Although this is the classic placement position, there are complications such as entropion and visibility associated with pretarsal weight placement. In the postseptal position, the septum is incised and the weight is placed immediately superior to the tarsus. In this position, complications are diminished; however, the weight chosen should be 0.2 g heavier than the preoperatively estimated weight.

Quantifiable complications such as hematoma and flap failure in facial reanimation are rare. However, qualitative and aesthetic issues such as incomplete correction, lack of strength in smile, asymmetry, and lack of spontaneity are frequently present. The recent advent of more objective methods of analysis such as the FACE-gram, an automated, objective assessment of facial movement, will likely assist in assessing surgical outcomes.[46]

Dermoid Cyst

Definition and Clinical Findings

Congenital facial dermoid cysts are benign, developmental malformations formed by inclusion of ectodermal elements.[47,48] Dermoid cysts are differentiated from the typical epidermoid cysts by the presence of mature adnexal structures such as hair and glands. Because of the process of formation, dermoid cysts are frequently, if not always, associated with some type of skeletal abnormality. Dermoid cysts are more common in females than in males.

Craniofacial dermoid cysts can be generally divided into lateral and midline. Lateral cysts may be further subdivided into the frontotemporal region and the orbit. By far, lateral dermoid cysts of the frontotemporal region are the most common type of craniofacial dermoids with the majority near the lateral eyebrow (**Figure 35.13**). The lesion is usually deep to the skin such that there is usually no evidence of sinus ostia. The lesions are typically firm and present as a discreet nodule. Dermoids within this region are rarely associated with intracranial extension and thus do not warrant imaging before surgical resection without additional clinical suspicion.

The orbit is the second anatomical subdivision of lateral cysts and accounts for the second most common area for dermoid cysts of the face. Extraocular mobility is typically not affected by orbital cysts; however, depending on the size, visual obstruction may occur (see Figure 35.13.A). Unlike epidermoid cysts, dermoid cysts are frequently found with skeletal abnormalities. Although the skeletal anomaly in the lateral brow dermoids is simple depressions within the frontal bone, orbital dermoids frequently traverse sutures, such as the frontozygomatic suture (see Figure 35.13.B). In such cases, the dermoid has an intraorbital component and an extraorbital component.

Unlike lateral orbital cysts, the midline dermoid cysts may have more extensive and potentially intracranial involvement. The estimated incidence of intracranial involvement ranges around 19% of all nasal dermoids.[49] Midline dermoids may be found in the upper, middle, or lower face. In all cases, because of the potential for intracranial extension, a CT scan and/or MRI is necessary to define the limits of the dermoid. Within the nasoethmoid region, the external clinical manifestations may be particularly mild. A small punctum, bulge of the glabella, or widening of the nasal dorsum may be seen. However, mild clinical presentations may portend extensive involvement of internal structures and intracranial involvement. Additionally, unlike the lateral dermoids, midline dermoids have a higher propensity to display puncta and sinus ostia. Owing to the presence of adnexal structures, dermoid cysts have the capability of enlarging over time. Although rare, complications of dermoid cysts include infection, with several instances of calvarial osteomyelitis reported in the literature.[47]

Etiology and Pathogenesis

Dermoid cysts are most often found as isolated entities and very rarely found in families. Formation of dermoid cysts is found at the embryologic fusion planes. For example, the lateral brow dermoid is found at the frontotemporal suture; the lateral orbital dermoid is found at the frontozygomatic suture; and the nasoglabellar suture is found at the frontonasal junction. In the circumstances of intracranial extension of dermoid sinuses and cysts, the development can be traced back to 8 weeks of gestation. During this time, the developing nasal and frontal bones are separated by dural extensions through the fonticulus nasofrontalis anteriorly and through the frontal bones into the prenasal space inferiorly. As the frontal bones grow, the dura migrates into the cranium and the fonticulus nasofrontalis fuses with the foramen cecum to become the cribriform plate. When this process is incomplete, the dura remains extracranial and becomes a cyst or sinus.

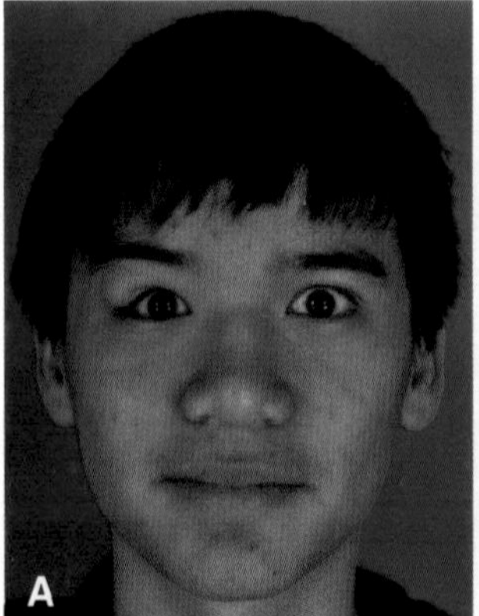

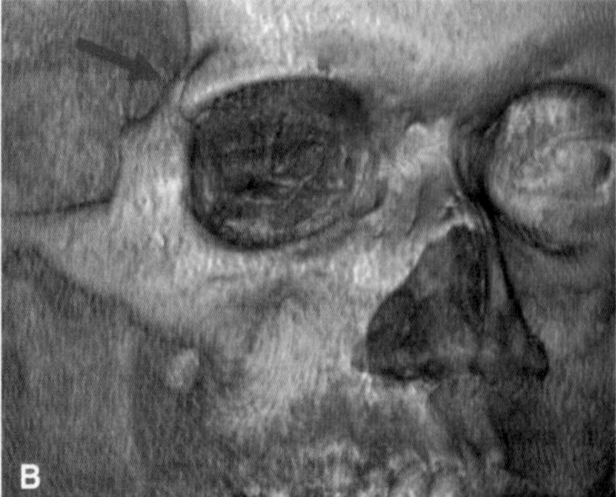

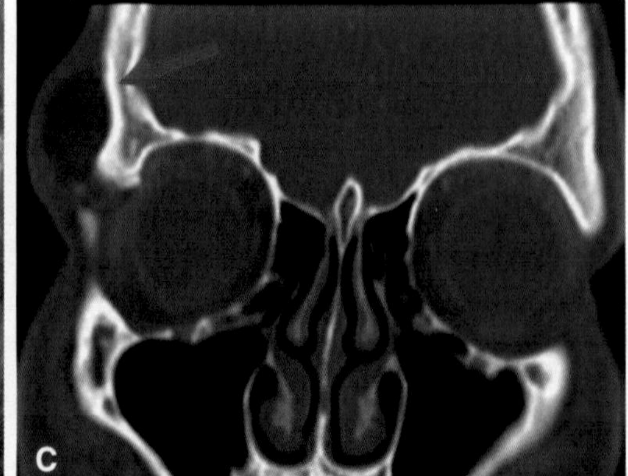

FIGURE 35.13. Dermoid cyst right lateral orbit. **A.** Preoperative image shows 2 cm mass. **B.** 3D CT scan shows erosion of lateral orbit from dermoid mass (arrow). **C.** CT scan coronal view shows dermoid mass distorting bone from lateral orbital rim (arrow). (Courtesy of J.C. Lee.)

Treatment and Complications

Surgery is the only treatment available for dermoids. In lateral dermoids of the frontotemporal or orbital region, excision can be approached with an incision directly over the dermoid or hidden in the supratarsal fold. Because the embryologic origins of the cyst formation, dissection of the cyst should be through the soft tissues to the periosteum; this dissection is distinguished from that of the dissection of a simple epidermal cyst. Additionally, a skeletal depression will be frequently found underneath the cyst.

In nasal dermoids, diagnosis requires imaging with an initial fine-cut CT scan. The two signs on CT scan suggestive of intracranial extension are a patent foramen cecum and a bifid crista galli. If either finding is present or suspicious for intracranial extension, an MRI should be performed next. If the MRI is negative, simple excision may be performed as above for glabellar dermoids. In nasal dermoids positioned more inferiorly, an open rhinoplasty approach should be considered.

If the MRI is positive for intracranial extension, excision of the dermoid requires neurosurgical involvement. Coronal incision access is used for the frontal craniotomy. Dissection of the cyst requires an osteotomy of the frontal bone which may be performed in the *keystone* technique with paramedian osteotomies of the frontal and nasal bones.[50] By removing this V-shaped piece of bone, the dermoid cyst can be better visualized for full excision.

Complications for extracranial dermoid excisions are rare but may include incomplete excision, recurrence, or infection. Resection of dermoids with intracranial extension may be complicated with osteomyelitis, incomplete resection, or cerebrospinal fluid leak.

REFERENCES

1. Cohen SR, Bartlett SP, Whitaker LA. Reconstruction of late craniofacial deformities after irradiation of the head and face during childhood. *Plast Reconstr Surg.* 1990;86:229-237.
2. Chen YR, Chang CN, Tan YC. Craniofacial fibrous dysplasia: an update. *Chang Gung Med J.* 2006;29:543-549.
   This up-to-date review documents the variation of fibrous dysplasia involvement as mild to severe in the craniofacial skeleton. This center has a broad experience and documents their care protocols in treating this disorder and dealing with monostotic and polyostotic cases.
3. Weinstein LS, Shenker A, Gejman PV, et al. Activating mutations of the stimulatory G protein in the McCune-Albright syndrome. *N Engl J Med.* 1991;325:1688-1695.
4. Posnick JC. Fibrous dysplasia of the craniomaxillofacial region: current clinical perspectives. *Br J Oral Maxillofac Surg.* 1998;36:264-273.
5. Moore AT, Buncic JR, Munro IR. Fibrous dysplasia of the orbit in childhood: clinical features and management. *Ophthalmology.* 1985;92:12-20.
6. Sassin JF, Rosenberg RN. Neurological complications of fibrous dysplasia of the skull. *Arch Neurol.* 1968;18:363-369.
7. Hunt JA, Hobar PC. Common craniofacial anomalies: conditions of craniofacial atrophy/hypoplasia and neoplasia. *Plast Reconstr Surg.* 2003;111:1497-1508.
8. Simpson AH, Creasy TS, Williamson DM, et al. Cystic degeneration of fibrous dysplasia masquerading as sarcoma. *J Bone Joint Surg Br.* 1989;71:434-436.
9. Gabbay JS, Yuan JT, Andrews BT, et al. Fibrous dysplasia of the zygomaticomaxillary region: outcomes of surgical intervention. *Plast Reconstr Surg.* 2013;131:1329-1338.
   This article compares surgical strategy for a known region of involvement (zygomatic maxillary complex) for fibrous dysplasia. This comparative study showed that near-total excision with bone graft reconstruction had decreased recurrence but was more morbid than in situ contouring with a bur.
10. Chen YR, Breidahl A, Chang CN. Optic nerve decompression in fibrous dysplasia: indications, efficacy, and safety. *Plast Reconstr Surg.* 1997;99:22-30.
11. Slack GC, Tabit CJ, Allam KA, et al. Parry-Romberg reconstruction: optimal timing for hard and soft tissue procedures. *J Craniofac Surg.* 2012;23:S27-S31.
   For Parry-Romberg, both hard and soft tissue reconstruction is needed in moderate to severe cases, and this article illustrates how an accepted treatment strategy is beneficial for patients. Most staged reconstruction involves soft tissue and fat/dermal grafts; however, osteotomies and bone grafting is sometimes needed.
12. Stone J. Parry-Romberg syndrome: a global survey of 205 patients using the Internet. *Neurology.* 2003;61:674-676.
13. Gorlin RCN, Hennekam R. *Syndromes with unusual facies: well-known syndromes.* In: *Syndromes of the Head and Neck.* 4th ed. New York, NY: Oxford University Press; 2001:977-1038.
14. Saadeh P, Reavey PL, Siebert JW. A soft-tissue approach to midfacial hypoplasia associated with Treacher Collins syndrome. *Ann Plast Surg.* 2006;56:522-525.
   This article documents a microsurgical solution to soft tissue fill with a parascapular (or IMECS) flap after hard tissue reconstruction.
15. Kumar A. Treacher-Collins syndrome. In: Thaller SR, Garri JI, eds. *Craniofacial Surgery.* New York, NY: CRC Press; 2008:273-281.
16. Trainor PA, Dixon J, Dixon MJ. Treacher Collins syndrome: etiology, pathogenesis and prevention. *Eur J Hum Genet.* 2009;17:275-283.
17. Posnick JC, Tiwana PS, Costello BJ. Treacher Collins syndrome: comprehensive evaluation and treatment. *Oral Maxillofac Surg Clin North Am.* 2004;16:503-523.
   Treacher Collins reconstruction is multistaged and challenging, and this paper offers acceptable evaluation and treatment that is time-tested and accepted by multidisciplinary teams.
18. Trainor PA. Craniofacial birth defects: the role of neural crest cells in the etiology and pathogenesis of Treacher Collins syndrome and the potential for prevention. *Am J Med Genet A.* 2010;152a:2984-2994.
19. Dai J, Si J, Wang M, et al. Tcof1-related molecular networks in Treacher Collins syndrome. *J Craniofac Surg.* 2016;27:1420-1426.
20. Splendore A, Jabs EW, Felix TM, Passos-Bueno MR. Parental origin of mutations in sporadic cases of Treacher Collins syndrome. *Eur J Hum Genet.* 2003;11:718-722.
21. Konofaos P, Arnaud E. Early fat grafting for augmentation of orbitozygomatic region in Treacher Collins syndrome. *J Craniofac Surg.* 2015;26:1258-1260.
22. Fan KL, Federico C, Kawamoto HK, Bradley JP. Optimizing the timing and technique of Treacher Collins orbital malar reconstruction. *J Craniofac Surg.* 2012;23:2033-2037.
   This comparative outcomes study is one of the few that critically looks at the timing of bone graft reconstruction for the malar region. It discusses the psychosocial balance with timing of surgery to avoid reoperations. If in-lay cranial bone grafting is performed less than 5 years of age, it will resorb.
23. Hopper RA, Kapadia H, Susarla S, et al. Counterclockwise craniofacial distraction osteogenesis (C3DO) for tracheostomy-dependent children with Treacher Collins syndrome. *Plast Reconstr Surg.* 2018;142(2):447-457.
   Mandibular distraction and orthognathic reconstruction is challenging with Treacher Collins patients because of the abnormal mandibular shape and short cranial base. This paper illustrates a unique way of using distraction osteogenesis to lengthen the posterior midface and mandible with a counterclockwise rotation.
24. Heller JB, Gabbay JS, Kwan D, et al. Genioplasty distraction osteogenesis and hyoid advancement for correction of upper airway obstruction in patients with Treacher Collins and Nager syndromes. *Plast Reconstr Surg.* 2006;117:2389-2398.
25. Hennekam RCM, Gorlin RJ, Allanson JE, Krantz ID. *Gorlin's Syndromes of the Head and Neck. Neurofibromatosis.* 5th ed. New York, NY: Oxford University Press; 2010.
26. Jackson IT, Carbonnel A, Potparic Z, Shaw K. Orbitotemporal neurofibromatosis: classification and treatment. *Plast Reconstr Surg.* 1993;92:1-11.
27. Greenwell TH, Anderson PJ, Madge SK, et al. Long-term visual outcomes in patients with orbitotemporal neurofibromatosis. *Clin Exp Ophthalmol.* 2014;42:266-270.
28. Hivelin M, Wolkenstein P, Lepage C, et al. Facial aesthetic unit remodeling procedure for neurofibromatosis type 1 hemifacial hypertrophy: report on 33 consecutive adult patients. *Plast Reconstr Surg.* 2010;125:1197-1207.
29. Munro IR, Martin RD. The management of gigantic benign craniofacial tumors: the reverse facial osteotomy. *Plast Reconstr Surg.* 1980;65:776-785.
30. Robin P. Glossoptosis due to atresia and hypotrophy of the mandible. *Am J Dis Child.* 1934;48:541-547.
31. Hanson JW, Smith DW. U-shaped palatal defect in the Robin anomalad: developmental and clinical relevance. *J Pediatr.* 1975;87:30-33.
32. Vyas RM, Dipple KM, Head C, et al. Management of neonatal upper airway obstruction: decreased morbidity by utilizing a decision tree model with mandibular distraction osteogenesis. *J Neonat Perinat Med.* 2008;1:21-29.
   Neonatal mandibular distraction for airway obstruction is an effective treatment, but determining the indications for this procedure may be challenging. This algorithm study proves that a multidisciplinary team may treat neonatal upper airway obstruction with the correct modality when the evaluations are performed immediately and carefully.
33. Izadi K, Yellon R, Mandell DL, et al. Correction of upper airway obstruction in the newborn with internal mandibular distraction osteogenesis. *J Craniofac Surg.* 2003;14:493-499.
34. Kohan E, Hazany S, Roostaeian J, et al. Economic advantages to a distraction decision tree model for management of neonatal upper airway obstruction. *Plast Reconstr Surg.* 2010;126:1652-1664.
35. Mofid MM, Manson PN, Robertson BC, et al. Craniofacial distraction osteogenesis: a review of 3278 cases. *Plast Reconstr Surg.* 2001;108:1103-1114.
36. Fan K, Andrews BT, Liao E, et al. Protection of the temporomandibular joint during syndromic neonatal mandibular distraction using condylar unloading. *Plast Reconstr Surg.* 2012;129:1151-1161.
37. Hennekam RCM, Gorlin RJ, Allanson JE, Krantz ID. *Gorlin's Syndromes of the Head and Neck. Moebius Syndrome.* New York, NY: Oxford University Press; 2010.
38. Terzis JK, Noah EM. Möbius and Möbius-like patients: etiology, diagnosis, and treatment options. *Clin Plast Surg.* 2002;29:497-514.
   This article documents the important diagnosis and technical details in dealing with and treating Möebius patients.
39. McGillivray BC, Lowry RB. Poland syndrome in British Columbia: incidence and reproductive experience of affected persons. *Am J Med Genet.* 1977;1:65-74.
40. McClure P, Kilinc E, Oishi S, et al. Mobius syndrome: a 35-year single institution experience. *J Pediatr Orthop.* 2017;37:e446-e449.
41. Pastuszak AL, Schüler L, Speck-Martins CE, et al. Use of misoprostol during pregnancy and Möbius' syndrome in infants. *N Engl J Med.* 1998;338:1881-1885.
42. Rozen SM. Facial reanimation: basic surgical tools and creation of an effective toolbox for treating patients with facial paralysis. Part A functional muscle transfers in the long-term facial palsy patient. *Plast Reconstr Surg.* 2017;139:469-471.
43. Rozen S. Facial palsy in children and young adults. In: Lee JC, ed. *Craniosynostosis and Rare Craniofacial Clefts.* New York, NY: Nova Science Publishers; 2016:223-247.

44. Labbé D, Huault M. Lengthening temporalis myoplasty and lip reanimation. *Plast Reconstr Surg*. 2000;105:1289-1297.
This article documents a better option for facial reanimation for many patients. It describes the details of the lengthening temporalis myoplasty procedure and outcomes.
45. Rozen S, Lehrman C. Upper eyelid postseptal weight placement for treatment of paralytic lagophthalmos. *Plast Reconstr Surg*. 2013;131:1253-1265.
46. Bhama PK, Weinberg JS, Lindsay RW, et al. Objective outcomes analysis following microvascular gracilis transfer for facial reanimation: a review of 10 years' experience. *JAMA Facial Plast Surg*. 2014;16:85-92.
47. New GB, Erich JB. Dermoid cysts of the head and neck. *Surg Gynecol Obstet*. 1937;65:48-55.
48. Bartlett SP, Lin KY, Grossman R, Katowitz J. The surgical management of orbitofacial dermoids in the pediatric patient. *Plast Reconstr Surg*. 1993;91:1208-1215.
This article presents a clear process for treating dermoids in the head and neck region in the pediatric population, going over the need for imaging, the surgical approach, and ususual variants.
49. Pensler JM, Bauer BS, Naidich TP. Craniofacial dermoids. *Plast Reconstr Surg*. 1988;82:953-958.
50. van Aalst JA, Luerssen TG, Whitehead WE, Havlik RJ. "Keystone" approach for intracranial nasofrontal dermoid sinuses. *Plast Reconstr Surg*. 2005;116:13-19.

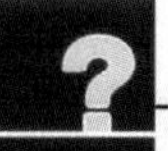

QUESTIONS

1. **A 40-year-old woman diagnosed with fibrous dysplasia is noted on CT scan to have extension of the abnormal osseous growth into the greater wing of the sphenoid bone close to the optic nerve. Which statement about treatment decision is true?**
   a. Optic nerve decompression should be performed with definitive radiographic evidence of fibrous dysplasia around or near the optic nerve.
   b. Optic nerve decompression may result in worsening of vision because of heat injury and therefore should not be performed.
   c. Optic nerve decompression should be performed when there is the beginning of visual changes.
   d. Bisphosphonates, steroids, and tamoxifen are the treatment of choice when visual changes occur because surgery is too risky.

2. **For patients with Pierre Robin sequence (PRS), both mandibular distraction and glossopexy address upper airway obstruction with improvement in which of the following?**
   a. Laryngomalacia
   b. Tracheomalacia
   c. Vascular webs
   d. Retroposition of the tongue base
   e. Chin position

3. **Which of the following about the treatment of Parry-Romberg syndrome is true?**
   a. The fat grafting for the Romberg patients is not advised because the *take* in the diseased Romberg region is less than the *take* in normal regions for cosmetic procedures.
   b. The classic *coup de sabre* sign means there is deeper, bony involvement and osseous correction will also be needed.
   c. Because Romberg disease *burns out* in puberty, observation is recommended, as most cases improve over time without treatment.
   d. For adults with severe soft tissue deficiencies, the parascapular free flap is recommended over the anterolateral thigh free flap because of the better adipose-fascial fill and sculpting.
   e. Dermal fat grafts have fallen out of favor because of the high infection rate.

4. **For Treacher Collins syndrome, orbitomalar reconstruction should not be attempted too early because:**
   a. premature absorption of orbital zygomatic bone grafts may occur.
   b. zygomatic body growth should be completed before custom implant placement.
   c. correction of malocclusion should be the paramount concern.
   d. all stages of total ear reconstruction should be completed first.
   e. bone graft take is more reliable at an older age.

5. **Which is true in facial plexiform neurofibromas with hemifacial hypertrophy?**
   a. The buccal fat is typically the most involved and should be radically resected.
   b. Multiple small resections are often recommended for large tumors to avoid bleeding and injury to vital structures.
   c. It is sometimes necessary to resect all the soft tissue between the skin and bone including the facial nerve and perform a reanimation procedure.
   d. All aesthetic units are distorted by large tumor masses so do not need to be considered.
   e. When considering risk/benefit, face transplantation is ultimately recommended for the best overall result.

1. **Answer: c.** Optic nerve decompression for optic canal involvement is controversial but should be reserved for patients with both definitive radiographic evidence of fibrous dysplasia around or near the optic nerve and the beginning of visual changes. Optic nerve decompression is deemed too risky with normal vision even with radiographic evidence of involvement.

2. **Answer: d.** PRS is a manifestation of triad of micrognathia, glossoptosis, and upper airway obstruction. Both mandibular distraction and glossopexy (tongue-lip adhesion) improve the retroposition of the tongue base. Laryngomalacia, tracheomalacia, and vascular webs may all obstruct the airway but neither mandibular distraction nor glossopexy will correct these lesions. The retroposition of the chin, seen in PRS, will be improved by mandibular distraction lengthening, not tongue-lip adhesion.

3. **Answer: d.** Although fat graft ***take*** in Romberg regions is diminished, it is still a worthwhile treatment. The ***coup de sabre*** sign may just involve skin and fat hypoplasia but not necessarily bone. Unlike hemangioma cases, Romberg hypoplasia does not get better with time. The back region provides better adipose-fascial fill for facial contouring than that of other free flaps.

4. **Answer: a.** If orbitomalar bone graft reconstruction is performed before the age of 8 to 10 years, premature bone absorption is likely. Alloplastic implants are not recommended for Treacher Collins reconstruction in children. Malocclusion and ear reconstruction issues are independent of the timing of orbitomalar reconstruction. Even with good initial bone healing and bone graft ***take***, absorption can still occur if performed early.

5. **Answer: c.** In the treatment of hemifacial hypertrophy, it is often necessary to sacrifice a certain amount of normal soft tissue structures and even the facial nerve, as it is usually poorly functioning and not possible to separate from the neurofibroma. Thus, smaller procedures with a goal of saving the facial nerve may be unrewarding. For severe cases, face transplantation has been performed but carries long-term risks associated with immunosuppression.

CHAPTER 36 Facial Fractures and Soft Tissue Injuries

Christine M. Jones and John A. van Aalst

KEY POINTS

- The patient with facial fractures is a trauma patient and requires a comprehensive evaluation for calvarial, intracranial, and cervical spine injuries.
- Impending optic nerve injury can be recognized early by examining for red desaturation.
- Entrapment of the extraocular muscles and septal hematoma are two surgical emergencies in facial trauma.
- Restoration of facial height, width, and projection is accomplished through rebuilding the facial buttresses in the vertical, horizontal, and sagittal dimensions.
- Achieving normal occlusion is of primary importance in the reduction of maxillary and mandibular fractures.
- Sequencing should build from known to unknown in panfacial fractures in a *top-down*, *bottom-up*, or *inside-out* fashion.

Facial trauma is one of the most common reasons for consultation with a plastic surgeon; an estimated 407,000 emergency department visits occur annually for facial fractures alone.[1] Appropriate evaluation and treatment is a fundamental skill for trainees. The principles learned in approaching and stabilizing fractures serve as a foundation for building more advanced concepts in soft tissue handling and orthognathic surgery.

CONCEPTS IN FACIAL TRAUMA

Mechanisms of injury vary and patients must first be considered from a comprehensive trauma standpoint. Each patient must undergo a thorough trauma evaluation for concomitant injuries, beginning with airway assessment, breathing, and circulation. Over 45% of patients with facial fractures have concomitant intracranial injury and nearly 10% have cervical spine injuries.[2] With areas of thin bone and sinuses, the face is designed to act as a shock absorber to help prevent trauma to these critical neurologic structures.

Stability of the Craniofacial Skeleton

The height, width, and projection of the facial skeleton is stabilized by facial buttresses, which are areas of thick bone that act as scaffolds in the vertical and horizontal dimensions (**Table 36.1**). Horizontal facial buttresses are divided into coronal and sagittal types (**Figure 36.1**). Fractures extending through these buttresses are more likely to be clinically significant; proper reduction restores alignment and stability in these areas. Whereas the frontal bone and mandible display stability in each plane, the midface lacks sagittal support, lending it particularly susceptible to flattening after attempts at reconstruction, especially centrally.[3]

Facial Examination

To avoid missing injuries, the face should be systematically examined through inspection, palpation, and evaluation of range of motion. Beginning in the upper third, the scalp should be inspected for lacerations and foreign bodies. Scalp lacerations are obscured by hair, positioning, or cervical collars and can bleed significantly. Moving onto the face, the soft tissue, including the auricle, external auditory canal, and nose, including the septum, are inspected for lacerations and foreign bodies. Prompt recognition of both auricular and septal hematomas is critical. Examination progresses to systematic palpation of bony prominences to determine the presence of step-offs, instability, or crepitus; sites of examination include the supraorbital ridge, lateral orbital walls, infraorbital rims, nasal bones, zygomatic arches, maxilla, and mandible. Maxillary stability is determined by stabilizing the head at the nasofrontal junction with one hand and using the examining hand to rock the maxillary alveolus in a forward-backward and medial-lateral motion (**Figure 36.2**).

Ocular examination begins with inspection of the conjunctiva for hemorrhage, assessment of the lids and canaliculi for lacerations, inspection for foreign bodies, and visualization of penetrating injuries. Pupillary examination is performed with a flashlight to compare pupillary size at rest and direct and consensual responses to light. The swinging flashlight test distinguishes afferent pupillary defects

TABLE 36.1. BUTTRESSES OF THE CRANIOFACIAL SKELETON[3,4]

Buttress	Purpose
Vertical	Maintain facial height
Orbital	
Nasofrontal	
Zygomatic	
Pterygomaxillary	
Mandible	
Horizontal	
Coronal	Maintain facial width
Supraorbital	
Infraorbital rim	
Transverse maxillary	
Mandible	
Sagittal	Maintain facial projection
Frontal bone	
Zygomatic arch	
LeFort I segment	
Mandibular body	

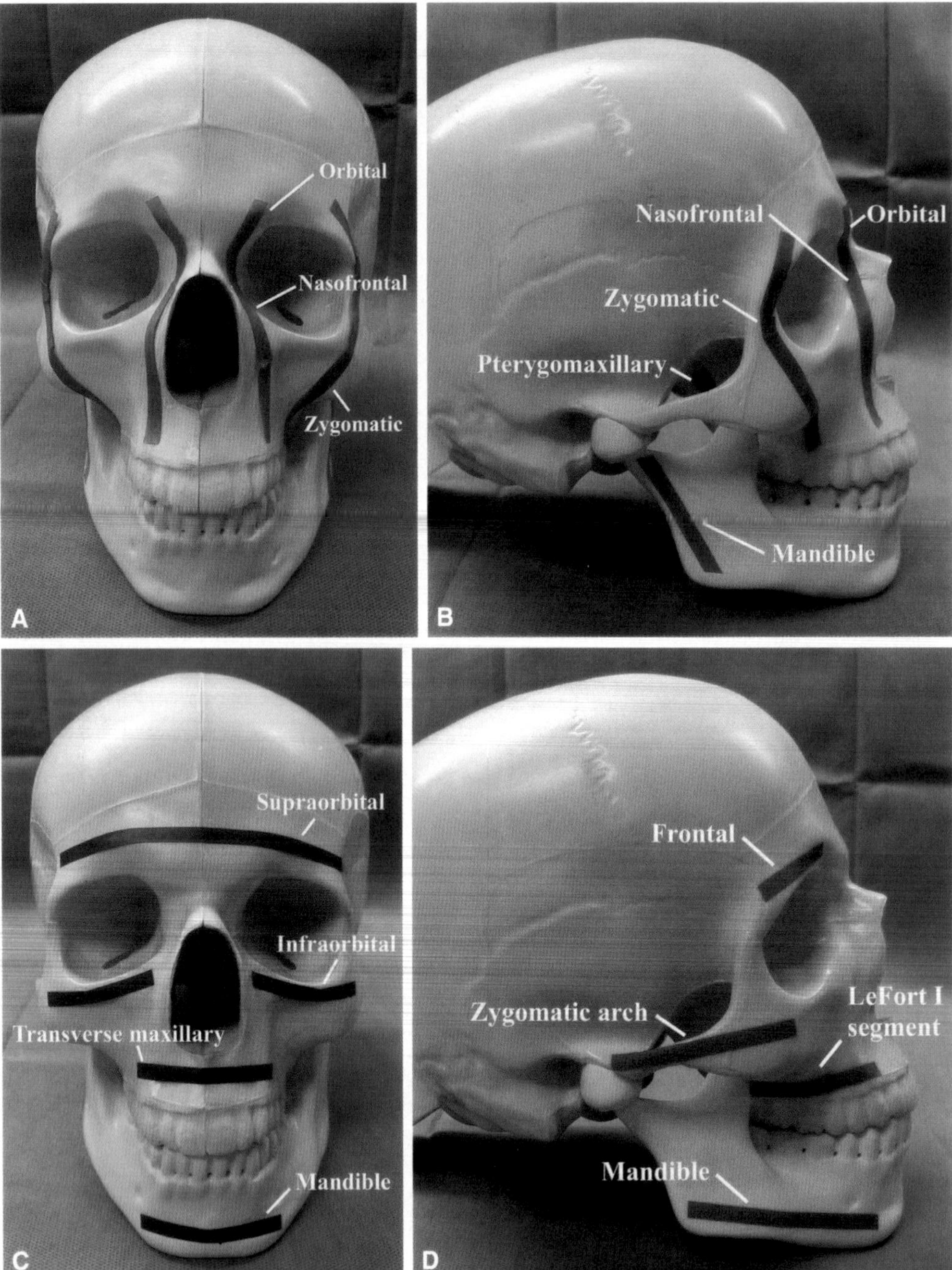

FIGURE 36.1. Buttresses of the craniofacial skeleton are divided into vertical **(A,B)** and horizontal **(C,D)** supports. Horizontal buttresses are further subdivided into coronal **(C)** and sagittal **(D)** types.

from an oculomotor nerve injury: an eye that has lost vision will lack the ability to constrict with direct light but will still display a consensual response when light is shone in the opposite pupil. Extraocular muscle excursion should be examined by asking the patient to look in each of the cardinal directions. In an unresponsive patient, forced duction testing rules out entrapment (Figure 36.3). Monocular and binocular vision is examined; the presence of diplopia is recorded. Because red desaturation is one of the earliest signs of visual loss, each patient is asked to compare a red object with both the affected and unaffected eye. A brief visual field examination reveals the presence of gross field cuts. Globe position is examined for early enophthalmos, which reliably indicates the need for orbital floor fracture correction because swelling usually masks enophthalmos in the acute setting.

Moving to the middle third, the nasal septum is examined for boggy mucosal swelling, indicative of a septal hematoma. An otoscope is useful for this step if a nasal speculum is not available. Hematoma can be distinguished from septal deviation by probing with forceps and assessing for ballotability.

The temporomandibular joint (TMJ), positioned directly anterior to the tragus and under the zygomatic arch, is evaluated for tenderness or deformity. The articular disc can be assessed by palpating anteriorly from within the external auditory canal while the patient gently opens her mouth. Maximal interincisal opening should be recorded.

Intraoral lacerations, open fractures, and loose or avulsed teeth should be noted. If a tooth is missing, ensure that it is not retained within the oral cavity where it presents an aspiration risk. Dental

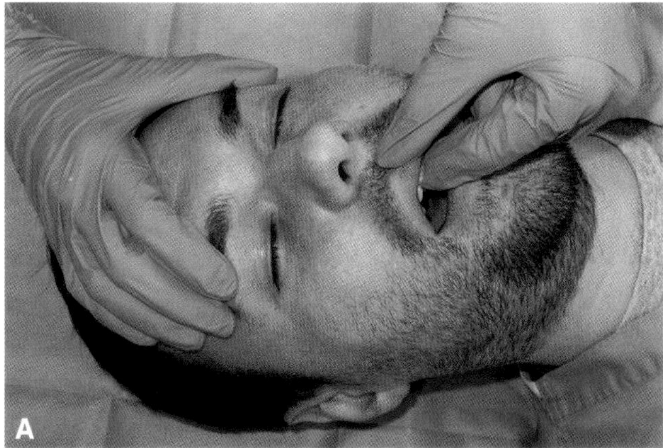

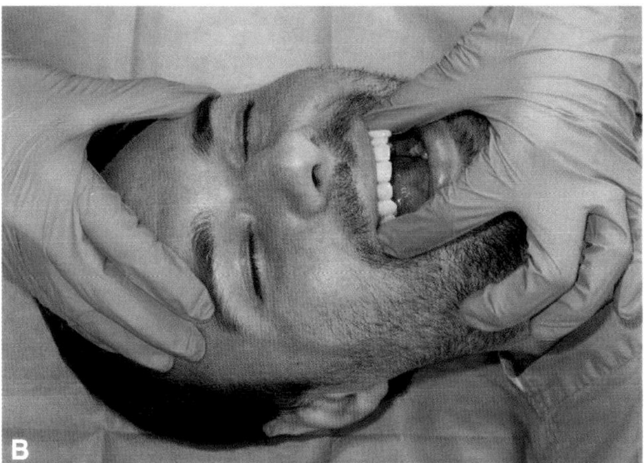

FIGURE 36.2. Testing maxillary stability helps diagnose LeFort I, II, or III fractures. The face is stabilized at the forehead while the dominant hand grasps the anterior maxilla and attempts to displace it in an anteroposterior **(A)** and lateral direction **(B)**.

hygiene should be noted, as this affects the success of maxillomandibular fixation. The patient's occlusion is recorded, including the presence of cross-bite or open-bite deformities.

Cranial nerve (CN) function is examined by testing sensation to light touch in the V1, V2, and V3 distributions, comparing sensitivity with the contralateral side and with baseline. Each branch of the facial nerve is tested by asking the patient to raise the eyebrows (temporal branch), close the eyes tightly (zygomatic), puff the cheeks (buccal), smile (marginal mandibular), and purse the lips (cervical). Loss of lip depression while smiling can result from injury to the ipsilateral marginal mandibular nerve or cervical branch, as the platysma (cervical branch innervation) can cofunction with the depressor anguli oris (marginal mandibular innervation) to display a full denture smile. These can be distinguished by asking the patient to evert her lower lip: with a cervical branch injury, eversion is preserved because of intact mentalis function. The tongue should protrude at midline (CN XII), the palate should elevate symmetrically (CN IX, X), hearing should be grossly symmetric (CN VIII), and the shoulders should be able to shrug (CN XI).

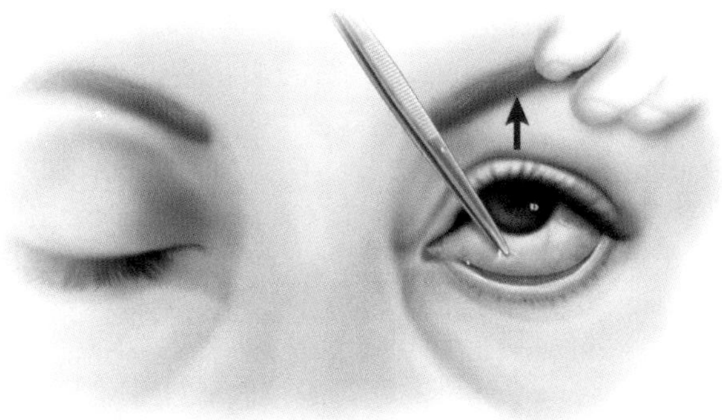

FIGURE 36.3. To test for entrapment in an unresponsive patient, several drops of ophthalmic tetracaine are instilled into each eye. The bulbar conjunctiva is grasped with toothed forceps near the inferior fornix and the globe is rotated upward, downward, medially, and laterally. Excursion is compared with the contralateral side.

Radiographic Evaluation

Thin-slice CT scan should be obtained for patients whose mechanism of injury or examination suggests facial fractures. Cuts should be 1 mm or finer. X-rays are rarely useful. CT scans should be examined in each plane of section to rule out skeletal injuries.

Regional Blocks

Small lacerations are managed by injecting local anesthetic at the site of injury. A 25-gauge needle is used to inject through existing laceration; inject slowly using buffered anesthetic to minimize patient discomfort. Larger areas of the face can be treated with regional blocks (Figure 36.4).[5]

Access Incisions

Numerous incisions are available to access various regions of the facial skeleton (Figure 36.5).[6] Lacerations from the injury can also be used to further improve access. For optimal access to correct bony injuries, edema should be allowed to subside for 7 to 10 days. Scars should be placed in concealed locations whenever possible; the transconjunctival and upper and lower buccal sulcus incisions are good examples. Whenever a skin incision is made, it should be placed in the relaxed skin tension lines (Table 36.2). For access to the midface in particular, multiple simultaneous incisions are often necessary.

Antibiotic Prophylaxis

Evidence supporting the use of perioperative antibiotics for the treatment of facial fractures is of low quality. However, routine antibiotic prescription is a common practice, with penicillin, cephalosporins, and clindamycin being the most commonly prescribed antimicrobials.[7,8] In a seminal article, two perioperative doses of cefazolin reduced infection risk from 42% to 8.9%.[9] Current literature supports the use of perioperative antibiotics (beginning < 60 minutes prior to incision and ending within 24 hours) for operative facial fractures, especially those that involve transmucosal access incisions with clean-contaminated surgical fields.[7,10] However, data describing use of antibiotics beyond this time period is inconclusive.

Although infection is rare, it can have serious consequences. Transmigration of sinus bacteria into the periorbital soft tissue can result in orbital cellulitis, leading to optic neuritis, optic nerve atrophy blindness, cavernous sinus thrombosis, or meningitis.[11] An unclear risk-benefit ratio for the use of antibiotics in facial trauma continues to make this a hotly debated topic.

Soft Tissue Injuries

Plastic surgeons are often consulted for complicated facial lacerations. In these cases, tissue debridement should be limited to only that which is clearly nonviable. The rich vascularity of the face allows partially compromised tissue to survive. Wounds should be meticulously debrided of gravel, glass, or other debris, using loupe magnification if needed. Copious irrigation with normal saline helps prevent infection. Closure should be completed in layers, minimizing buried dissolvable sutures that may incite

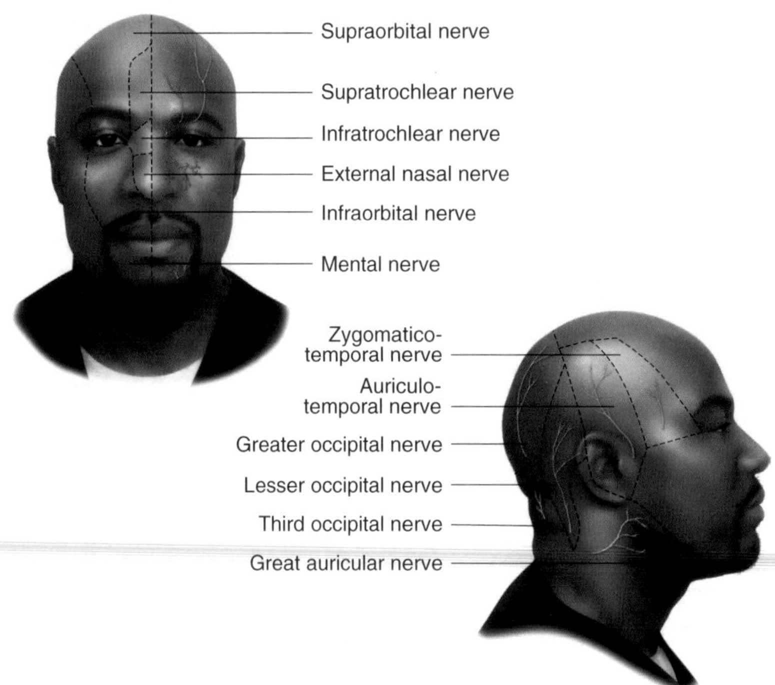

FIGURE 36.4. Multiple blocks are available to provide regional anesthesia for the face.

inflammatory and infectious responses in a contaminated field. Typically, 6-0 nylon or polypropylene suture is used in high-profile areas of the face and 5-0 for more concealed areas. In children, 6-0 plain or fast gut obviates the need for suture removal and provides acceptable appearance. Excellent blood supply to the face results in rapid healing. Permanent sutures should be removed within 5 to 7 days to prevent the *train track* scars that occur when epithelial cells migrate along sutures that are retained for greater than 7 to 10 days.

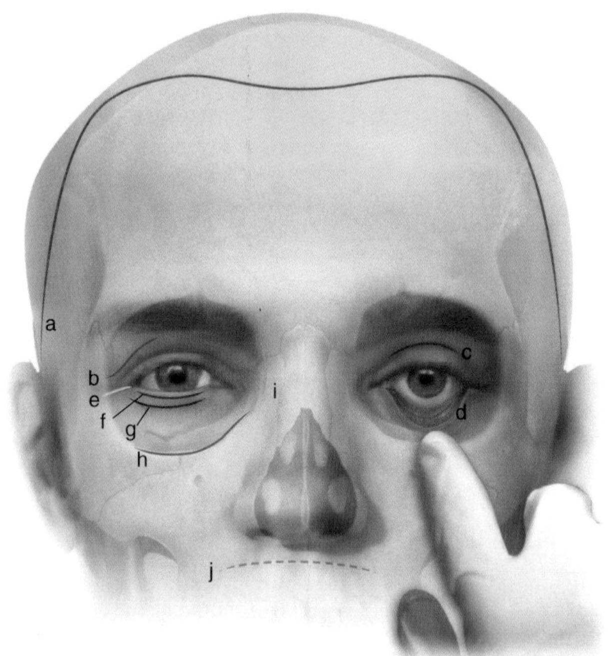

FIGURE 36.5. Selected incisions for periorbital and midface skeletal access: coronal **(a)**, Wright **(b)**, upper lid crease **(c)**, transconjunctival **(d)**, lateral canthotomy **(e)**, subciliary **(f)**, subtarsal/midlid **(g)**, infraorbital **(h)**, Lynch **(i)**, and upper buccal sulcus **(j)**.

Accurate tissue reapproximation is the most important step after wound debridement. Key sutures should be placed first in the areas where minor discrepancies of alignment would be most notable, for example, in the eyebrow margin or at the vermillion border.

Facial Nerve Injury

An accurate assessment of facial nerve function should be completed before injecting local anesthetic. Frontal branch injuries are most likely to occur when a laceration crosses the line described by Pitanguy, drawn from a point 0.5 cm inferior to the tragus to a point 1.5 cm superior to the lateral eyebrow. Neurologic deficits from zygomatic and buccal branch injuries are less common, particularly when lacerations occur medial to the lateral canthus because of the arborization that occurs medially, with multiple nerve endings innervating a muscle. Buccal branch injuries are most likely to occur with large, midcheek lacerations. Concomitant parotid duct injuries are common. The marginal mandibular nerve has little redundancy and is most commonly injured as it crosses the inferior border of the mid-mandibular body. Cervical branch injuries are less common and also exhibit crossover from multiple sub-branches.

If facial nerve injury is suspected within a laceration, the wound should be explored in an attempt to tag the cut ends proximally and distally. Stimulation of the distal cut end is possible up to 72 hours postinjury; after this period of time, depletion of acetylcholine makes further stimulation impossible.

Auricular Cartilage Injury

Lacerations that penetrate the auricular cartilage must take into account the limited vascularity of the cartilage and the need to restore stability. Nonviable segments of cartilage or skin should be minimally debrided and thoroughly irrigated. The cartilage and skin can usually be reapproximated in a single layer due to the firm adherence of the skin to the cartilage. In adults, 5-0 polypropylene is an appropriate suture choice, with 5-0 fast-absorbing gut reserved for children.

Hematoma and chondritis are two major concerns with ear injuries. Hematomas can be seen as ballotable fluid collections between the perichondrium and cartilage. Prompt drainage is essential to avoid necrosis, fibrosis, and deformed neocartilage formation, commonly known as *cauliflower ear*. After repair of an auricular

TABLE 36.2. SELECTED FACIAL ACCESS INCISIONS

Skeletal Access	Incision	Benefits	Drawbacks
General	Lacerations	No new facial scars	Limited control over which parts of skeleton are accessible
Frontal bone, midface	Bicoronal	Wide access to frontal bone and midface	Conspicuous scar
Orbital floor	Transconjunctival, preseptal	Hidden; avoids protrusion of orbital fat	Tedious dissection through lower lid
	Transconjunctival, post-septal	Hidden; ease	Orbital fat must be retracted during surgery
	Subciliary	Scar blends with resting tension lines	High risk of ectropion
	Subtarsal	Scar blends with resting tension lines	High risk of ectropion
	Infraorbital	Ease	Conspicuous scar, risk of ectropion
Zygomatic arch	Gillies	Hidden in scalp	Utility limited to arch alone; blind
Midface	Upper buccal sulcus	Ease, affords wide access, hidden	Risk of gingival retrusion
Mandible	Lower buccal sulcus	Wide applications	Risk of mental nerve injury; higher risk of infection for highly comminuted fractures or poor oral hygiene
	Risdon	Lower risk of infection, easier reduction for highly comminuted fractures, edentulous patients, poor oral hygiene	Risk of marginal mandibular nerve injury; conspicuous scar

laceration or drainage of a hematoma, the ear should be bolstered for 5 to 7 days to prevent hematoma formation or recurrence. A roll of petroleum-impregnated gauze placed on either side of the ear and secured in place with polypropylene or nylon mattress sutures serves as an appropriate bolster. Penetrating auricular injuries should receive 7 to 10 days of antibiotic prophylaxis, typically with ciprofloxacin, to prevent chondritis.[12]

Canalicular Injury

Lacerations near the medial canthus of the eyelid should raise suspicion for injury to the superior and inferior canaliculi. In these cases, consultation with ophthalmology is warranted. The canaliculi should be probed acutely to determine if injury is present. Suture repair and stenting are commonly used techniques for treatment.

Septal Hematoma

Because cartilage receives its blood supply from the perichondrium, any collection of fluid between the perichondrium and the cartilage will lead to cartilage destruction. The septum should always be inspected with a nasal speculum and good lighting to evaluate for hematoma. A septal hematoma will appear as a bulging, fluctuant collection along the septum. The collection should be aspirated with an 18-gauge needle or lanced with an 11-blade scalpel, and nasal packing should be placed to prevent fluid reaccumulation.

Parotid Duct Injury

The parotid duct (Stenson duct) travels horizontally within the cheek, allowing the parotid gland to drain intraorally through an opening on the buccal side of the second maxillary molar. Injury should be suspected with lacerations to the cheek, particularly those that injure the buccal branch of the facial nerve, as the nerve and duct travel in close proximity. A high index of suspicion is needed, because no immediate signs of duct injury exist; the injury is usually noted days later when saliva begins draining from the laceration. The intraoral orifice of the parotid duct can be cannulated with a pediatric intravenous catheter and injected with methylene blue or saline to examine for injury. If the duct is lacerated, repair should be conducted over a small-caliber pediatric feeding tube. The tube should be left in place as a stent for 14 days. A subcutaneous drain left in place for 1 week and facial wrap providing external pressure for the first 48 hours may also help prevent sialocele (Figure 36.6).[13]

SKELETAL INJURIES

Upper Facial Fractures

Frontal Sinus Fractures

The frontal bone is a particularly strong structure and is capable of withstanding more force than the other facial bones. For this reason, frontal bone fractures signify high-energy traumatic mechanisms and are often associated with intracranial injury.

Pneumatization of the frontal sinus begins around the age of 2 years and is completed by 12 years. Because the bone is thicker in childhood, frontal sinus fractures are not commonly seen. In

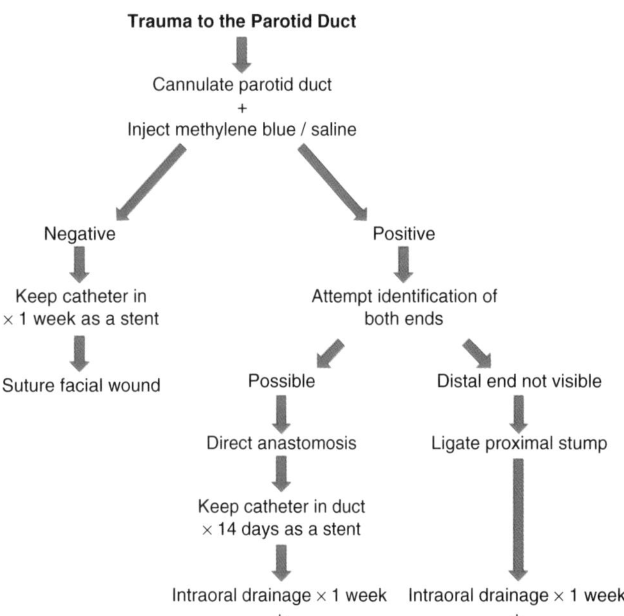

FIGURE 36.6. Suspected parotid duct injuries should be explored and repaired over a catheter if possible. (Adapted with permission from Lewkowicz AA, Hasson O, Nahleili O. Traumatic injuries to the parotid gland and duct. *J Oral Maxillofac Surg.* 2002;60:676-680.)

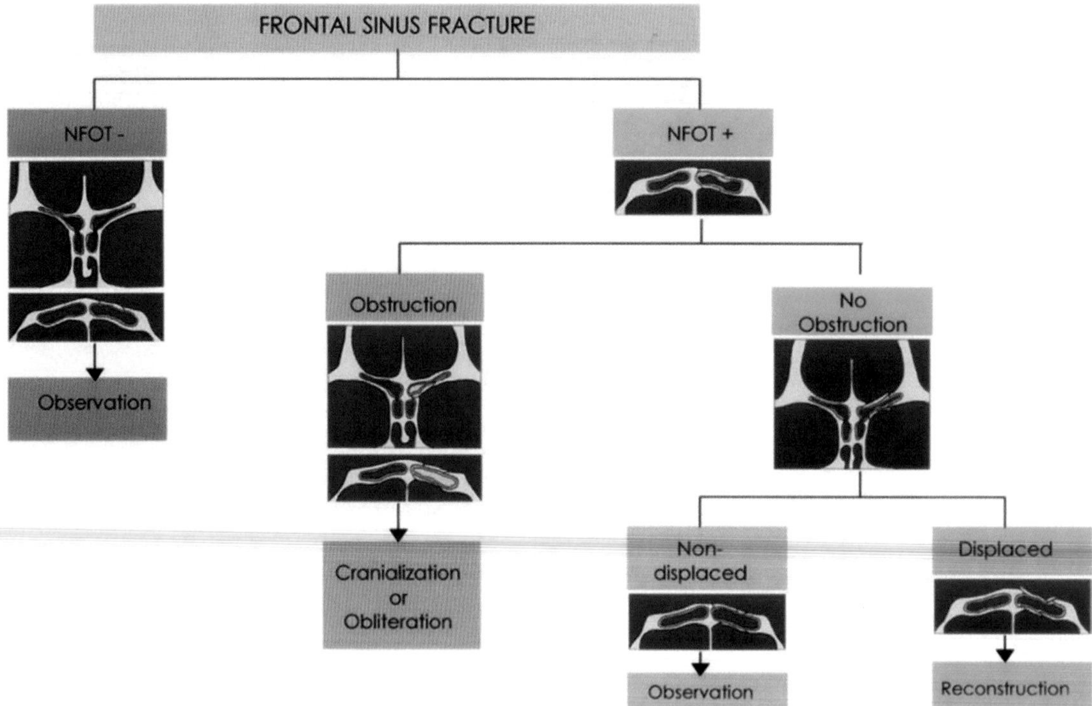

FIGURE 36.7. Management of frontal sinus fractures. NFOT, nasofrontal outflow tract. (Reproduced with permission from Rodriguez ED, Stanwix MG, Nam AJ, et al. Twenty-six-year experience treating frontal sinus fractures: a novel algorithm based on anatomical fracture pattern and failure of conventional techniques. *Plast Reconstr Surg*. 2008;122:1850-1866.)

adults, management of frontal sinus fractures depends on whether the fracture extends through the anterior or posterior table or both, the degree of displacement, and the likelihood of nasofrontal outflow tract obstruction (**Figure 36.7**).

Fractures of the anterior table may lead to visible or palpable contour irregularities of the forehead or instability of the supraorbital bar. Posterior table fractures have the potential for dural tear, cerebrospinal fluid leak, persistent pneumocephalus, or meningitis.

The nasofrontal outflow tract courses from the inferomedial frontal sinus in the most anterior and superior extent of the anterior ethmoidal complex to exit in the middle nasal meatus at the hiatus semilunaris. The nasofrontal outflow tract is likely to be injured with fractures to the inferomedial frontal bone and the floor of the sinus. The tract may become obstructed with injury, leading to abscess or sinusitis. Evaluation of the fracture pattern and location on CT scan will indicate the likelihood of nasofrontal tract involvement. Nasofrontal outflow tract involvement with obstruction is strongly correlated with a higher degree of fracture displacement.[14]

Several options for management exist. Nonoperative observation should include serial examinations and CT scans to evaluate for mucocele or persistent pneumocephalus. Obliteration requires surgical curettage of the sinus mucosa, burring of the sinus bone to remove any invaginations of mucosa, surgical occlusion of the nasofrontal ducts, and placement of bone, muscle, fat, pericranial, or galeal flaps. Cranialization is performed by removing the posterior table so the sinus and the anterior cranial fossa are contiguous. The sinus mucosa must be carefully curetted, the inner portion of the anterior table bone burred away, and the nasofrontal duct occluded with bone graft. The brain is allowed to fill what was formerly the frontal sinus space over subsequent months.

Nondisplaced fractures of the anterior table or combined anterior and posterior tables without nasofrontal outflow tract obstruction should be observed. Displaced fractures of only the anterior table generally require operative reduction and fixation with low-profile miniplates to restore forehead contour.

In posterior table fractures, the degree of displacement and presence of a cerebrospinal fuild (CSF) leak dictate management. Displaced fractures carry a higher risk of dural tear, CSF leak, and meningitis. These complications are minimized with obliteration for less severe fractures or cranialization for more displaced or comminuted fractures.

With obstruction of the nasofrontal outflow tract in either anterior or posterior table fractures, the sinus must be obliterated or cranialized regardless of the degree of fracture displacement.[14]

Complications

Abscesses can occur in acute or delayed fashion and can range from subcutaneous to intracranial. These are managed with repeat surgical debridement and obliteration or cranialization. Mucoceles result from the indolent overgrowth of residual basilar sinus mucosa from the diploic veins of Breschet, which are small mucosal crypts that invaginate into the bone. Mucoceles typically present in a delayed fashion with chronic headaches, mass effect, visual disturbance, nasal obstruction, or erosion of the frontal bone. Mucoceles are difficult to treat; therefore, prevention is of primary importance.

Midfacial Fractures

Orbital Fractures

The orbit is a thin-walled, conical, bony box in which the globe rests. Its structure is designed to support the vertical and sagittal position of the globe, and to absorb blunt trauma to the upper midface to prevent globe injury. With fractures to the medial wall or floor, the orbital space becomes contiguous with the ethmoid or maxillary sinus, respectively, and the position of the globe may change. Fractures often increase orbital volume, causing diplopia when the globe descends (vertical dystopia) or becomes positioned deeper within the orbital cavity (enophthalmos).

Particularly in children, greenstick fractures of the floor can occur, allowing the inferior rectus muscle to prolapse into the maxillary sinus with the bony fragment snapping back up into near original position because of periosteal recoil. This muscular entrapment is a surgical emergency because the prolapsed portion of the muscle quickly becomes ischemic. If the muscle is not released within 6 to

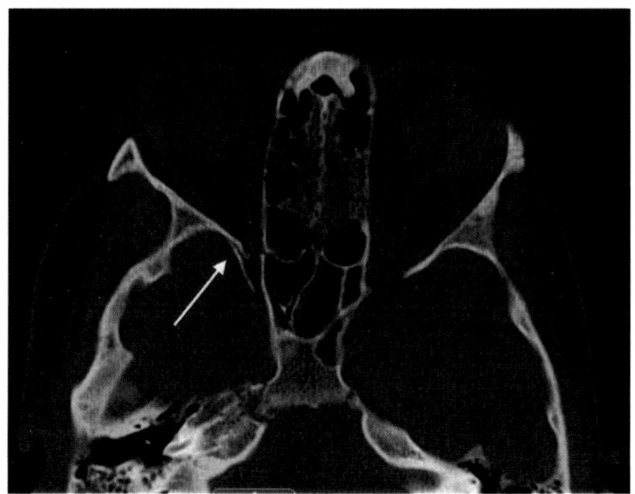

FIGURE 36.8. In this patient with a small fracture of the orbital roof and lateral wall, the bone fragment caused orbital apex syndrome with resultant blindness.

8 hours, it will become fibrotic with a high risk of permanent diplopia. Retrobulbar hematoma can acutely increase intraorbital pressure and quickly lead to optic nerve damage if not promptly diagnosed. Superior orbital fissure and orbital apex syndromes can be associated with direct injury from fractured bone fragments or with the subsequent retrobulbar hemorrhage (Figure 36.8; Table 36.3). Surgical reduction of these posterior fracture fragments is generally met with limited success. Because the compression is often from soft tissue, treatment is primarily medical, using high-dose corticosteroids. Some cases may resolve spontaneously as edema subsides.[15]

Orbital fractures should be suspected with any substantial blunt trauma to the face, including a fall from standing, blow to the face, or motor vehicle collision. Facial CT is the only method of ensuring accurate diagnosis. Alignment of the orbital floor should be evaluated on coronal and sagittal cuts, and the dimensions of the fracture in the anteroposterior and mediolateral directions should be measured. The extraocular muscles can be examined on soft tissue windows to evaluate for entrapment; however, the only way to accurately diagnose entrapment is by physical exam.

Diplopia is the primary surgical indication in orbital floor and medial wall fractures. Diplopia is more likely to occur with larger fractures exceeding 1 to 2 cm^2.[16,17] Often, when examined in the emergency room, patients have already developed substantial periorbital edema masking the enophthalmos and vertical dystopia that will result over time. Patients should be reexamined in 7 to 10 days, after the swelling has subsided, to determine need for surgical intervention.

Once an incision is selected (Figure 36.9), dissection proceeds to the infraorbital rim; the periosteum of the orbital floor and involved medial wall is lifted. At this point, an elevator can be used to identify the borders of the fracture and a rim of stable bone surrounding the fracture (Figure 36.10). The optic nerve is located approximately 32 to 42 mm posterior to the infraorbital rim[18]; as dissection proceeds deeper into the orbit, caution is used to avoid nerve injury. The elevator can be periodically removed to check the position of its tip by grasping it at the infraorbital rim and measuring the distance from the tip to the surgeon's fingertip.

A plate should be selected based upon fracture characteristics (Table 36.4). Complete coverage of the defect is needed for larger fractures; an anatomic titanium plate with medial extension is often appropriate for orbital floor fractures extending into the medial wall.

With orbital roof fractures, the most pertinent concern is risk of a growing skull fracture in children who have years of craniofacial growth ahead of them. Pulsation of the dura at the site of the fracture may impair normal bone healing, allowing the fracture to expand with growth. In adults, indications for reduction of orbital roof fractures are limited to patients with dural tears or orbital apex syndrome that does not respond to medical therapy.

Complications

Continued diplopia can result from inadequate reduction, or more specifically, inadequate restoration of orbital volume. The orbital fat that prolapses into the maxillary sinus must be lifted back into the orbit before placement of the plate to properly support the normal position of the globe. Diplopia can also result from fibrosis of extraocular muscles or necrosis of the intraorbital fat from manipulation.[17]

Lower eyelid malposition can include ectropion, scleral show, and entropion. Risk of ectropion and scleral show increases with use of a transcutaneous incision; ectropion can complicate 14% of orbital floor repairs approached through a subciliary incision.[20] A Frost stitch, placed through the lower lid tarsus and secured to the forehead, helps elevate the lower lid for the first several days until edema subsides. Although the Frost stitch can prevent acute globe exposure from chemosis, it has not been shown to prevent ectropion.[21]

Zygomaticomaxillary Complex and Zygomatic Arch Fractures

Fractures of the zygomaticomaxillary complex (ZMC) are also referred to as *tripod fractures*. In fact, the zygoma is a tetrapod structure that is stabilized by the zygomaticofrontal suture, zygomaticotemporal suture, zygomaticomaxillary buttress, and the zygomaticosphenoid suture.[22] The zygomatic bone sets the width and projection of the midface. Fractures typically displace the

TABLE 36.3. SEQUELAE OF INJURIES TO PERIORBITAL STRUCTURES ASSOCIATED WITH ORBITAL FRACTURES

Clinical Case	Presentation	Structures Involved
Entrapment	Pain during attempted upward gaze	Inferior oblique
Superior orbital fissure (SOF) syndrome	Ptosis	CN III to levator palpebrae superioris
	Proptosis	CN III; loss of retraction forces and bulge of flaccid extraocular muscles
	Ophthalmoplegia	CN III, IV, VI
	Pupillary dilation, with loss of direct and consensual light reflexes	Parasympathetic fibers of CN III
	Loss of forehead sensation	V1 supratrochlear and supraorbital nerves
	Loss of corneal sensation	V1 nasociliary branch
Orbital apex syndrome	Same as SOF syndrome, with the addition of blindness	Same as SOF syndrome, with the additional involvement of optic nerve (CN II)

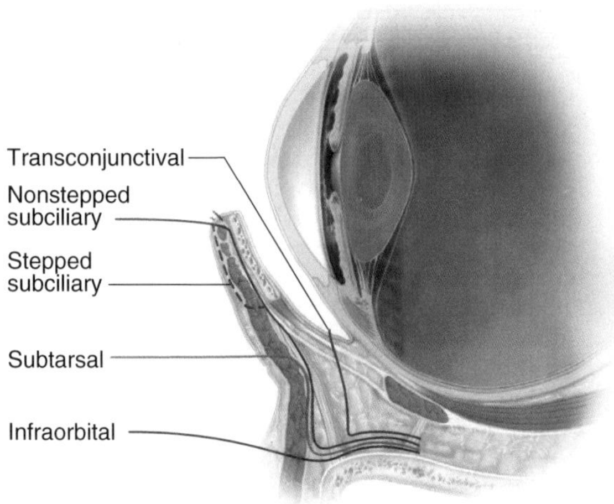

FIGURE 36.9. Cross-sectional view of incisions for orbital floor exploration.

TABLE 36.4. OPTIONS FOR ORBITAL IMPLANTS[19]

Type	Benefit	Drawback
Autologous bone	Biocompatible	Requires additional surgery at donor site Unpredictable resorption Inflexible; difficult to contour
Silastic sheets, silicone	Flexible Easy to use	Forms capsule prone to infection, seroma, cysts, and sinus tracts
Porous polyethylene	Flexible Easy to use Tissue ingrowth Reduces foreign body reaction	Risk of infection Difficult removal with tissue ingrowth
Titanium	Rigid, yet malleable Able to osseointegrate	Risk of infection

zygoma inferiorly, laterally, and posteriorly, widening and flattening the face. Reduction is of paramount importance to restore midface structure; therefore, most displaced fractures meet operative criteria. In addition, displacement of the zygoma can impinge upon the coronoid process of the mandible and its associated muscles of mastication, causing trismus, a limiting of mandibular excursion. Appropriate reduction alleviates muscular impingement and restores mandibular motion.

The ZMC can be approached through transconjunctival and upper buccal sulcus incisions. Sometimes a lateral canthotomy or an upper lid/lateral blepharoplasty incision is necessary as well, depending on the degree of displacement. Reduction can be performed by placing an elevator or curved bone hook under the body of the zygoma via the upper buccal sulcus incision and lifting the bone from its impacted position. Alternatively, a Carroll-Girard bone screw (Figure 36.11) can be inserted percutaneously and used to *joy-stick* the fracture into the desired position. Alignment must be determined at the zygomaticofrontal, zygomaticomaxillary, and zygomaticosphenoid articulations. Of these, the zygomaticosphenoid buttress is most important in verifying accurate realignment of the zygoma. The zygomaticosphenoid buttress can be visualized through a lateral canthotomy extension of a transconjunctival incision, or through a separate lateral rim incision. The buttresses are then stabilized with titanium miniplates.

In many cases, ZMC fractures are associated with fractures of the orbital floor. The ZMC must be reduced first, as its alignment will be based on intact bone at the buttresses described above. The orbital floor should then be checked for unmasking or widening of a fracture. Any significant fracture should be repaired as previously described.

Isolated fractures of the zygomatic arch are problematic if they are depressed enough to affect facial contour or cause trismus. Direct exposure cannot be achieved through limited incisions, given the conspicuous location and close association with the temporal branch of the facial nerve. For badly displaced and comminuted fractures a coronal incision must be used, because this is the only approach for the necessary access for plate fixation.

For depressed fractures with inherent stability, a Gillies approach may be used to reduce the fracture. A 2-centimeter horizontal incision is made within the hair-bearing portion of the temporal region 2.5 cm anterior and superior to the helical root, after palpating and avoiding the temporal artery. Dissection proceeds to the deep layer of the deep temporal fascia, which directly overlies the temporalis muscle. The fascia is then incised, exposing the muscle. An elevator is inserted and directed inferiorly, just under the zygomatic arch. Application of manual pressure reduces the fracture through this minimal access technique.

Alternatively, the arch can be approached from a 2-centimeter upper buccal sulcus incision (Keen incision) at the base of the

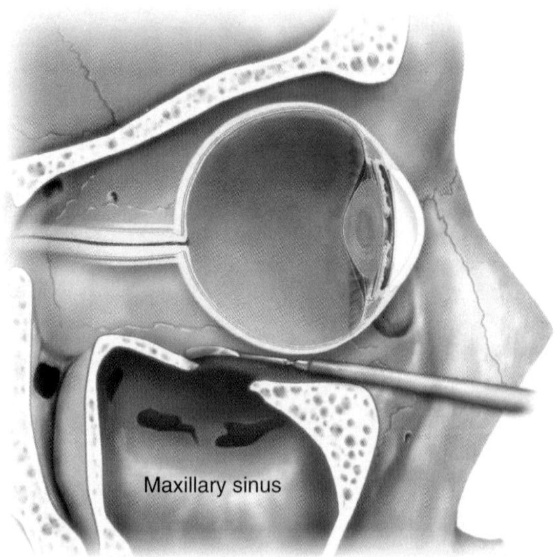

FIGURE 36.10. When identifying the borders of an orbital floor fracture, an elevator can be used to palpate medially, laterally, and posteriorly for a stable rim of bone.

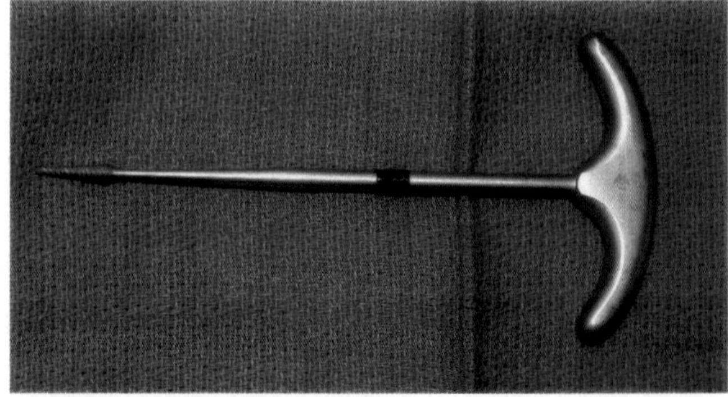

FIGURE 36.11. The Carroll-Girard screw can be anchored into the zygoma percutaneously and used to manipulate the bone.

zygomaticomaxillary buttress. The incision is made through the mucosa only, allowing an elevator to be passed under the zygomatic arch that is in direct proximity to the incision.

Nasal Bone Fractures

The nasal bones are the most commonly fractured facial bones,[23] accounting for over 55% of facial fractures.[1,23] The nose serves both aesthetic and functional purposes, and dissatisfaction with nasal appearance (13%–32%) and/or nasal airway patency (14%–36%) is high after fracture.[23]

Fractures of the cartilaginous septum are particularly prone to nasal deformity and airway obstruction. Even after closed reduction of the nasal bones, in the presence of an incomplete septal fracture, the bones will tend to deviate toward the displaced portion of the septum during the healing process.[24] In addition to restoring architecture of the nasal airway, reduction of the cartilaginous septum counteracts this deforming force of the septum on the nasal bones and improves final alignment.

The nasal bones and septum can be reduced under local anesthesia depending on fracture complexity and patient cooperation. Closed nasal reduction under general anesthesia has not been shown to have superior outcomes to that under local anesthetic,[23] but may be more appropriate for anxious or young patients, or more severely displaced fractures.

Regardless of the setting, the equipment and technique for closed nasal reduction are the same (Figure 36.12). Local anesthetic is injected within the soft tissue of the nasal dorsum to anesthetize the infratrochlear nerves, around the infraorbital nerve, and along the base of the columella and nasal floor (branches of the anterior and posterior ethmoidal nerves and sphenopalatine ganglion). Nasal pledgets impregnated with a topical vasoconstrictor such as oxymetolazone or cocaine are inserted into each nostril for 10 minutes and vasoconstriction is allowed to occur. To prevent inadvertent intracranial injury, the distance from the external nasal aperture to the displaced nasal bone is measured by holding an elevator on the exterior of the nose and grasping the distal portion of the elevator at the naris. The elevator is then inserted and manual pressure applied while stabilizing the head and palpating the displaced bones externally with the other hand. Once the nasal bones are reduced, the septum can be grasped with Asch forceps and manipulated to its anatomic, median position.

After manipulation of the septum, pressure should be applied to prevent septal hematoma. This can be done by transseptal mattress sutures, or with Vaseline-impregnated gauze packing that is left in place for 24 hours. Alternatively, silicone septal splints, such as Doyle or bivalve splints, can be sutured in place for 5 to 7 days. The nasal dorsum should be stabilized with an external thermoplastic splint. Curing of the thermoplastic material is an exothermic process, so the thin nasal skin should be protected with a layer of surgical tape to prevent skin burns. Because the nasal bones are reduced but not fixated, a too-tight splint may cause bony displacement.

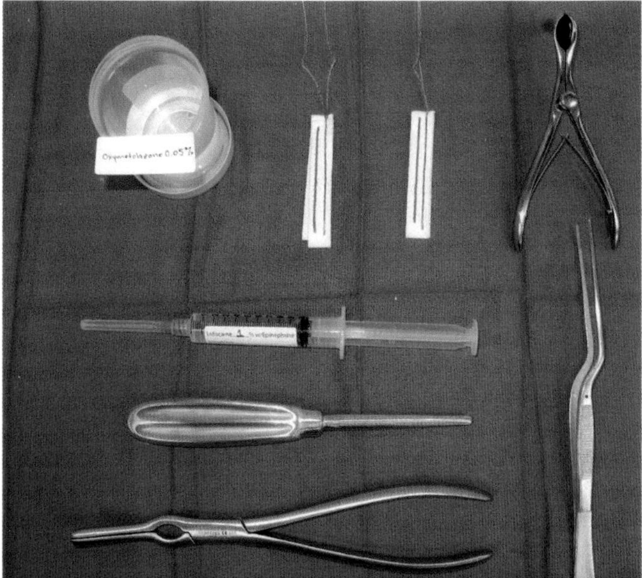

FIGURE 36.12. Closed nasal reduction can be accomplished with simple tools, including local anesthetic, oxymetolazone- or cocaine-soaked pledgets, bayonet forceps, Killian nasal speculum, Boies elevator, and Asch forceps.

Nasoorbitoethmoidal Fractures

The nasoorbitoethmoidal (NOE) complex is an area of thin bone in the upper midface that encompasses the superior nasal cavity and ethmoidal air cells. It is bordered superiorly by the frontal sinus, cribriform plate, and anterior skull base; anteriorly by the nasal bones, frontal process of the maxilla, and nasal process of the frontal bone; laterally by the lacrimal bone and lamina papyracea of the ethmoid bone; and medially by the septum and the perpendicular plate of the ethmoid. The thin bones of the anterior cranial fossa at the fovea ethmoidalis and the tight dural adhesion at the cribriform plate make NOE fractures particularly susceptible to CSF leak. The medial canthal tendon attaches the tarsal plates and the orbicularis oculi to the medial orbital wall, inserting onto the anterior and posterior lacrimal crests. The medial canthal tendon sets the intercanthal distance and the angle of the palpebral fissure.

NOE fractures are often the result of high-impact injuries to the midface. Comminution and instability are typical. Classification is based upon the involvement of the *central fragment*, or the fragment of bone to which the medial canthal tendon attaches.[25] Class I NOE fractures involve a single central fragment with relative stability (Figure 36.13A). In class II NOE fractures comminution is present, but the medial canthal tendon remains attached to a central fragment that is large enough for stabilization with a miniplate or microplate (Figure 36.13B). Class III fractures are characterized by detachment of the medial canthal tendon from bone, extensive bony loss, or a high degree of bony comminution such that fixation cannot be accomplished with traditional measures (Figure 36.13C).

Management is dictated by the fracture type. Class I fractures are stabilized with miniplates at the frontomaxillary, zygomaticomaxillary, and medial maxillary buttresses. Placement of miniplates for class II fractures is similar to class I, with the addition of miniplates or microplates for stabilization of the central fragment. In some class II and all class III fractures, instability of the medial canthal tendon requires transcanthal wiring. A 3-0 stainless steel wire is passed from a point superior and posterior to the medial canthal attachment through holes drilled to the contralateral medial orbital wall. In some cases, placement of a bone graft is necessary beforehand to attain bony stability sufficient to support the wire. Adequate restoration of the tendon attachment is critically important to avoid alteration of the palpebral fissure or telecanthus. Vertical asymmetry of as little as 2 mm is noticeable at conversational distance. The medial canthi should be positioned no more than 25 mm apart. Transcanthal wires placed anterior to the medial canthal attachment site will not prevent lateral migration of the canthus, thus leading to permanent telecanthus and a broad nasal base. Often, multiple surgical approaches are necessary to attain proper fracture reduction.

Management of soft tissue edema is of equal importance as bony reduction. Subperiosteal seroma, hematoma, or postoperative edema can lead to permanent soft tissue thickening, which effaces the normal contours of the nasoorbital region. Splinting with a padded metal bolster is recommended. The splint is fixated with transcanthal wires designed for soft tissue support alone. Careful monitoring is required to avoid soft tissue pressure injury during the period of postoperative edema.

Maxillary Fractures

The French surgeon René Le Fort classified three patterns of maxillary fractures that result from blunt trauma to the adult facial

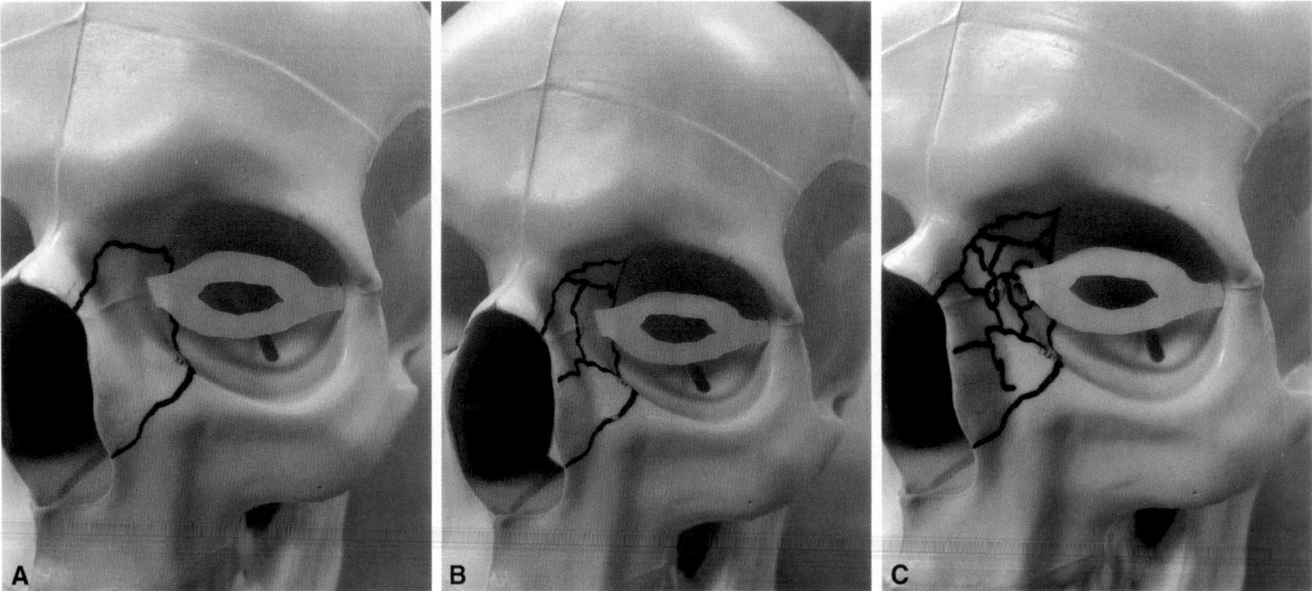

FIGURE 36.13. Nasoorbitoethmoid fractures can be divided into types I (A), II (B), and III (C).

skeleton. A key component of each fracture type is the disruption of the ipsilateral pterygoid plates, which are a major source of midfacial stability. The LeFort fracture classification scheme should be used as a guideline, as true fracture patterns are often combinations of the classic patterns and are most accurately described using anatomic terms. Fracture patterns may differ on each side of the face. In these cases, the term *hemi-LeFort* is often used.

LeFort I fractures occur in a horizontal pattern parallel to the occlusal plane, extending from the piriform aperture laterally through the pterygomaxillary junction (Figure 36.14). LeFort II fractures are pyramidal, extending from the pterygomaxillary junction through the zygomaticomaxillary buttress and orbital floor obliquely to the nasofrontal junction. LeFort III fractures are horizontally-oriented fractures through the upper midface that produce a separation of the cranium from the face, termed craniofacial disjunction. These fractures extend from the zygomatic arch, through the pterygomaxillary junction, lateral orbital rim and orbital roof, to the nasofrontal junction.

Although LeFort I fractures may be treated through an upper buccal sulcus incision, LeFort II and III fractures benefit from the exposure of a coronal approach. Reduction can be accomplished with Rowe disimpaction forceps. Restoring normal occlusion is the primary goal of reduction; normal facial width, height, and projection should follow secondarily. Facial stability is restored by placing plates along the involved facial buttresses. LeFort fractures are typically the result of high-energy trauma and are rarely isolated fractures. In these cases, sequencing of fracture reduction becomes an important consideration.

Palatal fractures usually occur in the sagittal plane, splitting the alveolar ridge between the central incisors or between the lateral incisor and canine. Alternatively, the maxillary tuberosity containing the molars may be split from the rest of the alveolar ridge. Palatal fractures often occur in conjunction with LeFort I fractures. After reduction, stability can be restored anteriorly with a miniplate in the area of the piriform, and posteriorly with a plate across the palatal concavity for maintenance of palatal width.

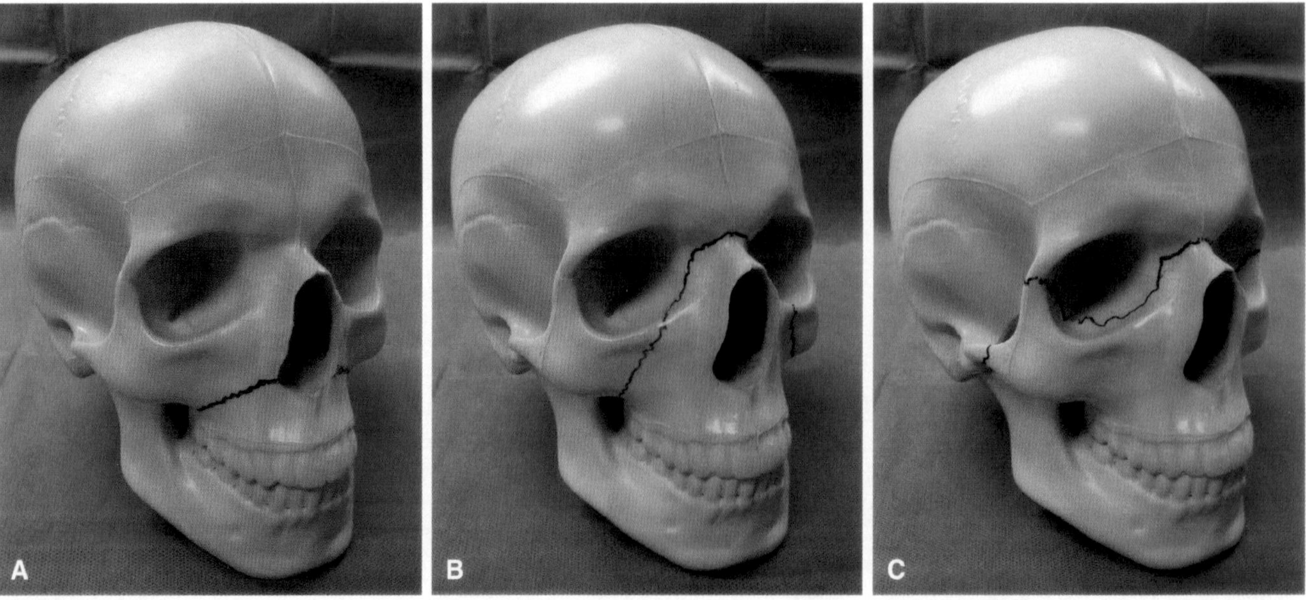

FIGURE 36.14. **A.** LeFort I fractures occur transversely across the maxilla. **B.** LeFort II fractures have a pyramidal pattern. **C.** LeFort III fractures represent a craniofacial disjunction.

Lower Facial Fractures: The Mandible

Biomechanics

The biomechanical properties of the mandible are the most complex of the facial skeleton. The mandible acts as a curved beam, supported on its ends by the muscular pterygomasseteric sling. The masseter and temporalis function to elevate the mandible and create a strong bite force. The medial and lateral pterygoids protrude the mandible and help with opening, or excursion. The suprahyoid muscles, comprised of the digastric, stylohyoid, mylohyoid, and geniohyoid muscles, function to elevate the hyoid and base of tongue during deglutition, and depress the mandible. In the fractured mandible, the muscles of mastication displace the posterior segment superiorly, whereas the suprahyoid muscles pull the anterior segment inferiorly.[26]

During mastication, external downward forces exerted by tooth-to-tooth contacts cause surrounding areas of compression balanced by the tension created either contralaterally or posteriorly by the upward pull of the muscles of mastication. The areas of tension and compression are dependent on the site of mandibular loading.

The mandible can also be thought of as a ring structure, articulating with the temporal bone at the TMJs. Similar to opening the rings of a binder, the mandibular *ring* is often disrupted through faults created in at least two areas. About 1/2 to 2/3 of mandibular fractures involve fractures at multiple sites.[27,28] Commonly, an anterior impact such as in a motor vehicle collision will result in condylar, symphyseal, and parasymphyseal fractures, whereas a lateral impact from assault will fracture the body and contralateral angle.[27]

Principles of Management

The most important objective in treating mandibular fractures is restoration of normal occlusion; anatomic reduction is a secondary goal. Stable, nondisplaced fractures may be treated nonoperatively with a soft diet. Sometimes, partially luxated teeth will prevent fracture reduction and will obscure normal occlusion; in these cases, teeth in the line of the fracture must be extracted. Tooth extraction is also recommended whenever the tooth roots are fractured.

Given the normal biomechanical loads exerted on the mandible, types of fixation fall into two categories: rigid and functionally stable. In rigid fixation (load-bearing), no micromotion is translated through the fracture site and primary bone healing occurs. This type of fixation bears more mechanical forces of the mandible and is useful if healing is delayed, such as in atrophic bone, bony defects, smokers, poor oral hygiene, or patients with multiple comorbidities. An example is a reconstructive plate applied to the inferior mandibular border. In functionally stable fixation (load-sharing), micromotion is allowed at the fracture site, and a bony callus forms during the process of secondary bone healing. Miniplates rely on the accumulation of bone at the fracture site to share mandibular loading before they become prone to fatigue failure. Examples of load-sharing fixation include a Champy plate along the external oblique ridge, a lower border miniplate with maxillomandibular fixation (MMF), or upper and lower border miniplates with monocortical screw fixation. In addition to plates, MMF uses contact at the apices of the teeth to serve as another point of functionally stable fixation.[28] In the multiply fractured mandible, at least one fracture site should be treated with heavier, more rigid plates due to the increased complexity of biomechanical stress forces.

Because of the curved nature of the mandible, locking plates are often desirable. Screws that lock to the plate fixate the plate in the position in which it was placed by the surgeon with lower risk of displacing the fracture fragments. Conversely, nonlocking screws can lag the plate into closer coaptation with the bone. Although the lag concept is useful in other anatomic areas, its use in the mandible can displace the fracture of the curvilinear bone and lead to malocclusion. Non-locking screws are typically only used in oblique mandibular fractures, and lag screws are usually only used at the symphysis.

Symphyseal and Parasymphyseal Fractures

The mandibular symphysis lies between the apices of the central incisors and is characterized by thick bone and short incisor tooth roots. The parasymphysis is defined by the lateral border of the central incisor root and the lateral border of the canine. A fixation technique unique to the symphysis is the placement of two bicortical lag screws in the coronal plane, perpendicular to the line of the fracture. A lower border plate is a common method of symphyseal or parasymphyseal fixation. This can be placed with bicortical screws below the level of the tooth apices for added stability. Rigid fixation can be attained with the addition of an upper border plate with monocortical screws. MMF is usually preferable as an extra point of stability.

Body and Angle Fractures

The mandibular body extends from the lateral canine to the medial border of the third molar. The body conducts the inferior alveolar nerve to the mental foramen, typically located between the first and second premolars where it exits as the mental nerve. The body contains longer tooth roots, the longest of which is the canine. During fracture fixation, avoiding injury to the inferior alveolar nerve and tooth roots is critical.

The angle contains the third molars and connects the body with the ramus. The body and angle experience tensile forces along the upper border and compression along the inferior border under axial loads. A neutral zone exists centrally, along the neurovascular canal. Methods of fixation take these biomechanical properties into account (Table 36.5). Fractures of the angle have the highest incidence of complications, particularly in the presence of partially erupted or impacted third molars.[28,29]

Subcondylar and Condylar Fractures

Fractures of the condylar head and subcondylar region are common, accounting for 25% to 35% of mandibular fractures in adults.[26] Loss of condylar height presents with early posterior tooth contact ipsilaterally and an anterior open bite. Risks of open treatment include facial nerve palsy, scarring, and inadequate reduction. Due to the high incidence of stiffness with an open approach, condylar and subcondylar fractures are often treated in a closed fashion. Normal

TABLE 36.5. OPTIONS FOR MANDIBULAR FIXATION. BY CONVENTION, PLATES ARE NAMED ACCORDING TO THE OUTER DIAMETER OF THE SCREWS THEY ACCOMMODATE

Region	Rigid Fixation	Functionally Stable Fixation
Symphysis, parasymphysis	Locking reconstructive plate (2.8 mm)	Two lag screws (2.4 mm)
		Lower border plate + upper border plate (2.0 mm each)
Body		Lower border plate (2–2.4 mm) + maxillomandibular fixation (MMF)
		Lower border plate + upper border plate (2 mm each) ± MMF
		Single monocortical miniplate in the central neutral zone (2 mm) + MMF
Angle		Champy plate (2 mm tension band across oblique ridge) + MMF
		Champy plate + lower border plate (2 or 2.4 mm) ± MMF
Condyle, subcondylar region	N/A	MMF
		Two miniplates (1.5 or 2 mm)

HEAD AND NECK

occlusion is established and stabilized with MMF for 2 to 3 weeks. Open treatment is best reserved for displaced fractures without comminution and requires specific training and experience on the part of the surgeon.

Complications

Malocclusion can result from insufficient reduction or loss of reduction during the healing process due to inadequate fixation, poor bone quality, or suboptimal patient compliance. This may cause malunion or nonunion. Injury to tooth roots can occur from drilling or placement of bone screws. Facial nerve injury may result from a Risdon incision (marginal mandibular nerve) or condylar approaches (main trunk or any of its branches). Paresthesias can occur if the inferior alveolar or mental nerves are injured; even without transection, neuropraxia is common due to traction of the nerve. Stiffness of the TMJ can result from inadequate seating of the condyle during fixation, condylar head fracture, or prolonged MMF. Hardware infection may be managed with a period of observation and antibiotics with or without surgical irrigation; ideally, hardware removal is delayed until union occurs.

Panfacial Fractures

The definition of panfacial fractures is variable in the literature, at times referring to fractures spanning each third of the face, and at other times indicating fractures involving the maxilla, mandible, and ZMC.[30,31] With panfacial fractures, the face assumes a spherical shape, with loss of vertical height, reduction in anteroposterior projection, and increase in facial width. Extensive facial fractures are the result of high-energy trauma, and comminution is expected. Plastic surgeons must recognize mechanisms of injury that suggest risk of concomitant injuries and consult the trauma team when warranted.

Restoration of facial dimensions must build from a stable, known skeletal base as a reference point. This can be sequenced in a *top-down*, *bottom-up*, or *inside-out* fashion. The most common sequence involves rebuilding the skeleton upwards after restoring mandibular stability. Restoring the preinjury occlusion with MMF allows the occlusal subunit to function as one, and ZMC and NOE fractures can be reduced from this reference point. Alternatively, the surgeon can work downwards from a noninjured cranial base and zygomaticofrontal suture. Primary bone grafting may be necessary to replace devitalized or highly comminuted bone.

REFERENCES

1. Allareddy V, Allareddy V, Nalliah RP. Epidemiology of facial fracture injuries. *J Oral Maxillofac Surg*. 2011;69:2613-2618.
2. Mithani SK, St Hilaire H, Brooke BS, et al. Predictable patterns of intracranial and cervical spine injury in craniomaxillofacial trauma: analysis of 4786 patients. *Plast Reconstr Surg*. 2009;123:1293-1301.
3. Manson PN, Clark N, Robertson B, et al. Subunit principles in midface fractures: the importance of sagittal buttresses, soft-tissue reductions, and sequencing treatment of segmental fractures. *Plast Reconstr Surg*. 1999;103:1287-1306.
   The authors present a classic description of how facial buttresses influence the technique and outcome of midfacial fracture reduction. Common pitfalls are addressed with recommendations as to how secondary complications can be avoided.
4. Manson PN, Hoopes JE, Su CT. Structural pillars of the facial skeleton: an approach to the management of Le Fort fractures. *Plast Reconstr Surg*. 1980;66:54-61.
5. Zide BM, Swift R. How to block and tackle the face. *Plast Reconstr Surg*. 1998;101:840-851.
6. Eppley BL, Custer PL, Sadove AM. Cutaneous approaches to the orbital skeleton and periorbital structures. *J Oral Maxillofac Surg*. 1990;48:842-854.
7. Mundinger GS, Borsuk DE, Okhah Z, et al. Antibiotics and facial fractures: evidence-based recommendations compared with experience-based practice. *Craniomaxillofac Trauma Reconstr*. 2015;8:64-78.
8. Brooke SM, Goyal N, Michelotti BF, et al. A multidisciplinary evaluation of prescribing practices for prophylactic antibiotics in operative and nonoperative facial fractures. *J Craniofac Surg*. 2015;26:2299-2303.
9. Chole RA, Yee J. Antibiotic prophylaxis for facial fractures: a prospective, randomized clinical trial. *Arch Otolaryngol Head Neck Surg*. 1987;113:1055-1057.
10. Ellis E. Antibiotics and mandibular fracture update. *J Oral Maxillofac Surg*. 2016;74:1911-1912.
11. Zix J, Schaller B, Iizuka T, Lieger O. The role of postoperative prophylactic antibiotics in the treatment of facial fractures:a randomised, double-blind, placebo-controlled pilot clinical study. Part I: orbital fractures in 62 patients. *Br J Oral Maxillofac Surg*. 2013;51:332-336.
12. Thill MP, Horoi M, Ostermann K, et al. Acute external ear lesions: clinical aspects, assessment, and management. *B-ENT*. 2016;26:155-171.
    This article provides a detailed, comprehensive approach to auricular hematoma, perichondritis, laceration, and burn with treatment algorithms for each clinical problem.
13. Lewkowicz AA, Hasson O, Nahleili O. Traumatic injuries to the parotid gland and duct. *J Oral Maxillofac Surg*. 2002;60:676-680.
    A literature review was conducted to supplant the experience of a single center in treating traumatic injuries to the parotid duct. An algorithm for treatment is proposed.
14. Rodriguez ED, Stanwix MG, Nam AJ, et al. Twenty-six-year experience treating frontal sinus fractures: a novel algorithm based on anatomical fracture pattern and failure of conventional techniques. *Plast Reconstr Surg*. 2008;122:1850-1866.
    This article reviews 857 cases of frontal sinus fractures treated at a tertiary hospital. A treatment algorithm is proposed, and the incidence of complications is described within the framework of the proposed algorithm.
15. Chen CT, Chen YR. Traumatic superior orbital fissure syndrome: current management. *Craniomaxillofac Trauma Reconstr*. 2010;3:9-16.
16. Manson PN, Grivas A, Rosenbaum A, et al. Studies on enophthalmos: II. the measurement of orbital injuries and their treatment by quantitative computed tomography. *Plast Reconstr Surg*. 1986;77:203-214.
17. Chaudry O, Isakson M, Franklin A, Maqusi S, El Amm C. Facial fractures: pearls and perspectives. *Plast Reconstr Surg*. 2018;141:742e-758e.
    This review article discusses concepts in treating facial fractures primarily and managing secondary complications. Multiple videos are available online with further detail on fracture management and surgical techniques.
18. Danko I, Haug RH. An experimental investigation of the safe distance for internal orbital dissection. *J Oral Maxillofac Surg*. 1998;56:749-752.
19. Mok D, Lessard L, Cordoba C, et al. A review of materials currently used in orbital floor reconstruction. *Can J Plast Surg*. 2004;12:134-140.
20. Al-Moraissi EA, Thaller SR, Ellis E. Subciliary vs. transconjunctival approach for the management of orbital floor and periorbital fractures: a systematic review and meta-analysis. *J Craniomaxillofac Surg*. 2017;45:1647-1654.
21. Bartsich S, Yao CA. Is frosting effective? The role of retention sutures in posttraumatic orbital reconstruction surgery. *J Plast Reconstr Aesthet Surg*. 2015;68:1683-1686.
22. Lee EI, Mohan K, Koshy JC, Hollier LH. Optimizing the surgical management of zygomaticomaxillary fractures. *Semin Plast Surg*. 2010;24:389-397.
23. Basheeth N, Donnelly M, Smyth D, Shandilya M. Acute nasal fracture management: a prospective study and literature review. *Laryngoscope*. 2015;125:2677-2684.
24. Rohrich RJ, Adams WP. Nasal fracture management: minimizing secondary nasal deformities. *Plast Reconstr Surg*. 2000;106:266-273.
25. Markowitz BL, Manson PN, Sargent L, et al. Management of the medial canthal tendon in nasoethmoid orbital fractures: the importance of the central fragment in classification and treatment. *Plast Reconstr Surg*. 1991;125:843-853.
    This landmark article describes the classification system for NOE fractures and a detailed treatment strategy for reduction and fixation of each type.
26. Morrow BT, Samson TD, Schubert W, Mackay DR. Evidence-based medicine: mandible fractures. *Plast Reconstr Surg*. 2014;134:1381-1390.
27. King RE, Scianna JM, Petruzzelli GJ. Mandible fracture patterns: a suburban trauma center experience. *Am J Otolaryngol*. 2004;25:301-307.
28. Ellis E, Miles BA. Fractures of the mandible: a technical perspective. *Plast Reconstr Surg*. 2007;120:76S-89S.
    This introductory article describes the biomechanics of the mandible as related to fracture fixation. Techniques of osteosynthesis in each region of the mandible are discussed in detail, along with depictive photographs and radiographs.
29. Chuong R, Donoff RB, Guralnick WC. A retrospective analysis of 327 mandibular fractures. *J Oral Maxillofac Surg*. 1983;41:305-309.
30. He D, Zhang Y, Ellis E. Panfacial fractures: analysis of 33 cases treated late. *J Oral Maxillofac Surg*. 2007;65:2453-2465.
31. Kelly KJ, Manson PN, Vander Kolk CA, et al. Sequencing LeFort fracture treatment (organization of treatment for a panfacial fracture). *J Craniofac Surg*. 1990;1:168-178.

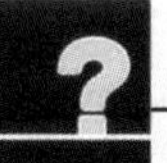

QUESTIONS

1. **A 14-year-old boy presents to the emergency department after an unwitnessed ATV accident in which he was found lying without a helmet on the trail. He complains of jaw pain and his right eye is swollen shut. What is the best next step in management?**
   a. Maxillofacial CT scan with 1.0 mm cuts
   b. Evaluation of extraocular motions to rule out entrapment
   c. Adherence to spinal precautions and palpation of the neck for tenderness
   d. Checking occlusion to compare to the patient's baseline

2. **Which of the following is most likely to lead to late deformity?**
   a. Bilateral subcondylar mandible fractures
   b. Comminuted nasoorbitoethmoidal fracture with canthal bowstringing
   c. Nasal bone fracture with septal deviation
   d. Zygomaticomaxillary complex fracture without displacement at the lateral orbital rim

3. **A 23-year-old man presents to the emergency department with multiple stab wounds. His facial lacerations were not fully evaluated during his workup. Which of the following are appropriate combinations of injury location and long-term complications?**
   a. Floor of mouth; Stenson duct leak
   b. 1 cm inferior to the auricular lobule; lack of ipsilateral lower lip depression while smiling
   c. Lateral infraorbital rim; inability to elevate ipsilateral eyebrow
   d. Central and medial lower eyelid; epiphora

4. **Which fracture is most likely to require operative intervention?**
   a. Anterior table frontal sinus fracture with obstruction of the nasofrontal duct
   b. Orbital roof fracture extending into the lateral wall
   c. Orbital floor fracture 1 cm in diameter in a patient without diplopia
   d. Concomitant LeFort I and ipsilateral ZMC fractures with normal occlusion

5. **A 50-year-old woman sustains panfacial fractures in a high-speed motor vehicle collision in which she was the unrestrained passenger. Which is the most appropriate sequencing of fracture reduction and fixation?**
   a. ZMC, orbital floor, mandibular angle, LeFort I, anterior table of the frontal sinus
   b. Anterior table of the frontal sinus, LeFort I, mandibular angle, orbital floor, ZMC
   c. Mandibular angle, LeFort I, ZMC, orbital floor, anterior table of the frontal sinus
   d. Anterior table of the frontal sinus, orbital floor, ZMC, LeFort I, mandibular angle

6. **You are reviewing the postoperative course of your most recent four operative mandible fractures. Which patient is the most likely to have had complications?**
   a. 21-year-old man with right angle fracture sustained during an altercation
   b. 34-year-old woman with bilateral subcondylar fractures from a motor vehicle accident
   c. 18-year-old boy with symphyseal fracture after an ATV accident
   d. 31-year-old man with subcondylar and contralateral body fracture after falling from a roof

1. **Answer: c.** Many patients whose mechanism of injury is sufficient to produce facial fractures are also at risk of more significant multisystem traumatic injuries. Evaluation must first focus on airway, breathing, circulation, and disability. Almost 10% of patients with facial fractures will have concomitant cervical spine injuries. Protecting the spine in at-risk patients must be a priority until the spine can be cleared. The remaining actions would be appropriate after serious concomitant injuries are ruled out. Priority should be placed on ruling out plastic surgical emergencies, including entrapment of the extraocular muscles which is diagnosed clinically by physical exam. Workup would also include a careful examination to determine occlusion status and a maxillofacial CT scan with thin cuts.

2. **Answer: b.** NOE fractures are notoriously difficult to treat. The central midface lacks sagittal buttresses to support adequate projection, giving the region a high propensity to heal in a depressed position. The medial canthal tendon inserts into the thin bone of the medial orbit and establishes the appropriate intercanthal distance. When canthal bowstringing is present, the surgeon must determine whether the bone fragment to which the medial canthal tendon attaches is stable enough to fixate with miniplates. If the fragment is too small or comminuted transcanthal wiring will be necessary, with or without primary bone grafting. NOE fractures have a high incidence of late deformity. Bilateral subcondylar mandible fractures are commonly treated with maxillomandibular fixation, with the greatest concern of inadequate treatment being a late anterior open bite. Both nasal bone and septal fractures can be reduced and stabilized more easily than the thin bones of the NOE region. The ZMC is unlikely to be displaced if the zygomaticofrontal buttress at the lateral orbital rim remains well aligned.

3. **Answer: d.** Lacerations of the medial upper or lower eyelid may involve the canalicular system. If canalicular injury is suspected, ophthalmologic consultation is warranted to probe and repair or bypass the ductal system. Untreated canalicular injury may lead to excessive eye tearing, or epiphora. Injury to the parotid duct (Stenson duct) should be suspected with deep cheek lacerations. The duct travels from the anterior parotid gland through the midcheek in close proximity to the buccal branch of the facial nerve to open into the oral cavity adjacent to the second maxillary premolar. A laceration to the floor of the mouth would risk injuring other salivary glands but the Stenson duct. Inability to depress the lower lip while smiling is characteristic of a marginal mandibular nerve injury. This branch of the facial nerve exits with the main trunk from the stylomastoid foramen 1 cm anterior and inferior to the tragal pointer. It is part of the inferior or cervicofacial division that separates from the temporofacial division within the parotid gland and then divides from the cervical branch at the pes anserinus. The nerve travels anteriorly along the mandibular body or 1 to 2 cm below the lower mandibular border to innervate the mentalis and produce lower lip depression. A laceration directly inferior to the lobule would be too posterior to injure this branch. The temporal branch of the facial nerve innervates the frontalis and is responsible for brow elevation. This branch separates from the main trunk as part of the temporofacial division. The temporal branch is at highest risk of injury along a line drawn from 0.5 cm inferior to the tragus to 1.5 cm superior to the lateral eyebrow, known as the Pitanguy line. A laceration at the lateral infraorbital rim would be too medial to injure this branch.

4. **Answer: a.** Frontal sinus fractures that involve the nasofrontal duct have a high incidence of complications. These fractures should be treated by cranialization or obliteration to avoid

mucocele or abscess formation. Orbital roof fractures are often managed nonoperatively, unless they create dural tears and cerebrospinal fluid leaks at the anterior cranial base. Indications for orbital floor repair include diplopia and entrapment. No definitive size cutoff exists over which an operative floor fracture requires fixation, although fractures larger than 1 to 2 cm^2 are more likely to be associated with persistent diplopia. Maxillary fractures meet operative criteria if they are displaced or unstable. A primary indication of displacement is malocclusion. Nondisplaced LeFort I and ZMC fractures can be managed with a soft diet and close observation.

5. Answer: c. Panfacial fractures distort many of the landmarks typically used for fracture reduction, so sequencing fracture reduction and fixation is critical. Strategies that build from known to unknown in a top-down or bottom-up fashion are most likely to be successful. In the patient presented, the mandibular condyles can be used as stable reference points to reduce the mandibular angle fracture; then place the patient in MMF and reduce the LeFort I fragment using the teeth as a point of reference. Of note, the ZMC should be reduced and fixated prior to the orbital floor because ZMC reduction may change the size and orientation of the orbital floor fracture but not vice versa. In this patient, a top-down strategy would also be effective, but the ZMC must be addressed before the orbital floor fracture.

6. Answer: a. Multiple studies have demonstrated that fractures of the mandibular angle have the highest incidence of complications. The presence of the inferior alveolar nerve, impacted third molars, and opposing muscle forces make this region more challenging to treat. Risk of infection is slightly heightened if a wisdom tooth is present within the fracture line. The other fracture patterns are not specifically associated with an increased risk of complications. Complications are also more likely to be experienced in ballistic injuries, edentulous patients, and smokers.

CHAPTER 37 Head and Neck Cancer and Salivary Gland Tumors

Head and Neck Cancer and Salivary Gland Tumors

Matthew M. Hanasono and Brian A. Moore

KEY POINTS

- Alcohol and tobacco use are the two most important risk factors for head and neck cancer, particularly cancers of the oral cavity, oropharynx, hypopharynx, and larynx, whereas human papillomavirus is increasingly recognized as a risk factor for oropharyngeal cancer.
- Treatment for head and neck cancer depends on the location of the tumor and the stage and can include surgery, radiation, chemotherapy, and/or targeted therapy.
- Cervical lymphadenectomy (neck dissection) is indicated for nodal disease and cancers at high risk for regional spread.
- About 80% of salivary gland tumors occur in the parotid glands, followed by the submandibular and minor salivary glands, and only about 1% occur in the sublingual glands.
- About 80% of parotid gland tumors are benign, and the parotid gland is the most common location for salivary gland malignancies; about 50% of submandibular gland tumors and 80% of minor salivary gland tumors are malignant.

This chapter will provide an overview to cancer staging and treatment of the upper aerodigestive tract (UADT), including the oral cavity, pharynx, and larynx, and the salivary glands. Although a comprehensive text is not possible in this space, our goal is to provide the reconstructive surgeon with adequate knowledge to communicate with the ablative surgeon and anticipate the surgical defect. Being able to predict the surgical defect helps the reconstructive surgeon to plan the reconstruction appropriately. Furthermore, knowledge of the cancer's biology and current recommended treatment assists the surgeon to factor in the possible need for adjuvant therapy, such as radiation, as well as get a sense of the patient's prognosis, both of which may affect choice of reconstructive techniques to be performed.

UPPER AERODIGESTIVE TRACT CANCERS

Over 95% of UADT tumors are squamous cell carcinomas (SCCs).[1] Overall, 5-year survival for these cancers is about 65% but varies substantially based on site, stage, and histologic findings.[2] Other cancers affecting the UADT include salivary gland malignancies, sarcomas, mucosal melanomas, and lymphomas.

Anatomy

The anatomic subsites of the oral cavity include the labial mucosa, buccal mucosa, floor of mouth, alveolar ridge and gingiva, anterior two-thirds of the tongue (anterior to the circumvallate papillae), hard palate, and retromolar trigone (Figure 37.1). The oropharynx lies posterior to the oral cavity and consists of the soft palate, base of tongue (posterior to the circumvallate papillae), palatine tonsils, palatoglossal folds, valleculae, and posterior pharyngeal wall. The nasopharynx is superior to the oropharynx and includes the mucosa over the posterior body of the sphenoid and basilar part of the occipital bone superiorly, the adenoids and pharyngobasilar fascia posteriorly, and the Eustachian tubes and the lateral pharyngeal recesses (fossae of Rosenmüller) laterally. The hypopharynx

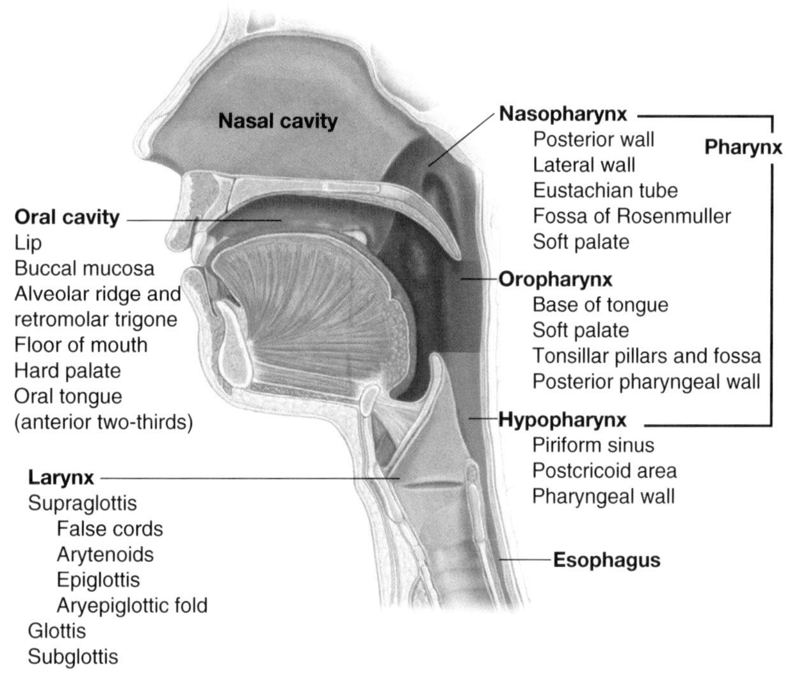

FIGURE 37.1. Upper aerodigestive tract (UADT) sites and subsites.

spans from the hyoid bone down to the inferior cricoid cartilage and includes the piriform sinuses, postcricoid area, and the pharyngeal wall. The larynx comprises the supraglottis, glottis (vocal folds), and subglottis.

Incidence and Risk Factors

Tobacco is a major risk factor for UADT SCC. A meta-analysis by Gandini et al.[3] found a relative risk of 3.4 for oral cavity and 6.8 for oropharynx SCC in current tobacco smokers compared with nonsmokers. Tobacco and concomitant alcohol consumption synergistically increase the risk 10- to 15-fold. Alcohol has also been shown by many studies to be an independent risk factor.[4] Smokeless tobacco and betel nut also significantly increase the risk for oral cavity cancers. Although lip cancers are included in the oral cavity cancer staging system, they are different in that sun exposure is highly correlated with their development. Leukoplakia (white patches) and erythroplakia (red patches) in the oral cavity are considered premalignant lesions but may harbor dysplasia or malignancy on histology evaluation up to 20% and over 50% of the time, respectively.[4]

Besides tobacco and alcohol, human papillomavirus (HPV) has been recognized as a major etiologic factor in SCCs of the oropharynx and is felt to be the cause of the rise in incidence of this cancer over the past 20 years. Recent studies suggest that HPV-associated cancers account for 73% of oropharyngeal SCCs, representing an increase of 225% between 1988 and 2004.[5,6] Compared with patients with HPV-negative tumors, patients with HPV-associated cancers tend to be younger, healthier, and have a better prognosis; middle-aged men with limited to no smoking history constitute the most commonly affected demographic.[7] HPV is the most common sexually transmitted infection, and certain subtypes, most commonly HPV-16, are associated with the development of malignancy in the oropharynx as well as of the cervix and anogenital tract. SCCs of the oropharynx can be tested for HPV positivity using immunohistochemical stains to identify p16 protein (cyclin-dependent kinase 2A, a tumor suppressor protein that is overexpressed in HPV-associated oropharyngeal cancer) or HPV DNA or RNA to help convey prognostic information to the patient. Because of its lower cost and ease of testing, p16 immunohistochemistry has evolved as an acceptable surrogate marker for HPV-associated cancers.[8] HPV vaccination in adults after the diagnosis of HPV-positive oropharyngeal SCC is not felt to be of any benefit, but there is apparent benefit in primary disease prevention if administered to boys and girls according to established guidelines.[7,9]

Nasopharyngeal cancer (NPC) is most common in southern China and other parts of Southeast Asia and, in endemic regions, is strongly associated with the presence of Epstein-Barr virus (EBV). Salt-cured fish and meats, rich in nitrosamines, which are popular in some Asian countries, have also been linked to NPC. Tobacco and alcohol use may also be risk factors, but the link is less clear.

Preoperative Considerations

Biopsies, Imaging, and Metastatic Workup

Following thorough history and physical examination, suspicious lesions of the UADT should be biopsied. Because of the relatively high risk of synchronous primary cancers, panendoscopy (laryngoscopy, bronchoscopy, and esophagoscopy) is often performed as part of the workup. Computed tomography (CT) helps identify nodal metastases as well as bony invasion, which is important for staging and surgical planning. If there is a question regarding the extent of soft tissue involvement or perineural spread, magnetic resonance imaging (MRI) may be preferred or obtained in addition to CT. Positron emission tomography (PET) and PET-CT may be used to look for distant metastases and second primary cancers. A metastatic workup should include a chest X-ray for early-stage/low-risk lesions or a chest CT or PET scan in advanced-stage cancers, as well as liver function tests.

Staging

In broad terms, small tumors without obvious nodal metastases represent early stage I and II cancers, whereas larger, more extensive tumors and/or the presence of cervical nodal metastases represent advanced stage III and IV cancers. Factors that have been linked to poorer outcomes include advanced-tumor stage, increased soft-tissue depth of invasion, presence of nodal metastases, perineural invasion, lymphovascular invasion, and extranodal extension (ENE).[4] These factors are used to guide treatment and provide patients with prognostic information. As a general rule, the presence of nodal metastases reduces survival by 50%, except in HPV-associated (p16-positive) oropharyngeal cancer.[10]

The TNM classification, based on the extent of the tumor (T), spread to the lymph nodes (N), and the presence of metastasis (M), is used to communicate information about tumor size and spread as well as provide prognostic data. At the time of this writing, the eighth edition of the American Joint Committee on Cancer (AJCC)/International Union Against Cancer (UICC) staging system has replaced the seventh edition.[11] For oral cavity cancers, the depth of invasion is now incorporated into the T classification because of the negative effect this parameter has on prognosis. Similarly, ENE has a profound adverse effect on the prognosis and is now part of the N classification. Another major difference is the division of oropharyngeal cancer classifications based on HPV positivity, because HPV-associated oropharyngeal cancer is markedly different in prognosis and behavior from non-HPV–associated cancer. Staging based on clinical and pathologic information is denoted by a "c" or "p" because surgical pathologic data, such as the number of involved lymph nodes or microscopic ENE, provide greater detail regarding adverse features with significant prognostic impact.

Sites

Oral Cavity Cancer

The oral cavity is the most common site for SCC of the head and neck (**Figure 37.2**). Most oral cavity cancers are treated surgically with the goal of achieving clear 1 to 2 cm margins.[10] Neck dissection is performed when lymph node metastases are detected or when there is elevated risk of occult lymph node metastases, and there is growing evidence to support sentinel lymph node biopsy for oral cavity malignancies.[12] Radiation can be used as definitive treatment; however, it is not routinely used because of the elevated rates of osteoradionecrosis associated with the higher therapeutic doses required for definitive versus adjuvant treatment. Advanced-stage cancer is usually treated with surgery and adjuvant radiation or combined chemotherapy and radiation when there are adverse findings (e.g., positive margins,

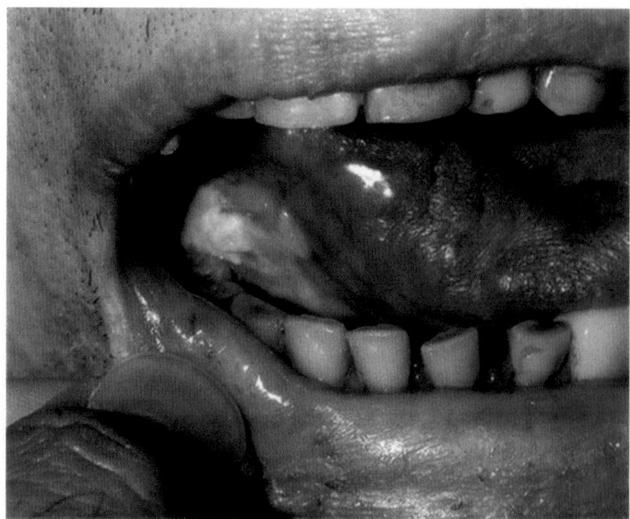

FIGURE 37.2. Cancer of the oral tongue seen on the right lateral tongue.

locally advanced disease, perineural or lymphovascular invasion, N2 or N3 nodal disease, and ENE).[13–16] Most surgery is performed transorally, except for very posterior lesions, which may require a mandibulotomy or a transcervical approach.

Oropharyngeal Cancer

Oropharyngeal cancer is distinctly different from oral cavity cancer, although here too SCC predominates, accounting for approximately 90% of cases.[5,7,17] The tonsillar region and base of tongue are the most common sites for oropharyngeal cancer, and specimens should be tested for p16 protein or HPV DNA or RNA for staging.[17]

Compared with treatment of oral cavity SCC, management of oropharyngeal SCC is more controversial. For early stage cancers, surgery alone or radiation alone results in comparable overall survival. Radiation has been favored at many centers to preserve speech and swallowing function.[18] However, transoral laser microsurgery (TLM) and transoral robotic surgery (TORS) have emerged as alternatives with improved functional outcomes over traditional open techniques.[19] For advanced cancers, current evidence supports the use of either combined chemotherapy and radiation therapy or surgery.[18] If surgery is performed, it may be followed by adjuvant therapy depending on the pathologic findings and stage.

Nasopharyngeal Cancer

The World Health Organization (WHO) classifies NPC into three subtypes[20]:

Type I: Keratinizing squamous cell carcinoma
Type II: Nonkeratinizing squamous cell carcinoma
Type III: Undifferentiated carcinoma

It is type III that accounts for over 95% of nasopharyngeal carcinomas in high-incidence areas, specifically southern China and Southeast Asia, with a strong association with EBV.[20] Presenting symptoms are often confused with benign and infectious processes, potentially leading to late diagnosis, and include a neck mass from nodal metastasis, middle ear effusion with hearing loss (from Eustachian tube obstruction), nasal obstruction, and sore throat. Flexible fiberoptic nasopharyngoscopy is performed to visualize the nasopharynx in patients suspected of NPC.

NPC is a radiosensitive malignancy, and radiation therapy to the primary and to the neck with or without concurrent chemotherapy is the mainstay of treatment for all types of NPC.[20,21] Neck dissection is performed for residual neck disease or resectable regional recurrence. Surgery with or without reirradiation is performed for resectable local recurrences.[20] Surgery of nasopharyngeal tumors can be complex because of limited access and perilous because of risk to the optic nerves as well as the internal carotid artery and cavernous sinus. Targeted treatment for NPC with monoclonal antibodies such as cetuximab, pembrolizumab, and nivolumab is being actively investigated.[20,21]

Hypopharyngeal Cancer

Hypopharyngeal and laryngeal cancers are often contiguous with each other as well as with the cervical esophagus. Additionally, many of these tumors are multicentric. Early stage hypopharyngeal cancers can be treated by surgery alone or radiation alone with comparable 5-year survival and local disease control.[4] Surgical approaches are most commonly transoral for early stage cancers, including robotic and laser resections, and transcervical for late stage cancers.[22] Advanced-stage piriform sinus cancers usually require a total laryngectomy and pharyngectomy (Figure 37.3). Advanced-stage cancers are given postoperative radiation. Alternately, they may be treated with combined chemotherapy and radiation with surgery reserved for salvage of residual or recurrent disease. As with laryngeal cancer, organ preservation (i.e., larynx preserving) protocols (induction chemotherapy followed by radiation with surgery reserved for salvage or concurrent chemoradiation therapy) have shown equivalent overall survival to the traditional approach of surgery and adjuvant radiation; therefore, many centers favor chemoradiation as the initial treatment for most hypopharyngeal cancers, although the prognosis for hypopharynx cancer remains grim.[22] The prevalence of neck metastases on presentation of hypopharyngeal cancers is 65% to 80%, and hypopharyngeal cancer is associated with the worst prognosis of all UADT SCCs, with an overall 5-year survival of around 35%.[21]

Laryngeal Cancer

Most laryngeal cancers occur in the glottis (64%), followed by the supraglottis (34%), and only rarely in the subglottis (2%).[4] Only about 5% of laryngeal SCCs occur in nonsmokers and nondrinkers.[4] HPV has been reported to be associated with laryngeal cancer but with much less frequency than in oropharyngeal SCC. The incidence and pattern of nodal spread varies with the location of the primary tumor. Lymphatic drainage of the glottis is sparse, and early stage primary cancers rarely spread to the lymph nodes. Also, because hoarseness is an early symptom, most glottic cancers are diagnosed at an early stage. Thus, cancer of the glottic larynx has an excellent average cure rate of 80% to 90%.[4]

TLM and TORS can be used for early stage glottic and supraglottic tumors if adequate visualization of the tumor can be achieved. Early stage glottic tumors are frequently treated with TLM or open cordectomy. If there is extension to the arytenoids, then a hemilaryngectomy can be performed. Such surgeries are aimed at preserving the laryngeal functions of phonation and airway protection.

Advanced laryngeal cancers are treated with total laryngectomy or combined chemotherapy and radiation therapy. Chemoradiation is usually the preferred initial treatment modality based on the results of the landmark Veterans Administration Laryngeal Cancer Study and subsequent RTOG 91-11 study, which showed comparable survival for patients treated with total laryngectomy versus an organ preservation protocol with surgical salvage. In this study, the laryngeal preservation rate was 67%.[23,24] Subsequent studies have confirmed these findings and have established concurrent chemotherapy with cisplatin and radiation therapy as the standard of care.[25–27] Bulky T4 cancers with either thyroid cartilage penetration or ≥1 cm base of tongue extension are an exception and should be treated with surgery. Also, patients with laryngeal dysfunction prior to treatment should not undergo organ preservation treatments because laryngeal preservation is valuable only if the core functions of breathing, speech, and airway protection during swallowing are preserved.[27]

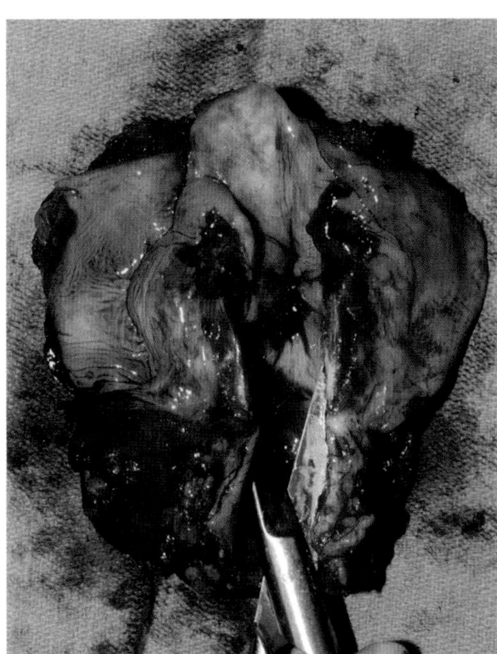

FIGURE 37.3. Laryngopharyngectomy specimen from a patient with hypopharyngeal cancer.

HEAD AND NECK

Unknown Primary Cancer

Neck metastases without a primary tumor that can be localized by physical examination or radiographic imaging are known as unknown primary or occult primary cancers. Unknown primary cancers account for 1% to 4% of head and cancers.[28] A painless neck mass in an adult should be considered a malignancy until proven otherwise. Fine-needle aspiration (FNA) is used to confirm the diagnosis. Metastatic UADT SCC is the most common cancer presenting as an unknown primary neck mass, followed by papillary thyroid cancer and cutaneous SCC.[28] The oropharynx is most frequently the origin of cancer in patients presenting with a cervical metastasis and an unknown primary. HPV detected in FNA specimens suggests an oropharyngeal primary, most commonly arising from either the tonsil or base of tongue. Further workup consists of imaging with CT or MRI and panendoscopy with directed biopsies, usually including the nasopharynx, both sides of the base of tongue (including potential lingual tonsillectomy), bilateral tonsillectomies, and both piriform sinuses, although biopsy sites may be selected based on the level(s) of neck disease and can vary slightly from institution to institution.[28,29]

When the primary remains unknown despite complete workup, most patients are treated with multimodality therapy, either resection (neck dissection) followed by adjuvant radiation with or without chemotherapy, or primary chemoradiation with or without posttherapeutic neck dissection. Radiation is usually given to both sides of the neck and to the nasopharynx, oropharynx, and hypopharynx/larynx. An exception is early stage cancers (T0N1 and HPV-associated T0N2a without other risk factors), which are usually treated with a single modality consisting of either surgery alone or radiation alone.[28]

Treatment

In general, early-stage tumors are treated with single modality therapy and late-stage tumors are treated with multimodality therapy, usually surgery followed by adjuvant radiation with or without chemotherapy with the exceptions noted earlier.

Surgery

Surgery is the mainstay for initial treatment of oral cavity cancer.[10,30] Most oral cavity lesions can be accessed transorally. A mandibulotomy with a lip-splitting incision may be used for very posterior lesions as well as oropharyngeal lesions. Transcervical resection may also be performed for oropharyngeal tumors. TORS is also an option for posterior oral cavity, oropharyngeal, and early-stage hypopharyngeal resections. For most sites, adequate surgical margins are defined in the National Comprehensive Cancer Network (NCCN) guidelines as ≥5 mm or more on final pathology, with close margins defined as anything <5 mm.[30] Early-stage laryngeal cancers may be treated microsurgically with or without CO_2 laser excision aiming for 1 to 2 mm margins in an effort to preserve vocal cord function because most data show that local control is equivalent to wider margins in this area.[30] Most surgeons rely on frozen section examination to facilitate complete tumor removal with a clear surgical margin followed by immediate flap reconstruction if needed.[31]

Indications for Marginal and Segmental Mandibulectomy

Preoperative imaging is used to determine the extent of bony involvement of the mandible or maxilla. Intraoperatively, the periosteum may be stripped in tumors abutting the mandible to inspect the underlying bone. When bone invasion is limited to the periosteum or there is minimal cortical involvement, a marginal mandibulectomy (single cortex) may be performed, but medullary invasion requires a segmental (full thickness) mandibular resection (**Figure 37.4**).[10]

Cervical Lymphadenectomy

Cervical lymphadenectomy or neck dissection has evolved over the past several decades.

- *Radical neck dissection* (RND): *en bloc* removal of lymph nodes from levels I-V along with the sternocleidomastoid muscle (SCM), internal jugular vein (IJV), and spinal accessory nerve (SAN) (**Figure 37.5**)
- *Modified radical neck dissection* (MRND): removal of all lymph node groups removed in a RND, but with preservation of one or more nonlymphatic structures (SCM, IJV, and SAN). Sparing of all three of these nonlymphatic structures is sometimes referred to as a *functional neck dissection.*
- *Selective neck dissection* (SND): cervical lymphadenectomy with preservation of one or more lymph node groups that are routinely removed in an RND or MRND

Regional control and survival rates have not been found to decrease with selective approaches, particularly with the addition of adjuvant therapies to manage microscopic residual disease.[32] Increasingly, lymph node yield and lymph node density are emerging as valuable quality indicators for neck dissection, with potential prognostic implication.[33]

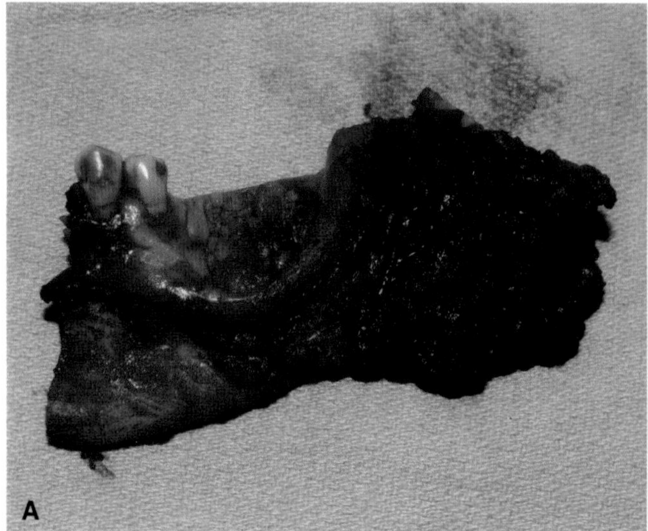

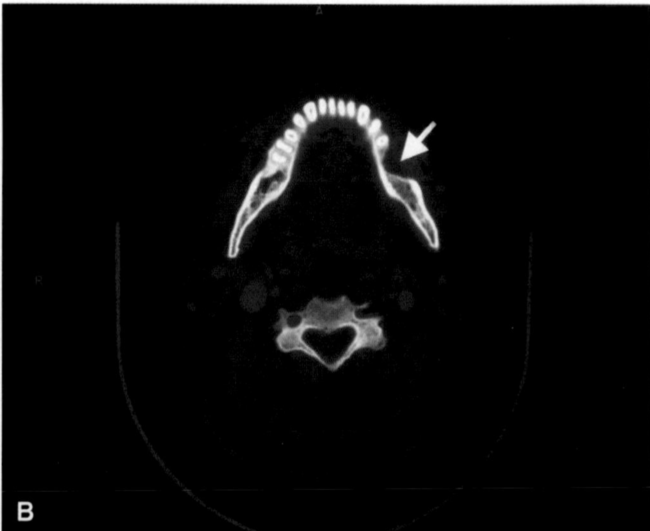

FIGURE 37.4. Gingival cancer invading the mandible seen in a surgical specimen **(A)**. Computed tomography (CT) scan demonstrating mandibular invasion of the buccal cortex extending to the medullary cavity (arrow) **(B)**.

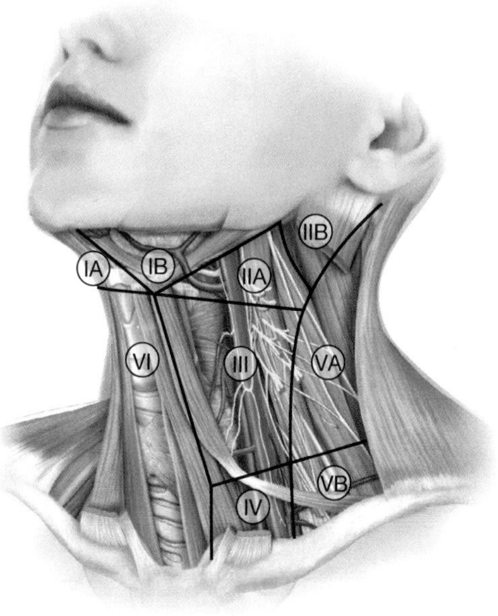

FIGURE 37.5. Levels of the neck. Level I is the submental and submandibular triangles. Level II, the upper jugular group, extends from the skull base to the carotid bifurcation (surgical landmark) or hyoid bone (clinical landmark). Level III, the middle jugular group, extends from the carotid bifurcation/hyoid bone to the omohyoid muscle (surgical landmark) or cricothyroid notch (clinical landmark). Level IV, the lower jugular group, extends from the omohyoid muscle to the clavicle. Level V is the posterior triangle bounded by the posterior border of the sternocleidomastoid muscle, the anterior border of the trapezius, and the clavicle. Level VI is the anterior (central) compartment.

Lymphatic drainage of the oral cavity usually occurs first to levels I-III or I-IV. Thus for oral cavity cancers, SND (I-III) or SND (I-IV) is commonly performed; more midline structures such as the lip and anterior oral tongue may spread to ipsilateral or contralateral nodes, so both necks should be investigated for such primary lesions.[10,30] SND (I-III) is also known as a supraomohyoid neck dissection. Sentinel lymph node biopsy for oral cavity cancer seems to be a safe and reliable technique to stage the N0 neck in oral cavity cancers, although further studies are ongoing.[12,34] For oropharyngeal, hypopharyngeal, and laryngeal cancers, SND (II-IV) is the procedure of choice.[30]

In patients with early-stage tumors that are clinically N0, the decision to proceed with neck dissection is based on having a probability of >20% of occult lymph node metastases. Bilateral neck dissections may be indicated when nodal metastases are present bilaterally or when a large midline primary tumor is present and there is a high probability of bilateral occult metastases (e.g., in the base of the tongue, the supraglottis, or the floor of the mouth).[10,30] RND and MRND are usually reserved for advanced nodal disease and disease extending into level V or invasion of critical structures in the neck.[30]

Adjuvant Therapy

As mentioned, surgery with postoperative radiation or combined radiation and chemotherapy has become the accepted treatment for high-stage head and neck cancers and those with adverse prognostic risk factors.[35] During the past decade, intensity-modulated radiation therapy has replaced standard delivery radiotherapy with decreased radiation-associated toxicity, particularly xerostomia.[36] It is an advanced form of radiation therapy that uses multiple radiation beams of varying intensities coming from different angles to precisely irradiate a tumor and avoid or reduce exposure of healthy tissue. More recently, intensity-modulated proton therapy (IMPT) has been used in head and neck cancer.[37] It may further reduce radiation-associated toxicity because of the decreased dose of radiation distal to the planned target. Besides xerostomia, other side effects of all forms of radiation include dermatitis, nausea and vomiting, fatigue, mucosal sores, hoarseness, and loss of taste.[37] Long-term problems may include dental decay, osteoradionecrosis, hypothyroidism, vascular disease, hypopituitarism if the pituitary gland is irradiated, and decreased hearing or vision when the orbits or middle ear/temporal bone are irradiated.[35]

Cisplatin is the chemotherapeutic drug most commonly used in head and neck cancer treatment regimens. It may be used alone or may be combined with 5-fluorouracil if given after radiation. Other agents include carboplatin, doxorubicin, epirubicin, paclitaxel, docetaxel, gemcitabine, bleomycin, and methotrexate. Combinations of two or more of these drugs are often used. Cisplatin is associated with neuropathies, especially peripheral neuropathy and hearing loss. Other side effects of chemotherapy agents include hair loss, mouth sores, loss of appetite, nausea and vomiting, diarrhea, immunosuppression, thrombocytopenia, and anemia.[4]

Targeted therapy works differently from standard chemotherapy drugs and often has different side effects. Targeted therapies consist of monoclonal antibodies that target specific protein receptors involved in the cancer pathway. Cetuximab effectively targets the epidermal growth factor receptor, a transmembrane tyrosine kinase receptor that is overexpressed in the majority of head and neck cancers and leads to division, angioinvasion, and metastasis through Ras and PI3K. Cetuximab has been demonstrated to be superior to radiation therapy alone and has become an integral component of systemic therapy for UADT SCC, although its efficacy remains undetermined compared with platin-based regimens.[38–40] Recently, immunotherapy with agents targeted against the PD-1 or PD-L1 checkpoint, such as pembrolizumab and nivolumab, has demonstrated prolonged disease-free survival in a subset of patients with recurrent or refractory head and neck cancer.[41,42]

SALIVARY GLAND TUMORS

Salivary gland tumors represent a diverse group of neoplasms involving the major and minor salivary glands. Tumors may arise from the various myoepithelial, ductal, and acinic components of the gland. Besides salivary gland epithelial neoplasms, the differential diagnosis for swelling in the region of the major glands includes metastatic cutaneous carcinoma (melanoma or SCC), lymphoma, hemangioma, tuberculosis, HIV, and lymphadenopathy.[43]

Anatomy

Salivary glands include the parotid, submandibular, and sublingual glands (Figure 37.6). There are 800 to 1000 minor salivary glands located throughout the oral cavity beneath the buccal, labial, and lingual mucosa; the soft palate; the lateral parts of the hard palate; and the floor of the mouth or between muscle fibers of the tongue. The minor salivary glands are 1 to 2 mm in diameter and, unlike the major glands, are not encapsulated by connective tissue, only surrounded by it.

Incidence and Risk Factors

Salivary gland tumors are rare, with fewer than 15 cases per 100,000 individuals annually.[43] About 80% of salivary gland tumors are benign.[43] Primary salivary gland malignancies represent less than 5% of all new head and neck cancers. About 80% of salivary gland tumors occur in the parotid glands, followed by the submandibular and minor salivary glands, and only about 1% occur in the sublingual glands. About 80% of parotid gland tumors are benign, and the parotid gland is the most common location for salivary gland malignancies; about 50% of submandibular gland tumors and 80% of minor salivary gland tumors are malignant.[43]

Rapid growth as well as pain and/or paresthesias caused by perineural invasion are associated with malignancy. In the parotid

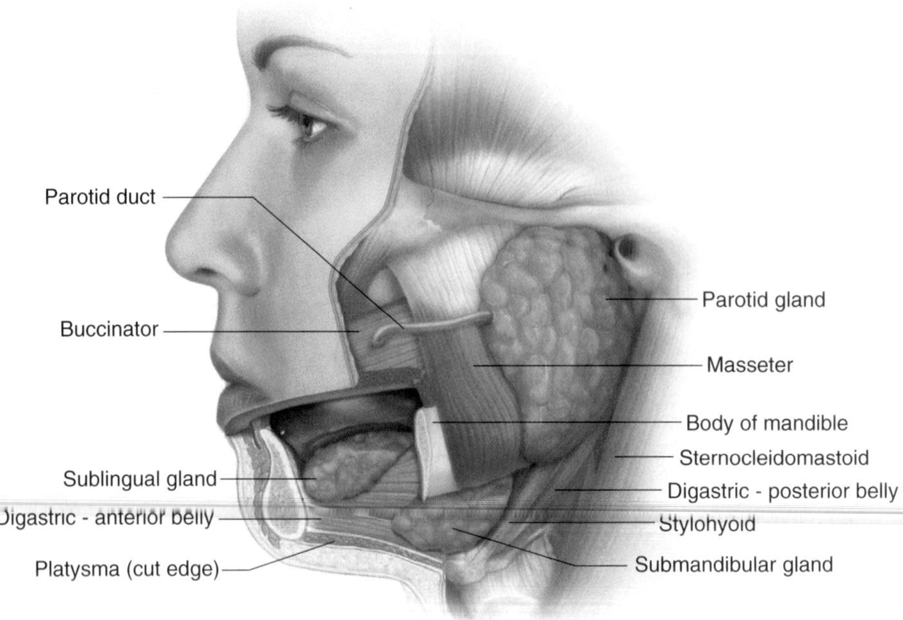

FIGURE 37.6. Anatomy of the major salivary glands, showing the parotid, submandibular, and sublingual glands.

gland, facial paralysis may be indicative of facial nerve invasion of a malignant tumor. Nodal metastases may also be seen in malignant tumors.

Preoperative Considerations

Biopsies, Imaging, and Metastatic Workup

Ultrasound, CT, and MRI are commonly used to evaluate salivary gland lesions. Contrast enhancement does not distinguish between benign versus malignant tumors but can delineate the extent of the lesion. Irregular margins, bony invasion, and the presence of metastatic lymph nodes or perineural spread can all be signs of malignancy; perineural spread may be apparent by widening of a nerve or neural foramina/space on CT scan, as well as by asymmetric enhancement or thickening on MRI. PET-CT is helpful for detecting disease recurrence and distant metastases.[44]

Ultrasound-guided FNA cytology is widely used but controversial because it has different levels of accuracy based on tumor type. FNA is reported to correctly diagnose tumor type in 61% to 94% of cases and differentiate between benign and malignant tumors in 81% to 98% of cases.[45,46] Because of this lack of complete accuracy, FNA alone should not be used to dictate the extent of surgery, such as radical resection or cervical lymphadenectomy. Some clinicians will choose to observe a lesion that is benign by FNA in patients deemed poor candidates for surgery. In all other patients, surgery is usually indicated for salivary gland neoplasms regardless of FNA results. The challenge for the extirpative surgeon is to correctly determine the appropriate extent of surgical treatment, taking into account not only results from FNA but also the preoperative and intraoperative findings, including those of frozen section examination, which has limitations in terms of making an accurate diagnosis as well. When the exact diagnosis is equivocal, the full scope of treatment should not be determined until final diagnosis has taken place.

Common Tumor Types

Most (≥95%) salivary gland neoplasms are of epithelial origin.[47] The WHO recognizes 11 benign and 22 malignant epithelial subtypes of salivary tumors, which are in turn characterized by marked biologic heterogeneity.[47] High-grade mucoepidermoid carcinomas (MECs), salivary ducts carcinomas, malignant mixed tumors, and high-grade adenocarcinomas have the most aggressive clinical course with early regional and distant metastases. The most common tumors are briefly discussed in the following sections. Metastatic skin cancer (most frequently SCC) is also an increasing concern, particularly, in elderly or immunocompromised patients, such as patients with chronic lymphocytic leukemia or organ transplant recipients.[48]

Pleomorphic Adenoma

Pleomorphic adenoma, also known as benign mixed tumor, is the most common salivary gland epithelial tumor in both adults and children and comprises one-half to two-thirds of all benign salivary gland tumors.[49] About 80% of pleomorphic adenomas are found in the parotid gland.[49] Tumors are most common in the fourth to fifth decade. Pleomorphic adenomas are well circumscribed and are grossly lobular and gray in appearance, although myxoid variants are more gelatinous, whereas cellular variants are firm and may appear tan-white. This tumor is histologically characterized by epithelial and connective tissue elements, with stellate and spindle cells interspersed within a myxoid background.

Pleomorphic adenomas are treated by surgical excision and are associated with very low recurrence rates (0%–5%).[49,50] Incomplete excision is the main risk for recurrence. For parotid tumors, pseudopodia pose a theoretic risk for recurrence when margins are narrow. Left untreated, up to 15% of pleomorphic adenomas may undergo malignant transformation into a lesion known as carcinoma ex pleomorphic adenoma, which is why resection is recommended.[49]

Warthin Tumor

Warthin tumor (papillary cystadenoma lymphomatosum) is the second most common tumor of the parotid gland and is benign. Warthin tumors predominantly occur in males of 50 to 70 years of age, most frequently smokers, and are the most common bilateral salivary gland tumors (5%–14%).[49] The histologic appearance of this tumor is characteristic, consisting of papillary cysts and mucoid fluid as well as nodules of lymphoid tissue. Because of the mitochondrial concentrations in oncocytes, Warthin tumors do not infrequently demonstrate fluorodeoxyglucose uptake on PET scan, potentially leading to a false-positive study.[50]

Mucoepidermoid Carcinoma

MEC is the most common salivary gland malignancy (about 35% of salivary gland cancers) and consists of mucin-secreting, intermediate, and epidermoid cells.[43] The histologic grade (low, intermediate, high) of MEC has prognostic value and dictates the need for adjuvant radiation therapy. Low- and intermediate-grade tumors often present as asymptomatic slow-growing, solitary masses. High-grade tumors may progress rapidly and present with symptoms including pain, nerve deficits, and local soft tissue invasion. Overall survival is 80% to 90% for low- and intermediate-grade tumors, whereas high-grade tumors have an overall survival of 40% to 50% at 5 years.[43,51] Elective node dissection is often recommended for high-grade tumors; however, histologic grade is seldom known preoperatively.

Acinic Cell Carcinoma

Acinic cell carcinoma accounts for 8% to 14% of salivary gland cancers.[43,51] The parotid is the most commonly involved salivary gland and usually presents as a slow-growing solitary mass. Tumor cells have a granular, metachromatic cytoplasm, resembling that seen in the serous acinar cells of salivary glands. Acinic cell carcinomas tend to behave indolently. Survival is 97%, 93%, and 89% at 5, 10, and 15 years, respectively.[51]

Adenoid Cystic Carcinoma

Adenoid cystic carcinoma (ACC) is the second most common malignancy of the salivary glands after MEC and exhibits a propensity for perineural invasion. There are three histologic subtypes: cribriform, tubular, and solid. The cribriform pattern has a classic *Swiss cheese* appearance with cells arranged in nests separated by round or oval spaces. The tubular pattern has a glandular architecture, whereas the solid (or basaloid) pattern has sheets of cells with little or no luminal spaces.[43]

ACC shows a slow but relentless progression. Five-year survival is as high as 90%, but 15-year survival is less than 70% and decreases substantially after this with a 20-year survival of 28%.[43,51] ACCs usually have an indolent natural history although high-grade transformation with markedly worse prognosis (median survival of 12–36 months) can occur.[43] The risk for regional spread is low (about 5%–20%), but these cancers have a propensity for local and distant recurrence even 10 to 15 years after initial treatment.[43] Most commonly, spread is to the lungs, bone, and brain. The development of asymptomatic, slowly growing pulmonary metastases can often be observed for years.

Malignant Mixed Tumors

Malignant mixed tumors of the salivary glands include carcinoma ex pleomorphic adenoma (the most common variant), intracapsular carcinoma ex pleomorphic adenoma, metastasizing pleomorphic adenoma, and carcinosarcoma.[51] Carcinoma ex pleomorphic adenoma presents in a preexisting pleomorphic adenoma with accelerated growth and new-onset pain and/or neuropathy. Nodal metastasis may be an early finding. Adjuvant radiation following surgery to the primary site and nodal basins may improve local control rates, although overall survival is poor (about 40% 5-year survival).[51] Intracapsular carcinoma ex pleomorphic adenoma shows evidence of malignancy cytologically but is confined within the capsule of a preexisting pleomorphic adenoma and generally has better prognosis than invasive variants. Metastasizing pleomorphic adenomas show histologic features of benign pleomorphic adenoma but present with distant metastases and local recurrences. Treatment involves surgical resection of the involved sites when possible. Prognosis is favorable despite metastases. Carcinosarcomas are rare and associated with frequent recurrences, distant metastases, and poor overall survival.

Treatment

Complete surgical excision is curative for benign tumors and malignancies when the tumor is small and low grade. Larger tumors and those with aggressive histologic type and/or high grade are usually treated with surgery and adjuvant radiation therapy.

Parotidectomy

A superficial parotidectomy is considered the treatment of choice for benign and most malignant tumors in the superficial lobe of the gland.[43,49] A less than complete superficial parotidectomy that still removes the entire tumor with a negative margin is referred to as a partial parotidectomy. Total parotidectomy, sparing the facial nerve if uninvolved, is indicated for deep lobe tumors and, increasingly, for metastatic cutaneous malignancy (Figure 37.7).[52] Preoperative weakness or invasion based on imaging may require one or more branches of the facial nerve to be sacrificed. The nerve may also need to be sacrificed if preservation would lead to grossly positive margins or tumor spillage. Radical parotidectomy involves total parotidectomy with facial nerve sacrifice. If adjacent structures such as the skin, mandible, or temporal bone are involved, an extended radical parotidectomy may be indicated. Mastoidectomy/lateral temporal bone resection may also be indicated to identify and/or resect the facial nerve proximally if the tumor abuts the mastoid bone or stylomastoid foramen or invades the nerve.[43]

Enucleation, which requires simple removal of the mass, is not indicated for malignant tumors and is controversial for benign tumors, with some surgeons advocating against it.[43,49] For those who consider enucleation, resection should include the capsule of the tumor (extracapsular enucleation), and it should be reserved for benign superficial tumors less than 4 cm in diameter.[49]

Submandibular, Sublingual, and Minor Salivary Gland Excision

Benign neoplasms of the submandibular gland are treated with submandibular gland excision. For malignant lesions, level I lymph nodes and possibly other cervical levels are dissected in continuity. Sublingual gland malignancies are often managed transorally and may include the floor of mouth mucosa if it is involved or close to the tumor. Obtaining negative margins in sublingual gland surgery can be challenging because it is not encapsulated by fascia and may invade the mandible, lingual nerve, or duct of the submandibular gland.[43] Resection of minor salivary gland tumors depends on their location. Wide local excision is usually performed with the goal of achieving clear margins of at least 5 mm. Resection of palatal and base of tongue tumors can affect speech, swallowing, and velopharyngeal competence.[43]

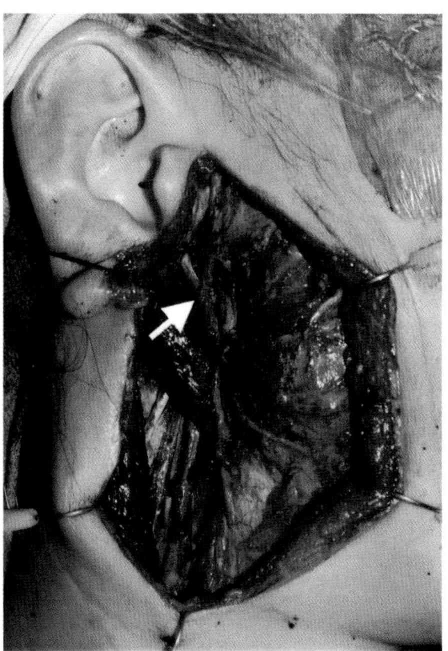

FIGURE 37.7. A total parotidectomy has been performed in which both the superficial and deep lobes of the parotid gland have been removed. The facial nerve (white arrow) is indicated and can be seen arising from the stylomastoid foramen, above of the posterior belly of the digastric muscle.

Cervical Lymphadenectomy

Known cervical metastases should be treated with cervical lymphadenectomy. In the clinically node-negative neck, the decision between observation and treatment via elective neck dissection or prophylactic radiation is made based on the likelihood for occult metastases. Risk factors for nodal spread include histological evidence of perineural invasion, lymphovascular invasion, and extracapsular spread, as well as high-grade histologic subtypes.[53,54] The most frequently involved nodal levels primarily depend on the site of the primary tumor.

Adjuvant Therapy

Unresectable locally advanced tumors with skull base or carotid involvement or those occurring in patients who are not able to tolerate surgery may be managed with primary radiation therapy. Undifferentiated and high-grade tumors, advanced-stage tumors, including those with facial nerve and deep lobe involvement, tumors with lymphatic or vascular invasion, and tumors with positive margins are usually treated with surgery and adjuvant radiation therapy to prevent locoregional recurrence. Systemic chemotherapy is considered for patients who have recurrence or metastatic disease who are not candidates for surgical or radiation treatment.[55] Differing histotypes and heterogeneity within histotypes make it difficult to standardize systemic treatment. Methotrexate, cisplatin, paclitaxel, epirubicin, and vinorelbine have been used in advanced salivary gland cancers, although not routinely.[55] Targeted therapy may also have a role in specific salivary gland malignant subtypes, and research is ongoing.

REFERENCES

1. American Cancer Society. *Cancer Facts and Figures 2013*. Atlanta, GA: American Cancer Society; 2013.
2. Porceddu SV, Veness MJ, Guminski A. Non-melanoma cutaneous head and neck cancer and Merkel cell carcinoma: current concepts, advances, and controversies. *J Clin Oncol*. 2015;33:3338-3345.
3. Gandini S, Botteri E, Iodice S, et al. Tobacco smoking and cancer: a meta-analysis. *Int J Cancer*. 2008;122:155-164.
4. Belcher R, Hayes K, Fedewa S, Chen AY. Current treatment of head and neck squamous cell cancer. *J Surg Oncol*. 2014;110:551-574.
5. Mehanna H, Oyaleye O, Licitra L. Oropharyngeal cancer: is it time to change management according to human papilloma virus status? *Curr Opin Otolaryngol Head Neck Surg*. 2012;20:120-124.
6. Chaturvedi AK, Engels EA, Pfeiffer RM, et al. Human papillomavirus and rising oropharyngeal cancer incidence in the United States. *J Clin Oncol*. 2011;29:4294-4301.
7. Deschler DG, Richmon JD, Khariwala SS, et al. The "new" head and neck cancer patient–Young, nonsmoker, nondrinker, and HPV positive: evaluation. *Otolaryngol Head Neck Surg*. 2014;151(3):375-380.
8. Hayes DN, Van Waes C, Seiwert TY. Genetic landscape of human papillomavirus-associated head and neck cancer and comparison to tobacco-related tumors. *J Clin Oncol*. 2015;33:3227-3234.
9. Mirghani H, Jung AC, Fakhry C. Primary, secondary and tertiary prevention of human papillomavirus-driven head and neck cancers. *Eur J Cancer*. 2017;78:105-115.
10. Chinn SB, Myers JN. Oral cavity carcinoma: current management, controversies and future directions. *J Clin Oncol*. 2015:33;3269-3276.
11. Lydiatt WM, Patel SG, O'Sullivan B, et al. Head and neck cancers: major changes in the American Joint Committee on Cancer Eighth Edition Cancer Staging Manual. *CA Cancer J Clin*. 2017;67:122-137.
Significant changes to head and neck cancer staging were introduced in 2017. The most important changes include the creation of a separate staging algorithm for HPV-associated cancer of the oropharynx; changes to the tumor (T) categories for oral cavity, skin, and nasopharynx cancer; and the addition of ENE to the lymph node category (N) in most head and neck subsite classifications.
12. Civantos FJ, Zitsch RP, Schuller DP, et al. Sentinel lymph node biopsy accurately stages the regional lymph nodes for T1-T2 oral squamous cell carcinomas: results of a prospective multi-institutional trial. *J Clin Oncol*. 2008;28:1395-1400.
13. Bernier J, Domenge C, Ozashin M, et al. Postoperative irradiation with or without concomitant chemotherapy for locally advanced head and neck cancer. *N Engl J Med*. 2004;350:1945-1952.
14. Cooper JS, Pajak TF, Forastiere AA, et al. Postoperative concurrent radiotherapy and chemotherapy for high-risk squamous cell carcinoma of the head and neck. *N Engl J Med*. 2004;350:1937-1944.
15. Cooper JS, Zhang Q, Pajak TF, et al. Long-term follow-up of the RTOG 9501/intergroup phase III trial: postoperative concurrent radiation therapy and chemotherapy in high-risk squamous cell carcinoma of the head and neck. *Int J Radiat Oncol Biol Phys*. 2012;84:1198-1205.
16. Pfister DG, Spenser S, Brizel DM, et al. Head and neck cancers, Version 2.2014. Clinical practice guidelines in oncology. *J Natl Compr Cancer Netw*. 2014;12:1454-1487.
17. Guo T, Goldenberg D, Fakhry C. AHNS Series: do you know your guidelines? Management of head and neck cancer in the era of human papillomavirus. *Head Neck*. 2017;39:833-839.
18. Parsons JT, Mendenhall WM, Stringer SP, et al. Squamous cell carcinoma of the oropharynx: surgery, radiation therapy, or both. *Cancer*. 2002;94(11):2967-2980.
19. Holsinger FC, Ferris RL. Transoral endoscopic head and neck surgery and its role within the multidisciplinary treatment paradigm of oropharynx cancer: robotics, lasers, and clinical trials. *J Clin Oncol*. 2015;33:3285-3292.
20. Lee AW, Ma BB, Ng WT, et al. Management of nasopharyngeal carcinoma: current practice and future perspective. *J Clin Oncol*. 2015;33:3356-3364.
21. Gooi Z, Richmon J, Agarwal N. AHNS series: do you know your guidelines? Principles of treatment for nasopharyngeal cancer a review of the national comprehensive cancer network guidelines. *Head Neck*. 2017:39;201-205.
22. Dziegielewski PT, Kang SY, Ozer E. Transoral robotic surgery (TORS) for laryngeal and hypopharyngeal cancer. *J Surg Oncol*. 2015;112:702-706.
23. Department of Veterans Affairs Laryngeal Cancer Study Group, Wolf GT, Fisher SG, et al. Induction chemotherapy plus radiation compared with surgery plus radiation in patients with advanced laryngeal cancer. *N Engl J Med*. 1991;324:1685-1690.
This landmark study compared induction chemotherapy with definitive radiation therapy with conventional laryngectomy and postoperative radiation for patients with laryngeal cancer. Surgical salvage was performed for chemoradiotherapy-treated patients who recurred locally. Using this strategy, they reported a high rate of laryngeal preservation without compromising overall survival. This study changed the treatment paradigm for laryngeal cancer at many centers throughout the country and across the world.
24. Forastiere AA, Zhang Q, Weber RS, et al. Long-term results of RTOG 91-11: a comparison of three nonsurgical treatment strategies to preserve the larynx in patients with locally advanced larynx cancer. *J Clin Oncol*. 2013;31:845-852.
25. Forastiere AA, Weber RS, Trotti A. Organ preservation for advanced larynx cancer: issues and outcomes. *J Clin Oncol*. 2015;33:3262-3268.
26. Chen AY, Halpern M. Factors predictive of survival in advanced laryngeal cancer. *Arch Otolaryngol Head Neck Surg*. 2007;133:1270-1276.
27. Gourin CG, Conger BT, Sheils C, et al. The effect of treatment on survival in patients with advanced laryngeal carcinoma. *Laryngoscope*. 2009;119:1312-1317.
28. Galloway TJ, Ridge JA. Management of squamous cancer metastatic to the cervical nodes with an unknown primary site. *J Clin Oncol*. 2015;33:3328-3337.
29. Byrd JK, Smith KJ, de Almeida JR, et al. Transoral robotic surgery and the unknown primary: a cost-effectiveness analysis. *Otolaryngol Head Neck Surg*. 2014;150(6):976-982.
30. Miller MC, Goldenberg D. AHNS series: do you know your guidelines? Principles of surgery for head and neck cancer a review of the National Comprehensive Cancer Network guidelines. *Head Neck*. 2017;39:791-796.
31. Maxwell JH, Thompson LD, Brandwein-Gensler MS, et al. Early oral tongue squamous cell carcinoma: sampling of margins from tumor bed and worse local control. *JAMA Otolarygol Head Neck Surg*. 2015;141(12):1104-1110.
32. Mukhija V, Gupta S, Jacobson AS, et al. Selective neck dissection following adjuvant therapy for advanced head and neck cancer. *Head Neck*. 2009;1(2):183-188.
33. Cheraghlou S, Otremba M, Kuo Yu P, et al. Prognostic value of lymph node yield and density in head and neck malignancies. *Otolaryngol Head Neck Surg*. 2018;158(6):1016-1023.
34. Schilling C, Stoeckli SJ, Haerle SK, et al. Sentinel European Node Trial (SENT): 3-year results of sentinel node biopsy in oral cancer. *Eur J Cancer*. 2015;51(18):2777-2784.
35. Gooi Z, Fakhry C, Goldenberg D, et al. AHNS series: do you know your guidelines? Principles of radiation therapy for head and neck cancer a review of the National Comprehensive Cancer Network guidelines. *Head Neck*. 2016;38:987-992.
36. Chen WC, Hwang TZ, Wang WH, et al. Comparison between conventional and intensity modulated post-operative radiotherapy for stage III and IV oral cavity cancer in terms of treatment results and toxicity. *Oral Oncol*. 2009;45:505-510.
There has been a dramatic rise in oropharyngeal SCC in recent years because of HPV infection. Patients with HPV-related oropharynx cancers are younger and lack traditional risk factors such as tobacco and alcohol use. Biologically, these HPV-related oropharyngeal cancers behave differently, necessitating new treatment algorithms and staging systems.
37. Van de Water TA, Bijl HP, Schilstra C, et al. The potential benefit of radiotherapy with protons in head and neck cancer with respect to normal tissue sparing: a systematic review of literature. *Oncologist*. 2011;16:366-377.
38. Bonner JA, Harari PM, Giralt J, et al. Radiotherapy plus cetuximab for squamous-cell carcinoma of the head and neck. *N Engl J Med*. 2006;354:567-578.
39. Buglione M, Maddalo M, Corvò R, et al. Subgroup analysis according to human papillomavirus status and tumor site of a randomized phase II trial comparing cetuximab and cisplatin combined with radiation therapy for locally advanced head and neck cancer. *Int J Radiat Oncol Biol Phys*. 2017;97(3):462-472.
40. Magrini SM, Buglione M, Corvò R, et al. Cetuximab and radiotherapy versus cisplatin and radiotherapy for locally advanced head and neck cancer: a randomized phase II trial. *J Clin Oncol*. 2015;34:427-435.
41. Seiwert TY, Burtness B, Mehra R, et al. Safety and clinical activity of pembrolizumab for treatment of recurrent or metastatic squamous cell carcinoma of the head and neck (KEYNOTE-012): an open-label, multi-centre, phase 1b trial. *Lancet Oncol*. 2016;17:956-965.

42. Ferris RL, Blumenschein G Jr, Fayette J, et al. Nivolumab for recurrent squamous-cell carcinoma of the head and neck. *N Engl J Med*. 2016;375:1856-1867.
43. Rodriguez CP, Parvathaneni U, Méndez E, Martina RG. Salivary gland malignancies. *Hematol Oncol Clin North Am*. 2015;29:1145-1157.
44. Dercle L, Hartl D, Rozenblum-Beddok L, et al. Diagnostic and prognostic value of 18F-FDG PET, CT, and MRI in perineural spread of head and neck malignancies. *Eur Radiol*. 2018;28(4):1761-1770.
45. Siewert B, Kruskal JB, Kelly D, et al. Utility and safety of ultrasound-guided fine-needle aspiration of salivary gland masses including a cytologist's review. *J Ultrasound Med*. 2004;23(6):777-783.
46. Seethala RR, LiVolsi VA, Baloch ZW. Relative accuracy of fine-needle aspiration and frozen section in the diagnosis of lesions of the parotid gland. *Head Neck*. 2005;27(3):217-223.
Use of FNA and frozen section in the diagnosis of salivary gland lesions are a subject of debate because of less than perfect accuracy. FNA was found to have a sensitivity of 86% and specificity of 92%. Frozen section was found to have a sensitivity of 77% and a specificity of 100%. The authors suggest that frozen section may be useful if FNA is nondiagnositc and may confirm or refute malignancy in some cases.
47. Seethala RR, Stenman G. Update from the 4th edition of the World Health Organization classification of head and neck tumors: tumors of the salivary gland. *Head Neck Pathol*. 2017;11:55-67.
48. O'Brien CJ. The parotid as a metastatic basin for skin cancer. *Arch Otolaryngol Head Neck Surg*. 2005;131(7):551-555.
49. Zhan KY, Khaja SF, Flack AB, et al. Benign parotid tumors. *Otolaryngol Clin North Am*. 2016;49:327-342.
50. Rassekh CH, Cost JL, Hogg JP, et al. Positron emission tomography in Warthin's tumor mimicking malignancy impacts the evaluation of head and neck patients. *Am J Otolaryngol*. 2015;36(2):259-263.
51. Guzzo M, Locati LD, Prott FJ, et al. Major and minor salivary gland tumors. *Crit Rev Oncol Hematol*. 2010;74:134-148.
52. Thom JJ, Moore EJ, Price DL, et al. The role of total parotidectomy for metastatic cutaneous squamous cell carcinoma and malignant melanoma. *JAMA Otolaryngol Head Neck Surg*. 2014;140(6):548-554.
53. Breen B, Rahimi S, Brennan. Current management of the neck in salivary gland carcinomas. *J Oral Pathol Med*. 2017;46:161-166.
54. Wang YL, Lin DS, Gan HL, et al. Predictive index for lymph node management of major salivary gland cancer. *Laryngoscope*. 2012;122;1497-1506.
This study examines predictive factors for spread of salivary gland cancer to regional lymph nodes. Tumor- and patient-related factors were used to determine the relative risk for lymph node metastases to guide the indications for elective neck dissection.
55. Laurie SA, Licitra L. Systemic therapy in the palliative management of advanced salivary gland cancers. *J Clin Oncol*. 2008;24:2673-2678.

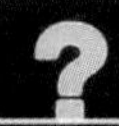

QUESTIONS

1. **A 40-year-old man presents with a neck mass that is found to be SCC on FNA biopsy. Subsequent examination demonstrates that he has a tonsillar primary cancer that is positive for HPV on biopsy. Which of the following statements are true regarding HPV-positive oropharyngeal cancer?**

   a. The cancer is contagious.
   b. The patient should get an HPV vaccination.
   c. The patient's spouse should get an HPV vaccination.
   d. The patient's children should get HPV vaccinations.
   e. This cancer is also frequently related to EBV infection.

2. **A 60-year-old woman presents with a 1.5 cm SCC of the right lingual mandibular gingiva and an upper cervical neck mass. Full-thickness cortical invasion of the tumor into the mandible is observed on computed tomography (CT) scan. In addition to neck dissection, the most appropriate surgical treatment is:**

   a. Wide local excision
   b. TORS
   c. Transoral laser surgery
   d. Marginal mandibulectomy
   e. Segmental mandibulectomy

3. **A 47-year-old Asian man presents with decreased hearing and a sense of fullness in the right ear of 3 months duration. Otoscopy demonstrates a middle ear effusion. He is otherwise asymptomatic. What is the next appropriate step in management?**

   a. Placement of a pressure equalization tube
   b. Referral for a hearing aid
   c. Trial of an oral penicillin
   d. Fiberoptic examination of the nasopharynx
   e. Serum blood work for EBV antigens

4. **A 40-year-old man presents with a 2 cm mass behind the angle of his right mandible. On examination, he has weakness of his facial muscles on the side of the tumor. A parotidectomy is performed, and pathology demonstrates a mixed population of predominantly poorly differentiated epithelial cells and intermediate cells with occasional mucous-secreting cells and neural invasion. The most likely diagnosis is:**

   a. MEC
   b. Pleomorphic adenoma
   c. Warthin tumor
   d. SCC
   e. Hemangioma

5. **A 55-year-old man presents with a 2.5 cm right lateral oral tongue squamous cell cancer and a single palpably enlarged jugulodigastric lymph node (clinically staged T2N1M0). In addition to partial glossectomy, what is the most appropriate treatment for the metastatic lymph node?**

   a. RND
   b. MRND
   c. SND of levels I-III and total parotidectomy
   d. SND of levels I-IV
   e. Observation with possible postoperative radiation depending on the final pathology of the tongue tumor

1. **Answer: d.** In recent years, HPV has been recognized as an etiologic factor in oropharyngeal SCC. Because such cancers have a more favorable prognosis than HPV-negative cancers, testing FNA biopsies and tumor specimens for HPV is recommended. The cancer cannot be transmitted to another person. Vaccination has no role in treating patients who are already infected and have no current role in cancer treatment. Vaccination is not recommended for adults who have already been sexually active for a number of years. Vaccination is recommended for all adolescents and young adults (not only children of patients with oropharyngeal SCC), aged 9 to 25, ideally prior to the onset of sexual activity. The vaccine provides protection against the four strains for HPV most commonly associated with cervical and oropharyngeal SCC, including HPV-16. EBV is associated with nasopharyngeal carcinoma in endemic regions and has no known association with HPV-related oropharyngeal SCC.

2. **Answer: e.** For transcortical invasion of the mandible, a segmental mandibulectomy, in which a full-thickness portion of the mandible is excised, is the most appropriate surgical treatment. Marginal mandibulectomy is reserved for cases in which the cancer stops at the periosteum or does not penetrate full-thickness through the cortex of the mandible. Wide local excision, TORS, and transoral laser surgery are not adequate treatment for this lesion. Immediate reconstruction of the mandible with an osteocutaneous free flap is usually indicated, as is postoperative radiation therapy for this advanced-stage cancer.

3. **Answer: d.** A serous middle ear effusion in an adult should raise the suspicion for an NPC causing Eustachian tube dysfunction. Nasopharyngoscopy with a flexible fiberoptic scope should be performed as the next step in management. NPC is one of the most common cancers in parts of Asia, most notably southern China, and is associated with EBV seropositivity. If no masses are seen, it would be reasonable to try an oral antibiotic but also to continue further workup with an imaging study (CT or MRI) as well as consider biopsy of the nasopharynx. A pressure equalization tube will allow drainage of the effusion and aeration of the middle ear, restoring hearing and making a hearing aid unnecessary.

4. **Answer: a.** Only about 20% of parotid gland tumors are malignant. Malignant tumors may invade the facial nerve causing facial paralysis. Malignant tumors may also metastasize to the regional lymph nodes and to distant sites. MECs are the most common malignancy of the parotid gland.

5. **Answer: d.** Based on the clinical diagnosis of a metastatic lymph node to the ipsilateral neck, a cervical lymphadenectomy should be performed. RND includes removal of neck lymph nodes in levels I to V as well as the SCM, IJV, and SAN.

CHAPTER 38 Reconstruction of the Scalp, Forehead, Calvarium, Skull Base, and Midface

Alexander F. Mericli, Jesse C. Selber, and Matthew M. Hanasono

KEY POINTS

- Locoregional or free flaps are usually required for scalp defects that include the pericranium.
- Unlike other head and neck sites, tissue expansion may play a role in reconstruction of the scalp.
- Resection of skull base tumors may be associated with significant complications including cerebrospinal fluid leak and cranial nerve deficits.
- The location of the skull base tumor determines the approach to resection and dictates the reconstructive needs.
- Maxillary defects are usually complex; prosthetics, soft tissue flaps, and/or bone grafts and flaps may play a role in reconstruction.

Defects involving the scalp, forehead, calvarium, skull base, and maxilla are among the most challenging reconstructions in our specialty. Although these structures are adjacent anatomically, their reconstructive requirements are vastly different given the multiple specialized functions located within the head and neck. The techniques employed to restore these anatomic regions are complex, nuanced, and frequently necessitate microsurgery. Furthermore, defects involving the calvarium, skull base, and maxilla are especially challenging because of the potential for major, life-threatening complications that may occur should the reconstruction fail, such as brain exposure and neurologic injury, blindness, cerebrospinal fluid (CSF) leak, meningitis, and osteomyelitis.

SCALP, FOREHEAD, AND CALVARIUM

Scalp and forehead tissue is intrinsically inelastic, limiting the application of primary closure and local flaps. Skin grafts are possible when the pericranium is intact, and a variety of local flaps can be designed. There are only three regional flaps (pericranium, temporoparietal fascia, and temporalis muscle), all of which have a limited arc of rotation thereby minimizing their utility; therefore, microvascular free tissue transfer is commonly required for durable reconstruction in this area of the body for sizable defects. Calvarial reconstruction can include alloplastic materials, customized implants, and bone grafting, depending on the circumstances.

Anatomy

The frontalis muscle overlies the frontal bone and is connected to the occipitalis muscle posteriorly, through the galea aponeurotica. The blood supply of the forehead and scalp is robust and consists of the paired supraorbital, supratrochlear, superficial temporal (ST), posterior auricular, and occipital vessels. The sensory nerves are also paired and include the supraorbital, supratrochlear, zygomaticotemporal, auriculotemporal, lesser occipital, and greater occipital nerves. The most clinically significant motor nerve is the temporal branch of the facial nerve, which innervates the frontalis muscle. This branch is located on the deep surface of the temporoparietal fascia and follows a course approximated by a line extending from 0.5 cm inferior to the external auditory meatus to a point 1.5 cm superior to the lateral eyebrow. Dissection in this area is occasionally needed to access the zygomatic arch for reduction and internal fixation or to raise a temporalis muscle flap. To avoid injury to this important nerve, dissection is performed in a plane deep to the superficial layer of the deep temporal fascia. The calvarium is covered by thick periosteum oftentimes called pericranium, which can be utilized as a local flap. Structurally, the calvarium is comprised of three layers: an outer table, a diploic space, and an inner table.

Forehead and Scalp Reconstruction

Nonmicrosurgical Techniques

The skin of the scalp is among the thickest in the body, measuring 3 to 8 mm. This thickness, as well as the fibrous galea aponeurotica, limits the pliability of the scalp. Although primary closure with adjacent hair-bearing tissue is the preferred wound closure technique in the appropriate scenario, this approach is typically limited to defects no greater than 3 cm in diameter. Tension should be avoided to prevent skin dehiscence or alopecia. There are several techniques that can be employed to reduce tension when reconstructing a scalp defect via primary repair or adjacent tissue rearrangement. First, the resection can be designed so that the closure is oriented perpendicular to the relaxed skin tension lines; this tends to be in a sagittal direction on the scalp and in a transverse direction on the forehead. Second, wide undermining in the subgaleal layer along the circumference of the defect can reduce tension. Finally, galeal scoring is an adjunctive technique that can increase scalp pliability and reduce closure tension. The scores should be designed in parallel with the leading edge of the flap, be spaced no closer than 1 cm apart, and only divide the galea. Scores deeper than the galea will disrupt the random pattern blood supply of the scalp. Each galeal incision increases the length of the scalp 1.67 mm; therefore, multiple incisions can substantially minimize tension and maximize pliability.[1]

If the scalp defect is too wide to permit primary closure and the underlying calvarium is not exposed, the wound can be closed with a split- or full-thickness skin graft. Alternatively, if the calvarium is exposed, burring the outer table with entry into the vascular diploic space can facilitate skin graft adherence. This can be performed immediately or with an intermediate stage using a dermal substitute; however, this often results in an unstable skin graft and is not recommended as a long-term solution or in the context of radiation. In any situation, once healed, the graft will not bear hair. Additionally, because of the difference in thickness between the native scalp and a skin graft, a noticeable contour deformity will be present.

One of the central tenets of reconstructive surgery—replacing like with like—is evident in the use of local flaps for scalp reconstruction. This technique will maintain the thickness of the scalp as well as the ability to bear hair. In situations where the calvarium is exposed at the base of the wound, reconstruction with vascularized tissue, such as a local flap, is required. Most local flaps are designed using the rotation-advancement principle and should be oriented to recruit tissue from areas of the scalp with laxity, such as the parietal and temporal regions. The meticulous plastic surgeon will attempt to match hair follicle direction with the flap and will also bevel the incision parallel to the angle of the hair follicles to minimize scar alopecia. In smaller defects, the local flap donor site can be closed primarily (**Figure 38.1**); however, reconstruction of larger defects may require elevating the local flap in the subgaleal plane and maintaining the pericranium so that the donor site can then be closed with a skin graft (back grafting). The skin graft can then be serially excised secondarily

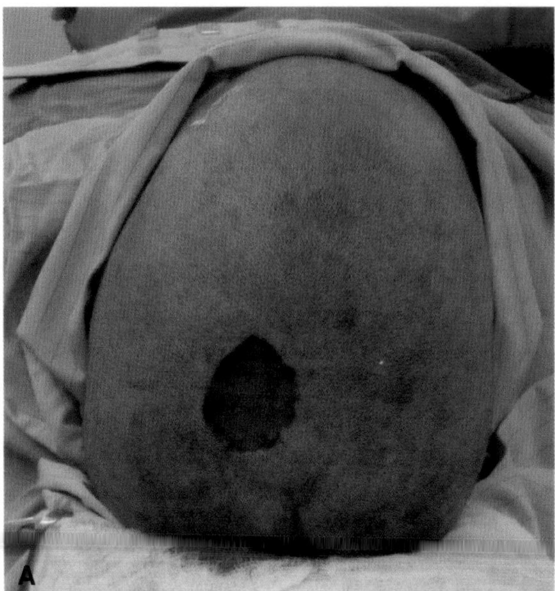

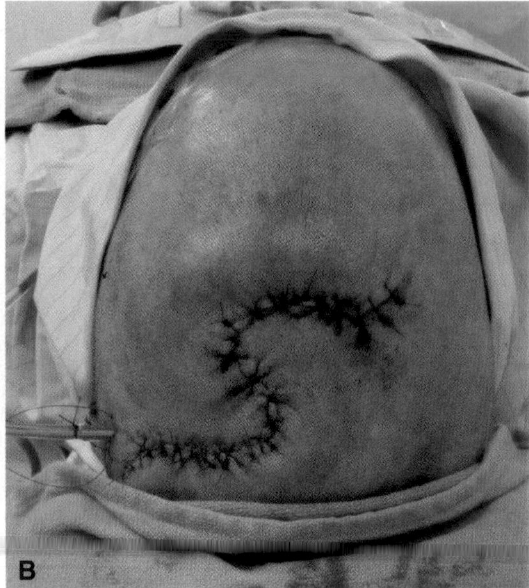

FIGURE 38.1. **A.** A 4-cm diameter defect of the vertex scalp reconstructed with bilateral rotation-advancement flaps. **B.** The flaps are advanced and the donor site is closed primarily.

or the remaining scalp tissue expanded and the skin graft excised, to improve appearance. Larger configurations of multiple flaps, such as the Orticochea flap, are well described but unpopular because of the high rate of partial flap necrosis.[2]

Unlike the scalp, additional attention is required when addressing a forehead wound so that the closure does not distort the brow or anterior hairline. This is often at odds with the direction of tissue laxity along the forehead; however, brow or hairline symmetry must never be compromised for primary closure; a local flap or graft, or even a free flap, is preferred. Because the forehead is a visible area as compared with the hair-bearing scalp, color match and incision orientation require careful planning. The aesthetic subunit principle should be followed to make the reconstruction as inconspicuous as possible.[3] Whenever possible, skin grafts should be harvested from a location above the clavicles to achieve a good color match. Incisions should be designed within the transverse forehead rhytids or along the anterior hairline or browline (Figure 38.2). For limited defect size, healing by secondary intention can have a better cosmetic outcome than skin grafting, as can be frequently seen in the treatment of donor defects for forehead flaps.[4] When operating anywhere around the forehead or brow, care should be taken to avoid injury to the temporal branch of the facial nerve. A variety of local flaps have been described for reconstruction of small forehead wounds, such as in the setting of Mohs surgery; these techniques are addressed elsewhere in this book.

Tissue expansion is useful in reconstructing scalp and forehead wounds due to trauma, burns, or congenital lesions. It is less germane in the oncologic setting when there is typically an urgent need for resection, thus eliminating the possibility of pre-expansion prior to resection and reconstruction. Additionally, a history of radiation therapy or the anticipated need for adjuvant radiation precludes the use of tissue expansion, as the associated complication rate is prohibitively high.[5] When appropriately implemented, tissue expansion is a powerful technique in scalp reconstruction, permitting reconstruction of an area up to 50% of the total surface area of the scalp with hair-bearing tissue of a similar thickness. Expanders come in a variety of shapes and sizes, allowing the surgeon to match the desired vector of expansion. Typically, the expander is placed in the subgaleal plane deep to the healthy scalp. The incision used to place the expander should be designed in the area of scalp that will be excised and should be oriented perpendicular to the axis of expansion to help prevent incisional dehiscence and exposure of the device. In large defects, multiple expanders can be placed; ports are typically remote.

Regional flaps are, in general, infrequently used in scalp reconstruction because of the limited number of donor flaps in close proximity. The temporoparietal fascial flap and temporalis muscle flap can be used for defects within or adjacent to the temporal area or lateral forehead and are usually combined with a skin graft. The trapezius muscle can be designed as either a muscle or myocutaneous flap and can be used to reconstruct the occipital scalp.

Microsurgical Techniques

Free flap reconstruction of the scalp is necessary when local options or skin grafting are inadequate. This may be because of defect size and depth, the anticipated need for radiation therapy, prior radiation therapy, or extensive scarring from past surgeries. Preoperatively, a thoughtful reconstructive plan should be devised that includes selection of an appropriate flap and options for recipient vessels.

Recipient vessels should have a similar caliber as those of the flap and should be in close proximity to the defect. For the scalp, the ST vessels are the typical first-line option.[6] Using the ST vessels is associated with a high flap success rate (96%) and compatibility with a variety of free flaps and defects.[6] The patency of these vessels should be evaluated preoperatively by gently palpating the preauricular area bilaterally to feel a pulse; alternatively, a pencil Doppler ultrasound can be used.

There are several technical points that must be understood to achieve success with the ST vessels. The ST artery and vein are located anterior to the ear and represent the distal extent of the external carotid system (Figure 38.3). Ideally, the anastomosis should be performed at the level of the tragal notch where the vessels emerge from the parotid. This portion of the artery has the greatest diameter and least tortuosity. The artery tends to be more superficial and posterior, whereas the vein may exist in a slightly deeper plane and more anterior. The vein is notoriously thin walled and prone to inadvertent twisting, so special care must be observed. Because of these anatomical nuances, many find it helpful to perform the majority of this recipient vessel dissection under the operating microscope or high-power loupe magnification.

If the ST vessels are not available or insufficient, the neck provides a multitude of options: facial, lingual, superior thyroid, etc. The pedicle length required to travel from the neck to the scalp almost always necessitates the use of a vein graft. Special care must be taken to avoid kinking or twisting the vein graft or pedicle, particularly with head turning. The vein grafts should be placed beneath a widely

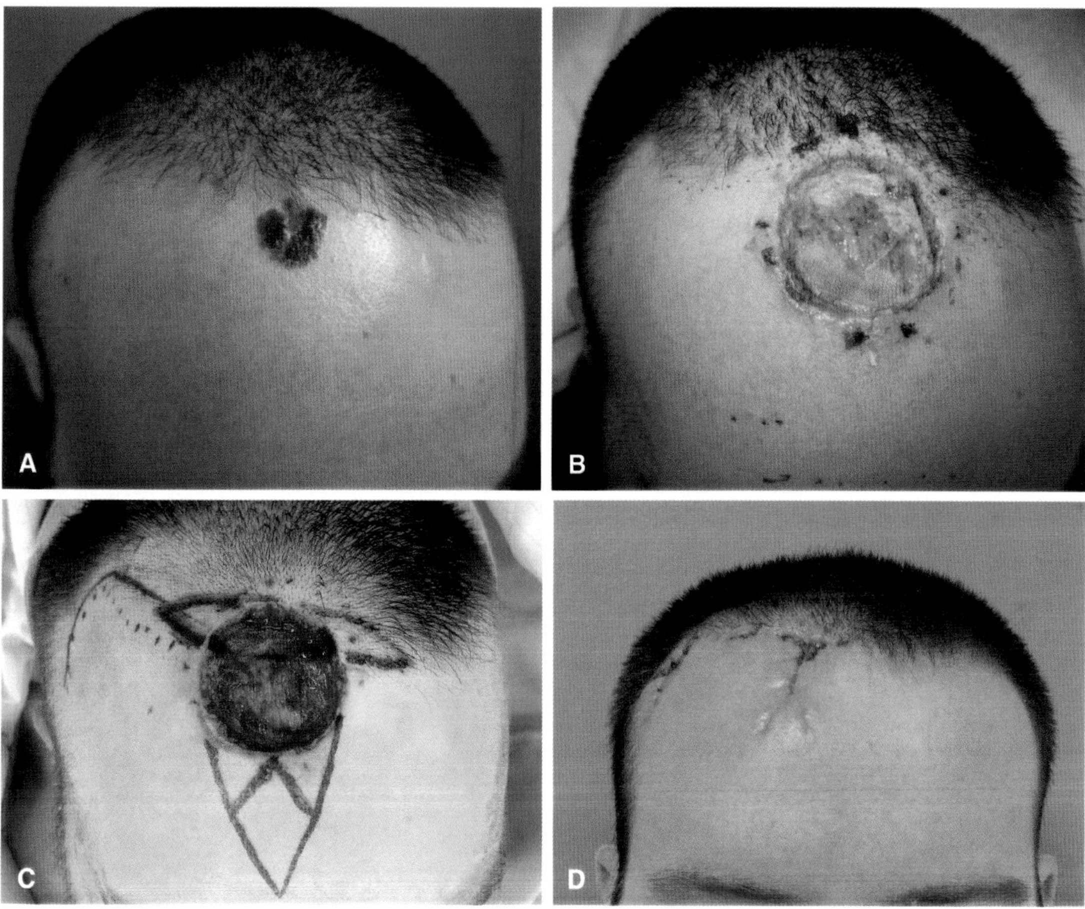

FIGURE 38.2. **A,B.** 5 cm defect after resection of forehead invasive melanoma. Delayed reconstruction performed after negative final margins. **C.** Scalp advancement flap to recreate anterior hairline, forehead rotation flap with *W-plasty* closure of dogear to limit the inferior extent of the scar. **D.** Retroauricular full-thickness skin graft used to close donor site along temporal scalp/forehead.

undermined cutaneous tunnel, and the patient should be prevented from wearing eyeglasses during the immediate postoperative period to avoid compression.

Many flaps have been described for use in microsurgical scalp reconstruction[6–8] (**Table 38.1**). The incidence of cutaneous malignancies located on the scalp is higher in elderly patients and continues to rise after age 65 years. Therefore, it is not uncommon for septua- and octogenarians (or older) to require extensive scalp resections. It is important to emphasize that age is not a contraindication to microsurgical scalp reconstruction, as has been demonstrated in several studies.[9,10] Muscle flaps covered with a skin graft as well as fasciocutaneous flaps have been repeatedly and successfully used for scalp reconstruction. Muscle flaps are bulky initially, but will atrophy over time; this effect is accelerated if postoperative radiation is given (see Figure 38.3). Once the flap atrophies, it contours nicely along the underlying skull. When insetting a muscle flap, it is prudent to inset the flap in a *vest-over-pants* fashion, with the flap tucked under the remaining scalp so that when the flap atrophies, it is less likely to pull away from the native scalp and cause exposure of the skull (see Figure 38.3). Flaps with a skin paddle are thought to be more durable and may be preferred in situations where the flap is covering a cranioplasty. The disadvantage to a skin paddle is that it may require a secondary debulking procedure to improve the contour, as these flaps are less likely to atrophy.

Reconstruction of the Calvarium

Resection of primary bone malignancies, bone metastases, osteoradionecrosis, traumatic defects, or soft tissue tumors of the scalp that involve the underlying calvarium can result in a bony defect. The goals of calvarial reconstruction are both functional and cosmetic, protecting the central nervous system as well as restoring the normal contour of the skull. Calvarial reconstruction is usually recommended for any full-thickness defect greater than 6 cm^2.[11]

Alloplastic Materials

Calvarial reconstruction is most commonly performed using alloplastic materials (**Table 38.2**). Alloplastic materials are abundant in supply and have no donor site morbidity, but may be more prone to infection than autologous bone grafts, which may preclude their use in infected or irradiated fields. The ideal alloplastic implant is compatible with surrounding bone and soft tissue, resistant to infection, strong, easily shaped, and remains stable over time. Numerous materials have been described, including titanium mesh, polymethyl methacrylate, porous polyethylene, calcium phosphate cement, and polyetheretherketone (PEEK)[12–14] (**Figure 38.4**). Many biomaterials can be produced using computer-aided design/computer-aided modeling (CAD/CAM) techniques to exactly match the dimensions of the existing or anticipated cranial defect. CAD/CAM technology is available for titanium, porous polyethylene, and PEEK implants.[14,15] Lee and colleagues evaluated their extensive experience in oncologic calvarial reconstructions and identified prior surgery, infection, radiation, and concurrent free tissue transfer to be associated with complications.[12] The type of alloplastic material used was not found to be an independent risk factor for complications on multivariate analysis.

Autologous Techniques

Autologous reconstruction of the calvarium involves the use of either vascularized or nonvascularized bone. Several options have been described, including split calvarial or iliac grafts, vascularized or nonvascularized rib, and vascularized fibula.[16–18]

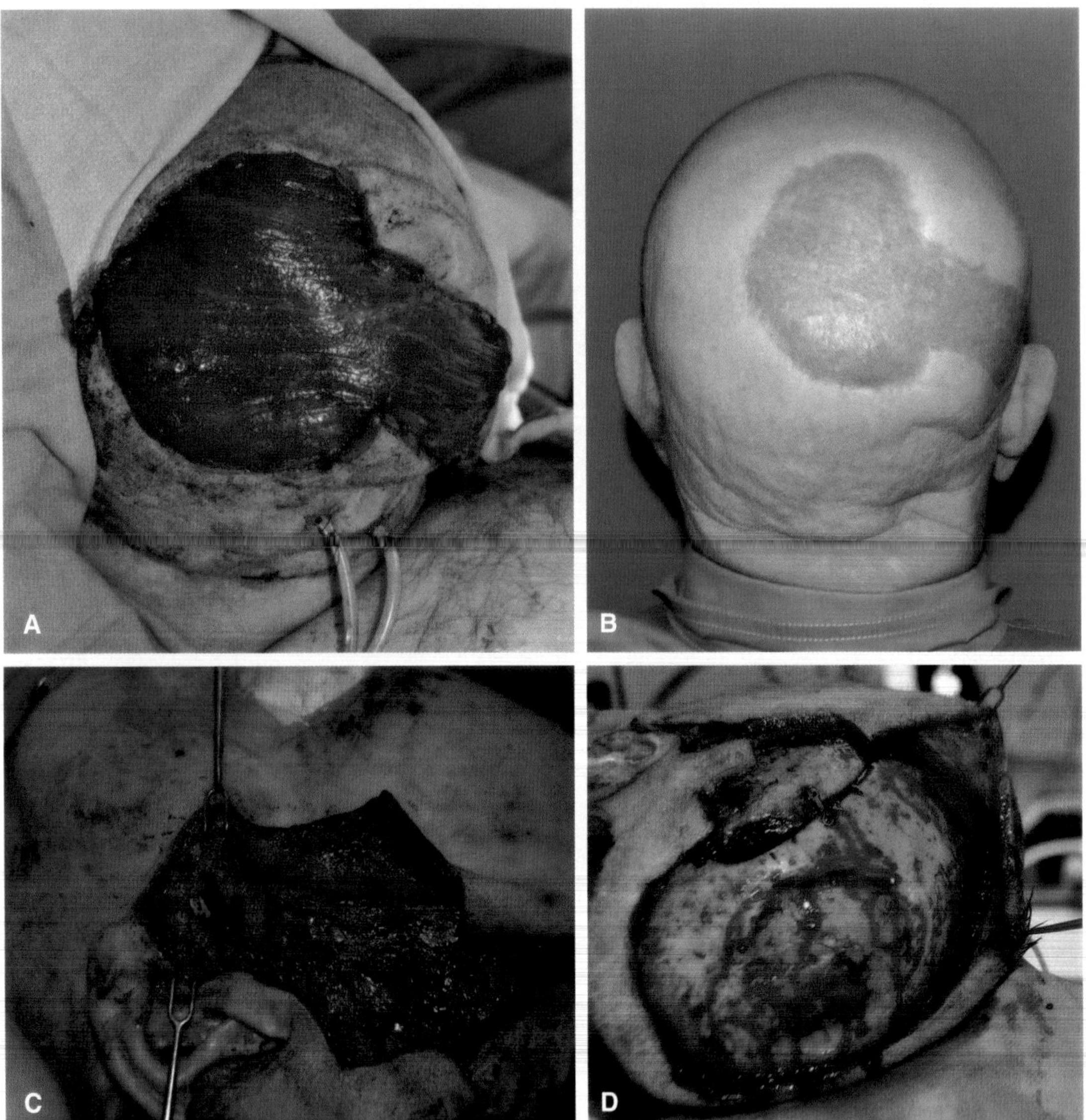

FIGURE 38.3. **A.** Large scalp defect reconstructed with free latissimus dorsi muscle flap and split-thickness skin graft. Microvascular anastomoses were performed to the superficial temporal artery and vein. **B.** Note the significant atrophy of the bulky muscle flap and its improved contour after radiation therapy 10 months after surgery. **C.** The superficial temporal artery and vein are commonly used as recipient vessels in microvascular reconstruction of the scalp. The anastomosis should be performed at the level of the tragal notch, where the vessels emerge from within the parotid gland. **D.** When insetting a free muscle flap for scalp reconstruction, the native scalp should be undermined circumferentially so that the flap can be inset in a vest-over-pants fashion.

Split calvarial grafts should be harvested from the parietal bone where the skull is the thickest. The graft site should not extend any further medially than 1.5 cm lateral to midline, to avoid inadvertent injury to the sagittal sinus. Calvarial bone can be harvested using an in situ technique or an extracranial approach. In the in situ technique, a trough is burred around the outline of the graft until the diploic space is reached. A saw or osteotome is then used to remove the outer table of the skull as a graft. The advantage of this technique is that it avoids accessing the intracranial space. Disadvantages include the creation of a depression contour deformity along the skull; additionally, the size of the graft is limited. In the extracranial approach, a craniotomy is performed and a full-thickness section of the calvarium is removed. On the back table, a saw or osteotome is then used to separate the inner and outer tables through the diploic space. The inner table is then plated back onto the donor site, flush with the adjacent calvarium, to avoid a contour depression. The external table is then used as a graft. Because of the need for a craniotomy, the extracranial technique is usually performed by a neurosurgeon.

Compared with calvarial bone grafts, larger defects can be repaired using rib. The seventh and eighth ribs are most commonly used; in men, rib graft is harvested through an incision directly over the rib, whereas in women, an inframammary fold incision is better camouflaged. No more than two or three ribs can be harvested, to maintain chest wall stability. Ribs are harvested in a subperiosteal plane to avoid pleural injury. Grafts can be shaped with a rib bender and plated to the calvarium. Gaps between the rib grafts can be filled with either particulate cadaveric allograft bone, calcium phosphate bone cement, or hydroxyapatite putty.

Vascularized bone flaps are useful for smaller calvarial defects within a hostile wound bed. Wounds exposed to radiation or chronic infection are particularly good candidates. A serratus anterior or chimeric latissimus-serratus anterior flap can be designed with vascularized rib and covered with a skin graft, thereby reconstructing an osseous and soft tissue defect with a single flap.[19] A chimeric scapular/parascapular flap has also been described for this purpose, but with using a segment of scapula bone for calvarial defect.[20] The ever-versatile free fibula flap has also been described for calvarial reconstruction—specifically for replacing the anterior table of the frontal sinus in the setting of a chronic mucocele.[18]

TABLE 38.1. COMMON FLAPS USED FOR MICROSURGICAL SCALP RECONSTRUCTION

Flap	Type	Size	Pedicle	Notes
Latissimus dorsi	Muscle or myocutaneous	25 × 35 cm	Thoracodorsal	■ Can be combined with the serratus muscle to make a chimeric flap able to resurface a larger area ■ Insertion area of the muscle overlying the pedicle should be transected obliquely to allow for a better, less bulky contour
Serratus anterior	Muscle	10 × 15 cm	Thoracodorsal or lateral thoracic	■ Only inferior 3 or 4 slips are harvested to prevent winging of the scapula ■ Pedicle is on anterior surface of the muscle; care must be taken during exposure
Rectus abdominis	Muscle or myocutaneous	25 × 6 cm	Deep inferior epigastric	
Deep inferior epigastric perforator	Fasciocutaneous perforator	40 × 15 cm	Deep inferior epigastric	■ Large surface area ■ Bulky flap limited by patient's habitus ■ Potentially long pedicle
Vastus lateralis	Muscle	20 × 10 cm	Descending branch of lateral femoral circumflex	■ Small muscle flap with limited donor site morbidity ■ May be useful when use of a fasciocutaneous ALT flap is precluded by habitus
Anterolateral thigh (ALT)	Fasciocutaneous or myocutaneous	20 × 9 cm	Descending branch of lateral femoral circumflex	
Radial forearm	Fasciocutaneous	15 × 8 cm	Radial artery	■ Small thin flap for modest defects ■ Long pedicle ■ Similar thickness as native scalp
Omentum	Visceral adipose tissue	25 × 35 cm	Gastroepiploic	■ Potential for significant donor site morbidity ■ Can be harvested robotically or laparoscopically ■ Usually atrophies significantly over time ■ Variable skin graft take

Management of the Infected Cranioplasty

Because of their robust vascularity, infection is fortunately uncommon in the scalp and calvarium. Infection of alloplastic cranioplasties and cranial *bone flaps* following craniotomy can be clinically challenging and place the patient at risk for meningitis or brain abscess. If there are signs of infection, the patient should first be treated with empiric, broad-spectrum intravenous antibiotics. If there is no significant clinical improvement, the patient may need to have the cranioplasty or bone flap explanted. This is a serious complication because a redo cranioplasty cannot be performed until the infection has fully cleared. During this period of time, the scalp will shrink in size and conform to the concave contour of the bony defect. Furthermore, if

TABLE 38.2. ALLOPLASTIC MATERIALS USED FOR CALVARIAL RECONSTRUCTION

Material	Structure	Structural Integrity	Infection Risk	Intraoperative Contouring	CAD/CAM	Advantages	Disadvantages
Titanium mesh	Metal alloy	Strong	Low	Yes	Yes	Readily available	Imaging artifact
Polymethyl methacrylate	Acrylic-based resin	Moderate; can be brittle	Moderate; becomes encapsulated	Yes	No	■ Easily moldable intraoperatively ■ Can be combined with titanium plate for increased strength	■ Cures by exothermic reaction that can damage surrounding tissue ■ Infection risk
Porous polyethylene	Porous hydrocarbon	Strong	Low; pores encourage tissue ingrowth	Yes	Yes	■ Pores mitigate infection risk	■ Pores make removal difficult
Calcium phosphate	Bone cement putty	Weak	High late infection risk	Yes; moldable	No	■ Best for small defects ■ Osteoconductive	■ Brittle ■ Use limited to smaller defects
Polyetheretherketone	Aromatic polymer	Strong	Moderate-becomes encapsulated	Minimal; edges can be burred	Yes	■ Radiolucent	■ Becomes encapsulated ■ Little ability to adjust intraoperatively

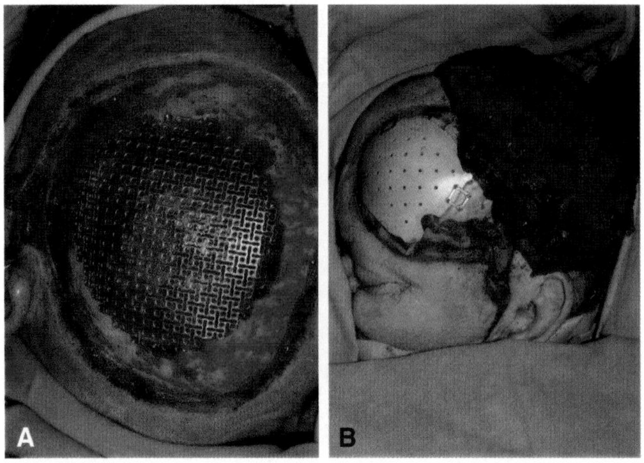

FIGURE 38.4. **A.** Titanium mesh calvarial reconstruction. **B.** Polyetheretherketone cranioplasty.

treatment of the infected cranioplasty requires debridement of devitalized scalp, there may be a significant soft tissue deficiency.

If after removal of the cranioplasty and debridement, the scalp cannot be closed primarily, the patient will require a soft tissue flap. In this situation, a well-vascularized free myocutaneous flap or muscle flap with skin graft is preferable. It is important for the patient to understand that he or she will have no skull in this area and will be vulnerable to intracranial injury during this period of time. Free flaps are purposefully made redundant for later placement of a convex cranioplasty. After the infection has been adequately treated, an elective cranioplasty can be performed by elevating the free flap and scalp off of the dura with the help of a neurosurgeon.

The Role of Composite Tissue Allograft Transplantation in Reconstruction of the Scalp and Calvarium

A recent addition to the reconstructive ladder in the treatment of scalp and calvarial wounds is vascularized composite allograft (VCA) transplantation.[21,22] Although not commonly employed, situations do exist in which VCA is a reasonable reconstructive option. One such scenario includes transplant patients with large, invasive, and diffuse malignancies of the scalp. These are more common than one may think, as invasive skin cancers of the head and neck occur frequently in the transplant population. For these patients, a transplant that includes scalp and calvarium can be based on ST vessels without the addition of alloplastic materials or donor site defects. A recent case involved a patient who was a previous recipient of a kidney-pancreas transplant, who was in need of a second transplant (**Figure 38.5**). As a result of his longstanding immunosuppression, he developed a leiomyosarcoma of the scalp, treated with excision and radiation therapy. He then developed an unstable scalp wound with underlying osteoradionecrosis of the skull; this chronic wound precluded him from being included on the transplant list for a repeat kidney-pancreas transplant. A single organ donor was acquired for simultaneous transplantation of the kidney, pancreas, skull, and scalp, thereby addressing all needs in one operation. VCA is an

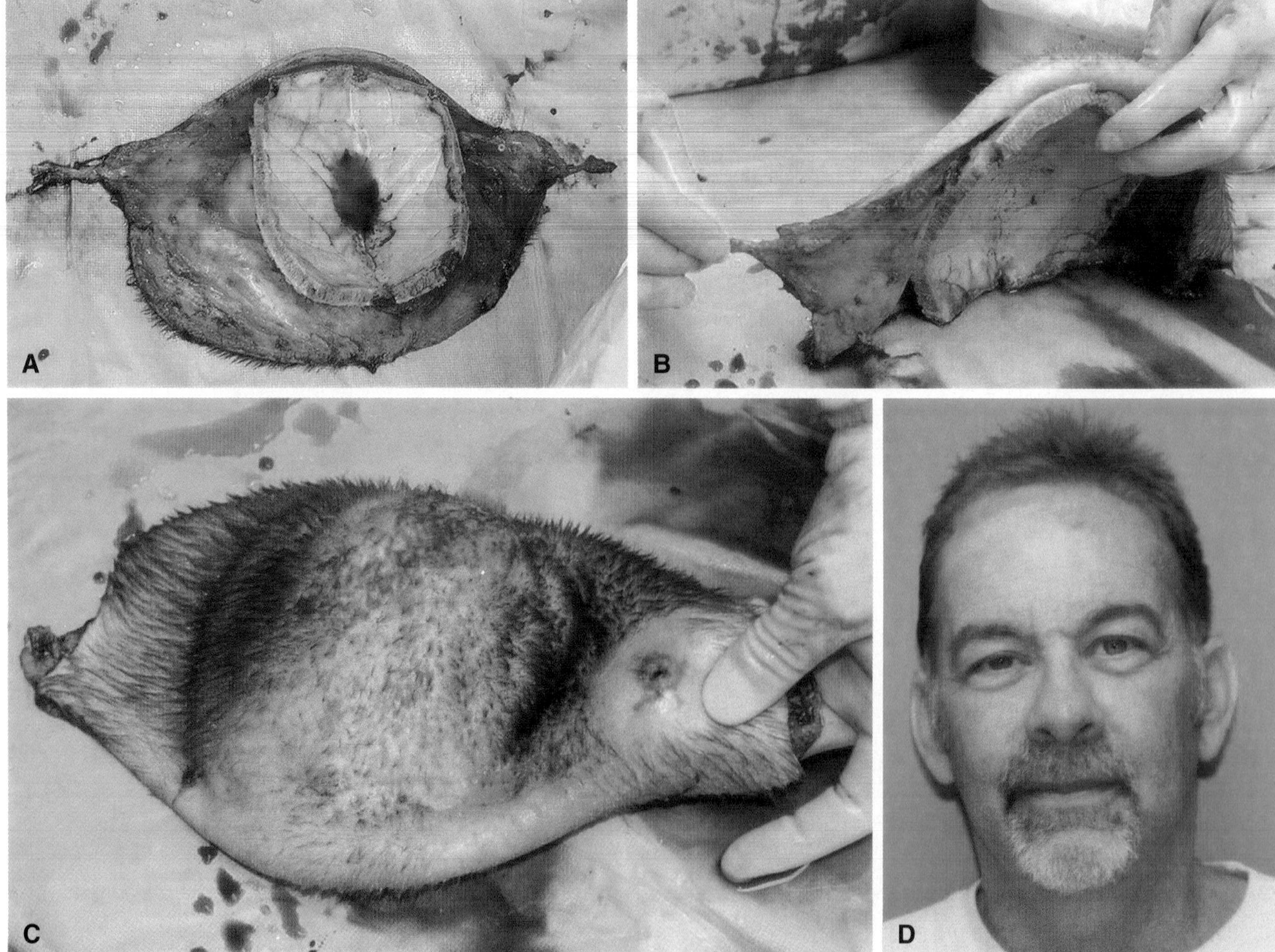

FIGURE 38.5. **A–C.** Vascular composite allograft transplant including scalp and skull. Donor specimen was harvested en block and supplied by the bilateral superficial temporal vessels. **D.** One-year postoperative result.

emerging field and can be a useful solution to complex problems in select transplant patients with extensive, composite head and neck defects.

SKULL BASE RECONSTRUCTION

Except for lesions removed via an endoscopic approach, reconstruction may play a major role in the treatment of skull base tumors because of the substantial anatomic and functional deficits that can result following resection of various craniofacial structures. Although historically, skull base resections have been associated with poor outcomes, advances in reconstruction, which minimize complications, loss of function, and disfigurement, concomitant with advances in oncologic treatment, have substantially decreased the morbidity resulting from the treatment of these tumors.

Anatomy

The Irish classification system, based on the relationship of the tumor to the anterior, middle, and posterior cranial fossae, is most useful for describing the clinical anatomy of the resection and associated reconstructive options[23] (Figure 38.6). These resections involve removal of skull base bone with or without the removal of the underlying dura.

Region I involves the anterior skull base; these tumors typically arise from in and around the orbits, nose, sinuses, or cribriform plate. Region II involves the lateral skull base; these tumors arise from the infratemporal or pterygopalatine fossae extending to the middle cranial fossa and can include nasopharyngeal carcinoma, juvenile nasopharyngeal angiofibroma, and locally advanced parotid tumors. Region III involves the temporal bone and posterior cranial fossa; these tumors typically arise from the ear, parotid, or temporal bone.

Reconstructive Approach

Cranial nerve deficits should be anticipated based on the location of the tumor and discussed with the patient preoperatively. Possible functional deficits after skull base surgery may include facial nerve paralysis, dysphagia, and dysarthria due to hypoglossal nerve palsy, and/or shoulder asymmetry due to transection of the spinal accessory nerve. If the facial nerve is removed with a portion of the tumor, then consideration should be given to the reconstruction of the nerve gap with an interposition cable graft. Static and dynamic procedures for facial nerve paralysis should be considered. A detailed discussion of treatment for facial nerve paralysis is addressed elsewhere in this book.

Given the paucity of local flap options in this anatomic area, free tissue transfer is frequently required for reconstruction. If the ST vessels are no longer present because of previous use, radiation-related changes, or resection, then the neck provides a multitude of recipient options. Unfortunately, the pedicle length required to reach the neck from the skull base may necessitate vein grafts; this should be recognized preoperatively and incorporated into the reconstructive plan prospectively.

The need or desire for an orbital or auricular prosthesis should be discussed preoperatively because this may influence flap design and reconstructive staging. Facial prostheses are created by an anaplastologist and can be secured with adhesive or through the use of osseointegrated anchors. Additionally, if the skull base resection includes removal of the middle ear components, an otologist should be involved preoperatively for placement of a bone-anchored hearing aid (BAHA). Osseointegrated implants and BAHAs have a higher failure rate when placed into irradiated bone; therefore, if radiation is anticipated, consideration should be given to immediate placement of the device.

Because use of either a regional or free flap may limit the utility of physical examination to detect local recurrence, serial imaging is mandatory for disease surveillance and should be incorporated into the survivorship plan.

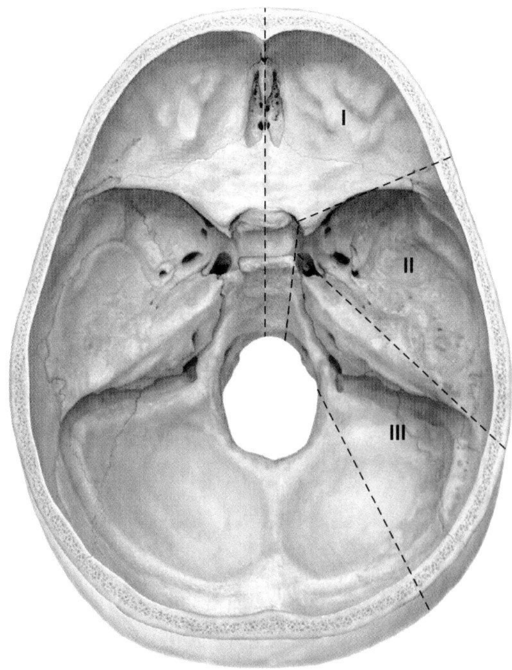

FIGURE 38.6. Skull base regions. (Adapted from Irish JC, Gullane PJ, Gentili F, et al. Tumors of the skull base: outcome and survival analysis of 77 cases. *Head Neck*. 1994;16(1):3-10. Copyright © 1994 Wiley Periodicals, Inc., A Wiley Company. Reprinted by permission of John Wiley & Sons, Inc.)

Region I

Midline region I tumors are usually resected with an anterior craniofacial approach, resulting in communication of the nasal cavity with the intracranial space. If the defect is small and limited to the upper nasal cavity, the intracranial space can be separated from the sinuses with a pedicled pericranial flap or galea frontalis flap, both of which derive their blood supply from the supratrochlear and supraorbital vessels. In situations where these blood vessels have already been transected, or in larger defects involving the external nose, forehead, and/or orbit, a free flap may be necessary (Figure 38.7). If there is no skin defect and the flap is only needed to separate the intracranial space, then the free flap may be buried and monitored with an implantable Doppler probe. The rectus abdominis, vastus lateralis, and serratus anterior muscle flaps are good options in this situation.

Lateral region I defects frequently involve orbital exenteration. If the resection spares the medial and inferior walls of the orbit, it is well suited for the eventual use of a prosthesis. To accommodate a prosthesis, the orbit must be resurfaced with a thin, pliable, well-vascularized tissue that will maintain the concave shape of the cavity. This can be achieved with a free radial forearm flap or pedicled temporalis muscle or temporoparietal fascia flap with a skin graft. If the orbital exenteration results in communication with the sinuses or nasal cavity, then a bulkier myocutaneous free flap is preferred. The anterolateral thigh (ALT) and rectus abdominis myocutaneous (RAM) flaps are highly customizable and allow for the design of flap with a variable amount of muscle, tailored to the defect's requirements. The muscle conforms to the complex geometry of the defect, sealing exposed dura and/or sinonasal cavities. This feature helps to minimize the occurrence of a sinocutaneous fistula; such fistulae are exceedingly difficult to heal owing to persistent pressure from nasal airway.

Region II

Resection of region II tumors, frequently, is performed through an anterior transmaxillary approach. After resection of the middle cranial fossa, the dura will be in direct communication with the nasopharynx; if the resection also necessitates a maxillectomy, then the oral cavity and oropharynx will be in direct communication with the intracranial space as well (Figure 38.8). The temporalis muscle may reach this area

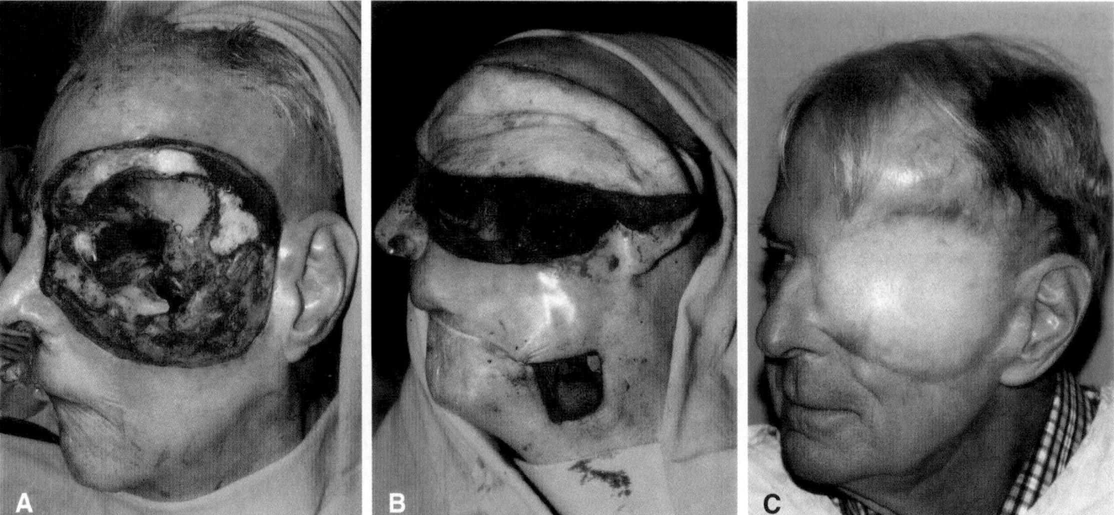

FIGURE 38.7. **A.** Zone I skull base defect following a left extended orbital exenteration resulting in communication with the anterior cranial fossa. **B.** Reconstruction with an anterolateral thigh myocutaneous free flap. The muscle (vastus lateralis) is placed against the dural patch to help prevent cerebrospinal fluid leaks and is also used to obliterate possible communication with the nasal cavity and paranasal sinuses. **C.** Postoperative result.

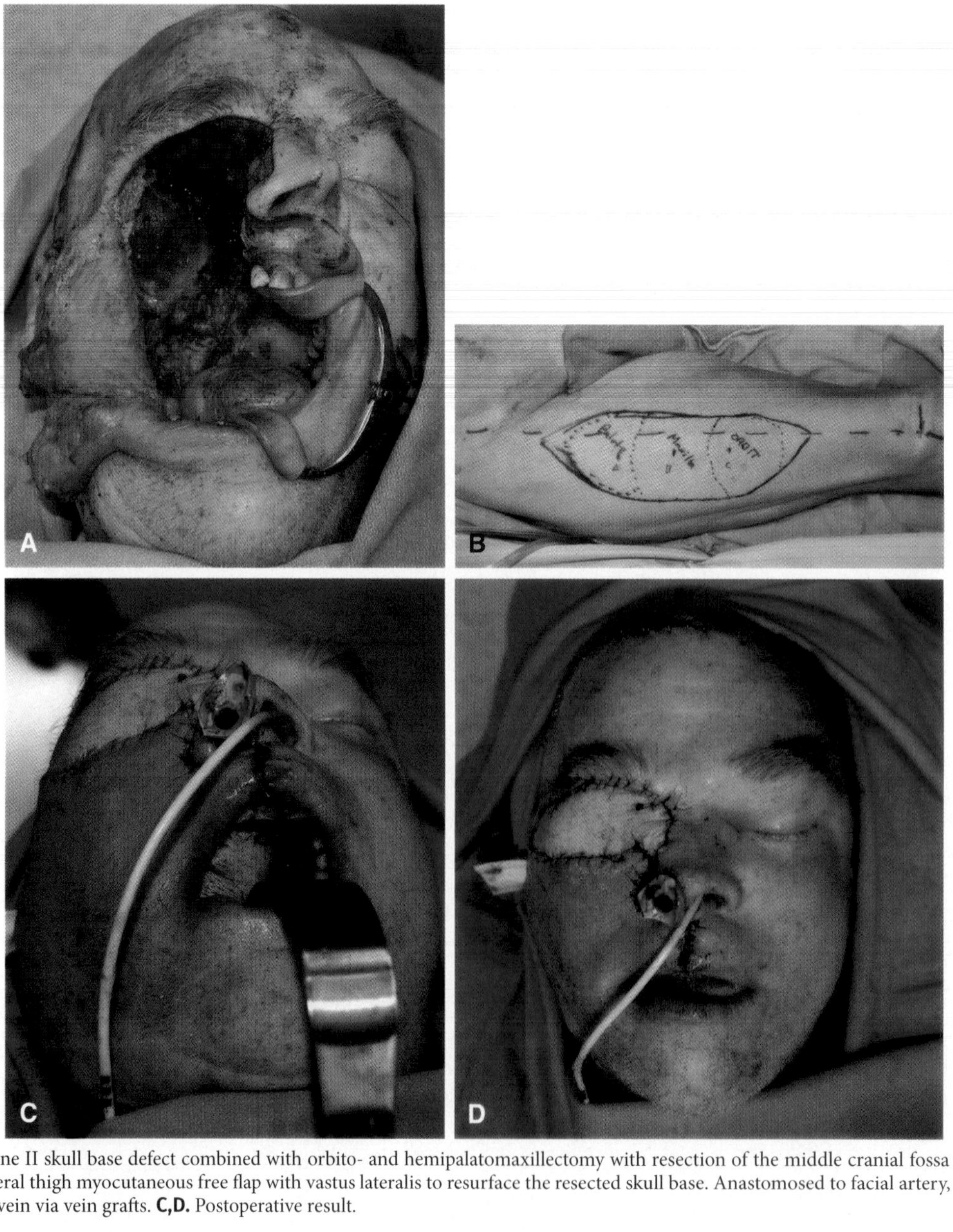

FIGURE 38.8. **A.** Zone II skull base defect combined with orbito- and hemipalatomaxillectomy with resection of the middle cranial fossa skull base. **B.** Multi-paddle free anterolateral thigh myocutaneous free flap with vastus lateralis to resurface the resected skull base. Anastomosed to facial artery, common facial vein, and external jugular vein via vein grafts. **C,D.** Postoperative result.

but often does not provide adequate bulk, especially after radiation-related atrophy occurs. In such cases, a bulky myocutaneous flap, such as the ALT or RAM free flaps, has great utility. When there is no oral mucosal, palatal, or external cheek defect, the skin paddle of the free flap can be de-epithelialized and the entire flap buried. The adipodermal component of the flap provides bulk, which is less prone to radiation atrophy than muscle; the muscle component serves as an adequate seal against exposed dura mater. Persistent bulk and volume maintenance is important in these reconstructions to not only maintain facial contour but also to adequately support the skull base so as to prevent herniation of the intracranial contents into the pharynx or oral cavity.

As in reconstruction of the maxillectomy defect, if the orbital floor is resected and the globe is spared, then skeletal reconstruction of the orbital floor is mandatory. Failing to reconstruct the orbital floor or performing an inaccurate reconstruction can result in enophthalmos, vertical dystopia, or diplopia. Various alloplastic materials are commercially available; alternatively, an autologous calvarial or iliac crest bone graft can be used. Although autologous grafts can be revascularized, our own experience does not support the use of one material over another.[24] However, evidence does strongly emphasize the importance of covering the entire implant or graft with well-vascularized tissue if adjuvant radiation is anticipated. If the globe is removed as well as the bony orbit, as in the case of an orbitomaxillectomy, then reconstruction of the floor is not necessary nor is maintaining a concave orbital cavity. In these situations, the reconstructive priority is filling the volume of the resected orbit and maxilla with vascularized tissue, sealing the exposed dura, and replacing any missing skin (see Figure 38.8).

Region III

Region III defects will often include parotidectomy or a lateral temporal bone resection in addition to removal of a portion of the posterior cranial fossa. Larger, bulky flaps, such as the ALT or RAM, are frequently required; if an oral cavity defect is anticipated, then two skin paddles may be needed. If a lateral temporal bone resection and/or mastoidectomy is performed, well-vascularized muscle is helpful to obliterate the middle ear and seal off any exposed dura and/or exposed mastoid air cells[25,26] (Figure 38.9). If resection of the middle ear is anticipated, upfront BAHA placement should be considered. If the external ear is resected, reconstruction is best addressed separately in a delayed manner. Prosthetic rehabilitation is the mainstay for oncologic auricular reconstruction; these prostheses can be secured with an adhesive or through the use of osseointegrated implants, provided adequate bone stock remains available to stabilize the implants.

Postoperative Care and Management of Complications

The principal goal of reconstruction of the resected skull base is to separate the aerodigestive tract from the brain and intracranial contents. Consequently, meticulous isolation of the dura and brain by well-vascularized soft tissue flaps is necessary to prevent meningitis, cerebritis, brain abscesses, neurologic injury, and death. Postoperatively, the patient should be maintained on prophylactic intravenous antibiotics with empiric coverage of normal sinonasal flora. If the dura has been resected, consideration should be given for antibiotics that can penetrate the blood-brain barrier. In addition to flap monitoring, frequent neurologic examinations should be conducted. Postoperative computed tomography (CT) or magnetic resonance imaging scans are obtained according to the recommendations of a neurosurgeon. Although it is not uncommon to see intracranial air on imaging in the early postoperative period, increasing pneumocephalus or any change in the clinical neurologic examination should trigger a prompt return to the operating room. Such findings could suggest a number of complications, including infection, flap dehiscence, hematoma, or intracranial bleed. Any concern for a CSF leak should be evaluated and confirmed with a beta-2 transferrin test. Most minor CSF leaks can be effectively treated conservatively with antibiotic prophylaxis and bed rest. Lumbar drains, externalized ventricular drains, or dural repair are more invasive options for recalcitrant leaks. If a portion of the orbit has been reconstructed, visual acuity and extraocular muscle function should be frequently examined postoperatively. Any concern for decreased visual acuity should prompt an ophthalmologic examination and imaging. Impingement of the optic nerve or entrapment of an extraocular muscle by the reconstruction usually requires a return to the operating room.

RECONSTRUCTION AFTER MAXILLECTOMY

Management of the maxillectomy defect is a particularly complicated and controversial field within head and neck oncologic reconstruction. Options include the use of prosthetic obturators, soft tissue free flaps, osseous free flaps, alloplastic implants, and autologous grafts. Reconstructive algorithms can be complex and must take into account a variety of considerations. Multiple approaches have been described and differ based on the prioritization of defect characteristics and reconstructive techniques.[27–31]

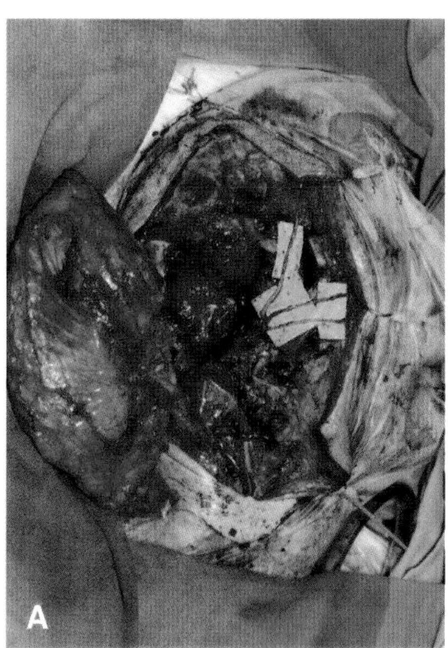

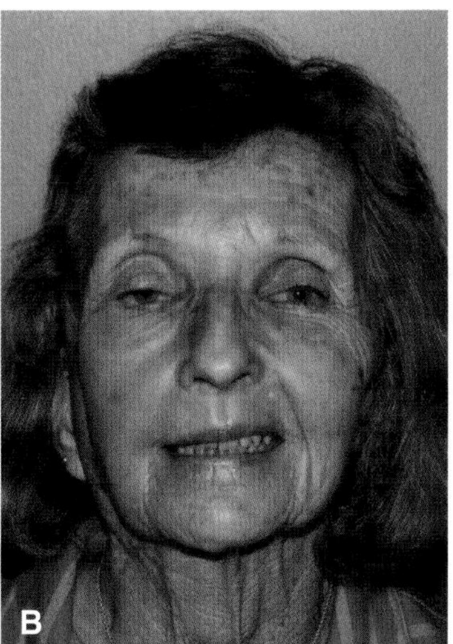

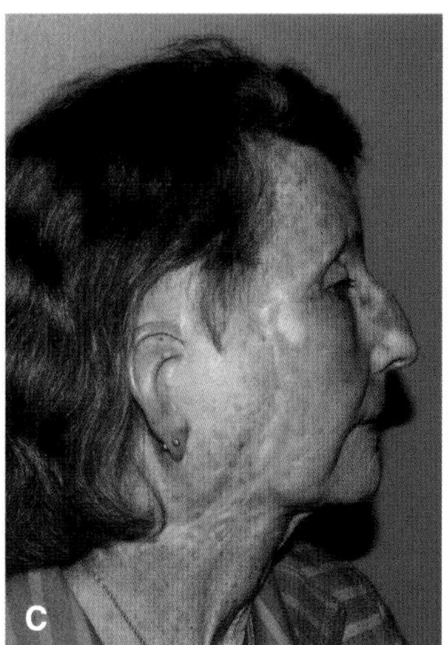

FIGURE 38.9. **A.** Zone III skull base defect following a right lateral temporal bone resection including division of the facial nerve. The defect is reconstructed with an anterolateral thigh myocutaneous free flap, with muscle placed into the deepest portion of the defect and obliterates the Eustachian tube orifice. Several cable nerve grafts were performed in conjunction with static facial reanimation to restore facial nerve function. **B,C.** Postoperative result. Note return of motor nerve function following cable nerve grafting, approximately 12 months after the reconstruction.

One of the fundamental problems with reconstructing the midface is that the defects created by oncologic resection are highly variable. Such defects usually involve not only the maxillary bones but may also include a number of adjacent facial and cranial bones, as well as soft tissues of the face, palate, and orbit. Several classification systems have been introduced and can be helpful in guiding reconstruction.[27-29]

Anatomy and Nomenclature

The maxilla contributes to forming the boundaries for three cavities: the roof of the mouth, the floor and lateral nasal walls, and the floor and medial orbital walls. Each maxilla articulates with the zygomatic, frontal, ethmoid, nasal, lacrimal, palatine, and vomer bones. Many maxillary tumors extend into or arise from the orbit. Therefore, a maxillectomy may be combined with an orbital floor resection or an orbital exenteration. The orbital roof consists of the frontal bone and separates the intracranial contents from the orbit; the floor is made up of the maxilla, palatine, and zygomatic bones; the medial wall consists of the frontal, lacrimal, and ethmoid bones; the lateral wall includes the zygomatic and sphenoid bones.

Spiro and colleagues categorized maxillectomies according to the number of walls resected, dividing them into *limited*, *subtotal*, and *total* subtypes.[30] Unfortunately, this algorithm is relatively simplistic and does not help to guide the reconstruction. Although several other classification systems have been described, we prefer a classification system that provides for an anatomic description of the defect[27-29] (**Table 38.3**). Orbital exenteration, which includes removal of the globe as well as the other orbital contents in contrast to enucleation which refers to globe removal only, may be included with the maxillary resection.

Medial maxillectomy involves resection of the medial wall of the maxilla and inferior turbinate. This surgery is usually indicated for tumors arising from the lateral nasal wall or lacrimal system. This resection may be performed through a lateral rhinotomy incision or, more recently, endoscopically. Reconstruction is only necessary if the skin of the medial canthal area or lateral nasal sidewall has been removed with the maxilla (**Figure 38.10**). In this situation, a paramedian forehead flap or radial forearm free flap can be used to resurface the medial canthus skin; a portion of the flap can be de-epithelialized and buried deep to the lateral rhinotomy incision to prevent fistula formation.

Suprastructure maxillectomies involve the orbital floor but do not involve the palate. In these cases, the orbital floor is reconstructed with an alloplast such as titanium mesh or bone graft from the calvarium or ilium. The nonvascularized orbital floor reconstruction and cheek are supported by a bulky soft tissue free flap with a de-epithelialized skin paddle, such as the ALT or RAM free flaps, or a pedicled temporalis muscle flap if the reach and volume appear to be adequate for the defect. If facial skin is also

TABLE 38.3. MAXILLECTOMY CLASSIFICATION SYSTEMS AND RECONSTRUCTIVE TECHNIQUES

Hanasono	Cordeiro	Brown	Resection Description	Resection Depiction	Reconstruction
Suprastructure	I	I	Any part of maxilla not including the palate or alveolus		No treatment versus soft tissue flap if skin resected (ALT/RAM/RFF)
Premaxillary	–	–	Central alveolus between canines ± primary palate		Obturator versus osteocutaneous flap (RFOC/FOC)
Unilateral posterior Palatomaxillectomy	IIa	IIb	Alveolus distad to canine, palate, and one or more walls of the maxilla		Obturator versus ALT/RAM/RFF
Unilateral hemipalatomaxillectomy	IIa	IIb	Entire hemipalate and maxilla		ALT/RAM versus FOC
Bilateral palatomaxillectomy	IIb	IId	Bilateral palate and maxilla		FOC
Maxillectomy with orbital floor resection	IIIa	IIIb	Any maxillectomy + orbital floor resection		Choice of flap based on maxillectomy defect; orbital floor reconstructed with alloplastic implant versus autologous bone graft (iliac crest versus split calvarial)
Orbitomaxillectomy	IV	V	Any maxillectomy + orbital exenteration		ALT/RAM versus ALT/RAM + FOC versus chimeric scapula osteomyocutaneous flap

ALT, anterolateral thigh; RAM, rectus abdominis myocutaneous.

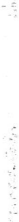

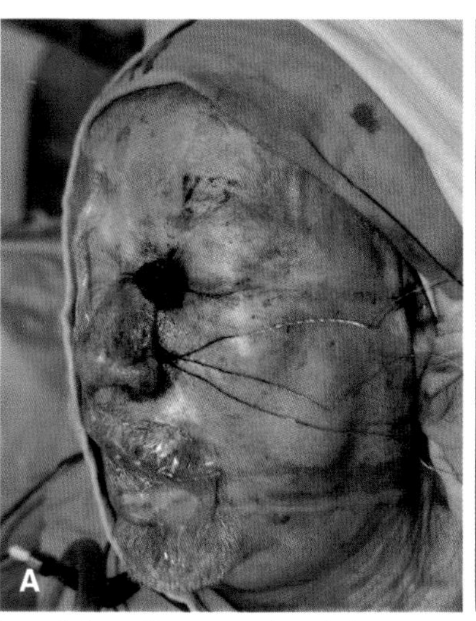

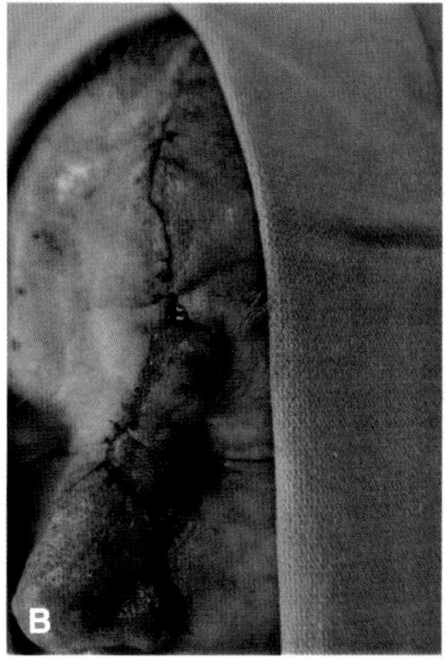

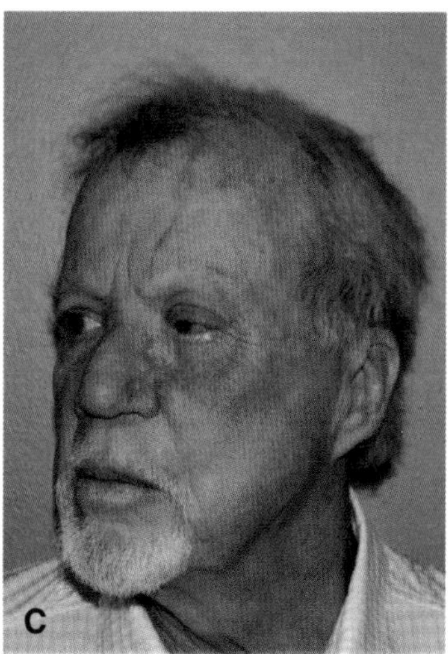

FIGURE 38.10. Medial maxillectomy via lateral rhinotomy incision. **A.** Defect involves resection of skin overlying the medial canthus and superior lateral nasal sidewall as well as medial maxillary wall. **B.** Reconstructed with paramedical forehead flap; distal aspect of flap de-epithelialized and buried to reinforce the inferior aspect of the incision. **C.** Postoperative result after pedicle transection and radiation therapy.

resected, cheek reconstruction becomes necessary and is usually best accomplished using a myocutaneous free flap, such as the ALT or RAM.

For maxillectomies that involve removal of some or all of the palate, the amount of hard and soft palate resected, as well as the plan for dental restoration, will dictate whether a prosthetic obturator is indicated or if a flap should be performed. Okay and colleagues provide a set of guidelines based on what defects are compatible with a prosthetic obturator.[32] In general, palatoalveolar defects that spare both canine teeth can be successfully treated with an obturator (Table 38.3). In these cases, cantilever forces resulting in unstable prosthetic retention are minimized because of the favorable root morphology of the canine adjacent to the obturator and the generous arch length provided by the remaining alveolus. Obturators are inappropriate for maxillectomy defects that include a concurrent resection of the skull base, orbital floor, orbital contents, or facial skin, regardless of the remaining dentition and alveolar arch. Additionally, some patients may not like certain features of an obturator, such as the fact that it must be removed and cleaned regularly and periodically adjusted or replaced for fit, wear and tear, and/or fungal colonization.

When an obturator cannot be used either because of defect geometry or patient preference, a soft tissue free flap can be used to replace the missing palate and support the soft tissues of the face for palatoalveolar defects posterior to the canine tooth. The ALT or RAM free flaps are well suited for this indication. In obese patients, the radial forearm fasciocutaneous flap can be used. In any palatal defect reconstructed with a flap, meticulous surgical technique must be practiced when insetting the flap to the remaining palate. We recommend resecting additional palatal mucosa so that the flap-palate seam is positioned over bone, thus minimizing the chance of an oronasal fistula should an incisional dehiscence occur.

When reconstructing any variety of midface defect with a free flap, achieving adequate pedicle length can be challenging. In general, either the ST vessels or any branch from the external carotid artery in the neck will serve as an adequate recipient. The vein corresponding to the selected recipient artery, or an end-to-side anastomosis to the internal jugular vein, will suffice for drainage. If a neck recipient is used, the pedicle will need to be tunneled from the midface, where the flap is inset, into the neck. This is typically done through a subcutaneous tunnel within the cheek and over the mandible into the neck. This should prevent injury to the distal branches of the facial nerve; care should be taken to avoid Stensen duct when creating the tunnel. When designing the flap, every effort should be made to design the skin paddle as distal as possible from the pedicle to maximize length. If the pedicle cannot reach the chosen recipient, then an interposition vein graft should be used to lengthen the pedicle.

It is difficult to use an obturator when the palatal-alveolar defect extends mesial to the ipsilateral canine tooth. In this geometry, there are greater cantilever forces acting on the prosthesis, which must also rely on less dentition for retention. There are a variety of flap options for reconstruction following hemipalatomaxillectomy, which results in a defect that extends to the midline. Soft tissue free flaps, such as the ALT or RAM, will provide adequate bulk to obliterate the maxillary sinus, support the cheek, and provide skin for reconstruction of the palatal defect (Figure 38.11). Unfortunately, they do not provide a rigid skeletal framework. Over time, this may contribute to loss of anterior maxillary projection on the side of the flap. Although surgery is usually more technically challenging, osteocutaneous free flaps can provide skeletal support and also facilitate dental rehabilitation via osseointegrated implants; we prefer this reconstructive technique for hemipalatomaxillectomy defects in highly functional, compliant patients with good oncologic prognosis (Figure 38.12). One caveat is that we have found that placement of osseointegrated implants in an irradiated bone flap is prohibitively dangerous, associated with a high rate of infection, osteoradionecrosis, and loss of the reconstruction. Therefore, if an osteocutaneous free flap is used for reconstruction and the patient receives postoperative radiation therapy, then one of the main purposes for using a bony reconstruction is obviated. In such cases, temporary placement of an obturator or soft tissue flap followed by delayed conversion to an osseous flap after radiation therapy is an option.

Premaxillary defects usually arise from resection of lip or nasal pathologies. Most defects are relatively small and amenable to obturation alone. However, if the patient does not prefer an obturator, reconstruction must be performed to support the upper lip and nasal tip, replace the nasal floor and primary hard palate, and serve as a site for future dental implantation. Although the bony defect is relatively small, it can be challenging to reconstruct. An osteocutaneous free radial forearm or fibula flap can be used to replace the missing alveolus, serve as a rigid skeletal framework to support the lip and nose, and replace the resected palate. A premaxillary maxillectomy is one of the rare circumstances in which an osteocutaneous radial forearm flap can be considered a first-line option. Ahmad and colleagues provide an excellent description of their experience and surgical technique for using this flap for this particular defect.[33]

A prosthetic obturator is not an option for bilateral palatomaxillectomy defects because of lack of support, and soft tissue flaps lack the rigidity to prevent midfacial collapse.[31,32] These defects require bony reconstruction to maintain midface height, width, and projection, as well as to house dental implants. A bilateral palatomaxillectomy requires a long length of bone, typically 14 to 16 cm, making the fibula the most appropriate choice.

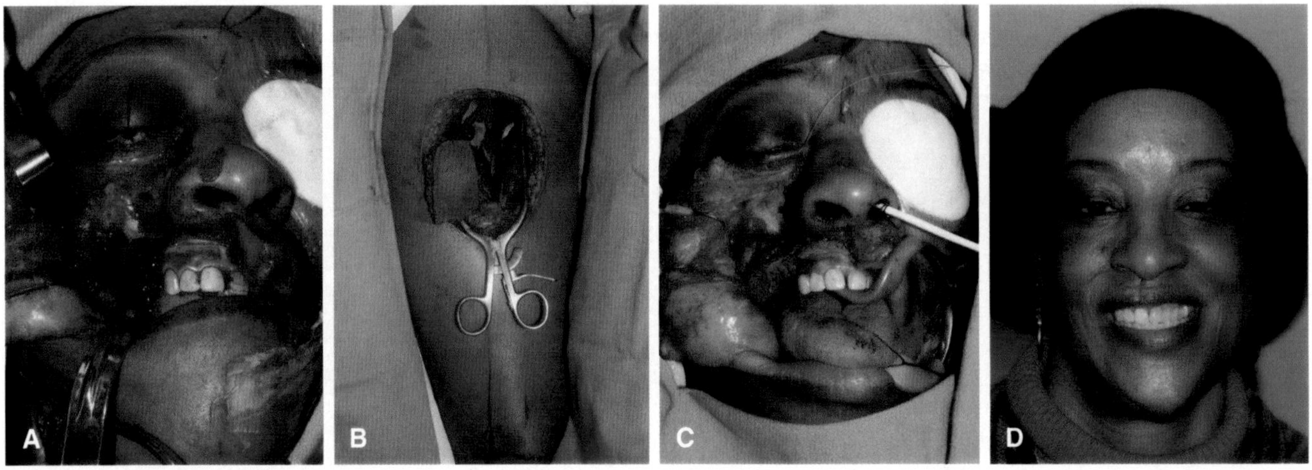

FIGURE 38.11. **A.** Posterior palatomaxillectomy defect. **B.** Anterolateral thigh perforator flap harvest. **C.** Closure of the palatomaxillary defect. **D.** Postoperative result showing good facial symmetry.

The leg that is ipsilateral to the side of the planned microvascular anastomosis is selected for fibula harvest. When the bony defect extends more laterally or posteriorly on one side than another, that side is usually preferred for the anastomosis because of the closer proximity to the neck. Alternatively, the side of the neck with better recipient blood vessels, if any, is used. In any bilateral palatomaxillectomy reconstruction, there is a strong possibility of requiring vein grafts to reach the recipient vasculature; this should be anticipated and planned appropriately. Typically, the fibula flap is shaped similarly to the Greek letter *omega* in the transverse plane (**Figure 38.13**). This configuration approximates the width and projection of the native maxilla. The lateral portions of the fibula replace the anterior wall of the maxillary sinus and malar eminence, if resected. The width of the fibula bone replaces the midfacial height. The middle portion of the flap restores the anterior projection and alveolus. A portion of soleus or flexor hallucis longus muscle is included with the fibula flap to fill the maxillary sinus. The skin paddle is designed to reconstruct the palatal defect.

There are a number of CAD/CAM systems available to assist with osseous flap planning, such as that required for maxillectomy reconstruction (see Figure 38.13).[34] For these highly complex, challenging surgeries, CAD/CAM and the advent of virtual surgical planning can improve accuracy of the reconstruction and reduce operative time. Using preoperative CT scans of the facial skeleton combined with a CT angiogram of the lower extremity, the exact location and angles of the osteotomies can be preplanned and designed according to the location of the patient's fibula perforators. These data are then translated to three-dimensionally printed cutting guides for both the fibula and the maxilla for an accurate and precise fit. Recently, using this same CT data, technology has been developed to create a milled titanium plate, corresponding to the exact shape of the reconstruction. CAD/CAM can increase the accuracy of the reconstruction, better approximating the patient's premorbid occlusion and craniofacial dimensions, translating to a better functional and cosmetic result.

Dental restoration with osseointegrated implants is performed 3 to 6 months after flap reconstruction. In patients with significant subcutaneous adipose tissue in the flap skin paddle, thinning of the flap is usually performed concurrently with implant placement. Removal of a portion of the plate or screws may be necessary for the fibula to accommodate the implants; therefore, bony union of the fibula at all osteotomy sites and to the native facial skeleton must be confirmed preoperatively.

Maxillectomy With Orbital Floor Defect

The orbital floor can be successfully reconstructed with a variety of alloplastic materials as well as autologous bone grafts, most commonly harvested from either the iliac crest or outer table of the calvarium. Many surgeons believe that bone grafts are more resistant to radiation-induced complications; however, our own experience does

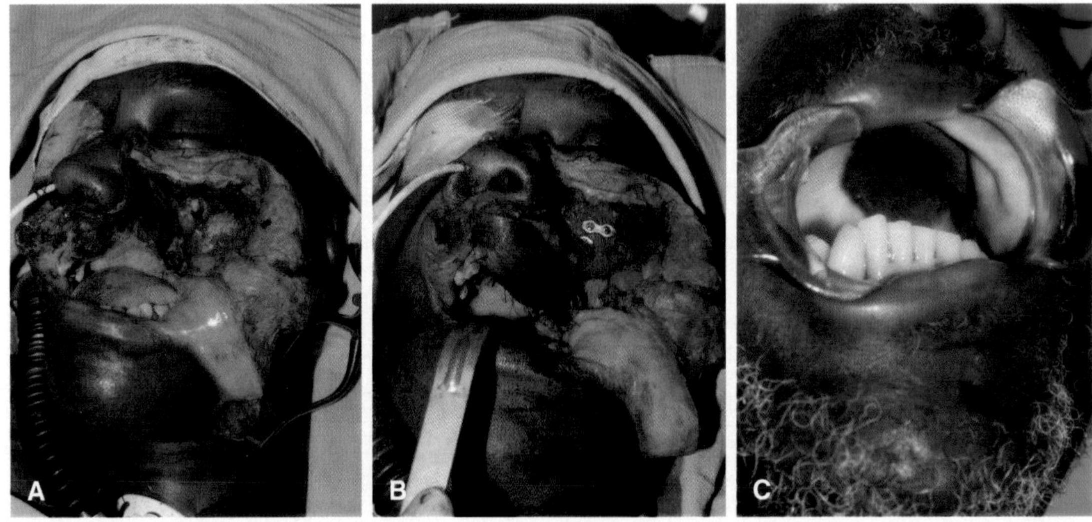

FIGURE 38.12. **A.** Left hemipalatomaxillectomy defect. **B.** A fibula osteocutaneous free flap was chosen so that osseointegrated implants could later be placed for dental restoration. **C.** Postoperative result, showing fibula skin paddle used to close the palatal defect.

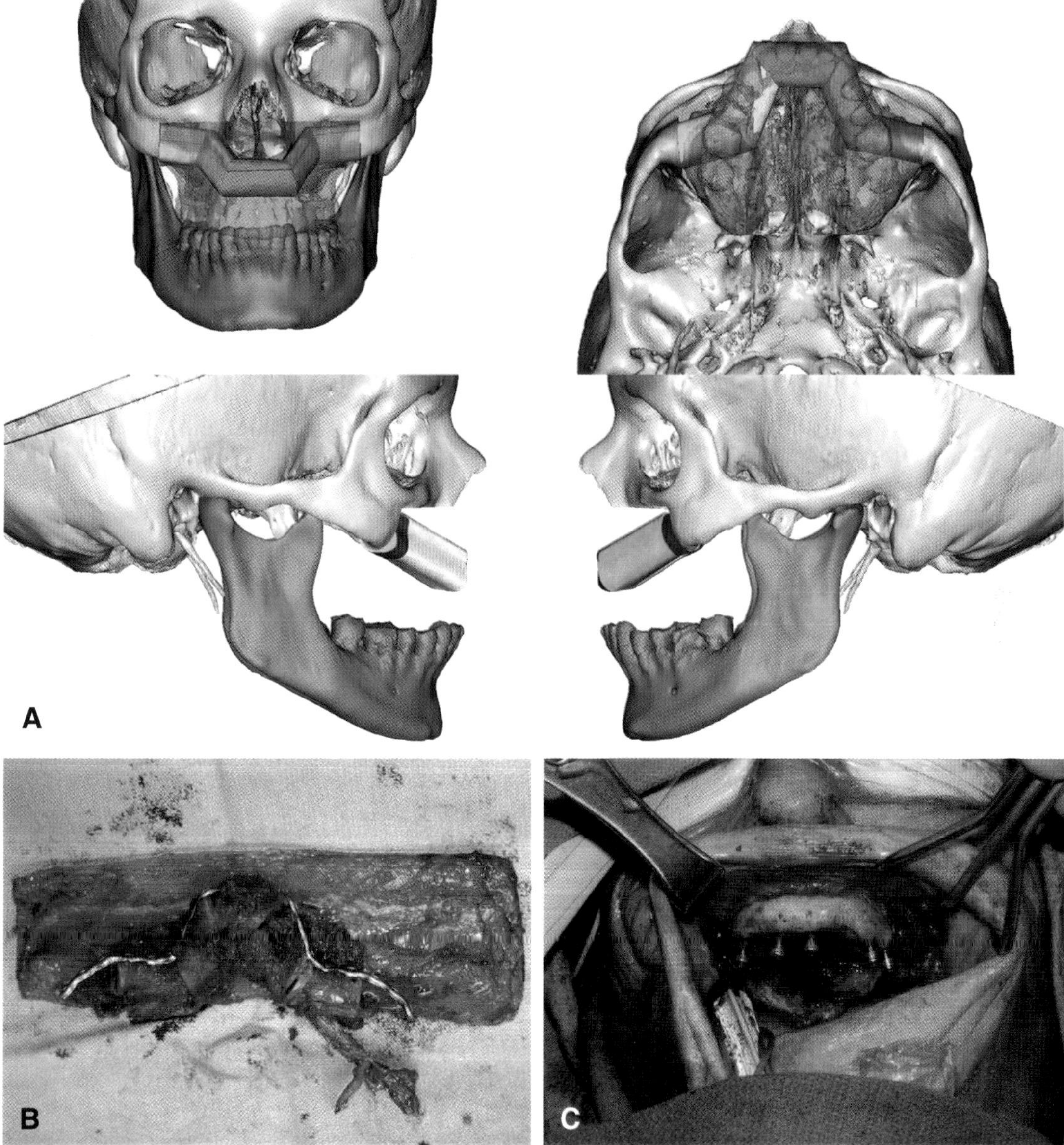

FIGURE 38.13. **A.** Computer modeling of a fibula reconstruction for a bilateral palatomaxillectomy defect. **B.** Fibula free flap after osteotomies for reconstruction of a bilateral palatomaxillectomy defect. **C.** The fibula can accommodate osseointegrated implants for dental restoration.

not support their use over alloplasts.[24,28] Kirby and colleagues found that bone grafts were more likely to be complicated by orbital dystopia and enophthalmos compared with alloplastic materials.[35] Indeed, shaping an autologous graft is more challenging than shaping titanium mesh; this feature likely contributed to the adverse outcomes discussed in this paper. When using a fibula osteocutaneous free flap to reconstruct a hemipalatomaxillectomy or bilateral palatomaxillectomy with an orbital floor defect, we will include soleus or flexor hallucis longus muscle to support the alloplast or bone graft. We believe it is imperative that the reconstructed orbital floor be in direct continuity with well-vascularized tissue to minimize complications.

Maxillectomy With Orbital Exenteration

When an orbital exenteration is performed in isolation and no aspects of the maxilla or skull base are removed, and there is no history of radiation or no anticipation of radiation, the reconstruction can be very simple. In this situation, the goal is to provide a deep, concave orbit lined with durable skin able to accept a prosthesis. A split-thickness skin graft lining the orbital cavity fulfills these criteria well. It may be helpful to allow for a period of secondary intention healing and dressing changes to build granulation tissue, prior to placing the skin graft. Other options include a local flap such as a temporalis muscle or temporoparietal fascia flap with a skin graft or a thin fasciocutaneous free flap such as a radial forearm flap. The temporalis muscle flap is thin enough to permit a secure prosthesis fit but results in a depression at the donor site. Such a depression can be easily corrected with either fat grafting or placement of a high-density porous polyethylene implant.[36] Rotation of either of these flaps may require removal of the lateral orbital wall to achieve the length needed to reach the medial aspect of the orbit; this also creates a significant contour deformity.

The complexity of the reconstruction increases significantly when the inferior, medial, or superior walls of the orbit have been removed. In this more complicated scenario, the primary goals of reconstruction are to line the orbital cavity with durable tissue, to exclude the nasal or sinus cavities, and to protect the brain when the orbital roof has been removed. If the bony resection is limited, the radial forearm free flap may still be a reliable option; this thin flap will accommodate an orbital prosthesis without revision surgery. In cases when the bony resection is more extensive, such as an orbitomaxillectomy, a bulky flap is preferred. The ALT or RAM flaps are good options in this scenario. Either flap can be designed with both a muscle component and fasciocutaneous segment; the muscle is used to fill the sinuses, thus preventing infection with sinonasal flora or fistula formation, and the skin portion is used to resurface the orbit. The added flap bulk is also required to restore midfacial volume and cheek contour. The orbital contour is usually convex in these cases, and the reconstruction will require a revision at a later date if an orbital prosthesis is desired.

Defects involving both an orbital exenteration and a palatomaxillectomy are best reconstructed with flaps with multiple skin paddles to close these three defects (orbit, cheek/sinuses, and palate). Both the RAM and ALT are good choices. In cases where the perforator anatomy is not compatible with multiple separate skin paddles, a portion of the flap can be de-epithelialized for reconstruction of multiple surfaces. It is the authors' preference to leave a noncutaneous flap surface facing the nasal cavity to spontaneously mucosalize around a soft silicone nasopharyngeal trumpet; this process takes 2 to 3 weeks.

REFERENCES

1. Raposio E, Santi P, Nordström RE. Effects of galeotomies on scalp flaps. *Ann Plast Surg*. 1998;41:17-21.
2. Orticochea M. Four flap scalp reconstruction technique. *Br J Plast Surg*. 1967;20:159-171.
3. Muresan C, Hui-Chou HG, Dorafshar AH, et al. Forehead reconstruction with microvascular flaps: utility of aesthetic subunits. *J Reconstr Microsurg*. 2012;28:319-326.
4. Menick FJ. A 10-year experience in nasal reconstruction with the three-stage forehead flap. *Plast Reconstr Surg*. 2002;109:1839-1855.
5. Kane WJ, McCaffrey TV, Wang TD, Koval TM. The effect of tissue expansion on previously irradiated skin. *Arch Otolaryngol Head Neck Surg*. 1992;118:419-426.
6. Hansen SL, Foster RD, Dosanjh AS, Mathes SJ, Hoffman WY, Leon P. Superficial temporal artery and vein as recipient vessels for facial and scalp microsurgical reconstruction. *Plast Reconstr Surg*. 2007;120:1879-1884.
   The superficial temporal artery and vein have historically not been considered adequate for microsurgical reconstruction and have rarely been described as recipient vessels.
   The authors demonstrate that the superficial temporal artery and vein for scalp and face reconstruction are reliable and safe and state that they should be considered as primary recipient vessels in microsurgical reconstruction of the upper two-thirds of the face and/or scalp.
7. Hussussian CJ, Reece GP. Microsurgical scalp reconstruction in the patient with cancer. *Plast Reconstr Surg*. 2002;109:1828-1834.
8. Sosin M, De la Cruz C, Bojovic B, et al. Microsurgical reconstruction of complex scalp defects: an appraisal of flap selection and the timing of complications. *J Craniofac Surg*. 2015;26:1186-1191.
9. Sosin M, Schultz BD, De La Cruz C, et al. Microsurgical scalp reconstruction in the elderly: a systematic review and pooled analysis of the current data. *Plast Reconstr Surg*. 2015;135:856-866.
10. Simunovic F, Eisenhardt SU, Penna V, et al. Microsurgical reconstruction of oncological scalp defects in the elderly. *J Plast Reconstr Aesthet Surg*. 2016;69:912-919.
11. Chao AH, Yu P, Skoracki RJ, et al. Microsurgical reconstruction of composite scalp and calvarial defects in patients with cancer: a 10-year experience. *Head Neck*. 2012;34:1759-1764.
12. Lee EI, Chao AH, Skoracki RJ, Yu P, DeMonte F, Hanasono MM. Outcomes of calvarial reconstruction in cancer patients. *Plast Reconstr Surg*. 2014;133:675-682.
   Retrospective review of 289 calvarial reconstructions in cancer patients. The authors demonstrate a similar complication profile in a variety of alloplasts with the exception of calcium phosphate, which was found to have a high infection rate.
13. Rubin JP, Yaremchuk MJ. Complications and toxicities of implantable biomaterials used in facial reconstructive and aesthetic surgery: a comprehensive review of the literature. *Plast Reconstr Surg*. 1997;100:1336-1353.
14. Hanasono MM, Goel N, DeMonte F. Calvarial reconstruction with polyetheretherketone implants. *Ann Plast Surg*. 2009;62:653-655.
15. Kumar AR, Bradley JP, Harshbarger R, et al. Warfare-related craniectomy defect reconstruction: early success using custom alloplast implants. *Plast Reconstr Surg*. 2011;127:1279-1287.
16. Moreira-Gonzalez A, Jackson IT, Miyawaki T, et al. Clinical outcome in cranioplasty: critical review in long-term follow-up. *J Craniofac Surg*. 2003;14:144-153.
17. Netscher D, Alford EL, Wigoda P, Cohen V. Free composite myo-osseous flap with serratus anterior and rib: indications in head and neck reconstruction. *Head Neck*. 1998;20:106-112.
18. Sinno S, Rodriguez ED. Definitive management of persistent frontal sinus infections and mucocele with a vascularized free fibula flap. *Plast Reconstr Surg*. 2017;139:170-175.
19. Lee JW, Hsueh YY, Lee JS. Composite skull and dura defect reconstruction using combined latissimus dorsi musculocutaneous and serratus anterior muscle-rib free flap coupled with vascularized galea transfer: a case report. *Microsurgery*. 2010;30:632-635.
20. Hasan Z, Gore SM, Ch'ng S, et al. Options for configuring the scapular free flap in maxillary, mandibular, and calvarial reconstruction. *Plast Reconstr Surg*. 2013;132:645-655.
21. Selber JC, Chang EI, Clemens MW, et al. Simultaneous scalp, skull, kidney, and pancreas transplant from a single donor. *Plast Reconstr Surg*. 2016;137:1851-1861.
   The first report of a simultaneous scalp, skull, kidney, and pancreas transplant from a single donor. The case was successful and established vascularized composite tissue allograft reconstruction of the scalp and skull as a potential option in the appropriate clinical scenario.
22. Sosin M, Ceradini DJ, Levine JP, et al. Total face, eyelids, ears, scalp, and skeletal subunit transplant: a reconstructive solution for the full face and total scalp burn. *Plast Reconstr Surg*. 2016;138:205-219.
23. Irish J, Gullane PJ, Gentili F, et al. Tumors of the skull base: outcome and survival analysis of 77 cases. *Head Neck*. 1994;16:3-10.
   This seminal article introduces the classification schema commonly used when describing skull base resections and reconstructions.
24. Hanasono MM, Lee JC, Yang JS, et al. An algorithmic approach to reconstructive surgery and prosthetic rehabilitation after orbital exenteration. *Plast Reconstr Surg*. 2009;123:98-105.
25. Rosenthal EL, King K, McGrew BM, et al. Evolution of a paradigm for free tissue transfer reconstruction of lateral temporal bone defects. *Head Neck*. 2008;30:589-594.
26. Hanasono MM, Silva AK, Yu P, Skoracki RJ, Sturgis EM, Gidley PW. Comprehensive management of temporal bone defects after oncologic resection. *Laryngoscope*. 2012;122:2663-2669.
27. Brown JS, Shaw RJ. Reconstruction of the maxilla and midface: introducing a new classification. *Lancet Oncol*. 2010;11:1001-1008.
   Seminal article introducing a widely accepted maxillectomy classification system.
28. Hanasono MM, Silva AK, Yu P, Skoracki RJ. A comprehensive algorithm for oncologic maxillary reconstruction. *Plast Reconstr Surg*. 2013;131:47-60.
   Seminal article describing an anatomic description and classification system for maxillectomy defects, as well as reconstructive options organized by defect classification.
29. Cordeiro PG, Santamaria E. A classification system and algorithm for reconstruction of maxillectomy and midfacial defects. *Plast Reconstr Surg*. 2000;105:2331-2346.
   Seminal article describing an important classification system for maxillectomy defects. It establishes that free tissue transfer provides the most effective and reliable form of immediate reconstruction for complex maxillectomy defects.
30. Spiro RH, Strong EW, Shah JP. Maxillectomy and its classification. *Head Neck*. 1997;19(4):309-314.
31. Moreno MA, Skoracki RJ, Hanna EY, Hanasono MM. Microvascular free flap reconstruction versus palatal obturation for maxillectomy defects. *Head Neck*. 2010;32:860-868.
32. Okay DJ, Genden E, Buchbinder D, Urken M. Prosthodontic guideline for surgical reconstruction of the maxilla: a classification system of defects. *J Prosthet Dent*. 2001;86:352-363.
33. Ahmad FI, Means C, Labby AB, et al. Osteocutaneous radial forearm free flap in nonmandible head and neck reconstruction. *Head Neck*. 2017;39:1888-1893.
34. Chang EI, Hanasono MM. State-of-the-art reconstruction of midface and facial deformities. *J Surg Oncol*. 2016;113:962-970.
35. Kirby EJ, Turner JB, Davenport DL, Vasconez HC. Orbital floor fractures: outcomes of reconstruction. *Ann Plast Surg*. 2011;66:508-512.
36. Mericli AF, Gampper TJ. Treatment of postsurgical temporal hollowing with high-density porous polyethylene. *J Craniofac Surg*. 2014;25:563-567.

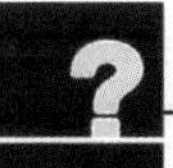

QUESTIONS

1. A 57-year-old man presents with a 6 cm ameloblastoma of the hard palate. He undergoes bilateral maxillectomy, including total removal of his hard palate and alveolar ridge. What is the most appropriate reconstructive technique?
   a. Prosthetic obturator
   b. Temporalis muscle pedicled flap
   c. Iliac crest bone graft
   d. ALT free flap
   e. Fibula osteocutaneous free flap

2. A 92-year-old man is diagnosed with diffuse squamous cell carcinoma of the scalp, metastatic to the cervical lymph nodes. He is healthy other than the fact that he has a BMI of 35 and requires corrective lenses in order to achieve normal vision. A 20-cm diameter excision, including the pericranium, of the scalp and cervical lymphadenectomy is planned. What is the most appropriate method of reconstruction?
   a. Latissimus dorsi myocutaneous flap with anastomosis to the ST vessels
   b. Vascularized composite tissue allograft of the scalp with anastomosis to the bilateral terminal external carotid arteries and end-to-side anastomosis to the internal jugular veins
   c. Latissimus dorsi muscle flap and skin graft with anastomosis to the ST vessels
   d. ALT fasciocutaneous flap to facial vessels
   e. Vastus lateralis muscle flap and skin graft with anastomosis to the ST vessels

3. A 37-year-old woman is diagnosed with osteosarcoma of the skull. The lesion has eroded through the scalp and the patient has been treated preoperatively with radiation. A 7 cm^2 diameter craniectomy and scalp resection is planned. The neurosurgeon tells you he is very worried about recurrence. What is the most appropriate material for the reconstruction of the calvarium?
   a. PEEK
   b. Titanium mesh
   c. No calvarial reconstruction necessary
   d. Bone allograft with bone morphogenic protein
   e. Calcium phosphate

4. A 42-year-old man undergoes resection of the anterior skull base to remove an esthesioneuroblastoma. He has a history of a significant laceration to the left preauricular area. The skull base surgeon reconstructs the missing anterior cranial fossa with a pedicled pericranium flap. Postoperatively, the patient develops CSF rhinorrhea. He is placed on prophylactic antibiotics with his head of bed elevated, but the leak persists even after 5 days. The neurosurgeons place a lumbar drain, but clear fluid continues to drain through the patient's nose. The plastic surgeon is consulted for recommendations. What is the most reasonable treatment option?
   a. Continue conservative management
   b. Return to the operating room for exploration, dural repair by neurosurgery, and re-inset of the pericranial flap
   c. Return to the operating room for exploration, dural repair by neurosurgery, and resurfacing the resected skull base with a buried vastus lateralis muscle flap.
   d. Return to the operating room for exploration, dural repair by neurosurgery, and resurfacing the resected skull base with a pedicled left temporalis major muscle flap
   e. Return to the operating room for exploration, dural repair by neurosurgery, and resurfacing the resected skull base with a free buried omentum flap

5. A 67-year-old man with an HbA1c of 11 mg/dL, dialysis-depended end-stage renal disease, and an ejection fraction of 20% is diagnosed with a squamous cell carcinoma eroding through the hard palate. An infrastructure palatomaxillectomy is planned with resection of the hard palate and left maxillary alveolus. The ipsilateral canine tooth and all teeth mesial to it will be spared. What is the most appropriate method of reconstruction?
   a. Free fibula osteocutaneous flap
   b. Radial forearm osteocutaneous flap
   c. Radial forearm fasciocutaneous flap
   d. Prosthetic obturator
   e. ALT flap

1. **Answer: e.** Several techniques are used in palatomaxillary reconstruction. Palatal obturators are acceptable for small defects. However, prosthetic retention can be difficult or impossible in sizable defects, particularly when there are few teeth to stabilize the prosthesis. The temporalis muscle flap can be rotated into the oral cavity and is useful for closing isolated defects of the midpalate. However, this flap would not provide the structural support necessary to maintain the shape of the midface. Iliac crest bone grafts stabilized with titanium hardware can be used for some posttraumatic defects but are prone to infection, extrusion, and nonunion in radiated patients, particularly when the defect is as extensive as this one. The ALT free flap can close the palatal defect and restore shape to the cheek in patients with a unilateral maxillectomy. However, in anterior and bilateral defects, such as this one, a myocutaneous free flap, like the temporalis muscle flap, would not restore the height, width, and projection of the anterior midface. The fibula osteocutaneous free flap and other vascularized bone flaps can be shaped to restore the skeletal support of the midface in extensive, bilateral maxillary defects. The skin paddle of the flap can be used to close the palatal defect to restore speech and swallowing function. Also, the fibula osteocutaneous free flap can accept osseointegrated implants for dental restoration because of the good quality of bone stock associated with this flap.

2. **Answer: c.** The extent of the planned resection will require a free tissue transfer because of lack of available locoregional options. A skin graft alone would be inappropriate considering the anticipated resection will include the pericranium. Using a latissimus myocutaneous flap for a 20-cm wide defect is possible, but the donor site would not be able to close primarily, requiring a skin graft. Additionally, with a BMI of 35, the thickness of the skin paddle would likely require multiple revisionary procedures to achieve an acceptable appearance; it is best to avoid procedures that will necessitate revision in the elderly. An ALT fasciocutaneous flap or vastus lateralis muscle flap will not be large enough to fully reconstruct the defect. The ST vessels are the recipient vessels of choice in any scalp reconstruction. Any patient that wears glasses should be instructed to not wear them postoperatively to avoid inadvertent pedicle compression. The facial vessels will likely be exposed, considering the need for a neck dissection in this patient. However, a vein graft is likely necessary to achieve the required pedicle length to reach the neck; if the ST vessels are adequate and available, they are preferred.

3. Answer: a. Titanium mesh is an effective material for craniectomy reconstruction; however, it is associated with significant imaging artifact, marking radiologic surveillance of disease recurrence challenging. Any calvarial defect greater than 6 cm^2 should be reconstructed. PEEK implants are radiolucent and can be customized to the patient, based on the planned resection and preoperative imaging data. In this scenario, given the other available answer choices, a PEEK reconstruction is most appropriate. Bone morphogenic protein is a morphogen and should be avoided in cases of malignancy. Calcium phosphate is useful for smaller calvarial defects; however, it carries a high late infection risk; therefore, it should be avoided in this patient with a history of preoperative radiation.

4. Answer: c. The CSF leak is unlikely to resolve with continued conservative management at this point. Re-inset of the pericranial flap is unwise considering it failed in initially preventing the leak. Although a temporalis muscle flap may reach the anterior skull base, the patient's prior left preauricular injury may be damaging the muscle's blood supply, obviating its use as a flap. The vastus lateralis muscle flap is a good option in this scenario; it is well vascularized and conforms to the shape of the skull base, easily sealing off the intracranial space from the sinonasal cavity. The muscle can be buried and monitored with an implantable Doppler probe. The omentum could be used; however, few plastic surgeons would consider it a first-line option given the need for a laparotomy to harvest it.

5. Answer: d. This patient with multiple medical comorbidities is not a good candidate for a free tissue transfer. An obturator is an excellent option for reconstruction of limited palatal defects. The extent of the remaining alveolar dentition is sufficient to counteract the substantial cantilever forces that will be imparted to the obturator.

CHAPTER 39 Reconstruction of the Eyelids, Correction of Ptosis, and Canthoplasty

Benjamin P. Erickson and Derrick C. Wan

KEY POINTS

- Comprehensive understanding of eyelid anatomy, coupled with careful assessment of individual patient factors, guides diagnosis, and selection of appropriate procedures.
- Divide upper and lower eyelid defects into anterior lamellar (partial-thickness and full-thickness defects), then by size to select reconstructive options.
- Full-thickness defects are reconstructed in layers, restoring a mucosalized posterior lining, structural support layer, and anterior skin/muscle layer. At least one lamella must have an intact blood supply.
- Avoid undue vertical tension while appropriately correcting horizontal laxity to minimize the risk of postoperative eyelid malposition. When necessary, use a wedge excision with the apex pointing away from the lid margin to approximate a pentagon to avoid dog-ears and notching.
- Repair of eyelid ptosis requires an understanding of the possible etiologies and full preoperative evaluation, including assessment of lid position and levator function.
- Lower eyelid malposition and lid laxity can be treated with a lateral canthoplasty (division of the canthus and repositioning) or canthopexy (redirection of intact canthal tendon). Procedures to shorten and provide lower eyelid support depend on the severity of lid laxity.

The eyelids are complex lamellar structures that function to protect the anterior globe from injury and maintain ocular surface integrity. They also aid in regulating light exposure to the eye and distribute the tear film over the cornea during blinking. Primary goals of any surgical procedure to reconstruct or modify the eyelids must focus on establishing or preserving a stable structure with adequate height and functional closure, and on maintaining a nonkeratinized mucosal posterior surface to avoid abrasion to the underlying cornea. Restoration of symmetry and appearance remain secondary goals. Understanding the anatomic architecture of the upper and lower eyelid is critical to achieving satisfactory functional and cosmetic outcomes.

EYELID ANATOMY

Lamellar Structure and Surface Anatomy

The upper and lower eyelids are composed of the skin, minimal subcutaneous tissue, orbicularis oculi muscle, submuscular areolar tissue, a fibrous layer consisting of orbital septum and tarsal plate, retroseptal fat pads, lid retractors, and conjunctiva (Figure 39.1). For conceptual purposes, however, these structures are divided into anterior and posterior lamellae, with the tarsofascial layer in between. The upper eyelid extends from the lid margin inferiorly to the eyebrow superiorly, which demarcates it from the forehead. The natural curvature of the lid is generated by the shape of the tarsal plate as well as coaptation to the curvature of the globe beneath. In the upper

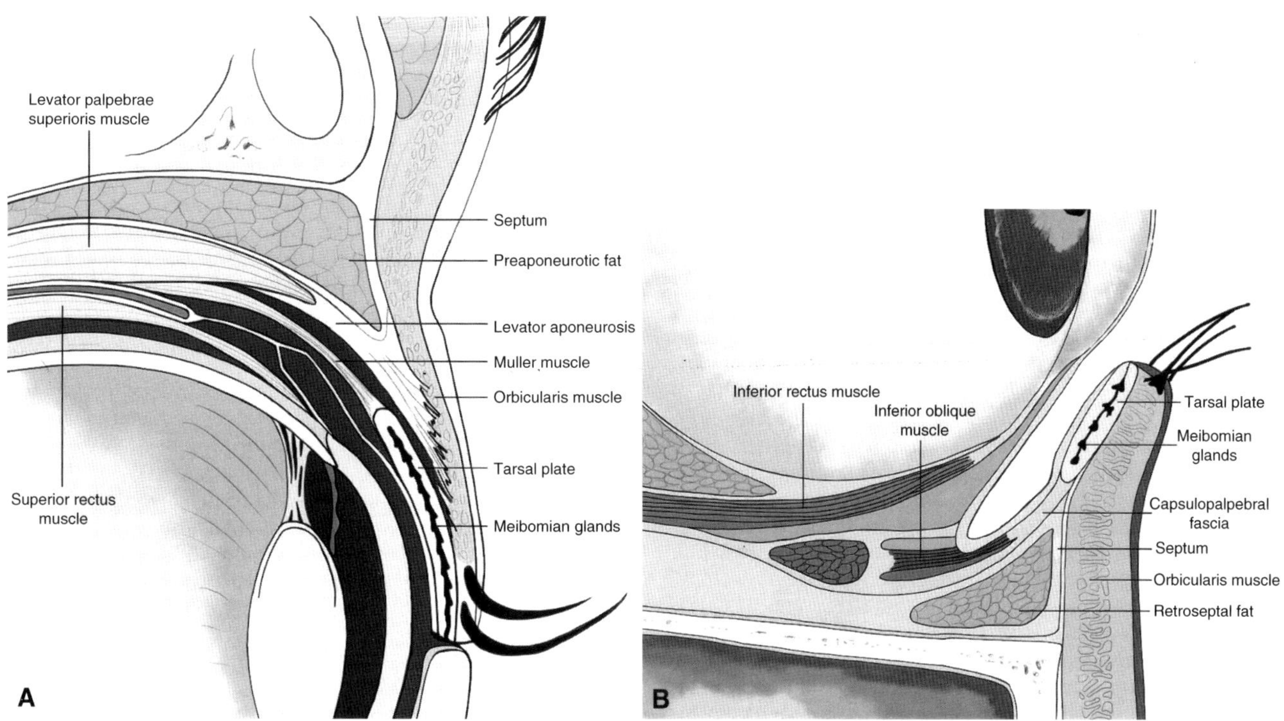

FIGURE 39.1. Cross-sectional schematic of upper **(A)** and lower **(B)** eyelid anatomy.

lid, a skin crease can be found approximately 8 to 9 mm superior to the eyelid margin in men and 9 to 11 mm in women, though in the Asians this lid crease can be found significantly lower. The inferior eyelid extends from the lid margin superiorly to the malar fold below, which runs from the medial canthal region inferomedially to the nasojugal fold and serves to delimit the lower lid from the cheek. A lower eyelid fold, particularly in children, can also be found approximately 3 to 5 mm from the lid margin.

With the eye open, the palpebral fissure measures 28 to 30 mm in length and approximately 9 mm in height. The highest point of the upper lid is typically found just medial to the center of the pupil, with the lid margin resting 1 to 2 mm below the superior limbus in adults. The lowest point of the lower eyelid can be found lateral to the center of the pupil, with the margin at the inferior limbus. Finally, in Caucasians, the lateral canthus is positioned 2 mm higher than the medial canthus, whereas in Asians this can be found 3 mm higher.

Eyelid Skin

The skin of the upper and lower eyelids is among the thinnest in the body, measuring less than 1 mm thick. A greater number of sebaceous glands can be found in the nasal portion of the lids, making these regions smoother and oilier than temporal eyelid skin. There is relatively minimal subcutaneous fat in the eyelids, which can mostly be found beneath preorbital and preseptal skin. Beneath pretarsal skin, as well as laterally over the medial and lateral canthal ligaments, the underlying fat is absent. This anatomic relationship facilitates motility, but also contributes to disproportionate redundancy with aging. Of note, descent of the brow fat pad into the lateral upper lid is common, and it should not be confused with retroseptal fat.

Eyelid Muscles

Muscles of the eyelids can be divided into protractors, which close the eyes, and retractors, which open them. The orbicularis oculi muscle is the primary protractor and is divided into orbital, preseptal, and pretarsal portions. Fibers of the orbital portion originate from the medial orbital margin and medial canthal tendon and sweep around the orbit in horseshoe fashion to insert back on the medial canthus. The preseptal and pretarsal subunits originate from the medial canthal tendon and insert on the lateral horizontal raphe. The orbital subunit functions in forced closure, whereas the preseptal and pretarsal subunits are employed for blinking and voluntary winking. Temporal, zygomatic, and buccal branches of the facial nerve innervate the muscle from the undersurface.

Eyelid retractors consist of the levator palpebrae superioris and Müller muscle in the upper lid, and capsulopalpebral fascia in the lower lid. The levator palpebrae superioris arises from the orbital apex and terminates in an aponeurosis, which fuses with the orbital septum anteriorly prior to attaching to the superior tarsal plate posteriorly. It is innervated by the oculomotor nerve and serves as the principal upper lid retractor. An anterior extension from the levator can be found inserting into the pretarsal orbicularis oculi muscle and skin, forming a skin crease in the upper eyelid. Dehiscence of the levator muscle from the tarsal plate with age or trauma results in blepharoptosis and elevation of the lid crease. In concert with the levator palpebrae superioris, the sympathetically innervated Müller muscle contributes an additional 2 to 3 mm lid elevation. It originates from the undersurface of the levator muscle and inserts on the superior margin of the tarsal plate. With decreased sympathetic tone, as in Horner syndrome, loss of this muscle function results in mild ptosis.

In the lower eyelid, fascial extensions of the inferior rectus muscle continue anterosuperiorly to form the capsulopalpebral fascia. This primarily inserts on the inferior border of the lower tarsal plate, though minor fibers also insert on the conjunctiva of the inferior fornix, facilitating lower lid descent with downward gaze. Analogous to the upper eyelid, sympathetically innervated fibers are intimately involved with the posterior surface of the capsulopalpebral fascia, although they are typically not identifiable as a distinct anatomical layer. The orbital septum in the lower eyelid also fuses with the capsulopalpebral fascia in similar fashion to the upper lid.

Orbital Septum

The orbital septum is a thin layer of connective tissue that separates the eyelid from the anterior orbit. It is continuous with the periosteum along the orbital rim (arcus marginalis) and attaches to the tarsal plates through fusion with the levator palpebrae superioris in the upper lid and capsulopalpebral fascia in the lower lid. Variable indistinct fusion, however, can result in more prominent orbital fat projection in different ethnicities, and with age, thinning of the septum can also lead to more noticeable fat descent. The orbital septum has considerable laxity, but scarring of the septum from trauma or surgical intervention can precipitate lid retraction.

Fat Pads

Adipose tissue in the upper eyelid is divided into two components, the central (preaponeurotic) fat pad and the medial fat pad. The central fat pad is broad and yellow secondary to higher levels of carotenoids and is found in between the orbital septum and levator aponeurosis. The medial fat pad, which is more pale yellow or white in color, is located in the same plane and is separated from the central fat pad by the trochlea of the superior oblique muscle. Finally, the lacrimal gland occupies the lateral compartment in the upper eyelid. It is firmer to palpation, pink in color, and may become more prominent on upper lid examination with age due to prolapse.

The lower eyelid contains three retroseptal fat compartments known as the lateral, central, and nasal fat pads. The inferior oblique muscle separates the medial and central fat pads, whereas the arcuate expansion extending from the capsulopalpebral fascia separates the medial and lateral fat pads. As the fat pads reside behind the septum, insertion of this fascial layer outside the orbital rim laterally creates the recess of Eisner into which a portion of the lateral fat pad sits. Because of the intimate association of the inferior oblique muscle with lower lid fat, injury to this muscle during surgical dissection can result in torsional diplopia.

Tarsoligamentous Sling

The tarsal plates comprise the fibrous skeleton of the upper and lower eyelids and provide structural integrity. The superior tarsal plate is typically 10 to 12 mm in height centrally, narrowing medially, and laterally to assume a crescentic shape. The inferior tarsal plate is more rectangular and measures approximately 4 mm in height centrally. The maximum thickness is 1 mm and each tarsus is approximately 30 mm long. Within the upper and lower eyelid, tarsus can be found 25 to 40 sebaceous meibomian glands. These empty at the lid margin posterior to the gray line and are responsible for the oily layer of the tear film.

Each tarsus tapers medially and laterally, joining to form canthal tendons. Together with the tarsal plates, they form the tarsoligamentous sling, which maintains lid-globe apposition. The medial canthal tendon is intricately related to the orbicularis oculi muscle and splits to form anterior and posterior limbs that insert into the anterior and posterior lacrimal crest, respectively. The lateral canthal tendon passes deep to the orbital septum and inserts 2 mm posterior to the lateral orbital rim on a bony prominence known as Whitnall tubercle. Proper attachment of canthal tendons both medially and laterally is responsible for preserving sharp canthal angles and maintaining lid-globe apposition.

Conjunctiva

The conjunctiva is a smooth, translucent, nonkeratinized mucous membrane that can be divided into palpebral, forniceal, and bulbar components. The palpebral conjunctiva lines the posterior surface of the upper and lower eyelid and is firmly adherent to the tarsal plates. This continues into the upper and lower fornices where there is redundant tissue to facilitate free motility of the eye. Beyond the forniceal conjunctiva, reflection anteriorly forms the bulbar conjunctiva which coats the surface of the globe. Goblet cells within the conjunctiva produce mucin, whereas accessory lacrimal glands are responsible for basal secretion of aqueous tears. Conjunctival tissue loss can result in lid malposition and limitation in ocular motility, and decreased mucin or tear production can increase risk for ocular surface injury.

Lacrimal System

The lacrimal glands are situated in the superolateral region of each orbit and are responsible for reflex secretion of the aqueous layer of the tear film. Two lobes can be found, separated by the levator aponeurosis, with the orbital lobe residing within the lacrimal fossa and the smaller palpebral portion close to the eye along the inner surface of the eyelid. Aqueous tears drain into the superolateral fornix via ductules and the *wiper-blade* action of the orbicularis oculi and tarsal plates pushes tears medially.

In the normal setting, tears pass over the surface of the globe to reach lacrimal puncta at the inner corner of eyelids. These then pass tears through lacrimal canaliculi and ducts into the lacrimal sac, which turns into the nasolacrimal duct to provide drainage into the inferior nasal meatus. The lacrimal sac sits within the lacrimal fossa which is enveloped by the orbicularis oculi and medial canthal tendon. Contraction of the orbicularis muscle during blinking drives the pumping mechanism of the lacrimal sac, which draw tears into the puncta and propels them through the nasolacrimal duct. Decreased tear production can lead to keratoconjunctivitis sicca, with persistent dryness and burning of the eyes, whereas excess tear production with disruption of the lacrimal drainage system at any level may result in epiphora, or overflow of tears onto the face.

Blood Supply and Lymphatics

The eyelids contain a rich anastomotic blood supply derived from both the internal and external carotid arteries. The internal carotid arterial supply arises from terminal branches of the ophthalmic artery, which supply the medial palpebral vessel directly and the lateral palpebral vessel via the lacrimal artery. In the upper eyelid, a marginal arcade can be found on the anterior tarsal surface, approximately 2 to 4 mm above the lid margin. A second peripheral arcade can be found above the tarsal plate on the anterior surface of the Müller muscle, which can be susceptible to injury during eyelid surgery. In the lower eyelid, only one, more rudimentary arcade can be found approximately 2 mm below the inferior tarsal margin. External carotid artery supply arises from anastomotic branches of the angular artery, the superficial temporal artery, and the maxillary artery. Rich lymphatic drainage can be found for the eyelids and the conjunctiva. The lateral two-thirds of the upper lid and lateral half of the lower lid drain primarily through the preauricular lymph nodes, whereas the medial portion of the upper and lower lid drain through the submandibular lymph nodes. Persistent lymphedema of the eyelids can be functionally and cosmetically debilitating, with high rates of recurrence after surgical revision, but is fortunately a rare complication.

PREOPERATIVE AND POSTOPERATIVE CONSIDERATIONS

Defects of the upper or lower eyelids can result from congenital anomalies, trauma, or tumor resection. Irrespective of etiology, however, structures of the eyelid, including skin, muscle, tarsoligamentous sling, and conjunctiva must be fully evaluated and, if deficient, must be addressed in operative planning. Evaluation with respect to location and extent of tissue involvement (partial- or full-thickness) may also help to guide reconstructive planning. For congenital defects, such as with colobomas seen in paramedian clefts, Treacher Collins syndrome, or Goldenhar syndrome, a full evaluation for other associated anomalies must be performed. For postoncologic resection defects, knowledge of the histologic diagnosis and resection margin status should be obtained prior to proceeding with reconstruction. Along with these concerns, a full ophthalmologic history and examination should be performed. Prior ocular injuries, surgery, or history of inflammation may alter anatomic relationships and need to be recognized prior to surgery to reduce risk of postoperative complications.

Malposition of the eyelid can be seen with entropion, ectropion, or lid retraction. A snap-back test is crucial for evaluation of laxity in the setting of eyelid malposition. The lower eyelid is pulled down and away from the globe to determine how long it takes to return to the original position without blinking. In the normal lower eyelid (Grade 0), it should spring back immediately to the original position, whereas a delay is observed with lid laxity. Grade I laxity is observed with 2 to 3 second delay, Grade II laxity with 4 to 5 seconds delay, and Grade III laxity with >5 seconds delay and return to position with blinking. Finally, with Grade IV laxity, frank ectropion is maintained without return to the original position. Importantly, though lid laxity must be addressed in successful periocular Mohs reconstruction, preoperative laxity may be beneficial and should therefore be treated conservatively until after definitive excision and repair is planned.

The patient must also be evaluated prior to surgery for signs and symptoms of dry eye or blepharitis, as these may be exacerbated postoperatively. Adequate tear film production can be assessed with a Schirmer's test, in which a filter paper strip is inserted into the lower sulcus for 5 minutes to measure moisture. Tear production is considered to be diminished with less than 15 mm in the absence of a topical anesthetic and with 5 to 10 mm when a topical anesthetic is given. Alternatively, tear production can also be evaluated by administering fluorescein eye drops to determine whether there is interpalpebral staining of the cornea.

For patients with excess tear accumulation or epiphora, a dye disappearance test or dilation and irrigation can be performed. While under sedation and anesthetic, a No. 00 Bowman probe can also be passed through the lacrimal drainage system to determine the precise locus of obstruction. Typical distances in an adult are 8 to 10 mm to the common canaliculus, 10 to 12 mm to the lacrimal sac, and 24 mm to the proximal end of the nasolacrimal duct.

UPPER EYELID RECONSTRUCTION

Defects of the upper eyelid may arise from various causes, but tissue loss following tumor resection is the most common indication for reconstruction. Mohs micrographic surgery is frequently employed in the periorbital region, and this technique provides increased certainty of negative margins prior to reconstruction. Less frequently, substantial tissue deficit arising from developmental anomalies or trauma may need to be addressed. As the upper eyelid covers a greater portion of the cornea, it serves a more important role in globe protection than the lower eyelid. Consequently, eyelid reconstruction is indicated in all but a few instances, such as when small defects <5 mm that do not involve the lid margin or canthus may be left to heal.[1] The type of reconstruction strategy employed depends on recognition of anatomic deficits, including vertical and horizontal dimensions, as well as depth. Careful assessment of regional and distant tissue availability is also critical. To approach upper lid reconstruction in an organized manner, eyelid defects are divided into anterior lamellar (partial-thickness) and full-thickness defects according to size.

Anterior Lamellar and Partial-Thickness Defects

The anterior lamella includes the skin and orbicularis oculi muscle of the eyelid, and small defects <5 mm involving only these structures can heal well by secondary intention.[1] Larger defects may result in contracture and lid deformity, necessitating further surgery to address lid retraction or ectropion. For partial-thickness defects involving less than 50% of the upper eyelid, primary closure is ideal, particularly when there is redundant skin adjacent to the defect. When more tissue recruitment is necessary, undermining of the skin and orbicularis muscle with advancement of local myocutaneous flaps are preferred, as they provide optimal color and texture match. Incisions should be concealed in relaxed skin tension lines when this does not result in significant vertical shortening of the anterior lamella, which can produce postoperative eyelid malposition. Vertical scars generally heal well when confined to the eyelid proper and are sometimes necessary to ensure that tension is distributed horizontally rather than vertically within the eyelids.

Primary closure is not typically feasible for larger partial-thickness defects involving greater than 50% of the upper eyelid. In this setting, skin grafts offer adequate replacement of eyelid skin. Full-thickness skin grafts are preferable to split-thickness skin grafts due to less contracture postoperatively. The optimal skin graft donor site for upper eyelid defects is the contralateral upper lid, as this provides skin with thin dermis, minimal hair, and excellent color/texture match. The skin graft can be harvested through a standard blepharoplasty incision, employing nontoothed forceps to pinch excess skin and determine the amount that can be removed safely. Incisions are made with a #15 blade, and Westcott scissors are used to elevate the skin off the orbicularis muscle. After hemostasis is obtained, the donor site is closed with running monofilament sutures and the skin graft is thinned to the rete ridges. Fenestrations or quilting sutures can be placed to prevent accumulation of serosanguinous fluid. The skin graft is secured with interrupted 6-0 or 7-0 absorbable sutures and a skin graft bolster dressing is kept in place for several days. Importantly, grafts may be oversized by approximately 30%, particularly over the preseptal lid to allow for contracture.[2] When there is insufficient contralateral upper eyelid skin, other secondary sites for skin harvest include the preauricular or postauricular region, supraclavicular region, and upper inner arm. Although color and texture match may be less ideal with some of these alternative donor sites, satisfactory results have been reported in up to 95% of patients with only mild complications reported, including hypertrophic scarring in 23% and hypopigmentation in 6%, particularly with supraclavicular and inner arm donor sites.[3]

Full-Thickness Defects

Depending on laxity, full-thickness defects of the upper lid up to 25% of the horizontal length may be closed primarily, though in older patients defects up to 1/3 may be treated in this fashion. Assessment includes pulling the edges together to confirm adequate closure under minimal tension, and if present, consideration can be made to include a lateral canthotomy and cantholysis. Prior to closure, defect margins should be trimmed to create sharp, perpendicular tarsal borders. A wedge can be resected superiorly to create a pentagonal defect with its apex pointing away from the lid margin to allow ends to meet appropriately without lid notching.[4] The lid margin is approximated with 5-0 or 6-0 silk vertical mattress suture placed through the meibomian gland orifices in a far-far, near-near fashion to help evert the wound edges. Three or four partial thickness 5-0 polyglactin sutures are then used to approximate the tarsus. Finally, the skin is closed over the repaired tarsus to complete the layered reconstruction.

Larger full-thickness defects of the upper lid involving 25% to 75% of the lid are typically not amenable to direct closure and are frequently reconstructed with a modified Hughes advancement/sliding tarsoconjunctival flap with skin graft or composite graft covered by a myocutaneous advancement flap. Key to any of these approaches is the re-establishment of a posterior mucosal layer, a structural support layer, and a well-vascularized covering anteriorly. Importantly, 4 mm of tarsus is necessary to maintain stability at the lid margin. If there is sufficient superior tarsus remaining above the defect, an advancement tarsoconjunctival flap may be used to reconstruct the upper lid. To accomplish this, the upper eyelid is everted, and relaxing incisions are made in the conjunctiva on either side of the defect. A tarsoconjunctival flap is then created by dissecting off the anterior orbicularis muscle, levator aponeurosis, and Müller muscle up to the superior fornix, leaving only the conjunctiva attached to the tarsus posteriorly. The flap is advanced inferiorly into the wound on a conjunctival pedicle and the edges are sutured to the marginal tarsus with 5-0 polyglactin sutures. A sliding tarsoconjunctival flap can also be elevated from either the medial or lateral eyelid remnant and swung into an adjacent defect using similar elevation of anterior tissue off the tarsus along with a horizontal relaxing incision in the conjunctiva. With either tarsoconjunctival flap technique, a full-thickness skin graft or a local myocutaneous flap is used for anterior coverage.

Alternatively, composite grafts combined with local myocutaneous advancement flaps can be utilized to address larger full-thickness upper eyelid defects.[5] A free tarsal graft with conjunctiva from the contralateral upper lid is preferred, as both nasal septal cartilage-mucosa and hard palate mucosa grafts are keratinized, potentially placing the cornea at risk of abrasion and damage until metaplasia has occurred. The donor area can be left to heal by secondary intention. Care must be taken, however, to preserve sufficient tarsus inferiorly, as well as to avoid damage to the upper eyelid retractors, as a donor-site complication in the contralateral normal lid could be devastating.

Once the composite graft is inset into the defect and anchored in lamellar fashion to the tarsal remnants and eyelid retractors, a vascularized myocutaneous advancement flap is used to address the anterior lamella. Commonly employed flaps include a sub-brow bipedicled skin-orbicularis oculi muscle flap, paramedian forehead flap, and modified Tenzel flap. The sub-brow myocutaneous orbicularis oculi flap yields excellent postoperative eyelid contour with the benefit of replacing deficient tissue with physiologically similar skin and muscle. It is also a single-staged procedure that maintains adequate eyelid closure due to preserved orbicularis oculi muscle function.[6] The resulting sub-brow defect at the donor site can be managed with a free skin graft obtained from the contralateral upper eyelid.

An inverted, modified Tenzel (semicircular) flap is another valuable single-stage myocutaneous advancement flap that is frequently utilized to close defects encompassing up to two-thirds of the upper eyelid. Extra skin is rotated from the lateral temple and the donor site is closed primarily. An incision is marked in a semicircular manner from the lateral canthus and extends inferiorly; the larger the diameter, the greater the advancement is possible. A skin-muscle flap is undermined in the preseptal plane and kept superficial beyond the orbital rim to avoid injury to the temporal branch of the facial nerve. After flap rotation, the primary defect is closed after removing a Burow triangle, as needed. Given the success of these procedures in reconstructing full-thickness defects of the upper lid, other historical techniques, including the Cutler-Beard flap, have fallen out of favor.

Full-thickness defects involving greater than 75% of the upper eyelid are among some of the most challenging problems to treat given limited donor options. Total or near-total upper eyelid reconstruction can often be approached using a mucosalized tarsal graft and overlying myocutaneous orbicularis oculi flap, as previously discussed, but the graft typically has insufficient horizontal length and needs to be combined with hinged periosteal flaps or other adjunctive techniques. This technique has been shown to result in excellent outcomes, with only occasional need for minor revision surgery necessary.[7]

Outcomes and Prognosis

Outcomes following reconstruction of the upper eyelid can be measured by both function and aesthetics. Asymmetric marginal position, though not a usually serious complication, can nonetheless be frustrating for both the patient and surgeon, and may require further procedures to correct. In most instances, ptosis following eyelid surgery should be monitored for 6 months for spontaneous recovery of function before considering additional revision surgery. The most frequent late complication in patients undergoing upper eyelid surgery is exposure keratopathy, which can be seen in 20%.[8] Other complications following upper eyelid reconstruction include lagophthalmos, lid ectropion, orbital hematoma, corneal injury, and conjunctival scarring/symblepharon. Although greater initial tissue deficits are generally associated with poorer outcomes, the above described techniques routinely yield satisfactory results, even with larger defects, if there is meticulous attention to detail.

LOWER EYELID RECONSTRUCTION

Reconstruction of the lower eyelid follows many of the same principles elaborated above for the upper eyelid. However, although there are many structural similarities between the upper and lower eyelid, special considerations arise specific to the lower lid. Anatomically, the lower eyelid is shorter in height and less mobile, and from a functional standpoint, it contributes minimally to closure. Nonetheless, the lower eyelid is critical for passive corneal coverage, and reconstruction must focus on appropriate lid position and tone. Surgical tension in the lower eyelid should also be directed horizontally in a superolateral direction. Vertical tension can result in entropion, ectropion, or retraction of the lower eyelid, all of which can be difficult to surgically correct secondarily. Finally, in the lower eyelid, attention must be paid to appropriate medial and lateral canthal fixation, which are essential for maintenance of position and contour and the nasolacrimal drainage system, which may need to be addressed in medial defects involving the lower eyelid. Much like the upper eyelid, defects can be considered based on the depth and size, both of which guide selection of the appropriate reconstructive strategy.

Anterior Lamella and Partial-Thickness Defects

Small partial-thickness defects involving the lower eyelid can generally be repaired primarily, although careful attention to the resulting vector forces is required to prevent postoperative eyelid malposition. Local tissue advancement with undermining of the skin and orbicularis muscle is helpful for tissue draping but does not reduce wound tension. Vertical closures should be avoided when possible, as previously discussed.

Larger partial-thickness defects involving greater than 50% of the lower eyelid cannot be closed primarily and require either skin grafting or a local myocutaneous flap. Similar to the upper eyelid, full-thickness skin grafting from the contralateral upper eyelid is preferred, as it contracts less than split-thickness skin grafts and provides for an excellent color and texture match. Alternative donor sites for skin graft harvest include pre- or postauricular and supraclavicular regions when the upper lid is not available. A Frost suspension suture can reduce downward pull on the lower eyelid during the early postoperative period.

Local myocutaneous transposition flaps are also useful to reconstruct larger anterior lamellar defects of the lower eyelid, and temporally hinged monopedicle or bipedicle (Tripier) flaps from the ipsilateral upper lid are two of the most commonly employed (Figure 39.2). The pedicle is kept as wide as possible laterally and should be at least 1:4 in base to length dimensions to preserve vascularity. For more extensive anterior lamellar defects, the myocutaneous transposition flap can be raised in a bipedicle fashion as a *bucket-handle* (Tripier flap).[9] For both techniques, good color match is achieved, donor sites can frequently be closed primarily, reconstruction can proceed without visual field obstruction, and second stage procedures are only occasionally needed.

Full-Thickness Defects

When faced with a full-thickness defect of the lower eyelid, replacement of the anterior and posterior lamella is required, just as in the upper eyelid, to restore adequate function. Lower lid defects in this category can be divided into small deficits involving less than 30% of the lower lid, moderate defects involving 30% to 50% of the lower lid, and large defects greater than 50% of the lower lid. Importantly, adjustments to these guidelines are often required based on the age and tissue characteristics of the individual.

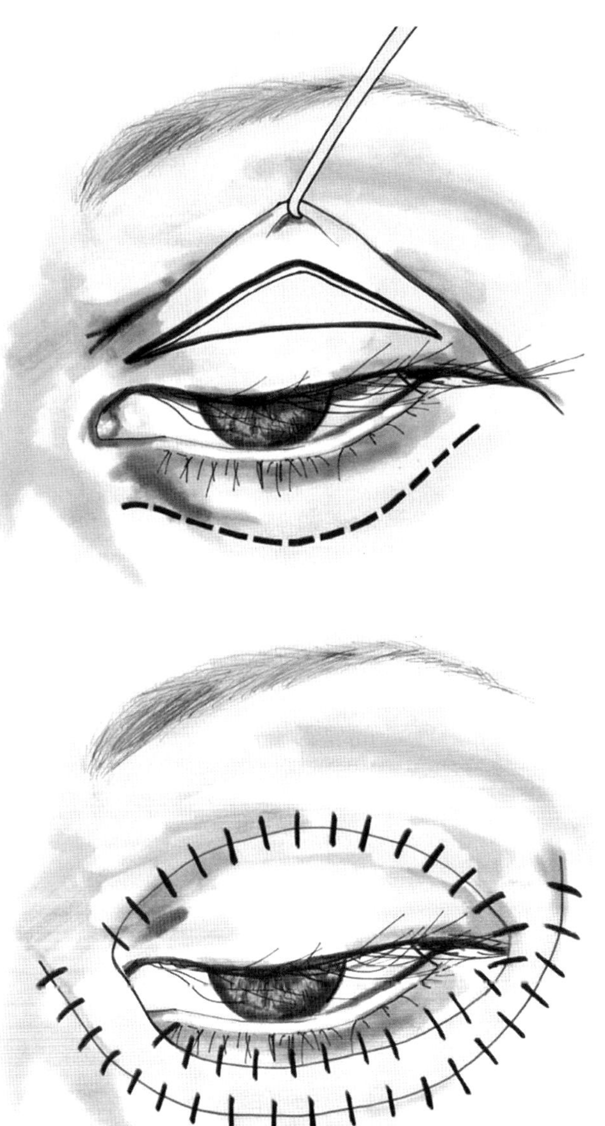

FIGURE 39.2. Schematic of bipedicled Tripier flap elevation from ipsilateral upper eyelid (top) and inset into lower eyelid (bottom).

With defects less than 30% of the eyelid width, primary closure can often be performed, though meticulous reapproximation of the lid margin is key to a satisfactory repair without lid notching. A pentagonal wedge resection with the apex directed inferiorly can be included to avoid a dog-ear deformity. Alternatively, a Burow triangle can be excised after posterior lamellar closure. Primary suture repair of the lower lid can be performed using analogous techniques and materials described for the upper eyelid. When excess tension is encountered, a lateral canthotomy and inferior cantholysis can be considered. The lateral canthotomy should initially be performed with relatively minimal external skin incision in the event that conversion to a Tenzel flap is required. The inferior crus of the split tendon can then be strummed with closed scissors and cut to release the lateral eyelid from the globe and complete the inferior cantholysis. Following the advancement of the lower eyelid, the canthal incision is closed with interrupted 7-0 sutures to reform the lateral canthal angle and prevent rounding of the palpebral fissure.

A Tenzel semicircular rotation flap is typically used to repair lower eyelid defects of moderate size. It involves rotation of a semicircular musculocutaneous tissue beginning at the lateral canthus and

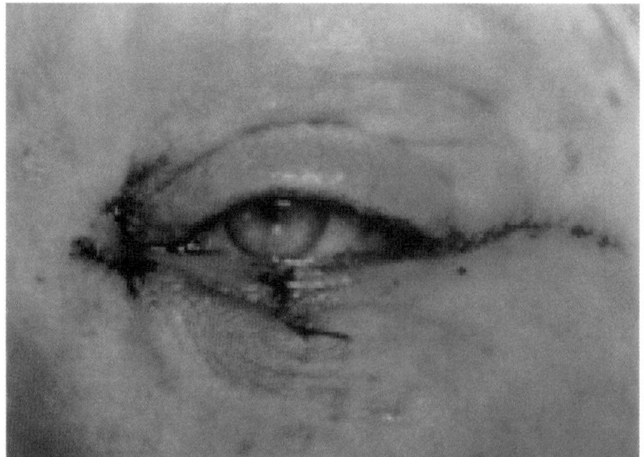

FIGURE 39.3. Photograph of patient following lower eyelid reconstruction with a Tenzel semicircular myocutaneous rotation flap.

extending upward in a semicircular fashion (Figure 39.3). Extensive lateral undermining of the flap with canthotomy and inferior cantholysis is also performed to facilitate the advancement of the eyelid and reapproximation of the tarsal defect with minimal tension. The canthal angle is then reformed by passing 4-0 Vicryl through the remaining superior canthal tendon/periosteum of the orbital rim and the orbicularis muscle on the deep margin of the flap. Other options for the closure include local myocutaneous transposition flaps, in concert with previously described composite grafts or a Hughes sliding tarsoconjunctival flap, although the latter may not be well suited for patients sighted only in the involved eye or in younger patients of amblyogenic age.[10,11]

The largest full-thickness defects of the lower eyelid, particularly those involving the entire lid or with a vertical dimension greater than the horizontal one, are best reconstructed using a Mustarde cheek rotation flap in conjunction with a composite graft or Hughes flap (Figure 39.4). This technique involves rotation of a large skin and muscle flap from the cheek, beginning at the lateral canthal angle and extending upward into the temple region. Marking the flap well above the level of the lateral canthus before extending to the periauricular skin is critical to correctly position the lateral canthal angle. When a Hughes flap is not used for posterior lamellar reconstruction, a temporary tarsorrhaphy is often useful during the initial phase of healing to combat the mechanical effect of edema. Posterior extension proceeds in the subcutaneous plane just anterior to the ear and then inferiorly across the mandible, as needed. A Burow triangle of the skin may need to be excised below the defect to facilitate the inset of the flap. Dermal anchorage of the Mustarde cheek flap to the lateral orbital rim periosteum is also key to minimizing vertical tension on the reconstructed lid.

Outcomes and Prognosis

Complications specific to lower eyelid reconstruction include lower lid laxity and lateral canthal dystopia, marginal ectropion, and lid retraction. These may all arise from inappropriate restoration of lid length or inadequate fixation. Lower lid laxity and lateral tissue sag may develop from overcorrection of horizontal length, as well as poor fixation at the lateral canthus. A lateral tarsal strip procedure or canthoplasty may be necessary to tighten the lower lid in these situations. With ectropion and lid retraction, vertical deficiency may be worsened by gravity and altered lid mobility. Early postoperative swelling can also contribute to mechanical ectropion. A Frost-style traction suture can be placed for 1 week to provide early postoperative lid support. Finally, with excessive scarring after reconstruction, cicatricial ectropion may be noted. This complication has been noted in 5% of patients undergoing lower eyelid reconstruction.[12] In general, scars should be allowed to mature and should not be surgically revised until 6 months or more postoperatively.

CANTHAL RECONSTRUCTION

Medial Canthal Reconstruction

Reconstruction of the medial canthal region is complex due to structures that may be involved and contours that are difficult to recreate. In addition, defects in this region are associated with a high incidence of lacrimal system injury, which may need to be repaired primarily or addressed in delayed fashion. For small defects limited to the anterior lamella, healing by secondary intention can be considered, though full-thickness skin grafting facilitates more expeditious healing. With larger defects, or those lacking sufficient vascularized tissue for skin grafting, a local medially based myocutaneous transposition flap from the upper eyelid can be performed. Alternatively, a glabellar rotation advancement flap may be employed (Figure 39.5).[13] Importantly, thicker flaps result in excess tissue bulk in the normally thin medial canthal region, and occasionally require thinning during a secondary procedure. When the medial canthal tendon is disrupted, fixation of the remaining portion is necessary to restore alignment and lower eyelid support. However, anterior fixation alone may not be adequate to restore lid-globe apposition. Suture fixation to posterior lacrimal crest, miniplate anchoring, or transnasal wiring may also be employed when there is more extensive disruption. Concomitant lacrimal probing or stent placement should be considered in select cases to reduce the risk of kinking the canaliculi and inhibiting lacrimal drainage.

Defects involving the lacrimal system should be fixed in concert with medial canthal reconstruction when possible with minimally invasive techniques. When a dacryocystorhinostomy with or without Jones tube is required, however, repair should be deferred until careful postoperative observation has ensured an acceptably low risk

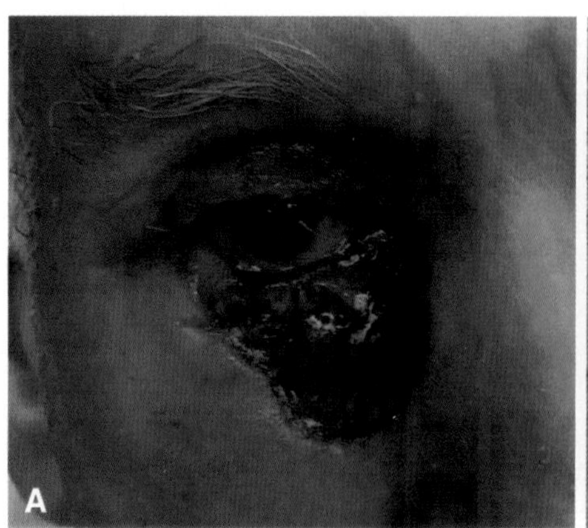

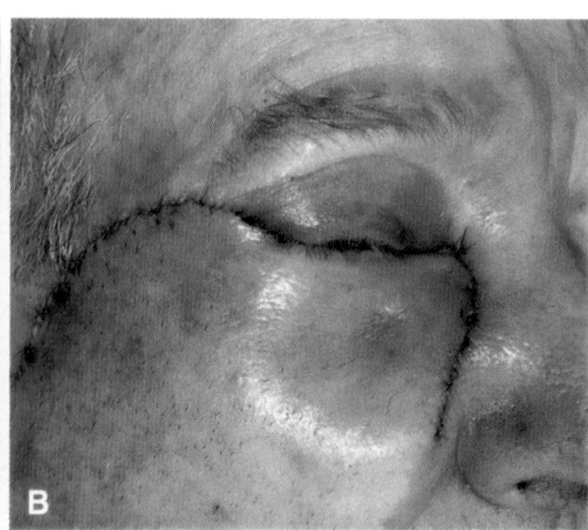

FIGURE 39.4. Lower eyelid Mohs defect **(A)** reconstructed with a Mustarde cheek rotation flap **(B)**.

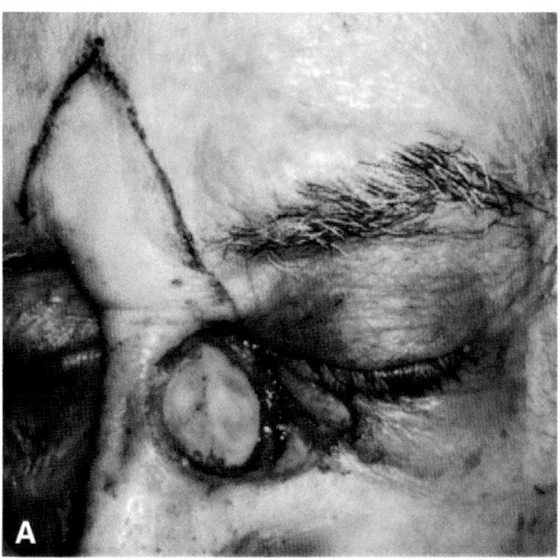

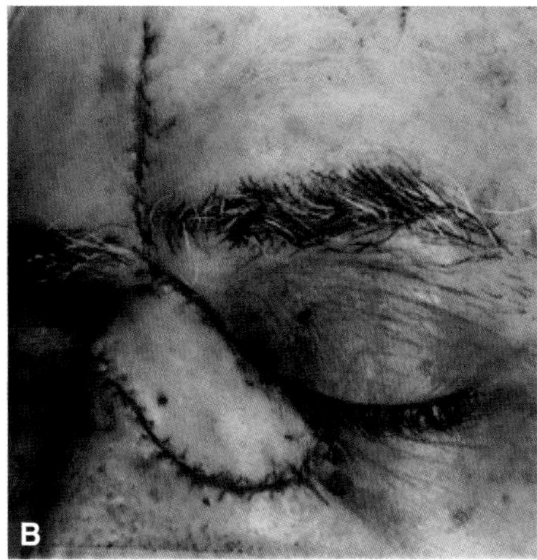

FIGURE 39.5. **A.** Medial canthal defect with glabellar flap marked. **B.** Elevation and inset of glabellar rotation flap into medial canthal defect.

of tumor recurrence has diminished. Partial interruptions of the canaliculus can be repaired over a monocanalicular or bicanalicular silicone stent, which is generally left in place for 3 months before removal. When primary reconstruction is deferred, follow-up evaluation is necessary to determine whether the patient develops epiphora.

Lateral Canthal Reconstruction

Defects in the lateral canthal region may include loss of skin and muscle as well as injury to the lateral canthal tendon. For tissue deficits limited to this region, the quantity of tissue that must be reconstructed is often minimal and may be addressed with full-thickness skin grafts or local advancement flaps. Color and texture match for full-thickness skin grafts can best be achieved by harvesting nearby tissue, and the postauricular donor site is frequently employed with minimal donor-site morbidity. A cheek flap, similar to that described above for lower eyelid defects, is also frequently employed, as are laterally based orbicularis oculi myocutaneous flaps from the upper eyelid region. Restoration of the lateral canthal tendon, if disrupted, is critical. Failure to adequately repair the lateral canthal tendon can result in rounding of the lateral canthus, shortening of the palpebral fissure, lower lid retraction, ectropion, lagophthalmos, and poor lacrimal pump function.[14] Simple disruptions may be primarily repaired with 4-0 polypropylene suture; however, larger defects in the lateral canthal tendon where the proximal end is lost may require suturing the periosteum at the level of Whitnall tubercle or through small drill holes in the lateral orbital rim.

CORRECTION OF EYELID PTOSIS

At rest, the normal upper eyelid position lies in between the pupillary aperture and the superior limbus. Ptosis describes an abnormally low upper eyelid margin in the relaxation, greater than 2 mm below the corneoscleral junction. This can arise from dysfunction of the levator complex (true ptosis) or abnormalities in surrounding anatomy (pseudoptosis), as can be seen in enophthalmos, brow ptosis, or hypertropia. True ptosis can be classified as congenital or acquired, and by etiology including aponeurotic, myogenic/neurogenic, or mechanical. For patients with congenital ptosis, fibrofatty dysgenesis of the levator complex is observed, and ptosis remains relatively constant throughout life until surgery is performed. Poor levator function and lagophthalmos is typically seen on examination of these patients. Various forms of acquired ptosis exist, with levator dehiscence the most common. Classically, ptosis seen from a dehisced levator aponeurosis is associated with a lid crease that is higher and an upper sulcus that is deeper than the uninvolved side. Aponeurotic dehiscence can also be seen following mild trauma or after cataract surgery. Myogenic/neurogenic causes of ptosis are associated with conditions such as myasthenia gravis, oculopharyngeal muscular dystrophy, and idiopathic late-onset familial ptosis. These etiologies are particularly difficult to treat as defects are progressive and ocular surface protective mechanisms function poorly, rendering these patients at heightened risk of corneal complications. Finally, for mechanical causes of ptosis, tumors of the upper eyelid or orbit may present with ptosis, and a careful evaluation of the entire orbit is thus necessary when examining the patient who presents for ptosis correction.

One situation that warrants individual consideration is ptosis seen with the Marcus Gunn jaw-winking phenomenon, which accounts for 2% to 13% of congenital ptosis.[15] Patients with this syndrome demonstrate both a variable degree of ptosis at rest and winking associated with jaw movement, sucking, or swallowing. These findings are as a result of aberrant connections between motor branches of CN V and the superior division of CN III. Both ptosis and winking can be disconcerting for the patient, and surgical approach is highly dependent on which component is responsible for the greater cosmetic defect. Although procedures that shorten the levator aponeurosis can improve the ptosis, patients must also be informed that concomitant increase in wink excursion may be noted. In contrast, severing the levator tendon can reduce winking, but requires placement of a frontalis sling, which will create other significant asymmetries that the patient must be prepared to accept.

Preoperative Evaluation

Examination of the patient who presents with ptosis should begin with a gross evaluation observing lid contour, eyelashes, and skin quality. Particular attention should be paid to the presence and position of the lid fold, as blunting can suggest poor lavatory function, whereas a deep, elevated fold suggests levator dehiscence. Inspection of the brow is also important, given that redundancy of tissue in this region may contribute to ptosis and that elevation can partially mask eyelid ptosis. Pupillary asymmetry (anisocoria) or deficiencies in extraocular muscle function may raise the suspicion of Horner syndrome or CN III palsy as a cause for ptosis. Possible myogenic causes should be pursued in patients with variable or fatigable ptosis. Palpation of the lid may reveal an orbital process, and computed tomography scanning should be considered in appropriate patients as part of a preoperative evaluation. An age-appropriate visual acuity and visual field test should be performed in all patients with ptosis who are able to cooperate. Additional evaluation should include testing orbicularis oculi function, corneal sensation, strength of Bell phenomenon, and in adults with dry eye symptoms, a Schirmer test for tear function. Though not an absolute contraindication to surgery, patients with poor orbicularis function, Bell phenomenon, or tear production may be at increased risk for keratitis following ptosis surgery as any lagophthalmos or corneal exposure may be worsened.

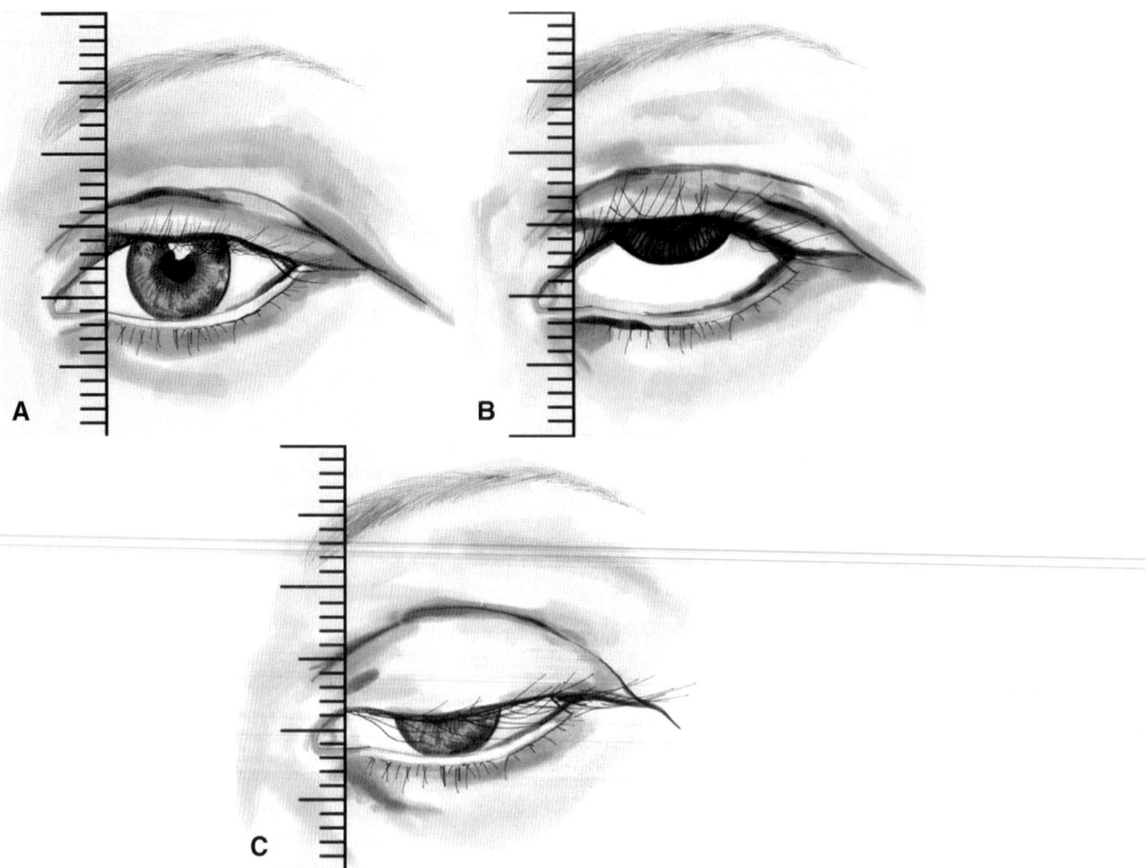

FIGURE 39.6. **A.** Upper eyelid ptosis evaluation with lid position noted first at rest. **B.** Using a ruler, levator excursion is then determined by measuring change in lid position between extreme upgaze **(B)** and extreme downgaze **(C)**.

Accurate quantification of lid ptosis and levator function is critical for selecting the correct surgical approach for ptosis repair. This begins with a measurement of the upper eyelid position in primary position with the brow relaxed (**Figure 39.6**). The adult cornea typically measures 11 mm in height, with the corneal light reflex serving as a useful reference midpoint. A normal upper eyelid margin rests 1 to 2 mm below the superior limbus, and a patient with 3.5 mm of ptosis would therefore be noted to have a resting lid margin at or just above the corneal light reflex. Severity of ptosis is classified as mild (1–2 mm), moderate (2–3 mm), or severe (≥4 mm). Levator function is next evaluated by stabilizing the patient's brow with the examiner's thumb. A ruler is then used to measure maximal excursion of the lid margin from extreme upgaze to extreme downgaze (see Figure 39.6). Normal excursion is usually greater than 12 mm. Levator function in the patient with ptosis is classified as good (≥8 mm), fair (5–7 mm), and poor (≤4 mm). Finally, evaluation of the sympathetically innervated Müller muscle function can be performed by instilling 2.5% phenylephrine eye drops and evaluating changes to marginal reflex distance after 10 minutes.[16] For patients with mild to moderate ptosis and good levator function, this test has been thought to accurately predict final eyelid position with a Müller muscle–conjunctiva resection.

The goals of surgical correction for ptosis are to elevate the lid position and restore the upper eyelid fold. Inherent anatomic defects, such as those seen in congenital ptosis, may limit the ability to achieve these goals, and an understanding of these constraints is necessary before proceeding with surgery. In children, general anesthesia is typically required, but in adults, local anesthesia may be preferred as it allows for patient cooperation in adjusting the lid height. Several procedures are routinely performed for correction of ptosis, including a Müller muscle–conjunctiva resection, levator advancement, and frontalis sling. The degree of eyelid ptosis and levator excursion measured preoperatively help to guide selection of proper surgical approach.

Müller Muscle–Conjunctiva Resection

Patients who demonstrate mild ptosis (2–3 mm), good levator excursion, and an appropriate phenylephrine test are good candidates for Müller muscle–conjunctiva resection. Posterior ptosis surgery was initially described by Fasanella and Servat, but subsequent modifications by Putterman have resulted in improved predictability and minimized anatomic disruption. In brief, the anesthetized eyelid is everted over a retractor, a graded quantity of conjunctiva and underlying Müller muscle are tented up and purchased with a Putterman clamp.[17] The edges are then sutured and the excess tissue excised. Importantly, although this technique offers a rapid approach to ptosis correction without need to significant dissection, there is little room for intraoperative adjustment and violation of the conjunctival surface may increase risk for postoperative corneal irritation. Consequently, proper patient selection for a modified Müller muscle–conjunctiva resection is critical.

Levator Advancement and Levator Repair

The levator advancement is a versatile procedure that can appropriately address patients with mild to moderate ptosis and fair to good levator excursion (≥5 mm). This approach is widely applicable to patients with senescent/involutional ptosis, traumatic ptosis, and even some with congenital ptosis who have some preserved levator function. A similar anterior approach is taken following placement of anesthetic eyedrops and injection of local anesthesia. The orbital septum is opened and the underlying preaponeurotic fat pad gently dissected from the underlying levator musculoaponeurotic complex.

The levator is then advanced and secured to the tarsal plate using interrupted lamellar mattress sutures. These are temporally tied and cooperative patient's lid height and contour can then be evaluated in a seated position with the operating room lights dimmed.

If epinephrine is used in the local anesthetic, an additional 1 to 1.5 mm of overcorrection may be necessary to account for Müller muscle stimulation. Once the lid position is set, the sutures are tied permanently. Restoration of the upper eyelid crease can be achieved through reattachment of the orbicularis muscle to the levator aponeurosis. Though this technique is quite versatile for treating many causes of ptosis, with overall success rates of 76% to 85% reported.[18,19] Both under- and overcorrection have been observed, with preoperative levator function, one of the most significant predictors of surgical outcome. Considerable dissection and consequent edema can also make intraoperative adjustments difficult. Of note, predictability for bilateral levator advancement is diminished due to Herring phenomenon, and postoperative surprises are more common.

Frontalis Sling

In patients with variable degrees of ptosis and poor levator excursion (≤4 mm), as can be seen in patients with congenital ptosis, elevation of the upper eyelid can best be accomplished through suspension to the frontalis muscle. Elevation of the lid is therefore coupled to elevation of the brow. A variety of materials can be used, with silicone, autologous fascia lata, and palmaris longus tendon among the more common choices.

Many different techniques have been described to create the frontalis sling, but the double rhomboid design remains the most often used (Figure 39.7). Three incisions are made in the brow in line with the lateral canthus, the center of the lid, and the medial canthus. Although analogous stab incisions may be made above the ciliary margin in young children, an open lid crease technique with tarsal dissection and sling fixation is typically performed in older patients. A Wright fascia needle is then passed starting from the brow incisions in a preperiosteal plane, exiting the lid incisions in the postorbicularis fascia plane. Care should be taken to avoid excessively superficial or deep passage.

Regardless of the material used and whether an open or closed lid technique, each rhomboid is independently tightened from the lateral or medial brow incision. Lagophthalmos is common and must be managed appropriately with liberal ocular surface lubrication. A temporary suture tarsorrhaphy, Frost suture, or bandage contact lens can be helpful in the early postoperative period. A recent review of studies evaluating treatment of unilateral congenital ptosis with fascia lata slings found good or excellent eyelid height in 85% of patients and excellent symmetry within 1 mm of the contralateral lid in 80% of patients.[20] However, lid lag was the most frequently noted complication present in 90%.[21]

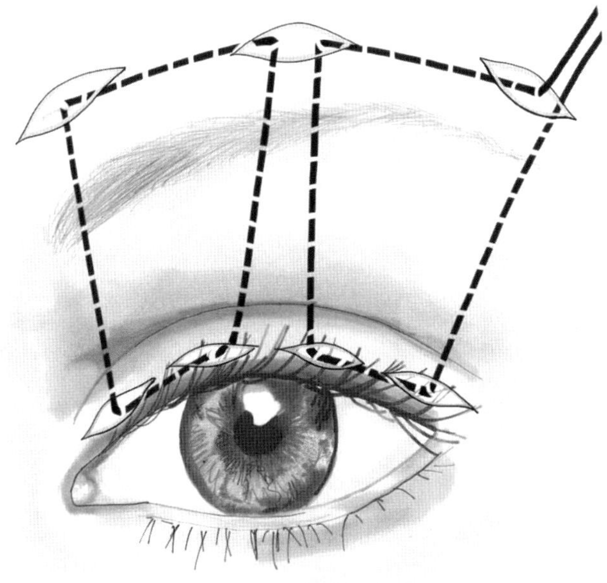

FIGURE 39.7. Schematic of the frontalis sling. Autologous fascia is tunneled in a preperiosteal plane using a double rhomboid design, coupling eyelid elevation with the brow.

Outcomes and Prognosis

Common complications following ptosis correction include eyelid asymmetry, which can result from undercorrection, overcorrection, or discrepancies in lid contour. Undercorrection is most frequently observed and may arise from inadequate advancement of the levator or postoperative relaxation of a frontalis sling. Early postoperative adjustment can be considered before tissue planes have healed. With undercorrection, the mechanical effect of lid edema must be factored into any decision to pursue correction, whereas some cases of less severe overcorrection can be managed conservatively with massage and stretching.

Lagophthalmos, exposure keratitis, and corneal abrasions are also quite common and must be managed appropriately to address patient discomfort and prevent ocular surface complications. In certain procedures, such as with a frontalis sling, persistent postoperative lagophthalmos is expected, and patients should be appropriately counseled. Transient and mild exposure keratitis is frequently noted after a variety of surgical procedures, and when symptomatic, liberal use of ointment is recommended. However, good to excellent results are frequently obtained with proper evaluation of the patient and selection of the procedure, and when surgeries are performed by experienced surgeons.

CANTHOPLASTY AND TREATMENT OF ECTROPION

The lower eyelid margin typically rests at or near the inferior limbus, with the nadir of the curvature slightly temporal to the midpupillary axis. In the normal setting, the lid rests in approximation with the globe, held by a balance of vector forces and tension. Malposition of the lid arises from an imbalance in these forces, and the most commonly resulting malposition is ectropion. This abnormal eversion of the lid margin away from the globe may lead to corneal exposure, keratinization of the conjunctiva, and in severe cases, corneal scarring or ulceration with vision loss. Patients with ectropion complain of eye irritation and tearing. Except when secondary to acute facial nerve palsy, patients may have symptoms for months or years before seeking treatment.

The incidence of lower lid ectropion has been estimated at 2.9%, and causes may be related to congenital or acquired conditions.[22] Congenital ectropion is rarely isolated and may be associated with blepharophimosis syndrome, microphthalmos, and ichthyosis. Acquired ectropion is most commonly involutional in nature, but paralytic, cicatricial, or mechanical causes may also result in lower lid malposition. Involutional ectropion occurs with increased horizontal lid laxity due to age-related weakness in canthal ligaments and pretarsal orbicularis muscle, often coupled with disinsertion of the capsulopalpebral fascia. Patients with negative orbital vectors are also at increased risk as 92% of eyelids with involutional ectropion have been noted to have this orbital relationship.[23] Other causes of acquired ectropion include facial nerve palsy, scarring of the anterior and/or midlamella, disinsertion of capsulopalpebral fascia, and lower eyelid tumors, such as neurofibromas.

Evaluation of the patient with lower lid malposition begins with a general appraisal of the patient's history, including symptoms, prior surgical scars or burns, and history of cancers, masses, or connective tissue disorders. Malar support should also be inspected, noting whether the patient has a *positive vector*, where soft tissues overlying the infraorbital rim project beyond the eye, or *negative vector*, where absence of rigid structural support and soft tissues in the lower lid produce a globe that is more prominent (Figure 39.8). Visual acuity

HEAD AND NECK

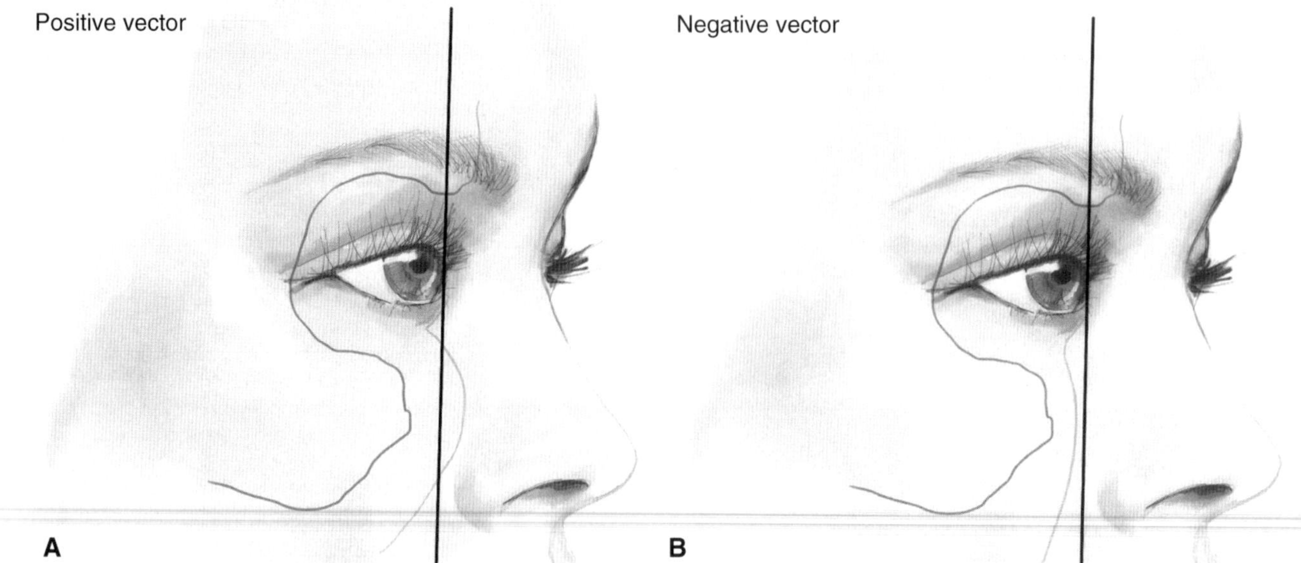

FIGURE 39.8. Schematics of patient with positive vector **(A)**, where soft tissues project beyond the eye, and negative vector **(B)**, where structural support and soft tissues are deficient resulting in more prominent globe.

should be documented, and examination of the cornea should be performed to identify signs of corneal exposure and conjunctival keratinization. A distraction test and snap-back test are also important components for evaluation of lower lid laxity.

Care for the patient with lower lid laxity begins with lubrication if significant corneal exposure is present. Taping of the inferolateral canthal skin in a superolateral direction may also provide temporary relief. Surgical correction of ectropion is dependent on the etiology of lid malposition and includes tarsal tuck, lateral tarsal strip, and canthoplasty/canthopexy procedures. Importantly, the terms canthoplasty and canthopexy describe distinct procedures. Though both are designed to provide support to the lower eyelid, canthopexy sutures tighten the lid without severing the lateral canthal tendon. In contrast, a lateral canthoplasty detaches part or all of the lateral canthal tendon to reposition the lower eyelid orientation and/or tighten the tendon. Although more powerful than a canthopexy, a canthoplasty may have greater risk of rounding at the reconstructed canthus.

Tarsal Tuck Canthopexy

The tarsal tuck procedure is simple canthopexy used to tighten and stabilize the lower eyelid in patients with mild lid laxity. Patients with minimal distensibility and a firm snap back of the lower lid may be candidates for this type of lid tightening. It provides support without shortening the lid and can be performed alone or in concert with other procedures such as lower lid blepharoplasty. Through a transcutaneous approach, such as a subciliary incision when combined with a blepharoplasty, or transconjunctival approach, the lateral tarsal plate is grasped and sutured to the periosteum on the inside aspect of the lateral orbital rim using 4-0 polydioxanone. In this fashion, the lateral tarsus is *tucked* inside the rim and the lateral canthus is elevated. In patients with mild lid laxity and an intact lateral canthal tendon complex, the tarsal tuck procedure can provide excellent results.[24] However, in patients with more significant lid laxity, increased tucking required may result in bunching of tissue and the lower lid may lose its apposition to the globe. In such patients, a lateral tarsal strip should instead be performed.

Lateral Tarsal Strip

The lateral tarsal strip canthoplasty is a useful technique to address most patients with involutional ectropion and may be an important adjunct in the treatment of lower lid laxity secondary to paralytic and cicatricial etiologies. Patients with greater lid distensibility and abnormal snap back are better candidates for canthoplasty procedures as opposed to canthopexy. Though many methods have been described for correction of significant lower lid laxity, including wedge resections and the Kuhnt-Szymanowski procedure, tightening with a lateral tarsal strip has gained ascendency due to restoration of a sharp lateral canthal angle and avoidance of layered closure of the lid margin, with associated risk of trichiasis and notching.

A lateral canthotomy and inferior cantholysis are first performed. The anterior and posterior lamella are then split along the gray line, and the mucocutaneous junction is then excised, forming a lateral tarsal strip (**Figure 39.9**). Tension is then assessed, and the strip shortened as needed. The lateral strip of tarsus is then secured

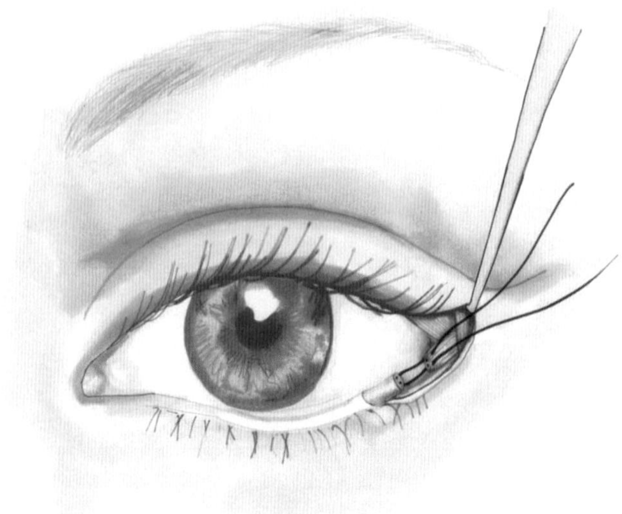

FIGURE 39.9. Schematic of lateral tarsal strip canthoplasty. The lateral portion of the lower eyelid tarsus is exposed, shortened, and secured to the inside aspect of the lateral orbit rim to increase lower lid tension.

to the inside aspect of the lateral orbital rim at Whitnall tubercle using 4-0 polypropylene with periosteal suture passes. A triangle of redundant anterior lamella and lashes is then excised and the lateral canthal angle reformed. Skin and orbicularis are then closed simultaneously. For repair of frank ectropion, reinsertion of the capsulopalpebral fascia via a transconjunctival approach is often required as well to produce a durable result. In cases of cicatricial malposition, adjunctive techniques such as sub-orbicularis fat lift, scar release with or without tissue transposition, or skin grafting may also be required.

The lateral tarsal strip is a well-recognized means for correcting lower lid laxity secondary to a wide array of etiologies and is the first-line procedure for involutional ectropion with excess horizontal lid laxity, although adjunctive procedures such as retractor reinsertion are necessary in some cases. The success rate for lateral tarsal strip canthoplasty alone has been reported to be 87%.[25] Complications associated with this procedure include lateral canthal irregularity with or without trichiasis and recurrence of laxity. In addition, when there is a failure to recognize concomitant involutional changes in the upper eyelid, tightening of the lower eyelid may result in the upper lid prolapsing over the lower lid margin and irritation of the upper eyelid palpebral conjunctiva from eyelashes. In these cases, the upper lid should be concomitantly shortened to avoid a lid length discrepancy.

Canthoplasty

Though the lateral tarsal strip canthoplasty remains one of the most frequently employed techniques to address lower lid laxity, a lateral canthoplasty may sometimes be necessary. Mobilization of both the upper crus and lower crus of the lateral canthal tendon can lengthen the palpebral fissure and reorient the position of the entire lateral canthus. Common approaches are via a temporal lid crease incision or transverse lateral canthal incision, the latter provides more clear exposure of the lateral canthal tendon complex but may be avoided when other surgical incisions are planned. Depending on the degree of tendinous laxity, division of the tendon body from the underlying periosteum may or may not be required. The crura of the tendon must be securely captured to reduce the risk of slippage. As with a lateral tarsal strip, periosteal anchoring is then performed well inside the lateral orbital rim to restore the vector forces for appropriate lid–globe apposition. In the reconstructive procedures where the soft tissue has insufficient integrity, a local periosteal flap or fascial graft can provide reinforcement.[26] Direct anchoring to bone is another alternative for fixation in these situations.[27] Complications following these procedures are infrequent and most commonly minor. Chemosis may occur but is generally short-lived and rarely requires a temporary tarsorrhaphy suture. Importantly, when an improper vector of fixation of established, lower eyelid displacement away from the globe may occur. Recurrence may occur in cases where robust tendon or periosteal fixation is not achieved, the eyelids are too lax to realistically be repositioned appropriately without a lateral tarsal strip procedure, or where other periocular vector forces are not fully addressed.

Outcomes and Prognosis

Complications following correction of lower lid laxity are primarily related to conjunctival and corneal exposure. Often temporary, these can nonetheless result in troublesome pain and epiphora, and it is not uncommon for patients to report discomfort at the lateral canthal region for several weeks following surgery. When severe, conjunctival keratinization and corneal breakdown can be noted. Other complications reported include hematoma, suture granulomas, and, rarely, wound infection. Recurrent lid malposition can be noted in up to 20% of patients, though this may be related to poor or inadequate repositioning of the lateral canthal tendon.[25]

REFERENCES

1. Lowry JC, Bartley GB, Garrity JA. The role of second-intention healing in periocular reconstruction. *Ophthalmic Plast Reconstr Surg*. 1997;13(3):174-188.
2. Morley AM, deSousa JL, Selva D, Malhotra R. Techniques of upper eyelid reconstruction. *Surv Ophthalmol*. 2010;55(3):256-271.
3. Rathore DS, Chickadasarahilli S, Crossman R, et al. Full thickness skin grafts in periocular reconstructions: long-term outcomes. *Ophthalmic Plast Reconstr Surg*. 2014;30(6):517-520.
4. Pham RT. Reconstruction of the upper eyelid. *Otolaryngol Clin North Am*. 2005;38(5):1023-1032.
5. Alghoul M, Pacella SJ, McClellan WT, Codner MA. Eyelid reconstruction. *Plast Reconstr Surg*. 2013;132(2):288e-302e.
6. Paarlberg JC, van den Bosch WA, Paridaens D. Reconstruction following subtotal full-thickness upper eyelid resection with preservation of the lid margin. *Orbit*. 2007;26(4):319-321.
7. Patrinely JR, O'Neal KD, Kersten RC, Soparkar CN. Total upper eyelid reconstruction with mucosalized tarsal graft and overlying bipedicle flap. *Arch Ophthalmol*. 1999;117(12):1655-1661.
8. Poh EW, O'Donnell BA, McNab AA, et al. Outcomes of upper eyelid reconstruction. *Ophthalmology*. 2014;121(2):612-613 e611.
This article reviewed 126 upper eyelid reconstructions following tumor resection to evaluate techniques used, outcomes, and postoperative complications. Tarsoconjunctival flaps were most frequently employed, as it avoided injury to the contralateral upper eyelid and can be performed as a single-stage procedure. The most common postoperative complications that the authors noted were exposure keratopathy and lagophthalmos. This article demonstrates the challenges in obtaining optimal functional results in reconstructing the upper eyelid and helps the clinician set postoperative expectations.
9. Elliot D, Britto JA. Tripier's innervated myocutaneous flap 1889. *Br J Plast Surg*. 2004;57(6):543-549.
10. Santos G, Goulao J. One-stage reconstruction of full-thickness lower eyelid using a Tripier flap lining by a septal mucochondral graft. *J Dermatolog Treat*. 2014;25(5):446-447.
11. Hawes MJ, Grove AS Jr, Hink EM. Comparison of free tarsoconjunctival grafts and Hughes tarsoconjunctival grafts for lower eyelid reconstruction. *Ophthalmic Plast Reconstr Surg*. 2011;27(3):219-223.
This study highlights the utility of free autogenous tarsoconjunctival grafts for reconstruction of mucosalized lining and structural support, as they possess normal eyelid features and lack keratinized mucosa which may irritate the cornea. Over a 15-year period, 70 patients with lower eyelid full-thickness defects were evaluated. Free tarsal grafts in association with myocutaneous advancement flaps were found to effectively reconstruct these defects and were less likely to require subsequent revision surgery compared to Hughes tarsoconjunctival flaps with skin grafts.
12. Fogagnolo P, Colletti G, Valassina D, et al. Partial and total lower lid reconstruction: our experience with 41 cases. *Ophthalmologica*. 2012;228(4):239-243.
13. Meadows AE, Manners RM. A simple modification of the glabellar flap in medial canthal reconstruction. *Ophthalmic Plast Reconstr Surg*. 2003;19(4):313-315.
14. Spinelli HM, Jelks GW. Periocular reconstruction: a systematic approach. *Plast Reconstr Surg*. 1993;91(6):1017-1024.
15. Sobel RK, Allen RC. Incidence of bilateral Marcus Gunn jaw-wink. *Ophthalmic Plast Reconstr Surg*. 2014;30(3):e54-e55.
16. Barsegian A, Botwinick A, Reddy HS. The phenylephrine test revisited. *Ophthalmic Plast Reconstr Surg*. 2018;34(2):151-154.
17. Putterman AM, Fett DR. Muller's muscle in the treatment of upper eyelid ptosis: a ten-year study. *Ophthalmic Surg*. 1986;17(6):354-360.
This study presents long-term outcomes for upper eyelid ptosis repair using a modified Fasanella-Servat tarsoconjunctival Müllerectomy, which is the most commonly employed technique for mild ptosis in patients responsive to phenylephrine eye drops. As described by Putterman, this simple approach removes 3 mm of Müller's muscle and 3 mm upper tarsal plate to achieve lid lifting, with minimal dissection required. In a ten-year study, Putterman found that lid position in 90% of patients with acquired ptosis and 100% of patients with congenital ptosis were still within 1.5 mm of the contralateral eyelid, demonstrating this strategy to be effective and the results durable.
18. Cates CA, Tyers AG. Outcomes of anterior levator resection in congenital blepharoptosis. *Eye (Lond)*. 2001;15(Pt 6):770-773.
19. Innocenti A, Mori F, Melita D, et al. Evaluation of long-term outcomes of correction of severe blepharoptosis with advancement of external levator muscle complex: descriptive statistical analysis of the results. *In Vivo*. 2017;31(1):111-115.
20. Bernardini FP, Cetinkaya A, Zambelli A. Treatment of unilateral congenital ptosis: putting the debate to rest. *Curr Opin Ophthalmol*. 2013;24(5):484-487.
This review elaborates relevant points on frontalis suspension with respect to selection of sling material, surgical steps, and techniques that can improve operative outcomes. It provides an analysis of sling materials, finding autologous fascia lata to be the gold standard material in patients with congenital ptosis and poor levator function. This article also highlights that preoperative spontaneous unilateral brow elevation is critical in achieving optimal surgical outcomes for unilateral congenital ptosis.
21. Bernardini FP, Devoto MH, Priolo E. Treatment of unilateral congenital ptosis. *Ophthalmology*. 2007;114(3):622-623.
22. Damasceno RW, Osaki MH, Dantas PE, Belfort R Jr. Involutional entropion and ectropion of the lower eyelid: prevalence and associated risk factors in the elderly population. *Ophthalmic Plast Reconstr Surg*. 2011;27(5):317-320.

This key ophthalmologic survey was performed on 24,565 patients to evaluate the prevalence of involutional entropion and ectropion, as well as symptoms and association with axial globe projection. The prevalence of involutional ectropion was found to be 2.9%: 5.1% in men and 1.5% in women. Chronic conjunctivitis was significantly more common in patients with involutional ectropion, as was axial ocular globe projection, which was noted to play a pathogenic role in involutional lower eyelid malposition. The findings in this study reinforce the importance of evaluating malar support in patients with lower lid laxity.

23. Rajabi MT, Gholipour F, Ramezani K, et al. The influence of orbital vector on involutional entropion and ectropion. *Orbit*. 2018;37(1):53-58.
24. Jordan DR, Anderson RL. The tarsal tuck procedure: avoiding eyelid retraction after lower blepharoplasty. *Plast Reconstr Surg*. 1990;85(1):22-28.
25. Kam KY, Cole CJ, Bunce C, et al. The lateral tarsal strip in ectropion surgery: is it effective when performed in isolation? *Eye (Lond)*. 2012;26(6):827-832.
26. McCord CD Jr, Ellis DS. The correction of lower lid malposition following lower lid blepharoplasty. *Plast Reconstr Surg*. 1993;92(6):1068-1072.
27. McCord CD, Boswell CB, Hester TR. Lateral canthal anchoring. *Plast Reconstr Surg*. 2003;112(1):222-237.

QUESTIONS

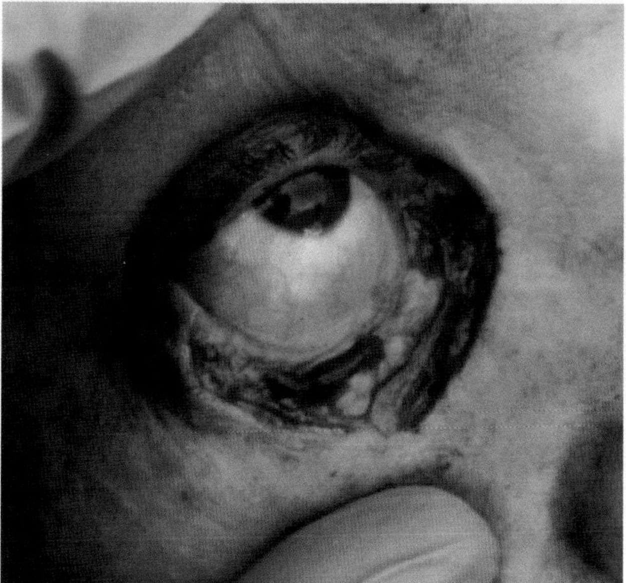

FIGURE 39.10.

1. **A 56-year-old man undergoes Mohs micrographic resection of a lower eyelid basal cell carcinoma and presents for reconstruction of the defect pictured in Figure 39.10. Which of the following reconstructive approaches will provide the best functional and aesthetic outcome for this patient?**
   a. Primary closure with resection of a Burow triangle
   b. Mustarde cheek advancement flap with composite graft
   c. Ipsilateral tarsal conjunctival graft and full-thickness skin graft
   d. Bipedicled Tripier flap from ipsilateral upper eyelid
   e. Cutler-Beard flap

2. **Among patients undergoing reconstructive surgery for upper eyelid defects, what is the most common late postoperative complication observed?**
   a. Corneal abrasion
   b. Wound dehiscence
   c. Exposure keratopathy
   d. Lagophthalmos
   e. Upper eyelid entropion

3. **A 58-year-old woman comes to the clinic for treatment of eyelid asymmetry. Her upper eyelid creases are asymmetric, with the left crease slightly higher than the right, and the left upper eyelid resting 4.5 mm below the superior limbus. Testing of levator excursion reveals 6 mm on the left. A levator advancement is performed, setting the upper eyelid at the level of the superior limbus. However, on postoperative examination, the patient is noted to have mild undercorrection. What is the most appropriate management?**
   a. Institute upper eyelid massage
   b. Surgical correction with levator recession
   c. Revision with frontalis sling
   d. Observation
   e. Liberal use of eye ointment

4. **A 7-year-old boy is brought to the office because of ptosis, which has been present since birth. On examination, the left upper eyelid is noted to rest 5 mm below the superior limbus and levator excursion is 4 mm. What is the most common complication seen following ptosis repair in this patient?**
   a. Peaking of the lid
   b. Lid lag
   c. Late granulomatous inflammatory reaction
   d. Exposure keratitis
   e. Ptosis relapse

5. **A 62-year-old woman comes to the office complaining of chronic right eye irritation and tearing. No prior surgical procedures have been performed on her eyelids. On examination, a snap-back test is performed, and the lower eyelid returns to its original position after 4 seconds. Malar support is found to be poor, and bony support and soft tissue are deficient, resulting in the patient's globe resting in a more prominent position. No visual abnormalities are noted on examination. What is the most appropriate management for this patient?**
   a. Temporary tarsorrhaphy
   b. Tarsal tuck procedure
   c. Lateral tarsal strip procedure
   d. Reorientation of the upper and lower canthal crus with direct bone anchoring
   e. Scar release with full-thickness skin grafting

1. **Answer: b.** In a defect involving both anterior and posterior lamella, a mucosalized posterior lining, structural support layer, and anterior skin must all be addressed. Among the choices, a Mustarde cheek advancement flap with composite graft best addresses the patient's lower eyelid tissue deficiencies. An ipsilateral tarsal conjunctival graft provides a mucosalized posterior surface and structural support whereas the Mustarde cheek advancement flap provides a vascularized replacement for the anterior skin. Primary closure is appropriate for small deficits involving less than 30% of the lower lid, and when employed, a Burow triangle may need to be excised inferiorly after closure of the posterior lamella. At least one lamella must have an intact blood supply when reconstructing either upper or lower eyelid, therefore an ipsilateral tarsal conjunctival graft and full-thickness skin graft would be inappropriate. A bipedicled Tripier flap from the ipsilateral upper eyelid may provide adequate vascularized tissue for anterior lamellar reconstruction but would still require posterior lining and structural support. Finally, a Cutler-Beard flap is a technique for addressing full-thickness defects of the upper eyelid using full-thickness skin, lid retractors, and conjunctiva from the lower eyelid, although this has fallen out of favor given the success of other procedures and the need for extended visual obstruction until the pedicle is divided.

2. **Answer: c.** In a retrospective multicenter study evaluating upper eyelid reconstruction following tumor excision, the most frequent late postoperative complication noted was exposure keratopathy.[8]

3. **Answer: d.** This patient most likely presents with involutional or senile ptosis. Levator advancement is a versatile approach that is frequently employed for such a patient with moderate ptosis (2–3 mm) and fair levator excursion (5–7 mm). Undercorrection is one of the most common complications following ptosis surgery, even when overcorrection is performed

intraoperatively to account for Müller muscle stimulation by local anesthetic with epinephrine. Preoperative levator function has been shown to be a significant predictor of surgical outcome with greater excursion associated with better outcomes. Patients with mild undercorrection noted in the immediate postoperative period can be managed with observation, as mild paresis of the levator muscle may occur following intraoperative manipulation, and these patients may note improvement with time. Significant undercorrection, however, can be adjusted in the early postoperative period within 48 to 72 hours before significant healing has occurred. Upper eyelid massage and surgical correction with levator recession are procedures used to address early and persistent overcorrection, respectively. Occasionally, when severe ptosis with poor excursion of the levator muscle is corrected with a levator advancement, a frontalis sling may be more appropriate and necessary in revision surgery when undercorrection remains persistent. Eye ointment can be used for patients with symptoms of exposure keratitis and lagophthalmos following eyelid surgery.

4. **Answer: b.** This patient presents with congenital ptosis classified as moderate (2–3 mm), as the normal upper eyelid margin rests 1 to 2 mm below the superior limbus and poor levator excursion (≤4 mm). In most cases, a myogenic developmental abnormality in the levator complex is the underlying cause, and the most frequently performed procedure for correction is frontalis suspension using fascia lata. A recent review of patients undergoing fascia lata sling noted lid lag in 90% of patients. Fortunately, in the pediatric population, this is well tolerated, and only 10% noted this to have an aesthetic impact.[20]

5. **Answer: c.** The patient's symptoms and presentation are consistent with involutional ectropion. This patient also has a negative vector. With a snap back test of 4 seconds, this patient has grade II laxity. A lateral tarsal strip procedure is one of the most useful techniques to address patients with involutional ectropion and moderate lid laxity on snap back. This technique restores a sharp lateral canthal angle without the need for layered lid margin closure and has reduced risk of trichiasis and notching. A temporary tarsorrhaphy is rarely required to address postoperative chemosis and does not address the underlying lower lid laxity in this patient. A tarsal tuck canthopexy can be appropriate for some patients with minimal distensibility and a firm snap back of the lower eyelid, although in this patient a tarsal tuck canthopexy would likely provide inadequate tightening. Reorientation of the upper and lower canthal crus and anchorage to bone may be necessary in reconstructive procedures where the soft tissue or local periosteal flap have insufficient integrity. Finally, a scar release with full-thickness skin grafting would be appropriate for patients with cicatricial ectropion.

CHAPTER 40 Nasal Reconstruction

Akhil K. Seth and Evan Matros

KEY POINTS

- The subunit concept is critical to consider in nasal reconstruction.
- Consider each nasal layer separately.
- Each anatomic area has a unique reconstructive solution (e.g. bilobed flaps are used on tip and ala, not the dorsum).
- The forehead flap is the workhouse for large and composite defect.

CONCEPTUAL CONSIDERATIONS

Nasal reconstruction represents one of the most nuanced fields within reconstructive plastic surgery. Globally, reconstruction of the nose can often require multiple stages of surgery and revision to achieve the desired final surgical result. Following restoration of nasal structural integrity, additional procedures may be required to improve appearance given the importance of the nose as a major esthetic unit of facial feature. Therefore, the plastic surgeon must be able to formulate a longitudinal vision for how to progressively execute each stage of reconstruction. Preoperative planning is the most important aspect of successful reconstruction. Also integral to this vision is its appropriate alignment with the goals and expectations of the patient. For a given nasal defect, a wide array of reconstructive options may be available to the patients, ranging from a skin graft to a forehead flap. Different reconstructive options must be considered and individualized to each patient following a thorough discussion of their priorities and willingness to invest in potentially multiple procedures. Successful nasal reconstruction requires that the surgical plan be formulated in conjunction with the patient throughout the reconstructive process.

Appropriate planning for any reconstructive procedure includes performing a thorough history and physical exam. A significant number of nasal reconstructions will be done following the resection of skin cancer, which is often associated with senescence. Therefore, review of any relevant medical comorbidities is important, including their impact on the patient's safety in the setting of general anesthesia. An active smoking history is of particular concern and should be a relative contraindication to certain forms of nasal reconstruction given the increased risk of wound complications. Previous facial surgery should be discussed, in particular an examination of any previous scars on the face or neck. In addition, any history of radiation to the region should be reviewed, as this can decrease the compliance of the surrounding soft tissue, thus precluding the use of local tissue for reconstruction. Physical exam, in addition to a thorough assessment of the nose and nasal defect itself, should include an assessment of forehead height and the surrounding skin quality and laxity.

In the patient with an oncologic defect, confirmation of final negative tumor margins is critical prior to beginning the reconstructive process. Temporary moist dressings can be placed on a defect until margin clearance is confirmed. In the setting of an aggressive tumor, the plastic surgeon should discuss with the oncologic surgeon regarding expectations for tumor clearance and recurrence as these may influence the choice of reconstruction. Strong consideration should be given to delaying the definitive reconstruction in those patients receiving adjuvant radiation therapy. In this setting, patients in whom a locoregional flap would be the appropriate definitive reconstruction can be temporized with a skin graft closure. For larger defects, such as a total rhinectomy, a nasal prosthesis can be constructed for temporary or permanent use.

SKIN QUALITY

The appropriate planning of any nasal reconstruction requires an understanding of the native skin of the nose. In particular, the nose is unique in that there are dramatic differences in skin quality over a relatively small surface area.[1] Cephalad, at the level of the radix and nasal dorsum, the skin is consistently thin with adequate compliance and pliability. This is in stark contrast to the caudal third of the nose, primarily the nasal tip and ala, which consist of thick, pitted, and sebaceous skin that lacks independent mobility from its underlying cartilaginous structure. These inherent differences in skin type can directly impact the final reconstruction, both in terms of the number and type of options available and the final esthetic result. This is conceptually demonstrated when comparing defects of comparable size located on the upper and lower nose. Small defects over the nasal dorsum and sidewalls can often be closed primarily without tension or disruption of the surrounding nasal and facial anatomy. Meanwhile, defects as small as a few millimeters on the nasal tip or ala can significantly distort a patient's appearance if closed without the recruitment of tissue from outside the area. Therefore, the relative location of a defect on the nose is a critical consideration in the nasal reconstruction algorithm.

THE SUBUNIT CONCEPT

The external anatomy of the nose is unique in each patient, directly impacting both its perceived appearance and the formulation of a reconstructive plan in the presence of a nasal defect. The underlying bony and cartilaginous architecture of the nose is unique to each individual. When combined with the progressive differences in skin quality along its entire surface, the nose has subtle but important convexities and concavities that should be noted and accounted for when performing nasal reconstruction. These subtleties create points of transition between adjacent areas of the nose that are historically defined as the subunits of the nose. Described by Burget and Menick, the nose possesses nine distinct esthetic subunits, including the dorsum, tip, columella and paired sidewalls, alae, and soft triangles[2] (Figure 40.1). Each subunit consists of a characteristic skin quality

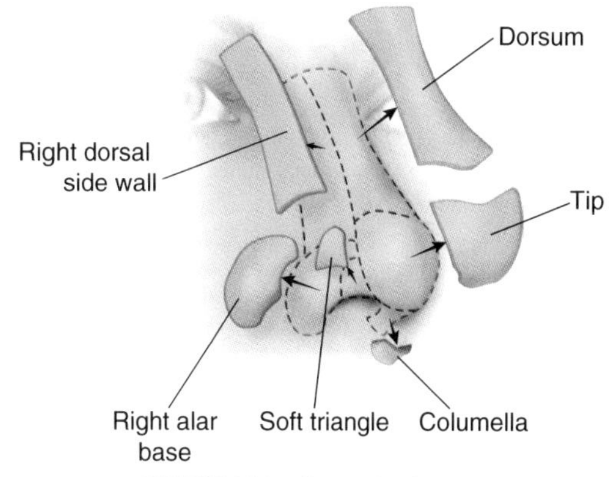

FIGURE 40.1. The nasal subunits.

and contour which impacts the way light is reflected and shadows are created. The shadows created between adjacent subunits represent areas in which incisions can be well hidden by the reconstructive surgeon. The extent of ambient light as well as patient positioning can impact the delineation of the borders of each subunit. Therefore, it is recommended that the relevant subunit anatomy be marked with the patient upright in the preoperative area rather than supine on the operating room table.

The subunit principle, as originally defined, has direct implications on how nasal defects are addressed. According to this principle, if more than 50% of a given subunit is involved in a nasal defect, the entire subunit should be excised prior to any reconstruction. Each patient has a uniquely shaped nose with different proportions and shape to the anatomical subunits, which help define a patient's normal external nasal appearance. Conceptually, replacement of a partial subunit rather than a complete subunit is considered less ideal as this often places a scar in the middle of a subunit, an area of convexity and high visibility, rather than hidden discreetly along its border. Therefore, removal of the remaining portion of the subunit facilitates a reconstruction that replaces the entire subunit, which can minimize the patch-like appearance of a partial subunit reconstruction. However, it is important to recognize that the application of the subunit principle in this manner is not universal for all patients and defects.[3-5] Consideration should be given to the impact of complete subunit excision on the available reconstructive options to the patient, as well as the patient's goals and expectations for nasal reconstruction. The subunit principle should be utilized as a tool to guide the reconstructive surgeon, rather than an absolute rule, and should be individualized for each patient.

An additional point of consideration relevant to the subunit concept is the physiologic concept of trapdoor healing. In general, myofibroblast cells are recruited to the areas of healing around a flap, which tends to create a bulging appearance. In the nose, this is often described as *pincushioning* of a locoregional flap relative to its surrounding native skin. This must be accounted for as part of the final reconstruction as it can detrimentally impact the final esthetic outcome. However, it is also important to recognize that this physiology can also be leveraged in areas that are naturally convex such as the alar or tip subunits. The pincushioning phenomenon can actually improve the final reconstructive contour in these areas by creating the needed convexity that was present in the native nasal subunit prior to excision. Ultimately this can improve the esthetic result when utilized selectively.

COVER, LINING, AND SUPPORT

In addition to its unique external anatomy, the nose can also be subdivided into three distinct anatomic layers: skin cover, cartilaginous or bony support, and nasal mucosal lining.[1] Conceptualizing the nose in this manner helps to recognize the specific considerations important to each layer while also facilitating the reconstructive process.

The subsurface bony and cartilaginous support structure of the nose are specific to each individual patient and can significantly impact the appearance of each nasal subunit.[6-8] Therefore, defects involving the support structure of nose require reconstruction with tissue of similar quality (*replacing like with like*) in order to maintain some semblance of normal appearance. For example, reconstruction of the nasal dorsum and sidewall subunits, because of their rigid structure and linear shape, are almost always replaced with grafts from the nasal septum or rib that have limited malleability. The nasal tip has a unique curved contour with an underlying native framework that is more compliant. In this region, cartilage grafts from the ear or nasal septum serve to provide the appropriate flexibility. The nasal alae lack any cartilaginous structure, instead consisting of fibrofatty tissue that has a curved appearance and also provides an inherent intrinsic rigidity that prevents external airway collapse during inhalation. Defects in this region often cause loss of this rigidity resulting in external valve collapse, requiring reconstruction with cartilage grafts placed nonanatomically to recreate the native alar structure.[6-8]

Nasal lining defects present distinct challenges to the reconstructive surgeon, in particular due to the limited availability of remaining native nasal lining that can be used to replace missing areas. Lining defects typically present as part of composite defects that require reconstruction of all three lamina, often dictating the use of a staged, algorithmic approach involving a combination of locoregional or free flaps, cartilage graft, and possible skin grafts.[7,9-13] With regards to available local flaps for lining reconstruction, a bipedicle bucket handle flap from high in the nasal vault may be used for small ala or alar margin lining defects. For mid-vault defects, the ipsilateral or contralateral septal lining can provide a large amount of mucosa for lining replacement.[7,9] When harvested from the ipsilateral nose, the lining flap is based anteriorly off of the labial artery via its columella branches. Alternatively, the septal mucosa from the contralateral nasal vault can be used as a turnover flap based on anterior ethmoidal artery branches.[10] It should be noted, however, that local mucosal flaps are technically challenging and can potentially be distorting to the remaining intact nasal anatomy. They also do not provide a sufficient amount of tissue for closure of largest lining defects, thus appropriate judgment, planning, and technical experience are required. Although many experts in the field at one time embraced lining-based flaps, these have been more recently replaced by the use of the folded forehead flap.[14]

For composite, trilamellar defects, a simple and reliable way to address the associated lining defects can be through the use of other locoregional flaps.[15] In the case of small- to moderate-sized defects, available options include the use of any remaining external skin as a turnover flap, or the use of a nasolabial or facial artery musculomucosal (FAMM) flap.[12] Ultimately, however, the workhorse flap for nasal reconstruction remains the forehead flap, which can be particularly useful for composite defects.[7,14,16,17] Beyond addressing the external skin cover, the forehead flap can be utilized to address the lining as well in one of two ways. The simplest of these is the placement of a skin graft on the undersurface of a forehead flap, either at the time of elevation and turning of the flap or in a separate preceding stage where the flap is prelaminated with the graft.[10] However, this technique comes with some drawbacks related to the skin graft itself. Secondary contracture of the graft can lead to distortion of the overlying skin envelope created by the forehead flap. Additionally, placement of cartilage grafts between the graft and forehead flap skin in a secondary stage can be difficult without devascularizing the graft. A more reliable utilization of the forehead flap for lining defects is the harvesting of additional distal tissue in the hair-bearing scalp, which can then be folded during inset of the flap for repair of the nasal lining. The flap is not thinned during this initial stage with the final reconstruction typically being completed in three distinct stages. Finally, for larger heminasal or subtotal lining defects, free tissue transfer such as a free radial or ulnar forearm flap is typically required[13,18] (**Figure 40.2**).

SURGICAL APPROACH AND ALGORITHM

In addition to an in-depth understanding of the relevant nasal anatomy, as previously discussed, a thoughtful preoperative reconstructive plan is integral to a successful nasal reconstruction.[1] The initial step in devising this plan is defining the nasal defect itself in terms of what is missing and what needs to be restored to achieve an appropriate nasal contour and an aesthetically acceptable nasal appearance. Defects should be characterized with regards to their absolute size, depth, orientation, and relative location on the nose. In the case of a delayed reconstruction, this may require recreating the original defect through the release of contractures and excision of previous scars in an effort to restore normal surrounding anatomy. The defect must also be clearly defined with regards to the soft tissue layers involved, particularly in larger or more complex defects where a composite and/or multistage reconstruction may be required. By understanding

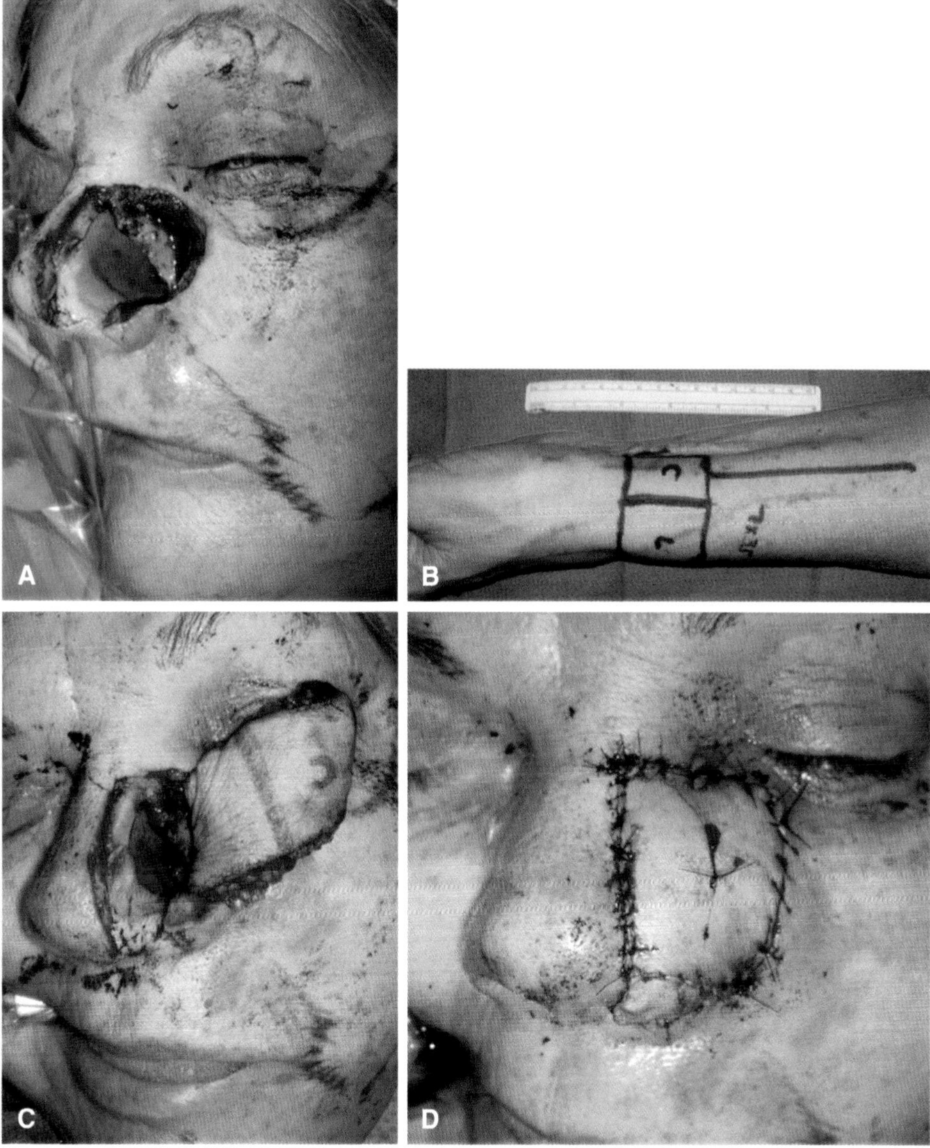

FIGURE 40.2. Radial forearm free flap for lining and soft tissue cover after a hemirhinectomy. The large lining and cover defects **(A)** are measured and transposed onto the arm, with the portions planned for lining and cover marked *L* and *C* **(B)**. The flap pedicle is tunneled in a subcutaneous tunnel to the left facial vessels for microvascular anastomosis **(C)** followed by final inset **(D)**.

the relative needs for replacement of skin cover, support, and/or lining, the reconstructive plan can then be similarly broken down into different components.

Finalizing the reconstructive plan also requires the identification of appropriate autologous tissue donor sites to meet the aforementioned needs. In general, missing tissue should be replaced in the exact amount that has been lost or removed. The associated contracture of skin grafts should be anticipated and accounted for when used. Flaps should not be made too small, as is commonly done in an effort to minimize the donor site. However, flap design should be done carefully to avoid distorting adjacent structures such as the eyelid, ala, and oral commissure.

Given the potential complexity associated with the variety of nasal defects a reconstructive surgeon may see in practice, it is useful to have and employ an algorithm for approaching nasal reconstruction. A commonly used algorithm for small- to medium-sized defects (1–2 cm) is described in detail by Parrett and Pribaz,[1] which involves division of the nose into thirds transversely, which helps to categorize defects based on location. This helps to further narrow and define defects, so that choosing a treatment plan is quicker and more simplified. With these defects being the most commonly seen in practice, this algorithm describes options for primary, skin graft, or local flap closure. Once defects exceed the 1.5 to 2-cm size mark, local flaps beyond the forehead flap are more difficult to utilize.

SECONDARY INTENTION, SKIN GRAFTS, AND LOCAL FLAPS

Delayed healing, or healing by secondary intention, which involves epithelialization, granulation tissue formation, and myofibroblast contraction, is a simple albeit slow way to close a small, superficial defect. A key concept to consider is that tissue will be drawn in equally and circumferentially from all directions around the defect. This minimizes distortion to any surrounding structures, in contrast to a linear closure, which recruits laxity from a single vector. Wounds due to a destructive process such as curettage, wound dehiscence, infection, or necrosis should be considered for delayed healing. Almost any wound will heal in this manner if other factors such as systemic illness, cost, or patient wishes prevent a more definitive repair. However, secondary healing should be avoided in wounds in which vital deep structures are exposed to prevent desiccation or trauma. Delayed healing can also be unpredictable with regards to the amount of contraction seen, which can distort surrounding anatomy. For example, secondary healing of wounds near the nasal tip or ala can result in esthetically unappealing nasal tip elevation. The quality of the resultant scar, which can be depressed or shiny in appearance, can also be hard to control (Figure 40.3). These imperfections should be avoided over convex nasal surfaces but may be imperceptible in flat or concave areas or within sun- or radiation-damaged skin. The medial canthal region and upper nasal sidewall are areas that generally have good outcomes using this approach. Assuming no significant distortion of the surrounding anatomy following delayed secondary healing, the resultant scars can be revised or excised with a more formal repair done at a later date.

Primary closure of defects is a viable option for defects that are less than 5 to 6 mm in size. This is particularly true in the upper two-thirds of the nose, where the overlying nasal skin is more compliant and mobile. In contrast, primary closure of defects in the lower third of the nose is challenging because of the thickness of the skin over the nasal tip and ala. Attempts at primary closure in this region can lead to wide, depressed scars as well unacceptable amounts of anatomic distortion.

Full-thickness skin grafts can be advantageous in that no additional scars are added to the area surrounding the defect, the amount of locally available tissue is not a limiting factor, and it is relatively quick and easy for the patient. Common donor sites include the preauricular, postauricular, supraclavicular, and forehead regions. However, skin grafts must be placed on a well-vascularized bed and should not be place over denuded cartilage or cartilage graft. For acute defects, it may be advisable to allow a wound to granulate for 7 to 10 days prior to definitive skin grafting. Alternatively, the placement of dermal regeneration template such as Integra® (Integra® Dermal Regeneration Template, Plainsboro, NJ) can be used as a bridge to generate a better soft tissue bed prior to delayed skin graft placement.[19] Traditional full-thickness grafts can do well in the thin-skinned areas of the dorsum or nasal sidewalls (Figure 40.4). However, grafts on the front of the nose on or near the nasal tip will often appear as depressed, off-colored patches that do not blend well with the surrounding skin. Skin grafts should be secured with sutures and a bolster dressing for a week.

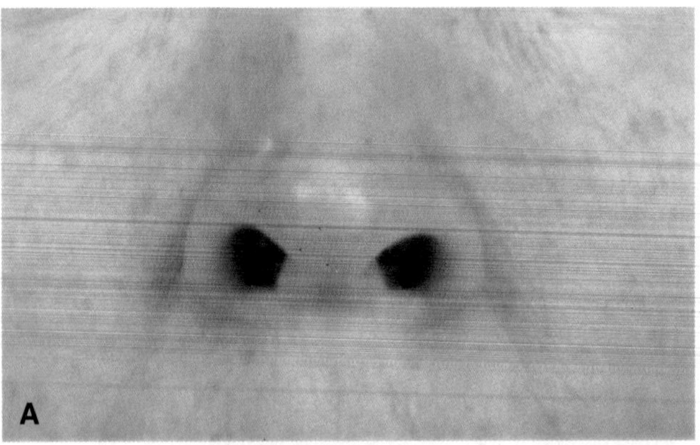

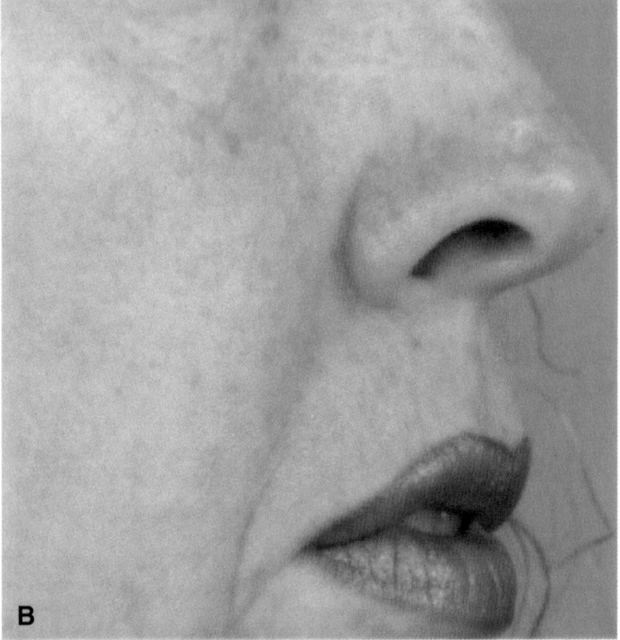

FIGURE 40.3. A,B. Healing of right alar defect with secondary intention. The resultant scar is often depressed and shiny in appearance.

Several local flap options have been described for nasal reconstruction, each of which is appropriate for particular types and locations of defects. The dorsal nasal flap, glabellar, Rieger, and miter flaps take advantage of the relative excess of tissue present in glabella and nasal dorsum regions and are useful for closure of defects in the proximal and middle third of the nose[20-22] (Figure 40.5). Supplied by the angular artery, these flaps are elevated as skin and subcutaneous tissue with or without muscle and rotated and/or advanced inferiorly toward the nasal tip. A standing cone, or dog-ear, is usually created along the nasal sidewall of the flap base and requires excision. The donor site is undermined laterally on each side for a tension-free primary closure. One common disadvantage of these flaps is the depressed transverse scar that is often apparent at the flap junction with the tip subunit.

The bilobed flap is a workhorse flap for defects of the thick, stiff skin of the distal third of the nose that are up to 1.5 cm in size.[23-25] Conceptually, the first lobe of the flap is designed over an area of excess skin adjacent to the nasal tip or alar defect (Figure 40.6). This lobe should be designed to replace the defect 1:1 to prevent tip or alar rim distortion. A smaller diameter second lobe, approximately 50% of the defect width, is designed in a vertical orientation within the more lax tissue of the upper nose. Traditionally, flaps were designed to require a 180° rotation, which created large dog-ears that, when excised, narrowed the flap's vascular base and thus jeopardized its viability. McGregor and Soutar,[23,24] and later Zitelli,[25] developed the aforementioned design to decrease the flap's rotation to 90° to 100°. The flap base should be positioned laterally and medially for tip and alar defects, respectively. It should not extend onto cheek or lower lid skin. As the primary lobe shifts to repair the defect, the second lobe resurfaces the defect from the primary lobe. The resultant tertiary defect from the second lobe is closed primarily utilizing the laxity of the upper nose. Resultant dog-ear excisions should be planned between the defect and the pivot point of the primary lobe to provide space for the flap to rotate and advance. These flaps are elevated with muscle immediately superficial to the periosteum or perichondrium with wide undermining of the adjacent skin to enable closure of the secondary and tertiary defects. Despite careful planning and design, postoperative distortion as well as a *pincushioning* appearance to the flap is not uncommon (Figure 40.7).

The V-Y flap is a relatively versatile local flap for small nasal defects that can be utilized throughout the nose.[26,27] In general, flaps can be designed immediately adjacent to the defect with an orientation such that the resultant Y scar is placed in a natural crease or concavity. For larger or rounder defects, extended flaps can be designed such that distal part of the flap includes the adjacent borders of the defect[27] (Figure 40.8). This portion of the flap can be elevated and rotated into the defect to extend the reach of the standard V-Y flap. In the proximal third of the nose, vertically oriented defects centrally can be reconstructed with V-Y flap from the nasal sidewall, whereas the nasal dorsum tissue can be utilized for more lateral defects. In the middle part of the nose, lateral defects that are vertically oriented can use a V-Y flap from the remaining

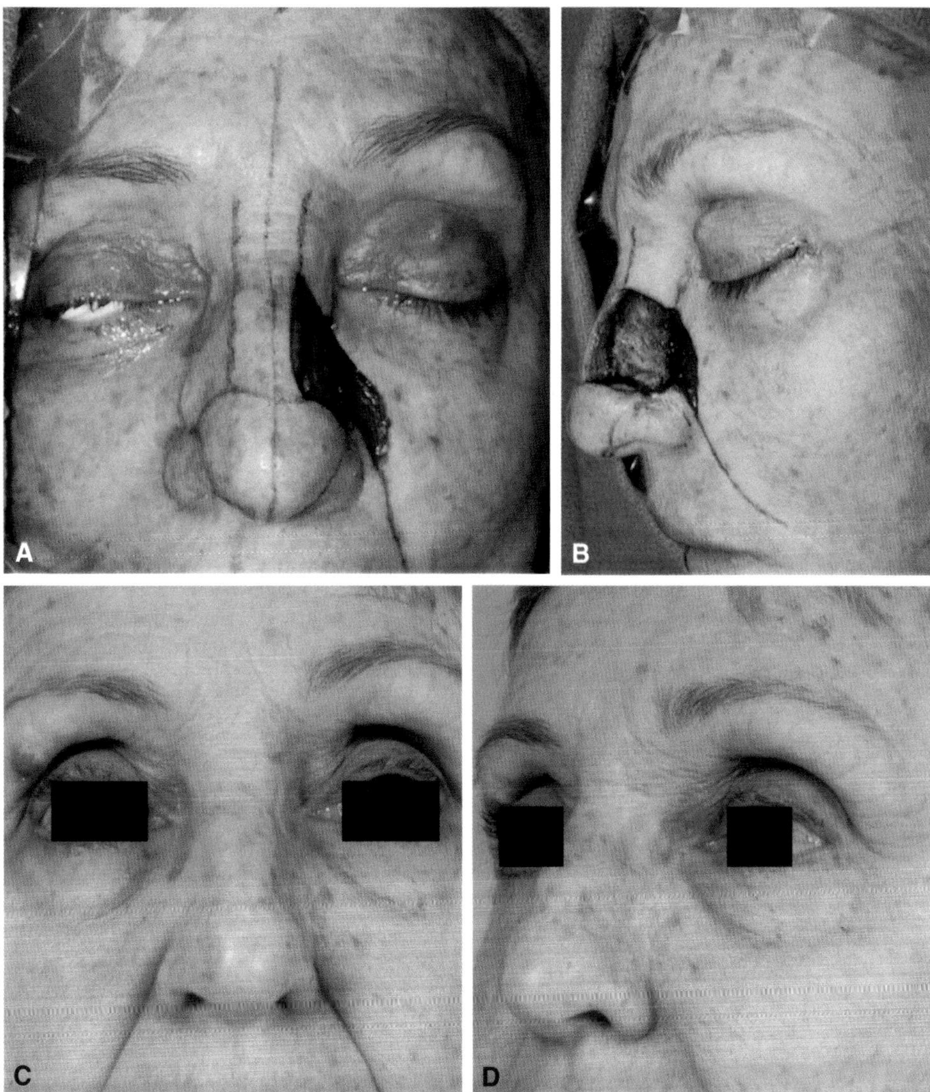

FIGURE 40.4. Full-thickness skin graft of a nasal sidewall defect. **A,B.** The defect includes both the left sidewall and a portion of the nasal-cheek junction. **C,D.** Final result is shown after left cheek advancement and full-thickness skin graft of the nasal sidewall.

sidewall extending onto the medial cheek. These flaps are based on the angular artery perforators, which can be isolated during flap elevation to provide greater mobility for flap advancement. The goal for inset should be that the flap is completely on the nose instead of straddling the nasal-cheek junction so as to not efface this natural crease. For the distal third of the nose, small alar defects sparing the nasal rim can be repaired with a V-Y advancement. In these cases, the flap should be designed above the alar groove and extending into the nasolabial area, again taking its blood supply from angular artery perforators.

Nasolabial flaps can be utilized for resurfacing defects of the nasal sidewall and ala. Because tissue is recruited from outside the nose itself, anatomic distortion is minimized enabling closure of larger nasal defects. These flaps can be based either superiorly or inferiorly and performed in one or two stages[28-30] (**Figure 40.9**). Whether or not to perform the flap in a single stage depends on a number of factors, including experience. For narrow flaps with a thin base, primary sculpting may not be safe so a second stage for additional contouring may be necessary. Another consideration is whether or not a skip area of remaining normal tissue is present between the flap base and defect. If soft tissue remains between the defect and flap base, the surgeon can simply remove the intervening tissue to perform the reconstruction in a single stage. Removal of intervening tissue is better tolerated at the nasal sidewall subunit, whereas defects of the ala, alar crease, and hairless triangle are a challenge to reconstruct. In this location, it is preferential to keep the intervening tissue with plans for division and inset 3 weeks later.

The nasal sidewall, residual ala, and nasolabial creases should be marked. Depending upon the size of defect and extent of alar distortion, a nonanatomic conchal cartilage graft can be harvested, positioned, and fixed into place to help prevent alar collapse. A template of the defect is created to delineate what is needed for coverage. For larger defect, such as whole alar replacement, the template is fashioned on the normal contralateral ala. Templates designed from the defect tend to underestimate the flap size because they do not account for convexity of the tissue removed. The width of the flap along the nasolabial crease has dimensions equal to the height of the defect. The flap is then elevated above the facial mimetic musculature to include small perforating branches of the facial artery. It is rotated into place. The cheek soft tissues are widely undermined and closed primarily, ensuring a tension-free flap inset. The nasolabial flap is laid into the defect, thinned and trimmed to fit, and inset.

The principal limitation of nasolabial flaps is the nature of pincushioning or trapdoor healing that occurs at the location of the ala.

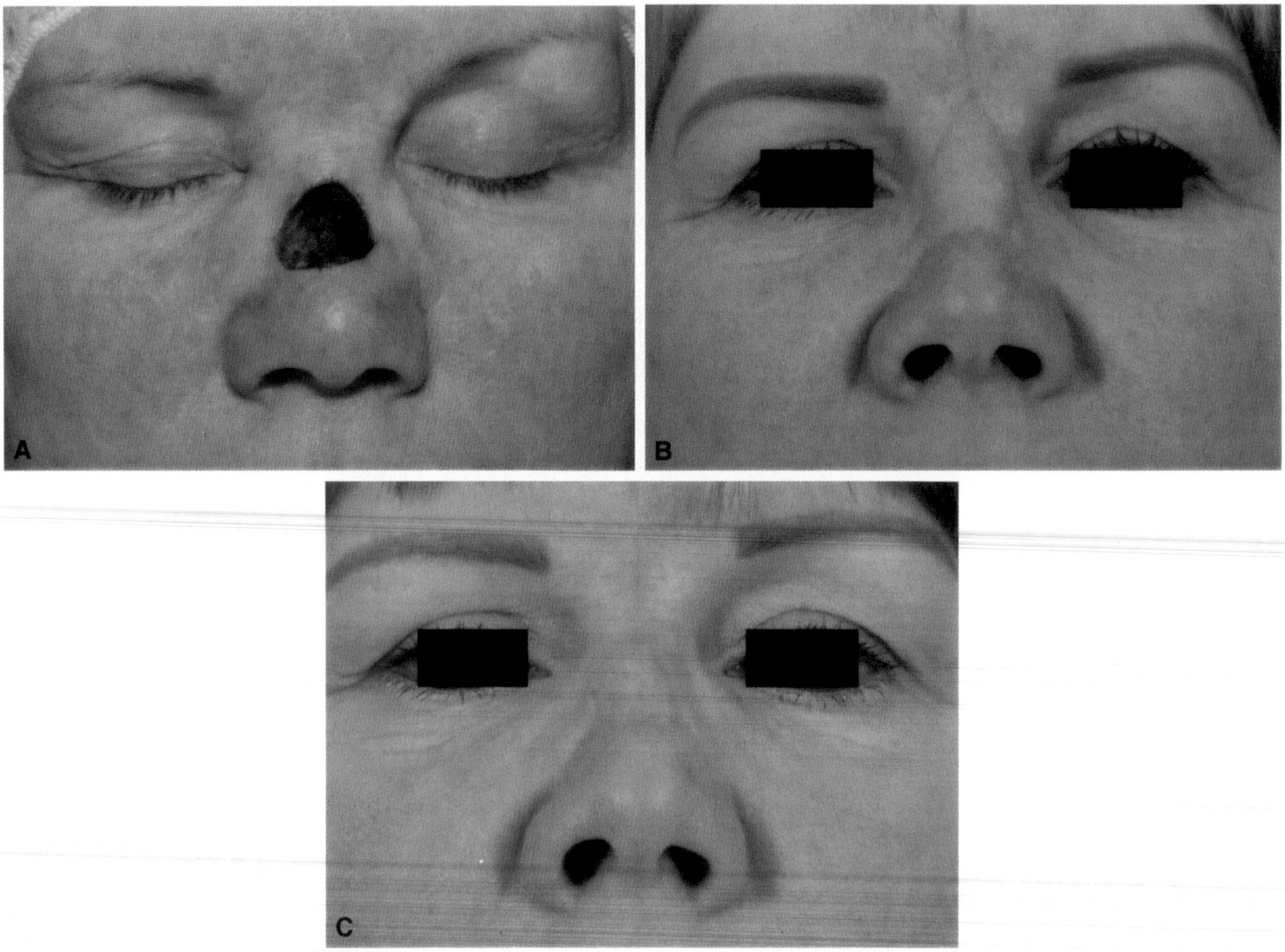

FIGURE 40.5. Miter flap for reconstruction of the nasal dorsum. Photographs demonstrate the defect within the dorsum **(A)**, initial result after primary flap inset **(B)**, and final result after revision to thin the flap for better contour **(C)**.

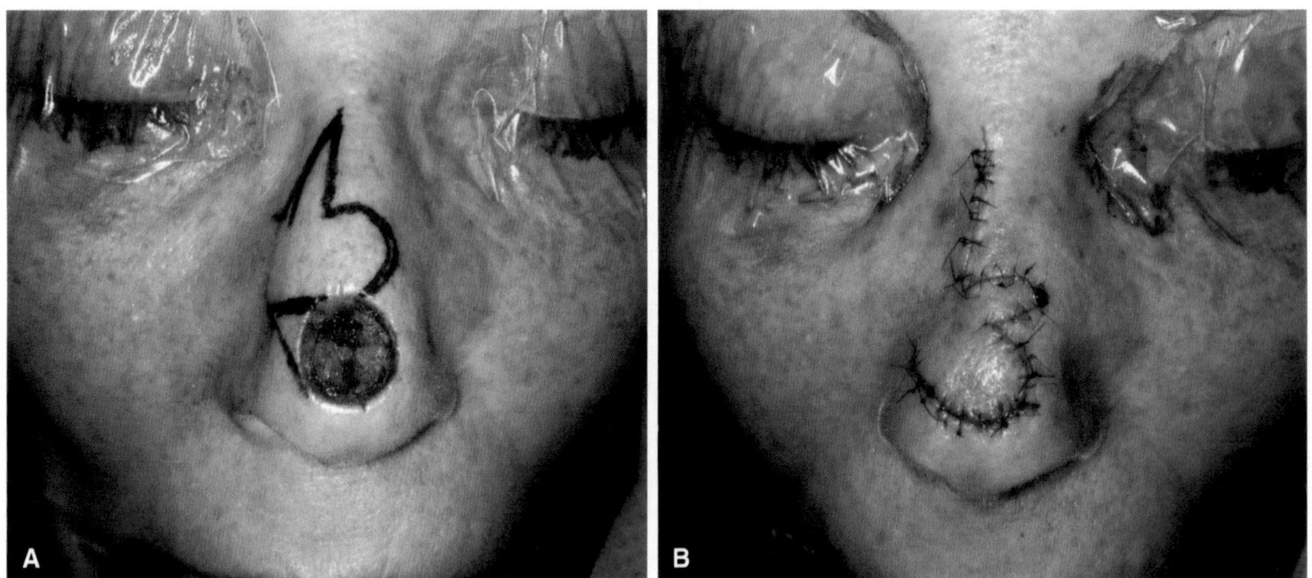

FIGURE 40.6. Bilobed flap for a nasal tip defect. Markings demonstrating two lobes of the flap at 90° angles with a vertical orientation of the second flap **(A)** and flap immediately after inset **(B)**.

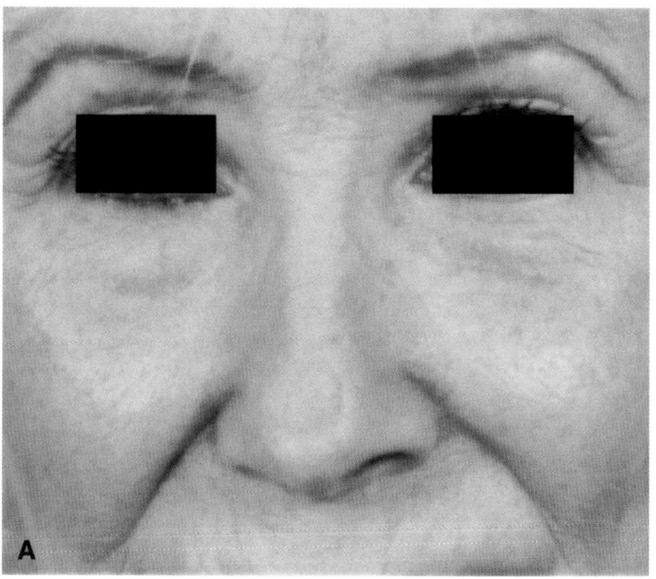

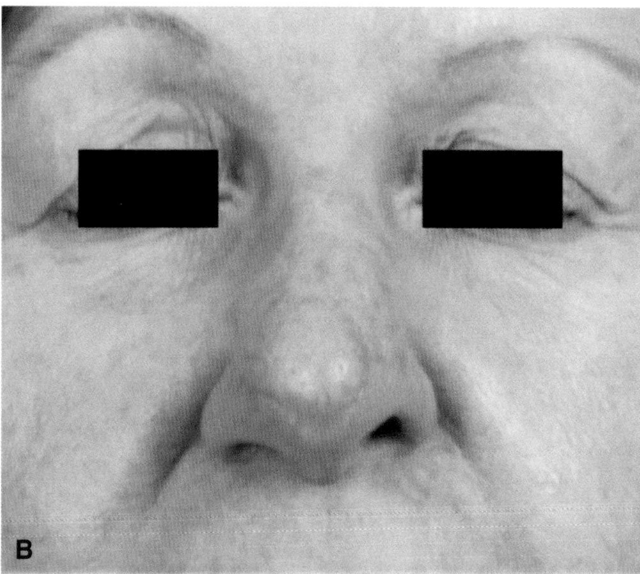

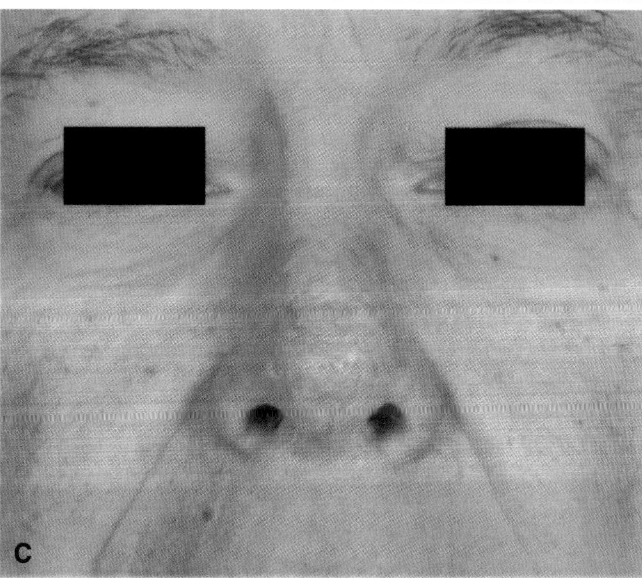

FIGURE 40.7. Final result after bilobed flaps for different nasal tip defects. The final appearance after bilobed flap can be unpredictable despite appropriate preoperative planning and markings. These can result in a distorted, indented **(A)** or *pincushioned* **(B)** appearance, or can provide an appropriate appearance and contour **(C)**.

Small defects, such as partial alar replacement, tend to create a patch-like appearance; therefore, the importance of the subunit concept should be strongly considered (Figure 40.10). Entire alar replacement is actually a much more predictable reconstruction than a 1-cm alar defect (Figure 40.11). For small defects, alternatives such as skin grafts should be discussed with the patient or consideration should be given to removal of the remainder of the subunit.

FOREHEAD FLAP

The forehead flap is acknowledged as the ideal donor site for nasal reconstruction due to its color, texture, and the ability to resurface part or all of the nose.[14,16] It is the workhorse flap for complex nasal reconstruction, with the most common iteration being the vertical paramedian forehead flap raised on the supratrochlear pedicle. The flap does tend to be thicker than nasal skin and so does need to ultimately be thinned to achieve the definitive reconstruction. The vertical paramedian forehead flap is typically designed to take skin from high on the forehead, beneath the hairline, with a narrow pedicle that can extend caudal to the ipsilateral medial eyebrow. The inferior aspect of the flap donor site can be closed primarily, typically with minimal eyebrow distortion, and the superior portion can be closed primarily or be allowed to heal secondarily through wound contracture and reepithelialization with good results. Skin grafting of the donor site should be avoided. Typically, midline nasal defects can be resurfaced using flaps based on either the left or right pedicle, whereas unilateral defects are reconstructed by flaps based on the ipsilateral pedicle to shorten the distance between the pivot point and the defect, assuming no previous scars in the area.

Indications for forehead flap reconstruction, in general, include defects larger than 1.5-cm that cannot be appropriately reconstructed with the aforementioned reconstructive techniques or those involving multiple subunits. Composite defects requiring lining and structural reconstruction can often benefit from the versatility and reliability that the forehead flap provides[14,16,31] (Figure 40.12). Forehead flap nasal reconstruction can be done in two or three stages depending on the complexity of the defect. For superficial defects that require primary resurfacing only, thinning of the flap can be accomplished at the time of rotation, eliminating the need for intermediate stage prior to pedicle division. However, in those cases for which cartilage

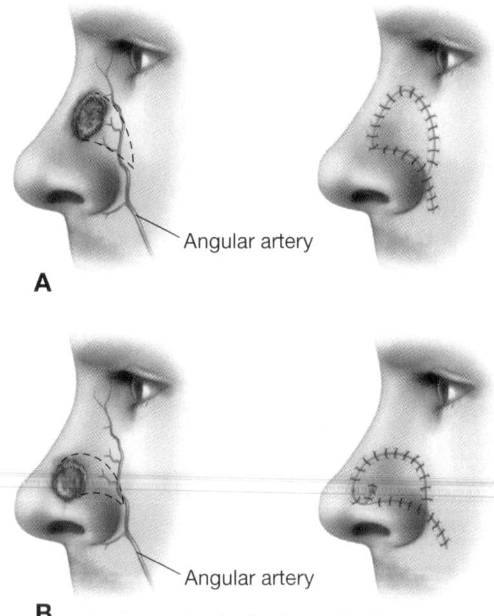

FIGURE 40.8. Design and inset of a V-Y flap **(A)** and an extended V-Y flap **(B)** for alar-nasal sidewall defects.

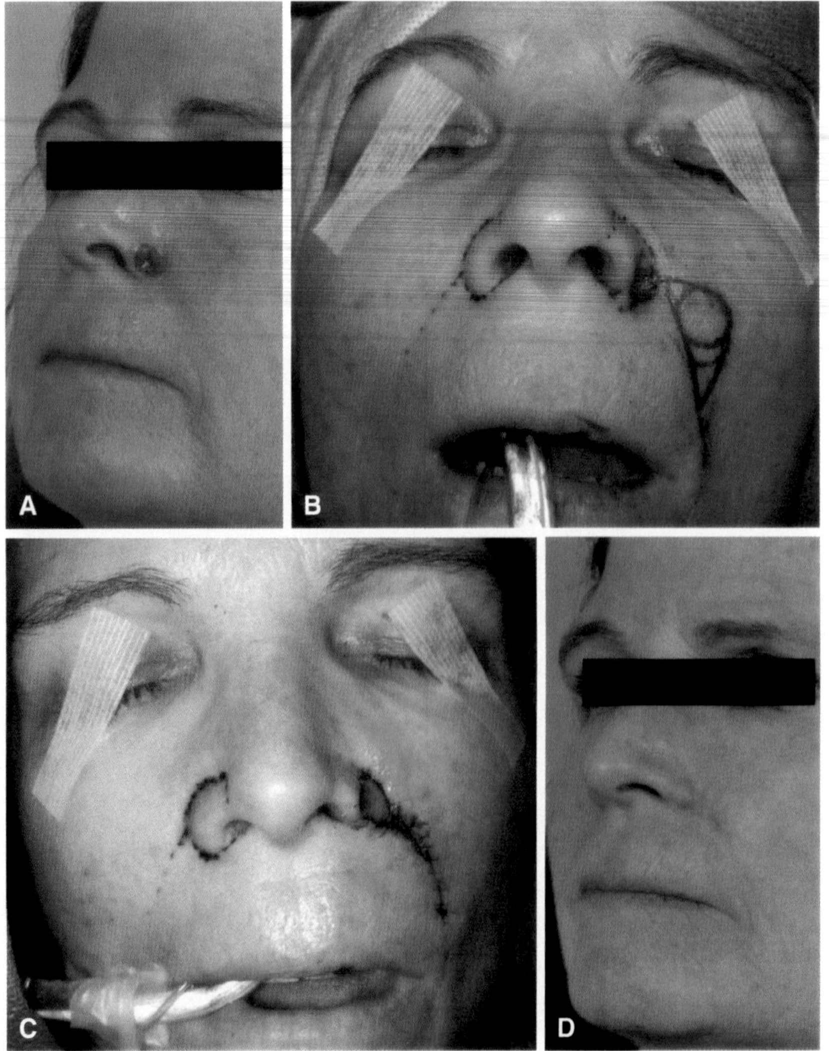

FIGURE 40.9. Single-stage nasolabial flap for lateral alar defect. The defect **(A)** is shown with minimal intervening tissue between it and the planned flap **(B)**, allowing for a single-stage reconstruction. Photographs are shown demonstrating the flap immediately after inset **(C)** and long-term result **(D)**.

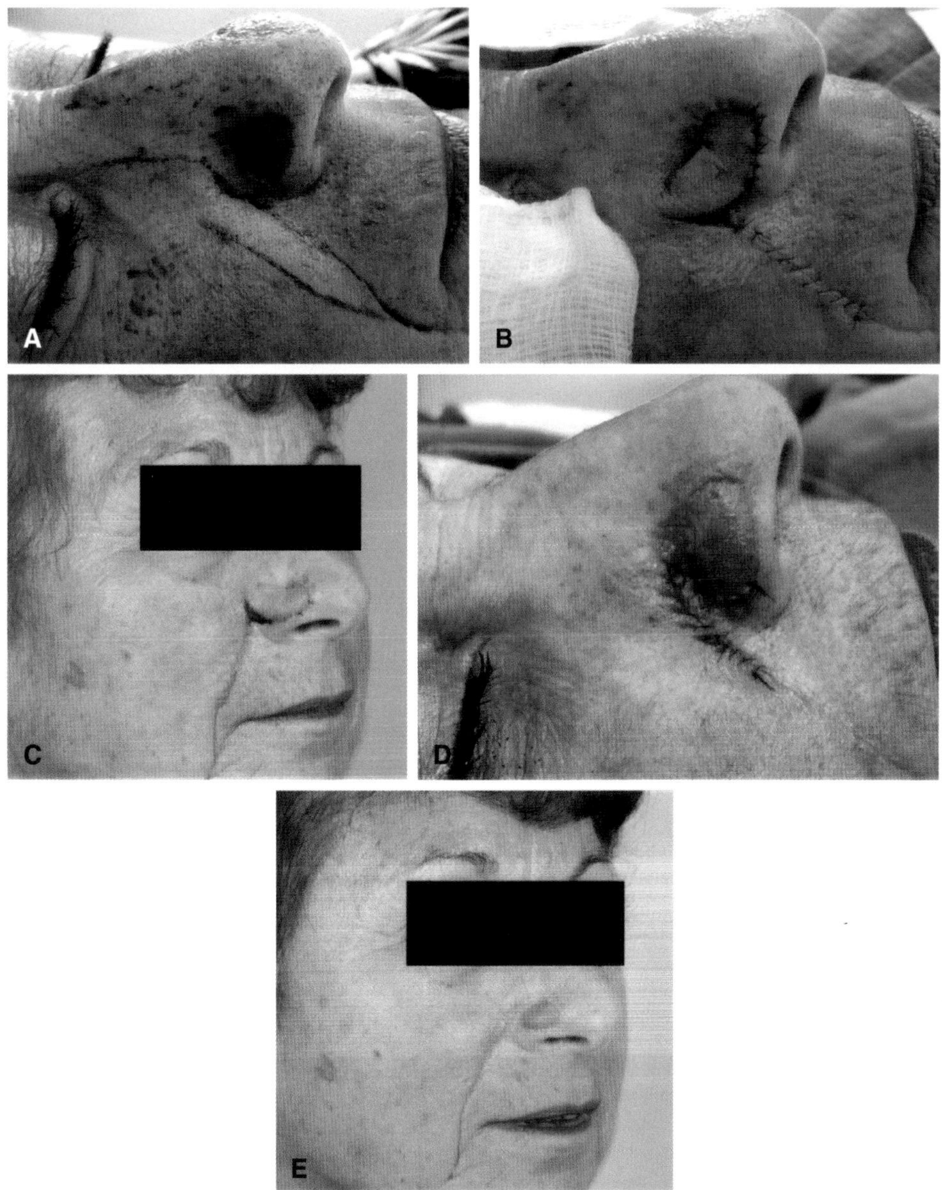

FIGURE 40.10. Two-stage nasolabial flap reconstruction for a lateral alar defect without completion subunit excision. Defect is shown **(A)**, followed by first-stage flap inset **(B,C)** and after second-stage division of flap **(D,E)**. Note the patchlike appearance of the flap due to incomplete excision of the right alar subunit.

placement or lining reconstruction through folding of the flap is being performed, an intermediate stage is necessary for contouring and/or separation of the skin cover and lining layers (**Figure 40.13**). When performing the reconstruction in three stages, there is no added benefit to thinning the flap during the initial stage, as this can be done more aggressively during the second stage when the flap is already delayed. In contrast, the two-stage approach can be limiting in terms of how much debulking can be done safely without compromising the vascularity of the flap. In trying to achieve an improved contour, occasional flap necrosis can be seen in two-stage reconstructions, particularly in smokers. For these reasons, the authors prefer a three-stage approach for the majority of cases given its vascular reliability and superior ability to achieve an appropriate contour during the intermediate stage.

The first stage of forehead flap nasal reconstruction involves defining the defect followed by elevation and inset of the flap. Defects must be defined utilizing the subunit principle as previously described, as well as with the removal and release of previous grafts or scar contractures. Consideration should be give to excisions so that final scar placement can be at the borders of adjacent subunits. A template of the defect should be transferred to the forehead as part of flap design. The contralateral uninvolved side of the nose can be used for templating of lateral defects; for central defects this can be more challenging as no normal structure exists. In these cases, templates must be based on borders of the defect as well surgical judgment to visualize the 3D aspect of the parts that are absent. A piece of bone wax can be used to build up the defect to more appropriately mimic the convexity of the missing subunit. For lining defects, additional templates can be made and transferred to the forehead if folding of the forehead flap is to be performed. The supratrochlear artery is identified with a Doppler probe near the corrugator frown crease, usually at the level of the medial canthus. The flap template is placed adjacent to or can cross into the hairline, as needed based on the length of the patient's forehead and length of flap needed to reach the defect. The flap is oriented vertically to maintain its axial blood supply and should be narrowed to 1.2 to 1.5 cm wide at its base, allowing the flap to rotate and transpose easily. Wider pedicles to capture additional blood supply are unnecessary and only serve to further limit the arc of rotation. Extending the flap base inferiorly across the orbital rim can be performed to

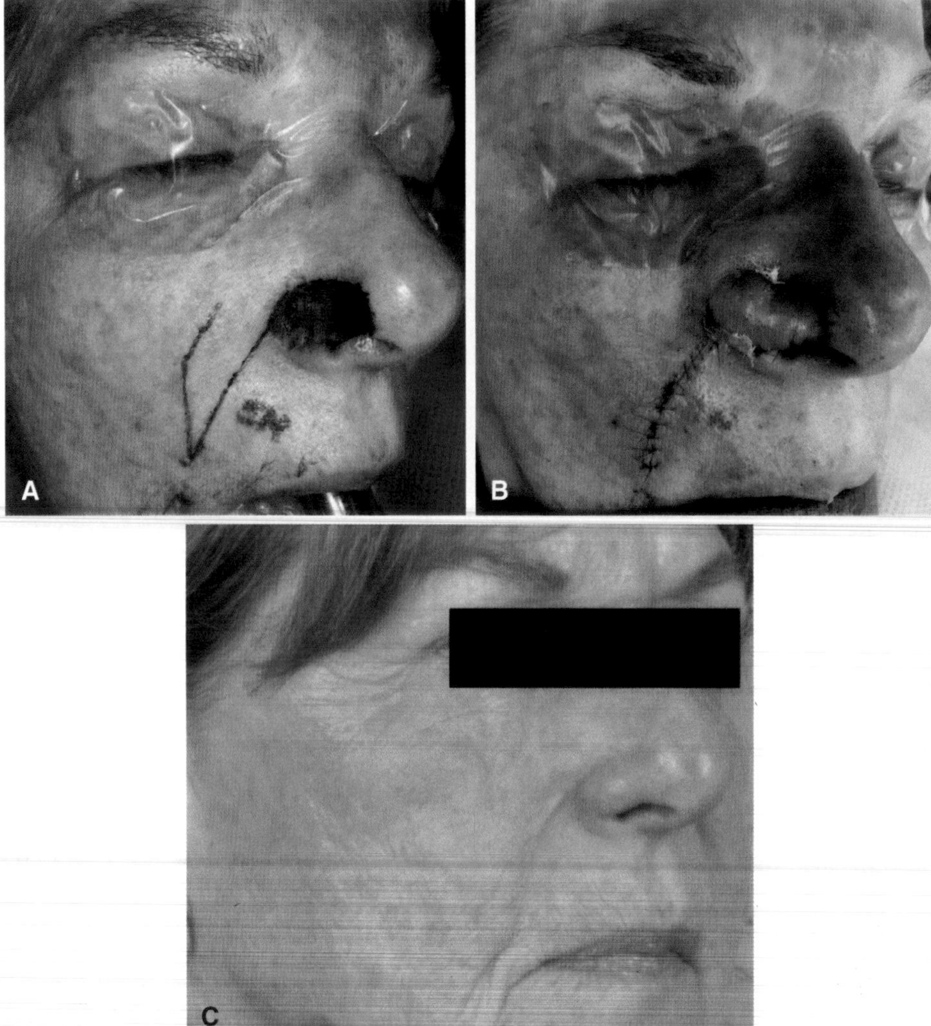

FIGURE 40.11. Two-stage nasolabial flap reconstruction for a lateral alar defect with completion subunit excision. Defect is shown **(A)**, followed by first-stage flap inset **(B)**. **C.** Long-term result after second-stage division of flap demonstrates an appropriate esthetic appearance and contour due to excision of the residual alar subunit prior to inset of the flap during the first stage.

gain additional flap length. The flap is elevated in the loose areolar plane above the periosteum so that frontalis muscle is included with the flap. Approximately 1 to 2 cm cephalad to the eyebrow, the plane of dissection proceeds deep to the periosteum to capture the supratrochlear vessels. The flap is rotated and transposed 180° and is inset with a single layer of fine permanent suture. The raw undersurface of the pedicle is dressed with a small piece of xeroform. The tissue surrounding the donor site is undermined and closed, often leaving the superior portion open for dressing changes and secondary intention healing.

The secondary or intermediate stage of the reconstruction should be performed at a minimum of 3 weeks after initial flap elevation and inset. During this stage, the forehead flap is elevated off of its nasal bed at a superficial subcutaneous level of 2 to 3 mm in thickness, leaving the supratrochlear pedicle intact. The residual excess subcutaneous fat and frontalis muscle left on the nasal substance are sculpted and thinned to create the desired contour. Cartilage grafts are placed for recreation of shape and to provide support as needed, depending upon the defect location. The flap is then re-inset over the newly contoured nasal structure. After an additional 3 weeks, the tertiary stage of the reconstruction can be performed, including pedicle division. Division is performed and the proximal portion of the pedicle, including scar, frontalis muscle, and excess fat, are debulked, and the medial brow skin is unfurled. This skin is then trimmed and inset into the medial eyebrow as an inverted V-shaped pennant. The forehead flap itself remains well vascularized by its distal attachments to the columella, alar rims, and nasal tip, for partial reelevation of the cephalad aspect of the flap to perform further thinning and contouring prior to its final inset.

SUBTOTAL OR TOTAL NASAL RECONSTRUCTION

Subtotal or total nasal reconstruction requires consideration of all three nasal layers and therefore typically involves a series of major reconstructive operations.[6,18] Careful preoperative planning is required and should not be embarked upon without appropriate experience and foresight by the reconstructive surgeon. Large, complex, central facial defects involving the nose and surrounding tissue usually require more tissue than that is available locally for reconstruction. A combination of free flap tissue transfer and locoregional tissue in the form of forehead flaps and cartilage grafts should be

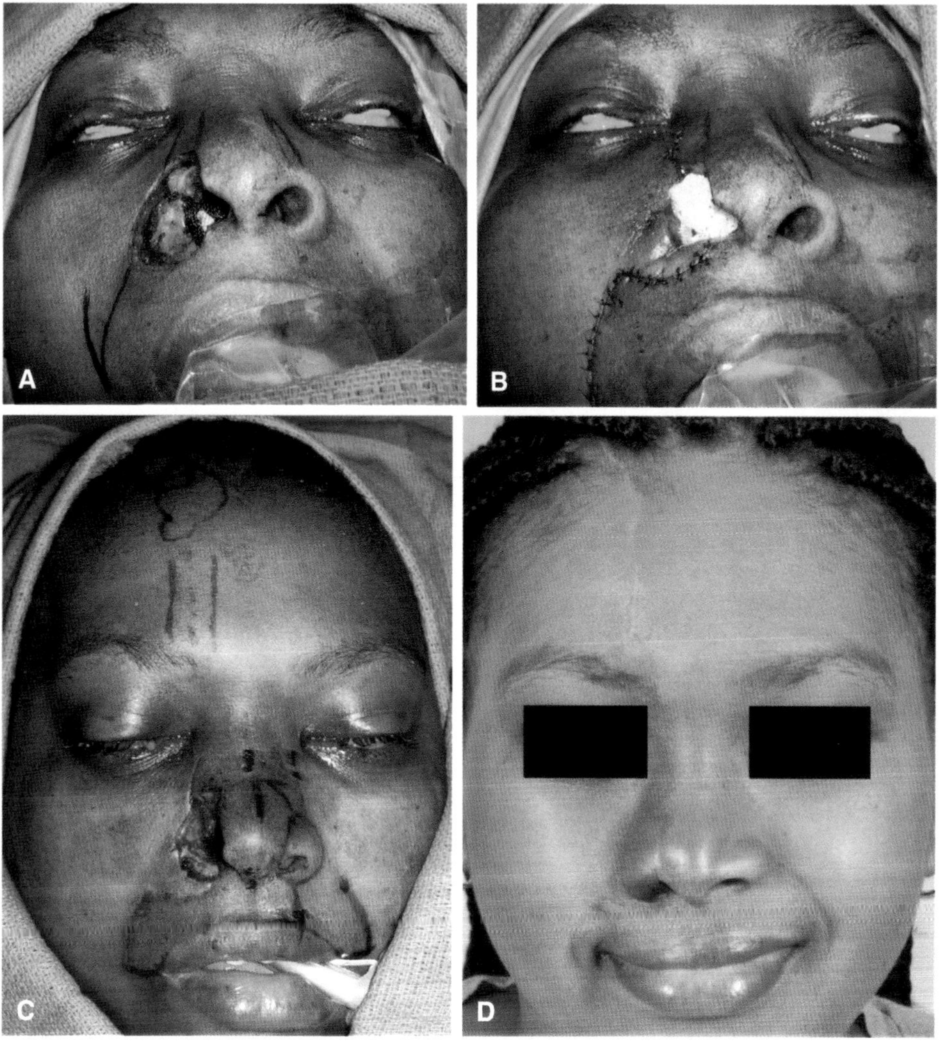

FIGURE 40.12. Three-stage folded forehead flap for reconstruction of composite right heminasal defect. Defect includes the nasal-cheek junction **(A)**, which is reconstructed with a nasolabial flap in an initial stage **(B)**, followed by folded forehead flap in three stages. Markings for the initial stage **(C)**, and final result **(D)** are shown.

employed in a sequential fashion with an expectation for multiple revisions. The aforementioned principles regarding skin cover, structural support, and lining should be followed. Alternatively, in the patient unwilling or unable to embark on a multistep reconstructive pathway, external nasal prosthetics have become more widely available and lifelike.[32,33]

COMPLICATIONS AND REVISIONS

Major complications following nasal reconstruction are generally rare. The abundant blood supply of the face helps to mitigate against ischemia or infection. Small areas of necrosis of lining or flaps can heal secondarily. However, larger areas of skin cover necrosis should be addressed early with debridement and replacement with vascularized tissue to prevent cartilage exposure and infection, as well as significant scarring or contracture. Cartilage exposed due to debridement of lining should be removed and banked if possible with placement of a skin graft for temporary lining. Infection, which is again rare, can occur in patients with a history of infection and/or multiple previous procedures or with contaminated wounds. Early debridement of any involved cartilage and culture directed antibiotic therapy should be initiated, with delay in replacement of any cartilage for at least 4 to 6 weeks. In general, every attempt should be made to save the repair or reconstruction, or at the very least to limit the damage.

Most complex reconstructions will require late revision to further improve the esthetic and functional outcome. Smaller local flap reconstructions may also require revision of surgical scars or any distortions of surrounding anatomy or contour. Revisions should be delayed until all tissue induration or swelling has resolved to accurately assess the current esthetic outcome and what is needed for improving that outcome. Over the course of a complex reconstruction, necessary revisions should be anticipated and discussed with the patient in advance. Revisions can range from minor ones needed to improve nasal definition and landmarks (e.g. intentional scar placement to mimic the alar crease) to more significant revisions for improving upon the dimension, volume, contour, or symmetry of the reconstruction. In cases in which the cover or lining are grossly deficient, such as after a postoperative complication, an additional reconstruction must be performed often with a secondary regional or distant tissue transfer.

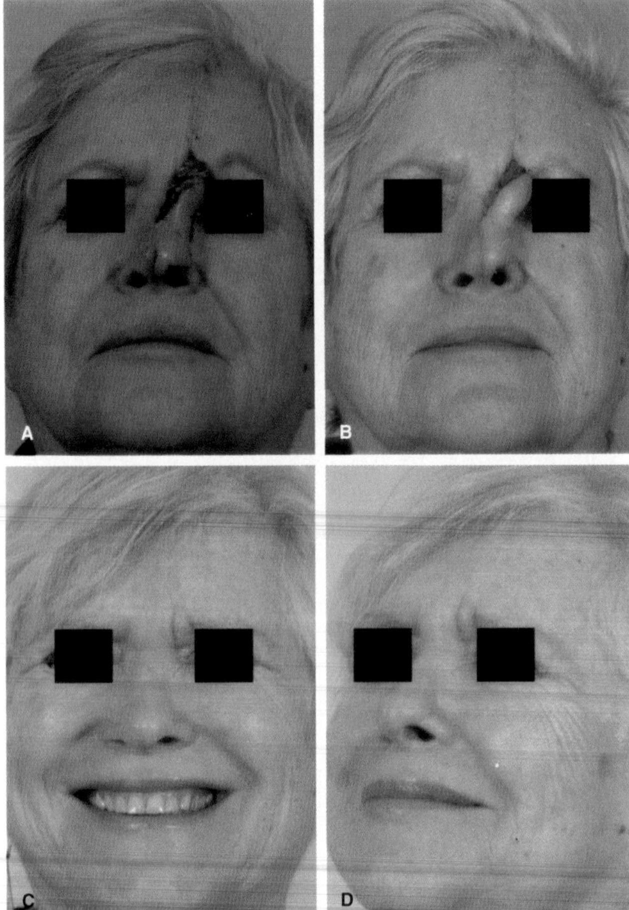

FIGURE 40.13. Three-stage forehead flap reconstruction of composite nasal tip and left ala. Photographs demonstrate appearance after first stage **(A)**, after second stage involving reelevation, thinning, and re-inset of flap with cartilage graft placement **(B)**, and long-term result after third-stage pedicle division **(C,D)**.

REFERENCES

1. Parrett BM, Pribaz JJ. An algorithm for treatment of nasal defects. *Clin Plast Surg.* 2009;36(3):407-420.
   This article presents an algorithmic approach to the appropriate reconstruction of nasal defects based on their location and orientation, focusing specifically on the commonly seen small defects seen after Mohs cancer excision. It helps to simplify the treatment selection in these patients, which can be worthwhile for the young reconstructive surgeon.
2. Burget GC, Menick FJ. Subunit principle in nasal reconstruction. *Plast Reconstr Surg.* 1985;76:239-247.
   This article introduced the concept of nasal subunits, in which the nose is divided into adjacent areas of characteristic surface quality, border outline, and three-dimensional contour. Using this subunit approach to nasal repair, scars can be positioned within the contours of the nasal surface and preference should be given to complete subunit resurfacing.
3. Singh DJ, Bartlett SP. Aesthetic considerations in nasal reconstruction and the role of modified nasal subunits. *Plast Reconstr Surg.* 2003;111(2):639-648.
4. Rohrich RJ, Griffin JR, Ansari M, et al. Nasal reconstruction—beyond aesthetic subunits: a 15-year review of 1334 cases. *Plast Reconstr Surg.* 2004;114(6):1405-1416.
5. Menick FJ. Aesthetic considerations in nasal reconstruction and the role of modified nasal subunits. *Plast Reconstr Surg.* 2003;111(2):649-651.
6. Taghinia AH, Pribaz JJ. Complex nasal reconstruction. *Plast Reconstr Surg.* 2008;121(2):15e-27e.
7. Burget GC, Menick FJ. Nasal support and lining: the marriage of beauty and blood supply. *Plast Reconstr Surg.* 1989;84(2):189-202.
8. Menick FJ. Anatomic reconstruction of the nasal tip cartilages in secondary and reconstructive rhinoplasty. *Plast Reconstr Surg.* 1999;104:2187-2198.
9. Burget GC, Menick FJ. Nasal reconstruction: seeking a fourth dimension. *Plast Reconstr Surg.* 1986;78:145-157.
10. Menick FJ. The use of skin grafts for nasal lining. *Clin Plast Surg.* 2001;28(2):311-321.
11. DeQuervain F. About partial lateral rhinoplasty. *Zentralbl Chir.* 1902;29:297-302.
12. Pribaz J, Stephens W, Crespo L, et al. A new intraoral flap: facial artery musculomucosal (FAMM) flap. *Plast Reconstr Surg.* 1992;90(3):421-429.
13. Walton RL, Burget GC, Beahm EK. Microsurgical reconstruction of the nasal lining. *Plast Reconstr Surg.* 2005;115(7):1813-1829.
14. Menick FJ. A 10-year experience in nasal reconstruction with the three-stage forehead flap. *Plast Reconstr Surg.* 2002;109:1839-1855.
   This article summarizes a comprehensive experience with the reconstruction of partial and full thickness defects of the nose using the three-stage forehead flap. A workhorse of nasal reconstruction, the forehead flap technique is thoroughly outlined including the advantages of the recommended three-stage approach.
15. Guo L, Pribaz JR, Pribaz JJ. Nasal reconstruction with local flaps: a simple algorithm for management of small defects. *Plast Reconstr Surg.* 2008;122(1):130-139.
16. Menick FJ. Nasal reconstruction: forehead flap. *Plast Reconstr Surg.* 2004;113(6):100E-111E.
17. Menick FJ. Nasal reconstruction CME. *Plast Reconstr Surg.* 2010;125:138e-150e.
18. Burget GC, Walton R. Optimal use of microvascular free flaps, cartilage grafts and a paramedian forehead flap for aesthetic reconstruction of the nose and adjacent facial units. *Plast Reconstr Surg.* 2007;120(5):1171-1207.
19. Burd A, Wong PS. One-stage Integra reconstruction in head and neck defects. *J Plast Reconstr Aesthet Surg.* 2010;63(3):404-409.
20. Marchac D, Toth B. The axial frontonasal flap revisited. *Plast Reconstr Surg.* 1985;76:686-694.
21. Reiger RA. A local flap for repair of the nasal tip. *Plast Reconstr Surg.* 1967;40:147-149.
22. Rohrich RJ, Muzaffar AR, Adams WP Jr, Hollier LH. The aesthetic unit dorsal nasal flap: rationale for avoiding a glabellar incision. *Plast Reconstr Surg.* 1999;104:1289-1294.
23. Zimany A. The bi-lobed flap. *Plast Reconstr Surg.* 1953;11:424-434.
24. McGregor JC, Soutar DS. A critical assessment of the bilobed flap. *Br J Plast Surg.* 1981;34:197-205.
25. Zitelli JA. The bilobed flap for nasal reconstruction. *Arch Dermatol.* 1989;125:957-959.
   This article describes the most recent modification to the technique for designing and raising a bilobed flap for nasal reconstruction. The Zitelli modification is now the most common manner in which the flap is designed, increasing its viability by decreasing the arc of flap rotation.
26. Zook EG, Van Beek AL, Russell RC, Moore JB. V-Y advancement flap for facial defects. *Plast Reconstr Surg.* 1980;65:786-797.
27. Pribaz JJ, Chester CH, Barrall DT. The extended V-Y flap. *Plast Reconstr Surg.* 1992;90:275-280.
28. Herbert DC, Harrison RG. Nasolabial subcutaneous pedicle flaps. *Br J Plast Surg.* 1975;28:85-89.
29. Herbert DC. A subcutaneous pedicle cheek flap for reconstruction of alar defects. *Br J Plast Surg.* 1978;31:79-92.
30. Hofer S, Posch N, Smit X. Facial artery perforator flaps for reconstruction of perioral defects. *Plast Reconstr Surg.* 2005;115:996-1003.
31. Menick FJ. The modified folded forehead flap for nasal lining—the Menick method. *J Surg Oncol.* 2006;94:509-514.
32. Malard O, Lanhouet J, Michel G, et al. Full-thickness nasal defect: place of prosthetic reconstruction. *Eur Ann Otorhinolaryngol Head Neck Dis.* 2015;132(2):85-89.
33. Menick FJ. Defects of the nose, lip, and cheek: rebuilding the composite defect. *Plast Reconstr Surg.* 2007;120:887-898.
   Composite defects of the midface are those that combine nasal, cheek, and lip. Their repair is especially difficult due to the complex aesthetics and tissue requirements. The basic principles of repair and current approaches are presented to satisfy the unique needs of these defects.

QUESTIONS

1. A 65-year-old man presents after undergoing Mohs micrographic surgery to remove a basal cell carcinoma of the nasal tip. On examination, the resulting defect measures 10 × 3-mm and is full thickness, with exposed, denuded lower lateral cartilages with no perichondrium. Which of the following is the most appropriate reconstruction option?

a. Healing by secondary intention
b. Skin graft
c. Bilobed flap
d. Glabella flap
e. Forehead flap

2. A 22-year-old woman is evaluated after a dog bite injury to the left nasal alar rim that she sustained 6 months ago. Examination shows full-thickness loss of the left alar and soft triangle subunits of her nose. Which of the following treatment options best addresses all of the missing components?

a. Composite helical root graft
b. Conchal cartilage graft and bilobed flap for coverage
c. Nasolabial flap with full-thickness skin graft for lining
d. Forehead flap with skin graft for lining and septal cartilage graft
e. Ulnar forearm free flap

3. An 80-year-old man undergoes resection of a melanoma on the right nasal sidewall. Final pathological margins are found to be free of tumor. Examination of the defect shows a 2 × 3-cm partial-thickness defect involving only the nasal sidewall subunit with intact perichondrium and soft tissue at the base. Which of the following methods of reconstruction is most appropriate for this defect?

a. Partial-thickness skin graft
b. Full-thickness skin graft
c. Bilobed flap
d. Cheek flap
e. Nasolabial flap

4. A 36-year-old woman is brought to the emergency department after sustaining a dog bite to the tip of the nose. Physical examination shows a 3-cm soft tissue deficit involving almost the entire nasal tip. In addition to resection of the remaining nasal tip, which of the following methods of reconstruction is most likely to provide the most satisfactory esthetic outcome?

a. Split-thickness skin graft
b. Full-thickness skin graft
c. Bilobed flap
d. Nasolabial flap
e. Forehead flap

5. What is the number of esthetic subunits that compose the surface anatomy of the nose?

a. Six
b. Seven
c. Eight
d. Nine
e. Ten

1. **Answer: c.** There are many methods to reconstruct this nasal tip defect. Denuded cartilage needs a flap for coverage. Healing by secondary intention or a skin graft would not be appropriate. As this patient's cartilages are intact, they do not need to be replaced. Smaller defects can be covered with a locally available flap. In this case, a forehead is not necessary, as it would result in more severe donor site morbidity. Bilobed flaps are ideal for distal nasal reconstruction, whereas the glabella flap is ideal for proximal reconstruction. A dorsal nasal flap, if large enough, may also be an option for reconstruction of the nasal tip.

2. **Answer: d.** Full-thickness nasal alar defects must be reconstructed with all missing lamellae including lining, support, and coverage in addition to all subunits that are missing. Although many reconstructive options exist, each with their respective benefits and drawbacks, only those options that provide lining, support, and coverage will successfully address the defect in question. Of the options listed, only a forehead flap and skin graft for lining with septal cartilage reconstructs all missing lamellae. Although a composite helical root graft comprises all three nasal lamellae, it is not big enough to address both the alar and the soft triangle nasal subunits.

3. **Answer: b.** In considering nasal reconstruction, the surgeon must understand the location of the defect relative to the nasal subunits involved as well as the nasal lamellae involved. The described defect is limited to the nasal sidewall and only involves the cover or skin. The defect described is too large to close with either a bilobed or nasolabial flap. A cheek flap would be inadequate for a sidewall defect because it would efface the important anatomic junction between the cheek and the nose. Though either a full-thickness or split-thickness skin graft could adequately close a sidewall defect, the increased thickness of a full graft would have a better esthetic result with less secondary contracture and distortion. Although local flaps are preferred on the face, the nasal sidewall is considered a privileged area for skin grafting because the native skin is thin and there is strong underlying bony structure to resist contractile forces of skin grafts. In other areas of the nose, skin grafts are generally avoided.

4. **Answer: e.** The subunit concept, as outlined by Burget and Menick, dictate that when greater than 50% of a subunit are involved in a defect, the best esthetic outcome will result when the entire subunit is resected and reconstructed. In particular, for the nasal tip, scars should be avoided directly on the tip itself. A skin graft will contract and show a different skin color and quality than the surrounding skin, making it less likely to be esthetically acceptable. A bilobed or nasolabial flap, whereas an appropriate choice for smaller defects and alar defects, is unlikely to be able to resurface the entire nasal tip. A forehead flap is a classic reconstructive option for nasal tip defects.

5. **Answer: d.** The nose has nine topographic subunits. These include the nasal dorsum, tip, and columella, as well as the paired sidewalls, ala, and soft triangle subunits. This system of classification of the nasal surface anatomy allows for greater ease of reconstruction because scars can be positioned between the subunits, where they will be less obvious. In addition, knowledge of the esthetics of each subunit helps in choosing replacement tissue of the appropriate contour and thickness. If a patient has a defect that encompasses more than one half of the esthetic subunit, it is best to reconstruct the entire subunit rather than to attempt to cover the defect.

CHAPTER 41 Reconstruction of Acquired Lip and Cheek Deformities

Ian C. Sando and David L. Brown

KEY POINTS

- The rich vascular supply of all structures of the face provides multiple options to reconstruct defects with like tissue.
- Incisions/scars should cross the vermilion-cutaneous junction (white roll) at 90° angles.
- Mark the white roll with parallel marks above and below this structure prior to infiltrating local anesthetic.
- Three considerations are essential in choosing a reconstructive method and orientation of a flap for cheek defects—where laxity exists and how to take advantage of it and where tension of the flap will affect surrounding structures; where resulting scars will lie (parallel to relaxed skin tension lines is best); and the need for excision of residual cutaneous deformities after flap transfer.
- Adjunctive lower lid procedures may be indicated to support the lid to minimize the risk of ectropion.

LIP RECONSTRUCTION

Aesthetic and Functional Considerations

The lips are the principal aesthetic unit of the lower third of the face. Even subtle changes to the intricate anatomy of the lips are readily visible. Alterations to normal lip appearance and motion can have a profound impact on patients' daily activities and psychosocial well-being. Although lip movement plays a pivotal role in verbal communication (e.g., bilabial plosives), the position, shape, and motion of the lips have equally important roles in nonverbal communication and expressions of emotion.[1] Arguably, however, the most important function of the lips is their role in deglutition and maintenance of oral competence. Goals of lip reconstruction are therefore aimed at restoring these diverse functions by maximizing lip aperture, mobility, sensation, and appearance.

Anatomy

The lips are laminar structures composed of four layers: skin, subcutaneous tissue, orbicularis oris muscle, and mucosa. The vermilion forms the major aesthetic feature of the upper and lower lips and is composed of keratinized squamous epithelium, a type of modified mucosa that lacks minor salivary glands. At the external junction of the vermilion and surrounding the lip skin is a pale ridge of tissue termed the white roll, which is formed by pars marginalis fibers of the orbicularis oris muscle. The white roll is most distinct centrally and tapers gradually toward the commissures. Intraorally, the vermilion transitions at the red line (i.e., wet-dry border) into nonkeratinized squamous epithelium of oral mucosa, which is where the upper and lower lips meet when the mouth is closed. Topographically, the upper lip extends from its cephalic border at the nostril sill and alar bases and terminates laterally at the nasolabial creases (**Figure 41.1**). The upper lip is further divided into three anatomic subunits by the philtral columns, which are ridges partially formed by decussation of the orbicularis oris muscle that cross midline to insert directly into the overlying dermis.[2,3] The central subunit is the soft tissue concavity between the philtral columns termed the philtral groove or dimple. Inferior to this is the most projecting portion of the vermilion, the tubercle. The remaining two lateral lip subunits on either side of the philtrum extend to the nasolabial folds. Cupid's bow is the term given to the contour along the vermilion-cutaneous junction between the philtral columns,[4] as its resembles the double-curved bow carried by the Roman god after which it was named. The upper and lower lips join at the commissures. The lower lip differs from the upper lip in that it is a single aesthetic unit. The borders of the lower lip include the nasolabial creases laterally and the labiomental crease inferiorly. The normal intercommissural distance in an adult at rest is 5 to 6 cm, and the relationship of the commissures to the medial limbus sets an aesthetic harmony to the vertical dimensions of the facial profile.

The bulk of the lips is composed of the orbicularis oris muscle, which is the most important muscle for oral competence. The orbicularis oris muscle is innervated by the buccal branch of facial nerve and originates at the modiolus, which is a complex interdigitation of perioral muscles that retract the corners of the mouth. Other muscles originating at the modiolus include the levator anguli oris, the risorius, and the depressor anguli muscles. The orbicularis oris muscle is arranged circularly around the mouth forming a functional sphincteric ring. It also sends fibers to the skin at the base of the ala, nasal sill, and septum. The orbicularis oris is composed of two components: the pars marginalis, which is mostly limited to the area deep to the vermilion; and the pars peripheralis, which lies deep to the pars marginalis at the vermilion and extends peripherally within the cutaneous portion of the lip. The remaining facial and perioral muscles are arranged into four layers based upon their relative depth to one another (**Figure 41.2**). With the exception of the deepest layer of muscles, which includes the mentalis, levator anguli oris, and buccinator muscles, all other facial muscles are innervated on their deep surfaces.[5] The muscles responsible for lip elevation include the paired levator anguli oris, levator labii superioris, levator labii superioris alaeque nasi, zygomaticus major, and zygomaticus minor muscles. These muscles are innervated by the zygomatic and buccal branches of the facial nerve. The mentalis muscles are primary elevators of the lower lip and help to coapt the upper and lower lips and push contents

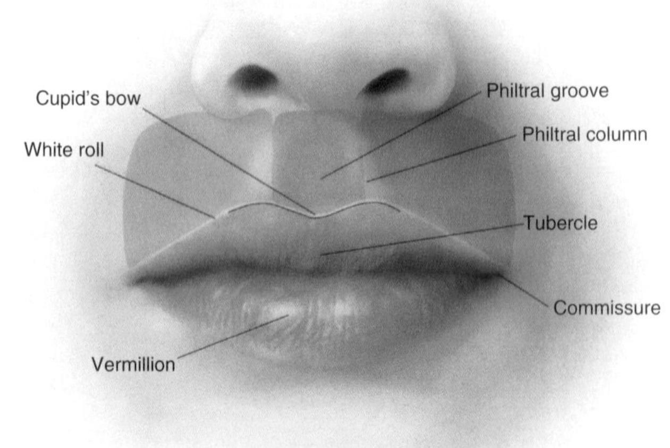

FIGURE 41.1. Topographic anatomy of the lips. Medial aesthetic subunit of the upper lip is depicted by the shaded red area, and the lateral aesthetic subunits are depicted by shaded blue areas.

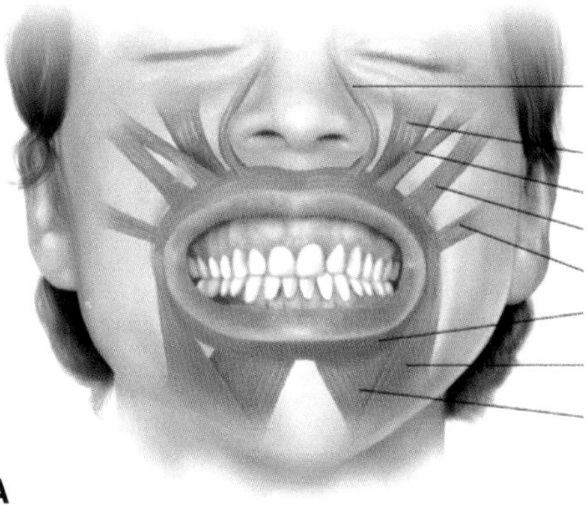

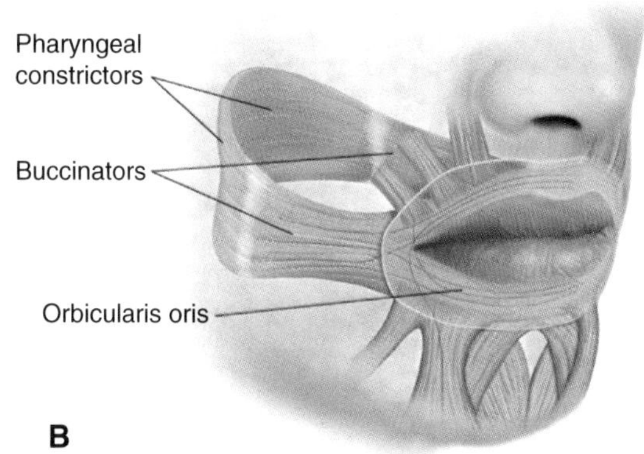

FIGURE 41.2. Muscles of facial expression. (Adapted from Neligan PC. *Plastic Surgery*. 3rd ed. London, UK: Elsevier Saunders; 2013. Copyright © 2013 Elsevier. With permission.)

out of the gingivobuccal sulcus. They are innervated by the marginal mandibular branch of facial nerve and originate from mandible just inferior to the attached gingiva and insert into the chin pad inferior to the labiomental crease. The lip depressors include the depressor anguli oris, the depressor labii inferioris, and, to some degree, the platysma. With the exception of the platysma, which is innervated by the cervical branches of the facial nerve, the lower lip depressors are innervated by the marginal mandibular branch.

The primary arterial supply to the lips is from the superior and inferior labial arteries, which form a rich, 360° vascular network to facilitate the design of multiple flaps for lip reconstruction. The labial arteries arise from the facial artery approximately 1.5 cm lateral to the oral commissure and lie either within or lingual to the orbicularis oris muscle at the level of the red line.[6] The venous drainage does not mirror the well-formed arterial supply, but rather resembles a dense venous plexus that coalesces in the area of the major named arteries. The lymphatic drainage of the upper lip is primarily to the submandibular nodes with some drainage from the commissure to the ipsilateral preauricular nodes. The lower lip also drains to the ipsilateral submandibular nodes; however, there is more potential for crossover in the midline. The medial lower lip tends to drain into the ipsilateral or contralateral submental nodes, which in turn drain into the submandibular nodes. Sensation to the upper and lower lips is provided by the infraorbital (V2) and mental (V3) branches of the trigeminal nerve, respectively. Successful anesthesia without distortion of critical anatomic landmarks can be accomplished by placing small depots of local anesthetic either at the infraorbital foramen, 1 cm below the inferior orbital rim in line with pupil, or at the mental foramen at the depth of the gingivobuccal sulcus below the second premolar. The superior aspect of the philtrum is occasionally innervated by a branch of the nasopalatine and requires direct infiltration at the base of the columella.

Defect Etiology and Assessment

The primary etiology of acquired lip defects is malignancy. Over 90% of cases involve the lower lip, presumably due to its susceptibility to extensive sun exposure. Basal cell carcinoma is the most common malignancy involving the upper lip, and squamous cell carcinoma is the most common in the lower lip. The vast majority of patients with lip cancer are male (96%).[7] Other indications for lip reconstruction, in descending order of frequency, include trauma, burns, and vascular anomalies. When approaching lip reconstruction, one should first assess the lesion and attempt to determine the amount of skin, muscle, and mucosa that will be involved. Defects can be divided into superficial skin defects, vermilion-only defects, small defects involving less than one-third the total lip length, intermediate defects between one-third and two-thirds the lip length, and subtotal or total lip defects. Choices of donor tissue for lip reconstruction include the remaining lip segments, the opposite lip, the adjacent cheek, and distant sites. Goals of reconstruction are focused on providing complete skin coverage and oral lining, producing a semblance of a vermilion, creating an adequate stomal diameter, restoring sensation, and maintaining a competent oral sphincter.[8]

Superficial Cutaneous Defects

Options for closing superficial defects involving the cutaneous lip include primary closure, skin grafts, and local flaps. When closing defects primarily, dog-ears should be excised and oriented in a linear fashion along relaxed skin tension lines, ideally along anatomic boundaries (e.g., philtral column). Natural facial contours such as the nasolabial crease or alar groove are difficult to recreate. If possible, closures should be planned immediately adjacent to these contours to preserve their architecture and help camouflage scars. To avoid tissue redundancy, partial-thickness defects around the vermilion border are generally best managed by converting defects into full-thickness wedge excisions. Skin grafts are generally not required for superficial skin defects because adjacent soft tissue laxity permits the use of local flaps for primary closure. An exception to this includes defects of the central lip involving large portions of the philtral groove. Here, local flaps may cause distortion of Cupid's bow and the philtral columns. Instead, resurfacing the entire subunit with a full-thickness graft limits contraction and optimizes appearance. For smaller defects within the philtral groove, healing by secondary intention generally provides good results and avoids the patch-like appearance of a skin graft. Local tissue rearrangement techniques generally offer the best match in terms of tissue thickness, color, and texture, and are generally designed as either advancement or transposition flaps using cheek and/or adjacent lip tissue. Most common techniques include cheek advancement combined with perialar crescentic excisions, nasolabial flaps, and lateral V-Y advancement flaps (Figure 41.3). The nasolabial flap is a particularly good option for recreating a hair-bearing upper lip in male patients; however, the potential for horizontal hair orientation creates an unnatural appearance.

Vermilion Defects

The vermilion is a modified mucosal surface consisting of a thin layer of nonkeratinized epithelium that is devoid of hair follicles or sebaceous glands. Its unique color is produced by the dense capillary network sandwiched between the mucosa and underlying orbicularis oris muscle. The human eye is remarkably accurate at detecting subtle asymmetries, and the sharp juxtaposition of color at the vermilion-cutaneous junction makes step-offs as small as 1 mm noticeable at conversational distances. Alignment of the vermilion border and

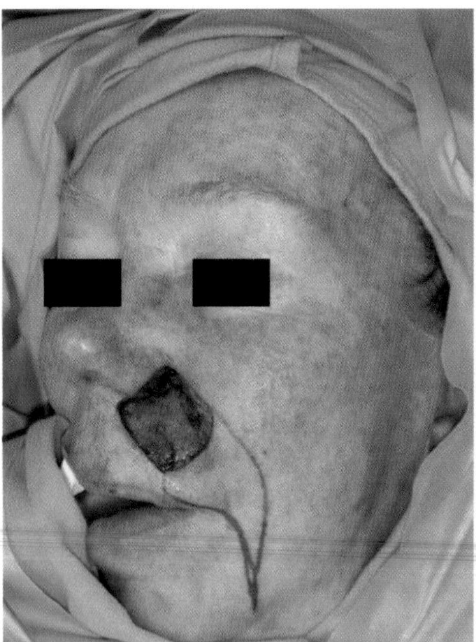
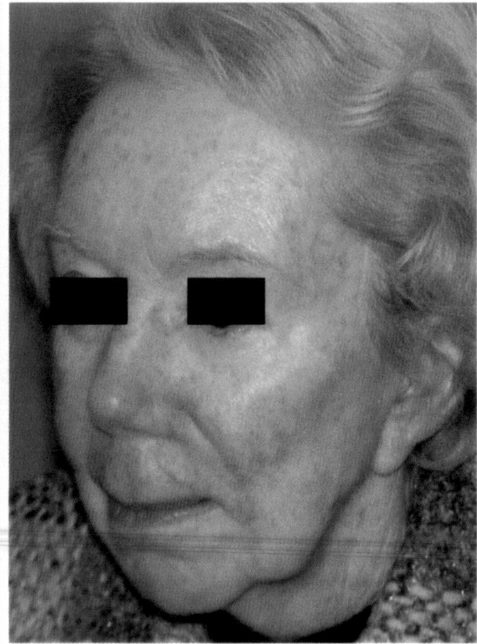

FIGURE 41.3. Reconstruction of left upper lip cutaneous defect with V-Y advancement flap.

white roll is essential in any lip procedure, from simple lacerations to complex reconstructions. To avoid misalignment from tissue distortion, regional nerve blocks (e.g., infraorbital nerve block) are preferred over direct infiltration. The fine anatomic borders of the uninvolved, marginal vermilion should be marked to facilitate precise repair. Small defects confined to the vermilion can be managed with musculomucosal V-Y advancement flaps designed horizontally. Lesions closer to the vermilion border are preferentially excised perpendicular to the white roll to facilitate alignment of this landmark. The simplest method for repair of larger, partial-thickness vermilion defects is undermining and advancement of adjacent buccal mucosa over the remaining orbicularis oris muscle to restore the mucocutaneous junction. This is often used for lip shave procedures resulting in loss of the entire lower lip vermilion. The major disadvantages of this technique are inward retraction and thinning of the lower lip due to mucosa retraction as well as decreased mucosal sensation.

For larger defects that do not involve the white roll, transposition or advancement flaps of vermilion are generally recommended. These include lip sharing procedures, such as the staged bipedicle mucosa flap, or the cross-lip mucosal flap (lip switch) (**Figure 41.4A**). For larger defects that include a portion of orbicularis muscle, myomucosal flaps of lateral lip vermilion based axially on the labial artery may be advanced to close the defect (**Figure 41.4B**). In addition, random buccal mucosal flaps or, more reliably, a facial artery musculomucosal (FAMM) flap can be rotated from intraorally to reconstruct defects of the vermilion.[9] The FAMM flap is an axial flap that includes part of the buccinator muscle and can be based inferiorly (antegrade) or superiorly (retrograde) on the facial vessels. Lastly, tongue flaps are another method for lip reconstruction and can provide significant bulk; however, they require a second stage for pedicle division and flap inset. Utilizing the lateral or ventral surfaces of the tongue avoids transferring the dorsal tongue papillae, which has a rough texture. The biggest drawback of any oral mucosal or tongue flap for lip reconstruction is the tendency for the tissue to desiccate.

Small Full-Thickness Defects

The elasticity of the upper and lower lips permits primary closure of small full-thickness defects in many instances. In the lower lip, 40% of the width can generally be reapproximated using layered closure, whereas in the upper lip, the distinct topographic landmarks (e.g., philtrum and Cupid's bow) can only tolerate primary closure of defects up to 25% without significant distortion. Defects should generally be converted into a shield excision design so that layered closure at the vermilion border is perpendicular to white roll for precise alignment. For larger defects, one is able to keep the scar above the labiomental crease using a W-plasty design (**Figure 41.5**). During closure, careful approximation of the mucosa, orbicularis oris muscle, and skin layers ensures a functional repair and good aesthetic result. Wound edge eversion is critical to prevent notching.

Intermediate-Sized Full-Thickness Defects

Intermediate-sized full-thickness defects represent the most complex decision-making challenge. For defects involving slightly greater than one-third the width of the lip, primary closure is possible if combined with perioral skin excisions. The Schuchardt procedure is a sliding lip reconstruction that combines medial advancement of the lower lip tissue with bilateral labiomental crease excisions.[10] The barrel-shaped incision may be extended all the way around the labiomental folds. For central upper lip defects, Webster's technique of crescentic perialar cheek excisions move the upper lip without disturbing lateral muscle function.[11] The Bengt-Johansson staircase technique is a useful, one-stage repair for central lower lip defects of intermediate width.[12,13] In this technique, neither the orbicularis oris muscle, opposite lip, nor the labiomental crease are violated. The design includes two to four small squares of the skin and subcutaneous tissue that are excised in a stair-step fashion descending from medial to lateral at 45° angles from the base of the defect. Thus, advancement of the flap in the direction of the defect proceeds with each succeeding higher step in the staircase.

Despite the advantages of these techniques, lip-switch flaps are arguably the best method for reconstructing full-thickness lip defects of intermediate width. These are axial flaps based on the labial arteries to reconstruct skin, subcutaneous tissue, muscle, and mucosa of one lip using the same composite tissue from the other. For defects of the central upper lip, excising the entire central subunit and interpolating an Abbe flap into the defect is an excellent option.[14] The Abbe flap is a two-staged lip-switch procedure where a full-thickness flap of up to one-third of the donor lip can be used to reconstruct up to two-thirds of the recipient lip (**Figure 41.6**). The flap is rotated 180° on its pedicle (labial artery) and remains for about 3 weeks, after which the pedicle is divided at a second stage. This technique is effective at recreating the philtral columns without flattening the

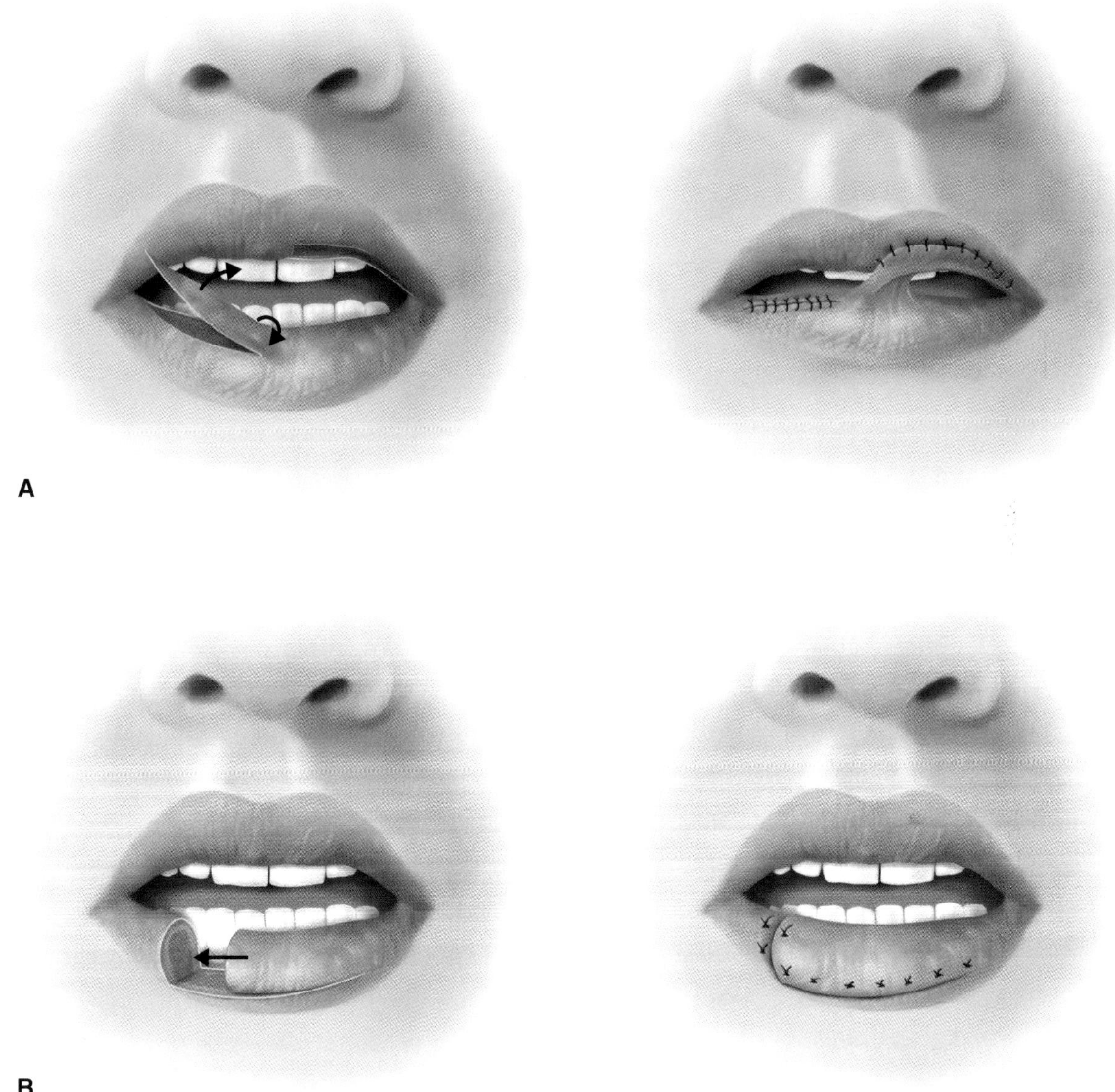

FIGURE 41.4. Vermilion reconstruction. **A.** Reconstruction of a partial-thickness upper lip defect using a unipedicle vermilion lip switch flap. The pedicle is divided 10 to 14 days later at a second-stage procedure. **B.** Laterally based vermilion musculomucosal advancement flap supplied by labial artery.

upper lip contour. Flaps are designed with their borders parallel to relaxed skin tension lines and can be based either medially or laterally on the labial arteries. The height of the flap should match that of the defect and the width of the flap and should be about half the width of the defect. The reverse Abbe flap based on the superior labial artery is useful for reconstructing lateral or midline lower lip defects. However, the central part of the upper lip should never be used for donor tissue, as the philtral columns and dimple are irreplaceable. Instead, a flap from the junction of the middle and lateral thirds of the upper lip should be used.

The Estlander flap is a full-thickness, medially based triangular flap from the upper lip used to reconstruct lateral lower lip defects when the oral commissure is involved (Figure 41.7).[15] Similar to the Abbe flap, it is designed so that its width equals half the width of the defect. Although incisions can be well-hidden within the nasolabial fold, the flap creates a rounded commissure and causes distortion of the modiolus. Therefore, secondary commissuroplasty is often required.

The Gillies *fan flap* is a modification of the cross-lip technique. It rotates tissue around the commissure similar to an Estlander flap, but it includes additional tissue from the nasolabial region. A quadrangular-shaped flap is designed and the incision is extended from the inferior aspect of the defect laterally around the commissure and superiorly into the melolabial crease. Modifications of this technique include the incorporation of a Z-plasty, which allows better turning of the pedicle around the commissure (Figure 41.8). Bilateral flaps are often required for large defects approaching up to 80% of the lip; however, undesirable sequelae of reconstructing such large defects include significant microstomia and oral incompetence due to denervation of the orbicularis oris muscle.

The Karapandzic flap is a musculocutaneous rotation advancement flap similar to the Gillies fan flap; however, with the Karapandzic flap, incisions are limited to the skin and subcutaneous and the neurovascular bundles are carefully dissected and preserved to maintain muscle function and lip sensation (Figure 41.9).[16,17] In addition, small separate mucosal-releasing incisions are made to create a

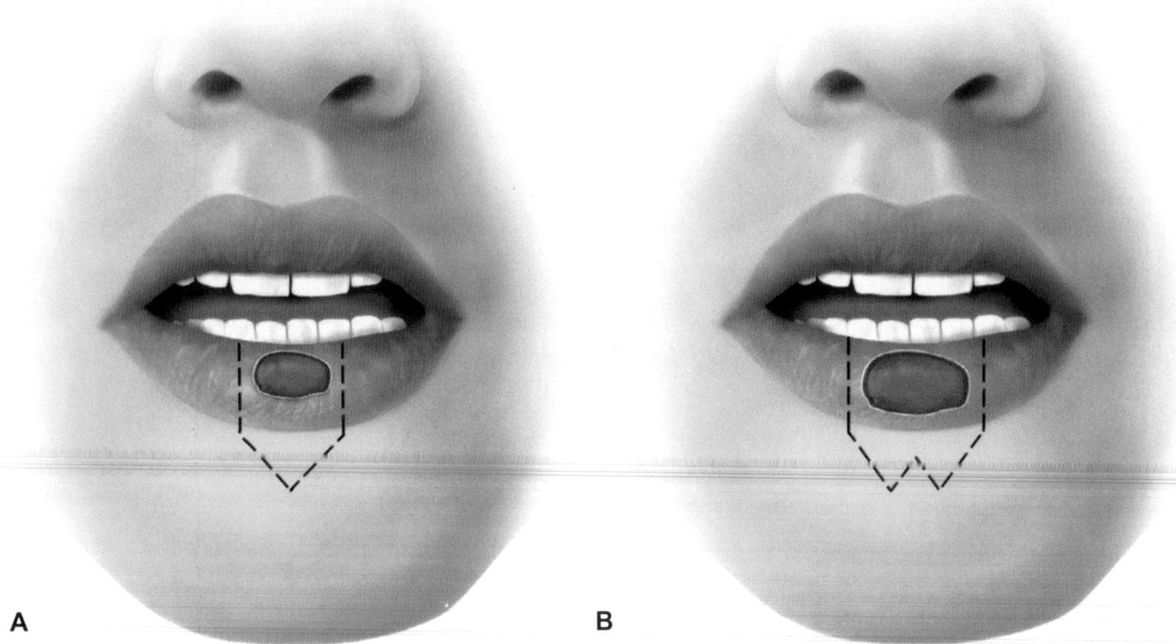

FIGURE 41.5. Wedge excisions of the lower lip using shield **(A)** and W-plasty designs **(B)**.

gingivobuccal sulcus, and redundant skin along the outer circumference generally requires excision as a Burow triangle. These flaps can be used for large central defects up to 80%; however, blunting of the commissures and microstomia may occur.

Subtotal or Total Lip Defects

Reconstructing lip defects over 80% is difficult to achieve with regional tissue alone. Attempts at reconstruction for these defects often leads to poor aesthetic outcome and compromised oral competence due to a denervated, adynamic lower lip. A number of eponyms exist for the bilateral opposing cheek advancement techniques described for reconstructing large lower lip defects.[18-21] All consist of horizontal advancement of cheek skin with removal of Burow triangles as originally described with the *Bernard cheiloplasty* in 1853. These techniques may be combined with a buccal mucosal advancement flap to reconstruct the vermilion. Webster's modification of the Bernard-Burow technique for lower lip reconstruction combines triangular skin excisions adjacent to the nasolabial folds with paramental triangular flaps (**Figure 41.10**). Benefits of this technique are the ability to produce good contour of the commissure, place scars within natural skin creases, and preserve the aesthetic region of the chin; however, drawbacks include incomplete recovery of sensation, vermilion color mismatch, and poor oral competence.[21,22] To overcome these limitations, current techniques excise the skin and subcutaneous only and preserve the neurovascular structures to maximize oral competence and sensation.

Various nasolabial flaps have been described for reconstruction of large upper and lower lip defects.[19,20,23] Long segments of skin and subcutaneous tissue based on perforators of angular artery are transposed to reconstruct full-thickness defects. Examples include Fujimori's *gate flap* design, which rotates two nasolabial island flaps 90° for reconstruction of lower lip defects,[23] and Von Brun interiorly based nasolabial flaps for reconstructing upper lip defects.[19] These designs pivot on the commissures and often require a skin graft to line the inner surface. Surgeons must account for significant

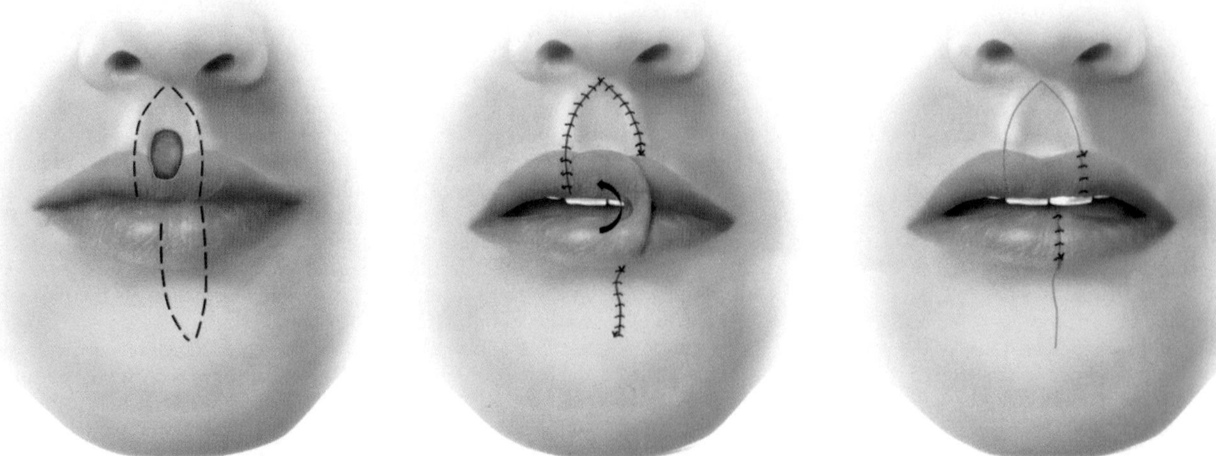

FIGURE 41.6. Full-thickness defect involving central upper lip reconstructed with an Abbe flap.

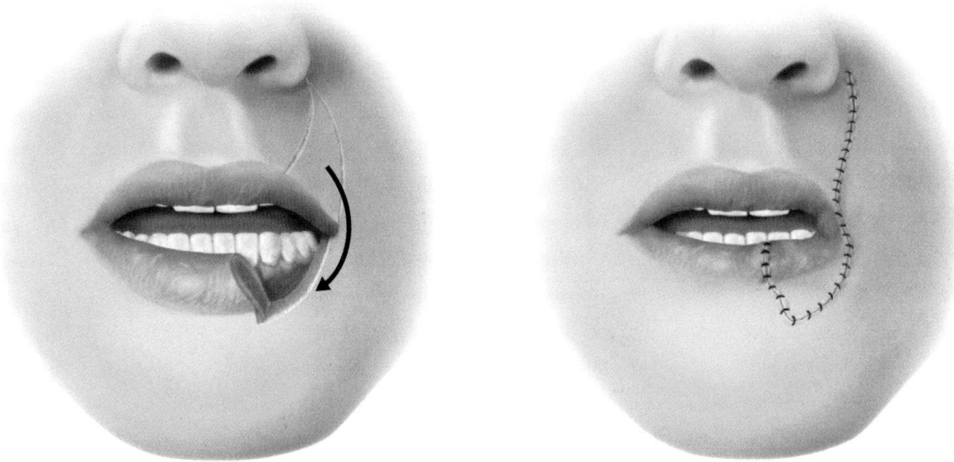

FIGURE 41.7. The Estlander flap rotates upper lip tissue to the lower but results in blunting of the commissure and loss of the normal taper of the vermilion.

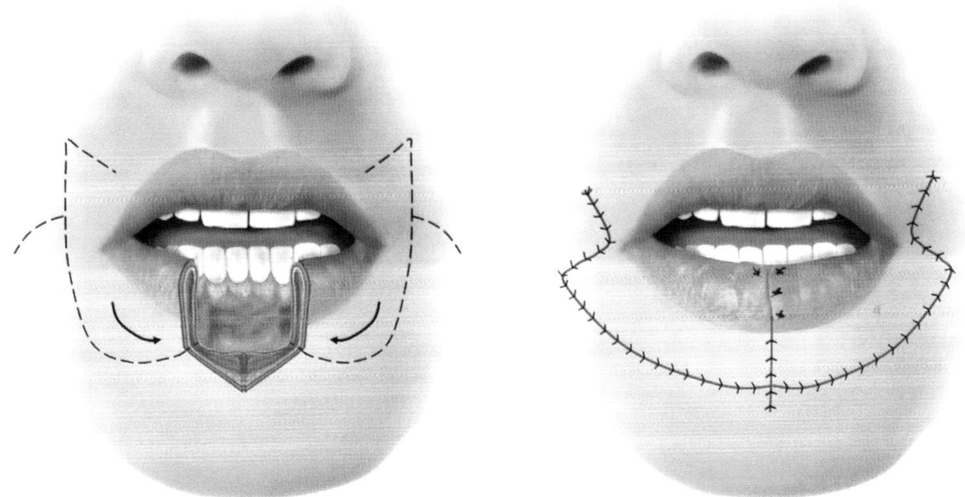

FIGURE 41.8. Z-plasty modification of the Gillies fan flap technique.

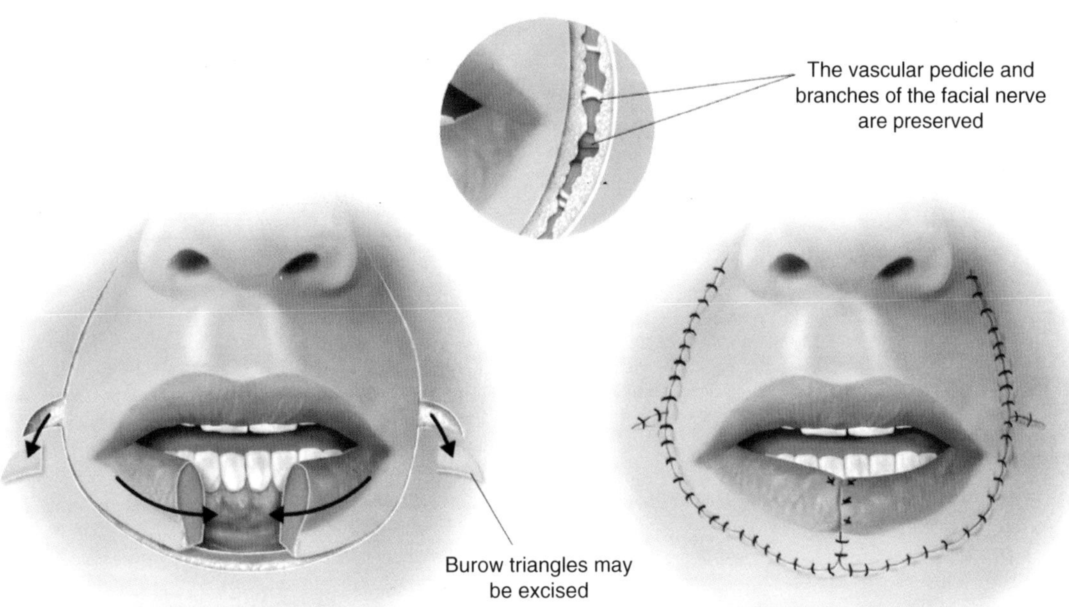
The vascular pedicle and branches of the facial nerve are preserved
Burow triangles may be excised

FIGURE 41.9. The Karapandzic technique.

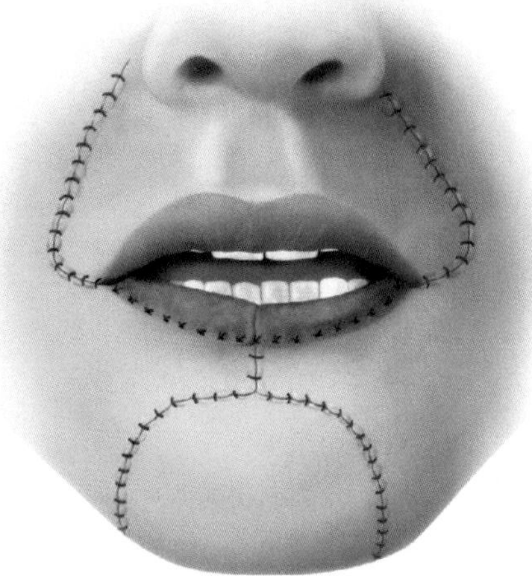

FIGURE 41.10. Webster modification of the Bernard-Burrow technique.

contraction and therefore flaps should be made larger than the lip defect. Reconstruction of the vermilion occurs at a second stage. Despite their ability to recruit large amounts of tissue, nasolabial flaps generally produce suboptimal oral competence and aesthetics, and the use of multiple local flaps is typically more effective.[24-26] For example, two reverse Abbe flaps of lateral upper lip tissue may be used to reconstruct the lower lip whereas perialar crescent excisions and cheek advancement are used to close the upper lip Abbe donor sites. For the upper lip, an Abbe flap from the lower lip may be used to reconstruct the philtrum and combined with bilateral perialar crescent excisions with cheek advancement.

Regional flaps and free tissue transfer are often employed for total or subtotal lip defects when recruitment of local tissue would result in significant microstomia. The submental flap based on the submental branch of the facial artery can be transferred as an island and interpolated to reconstruct upper or lower lip defects. This flap is reliable and offers good tissue match. The temporoparietal scalp flap is best suited for male patients when hair-replacement is desired.[27] The most commonly used free flap for total or near-total defects of the lower lip is the radial forearm free flap. This flap provides thin, pliable, hairless skin with reasonably good color match. Oftentimes, a palmaris longus tendon graft is incorporated with the flap and either attached to the modiolus or anchored to the malar eminence to act as a sling for oral competence.[28-30] This flap can be made sensate by coaptating the lateral antebrachial cutaneous nerve to the mental or inferior alveolar nerve. Another option for microvascular reconstruction is the free gracilis muscle flap. Some surgeons describe prelaminating the gracilis by incorporating a long strip of fascia lata tendon for lower lip support and placing a silicone sheet along the deep site of the muscle to create a neomucosal lining before final transfer.[31,32] The use of a reinnervated gracilis muscle free flap has also been described.[33] Symmetrical spontaneous and voluntary lower lip control was restored by coaptating the motor branch of the gracilis muscle to the marginal branch of the facial nerve. A regional mucosal flap (e.g., FAMM flap) is used to replace the vermilion and inner mucosa, and a skin graft is used to line the external surface of the gracilis muscle.

CHEEK RECONSTRUCTION

Preoperative Considerations

The cheeks represent a large proportion of the facial surface area and play an important role in the aesthetic relationships of the central face. Cheek reconstruction should be meticulously planned and executed to restore facial contours, camouflage scars, maintain hair patterns, minimize wound healing complications, and minimize tension to neighboring facial units (e.g., avoiding lower lid ectropion). Ideally, scars should be planned at the cheek margins or within relaxed skin tension lines.[34] Vertical incisions placed medial to a line drawn from the lateral canthus remain obvious on frontal view and ideally should be replaced by incisions along the nasolabial fold or by blepharoplasty incisions. Care should be taken to avoid placement of hair-bearing skin into non-hair-bearing areas and vice versa. Patient factors such as smoking, diabetes, immunosuppression, history of radiation, and prior scars may compromise wound healing and should be considered when planning reconstruction. The potential need for facial nerve reconstruction should also be anticipated. Furthermore, patients should be counseled about the possible need for revision to improve contour irregularities, particularly for complex reconstructions.

Several authors divide the cheek into subunits based on anatomic characteristics and reconstructive needs, which may be helpful for preoperative planning.[35,36] However, the principles for subunit reconstructive (e.g., discarding remaining tissues of a subunit) are less applicable to cheek reconstruction. The central cheek has more complex and subtle contours compared to the lateral cheek. Because these contours are visually compared to the contralateral side in primary gaze, this region should have a high priority during reconstruction. On the other hand, because the lateral cheek does not play a role in framing the central facial units (nose, lips, and eyelids) and cannot be fully compared with the other cheek, exact symmetry is less important.

Anatomy

The cheek is bounded laterally by the preauricular skin, medially by the nasal sidewall and nasolabial fold, inferiorly by the mandibular border, and superiorly by the temple and lower eyelids. Sensory innervation is provided by the maxillary (V2) and mandibular (V3) divisions of the trigeminal nerve and from small contributions from the anterior cutaneous nerve of the neck and great auricular nerve. Motor innervation of the mimetic facial muscles is provided by the facial nerve and its main branches, whereas the masseter and temporalis muscles are innervated by the trigeminal nerve. The facial nerve is located deep to superficial lobe of parotid. Beyond this, the distal branches are found just deep to the parotid masseteric fascia. Perfusion of the cheek is robust and affords the ability to reliably elevate large, random-pattern flaps for reconstruction of large defects. The arterial supply of the cheek is predominantly provided by the facial artery, which gives off the angular artery that anastomoses with the infraorbital artery and infratrochlear artery distally. The superficial temporal artery and the transverse facial artery supply the superior aspect of the cheek. The lymphatic drainage is via lymphatic channels within the parotid nodes and those along the facial vessels to the submandibular nodes.

The retaining ligaments of the face are fascial condensations that anchor the superficial tissues to the facial skeleton and deep fascia. The zygomatic ligaments (McGregor patch) anchor the skin of the cheek to the inferior border of the zygoma just posterior to the origin of the zygomaticus minor muscle. The mandibular ligaments tether the overlying skin to the anterior mandible.[37] These ligaments resist advancement of cheek skin and may require release to mobilize skin flaps for closure of cheek defects.

Reconstructive Options

Healing by Secondary Intention

The simplest method for closing cheek defects is healing by secondary intention. This is most useful for small, superficial defects, in inconspicuous areas such as the temple or preauricular region. Concave areas heal exceedingly better than areas of convexity because of tension and skin laxity and provide better outcomes as well due to shadows produced by adjacent tissue contours. Larger defects left to heal by secondary intention are prone to significant scar contraction causing distortion of surrounding structures and contour irregularities.

Primary Closure

Primary closure is the best option as long as tension and distortion of surrounding facial units is avoided. The size of the defect that can be closed primarily depends on location, degree of surrounding skin laxity, amount of skin undermining that can be performed, and the tolerable length of the linear scar. Elderly patients demonstrate significant skin laxity, and therefore primary closure is often appropriate even for larger cheek defects. Scars are ideally placed along relaxed skin tension lines or within natural skin contours. Scars are not well *hidden* in structures such as the nasolabial or preauricular crease and instead obliterate these natural landmarks. Placing incisions/scars immediately adjacent to them (1 mm away and parallel) is best.

Skin Grafts

Skin grafts are occasionally used for cheek reconstruction. They are one of the most effective techniques for covering large defects but may be associated with shiny, patch-like reconstructions with poor color match and contour deformity. Skin grafts are useful in patients with significant comorbidities and in patients who require surveillance for recurrence of aggressive tumors. They are primarily reserved for resurfacing less-critical areas of the cheek, such as the preauricular region. Full-thickness skin grafts result in less secondary contracture and less contour deformity. A better color match is more often achieved if skin grafts are harvested from the supraclavicular or preauricular/postauricular skin.

Local Tissue Rearrangement

Transposition flaps such as banner flaps, bilobed flaps, and rhomboid flaps exploit the mobility of the cheek to close many medium to large size defects of the cheek. Skin and subcutaneous tissue from adjacent areas is transferred into the defect and the donor site is closed primarily. Drawbacks include complex scars, pincushioning, trapdoor scarring, and alterations in hair patterns; however, good results can be obtained with careful design to place scars within relaxed skin tension lines or adjacent to natural creases. Banner flaps are the simplest form of transposition flap and are typically used to transfer skin from the preauricular or nasolabial area to close a defect. The apex of the banner flap is excised to avoid a standing cutaneous deformity. Bilobed flaps are modified banner flaps that use a secondary flap to help close the donor site of the primary flap. Flaps are typically designed at 45° angles to one another and are pivoted on arcs of rotation between 90° and 100°. Scarring from bilobed flaps is complex and pincushioning can be a problem. Because of the laxity of the cheek and the ability to use flaps that produce more inconspicuous scar patterns, bilobed flaps are generally not a first choice in cheek reconstruction. Rhomboid flaps are another modification of the banner flap that are commonly used for coverage of lateral lower cheek or temporal defects. The classic rhomboid flap requires an excision of a rhombus defect with 60° and 120° angles. The donor flap bisects one of the 120° angles and is designed so that the vector of maximum tension is in the direction of adjacent cheek laxity, so distortion of surround structures is avoided (Figure 41.11). In addition, the flap is planned so that the donor scar is placed within a relaxed skin tension line or facial crease. Drawbacks with the rhomboid flap are that they have a tendency to pincushion and the need for multiple incisions creates one or more scars that lie perpendicular to lines of relaxed skin tension.

Advancement flaps are particularly useful for preauricular or superomedial defects in patients with significant skin laxity. A flap of cheek tissue can be directly advanced into the defect with excision of a Burow triangle at the base. First described by Esser, V-Y flaps have more recently become a workhorse flap for cheek reconstruction.[38,39] They are useful for defects of the medial cheek, alar base, and along the nasolabial fold and provide excellent color and texture match for reconstruction. V-Y flaps have been shown to provide excellent outcomes in even large, superior cheek/lower eyelid defects, with less undermining required and improved rates of ectropion compared to Mustarde-type cheek flaps.[40] V-Y flaps survive on perforators within the subcutaneous pedicle and are designed with curved limbs that follow the relaxed skin tension lines. One of the limbs is planned along the nasolabial fold for concealed scar placement. Performing a subcutaneous dissection around the V-Y flap, designing an appropriately sized flap, and meticulous closure of the donor defect achieves good mobilization for closure with minimal tension on the closure.

Regional Flaps

The most common method for reconstructing medium to large defects of the cheek is medially or laterally based cheek rotation advancement flaps. These flaps utilize loose preauricular and neck skin and are most useful for defects in the superior medial region of the cheek. Various designs exist depending on the size and location of defect (Figure 41.12). Wide subcutaneous undermining enables advancement and rotation, and flap anchoring to the deep fascia helps reduce tension on the repair and to prevent distortion of surrounding facial units. Standing cutaneous deformities often develop and require excision of a Burow triangle. Incisions crossing the mandibular border tend to be noticeable and may develop scar contracture. Here, inclusion of a Z-plasty helps to minimize these issues. Resections performed close to the lower eyelid are at risk for lower lid edema and ectropion, and concomitant lower eyelid-tightening procedures should be performed in select patients. Ischemia of the distal flap is the most common complication and is more likely in smokers. A deep plane approach with composite elevation of the skin, subcutaneous tissue, superficial muscular aponeurotic system, and platysma improves flap vascularity and is useful in those at risk for distal flap ischemia; however, facial nerve injury is a significant risk.

Cervicopectoral flaps recruit skin of the neck and chest to cover large cheek defects requiring significant advancement and rotation of donor tissue.[41-43] The upper border of defects suitable for cervicopectoral flap reconstruction can be estimated by drawing a line connecting the tragus to the lateral commissure; otherwise, skin necrosis may result. Anteriorly based flaps based on internal mammary perforators are raised deep to the platysma muscle and include deltoid and pectoral fascia and are used for reconstructing large defects of the posterior and lower cheek. Posteriorly based flaps are based on blood supply from the superficial temporal, occipital, transverse cervical, and thoracoacromial vessels and are used for large anterior cheek defects. These flaps are designed by extending the cervicofacial incision inferiorly along the sternum, then laterally down across the chest above the nipple-areola complex. Skin grafting of the donor site is occasionally required to minimize tension on the closure. Other regional flaps to consider in the armamentarium for cheek reconstruction include the pectoralis major, trapezius, and supraclavicular flaps, which are useful for lower lateral cheek defects, as well as the submental artery flap for central cheek defects.

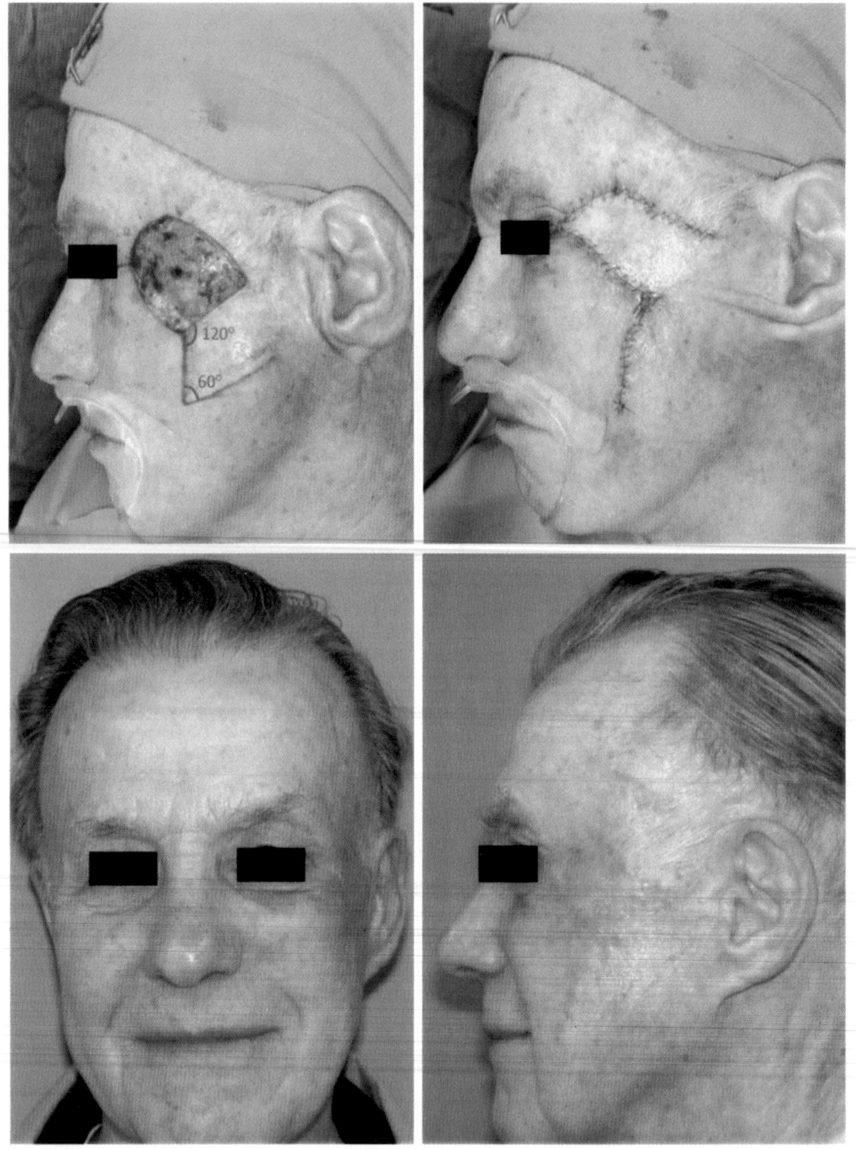

FIGURE 41.11. Rhomboid flap for reconstruction of a left temple defect.

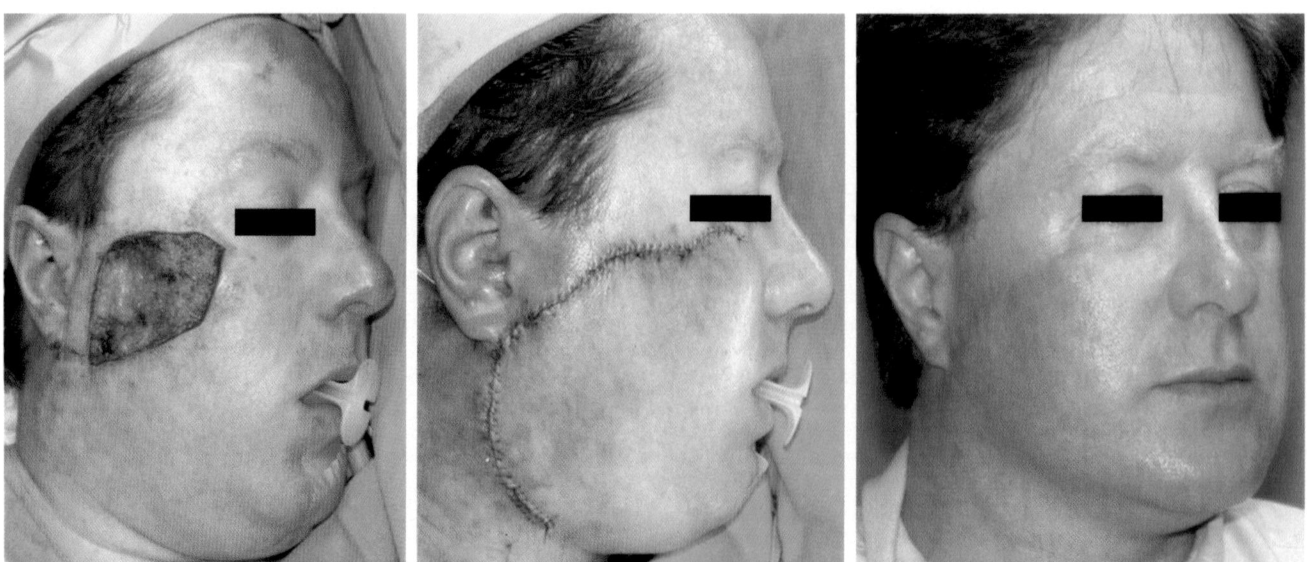

FIGURE 41.12. Inferiorly based cervicofacial advancement flaps for reconstruction of a lateral cheek defect.

Tissue Expansion

Tissue expansion has the benefit of transferring well-vascularized skin with similar color, texture, and hair-bearing status for resurfacing large cheek defects with the least number of additional incisions. It is particularly useful in secondary revision of existing scars, large benign skin lesions, skin grafts, or skin paddles of previously performed free flaps. However, tissue expansion in the head and neck region is associated with high complication rates.[44-46] Good patient selection and careful consideration of the expander size, placement of incisions, expander pocket location, position of the expander fill-valve, and ultimate fill volume are keys to success.

Free Tissue Transfer

Though technically challenging, free flaps are the first choice for complex defects involving multiple tissue layers. They are also useful for resurfacing large skin defects for patients in whom local flaps are not available (e.g., facial burns) or advisable (e.g., history of radiation). Commonly used options include the radial forearm flap, scapular/parascapular flap, anterolateral thigh flap, rectus abdominis myocutaneous flap, and fibula osteocutaneous flap. The choice of free flap depends on the external skin, intraoral lining, skeletal stability, and soft tissue contour requirements. Limitations of free flap coverage include the inability to provide color- and texture-matched skin and the propensity for bulky reconstructions.

REFERENCES

1. Neligan PC. Strategies in lip reconstruction. *Clin Plast Surg.* 2009;36(3):477-485.
2. Briedis J, Jackson IT. The anatomy of the philtrum: observations made on dissections in the normal lip. *Br J Plast Surg.* 1981;34(2):128-132.
   The anatomical basis of the phitrum are investigated in this anatomic study. The authors discuss the contribution of the vertical fibers of the orbicularis oris muscle, the intricate intradermal collagen network, the high concentration of elastin fibers, and underlying dentoskeletal framework to the normal architecture of the philtrum.
3. Burget GC, Menick FJ. Aesthetic restoration of one-half the upper lip. *Plast Reconstr Surg.* 1986;78(5):583-593.
   In this article, the authors describe the anatomic subunits of the upper lip, which include the philtrum and the lateral lip elements. They suggest that defects involving greater than half of a topographic subunit necessitate removal of the entire subunit and reconstruction with local flaps of like tissue.
4. Mulliken JB, Pensler JM, Kozakewich HP. The anatomy of Cupid's bow in normal and cleft lip. *Plast Reconstr Surg.* 1993;92(3):395-403.
5. Freilinger G, Gruber H, Happak W, Pechmann U. Surgical anatomy of the mimic muscle system and the facial nerve: importance for reconstructive and aesthetic surgery. *Plast Reconstr Surg.* 1987;80(5):686-690.
6. Schulte DL, Sherris DA, Kasperbauer JL. The anatomical basis of the Abbe flap. *Laryngoscope.* 2001;111(3):382-386.
7. Zitsch RP 3rd, Park CW, Renner GJ, Rea JL. Outcome analysis for lip carcinoma. *Otolaryngol Head Neck Surg.* 1995;113(5):589-596.
8. Tobin GR, O'Daniel TG. Lip reconstruction with motor and sensory innervated composite flaps. *Clin Plast Surg.* 1990;17(4):623-632.
9. Pribaz JJ, Meara JG, Wright S, et al. Lip and vermilion reconstruction with the facial artery musculomucosal flap. *Plast Reconstr Surg.* 2000;105(3):864-872.
   The composite facial artery musculomucosal (FAMM) flap for lip reconstruction is described in this article. The axial pattern blood supply for both superiorly and inferiorly based flaps is detailed. The buccal mucosa included with the FAMM flap has many similarities to the vermillion, and the buccinator muscle adds additional bulk for more convexity, which makes the flap an excellent option for lip reconstruction.
10. Schuchardt K. Surgery as an aid to orthodontics. *Osterr Z Stomatol.* 1954;51(11):563-565.
11. Webster JP. Crescentic peri-alar cheek excision for upper lip flap advancement with a short history of upper lip repair. *Plast Reconstr Surg.* 1955;16(6):434-464.
12. Blomgren I, Blomqvist G, Lauritzen C, et al. The step technique for the reconstruction of lower lip defects after cancer resection: a follow-up study of 165 cases. *Scand J Plast Reconstr Surg Hand Surg.* 1988;22(1):103-111.
13. Johanson B, Aspelund E, Breine U, Holmstrom H. Surgical treatment of non-traumatic lower lip lesions with special reference to the step technique: a follow-up on 149 patients. *Scand J Plast Reconstr Surg.* 1974;8(3):232-240.
14. Abbe R. A new plastic operation for the relief of deformity due to double harelip. *Med Rec.* 1898;53:477.
    In this report, the American surgeon Robert Abbé (1851–1928) publishes on the transposition labial flap harvested from the lower lip for cleft lip repair. This flap is not only the first musculocutaneous flap described but also the first flap based on a defined vascular supply, the labial vessels. It should be noted that Italian surgeon, Pietro Sabattini, first performed this operation in 1837 to repair a posttraumatic upper lip defect using composite tissue from the lower lip.
15. Estlander JA. Eine methode aus er einen ippe substanzverluste der anderen zu ersetzein. *Arch Klin Chir.* 1872;14:622.
16. Karapandzic M. Reconstruction of lip defects by local arterial flaps. *Br J Plast Surg.* 1974;27(1):93-97.
    Dr. Miodra Karapandzic reports his experience reconstructing large lower lip defects in 58 patients between 1967 and 1972 using his modification of the Gillies fan flap. He describes designing a musculocutaneous rotation advancement flap with careful dissection and preservation of facial artery branches and sensory and motor nerves to ensure a dynamic reconstruction with good sensation.
17. Jabaley ME, Clement RL, Orcutt TW. Myocutaneous flaps in lip reconstruction. Applications of the Karapandzic principle. *Plast Reconstr Surg.* 1977;59(5):680-688.
18. Ducic Y, Athre R, Cochran CS. The split orbicularis myomucosal flap for lower lip reconstruction. *Arch Facial Plast Surg.* 2005;7(5):347-352.
19. Hauben DJ. Victor von Bruns (1812–1883) and his contributions to plastic and reconstructive surgery. *Plast Reconstr Surg.* 1985;75(1):120-127.
20. Dieffenbach JF. *Die Operative Chirurgie.* Leipzig: FA Brockhaus; 1845.
21. Webster RC, Coffey RJ, Kelleher RE. Total and partial reconstruction of the lower lip with innervated musclebearing flaps. *Plast Reconstr Surg Transpl Bull.* 1960;25:360-371.
22. Seo HJ, Bae SH, Nam SB, et al. Lower lip reconstruction after wide excision of a malignancy with barrel-shaped excision or the webster modification of the bernard operation. *Arch Plast Surg.* 2013;40(1):36-43.
23. Fujimori R. "Gate flap" for the total reconstruction of the lower lip. *Br J Plast Surg.* 1980;33(3):340-345.
24. Williams EF 3rd, Setzen G, Mulvaney MJ. Modified Bernard-Burow cheek advancement and cross-lip flap for total lip reconstruction. *Arch Otolaryngol Head Neck Surg.* 1996;122(11):1253-1258.
25. Kroll SS. Staged sequential flap reconstruction for large lower lip defects. *Plast Reconstr Surg.* 1991;88(4):620-625; discussion 6–7.
26. Kiyokawa K, Takagi M, Fukushima J, Kizuka Y, Inoue Y, Tai Y. Surgical treatment following huge arteriovenous malformation extending from the lower lip to the chin: combination of embolization, total resection, and a double cross lip flap. *J Craniofac Surg.* 2005;16(3):443-448.
27. Chang KP, Lai CS, Tsai CC, Lin TM, Lin SD. Total upper lip reconstruction with a free temporal scalp flap: long-term follow-up. *Head Neck.* 2003;25(7):602-605.
28. Sadove RC, Luce EA, McGrath PC. Reconstruction of the lower lip and chin with the composite radial forearm-palmaris longus free flap. *Plast Reconstr Surg.* 1991;88(2):209-214.
29. Jeng SF, Kuo YR, Wei FC, Su CY, Chien CY. Total lower lip reconstruction with a composite radial forearm-palmaris longus tendon flap: a clinical series. *Plast Reconstr Surg.* 2004;113(1):19-23.
30. Carroll CM, Pathak I, Irish J, Neligan PC, Gullane PJ. Reconstruction of total lower lip and chin defects using the composite radial forearm–palmaris longus tendon free flap. *Arch Facial Plast Surg.* 2000;2(1):53-56.
31. Lengele BG, Testelin S, Bayet B, Devauchelle B. Total lower lip functional reconstruction with a prefabricated gracilis muscle free flap. *Int J Oral Maxillofac Surg.* 2004;33(4):396-401.
32. Jeng SF, Kuo YR, Wei FC, Su CY, Chien CY. Reconstruction of extensive composite mandibular defects with large lip involvement by using double free flaps and fascia lata grafts for oral sphincters. *Plast Reconstr Surg.* 2005;115(7):1830-1836.
33. Ninkovic M, Spanio di Spilimbergo S, Ninkovic M. Lower lip reconstruction: introduction of a new procedure using a functioning gracilis muscle free flap. *Plast Reconstr Surg.* 2007;119(5):1472-1480.
34. Menick FJ. Reconstruction of the cheek. *Plast Reconstr Surg.* 2001;108(2):496-505.
35. Zide B, Longaker M. Cheek surface reconstruction: best choices according to zones. *Oper Tech Plast Reconstr Surg.* 1998;5:26.
36. Chandawarkar RY, Cervino AL. Subunits of the cheek: an algorithm for the reconstruction of partial-thickness defects. *Br J Plast Surg.* 2003;56(2):135-139.
37. Furnas DW. The retaining ligaments of the cheek. *Plast Reconstr Surg.* 1989;83(1):11-16.
38. Pontes L, Ribeiro M, Vrancks JJ, Guimaraes J. The new bilaterally pedicled V-Y advancement flap for face reconstruction. *Plast Reconstr Surg.* 2002;109(6):1870-1874.
39. Esser FJS. Island flaps. *NY State J Med.* 1917;106:264-267.
40. Sugg KB, Cederna PS, Brown DL. The V-Y advancement flap is equivalent to the Mustardé flap for ectropion prevention in the reconstruction of moderate-size lid-cheek junction defects. *Plast Reconstr Surg.* 2013;131(1):28e-36e.
41. Dyer PV, Irvine GH. Cervicopectoral rotation flap. *Br J Plast Surg.* 1994;47(1):68-69.
42. Becker DW Jr. A cervicopectoral rotation flap for cheek coverage. *Plast Reconstr Surg.* 1978;61(6):868-870.
43. Anand AG, Amedee RG, Butcher RB II. Reconstruction of large lateral facial defects utilizing variations of the cervicopectoral rotation flap. *Ochsner J.* 2008;8(4):186-190.
44. McIvor NP, Fong MW, Berger KJ, Freeman JL. Use of tissue expansion in head and neck reconstruction. *J Otolaryngol.* 1994;23(1):46-49.
45. Argenta LC, Watanabe MJ, Grabb WC. The use of tissue expansion in head and neck reconstruction. *Ann Plast Surg.* 1983;11(1):31-37.
46. Antonyshyn O, Gruss JS, Zuker R, Mackinnon SE. Tissue expansion in head and neck reconstruction. *Plast Reconstr Surg.* 1988;82(1):58-68.

QUESTIONS

1. A 68-year-old man undergoes wide local excision of a squamous cell carcinoma of the lower lip resulting in a full-thickness defect of the central two-thirds. Margins are free of involvement. Reconstruction using which of the following techniques is most appropriate?

   a. Primary closure
   b. Estlander flap
   c. Karapandzic flap
   d. Nasolabial flap
   e. Submental artery island flap

2. A 40-year-old man sustains complete loss of the lower lip following a traumatic blast injury. Which of the following treatment plans is most likely to restore a competent lower lip with adequate aperture?

   a. Karapandzic flap
   b. Innervated anterolateral thigh flap
   c. Gillies fan flap
   d. Radial forearm flap with tendon graft
   e. Prosthetic lower lip appliance

3. A 66-year-old woman is evaluated for reconstruction of a full-thickness defect of the right lateral lower lip and commissure following resection of a 2.5 cm lesion with clear margins. Which of the following flaps is most appropriate?

   a. Gillies
   b. Webster-Bernard
   c. Abbe
   d. Karapandzic
   e. Estlander

4. A 58-year-old man undergoes resection of a basal cell carcinoma of the upper lip with negative margins, resulting in a full-thickness defect involving three-fourths of the upper central lip. Which of the following is the most appropriate method of reconstruction?

   a. Bilateral Karapandzic flaps
   b. Estlander flap only
   c. Abbe flap only
   d. Bilateral Karapandzic flaps with an Abbe flap
   e. Bilateral Estlander flaps with an Abbe flap

5. A 68-year-old woman has a 6.0 cm defect of the central left cheek just below the eyelid after excision of a lentigo maligna melanoma with clear margins. Which of the following is the most appropriate method for management?

   a. Free anterolateral thigh flap
   b. Cervicofacial advancement flap
   c. Primary closure
   d. Healing by secondary intention
   e. Full-thickness skin grafting

1. Answer: c. Karapandzic flaps are appropriate for reconstruction of defects involving one- to two-thirds of the lower lip, such as in this case. Attempts to reconstruct defects larger than 80% of the lower lip often leads to microstomia. The one-stage technique involves performing circumoral incisions and mobilizing the orbicularis oris muscle, while preserving its innervations and vascular supply. The main advantage of this technique is that a continuous sphincter of functional orbicularis muscle is created, helping to restore oral competence. Primary closure of such a defect would likely result in significant microstomia and is primarily indicated for defects involving less than one-third of the lower lip. The Estlander flap is a full-thickness, cross-lip transposition flap designed to reconstruct lateral defects of the lower lip (one- to two-thirds) requiring recreation of the oral commissure. Nasolabial flaps can be used to reconstruct large full-thickness lower lip defects. However, they require grafting of the deep surface of the flap, do not provide a functional muscular oral sphincter, and have a less reliable random blood supply. The submental artery island flap is based on the submental branch of the facial artery. A paddle of skin and subcutaneous tissue harvested from the submental area can be used for coverage of large lower lip defects; however, it is does not contribute to a functional muscular oral sphincter.

2. Answer: d. Functional restoration of a competent and dynamic lower lip is challenging. A prosthetic lower lip appliance may have an acceptable appearance but does not provide dynamic function and generally does little to provide oral competence. Gillies fan flaps and innervated regional advancement flaps such as the Karapandzic flap are not indicated for total lip loss and would lead to significant microstomia. An innervated anterolateral thigh flap may allow for some degree of sensory restoration, but it would be bulky and adynamic. Radial forearm flaps with tendon grafts are capable of achieving oral competence without risking significant microstomia. They can also be made sensate by coapting the lateral antebrachial cutaneous nerve to the mental or inferior alveolar nerve.

3. Answer: e. In this scenario, reconstruction of both the lower lip and commissure is required. The most appropriate flap for reconstruction of the defect is the Estlander flap, which is an upper lip-switch flap used to reconstruct defects involving the commissure. However, rotation of upper lip to the lower lip results in a rounded commissure, and often requires additional surgery. The Abbe flap is a two-staged lip-switch procedure where a full-thickness segment of the lower lip based on the inferior labial artery is used to fill a central upper lip defect. The Abbe flap can be used to reconstruct defects up to two-thirds of the upper lip and is designed in the center of the lower lip, thereby preserving innervation to the orbicularis oris muscle lateral to the defect. The Karapandzic and Gillies flaps are advancement flaps of the remaining lower lip and are most useful for central defects of the lower lip. The Karapandzic flap differs from the Gillies flap in that branches of the facial nerve are dissected and preserved, thereby preserving facial nerve function. Webster-Bernard flap is also used for reconstruction of central lip defects by removing Burrow triangles bilaterally and advancing cheek skin toward the midline.

4. Answer: d. In this scenario, the patient has a large resection of the central upper lip. The Abbe flap alone is insufficient to close a defect this large and the Estlander flap is reserved for reconstruction of commissure defects, not central defects. The best choice for reconstruction is closure with bilateral Karapandzic flaps with a central Abbe flap for philtral reconstruction. Inferiorly based Karapandzic flaps enable transfer of the remaining upper lip while preserving its neurovascular supply. Although bilateral Karapandzic flaps alone may be useful for defects up to 80% of the width of the upper lip, they are not an ideal choice in this case because of the concern for microstomia. Furthermore, loss of the philtrum would result in significant cosmetic deformity.

5. **Answer: b.** The cervicofacial flap is an inferomedially based flap that transfers large amounts of cutaneous and subcutaneous soft tissues from the loose preauricular and neck regions to the medial cheek. By utilizing tissue adjacent to the defect, the flap provides excellent color and texture match for cheek reconstruction. The incision begins at the superior margin of the defect and extends in a superolateral vector along the outer canthus toward the zygoma and down the preauricular crease. The incision ends in the retroauricular hairline or curves anteriorly in the region of the neck. The flap is advanced and rotated into the defect, and primary closure of the donor site can usually be achieved via wide subcutaneous undermining. Anchoring of the flap to the zygoma reduces tension on the lower eyelid and minimizes the risk of ectropion, which is particularly important in this case.

Primary closure is an effective method for reconstructing small defects of the cheek. Orienting the incision along lines of minimal tension or natural cheek contours often provides inconspicuous scars. However, for such a large defect, primary closure cannot be achieved without significant wound tension and distortion of surrounding structures. Closure by secondary intention would require a prolonged period of healing. In addition, it would result in significant scar contracture and likely lower lid ectropion. Full-thickness skin grafts tend to appear patchlike and shiny with a poor contour match. Free tissue transfer for reconstruction of the aforementioned defect is unnecessary, would create excessive bulk, and likely result in poor color and texture match.

CHAPTER 42 Facial Paralysis

Leahthan F. Domeshek and Gregory H. Borschel

KEY POINTS

- A multidisciplinary approach to the patient with facial paralysis is required to optimize outcomes.
- Ocular protection is of utmost importance in patients with facial paralysis. Appropriate conservative measures must be undertaken and initiated early to protect ocular integrity in setting of exposure.
- In traumatic/iatrogenic cases of facial paralysis in which distal nerve stumps are available, nerve repair or transfer is best performed within 72 hours of injury, prior to depletion of neurotransmitter in the distal stump.
- The standard technique for smile reanimation remains free functional muscle transfer in children. Local muscle transfers reliably improve resting tone and appearance (in both children and adults) but ability to animate remains variable and often inferior to that provided by free functional muscle transfer.
- Both nerve to masseter and cross-facial nerve grafts can be used with free functional muscle transfers to generate powerful, reliable smile. However, only use of cross-facial nerve grafts can lead to smile under emotional control.
- Bell palsy is the most common diagnosis for facial paralysis in adults. It is a diagnosis of exclusion and likely caused by a latent herpes simplex virus infection. In children, paralysis is more often due to infection or trauma.

BACKGROUND

Facial paralysis is a complicated and potentially devastating condition. It occurs in both the adult and pediatric populations, may be congenital or acquired, and can present uni- or bilaterally. A myriad of etiologies exist, including infectious, autoimmune, oncologic, iatrogenic, traumatic, congenital, and idiopathic. Depending on the cause, paralysis ranges from self-limited to irreversible.

Palsy generates cosmetically disruptive facial asymmetry and impairs facial functions, hampering nonverbal communication and inhibiting social interactions. The result may be significant psychosocial distress.

Care of these patients is complex and best approached from a multidisciplinary standpoint, including therapeutic, medical, and surgical disciplines. In patients who do not recover function with conservative measures, surgical reanimation should be considered.

ANATOMY AND FUNCTION OF THE FACIAL NERVE

Functional Components

Functionally, the facial nerve consists of four components[1]:

- *Branchial motor* (from the motor nucleus): Accounts for most of the axons of the facial nerve. Innervates the mimetic musculature of the face as well as the stylohyoid, stapedius, and posterior belly of the digastric.
- *Visceral motor* (superior salivatory nucleus): Provides parasympathetic control to multiple glands and mucosal elements of the face. The submandibular and sublingual glands receive fibers via the chorda tympani. The lacrimal gland and nasal mucosa receive fibers via the pterygopalatine ganglion.
- *General sensory* (sensory nuclei of the trigeminal nerve): Provides sensation to the external auditory canal and the concha.
- *Special sensory* (solitary nucleus): Contributes taste to the anterior two-thirds of the tongue (via the chorda tympani).

The facial nerve consists of intracranial, intratemporal, and extracranial components.

Intracranial Facial Nerve

The motor nucleus of the facial nerve lies in the pons. Upper motor neuron control derives from the cortex and differs from upper and lower facial functions. Input to the motor nucleus for upper facial function is from bilateral motor cortices. Control of lower facial function comes from only the contralateral motor cortex. For this reason, upper motor neuron lesions generally lead to contralateral lower facial paralysis with preserved forehead function. Distal to the motor nucleus, lesions of the facial nerve result in paralysis of all ipsilateral distributions.

Intracranially and proximally within the temporal bone, the motor component of the facial nerve runs separately from the visceral motor, general sensory, and special sensory fibers. These latter three components combine to form the nervus intermedius, which exits the brainstem between the pons and inferior cerebellar peduncle, lateral to the motor component.

The motor component and nervus intermedius run in loose approximation from the brainstem toward the internal auditory meatus, through which they enter the temporal bone.

Intratemporal Facial Nerve

The intratemporal course of the facial nerve is divided into three segments (**Table 42.1** and **Figure 42.1**). The most proximal is the labyrinthine, spanning from the fallopian canal to the geniculate ganglion (which contains taste and sensory nerve cell bodies). At the level of the geniculate ganglion, the nervus intermedius and the motor component join together. Within this segment, the facial nerve gives off three branches. The diameter of the labyrinthine segment is small compared with that of the facial nerve, placing the nerve at risk for compression.

The facial nerve proceeds to the tympanic segment, which extends to the semicircular canal. The labyrinthine and tympanic segments meet at an acute angle that is a common location for shearing injuries to the nerve in trauma involving the temporal bone.

Finally, the nerve enters the mastoid segment, within which the nerve to the stapedius, the sensory branch to the external auditory canal, and the chorda tympani arise. At the end of the mastoid segment, the nerve exits the skull base through the stylomastoid foramen.

Extratemporal Facial Nerve

In adults, the facial nerve is relatively protected by the mastoid tip, tympanic ring, and mandibular ramus, as it emerges from the stylomastoid foramen. In children, it is more superficial, lacking this bony protection, and thus more susceptible to trauma in this area.

On exiting the skull base, the facial nerve can be identified in relationship to specific landmarks. It is located medial to the tympanomastoid suture, running lateral to the styloid process, roughly midway between it and the posterior belly of the digastric muscle. Additionally, it can be identified in relation to the tragal pointer (to which it lies 1 cm deep, and just inferomedially).

Prior to coursing anteriorly around the earlobe, the facial nerve gives off branches to the stylohyoid muscle and the posterior belly of the digastric muscle as well as to the occipitalis and the auricularis muscles.

TABLE 42.1. INTRATEMPORAL FACIAL NERVE BRANCHES

Nerve	Intratemporal Segment of Origin	Function
Greater petrosal nerve	Labyrinthine (Geniculate ganglion)	Parasympathetic innervation to nasal, palatine, lacrimal, and pharyngeal glands, as well as to the sphenoid, frontal, maxillary, and ethmoid sinuses, and nasal cavity Taste fibers for the palate (via greater and lesser palatine nerves)
External petrosal nerve *(variably present)*	Labyrinthine (Geniculate ganglion)	Sympathetic innervation to middle meningeal artery
Lesser petrosal nerve	Labyrinthine (Geniculate ganglion)	Parasympathetic fibers to the parotid gland (via the glossopharyngeal nerve)
Nerve to stapedius	Mastoid	Motor nerve helps to dampen loud noises (innervates stapes muscle). *Of note, cell bodies for this nerve are not located in the motor nucleus and therefore function is spared in congenital palsies such as Mobius syndrome.*
Sensory	Mastoid	Sensation to the external auditory canal *Hitselberger sign: hypesthesia of the external auditory canal (i.e., from tumors generating mass effect on these fibers)*
Chorda tympani	Mastoid	Taste to anterior two-thirds of tongue Parasympathetics to salivary glands

The Facial Nerve in the Face

Preauricularly, the facial nerve enters the parotid gland, where it travels between the deep and superficial lobes. Within the gland, the nerve divides into two main branches—the temporofacial superiorly and the cervicofacial inferiorly. These quickly divide into multiple branches that exit the parotid to run deep to the superficial musculoaponeurotic system (SMAS) (**Table 42.2**, **Figure 42.2**).

Conceptually, the facial nerve is divided into five divisions with distinct functions: temporal, zygomatic, buccal, marginal mandibular, and cervical. Realistically, however, branching patterns are complex. The facial nerve exits the parotid as eight to 15 branches, which arborize and communicate as they continue distally. There is significant functional crossover between terminal branches. Some generate multiple movements (i.e., eye closure and smile) and there exists considerable redundancy in function. As a result, distal injury to individual branches may not produce significant functional deficits. This also permits utilization of distal branches as donors for facial reanimation.

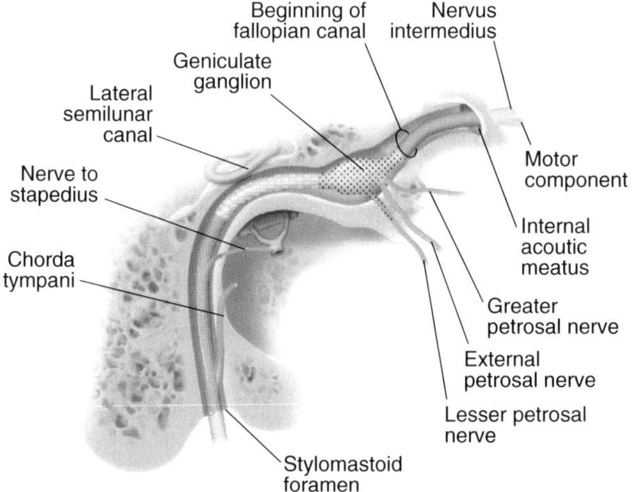

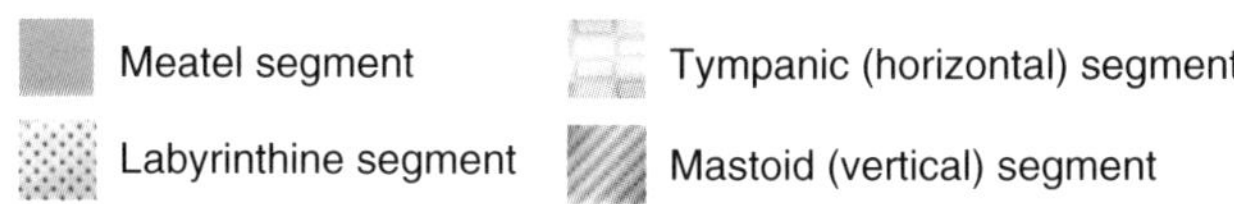

FIGURE 42.1. Anatomy of the intratemporal facial nerve. The intratemporal portion of the facial nerve is comprised of three segments: labyrinthine, tympanic, and mastoid. In both the labyrinthine and mastoid segments, the facial nerve gives off branches as illustrated.

Despite variability among patients, some general anatomic characteristics are recognized for the main divisions of the facial nerve. These characteristics are useful clinically for identifying and protecting the nerves in surgery.

Temporal Division

The course of the temporal branches roughly follows Pitanguy's line, which extends from a point 0.5 cm inferior to the tragus to a point 1.5 cm superior to the lateral extent of the eyebrow.[2] As the branches travel distally, they become superficial.

After exiting the parotid, the nerves travel within the parotidomasseteric fascia. They remain in this plane as they reach the zygomatic arch, traveling within the innominate fascia (contiguous with the parotidomasseteric fascia). Two to four branches cross the arch, spanning up to 50% of its length.[3] Crossing the arch, they move superficially, coursing on the undersurface of the superficial temporal fascia.[4]

Zygomatic and Buccal Division

Although conceptually divided into separate divisions, zygomatic and buccal branches can be, in practice, very difficult to distinguish from one another both anatomically and functionally and are often considered together as a single component (the zygomaticobuccal division).

Generally, one to three zygomatic branches exist. The zygomatic and buccal branches run in close approximation as they exit the parotid, and may emanate from a common trunk. In approximately 10% of the population, the lower zygomatic branch joins with buccal branches to create a zygomaticobuccal plexus.[5]

The buccal branch(es) run in close proximity to the parotid duct. Most often, the nerve travels inferiorly, but can be located superior to or, when multiple nerve branches are present, flanking the duct.[6]

Identification of the branch of the zygomaticobuccal branch that innervates the zygomaticus major (integral in generation of smile) can be facilitated through use of Zuker's point.[7] This is a surface landmark – the midpoint of the line drawn from the root of the helix to the oral commissure. Generally, the branch to zygomaticus major will be found within 2.3 mm of this location. This is particularly helpful in identification of donors for cross-facial nerve grafting (described below) and in identifying a *danger zone* in other facial procedures that require dissection in this region.

Marginal Mandibular Division

The marginal mandibular division runs as two to four branches.[8] They descend from the parotid, commonly running to a position below the body of the mandible, deep to the platysma.[9] The branches

TABLE 42.2. FACIAL NERVE BRANCHES, MUSCULAR TARGETS, AND FUNCTIONS

Facial Nerve Division	Injury	Muscle	Function
Temporal	Inability to raise or furrow brows, impaired blink	Frontalis	Brow elevation
		Corrugator supercilii	Medial and inferior movement of eyebrows (generate vertical glabellar rhytids)
		Procerus	Inferior movement of eyebrow (horizontal glabellar rhytids)
		Orbicularis oculi	Eyelid closure
Zygomatic	Impaired smile and blink	Orbicularis oculi	Eyelid closure
		Zygomaticus major	Elevation of commissure (instrumental in smile)
Buccal	Impaired smile, difficulty chewing, impaired speech, nasal airway obstruction, impaired oral competence	Zygomaticus major	Elevation of commissure (instrumental in smile)
		Zygomaticus minor	Upper lip elevation
		Levator labii superioris	Upper lip elevation
		Levator labii superioris alaeque nasi	Flaring of nasal ala Elevation of nasolabial fold
		Risorius	Assists smile
		Buccinator[a]	Instrumental in chewing (maintaining food bolus centrally in mouth for effective mastication)
		Levator anguli oris[a]	Superior and medial migration of commissure
		Nasalis	Dilator component: alar flaring Compressor component: compresses nostrils
		Orbicularis oris	Lip closure/compression
		Depressor anguli oris	Frowning/inferior pull at commissure
Marginal mandibular	Impaired lower lip depression (decreased lower dentition show on full-denture smile), drooling, inability to evert lip (asymmetric pout)	Depressor anguli oris	Frowning/inferior pull at commissure
		Depressor labii inferioris	Lower lip depression
		Mentalis[a]	Lower lip eversion, pout Lower lip elevation
Cervical	Impaired lower lip depression (decreased lower dentition show on full-denture smile)	Platysma	Depression of lower lip

[a]These muscles are deep and are innervated on their superior surface. All other mimetic muscles are innervated from their deep surfaces.

then turn to travel superiorly, across the inferior border of the mandible to innervate their target musculature. The nerves run superficial to the facial vessels.

Cervical Division

Unlike the other divisions, which exist as multiple branches in the face, generally only one cervical branch is present. It exits the parotid anterior to the angle of the mandible and does not divide until it passes inferior to the mandibular border.[10] It innervates the platysma from its undersurface, near the junction between its cranial and middle thirds.[11]

CAUSES OF FACIAL PARALYSIS

Causes of facial paralysis are many and varied (**Table 42.3**). Multiple studies have examined relative frequencies of different diagnoses. In general, Bell palsy is accepted as the most common diagnosis in adults. It is an acquired, idiopathic palsy of sudden onset and is a diagnosis of exclusion. Other diagnoses must be ruled out before settling on Bell palsy, as other etiologies may warrant different intervention and be at risk for progression if not addressed. Bell palsy is less likely to be the diagnosis in the setting of bilateral palsy, paralysis of insidious onset, or palsy that is waxing and waning.

The underlying etiology of Bell palsy is likely a latent herpes virus. The mainstay of treatment is a course of corticosteroids (most effective when instituted within 24 hours of symptom onset) and antivirals, which may help to improve recovery. Most patients begin to experience recovery within 3 weeks of symptom onset, although some may not see signs of returning function for up to 3 to 6 months. Approximately 75% of patients experience full resolution of symptoms. The remaining patients suffer from varying degrees of lasting weakness, spasm, and synkinesis.

The relative frequencies of other etiologies of paralysis vary by report, likely because of specific populations examined and variable referral patterns among institutions. Infection, trauma, and iatrogenic injury are often considered the next most common causes of acquired paralysis. However, evaluation of diagnoses in a series of patients at a facial nerve center with a specialized referral base identified resection of acoustic neuromas, head and neck malignancies, and iatrogenic injuries to be the most common etiologies after Bell palsy.[12]

Facial paralysis attributed to acoustic neuromas and malignancies is most often secondary to resection, although palsy may follow radiotherapy or may be noted pretreatment. Parotid tumors, through mass effect or direct neural invasion, are the malignancies most commonly directly responsible for paralysis.

Iatrogenic injury to the facial nerve at nearly any point along its course may occur following a variety of head and neck procedures, especially temporomandibular joint surgery and parotidectomy.

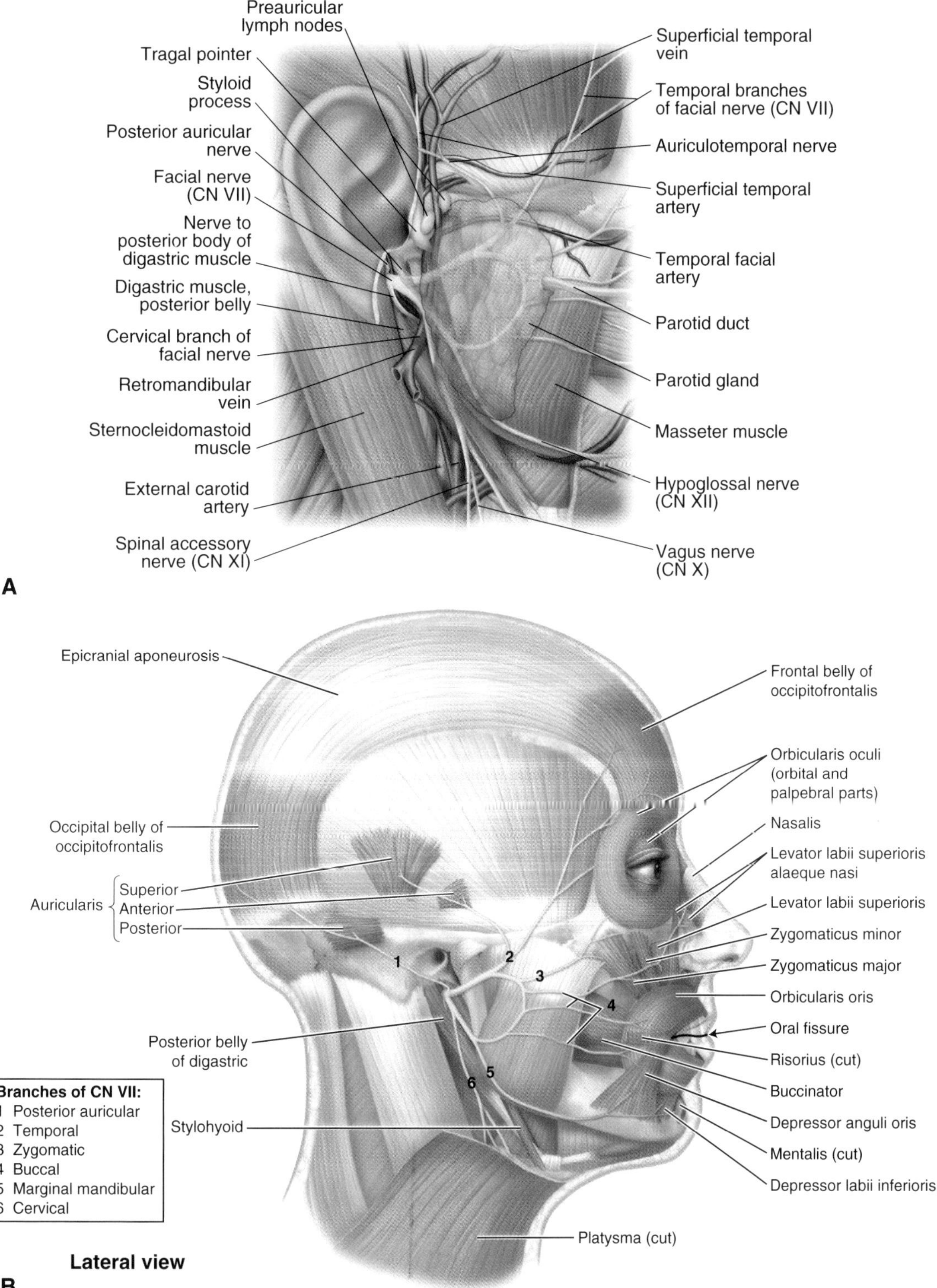

FIGURE 42.2. Facial nerve and mimetic musculature. **A.** The facial nerve exits the skull base through the stylomastoid foramen to run between the styloid process and the posterior belly of the digastric muscle prior to coursing anteriorly around the ear to run between the deep and superficial lobes of the parotid gland to reach the facial musculature. **B.** The facial nerve gives off the posterior auricular branch posteriorly. Traveling anteriorly, the facial nerve broadly divides into five main distributions to innervate the mimetic musculature of the face. (**B.** Reproduced with permission from Moore KL. *Essential Clinical Anatomy*. 5th ed. Philadelphia, PA: Wolters Kluwer Health; 2014. Figure 9-11.

Resection of a variety of benign and malignant processes both intra- and extracranially may result in iatrogenic injury. Distally, terminal branches are at risk during facial cosmetic procedures and treatment of facial fractures.

Viral, rickettsial, and bacterial infections may also lead to facial paralysis. Varicella zoster virus–associated facial paralysis may occur with (Ramsay Hunt Syndrome) or without documented prior vesicular outbreak. Paralysis following acute otitis media is a particularly common finding in pediatric patients. Lyme disease is a common diagnosis in bilateral paralysis.

Both blunt and sharp trauma may affect the facial nerve. Temporal bone fractures can result in compression or shearing injury.

TABLE 42.3. ETIOLOGICAL CLASSIFICATION OF FACIAL PARALYSIS WITH EXAMPLES

Congenital	
Syndromic	Hemifacial microsomia (unilateral; may be associated with abnormalities of ear, mandible, orbit, soft tissues of face) Mobius syndrome (bilateral; cranial nerve (CN) VI palsy, Poland's; talipes equinovarus)
Traumatic	Use of forceps
Other	Congenital unilateral lower lip paralysis (CULLP)
Acquired	
Traumatic	
Blunt	Temporal bone fractures Neurapraxic injuries to extracranial nerve
Sharp	Direct laceration to distal branches
Other	Cerebral event
Idiopathic	Bell palsy (frequently associated with pregnancy, at least partial recovery expected) Melkersson-Rosenthal syndrome (recurrent facial paralysis, orofacial swelling, fissured tongue)
Infectious	
Viral	HSV, EBV, VZV Ramsay-Hunt syndrome (VZV, sudden onset paralysis, hearing loss, severe pain, ±vesicular rash) HIV (often bilateral)
Bacterial	Otitis media
Rickettsial	Lyme disease (bilateral)
Autoimmune	Guillain-Barre syndrome (bilateral)
Tumor	Acoustic neuroma (bilateral in NF2), meningioma, cerebellopontine tumors (intracranial) Cholesteatoma (intratemporal) Parotid mass (extracranial)
Iatrogenic	Management of facial trauma (especially mandibular fractures) TMJ surgery Aesthetic procedures Resection of intracranial, intratemporal, or extracranial masses Middle ear surgery
Neuromuscular	Myesthenia gravis

EBV, Epstein-Barr virus; HIV, human immunodeficiency virus; HSV, herpes simplex virus; NF2, neurofibromatosis type 2; TMJ, temporomandibular joint; VZV, varicella zoster virus.

Extracranially, laceration from penetrating trauma is a risk, and blunt trauma may directly generate a neurapraxic injury or lead to compression effect on the nerve from soft tissue changes (i.e., hematoma).

Autoimmune diseases generally lead to bilateral, rather than unilateral facial paralysis, and they can be recurrent. The most common of these processes is Guillain–Barre syndrome.

The distribution of etiologies in children is different from that in adults. Infectious, traumatic, and iatrogenic sources have been found to occur more frequently than Bell palsy in the pediatric population. Additionally, congenital facial paralysis accounts for a larger portion of diagnoses in children compared with adults.

The most common cause of congenital facial paralysis is birth trauma, frequently from the use of forceps. Often, these cases resolve fully by 1 month of age. Congenital unilateral lower lip paralysis (CULLP) is an isolated dysfunction of a unilateral marginal mandibular nerve. In CULLP, also referred to as *asymmetric crying facies*, there is generally no significant asymmetry noticed at rest, but obvious deficit of lower lip depression on the affected side in crying. Etiology can include ante- or intrapartum compression on the marginal mandibular branch. Syndromic sources of paralysis include hemifacial microsomia (most commonly) and Mobius syndrome.

Although many diagnoses are shared between unilateral and bilateral facial paralysis, relative frequencies differ. Although unilateral facial paralysis is most often attributed to Bell palsy, bilateral paralysis most commonly has an identifiable cause.[13] A recent study of etiologies at a large referral center for facial palsy found that Bell palsy accounted for approximately one-third of their cases.[13] Among the more common identified causes were Lyme disease, Mobius syndrome, Guillain–Barré syndrome, benign neoplastic processes (i.e., neurofibromatosis type 2), vascular malformations, and trauma.

Mobius syndrome is the most common congenital cause of bilateral paralysis. With an incidence of approximately 1 in 50,000 live births, it involves chest wall and limb anomalies in addition to variable involvement of other cranial nerves. Poland syndrome and talipes equinovarus are among the more commonly associated findings. The most commonly involved cranial nerves are the sixth (abducens) and seventh (facial). The hypoglossal nerve (cranial nerve [CN] XII) is the third most commonly affected, and the third, fourth, fifth, ninth, and tenth cranial nerves may also be. Although facial paralysis is most commonly bilateral, it is variable, and may be unilateral. The etiology of Mobius syndrome is unclear, but it may be ischemic/hypoxic events during development that affects the distribution of the subclavian artery. Both genetic[14] as well as acquired causes exist. Misoprostol exposure in utero has been identified as a risk factor for the latter.[15]

EFFECTS OF FACIAL NERVE PARALYSIS

Upper Face

Ocular damage and degradation of vision from corneal exposure is the biggest concern. Lagophthalmos results from abnormalities of both the upper and lower eyelids. In the upper lid, unopposed function of the levator palpebrae superioris (innervated by the oculomotor nerve) impairs downward excursion, leading to failure to contact lower lid in attempted closure.

Additionally, because the upper facial divisions of the facial nerve are responsible for the efferent component of the blink reflex (the trigeminal nerve is responsible for the afferent component), decreased blinking is observed in facial paralysis and impairs the maintenance of tear film over the cornea.

Paralytic ectropion may result over time with the effects of gravity on a paralyzed lower eyelid. With increasing laxity, the lid everts and falls away from the globe, pulling the canalicular punctum away as well. The result is increased exposure and lacrimal pump failure, which exacerbates exposure and leads to excessive tearing (epiphora).

Risk of corneal damage is increased in patients who lack a Bell phenomenon (reflexive upward rotation of the eye with eye closure or blink) and in patients who have concomitant injury to the ophthalmic division of the trigeminal nerve (responsible for corneal sensation and epithelial maintenance).

Lower Face

The greatest concerns are impaired speech (especially difficulty with *p* and *b* sounds), difficulty eating, excessive drooling, and inability to smile. Eating difficulties arise in part from denervation of the buccinator which impairs control of food boluses during chewing can lead to sequestration of food into the buccal sulcus.

Loss of smile can have significant implications for nonverbal communication and psychosocial well-being. This inability is one of the most frequent complaints of patients, and a common indication for surgery in patients. In children, especially those with bilateral paralysis (i.e., Mobius syndrome), this is particularly concerning, as inability to emote can seriously impact propensity for social integration.

Other dysfunctions may also present. Nasal airway obstruction results in part from denervation of nasalis and levator labii superioris alequae nasi, which may lead to collapse of the affected ala. In the setting of unilateral facial paralysis, this external nasal valve collapse is accentuated by deviation of the nasal tip to the unaffected side, further obstructing airflow.

In older patients, frontalis dysfunction in the setting of a heavy brow results not only in stark visible asymmetry, but can contribute to ptosis and impaired field of vision.

Synkinesis may be observed in patients recovering from facial paralysis. As they perform one action (i.e., smiling), a second undesired action occurs in tandem (i.e., blinking). This can be quite distressing to patients and, as with paralysis itself, can have significant psychosocial impacts. Synkinesis likely results from aberrant axonal sprouting into incorrect muscles, as nerves regenerate following paralysis. It may also be related to central changes that take place as reinnervation occurs.

PREOPERATIVE EVALUATION

A thorough history and physical examination are necessary. Determination of the underlying etiology informs on potential treatments and likelihood of recovery of facial function. **Tables 42.4** and **42.5** include the key components of patient history and evaluation.

Duration of symptoms and characteristics of onset can help determine the need for adjunctive diagnostic tools (i.e., blood tests for infectious or immunologic etiologies, imaging in the setting of trauma, or suspicion of central nervous system disorders) and involvement of additional specialists in management of the patient. Electrodiagnostic studies are not commonly utilized, but for select patients may provide information regarding expected recovery (electrodiagnostics are not generally used in pediatrics). In the setting of suspected Bell palsy (low suspicion for ominous or medically/surgically reversible etiology), it is advisable to wait 3 weeks prior to obtaining electrodiagnostics (for prognostication) or delving into in-depth workup. This is because most patients with Bell palsy will regain some function within this time, precluding the need for invasive and time-consuming tests that may be unnecessary.

Specific functional deficits must be elicited. Regardless of potential for spontaneous recovery of function, conservative (especially physical therapy) or medical approaches are often used either as sole treatment or as adjuncts to surgery.

Multiple grading systems have been developed for description of symptom severity and to assist with reporting on facial paralysis. The most commonly used system is the House–Brackmann scale.[16] This scale, however, does not differentiate between dysfunction of specific divisions of the facial nerve and really has little ability to describe pre- and postoperative movement; other scales, such as the Sunnybrook scale and the Yanagihara scale (popular in Japan), do.

MANAGEMENT OF FACIAL PARALYSIS

A multidisciplinary approach to the patient with facial paralysis is critical to optimize outcomes. The medical team varies depending on the etiology of the paralysis and the affected functions (i.e., the need for infectious disease, rheumatologic, oncologic treatment, etc). Ophthalmologic intervention should occur early in the setting of upper facial paralysis. All patients, regardless of their need for surgical intervention, should undergo physical therapy to maximize their functional recovery. Finally, psychologic and social work services often play a central role in the care of patients. The psychosocial effects of facial paralysis should not be underestimated, especially in the congenital population, and they must be addressed to minimize implications for social function and psychologic well-being.

Conservative Management

Medical Management and Watchful Waiting

For certain etiologies, such as infectious, autoimmune, and idiopathic, conservative management may be warranted prior to consideration of surgical treatment. Medical management will be directed by appropriate specialists depending on diagnosis. Infectious etiologies (bacterial or rickettsial) may benefit from antibiosis. Patients with Bell palsy or autoimmune etiologies may benefit from steroids, as may patients with viral causes (with or without the addition of antivirals). Additionally, for all patients, physical therapy by specially trained therapists can help recovering patients strengthen and relearn specific movements such as eye closure and smile.

Ocular Protection

Many nonsurgical modalities are used for eye protection, including:

- Exogenous lubrication (drops and ointments)
- Closure assistance (eyelid taping, especially at night)
- External protective devices (protective chambers, eye patches)
- Soft contact lenses

These serve as temporizing measures for patients who recover function as well as adjuncts to surgery when operative intervention is indicated.

Synkinesis

Management of synkinesis requires denervating the muscle that activates inappropriately or retraining it to inhibit unwanted movement. The former is accomplished through the use of botulinum toxin, and the latter through specialized physical therapy. Therapeutic techniques generally focus on the use of biofeedback through tools such as mirror training and electromyographic feedback.

Surgical Management

Surgical intervention may be pursued when facial paralysis is congenital, secondary to trauma or iatrogenic injury, or when conservative/medical management of potentially recoverable cases fails to generate satisfactory facial movement or tone. The choice of procedure depends on specific functional deficits, patient desires, and suitability of the patient to undergo various surgeries.

Procedures can be classified as static or dynamic. Static procedures do not produce new motion, but through suspension or repositioning of tissues, improve symmetry, appearance, and sometimes function. Dynamic procedures generate new movement under emotional and/or volitional control.

Static Procedures (Table 42.6)

Static procedures around the eye aim to improve lid closure and protect the cornea. Procedures can target either the upper lid (enhance downward excursion) or the lower lid (ectropion repair to better appose lid to globe). Placement of gold weights[17] **(Figure 42.3)** or platinum chain weights overlying the tarsus within the upper lid is a popular procedure to enhance closure. Implants are available in a range of weights such that the most appropriate one may be selected for each patient depending on their functional deficiency.

Both the upper and lower eyelids may be operated on simultaneously. When done, the upper lid should be corrected first to assist in determination of the appropriate degree of lower lid tightening.

Although static procedures in the lower face cannot generate smile, they improve appearance and oral competence. These techniques are avoided in the pediatric population because of the success of dynamic procedures in children, and in whom the ability to emote is particularly important for social integration.

Contralateral Defunctioning

When asymmetry between the normal and paralyzed sides is the primary aesthetic concern, defunctioning of the normal side, through

TABLE 42.4. KEY POINTS IN HISTORY AND POSSIBLE IMPLICATIONS OF FINDINGS

Category	Directed Questions/Specific Concerns
Related Events	
Recent infections	Viral illnesses Otitis media
Potential exposure to ticks	Lyme disease
Oncologic history	Space-occupying lesions Intraneural tumor
Trauma	Blunt (skull base fracture; distal neurapraxic injury) Sharp (direct laceration to facial nerve)
Iatrogenic injury	Tumor resection Radiotherapy Other craniofacial procedures (i.e., facelift)
Congenital	Birth history—trauma from forceps Associated anomalies (concern for syndromic etiology)
Characteristics of Paralysis	
Circumstances of onset	Sudden (Bell palsy, trauma, iatrogenic, cerebrovascular accident, infection) Gradual (oncologic, systemic) Congenital
Duration of symptoms	<12 months Long (concerning for irreversible muscle fibrosis/atrophy)
Waxing/waning/resolution	Improvement or plateau of recovery and time over which symptoms changed (even in the setting of self-limited processes, improvement is often slow, occurring over several months)
Recurrent	Concerning for Guillain-Barre syndrome, Melkersson-Rosenthal
Specific Deficits	
Bilateral/unilateral	Bilateral (more likely to be Lyme disease, Guillain-Barre syndrome, benign neoplastic processes)
Eye	Altered blink/eye closure Change in lower lid position (paralytic ectropion) Symptoms of corneal exposure (corneal exposure/degradation of vision/dry eyes/excessive tearing) Double vision
Nasal airway	Collapse, difficulty breathing
Lower face	Altered smile Altered speech (particularly difficulty with bilabial consonants, such as *p* and *b* sounds) Drooling Difficulty eating/cheek biting with chewing Isolated asymmetric lower lip depression
Other	Altered taste Hyperacusis (paralysis of stapedius) Dry mouth (may indicate proximal facial nerve injury)
Associated palsies of other cranial nerves	Deviation of tongue to one side (CN XII) Loss of facial sensation (CN V, especially corneal sensation; CN VI) Abducens (CN VI, concern for Mobius syndrome)
Psychosocial effects	Self-consciousness, difficulty with social interactions, depression, anxiety
Comorbidities	
Overall health	Ability to tolerate surgical reconstruction (i.e., long procedures, suitability of vessels for microvascular reconstructions)
Prior surgeries	Potential for iatrogenic injury (see above) Potential effects on reconstructive options (i.e., destruction of neurovascular pedicle to temporalis; destruction of facial vessels)

TABLE 42.5. KEY POINTS OF PHYSICAL EXAMINATION

Basic movements	Evaluate key facial movements that indicate function of the major divisions of the facial nerve. note presence/absence of function and symmetry: ■ Elevate Brows (frontalis) ■ Close Eyes (orbicularis oculi) ■ Smile (zygomaticus major, zygomaticus minor) ■ Purse Lips (orbicularis oris)
Detailed findings	Note right-left asymmetries. Evaluate the face in repose and animation ■ Brow ptosis (assess for visual field impairment) ■ Eye □ Height of palpebral aperture in rest and maximal eye closure □ Presence of Bell phenomenon □ Position of lower lid (paralytic ectropion) – snap test and comparison to contralateral side □ Corneal examination (sensory examination; assess for damage/irritation) ■ Mouth □ Symmetry at rest □ Dynamic ● Ability to smile and symmetry thereof ● Oral competence (drooling, eating) ● Speech intelligibility ■ Nasal airway □ Collapse of nasal airway with forced inspiration ■ Presence of synkinesis
Associated palsies	Cranial nerves III, V, VI, XI, XII

neurectomy/myectomy or chemodenervation (botox), may be considered. These techniques are commonly used with good results in CULLP and in adult patients with acquired unilateral lip depressor dysfunction.[18,19]

TABLE 42.6. COMMONLY USED STATIC PROCEDURES THROUGHOUT THE FACE

Focus	Static Options
Eye (lagophthalmos)	Upper lid ■ Gold weights/platinum chain weights ■ Palpebral springs Lower lid ■ Canthoplasty/canthopexy (mild to moderate deformity) ■ Fascial slings (severe deformity) ■ Tarsorrhaphy (when other techniques fail to protect the cornea)
Ptosis	Brow lift
Nasal airway collapse	Alar base fixation and periosteal anchoring (mild to moderate deformity) Alar base elevation and support via tendon sling (severe deformity)
Resting tone of mouth/lower face, oral incompetence	Dermal or fascial slings for suspension of oral commissure (often use tensor fascia latae or tendon—palmaris, plantaris, extensor digitorum longus) Facelift

Dynamic Procedures

Multiple procedures offer restoration of function. The most appropriate procedure for a given patient depends on the circumstances of paralysis as well as patient desires and suitability for surgery.

The state of both nerves and musculature dictates reconstructive options (**Table 42.7**). When paralysis results from trauma or iatrogenic nerve injury, with relative sparing of muscle, reinnervation (via nerve repair or transfer) of affected musculature may be an option when performed in a timely fashion. When viable muscle is not present because of prolonged denervation (after approximately 24 months of denervation, the muscles undergo irreversible atrophy and fibrosis), traumatic destruction, or agenesis, dynamic reconstructive options include free or local muscle transfer.

Following traumatic/iatrogenic damage to the facial nerve in which both proximal and distal stumps are identified, nerve repair may be possible. If the ends can be approximated without tension, primary repair is favored. Otherwise, interpositional grafting (usually sural) is required. Although results are reliable following repair up to 12 to 18 months following injury, ideally, nerves are repaired within 72 hours. This allows for intraoperative stimulation of distal stumps to assist in identification. After 72 hours following injury, neurotransmitter reserves in the distal stumps become too depleted to reliably generate muscular activity.

Nerve Transfer

When injury leaves viable distal nerve stumps/musculature but no proximal nerve stumps, nerve transfer is an option.[20] As with nerve repair, transfer should be performed as early as possible. Multiple donor nerves exist (**Table 42.8**). In unilateral palsy with normal contralateral facial nerve function, cross-facial nerve grafting from the corresponding contralateral facial nerve branch (**Figure 42.4**) is favored (when performed within 6–12 months of injury). Twelve to eighteen months following injury, direct transfer from physically closer nerves (i.e., nerve to masseter) is favored to shorten time to reinnervation.

When cross-facial nerve grafting is unavailable (i.e., bilateral palsy), other donor nerves may be used. Selection depends on donor availability, proximity to target (with the goal of decreasing the length or need for interpositional grafts), and surgeon preference. Cranial nerve V (specifically, nerve to masseter) is often a favorable choice because of proximity to targets and reliable anatomy. If a single donor nerve is used to reinnervate multiple functions (i.e., smile and blink), synkinesis results.

Muscle Transfer

When viable mimetic musculature is not available for reinnervation, animation can be achieved by transfer of a functioning muscle, either local or free.

Local muscle transfer most commonly reroutes all or part of the temporalis and/or masseter for generation of smile and/or blink. This can be a good option for patients who are not suitable candidates for (or who do not wish to undergo) free muscle transfer.

Multiple techniques exist for transfer of all or part of the masseter to generate smile and/or blink.[21] For smile, transfer may be performed through an intraoral approach, sparing the patient external scars. In the lower face, masseter transfers reliably improve static tone, but results for animation are less consistent. Functional smile may be achieved, but the vector of pull through many techniques of transfer leads to a smile of unnatural appearance.

The temporalis transfer (**Figure 42.5**), as described by Labbe,[22] disinserts the temporalis from the coronoid and transfer of the insertion to the commissure (for smile) or, in other descriptions, to the periorbital region (for blink). As with masseteric transfers, temporalis transfer reliably provides static support, although excursion is variable.[23] Additionally, depending on technique, temporal hollowing can occur.

Temporalis transfer may not be possible for some patients who have undergone neurosurgical procedures that require access through the temporal region because of potential disruption of the neurovascular pedicle.

HEAD AND NECK

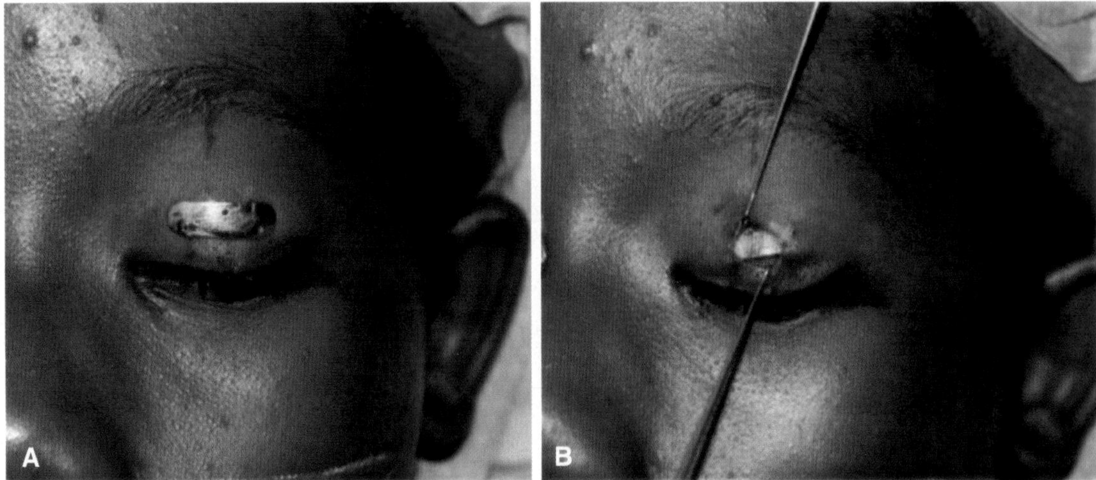

FIGURE 42.3. An appropriately sized gold weight is selected based on the weight needed to achieve lid closure and size of the eyelid **(A)**. It is centered over midline and affixed over the superior portion of the tarsus **(B)**.

TABLE 42.7. RECONSTRUCTIVE OPTIONS FOR REANIMATION BASED ON NERVE AND MUSCLE VIABILITY

	Proximal Stump Present	Proximal Stump Absent
Muscle viable with usable distal nerve stump (i.e., early traumatic/iatrogenic paralysis)	Nerve repair ■ Primary (if no tension between nerve ends) ■ Interpositional graft (if tension between ends or if they do not approximate)	Paralysis of <18 months duration ■ Cross-facial nerve graft (transfer from contralateral facial nerve) ■ Nerve transfer from alternate donor (see **Table 42.8**) Paralysis of 18–24 months' duration Nerve grafting from alternate donor, without need for interpositional graft ■ Nerve to masseter ■ Hypoglossal nerve
Muscle not viable (or no distal nerve stump, i.e., late paralysis; agenesis)	Free functional muscle transfer, innervated by proximal stump Local muscle transfer	Free functional muscle powered by cross-facial nerve graft or alternate donor (see **Table 42.9**) Local muscle transfer

TABLE 42.8. DONOR NERVES FOR NERVE TRANSFER AND INNERVATION OF FREE FUNCTIONAL MUSCLE TRANSFERS

Nerve	Advantages	Disadvantages
Contralateral facial nerve (via cross-facial nerve graft)	■ The only donor capable of generating emotional control of smile ■ Capable of generating good excursion in smile ■ Can use corresponding contralateral branches for blink ■ No significant donor deficit	■ Not available in bilateral cases ■ Requires two-stage procedure when used in innervation of free muscle transfers ■ In the setting of reinnervation of native mimetic musculature through nerve transfer, the need for long nerve graft may preclude use in paralysis of greater than 12 months duration owing to time for neural regeneration through graft
Nerve to masseter	■ Reliable donor (even in patients with Mobius syndrome) ■ Capable of generating good excursion in smile (can show greater excursion than that achieved via cross-facial nerve grafting) ■ Consistent anatomy ■ No significant donor deficits ■ Generally close enough to recipient nerve to avoid an intervening nerve graft	■ Volitional rather than emotional control
Hypoglossal	■ Capable of producing powerful smile	■ Third most commonly affected cranial nerve in Mobius syndrome—unreliable source of innervation in these patients and use may impair speech and ability to swallow ■ Volitional rather than emotional control
Spinal accessory	■ Often available when other cranial nerves may not be	■ Distance from target often necessitates use of intervening nerve graft ■ Volitional rather than emotional control

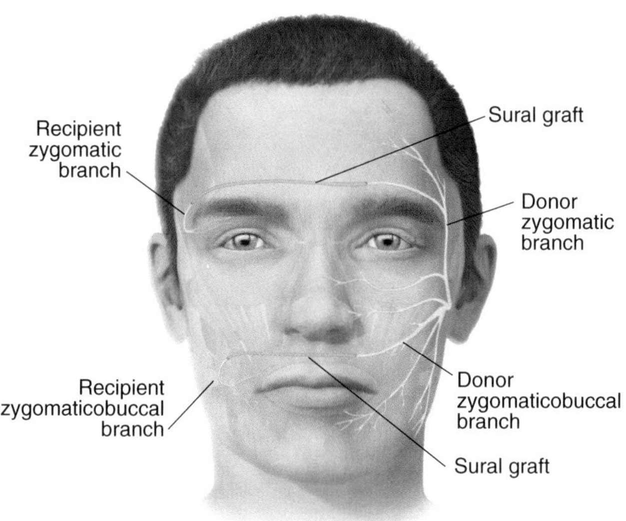

FIGURE 42.4. Cross-facial nerve graft for reinnervation of contralateral facial nerve. When distal facial nerve stumps are available for reinnervation on the injured side, contralateral (functional) facial nerve stumps can be transferred (via cross-facial nerve graft) to the corresponding viable nerve stumps for neural input. Here, cross-facial nerve grafting for both blink and smile are shown.

Free Functional Muscle Transfer

Free functional muscle transfer is often considered the standard for smile reanimation, particularly in children. Generally, these transfers produce superior commissure excursion (in terms of magnitude and direction) compared with local muscle transfer. In children, these are nearly always the procedure of choice for reanimation because of reliability in the younger population.

Options exist for both upper and lower facial reanimation. Many muscles have been utilized for smile (**Table 42.9**).[24-29] Similarly, options exist for blink reinnervation[30] – most commonly either a segment of gracilis or a slip of platysma.

As with selection for muscle transfer, there are choices for neural input. Options are the same as those for nerve transfer above[31] (see **Table 42.8**). Two of the most commonly used nerves are the contralateral facial nerve (via cross-facial nerve graft) and the ipsilateral nerve to masseter. Both have been proven to generate reliable, satisfactory smile excursion when powering free functional muscles. Each technique has advantages and disadvantages.

Cross-Facial Nerve Grafting

As with nerve transfers to reinnervate native mimetic musculature, emotional control of a free muscle can be achieved only through use of the contralateral facial nerve as donor. This method of reconstruction is performed in two stages (**Figure 42.6**). In the first stage, a cross-facial nerve graft (generally sural) is coapted to the donor facial nerve and tunneled toward the affected side. The specific donor nerve branches are selected through intraoperative nerve stimulation to identify those that produce commissure and upper lip movement—most consistent with the smile to be reconstructed on the affected side. These branches are then transected and coapted to the nerve graft, which is tunneled through the upper buccal sulcus for later coaptation to the nerve to the transferred muscle.

The technique for generation of eye closure is similar. Instead of selecting donor branches that generate smile, donors are selected on their ability to produce desired blink. Rather than tunneling through the upper buccal sulcus, the graft is tunneled supraorbitally, across the nasal bridge, into the region of the affected orbicularis oculi muscle.

In the second stage, performed approximately 12 months following the first (adequate time between procedures is dictated by the presence of an advancing Tinel sign along the nerve graft, indicating the distal extent of neural regeneration), free muscle transfer is performed and neurotized by the cross-facial nerve graft that was previously placed.

Nerve to Masseter

Unlike with cross-facial nerve grafting, reanimation is accomplished in a single stage,[32] making it a good choice for patients who wish to avoid two procedures. Additionally, it can be used in patients with bilateral paralysis, in whom the contralateral facial nerve is not available. The nerve to masseter is almost always unaffected in patients with Mobius syndrome, making it a reliable choice in this population[26] (its function

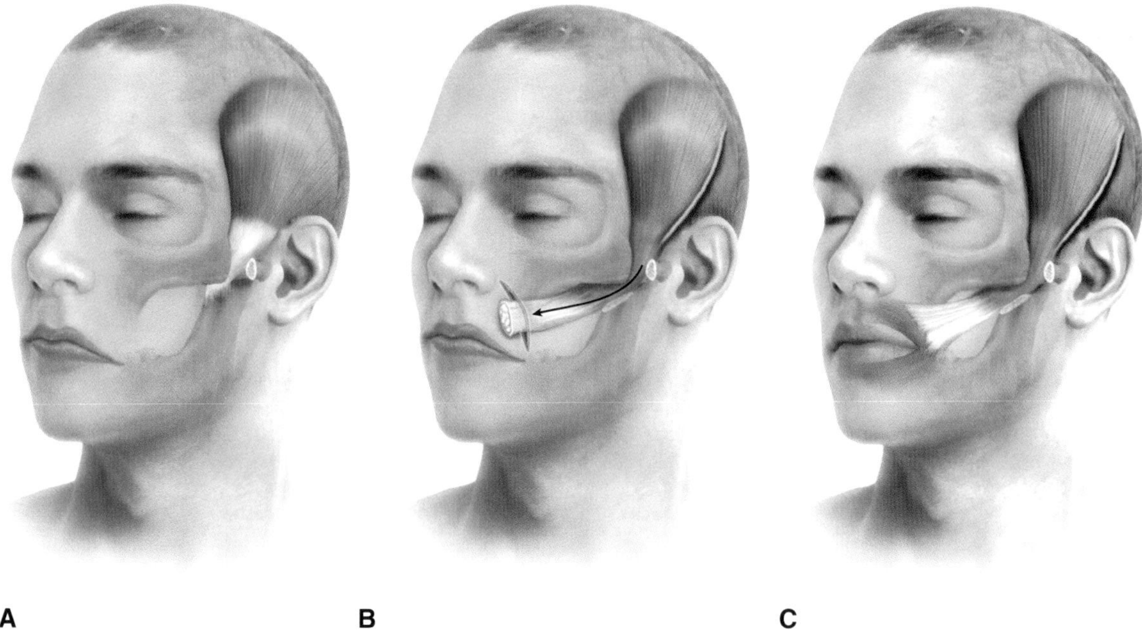

FIGURE 42.5. The temporalis transfer as described by Labbe involves a coronoid osteotomy for ease of repositioning of the temporalis tendon **(A)**, zygomatic arch osteotomy for enhanced accessibility to the temporalis **(B)**, elevation and repositioning of the entire temporalis muscle, and insertion of the temporalis tendon (stripped from the coronoid) to the oral commissure **(C)**. (Reproduced with permission from Panossian A. Temporalis flap and lengthening temporalis myoplasty for facial paralysis. In: Chung KC, ed. *Operative Techniques in Plastic Surgery*. Philadelphia, PA: Wolters Kluwer; 2019. Part 3, Figure 50-2.)

TABLE 42.9. COMMONLY USED MUSCLES USED FOR FREE FUNCTIONAL TRANSFERS

Muscles Free Functional Transfers	Advantages	Disadvantages
Gracilis	■ Consistent, reliable anatomy/pedicle ■ Can harvest with two-team approach in facial reanimation ■ Can be transferred with minimal bulk ■ Minimal donor morbidity	
Pectoralis minor	■ Can be transferred with minimal bulk ■ Minimal donor morbidity	■ Pedicle variable ■ Two-team approach difficult in facial reanimation
Latissimus dorsi	■ Reliable donor	■ Often bulky ■ Two-team approach difficult in facial reanimation
Extensor carpi radialis brevis	■ Can be transferred with minimal bulk ■ Minimal donor morbidity	■ Results often inferior to use of other muscles

can be verified by asking the patient to clench their masseter muscle). The nerve to masseter is large and can donate more axons to the recipient free muscle than can a cross-facial nerve graft. This may manifest functionally as greater commissure excursion resulting from use of nerve to masseter as compared with cross-facial nerve grafting.[33]

REANIMATION IN CHILDREN

Ideally, smile reanimation should be completed by school age. In the setting of bilateral paralysis, this ideally the first muscle transfer is not performed prior to the age of 4 years. This allows sufficient growth of anatomic structures (i.e., neurovascular pedicles) and increases the likelihood of sufficient maturity on the part of the patient for them to actively participate in postoperative rehabilitation and flap care. Reanimation can be performed either simultaneously or staged (one side at a time, spaced 3 months apart).

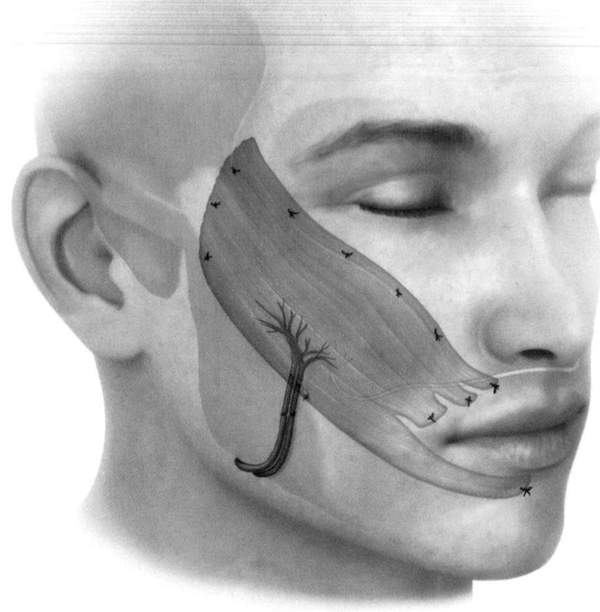

FIGURE 42.6. Free gracilis transfer powered by cross-facial nerve graft. The gracilis has been inset in the vector required to produce a smile in the desired vector. The obturator nerve has been coapted to a cross-facial nerve graft, and the vascular pedicle is receiving supply from the facial vessels. (Reproduced with permission from Sugg KB. Facial paralysis. In: Brown DL, Borschel GH, Levi B, eds. *Michigan Manual of Plastic Surgery*. 2nd ed. Philadelphia, PA: Wolters Kluwer Health; 2014:239. Figure 24-3.)

SUMMARY

Facial paralysis is a complex problem that can have significant functional as well as psychosocial effects. Multiple etiologies exist, and proper diagnosis is essential to multidisciplinary care to ensure appropriate treatment is offered. For those patients who will not regain adequate function with conservative management, surgical intervention for improvement of static symmetry or restoration of function may be indicated. All patients, regardless of surgical status, should undergo physical therapy. Retraining of musculature can be laborious and slow, and targeted therapy directed to trained therapists is essential for optimizing function.

REFERENCES

1. Myckatyn TM, Mackinnon SE. A review of facial nerve anatomy. *Semin Plast Surg*. 2004;18(1):5-12.
2. Pitanguy I, Ramos AS. The frontal branch of the facial nerve: the importance of its variations in face lifting. *Plast Reconstr Surg*. 1966;38(4):352-356.
3. Gosain AK, Sewall SR, Yousif NJ. The temporal branch of the facial nerve: how reliably can we predict its path? *Plast Reconstr Surg*. 1997;99(5):1224-1236.
4. Agarwal CA, Mendenhall SD, Foreman KB, Owsley JQ. The course of the frontal branch of the facial nerve in relation to fascial planes: an anatomic study. *Plast Reconstr Surg*. 2010;125(2):532-537.
5. Saylam C, Ucerler H, Orhan M, Ozek C. Anatomic guides to precisely localize the zygomatic branches of the facial nerve. *J Craniofac Surg*. 2006;17(1):50-53.
6. Saylam C, Ucerler H, Orhan M, Ozek C. Anatomic landmarks of the buccal branches of the facial nerve. *Surg Radiol Anat*. 2006;28(5):462-467.
7. Dorafshar AH, Borsuk DE, Bojovic B, et al. Surface anatomy of the middle division of the facial nerve: Zukerês point. *Plast Reconstr Surg*. 2013;131(2):253-257.
This study validates the use of Zuker's point as an anatomic landmark for identification of the branches of the facial nerve that generates smile (i.e., for use in cross-facial nerve grafting).
8. Davies JC, Ravichandiran M, Agur AM, Fattah A. Evaluation of clinically relevant landmarks of the marginal mandibular branch of the facial nerve: a three-dimensional study with application to avoiding facial nerve palsy. *Clin Anat*. 2016;29(2):151-156.
9. Nelson DW, Gingrass RP. Anatomy of the mandibular branches of the facial nerve. *Plast Reconstr Surg*. 1979;64(4):479-482.
10. Chowdhry S, Yoder EM, Cooperman RD, et al. Locating the cervical motor branch of the facial nerve: anatomy and clinical application. *Plast Reconstr Surg*. 2010;126(3):875-879.
11. Terzis JK, Kalantarian B. Microsurgical strategies in 74 patients for restoration of dynamic depressor muscle mechanism: a neglected target in facial reanimation. *Plast Reconstr Surg*. 2000;105(6):1917-1931.
12. Hohman MH, Hadlock T. Etiology, diagnosis, and management of facial palsy: 2000 patients at a facial nerve center. *Laryngoscope*. 2014;124(7):E283-E293.
13. Gaudin RA, Jowett N, Banks CA, et al. Bilateral facial paralysis: a 13-year experience. *Plast Reconstr Surg*. 2016;138(4):879-887.

14. Kadakia S, Helman SN, Schwedhelm T, et al. Examining the genetics of congenital facial paralysis—a closer look at Moebius syndrome. *Oral Maxillofac Surg.* 2015;19(2):109-116.
15. Pastuszak AL, Schuler L, Speck-Martins CE, et al. Use of misoprostol during pregnancy and Mobius' syndrome in infants. *N Engl J Med.* 1998;338(26):1881-1885.
16. House JW, Brackmann DE. Facial nerve grading system. *Otolaryngol Head Neck Surg.* 1985;93(2):146-147.
17. Manktelow RT. Use of the gold weight for lagophthalmos. *Oper Tech Plast Reconstr Surg.* 1999;6(3):157-158.
18. Lindsay RW, Edwards C, Smitson C, et al. A systematic algorithm for the management of lower lip asymmetry. *Am J Otolaryngol Head Neck Med Surg.* 2011;32(1):1-7.
19. Hussain G, Manktelow RT, Tomat LR. Depressor labii inferioris resection: an effective treatment for marginal mandibular nerve paralysis. *Br J Plast Surg.* 2004;57(6):502-510.
This article describes deformity related to dysfunction of the marginal mandibular nerve and details myectomy for treatment of asymmetry.
20. Conley J, Baker DC. Hypoglossal–facial nerve anastomosis for reinnervation of the paralyzed face. *Plast Reconstr Surg.* 1979;63(1):63-72.
21. Baker DC, Conley J. Regional muscle transposition for rehabilitation of the paralyzed face. *Clin Plast Surg.* 1979;6(3):317-331.
22. Labbé D, Huault M. Lengthening temporalis myoplasty and lip reanimation. *Plast Reconstr Surg.* 2000;105(4):1289-1297.
23. Bos R, Reddy SG, Mommaerts MY. Lengthening temporalis myoplasty versus free muscle transfer with the gracilis flap for long-standing facial paralysis: a systematic review of outcomes. *J Craniomaxillofac Surg.* 2016;44(8):940-951.
24. Terzis JK. Pectoralis minor: a unique muscle for correction of facial palsy. *Plast Reconstr Surg.* 1989;83(5):767-776.
25. Dellon AL, Mackinnon SE. Segmentally innervated latissimus dorsi muscle. Microsurgical transfer for facial reanimation. *J Reconstr Microsurg.* 1985;2(1):7-12.
26. Zuker RM, Goldberg CS, Manktelow RT. Facial animation in children with Mobius syndrome after segmental gracilis muscle transplant. *Plast Reconstr Surg.* 2000;106(1):1-8.
This article describes techniques of reanimation in children with Mobius. It describes key considerations in this patient population from a surgical standpoint and describes a technique for reanimation.
27. Yang D, Morris SF, Tang M, Geddes CR. A modified longitudinally split segmental rectus femoris muscle flap transfer for facial reanimation: anatomic basis and clinical applications. *J Plast Reconstr Aesthet Surg.* 2006;59(8):807-814.
28. Liu AT, Lin Q, Jiang H, et al. Facial reanimation by one-stage microneurovascular free abductor hallucis muscle transplantation: personal experience and long-term outcomes. *Plast Reconstr Surg.* 2012;130(2):325-335.
29. Sugg KB, Kim JC. Dynamic reconstruction of the paralyzed face, part II: extensor digitorum brevis, serratus anterior, and anterolateral thigh. *Oper Tech Otolaryngol Head Neck Surg.* 2012;23(4):275-281.
30. Terzis JK, Karypidis D. Blink restoration in adult facial paralysis. *Plast Reconstr Surg.* 2010;126(1):126-139.
31. Borschel GH, Kawamura DH, Kasukurthi R, et al. The motor nerve to the masseter muscle: an anatomic and histomorphometric study to facilitate its use in facial reanimation. *J Plast Reconstr Aesthet Surg.* 2012;65(3):363-366.
This article describes the technique for identifying the nerve to masseter through the use of surface landmarking: 3 cm anterior to the tragus and 1 cm inferior to the zygomatic arch.
32. Klebuc MJA. Facial reanimation using the masseter-to-facial nerve transfer. *Plast Reconstr Surg.* 2011;127(5):1909-1915.
33. Bae YC, Zuker RM, Manktelow RT, Wade S. A comparison of commissure excursion following gracilis muscle transplantation for facial paralysis using a cross-face nerve graft versus the motor nerve to the masseter nerve. *Plast Reconstr Surg.* 2006;117(7):2407-2413.
This study compares results of innervation of free gracilis transfer for smile using nerve to masseter and cross-facial nerve grafting to power the transfer. It finds that excursion is greater following transfer from nerve to masseter.

QUESTIONS

1. A 4-year-old girl with congenital bilateral facial paralysis and palsy of bilateral abducens nerves presents for smile reanimation. She was told that she would undergo reanimation for the right and left sides at separate surgeries. What is the most appropriate surgical method of smile reanimation in this patient?

a. Bilateral gracilis free muscle transfers powered by cross-facial nerve grafts
b. Bilateral gracilis free muscle transfers powered by nerve to masseter
c. Bilateral gracilis free muscle transfers powered by the hypoglossal nerve
d. Bilateral temporalis transfers
e. She is not a candidate for smile reanimation.

2. A 22-year-old woman was stabbed in the cheek during an altercation and brought immediately to the emergency room. She has unilateral difficulty with smiling. You suspect that she has suffered sharp laceration to zygomaticobuccal branches of the facial nerve on that side. She has no other obvious injuries. Ideally, the longest you should wait before bringing her to the operating room for exploration and repair is:

a. 24 hours
b. 72 hours
c. 1 week
d. 6 months
e. 36 months

3. A 6-year-old girl with hemifacial microsomia presents for smile reanimation. She and her parents wish for whatever procedure will produce the most favorable, natural appearing results. The procedure that you will recommend to her is:

a. Temporalis transfer
b. Free gracilis transfer powered by the ipsilateral nerve to masseter
c. Free gracilis transfer powered by a cross-facial nerve graft
d. Chemodenervation of the contralateral zygomaticus major
e. Cross-facial nerve graft (nerve transfer) directly to a native zygomaticobuccal branch on the paralyzed side
f. Nerve transfer from ipsilateral nerve to masseter directly to zygomaticobuccal branch on the paralyzed side

4. A 56-year-old woman presents with lower lip dysfunction following a facelift. You wish to determine which facial nerve branches may have been injured. You ask her first to perform a full-denture smile and notice greater lower tooth show on the left. You then ask her to pout and notice significant asymmetry, with no eversion on the right. Based on these findings, you can conclude:

a. The right marginal mandibular branch has been injured
b. The right cervical branch has been injured
c. The left marginal mandibular branch has been injured
d. The left cervical branch has been injured
e. Both the marginal mandibular and cervical branches have been injured

5. A 32-year-old male presents to clinic 1 week after a deep laceration to the midcheek that was initially quickly irrigated and closed without exploration. You notice significant swelling on that side consistent with a sialocele and suspect that a parotid duct injury may have gone undetected. Which branch of the facial nerve is most likely to have also suffered injury in this patient?

a. Temporal
b. Zygomaticobuccal
c. Marginal mandibular
d. Cervical
e. All equal likelihood

1. **Answer: b.** Based on the description of the patient, she most likely has Mobius syndrome. There is no reason to expect that she would not be a candidate for smile reconstruction. In the pediatric population, local muscle transfers are not generally used as first-line strategies for reanimation because of the success of free functional muscle transfers. In patients with Mobius (or indeed bilateral paralysis in general), the contralateral facial nerve is not available as a donor. The hypoglossal nerve is the third most commonly affected cranial nerve in these patients and is not a reliable donor, such that use may lead to poor reanimation outcomes and may also generate significant donor deficits (i.e., impaired speech and eating). The best choice for these patients is bilateral free functional gracilis transfer powered by the nerve to masseter, which is nearly always sufficient in this patient population.

2. **Answer: b.** Facial nerve lacerations (as with motor nerve lacerations throughout the body) should ideally be explored and repaired within 72 hours of injury. This allows the distal nerve stumps to be stimulated to help in intraoperative identification. After 72 hours, neurotransmitter stores in the distal stumps are generally too depleted to activate muscular contraction with stimulation.

3. **Answer: c.** In patients with hemifacial macrosomia, there is no viable recipient nerve or normal musculature available for reinnervation (ruling out answers E and F). Local muscle transfers are not considered first-line options for reanimation in children given success with free muscle transfers. A free gracilis transfer is ideal for smile reanimation in patients who lack viable mimetic musculature, especially children, with facial paralysis. Although both cross-facial nerve grafts and nerve to masseter are both reliable donors for free functional muscle transfers, only use of cross-facial nerve graft will permit emotional smile. Additionally, use of cross-facial nerve grafts will also generate some resting tone, which does not occur with reinnervation using nerve to masseter.

4. **Answer: a.** Injury to cervical and marginal mandibular branches can look quite similar. Both may result in weakness of lower lip depression (although it is possible to have intact depression with isolated injury to cervical branches depending on the patient). Only injury to the marginal mandibular branch, however, because of its innervation of the mentalis, will leave a patient unable to evert their lower lip. It is possible that this patient has injured both branches. However, based on the information given, the only absolute conclusion that may be drawn is that the right marginal mandibular branch is not working.

5. **Answer: b.** Despite variations in branching patterns of the facial nerve, it is generally accepted that the zygomaticobuccal branch runs in close approximation to the parotid duct. Although it is certainly possible to injure multiple nerve branches with a laceration to the midcheek that also injures the parotid duct, the proximity of the zygomaticobuccal branch makes it the most likely to be involved.

CHAPTER 43 Mandible Reconstruction

Mark W. Stalder and Chad A. Perlyn

KEY POINTS

- The ideal donor site for nonvascularized bone grafts is from the ilium, whereas the free fibula flap remains the standard for vascularized reconstruction of critical mandibular defects.
- Rigid fixation of bone grafts, both vascularized and nonvascularized, is essential for optimum healing and integration.
- An essential component of bony reconstruction of the mandible, particularly with nonvascularized grafts, lies in having a healthy bed of soft tissue to receive the graft.
- In reconstruction of major posttraumatic defects of the mandible, it is advisable to set the occlusion temporarily and delay reconstruction until the soft tissue has had adequate time to heal.
- In cases of postoncologic reconstruction, the surgeon must be cognizant of the likely need for radiation, and thus vascularized bone is essential to maintain support of the soft tissue and viability of bone.
- In cases of osteoradionecrosis of the mandible, radical debridement of any involved tissue to that which is obviously healthy and bleeding, and beyond—both soft tissue and bone—is essential to prevent future complications and/or a failed reconstruction.
- The surgeon must not hesitate to use multiple free flaps, if necessary, to attain the necessary volume of healthy tissue in cases of massive tissue loss or resection.
- Preoperative virtual surgical planning offers an ideal option for improving accuracy of bony reconstruction, as well as the efficiency of intraoperative maneuvers.

The mandible is one of the primary structural components essential to mastication and maintenance of a patent airway, as well as an essential component of the aesthetic balance and appearance of the lower third of the face. As such, traumatic, ablative, and congenital defects of the bony mandible confer significant physical and psychosocial impediments in the daily lives of affected patients. Restoration of this structure is essential to providing a sense of normalcy to these patients, allowing them to eat, speak, and interact socially without undue disruption and stigmata of deformity.

Objectives of mandibular reconstruction are clear: restoration of premorbid form and function. This ideally includes an intact and functional bony construct capable of supporting normal dental occlusion, through osseointegrated dental implants, dental bridge, or dentures. Optimally the patient should be capable of eating a regular diet postoperatively. Additionally, the postoperative result should attempt to restore or maintain the appearance of the soft tissue envelope of the lower face by providing appropriate bony support.

Successful reconstruction is strongly contingent upon patient optimization, donor site selection, surgical technique, and reconstructive timeline, as well as the surgeon's experience and aptitude at evaluating those factors and establishing the appropriate conditions that promote a successful surgical effort. The mandible presents several challenges to the reconstructive surgeon that may affect outcomes. It is a mobile, load-bearing structure that requires proper fixation to promote adequate healing. Additionally, its adjacent position to the oral cavity increases the risk for bacterial contamination and salivary leakage into the surgical site. If these factors can be properly mitigated, surgical outcomes can be suboptimal. Prior to the rise of vascularized free tissue transfer techniques, the primary method of bony reconstruction of the mandible used nonvascularized autologous bone grafting and often included nonrigid fixation that had high potential for failure or suboptimal outcomes. However, due to the continued advancement of technological and surgical techniques, reconstructive surgeons currently can treat mandibular defects with high reliability, achieving excellent short- and long-term functional and aesthetic results.

INDICATIONS FOR RECONSTRUCTION

Trauma

Traumatic injury with associated segmental bony loss represents a relatively smaller component of the overall volume of reconstructive procedures of the mandible that are performed each year. There are three main classifications of traumatic etiology affecting the mandible: low-energy blunt trauma, high-energy blunt trauma, and ballistic trauma. Low-energy blunt trauma involves simple assault or falls from standing height and typically results in simple fractures that are easily treated with closed reduction or simple open reduction and fixation. Generally these injuries do not include soft tissue loss, comminution, periosteal stripping, or devascularization of bony fragments. High-energy blunt trauma includes motor vehicle collisions, motorcycle accidents, assault with a blunt object, or falls from significant height. These are generally more serious injuries and frequently cause comminuted fractures that may result in small segmental bony defects and damage to soft tissue that can impact both the viability of the bony fragments as well as the techniques that must be considered for adequate coverage of any internal hardware or efforts at bony reconstruction. Ballistic injury from gunshot wounds or explosive events can cause devastating damage to the mandible and surrounding soft tissue. Fractures are commonly comminuted, often with acute segmental loss of bone and frequently include significant soft tissue damage or loss. These severe injuries require careful planning to achieve functional mandibular reconstruction and are the most likely to require bony reconstruction.

Regardless of the nature of the injury, the approach for treating traumatic injuries of the mandible remains the same, following established stepwise principles for optimum outcomes. Fractures should be stabilized acutely—either by closed reduction and maxillomandibular fixation or open reduction with internal fixation—to reestablish premorbid occlusion, or in the event of poor dentition, anatomic alignment of the bony framework. For simple fractures without loss of bone, this is likely the definitive treatment. For more serious injuries that include segmental loss of bone, acute reduction and fixation achieve optimal healing of the larger fractured segments, while permitting interval healing of damaged soft tissue so that there may be an adequate envelope of vascularized tissue to provide a healthy recipient bed for nonvascularized bone grafts without undue contraction of the defect. Likewise, if possible, delayed reconstruction using vascularized bone allows for demarcation of tissue injury and a healthy recipient site, as well as resolution of edema and inflammatory processes. It also gives time for careful preoperative planning using virtual surgical planning (VSP) techniques.

Stabilization under these circumstances is typically performed with a defect-spanning reconstruction plate for load-bearing fixation for early mobilization and prevention of ankylosis of the temporomandibular joint. If there is significant loss of soft tissue associated with a segmental loss of bone, vascularized tissue transfer is required in addition to any bony reconstruction (vascularized or nonvascularized) to provide adequate coverage and healing of the construct.

Primary Oncologic Resection

Reconstruction of mandibular defects secondary to oncologic ablation represents a much larger percentage of the overall volume of bony reconstructive cases involving the mandible. These patients also present a very different set of circumstances that must be considered relative to the trauma patient. On one hand, these cases are typically planned in advance with the ablative surgeon, to achieve patient's physical status and set expectation, as well as VSP for improved efficiency in the operating room (OR) and accuracy of the reconstruction. There is also the advantage of controlling damage to the surrounding soft tissue envelope (if the patient has not been radiated), so edema and inflammatory processes are minimized. Having said that, these patients are typically older, have a long history of tobacco and sometimes alcohol abuse, commonly do not have an optimized nutrition status, and most importantly are often radiated either preoperatively or postoperatively. The significance of the damage to the surrounding soft tissue envelope due to radiation cannot be overstated. The implications for healing can result in an array of postoperative complications ranging from small wounds to total graft failure or even life-threatening medical complications.

The vast majority of these patients (radiated or not) will require vascularized bone for optimum functional and aesthetic reconstructive results. Under no circumstances should a nonvascularized bone graft be placed either in a radiated soft tissue envelope or in a patient who will require postoperative radiation therapy. Additionally, the impaired nutrition and continued tobacco use in many of these patients can impede proper healing of nonvascularized grafts. If possible, advanced preoperative placement of a feeding tube should be considered to ameliorate nutritional deficiencies with supplementation of oral intake for improved healing.

As with trauma patients, fixation of the bony construct should be performed with load-bearing plates, as early mobilization remains important. These patients will also require a temporary tracheostomy to maintain an established airway postoperatively during the acute phase of edema, for unencumbered access to the operative field during the procedure. If there are no significant postoperative concerns, the patient can typically be decannulated prior to discharge.

Osteoradionecrosis

Likely, the most complex patients undergoing bony reconstruction of the mandible are those who suffer from osteoradionecrosis. These patients have the unfortunate circumstance of having suffered from an oral malignancy as well as having been treated with radiation and experiencing all of the negative sequelae inherent to that process. Mandibular bone death occurs due to the resulting localized hypovascularity, hypocellularity, and hypoxia from radiation. In these patients, it is the treatment that has caused their insidious and progressive pathology. The extent of disease is commonly not obvious on imaging or examination and often involves the soft tissue. When the patient demonstrates pathologic fracture or extensive segmental disease, the appropriate treatment is aggressive resection of the involved mandible and reconstruction with vascularized bone. Use of nonvascularized bone grafts under these circumstances is wholly unsuitable for the problem at hand, as the radiated tissue bed will not permit appropriate healing. These patients will often require a soft tissue free flap in addition to vascularized bone to achieve a proper result.

As these are very complicated patients, VSP is a key component for obtaining an accurate bony reconstruction while improving the patient's chances for a long-lasting result. Resection of the diseased bone should be planned based on computed tomography (CT) imaging and extend at least 1 cm beyond the edges of the lesion to assure the presence of healthy bone stock at the margins of the reconstruction. Not only will this improve the chances of a successful bony union, but also diminishes the risk of leaving behind occult disease that could cause failure of the reconstructive effort.

NONVASCULARIZED BONE GRAFTS

A long-standing technique for the reconstruction of noncritical bony defects of the mandible is the use of nonvascularized bone grafts. This is an effective strategy for patients who have not suffered devastating traumatic soft tissue injury, have not undergone prior radiation treatment for malignancy, or who will not undergo postoperative radiation treatment following ablative surgery. These grafts are commonly used after ablation of benign tumors of the mandible or localized malignancies with nonaggressive features where the bony resection is less and there is minimal disruption of the surrounding tissue envelope.

There are numerous reports of the successful use of nonvascularized grafts for mandibular defects greater than 6 cm; however, the risk for failure becomes significantly greater as defect size increases, and it is generally recommended to avoid this technique beyond that length.[1-4] The main factors resulting in graft failure include bony resorption, infection, and defect length. Above all else, the use of nonvascularized grafts requires a healthy, well-vascularized recipient bed of surrounding soft tissue, and healthy adjacent mandibular bone at the margins of the defect to achieve an osseous union and reestablish effective bony structural support. As such, it can be advantageous to delay grafting for soft tissue healing to occur.[2,3,5] As with any procedure designed to reestablish the bony structure of the mandible, proper fixation techniques are essential for a successful bony union, and an extraoral approach is often recommended to avoid undue salivary contamination and mitigate the risk of infection.

There is an abundance of potential donor sites from which to harvest bone grafts that can be used for this purpose, and most trained reconstructive surgeons can successfully perform these procedures. By far, the most common site for graft harvest is the ilium. The iliac crest, both anterior and posterior, is an ideal donor for intact corticocancellous grafts that immediately provide inherent structural support for the reconstruction, as well as purely cancellous or particulate corticocancellous grafts that, while offering no immediate structure, are able to be manipulated and molded to provide ideal aesthetic reconstructive outcomes.[2,5,6] After adequate healing and ossification of these grafts, they can also serve as a base for dental restoration using osseointegrated implants, though without the same degree of success seen with vascularized bone grafts.[2,3,5] Additional possible nonvascularized bone grafts that can be used successfully for mandibular defects are rib grafts, fibular grafts, tibial grafts, and split calvarial grafts. These sites are used less frequently than the ilium but offer adequate alternatives should the need arise.[4,6,7]

VASCULARIZED FREE TISSUE TRANSFER

As microsurgical techniques and surgical efficiency continue to improve over the last two decades, the use of vascularized bone flaps has become the standard for reconstruction of critical segmental defects of the mandible. Though these procedures have a big learning curve and require specialized training and experience, there is simply no better substitute than living, vascularized bone in most complex reconstructive cases. The time to bony union is significantly faster than with nonvascularized grafts, the risk of infection is considerably lower. Because these flaps do not depend upon an optimized wound bed, they can be transferred with the addition of healthy, vascularized soft tissue, and can achieve successful reconstruction of the entire length of the mandible in a single procedure. More specifically, any defect greater than 6 cm and any patient who has been radiated or will be radiated should be considered a prime candidate for vascularized bone reconstruction.

Deep Circumflex Iliac Artery Free Flap

The deep circumflex iliac artery (DCIA) flap offers vascularized iliac crest bone stock of moderate length (though up to 16 cm has been reported) as a reconstructive option for shorter straight-segment bony defects of the mandible. Its advantage over nonvascularized iliac crest grafts is quicker healing, improved resistance to infection, and the possibility of simultaneous transfer of vascularized soft tissue if need be. Because of its shape and relatively limited length, this flap is more suited for lateral segmental defects as opposed to anterior or ramus/angle defects that might require multiple osteotomies for adequate contouring. It can be harvested as an osteocutaneous flap if skin is required, or along with a segment of internal oblique muscle based off of a perforating vessel from the main pedicle that can be used for intraoral lining (Figure 43.1). The bone stock can provide good matching height to the native mandible and is capable of accepting osseointegrated implants for dental restoration, with excellent long-term retention of upwards of 96% reported.[8-11]

Downsides of this vascularized option include a relatively short pedicle that may require the use of vein grafts for anastomosis, an inability to effectively perform segmental osteotomies for purposes of multisegment reconstruction of the mandible, and a general lack of available bony length.[10] Additionally, donor site morbidity can include an increased risk for abdominal wall hernias, persistent pain, gait disturbances, and sensory alteration.[12] Because of these factors and the advantages offered by the free fibula flap, the DCIA flap is employed less frequently for purposes of mandibular reconstruction. However, it can be useful for moderate length lateral segmental traumatic defects that also require soft tissue coverage, or similar defects that occur in a radiated field. From a perspective of functional and aesthetic restoration, the DCIA offers similar outcomes when compared to the fibula flap with regard to appearance, speech, and oral continence.[11]

Scapula Free Flap

The free scapula bone flap is another less-frequently used vascularized option for reconstruction of critical mandibular defects. Based off of the circumflex scapular (lateral border of the scapula) or angular (scapular tip) arteries from the subscapular system, this flap offers a segment of bone of moderate length—up to 13 cm long at the upper end of its range—though only 1 to 2 cm wide and somewhat thin (Figure 43.2). The scapular tip has been shown to be useful in the reconstruction of short-segment defects and isolated angular defects, whereas the lateral border provides more length in cases of longer defects of the body. This is also an excellent option in revision procedures and conveys the versatility inherent to its root vascular supply, namely the opportunity to be harvested along with one of a number of other tissue flap options as a chimera with a single common vascular pedicle of significant length. This facilitates the transfer and inset of a variety of skin or muscle flaps if soft tissue is required for the reconstruction and without the need for a second microvascular anastomosis. Additionally, when treating older patients, use of this vascular system can mitigate the issues inherent to the lower extremity peripheral vascular disease often present in this population.[13]

Although the scapula flap does present a viable option for successful restoration of mandibular form and function, including osseointegrated implant-based dental prostheses, there are disadvantages that diminish its usefulness as a primary choice for these cases. Intraoperative logistics can sometimes be difficult due to the required lateral positioning of the patient, which can prevent a simultaneous two-surgeon approach to the case. The need to reposition after harvest of the flap can negatively influence efficiency and increase surgical times. Reported complication rates associated with the scapula flap vary, and in some cases are suggested to be more favorable relative to the free fibula flap with regard to donor site healing, but can cause some degree of long-term shoulder dysfunction.[14]

Fibula Free Flap

The free fibula flap, first described in the late 1980s by Hidalgo, has since become the standard for vascularized bony reconstruction of critical defects of the mandible.[15] This flap offers numerous advantages over all other vascularized options that make it the primary choice for almost all cases including traumatic and primary ablative defects, as well as for reconstruction of osteoradionecrosis (Figures 43.3–43.5). Its ample length of up to 26 cm (depending upon the patient) and consistent shape make it incredibly versatile, capable of recreating any segment of the mandible, including defects of the condyle, body, or anterior segment. This flap is also highly reliable, with numerous published reports demonstrating up to 100% flap survival.[16,17] Morbidity of the donor site is also within acceptable limits. At times there can be incisional wound breakdown when a large skin paddle is taken and there is too much tension on the closure. Additionally, some patients can experience a slightly altered gait, or reduced ability to participate in strenuous physical activity.[18] However, most patients do not experience significant postoperative complications.[16]

Based off the peroneal artery, the vascular pedicle can provide excellent length often required in head and neck reconstruction. Though the peroneal provides an endosteal blood supply through a large nutrient artery, when transferred as a free flap, the bone stock is usually dependent on the robust periosteal circulation, as this allows for multiple segmental wedge osteotomies for incredibly versatile shaping and manipulation. This permits simultaneous reconstruction of straight segments as well as the curved structures of the mandible at the angle and the parasymphysis anteriorly. Though the surgeon must bear in mind that to optimize viability, it is generally accepted that each segment must maintain at least 2 cm in length. Likewise, although the bone stock does not necessarily possess ideal height, it can be cut for a stacked or double-barreled technique that can adequately recreate the shape of the native mandible and provide for an optimum aesthetic restoration of the lower third of the face.

Although not all cases of mandibular reconstruction require additional soft tissue coverage, it is often necessary to achieve a watertight intraoral closure, which is essential to prevent salivary leakage onto the vascular pedicle. The fibula flap, again, offers great versatility in this regard, as it can be harvested either as an osteocutaneous flap, or more commonly, along with a skin paddle based off the perforating vessels of the peroneal artery. Though there is not an ample volume of excess skin of the lower leg, flaps of up to 5 cm wide and traversing the entire length of the bone flap can be harvested based on these perforators and still closed primarily. If a skin paddle of greater width is required, the donor site can be readily closed with a skin graft. The advantage of the perforator-based skin paddle is that it offers flexibility of inset, with the surgeon able to manipulate positioning with relative ease. These cutaneous flaps can also be used to provide external coverage if needed. And if the patient requires a very large volume of soft tissue, or both intraoral and external coverage, the distal end of the peroneal pedicle can provide excellent flow through vessels for transferring a second fasciocutaneous free flap in series.

As restoration of function is of primary importance, dental restoration is an important consideration for these patients. The fibula provides excellent bone stock for this purpose with the use of osseointegrated implants and subsequent design and placement of a dental prosthesis. Numerous studies have confirmed both the excellent success rates and quality of life measures when dental restoration is pursued in conjunction with a free fibula reconstruction of the mandible. Additionally, when required, and with proper contouring, the fibula provides the opportunity for condyle reconstruction, a relative limitation of the other vascularized bone options.

From a technical perspective, though the basic dissection of the fibula flap is relatively straight forward (Figure 43.4), the level of complexity can quickly become overwhelming for the inexperienced surgeon in cases of composite tissue or multisegmental defects. This can become readily apparent when the need arises for multiple osteotomies or the addition of perforator-based skin paddles or a simultaneous second fasciocutaneous free flap. Keeping this in mind, the regular use of virtual surgical planning, three-dimensional-printed osteotomy guides, and predesigned patient-specific reconstruction plates can significantly reduce the risk of a poor outcome and greatly increase surgical efficiency in the OR. The addition of a second surgeon to prepare simultaneously the recipient site and vessels is also highly recommended.

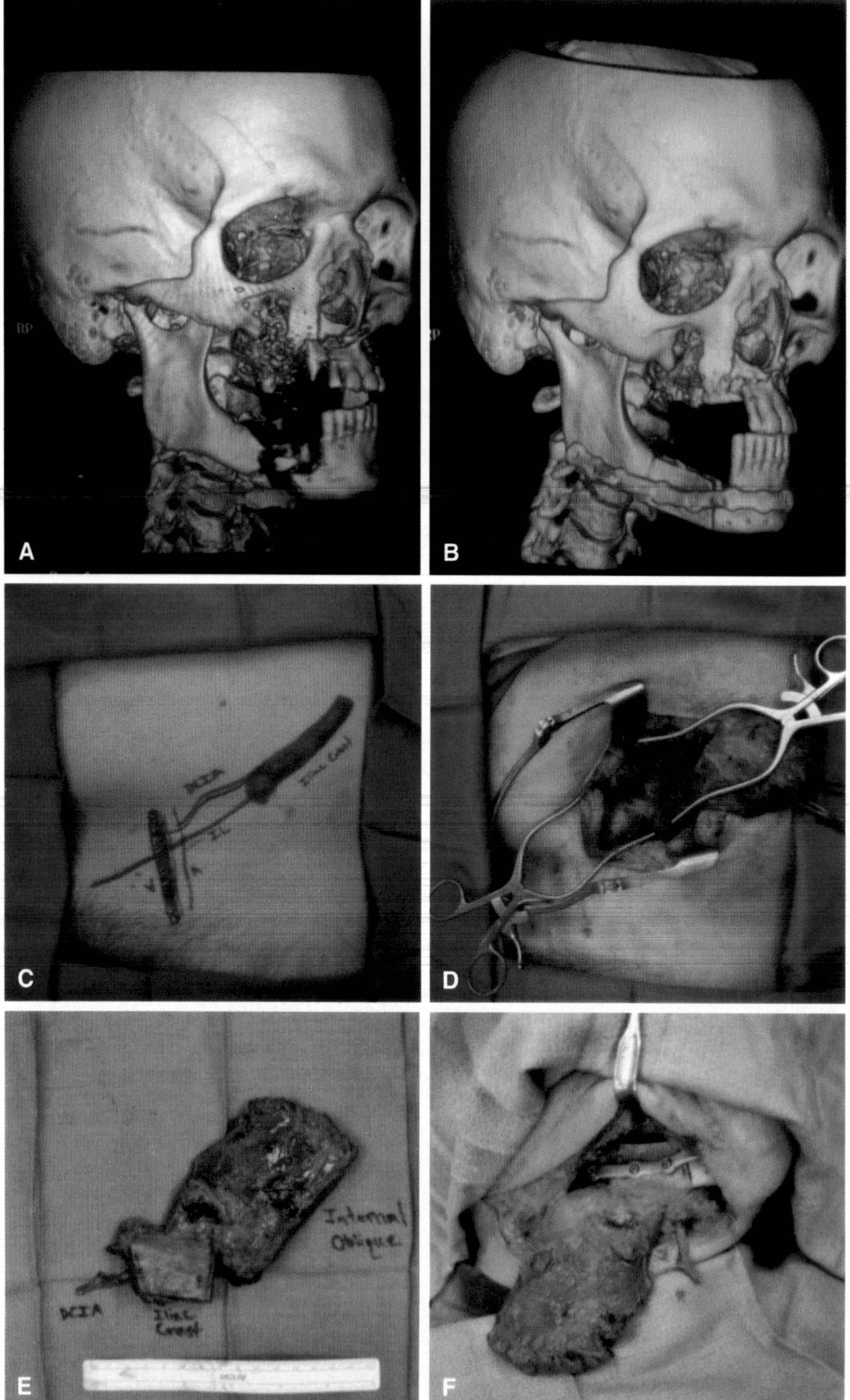

FIGURE 43.1. This patient suffered a self-inflicted gunshot wound to the face. **A.** Resultant injuries included a comminuted fracture with segmental loss of the right mandibular body and loss of intraoral mucosal coverage of that area. He underwent initial debridement and stabilization of the mandible with a defect-spanning reconstruction plate in preparation for a delayed definitive reconstruction. Subsequent reconstruction was performed using a vascularized segment of the anterior iliac crest based off the deep circumflex iliac artery (DCIA). **C.** Dissection proceeded through an incision along the length of the vessel and iliac crest as marked. **D.** A flap of internal oblique muscle based off an ascending perforator from the main vascular pedicle was included in order to provide intraoral coverage with vascularized soft tissue. **E.** Ultimately the dissection yielded about 5 cm of bone, along with the vascularized muscle on a short but adequate vascular pedicle. The flap was inset into the defect using a custom-milled plate designed through the virtual surgical planning process, and the muscle flap was wrapped around the construct intraorally **(F)** to provide an excellent reconstruction of the mandible with matching height and good contour of the mandibular border **(B)**.

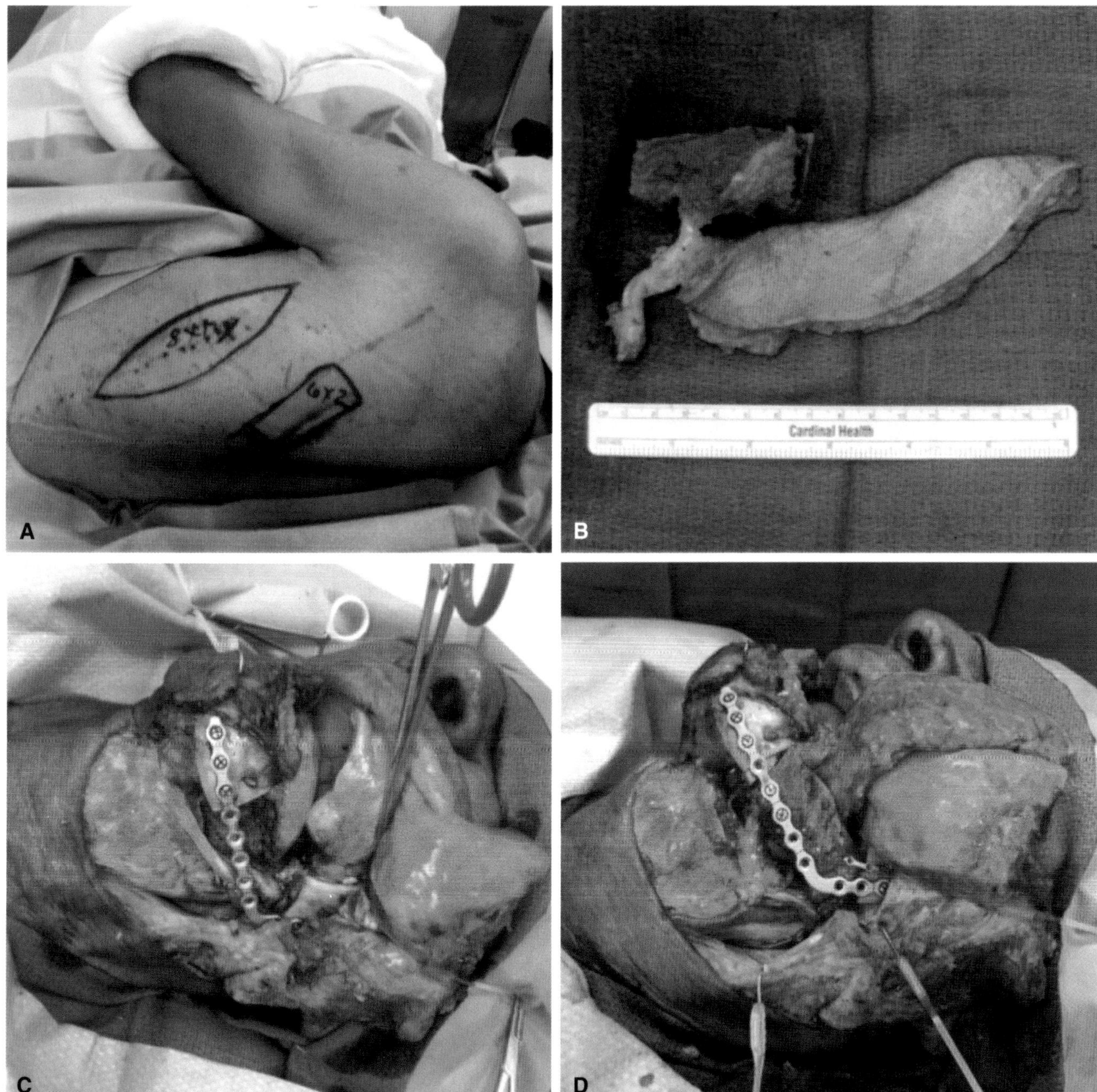

FIGURE 43.2. This patient underwent primary resection of an oral malignancy that involved segmental resection of the left mandibular body and associated mucosa. Reconstruction of the mandibular defect was undertaken using a vascularized bone flap from the lateral border of the scapula based off the circumflex scapular artery from the subscapular system. Additionally, a skin paddle was planned for intraoral coverage based off perforators of the thoracodorsal artery leading back to the common subscapular vascular pedicle. **A.** After the ablative procedure was complete, the flap harvest necessitated placing the patient in the lateral decubitus position. Once the chimeric flap had been harvested **(B)**, the patient was placed back into the supine position, and a load-bearing reconstruction plate was shaped and fixed into position at the inferior border of the mandible **(C)**. **D.** The bone flap was subsequently inset into the defect, and the skin paddle positioned intraorally for coverage of the construct. Microvascular anastomosis was performed using the facial artery and vein as recipient vessels.

Virtual Surgical Planning

One of the more recent and useful technological developments that has helped to shape present day reconstructive efforts is VSP. VSP offers the opportunity to precisely plan the bony mandibular reconstruction well in advance of the actual procedure using computer-generated three-dimensional reconstructions of the patient's anatomy with imported CT imaging files (Figure 43.5). This allows the surgeon to enter the OR with the details of the procedure having already been thought out and virtually played out in a stepwise manner. Beyond that, the most practical aspect of this technology is the design and production of three-dimensional-printed patient-specific guides for use when performing osteotomies. These guides can be used both to guarantee an accurate bony resection at the recipient site, as well as on the donor flap to permit accurate and efficient shaping of the bony construct to maximize bony contact of the osteotomized segments. The potential benefits of regular utilization of VSP are significant. Published reports demonstrate significantly diminished operative times, more accurate bony reconstructions, and increased complexity of the cases that can be performed.[19-23]

An even more recent addition to this technology is the advent of patient-specific reconstruction plates. These plates are typically produced through a custom milling process. The surgeon is able to design the length and screw-hole placement, as well as bends in the

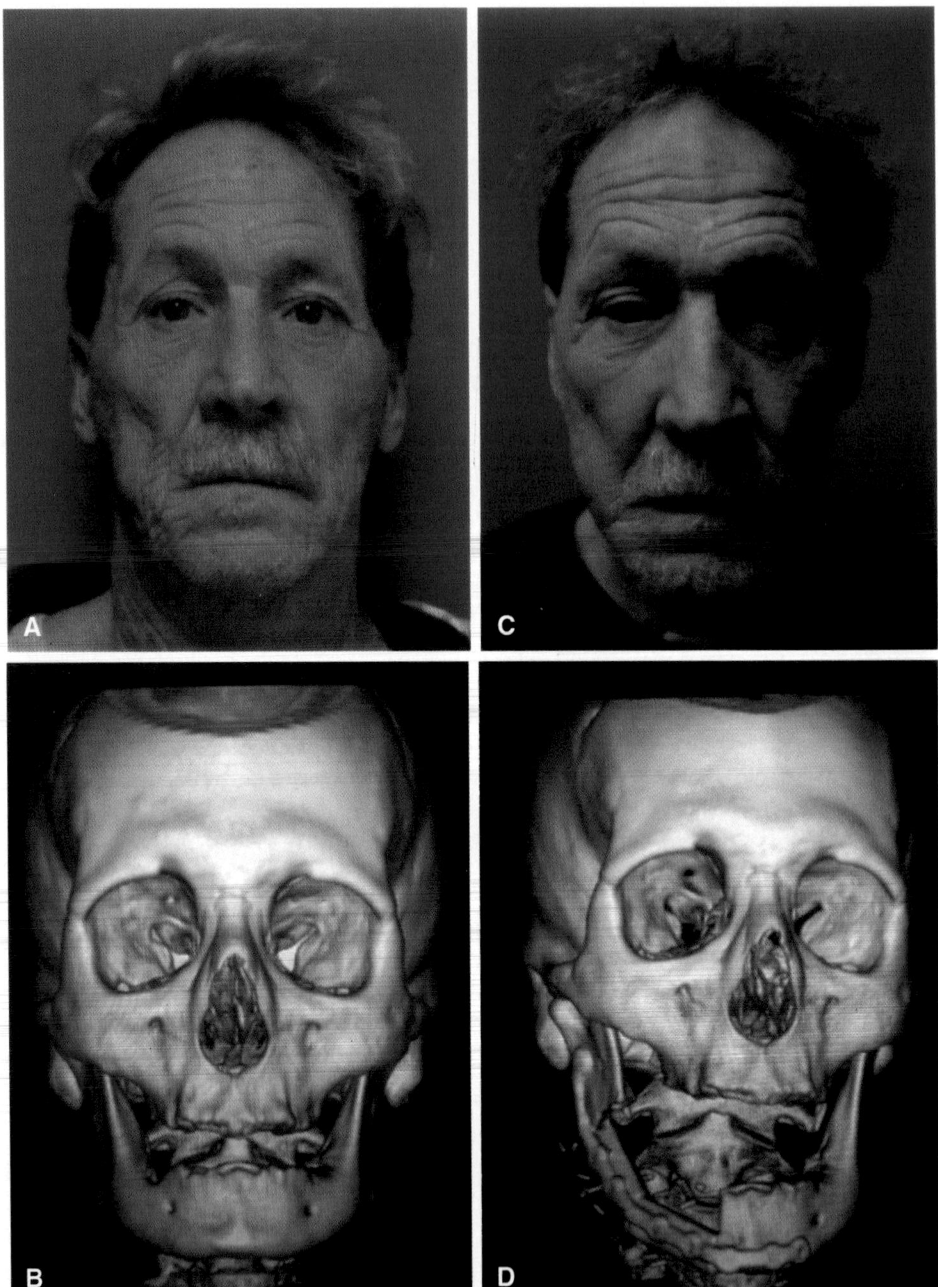

FIGURE 43.3. This patient previously underwent radiation therapy to treat an oral malignancy but subsequently developed osteoradionecrosis of the right mandibular body. Virtual surgical planning was used to design the appropriate resection of the diseased bone and to plan for reconstruction using a vascularized free fibula flap with a perforator-based skin paddle for intraoral coverage. These preoperative **(A,B)** and 3-month postoperative **(C,D)** images demonstrate the ability of this technique to restore bony structure and continuity to the mandible and maintain an aesthetic appearance of the lower third of the face with almost no stigmata of surgery.

plate specific to the needs of the individual reconstructive procedure. Based on the CT imaging, the plate is contoured precisely to fit the patient's native mandible and the designed bony construct to be used in reconstructing the segmental defect. This additional tool further reduces operative time by preventing the need for intraoperative design and plate contouring, and the accuracy is unmatched.

At the present time, VSP should be considered for essentially all but the simplest straight-segment cases of mandible reconstruction employing free osseous flaps. The time saved in the OR as well as the improvements in accuracy of the reconstruction and plating design justify and make up for the added expense. Use of this technology is rapidly becoming the de facto standard of care for these procedures.

Single-Stage Comprehensive Mandibular Restoration

The jaw-in-a-day procedure, as it is popularly known, is the penultimate technique for mandibular reconstruction. This procedure fully implements currently available state-of-the-art technology and surgical techniques by virtually planning vascularized fibula flap reconstruction of mandibular defects in conjunction with simultaneous osseointegrated implant-based dental prosthetic restoration. Printed osteotomy guides are used to create a precise bony defect, as well as to accurately shape the fibula bone flap. Additionally, the virtual planning process allows for the preplanned placement of implants prior to transfer of the flap, as well as prefabricated prosthetic dentition. The patient awakens from

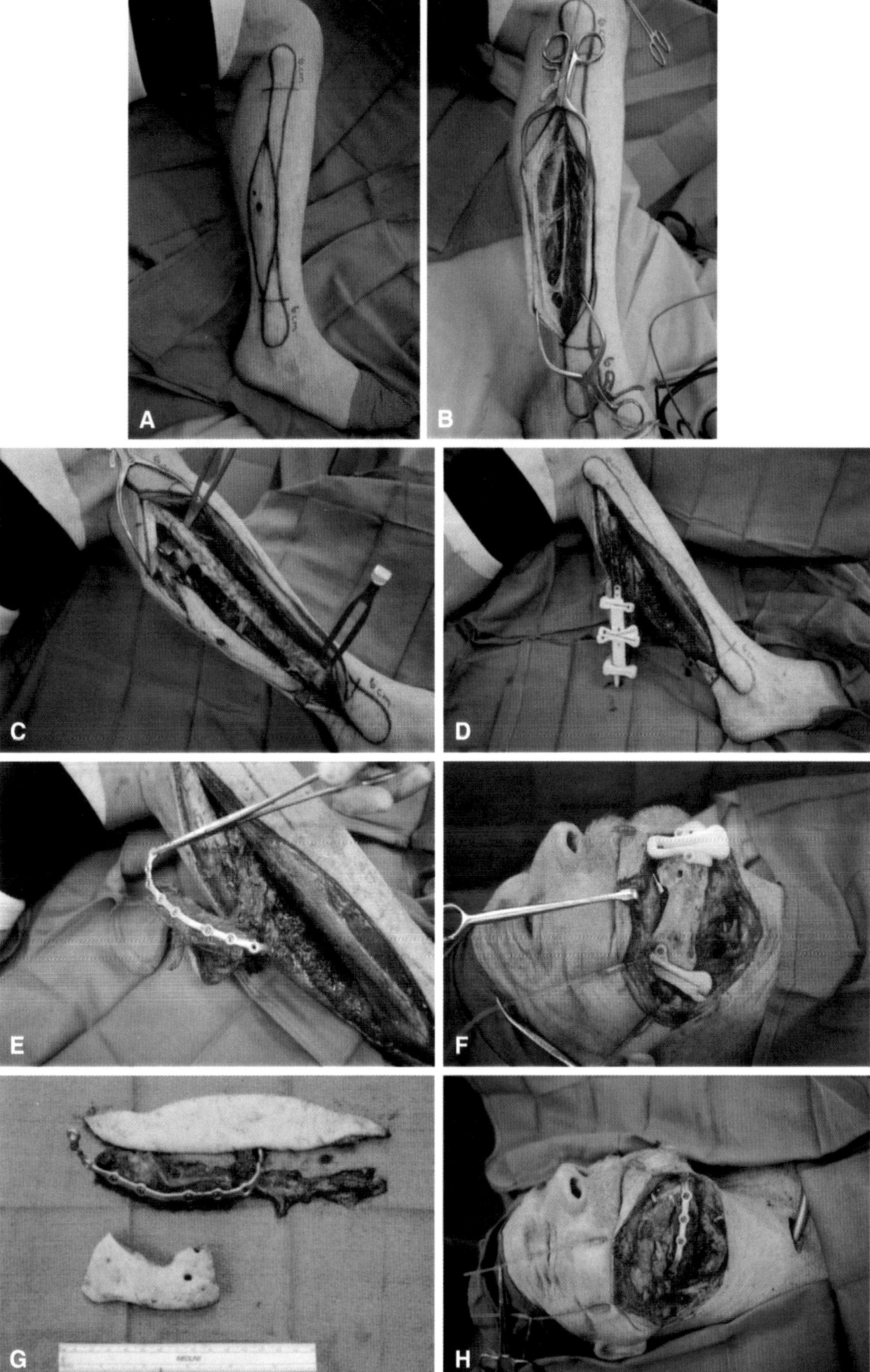

FIGURE 43.4. The dissection shown in these images was undertaken to reconstruct the segmental mandibular defect for the patient in Figure 43.3. This is performed under tourniquet to facilitate visualization and speed of the dissection in a bloodless field. **A.** The fibula is marked preoperatively, taking care to preserve 6 cm of proximal and distal bony length in order to protect joint integrity and important neurologic structures. Additionally, a handheld Doppler device is used to identify perforators along the posterior border of the fibula and the skin paddle designed based off one or more of these vessels. **B.** An incision is made along the axis of the fibula contiguous with the anterior edge of the designed skin paddle, and dissection proceeds until the appropriate perforating vascular bundle is identified and adequate length is obtained. Once the perforator dissection is complete, the harvest then continues anteriorly along the length of the fibula, taking care to leave a couple of millimeters of muscle attached to the bone so as not to disrupt the vascular supply from the periosteum. This is taken to the interosseous membrane, and then proceeds along the posterior aspect of the fibula in a similar fashion. **C.** At this point, the periosteum is dissected away from the bone circumferentially at the proximal and distal sites of the planned osteotomies. A retractor is placed between the fibula and the peroneal vessels to protect them during the osteotomies. Once these have been made, the interosseous membrane is divided, exposing the length of the vascular pedicle and giving freedom of movement so that the vessels can be released from the surrounding tissue and its branches from distal to proximal. **D.** The tourniquet is then released to allow perfusion of the flap while the printed osteotomy guide is positioned in situ along the fibula. **E.** Once the closing osteotomies are made, the patient-specific plate can be applied, completing the planned construct. **F,G.** Meanwhile, the printed osteotomy guides for the resection are positioned on the mandible, the diseased portion of bone is removed, and the flap construct can be fully harvested. **H.** The flap is then fixed into place at the recipient site using preplanned screw holes for the custom plate, and the skin paddle is inset intraorally to obtain a watertight closure. Microvascular anastomosis in this patient was performed using the ipsilateral facial vessels.

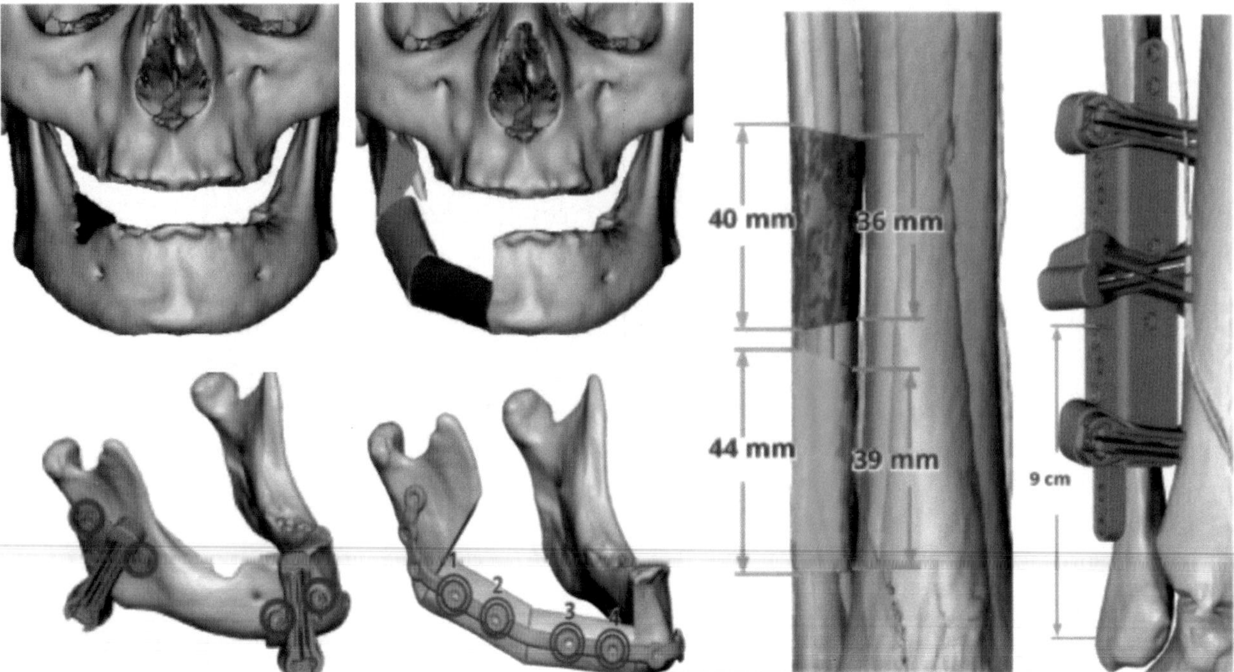

FIGURE 43.5. Virtual surgical planning was performed preoperatively for the patient shown in Figures 43.3 and 43.4. This process allows the surgeon to identify the segment of the mandible to be resected/reconstructed and design an exact-fitting construct from the fibula. Patient-specific osteotomy guides can then be printed for precise cuts at both the mandible and at the fibula. Additionally, custom-milled reconstruction plates can then be designed to the surgeon's specifications and fitted to the contour of the patient's mandible.

surgery and has a fully functional lower jaw. This technique successfully omits the time gap between reconstruction and dental rehabilitation under the presumption that early restoration of form and function is psychologically beneficial for patients by allowing them to seamlessly maintain normal daily activities and social interactions.[19,20,24,25]

This is a highly complex and sophisticated procedure that, at present, is only available at relatively high-volume centers of microsurgical head and neck reconstruction and requires the availability of several different specialists to optimize outcomes. Of note, funding is often a significant barrier for obtaining the implant-based dental prostheses for these patients, limiting the overall number of these cases that are performed.

PEDIATRIC CONSIDERATIONS

Pediatric mandibular reconstruction is performed for congenital anomalies of the lower jaw. Congenital differences include micrognathia, retrognathia, asymmetries, or absence of the mandible or its components. These issues are commonly associated with diagnoses, including hemifacial or craniofacial microsomia, Treacher Collins syndrome, Pierre Robin sequence, and Nager syndrome.[26]

Though most children with congenital mandibular issues do not require intervention in early infancy, the exception is the infant with acute respiratory distress who does not respond to conservative measures such as repositioning or nasal trumpet. Rather than directly proceeding to tracheostomy, mandibular lengthening can be performed with distraction osteogenesis to improve the upper airway and airflow resistance, thereby avoiding the need for a surgical airway. Upper airway volume expansion via distraction has been shown to be able to decrease the flow resistance over the length of the airway, presumably secondary to an increase in the average cross-sectional area.[26]

Those patients with absence of the vertical ramus, condyle, and temporomandibular joint may require costochondral grafting. Timing for this procedure is typically between 3 and 6 years of age, as this allows for a more robust donor rib and improved postoperative cooperation.[27] The donor site harvest is not technically demanding, and after the donor rib has been secured (along with a cartilaginous cap) the graft is fixed in an overlap fashion to the native mandible using either a lag screw technique or conventional screws with a piece of titanium plate cut to act as a *washer* to prevent fracture of the graft. The major goals of reconstruction in these patients should be alignment of the maxillary and mandibular dental midlines with the midsagittal plane, a correction/leveling of the mandibular cant, and restoration of facial symmetry. Published reports have demonstrated the effectiveness of this technique at improving both functional outcomes (chewing and better oral opening) and aesthetic facial appearance.[28,29] As an additional consideration, though costochondral grafts can have excellent growth with time, occasionally additional length is still necessary as the child grows. In these cases, distraction of the rib graft can achieve the desired symmetry.[30]

Mandibular reconstruction following ablative surgery is uncommon in the pediatric patient. When necessary, the techniques described above, as well as those presented previously in this chapter, can be applied. Autologous material is preferred and the amount of hardware should be limited and/or subsequently explanted in the growing child. And consideration of the developing tooth root anatomy must be considered when using plates on the mandible of a child.[31]

ACKNOWLEDGMENTS

Hugo St. Hilaire, DDS, MD, assisted on the cases presented within this chapter, and also contributed expert insight to the material of the text. Camille Rogers, PhD, contributed significantly in the collection and organization of background information and bibliographical sources.

REFERENCES

1. Akinbami BO. Reconstruction of continuity defects of the mandible with non-vascularized bone grafts. Systematic literature review. *Craniomaxillofac Trauma Reconstr*. 2016;9(3):195-205.
2. Pogrel MA, Podlesh S, Anthony JP, Alexander J. A comparison of vascularized and nonvascularized bone grafts for reconstruction of mandibular continuity defects. *J Oral Maxillofac Surg*. 1997;55(11):1200-1206.

3. Foster RD, Anthony JP, Sharma A, Pogrel MA. Vascularized bone flaps versus nonvascularized bone grafts for mandibular reconstruction: an outcome analysis of primary bony union and endosseous implant success. *Head Neck.* 1999;21(1):66-71.
This study elucidates the clear superiority of vascularized bone grafts versus nonvascularized bone grafts for critical defects in mandible reconstruction, demonstrating a significantly higher rate of bony union, fewer operations required, and significantly higher rate of endosseous implant success. These results were seen despite reconstructing larger average bony defects, and often in radiated patients.
4. Moura LB, Carvalho PH, Xavier CB, et al. Autogenous non-vascularized bone graft in segmental mandibular reconstruction: a systematic review. *Int J Oral Maxillofac Surg.* 2016;45(11):1388-1394.
5. van Gemert JT, van Es RJ, Van Cann EM, Koole R. Nonvascularized bone grafts for segmental reconstruction of the mandible—a reappraisal. *J Oral Maxillofac Surg.* 2009;67(7):1446-1452.
6. Ferretti C, Muthray E, Rikhotso E, et al. Reconstruction of 56 mandibular defects with autologous compressed particulate corticocancellous bone grafts. *Br J Oral Maxillofac Surg.* 2016;54(3):322-326.
7. Gadre PK, Ramanojam S, Patankar A, Gadre KS. Nonvascularized bone grafting for mandibular reconstruction: myth or reality? *J Craniofac Surg.* 2011;22(5):1727-1735.
8. Kniha K, Möhlhenrich SC, Foldenauer AC, et al. Evaluation of bone resorption in fibula and deep circumflex iliac artery flaps following dental implantation: a three-year follow-up study. *J Craniomaxillofac Surg.* 2017;45(4):474-478.
9. Möhlhenrich SC, Kniha K, Elvers D, et al. Intraosseous stability of dental implants in free revascularized fibula and iliac crest bone flaps. *J Craniomaxillofac Surg.* 2016;44(12):1935-1939.
10. Chen S, Chen H, Horng S, et al. Reconstruction for osteoradionecrosis of the mandible: superiority of free iliac bone flap to fibula flap in postoperative infection and healing. *Ann Plast Surg.* 2014;73(suppl 1):S18-S26.
11. Shpitzer T, Neligan PC, Gullane PJ, et al. The free iliac crest and fibula flaps in vascularized oromandibular reconstruction: comparison and long-term evaluation. *Head Neck.* 1999;21(7):639-647.
12. Schardt C, Schmid A, Bodem J, et al. Donor site morbidity and quality of life after microvascular head and neck reconstruction with free fibula and deep-circumflex iliac artery flaps. *J Craniomaxillofac Surg.* 2017;45(2):304-311.
13. Dowthwaite SA, Theurer J, Belzile M, et al. Comparison of fibular and scapular osseous free flaps for oromandibular reconstruction: a patient-centered approach to flap selection. *JAMA Otolaryngol Head Neck Surg.* 2013;139(3):285-292.
14. Fujiki M, Miyamoto S, Sakuraba M, et al. A comparison of perioperative complications following transfer of fibular and scapular flaps for immediate mandibular reconstruction. *J Plast Reconstr Aesthet Surg.* 2013;66(3):372-375.
15. Hidalgo DA. Fibula free flap: a new method of mandible reconstruction. *Plast Reconstr Surg.* 1989;84(1):71-79.
This is the landmark article that first described the use of the vascularized fibula flap for mandibular reconstruction. Dr. Hidalgo performed 12 successful reconstructions of large bony defects in this series, and also demonstrated the ability to perform segmental osteotomies on the fibula construct while still maintaining vascularity. The fibula flap has since become the workhorse free flap for reconstruction of large segmental bony defects of the mandible.
16. Hidalgo DA, Rekow A. A review of 60 consecutive fibula free flap mandible reconstructions. *Plast Reconstr Surg.* 1995;96(3):585-596.
17. Cordeiro PG, Disa JJ, Hidalgo DA, Hu QY. Reconstruction of the mandible with osseous free flaps: a 10-year experience with 150 consecutive patients. *Plast Reconstr Surg.* 1999;104(5):1314-1320.
18. Feuvrier D, Sagawa Y Jr, Béliard S, et al. Long-term donor-site morbidity after vascularized free fibula flap harvesting: clinical and gait analysis. *J Plast Reconstr Aesthet Surg.* 2016;69(2):262-269.
19. Avraham T, Franco P, Brecht LE, et al. Functional outcomes of virtually planned free fibula flap reconstruction of the mandible. *Plast Reconstr Surg.* 2014;134(4):628e-634e.
This article describes the outcomes of mandible reconstruction with free fibula flaps performed with the assistance of virtual surgical planning (VSP) and printed cutting guides in a high-volume center. While the accuracy of the reconstructions were similar, cases performed with VSP were overall more complex (with more average osteotomies performed), and were performed significantly faster in the operating room (163 minutes faster on average). These results demonstrate how VSP technology can be harnessed to enhance the surgeon's ability to improve upon reconstructive outcomes.
20. Monaco C, Stranix JT, Avraham T, et al. Evolution of surgical techniques for mandibular reconstruction using free fibula flaps: the next generation. *Head Neck.* 2016;38(suppl 1):E2066-E2073.
21. Metzler P, Geiger EJ, Alcon A, et al. Three-dimensional virtual surgery accuracy for free fibula mandibular reconstruction: planned versus actual results. *J Oral Maxillofac Surg.* 2014;72(12):2601-2612.
22. Craig ES, Yuhasz M, Shah A, et al. Simulated surgery and cutting guides enhance spatial positioning in free fibular mandibular reconstruction. *Microsurgery.* 2015;35(1):29-33.
23. Chang EI, Jenkins MP, Patel SA, Topham NS. Long-term operative outcomes of preoperative computed tomography-guided virtual surgical planning for osteocutaneous free flap mandible reconstruction. *Plast Reconstr Surg.* 2016;137(2):619-623.
24. Levine JP, Bae JS, Soares M, et al. Jaw in a day: total maxillofacial reconstruction using digital technology. *Plast Reconstr Surg.* 2013;131(6):1386-1391.
The patient series described in this article demonstrates the penultimate example of mandible reconstruction—restoration of full functional dentition performed simultaneously with vascularized free fibula reconstruction of a critical mandibular defect. This procedure would not be possible without the use of VSP, again demonstrating the power of this technology to enhance our outcomes as surgeons.
25. Qaisi M, Kolodney H, Swedenburg G, et al. Fibula jaw in a day: state of the art in maxillofacial reconstruction. *J Oral Maxillofac Surg.* 2016;74(6):1284.e1-1284.e15.
26. Perlyn CA, Schmelzer RE, Sutera SP, et al. Effect of distraction osteogenesis of the mandible on upper airway volume and resistance in children with micrognathia. *Plast Reconstr Surg.* 2002;109:1809-1818.
27. Singhal V, Hill E. *Craniofacial macrosomia and craniofacial distraction.* In: *Principles and Practice of Pediatric Plastic Surgery.* St Louis, MO: Quality Medical Publishing; 2008:755-800.
28. Goerke D, Sampson DE, Tibesar RJ, Sidman JD. Rib reconstruction of the absent mandibular condyle in children. *Otolaryngol Head Neck Surg.* 2013;149(3):372-376.
29. Tahiri Y, Chang CS, Tuin J, et al. Costochondral grafting in craniofacial microsomia. *Plast Reconstr Surg.* 2015;135(2):530-541.
30. Stelnicki EJ, Hollier L, Lee C, et al. Distraction osteogenesis of costochondral bone grafts in the mandible. *Plast Reconstr Surg.* 2002;109(3):925-933.
31. Adolphs N, Liu W, Keeve E, Hoffmeister B. Craniomaxillofacial surgery planning based on 3D models derived from cone-beam CT data. *Comput Aided Surg.* 2013;18:101-108.

QUESTIONS

1. A 57-year-old man with a history of oral squamous cell carcinoma treated initially with radiation therapy is referred to your office with complaints of recent development of a draining wound to his left cheek and difficulty chewing food. Examination shows poor dentition. Panorex imaging demonstrates pathologic fracture at the angle of the left side of the mandible. What is the appropriate course of treatment?

   a. a. A 10-day course of oral amoxicillin/clavulanate
   b. Debridement and closure of the cutaneous wound and open reduction/internal fixation (ORIF) of the angle fracture via extraoral approach
   c. Closed reduction of the angle fracture and placement in maxilla-mandibular fixation
   d. Radical debridement of the fractured segment of the mandible and free tissue transfer to reconstruct the angle and involved soft tissue
   e. Open debridement of the involved bone and cutaneous tissue and reconstruction with iliac bone graft

2. A 22-year-old male patient presents to the emergency department having suffered a gunshot wound to the face. His airway is stable, and there is no active hemorrhage. On physical examination, there is a contour deformity of the lower face with moderate-sized stellate soft tissue injury to the lateral cheek. There is significant loss of mucosa on intraoral examination, with multiple mobile segments of mandibular bone. CT scan shows severely comminuted fractures of the right body and parasymphysis, with readily apparent loss of bone. What is the most appropriate sequence of events in the treatment of this patient's injury?

   a. Operative washout and debridement with delayed ORIF of the fractures using load-bearing fixation
   b. Immediate load-bearing fixation of the mandible fractures with primary nonvascularized bone graft from the iliac crest
   c. Operative washout and debridement with immediate load-bearing fixation of the mandibular segments, followed by delayed reconstruction using a vascularized fibula flap including a skin paddle based off a peroneal artery perforator
   d. Operative washout and debridement with immediate load-bearing fixation of the mandibular segments, followed by delayed reconstruction using an osteocutaneous DCIA flap
   e. Operative washout and debridement with maxillomandibular fixation

3. A 54-year-old woman presents to the emergency department having been involved in a motor vehicle accident in which she was unrestrained and thrown from the vehicle. She has suffered multiple injuries including multiple rib fractures, a fractured humerus, a subdural hematoma, complex lacerations to the face, and multiple facial fractures. CT imaging demonstrates a severely comminuted fracture of the mandible involving the left mandibular body and a displaced right subcondylar fracture. On intraoral examination the mucosa is lacerated, but appears to be mostly intact. After initial debridement and stabilization of the mandible with a load-bearing plate, subsequent washouts demonstrate a 2-cm segmental defect due to removal of nonviable bone fragments. The complex cutaneous lacerations have been repaired, but are located immediately adjacent to the site of bone loss. What is the most appropriate course of treatment for this patient's mandible injury?

   a. Immediate reconstruction with nonvascularized corticocancellous iliac crest bone graft
   b. Delayed reconstruction with nonvascularized corticocancellous iliac crest bone graft
   c. Delayed reconstruction with a vascularized free fibula flap, including a perforator-based skin paddle for intraoral coverage
   d. Delayed reconstruction with nonvascularized split calvarial bone graft
   e. Immediate reconstruction with a vascularized DCIA iliac crest bone flap

4. A newborn infant is born with severe micrognathia. There is significant respiratory distress and conservative measures to improve the airway have not been tolerated. The jaw is symmetrical with formed condyles, but extremely small. The baby is intubated by the neonatologist and the Plastic Surgery team is consulted. There are no intrinsic airway anomalies. The next step in the management of this infant should be:

   a. bilateral costochondral grafts for mandibular lengthening
   b. bilateral distraction osteogenesis for mandibular lengthening
   c. tracheostomy
   d. tracheostomy followed by immediate distraction osteogenesis

5. A 16-year-old female presents to the emergency department with a large mass in the mandible. It has been growing slowly for several years. Imaging shows an expansile lesion with multilocular lytic lesion and *soap bubble* appearance, and the diagnosis of ameloblastoma is made. Following segmental resection, the patient has a mandibular defect of approximately 65%. What is the most appropriate reconstructive option?

   a. Reconstructive plate
   b. Costochondral graft
   c. Mandibular distraction
   d. Free fibular flap
   e. Iliac crest bone graft and bone morphogenic protein

1. **Answer: d.** This patient who has been previously treated with radiation for his oral cancer now developed osteoradionecrosis of the mandible with loss of structural integrity and orocutaneous fistula. At this stage of disease, the tissue exhibits severe radiation damage and no longer has the ability to properly heal. The major principles in treating this patient require replacing the unhealthy, radiation-damaged tissue (both bone and soft tissue), and reestablishing the structural and functional integrity of the mandible. This can only be done with wide debridement of the involved bone and soft tissue and free tissue transfer using the fibula, and quite possibly a second fasciocutaneous free flap for adequate healthy soft tissue coverage. A course of antibiotics will not repair or replace the radiation-damaged tissue. ORIF of this pathologic fracture is not an adequate plan for this patient, as the bone will not have the localized blood supply/tissue oxygenation necessary to heal and is essentially dead at this point. Likewise, placing the patient in maxilla-mandibular fixation may reestablish premorbid occlusion, but adequate healing will not take place.

Nonvascularized bone graft will not be adequate to reconstruct what will likely be a large segmental loss of the mandible, nor will the graft have an adequate recipient site with the healthy soft tissue necessary to integrate and heal.

2. **Answer: c.** This patient has suffered a high-energy ballistic injury to the face with significant intraoral soft tissue loss and segmental loss of the mandible, likely including the body and the parasymphysis. Immediate washout and debridement of the site of injury is required, along with stabilization of the fractured mandible. If he has adequate dentition remaining, maxillomandibular fixation may be possible as a stabilization technique, but this is highly unlikely considering the nature of the injury. A

load-bearing, segment-spanning reconstruction plate is the best choice for stabilizing this patient's mandible based on the information at hand. This approach will temporize the reconstruction by allowing additional debridements as the injured tissue declares itself and time for adequate soft tissue healing and resolution of edema. The patient is most likely to require a free fibula for bony reconstruction due to the multisegment involvement of the injury and will also need intraoral soft tissue coverage of the construct with a perforator-based skin paddle due to the loss of mucosa. Immediate nonvascularized bone grafting would not be appropriate in this patient due to the inadequate bed of soft tissue at the site of injury. Reconstruction with a DCIA iliac crest flap will not provide adequate length or the ability to reliably perform osteotomies to reconstruct the involved body and parasymphyseal segments. Maxillomandibular fixation is likely not possible in this patient based on the description of his injury, as there will probably not be adequate dentition. Additionally, the patient has segmental loss of bone and will require additional bone stock for a proper reconstruction.

3. **Answer: b.** This patient has a noncritical segmental defect of the mandible with intact, but suspect soft tissue coverage. After stabilization of the fractures with load-bearing fixation, the site of injury should be permitted time to properly heal to receive a bone graft later. In this case, due to the small size of segmental loss, a vascularized bone flap is not likely to be necessary, and a structurally sound nonvascularized corticocancellous graft from the iliac crest should be adequate, and represents the simplest option. Immediate reconstruction with a nonvascularized bone graft should not be performed in this patient with questionable soft tissue at the recipient site. A free fibula flap is not necessary in this patient with a 2-cm segmental defect.

Split calvarial bone graft is not the best option available for this patient compared to the iliac crest, as it would not provide the same level of structural support. A vascularized DCIA iliac crest graft is not necessary in this patient with a 2-cm segmental defect.

4. **Answer: b.** Bilateral distraction osteogenesis for mandibular lengthening. This technique has been shown to be effective at lengthening the mandible, alleviating airway obstruction and preventing tracheostomy. The infant should remain intubated during the distraction period and extubated once the jaw has been brought to length. Bilateral costochondral grafts for mandibular lengthening is not indicated in the newborn, nor is it necessary given that there are formed vertical rami and condyles. Tracheostomy may be avoided if successful mandibular lengthening can be achieved with distraction. While it may still be necessary, an attempt to avoid a tracheostomy would be of benefit to the newborn given the associated comorbidities. If a tracheostomy is performed, it typically is left in place until the child is at least 1 year of age before consideration is given to removing it. As such, it would be prudent to wait until the child was older before performing the distraction.

5. **Answer: d.** A free fibula flap is the most appropriate choice for a defect of this size. In addition, a free fibular flap can be designed to restore the normal contour of the mandible. It also will have the viability and durability to accept osseointegrated implants. With proper planning, these implants can be placed prior to flap elevation. The defect is too large for a costochondral graft or iliac crest bone graft. In addition, bone morphogenic protein is not indicated in the pediatric patient population. Mandibular distraction is a possibility, but it is difficult to obtain the natural contour of the mandible and will likely not be effective for reconstruction of this type of defect. A free fibula would be a much more appropriate choice.

CHAPTER 44 Reconstruction of the Oral Cavity, Pharynx, and Esophagus

Carrie K. Chu and Peirong Yu

KEY POINTS

- Buccal defects are best reconstructed with a thin flap that does not protrude into the oral cavity.
- Floor-of-mouth defects with a neck dissection create a large fistula to the neck. Flap reconstruction with obliteration of dead space is essential to avoid infection and fistula formation.
- Goal of hemiglossectomy reconstruction is to preserve the function of the remaining tongue. A thin and pliable flap is preferred.
- Total and subtotal glossectomy reconstruction requires a bulky flap so that the neotongue can touch the palate to achieve reasonable speech and swallowing functions and avoid aspiration.
- Common complications following pharyngoesophageal reconstruction include fistula and strictures. Appropriate flap choice and inset are important to minimize these complications.
- The transverse cervical vessels are excellent recipient vessels in an otherwise vessel-depleted neck due to surgeries and radiation. The combination of multiple skin island anterolateral thigh (ALT) flaps and the use of transverse cervical vessels provides a straightforward reconstruction in an otherwise impossible neck.
- Tracheoesophageal puncture (TEP) is the standard for speech rehabilitation following a laryngopharyngectomy.
- The indications for the supercharged jejunal flap for total esophageal reconstruction include the absence of stomach, radiated stomach, and a combined total laryngopharyngectomy and total esophagectomy in which the stomach would not reach.

Defects of the oral cavity, pharynx, and esophagus result most frequently from oncologic resections, though traumatic and congenital etiologies may also lead to extensive defects requiring complex reconstruction. These anatomic regions support critical functions related to speech, feeding, and respiration. Further, vital structures such as the great vessels and trachea occupy close proximity to the oropharynx and esophagus where they remain susceptible to injury. These considerations present unique challenges for functional restoration while maintaining quality of life, providing reasonable appearance and minimizing morbidity. Without the plastic surgeons' reconstructive armamentarium, resections in these organ systems would often not be feasible. Reconstructive failures in turn may be debilitating or even life-threatening. Therefore, familiarity with the principles and techniques for oropharyngeal and esophageal reconstruction is essential.

ORAL CAVITY RECONSTRUCTION

Anatomy of the Oral Cavity

The oral cavity consists of the lips, buccal mucosa, maxillary and mandibular alveolar ridges, retromolar trigone, floor of mouth, hard palate, and the anterior (oral or mobile) tongue (**Figure 44.1**).

The tongue plays the foremost role in speech, swallow, and airway protection. The anterior tongue in particular is critical for articulation, taste, and food manipulation. Intrinsic motor innervation is provided by the hypoglossal nerve. The lingual nerve supplies general sensation to the anterior two-thirds of the tongue, whereas the chorda tympani (through cranial nerve VII while accompanying the lingual nerve) is responsible for taste. The V2 and V3 divisions of the trigeminal nerve provide general sensation to the remainder of the oral cavity. Stenson duct drains salivary production from the parotid duct into the oral cavity via an orifice opposite the second maxillary molar.

Common Defects

Typical oral cavity defects include the buccal mucosa, retromolar trigone, floor of mouth, and varying extents of the tongue including partial, subtotal, and total glossectomy. Composite defects are common with inclusion of multiple oral cavity components, and may also involve the palate, oropharynx, mandible, and lips. Reconstruction of these more complex defects requires additional functional and aesthetic considerations, but the basic reconstructive principles of the oral cavity and pharyngeal components are reviewed for this chapter.

BUCCAL AND RETROMOLAR TRIGONE RECONSTRUCTION

Goals of Reconstruction

The buccal mucosa serves as a barrier of oral cavity contents from the facial musculature and nerves, which are protected from mechanical trauma during mastication and speech. Its pliability allows for unrestricted mouth opening during these functions. In addition to its functions related to vocalization, suckling, and smile, the buccinator muscle and the buccal fat pad contribute to the contour and symmetry of the cheek. Reconstructive goals for defects involving the buccal mucosa should address these considerations.

Flap Choices and Technique

Small buccal defects restricted to the mucosal layer may heal with secondary intention, or may be reconstructed with skin grafts or skin-substitute matrices. Alternatively, locoregional options such as the facial artery musculomucosal, buccal, tongue, submental, or supraclavicular flaps may be suitable.[1] As is often the case, however, preoperative radiation exposure and/or concomitant neck dissection with sacrifice of facial or lingual vessels may render locoregional options unavailable. A larger defect or one that extends to include the floor of mouth or exposes the mandible or palate typically benefits from free tissue transfer using a thin, pliable fasciocutaneous flap. Flaps with excessive bulk will protrude into the oral cavity, thereby interfering with speech and swallow or potentially obstructing the airway. Forearm free flaps based off of either the radial or ulnar pedicles are the classic donor sites for these defects. However, depending on body habitus and pedicle length requirements, the anterolateral thigh, profunda artery perforator, lateral arm, and medial sural artery perforator flaps represent suitable alternatives, especially if the buccinator and/or the buccal fat are resected resulting in deficient cheek contour (**Figure 44.2**).[2,3] Radiation will result in further flap volume atrophy by up to 44%.[4] Occasionally, a full thickness cheek defect that includes skin loss may require double-skin island reconstruction. These may be thoughtfully designed using multi-perforator flaps such as the ALT or forearm flaps.

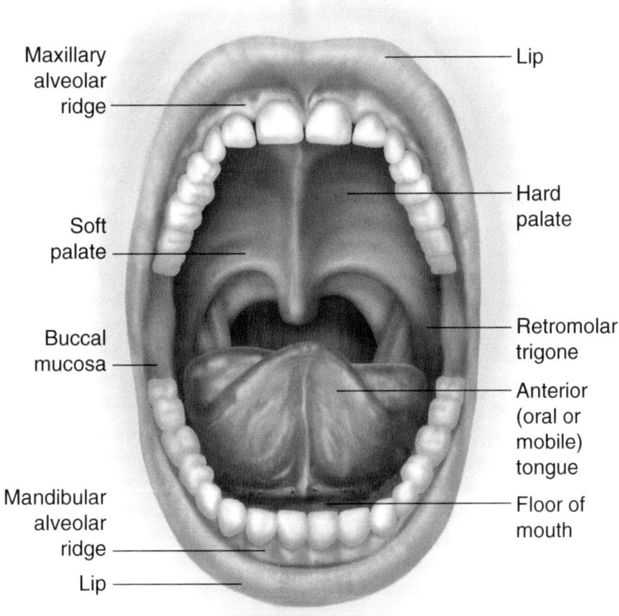

FIGURE 44.1. Graphical depiction of the structures of the oral cavity.

The most commonly used recipient vessels are the facial artery and facial vein. The passage of the pedicle for buccal defects should be carefully planned. In the absence of a floor-of-mouth component of the defect, the pedicle is passed through a subcutaneous tunnel and anteriorly over the intact mandibular body into the neck. These pedicles may be more subject to compression with mouth opening and animation, and adequate pedicle length should be harvested to avoid compromise. In the presence of a floor-of-mouth defect component, which often requires marginal mandibulectomy and a neck dissection, the vascular pedicle may be brought through the floor of mouth to the neck.

FLOOR OF MOUTH RECONSTRUCTION

Analysis of Defect

The floor of mouth segregates the oral cavity from the sterile contents of the neck. Isolated floor-of-mouth defects are relatively rare. More commonly, defects are also associated with glossectomy and/or mandibulectomy. These larger defects lead to fistulous communication between the oral cavity and the neck, and the reconstruction must prevent leakage of saliva and other oral cavity content into the neck, where infection may threaten great vessel integrity or manifest as external cutaneous fistulae.

Flap Choices

When a small floor of mouth defect exists that does not violate the suprahyoid musculature, skin graft or skin substitute matrix application are suitable solutions. Alternatively, locoregional options such as the facial artery musculomucosal flap or the submental flap may be considered.[1] However, concomitant neck dissection typically sacrifices the facial artery, which serves as the pedicle for both of these flaps. The supraclavicular flap has enjoyed increased recent popularity in both oral cavity and external neck skin reconstruction, as its pedicle origin from the transverse cervical artery typically remains intact following oncologic neck dissection.

For large full thickness defects of the floor of mouth, resections that include concurrent mandibulectomy or partial glossectomy, or reconstruction in the setting of previous radiotherapy, free tissue transfer remains the most definitive option. The amount of dead space requiring soft tissue obliteration should dictate optimal flap selection. A radial forearm or ulnar artery perforator flap provides a thin and supple lining that can be folded to provide coverage for the ventral tongue or to recreate the lingual sulcus (Figure 44.3).[5] Recreation or maintenance of the sulcus is critical for tongue mobility and minimize tethering. Other thicker fasciocutaneous flaps may be selected if greater bulk is desirable to fill the upper neck; the lateral arm, anterolateral thigh, and profunda artery perforator flaps are reasonable choices depending on individual body habitus. Chimeric muscle components may also be harvested with fasciocutaneous flaps for dead space filling. The addition of vascularized muscle has the added benefit of buttressing the flap skin island suture line to avoid salivary leakage. Pedicle length is not typically a critical flap selection factor, because the proximity of floor of mouth defects to the neck allows for shorter flap pedicle lengths in general.

The pedicled pectoralis major muscle or myocutaneous flap remains an alternative solution for floor of mouth defects. With improved microsurgical capabilities, however, the donor site morbidity, propensity for neck contracture, and poor aesthetic associated with the pectoralis flap limit its use in our practice to high risk patients or to salvage scenarios of free flap failure or fistulae.

Technical Details

Meticulous flap inset is of paramount importance, as small salivary leaks into the neck can result in serious infection. If the remaining alveolar mucosal cuff is inadequate following the ablative procedure, options include circumdental suturing (most common), continued elevation of a buccal mucosal edge around the alveolus, or bony suture anchoring devices. Pedicle passage into the neck must be atraumatic, tension-free, and accurately oriented. In most cases, the pedicle can be directly passed through the floor of mouth.

GLOSSECTOMY RECONSTRUCTION

Analysis of Defect and Goals of Reconstruction

The most common defects of the oral cavity requiring reconstruction are glossectomy defects. Glossectomy compromises tongue function including speech, deglutition, and taste. The base of the tongue is more important for swallowing function, whereas the oral tongue is critical for speech and food manipulation. Restoration of these

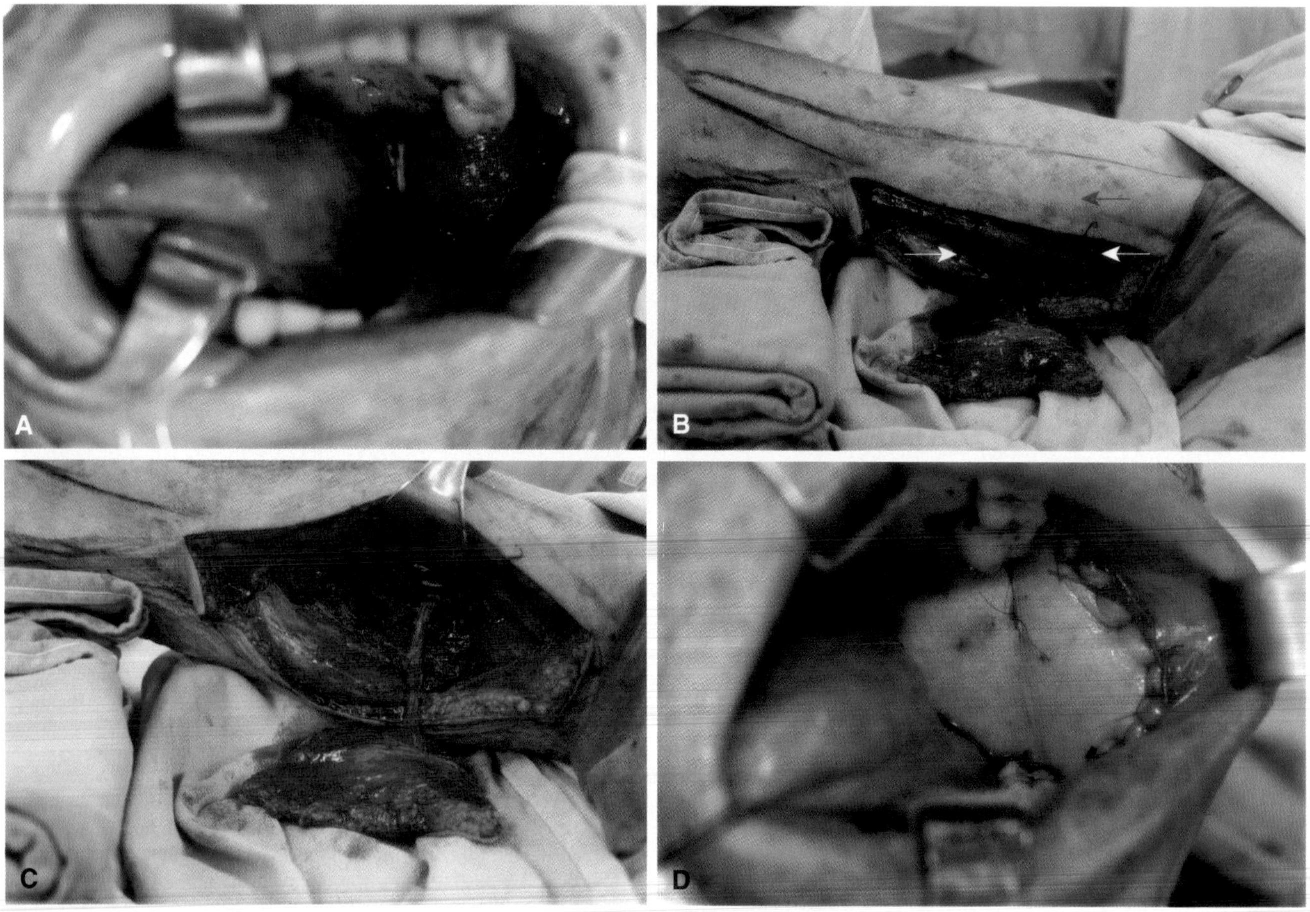

FIGURE 44.2. **A.** Buccal mucosal defect following excision of squamous cell carcinoma with loss of buccinator muscle and exposure of buccal fat pad. **B.** Surface landmarks for harvest of the profunda artery perforator flap include the adductor longus *(red arrow)* and gracilis *(white arrow)* muscles. The intramuscular pedicle is dissected through the fibers of the adductor magnus *(yellow arrow)*. **C.** Completed dissection of the musculocutaneous perforator pedicle of the profunda artery perforator flap through the adductor magnus muscle. **D.** Completed inset and revascularization of flap for buccal mucosal defect.

functions while preserving airway patency represents the main objectives of tongue reconstruction.

The amount of remnant native tongue musculature is the foremost determinant of future tongue function.[6] The distinction among partial, hemi, subtotal, and total glossectomy types translates to disparate reconstructive goals. Partial glossectomy typically implies resection of less than one-third of the tongue, whereas hemiglossectomy describes loss of up to half of the tongue. Subtotal glossectomy removes up to three-fourths of the tongue. Preservation of native tongue function is the primary goal after partial and hemiglossectomy; reconstructive flaps need to be thin, supple, and pliable to avoid tethering or displacement of the native tongue range of motion. By contrast, reconstruction after subtotal or total glossectomy requires recreation of bulk for contact of the flap with the palate, thereby generating acceptable speech and swallow while avoiding aspiration. The tissue bulk also serves to divert saliva and food to the lateral gutters during swallowing to minimize aspiration.

Defect assessment should include the percentages of the anterior and base of tongue resected. The length of the resection defect is measured from the tip of the remnant tongue to the tongue base. More extensive posterior defects may extend to the epiglottis and/or the lateral pharyngeal wall. Contiguous loss of floor of mouth and lingual

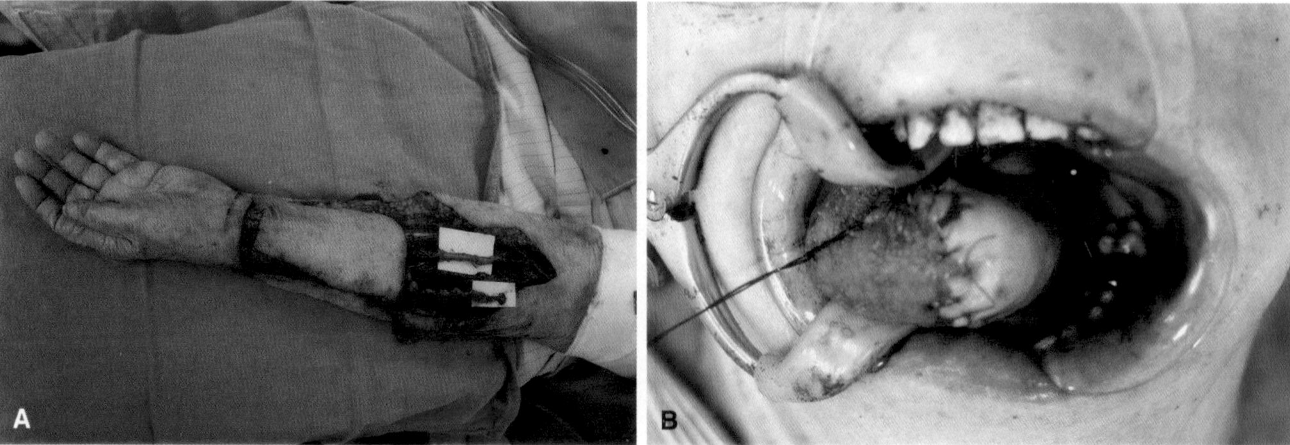

FIGURE 44.3. **A.** Harvested radial forearm flap with inclusion of the cephalic vein. **B.** Radial forearm flap inset following hemiglossectomy. Care is taken to preserve the lingual sulcus for tongue mobility.

alveolar mucosa should also be noted. Composite segmental mandibular resection can mandate a second osseous or osteocutaneous flap reconstruction.

Flap Choices for Partial and Hemiglossectomy With Technical Details

Partial glossectomy defects that preserve up to two-thirds of the tongue with minimal violation of the floor of the mouth may be closed primarily or reconstructed with a skin graft. However, resection of the floor of the mouth combined with a neck dissection often creates a wide communication between the oral cavity and the neck. These defects, even if they involve less than one third of the tongue, are best reconstructed with a flap to minimize the risk of fistula, which can in turn delay adjuvant therapies.

Thin, pliable fasciocutaneous flaps that fold easily are optimal for partial or hemiglossectomy reconstruction. Folding creates the ventral and dorsal tongue surfaces, as well as formation of the lingual sulcus extending onto the floor of mouth. Reproduction of this anatomy at the time of the initial reconstruction is important for uninhibited tongue function; delayed revision to produce the sulcus is challenging. For a hemiglossectomy, flap width of 6 to 8 cm usually provides adequate surface area, though recreation of the lingual sulcus should be included in the three-dimensional defect measurement. Radial and ulnar artery free flaps are most suitable for this purpose. The ulnar artery perforator flap has been demonstrated to be a reliable alternative to its radial counterpart.[5] Flap dissection requires meticulous attention to the safety of the ulnar nerve and generates a shorter length pedicle. However, the ulnar forearm provides a more cosmetically-favorable donor site, and long-term hand function is uncompromised.

For hemiglossectomy in thin patients, thigh-based options such as the anterolateral thigh (ALT) and profunda artery perforator (PAP) flaps are viable alternatives (Figure 44.4). Pedicle length and flap width for the two flaps are generally comparable, and some published evidence shows greater pliability of the medial thigh tissue of the profunda artery perforator (PAP) flap that may be more amenable to folding.[3,7,8] The lateral arm is another fasciocutaneous option that often yields a pliable and relatively thin subcutaneous adipose layer suitable for hemiglossectomy reconstruction.[2,9] With facile perforator dissection techniques and improved knowledge of angiosome anatomy, microsurgeons have a large flap armamentarium from which tailored flap selection can be individualized based on defect features, pedicle length, and regional body habitus.

Flap inset, in particular where the defect is posterior and includes the lateral pharyngeal wall, can be challenging. Posterior inset should be performed first, preferably preceding flap reperfusion, in order to maximize visualization. This can be accomplished through the neck exposure until the inset reaches the mandible. Parachuting suture techniques are often helpful. The rest of the flap inset is completed through the intraoral approach. It is essential to obliterate the submandibular dead space either with a small amount of muscle (with ALT flap) or adipofascial tissue from the proximal forearm to minimize the risk of infection.

In salvage scenarios following free flap failure or other high-risk settings where free flaps are contraindicated, the pectoralis major muscle or myocutaneous flap may provide basic coverage.[10] Sufficient mobilization of the flap to ensure adequate cephalad reach requires at times division of the clavicle. The flap can be islanded to avoid bulk in the lower neck. In some cases, muscle only may be used to obliterate the floor-of-mouth defect, leaving the mucosal defect to heal secondarily or to be skin grafted. This method obviates the need of a bulky skin island, and minimizes tethering of the tongue remnant.

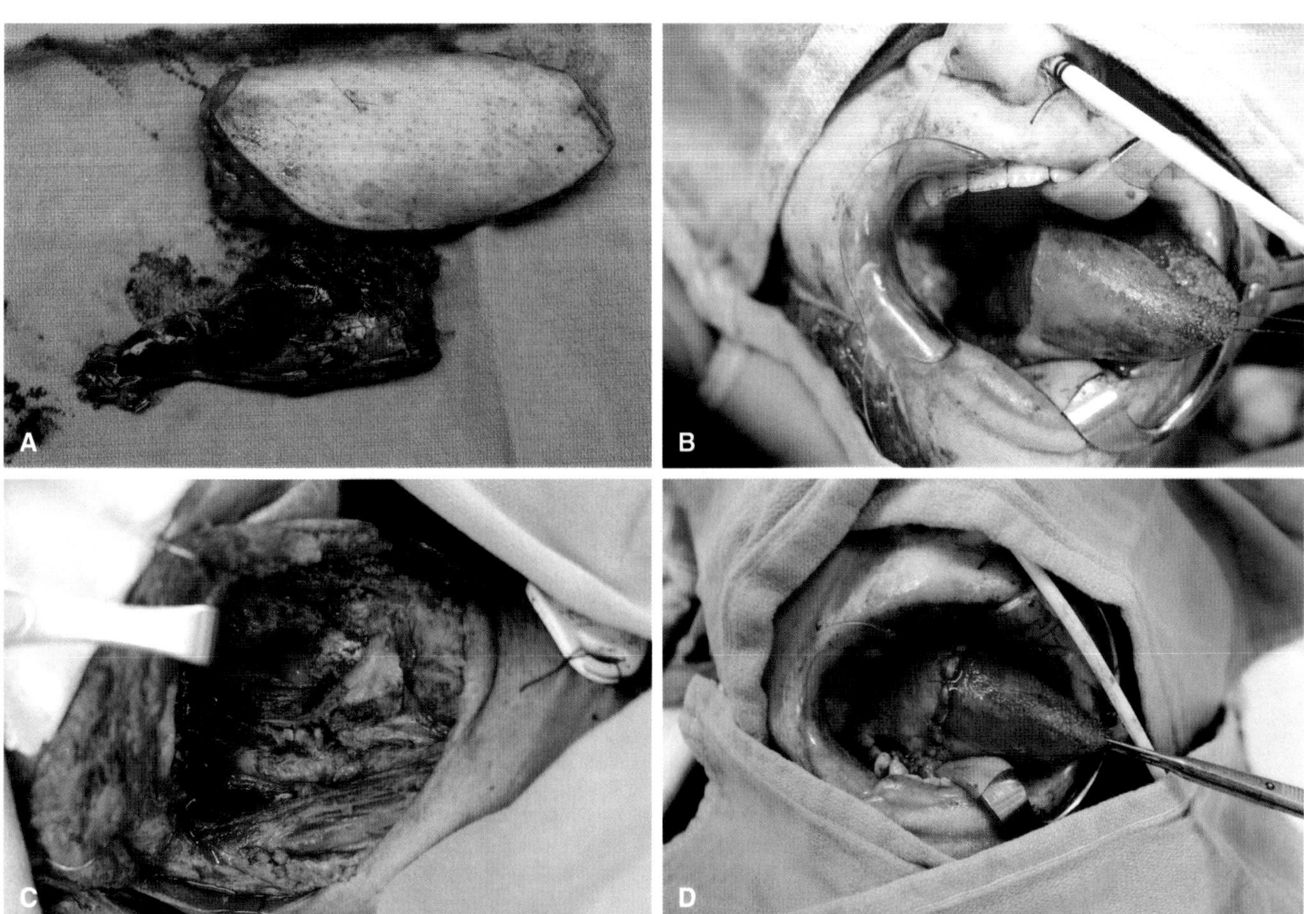

FIGURE 44.4. **A.** A thin anterolateral thigh flap is also suitable for hemiglossectomy defects. Flap dimensions may be more suitable for creation of larger skin islands for reconstruction of defects that extend into the lateral pharyngeal wall posteriorly. Chimeric muscle components may also be useful to buttress friable suture lines or provide additional tongue base bulk as necessary. **B–D.** A posterior partial glossectomy defect with contiguous lateral pharyngeal defect is reconstructed with an anterolateral thigh flap.

Flap Choices for Subtotal and Total Glossectomy With Technical Details

The amount of flap bulk necessary for contact with the palate after a subtotal or total glossectomy can be substantial, because the floor-of-mouth musculature is often included in the resection. A thick fasciocutaneous or myocutaneous flap is desirable. The anterolateral thigh flap with some vastus lateralis muscle is a versatile option.[11-13] Again, the muscle can be helpful for obliteration of the dead space. In the morbidly obese population, muscle-only free flaps with skin grafting remain a reasonable alternative, but such options are subject to atrophy with time and radiation, and speech and swallow functions may decline as a result. The forearm flaps are quite thick in these patients and may be a better choice. A summary of common free flaps used for oral cavity reconstruction is listed in **Table 44.1** with a summary of advantages and disadvantages. The pedicled pectoralis major flap may be used in poor candidates for free tissue transfer or in cases of free flap failure.

Flap inset may present challenges due to paucity of remaining mandibular gingiva of suitable substance. Interdental fixation or suturing the lower buccal mucosa may be necessary, rendering impossible the recreation of any lingual sulcus. Trismus related to previous radiation may also limit visualization and access. Proper flap planning to optimize muscle inclusion during harvest can limit risk of fistula or infection into the neck by buttressing skin island suture lines. At the completion of flap inset, the bulk of the flap should come into contact with the palate with the mouth closed (**Figure 44.5**).

Because the suprahyoid musculature is removed during total and subtotal glossectomy, hyoid bone resuspension is necessary to minimize aspiration risk. Circumhyoid sutures (0-Prolene) may be placed through drill holes in the mentum on the mandible on both sides of the midline. The distance between the hyoid bone and the mentum is approximately 4.5 to 5 cm. Care should be taken to avoid compression of the vascular pedicle by these suspension sutures.

Recipient Vessel Selection

A virgin neck presents numerous recipient vessel options (**Figure 44.6**). The facial artery and common facial vein are typically the primary candidates. Facial arterial lie may benefit from proximal dissection and vessel transposition around the posterior digastric muscle belly, or the muscle may require division to ensure absence of pedicle compression. The common facial vein is typically of excellent diameter to serve as outflow. Secondary inflow options include the lingual and the superior thyroid arteries. The middle thyroid vein and any other internal jugular venous branches are also outflow alternatives. In the absence of venous branches off the internal jugular, an end-to-side anastomosis may be performed. The external jugular may be used if the deep system is unavailable, but it is prone to twisting and kinking. It should be carefully positioned before closing the incision and care should be taken postoperatively to avoid extrinsic compression from neck malposition or devices such as tracheostomy collars.

The radiated or reoperative neck presents increased challenges due to vessel depletion.[14] Arterial walls become notoriously friable. The

TABLE 44.1. COMMON FREE FLAPS FOR ORAL CAVITY RECONSTRUCTION

Flap Type	Pedicle	Innervation Potential	Advantages	Disadvantages
Radial forearm	Radial artery and venae comitantes, cephalic vein	Sensory (lateral antebrachial cutaneous)	■ Long pedicle length ■ Large arterial vessel caliber ■ Thin pliable skin island amenable to folding ■ No need for perforator dissection ■ Rapid harvest time	■ Venae comitantes can be small in diameter, and may need to include cephalic vein ■ Unaesthetic donor site ■ Typically require skin graft reconstruction of donor site
Ulnar artery perforator	Ulnar artery and venae comitantes, basilica vein	Sensory (medial antebrachial cutaneous)	■ Shorter pedicle length compared with radial forearm flap ■ Thin pliable skin island amenable to folding ■ Venae comitantes often larger than radial venae comitantes. ■ Better hidden donor site than radial forearm	■ Close proximity and potential injury to ulnar nerve ■ Perforator vessels more subject to shear than radial forearm. ■ Typically require skin graft reconstruction of donor site
Anterolateral thigh	Descending branch of the lateral femoral circumflex artery and venae comitantes	Sensory (lateral femoral cutaneous) and motor (motor branch to vastus lateralis)	■ Relatively long pedicle length ■ Versatile flap design including skin island size, possible chimeric design (muscle, multiple skin islands) ■ Primary donor site closure usually feasible	■ Variable septocutaneous and musculocutaneous perforator course ■ Proximal perforator may arise from the transverse branch of the lateral femoral circumflex. ■ Variable thickness depending on body habitus
Profunda artery perforator	Perforating vessels off of the profunda femoral artery and venae comitantes	None	■ Relatively long pedicle length ■ Versatile transverse or longitudinal design depending on laxity ■ Consistent anatomy ■ Primary donor site closure usually feasible	■ Positioning difficulty for dissection and closure ■ Extended intramuscular dissection of perforator ■ Variable thickness depending on body habitus ■ Less versatile than ALT flap when chimeric flap is needed.
Lateral arm	Posterior radial collateral and venae comitantes	Sensory (posterior cutaneous nerve of forearm)	■ Aesthetic donor site with primary closure usually feasible	■ Short pedicle length and small artery ■ Flap size limitation for primary donor site closure. ■ Potential injury to radial nerve. ■ Variable thickness depending on body habitus

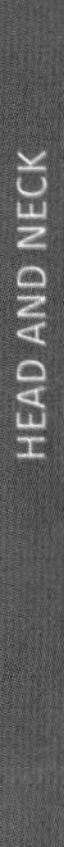

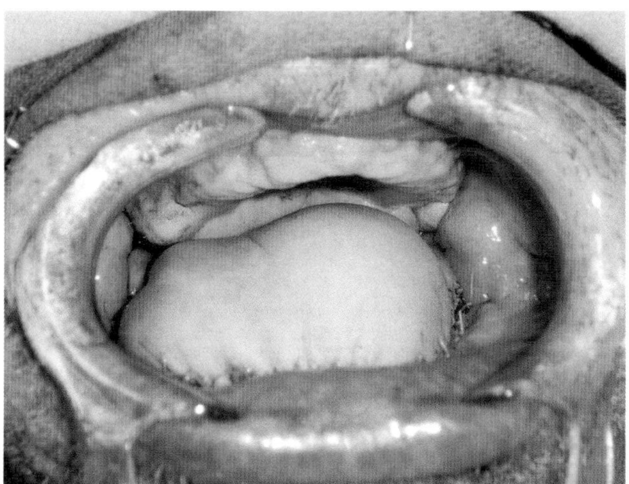

FIGURE 44.5. Flap inset following total glossectomy should allow for contact with the palate during mouth closure to ensure adequate bulk.

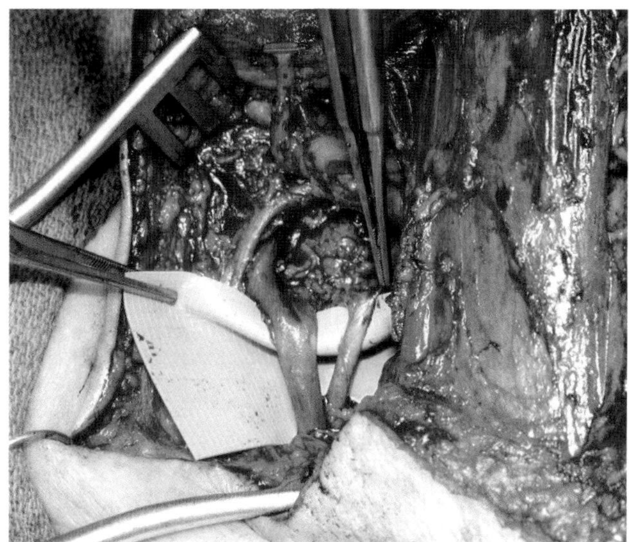

FIGURE 44.7. The transverse cervical artery and external jugular are good recipient vessel alternatives in the vessel-depleted neck.

transverse cervical artery which lies posterior to the sternocleidomastoid at the base of the neck is usually spared after neck dissection, and in the majority of cases can provide reliable inflow in an otherwise vessel-depleted neck (Figure 44.7).[15] Its transverse course rests just deep to the posterior belly of the omohyoid muscle, which may be divided for exposure. The adjacent vena comitans may or may not be of suitable caliber for outflow, but the external jugular vein at this level near its convergence with the subclavian vein is another corresponding option, as compression is unlikely at this depth. Further choices for the artery include end-to-end or end-to-side anastomoses to the external carotid artery. The contralateral neck may yield vessel options, although a vein graft is often necessary for reach. As a last resort, the internal mammary vessels have been used in head and neck surgery in conjunction with vein grafts.[16] The cephalic vein may also be fully mobilized along the length of the upper extremity and turned up into the neck for venous outflow. The need for and use of vein grafts alone are not necessarily predictive of increased risk of flap compromise; studies that do demonstrate an association may merely reflect the overall increased complexity of such cases.[17]

Sensory and Motor Innervation

As a branch of the mandibular division of the trigeminal nerve, the paired lingual nerves supply sensory innervation to the anterior two-thirds of the tongue. Fibers from the facial nerve via the chorda tympani also course along the lingual nerve to generate taste from the anterior two thirds of the tongue. The lingual nerve is typically cut during hemiglossectomy, and provides a potential target for sensory reinnervation. Typically 2 mm in diameter, the nerve stump is located adjacent to the lingual cortex of the mandible anterior to the angle. Some of the aforementioned common flap choices may be readily harvested with inclusion of a sensory branch for reinnervation.[18] The anterolateral thigh flap has the lateral femoral cutaneous nerve, the radial forearm or ulnar artery perforator flap may include an antebrachial cutaneous nerve, and the rectus abdominis myocutaneous flap may be harvested with an intercostal sensory nerve branch. Although spontaneous sensory recovery has been described without nerve reconstruction, recovery is typically incomplete. A study of 21 patients who underwent glossectomy reconstruction with the anterolateral thigh flap including 11 that had reinnervation using the lateral femoral cutaneous nerve showed not only meaningful recovery of two-point discrimination, pain and temperature sensation by 1 year after surgery, but also improved speech function in the sensory reinnervated group. Although radiation delayed regaining of sensory function, differences were not observed following 1 year.[18]

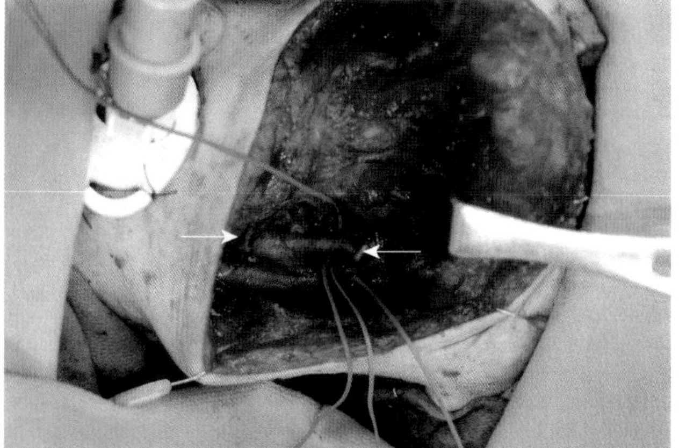

FIGURE 44.6. Common recipient arteries include the facial, lingual, and superior thyroid arteries, which are all branches off the external carotid artery *(red vessel loop)*. The common facial *(blue vessel loop)* and middle thyroid *(yellow arrow)* veins provide suitable venous outflow. Note the location of the hypoglossal nerve *(white arrow)*.

Although sensory reinnervation is achievable,[19] dynamic reanimation of the reconstructed tongue is much more unpredictable. The complexity of the interactive functions among the intrinsic and extrinsic tongue musculature is technically impossible to fully reproduce. For speech, contact of the tongue tip with the roof of the mouth is critical but achievable with passive movement of the reconstruction by the native remnant tongue. For swallow and prevention of aspiration, intricate tongue motor actions are hard to mimic with a single piece of muscle with linear contractility. Attempts at neurotized muscle flap reconstruction with use of the hypoglossal nerve, in particular in the setting of radiation, have been generally unsuccessful. Muscle fibrosis typically develops prior to reinnervation. Although innervation may in some cases prevent muscle flap atrophy, there is no existing evidence that functional muscle transfer for glossectomy leads to meaningfully improved function. In general, functional muscle transfer is not indicated for partial glossectomy reconstruction. In total glossectomy cases, consideration may be given to use of the anterolateral thigh flap, as this chimeric flap is unique in that concurrent motor and sensory reinnervation is anatomically feasible using the motor branch to the vastus lateralis and the lateral femoral cutaneous nerve.

Postoperative Care and Complication Management

Patients typically undergo concurrent tracheostomy for airway protection. Nasogastric feeding tubes are inserted for enteral nutrition while allowing for intraoral suture line healing. In the absence of medical risk factors or other mitigating circumstances, spontaneous respiration is preferable with hourly flap monitoring by nursing. With appropriate staff training, intensive care monitoring can be obviated. Enhanced recovery protocols include minimization of narcotic use and early ambulation, including in cases of lower extremity flap harvest. Care is taken to maintain neutral neck positioning to avoid pedicle compression. By postoperative day one, tube feeding may be initiated along with pharmacologic thromboembolic prophylaxis. A low threshold should be maintained for treatment of delirium tremens or other symptoms of alcohol withdrawal, which is prevalent in this patient population. Though vascular compromise of the flap is of utmost concern during the first 72 hours, vigilant monitoring for signs or symptoms of infection should take place thereafter, as late flap loss is typically associated with infection. Perioperative antibiotic prophylaxis beyond the initial 24 hours after surgery has not been shown to reduce infectious complications, although the use of extended antibiotics remains common but varied.[20,21] Oral hygiene with gentle suture line cleansing and oral rinses should be diligently performed.

Swallow assessment with a modified barium test may be performed at 7 to 14 days after surgery, but a more conservative 6-week waiting period of nothing by mouth may be more appropriate for radiated defects extending to the hyoid bone. If a clinically-silent leak is detected, oral intake should be delayed for 1 to 2 weeks before radiographic reassessment.

The overall complication rate following glossectomy reconstruction is 15% to 25%.[22] Respiratory complications including pneumonia and respiratory failure are the most common, highlighting the importance of appropriate pulmonary toilet and avoidance of prolonged ventilatory support where possible. Surgery-specific complications include neck infection, which should be treated early and aggressively with operative washout, debridement, and drain placement. Neglected infection not only threatens flap viability, but also poses risk to radiated great vessels of the neck that are susceptible to catastrophic blowout. Persistent infection may also delay adjuvant therapies that need to be delivered within a critical postoperative window. Any dead space or communication with the carotid or internal jugular may be obliterated or covered with a pedicled pectoralis muscle flap; reservation of this flap for secondary salvage is therefore beneficial.

When faced with a neck infection, careful intraoral examination must be performed for leak, dehiscence, or fistula as the source of infection. Suture error, compromised tissue quality due to smoking or radiation, and wound infection may all lead to dehiscence and leak. Proper flap inset is an exercise in balance between appropriate suture spacing to allow for watertight closure and avoidance of tissue edge ischemia with excessive numbers of small stitches. Pectoralis major muscle flaps are similarly useful for early postsurgical and postradiation fistulae.

Flap failure due to arterial or venous thrombotic complications are reported at 1% to 2% in high-volume centers.[17,23] Root cause analysis should be performed to determine the corrective course of action. If a technical error can be identified, a second free flap reconstruction may be undertaken. Suspicion for underlying hypercoagulability often may not be confirmed immediately, as these results may be delayed or confounded by therapeutic anticoagulation. Judicious use of systemic anticoagulation is appropriate in reoperative free flap cases, but there is a paucity of evidence for effective algorithmic anticoagulation use in free flap surgery.[24]

Functional Outcome

Functional outcome following glossectomy directly correlates with the amount of preserved native tongue tissue. Partial and hemiglossectomy reconstructive results are quite satisfactory in both speech and swallow. Over 90% of patients are able to resume an oral diet without supplementary tube feeding. Close follow-up with speech pathology and compliance with a dedicated training program can optimize outcomes. On a standardized speech intelligibility and deglutition scale, all hemiglossectomy patients should be able to achieve scores of 4 or 5 following rehabilitation.[25]

Speech intelligibility scale:

1. Gross errors, unintelligible speech
2. Multiple errors, intelligible speech if the subject is known to the listener
3. Multiple errors, intelligible speech if the subject is unknown to the listener
4. Minor errors, acceptably intelligible speech
5. No errors, normal intelligible speech

Deglutition scale:

1. Severe dysphagia, nonoral feeding only
2. Partial oral, partial nonoral feeding
3. Liquid diet only
4. Pureed or soft mechanical diet
5. Regular diet

By contrast, outcomes following total glossectomy are much less favorable.[6] Over half of these patients in long term are unable to rely solely on oral intake for nutrition and require tube feed supplementation. Speech intelligibility is often poor; most patients achieve 2 or 3 on the intelligibility scale at best.

PHARYNGOESOPHAGEAL RECONSTRUCTION

Anatomy of the Pharynx

The pharynx is the anatomic region that provides aerodigestive continuity between the oral and nasal cavities and the esophagus (**Figure 44.8**). The pharynx is subdivided into the nasopharynx, oropharynx, and hypopharynx. Posterior to the nasal cavity, the nasopharynx is superiorly bordered by the skull base and inferiorly by the nasal surface of the soft palate. The pharyngeal tonsils are located on the posterior wall of the nasopharynx. Posterior to the oral cavity lies the oropharynx, which begins at the uvula. The base of the tongue serves as the anterior wall of the oropharynx. The hyoid bone represents the inferior limit of the oropharynx. At this level, the epiglottis is an anterior-based connective tissue flap that seals the entrance into the larynx during swallow, thus preventing aspiration. The hypopharynx (or laryngopharynx) provides the final route of passage of food into the cervical esophagus. The hypopharynx lies posterior to the larynx, the musculo-cartilaginous organ that transmits air from the hypopharynx to the trachea for phonation. Extending from the level of the hyoid bone to the lower border of the cricoid cartilage, the hypopharynx is a critical area responsible for airway protection, swallow, and speech.

LARYNGOPHARYNGEAL RECONSTRUCTION

Defect Analysis and Goals of Reconstruction

Most pharyngeal defects are created following total laryngectomy, which violates the anterior wall of the hypopharynx to varying degrees.[10,26] Indications for total laryngectomy have narrowed as trends have favored chemoradiation therapy with partial organ preservation for early-stage disease. These indications include advanced primary laryngeal tumors with aggressive local spread, advanced hypopharyngeal cancer, cancer recurrence or persistence after chemoradiation, and laryngeal failure with severe aspiration following radiation. Although the frequency of total laryngectomies has decreased with time, the difficulty of the cases encountered has increased with previous radiation exposure, reoperation, and other high-risk factors. At the conclusion of the resection, assessment of the extent and viability of any pharyngeal remnant should be made. Any devitalized edges should be sharply trimmed to avoid partial necrosis resulting in a leak. The reconstructive goals following total laryngectomy include restoration of digestive tract continuity from

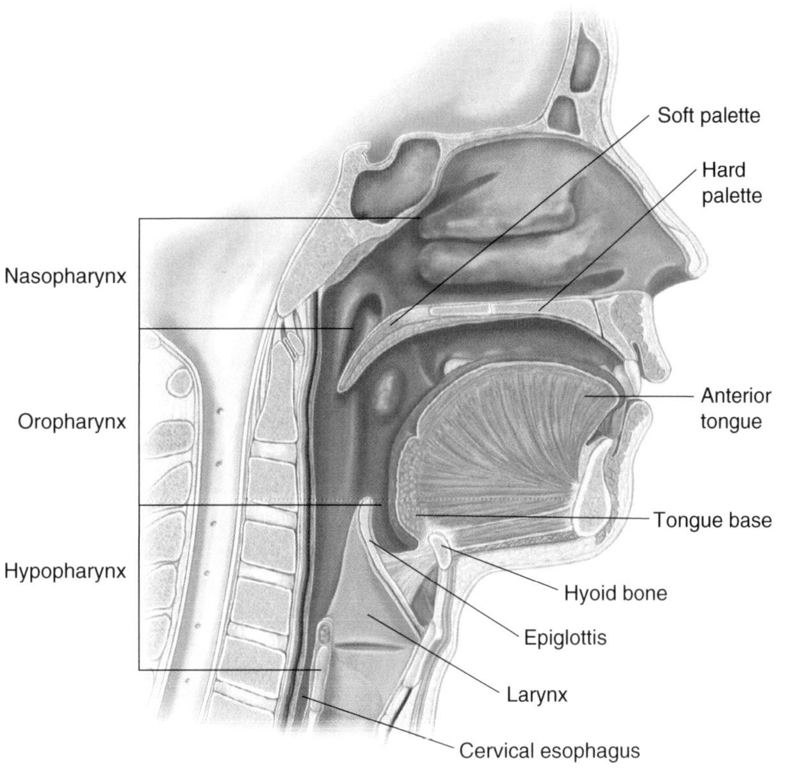

Nasopharynx
Oropharynx
Hypopharynx
Soft palette
Hard palette
Anterior tongue
Tongue base
Hyoid bone
Epiglottis
Larynx
Cervical esophagus

FIGURE 44.8. Sagittal cross section anatomy of the nasopharynx, oropharynx, hypopharynx, and larynx.

the tongue base to the cervical or thoracic esophagus without leak, stabilization of airway with a secure tracheostoma, protection of the great vessels of the neck, dead space obliteration, and possible external neck resurfacing.

Flap Choice for Partial Defects

Partial pharyngectomy defects are characterized by preservation of a posterior strip of viable pharyngeal mucosa (Figure 44.9). The width of the mucosal strip should be measured; the flap should be designed such that the flap width plus the mucosal strip width equals approximately 9.4 cm.[27] A radial forearm flap skin island provides an excellent anterior patch that replaces the anterior pharyngeal wall. However, the flap provides little soft tissue excess for reinforcement of the suture line against leak, and dead space obliteration is challenging. The anterolateral thigh flap may be similarly used as an anterior patch.[28] The versatility of this flap is fully demonstrated with pharyngoesophageal reconstruction. The fascial dimensions may be designed slightly larger than the skin island so that a second layer of coverage can be created to protect the inset suture line, limiting the risk of salivary leak. Portions of the vastus lateralis muscle may be harvested to fill dead space, buttress suture lines, and to provide coverage over the great vessels of the neck. If perforator anatomy is suitable, a second skin island may be used to resurface the peristomal skin (Figure 44.10). The pedicled pectoralis major muscle or myocutaneous flap remains an option for partial pharyngoesophageal reconstruction. Its disadvantages include neck contracture and poor appearance, and its primary use eliminates it as a potential source of salvage in the event of leak, fistula, or infection.

Flap Choice for Circumferential Defects

Traditionally, the jejunum free flap was the primary choice for circumferential defects of the pharyngoesophagus. The anterolateral thigh has since supplanted the free jejunum flap as the optimal donor site for this indication.[29] Table 44.2 is a comparison of free anterolateral thigh and jejunal flaps for hypopharyngeal reconstruction. In most patients, the fasciocutaneous flap can be sutured into a cylindrical tube using a 9.4 cm wide flap (Figure 44.11). In morbidly obese patients in whom tubular fasciocutaneous flaps are prohibitive,[30] the jejunum flap may be the preferred option.

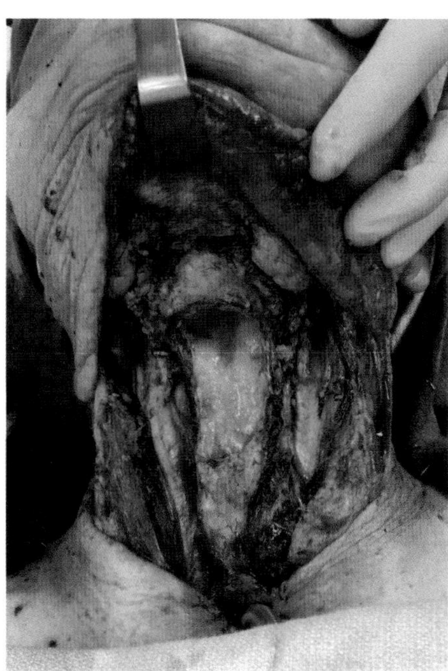

FIGURE 44.9. Partial pharyngectomy defects following laryngectomy preserve a posterior strip of viable pharyngeal mucosa.

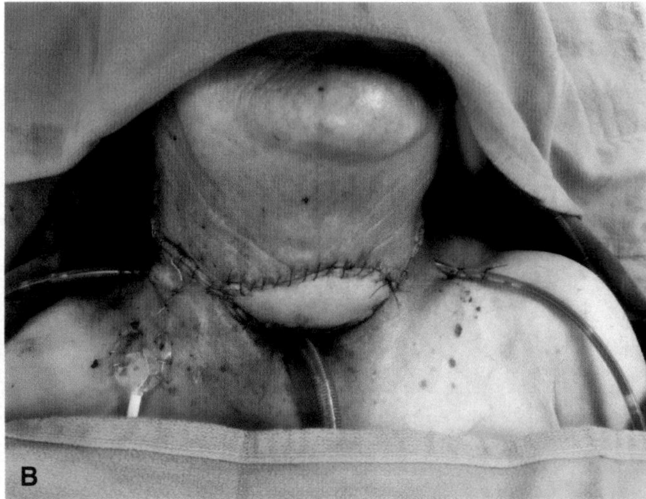

FIGURE 44.10. **A.** Anterolateral thigh flaps often have multiple perforators to allow for a second, distal skin island that can be used to resurface neck skin around the tracheostoma. The proximal skin island is used for pharyngeal reconstruction. The V-shape addition allows for spatulation of the distal neopharynx reconstruction. **B.** The distal skin island of the anterolateral thigh flap is used for neck resurfacing.

Reconstruction of Simultaneous Pharyngoesophageal and Tracheostomal Defects

The upper neck skin flap on an apron incision typically used for laryngopharyngectomy is often compromised by radiation exposure or even direct tumor invasion. The radiated skin lacks normal compliance, and the neck may be contracted at baseline. Once the skin is elevated and the neck opened, skin deficiency may present a challenge. Even without skin loss, direct closure of the upper skin flap to the superior half of the tracheostoma may result in excess tension and delayed healing of the site. There are four main methods to address the skin resurfacing needs. First, if the flap perforator anatomy is amenable to creation of a second skin island, the latter may be used to secure the tracheostoma from 3 to 9 o'clock. If no second perforator is available, muscle may be harvested as a chimeric flap component and covered with skin graft. These two techniques provide an externalized flap portion for monitoring of an otherwise buried flap.[10] Finally, if the skin loss is extensive, or if a jejunal flap reconstruction is completed, a second fasciocutaneous free flap or a pectoralis flap may be used.

Pharyngoesophageal Reconstruction in a Vessel-Depleted Neck

Typical recipient vessel choices in head and neck reconstruction are often unavailable following laryngectomy performed in the setting of reoperation and radiotherapy. Dissection and control of the external carotid and internal jugular for end-to-side anastomoses is technically feasible but fraught with risk of catastrophic hemorrhage. The transverse cervical vessels become critically useful under such circumstances, because they are available in at least 92% of patients and are typically spared during most neck dissections and radiation fields.[15] Located within the supraclavicular fossa posterolateral to the base of the sternocleidomastoid muscle, exposure is relatively straightforward. The phrenic nerve should be preserved, and the thoracic duct should be avoided in the vicinity on the left. The transverse cervical, external jugular, or even stump of a ligated internal jugular vein may provide outflow options. The external jugular near its confluence with the subclavian at this level is resistant to compression and typically provides excellent vessel caliber. With proper flap planning, skin island orientation, and adequate pedicle harvest, avoidance of vein graft even in the common setting of vessel depletion can be achieved.

TABLE 44.2. COMPARISON OF FREE ANTEROLATERAL THIGH AND JEJUNAL FLAPS FOR HYPOPHARYNGEAL RECONSTRUCTION

	Jejunal Flap	Anterolateral Thigh Flap
Defect type	Circumferential defects only	Circumferential or noncircumferential Allows preservation of posterior pharyngeal cuff
Flap harvest difficulty level	High	Moderate; requires perforator dissection
Donor site morbidity	Requires laparotomy with enteral reconstruction	Primary closure typically feasible
Ischemia time tolerance	60 min	4 or more hours
Potential for external neck resurfacing	None; requires second flap	High; may use second perforator for additional skin island or chimeric muscle with skin graft
Leak	Prone to leak at proximal anastomosis, 2%	Distal anastomosis most prone to leak, 1%
Fistula	3%[a]	7%[a]
Stricture	2%[a]	4%[a]
Speech fluency	50%–75%	80%–100%
Use of tracheoesophageal speech	25%	60%–100%
Return to oral diet	73%	91%
Tube feeding dependence	27%	9%

[a] Not statistically significant.

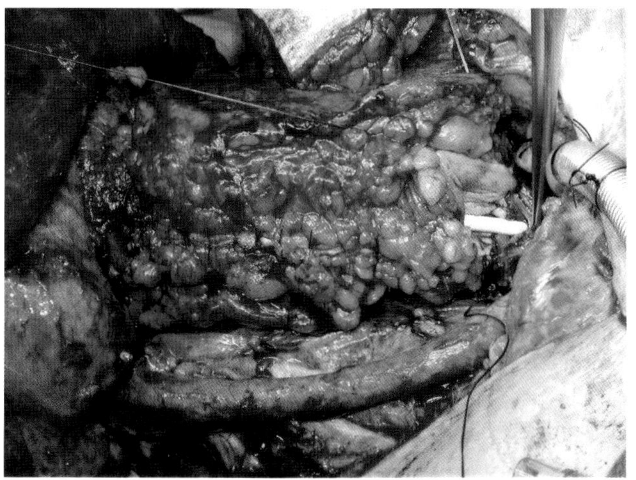

FIGURE 44.11. Anterolateral thigh flap sutured as a cylindrical tube for circumferential pharyngeal reconstruction.

Flap Inset and Technical Details

The authors use a single-layer flap inset with interrupted 3-0 Vicryl. Precise flap inset with edge eversion is key. Optimal suture placement and spacing balances water-tight closure with marginal ischemia. In tube-flap reconstructions, the T-junctions and proximal and distal anastomoses deserve special attention as potential sites of leak. The authors prefer posterior orientation of the longitudinal suture line over the prevertebral fascia to avoid any direct salivary leakage into the neck. Where possible, a second layer of fascial wrap secured to the prevertebral fascia can serve to confine and limit any small dehiscence. Further comprehensive detailing of the steps of completion of the individual flaps is beyond the scope of this chapter, but is described in published journal articles.[27]

Minimizing Fistula and Stricture

Although older data demonstrate high complication profiles associated with laryngopharyngectomy reconstruction, fistula and stricture rates can be as low as 6% and 19%, respectively, with appropriate technical considerations and maneuvers.[10,26,27] Pharyngocutaneous fistula tends to manifest the first and fourth weeks after surgery, but may also present in late stages following radiation. Smoking and radiation increase fistula risk, but modifiable risk factors including technical error and inadequate debridement of devitalized mucosal edges should be minimized. Proper eversion of tissue edges into the lumen of the neopharynx with simple interrupted absorbable suture spaced 5 to 7 mm apart is optimal. Suture line coverage with a wider fascial cuff or muscle offer added protection.

Any pharyngeal reconstruction is subject to postoperative scarring that may lead to long-term stricture formation. Radiation is an exacerbating factor. The distal suture line near the cervical esophageal inlet is particularly susceptible, as a natural funnel shape occurs at the normal pharyngoesophageal transition. The upper esophageal sphincter, or the cricopharyngeus muscle, may be divided anteriorly with a longitudinal myotomy.[10] This spatulating effect will then accommodate flap inset with a built-in V shape to maintain width of the distal reconstruction. In extremely high-risk cases such as a low distal anastomosis to the upper limit of the thoracic esophagus, an area that is particularly prone to stricture, placement of a Montgomery salivary bypass tube with a 14 mm diameter within the tubed neopharynx extending across the distal anastomosis may be helpful to reduce fistula and stricture. The tube may be left in place while secured to the cheek for 2 to 4 weeks depending on patient tolerance.

Postoperative Care and Management of Complications

Prolonged mechanical ventilation following laryngopharyngectomy reconstruction is not necessary. Spontaneous breathing via the newly secured tracheostomy is desirable. Flap monitoring protocols will depend on availability of external monitoring segments or placement of internal flow monitors for buried flaps. Nasogastric or percutaneous gastrostomy feeding can be started on postoperative day one. Mean length of stay based on our experience is 8 days. Modified barium swallow is performed at 2 weeks postoperatively, or 6 weeks for radiated patients.

Infections of the neck should be aggressively treated with washout and antibiotics, and a low suspicion for leak or fistula should be maintained. Infection can compromise flap viability leading to flap loss. Small subclinical fistulae noted on swallow evaluation will typically heal within 2 weeks with continued avoidance of oral intake. The swallow evaluation can be repeated to confirm resolution. Larger fistulas usually require reoperation. The infection should be thoroughly debrided. The site of leak should be identified. Upper endoscopy may facilitate intraoperative identification of the fistula if it is not immediately apparent within the inflamed neck. Although attempt at debridement and reclosure of edges may be possible, the tissue friability, dead space, and threat to great vessels associated with these cases often mandates use of a pectoralis muscle flap. Persistent nonhealing fistulae should raise suspicion for disease recurrence and/or distal obstruction due to stricture.

New onset dysphagia or regurgitation during long-term follow-up warrants work up for stricture or recurrence. Modified barium swallow can localize the stricture, and endoscopic biopsy or balloon dilation may be performed as indicated. Severe strictures that do not respond to dilation may ultimately require excision and free fasciocutaneous flap reconstruction. Cases of reconstructive failure may rarely be palliated with salivary diversion using a spit fistula at the neck, esophageal ligation, and gastrostomy or jejunostomy feeding.

Tracheoesophageal Speech

Following removal of the larynx, the patient becomes aphonic. Esophageal speech is where patients use swallowed air to create esophageal oscillation that is typically softer and less precise than vocal cord phonation. An electrolarynx is a device that can be used to transmit esophageal vibrations through neck skin to generate speech. Use of the electrolarynx may be introduced during the early postoperative period, but a period of rehabilitation to achieve familiarity and efficiency with the device is typically necessary. A better alternative, the tracheoesophageal puncture, is a surgical procedure that may be performed primarily at the time of laryngectomy with flap reconstruction or as a secondary operation. A controlled communication is created by puncture through the trachea into the esophagus. Once the tract size stabilizes and becomes optimized, an indwelling prosthetic device may be applied by speech pathology. Fluent intelligible speech is achieved in 63% to 89% of patients.[31] Use of a fasciocutaneous flap provides some advantages for postoperative speech intelligibility; speech after jejunal reconstruction is typically characterized as sounding "wet" with diminished clarity.

TOTAL ESOPHAGEAL RECONSTRUCTION

Indications

Indications for total esophagectomy include extensive tumor, radiation-related stricture or other injury, ingestion injuries, direct trauma, or congenital and autoimmune disease. Restoration of digestive tract continuity while limiting reflux and aspiration is the primary reconstructive goal, but such should be accomplished while diminishing risk to the numerous vital structures of the mediastinum and neck and minimizing donor site morbidity. The primary reconstructive option is the gastric pull-up procedure where the stomach is mobilized based on its blood supply from the right gastric and right gastroepiploic pedicles. The stomach is then advanced into the thoracic cavity to achieve anastomosis to the proximal esophageal remnant. The reach of the stomach is limited by its pedicled blood supply; the cephalad position of the cervical esophagus and hypopharynx exceed the advancement capacity of the gastric pull-up procedure.

In this scenario and in other cases in which the stomach is unavailable (gastric or lower esophageal radiation, previous gastrectomy, tumor invasion of the stomach, or other contraindicating abdominal surgical history), the colonic interposition and the supercharged jejunum flap are viable alternatives. The colonic interposition flap typically makes use of the descending colon, which is segmentally discontinued from the remaining colon and transposed to the esophagectomy defect while vascularized by the left colic vessels. Proximal and distal anastomoses are then required for colonic interposition inset, in addition to a third anastomosis for colon continuity. The main cited advantage of the colonic interposition over the supercharged jejunum flap is the lack of need for a microsurgical anastomosis. Many thoracic surgeons therefore favor colonic interposition when the gastric conduit is unavailable. However, adequate colonic mobilization sometimes compromises anastomotic perfusion at the proximal and distal limits of the segment. Over time, colonic interposition flaps are prone to dilation and redundancy, leaving a defunctionalized conduit that may compromise dietary intake. The colon is also a common site for diverticula, cancer, and polyps, whereas the jejunum is typically disease-free.

Technique of the Supercharged Jejunum Flap

The supercharged jejunum flap is a long-segment jejunal flap (Figure 44.12).[32] Via an open laparotomy, the ligament of Treitz is identified. The small bowel mesentery is transilluminated for identification of the second vascular arcade off of the superior mesenteric artery. The first arcade is preserved for perfusion of the proximal jejunum for eventual Roux-en-Y reconstruction. The second arcade is completely dissected toward its superior mesenteric artery origin and divided. The bowel is mobilized along the marginal vessels along the length of the flap. The third arcade is usually divided to achieve further length. The fourth arcade is typically preserved, serving as the actual pedicle to the flap. The bowel is then divided at the proximal limit of perfusion of the second arcade, which will be used for microvascular supercharging. This location typically measures between 30 and 40 cm from the ligament of Treitz. The jejunal flap is then passed either retrocolic along the posterior mediastinum or antecolic through the retrosternal space. Working space and visualization are typically enhanced with manubriectomy and resection of the medial clavicular head and the first rib at the costosternal junction which also exposes the internal mammary vessels to serve as excellent recipient vessels. The transverse cervical vessels are within easy reach and are the authors' second choice. Using branches of the external carotid artery mandates vein grafting. The jejunum is notoriously intolerant of prolonged ischemia, and facile and expedient technique is paramount to success.

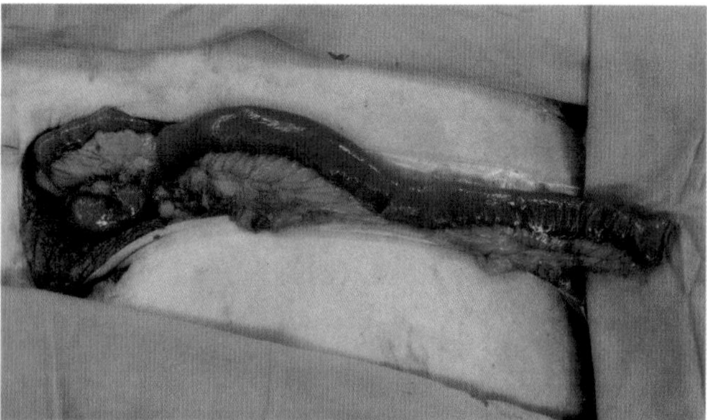

FIGURE 44.12. Supercharged jejunum flap harvested for total esophagectomy reconstruction.

After the anastomoses are completed, the requisite length for the jejunal segment to achieve tension-free proximal anastomosis while providing a straight, nonredundant conduit is determined. A short segment of the most proximal portion of the flap is divided and externalized as a monitoring segment. A healthy jejunal segment is light pink without congestion or edema, and maintains briskly peristaltic to mechanical stimulation. A Doppler signal should be detectable both intrinsically and within its mesentery. The remaining jejunal stump may then be anastomosed to the tongue base or hypopharynx, typically using a hand-sewn two-layer technique. The distal aspect of the isoperistaltic flap is anastomosed to the stomach or another small bowel segment to restore alimentary continuity. The biliary limb is also reconstructed, typically in Roux-en-Y fashion. A feeding jejunostomy is placed. Cautious neck drain placement is performed to avoid direct contact against vascular and enteric anastomoses.

Postoperatively, the externalized segment is monitored using free flap protocols. Meticulous pulmonary toilet should be instituted to avoid prevalent pulmonary complications. Signs of early leak may manifest as tachycardia or other cardiac arrhythmia. Barring unexpected deviation from the recovery course, the monitoring segment may be ligated and excised at bedside before discharge. Swallow evaluation may take place at 2 to 6 weeks.

Outcomes

In the largest published experience of supercharged jejunal flaps for total esophagectomy reconstruction, 51 patients underwent the procedure with 94% flap success rate.[32,33] Overall complication rate was 65%, with intraabdominal and respiratory morbidity being most prevalent. Twelve percent of patients experienced subclinical leaks that healed spontaneously. More clinically significant esophagocutaneous fistulae occurred in 14% of patients, of which almost half healed spontaneously. Anastomotic stricture rate was 10%. Two patients died during their prolonged hospitalizations, reflecting the complexity of the procedure and the severity of complicating comorbid conditions. Overall, 90% were able to achieve a regular diet, while 80% were able to discontinue enteral tube feeding.

COMBINED ESOPHAGEAL AND TRACHEAL RESECTIONS

Combined esophageal and tracheal resections for locally aggressive cancers complicated by tracheoesophageal fistula presents a tremendous reconstructive challenge.[34] Though convention suggests that such advanced disease contraindicates resection, successful reconstruction may provide good quality of life and palliation. The esophagectomy component may be reconstructed using a supercharged jejunum, and the tracheal resection may be reconstructed with a tubed fasciocutaneous flap, such as the anterolateral thigh flap. The fasciocutaneous flap may also be extended to help create the tracheostoma as previously described, as the neck skin is often deficient. The primary surgical goals in these cases include provision of airway safety and stability as well as infection control. Consideration may be given to delay of the esophageal component of the reconstruction with temporary diversion in order to limit operative time and to allow for improved nutritional and functional status prior to staged reconstruction.

SUMMARY

Oral cavity, pharyngeal, and esophageal reconstruction present challenges to the reconstructive surgeon.[35] Free tissue transfer remains the most predictable means of reconstruction for these complex defects that are often further complicated by risk factors such as radiation injury and patient comorbidities. Optimal flap selection with a clear knowledge of reconstructive goals along with preemptive measures to avoid common complications can increase the likelihood of success. With knowledge expertise and meticulous execution, good functional outcomes are achievable while minimizing morbidity and maximizing quality of life.[36]

REFERENCES

1. Patel UA, Hartig GK, Hanasono MM, et al. Locoregional flaps for oral cavity reconstruction: a review of modern options. *Otolaryngol Head Neck Surg.* 2017;157(2):201-209.
2. Chang EI, Ibrahim A, Papazian N, et al. Perforator mapping and optimizing design of the lateral arm flap: anatomy revisited and clinical experience. *Plast Reconstr Surg.* 2016;138(2):300e-306e.
3. Wu JC, Huang JJ, Tsao CK, et al. Comparison of posteromedial thigh profunda artery perforator flap and anterolateral thigh perforator flap for head and neck reconstruction. *Plast Reconstr Surg.* 2016;137(1):257-266.
4. Tarsitano A, Battaglia S, Cipriani R, Marchetti C. Microvascular reconstruction of the tongue using a free anterolateral thigh flap: three-dimensional evaluation of volume loss after radiotherapy. *J Craniomaxillofac Surg.* 2016;44(9):1287-1291.
5. Yu P, Chang EI, Selber JC, Hanasono MM. Perforator patterns of the ulnar artery perforator flap. *Plast Reconstr Surg.* 2012;129(1):213-220.
6. Manrique OJ, Leland HA, Langevin CJ, et al. Optimizing outcomes following total and subtotal tongue reconstruction: a systematic review of the contemporary literature. *J Reconstr Microsurg.* 2017;33(2):103-111.
7. Fernandez-Riera R, Hung SY, Wu JC, Tsao CK. Free profunda femoris artery perforator flap as a first-line choice of reconstruction for partial glossectomy defects. *Head Neck.* 2017;39(4):737-743.
8. Ito R, Huang JJ, Wu JC, et al. The versatility of profunda femoral artery perforator flap for oncological reconstruction after cancer resection: clinical cases and review of literature. *J Surg Oncol.* 2016;114(2):193-201.
9. Yang XD, Zhao SF, Wang YX, et al. Use of extended lateral upper arm free flap for tongue reconstruction after radical glossectomy for tongue cancer. *Aesthetic Plast Surg.* 2015;39(4):562-569.
10. Sharaf B, Xue A, Solari MG, et al. Optimizing outcomes in pharyngoesophageal reconstruction and neck resurfacing: 10-year experience of 294 cases. *Plast Reconstr Surg.* 2017;139(1):105e-119e.
Recent update of the MD Anderson Cancer Center experience on reconstruction after laryngopharyngectomy in a large series of patients.
11. Selber JC, Robinson J. The manta ray flap: a technique for total glossectomy reconstruction. *Plast Reconstr Surg.* 2014;134(2):341e-344e.
12. Paydarfar JA, Freed GL, Gosselin BJ. The anterolateral thigh fold-over flap for total and subtotal glossectomy reconstruction. *Microsurgery.* 2016;36(4):297-302.
13. Longo B, Pagnoni M, Ferri G, et al. The mushroom-shaped anterolateral thigh perforator flap for subtotal tongue reconstruction. *Plast Reconstr Surg.* 2013;132(3):656-665.
14. Hanasono MM, Barnea Y, Skoracki RJ. Microvascular surgery in the previously operated and irradiated neck. *Microsurgery.* 2009;29(1):1-7.
15. Yu P. The transverse cervical vessels as recipient vessels for previously treated head and neck cancer patients. *Plast Reconstr Surg.* 2005;115(5):1253-1258.
Description of the transverse cervical vessels as a useful option for microsurgical recipient targets in the vessel-depleted neck.
16. Roche NA, Houtmeyers P, Vermeersch HF, et al. The role of the internal mammary vessels as recipient vessels in secondary and tertiary head and neck reconstruction. *J Plast Reconstr Aesthet Surg.* 2012;65(7):885-892.
17. Yu P, Chang DW, Miller MJ, et al. Analysis of 49 cases of flap compromise in 1310 free flaps for head and neck reconstruction. *Head Neck.* 2009;31(1):45-51.
18. Yu P. Reinnervated anterolateral thigh flap for tongue reconstruction. *Head Neck.* 2004;26(12):1038-1044.
19. Namin AW, Varvares MA. Functional outcomes of sensate versus insensate free flap reconstruction in oral and oropharyngeal reconstruction: a systematic review. *Head Neck.* 2016;38(11):1717-1721.
20. Dort JC, Farwell DG, Findlay M, et al. Optimal perioperative care in major head and neck cancer surgery with free flap reconstruction: a consensus review and recommendations from the Enhanced Recovery After Surgery Society. *JAMA Otolaryngol Head Neck Surg.* 2017;143(3):292-303.
21. Haidar YM, Tripathi PB, Tjoa T, et al. Antibiotic prophylaxis in clean-contaminated head and neck cases with microvascular free flap reconstruction: a systematic review and meta-analysis. *Head Neck.* 2018;40(2):417-427.
22. Chang EI, Yu P, Skoracki RJ, et al. Comprehensive analysis of functional outcomes and survival after microvascular reconstruction of glossectomy defects. *Ann Surg Oncol.* 2015;22(9):3061-3069.
A large single-institution experience examining long term outcomes of free flap reconstruction after glossectomy.
23. Chang EI, Zhang H, Liu J, et al. Analysis of risk factors for flap loss and salvage in free flap head and neck reconstruction. *Head Neck.* 2016;38(suppl 1):E771-E775.
24. Wang TY, Serletti JM, Cuker A, et al. Free tissue transfer in the hypercoagulable patient: a review of 58 flaps. *Plast Reconstr Surg.* 2012;129(2):443-453.
A frequently cited article describing the use of free tissue transfer in patients with hypercoagulable conditions.
25. Dzioba A, Aalto D, Papadopoulos-Nydam G, et al. Functional and quality of life outcomes after partial glossectomy: a multi-institutional longitudinal study of the head and neck research network. *J Otolaryngol Head Neck Surg.* 2017;46(1):56.
26. Selber JC, Xue A, Liu J, et al. Pharyngoesophageal reconstruction outcomes following 349 cases. *J Reconstr Microsurg.* 2014;30(9):641-654.
27. Yu P, Hanasono MM, Skoracki RJ, et al. Pharyngoesophageal reconstruction with the anterolateral thigh flap after total laryngopharyngectomy. *Cancer.* 2010;116(7):1718-1724.
With its proposal of the anterolateral thigh flap for laryngopharyngectomy reconstruction, this study was key in the popularization of the reconstructive technique as potentially advantageous over the more conventional use of jejunal flaps previously.
28. Yu P, Robb GL. Pharyngoesophageal reconstruction with the anterolateral thigh flap: a clinical and functional outcomes study. *Plast Reconstr Surg.* 2005;116(7):1845-1855.
29. Yu P, Lewin JS, Reece GP, Robb GL. Comparison of clinical and functional outcomes and hospital costs following pharyngoesophageal reconstruction with the anterolateral thigh free flap versus the jejunal flap. *Plast Reconstr Surg.* 2006;117(3):968-974.
This study was key in direct comparison of speech and swallow outcomes after anterolateral thigh and jejunal free flap reconstruction after pharyngoesophageal reconstruction, demonstrating several advantages of the anterolateral thigh option.
30. Yu P. Characteristics of the anterolateral thigh flap in a Western population and its application in head and neck reconstruction. *Head Neck.* 2004;26(9):759-769.
31. Lewin JS, Barringer DA, May AH, et al. Functional outcomes after circumferential pharyngoesophageal reconstruction. *Laryngoscope.* 2005;115(7):1266-1271.
32. Poh M, Selber JC, Skoracki R, et al. Technical challenges of total esophageal reconstruction using a supercharged jejunal flap. *Ann Surg.* 2011;253(6):1122-1129.
A high-impact article that describes use of the supercharged jejunal flap as an alternative for esophageal reconstruction.
33. Blackmon SH, Correa AM, Skoracki R, et al. Supercharged pedicled jejunal interposition for esophageal replacement: a 10-year experience. *Ann Thorac Surg.* 2012;94(4):1104-1111.
34. Ghali S, Chang EI, Rice DC, et al. Microsurgical reconstruction of combined tracheal and total esophageal defects. *J Thorac Cardiovasc Surg.* 2015;150(5):1261-1266.
35. Vosler PS, Orsini M, Enepekides DJ, Higgins KM. Predicting complications of major head and neck oncological surgery: an evaluation of the ACS NSQIP surgical risk calculator. *J Otolaryngol Head Neck Surg.* 2018;47(1):21.
36. Cohen WA, Albornoz CR, Cordeiro PG, et al. Health-related quality of life following reconstruction for common head and neck surgical defects. *Plast Reconstr Surg.* 2016;138(6):1312-1320.

QUESTIONS

1. A 59-year-old woman initially presented with a squamous cell carcinoma in the right oral tongue and underwent partial glossectomy with skin grafting, right neck dissection, and postoperative radiotherapy 2 years ago. Approximately 3 months ago, she developed an ulcer in the remaining tongue that grew quickly to involve much of the remaining tongue including the tongue base. CT of head and neck suggested recurrence of tongue cancer. Subsequent biopsy confirmed squamous cell carcinoma. There was no evidence of bone involvement. Her BMI is 28. On physical examination, she has severe scarring in the right neck. All extremities are well perfused. She has very thin forearms and moderate thickness in the thighs, estimated 2 cm thickness of subcutaneous fat. There are no surgical scars in the abdomen. Which of the following is the most appropriate treatment option?

   a. A partial glossectomy with split thickness skin grafts
   b. A total glossectomy with a thin radial forearm flap
   c. A total glossectomy with an anterolateral thigh flap
   d. A subtotal glossectomy with a free jejunal flap
   e. A subtotal glossectomy with a submental flap

2. A 65-year-old man status post laryngopharynectomy with tubed anterolateral thigh flap reconstruction 4 weeks ago presents to the emergency department with persistent drainage from a small opening on the neck skin. He has a history of preoperative radiation. CT scan is pending. He also reports that earlier that day, he noticed a small amount of bloody drainage around his tracheostoma that spontaneously subsided in a few minutes. His vital signs are normal, and he feels overall well. There is no ongoing bleeding on exam. What is the most appropriate course of action next?

   a. Perform bedside incision and drainage of suspected neck abscess under local anesthesia
   b. Obtain a complete blood count and coagulation panel to quantify amount of bleeding
   c. Occlude the tracheostoma with a finger to prevent hemorrhage
   d. Prepare for emergent operative treatment with or without angiography
   e. Obtain a modified barium swallow evaluation to look for leak or fistula

3. A 48-year-old woman previously underwent a partial glossectomy and bilateral neck dissection for squamous cell cancer. Reconstruction was performed with skin graft only. Postoperatively, she received adjuvant radiation treatment. One year later, she presents with a local recurrence. During free flap reconstruction for the defect after subtotal glossectomy, the right neck is explored for vessels. The external carotid artery was injured during exploration and required ligation at the carotid bifurcation. The left neck has not been opened, but the skin is densely scarred. Which blood vessel should be explored next as a microsurgical recipient artery for free flap reconstruction?

   a. Right internal carotid artery
   b. Left facial artery
   c. Right facial artery
   d. Left transverse cervical artery
   e. Right transverse cervical artery

4. During exploration of the neck for possible recipient vessels for free flap reconstruction of a floor-of-mouth defect, a linear structure is encountered emerging from behind the posterior belly of the digastric muscle inferior to the border of the mandible. The structure may be followed proximally between the internal carotid artery and the internal jugular vein, and more distally crosses anterior to the lingual artery. What is this structure?

   a. Hypoglossal nerve
   b. Lingual nerve
   c. Facial artery
   d. Spinal accessory nerve
   e. Great auricular nerve

5. A 71-year-old man has a history of perforated colonic diverticulitis requiring segmental colectomy. He now presents with cervicothoracic esophageal carcinoma requiring transhiatal esophagectomy of the proximal two-thirds of the esophagus with resection of the pharynx to the base of tongue. What is the best option for reconstruction?

   a. Tubed anterolateral thigh flap
   b. Free jejunal interposition flap
   c. Supecharged jejunal flap
   d. Colonic interposition
   e. Gastric pull-up

1. **Answer: c.** In this patient with massive recurrence, a total glossectomy is required to remove the cancer. The goal of total glossectomy reconstruction is to provide enough bulk with a rather thick flap so that the reconstructed neotongue can touch the palate to improve speech quality. The bulk is also necessary to divert the food and saliva to the lateral gutters to avoid "dumping" of food and liquid into the airway causing aspiration. A partial glossectomy would not be able to remove all the cancer. Skin grafting in a previously radiated area, especially in the oral cavity will likely to fail, resulting a massive orocutaneous fistula. A thin radial forearm flap would not provide enough bulk for the neotongue. In fact, it will only provide lining with no bulk at all. Such a reconstruction will create a "funnel" in the oral cavity causing massive aspiration and unintelligent speech. Frequent aspiration pneumonias can be fatal and often require a total laryngectomy. A free jejunal flap is not indicated for tongue reconstruction. The jejunal flap is often used to reconstruct a circumferential pharyngoesophageal defect from a total laryngopharyngectomy. The submental flap is often unavailable in a radiated and previously operated neck. The vascular supply of the submental flap is a branch of the facial artery. During a neck dissection, the facial artery is often ligated and divided. Even with the contralateral facial artery intact, previous radiotherapy will significantly compromise the flap viability. In addition, the radiated and operated neck is firm and tight, and will not have enough skin laxity. The flap is also not bulky enough for subtotal glossectomy reconstruction.

2. **Answer: d.** The patient reports symptoms consistent with a sentinel bleed, a possible innocuous sign of impending catastrophic hemorrhage from carotid blowout. Risk factors include radiation, reoperation of the neck, and concomitant infection. The additional presenting symptoms are also concerning for fistula and infection. Assessment and preparation for either angiographic and/or open surgical treatment of arterial hemorrhage should immediately be initiated. This patient has ongoing infection that will also require operative washout, and adequate vascular control of the great vessels of the neck need to be obtained given the likelihood of carotid blowout. Bedsides, incision and drainage of the infection may result in uncontrolled hemorrhage compromising airway and circulation leading to a potentially fatal outcome. The likely cause of bleeding is not coagulopathy, and a normal complete blood count does not rule out the possibility of impending massive hemorrhage. There is no ongoing

bleeding site that requires direct digital pressure. Empiric occlusion of the tracheostoma obstructs the permanent airway after total laryngectomy, and leads to asphyxiation. A modified barium swallow evaluation does not adequately address the sentinel bleed and probable impending hemorrhage.

3. **Answer: e.** The transverse cervical artery is located within level Vb of the neck, which is not typically routinely dissected during cervical lymphadenectomy for cancers of the anterior tongue. Experience shows that, despite previous surgery and radiation the transverse cervical artery is available in over 90% of patients, making the vessel suitable to serve as a microsurgical recipient target. The internal carotid artery perfuses the brain and should not be used as an inflow vessel for free flap reconstruction of the head and neck. The transverse cervical artery should be explored in the open neck prior to attempted opening and investigation of the contralateral neck. In the setting of previous neck dissection and radiation, the left neck may be similarly hostile, and another vascular or nerve injury is possible. The facial artery is a branch of the external carotid artery, which has already been ligated.

4. **Answer: a.** The anatomic description corresponds with the extracranial course of the hypoglossal nerve. This structure is divided during hemiglossectomy on the ipsilateral side, but should be preserved for motor function of the tongue (deviation to the ipsilateral side) during vessel exploration for a floor-of-mouth reconstruction. The lingual nerve is encountered higher in the neck, typically posterior to the lingual surface of the mandible. Knowledge of the lingual nerve anatomy is useful for sensory reinnervation of glossectomy reconstructions. Although the facial nerve courses deep to the posterior belly of the digastric, it originates from the external carotid artery and does not course between the external and internal carotid arteries. The spinal accessory nerve crosses the internal jugular vein around the level of the posterior belly of the digastric, crosses posteriorly over the spinal accessory muscle, and continues into the posterior neck to reach the trapezius muscle. The great auricular nerve is located in the posterior neck, coursing around the posterior border of the sternocleidomastoid and running on its anterior surface to provide sensation to the skin over the mastoid and parotid region.

5. **Answer: c.** The procedure allows for diversion of the oropharyngeal lumen into a limb of mobilized jejunum that remains in continuity distally. While the more distal jejunum remains vascularized via the intact superior mesenteric blood supply and marginal arcade, the more proximal stump that is pulled into the neck is revascularized with microsurgical supercharging of the second mesenteric arcade stump which requires division to gain adequate mobilization into the neck. When the gastric pull-up procedure is unavailable or insufficient for superior reach, an alternate means of reconstruction needs to be selected. A tubed anterolateral thigh flap is unlikely to be of sufficient length to allow for complete replacement of the long segment of resected esophagus. Inset would also require an intrathoracic anastomosis that is challenging during a transhiatal approach and subject to intrathoracic leak. An intrathoracic anastomosis would also be required for a free jejunum interposition. This anastomosis can be avoided with other options. The jejunum is poorly tolerant of ischemia, but complete ischemic rendering of this flap is necessary. The supercharged jejunum flap avoids total flap ischemia, and only requires revascularization of the most proximal aspect of the mobilized stump. The patient has a history of perforated colonic diverticulitis that required segmental colectomy. Use of the colon would be inappropriate in this scenario. Absent this circumstance, some centers favor the colonic interposition procedure over the supercharged jejunum flap when the gastric pull-up procedure is not feasible. While the gastric pull-up procedure is the primary reconstructive option following esophagectomy, the stomach typically cannot be mobilized to reach the base of tongue without devascularization.

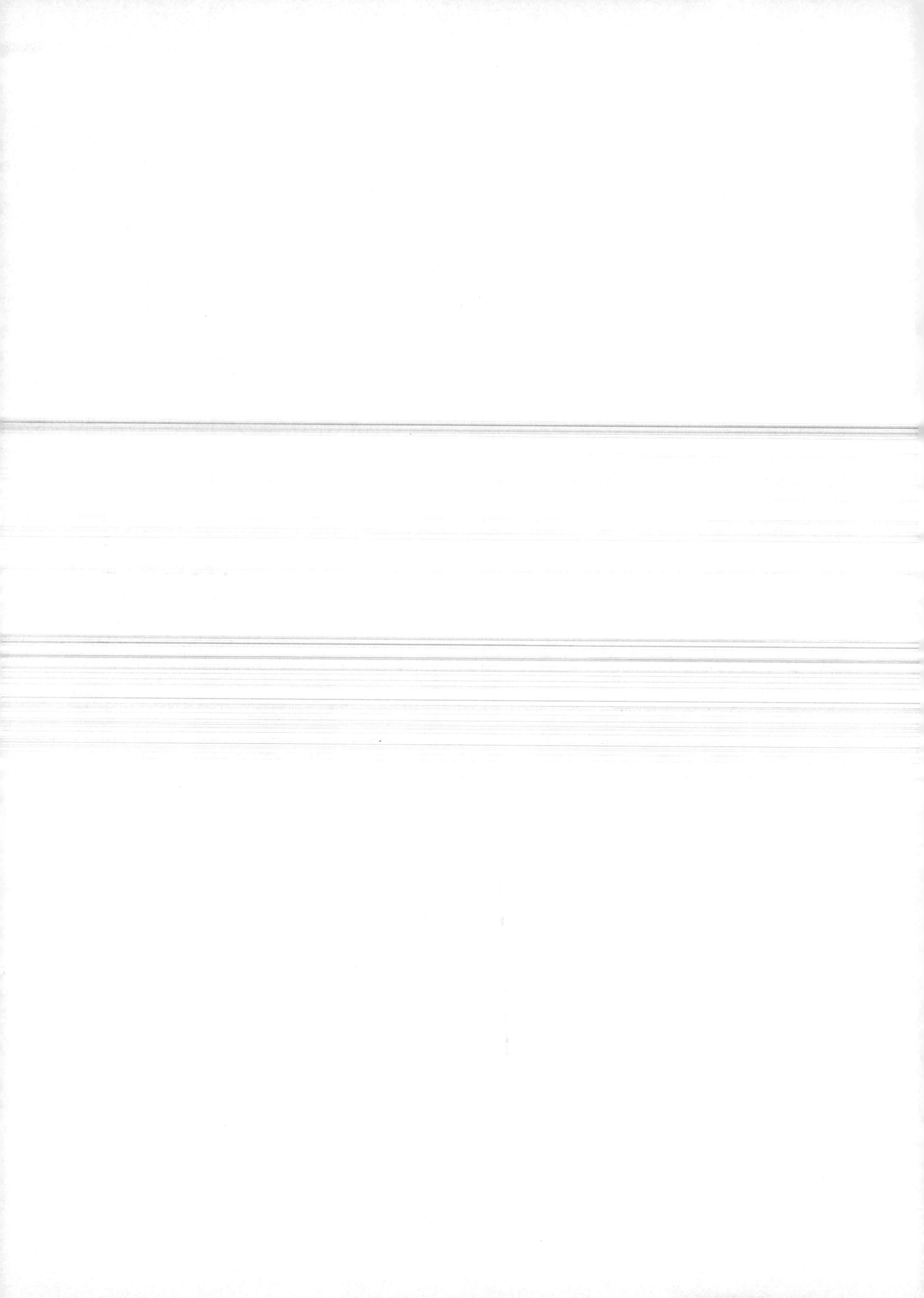

PART V

■ AESTHETIC SURGERY

CHAPTER 45 Nonsurgical Facial Rejuvenation and Skin Resurfacing

Deniz Basci and Jeffrey Kenkel

KEY POINTS

- Ablative resurfacing techniques rely on controlled injury to targeted layers of the epidermis and dermis, followed by healing and replacement of the ablated tissue with normal tissue.
- Various resurfacing modalities produce similar injuries; the appropriate treatment should be chosen based on patient evaluation, their specific goals, and physician comfort with the procedure.
- Aesthetic benefit, complication risk, prolonged erythema, and hypopigmentation are directly related to depth of injury and target tissue specificity.
- Treatment of skin wrinkles requires ablative therapy through the dermal-epidermal junction into a variable depth of the papillary dermis.
- The precision and outcomes of chemical peeling and dermabrasion are more technique dependent than their laser counterparts.
- Pretreatment with tretinoin or hydroquinone is recommended prior to chemical resurfacing, for even depth of penetration and a reduction in associated morbidity.
- Protection from the sun before and after treatment is mandatory for all resurfacing modalities, especially when light amplification is being used to prevent burns, hyperpigmentation, and recurrence.
- Selective photothermolysis targets chromophores melanin, hemoglobin, or water in the skin to deliver targeted thermal injury. The ideal treatment parameters remain controversial.
- Fractionated lasers are designed to keep the stratum corneum largely intact while ablating a variable amount of dermis depending on the physicians' preferred density.

Nonsurgical treatments to reverse the signs of aging are in increasingly high demand and continue to evolve rapidly as new technology develops. The American Society of Aesthetic Plastic Surgery 2017 survey data show that noninvasive procedures have risen 38% since 2012 and have increased 4.4-fold since 1997.[1]

Irregularities in surface texture, pigmentation, and wrinkling are hallmarks of aged skin. Classically, mechanical, chemical, and photodynamic injuries to the skin have been used in a controlled fashion to elicit desired changes. Cutaneous resurfacing targets abnormal skin structures at specific depths causing the body to replace the desired areas with normal healthy tissue to achieve aesthetic goal. The face, neck, décolletage, and hands are subject to the most sun exposure over a lifetime and are the most frequent sites of skin resurfacing.

Although multiple modalities exist to achieve similar injury patterns, patients present different challenges to achieving the desired aesthetic result. To minimize the risk of complications, an understanding of skin anatomy as it relates to aging and a logical approach to selecting an intervention are of the utmost importance.

ANATOMY

The skin is composed of an outer epidermis, a deeper dermal layer, and subcutaneous fat. The epidermis is principally responsible for protection from the sun and acts as a lipid barrier for water exchange. The superficial-most layer of the epidermis, the stratum corneum, is composed of devitalized cells that are continually replaced by precursor cells migrating from the dermal-epidermal junction (DEJ). The underlying dermis is itself divided into a superficial papillary layer and a deeper reticular dermis (**Figure 45.1**). The papillary dermis begins at the type III collagen–rich basement membrane and is composed of loose areolar tissue with a dense capillary network that nourishes the overlying epidermis. This capillary network is also important for heat exchange with the environment and helps distinguish this layer from the underlying reticular layer. The reticular dermis, primarily composed of type I collagen, accounts for the majority of skin thickness. Fibroblasts, macrophages, and mast cells are all found in the reticular layer and are key players in skin healing. Dermal appendages, including hair follicles and sebaceous glands, are important for re-epithelialization. These adnexal structures are found in higher concentration in the papillary dermis. Thus, efficiency of healing is inversely related to depth of injury.

Total skin thickness varies at any given anatomical site on the face and neck. The thinnest skin is found at the upper eyelid and neck whereas the thickest skin overlies the nasal tip.[2] Recently, high-resolution ultrasound has been used to map the varying dermal and epidermal thickness of the face and neck. Notably, skin depth was measured at 0.2 cm at the forehead, 0.5 cm at the menton, and 0.1 cm at the zygomatic process and cheek and nasolabial fold regions.[3]

AGING SKIN

Common age-related skin changes include skin laxity, pigment changes, keratoses, and wrinkles. Identification and diagnosis of the target skin malady guide treatment toward options aimed at reversing these changes.

Solar damage causes actinic irregularities that are characterized histologically by epidermal hyperplasia and keratinocyte proliferation forming seborrheic and actinic keratoses. These may be individually treated with curettage and cryotherapy if they are isolated or more broadly targeted with full facial resurfacing in the form of a chemical peel, mechanical dermabrasion, or ablative technologies when appropriate.[4]

Age and photodamage cause asynchronous melanin distribution and basilar hyperpigmentation or dyschromias. Melanocytes along the basement membrane, which normally produce and distribute melanin to 15 to 18 keratinocytes, are disrupted leading to collections of excess pigment (lentigines). Both an increased number of basal melanocytes and increased deposition of melanin in keratinocytes are observed. Elimination of these pigmented lesions requires targeted destruction of melanocytes in the basal layer of

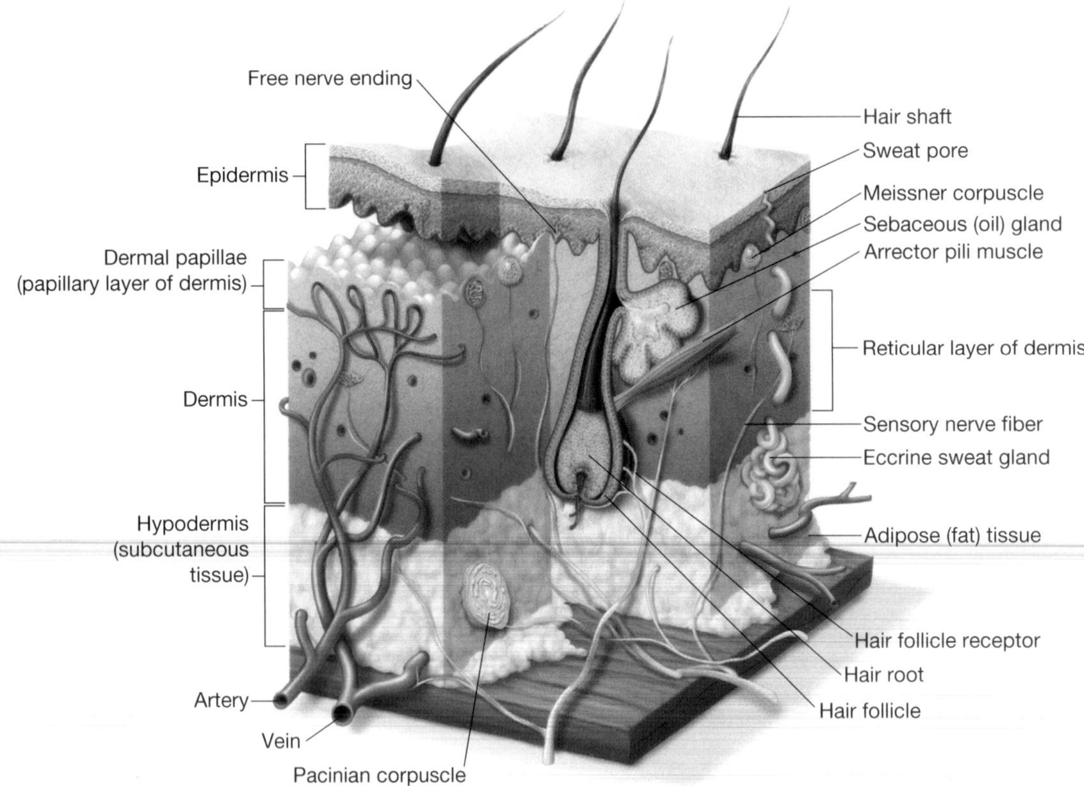

FIGURE 45.1. Cross section of skin elements.

the epidermis. Treatment options include trichloroacetic acid (TCA) peels, lasers that are absorbed by melanin, or intense pulsed light (IPL).[5,6]

Melasma is a condition characterized by symmetric hyperpigmented patches with an irregular outline, commonly occurring on the face that is important to differentiate from other pigmented lesion. It is most prevalent in young females and is exacerbated by sun exposure, pregnancy, and use of oral contraceptives. The condition is unpredictable, usually recalcitrant to treatment and prone to recurrence. A Wood lamp can help distinguish melasma from other more superficial skin pigmented lesions. The Wood lamp enhances superficial pigment and leaves deeper dermal pigment, as seen in melasma, unchanged. The treatment of melasma is targeted at blocking melanin production with topical tretinoin, hydroquinone (HQ) 2% to 4%, and topical corticosteroids. Additionally, dermal chemical peels, IPL, and nonablative and ablative laser treatments may improve but not fully eliminate melasma.

The etiology of static and dynamic rhytids is multifactorial. Atrophy of all layers of the skin progresses over time resulting in thinning and deflation. The protective stratum corneum of the epidermis becomes loose and disorganized. Loss of elastic fibers in the superficial dermis and elastotic thickening of the remaining elastic fibers gives the skin a thickened and fissured appearance. Degeneration of collagen fibers and reduction in glycosaminoglycans in the reticular dermis contributes to dermal thinning. A loss of oxytalan fibers at the DEJ that normally form vertical attachments between the two layers of skin leads to laxity and also contributes to cutaneous lines.[7-9] Telangiectasias form from weakened and dilated blood vessels. Finally, underlying bony resorption, soft tissue volume loss, and weakened osseocutaneous connections result in deflation and, thus, the more prominent appearance of wrinkles.

Although many factors have yet to be elucidated, what remains clear is that the treatment of skin wrinkles requires ablative therapy of the DEJ into the papillary dermis.[8,9]

PATIENT SELECTION

Patient evaluation including a thorough history and clinical examination is required for patients seeking skin rejuvenation. The aim should be to establish patient goals and set clear expectations of outcomes. Photographic documentation is critical to assess treatment response.

Arguably the most important factor to consider in patients seeking skin rejuvenation is Fitzpatrick skin type (**Table 45.1**). It is prognostic of developing signs of photoaging. Alternatively, the Glogau skin scale separates patients into four categories based on cumulative sun exposure (**Table 45.2**). Although both of these classification systems are useful, they do not provide the physician with all the information needed to select the ideal patient-specific treatment. They precede the advent of nonablative and fractional ablative technologies and fall short in addressing patients with thicker and darker skin types.

Other factors to consider and discuss with the patient before treatment include

- Skin tone, pore size, pore density, amount of sebaceous secretions
- Degree of actinic damage

TABLE 45.1. FITZPATRICK SKIN TYPE

Type I	Always burns, never tans, extremely fair complexion
Type II	Always burns, sometimes tans, fair complexion
Type III	Sometimes burns, always tans, medium complexion
Type IV	Rarely burns, always tans, olive complexion
Type V	Never, burns, always tans, medium brown complexion
Type VI	Never burns, always tans, markedly dark brown/black complexion

TABLE 45.2. GLOGAU SCALE

Mild	No wrinkles	No keratosis Wears little to no makeup
Moderate	Wrinkles in motion	Early keratosis, sallow complexion Usually needs makeup
Advanced	Wrinkles at rest	Many actinic keratosis, telangiectasia Always wears makeup
Severe	All wrinkles	Severe keratosis, severe photoaging Wears makeup with poor coverage

- Depth, location and severity of wrinkles (static versus dynamic rhytids)
- History of pathologic scarring
- Isotretinoin, HQ, SPF use within the past 6 months
- Previous surgeries, dry eyes
- Color of dyschromia (brown versus red lesions)
- Patient's lifestyle, expectations, and acceptable downtime

Special attention should be taken while treating patients with freckles, melasma, or postinflammatory hyperpigmentation (PIH). Regardless of ethnic background or skin type, a history of these signs heralds the risk of PIH.

BIOLOGY OF WOUND HEALING FOLLOWING RESURFACING PROCEDURES

Resurfacing treatments rely on controlled destruction of targeted layers of the skin past the level of the abnormality, followed by healing and replacement with healthy tissue. The goal is to optimize healing and minimize scarring. The limits of the body's normal healing capacity are unknown. Deeper injuries carry higher risk of scarring. However, the mechanism and depth of insult after which permanent scarring occurs remain unclear and vary by modality.

If the injury is isolated to the epidermal layer, an intact basal layer is capable of re-epithelialization without involvement of the underlying dermis. Insults extending into the superficial layer of the dermis repopulate the epidermis in two mechanisms—vertical migration of epithelial cells within dermal appendages (hair follicles and sweat glands) and lateral migration of keratinocyte from adjacent epidermal edges. Deeper injuries within the dermal layer stimulate fibroblast production of new collagen via the classic inflammation, proliferation, and remodeling phases of wound healing. Appropriate remodeling and reorganization of the collagen deposited can result in skin tightening and the decreased appearance of fine lines.[10,11]

Areas prone to scar include the neck and mandibular border that have thinner underlying dermis and fewer adnexal skin structures for efficient re-epithelialization.

CHEMICAL PEELS

Epidermal Targets

The targets of epidermal treatments are excess accumulation of keratinocytes, pigmented lesions, and actinic keratoses. Complete treatment of an area is safe and effective, as the epidermal basement membrane remains intact for rapid re-epithelialization.

Skin Preconditioning

Skin conditioning should begin at least 6 weeks (or 8–12 weeks in darker individuals) prior to chemical resurfacing.[8] Topical tretinoin 0.05% to 0.1% is used in conjunction with HQ 4% cream to restore even epidermal thickness and improve solar elastosis.

Vitamin A and its derivatives (tretinoin) are effective for reversing actinic sun damage, reducing fine lines, improving skin texture, and increasing collagen synthesis.[12] On a cellular level, there is increased epithelial cell turn over, decreased thickness of stratum corneum keratinized cells, and decreased adherence of epithelial cells within dermal appendages. Additionally, tretinoin suppresses melanocyte activity.[12-14] It is often used as pretreatment for chemical peels to ensure even depth of treatment penetration and faster postprocedure healing.[15]

Many retinoids are photolabile. It is suggested that they be applied at night and to the entire face (avoiding the corners of their mouth and eyelids). Treatment begins with either 0.025% or 0.05% tretinoin cream every other night and can be increased to nightly application if tolerated. Side effects include dry skin, peeling, and erythema similar to a sun burn and hypersensitivity to the UV rays—collectively referred to as *retinoid dermatitis*. It is the only therapy proven to repair photodamage with benefits persisting even after discontinuation of use (Figure 45.2).

A topical 4% HQ may be added for darker skin patients twice daily to decrease melanin production. A 6- to 12-week pretreatment with tretinoin and HQ can help prevent pigmentation irregularities following a chemical resurfacing procedure.

Superficial Peels

α-Hydroxy Acids

α-Hydroxy acids (i.e., glycolic, lactic, malic, tartaric, and citric acids) occur naturally in milk products and fruit. Treatment end point for α-hydroxy acids is an indistinct *frosting* followed by water rinse. Glycolic is the most widely used acid of the group because it penetrates the epidermis most easily owing to the fact that it is a small molecule (two carbon chain). The Food and Drug Administration suggests a limit of 30% concentration, but it has been used off label as high as 50%, and the recommended lower limit of the pH is 3. Both the concentration and pH affect penetration depth. α-Hydroxy acids are usually applied in a gel base for more even epidermal penetration to avoid patchy peeling.[16]

β-Hydroxy Acids

β-Hydroxy acids differ from the α-hydroxy acid group on a molecular level owing to two carbons separating the hydroxyl groups instead of one. Salicylic acid is the most commonly used acid in this group and usually dosed up to a concentration of 30%. There is a risk of tinnitus at higher concentrations. The treatment end point for salicylic acid is a much more distinct white frost, and it has demonstrated particular effectiveness in acne patients. The white frost is a byproduct of coagulation of keratinocyte proteins.[16]

Jessner Solution

Jessner solution (formerly Coombs; resorcinol 14 g, salicylic acid 14 g, lactic acid 14 mL and OS ethanol 100 mL) is the most commonly used superficial peeling agent.[17] It combines both α-hydroxy and β-hydroxy acids in low concentrations to take advantage of the benefits of each while limiting side effects. There is a clear light frost end point, and it does not require neutralization owing to its rapid volatility. The depth of treatment is controlled by number of layers applied. Jessner solution can be used in isolation as a superficial chemical peel or as a prelude to a deeper peel, such as TCA. Preemptive Jessner dekeratinization of the cutaneous surface promotes a more even and more intense depth of penetration with a TCA peel.

Medium-Depth Peels

Trichloroacetic Acid

Trichloroacetic acid (TCA) is a derivative of acetic acid that has been used since the 1960s for resurfacing of aging skin. As it penetrates the skin, TCA causes protein coagulation and denaturation and can be used to reach a variety of depths. It is self-neutralizing and will

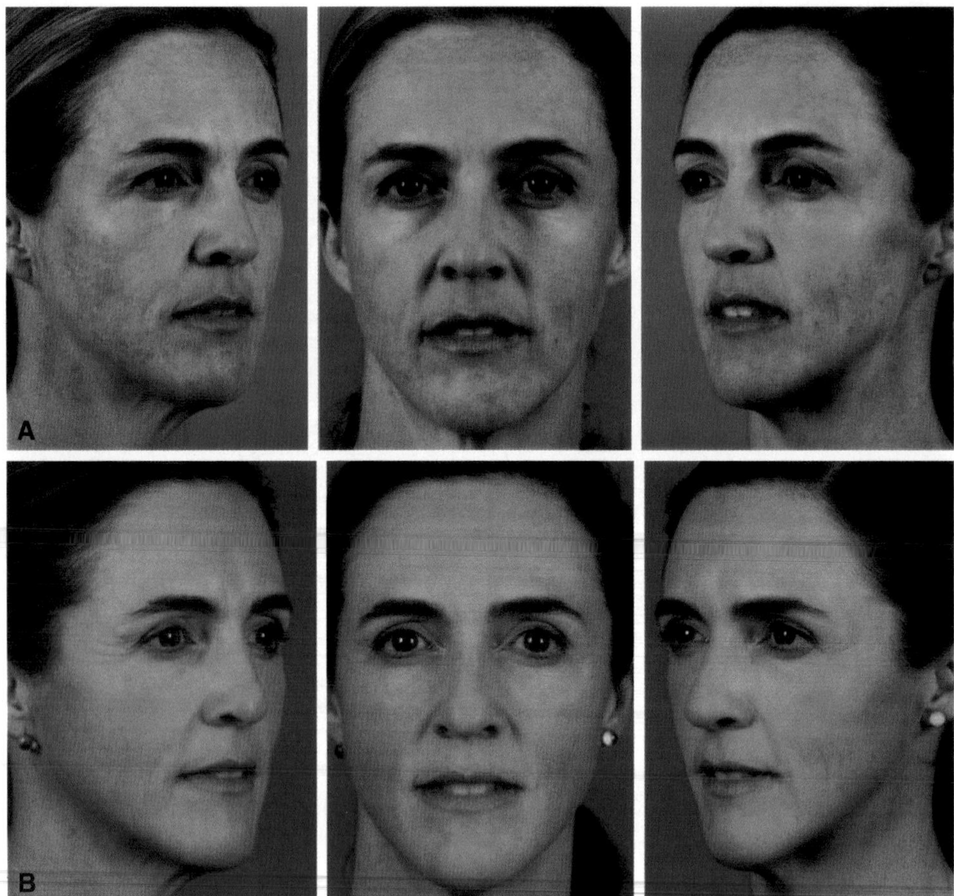

FIGURE 45.2. Patient with sun-damaged skin before **(A)** and 7 months after **(B)** beginning topical skin conditioning with 0.05% tretinoin and 4% hydroquinone.

keep penetrating until the acid has been used up by a certain amount of protein. Therefore, regardless of concentration, the acid can drive deeper into the skin with repeated application. For this reason, it is important to monitor clinical depth signs during the peeling process to achieve safe and reproducible depths of peel. TCA peel depth and clinical end points are as follows[18]:

- Partial-depth epithelial: light white frost with stable epidermis
- Full-thickness epithelial: light white frost with epidermal sliding
- Papillary dermis: white frost with pink beneath
- Reticular dermis: opaque white frost

The TCA solution is applied with sweeping brush strokes to regional facial units and allowed to sit for one to 2 minutes until the characteristic white frost develops. Pretreatment with a keratolytic agent like Jessner solution will degrease the skin just before the peel for more uniform treatment with increased depth of TCA penetration. The progression of the frosting color from pink to uniform white signifies entry into the papillary dermis, and the subsequent gray hued frost denotes the reticular dermis. Once the desired depth of peel is reached, the acid is diluted with water, which helps to dissipate the heat generated. A fan may be helpful for patient comfort to further diffuse the heat.[17,19]

Special care must be taken with thin, dry, crepey skin. Ultimately, practitioner experience is the best judge of safety. Experience, technique and attention to subtle differences in the desired end points help optimize maximum treatment efficacy while minimizing the risk of scarring.

After 24 hours, the skin will feel tight and darken. The patient should cleanse daily with water and apply ointment to help promote re-epithelialization. Once desquamation is completed after 5 to 7 days, the patient may begin to use moisturizer and even makeup. Erythema may persist for several months while collagen remodeling proceeds (**Figure 45.3**).

Deep Peels

Phenol, or carbolic acid, causes rapid coagulation and destruction of surface keratin. It predictably penetrates the upper reticular dermis for a relatively deep chemical peel to treat fine lines, wrinkles, and dyschromias. In the 1960s, Baker-Gordon popularized a formula mixing phenol with croton oil for severely sun-damaged and thickened skin.[20] Further investigation by Hetter demonstrated that croton oil was

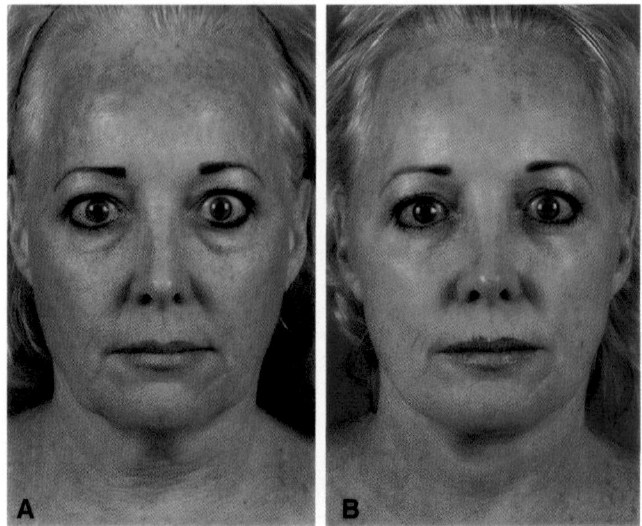

FIGURE 45.3. Patient with sun-damaged skin before **(A)** and 1 year after **(B)** face and neck lift with 30% trichloroacetic acid (TCA) peel.

TABLE 45.3. PHENOL PEEL FORMULAS[22]

Hetter Formulas		
Heavy Peel	**Medium-Light (most common)**	**Very Light (for eyelids and neck)**
■ 33% phenol □ 4 mL phenol 88% □ 6 mL water □ 16 drops septisol ■ 1.1% croton oil □ 3 drops croton oil	■ 33% phenol □ 4 mL phenol 88% □ 6 mL water □ 16 drops septisol ■ 0.35% croton oil □ 1 drop croton oil	■ 27.5% phenol □ 2 mL phenol 88% □ 5 mL water

the active ingredient for deep peeling in the Baker-Gordon formula, and he suggested concentrations for different depths[21,22] (**Table 45.3**).

Follow-up studies by Stone suggest that friction during application is the major factor in treatment depth and efficacy.[23] The end point for phenol/croton oil is similar to the TCA frosting, but it appears more gray-white. Of note, the croton oil elicits an erythematous response, which can skew the appearance of the frost. The phenol/croton oil peel is the most aggressive and most efficacious peel for deep set and perioral rhytids. Owing to its depth of penetration, it also carries the highest risk of scarring and hypopigmentation. It should be performed with extreme care and caution not to exceed the slightly gray-white frost end point. Completely gray could indicate full thickness skin destruction. Additionally, care must be taken to make sure the solution does not inadvertently drip onto the patient, as this can lead to uneven peels.

Posttreatment care is much like that of the TCA peel. Patients should use wet dressings for several hours until hemostasis sets in, followed by ointment until re-epithelialization in 10 to 14 days. Erythema persists for several months while collagen is remodeled.

Complications of Peels

A common complication from TCA peels is PIH especially in darker skinned patients. This is thought to be due to over production of melanin from newly regenerated melanocytes. Patients with a history of herpes are at risk for outbreak during the peeling process and should be prophylactically treated with antivirals. Pretreatment with isotretinoin (Accutane) may increase the risk of hypertrophic scarring because it interferes with the re-epithelialization process and keratinocyte adherence along dermal adnexal structures (hair follicles and sweat glands).

Complications of phenol/croton peels include hypopigmentation due to decreased melanocytes. Following treatment, PIH may occur while neomelanocytes are especially sensitive to sunlight stimulation. Sunscreen must be used regularly. Rarely wound infections with yeast or staphylococcus and streptococcus can occur and must be treated immediately. Cardiac monitoring and easily accessible resuscitation equipment are recommended in case of arrhythmia for phenol peels.

DERMABRASION

Mechanical injury from surgical sanding or dermabrasion is thought to be one of the first resurfacing techniques, which was developed as early as the 1940s. The treatment involves mechanical abrasion and complete obliteration of the epidermis with varying depth of dermal penetration depending on the desired effect. Depth of treatment is determined through reliable end points:

- DEJ: uniform pink
- Superficial papillary dermis: punctate bleeding, transudate
- Midpapillary dermis: confluent bleeding
- Deep papillary dermis: scattered bleeding

Dermabrasion is most commonly used to reduce raised scars, especially acne scars, to bring them to the same level as the surrounding skin. Baker described the current technique for microdermabrasion in 1998, which uses course crystals, diamond fraise, or a wire brush in lieu of sand paper to exfoliate the epidermis.[24] Histological studies have demonstrated permanent reduction in dermal thickness following dermabrasion, which is distinct from the compensatory dermal thickening that occurs following chemical peels and coagulative lasers.[24-27]

Dermabrasion patients receive pretreatment nerve blocks, intravenous sedation, and/or general anesthesia for comfort. Rhytids are marked prior to treatment. The hand-held power dermabrading instrument spins at 12,000 to 15,000 rpm. Gentle pressure is applied to the tissue until the proper depth is achieved. Treatment end points for dermabrasion depend on the desired depth of treatment based on the predetermined depth of the wrinkle. There is a notable color transition from white in the epidermal layer to the pink DEJ. The papillary dermis layer demonstrates a progression from punctate to an almost confluent bleeding pattern with a fine lattice. Deeper reticular dermal bleeding becomes sparser with the points spread out wider.

The challenge with dermabrasion is the technical demands of uniform treatment. It is excellent for isolated scars or the lip borders, but it is difficult to stabilize the tissue for even sanding with the power rotary device. This can be problematic particularly around the eyes. Temporary freezing techniques may increase tissue stiffness to facilitate ease of treatment.[26]

Following treatment, a wet dressing is applied until the bleeding stops a few hours later. Once the wound bed is hemostatic, a thin layer of ointment is applied and either covered with a semiocclusive xeroform gauze or left uncovered until re-epithelialization is complete.

LASER RESURFACING

Laser technology began to develop in the 1960s. The devices use light energy and are classified by wavelength on the electromagnetic spectrum (**Figure 45.4**). Discovery of *selective photothermolysis*, or the specific affinity of certain wavelengths for different biologic targets or *chromophores*, ultimately made way for the advent of cutaneous laser resurfacing in the 1980s.[22] The chromophore or target in the treatment of skin resurfacing for fine lines and rhytids is water. Other chromophores that are popular targets include melanin and dermal hemoglobin. Selective photothermolysis uses a wavelength that reaches and is preferentially absorbed by the desired chromophore (**Figure 45.5**). The tissue is then exposed to the energy for a duration equal or less than the time it takes for the target structures to cool, which is called the thermal relaxation time. Sufficient energy must be delivered to damage the target. Laser treatments targeting water produce histological changes similar to those of phenol peels, although the permanence of skin changes following laser treatment remains controversial.[23] Complete photorejuvenation requires targeting water, hemoglobin, and melanin. No one laser or wavelength meets all of those objectives on its own.

All lasers have four basic components: an active medium, an energy source, a rear reflective mirror, and a partially reflective mirror/output coupler (**Figure 45.6**). Laser light differs from ordinary light in that it is more organized. Laser light is monochromatic (all photons in the laser beam exhibit the same color wavelength), collimated (all photons travel in parallel), and coherent (all photons are in phase and travel in the same direction).[28]

There are several basic parameters that should be considered when performing a procedure using light.[29] Light interaction with tissue is based on absorption and scattering. A beam of light weakens as it moves through scattering surfaces. The dermis is white making it a strongly scattering surface. In general, shorter wavelengths have a higher absorption coefficient and penetrate more superficially compared with longer wavelengths (**Figure 45.7**). Wavelengths in the near-infrared spectrum (740–1300 nm) are absorbed by the darkest

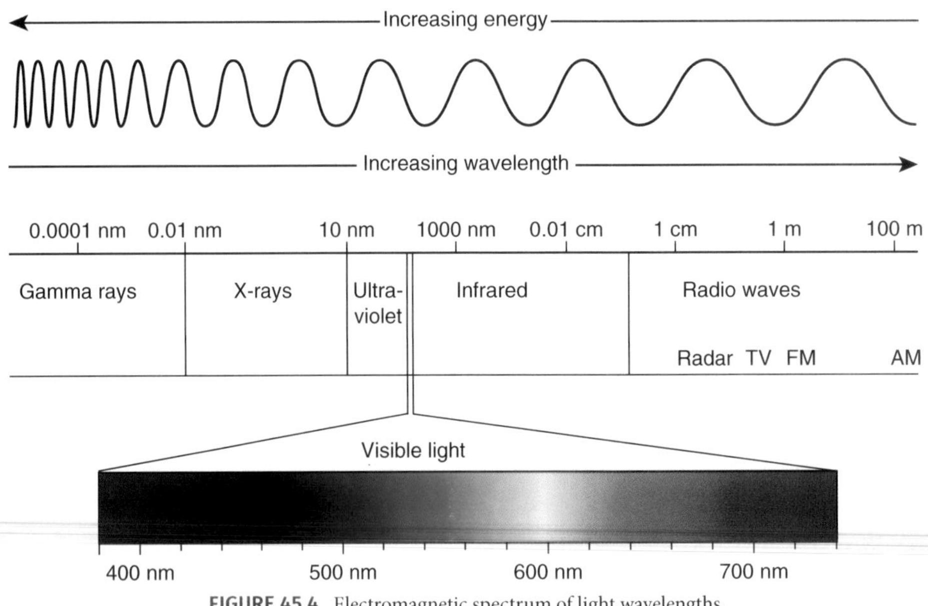

FIGURE 45.4. Electromagnetic spectrum of light wavelengths.

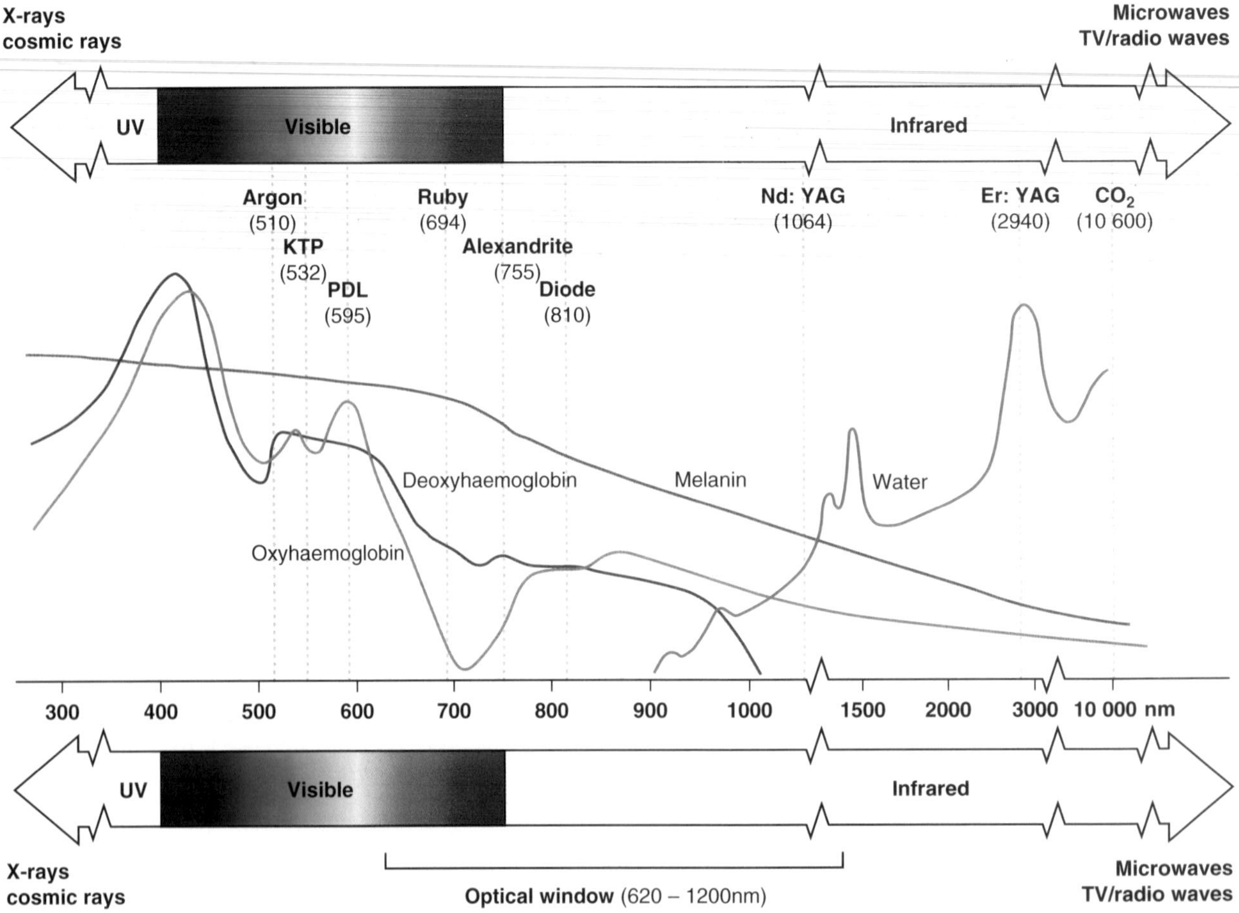

FIGURE 45.5. Chromophore absorption spectrum, illustrating which wavelengths are preferentially absorbed by specific components of the skin.

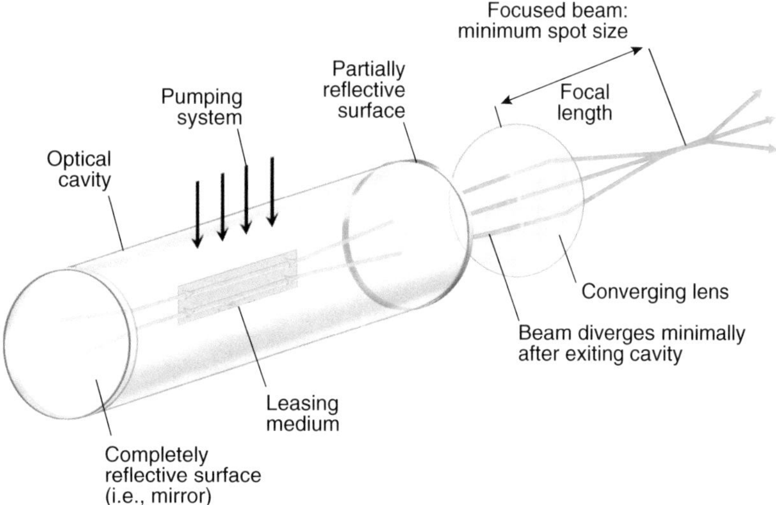

FIGURE 45.6. Components of a laser. The external power source excites the medium, which stimulates photon emission. These photons collide with surrounding atoms that release more photons all of which are reflected between the mirrors at either end of the optical chamber. Opening the output coupler allows emission of the laser beam.

shade of gray present in tissue and far infrared spectrum (1300 nm+) wavelengths are absorbed by water as opposed to pigment.

For continuous wave lasers, important factors include power, time, and spot size, while for pulsed lasers, parameters include energy per pulse, pulse duration, spot size, fluence, and repetition rate. Energy is measured in joules (J). Power is the rate of energy delivered and is measured in Watts (W = J/s). Spot size (cm^2) is the area over which the laser energy is delivered. Power density (power/spot size or W/cm^2) can be controlled in a manner similar to a magnifying glass by concentrating a given number of photons over a smaller area to

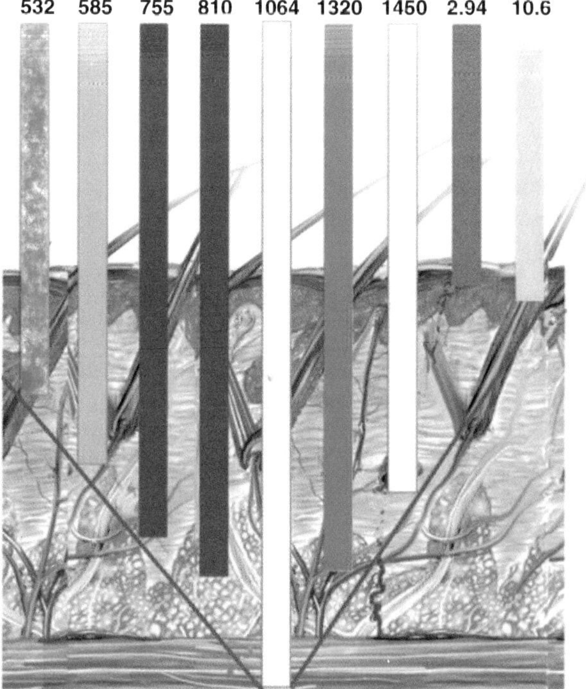

FIGURE 45.7. Illustration demonstrating the inverse relationship between wavelength and depth of penetration. (From Farkas JP, Hoopman JE, Kenkel JM. Five parameters you must understand to master control of your laser/light based devices. *Aesthet Surg J.* 2013;33(7):1059-1064. Reproduced by permission of The American Society for Aesthetic Plastic Surgery, Inc.)

increase thermal effect on a target tissue. Thus, decreasing the spot size will increase the power density. However, decreasing spot size also decreases depth of penetration and increases scatter. To maintain the depth of thermal energy delivered, one must increase the power (rate of energy delivered) as one decreases the spot size (Figure 45.8). For example, a 6 mm spot size and 90 J/cm^2 may be needed to close a vessel; if you increase the power density and use a 3 mm spot size instead, the energy needed would increase to 190 J/cm^2 to have a similar effect.

Finally, pulse width is the time over which the energy is delivered and represents the duration of laser exposure. The energy must be deposited in the target before the target has time to cool. Thermal relaxation time is how long it takes for a target chromophore to release over half of the temperature rise after laser exposure. Larger targets take longer to cool. For example, a 200 to 300 μm hair follicle has a thermal relaxation time of 10 to 100 ms, whereas a 100 μm blood vessel has a thermal relaxation time of 5 ms. Assuming equal power densities are applied, longer pulse durations cause greater collateral damage.[30]

The degree of thermal injury and thus tissue response are related to the duration and temperature of exposure. Cell death is more sensitive to temperature than time, as seen when protein denaturation increases linearly with time and exponentially with temperature.[31] Most resurfacing devices convert light or electrical energy to heat. Under 43°C, the skin remains unharmed for as long as 20 minutes. Molecular structural changes occur at temperatures from 43 to 50°C. High temperatures at shorter times (>100°C for 1 ms) can induce cell death as well.[22]

Effective laser therapy aims to maximize thermal effect on specific targets while minimizing collateral damage. Selective photothermolysis aims to deliver thermal energy to targets with a higher absorption coefficient than the surrounding tissue to minimize damage to *innocent bystanders*.[31] When the ratio of light absorption between the chromophore and surrounding tissue is large (>10), there is a desirable advantage. However, when the target is water, which constitutes 65% of the dermis, differential light absorption cannot be manipulated to protect neighboring structures. Other ways to localize temperature elevation to specific targets is to cool surrounding areas or deliver very small beams (fractional methods).[32]

Surface cooling methods have helped deliver higher energy to targets with less risk of collateral damage and at a deeper depth. Epidermal damage is most likely with visible light (green-yellow, IPL) treatments targeting dermal hair follicles and blood vessels. Cooling is also important in infrared laser technology to prevent bulk heating of deep tissues. When water is the chromophore, even at low power density, the ubiquitous nature of the target creates the

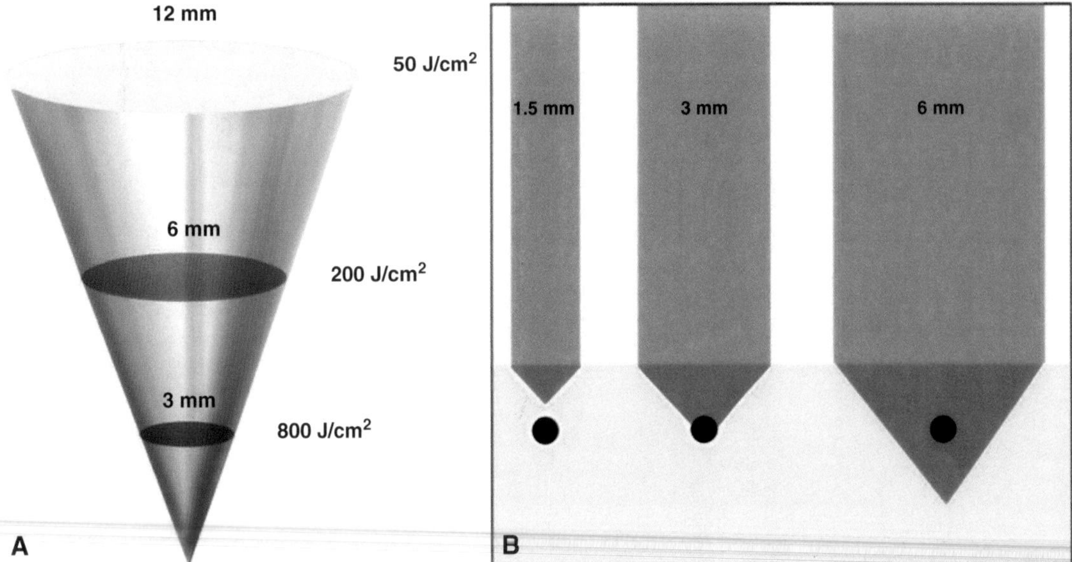

FIGURE 45.8. A. Power density equals power multiplied by spot size. A given number of photons are concentrated into an area or spot size. As the spot size decreases, the power density increases. **B.** Effective treatment zones versus spot size. Depth of penetration is proportionally related to spot size: larger spot sizes allow for deeper absorption of a given wavelength. (From Farkas JP, Hoopman JE, Kenkel JM. Five parameters you must understand to master control of your laser/light based devices. *Aesthet Surg J*. 2013;33(7):1059-1064. Reproduced by permission of The American Society for Aesthetic Plastic Surgery, Inc.)

risk of catastrophic tissue damage. Cooling or fractionated techniques must be used to avoid laser-induced top to bottom skin injury.

Generally speaking, lasers used in skin resurfacing are either ablative or nonablative and can be full field or fractionated. Ablation refers to the uniform destruction of tissue within the epidermis and/or papillary dermis. Nonablative resurfacing spares epidermal destruction, targeting deeper structures within the dermis. This triggers collagen remodeling during the process of healing. Fractional photothermolysis delivers treatment in core sections or microthermal zones, leaving untreated areas in the skin to promote more rapid healing.

A word about safety: Appropriate laser safety precautions include wavelength-appropriate eyewear, appropriate signage, and smoke evacuation.

Types of Lasers

Ablative Lasers

There are two ablative lasers with the highest affinity for water, and those are erbium:YAG and carbon dioxide (CO_2). Both of these have wavelengths in the infrared portion of the electromagnetic spectrum.

CO_2 Laser

The earliest CO_2 (10,600 nm) lasers used continuous wave to heat water in the skin to ablate fine lines. The primary chromophore is water, and the depth of penetration can be controlled by altering power, density, or duration of exposure.[33] The threshold for tissue ablation has been calculated to be 5 J/cm^2. Below this, the tissue is not vaporized but rather coagulated which is also useful to trigger skin remodeling. At high powers and short exposures, the CO_2 laser can be used for tissue cutting (depth of 100–150 microns).[34] Significant variability in depth of injury exists among different CO_2 lasers and carries with energy and pulse duration.

Continuous CO_2 laser resurfacing remains the most effective method of wrinkle removal. It is effective against deep coarse fixed perioral and periorbital rhytids.[35] Redundant skin is tightened by thermal coagulation, wound healing, and collagen contraction. These dramatic results come at the expense of slow healing, painful recovery, prolonged erythema (6+ months), and permanent hypopigmentation which has decreased the CO_2 modality's popularity.[36]

Erbium-Yttrium-Aluminum-Garnet Laser

The next major advancement was the development of the erbium-yttrium-aluminum-garnet (Er:YAG) 2940-nm wavelength laser. The 2940 nm wavelength has an affinity for water that is nearly 12 to 15 times higher than that of the CO_2 laser. This affinity allows Er:YAG to deliver energy to specific depths in the skin without heating the surrounding tissue, thus causing less collateral damage. However, the limited photothermal effects of this laser also lead to significantly reduced collagen contraction. Newer Erbium devices have lengthened the laser pulse duration to induce better tissue contraction.[37] The Er:YAG laser can be used to deliver either coagulation or cool ablation. This is a solid-state laser with a solid rod through which the light is passed. This is different from the CO_2 laser that is only a heat-coagulative ablative technology. The cool ablation mode produces a result similar to dermabrasion. In the cool ablative mode, the resulting skin may have thinner dermis, as with dermabrasion. Erbium and CO_2 lasers have similar resurfacing results with settings of 50% overlap, 25 to 100 microns of ablation, and 50 to 100 microns of coagulation.[38]

The clinical end point of using the CO_2 laser is a chamois color seen with ablation of the papillary dermis and *waterlogged cotton thread* appearance upon penetration into the reticular dermis.[39] With each additional pass of the CO_2 laser, there is a diminishing or plateaued response because the residual carbonized tissue acts as a heat sink.[40] Erbium lasers create less coagulated tissue to absorb heat and make it is easier to drill deeper wounds into the skin with each pass. Following CO_2 laser treatment, the desiccated tissue should be wiped off; however, after erbium laser treatment, the barrier is left in place for faster healing and decreased posttreatment pigmentary changes. A split-face study of CO_2 and Er:YAG laser resurfacing study demonstrated a 63% improvement on the CO_2 laser side with 7.7 days of crusting compared with 48% improvement on the Er:YAG side with 3.4 days of crusting, although these results are highly dependent on depth of treatment and energy used.[41,42]

Ablative lasers are also commonly used to treat acne scarring. Specifically, elevated acne scars are more amenable to ablative resurfacing than ice-pick or nondistensible surface irregularities. Benign hyperplasias such as rhinophyma and other epidermal proliferations (seborrheic keratosis, actinic keratosis, xanthomas) can be treated with ablative laser therapy. Of note, ablative laser therapy carries the risk of infection (bacterial, viral, and fungal) due to the absence of the protective epidermal barrier. All patients should be treated prophylactically with antiviral medications to prevent herpetic infection

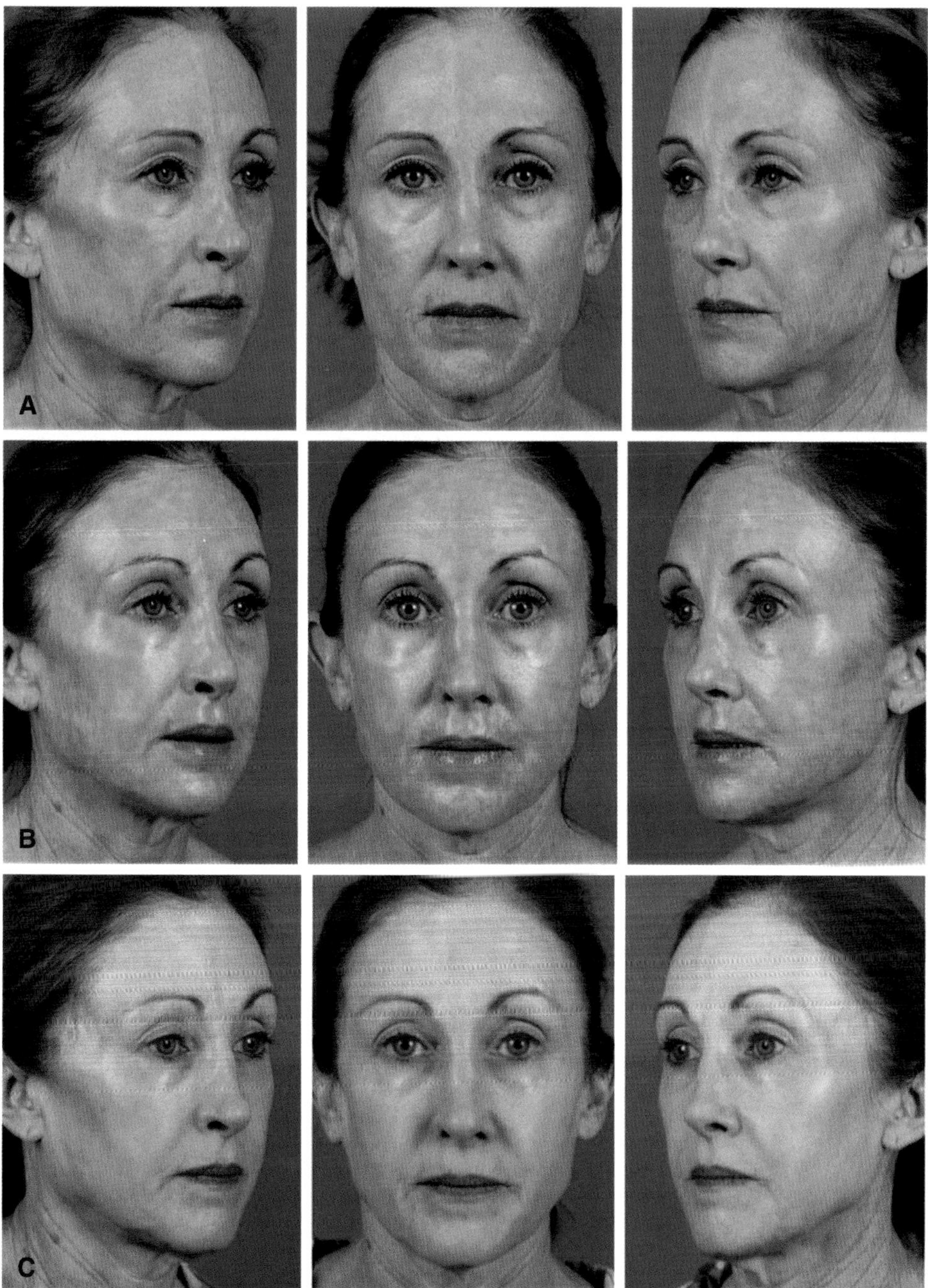

FIGURE 45.9. Patient with sun-damaged skin before **(A)** and 7 days **(B)** and 1 year **(C)** after erbium laser ablative resurfacing.

of the denuded skin. This treatment should begin 1 or 2 days before laser treatment and continue for 2 weeks following (Figures 45.9 and 45.10).

Fractionated Photothermolysis Lasers

Fractionated lasers first became available in 2003 to preserve dermal appendages for more efficient healing. They are designed to keep the stratum corneum largely intact, delivering thousands of microscopic ablative injuries surrounded by healthy tissue. Fractionated lasers ablate a variable amount of dermis depending on the physician's preferred density.[43] The laser creates an array of microthermal treatment zones. These columns of thermally denatured collagen that vary in size and density are scattered between islands of untreated skin to maintain the skin's barrier function and act as a reservoir for healing to speed re-epithelialization.[44] The advent of fractionated photothermolysis, in theory, allows a more aggressive depth of treatment with a better safety profile to the predecessor ablative lasers. These devices can safely be used on darker skinned patients. The skin surface usually heals within 7 days; however, the recovery and downtime for patients remains significant with prolonged erythema and swelling for several months post treatment. The best parameters for optimal outcomes remain the subject of ongoing debate.

There are multiple ablative and nonablative fractional lasers available commercially. They differ based on spot sizes, depth of treatment, energy delivered, and mode of delivery. One of the first clinical applications of fractionated laser therapy was treatment of facial melasma. Initial results suggested resolution of the deep pigment; however, lengthy follow-up demonstrated a tendency of the melasma to recur. Fractionated treatments have led to less dramatic results than the nonfractionated ablative devices, with noticeable improvement of periorbital rhytids in only 30% of patients in one study, which improved to 54% improvement after four treatments.[45]

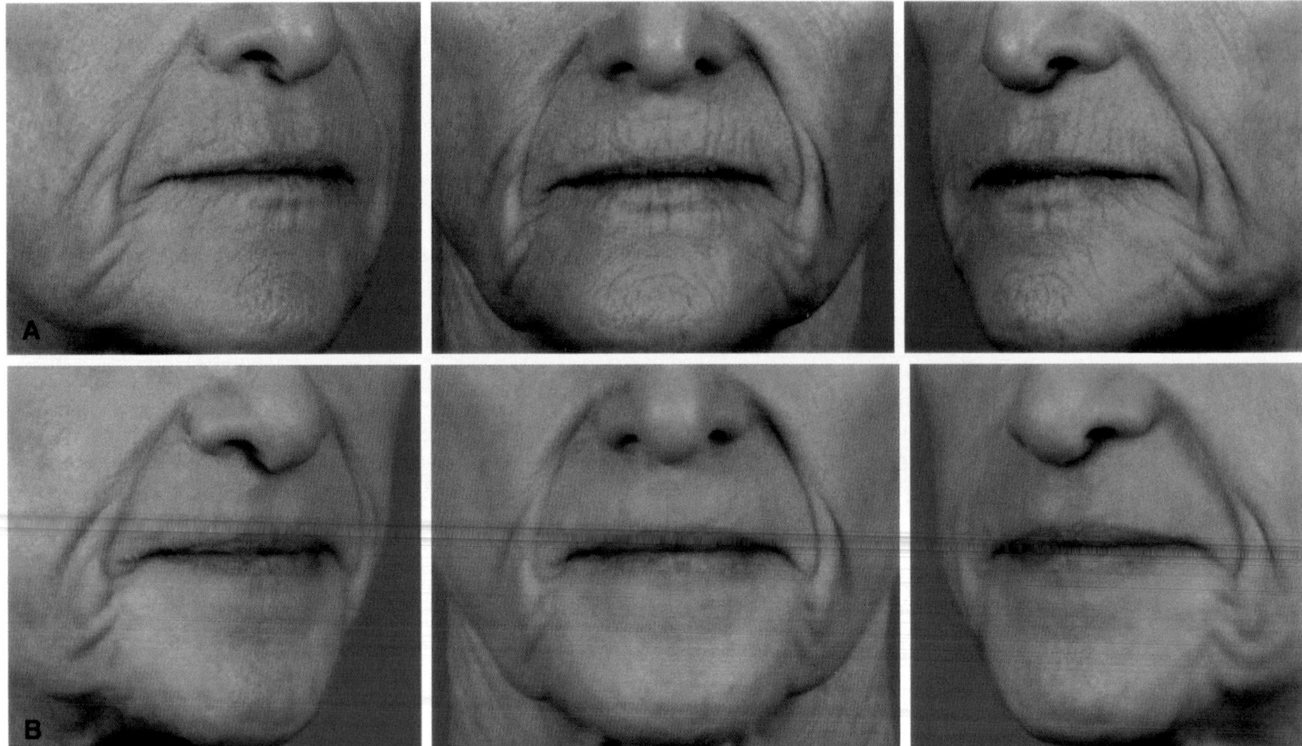

FIGURE 45.10. Patient with deep perioral static rhytids before **(A)** and 9 months after **(B)** erbium laser ablative resurfacing.

These results are highly dependent on depth of treatment, density of microthermal treatment zones, and energy used. Fractionated ablative treatments have also proven to be relatively safe in notoriously difficult to rejuvenate areas such as the neck and décolletage because the areas of undamaged skin left behind aide in efficient healing.

Hybrid Fractionated Lasers

Dual wavelength hybrid fractional lasers use both fractionated Er:YAG 2840 nm to deliver epidermal ablation up to 100 μm and diode laser 1470 nm to cause dermal coagulation from 100 to 700 μm.[46] In doing so, there is simultaneous treatment of the epidermis and dermis, but the fractional component allows more efficient healing over an intact dermis. The epidermis is able to regenerate in 24 hours following ablation to 100 μm. The underlying coagulated dermis heals more slowly over 1 week. This dual technology takes advantage of ablative and nonablative technology to obtain more dramatic ablative type results with shorter nonablative type healing times. Early studies suggest improvement in skin texture, pigment, pore size, and number; additional studies are ongoing.[47]

Nonablative Lasers

Nonablative facial skin rejuvenation refers to interventions that preserve the epidermis and generate selective dermal heating for wrinkle reduction. These so called *subsurface remodeling* include electrical, light, and ultrasound modalities to induce selective dermal injury and remodeling.[48] Nonablative devices include neodymium-doped yttrium aluminum garnet (Nd:YAG), pulsed dye laser (PDL), IPL, and potassium-titanyl-phosphate (KTP). Their applications are wide, including acne scars, dyschromias, and vascular lesions.

Laser Treatment of Vascular Lesions

Blood vessels can be heated by three different techniques:

- Visible light: 520 to 600 nm
- Near-infrared I: 755, 700 nm
- Near-infrared II: 940, 980, 1064 nm

The chromophore target oxyhemoglobin has absorption peaks at 418, 542, and 577 nm. Using any of these wavelengths when treating lesions with high hemoglobin concentration (telangiectasias) relative to their surrounding tissue induces intravascular thrombosis and subsequent fibrosis of the target vessel. This leads to an immediate purpuric reaction, which can be avoided by delivering longer pulse widths (>6 ms) to gently heat the vessel and avoid bruising.

Visible light (520–600 nm) has a very strong affinity for hemoglobin and melanin, whereas infrared technology has progressively weaker affinity. Specifically, infrared II has the weakest affinity for melanin rendering it safer to use in patients with higher Fitzpatrick types.

Treatment considerations when selecting a device include blood vessel depth and thickness and patient skin type. Equally important considerations include hair follicles, melanin content of skin, and other structures that may unintentionally absorb light energy. It is important not to compress the target vessel, as compression of the vessels can exclude blood and decrease the laser target. Conversely, vasodilatory anesthetics should be avoided in the treatment of vascular lesions.

Pulsed Dye

The pulsed dye laser (PDL) emits a wavelength of 577 nm or 585 and 595 nm for deeper tissue penetration up to 1.2 mm. These wavelengths target hemoglobin as the chromophore and make the PDL an effective laser choice for treating vascular lesions (telangiectasias, capillary malformations, rosacea). Short pulse durations (0.45–3 ms) have been shown to cause a bruised appearance related to intravascular coagulation and vessel leakage. Longer pulse durations (6–10 ms) are less effective, but when multiples passes are employed (*pulse stacked*) purpura-free results can be achieved.

The 577 to 595 nm wavelengths are also absorbed by melanin to a lesser degree than hemoglobin. This device should be used with caution in patients with darker skin, as they may be prone to burns and depigmentation. The treatment has been described as a *hot rubber band* snapping on the skin and is generally well tolerated by adults.

Potassium-Titanyl-Phosphate

Potassium-titanyl-phosphate (KTP) lasers have a wavelength of 532 nm and are popular for treatment of fine facial capillaries, small leg veins, capillary malformations, and rosacea. The wavelength closely corresponds to hemoglobin absorption peak at 542 nm. This device is safest in patients with skin phototypes I-III as the wavelength is also absorbed by melanin. Patients usually require 6 to 12 serial treatments under general anesthetic with this laser to adequately treat their vascular lesions. The KTP laser is associated with a fleeting stinging sensation and is generally well tolerated by adults.[49]

Nd:YAG

The Nd:YAG (1064 nm) penetrates deeper than the 532 nm wavelength. The darkest target in the field absorbs this wavelength; it is not attracted to a specific chromophore. The 1064 nm wavelength has much less affinity for hemoglobin than the KTP and PDL lasers, but its absorption by melanin is also limited, making it relatively safer to use in darker skinned patients. With a longer wavelength, this laser can be used to treat deeper vascular lesions. Higher energy and longer pulse widths are required when using this wavelength because of its relatively low absorption coefficient by hemoglobin, making it potentially painful and with a narrow window of safety.[50]

Intense Pulsed Light

Intense pulsed light (IPL) is a filtered flash lamp that emits noncoherent, noncollimated, polychromatic light at a range of 420 to 1300 nm. These devices are not lasers, much like a laser an IPL device can be fitted with filters to eliminate unwanted wavelengths and target more specific chromophores. A 550 nm filter will block all wavelengths from 420 to 550 nm, delivering only wavelengths of 551 to 1200 nm to the tissue. Similar to penetration of laser light, longer IPL wavelengths penetrate deeper into the tissue for treatment of deeper targets. Different filters serve different purposes (i.e., vascular lesions, pigmented lesions, and hair removal).

Two to three passes of this device to the particular treatment area are performed in different orientations help produce uniform treatment without zebra-like pigmentary irregularities and skipped areas. Clinical end points vary with target chromophore. They may include darkening of the pigmented lesions and disappearance or dark blue appearance of the telangiectasias. IPL is safest to use in patients with skin phototypes I-III. Care must be taken to avoid photoepilation of eyebrows or bearded skin.[51]

Melanin-Containing Lesions

Melanin has a broad spectrum of absorption. Many different lasers and wavelengths can treat melanin-containing lesions. The depth of the pigment is important in selecting the appropriate treatment modality. The KTP laser can effectively target epidermal and papillary dermal pigment in most skin types with limited recurrence.[52] PDL at 595 nm has affinity for both hemoglobin and melanin. By manually compressing the skin with the laser hand piece, the vasculature blanches removing the hemoglobin chromophore, and melanin-containing lesions absorb the light. Q-switched Nd:YAG laser with a wavelength of 1064 nm is much less well absorbed by melanin than the aforementioned devices, but it reaches deeper tissue and can treat dermal pigmented lesions.

Melasma is difficult to predictably treat with laser resurfacing. Er:YAG and Q-switched lasers can lead to temporary improvement followed by problematic PIH.[53] The aforementioned topical modalities remain the mainstay treatment.

Postprocedural Care

Meticulous postprocedural care is paramount for optimal results. Open or closed dressings may be used to dress the patient. Potential advantages to open dressings include fewer wound infections, ability to survey the resurfacing process, and decreased maceration. Pain is a frequent patient complaint when open dressings are used in ablative therapy. Immediately after ablative therapy, serous drainage is expected. Keratinaceous crust forms over 24 to 48 hours. If the open wound care regimen is selected, the patient must frequently wash with normal saline or 0.25% acetic acid (dilute vinegar) soaks followed by gentle blotting for exfoliation. Moisturizer is applied during re-epithelialization.

Numerous studies have shown that occlusive dressings may speed re-epithelialization and decrease discomfort, erythema, and edema. These occlusive dressings (e.g., Biobrane, Flexzan) can be used for 1 to 3 days and then left open to air.

Edema and erythema of treated skin is common following both ablative and nonablative therapies, although they are more pronounced and longer lasting in ablative procedures.[54] Nonablative edema and erythema can resolve in 24 to 48 hours following treatment. Most patients are able to return to normal activities and apply makeup in 7 to 10 days. Delayed hypopigmentation or PIH are feared complications of laser resurfacing.[55] Lines or demarcation of treated areas can be avoided by feathering and crosshatching during nonablative laser treatment. Caution must be taken when overlapping treatments during ablative therapy. Decreasing the density and/or energy may allow for this without focused areas of deeper injury.

Infection must be recognized and treated early. Staphylococcal, viral, or fungal infections are all possible following ablative treatments. The use of prophylactic antivirals is recommended from the day before the procedure to up to 2 weeks after. Antibiotics and antifungal treatment can be utilized on a case by case basis, although they are not routinely administered.

Scarring following laser therapy is a risk that is especially pronounced in the neck and chest. It is important to make sure the patient has not had any sun exposure in the 2 weeks leading up to light energy treatment, increasing risk of burns and dyspigmentation. PIH can occur in the months following treatment when new repopulating melanocytes are extrasensitive to sunlight. It can be seen can be seen in any patient who has had an energy-based treatment. Use of 4% HQ cream and sun avoidance help decrease the risk of PIH.

CONCLUSION

A wide range of resurfacing techniques from peels to mechanical dermabrasion to selective photothermolysis can all be employed to achieve predictable and safe results. Careful patient selection and meticulous tailoring of resurfacing modalities based on individual needs is of the utmost importance to achieve predictable, safe, and appreciable results. These noninvasive techniques are never a replacement for surgical intervention but can be extremely powerful adjuncts to help ensure the most satisfied patients.

AESTHETIC SURGERY

REFERENCES

1. American Society of Aesthetic Plastic Surgeons. *Cosmetic Surgery National Data Bank Statistics*; 2017. Available at https://surgery.org/sites/default/files/ASAPS-Stats2017.pdf.
2. Ha RY, Nojima K, Adams WP Jr, Brown SA. Analysis of facial skin thickness: defining the relative thickness index. *Plast Reconstr Surg*. 2005;15(6):1769-1773.
3. Iyengar S, Makin IR, Sadhwani D, et al. Utility of a high-resolution superficial diagnostic ultrasound system for assessing skin thickness: a cross-sectional study. *Dermatol Surg*. 2018;44:855-864.
4. Ortonne JP, Pandya AG, Lui H, Hexsel D. Treatment of solar lentigines. *J Am Acad Dermatol*. 2006;54:S262.
5. Weiss RA, Weiss MA, Beasley KL. Rejuvenation of photoaged skin: 5 years results with intense pulse light of the face, neck and chest. *Dermatol Surg*. 2002;28:1115.
6. Kilgman DE, Zhen Y. Intense pulsed light treatment of photoaged skin. *Dermatol Surg*. 2004;30:1085.
7. Bosset S, Barré P, Chalon A, et al. Skin aging: clinical and histopathologic study of permanent and reducible wrinkles. *Eur J Dermatol*. 2002;12:247.
8. Smith L. Histopathologic characteristics and ultrastructure of aging skin. *Cutis*. 1989;43:414.
9. Lee JY, Kim YK, Seo JY, et al. Loss of elastic fibers causes skin wrinkles in sun-damaged human skin. *J Dermatol Sci*. 2008;50:99.

10. Janis JE, Harrison B. Wound healing: part 1. Basic science. *Plast Reconstr Surg*. 2014;133(2):199e-207e.
11. Janis JE, Harrison B. Wound healing: part 2. Clinical applications. *Plast Reconstr Surg*. 2013;133(3):383e-392e.
12. Kligman AM, Grove GL, Hirose R, Leyden JJ. Topical tretinoin for photoaged skin. *J Am Acad Dermatol*. 1986;15:836-859.
13. Giguere V, Ong ES, Segui P, Evans RM. Identification of a receptor for the morphogen retinoic acid. *Nature*. 1987;330:624-629.
14. Petkovich M, Brand NJ, Krust A, Chambon P. A human retinoic acid receptor which belongs to the family of nuclear receptors. *Nature*. 1987;330:444-450.
15. Hevia O, Nemeth AK, Taylor JR. Tretinoin accelerates healing after trichloroacetic acid chemical peel. *Arch Dermatol*. 1991;127:678-682.
16. Stagnone JJ. Superficial peeling. *J Dermatol Surg Oncol*. 2003;42:829.
17. Obagi ZE, Ichinose H, Obagi ZE, Laub DR. TCA-based blue peel: a standardized procedure with depth control. *Dermatol Surg*. 1999;10:773-780.
18. Obagi ZE. *Obagi Skin Health Restoration and Rejuvenation*. New York, NY: Springer; 2000.
19. Johnson JB, Ichinose H, Obagi ZE, Laub DR. Obagi's modified trichloroacetic acid (TCA)-controlled variable-depth peel: a study of clinical signs correlating with histological findings. *Ann Plast Surg*. 1996;3:225-237.
20. Baker TJ, Gordon HL. The ablation of rhytids by chemical means: a preliminary report. *J Fla Med Assoc*. 1961;48:451.
The art and science behind chemical peeling is discussed. This landmark article came at the beginning of the development of chemical resurfacing techniques. Description of the technique for peeling is included.
21. Hetter GP. An examination of the phenol-croton oil peel. Part I: dissecting the formula. *Plast Reconstr Surg*. 2000;105:227.
22. Hetter GP. An examination of phenol-croton oil peel: face peel results with different concentrations of phenol and croton oil. *Plast Reconstr Surg*. 2000;105:1061.
23. Stone PA. Chemical peeling. In: Rubin MG, ed. *Chemical Peels*. Philadelphia, PA: Elsevier; 2007:87.
24. Baker TJ, Gordon HL. Chemical face peeling and dermabrasion. *Surg Clin North Am*. 1971;51:387.
25. Karimipour DJ, Karimipour G, Orringer JS. Microdermabrasion: an evidence-based review. *Plast Reconstr Surg*. 2010;125:372.
26. Poilos E, Taylor C, Solish N. Effectiveness of dermasanding (manual dermabrasion) on the appearance of surgical scars: a prospective, randomized blinded study. *J Am Acad Dermatol*. 2003;48:897.
27. Gold MH. Dermabrasion in dermatology. *Am J Clin Dermatol*. 2003;4(7):467.
28. Alster TS, Lupton JR: Lasers in dermatology: an overview of types and indications. *Am J Clin Dermatol*. 2001;2:291.
29. Farkas JP, Hoopman JE, Kenkel JM. Five parameters you must understand to master control of your laser/light based devices. *Aesthet Surg J*. 2013;33:1059-1064.
A review of the basic science behind laser- and light-assisted selective photothermolysis. This article reviews energy, power, fluence, spot size, and pulse width, as they relate to choosing appropriate settings for patients. Comprehensive explanations of the guiding principles of light energy.
30. Herd RM, Dover JS, Arndt KA. Basic laser principles. *Dermatol Clin*. 1997;5:355.
31. Anderson RR, Parish JA. Selective photothermolysis: precise microsurgery by selective absorption of pulsed radiation. *Science*. 1983;22:535.
32. Achauer BM. Lasers in plastic surgery: current practice. *Plast Reconstr Surg*. 1996;99:1442.
33. Walsh JT, Flotte TJ, Anderson RR, et al. Pulsed CO2 laser tissue ablation: effect of tissue type and pulse duration on thermal damage. *Lasers Surg Med*. 1988;8:108-118.
34. Newman JB, Lord JL, Ash K, et al. Variable pulse erbium:YAG laser skin resurfacing of perioral rhytides and side-by-side comparison with carbon dioxide laser. *Lasers Surg Med*. 2000;26:208-214.
35. Fitzpatrick RE, Goldman MP, Satur NM, et al. Pulsed carbon dioxide laser resurfacing of photo-aged facial skin. *Arch Dermatol*. 1996;132(4):395-402.
This is a blinded assessment of CO_2 *laser efficacy for periorbital and perioral rhytids. It was a landmark paper for selective photothermolysis and the clinical application of ablative facial resurfacing.*
36. Hunzeker CM, Weiss ET, Geronemus RG. Fractionated CO2 laser resurfacing: our experience with more than 2000 treatments. *Aesthet Surg J*. 2009;29:317-322.
37. Fitzpatrick RE, Rostan EF, Marchell N. Collagen tightening induced by carbon dioxide laser versus erbium:YAG laser. *Lasers Surg Med*. 2000;27:395.
38. Conn H, Nanda VS. Prophylactic fluconazole promotes reepithelialization in full-face carbon dioxide laser skin resurfacing. *Lasers Surg Med*. 2000;26:201-207.
39. Zachary CB. Modulating the Er:YAG laserModulating the Er:YAG laserModulating the Er:YAG laser. *Lasers Surg Med*. 2000;26:223-226.
40. Alster TS, Garg S. Treatment of facial rhytides with a high-energy pulsed carbon dioxide laser. *Plast Reconstr Surg*. 1996;98:791-794.
41. Manstein D, Herron GS, Sink RK, et al. Fractional photothermolysis: a new concept for cutaneous remodeling using microscopic patterns of thermal injury. *Lasers Surg Med*. 2004;34:426-438.
The first description of fractional laser treatment and microthermal zones are described. This was a landmark article for the introduction of fractional therapy. The first clinical applications of fractional photothermolysis followed.
42. Karsai S, Czarnecka A, Jünger M, Raulin V. Ablative fractional lasers (CO2 and Er:YAG): a randomized controlled double-blind split-face trial of the treatment of peri-orbital rhytides. *Lasers Surg Med*. 2010;42(2):160-167.
Well-designed study comparing fractional CO_2 *and Er:YAG outcomes in the treatment of periorbital rhytids. The study supports efficacy of both techniques. There is increased recovery and erythema as well as increased efficacy seen with* CO_2.
43. Manaloto RM, Alster T. Erbium:YAG laser resurfacing for refractory melasma. *Dermatol Surg*. 1999;25:121-123.
44. Laubach HJ, Tannous Z, Anderson RR, et al. Skin responses to fractional photothermolysis. *Lasers Surg Med*. 2006;38:142-149.
45. Pozner J, DiBernardo B. Laser resurfacing. *Clin Plast Surg*. 2016;43(3):515-525.
46. Bass LS, DelGuzzo M, Doherty S, et al. Combined ablative and non-ablative fractional treatment for facial skin rejuvenation. *Lasers Surg Med*. 2009;15(suppl):29.
47. Tanzi EL, Alster TS. Single-pass carbon dioxide versus multiple-pass Er: YAG laser skin resurfacing: a comparison of postoperative wound healing and side-effect rates. *Dermatol Surg*. 2003;29:80-84.
48. Ross EV, Sajben FP, Hsia J, et al. Nonablative skin remodeling:selective dermal heating with a mid-infrared laser and contact cooling combination. *Lasers Surg Med*. 2000;26(2):186-195.
49. Rashid T, Hussain I, Haider M, et al. Laser therapy of freckles and lentigines with quasi-continuous, frequency-doubled, Nd: YAG (532 nm) laser in Fitzpatrick skin type IV: a 24-month follow-up. *J Cosmet Laser Ther*. 2002;4:81-85.
50. Ozturk S, Hoopman J, Brown SA, et al. A useful algorithm for determining fluence and pulse width for vascular targets using 1064 nm Nd:YAG laser in an animal model. *Lasers Surg Med*. 2004;34(5):420-425.
51. Sadick NS. Update on non-ablative light therapy for rejuvenation: a review. *Lasers Surg Med*. 2003;32(2):120-128.
A review of nonablative skin resurfacing modalities is presented. A thorough look at the various modalities available and their indications.
52. Nanni CA, Alster TS. Complications of carbon dioxide laser resurfacing: an evaluation of 500 patients. *Dermatol Surg*. 1998;24:315-320.
53. Zenzie HH, Altshuler GB, Smirnov MZ, Anderson RR. Evaluation of cooling methods for laser dermatology. *Lasers Surg Med*. 2000;26:130-144.
54. Wanner M, Sakamoto FH, Avram MM, Anderson RR. Immediate skin responses to laser and light treatmentswarning endpoints: how to avoid side effects. *J Am Acad Dermatol*. 2016;74:807-819.
55. Grimes PE, Bhawan J, Kim J, et al. Laser resurfacing–induced hypopigmentation: histologic alterations and repigmentation with topical photochemotherapy. *Dermatol Surg*. 2001;27:515.

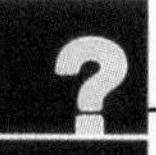

QUESTIONS

1. **What is the clinical end point for full-field CO_2 ablative facial resurfacing?**
   a. Punctate bleeding
   b. Subcutaneous fat
   c. Pale yellow coloration of the skin
   d. No clinical end point, settings determine therapy

2. **What is the clinical end point for full-field erbium:YAG ablative facial resurfacing?**
   a. Punctate bleeding
   b. Subcutaneous fat
   c. Pale yellow coloration of the skin
   d. No clinical end point, settings determine therapy

3. **Two days after full-face erbium laser resurfacing, a 54-year-old otherwise healthy woman with Fitzpatrick type II skin experiences facial pain and pruritus. She has been treated with occlusive dressing immediately post procedure. On examination, there is diffuse erythema and edema. Which of the following is the most likely diagnosis?**
   a. Allergic reaction
   b. Bacterial infection
   c. Fungal Infection
   d. Herpes simplex virus
   e. Normal healing

4. **Which of the following is the beneficial effect of pretreatment with tretinoin prior to facial chemical peel?**
   a. Decreased epidermal proliferation
   b. Decreased fibroblast deposition of glycosaminoglycans
   c. Increased epidermal melanin
   d. Increased transit rate of keratinocytes through the epidermis

5. **A patient returns to the office 2 weeks after full-face carbon dioxide ablative laser resurfacing with persistent erythema and edema. Which of the following topical treatments will decrease the patient's postoperative erythema?**
   a. Amoxicillin
   b. Ascorbic acid
   c. HQ
   d. Prednisone
   e. Valacyclovir

6. **A patient presents to your office with pigmented lesions of the face and desires fractional laser resurfacing. The patient is followed by a dermatologist and completed an oral course of isotretinoin 2 months ago. What is your next step?**
   a. Schedule fractionated laser treatment at next available appointment
   b. Contact the dermatologist and request his opinion on proceeding
   c. Wait 10 months and then schedule the procedure
   d. Begin a course of oral antivirals in preparation for procedure

7. **A patient with Fitzpatrick type III skin type undergoes CO_2 laser resurfacing for facial rhytides and acne scars. What is the patient most at risk for after the procedure?**
   a. Treatment failure
   b. PIH
   c. Infection
   d. Scarring
   e. Hypopigmentation

1. **Answer: c.** Color indicators help define clinical end points for CO_2 ablative laser. Vaporization limited to the epidermis results in an opalescent hue with a cracking sound. Entering the superficial papillary dermis is characterized by a flat smooth pink color with punctate bleeding that progresses to confluent bleeding. Further vaporization into the deeper papillary dermis has a characteristic yellow ***chamois skin*** color, which is the common end point for treatment. Finally, the reticular dermis has a ***waterlogged*** cotton thread appearance.

2. **Answer: a.** Erbium ablative therapy is optimal for fine and superficial skin resurfacing. The goal of treatment is a depth just past the DEJ. This depth is characterized by pinpoint bleeding, which usually is the clinical sign to stop treatment.

3. **Answer: e.** Erythema and edema are expected for routine healing at 48 hours following an ablative laser resurfacing. Desquamation can last anywhere from 5 to 7 days, after which the skin should re-epithelialize. Abnormal postoperative infections would be marked by increased pain, increased drainage, and possible blisters or vesicles if herpes simplex is suspected.

4. **Answer: d.** Tretinoin is one of the most studied resurfacing agents on the market. At a histological level it has been shown to improve the appearance of fine lines by increased glycosaminoglycan content of the skin, decrease melanocyte activity, and increase epidermal proliferation. Epidermal cells have a faster turn over rate as they travel from the basement membrane to the surface.

5. **Answer: b.** Vitamin C, L-ascorbic acid, is powerful antioxidant normally found in the skin. It is rapidly depleted during the inflammatory state. It is readily absorbed transcutaneously and has been shown to decrease both the degree and duration of post–CO_2 laser erythema. It is essential for collagen synthesis and also has photoprotective qualities.

6. **Answer: c.** Isotretinoin, 13-cis-retinoic acid, use has been shown to cause delayed wound healing and potentially abnormal scarring. The mechanism is thought to be related to disruption of keratinocyte adherence along dermal adnexal structures interfering with the skin's ability to re-epithelialize. It is recommended that treatment with isotretinoin be stopped 6 to 12 months prior to any elective cosmetic laser resurfacing procedure to avoid potential complications.

7. **Answer: b.** PIH tends to affect darker skinned patients with greater frequency. It is an acquired hypermelanosis following cutaneous inflammation or injury. Patients with higher Fitzpatrick skin type do not have an increased risk of treatment failure or infection with ablative procedures. They are more likely to develop hyperpigmentation than hypopigmentation.

CHAPTER 46 Dermal and Soft-Tissue Fillers: Principles, Materials, and Techniques

Ivo A. Pestana and Malcolm W. Marks

KEY POINTS

- The use of injectable fillers for tissue augmentation is increasing.
- The most common indication for the use of injectable fillers is minimizing the stigmata of aging.
- Each injectable filler has its own biophysical properties and risk/benefit profile, making an understanding of these characteristics, as well as injection techniques for their application, critical to the safe use of these products.

Soft-tissue augmentation with injectable fillers is one of the most common minimally invasive interventions employed for cosmetic facial and body rejuvenation. According to the American Society of Plastic Surgeons (ASPS) *National Plastic Surgery Statistics*, 2.7 million soft-tissue filler procedures were performed in 2017. This is over a 300% increase compared with the year 2000.[1]

The dramatic increase in the number of filler procedures performed over the years is multifactorial and includes improved access to physicians and physician extenders who perform filler procedures, increased understanding of soft tissue and bone volume alterations associated with the aging process, and improved product quality and marketing. As injectable products and their use rapidly expand, a comprehensive knowledge of indications for filler use, of available filler products and their biologic properties, and of filler complications and their management is essential for the safe execution of soft-tissue filler procedures.

HISTORICAL PERSPECTIVE

Similar to other reconstructive and cosmetic procedures, injectable filler use has its origin in Europe. The first soft-tissue filler employed was autologous free fat. The German surgeon Gustav Adolf Neuber in 1893 harvested several small fat grafts from the arms to fill a soft-tissue depression of the face in a 20-year-old man.[2] Vaseline and paraffin injections for cosmetic purposes were described in 1899 by the Austrian surgeon Robert Gersuny who injected these materials into the scrotum of a man to improve the appearance of the genitals after castration for tuberculous epididymitis.[3] Vaseline, paraffin, and mineral oil remained popular in both Europe and the United States until the early 1900s. Liquid silicone use was popularized for cosmetic purposes in the 1940s and used through the 1970s. Liquid silicone use was associated with multiple complications such as migration of the material, hepatic granulomas and hepatitis, and even death.[4,5]

Because of the problems associated with silicone and other nonautologous fillers, use of autologous fat was revitalized and improved by the invention of the liposuction technique by Fischer in 1974. Later in 1978, French physicians, Illouz and Fournier, further developed the liposuction procedure and introduced it to clinical practice such that by 1980 liposuction was becoming extremely popular in the United States. Subsequently, in 1986, Illouz described the reinjection of fat from liposuction to fill soft-tissue defects.[6]

Nonautologous fillers also advanced in the 1980s with introduction of bovine collagen for the treatment of wrinkles, perioral lines, and certain scar types in 1981. Human-derived collagen and hyaluronic acid (HA) fillers were introduced in the early 2000s. Since that time, modification of HAs fillers and introduction of other filler materials—including poly-L-lactic acid (PLLA) in 2004, calcium hydroxylapatite (CaHA) in 2006, polymethylmethacrylate (PMMA) in 2006, and porcine collagen in 2008—have come to characterized the injectable filler market.

INDICATIONS FOR FILLER USE

Amelioration of the stigmata of aging is the most common indication for the use of injectable fillers. This indication extends to the most visible portions of the human body including the head and neck and, most recently, the hands.[7,8]

The effects of gravity on the skin and muscle in conjunction with extrinsic factors, such as smoking and sun exposure, has been the leading theory that accounts for the aged appearance. Thinning of the skin because of dermal collagen reduction, elastosis, and lipoatrophy has been demonstrated in aging skin and results in characteristic appearance changes (**Figure 46.1**). Common appearance complaints associated with aging are static rhytids of the midface and lower face, drooping of the malar soft tissues, increased prominence of the nasolabial folds, jowl development, and atrophy and actinic changes of the lips including the vermillion border resulting in downturning of the oral commissures.

Recently, vertical descent of the skin and subcutaneous tissue as the main component of aging has been challenged.[9,10] Using computed tomography (CT), Pessa et al. demonstrated a posterior and inferior rotation of the facial skeleton and bony remodeling contributing to the loss of midface projection seen with aging. Alteration in ligamentous support or ligament-resting vectors may also contribute to the characteristic changes seen in the aged individual.[11] Based on the above, it appears that composite tissue (skin, subcutaneous tissue, ligamentous structures of the midface, and bone) changes over time may explain the aged appearance as well as support the benefits of volume restoration provided by filler procedures.[12]

PATIENT SELECTION

Cosmetic filler use is an elective procedure asked for by the patient and therefore careful consideration must be employed prior to the procedure to maximize patient satisfaction and minimize procedure-related complications. In addition to physical examination, a comprehensive medical history, including previous cosmetic procedures (injectables, implants), allergic reactions and sensitivities, acne, keloids, viral infections or dental infections, and immunocompromised states should be obtained to prevent treatment of patients with preexisting conditions that are contraindications to the use of soft-tissue augmentation with injectable fillers.

A critical element of the preprocedural interview must include a discussion of the patient's procedural expectations. These expectations must be thoroughly understood and managed to prevent the expectation of an unrealistic outcome. Each patient must be made aware of the limitations and risks associated with the planned filler as well as the financial commitment associated with injectables because of their finite duration in some cases. Caution should be exercised when caring for an individual who demonstrates signs of underlying mental health disturbances.

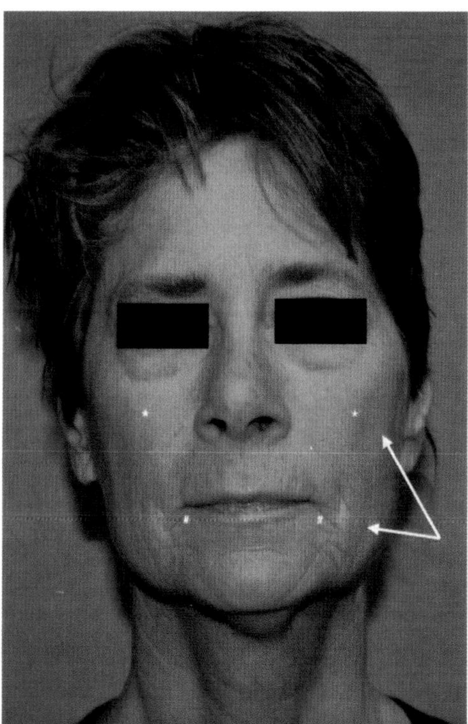

FIGURE 46.1. A 60-year-old woman demonstrating characteristic age-related facial changes. Arrows indicate static rhytids of the midface and lower face. Asterisks mark the drooping of the malar soft tissues. Hashtags indicate atrophy and actinic changes of the lips including the vermillion border resulting in downturning of the oral commissures. The patient also demonstrates visible tear trough deformity at the lower eyelid-cheek junction and increased prominence of the nasolabial folds with associated jowl development.

Patients should be advised that, if medically appropriate, they should stop anti-inflammatory and antiplatelet agents a week prior to treatment to minimize bruising. If this is not possible, the American College of Chest Physicians recommends continuation of anticoagulation for minor skin procedures with low risk of bleeding. Today, there are more than 20,000 herbal supplements/medicines on the market and their use has dramatically increased in the past 2 decades. Common supplements like arnica, bromelain, dong quai, feverfew, garlic, ginger, ginseng, and saw palmetto may increase bleeding; therefore, patients utilizing these products should stop their use 1 to 2 weeks prior to the procedure.[13] As the number of supplements available is vast and difficult to cover completely in a clinic visit, patients may benefit from a list of foods, herbal supplements, and over-the-counter medications to avoid to minimize postprocedural problems or complaints.[14]

PERI-INJECTION PRACTICES AND INJECTION TECHNIQUES

Preinjection

As for all procedures involving the implantation or injection of foreign materials, avoidance of contamination is critical. Practices such as hand cleansing, makeup removal and delay of its reapplication for several hours, skin preparation prior to injection, sterile technique for product reconstitution and dilution, and glove changes after contact with contaminated surfaces or cavities should be employed by all practitioners performing soft-tissue augmentation with fillers. Injection of foreign materials during active skin infections of the planned injection area, or infection in the close vicinity, should be avoided. Patient with infections such as periodontal disease, ear-nose-throat (ENT) infections, or dental abscesses should not be treated until the process has resolved.[15]

Practices to reduce pain associated with filler procedures abound to maximize patient satisfaction with the entire process of filler injection. Ice anesthesia, topical anesthetic mixtures, nerve blocks, and local anesthetic administration to the planned injection area followed by filler injection can be employed. Because of the increased time associated with the above anesthetic practices, concomitant injection of local anesthetic and filler has been described,[16] and filler companies have released products that contain a mixture of the filler and a local anesthetic. Similarly, smaller needles may be associated with reduced pain by minimizing injection site trauma, adjacent soft-tissue trauma, and risk of infection. In general, the smallest needle that allows safe passage of the filler material and affords accurate injection should be utilized. Fillers with low viscosity may be safely injected with 30-gauge needles whereas more viscous fillers should be injected with larger bore needles such as a 27-gauge needle (e.g., CaHA) or 25-gauge needle (e.g., PLLA) to avoid clumping of the material or clogging of the needle itself.

Injection

Commonly described injection techniques include: *serial puncture and droplet technique*, *linear threading*, and *fanning and/or cross-hatching*. The serial puncture and droplet technique requires multiple injections along an area of tissue deficit and deposition of small aliquots of filler material. The injection sites are located in close proximity to allow the material to meld into a continuous line filling and lifting the deficient area. In contradistinction, linear threading deposits filler material in a continuous line. Anterograde and retrograde linear threading have been described, each with their own benefits and drawbacks. Anterograde technique, due to hydrodissection of the planned filler trajectory, may be associated with less bruising as vascular structures in the area may be displaced out of the way of the needle. Retrograde injection of filler as the needle is withdrawn may minimize the risk of intravascular injection and diminish accessory dissected regions, as hydrodissection is not an important component of this technique. Fanning and cross-hatching employ multiple distinct passes of the needle with an administration of filler in different patterns (fan pattern versus grid pattern, respectively) in multiple planes allowing for three-dimensional filling.

Although different products are recommended to be injected at different soft-tissue depths, the majority of product injected is found in the subcutaneous tissues despite use of general visual cues guiding needle depth and use of the various injection techniques.[17] Moreover, certain technique may be associated with the occurrence of local adverse events. Techniques that produce higher levels of subepidermal injury and dissection (fanning, rapid injections, high-injection flow rates, and larger volume filler injections) are associated with higher incidence of local adverse events. On the other hand, techniques that produce more epidermal injury (multiple punctures as in serial puncture or cross-hatching techniques) do not seem to increase the occurrence of adverse events.[18]

Postinjection

Postprocedure management is also important because it may improve the patient's overall experience with the filler visit as well as improve the patient's cosmetic outcome. Distribution and blending of the filler material into the surrounding nontreated areas is assisted by digital molding and massage. Once molding is completed, cold compresses or ice therapy helps reduce swelling and tenderness and is commonly employed to limit early injection site reactions. Finally, reduction in facial expressions for the first 48 hours may be associated with decreased filler material migration and improved patient's cosmetic outcomes.[19]

BIOSCIENCE OF INJECTABLE FILLERS

The number of available injectable filler products, each with its own risk/benefit profile, continues to rapidly expand. Injectable fillers can be broadly grouped into biologic fillers (including autologous tissues) and synthetic fillers (**Table 46.1**).

TABLE 46.1. SOFT TISSUE FILLERS AND THEIR CATEGORIZATION, DURATION OF EFFECT, NEED FOR ALLERGY SKIN TESTING, AND RECOMMENDED DEPTH OF INJECTION

Biologic Fillers	Trade Name	Skin Test	Duration	Depth of Injection
Autologous			Years	Subdermal or subcutaneous
Fat				
Dermis				
Fascia				
Nonautologous				
Collagen			3–6 months	Mid to deep dermis
Bovine	Zyderm 1	X		
	Zyderm 2	X		
	Zyplast	X		
Porcine	Evolence			
	Fibrel			
Human	Cosmoderm 1			
	Cosmoderm 2			
	Cosmoplast			
Hyaluronic acid (HA)			6–12 months	Mid to deep dermis
	Restylane			
	Perlane			
	Juvederm			
	Prevelle Silk			
	Puragen			
	Captique			
	Hylaform			
	Belotero Balance			
	Elevess			
Acellular dermal matrix (ADM)			Years	Subdermal or subcutaneous
	Alloderm			
	Cymetra			
Synthetic				
Poly-L-lactic acid (PLLA)	Sculptra		24 months	Subdermal or subcutaneous
Calcium hydroxylapatite (CaHA)	Radiesse		18 months	Subdermal or subcutaneous
Polymethylmethacrylate (PMMA)	Artefill/Bellafill	X	Permanent	Subdermal or subcutaneous
Silicone			Permanent	Not FDA approved for soft-tissue augmentation
Polytetrafluoroethylene (PTFE)	Gore-Tex		Permanent	Subdermal or subcutaneous

Biologic Fillers

Autologous Biologic Fillers

Autologous tissues continue to be used for soft-tissue augmentation of the face and other locations of the body. Tissues currently employed for soft-tissue volume augmentation include fat, dermis, and fascia.

Despite being the first soft-tissue filler described, autologous fat remains a popular option for volume augmentation today. In the face, autologous fat is used to fill deep wrinkles, minimize soft-tissue depressions and skin folds, and improve regions of fat atrophy. In addition, this technique may be employed for augmentation of lip volume. Fat injection is advantageous because there is no risk of an allergic reaction or rejection of foreign material. Moreover, the injected fat tends to be longer lasting than foreign materials used for soft-tissue augmentation. A complete description of autologous fat grafting is beyond the scope of this chapter. Please see Chapter 48 *Fat Grafting in Plastic Surgery* for a more in-depth discussion of this technique.

Dermis and fascia are alternative autologous tissues used for soft-tissue augmentation. Both dermal and fascial grafts have incorporation rates equivalent to that of autologous fat and provide similar duration of improvement.[20,21] Because of advancement in lipofilling techniques as well as improvements in nonautologous filler products, autologous dermal and fascial grafting have been employed less frequently because they require excision of tissue for graft preparation.[22]

Nonautologous Biologic Fillers

Collagen

The bovine collagen filler Zyderm (Inamed Corp., Santa Barbara, Calif.) was the first nonautologous filler to be approved by the U.S. Food and Drug Administration (FDA). Because of its high immunologic reactivity, bovine collagen requires double skin testing consisting of injecting 0.1 mL of the product into the antecubital area and, 30 days later, injecting a separate body area with the product. A positive skin test is a local wheal-and-flare reaction within 48 to 72 hours. In general, less than 5% of patients will manifest a positive test. Furthermore, a negative skin test indicates less than 0.5% risk of allergic reaction to the bovine collagen product. Both human collagen products, Cosmoderm (Inamed) and Cosmoplast (Inamed), and porcine collagen products, called Evolence (Colbar LifeScience Ltd., Herzliya, Isreal) and Fibrel (Mentor Worldwide, LC, Santa Barbara, Calif.), have a low risk of allergic reaction and do not require skin testing prior to treatment.

Collagen injection has been demonstrated to improve nasolabial folds for a period of 3 to 6 months with a 75% loss of filler correction by 6 months after injection. Collagen injection for the improvement of wrinkles and nasolabial folds has been compared with other injectable fillers (most commonly HA) in randomized clinical trials. HA is equal to or superior to collagen in correcting nasolabial folds for longer periods of time.[23] Furthermore, HAs do not require allergy testing prior to injection. Because of the above, the manufacture of collagen-based fillers has largely been discontinued.

Hyaluronic Acid

Hyaluronic acids (HAs) are glycosaminoglycans which are natural components of connective tissue in living organisms. HAs are chemically identical in all species; therefore, no allergy skin testing is required prior to their use. A key feature of HA proteins is their hypdrophilic properties which act to maintain moisture within the dermis, therefore accounting for their capability of filling/lifting soft-tissue deficits. Regarding their production, HAs may be animal-based or non–animal-based. Animal-based HA fillers, which are no longer marketed in the United States, are derived from rooster combs whereas non–animal-based HAs are derived from bacterial fermentation of *Streptococcus equi*.

HAs have specific, modifiable characteristics that account for their biophysical properties. HA cross-linking, viscosity, and elastic modulus (G') account for the physiologic behavior of the filler. A greater degree of cross-linking correlates clinically with longer duration of effect of the filler. Use of other chemical compounds such as epoxides, which stabilize cross-links, or the incorporation of varying degrees of cross-linking in a single product, may contribute to prolong filler efficacy.[24] Viscosity refers to the ability of the gel to resist shear forces and the elastic modulus refers to the ability of the gel to resist deformation. Factors affecting viscosity include size and molecular weight of the HA particles. The G' level is determined by bond strength which, in turn, dictates the degree that bonds between particles stretch with applied forces. Clinically, variations in G' manifest as differential ability to lift tissue where higher G' translates into greater tissue lift but firmer feel. Higher viscosity is associated with decreased spread of the filler within tissues but also with decreased ease of injection.

The first HA filler to receive FDA approval for the correction of facial wrinkles was Restylane (Q-Med Esthetics, Uppsala, Sweden) in 2003. Since that time, HAs, particularly Restylane (Q-Med Esthetics) and Juvederm (Allergan, Inc., Irvine, Calif.), have been the most studied of the injectable fillers, and treatment regions included most commonly the nasolabial folds but also the lips, glabellar lines, the upper extremity (arm and hand), cheeks, and the chin. In general, randomized clinical trials demonstrated that HAs are equivalent or superior to human, bovine, and porcine collagen in correcting nasolabial folds as well as volume deficits at other sites including the dorsal hands.[25] In a prospective study from Canada, HAs were demonstrated to be a safe method to correct age-related lip complaints for over a 6-month period in some cases[26] (**Figure 46.2**). In other uncontrolled clinical trials, HAs have been safely utilized for cosmetic improvement of the chin and cheeks lasting up to 6 to 12 months.[27]

Since Restylane's FDA approval, other HA fillers have received similar approval in the United States and these include Perlane (Inamed), Juvederm Ultra and Ultra Plus (Allergan), Juvederm Volbella, Puragen and Prevelle Silk (Mentor Worldwide, LC, Santa

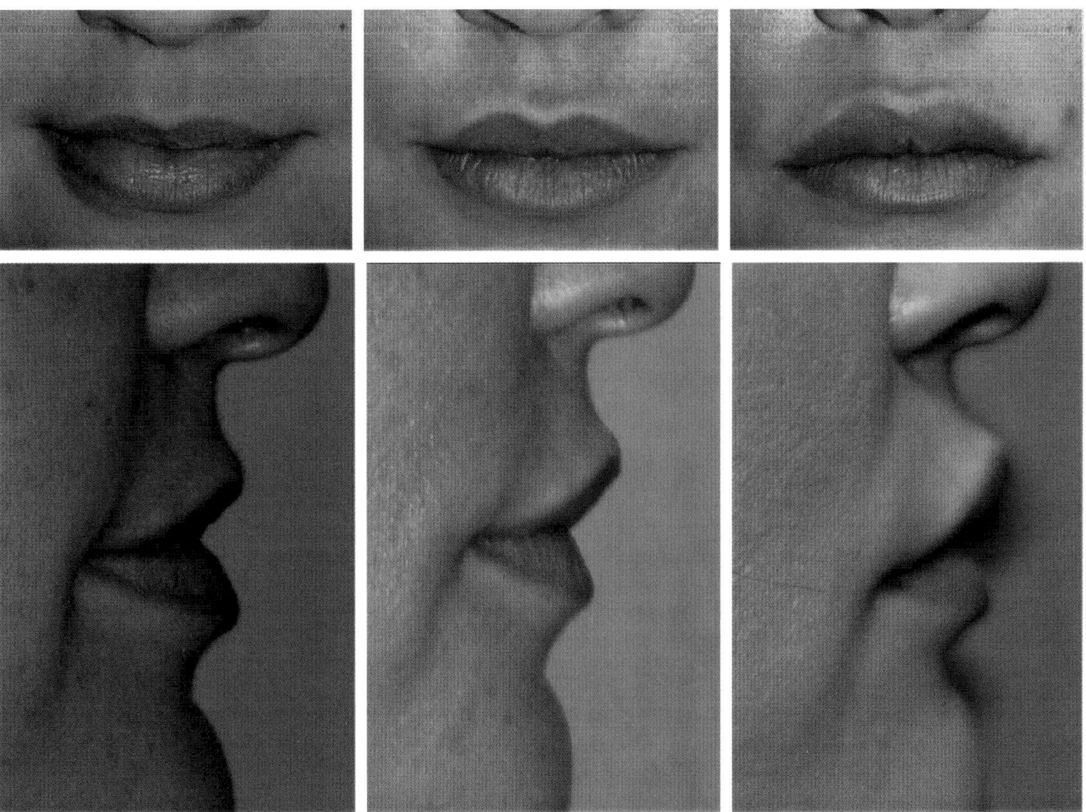

FIGURE 46.2. A 40-year-old woman with lip volume loss treated with hyaluronic acid filler (Juvederm Volbella). Note the significant improvement in upper lip *plumpness* and rotation of the upper lip in a cephalad direction producing an aesthetic improvement in lip appearance.

Barbara, Calif.), Captique and Hylaform (Genzyme Biosurgery), and Belotero Balance (Merz Aesthetics). HA fillers containing local anesthetics, such as Restylane Silk, Juvederm XC and Ultra Plus XC, Juvederm Voluma XC, Juvederm Volbella XC, Juvederm Vollure XC, and Elevess (Anika Therapeutics), are available and patients report less procedural pain when these formulations are utilized.[28]

Acellular Dermal Matrix

Subdermally implanted acellular dermal matrix (ADM) material has been described for soft-tissue volume augmentation. Sclafani et al. compared Alloderm (Lifecell) disks or micronized Alloderm to the bovine collagen product, Zyplast, in the postauricular region of adult patients. Alloderm's duration of persistence in this anatomic region was longer than that of bovine collagen and showed promise as an alternative filler not requiring skin testing.[29,30] An injectable acellular dermal graft (Cymetra; Lifecell Corp., Branchburg, N.J.) has been developed and demonstrated to be effective in improving upper lip volume and lower lip projection without local or systemic complications.[31]

Synthetic Fillers

Synthetic fillers are composed of biodegradable materials that stimulate endogenous tissue growth.

Poly-L-Lactic Acid

Derived from cornstarch, PLLA is a biodegradeable, nontoxic, and inactive material that has been utilized in the production of indwelling stents, suture material, and meshes. Sculptra (Galderma Laboratories, L.P., Fort Worth, Texas) was the first FDA-approved PLLA filler. In 2004, it was approved for the correction of facial lipoatrophy associated with treatment of human immunodeficiency virus (HIV). In contradistinction to HA fillers, PLLA is a hydrophobic compound and requires reconstitution with bacteriostatic water for a minimum of 3 hours prior to injection. In the body, PLLA is metabolized to carbon dioxide, glucose, and water for several months after injection, which accounts for the characteristic delayed achievement of the desired effect with use of this filler type. Once achieved, the filler effect has a duration of approximately 18 to 24 months which is due to fibroblast stimulation and deposition of type 1 collagen into the areas of PLLA microspheres.

PLLA correction of facial lipoatrophy in patients suffering the sequelae of antiretroviral agents has been demonstrated in randomized controlled clinical trials.[32] Regarding its use in non–HIV patients for cosmetic improvement of soft-tissue volume deficits of the face (cheeks, chin, perioral, and periorbital region), PLLA has improved cosmetic complaints for a duration of up to 24 months. Of note, use of the filler in the perioral and periorbital regions may be associated with an increase risk of skin papules or subcutaneous nodules; therefore, caution should be used or treatment avoided in these areas.[33]

Calcium Hydroxylapatite

Calcium hydroxylapatite (CaHA) is another highly biocompatible material naturally occurring in the human body as the mineral component of bone. Radiesse (Bioform Medical, Inc., San Mateo, Calif.) received FDA approval in 2006 for the correction of antiretroviral medication–associated facial lipoatrophy as well as for the cosmetic correction of facial wrinkles and folds. Because of CaHA's suspension in a cellulose gel, this product is highly viscous and deep injection is recommended.

CaHA as a cosmetic filler has been compared to collagen and HAs in randomized clinical trials. CaHA was noted to have significantly better nasolabial fold improvement at 8 months postinjection when compared to several HA fillers and to collagen products.[34,35] In other clinical trials, CaHA has been safely employed for malar soft-tissue augmentation with injection into the subdermal and subcutaneous planes.[36]

Polymethylmethacrylate

Polymethylmethacrylate (PMMA) is a permanent material that has been used in healthcare since its introduction in 1928. Applications have included bone surgery and cement, dental rejuvenation, and cardiac devices. Bellafill (Suneva Medical, San Diego, Calif.) is the FDA-approved version of this product, and it is approved for the correction of moderate to severe facial scars in patients over 21 years of age. Of note, this product contains bovine collagen; therefore, patients must undergo skin testing prior to its use.

Silicone

Injectable silicone is produced from silica and has many manufacturers and different manufactured viscosities. The use of this permanent product as an injectable filler for cosmetic purposes is considered off-label. Injectable silicone has been described for soft-tissue augmentation, but its use has been fraught with inconsistencies in terms of outcomes, the development of granulomas, product infection, and extrusion.

Gore-Tex

Polytetrafluoroethylene (PTFE), or Gore-Tex (W. L. Gore Associates, Flagstaff, Ariz.), is a permanent material that has been described for soft-tissue augmentation. Compared with silicone, this material allows higher levels of tissue ingrowth. Similar to silicone, it is prone to outcome inconsistencies, granuloma formation, infection, and extrusion.

ADVERSE EVENTS AND THEIR MANAGEMENT

Injectable fillers rarely have side effects such that most complications are procedural rather that product-related.

Superficial Filler Placement

Most injectable fillers are recommended to be placed into the deep dermis or deeper planes. Filler material in planes superficial to the deep dermis appear differently based upon the type of filler used.

HAs placed too superficially produce small lumps or visible bumps. These irregularities frequently appear quickly and may exhibit a bluish coloration that is called the Tyndall effect. This effect, named after the physicist John Tyndall, results from differing wavelengths of light scattering because of the filler particles in a very fine suspension underneath the superficial layers of skin. HAs placed excessively superficial can be managed immediately with a massage to distribute the filler more evenly in the soft-tissue region being treated. If this is inadequate, hyaluronidase may be administered. Hyaluronidase is an enzyme that metabolizes HA and this enzyme is commonly an animal-based preparation. Hyaluronidase is diluted, commonly with local anesthetic, prior to injection. Practitioners using hyaluronidase must be aware that, depending upon the preparation of hyaluronidase used, patients may have a reaction to the medication if it is animal-based and this likely results from a sensitivity to animal protein or thimerisol contained in the preparation. If hyaluronidase fails to correct the lumps or bumps resulting from HAs placed too superficially, incision and drainage with the use of an 18-gauge needle or no. 11 blade scalpel may be completed to express the product from the dermis.

CaHA placed superficial to the deep dermis appears as white nodules in the skin. As described above, incision and drainage may be required to correct the skin nodules created. Because of the biochemical properties of CaHA, the material when placed too superficially or in highly mobile regions (lips) tends to migrate and subsequently coalesce into nodules. Massage and incision/drainage have been described to treat this problem.

Available preparations of PMMA contain bovine collagen and superficial placement of this product is associated with pruritis, redness, and hypertrophic scarring.[37] Topical steroid use and intralesional corticosteroid administration may be employed to ameliorate these problems.

Hypersensitivity Reactions

Hypersensitivity to nonautologous filler material may range from mild skin irritation to anaphylaxis. These reactions can occur despite appropriate skin testing and meticulous filler selection individualized to the patient. HAs, despite their structure being identical in all species, have been associated with angioedema reactions when injected into the lips. Common manifestations of hypersensitivity reaction to injectable fillers include erythema, induration, burning, and subcutaneous lumps. The reactions may be managed with intralesional corticosteroids, oral antihistamines, or systemic steroids depending on the severity of symptomatology.

Nodule Formation (Acute Versus Delayed)

Nodule formation may be considered acute or delayed. Acute nodule formation is commonly a result of filler material placement superficial to the deep dermis (see earlier section Superficial Filler Placement). Delayed nodule formation may be attributed to a granulomatous reaction and occur several weeks after filler injection.[38] These nodules may present as painful, red, and inflamed bumps. The differential diagnosis for these findings includes allergic reaction, foreign body reaction, sterile abscess, or acute infection. Recently, biofilm-producing bacteria have been implicated in the development of delayed-presentation nodules after the use of dermal fillers leading to consideration of antibiotic use after a filler procedure.[39] Specific to the type of filler used, interventions to prevent and manage delayed nodules have been developed. Despite increasing reconstitution times and placement of this filler in deeper tissue planes, PLLA nodule risk remains. If PLLA nodules persist or present in a delayed fashion, management options include intralesional steroids alone or in combination with imiquimod or 5-fluorouracil. If PLLA nodules persist despite these interventions, surgical excision may be the only option to arrive at satisfactory result. Similar to PLLA, CaHA nodules can be managed with surgical excision. For HA-associated delayed nodules, hyaluronidase injection, empiric antibiotics, and incision and drainage are management options.

Skin Necrosis and Vision Loss

Vascular structure being compressed due to filler material or vessel occlusion due to intravascular injection of filler material may occur. Although rare, this may result in skin necrosis along the distribution of the compromised vasculature. The glabellar region is considered a high-risk area due to the small caliber of the supratrochlear vessels. Anatomic communication between the terminal branches of the angular artery and terminal branches of the ophthalmic artery (supratrochlear and supraorbital arteries) has been implicated in the occurrence of blindness after intraarterial injection of filler material in the dorsal nasal region and glabella.[40] Techniques and interventions to reduce the risk of skin injury or necrosis include aspiration prior to injection of the filler material, serial puncture technique use, antegrade or retrograde linear threading technique use, skin tenting prior to injection to allow accurate placement of filler superficial to arterial structures, and manual occlusion of larger vessels in the treatment zone prior to injection. If a vascular problem is identified, immediate action to augment blood flow is necessary to preserve tissue. These interventions include application of warm gauze, tapping the area to produce vasodilation, and use of nitroglycerin paste to the affected region. If a HA filler was utilized and the working diagnosis is external compression of the vessel or intraarterial injection, hyaluronidase injection in the previous injection site and along the affected vessels course is the mainstay of treatment. Treatment adjuncts may involve intraarterial hyaluronidase, hyperbaric oxygen therapy, and ancillary vasodilating agents such as prostaglandin E1.[41]

Scarring

Fortunately, scarring after filler procedures is rare. Multiple studies employing a variety of filler material, including longer-acting products, have not demonstrated increased risk of hypertrophic scarring or keloid formation, even when employed in Fitzpatrick skin types IV to VI.[42]

FUTURE OF SOFT-TISSUE AUGMENTATION

Multidisciplinary efforts to identify and develop the ideal soft-tissue augmentation material and technique of its application will continue. Because it is unrealistic to expect that one product will be applicable to all patients with an indication for filler use, the perfect filler material must continue to be individualized to the patient based upon the location of the volume deficit, potential for hypersensitivity reactions or complications, and desired duration of the filler's effect.

REFERENCES

1. American Society of Plastic Surgeons. *Plastic Surgery National Statistics*; 2017. Available from https://www.plasticsurgery.org/documents/News/Statistics/2017/plastic-surgery-statistics-report-2017.pdf.
2. Neuber F. Fettransplantation Bericht uber die Verhandlungen der Deutscht Gesellsch Chir. *Zentralblatt Chir*. 1893;22:66.
   Seminal article describing the harvest of several small fat grafts from the arms to fill a facial soft-tissue depression in a 20-year-old man. This is the first injectable filler *described in the medical literature.*
3. Gersuny R. Ueber eine subcutane Prothese. *Z Heilkd*. 1900:199-204.
4. Ellenbogen R, Rubin L. Injectable fluid silicone therapy: human morbidity and mortality. *JAMA*. 1975;234(3):308-309.
5. Achauer BM. A serious complication following medical-grade silicone injection of the face. *Plast Reconstr Surg*. 1983;71(2):251-254
6. Illouz YG. The fat cell "graft": a new technique to fill depressions. *Plast Reconstr Surg*. 1986;78(1):122-123
   Dr. Illouz's letter to the editor describing the use of fat harvested from liposuction for the correction of dimples, depressions, or hollows, or to fill in natural or accidental depressions *in 37 patients with good results.*
7. Butterwick KJ. Rejuvenation of the aging hand. *Dermatol Clin*. 2005;23(3):515-527.
8. Hoang D, Orgel MI, Kulber DA. Hand rejuvenation: a comprehensive review of fat grafting. *J Hand Surg Am*. 2016;41(5):639-644.
9. Pessa JE. An algorithm of facial aging: verification of Lambros's theory by three-dimensional stereolithography, with reference to the pathogenesis of midfacial aging, scleral show, and the lateral suborbital trough deformity. *Plast Reconstr Surg*. 2000;106(2):479-488.
10. Lambros V. Observations on periorbital and midface aging. *Plast Reconstr Surg*. 2007;120(5):1367-1376.
11. Muzaffar AR, Mendelson BC, Adams WP Jr. Surgical anatomy of the ligamentous attachments of the lower lid and lateral canthus. *Plast Reconstr Surg*. 2002;110(3):873-884.
12. Donath AS, Glasgold RA, Glasgold MJ. Volume loss versus gravity: new concepts in facial aging. *Curr Opin Otolaryngol Head Neck Surg*. 2007;15(4):238-243.
13. Broughton G II, Crosby MA, Coleman J, Rohrich RJ. Use of herbal supplements and vitamins in plastic surgery: a practical review. *Plast Reconstr Surg*. 2007;119(3):48e-66e.
14. De Boulle K, Heydenrych I. Patient factors influencing dermal filler complications: prevention, assessment, and treatment. *Clin Cosmet Investig Dermatol*. 2015;8:205-214.
15. Narins RS, Coleman WP III, Glogau RG. Recommendations and treatment options for nodules and other filler complications. *Dermatol Surg*. 2009;35(suppl 2):1667-1671.
16. Rohrich RJ, Herbig KS. Minimizing pain, maximizing comfort: a new technique for facial filler injections. *Plast Reconstr Surg*. 2009;124(4):1328-1329.
    One of the first descriptions of the combination of injectable filler and local anesthetic to improve patient comfort during filler procedures.
17. Arlette JP, Trotter MJ. Anatomic location of hyaluronic acid filler material injected into nasolabial fold: a histologic study. *Dermatol Surg*. 2008;34(suppl 1):S56-S62.
18. Glogau RG, Kane MA. Effect of injection techniques on the rate of local adverse events in patients implanted with nonanimal hyaluronic acid gel dermal fillers. *Dermatol Surg*. 2008;34(suppl 1):S105-S109.
19. Alam M, Gladstone H, Kramer EM, et al. ASDS guidelines of care: injectable fillers. *Dermatol Surg*. 2008;34(suppl 1):S115-S148.
20. Kempf KK, Seyfer AE. Facial defect augmentation with a dermal-fat graft. *Oral Surg Oral Med Oral Pathol*. 1985;59(4):340-343.
21. Erol OO. Facial autologous soft-tissue contouring by adjunction of tissue cocktail injection (micrograft and minigraft mixture of dermis, fascia, and fat). *Plast Reconstr Surg*. 2000;106(6):1375-1387.

22. Bassetto F, Turra G, Salmaso R, et al. Autologous injectable dermis: a clinical and histological study. *Plast Reconstr Surg*. 2013;131(4):589e-596e.
23. Baumann LS, Shamban AT, Lupo MP, et al. Comparison of smooth-gel hyaluronic acid dermal fillers with cross-linked bovine collagen: a multicenter, double-masked, randomized, within-subject study. *Dermatol Surg*. 2007;33(suppl 2):S128-S135.
    Multicenter, blinded, and randomized trial comparing hyaluronic acid (HA) to bovine collagen for nasolabial fold correction in 439 patients. This study demonstrated that HAs offer longer-lasting correction of the nasolabial folds when compared to collagen and the majority of test subjects preferred HAs to bovine collagen.
24. Wang F, Garza LA, Kang S, et al. In vivo stimulation of de novo collagen production caused by cross-linked hyaluronic acid dermal filler injections in photodamaged human skin. *Arch Dermatol*. 2007;143(2):155-163.
25. Man J, Rao J, Goldman M. A double-blind, comparative study of nonanimal-stabilized hyaluronic acid versus human collagen for tissue augmentation of the dorsal hands. *Dermatol Surg*. 2008;34(8):1026-1031.
26. Carruthers J, Klein AW, Carruthers A, et al. Safety and efficacy of nonanimal stabilized hyaluronic acid for improvement of mouth corners. *Dermatol Surg*. 2005;31(3):276-280.
27. DeLorenzi C, Weinberg M, Solish N, Swift A. The long-term efficacy and safety of a subcutaneously injected large-particle stabilized hyaluronic acid-based gel of nonanimal origin in esthetic facial contouring. *Dermatol Surg*. 2009;35(suppl 1):313-321.
28. Weinkle SH, Bank DE, Boyd CM, et al. A multi-center, double-blind, randomized controlled study of the safety and effectiveness of Juvederm injectable gel with and without lidocaine. *J Cosmet Dermatol*. 2009;8(3):205-210.
29. Sclafani AP, Romo T III, Jacono AA, et al. Evaluation of acellular dermal graft in sheet (AlloDerm) and injectable (micronized AlloDerm) forms for soft tissue augmentation: clinical observations and histological analysis. *Arch Facial Plast Surg*. 2000;2(2):130-136.
30. Sclafani AP, Romo T III, Jacono AA, et al. Evaluation of acellular dermal graft (AlloDerm) sheet for soft tissue augmentation: a 1-year follow-up of clinical observations and histological findings. *Arch Facial Plast Surg*. 2001;3(2):101-103.
31. Sclafani AP, Romo T III, Jacono AA. Rejuvenation of the aging lip with an injectable acellular dermal graft (Cymetra). *Arch Facial Plast Surg*. 2002;4(4):252-257.
32. El-Beyrouty C, Huang V, Darnold CJ, Clay PG. Poly-L-lactic acid for facial lipoatrophy in HIV. *Ann Pharmacother*. 2006;40(9):1602-1606.
33. Lowe NJ, Maxwell CA, Lowe P, et al. Injectable poly-l-lactic acid: 3 years of aesthetic experience. *Dermatol Surg*. 2009;35(suppl 1):344-349.
34. Moers-Carpi M, Vogt S, Santos BM, et al. A multicenter, randomized trial comparing calcium hydroxylapatite to two hyaluronic acids for treatment of nasolabial folds. *Dermatol Surg*. 2007;33(suppl 2):S144-S151.
35. Smith S, Busso M, McClaren M, Bass LS. A randomized, bilateral, prospective comparison of calcium hydroxylapatite microspheres versus human-based collagen for the correction of nasolabial folds. *Dermatol Surg*. 2007;33(suppl 2):S112-S121.
36. Beer K, Yohn M, Cohen JL. Evaluation of injectable CaHA for the treatment of mid-face volume loss. *J Drugs Dermatol*. 2008;7(4):359-366.
37. Lemperle G, Romano JJ, Busso M. Soft tissue augmentation with artecoll: 10-year history, indications, techniques, and complications. *Dermatol Surg*. 2003;29(6):573-587.
38. Lemperle G, Gauthier-Hazan N, Wolters M, Eisemann-Klein M, Zimmermann U, Duffy DM. Foreign body granulomas after all injectable dermal fillers: part 1. Possible causes. *Plast Reconstr Surg*. 2009;123(6):1842-1863.
39. Beer K, Avelar R. Relationship between delayed reactions to dermal fillers and biofilms: facts and considerations. *Dermatol Surg*. 2014;40(11):1175-1179.
40. Tansatit T, Moon HJ, Apinuntrum P, Phetudom T. Verification of embolic channel causing blindness following filler injection. *Aesthet Plast Surg*. 2015;39(1):154-161.
41. DeLorenzi C. Complications of injectable fillers, part 2: vascular complications. *Aesthet Surg J*. 2014;34(4):584-600.
42. Marmur ES, Taylor SC, Grimes PE, et al. Six-month safety results of calcium hydroxylapatite for treatment of nasolabial folds in Fitzpatrick skin types IV to VI. *Dermatol Surg*. 2009;35(suppl 2):1641-1645.

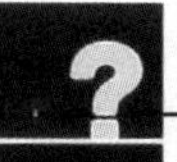

QUESTIONS

1. **Which of the following characteristics of hyaluronic acid dermal fillers may be modified to produce prolonged results?**
   a. Cross-linking
   b. Particle size
   c. Viscosity
   d. Gel hardness (G′)

2. **Accidental injection of hyaluronic acid filler into which of the following areas is most likely to cause blindness by retrograde occlusion of the central retinal artery?**
   a. Cheek
   b. Lip commissure
   c. Nasal dorsum
   d. Philtral column
   e. Nasolabial fold

3. **A 55 year-old woman receives an injection of 0.5 mL of hyaluronic acid filler into the nasolabial folds bilaterally. She returns to the office 30 minutes later because of moderate pain and mottled skin discoloration of the nasal tip and right side of her nose. Which of the following is the most appropriate next step in management?**
   a. CT angiogram of the face
   b. Prostaglandin E1 injection
   c. Lidocaine injection
   d. Massage
   e. Hyaluronidase injection

4. **A 40-year-old woman desires longer-lasting correction of her nasolabial folds. She has had excellent results previously with hyaluronic acid fillers. Calcium hydroxyapatite is injected and on follow-up examination 1 week later, the patient is unhappy with white nodules along the treated nasolabial folds. Which of the following is the least effective treatment option to address the white nodules?**
   a. Direct excision of the filler
   b. Injection of a corticosteroid
   c. Massage of the folds
   d. Needle disruption and unroofing of the lumps

5. **A 45-year-old woman comes to the office for consultation regarding correction of her deep nasolabial folds. Soft-tissue fillers are considered. Which of the following filler products is most likely to result in a hypersensitivity reaction?**
   a. Polymethylmethacrylate (Belafill)
   b. Calcium hydroxylapatite (Radiesse)
   c. Human collagen (CosmoPlast)
   d. Hyaluronic acid (Restylane)
   e. Porcine collagen (Evolence)

1. **Answer: a.** All hyaluronic acids (HAs) are hydrophilic polymers and in the United States, they are all produced from bacteria. HAs may be differentiated by their degree of cross-linking, viscosity, and gel hardness (elastic modulus or G′). Cross-linking produces a gel like product, and the degree of cross-linking is directly proportional to the products duration. Viscosity is affected by particle size and molecular weight. It is important when evaluating dermal fillers and relates more to ease of injection and depth of injection rather than persistence of the product. Larger particles must be injected deeper into the dermis or subcutaneously to avoid visibility. The elastic modulus level is determined by bond strength which, in turn, dictates the degree that bonds between particles can stretch with applied forces. Clinically, variations in G' manifest as differential ability to lift tissue where higher G' translates into greater tissue lift.

2. **Answer: c.** The glabellar region and the nasal dorsum are areas considered to be high-risk for resultant blindness after filler injection. Anatomic communication between the terminal branches of the angular artery and terminal branches of the ophthalmic artery (dorsal nasal artery, supratrochlear and supraorbital arteries) has been implicated in this process. During nasal dorsum augmentation, accidental injection of filler into the dorsal nasal artery under pressure can push the filler retrograde into the ophthalmic artery. The filler then can flow distally occluding the retinal artery and causing vision changes or blindness. Intravascular injection of fillers into the angular artery of the nasolabial fold can also cause blindness, although this would more commonly result in skin mottling and necrosis of the nasal tip skin. The cheek area, overlying the malar bone, is a safe place for injectable filler administration, as there are few deep vessels in this region.

3. **Answer: e.** This patient presents with signs and symptoms consistent with right-sided nasal vascular embarrassment due to hyaluronic acid (HA) filler injection. Because there are visible ischemic changes of the nasal tip and lateral nose, emergency treatment to restore circulation is required. Massage of the HA filler is usually inadequate for management of skin ischemia and pending necrosis. The mainstay of treatment for intraarterial injection of HA products is local injection of hyaluronidase into the site of injection and the local area of skin mottling. Other treatments used as adjuncts to hyaluronidase administration include massaging the area in order to promote distribution of hyaluronidase, warm compresses, and application of topical nitroglycerin paste. Intraarterial hyaluronidase, hyperbaric oxygen therapy, and other vasodilating agents such as prostaglandin E1 have been described as ancillary treatments in conjunction with hyaluronidase use. Imaging of the affected area with computed tomography angiography, magnetic resonance angiogram (MRA), or Doppler ultrasound would delay treatment and are not indicated.

4. **Answer: b.** Calcium hydroxyapatite (CaHA) is a highly biocompatible material naturally occurring in the human body as the mineral component of bone. It received FDA approval in 2006 for the correction of antiretroviral medication–associated facial lipoatrophy as well as for the cosmetic correction of facial wrinkles and folds. Because CaHA is suspended in a cellulose gel, this product is highly viscous and deep injection is recommended. In addition to injection below the dermis, safe injection of this material includes prevention of overcorrection, prevention of clumping of filler due to bolus injections, and use of postinjection massage. The patient described has an acute nodule formation after CaHA injection. If acute nodules form (which usually occur in areas of thin soft-tissue coverage such as the eyelids, lips, and nasolabial region), there are multiple described effective treatments, which include direct excision, observation to allow for the product to resorb, and needle disruption and unroofing. Intralesional corticosteroids are not effective in the management of acute nodule formation after CaHA injection.

5. **Answer: a**. Hypersensitivity reactions with soft-tissue fillers are relatively uncommon. Local reactions can occur with any of the fillers, but most reactions likely stem from local irritation associated with the technique of injection or quantity injected versus a true allergic reaction. In the case of Bellafill, because the preparation of polymethylmethacrylate (PMMA) contains bovine collagen, risk of allergic reaction is present; so skin testing is required prior to its use. The other fillers listed have much lower incidences of reactions. Thus, they do not require skin tests prior to injection. CosmoPlast is derived from a single human fibroblast cell culture and is treated with glutaraldehyde to decrease its immunogenicity. Evolence is a porcine-derived collagen. It is much less immunogenic than bovine collagen. During its preparation, it is treated to remove allergenic telopeptides. Restylane is a hyaluronic acid–based product. Because it is not derived from animals, it is also associated with a lower risk of allergic reactions than the bovine collagen–containing product.

CHAPTER 47 Botulinum Toxin

Scott T. Hollenbeck and David A. Brown

KEY POINTS

- Botulinum toxin is derived from the *Clostridium botulinum* bacterium and functions to inhibit acetylcholine release from the neuromuscular junction by targeting SNAP/SNARE receptors.
- Three commercial preparations of botulinum toxin A are currently available in the United States: Botox (onabotulinumtoxinA), Dysport (abobotulinumtoxin), and Xeomin (incobotulinumtoxinA).
- FDA-approved aesthetic indications for botulinum toxin use are glabellar lines and lateral canthal lines (crow's feet); off-label uses include forehead lines, lateral nasal lines, perioral rhytids, marionette lines, and platysmal bands.
- Recommended dosing for treatment of glabellar lines with Botox is 4 units intramuscularly into each of five sites in the corrugator and procerus muscles, for a total of 20 units.
- Aminoglycosides, penicillamine, quinine, and calcium channels may potentiate the effects of botulinum toxin; whereas choloroquine and hydroxychloroquine may reduce the effects.
- Absolute contraindications include known hypersensitivity reactions to any ingredient in the formulation, including lactose (Dysport) and albumin (all preparations), as well as preexisting infections at the injection sites.

The nerve conduction is brought by the toxin into a condition in which its influence on the chemical process of life is interrupted. The capacity of nerve conduction is interrupted by the toxin in the same way as in an electrical conductor by rust.

Justinus Kerner, *New Observations on the Lethal Poisoning Occurring so Frequently in Wurttemberg through the Consumption of Smoked Sausages* (1822).

HISTORY OF BOTULINUM TOXIN THERAPEUTIC USE

From a deadly food-borne neurotoxin that plagued the premodern era to a cosmetic surgery sensation, the story of botulinum toxin in human society is as fascinating in its detail as it is ironic in its history. Botulinum toxin type A is a zinc metalloprotease exotoxin derived from the gram-positive, spore-forming bacillus *Clostridium botulinum*; it is the agent responsible for the lethal paralytic condition known as botulism. The most toxic, known, naturally occurring substance, it is so poisonous that one-millionth of a gram can kill an adult, and a pint could kill every person on earth. In 2017, over 7 million medical procedures involving botulinum toxin are performed in the United States annually, with a staggering growth rate of 819% between 2000 and 2017. As the most frequently performed cosmetic procedure in the country, this specialty drug occupies a central place in the plastic surgery toolkit. The indications for botulinum toxin in medicine are ever-expanding, and it is anticipated that many readers of this chapter will continue to shape the evolution of this drug by contributing to its study across new frontiers in medicine. As we will elaborate in the following pages, botulinum toxin is a powerful, accessible, and productive treatment modality for a variety of applications in plastic surgery.

The disease was first described in Europe in 1735, named after the Latin word for sausage, *botulus*, as it was originally suspected of being acquired from German sausage. Throughout the 19th century, the epidemic of *sausage poisoning*stood as a major source of food poisoning in Europe.[1] Justinus Kerner, a German physician and romantic poet, was the first to conduct experiments on both animals and himself. Kerner observed that the toxin acts by interrupting signals in the somatic and autonomic nervous systems, though spares the central and sensory systems. He uncovered a number of highly relevant aspects of the toxin, including its lethality in very small dosages and its ability to develop in anaerobic conditions.[2] In a striking example of forethought, he even postulated the use of the toxin for therapeutic relevance over 150 years before its first clinical application.[3]

Over the next century, the bacterial origins of the toxin were demonstrated, along with strategies to mitigate growth of Clostridial bacteria in food. Military applications were also explored. According to a *New York Times* report in 1982, several nations produced botulism toxins during World War II as a potential biologic weapon.[4] The agent was even spray-tested over a section of Canadian wilderness, which reportedly killed all animals within 6 hours, although was never used in war. Today, botulism is relatively rare, owing to improved techniques of food preparation and storage that limit the growth of anaerobic organisms.[5]

Clinical use of botulinum toxin type A was pioneered by the ophthalmologist Alan Scott, who first tested the compound in primates[6] and later reported its use in a series of patients with strabismus[7] as an alternative to surgery. A decade later, Jean Carruthers, also an ophthalmologist, observed the auspicious ability of the toxin to ameliorate facial wrinkles in patients injected for essential blepharospasm. His findings were presented at the American Society for Dermatologic Surgery (ASDS) conference the following year, followed by a landmark publication in the *Journal of Dermatology and Surgical Oncology* entitled "Treatment of glabellar frown lines with C. botulinum-A exotoxin."[8] Although the initial publication only dealt with glabellar lines, testing was already underway for crow's feet, nasolabial folds, mental crease, and nasal flare. Two clinical trials followed that confirmed safety and efficacy of the method.[9] In 2002, the Food and Drug Administration approved its use for "temporary improvement in the appearance of moderate to severe glabellar lines associated with corrugator and/or procerus muscle activity." Since this time, the indications and familiarity of botulinum neurotoxins (BoNTs) in medicine have exploded. In plastic surgery, it is a well-established and efficacious treatment modality for facial rhytids, as well as a promising therapy for functional problems such as migraines, vasospastic disorders, and hypertrophic scars.

STRUCTURE, MECHANISMS OF ACTION, AND PHARMACOLOGY

Botulinum neurotoxins (BoNTs) are generally produced by the Clostridium genus of bacteria, most prominently *Clostridia botulinum*. BoNTs inhibit neurotransmitter release at peripheral cholinergic nerve terminals which results in the flaccid paralysis characteristic of botulism. Seven major serotypes of BoNT exist (designated A-G), with over 40 different subtypes identified.[10] The structure of the toxin, which is highly conserved between serotypes, has evolved to ensure rapid and efficient delivery to within the cytosol of target cells and execution of its neurotoxic effect.

Transcribed from one of several *bont* genes, the protein is a 150 kDa single-chain polypeptide that contains an N-terminal light chain, a C-terminal heavy chain, and a globular L domain that is responsible for the metalloprotease activity of the protein. The heavy chain (HC) domain, which binds specifically to unmyelinated areas of motor neurons, consists of an N-terminal portion that mediates translocation into the cytosol and a C-terminal portion that is essential for binding and endocytosis into the presynaptic neuron.[11] The L domain is a conserved sequence containing a Zn^{2+} atom bound to a conserved sequence motif, which is also shared with tetanus neurotoxin.[5] The unique substrates of the L domain are the three SNARE proteins: VAMP/synaptobrevin, SNAP-25, and syntaxin. SNARE proteins are involved in fusion of the synaptic vesicle with the plasma membrane and were the subject of the 2013 Nobel Prize in Physiology or Medicine awarded to James Rothman, Randy Schekman, and Thomas Südhof.

The mechanism of BoNTs can be grouped into five major steps[5]: (1) binding to skeletal and autonomic cholinergic nerve terminals that use acetylcholine (ACh), (2) endocytosis inside synaptic vesicles that require the ATPase proton pump, (3) translocation of the L chain across the vesicle membrane, (4) release of L chain in the cytosol and activation of the toxin, and (5) cleavage of SNARE proteins. Once the SNARE protein has been cleaved, it is unable to facilitate fusion of vesicles with the host cell membrane, preventing ACh release from axon endings. Signal transmission at the neuromuscular junction is interrupted, and the muscles are unable to respond to neuronal activity. Over time, regeneration of nerve activity occurs as the toxin loses its activity and the host cell replaces SNARE proteins.

Local movement of injected toxin can be characterized by two distinct phenomena: diffusion and spread.[12] Whereas diffusion refers to the concentration gradient–driven transport of the molecule through the tissue, *spread* portrays the initial extent of injection by the practitioner. Diffusion is largely a property of the initial concentration of toxin, as well as the water content of the tissue and efficiency of receptor binding and uptake. This process is mostly complete after 24 hours,[13] and no further diffusion to surrounding tissues should occur. Although there are theoretical differences in diffusivity because of the larger sizes of onabotulinumtoxinA (900 kDa) and abobotulinumtoxinA (500–900 kDa) versus incobotulinumtoxinA (150 kDa),[14] no differences in diffusion of the toxins have been observed in vivo.[15] Dilution of the toxin should also impact the extent of diffusion into surrounding tissue, though there is little evidence supporting this prediction either.[14] Spread is a much more controllable factor in the sense that distribution of the drug is accomplished by the pathway of the needle and egress into the tissue.

Importantly, BoNT does not appear to cross the blood-brain barrier, but modulatory effects on the central nervous system can occur. Migration of the toxin, defined as its movement to distant tissues, can occur either by neuroaxonal transport or hematogenously. Although BoNT primarily acts at the neuromuscular junction, there is reasonable evidence that BoNTA and BoNTE, injected at therapeutic dosages, undergo retrograde axonal transport from sites of injection to the spinal cord and motor cortex.[16] Several studies in stroke patients have observed reduced inhibition of antagonistic muscles after injection into a particular muscle group, indicating a centrally acting effect of the toxin.[17] An alternative explanation is that BoNT acts on intrafusal fibers that inhibit afferent nerves in the target muscle as well as Renshaw cells which also use acetylcholine as a neurotransmitter. This generates an inhibitory effect on alpha motor neurons, which could produce the same inhibition of antagonistic muscles as a centrally acting mechanism of the drug itself.[11]

COMMERCIAL PREPARATIONS

Currently there are four commercially available BoNT preparations available in Western nations (**Table 47.1**): Botox® (OnabotulinumtoxinA, Allergen Inc., Irvine CA), Dysport® (AbobotulinumtoxinA, Ipsen Ltd., Slough, UK), Xeomin® (IncobotulinumtoxinA, Merz Pharmaceuticals, Frankfurt, Germany), and MyoBloc® or NeuroBloc® (RimabotulinumtoxinB, US World Meds, Louisville, KY). Several other preparations are available in Asian countries, including Prosigne® (Lanzhou Biological Products, Gansu, China), Meditoxin® (Medy-tox, Seoul, Korea), and Botulax®(Hugel Inc., Chuncheon, Korea). Although all formulations of the compound have unique properties and clinical effects, we will focus on the four common Western formulations in this chapter. The properties of these formulations are outlined in **Table 47.1**. All formulations except incobotulinumtoxinA (Xeomin) contain complexing proteins. As the smallest of these formulations, incobotulinumtoxinA contains only the active 150 kDa neurotoxin responsible for the therapeutic effect and is the most stable of the commercially available preparations (3–4 year shelf life at room temperature).

CLINICAL APPLICATIONS

BoNTs were originally described for ophthalmologic conditions and perhaps best known by the public for aesthetic applications. However, the concept of injectable, longer-term, neuromuscular inhibition has proven a powerful therapeutic modality and has undergone a vast array of studies in the last 2 decades. BoNTs have been reported to be safe and effective in the treatment of oromandibular dystonia including bruxism and tremors including essential tremor, parkinsonian rest tremors, motor tics, overactive bladder, pain depression, and a number of other movement disorders (see Jankovic[11] for review). The most commonly used and most extensively tested of the formulations

TABLE 47.1. PROPERTIES OF COMMON BOTULINUM TOXIN PREPARATIONS[11,18]

	OnabotulinumtoxinA	AbobotulinumtoxinA	IncobotulinumtoxinA	RimabotulinumtoxinB
Manufacturer	Allergen Inc.	Ipsen Ltd.	Merz Pharmaceuticals	US World Meds
Trade name	BOTOX	Dysport	Xeomin	NeuroBloc/Myobloc
Approved indications in plastic surgery	Moderate to severe glabellar lines, canthal lines, and forehead lines	Moderate to severe glabellar lines and canthal lines	Moderate to severe glabellar lines and canthal lines, blepharospasm	None (cervical dystonia only)
Cleavage target	SNAP-25	SNAP-25	SNAP-25	VAMP
Molecular weight	900 kD	500–900 kD	150 kD	700 kD
Formulation	Vacuum-dried powder	Lyophilized powder	Lyophilized powder	Sterile solution
Shelf life	2–3 y	2 y	3–4 y	2 y
Storage temperature	2–8°C	2–8°C	Room temperature	2–8°C
Units per vial	50, 100, 200	300, 500	50, 100	2500, 5000, 10,000
Potency	154 U/ng	137 U/ng	227 U/ng	70–130 U/ng

is onabotulinumtoxinA, which will we refer to by its more commonly known trade name, Botox. Botox has been vetted by more than 60 randomized clinical trials in the last 2 decades and is approved in at least 85 countries for more than 27 indications.[19] In this chapter, we will focus on the plastic surgery applications of all BoNTs, which include facial rhytids, migraines (as diagnostic and therapeutic tool before migraine surgery), axillary hyperhidrosis, upper extremity vasospastic disorders, and hypertrophic scars.

Facial Rhytids

A detailed understanding of facial anatomy is critical to successful application of BoNTs. Muscles of facial expression are unique in that they attach to a fibrous soft-tissue support system, called the superficial muscular aponeurotic system, instead of bone. Contraction of facial muscles produces wrinkling of the overlying skin, which produces many of the rhytids associated with aesthetic dissatisfaction. In addition to the muscular targets of BoNT injection, the practitioner must have an understanding of surrounding anatomy to appreciate and anticipate potential off-target effects of injection. The FDA has approved the use of botulinum toxin for cosmetic treatment of three specific areas and the associated facial muscles, including:

- Glabellar lines associated with corrugator and/or procerus muscle activity
- Lateral canthal lines associated with orbicularis oculi activity
- Forehead lines associated with frontalis activity

Undoubtedly, a large number of clinicians use botulinum toxin to treat other facial muscles located in the eyebrow, midface, lower face, and neck.

When considering treatment with botulinum toxin, a discussion with the patient to identify goals and expectations is warranted. The temporary effect of botulinum toxin (3–4 months) should be emphasized as well as the risks of the procedure. Next, it is important to assess the patient's facial anatomy in the context of their expressed concerns. A consistent approach to examining the patient is helpful. This should include evaluation in natural repose position as well as during animation. It is helpful to ask the patient to frown and squint to accentuate facial lines. Eyelid and brow ptosis should be appreciated prior to injection. Once the examination is complete, a treatment plan can be discussed with the patient. Dosing calculations and drug reconstruction should occur just prior to injection. A 30 or 33 gauge needle is used in conjunction with a 1 cc syringe to deliver the drug.

Glabella

The glabella region was the first area to be treated with botulinum toxin for cosmetic purposes and remains a common target for therapy (Figure 47.1). Glabellar lines, or frown lines, are formed from a compound movement of the glabellar complex depressor muscles, which include the corrugator supercilii, procerus, and depressor supercilii. Contraction of this complex, as well as the orbicularis oculi, pulls the brow inferiorly and medially, which produces one or more vertical skin lines between the medial aspects of the eyebrows. Patients seeking treatment of glabellar lines often note that they are mistaken for being angry, fatigued, or stressed. Jean Carruthers, who initially reported the effects of botulinum toxin on facial rhytids, published a landmark clinic trial in *Plastic and Reconstructive Surgery* in 2003, which demonstrated a significant improvement in appearance of glabellar lines with Botox administration as judged by both blinded

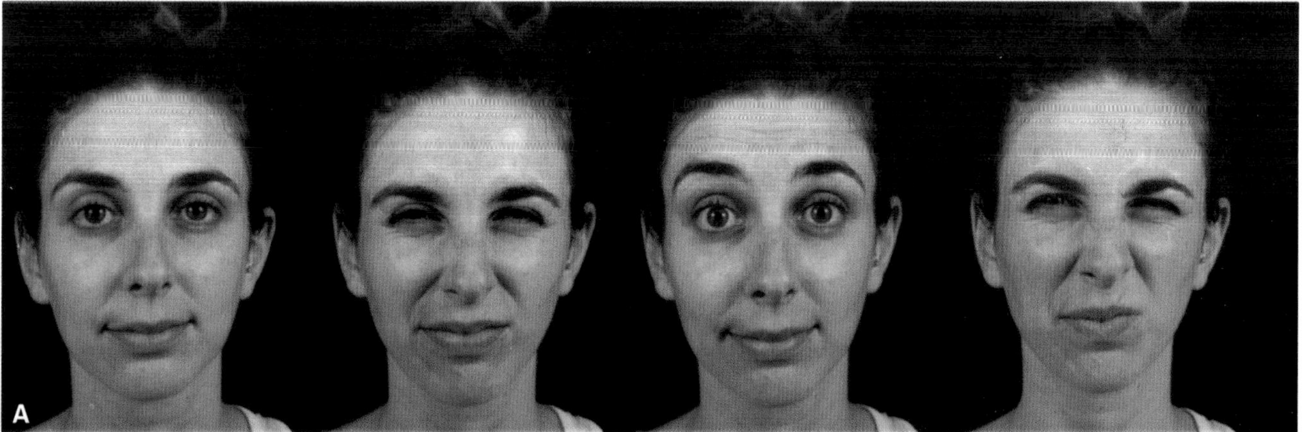

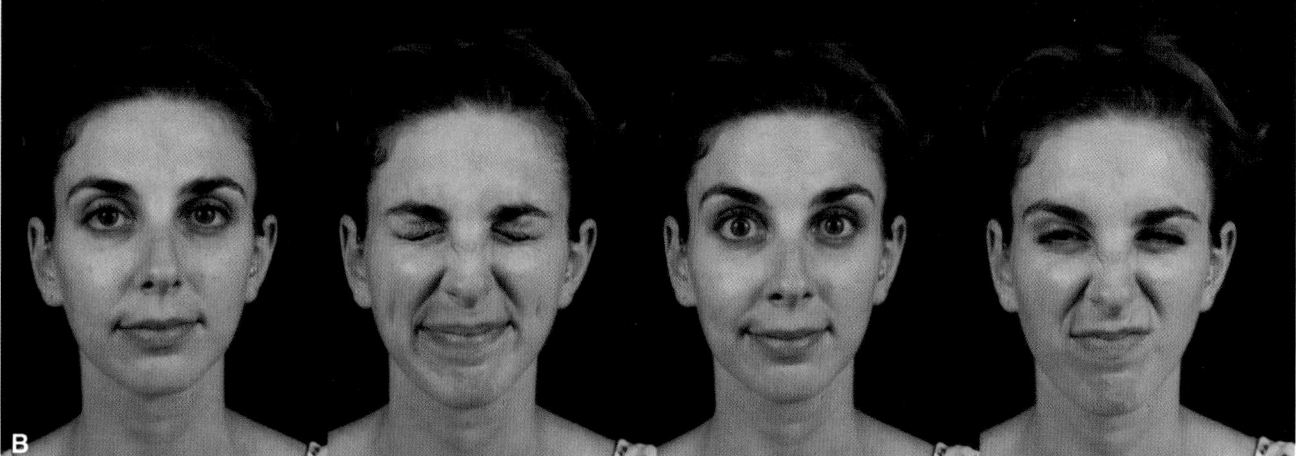

FIGURE 47.1. A 32-year-old woman underwent injection of 50 units of Botox, including 15 units to three sites in each of the glabella and corrugators, 7.5 units to three sites around each orbit, and 20 units to six sites on the forehead. Preinjection **(A)** and 8 days postinjection **(B)** photos are shown. Note the prominent reductions in forehead lines and lateral canthal lines during facial animation, which are not noticeable in repose.

physicians and the treated patients.[20] A number of supporting trials followed, and a 2015 meta-analysis confirmed the safe and effective dosing practice of 20 units for the glabellar region.[21]

Surgical approaches to treating glabellar lines exist and may be incorporated with other procedures. However, chemodenervation of the corrugator and/or procerus with botulinum toxin is effective toward achieving similar results to open surgical approaches.[22] If using Botox, five injections of 4 units (20 units total) are typically performed in this area: two injections into each corrugator muscle and one injection into the procerus muscle. The efficacy of botulinum toxin in treating glabellar lines is very high (60%–100%) with the most frequent adverse reaction noted as eyelid ptosis (about 3%).[21,23] To prevent this complication, avoid injection near the levator palpebrae superioris muscle and make lateral injections at least 1 cm above the supraorbital ridge. Signs of chemodenervation will begin to occur at 2 to 3 days after injections, increase in intensity over the first week, and usually persist for 3 to 4 months.

Lateral Canthal Region (Crow's Feet)

An appreciation for the extent of the lines associated with the orbicularis oculi muscle should be gained during the preinjection physical examination. This may include upper, lower, or a fanlike combination of lines throughout the lateral canthal region. These are best identified while asking a patient to smile. Lateral canthal lines arise predominantly from forceful contraction of the orbicularis oculi muscles, which originate from the lateral canthus.

An appreciation for the overlap between the orbicularis oculi muscle and the zygomaticus muscles should be established to avoid injecting the zygomaticus muscles. If using Botox, 4 units should be injected into three sites per side (six total injection points) for a total of 24 units. The injection sites for this area start in the lateral orbicularis oculi muscle, just temporal to the lateral orbital rim. The other areas are 1 cm superior and 1 cm inferior with a 30-degree angle toward the midline. Occasionally, the crow's feet lines will be more focused on the lower periorbital region and require a lower placement of injection sites. However, injections should not extend inferior to the maxillary prominence. The overall satisfaction of treating lateral canthal lines with botulinum toxin at 6 months is about 50%.[23] The most frequent adverse reactions following injection of botulinum toxin in the lateral canthal region are eyelid edema and bruising (about 1%).[19,20]

Forehead

The forehead lines can be evaluated by asking the patient to raise and lower their eyebrows. The extent of the frontalis muscle can be appreciated by visual inspection and palpation with the superior aspect extending just above the highest forehead crease. Typically, two treatment rows are used to treat the frontalis muscle. The lower treatment row will be halfway between the superior extent of the frontalis muscle and the eyebrow. The upper treatment row will typically be halfway between the superior aspect of the frontalis muscle and the lower treatment row. Forehead lines are typically treated in conjunction with glabellar lines using 40 units total, to minimize the possibility of brow ptosis. The most frequent adverse reactions following injection of botulinum toxin for forehead lines are headache (9%), brow ptosis (2%), and eyelid ptosis (2%).[19,20]

Brow Elevation

The use of botulinum toxin for treating brow ptosis and asymmetry has been somewhat challenging because there is no standard approach for achieving brow elevation. In general, the two muscles targeted for generating brow elevation are the frontalis and the orbicularis oculi. When the central and lateral portions of the frontalis are weakened, there is compensatory contraction of the frontalis muscle directly over the brow resulting in elevation. Likewise, injections directed toward the superolateral aspect of the orbicularis muscle can result in a significant increase in brow height without a significant risk of asymmetry.[24] Although the standard plane of injection is intramuscular, subcutaneous injections may be equally effective in achieving paralysis.[25]

Nasolabial Fold and *Gummy Smile*

The levator labii superioris alaeque nasi muscle is attached to the frontal process of the maxilla and attaches to the skin of the upper lip and lateral nostril. The muscle name translates to lifter of the upper lip and wing of the nose. The zygomaticus major also contributes the smile and nasolabial fold as it primarily pulls and elevates the oral commissure. In a classic article published in *Plastic and Reconstructive Surgery,* Leonard Rubin described three major smiling patterns (*Mona Lisa*, *Canine*, and *Gummy*) and the impact that each muscle has on the resulting appearance.[26] Botulinum toxin can be used to modify the appearance of the gummy smile by direct injection into the levator labii muscle which can be palpated during smiling along the lateral aspect of the piriform aperture. This can be accomplished typically with one injection on each side with a modest dose.[27] Excess gingival display (>2 mm) can be addressed with this approach, and further softening of the nasolabial folds can be achieved with targeting the zygomaticus muscles.

Neck

Visible bands in the neck resulting from platysma muscle attenuation can be a source of dissatisfaction for patients. Patients are evaluated by asking them to clench their necks and show their lower teeth. Hyperactive platysmal bands in the superficial subdermal space can be visualized and are the target of treatment. Numerous approaches to treating platysma bands with botulinum toxin have been reported with varying doses techniques.[28,29] It is well accepted that patients with excess skin laxity in the neck are not good candidates for this procedure as they have minimal overall improvement. In a recent study, patients were injected with botulinum toxin along the inferior border of the mandible and with the platysmal bands using a mean dose of 124.9 units.[30] The authors noted a significant improvement using this technique; however, some express concern given the high dose needed for effect and the potential risks of dysphagia and salivary gland dysfunction. Other more conservative approaches include direct platysmal band injection with 20 units of botulinum toxin.[29] Again, patient selection through proper physical examination is paramount for success in this approach.

Noncosmetic Uses

Axillary Hyperhidrosis

Hyperhidrosis is characterized by the excessive sweating without any specific cause and can be socially stigmatizing for patients. The axilla, palms, and soles are the most common sites for hyperhidrosis. A variety of topical agents have been used for hyperhidrosis as well as surgical sympathectomy, all with formidable downsides. In 2001, a multicenter trial utilizing botulinum toxin injections for axillary hyperhidrosis was performed.[31] In this randomized double-blinded study, participants received 200 units of botulinum toxin injected into one axilla in comparison to placebo injections into the other. Within 2 weeks, there was a noticeable drop in sweat production from the treatment side. This effect continued for 24 weeks, and patients were highly likely to recommend this treatment to other patients. Further validating this technique was a modeled comparison study between endoscopic thoracic sympathectomy and intradermal botulinum toxin published in 2016.[32] The authors concluded that treatment costs reached an equivalence at 13 years, yet because of the low risk of botulinum toxin injections, they would recommend this over surgical sympathectomy. With this approach, the duration of effect is typically 7 months, and high patient satisfaction is typical.[33] Although side effects remain somewhat uncommon in most studies, a low rate of compensatory sweating in other areas was noted to occur with some regularity.[34,35]

Chronic Migraines

An emerging treatment for chronic migraines lies in the neurolysis of sensory nerves of the head, which can be achieved by both surgical (decompression, neurolysis, and ablation) and chemical (BoNT injection) means. Chronic migraines affect over 3 million people in the US population and are distinguished from episodic migraine by a distinct frequency, epidemiology, pathophysiology, and response to treatment.[19] The effectiveness of BoNTs was incidentally discovered by William Binder, a facial plastic surgeon, who was conducting studies with Botox for aesthetic applications and noted a correlation between pericranial injections and alleviation of migraine symptoms.[36] He published the first open-label clinical trial on Botox for chronic migraines in 2000.[37]

The pathophysiology of chronic migraines is incompletely understood, and the knowledge base surrounding this issue exceeds the scope of this chapter. The current model of the disease process is based on abnormal excitability in both central and peripheral neurons, particularly in the trigeminal neurovascular bundles.[19] It is thought that peripheral sensitization occurs, in which the threshold of sensory neurons responses to external stimuli is altered because of various maladaptive processes, and the neurons become hyperexcitable. Botox is thought to interrupt both neurotransmitter and neuropeptide release from sensory neurons, which interrupts signal transmission to the central nervous system and mitigates the effects of peripheral sensitization.

Two phase III clinical trials were conducted that led to FDA approval of Botox for chronic migraines. The Phase III REsearch Evaluating Migraine Prophylaxis Therapy (PREEMPT 1[38]) and PREEMPT 2 trials[39] consisted of a multicenter, randomized, double-blind, placebo-controlled clinical trial of Botox for chronic migraines in both North America and Europe. The pooled analysis of 1384 patients randomized to Botox or placebo demonstrated that Botox significantly reduced the number of headache days per month (−8.4 days for Botox and −6.6 days for placebo, $P < 0.001$, 95% CI −2.52 to −1.13), as well as frequency of migraine days, moderate or severe headache days, cumulative hours of headaches, and other measures of migraine severity and frequency. Safety analysis from the trials also revealed no new concerns, with the percentage of adverse events similar between treatment and control groups.

Botox is currently indicated for the treatment of chronic migraines, defined as at least 15 days per month with headaches that last 4 hours or longer. The recommended dosage is 155 units administered intramuscularly, divided between seven sites in the head and neck: corrugators (5 U each side), procerus (5 U), frontalis (5 U each side), temporalis (5 U each side), occipitalis (15 U each side), cervical paraspinal muscles (10 U each side), and trapezius (15 U each side).

Upper Extremity Vasospastic Disorders

Patients with Raynaud phenomenon have abnormal vascular function in the hand who may develop chronic pain and ulceration. Botulinum toxin injections are a promising nonsurgical option for these difficult-to-manage patients. Prior to injection, patients should undergo vascular imaging studies to rule out occlusive disease. Neumeister et al. demonstrated improvements in hand pain, hand blood flow, and healing of chronic ulceration in a retrospective study evaluating the efficacy of botulinum toxin for patients suffering with Raynaud condition.[40] In this study, 50–100 units of Botox was injected into the palm directed toward the neurovascular bundles of the digits, and many patients demonstrated long-term relief of symptoms. Likewise, a study by Fregene et al. demonstrated similar improvements with pain and blood flow to the hand in patients with Raynaud conditions undergoing 100 unit Botox injections to the palm.[41] Side effects from this approach can include recurrence of pain and intrinsic muscle weakness.[40-42]

Hypertrophic Scarring

A fascinating application of BoNT lies in the treatment and prevention of hypertrophic scars. Because wound tension is known to lead to an exuberant and potentially pathologic fibrotic response, chemical paralysis of muscles surrounding a wound may reduce tension during the critical healing period. Although only smaller studies have been performed to date, a 2016 meta-analysis showed statistically significant differences in both scar width and patient satisfaction with the use of botulinum toxin type A[43] for head and neck scars. Future studies are needed to flesh out the clinical utility and generalizability of this practice.

CONTRAINDICATIONS AND WARNINGS

The absolute contraindications for BoNTs are only two: hypersensitivity to any BoNT preparation (including any component of the preparation) and infection at the injection site. However, there are a number of warnings and precautions issued by the FDA, as well as potential drug interactions of which the practitioner should be aware. The dosages of BoNTs, even of the same toxin family (e.g., OnabotulinumtoxinA and AbobotulinumtoxinA, or Botox and Dysport), are not interchangeable and cannot be compared. As described earlier, movement of toxin beyond the site of injection is always a concern, particularly when injecting the toxin around the airway muscles as is performed for spasticity. Although ongoing controversy exists about the retrograde migration of BoNTs to the central nervous systems (see above), no adverse events have been reported during dermatologic uses of BoNTs. The practitioner should be especially careful when treating patients with cardiovascular disease or neuromuscular disorders (e.g., myasthenia gravis or Lambert-Eaton), who should be monitored after treatment.

ADVERSE EFFECTS

As with any medical intervention, the side effects of treatment must be well understood by the clinicians prior to application. Distant spread of the effects of botulinum toxin may occur following local infections. These effects are reported to include generalized muscle weakness, diplopia, eyelid ptosis, dysphagia, dysphonia, urinary incontinence, and breathing difficulties. Symptoms may occur hours or even weeks after injection and are most common in children being treated for spasticity. Spread of the toxin effect during facial dermatologic treatments is unlikely when labeled doses are used. For Botox, this includes 20 units for glabellar lines, 24 units for lateral canthal lines, 40 units for forehead lines, 44 units for simultaneous lateral canthal and glabellar lines, and 64 units for simultaneous lateral canthal, glabellar, and forehead lines. Finally, treatment with botulinum toxin is contraindicated when there is an active infection at the injection site. Hypersensitivity to botulinum injections can occur and may include anaphylaxis and other forms of immediate allergic reactions.

Botulism-like symptoms have been reported in patients undergoing BoNT injections for dystonia,[44] hyperhidrosis,[45] and blepharospasm.[46] These symptoms included dry eyes and mouth, gastrointestinal disturbances, dysphagia, hoarseness, and breathing difficulties. Notably, it is suspected that an underlying condition of myasthenia gravis was not recognized in these patients,[46] and none of the patients received the drug for aesthetic indications. Dosages of the drugs were also far higher than used for typical aesthetic indications: 6.25 to 32 U/kg of Botox and 388 to 625 U/kg of MyoBloc. Nonetheless, practitioners injecting BoNTs for plastic surgery indications must be aware of the potential for serious adverse events, particularly in patients with preexisting cardiovascular conditions or compromised respiratory function.

ACKNOWLEDGMENTS

The authors thank Andre Marshall, MD, for his assistance with Figure 47.1.

REFERENCES

1. Erbguth FJ. Historical notes on botulism, *Clostridium botulinum*, botulinum toxin, and the idea of the therapeutic use of the toxin. *Mov Disord.* 2004;19(S8):S2-S6.
2. Patil S, Willett O, Thompkins T, et al. Botulinum toxin: pharmacology and therapeutic roles in pain states. *Curr Pain Headache Rep.* 2016;20(3):15.
3. Erbguth FJ, Naumann M. Historical aspects of botulinum toxin: Justinus Kerner (1786–1862) and the "sausage poison." *Neurology.* 1999;53(8):1850-1853.
4. Sterba JP. The history of botulism. *New York Times.* April 28, 1982.
5. Pirazzini M, Rossetto O, Eleopra R, Montecucco C. Botulinum neurotoxins: biology, pharmacology, and toxicology. *Pharmacol Rev.* 2017;69(2):200-235.
6. Scott AB, Rosenbaum A, Collins CC. Pharmacologic weakening of extraocular muscles. *Invest Ophthalmol.* 1973;12(12):924-927.
7. Scott AB. Botulinum toxin injection into extraocular muscles as an alternative to strabismus surgery. *J Pediatr Ophthalmol Strabismus.* 1980;17(1):21-25.
8. Carruthers JD, Carruthers JA. Treatment of glabellar frown lines with *C. botulinum*-A exotoxin. *J Dermatol Surg Oncol.* 1992;18(1):17-21.
   This publication represents the first report of BoNTs for facial rhytids (in this case glabellar lines). This article reflects the author's experience injecting BoNT for essential blepharospasm, and the serendipitous observation that glabellar lines were also reduced.
9. Giordano CN, Matarasso SL, Ozog DM. Injectable and topical neurotoxins in dermatology: basic science, anatomy, and therapeutic agents. *J Am Acad Dermatol.* 2017;76(6):1013-1024.
10. Peck MW, Smith TJ, Anniballi F, et al. Historical perspectives and guidelines for botulinum neurotoxin subtype nomenclature. *Toxins.* 2017;9(1):38.
11. Jankovic J. Botulinum toxin: state of the art. *Mov Disord.* 2017;285(8):1059.
12. Wortzman MS, Pickett A. The science and manufacturing behind botulinum neurotoxin type A-ABO in clinical use. *Aesthet Surg J.* 2009;29(6 suppl):S34-S42.
13. Tang-Liu DD, Aoki KR, Dolly JO, et al. Intramuscular injection of 125I-botulinum neurotoxin-complex versus 125I-botulinum-free neurotoxin: time course of tissue distribution. *Toxicon.* 2003;42(5):461-469.
14. Castaneda JR, Jankovic J, Comella C, et al. Diffusion, spread, and migration of botulinum toxin. *Mov Disord.* 2013;28(13):1775-1783.
15. Carli L, Montecucco C, Rossetto O. Assay of diffusion of different botulinum neurotoxin type a formulations injected in the mouse leg. *Muscle Nerve.* 2009;40(3):374-380.
16. Restani L, Giribaldi F, Manich M, et al. Botulinum neurotoxins A and E undergo retrograde axonal transport in primary motor neurons. *PLoS Pathog.* 2012;8(12):e1003087.
17. Mas M, Li S, Francisco G. Centrally mediated late motor recovery after botulinum toxin injection: case reports and a review of current evidence. *J Rehabil Med.* 2017;49(8):609-619.
18. Frevert J. Pharmaceutical, biological, and clinical properties of botulinum neurotoxin type A products. *Drugs Res Dev.* 2015;15(1):1-9.
19. Whitcup SM, Turkel CC, DeGryse RE, Brin MF. Development of onabotulinumtoxinA for chronic migraine. *Ann NY Acad Sci.* 2014;1329(1):67-80.
20. Carruthers JD, Lowe NJ, Menter MA, et al. Double-blind, placebo-controlled study of the safety and efficacy of botulinum toxin type A for patients with glabellar lines. *Plast Reconstr Surg.* 2003;112(suppl):21S-30S.
    This publication reports on the first major clinical trial of botulinum toxin A for glabellar lines. The trial involved blinded administration of the toxin and placebo. Results were evaluated by blinded physicians and patients. Both physician and patient ratings were significantly greater for the BoNT group over the placebo group, which peaked at 30 days after injection.
21. Guo Y, Lu Y, Liu T, et al. Efficacy and safety of botulinum toxin type A in the treatment of glabellar lines: a meta-analysis of randomized, placebo-controlled, double-blind trials. *Plast Reconstr Surg.* 2015;136(3):310e-318e.
22. Carruthers A, Kiene K, Carruthers J. Botulinum A exotoxin use in clinical dermatology. *J Am Acad Dermatol.* 1996;34(5):788-797.
23. Fagien S, Carruthers JDA. A comprehensive review of patient-reported satisfaction with botulinum toxin type A for aesthetic procedures. *Plast Reconstr Surg.* 2008;122(6):1915-1925.
24. Uygur S, Eryilmaz T, Bulam H, Yavuzer R, Latifoglu O. The quantitative effect of botulinum toxin A over brow height. *J Craniofac Surg.* 2013;24(4):1285-1287.
25. Gordin EA, Luginbuhl AL, Ortlip T, et al. Subcutaneous vs intramuscular botulinum toxin: split-face randomized study. *JAMA Facial Plast Surg.* 2014;16(3):193-198.
26. Rubin LR. The anatomy of a smile: its importance in the treatment of facial paralysis. *Plast Reconstr Surg.* 1974;53(4):384-387.
    This article describes three smile patterns ("Mona Lisa," "canine," and "gummy") and the impact that each muscle has on the resulting appearance. The Mona Lisa smile, for instance, involves the zygomaticus major muscles drawing the oral commissure upwards and outwards, along with elevation of the upper lip.
27. Nasr MW, Jabbour SF, Sidaoui JA, et al. Botulinum toxin for the treatment of excessive gingival display: a systematic review. *Aesthet Surg J.* 2015;36(1):82-88.
28. Matarasso A, Matarasso SL, Brandt FS, Bellman B. Botulinum A exotoxin for the management of platysma bands. *Plast Reconstr Surg.* 1999;103(2):645-652.
29. Kane MA. Nonsurgical treatment of platysmal bands with injection of botulinum toxin A. *Plast Reconstr Surg.* 1999;103(2):656-663.
30. Jabbour SF, Kechichian EG, Awaida CJ, et al. Botulinum toxin for neck rejuvenation: assessing efficacy and redefining patient selection. *Plast Reconstr Surg.* 2017;140(1):9e-17e.
31. Heckmann M, Ceballos-Baumann AO, Plewig G. Botulinum toxin A for axillary hyperhidrosis (excessive sweating). *N Engl J Med.* 2001;344(7):488-493.
32. Gibbons JP, Nugent E, O'Donohoe N, et al. Experience with botulinum toxin therapy for axillary hyperhidrosis and comparison to modelled data for endoscopic thoracic. *Surgeon.* 2016;14(5):260-264.
33. Rosen R, Stewart T. Results of a 10-year follow-up study of botulinum toxin A therapy for primary axillary hyperhidrosis in Australia. *Intern Med J.* 2018;48(3):343-347.
34. Naumann M, Lowe NJ. Botulinum toxin type A in treatment of bilateral primary axillary hyperhidrosis: randomised, parallel group, double blind, placebo controlled trial. *BMJ.* 2001;323(7313):596-599.
35. Scamoni S, Valdatta L, Frigo C, et al. Treatment of primary axillary hyperhidrosis with botulinum toxin type a: our experience in 50 patients from 2007 to 2010. *ISRN Dermatol.* 2012;2012(5):1-5.
36. Binder WJ, Blitzer A, Brin MF. Treatment of hyperfunctional lines of the face with botulinum toxin A. *Dermatol Surg.* 1998;24(11):1198-1205.
37. Binder WJ, Brin MF, Blitzer A, et al. Botulinum toxin type A (Botox) for treatment of migraine headaches: an open-label study. *Otolaryngol Head Neck Surg.* 2016;123(6):669-676.
38. Dodick DW, Turkel CC, DeGryse RE, et al. Onabotulinumtoxin A for treatment of chronic migraine: pooled results from the double-blind, randomized, placebo-controlled phases of the PREEMPT clinical program. *Headache.* 2010;50(6):921-936.
    This publication details the results of the PREEMPT 1 trial, which demonstrated improvement in headache scores of patients receiving onabotulinumtoxinA versus placebo. A total of 1384 adults were randomized. Those receiving the toxin reported a significant decrease in the number of headache days (−8.4 versus −6.6, $P < 0.001$) versus those receiving placebo.
39. Diener HC, Dodick DW, Aurora SK, et al. Onabotulinumtoxin A for treatment of chronic migraine: results from the double-blind, randomized, placebo-controlled phase of the PREEMPT 2 trial. *Cephalalgia.* 2010;30(7):804-814.
    The PREEMPT 2 trial was the second in a pair of studies evaluating the effect of onabotulinumtoxinA for treatment of chronic migraines. Like the PREEMPT 1 trial, this publication reported a significant a statistically significant reduction in frequency of headache days (the primary endpoint) in patients receiving toxin versus placebo. The PREEMPT 1 and 2 trials laid the evidence-based foundation for the clinical use of BoNTs for chronic migraines.
40. Neumeister MW, Chambers CB, Herron MS, et al. Botox therapy for ischemic digits. *Plast Reconstr Surg.* 2009;124(1):191-201.
41. Fregene A, Ditmars D, Siddiqui A. Botulinum toxin type A: a treatment option for digital ischemia in patients with Raynaud's phenomenon. *J Hand Surg.* 2009;34(3):446-452.
42. Eickhoff JC, Smith JK, Landau ME, Edison JD. Iatrogenic Thenar eminence atrophy after Botox A injection for secondary raynaud phenomenon. *J Clin Rheumatol.* 2016;22(7):396-397.
43. Zhang D-Z, Liu X-Y, Xiao W-L, Xu Y-X. Botulinum toxin type A and the prevention of hypertrophic scars on the maxillofacial area and neck: a meta-analysis of randomized controlled trials. *PLoS One.* 2016;11(3):e0151627.
44. Bhatia KP, Münchau A, Thompson PD, et al. Generalised muscular weakness after botulinum toxin injections for dystonia: a report of three cases. *J Neurol Neurosurg Psych.* 1999;67(1):90-93.
45. Tugnoli V, Eleopra R, Quatrale R, et al. Botulism-like syndrome after botulinum toxin type A injections for focal hyperhidrosis. *Br J Dermatol.* 2002;147(4):808-809.
46. Omprakash HM, Rajendran SC. Botulinum toxin deaths: what is the fact? *J Cutan Aesthet Surg.* 2008;1(2):95.

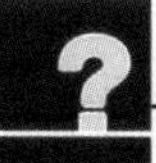

QUESTIONS

1. **A 44-year-old woman presents with unilateral ptosis 1 week after undergoing botulinum toxin injection for glabellar rhytids. Which of the following is the most likely explanation for this finding?**
   a. Horner syndrome
   b. Corrugator paralysis
   c. Levator palpebrae superioris paralysis
   d. Orbicularis oculi paralysis
   e. Incomplete administration of toxin

2. **A 49-year-old woman presents to your clinic with dissatisfaction of fine rhytids radiating outward from the lateral canthus. Twelve units of Botox are injected intramuscularly in regions of the lateral orbicularis oculi muscle on each side. The procedure is uncomplicated, although 3 days later the patient calls to state that she has minor bruising in the area and has no visible improvement in the rhytids. Which of the following factors is most likely contributing to the lack of effect?**
   a. Injection of improper anatomic region
   b. Inadequate dosage of injected toxin
   c. Failure to recognize underlying comorbidity
   d. Inadequate time for effect
   e. Wrong depth of injection

3. **A 25-year-old man reports migraine headaches that persist more than half the day and occur most days of the month. Symptoms are present diffusely, but predominantly localized to the frontal, temporal, and occipital regions. Ten units of Botox are injected intramuscularly in both the frontalis and temporalis muscles. Which of the following factors is most likely to contribute to a weaker effect of treatment?**
   a. Frequency of migraines
   b. Insufficient injection into the frontalis and temporalis muscles
   c. Lack of injection into other pericranial muscles
   d. a, b, and c
   e. b and c

1. **Answer: c.** The levator palpebrae superioris muscle is innervated by the superior division of the ipsilateral oculomotor nerve (cranial nerve III). Its function is to elevate and retract the upper eyelid. Loss of innervation, which may occur from botulinum toxin administration or trauma, will cause blepharoptosis. Although this is considered an adverse event in aesthetic botulinum toxin administration, purposeful levator chemodenervation has been used as a strategy to protect the cornea after facial nerve paralysis–induced lagophthalmos. Although ptosis may also result from inadvertent chemodenervation of the superior tarsal muscle (Müller muscle), Horner syndrome is defined by the classic constellation of ptosis, miosis, and anhidrosis. The latter symptoms are not present in this patient. Horner syndrome is due to lesions in the ipsilateral sympathetic pathway responsible for innervating the superior tarsal muscle. Symptoms can arise from the lesion at any point in the sympathetic nerve pathway including the hypothalamospinal tract, sympathetic trunk of the thoracic spinal cord, sympathetic chain, internal carotid plexus, or superior cervical ganglion. Botulinum toxin injected would not be expected to interrupt sympathetic nerve transmission at these locations. Corrugator paralysis is an anticipated and desirable effect of botulinum toxin injection for glabellar rhytids. Orbicularis oculi paralysis would result from facial nerve (cranial nerve VII) paralysis and cause lagophthalmos, an inability to close the eye. Incomplete administration of toxin would result in persistent rhytids and would not be expected to cause ptosis.

2. **Answer: d.** BoNTs typically demonstrate an effect between 3 and 7 days postinjection and persist for 4 to 6 months. If no visible improvement is seen after 3 days, the best course of action is to reassure the patient and reassess in another week. The correct anatomic region for lateral canthal lines (Crow's feet) is in the lateral orbicularis oculi region, within the muscle, as was done in this patient. A total of 24 units are recommended for lateral canthal lines (12 on each side). The injection sites for this area start in the lateral orbicularis oculi muscle, just temporal to the lateral orbital rim. The next areas are 1 cm superior and 1 cm inferior with a 30-degree angle toward the midline. A comorbidity that predisposes the patient to poor effect of the toxin is unlikely. Minor bruising is a common phenomenon after injections and usually resolves without intervention.

3. **Answer: c.** The recommended administration of Botox for chronic migraines is 155 units divided between seven sites on the head and neck (see text for specific dosages). The frontalis and temporalis muscles comprise two of these sites, which should both receive 5 units of toxin on each side, as was done for this patient. However, the patient's diffuse symptoms suggest that complete coverage of the seven sites is appropriate. Chronic migraines are defined as those occurring more frequently than 15 days per month with symptoms lasting at least 4 hours per episode. The patient in this question qualifies for this diagnosis and should benefit from Botox therapy.

CHAPTER 48 Fat Grafting in Plastic Surgery

Edward I. Chang

KEY POINTS

- Harvesting techniques have not been proven to increase fat graft take; however, the yield can vary based on handheld suction or power-assisted suction. In general, the less manipulation of the fat graft, the better the viability.
- Fat graft take following injection is never 100%, and therefore the process of fat grafting often needs to be repeated.
- The technique for injection is critical for maximizing outcomes and minimizing complications.
- Fat grafting into the breast following oncologic resection has not been associated with increased risks for tumor recurrence.
- Although early animal studies demonstrated potential benefits of adipose-derived stem cells in wound healing, the true clinical application of these has yet to be recognized.

The technique of autologous fat injection has grown in popularity over the years and has permeated nearly all aspects of plastic surgery. The first recorded use of fat grafting was performed in 1893 by Gustav Neuber who transferred autologous fat to correct periorbital scars.[1,2] However, since its first description, the use of autologous fat was fraught with controversy particularly when injecting into the breast. Concerns regarding breast cancer and possibilities of compromising detection of breast cancer prompted the American Society of Plastic and Reconstructive Surgeons to issue a formal statement cautioning the routine use of lipofilling.[3] Since this declaration, over a decade has passed before the concept witnessed a rebirth with the Coleman technique that ushered an emergence of novel applications and growing technologies by expanding its use in all aspects of plastic and reconstructive surgery.[4-8]

One of the defining characteristics of the field of plastic surgery is that it is not limited to a particular anatomic region and as such, the application of autologous fat grafting has also found utility in all areas of the body. The use of autologous fat, now termed fat grafting or lipofilling, has been described for cosmetic augmentation and rejuvenation of the face as well as reconstruction of facial deformities and for both cosmetic and reconstructive procedures over the entire body including the breast, gluteal region, and extremities. Although there are a number of synthetic tissue substitutes available, autologous fat represents one of the most popular fillers available to plastic and reconstructive surgeons.

INDICATIONS

Even before the American Society of Plastic Surgeons issued a new declaration regarding the safety of autologous fat transfer, using autologous fat as a filler was growing in popularity.[9] The concept of fillers is well accepted in the field of plastic surgery, and autologous fat is simply another filler that should be in the armamentarium of plastic surgeons. For most patients, there are ample donor sites with sufficient adiposity to provide injectable fat that can be obtained with low cost and also provides the added benefit of contouring and sculpting the donor site. The use of autologous fat grafting focuses on harvesting fat from one donor site and transferring the fat to a desired location for volume augmentation. Not surprising, fat grafting has found broad applications both in the cosmetic arena as well as in reconstructive operations. Plastic surgeons have employed lipofilling in facial rejuvenation and lip and cheek augmentation.[10-12] However, its applications and successes in facial plastic surgery have since been expanded into cosmetic augmentation of other anatomic regions, particularly the gluteal region, the calf, and even for penile enlargement.[13-16]

Not surprisingly, the concept of lipofilling as a natural filler and volume enhancer was immediately adopted for breast augmentation. Studies have demonstrated long-term efficacy in maintaining breast volume using autologous fat grafting.[17-19] The use of negative pressure systems such as BRAVA to augment vascularization and engrafting of autologous fat has also been reported, although it has not been widely adopted.[20,21] Lipofilling of the breast introduces a number of considerations and concerns that are unique to the breast. There is little doubt that the fat grafting can add volume to the breast, which obviates the need for a foreign body and the other potential complications associated with a breast implant. However, fat grafting does introduce questions regarding the ability to monitor and image the breast for malignancy and especially in the setting of breast reconstruction.

Nonetheless, the use of autologous fat grafting has found some of its greatest uses in plastic surgery not only in breast reconstruction but also in reconstruction of head and neck defects as well as for burns and scars.[22-24] The most widely used reconstructive application for fat grafting is for breast reconstruction.[25] Studies have demonstrated excellent volume retention, efficacy, and safety of autologous fat grafting for breast cancer patients without increased risks of recurrence.[26-29] Further studies focusing on patient-reported outcomes have also confirmed high patient satisfaction with lipofilling both as an adjunct in mastectomy reconstruction as well as for reconstruction of partial mastectomy defects in the setting of breast conservation.[29-31]

SURGICAL TECHNIQUE

Given the increasing utilization of autologous fat grafting, there are a number of variables that are involved in maximizing the take of the fat graft as well as acquiring the best quality fat for injection. These variables can be classified as technical variables and patient-related variables; however, within these broader categories, there are a number of components that also need to be considered including tumescent solution, harvest technique, processing technique, and injection technique. From the perspective of patient factors, there are also a number of considerations including the most optimal donor site and body habitus include body mass index, comorbidities, and smoking.[32,33]

Studies examining the wetting solution demonstrated a negative impact on adipocyte viability with the use of lidocaine. Because most grafts undergo a processing step that often includes washing the harvested fat, the effects of lidocaine are mitigated.[34] Another study found contradictory findings and demonstrated no impact of lidocaine or epinephrine or prilocaine on fat graft viability.[35] The technique for aspiration and injection has also been examined as a factor that could potentially impact fat graft viability to exert mechanical stress and pressure on the adipocytes. Studies found aspiration via handheld or with mechanical suction and centrifugation have little impact on fat graft viability; however, injection via slow, controlled pressure to minimize the shear stress and forces on adipocytes does improve adipocyte viability.[36,37] These additional steps are important to separate the adipocytes from the other constituents comprising the lipoaspirate. Although some believe there are benefits in preserving the potential growth factors contained in aspirate, there are also nonviable cells that have undergone cell lysis during the harvesting, liquefied fat, and hematocyte component comprised of blood cells and other contaminants. Others believe that one of the most valuable components of the lipoaspirate is the stromal cell fraction containing the adipose derive stem cells and other pluripotent stem cells that can enhance tissue recovery or augment fat graft take. A number of products and devices that will be described in the subsequent section have since come to market to streamline this process to maximize both efficiency and fat graft yield.

Aside from the technical aspects of autologous fat grafting, studies also aimed to examine patient-related factors that may influence graft yield and viability. Patient factors such as age have been found to have an impact on fat graft viability, and in general, younger patients tend to have superior fat viability compared to older patients. Interestingly, obesity was also found to be a factor; although a larger amount of fat can theoretically be harvested from a patient with a higher body mass index, the viability of the fat is actually compromised in obese patients. Finally, the ideal location of the donor site has also been an area of tremendous debate and investigation. Although some studies demonstrated the greatest yield and viability of adipocytes from the medial thigh, larger and more comprehensive studies have not found any significant benefits comparing one donor site to another.[38-40]

FAT GRAFT PROCESSING

Given the increasing popularity and applications for autologous fat transfer and lipofilling in plastic surgery, it is not surprising that commercialized products have emerged on the market to improve the adipocyte yield, enhance adipose-derived stem cell concentration, and maximize the efficiency of the process. In its original description, the autologous fat was harvested via syringe aspiration and then separated from the other constituents using centrifugation.[40,41] Most studies examining this process found this technique to be simple and atraumatic to the adipocytes; however, this is a relatively labor-intensive method for harvesting autologous fat graft. A number of other devices have been introduced to the market to streamline the harvesting and processing of the fat graft and have demonstrated tremendous potential with promising results. Some devices can be attached to power-assisted suction that decreases the energy expenditure in obtaining the fat graft and allow the fat graft to be washed while contained within a closed system to minimize risks of contamination or exposure to air. Another device utilizes centripetal forces to isolate the injectable fat from other contaminants and constituents of the lipoaspirate. One device passes the aspirate through a filtration system that separates the fat from the other components. All systems claim to provide superior adipocyte viability, fat graft yield, and stem cell composition, but no unbiased studies are available that have demonstrated superior outcomes compared to the traditional handheld syringe aspiration and centrifugation technique. Nonetheless, the increasing industry involvement in device development is a clear indication of the growing popularity and potential of lipofilling and fat grafting.[41-43]

Another trademark device that has been marketed to improve the take and engraftment of the injected fat cells is the BRAVA system. This device is solely promoted for lipofilling of the breast and is based on the premise that negative pressure applied to a recipient bed enhances the vascularity of the recipient site by promoting angiogenesis, which will support large volumes of fat. The product has merit because negative pressure wound dressings have been shown to increase neovascularization of wound, promoting granulation tissue and maximizing the wound healing process.

COMPLICATIONS

As with any surgical procedure, there are potential complications, and autologous fat grafting is no different. Although sound judgment and proper technique are paramount in avoiding complications, complications can occur either in the recipient site or the donor site. With regards to the recipient site, there are always risks of fat necrosis as fat retention following fat grafting is never 100%. Studies vary tremendously based on the percentage of viable adipocytes following fat grafting, but range from 50% to 70%.[44,45] The remaining injected fat often is reabsorbed; however, in other circumstances, it can lead to oil cysts or fat necrosis that can be palpable and cause discomfort or deformity for patients. This can be particularly worrisome in patients undergoing breast reconstruction because a palpable mass in the breast may require further diagnostic testing and potentially biopsies to confirm the mass is benign.[46,47] Although this can also occur in the face, the most dreaded complication following lipofilling of the face is blindness, which results if the fat graft is injected under pressure or while advancing the cannula leading essentially to a fat embolism in the ophthalmic or central retinal artery.[48,49] For these reasons, the fat graft should always be injected without excessive force and always while withdrawing the cannula.

CONTROVERSIAL ISSUES

As previously discussed, the stromal cell fraction of the lipoaspirate contains adipose-derived stem cells that can have tremendous potential benefits predominantly shown in animal models demonstrating improved angiogenesis and fat graft retention. Anecdotally, reconstructive surgeons noted improvements in tissue quality particularly following radiation and perhaps dramatic improvements in facial rejuvenation. These remarkable results can be attributed to the stem cell component of the autologous fat graft but remain to be proven.

Another area of great concern regarding lipofilling is the potential risk that adipose-derived stem cells and the associated angiogenesis can impact recurrence in patients who have undergone autologous fat transfer for breast cancer reconstruction. Complications with fat necrosis and oil cysts may mimic breast cancer, and imaging studies and a biopsy may be warranted to rule out recurrent disease. However, no studies have demonstrated a direct correlation with lipofilling and breast cancer recurrence. Large case-controlled studies comparing patients who underwent fat grafting to a control cohort of breast cancer patients demonstrated lipofilling to be a safe and effective technique in breast reconstruction without any association with breast cancer recurrence.[50-52]

SUMMARY

- Fat grafting is a powerful tool for volume augmentation both in cosmetic as well as reconstructive plastic surgery.
- Although a number of different techniques are available for harvesting and processing of the harvested fat, none are proven to provide superior outcomes or increased fat graft viability or fat graft take.
- There is no clinical evidence to correlate increased risks of breast cancer recurrence with lipofilling or autologous fat grafting into the breast.

REFERENCES

1. Billings E Jr, May JW Jr. Historical review and present status of free fat graft autotransplantation in plastic and reconstructive surgery. *Plast Reconstr Surg.* 1989;83(2):368-381.
2. Ersek RA, Chang P, Salisbury MA. Lipo layering of autologous fat: an improved technique with promising results. *Plast Reconstr Surg.* 1998;101(3):820-826.
3. Report on autologous fat transplantation: ASPRS Ad-Hoc Committee on new procedures, September 30, 1987. *Plast Surg Nurs.* 1987;7(4):140-141.
4. Ellenbogen R. Free autogenous pearl fat grafts in the face: a preliminary report of a rediscovered technique. *Ann Plast Surg.* 1986;16(3):179-194.
5. Hartrampf CR Jr, Bennett GK. Autologous fat from liposuction for breast augmentation. *Plast Reconstr Surg.* 1987;80(4):646
6. Coleman WP III. Autologous fat transplantation. *Plast Reconstr Surg.* 1991;88(4):736.
7. Coleman SR. Facial recontouring with lipostructure. *Clin Plast Surg.* 1997;24(2): 347-367.

AESTHETIC SURGERY

8. Coleman SR. Structural fat grafting: more than a permanent filler. *Plast Reconstr Surg*. 2006;118(3 suppl):108S-120S.
The study was one of the earliest studies that brought the resurgence of lipofilling and fat grafting into the modern era. While described much earlier, the concept of fat grafting gained in popularity with increasing applications, research, and innovations following based on the findings and contribution of this paper.
9. Gutowski KA; ASPS Fat Graft Task Force. Current applications and safety of autologous fat grafts: a report of the ASPS fat graft task force. *Plast Reconstr Surg*. 2009;124(1):272-280.
This study provides the ASPS evaluation regarding the introduction and safety of fat grafting. Although more recent studies have confirmed the findings of the ASPS task force, this study remains a landmark review of the emerging technology and safety of fat grafting.
10. Pezeshk RA, Stark RY, Small KH, et al. Role of autologous fat transfer to the superficial fat compartments for perioral rejuvenation. *Plast Reconstr Surg*. 2015;136(3):301e-309e.
11. Marten TJ, Elyassnia D. Fat grafting in facial rejuvenation. *Clin Plast Surg*. 2015;42(2):219-252.
12. Charles-de-Sá L, Gontijo-de-Amorim NF, Maeda Takiya C, et al. Antiaging treatment of the facial skin by fat graft and adipose-derived stem cells. *Plast Reconstr Surg*. 2015;135(4):999-1009.
13. Sinno S, Chang JB, Brownstone ND, et al. Determining the safety and efficacy of gluteal augmentation: a systematic review of outcomes and complications. *Plast Reconstr Surg*. 2016;137(4):1151-1156.
14. Rosique RG, Rosique MJ, De Moraes CG. Gluteoplasty with autologous fat tissue: experience with 106 consecutive cases. *Plast Reconstr Surg*. 2015;135(5):1381-1389.
15. Mundinger GS, Vogel JE. Calf augmentation and reshaping with autologous fat grafting. *Aesthet Surg J*. 2016;36(2):211-220.
16. Kang DH, Chung JH, Kim YJ, et al. Efficacy and safety of penile girth enhancement by autologous fat injection for patients with thin penises. *Aesthet Plast Surg*. 2012;36(4):813-818.
17. Coleman SR, Saboeiro AP. Fat grafting to the breast revisited: safety and efficacy. *Plast Reconstr Surg*. 2007;119(3):775-785.
18. Kerfant N, Henry AS, Hu W, et al. Subfascial primary breast augmentation with fat grafting: a review of 156 cases. *Plast Reconstr Surg*. 2017;139(5):1080e-1085e.
19. Serra-Mestre JM, Fernandez Peñuela R, Foti V, et al. Breast cleavage remodeling with fat grafting: a safe way to optimize symmetry and to reduce intermammary distance. *Plast Reconstr Surg*. 2017;140(5):665e-672e.
20. Khouri RK, Eisenmann-Klein M, Cardoso E, et al. Brava and autologous fat transfer is a safe and effective breast augmentation alternative: results of a 6-year, 81-patient, prospective multicenter study. *Plast Reconstr Surg*. 2012;129(5):1173-1187.
The use of large volume fat grafting and lipofilling for breast reconstruction was popularized and introduced using the BRAVA system. The concept has not only been adopted by numerous other plastic surgeons all over the world, but is responsible for the increasing use in augmentation of other areas of the body. Although this is not the most common or widely used technique for breast reconstruction, the BRAVA device and authors are pioneers in lipofilling increasing the public awareness and interest in fat grafting.
21. Del Vecchio DA, Bucky LP. Breast augmentation using preexpansion and autologous fat transplantation: a clinical radiographic study. *Plast Reconstr Surg*. 2011;127(6):2441-2450.
22. Haddock NT, Saadeh PB, Siebert JW. Achieving aesthetic results in facial reconstructive microsurgery: planning and executing secondary refinements. *Plast Reconstr Surg*. 2012;130(6):1236-1245.
23. Fredman R, Edkins RE, Hultman CS. Fat grafting for neuropathic pain after severe burns. *Ann Plast Surg*. 2016;76(suppl 4):S298-S303.
24. Klinger M, Caviggioli F, Klinger FM, et al. Autologous fat graft in scar treatment. *J Craniofac Surg*. 2013;24(5):1610-1615.
25. Khouri RK Jr, Khouri RK. Current clinical applications of fat grafting. *Plast Reconstr Surg*. 2017;140(3):466e-486e
26. Mirzabeigi MN, Lanni M, Chang CS, et al. Treating breast conservation therapy defects with brava and fat grafting: technique, outcomes, and safety profile. *Plast Reconstr Surg*. 2017;140(3):372e-381e.
27. Niechajev I, Sevćuk O. Long-term results of fat transplantation: clinical and histologic studies. *Plast Reconstr Surg*. 1994;94(3):496-506
28. Katzel EB, Bucky LP. Fat grafting to the breast: clinical applications and outcomes for reconstructive surgery. *Plast Reconstr Surg*. 2017;140:69S-76S.
29. de Blacam C, Momoh AO, Colakoglu S, et al. Evaluation of clinical outcomes and aesthetic results after autologous fat grafting for contour deformities of the reconstructed breast. *Plast Reconstr Surg*. 2011;128(5):411e-418e.
30. Bennett KG, Qi J, Kim HM, et al. Association of fat grafting with patient-reported outcomes in postmastectomy breast reconstruction. *JAMA Surg*. 2017;152(10):944-950.
31. Komorowska-Timek E, Turfe Z, Davis AT. Outcomes of prosthetic reconstruction of irradiated and nonirradiated breasts with fat grafting. *Plast Reconstr Surg*. 2017;139(1):1e-9e.
32. Sinno S, Wilson S, Brownstone N, Levine SM. Current thoughts on fat grafting: using the evidence to determine fact or fiction. *Plast Reconstr Surg*. 2016;137(3):818-824.
33. Nguyen A, Pasyk KA, Bouvier TN, et al. Comparative study of survival of autologous adipose tissue taken and transplanted by different techniques. *Plast Reconstr Surg*. 1990;85(3):378-386;
34. Moore JH Jr, Kolaczynski JW, Morales LM, et al. Viability of fat obtained by syringe suction lipectomy: effects of local anesthesia with lidocaine. *Aesthet Plast Surg*. 1995;19(4):335-339.
35. Livaoğlu M, Buruk CK, Uraloğlu M, et al. Effects of lidocaine plus epinephrine and prilocaine on autologous fat graft survival. *J Craniofac Surg*. 2012;23(4):1015-1018.
36. Lee JH, Kirkham JC, McCormack MC, et al. The effect of pressure and shear on autologous fat grafting. *Plast Reconstr Surg*. 2013;131(5):1125-1136.
37. Rohrich RJ, Sorokin ES, Brown SA. In search of improved fat transfer viability: a quantitative analysis of the role of centrifugation and harvest site. *Plast Reconstr Surg*. 2004;113(1):391-395.
38. Geissler PJ, Davis K, Roostaeian J, et al. Improving fat transfer viability: the role of aging, body mass index, and harvest site. *Plast Reconstr Surg*. 2014;134(2):227-232.
39. Strong AL, Cederna PS, Rubin JP, et al. The current state of fat grafting: a review of harvesting, processing, and injection techniques. *Plast Reconstr Surg* 2015;136(4):897-912.
40. Gir P, Brown SA, Oni G, et al. Fat grafting: evidence-based review on autologous fat harvesting, processing, reinjection, and storage. *Plast Reconstr Surg*. 2012;130(1):249-258.
With the increasing use of fat grafting in all aspect of plastic and reconstructive surgery, there is an increasing need and interest in optimizing outcomes. There are a number of important details that can impact fat graft yield and take, and few studies have provided such a comprehensive analysis of the different factors. References 39 and 40 are landmark studies in demonstrating which factors are important in maximizing fat graft yield and retention.
41. Fisher C, Grahovac TL, Schafer ME, et al. Comparison of harvest and processing techniques for fat grafting and adipose stem cell isolation. *Plast Reconstr Surg*. 2013;132(2):351-361.
42. Aronowitz JA, Ellenhorn JD. Adipose stromal vascular fraction isolation: a head-to-head comparison of four commercial cell separation systems. *Plast Reconstr Surg*. 2013;132(6):932e-939e.
43. Zhu M, Cohen SR, Hicok KC, et al. Comparison of three different fat graft preparation methods: gravity separation, centrifugation, and simultaneous washing with filtration in a closed system. *Plast Reconstr Surg*. 2013;131(4):873-880.
44. Harrison BL, Malafa M, Davis K, Rohrich RJ. The discordant histology of grafted fat: a systematic review of the literature. *Plast Reconstr Surg*. 2015;135(3):542e-555e.
45. Herly M, Ørholt M, Glovinski PV, et al. Quantifying long-term retention of excised fat grafts: a longitudinal, retrospective cohort study of 108 patients followed for up to 8.4 years. *Plast Reconstr Surg*. 2017;139(5):1223-1232.
46. Kim HY, Jung BK, Lew DH, Lee DW. Autologous fat graft in the reconstructed breast: fat absorption rate and safety based on sonographic identification. *Arch Plast Surg*. 2014;41(6):740-747.
47. Parikh RP, Doren EL, Mooney B, et al. Differentiating fat necrosis from recurrent malignancy in fat-grafted breasts: an imaging classification system to guide management. *Plast Reconstr Surg*. 2012;130(4):761-772.
48. Carruthers JD, Fagien S, Rohrich RJ, et al. Blindness caused by cosmetic filler injection: a review of cause and therapy. *Plast Reconstr Surg*. 2014;134(6):1197-1201.
49. Kim SM, Kim YS, Hong JW, et al. An analysis of the experiences of 62 patients with moderate complications after full-face fat injection for augmentation. *Plast Reconstr Surg*. 2012;129(6):1359-1368.
50. Kronowitz SJ, Mandujano CC, Liu J, et al. Lipofilling of the breast does not increase the risk of recurrence of breast cancer: a matched controlled study. *Plast Reconstr Surg*. 2016;137(2):385-393.
51. Petit JY, Maisonneuve P, Rotmensz N, et al. Fat grafting after invasive breast cancer: a matched case-control study. *Plast Reconstr Surg*. 2017;139(6):1292-1296.
52. Cohen O, Lam G, Karp N, Choi M. Determining the oncologic safety of autologous fat grafting as a reconstructive modality: an institutional review of breast cancer recurrence rates and surgical outcomes. *Plast Reconstr Surg*. 2017;140(3):382e-392e.

QUESTIONS

1. A 54-year-old woman underwent fat grafting to her breasts and had the fat graft harvested from her abdomen, hips, and flanks using tumescent fluid and suction-assisted cannulas. The patient wakes up from anesthesia and is disoriented, with slurred speech, and complaining of vertigo and tinnitus. What is the most appropriate next step in treatment?

a. Electrocardiogram
b. Administer intravenous intralipid
c. Ativan intravascular injection
d. Morphine intramuscular injection
e. Computed tomography (CT) scan of the head with and without contrast

2. A 62-year-old woman with a prior mastopexy and abdominoplasty undergoes an upper outer quadrantectomy for ductal carcinoma in situ and completed postoperative radiation 8 months earlier. She has a noticeable contour deformity from the resection in the upper pole of the breast. She is interested in reconstruction. Which is the most appropriate means of reconstruction?

a. Lipofilling
b. Shaped silicone breast implant
c. Pedicle thoracodorsal artery perforator flap
d. Free superficial inferior epigastric artery flap
e. Free omental flap

3. A 65-year-old man presents for facial rejuvenation and undergoes a rhytidectomy with a superficial musculoaponeurotic system plication, upper lid blepharoplasty, and autologous fat grafting. The fat is harvested from the abdomen, love handles, and flanks using tumescent solution. In the recovery room, the patient is complaining of severe abdominal pain. On examination, the pain is diffuse with guarding but no appreciable mass effect or significant bruising. What is the most appropriate next step in management?

a. Observation and trial of clear liquids
b. Narcotic pain medication
c. Abdominal binder and compression dressing
d. CT scan with and without intravenous contrast
e. Emergent reoperation

4. A 43-year-old man presents to the emergency center 1 day after autologous fat grafting to his calves for augmentation. The fat was harvested from the abdomen, hips, and flanks and processed through the Coleman technique and injected into both calves. A total of 120 cc was injected into the right side and 90 cc was injected into the left calf. The patient is having severe pain in both calves, more on the left than the right. There is postoperative swelling without evidence of a hematoma, with paresthesias and strongly palpable pulses on in both the dorsalis pedis and posterior tibial of both feet. What is the next most important step in the management of the patient?

a. Operating room for fasciotomies
b. Operating room for liposuction of calves
c. Interventional Radiology angiogram and angioplasty
d. Ultrasound to rule out deep vein thrombosis
e. Compression wrapping and elevation

5. A lawyer contacts you regarding a patient who underwent lipofilling to augment her breasts and is very displeased with her result 5 months following the operation. The lawyer states that there is asymmetry and lack of fullness in the upper portions of both breasts with insufficient cleavage to the patient's liking. The lawyer examined the operative notes and states that the fat graft was harvested from the abdomen, flanks, and upper arm and that 280 cc were injected into both breasts. The patient was reasonably pleased with the initial result but now feels that the breasts are not much different than prior to her fat grafting. What is the best explanation for the findings?

a. The plastic surgeon did not use tumescent solution.
b. A stem cell augmenting system should have been used.
c. The fat graft should have been harvested from the medial thigh.
d. A breast implant is always needed to supplement the procedure.
e. Some fat graft failed to survive the transfer.

6. A 54-year-old woman underwent bilateral skin-sparing mastectomies for a right-sided breast cancer treated with adjuvant chemotherapy and hormonal therapy. She then had reconstruction with shaped silicone implants and presents for autologous fat grafting to provide more upper pole fullness. Two years following three rounds of lipofilling to the upper pole, the patient was found to have a fluid collection with a nodule measuring 2.1 cm in the upper pole of the right breast. An ultrasound-guided biopsy demonstrates atypical cells with enlarged irregular nuclei and high mitotic figures. What is the diagnosis?

a. Fat necrosis from fat grafting
b. Oil cysts from resorbed fat graft
c. Breast implant–associated anaplastic large cell lymphoma
d. Recurrent invasive ductal carcinoma
e. Second primary invasive lobular carcinoma

1. **Answer: b.** The clinical presentation for this patient suggests that she had tumescent solution–assisted liposuction, which typically contains epinephrine and lidocaine in an isotonic solution. The symptoms presented are consistent with lidocaine toxicity. The next step in treatment is administration of intravenous intralipids to prevent the progression of toxicity, which includes seizures and arrhythmias.

2. **Answer: c.** For a partial mastectomy defect that involves a significant portion of the breast, lipofilling is an option but would likely require multiple rounds of autologous fat grafting to achieve a reasonable result, which is less optimal for a 62-year-old woman with prior radiation. A shaped implant would likely not provide her with the fullness in the upper pole, and a free tissue transfer would be an aggressive reconstruction for a partial mastectomy defect. Healthy vascularized tissue in the form of a local pedicle flap can provide sufficient volume in a single stage operation without the need for a free tissue transfer.

3. **Answer: d.** A patient with severe pain following liposuction for autologous fat grafting using the abdominal donor site should not be managed conservatively with observation or pain medication. Pain that is out of proportion to physical examination should raise the concern for puncturing the abdominal wall with a possible vascular injury or bowel injury. The most appropriate next step would be an imaging study to look for free air or active bleeding. Taking the patient back for exploration is likely necessary, but a CT scan should be performed prior to a return to the operating room.

4. **Answer: a.** The clinical picture presented is most consistent with compartment syndrome of the lower extremities following autologous fat grafting to the calves. The symptoms of pain, paresthesias with persistent pulses, is most consistent with compartment syndrome, which warrants immediate decompression with fasciotomies to prevent further ischemic damage and morbidity.

5. Answer: e. There is always some resorption of the fat graft following lipofilling as the ***take*** is never 100%. The different modalities for processing, use of wetting solutions, and the fat graft donor sites have not proved to be relevant in maximizing fat graft survival and take. The loss of volume from the initial postoperative period can be because of a combination of resolution from swelling and resorption of a portion of the fat graft.

6. Answer: c. There is no evidence to suggest that lipofilling is associated with recurrent breast cancer or an increased risk for developing breast cancer. A patient who has had shaped textured silicone implants and develops a delayed seroma with an associated mass should be suspected of having breast implant–associated anaplastic large cell lymphoma. The diagnosis is confirmed with staining for CD30, and the patient should be referred appropriately for proper treatment.

CHAPTER 49 Forehead and Brow Rejuvenation

Alan Matarasso and Darren M. Smith

KEY POINTS

- The forehead should be considered in any complete evaluation of the aging face.
- Changes in skin and muscle tone, volume, and activity contribute to the appearance of aging.
- Several techniques are available to treat this region.
- Successful treatment of the aging brow begins with an individualized, problem-based approach. Goals in brow rejuvenation can be summarized as restoring eyebrow height, maximizing symmetry, and minimizing the visual impact of rhytids.
- Forehead rejuvenation can be a powerful addition to other procedures such as a facelift for global facial rejuvenation.

It is common practice to focus more on the aging of the lower two facial thirds than on the uppermost facial third during an assessment of the aging face. This bias is further reflected by a parallel imbalance in the literature. This disproportionate distribution of clinical and academic interest is unfortunate, given the critical role the brow plays in interpersonal communication and overall facial appearance. Aging of the brow (progressive descent, deepening of rhytids, and upper lid hooding) classically connotes an angry or tired appearance.[1] Indeed, the eyes have been called the window of the soul, and as coined by the senior author, the brow is the curtain of emotion. Restoration of the brow to a rejuvenated state reverses this stigmatized default faces and instead frees the individual to express joy, surprise, and confusion with their upper facial third. Additionally, the proper position and tensioning of the brow has a significant effect on the appearance of adjacent structures. Consider, for example, the effects of a heavy brow on exaggerating dermatochalasis of the upper eyelids. It has also been noted that sagging glabellar skin can make the nose appear foreshortened; this phenomenon, in combination with a nasal tip elongated with age, can give the illusion of a nose situated too low on the face.[2]

Several approaches to the aging brow have evolved since the early 20th century, ranging from the least invasive (neurotoxin) to the most invasive (open brow lift). In our experience, invasiveness is not a proxy for effectiveness in brow lifting. Instead, the practitioner should assess the anatomical basis for the patient's presenting complaint and identify the appropriate intervention or set of interventions using a problem-based treatment plan. This plan must consider not only the brow but also surrounding structures to ensure that the upper facial third is rejuvenated as a cohesive expressive unit; unresolved dermatochalasis, for example, will undercut the most perfectly executed brow lift. Conversely, the forehead should be considered when assessing other elements of the upper face. An isolated upper blepharoplasty performed in the presence of brow ptosis can over time worsen that problem, as frontalis tone decreases with the elimination of the compensatory stimulus provided by hanging upper lid skin, resulting in increased brow ptosis.

Moreover, the proper approach must account not only for the patient's pathology but also for his or her desired outcome. For example, a publicly photographed female may benefit from more aggressive muscle interruption or resection to achieve a smoother brow; in contrast, an actor may be better off preserving more motility (less aggressive muscle intervention) to maximize remaining facial expression at the expense of a smoother brow.[2]

HISTORY

Aesthetic surgery of the brow has evolved considerably over time, as chronicled in detail by Paul[3] and summarized here. The earliest description of surgical brow rejuvenation can be credited to Passot in 1919 with his direct forehead skin excision designed to correct brow ptosis.[3] The idea of frontalis and corrugator modification to decrease muscle activity and thereby efface overlying dynamic rhytids gained favor in the 1960s.[4,5] Pitanguy expanded on these principles in the late 1970s and described his approach to coronal brow lifting, entailing wide exposure with muscle-weakening maneuvers and orbital rim soft-tissue release.[6] As more sophisticated techniques evolved, the indications for brow rejuvenation procedures expanded to include glabellar hyperactivity, transverse brow rhytids, upper eyelid aesthetics, and lateral brow laxity.[7] Until the mid-1990s, the coronal approach remained the form of brow lifting of choice. The mid-to-late 1990s saw the introduction of the endoscopic brow lift.[8,9] The open coronal procedure, though successful, lost favor primarily because of patient and surgeon resistance to the long incision and other issues, such as the potential for alopecia. Additionally, an increase in the popularity and effectiveness of neurotomies which addressed two of the more frequent complaints of patients seeking upper forehead rejuvenation—glabellar and forehead rhytids—further eroded the utility of open coronal techniques.[10] Additionally, brow lift procedures in general have always engendered notable reluctance by patients concerned with creating a look of surprise.

With interest waning in the coronal approach, practitioners began focusing on improving internal fixation methods for use with the endoscopic technique. Brow lifting went on to inspire more disagreement over a standard technique than most other facial rejuvenation operations. The endoscopic brow lift ultimately created some consternation with many surgeons, as definitive strategies to obtain fixation were not forthcoming, concerns over longevity of its results lingered, and the inability to apply this method to the high-forehead patient persisted.

In the context of these issues, alternative approaches to brow rejuvenation, including the lateral subcutaneous temporal brow lift (LTL) came to fruition. Our technique evolved from a biplanar dissection in a subperiosteal and subcutaneous plane before taking its current form as a lateral subcutaneous brow lift. Ultimately, the authors found the lateral temporal lift (with or without a corrugator excision as indicated) to offer the benefits of previous approaches with reduced morbidity, shorter incisions, no fixation device issues, reliable brow elevation, and consistent longevity.

ANATOMY

The normal anatomy of the forehead can be discussed in terms of skin, muscle, the innervation of that muscle, and fat. The skin of the brow is quite thin and tightly adherent, facilitating its transmission of the actions of the underlying muscles of facial expression. Surface landmarks are useful in assessing the degree of pathology present. The intersection of a vertical line drawn at the alar base and the supraorbital rim represents the medial extent of the brow. The brow extends laterally to an oblique line extending from the alar base through the lateral canthus. According to classic standards of beauty, the brow peaks (0.5–1 cm above the rim in women and at the height of the rim in men) at the junction of the middle and lateral third of its width, approximately at the lateral limbus.[1] By some standards in fashion, it may be more desirable for the brow to reach its vertical peak closer to the lateral canthus.[11]

The forehead musculature demonstrates the same agonist-antagonist configuration found throughout the body.[9] In the brow, these opposing forces take the form of the depressors (corrugators, procerus, orbicularis oculi) acting as a unified force to draw the brow inferiorly whereas the elevator (the frontalis) works to raise the brow. It is subtle variations in the strength of contractions that result in varying net vectors of skin motion and thereby the multitude of facial expressions produced or enhanced by brow appearance. The muscles of the brow are innervated by the temporal branch of the facial nerve, and this is the only motor nerve at risk during a brow lifting procedure. The temporal branch runs in the temporoparietal fascia and can be avoided by adhering to the deep temporal fascia during dissection and remaining more than 1.5 cm above the lateral orbital rim. Staying in the subcutaneous plane while dissecting the forehead avoids any possibility of motor nerve injury. The first two branches of the trigeminal nerve, the supraorbital nerve and the supratrochlear nerve, supply sensory innervation to the brow. The supraorbital nerve exits the supraorbital foramen in the mid-pupillary line. The supraorbital foramen can often be palpated and marked on the skin to assist in efforts to avoid the nerve during dissection. The supratrochlear nerve fibers are found in the substance of the corrugator muscle approximately 8 to 12 mm medial to the supraorbital nerve (**Figure 49.1**). The supraorbital nerve plays a far more significant role in brow innervation than the supratrochlear nerve. In the lateral temporal brow lift, these nerves should not be at risk.

There is minimal adiposity in the brow. Therefore, fat plays little role in the aging process of the brow, and volume redistribution does not enter into the discussion of brow rejuvenation techniques. This observation does not apply laterally as the brow gives way to the temple. Temporal hollowing can indeed play a significant role in aging the face, and volumetric restoration of this region with techniques ranging from autologous fat grafting to injection of various fillers can be an important part of a comprehensive rejuvenation strategy for the upper facial third. Additionally, the lateral temporal fat pad can descend and contribute to a ptotic brow appearance.

Finally, with reference to endoscopic brow lift techniques, mention must be made of the sentinel vein, a structure that lies 1.5 cm superior and lateral to the lateral canthus.[12] The sentinel vein represents an important landmark, as it can be used to establish the position of the temporal branch of the facial nerve (1 cm lateral and inferior to the sentinel vein) as well as the temporal line of fusion at the temporal crest.[1]

This anatomic background accounts for the changes in appearance associated with the aging brow. As gravity and the relatively stronger depressor muscles overpower the weaker brow elevators, a frown-muscle imbalance results in glabellar creases and central forehead furrows.[13] Compensatory frontalis hypertrophy may result, yielding transverse forehead rhytids. Therefore, it is interesting to note that whereas in the neck and midface it is skin laxity and loss of adipose volume that are the dominant forces in the aging process, muscle activity and imbalance of that activity over time play a greater role in the appearance of the brow in aging.[9] This explains why unlike antiaging procedures of the face and neck which are aimed at excising excess skin and repositioning or revolumizing underlying fat, brow rejuvenation procedures are focused more on rebalancing the underlying muscle equilibrium and repositioning ptotic tissue. This distinction does begin to fade further from the midline, as the frontalis muscle is attenuated at its lateral extent. This anatomical fact, together with the weaker attachments of skin to periosteum found in this region, accounts for early lateral brow laxity.[14,15] This laxity manifests as lateral orbital hooding and contributes to the formation of crow's feet.[1]

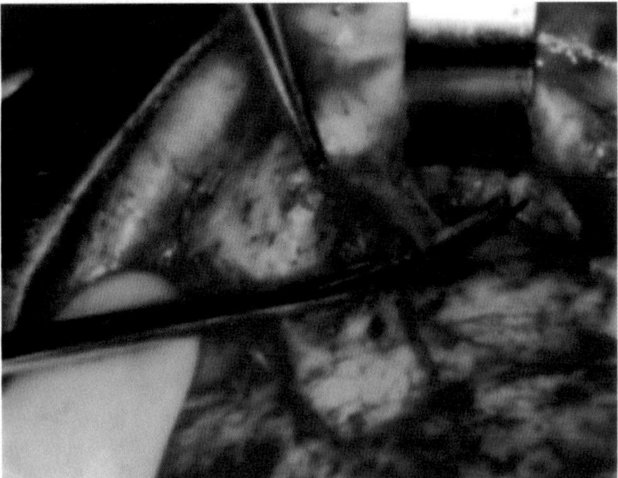

FIGURE 49.1. This dissection demonstrates the relationship of the corrugator (being dissected with the scissor) to the supraorbital nerve (at the fingertip). The retractor is at the nasal root.

Also of note, one must also consider the equilibrium that is present between the elevators and depressors of the brow when performing an evaluation for dermatochalasis. If the frontalis is being relied upon to compensate for upper eyelid ptosis, and an upper blepharoplasty is performed without regard for the state of the brow musculature, the appearance of the brow can be adversely impacted. An isolated upper blepharoplasty in the presence of brow ptosis may remove the stimulus for frontalis-based brow elevation and exacerbate glabellar furrows and eyebrow malposition because of unbalanced depressor activity. The presence of *compensated* brow ptosis must also be ruled out prior to performing an upper blepharoplasty. The examiner should be alerted to the presence of this condition when there are significant horizontal forehead rhytids at rest. These lines are indicative of a requirement for frontalis contraction to maintain brow height at baseline. The diagnosis of compensated brow ptosis is confirmed by having the patient close his or her eyes. If the frontalis relaxes and the brow drops, compensated brow ptosis is present. In addition, the patient should be examined for upper eyelid ptosis, which frontalis hyperactivity can camouflage. Isolated brow lifting procedures can unmask unrecognized upper eyelid ptosis and contribute to an appearance of *deep set* eyes.

MANAGEMENT OF THE AGING BROW

Correctable problems of the aging brow include forehead rhytids, glabellar creases (corrugator muscle hypertrophy), lateral brow laxity, and brow ptosis (including congenital and senescent subtypes). Congenital brow ptosis is beyond the scope of this chapter, which is addressed in discussions of congenital facial palsies. The senior author previously introduced an algorithm designed to aid in decision-making for brow rejuvenation from a perspective that considers the gamut of possible surgical and nonsurgical interventions with respect to the underlying anatomical problem at hand.[7] The following review of approaches to the aging brow takes its origins from the thought processes initially set forth in this algorithm. The options discussed below range from noninvasive (neuromodulators) to open approaches.

Neuromodulators are indicated in the treatment of isolated dynamic rhytids of the brow. There is also a preventive role for neuromodulators in deterring the eventual formation of static brow rhytids. The three neuromodulators currently in common use are botulinum toxin serotype A and include Botox (onabotulinumtoxin A, Dublin, Ireland), Dysport (abobotulinumtoxin A, Galderma, Lausanne, Switzerland), and Xeomin (incobotulinumtoxin A, Merz, Frankfurt, Germany). These products are all based on botulinum toxin's capacity to prevent nerves from releasing the neurotransmitter acetylcholine. Acetylcholine is the neurotransmitter responsible for mediating contraction of the muscles of facial expression. The inhibition of acetylcholine release, in turn, weakens contraction of the target muscles and thereby softens overlying dynamic rhytids.

In the upper face, neuromodulators are most frequently used at the glabella, the forehead, and the lateral canthal lines, or *crow's feet*. Vertical glabellar rhytids are caused by horizontal contractions of the corrugators, whereas transverse forehead rhytids are caused by vertical contractions of the frontalis, and radial lateral canthal rhytids are caused by concentric contractions of the orbicularis oculi. Decreasing motion in the underlying muscles with a neuromodulator softens the appearance of the corresponding rhytids running perpendicular to the axis of muscle contraction. The *frozen* appearance of complete paralysis is generally to be avoided, whereas measured softening of these rhytids is preferable. Though recommended doses by region are widely published, the key to an excellent outcome lies in understanding an individual patient's desires, prior experience, and understanding the patient's anatomy well enough to deliver a dose compatible with inducing a degree of paralysis consistent with those desires. One technique useful for beginning injectors is to employ a planned two-stage injection technique. At the first stage of treatment, a low dose of the desired neuromodulator is injected. The patient is seen back for a second visit once the initial dose has had time to reach maximal efficacy (10 days to 2 weeks is a reasonable window for this visit). The need for an additional neuromodulator is assessed at this visit, taking the patient's degree of residual muscle activity and his or her desired outcome into account. An additional neuromodulator is administered at this second stage as needed on the basis of this examination. The practitioner then knows the total dose required to reach a desired outcome for a given patient. This dose can be repeated in one session generally at 3 months later when the first treatment (delivered in two sessions) has worn off. Although botulinum toxin's effectiveness generally wears off gradually, efficacy is more rapidly lost in males.

It is critical to ensure appropriate dosing and placement of neuromodulators to achieve the desired effect and avoid adverse outcomes. Perhaps, the most common complication to occur with administration of a neuromodulator to the forehead is the *dropped brow* in which the eyebrows sag and brow (and often upper eyelid) ptosis is exaggerated. This results from placement of either too much neuromodulators, a proper dose of neuromodulator placed too far inferiorly, or a combination of both scenarios such that the frontalis is no longer properly tensioned to maintain the brow at an appropriate height.

When brow ptosis is present, a surgical brow lifting procedure is required. The concept of a chemical brow lift produces minimal brow elevation and is based on deactivating the depressors (corrugators, orbicularis oculi, and central frontalis muscles) while preserving sufficient muscle function to allow emotive facial expression. An open brow lift represents a reliable method to gain wide exposure and comprehensively address the anatomical problems responsible for aging brow appearance. It is generally done via a coronal (gull-wing) approach or modified centrally to the widow's peak hairline (anterior approach) in patients with a wide forehead. The latter approach will improve the appearance of a wide forehead. The choice of incision in an open brow lift is determined by the patient's forehead morphology. In patients with a wide forehead, defined as greater than 5 to 6 cm from hairline to brow, a hairline incision is used. In patients with *normal* brow width, a coronal incision is utilized and excess tissue is excised from the hair-bearing scalp.

Markings are made with the patient sitting upright. We use the landmarks noted above to mark the location of the nerves (motor and sensory), followed by the planned incision. It is helpful to mark the rhytids because they can become effaced by infiltration with local anesthetic solution, changes in position, decreased tone with anesthesia, and swelling. Either sedation or general anesthesia with infiltration of local anesthesia is utilized. We do not shave or trim any scalp hair. The incision is made as marked to the subgaleal plane in the central scalp and to the deep temporal fascia lateral to the line of temporal fusion. The scalp flap is elevated anteriorly using a combination of scalpel and finger dissection. Electrocautery is used cautiously in the vicinity of hair follicles. This plane of dissection is continued until 3 cm above the supraorbital rim, at which point the subperiosteal plane is sharply accessed with a knife and periosteal elevator, thereby staying deep to the temporal branch of the facial nerve. The supraorbital nerves are preserved. The corrugator muscles are resected carefully while dissecting and preserving the supratrochlear nerves. In patients with hyperactive frontalis muscles, a wedge of frontalis is marked and excised between the supraorbital nerves to preserve underlying fat. Connell has stated that it is important to perform this maneuver evenly and avoid completely denuded regions interposed with areas of untouched muscle, which would result in "islands of immobility surrounded by angry seas of muscle hyperactivity." The anterior flap is carefully draped over the incision to determine the appropriate degree of resection. The wound is closed with staples in the temporal hair and in two layers centrally.

With increasing familiarity and better anatomical understanding, the endoscopic brow lift evolved into an operation most believe capable of addressing the same issues that were previously the exclusive domain of open procedures. The endoscopic approach is especially suited to individuals with a low brow position, as the forehead with properly toned musculature can be expected, after wide elevation, to redrape to a favorably cephalic position with disruption of the depressors and incision of the periosteum for brow elevation. Further advantages of this technique are attributed to patients who are more apt to accept this procedure with its reduced scar burden, decreased risk of scalp paresthesias, and diminished postoperative edema.[1,16]

Many variations on this procedure have evolved. That presented here is the technical sequence preferred by the authors.[9] Again, markings are made with the patient sitting upright. The nerves, planned incisions, and rhytids can be marked. Local anesthesia is injected with or without the use of systemic anesthesia. The first incision is oriented vertically (this orientation minimizes the chance of nerve injury) in the hairline at the midline of the nose and is 3 cm in length. This is carried to the subgaleal plane. An incision is made on each side of the scalp lateral to the course of the supraorbital nerves, approximately at the superior extent of the temporalis muscle. These are carried down to the deep temporal fascia. This approach allows access to the forehead subgaleal plane as dissection is carried medially across the temporal crest. After the incisions are made, the dissection is continued anteriorly from each port to 2 cm proximal to the superior orbital rim and posteriorly as far as necessary to permit the requisite amount of skin redraping. The pockets from each dissection are then connected with one another. The subperiosteal plane is entered sharply, and the endoscope is then introduced into the cavity with overhead lights turned off. Periosteal elevators are employed to develop a subperiosteal plane. The muscles comprising the depressor apparatus including the orbicularis oculi, the procerus, and the corrugators are sectioned with a Takahashi forceps aided by electrocautery and external traction sutures. The eyebrow-supraorbital rim relationship is used as a reference as the skin is mobilized and redraped cephalically.

Several modalities of skin fixation have been described, encompassing both external (e.g., bolster sutures) and internal (e.g., fibrin glue or calvarial fixation) techniques. Calvarial fixation techniques include cortical tunnel fixation and anchoring devices. In the cortical tunnel technique, a guarded drill is used to create monocortical tunnels (**Figure 49.2**) through which sutures are passed to anchor the scalp flap. Anchoring devices, alternatively, are attached to the calvarium and provide a point of fixation for the scalp flap (e.g., MicroAire's [Charlottesville, Virginia] Endotine device). Though multiple strategies of scalp flap fixation exist, most would agree that the periosteum reattaches to the mobilized scalp flap rapidly regardless of the method of fixation that is employed.

Although the endoscopic brow lift effectively addresses central forehead and glabellar rhytids, lateral ptosis and crow's feet are not as readily addressed with this procedure.[1] Therefore, a conscious effort must be made in designing these procedures to provide maximal lateral lift when indicated. Moreover, a high hairline or an acutely sloped forehead can make this procedure technically difficult to perform

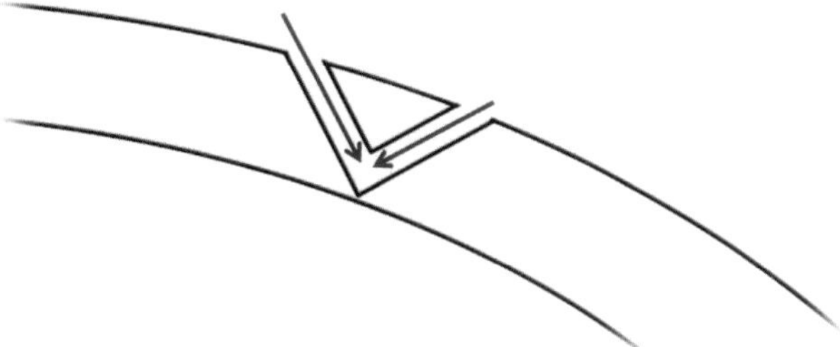

FIGURE 49.2. Cross-section of the outer table of the frontal bone. A guarded drill is used to create tunnels (direction of drilling indicated by arrows) that are angled such that they connect and allow for passage of a suture.

because of the curvature of the skull and the necessary vectors.[2] The degree of muscle disruption necessary to achieve the desired result can be more difficult to judge with the endoscopic approach, predisposing those starting with the procedure to be prone to corrugator over-resection and resultant widening of the space between the eyebrows.

The lateral temporal subcutaneous brow lift has evolved to become the authors' technique of choice for managing the aging lateral brow. The lateral temporal lift can be used reliably to achieve a significant improvement in brow ptosis with minimal morbidity. A medial subgaleal brow lift with corrugator muscle excision and procerus disruption can be done alone or in combination with a lateral temporal brow lift in patients with a low medial brow.

Lateral temporal brow lift markings are designed as follows. In the sitting position, the midline of the forehead is marked (the widow's peak is a good landmark if present). The midpupillary line, approximately 3.5 cm lateral to the midline, is then marked. After an extensive discussion of incision placement based on patient preference, brow pattern, hair density, and forehead width, an elliptical incision is demarcated that is 4 to 5 cm in length and 2 to 2.5 cm in width. The closer the incision is to the eyebrow and less ptotic the brow, the narrower is the planned excision. Conversely, the more ptotic the brow or farther away the incision is from the eyebrow, the wider the excision (**Figure 49.3**). The long axis of the ellipse generally runs parallel to the brow and is verified prior to surgery with the patient in the sitting position.

At the beginning of the procedure, the field is injected with a lidocaine and epinephrine-containing solution. The ellipse is preexcised (**Figure 49.4**). Dissection begins sharply toward the brow and ensues by finger-assisted (wrapped in gauze) dissection medially, laterally, and inferiorly. Scissor dissection is used as necessary at points of adherence. The dimensions of the dissection are confirmed, and hemostasis is obtained by electrocautery. The pocket is packed with a lidocaine with epinephrine-soaked gauze, and the procedure is repeated on the opposite side. At this point, we return to the first side and reinspect for hemostasis. After hemostasis is ensured, we prefer to spray Tisseel fibrin glue (Baxter International, Deerfield, IL) into the pocket, although this is not an essential component of the procedure (**Figure 49.5**). The wound edges are approximated, and gentle pressure is held on the flap for 3 minutes to allow the Tisseel to set. The wound is then closed with 3-0 monoderm Quill (Surgical Specialties Corporation, Tijuana, Mexico) and interrupted Prolene (Ethicon, New Brunswick, NJ) sutures. No dressing is used (**Figure 49.6**).

We have found this procedure to be reliable and safe over a decade-long experience encompassing more than 400 consecutive patients undergoing lateral temporal lifts as described here (**Figures 49.7** and **49.8**).[17] We have followed these patients for between 1 and 10 years. Those treated with this procedure were uniformly pleased with the results. The lateral temporal lift produces long-lasting results, with only one patient in this series requiring correction of relapse. Scar revisions were necessary in two patients. Late fluid collections containing serous fluid and old blood were identified in 3% of patients. These collections generally did not require a return to the operating room and could be aspirated in the office. Skin ischemia and necrosis occurred in two patients after the procedure. The incision from the lateral temporal lift heals quite well, and the resulting scars are often nearly imperceptible.

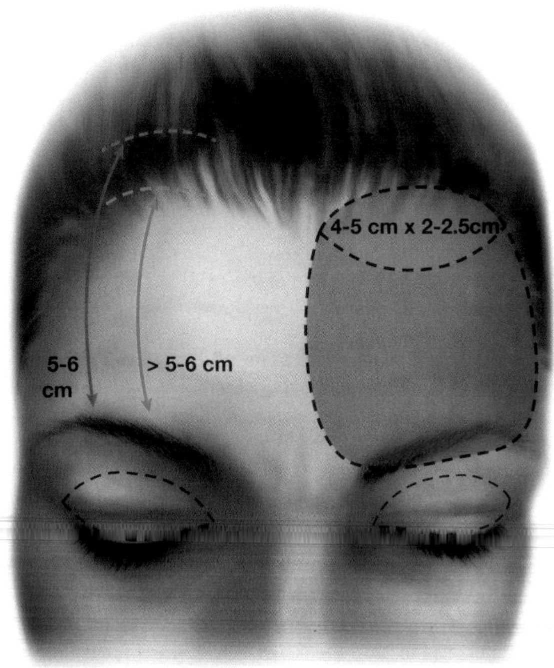

FIGURE 49.3. The curved arrows and corresponding hashed lines indicate possible incision positions. The red arrow and incision correspond to positioning in a lower brow (<5–6 cm), whereas the blue arrow and incision correspond to positioning in a higher brow (>5–6 cm). The ellipse (green) represents the skin excision, and the purple shading represents the area of undermining.

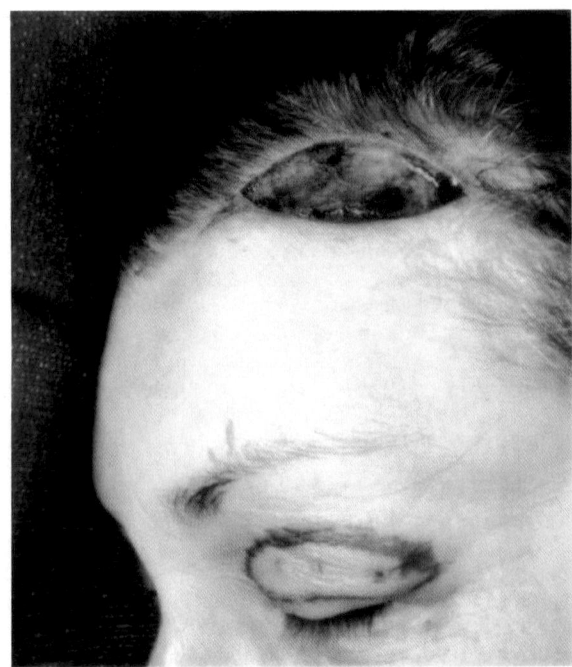

FIGURE 49.4. The skin ellipse has been preexcised.

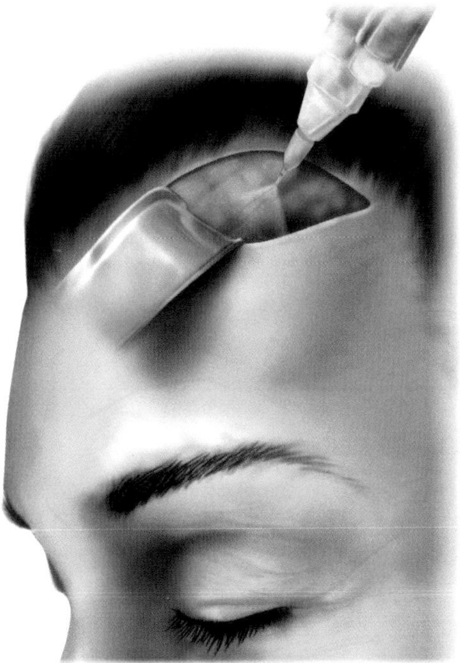

FIGURE 49.5. Fibrin glue is sprayed into the pocket, exposed here with a lighted retractor.

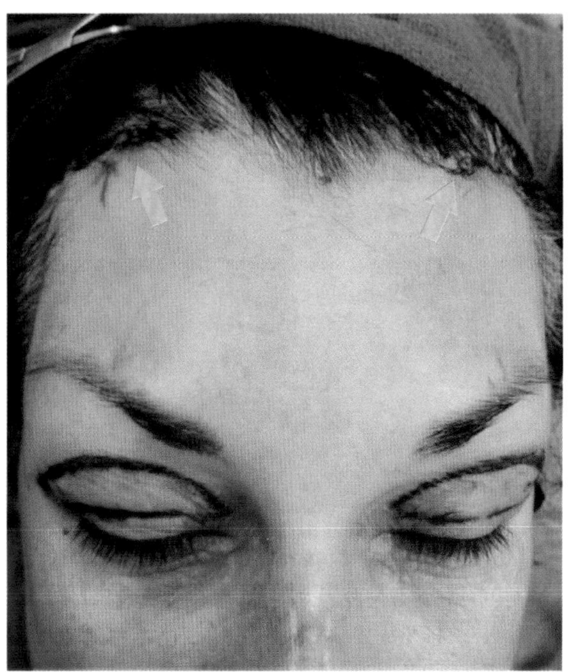

FIGURE 49.6. The appearance of the lateral temporal lift incision (arrows) immediately after closure.

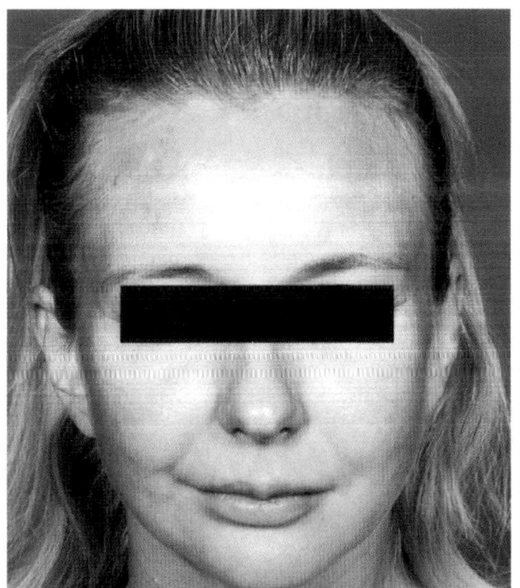

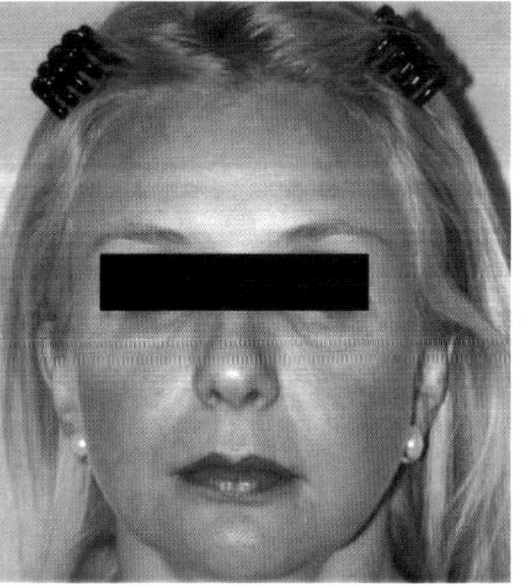

FIGURE 49.7. A 42-year-old woman is shown before and after a lateral temporal lift and upper and lower blepharoplasty.

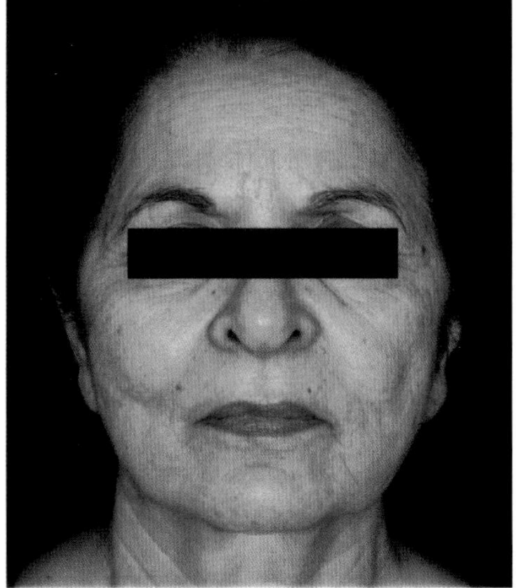

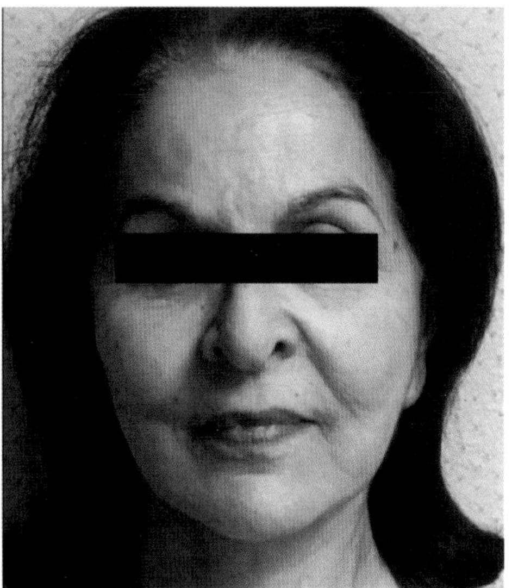

FIGURE 49.8. A 70-year-old woman is shown before and after a lateral temporal lift, facelift, and upper blepharoplasty.

SUMMARY

The aging forehead represents something of a paradox in aesthetic surgery. The upper facial third is critically important in facial expression, and the rhytids and ptosis associated with aging dramatically impact the ability of the brow to accurately express an individual's intended emotions. However, despite the forehead's important role in emotional communication and its great susceptibility to the passage of time, rejuvenation of the brow can be overlooked or minimized in consultations for facial rejuvenation. Similarly, the frequency with which the aging brow and strategies for its management are addressed in the literature pales in comparison to explorations of senescence and rejuvenation of the face's lower two-thirds. There are numerous options available to the surgeon looking to treat the aging brow. This includes surgical procedures and injectables that can be efficacious in addressing brow rhytids. These strategies may be used to address the aging brow alone or as part of a broader approach to facial rejuvenation. Ultimately, as in all procedures designed to reverse the changes of facial aging, it is an understanding of regional anatomy, the forces at play responsible for age-related changes, and the individual patient's desired outcome that are the ingredients essential to choosing and implementing an appropriate treatment plan for brow rejuvenation and achieving patient satisfaction.

REFERENCES

1. Codner MA, Kikkawa DO, Korn BS, Pacella SJ. Blepharoplasty and brow lift. *Plast Reconstr Surg.* 2010;126:1e-17e.
   This excellent article provides an anatomy-based approach to identifying problems and their solution in managing signs of aging in the upper facial third.
2. Connell BF, Lambros VS, Neurohr GH. The forehead lift: techniques to avoid complications and produce optimal results. *Aesthetic Plast Surg.* 1989;13:217-237.
3. Paul MD. The evolution of the brow lift in aesthetic plastic surgery. *Plast Reconstr Surg.* 2001;108:1409-1424.
4. Marino H, Gandolfo E. Treatment of forehead wrinkles. *Prensa Medica Argentina.* 1964;51:1368.
5. Uchida JI. A method of frontal rhytidectomy. *Plast Reconstr Surg.* 1965;35:218-222.
6. Pitanguy I. Section of the frontalis-procerus-corrugator aponeurosis in the correction of frontal and glabellar wrinkles. *Ann Plast Surg.* 1979;2:422-427.
   This seminal article clearly addresses the importance of muscle release in treating brow rhytids. The author's technique and experience are discussed.
7. Matarasso A, Hutchinson OH. Evaluating rejuvenation of the forehead and brow: an algorithm for selecting the appropriate technique. *Plast Reconstr Surg.* 2000;106:687-694.
   The aging brow is addressed from a functional anatomical perspective, and the management algorithm presented offers an excellent framework for considering strategies to address the changes of aging in this region.
8. Matarasso A, Matarasso SL. Endoscopic surgical correction of glabellar creases. *Dermatol Surg.* 1995;21:695-700.
9. Matarasso A. Endoscopically assisted forehead-brow rhytidoplasty: theory and practice. *Aesthetic Plast Surg.* 1995;19:141-147.
10. Matarasso A, Terino EO. Forehead-brow rhytidoplasty: reassessing the goals. *Plast Reconstr Surg.* 1994;93:1378-1389.
11. Daniel RK, Tirkanits B. Endoscopic forehead lift: an operative technique. *Plast Reconstr Surg.* 1996;98:1148-1157.
12. Trinei FA, Januszkiewicz J, Nahai F. The sentinel vein: an important reference point for surgery in the temporal region. *Plast Reconstr Surg.* 1998;101:27-32.
13. Duchenne de Boulogne GB. *The Mechanism of Human Facial Expression.* New York, NY: Cambridge University Press; 1990.
14. Gasperoni C, Salgarello M, Gargani G. Subperiosteal lateral browlift and its relationship to upper blepharoplasty. *Aesthetic Plast Surg.* 1993;17:243-246.
15. Lemke BN, Stasior OG. The anatomy of eyebrow ptosis. *Arch Ophthalmol.* 1982;100:981-986.
16. Mackay GJ, Nahai F. The endoscopic forehead lift. Operative techniques. *Plast Reconstr Surg.* 1995;2:137-144.
17. Matarasso A, Smith DM. The lateral temporal subcutaneous brow lift: a method for consistent, stable brow rejuvenation. *ISAPS News.* 2016;10:35.
    This article presents the technique of brow rejuvenation preferred by the authors of this chapter.

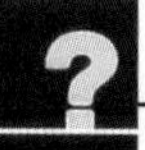

QUESTIONS

1. **Performing an isolated upper blepharoplasty in the context of brow ptosis is inadvisable primarily because:**
   a. The brow ptosis will remain uncorrected.
   b. The brow ptosis may worsen.
   c. Compensated lower lid ptosis may be unmasked.
   d. A *Spock-like* configuration of the brows may result.
   e. It is difficult to accurately plan the upper lid skin excision in the setting of brow ptosis.

2. **Deep horizontal forehead rhytids at rest should alert the examiner to the possible presence of:**
   a. Chronic frontalis over-treatment with botulinum toxin
   b. Dermal pathology requiring evaluation by a dermatologist
   c. Congenital brow furrows
   d. Compensated brow ptosis
   e. A hyperhydrotic brow

3. **The temporal branch of the facial nerve can be most practically avoided during brow rejuvenation procedures by:**
   a. Adhering to the deep temporal fascia during dissection
   b. Dissecting in the temporoparietal fascia
   c. Dissecting in the superficial temporal fascia
   d. Using a nerve stimulator during dissection
   e. Meticulous intramuscular dissection

4. **In a lateral temporal brow lift, a patient with a narrower brow:**
   a. Should always have a hairline incision
   b. Should always have an incision in the hair-bearing scalp
   c. Should have their incision placed based on a conversation with the patient to assess his or her preference and an evaluation of brow pattern, hair density, and forehead width
   d. Is more likely to have hypertrophic corrugator muscles
   e. Is less likely to have hypertrophic corrugator muscles

5. **The supratrochlear nerves:**
   a. Run in the substance of the frontalis muscles and are the dominant source of brow sensation
   b. Run in the substance of the frontalis muscles and the supraorbital nerve is the dominant source of brow sensation
   c. Run in the substance of the corrugator muscles and are the dominant source of brow sensation
   d. Run in the substance of the corrugator muscles and the supraorbital nerve is the dominant source of brow sensation
   e. Have a sensory and motor component

1. **Answer: b.** Hanging upper lid skin can provide a compensatory stimulus of frontalis contraction. In the ptotic brow, eliminating this compensatory stimulus may cause frontalis relaxation and worsening of the brow ptosis. There is no relevant phenomenon called compensated lower lid ptosis. A *Spock like* appearance results from unbalanced disruption of medial brow elevators, not isolated upper lid blepharoplasty.

2. **Answer: d.** Significant horizontal brow rhytids at rest could indicate that the frontalis is chronically contracting to compensate for a ptotic brow. This condition should be tested for in individuals with this presentation prior to upper blepharoplasty. The test is performed by having the patient close his or her eyes. If the brow drops, compensated brow ptosis is present. Chronic botulinum treatment would likely smooth brow rhytids. Dermatologic evaluation is not necessitated by this condition. Congenital brow furrows are not a commonly recognized occurrence. A hyperhydrotic brow is not related to the presence of brow rhytids.

3. **Answer: a.** The temporal branch of the facial nerve runs in the temporoparietal fascia (synonymous with the superficial temporal fascia). Dissecting in either of these planes risks damage to the nerve. Adhering to the deep temporal fascia during dissection is safe as the nerve runs superficial to this plane. Utilizing a nerve stimulator during dissection is unnecessary for this procedure given the clear anatomical relationships. The temporal branch of the facial nerve does not have an intramuscular course in the field of a brow lift

4. **Answer: c.** Although a patient with a narrower brow would likely benefit from an incision in the hair-bearing scalp, the factors mentioned in answer c must be taken into account. The degree of hypertrophy of the corrugator muscles is not related to the width of the brow.

5. **Answer: d.** The supratrochlear nerves run through the corrugators and should be avoided during corrugator resection. The supraorbital nerve is the dominant source of brow sensation. The supratrochlear nerve does not have a motor component.

CHAPTER 50 Blepharoplasty

Sheri Slezak and Katherine E. Duncan

KEY POINTS

- Functional assessment of the aging eye must check for visual acuity, eyelid ptosis, dry eyes, history of refractive surgery, asymmetry, thyroid disease, and eyelid tone.
- Cosmetic assessment of the aging eye should include the skin, brow, cheek, and tear trough as well as upper and lower lid skin redundancy, fat prominence, and muscle function.
- Upper lid blepharoplasty includes skin resection and limited or no muscle and fat excision. Fat is preserved or added rather that resected to avoid superior sulcus hollowing. Ancillary brow procedures may be needed.
- Lower lid blepharoplasty is performed through transcutaneous or transconjunctival incisions and resects minimal skin. It resects, repositions, releases, or adds fat, with lid support techniques as needed. The eyelid-cheek junction is modified as indicated.
- Ancillary procedures to orbital rejuvenation may include browlift, onabotulinum toxin, peels, laser, or fillers.
- Complications following upper lid surgery are rare but include lagophthalmos and dry eye. Lower lid surgery carries more risk, including ectropion, corneal abrasion, exposure keratopathy or dry eyes, diplopia, and chemosis. A retrobulbar hemorrhage can result in pain, proptosis, and vision loss and is a surgical emergency.

The eyes are a focal point of beauty and expression: art and literature is replete with images that allude to the importance of the eye. Saint Jerome said that "The face is the mirror of the mind, and eyes without speaking confess the secrets of the heart," Henry Thoreau wrote that "The eye is the jewel of the body," and Ralph Waldo Emerson said that "One of the most wonderful things in nature is a glance of the eye; it transcends speech; it is the bodily symbol of identity." We endow the eye with far more than its physiology: it is the pathway to the mind and the soul. Although 20/20 vision is desirable, the eye is also admired for its color, shape, expressiveness, lashes, and size. Therefore, it is not surprising that males and females of diverse backgrounds desire to change the appearance of their eyes to enhance their beauty and to avoid the signs of aging that are so evident around the eyes.

Periorbital aging causes predictable changes in the skin, fat, muscle, and bone. The brows descend, producing a sad or fatigued appearance. There is excessive skin in the upper lid that may cover the lid crease or the eyelashes and may obstruct the upper visual field. Lateral hooding due to excess skin and brow ptosis can cause a frowning look. The lacrimal gland may descend from attenuated ligaments. Fat may atrophy, producing superior sulcus hollowing, or the fat pads may herniate and protrude. The lower lids may become lax with increasing scleral show. The pretarsal roll in the lower lid descends and flattens. The septum attenuates and bulging of the lower eyelid fat is seen. Malar bulging with attenuated skin and muscle can be seen as the midface descends. The tear trough becomes more pronounced and the lateral canthus may become lax, causing lid malposition and rounding of the lateral commissure (**Figure 50.1**).

Blepharoplasty can reverse many of these undesired effects and restore the periorbital area to a more youthful state. Blepharoplasty is among the most common aesthetic procedures performed. According to American Society of Plastic Surgeons statistics, 209,571 blepharoplasties were performed in 2017, the 4th leading cosmetic procedure for plastic surgeons. Blepharoplasties are performed also by ophthalmologists and otolaryngologists, making it one of the most common aesthetic procedures. The goal of blepharoplasty is to restore a more youthful appearance without any compromise of physiologic function. Many successful techniques have been described and refined over time, and techniques vary with the patient's particular anatomy. Outcomes are usually excellent, and patients are happy with their improved aesthetics.

ANATOMY

Correction of the orbital aging process requires a firm knowledge of normal and abnormal anatomy. Different patients may demonstrate varying anatomical problems and concerns.

The upper and lower eyelids surround the palpebral fissure and meet at the medial and lateral canthi. The lateral canthus is 2 mm higher than the medial canthus. With the eye in primary position, the margin of the upper eyelid should cover the superior 1 to 2 mm of the cornea whereas the margin of the lower eyelid is usually within 2 mm of the inferior border of the cornea.

The brow should sit at the level of the supraorbital rim in men and above the rim in women. The peak of the brow is at the junction of middle and lateral thirds of the brow (**Figure 50.2**).

The most superficial layer of the upper and lower eyelids is skin. Eyelid skin is one of the thinnest in the body with little subcutaneous tissue. The orbicularis muscle is immediately under this layer of skin and is responsible for closure of the eyelids. It is innervated by the facial nerve (mnemonic OO7). The muscle consists of three concentric circles: pretarsal, preseptal, and orbital. The pretarsal portion is important for involuntary blinking. The preseptal and orbital portions of the orbicularis are involved with voluntary blinking and forced eyelid closure. The orbital portion of the orbicularis can cause brow depression in the upper lid, and attenuation of this muscle can contribute to festoons in the lower lid (**Figure 50.3**).

The orbital septum is contiguous with the periosteum of the orbit, and delineates the preseptal and postseptal space. Posterior to the bands of orbital septum are the fat pads of the orbit. Fat pads serve to cushion the eye, promoting smooth movement of the eyelids and eye muscles within the orbit. The upper lid has two fat compartments, the central and medial (or nasal) fat pad, separated by the superior oblique extraocular

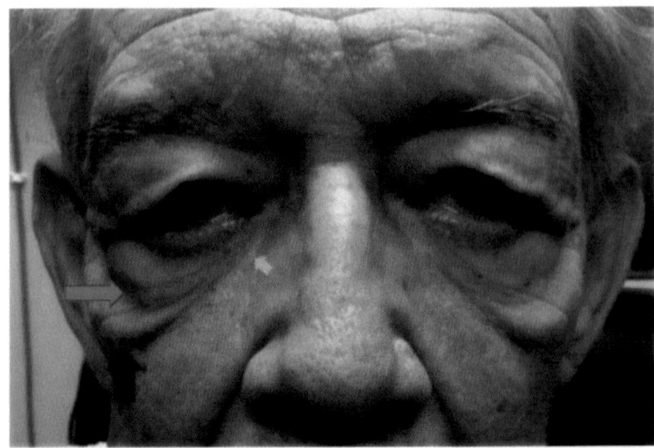

FIGURE 50.1. Characteristic signs of aging in the eyes. The blue arrow marks the orbitomalar ligament, the black arrow the zygomaticofacial ligament, and the yellow arrow the nasojugal groove.

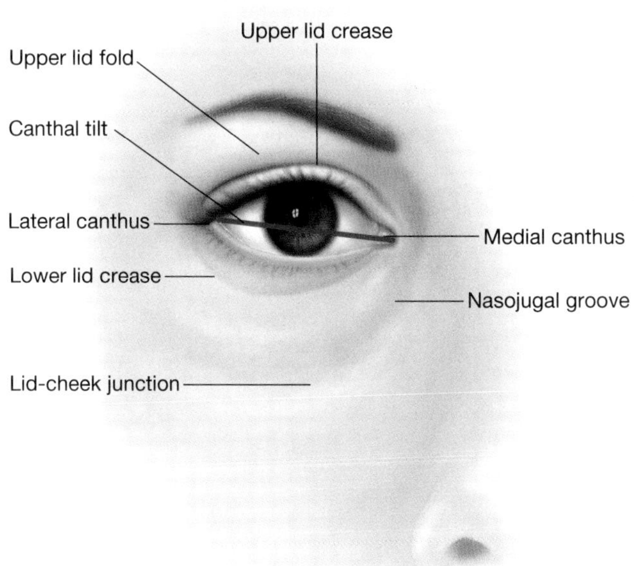

FIGURE 50.2. Surface anatomy of the upper eyelid, eyelid folds, and canthal tilt.

muscle. The medial fat pad is lighter in color than the central fat pad and sits near the supratrochlear nerve and vessels. Laterally, in a shallow fossa of the frontal bone lies the two lobes of the lacrimal gland (orbital and palpebral). When the ligaments that connect the glands to the bone (Sommering ligaments) attenuate, the palpebral lobe can cause a prominent fullness in the lateral upper lid fold (Figure 50.4).

The main retractors of the upper eyelids, the levator muscle and Müller muscle are posterior to the fat pads. The levator is innervated by cranial nerve III and Müller muscle is innervated by the sympathetic nervous system. The levator muscle has anterior fiber projections into the skin and orbicularis just above the tarsal plate, and this defines the lid crease. Typically, the lid crease is found 6 to 10 mm above the lid margin, near the most superior aspect of the tarsal plate. The lid crease is generally lower in men (6–8 mm) than women (8–10 mm; Figure 50.5).

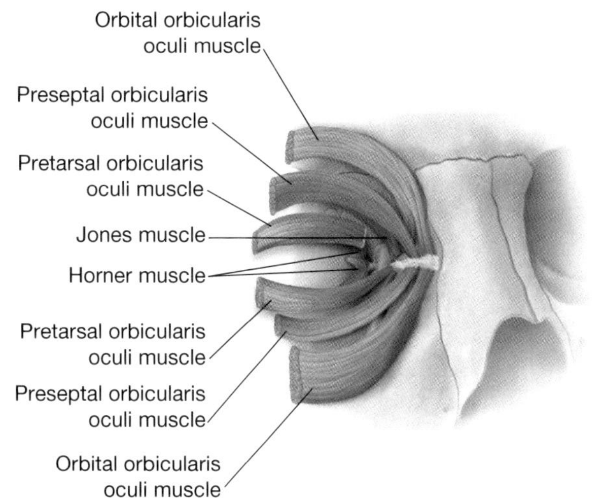

FIGURE 50.3. Muscle contributions to the medial canthus. The complex origin of the deep and superficial heads of the canthal portion of the orbicularis muscle.

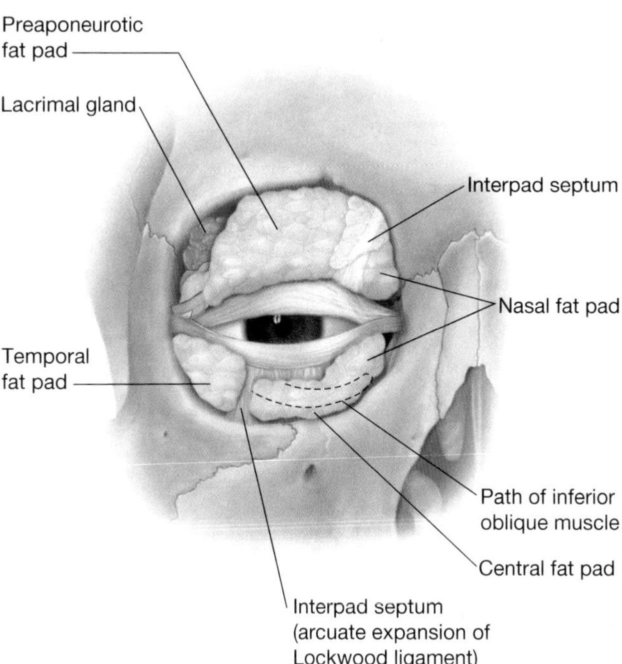

FIGURE 50.4. Anatomy of the orbital fat pads and the interpad septae that are addressed during blepharoplasty.

The tarsus, or tarsal plate, is the cytoskeleton structure of the eyelid. It is made up of connective tissue and Meibomian glands, which secrete an oil that prevents evaporation of the eye's tear film. The tarsus is usually 8 to 10 mm in height in the upper lid. The levator aponeurosis inserts onto the anterior surface of the tarsus. The palpebral conjunctiva is the most posterior layer of the eyelids continuous with the bulbar conjunctiva, forming the mucosal layer of the ocular surface. The superior tarsal conjunctiva contains an abundant number of goblet cells responsible for forming the mucous layer of the tear film.

The lower eyelid anatomy is similar to the upper eyelids, although some differences exist. The tarsal plate of the lower eyelid is shorter, only 3 to 4 mm in height. There are three orbital fat compartments in the lower lid: the lateral, central, and medial fat pads. The medial and central fat pads are divided by the inferior oblique extraocular muscle. The lower eyelid retractors include the capsulopalpebral fascia and inferior tarsal muscle, and are analogous to the levator and Müller muscle of the upper eyelid (Figure 50.6).

The orbital fat pads behind the septum are separated from the inferior fat pad by the orbitomalar ligament, which stretches from the bone through the muscle and attaches to the orbicularis and skin. The medial portion of this arc is called the tear trough or nasojugal groove and extends inferolaterally from the medial canthus to approximately the midpupillary line, where it connects with the orbitomalar ligament. The tear trough ligament is an osteocutaneous ligament between the palpebral and orbital portions of the orbicularis oculi muscle. A tear trough may become more prominent with age, as the tissue above this area is protruding (from fat pad herniation) and the area below it is descending (from malar fat pad descent or subcutaneous thinning; Figure 50.7).

Beneath the orbitomalar ligament is the prezygomatic space where the suborbicularis oculi fat resides. The inferior border of the prezygomatic space is defined by the zygomatical-facial (or cutaneous) ligament, which forms attachments from the bone to the dermis. This usually represents the lower edge of the orbicularis. Inferior to this ligament, the malar fat is present anterior to the facial muscles. This is the area where fat, excess skin, muscle, edema, and lymphatic swelling can cause malar mounds and festoons. Malar mounds are defined as chronic soft tissue edema between the infraorbital rim and the midcheek. If chronically and severely swollen, then the skin and muscle in this area may elongate and form permanent cascades called festoons (Figure 50.8).

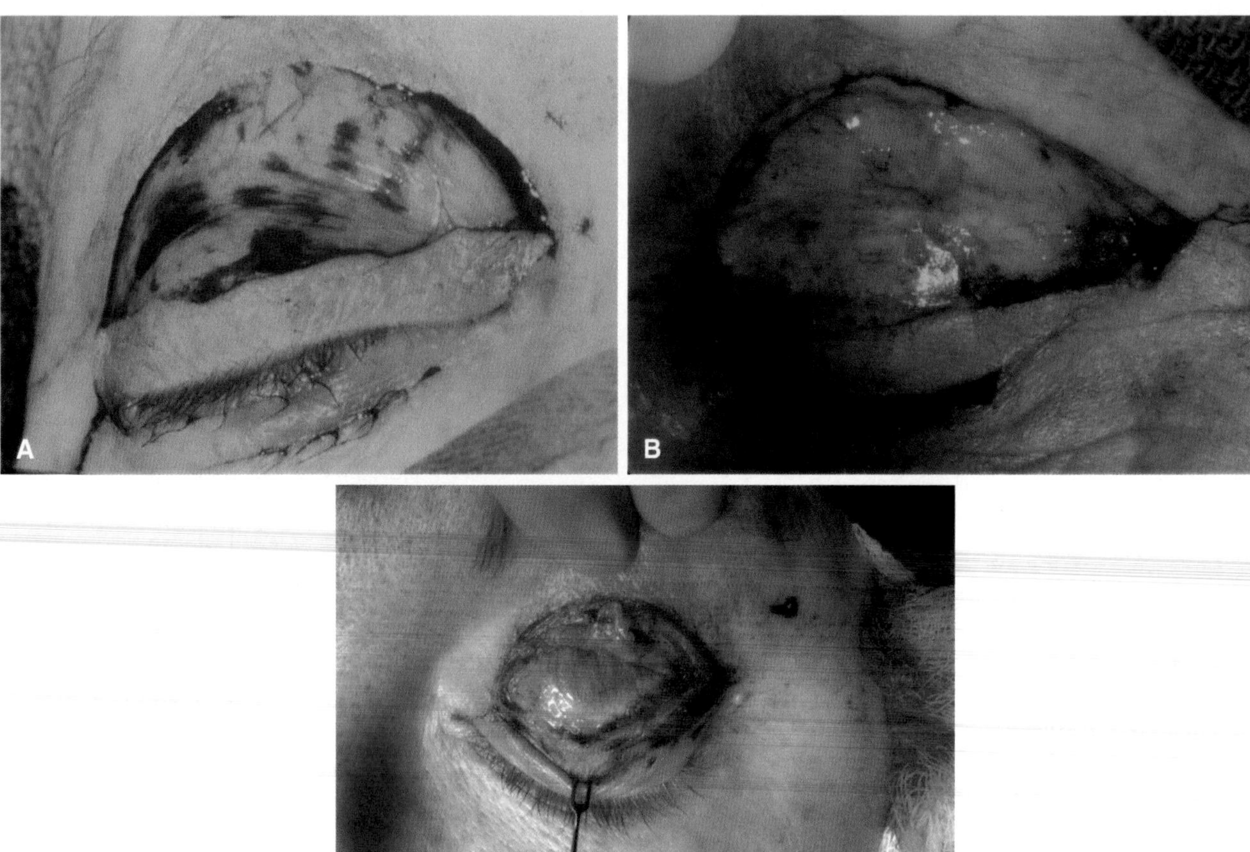

FIGURE 50.5. Layers of the upper eyelid: orbicularis muscle **(A)**, fat compartments **(B)**, and levator muscle and tendon **(C)**.

The lateral canthus is dense connective tissue running from the tarsus to the lateral orbit. It has a deep limb that attaches to a tubercle 1.5 mm posterior to the lateral orbital rim (Whitnall tubercle) as well as a superficial limb, which inserts on the rim. The tendon is approximately 10 mm in length. The medial canthus has a large anterior limb and a small posterior limb, inserting on the anterior or posterior lacrimal crest, respectively. They surround the lacrimal sac (**Figure 50.9**).

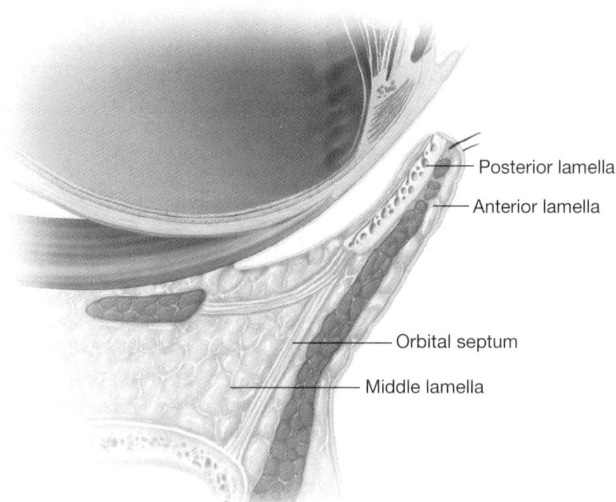

FIGURE 50.6. Cross section of the lower lid demonstrating the anterior and posterior lamella.

The vascular supply of the eyelids is formed by the anastomoses of the branches of the internal and external carotid arteries. The marginal arcade is usually found 2 to 3 mm from the lid margin on the anterior surface of the tarsus. The upper lid has an additional peripheral arcade, found on the anterior surface of the Müller muscle. The marginal arcade ought to be avoided during injection of local anesthetics to avoid a hematoma. The venous drainage follows the same pattern.

The Asian eyelid differs significantly from Caucasian anatomy. The upper lid crease may be absent, low, or present only laterally because of lack of connections between the skin and levator. A medial epicanthal fold may be present, and the upper tarsus may be shorter. The Asian upper lid has more fullness because of preaponeurotic fat that extends more caudally, and there is an upward lateral canthus tilt.

PREOPERATIVE EVALUATION

Patients seek blepharoplasty for many reasons. They complain of excess skin, fatty bags, wrinkles, and dark circles. They may have reduced visual fields and a tired or angry appearance. General aesthetic goals include a crisp upper crease with pretarsal show of 3 to 6 mm, a full orbital sulcus, and a brow in good position. Aesthetic features of the lower lid include pretarsal muscle fullness with a smooth lid-cheek junction, and a well-defined almond-shaped lateral commissure.

Determining the patient's motivations for surgery, goals and expectations is crucial to the success of any surgical intervention. For example, patients who are interested in restoring function will generally be satisfied with removal of vision-obstructing excess skin only; whereas, patients who want to improve their appearance may require a greater amount of skin removal, removal of prolapsed fat, and greater attention to symmetry to meet expectations. It is important

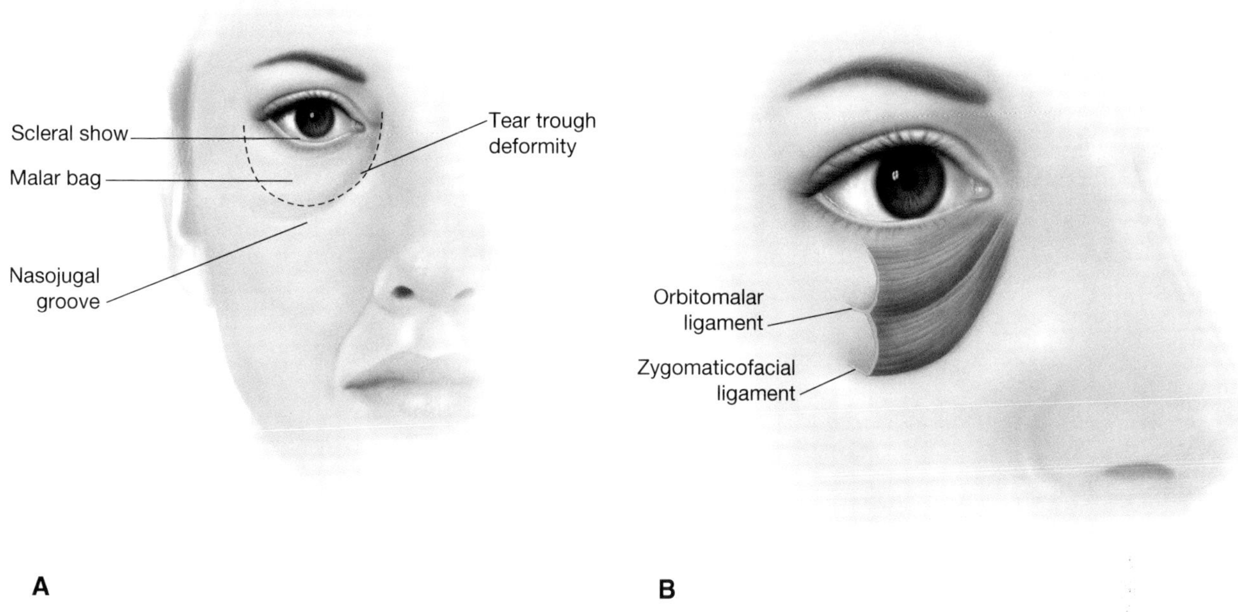

FIGURE 50.7. Lower lid ligaments. **A.** Surface anatomy of the tear trough deformity and midfacial aging. **B.** Three-dimensional anatomy of malar bags created by edematous soft tissue that is surrounded by the orbicularis oculi, the malar periosteum, and the zygomaticocutaneous and orbitomalar ligaments.

to impart to the patient a clear understanding of what goals and expectations can and cannot be achieved with surgery. Patients with unrealistic self-image or who are not capable of understanding the limitations of the procedure are poor surgical candidates.

Preoperative evaluation of the patient begins with taking a careful history. It is important to specifically ask about visual problems, ophthalmology visits, and prior refractive surgery. Blepharoplasty should not be considered within 6 months of refractive surgery as this predisposes the patient to dry eyes. The use of neurotoxin and/or fillers should be elicited as this can alter the physical examination. Specific questioning about coagulopathies, blood thinning medicines, herbal medicines, thyroid disease, allergies, high blood pressure, and glaucoma is required. Dry eye history is elicited by asking about blurry vision that clears with blinking, a burning or irritating feeling, conjunctival injection, the sensation of a foreign body in the eye, or frequent use of artificial tears.

Physical examination of the patient should focus on the structure, function, and appearance of the eyelids, eyebrows, cheeks, and

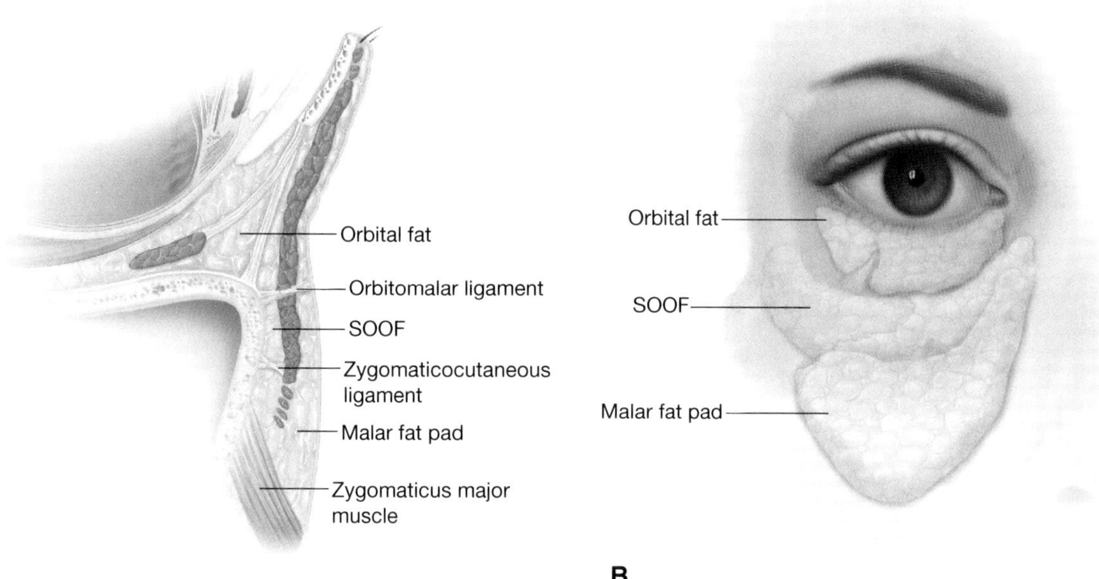

FIGURE 50.8. Lower lid fat compartments. **A.** Anatomy of the deep supporting structures of the posterior lamella, including the tarsoligamentous sling and the medial and lateral horns of the levator muscle. **B.** Three fat compartments in the periorbital region include the orbital, SOOF (suborbicularis oculi fat), and malar fat pads.

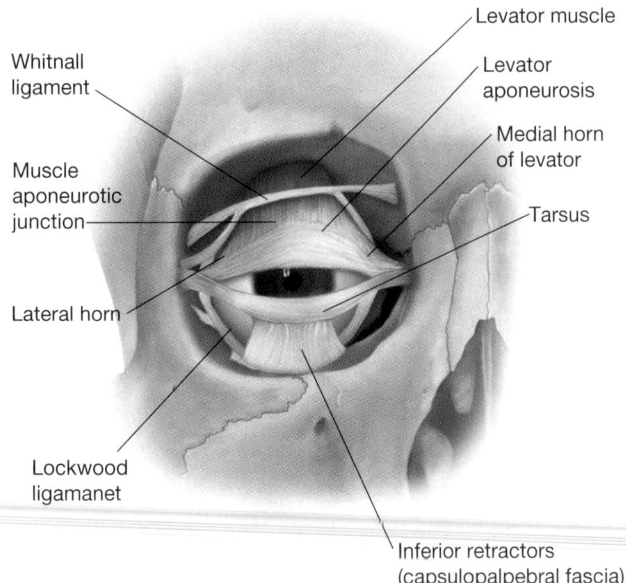

FIGURE 50.9. Anatomy of the deep supporting structures of the posterior lamella, including the tarsoligamentous sling, the medial and lateral horns of the levator muscle, medial and lateral canthi, and Whitnall and Lockwood ligaments.

forehead. Symmetry of the two eyes is also evaluated. This is very important as there is always some degree of asymmetry, but patients do not always recognize this preoperatively. Postoperatively, however, the patient may detect the smallest of differences. A preoperative picture is helpful in every patient, so that the presurgical state can be reviewed.

Careful attention should be given to the position of the eyebrows. The normal brow position in men is along the superior orbital rim. In females, the eyebrow sits slightly higher than the orbital rim, especially in the mid lateral area. Descent of the eyebrow position is an age related change than can make dermatochalasis more severe, and this can be treated surgically with a brow lifting procedure. When assessing eyelid and eyebrow position, it is important that the frontalis muscle is relaxed. Patients may compensate for eyebrow and eyelid ptosis by contracting the frontalis muscle, which can lead to subjective complaints of fatigue and heaviness of the eyelids.

The position of the eyelid margin should then be assessed. If the margin of the eyelid is more than 2 mm and lower than the superior limbus, the patient may have eyelid ptosis, typically caused by dehiscence or stretching of the levator aponeurosis. The margin to reflex distance (MRD1) can also be noted. This is the measurement in millimeters from the light reflex on the patient's cornea to the level of the center of the upper eyelid margin, with the patient gazing in the primary position. If the margin to reflex distance is 2 mm or less, the patient is considered to have visually significant ptosis. If present, ptosis can be corrected at the time of blepharoplasty. The amount of excess skin of the upper eyelid (dermatochalasis) should be assessed. If it overhangs the lid margin or sits on the eyelashes of the upper lid, it may be visually significant. Attention should also be given to any medial or lateral bulging: this may represent fat or lacrimal gland prolapse. Fat herniation can be accentuated by pushing gently on the globe.

In contrast to upper eyelid blepharoplasty, lower eyelid blepharoplasty is generally cosmetic. In assessing a patient for lower lid blepharoplasty, it is important to evaluate the amount of excess skin present, the presence of orbital fat prolapse, and the tear trough appearance. The position of the lower lid is recorded relative to the limbus. The degree of lower eyelid laxity is assessed by a snap back test. This is done by distracting the lower lid inferiorly from the globe and seeing how quickly it returns to its original position. A normal lid will snap back into its normal position instantaneously. A delay of 2 to 5 seconds for the lid to return to its native state or the need to blink to return to normal state is indicative of abnormal laxity. A lid distraction test pulls the lower lid from the globe anteriorly, and a distance of greater than 6 mm is considered abnormal. A squint test delineates the function of the lower orbicularis. The patient squeezes the eyelids tightly together and the orbicularis contracts. This gives the surgeon a sense of the muscle tone and location of fat (**Figure 50.10**).

The position of the globe relative to the orbital rim in noted. If the globe is more anterior than the orbital rim, this is called a positive vector and may suggest thyroid disease or a patient prone to dry eye problems. If the globe is posterior to the rim, this is called a negative vector.

Lastly, examination of the ocular surface for dryness is important as this can be exacerbated by surgical interventions. If patient complaints or exam findings suggest dryness, an objective test such as the Schirmer test can assess for quantity of tears present. This is done by placing a 5 by 35 mm strip of filter paper in the lateral conjunctival cul-de-sac, and waiting 5 minutes. Normal eyes show 10 or more mm of wetting of the filter paper. In clinical practice, Schirmer testing is infrequently used. Staining of the ocular surface with fluorescein dye and examination under blue light reveals punctate staining corneal erosions in patients with dry eyes. This examination is more efficient in identifying patients with dry eye and is preformed routinely in ophthalmology offices.

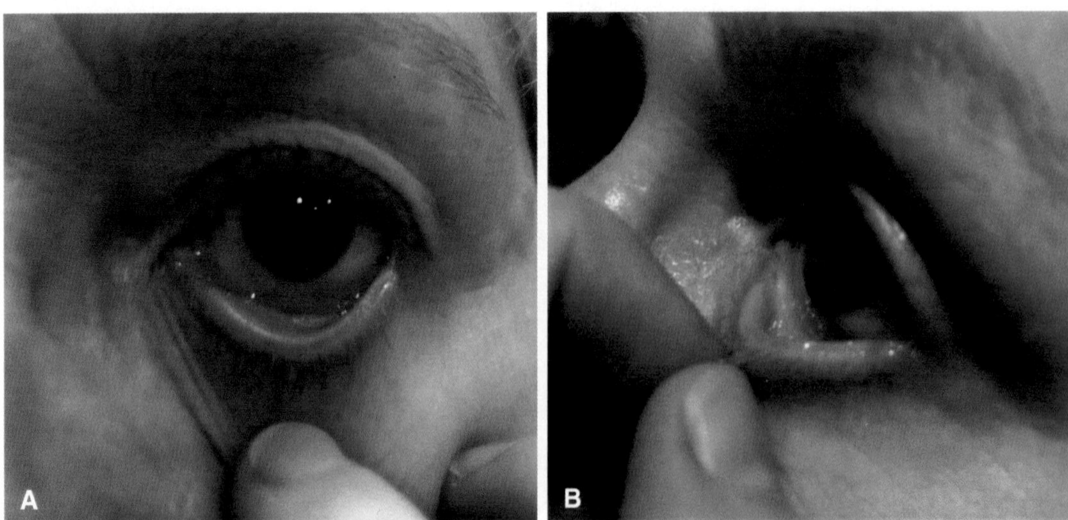

FIGURE 50.10. A. Snap back test. **B.** Distraction test.

TABLE 50.1. COMMON EYELID TERMINOLOGY

Anterior lamella—Skin and orbicularis
Posterior lamella—Tarsus and conjunctiva
Lower lid retractors—Made up of the capsulopalpebral fascia (a fibrous extension from the inferior rectus that inserts onto the inferior tarsus) and inferior tarsal muscle. Support normal lower lid position and provide 3–4 mm of inferior displacement of the lower lid margin with downgaze
Orbitomalar ligament—Cutaneous crease at the level of the orbital rim. Also called the orbicularis retaining ligament
Arcus marginalis—Thickening of the orbital septum where it fuses with the periosteum of the orbital rim
Lockwood ligament—Suspensory ligament that runs horizontally along the inferior orbit and supports the globe
Whitnall ligament—Dense white band of fibrous tissue running horizontally along the superior orbit. Supports the structures in this area and acts as a fulcrum for the levator muscle
Whitnall tubercle—Small elevation of the zygomatic bone just inside the lateral orbital rim that serves as the attachment point for the lateral canthal tendon, the lateral horn of the levator aponeurosis, the check ligament of the lateral rectus and Lockwood ligament
Suborbicularis oculi fat (SOOF)—Fat pad deep to the orbicularis oculi overlying the maxillary and zygomatic periosteum. Descends with aging
Retro-orbicularis oculi fat (ROOF)—Fat pad deep to the brow, which may also descend with aging
Dermatochalasis—Excess skin of the upper or lower eyelid, and may obstruct the upper visual field
Blepharochalasis—Excess skin caused by repeated episodes of edema
Steatoblepharon—Excess or protruding fat
Canthopexy—Tightening of canthus by suturing
Canthoplasty—Tightening of eyelid by division of the canthus and reinsertion
Ectropion—Outward turning of the eyelid margin, caused by aging, cicatrices, paralysis, or mechanical
Entropion—Inward turning of the eyelid margin, which can result in trichiasis (rubbing of the lashes against the eye) and corneal abrasions, due to age, cicatrices, or spasticity
Epiphora—Excessive tearing, often a result of a blockage in the nasolacrimal system
Festoon—Excessive skin and muscle with swelling below the orbitomalar ligament from long-term edema

A visual acuity examination of each eye individually should be performed. The presence or absence of the Bell phenomenon is also noted. This is done by forcibly holding the eyelids open as the patient tries to close them, and seeing if the globe rolls up to protect the cornea. Absence of this reflex puts the eye at risk for dryness and ulceration if postoperative lagophthalmos is present (**Table 50.1**).

OPERATIVE TECHNIQUE

In the past, operative techniques included aggressive fat and skin removal but this led to an unnatural, hollowed appearance. Modern techniques rely on a careful diagnosis of the patient, restoration of more youthful anatomy, and preservation of fat.

Upper Lid Techniques

Repair of dermatochalasis and ptosis can offer functional as well as aesthetic improvement. Functional benefits are noted for an MRD1 of 2 mm or less measured in primary gaze, superior visual field loss of 12 degrees or 24%, and downgaze ptosis impairing reading documented by MRD1 of 2 mm or less measured in downgaze. Improved qualitative findings have also been noted in patient-reported functional impairment from upper eyelid droop, head tilt induced by visual field impairment, and interference with occupational duties resulting from visual impairment caused by the upper lids.

The steps of the basic upper eyelid blepharoplasty are outlined next. Additional procedures involving the correction of brow ptosis or eyelid blepharoptosis are described elsewhere in this book.

Markings

Mark the patient in the sitting position. First, identify the natural upper lid crease. If the brow is ptotic, fix it in the intended position to mark. Less skin is taken if concomitant brow lift is performed. Measure the position of the lid crease centrally on each side with calipers. This should fall between 6 and 10 mm above the eyelid margin centrally. Men are in the lower range, and women will be on the upper range. The medial and lateral crease is generally 4 to 5 mm above the lid margin. If the position of the lid crease is different on each side, choose one crease height and mark symmetric incisions for each eyelid. If the crease is not obvious, manually move the eyelid up and down to better visualize the crease. The lateral edge of the mark should be extended to the orbital rim along a crow's foot crease, but no more than 10 mm beyond the canthus. Typically, one would want to place this 4 to 5 mm above the lateral canthus to avoid a lower lid incision. Placement of the incision along the lid crease results in a hidden scar. The medial marking should not extend beyond the punctum to avoid webbing.

After the lid crease has been marked, with the eyelids closed, use a smooth fine tipped forceps to pinch the excess skin. One tip of the forceps will grasp the skin along the marked lid crease, whereas the other end of the forceps is used to grasp the superior extent of the excess skin. Repeat this maneuver at several points along the eyelid and connect the points to outline the upper limit of skin to be removed. Eyelashes should just evert with this pinch. There should always be at least 10 mm of skin left below the brow. The superior extent line is then connected to the lid crease marking medially and laterally. The shape of the excision can be an ellipse or a scalpel shape with more lateral resection. A safe rule of thumb is that skin resection should preserve a brow to margin distance of at least 20 mm (**Figure 50.11**).

Anesthesia

Inject subcutaneous anesthetic superficially in the area to be resected. Upper lid blepharoplasty alone is generally done under local anesthesia but additional procedures or patients' characteristics may dictate the use of intravenous (IV) sedation or general anesthesia.

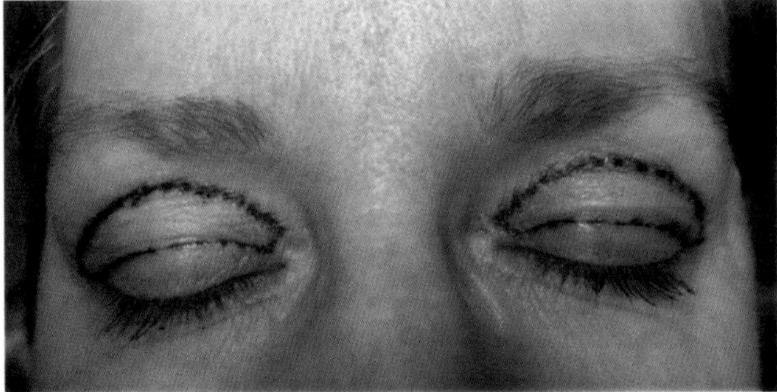

FIGURE 50.11. Upper eyelid markings.

Skin Resection

Incise the skin along the marked incision lines with a no. 15 blade. Some surgeons prefer to use a CO_2 laser or Colorado microdissection needle to incise the skin. Excise the marked area of skin by taking care to excise skin only and leaving the orbicularis intact.

Muscle Resection

Although not always needed, removal of muscle may be done to decrease fullness or to create a crisp supratarsal fold. A strip of 3 to 5 mm is removed, and cautery is used to achieve hemostasis from the muscle vessels.

Fat Removal

Fat removal may or may not be needed. If needed, the orbicularis and septum are opened with scissors or cautery to expose the fat pads. Gentle pressure on the globe will further prolapse the fat. The medial orbital fat pad typically requires debulking more often than the central pad. The fat can be resected with needle tip cautery or by clamping the fat with a hemostat, excising it and then cauterizing the cut end. Great care is taken to avoid any traction on the fat as this can lead to bleeding posterior to the septum and a retro-orbital hemorrhage. Aggressive fat debulking of the eyelids can result in a hollowed appearance and has fallen out of favor. Minimal conservative fat removal is recommended.

Some patients have a prominent fat fad under the lateral third of the brow, which is below the orbicularis. This is called retro-orbicularis oculi fat and can be resected at the time of blepharoplasty. Dissection is carried out superiorly beneath the orbicularis where the fat is resected. Browpexy may also be performed in this space by placing sutures to secure the lateral orbicularis and brow to the periosteum at the desired position at or above the superior orbital rim.

Lacrimal Gland

A prolapsed lacrimal gland presents as a mass below the brow and lateral orbital rim. Double armed sutures can be used to engage the inferior tip of the gland and secure it to the periosteum just inside the superior orbital rim at the lacrimal fossa. Excision of the gland tissue should be avoided, as this can lead to dry eye.

Skin Closure

Many different skin closures are successful; running or interrupted sutures and absorbable and nonabsorbable sutures can be used. Fine suture (6-0 to 8-0 suture) is used in a single layer, and sutures are typically removed 7 days after surgery (**Figure 50.12**).

Lower Lid Techniques

Unlike upper eyelid blepharoplasty, there are multiple approaches to a lower eyelid blepharoplasty. Variation in patient anatomy will influence the chosen technique. Older patients with excess skin may warrant a transcutaneous lower eyelid blepharoplasty. If lower eyelid laxity is also present, a lower eyelid tightening procedure (i.e., lateral tarsal strip) can be performed at the same time. Patients with fat prolapse or tear trough deformity and minimal excess skin can be approached with a transconjunctival lower lid blepharoplasty with fat excision or redraping. Different surgeons prefer different techniques.

Markings

A subciliary skin incision is marked 2 mm below the lower eyelid lashes. The marking is extended inferotemporally along a crow's foot crease to the lateral orbital rim. The lower incision should be 5 to 7 mm inferior to the upper lid incision. The location and the planned amount of fat pad resection is noted or marked. Fat pad anatomy can be better visualized by gentle pressure on the globe. The tear trough is marked.

Anesthesia and Shields

Various surgeons use local, IV sedation, or general anesthesia. A corneal shield may be used for lower lid surgery to protect the globe.

Transcutaneous Approach

The marked subciliary incision is made with a knife or sharp scissors. The incision is then *stairstepped* so that the muscle incision is made 5 mm below the lashes to spare the pretarsal orbicularis. A skin-muscle flap is dissected inferiorly to below the orbital rim. The orbitomalar ligament is completely released so that the skin is no longer fixed to the bone.

Fat Removal, Relocation, and Augmentation

The orbital septum may be opened with iris scissors or cautery to expose the lower eyelid fat pads. Fat may then be resected in a similar fashion as was described in the upper eyelid blepharoplasty or can be redraped over the inferior orbital rim to address any tear trough deformity. It may also be harvested to use as free fat grafts. Care must be taken to avoid injury to the inferior oblique muscle that divides the nasal and central fat pads.

Skin/Muscle Resection

The skin-muscle flap is then redraped superiorly and laterally and any excess overlapping skin and muscle is excised. It is important to be conservative in the amount of skin resected because this can cause retraction of the lower eyelid. Generally, only a few mm of skin is excised. Vicryl suture is used to resuspend the orbicularis to the soft tissue and periosteum in the area of the lateral orbital rim to provide mechanical support for the lower lid and prevent ectropion.

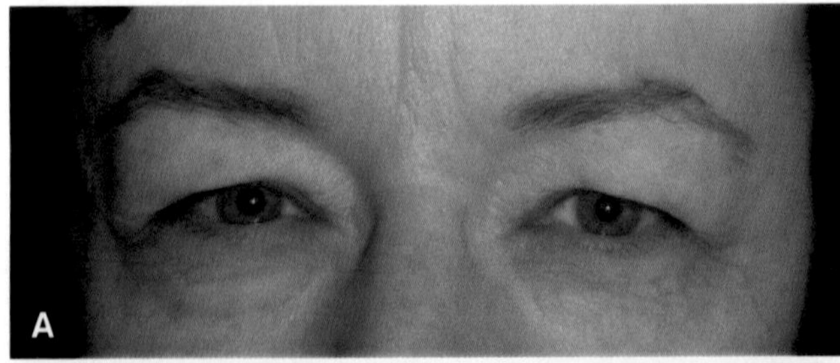

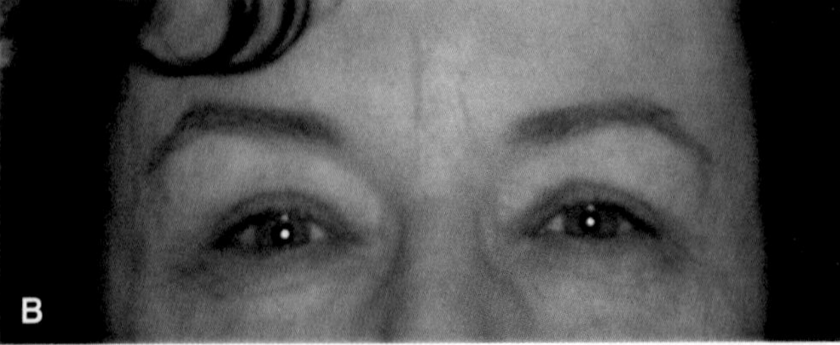

FIGURE 50.12. Upper lid blepharoplasty: preoperative **(A)** and postoperative **(B)**.

Lateral Canthal Tightening

If the patient was found to have significant lower eyelid laxity during the preoperative evaluation, they are at higher risk for ectropion with any skin resection and a lateral canthal tightening procedure should be performed. A canthopexy can be used for mild laxity. This is performed by placing a mattress suture through the edge of the tarsal ligament or tarsal plate and securing it to the periosteum inside the lateral orbital rim. A canthoplasty or lateral tarsal strip addresses moderate to severe lower lid laxity. A canthoplasty divides the tarsal ligament and reinserts it. In a lateral tarsal strip, the lid is redraped laterally. The anterior lamella and lid margin in the area of excess lid overlapping the lateral canthus is separated from the tarsus, and the extra lateral tarsus is removed. A mattress suture is then placed through the new lateral end of the shortened tarsus and secured to the periosteum. When placing the periosteal stitch, it is important to ensure proper height of the lateral canthus (2 mm above the medial canthus).

Closure

Close the skin with running fine suture (6-0 to 8-0). Sutures are removed in 7 days (**Figure 50.13**).

Transconjunctival Approach

The lower eyelid is retracted anteriorly to expose the palpebral conjunctiva. A scalpel or cutting cautery is used to incise the conjunctiva just below the tarsal plate. The lower eyelid retractors are divided. Dissection proceeds inferiorly, between the septum and orbicularis, to expose the fat pads and orbital rim. The orbital malar ligament is completely released. Fat resection or relocation proceeds as earlier. Some surgeons use a lower conjunctival incision, at about 4 to 5 mm below the tarsus, and go directly into the fat pads. Lateral canthal support is generally not needed in a transconjunctival approach, as the orbicularis is not weakened by division. If necessary, a small pinch of pretarsal skin can be resected. The conjunctival incision can be closed with two or three interrupted absorbable sutures or may be left open after the procedure.

Adjunct procedures, such as browlift, peels, laser, fillers, and muscle denervation can be added at the time of blepharoplasty or can be performed later in the office. Severe festoons may require muscle resection, redraping, or suspension along with midface lift, liposuction, or direct excision.

POSTOPERATIVE CARE

Patients are advised to elevate their heads and apply cool compresses or ice to the eyelids for the first 24 to 48 hours. They may apply antibiotic ointment to the surgical incisions twice daily for 1 week.

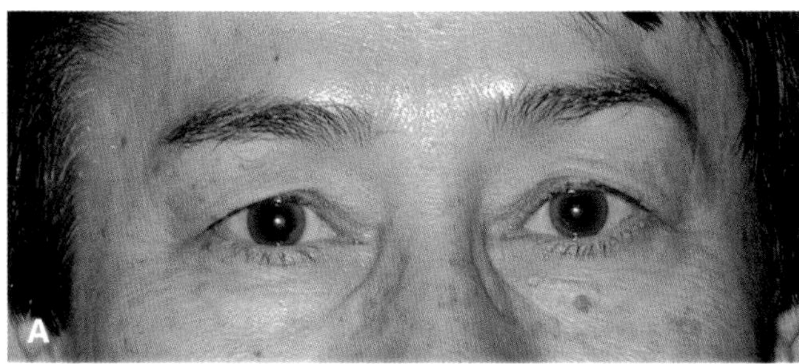

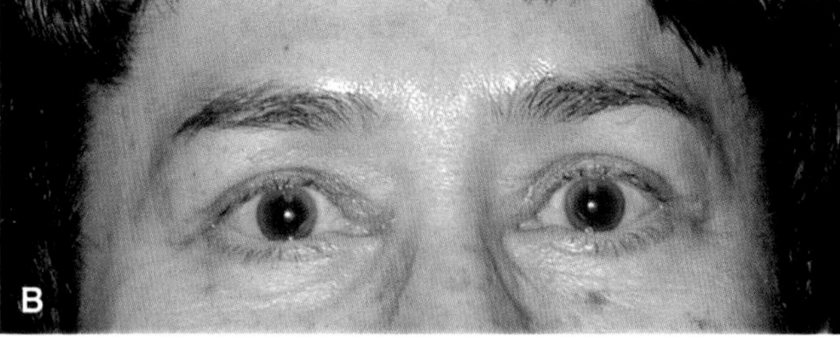

FIGURE 50.13. Four-lid blepharoplasty: preoperative **(A)** and postoperative **(B)**.

Patients should avoid strenuous activity or bending below the waist for 2 weeks. Nonabsorbable sutures can be removed 7 days after surgery. Patients should expect postoperative swelling and bruising to persist for up to 2 weeks after surgery.

Complications

Fortunately, complications are rare in blepharoplasty, but when present, can be devastating both aesthetically and functionally. A full discussion of possible complications with documentation in the record is prudent for every patient. Complications can be divided into acute and long-term risks.

Acute Complications

Orbital Hematoma

The most feared complication of eyelid surgery is hemorrhage behind the orbital septum, which can result in an orbital compartment syndrome and vision loss. Although rare, this needs immediate attention. It generally happens in the operating room or in the first 24 hours postop and presents as severe pain, pressure, and decreased vision. Examination is diagnostic as there is proptosis, limitation of extraocular movements, and increased intraorbital pressure. This complication can be averted by careful tissue handling to avoid traction of the fat pads and careful hemostasis of the base of the fat pad. Preoperative considerations such as control of hypertension and the avoidance of aspirin and blood thinners can decrease this risk as well. In the case of vision threatening hematomas, treatment is directed at urgent opening of the incision for evacuation of the hematoma. A lateral canthotomy can be performed to relieve intraorbital pressure. If the patient has developed vision loss, high-dose IV steroids should be initiated to maximize visual recovery. Operative drainage of the hematoma is a surgical emergency.

Small eyelid hematomas without vision changes can be treated conservatively with elevation and ice.

Corneal Abrasion

The patient presents immediately postoperatively with severe eye pain, tearing, and blurred vision with a foreign body sensation. Ophthalmology consultation may use fluorescein and a Wood's lamp to document an abrasion. Abrasions are treated with frequent use of ophthalmic antibiotic ointment. The use of scleral shields can help prevent this problem. Pain beyond 24 hours requires further ophthalmologic evaluation.

Lagophthalmos

Mild postoperative lagophthalmos (inability to completely close the eyes) is common and typically resolves in the first few days after surgery. This can be managed with lubrication of the eyes. If is present beyond the first week, it can typically be managed with ointment and massage of the upper eyelids. Persistent lagophthalmos is usually the result of aggressive skin removal or scarring of the orbital septum. Reoperation with lysis of scar tissue and/or skin grafting may be required in severe cases.

Chemosis

Conjunctival edema is common after surgery and is usually self-limited. Artificial tears and a steroid eyedrop/ointment can be prescribed if the swelling is severe. Topical ophthalmic steroid use should always be temporary or monitored by an ophthalmologist as it can lead to elevated intraocular pressures and glaucoma with long-term use.

Infection

Infection is rare because of the excellent vascularity of the face. Eyelid surgery is considered clean surgery and antibiotics are not generally used. Erythema and purulent discharge should be treated with antibiotics and culture, and computed tomography may be necessary to evaluate for an orbital abscess.

Corneal Exposure/Dry Eye

Dryness can be transient in the postoperative period and can be corrected with aggressive use of artificial tears and lubricating ointments.

Diplopia

The superior and inferior oblique muscles are the most commonly injured extraocular muscles in upper and lower blepharoplasty, respectively. They can be injured either during fat resection, transconjunctival dissection, or by traction. Diplopia is usually transient and is managed conservatively. Should it persists, ophthalmologic evaluation is needed. Strabismus surgery or prism glasses may be used to correct persistent diplopia.

Epiphora

Tearing can result from irritation, inflammation, or rarely injury to the puncta or the canalicular pump system. An altered lid position may also cause tearing. Tearing is usually transient.

Long-Term Complications

Asymmetry

Asymmetry of the lid position or contour can occur in the immediate postoperative period as a result of swelling and should be monitored initially. Asymmetry of the upper lid creases can be avoided by careful and equal marking of the eyelid crease at the beginning of the procedure as well as uniform dissection of fat.

Lid Malposition

Ptosis of the upper eyelids can occur because of injury to the levator aponeurosis if surgical dissection was carried too deep into the eyelid structures. Complications of lower eyelid blepharoplasty include lower eyelid retraction, ectropion, and inferior scleral show. These typically occur when there is excessive removal of skin and muscle. Upward massage of the lids can be attempted in the acute postoperative period. Persistent ectropion and/or retraction may require surgical revision with skin grafting.

Dry Eye Syndrome

Ocular surface irritation and dryness can persist despite good position of the lids and short-term use of artificial tears. In these situations, it would be most appropriate to refer the patient to an ophthalmologist for further evaluation and management.

Unsightly Scars

Careful camouflage of the incisions in the upper crease and close to the lower eyelid are key to avoid a noticeable scar. Medial scar extension can cause noticeable webbing.

OUTCOMES

Interestingly, there are few outcome studies from the patients' point of view. One outcome study used the Face Q. They reported that the most common patient-reported adverse effects after eyelid surgery included *obvious, noticeable, or uneven scars* (37%); *dry eyes* (35%), *eye irritation (itching or redness)* (33%); and *excessive tearing* (25%). This is significantly different from physician-reported complications, although global satisfaction is generally positive. Fortunately, most adverse effects are self-limited and fully resolve.

CONCLUSION

Blepharoplasty is a procedure that can improve both the function and the aesthetics of the eyelids. It is a short operation, often under local anesthesia, with generally acceptable risk. Success of the procedure is dependent on a detailed understanding of the eyelid anatomy as well as careful preoperative evaluation and planning. Meticulous surgical technique helps the surgeon to attain the desired goals while avoiding postoperative complications. Long-lasting improvement and satisfied patients make blepharoplasty a popular operation in men and women of many age groups.

BIBLIOGRAPHY

1. Cahill KV, Bradley EA, Meyer DR, et al. Functional indications for upper eyelid ptosis and blepharoplasty surgery: a report by the American Academy of Ophthalmology. *Ophthalmology*. 2011;118(12):2510.
   A review of 13 studies that demonstrate the improvement in vision, peripheral vision, and quality of life activities with repair of upper lid dermatochalasis and blepharoptosis.
2. Damasceno RW, Cariello AJ, Cardoso EB, et al. Upper blepharoplasty with or without resection of the orbicularis oculi muscle: a randomized double blind left right study. *Ophthal Plast Reconstr Surg*. 2011;27:195.
3. Drolet BG Sullivan PK. Evidence based medicine medicine: blepharoplasty. *Plast Reconstr Surg*. 2014;133:1195.
4. Espinoza GM, Holds JB. Evaluation and treatment of the tear trough deformity in lower. *Blepharoplasty Semin Plast Surg*. 2007;21:57.
5. Faigen S. Advanced rejuvenation upper blepharoplasty. *Plast Reconstr Surg*. 2002;110:278.
6. Fleury CM, Schwitzer JA, Hung RW, Baker SB. Adverse event incidences following facial plastic surgery procedures: incorporating FACE-Q data to improve patient preparation. *Plast Recosntr Surg*. 2018;141:28e.
7. Ghabrial R, Lisman R, Kane M, et al. Diplopia following transconjunctival blepharoplasty. *Plast Reconstr Surg*. 1998;102:1219.
8. Hashem AM, Couto RA, Waltzman JT, et al. Evidence-based medicine: a graded approach to lower lid blepharoplasty. *Plast Reconstr Surg*. 2017;139(1):139e-150e.
   Accurate diagnosis of the problems in the lower lids is used for a graded, individualized correction of fat excess, tear trough, lid-cheek junction abnormalities.
9. Hoorntje LE, Lei BV, Stollenwerck GA, Kon MJ. Resecting orbicularis oculi muscle in upper eyelid blepharoplasty: a review of the literature. *Plast Reconstr Aesthet Surg*. 2010;63(5):787-792.
10. Jindal K, Sarcia M, Codner M. Functional considerations in aesthetic eyelid surgery. *Plast Reconstr Surg*. 2014;134:1154.
11. Kiang L, Deptula P, Mazhar M, et al. Muscle-sparing blepharoplasty: a prospective left-right comparative study. *Arch Plast Surg*. 2014;41(5):576-583.
    A randomized prospective study of 22 patients with skin-only upper lip blepharoplasty on one side and muscle-skin resection on the other.
12. Kiranantawar K, Suhk JH, Nguyen AH. The Asian eyelid: relevant anatomy. *Semin Plast Surg*. 2015;29:158.
    Thorough discussion of the various types of Asian eye anatomy variations in crease, skin, fat, and epicanthal folds.
13. Korn BS, Kikkawa DO, Cohen SR. Transcutaneous lower eyelid blepharoplasty with orbitomalar suspension: retrospective review of 212 consecutive cases. *Plast Reconstr Surg*. 2010;125(1):315-323.
14. Kpodzo DS, Nahai FC, McCord CD. Malar mounds and festoons: review of current management. *Aesthet Surg J*. 2014;34(2):235.
    Reviews the terminology and anatomy of mounds and festoons, and gives a treatment algorithm for these difficult problems.
15. Friedland JA, Lalonde D, Rohrich R. An evidence-based approach to blepharoplasty. *Plast Reconstr Surg*. 2010;126:2222.
16. Lellli GJ, Lisman RD. Blepharoplasty complications. *Plast Reconstr Surg*. 2010;125:1007.
17. LoPiccolo MC, Mahmoud BH, Liu A, et al. Evaluation of orbicularis oculi muscle stripping on the cosmetic outcome of upper lid blepharoplasty: a randomized, controlled study. *Dermatol Surg*. 2013;39:739.
18. Miranda SG, Codner MA. Micro free orbital fat grafts to the tear trough deformity during lower blepharoplasty. *Plast Reconstr Surg*. 2017;139:1335.
19. Muzaffar AR, Mendelson BC, Adams WP Jr. Surgical anatomy of the ligamentous attachments of the lower lid and lateral canthus. *Plast Reconstr Surg*. 2002;110(3):873.
    Excellent cadaver study that describes the anatomy of the orbicularis retaining ligament (also called the orbitomalar ligament) and discusses its implications in the aging eyelid.
20. Pacella S, Codner M. Minor complications after blepharoplasty: dry eyes, chemosis, granulomas, ptosis, and scleral show. *Plast Reconstr Surg*. 2010;125:709.
21. Ramil M. Fat grafting in hollow upper eyelids and volumetric upper blepharoplasty. *Plast Reconstr Surg*. 2017;140:889.
22. Rohrich R, Pezeshk R, Sieber D. The six step lower blepharoplasty: using fractionated fat to enhance blending of the lid cheek junction. *Plast Reconstr Surg*. 2017;139:1381.
    A step-by-step guide to a lower lid blepharoplasty with additional video demonstrations.
23. Tonnard PL, Verpaele AM, Zeltzer AA. Augmentation blepharoplasty: a review of 500 consecutive patients. *Aesthet Surg J*. 2013;33(3):341.
    The modern concept of fat replacement rather than resection is highlighted here as fat obtained by liposuction is used as micrografts in 500 consecutive upper and lower blepharoplasties.
24. Wong CH, Mendelson B. Extended transconjunctival lower lid blepharoplasty with release of the tear trough ligament and fat redistribution. *Plast Reconstr Surg*. 2017;140:273.
25. Zoumalan CI, Roostaeian J. Simplifying blepharoplasty. *Plast Reconstr Surg*. 2017;137:196e.

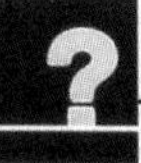

QUESTIONS

1. A 56-year-old woman who desires a blepharoplasty is evaluated for ptosis. With the eye in primary gaze, the margin of the upper lid should not be lower than which of the following positions?

a. 1 to 2 mm above the superior limbus
b. The level of the superior limbus
c. 1 to 2 mm below the superior limbus
d. The level of the superior pupil

2. A 39-year-old woman comes to the office complaining of dark circles under her lower eyelids that make her look tired. Physical examination shows a prominent tear trough. What is the anatomic basis of the tear trough?

a. Prominence of the orbital rim following ptosis of the malar fat pad
b. Osteocutaneous ligament between the palpebral and orbital parts of the orbicularis oculi
c. Herniation of the medial fat compartment over the arcus marginalis
d. Depression between the orbicularis oculi and levator labii superioris

3. As compared with an upper lid blepharoplasty with orbicularis muscle resection, a muscle sparing upper lid blepharoplasty results in which of the following?

a. Less lagophthalmos
b. Faster recurrence of blepharochalasis
c. A superior aesthetic result
d. More dry eye symptoms

4. A 49-year-old man complains of double vision 3 weeks after a four-lid blepharoplasty. On examination, he has vertical diplopia in primary gaze, and it increases in adducted upgaze. An injury to which of the following muscles is probable?

a. Superior oblique
b. Inferior oblique
c. Inferior rectus
d. Superior rectus

5. Three days after a four-lid blepharoplasty, a patient complains of excessive tearing. Physical findings include normal lid position and mild globe irritation without abrasion. The most appropriate next step in management is

a. Observation
b. Jones I test
c. Anticholinergic drops
d. Pensieve test

6. Canthoplasty is differentiated from canthopexy by which of the following?

a. Disinsertion of the lateral canthus
b. Tightening of the canthus
c. Corrects lower lid laxity
d. Use of suture fixation

7. A 69-year-old woman who underwent a four-lid blepharoplasty complains of left eye pain, pressure, and decreased vision in the recovery room. Examination shows left eye proptosis, limitation of extraocular movements, and increased intraorbital pressure. A retrobulbar hematoma is suspected. The sutures are released. Which of the following is the next most appropriate step?

a. Steroid bolus
b. Anterior compartment paracentesis
c. CO_2 inhalation
d. Lateral canthotomy

8. The threshold for adding a lid-supporting procedure to a lower lid blepharoplasty is a lower lid distraction test of which of the following?

a. 4 mm
b. 6 mm
c. 8 mm
d. 10 mm

1. **Answer: c.** The normal eyelid is 1 to 2 mm below the superior limbus. A lid that is lower than this needs to be recognized as ptotic, and this can be addressed surgically at the time of blepharoplasty. A higher lid position suggests thyroid disease.

2. **Answer: b.** The tear trough ligament is an osteocutaneous ligament between the palpebral and orbital portions of the muscle. It extends inferolaterally from the medial canthus to approximately the midpupillary line, where it connects with the orbitomalar ligament.

3. **Answer: a.** If muscle is not resected, there is less retraction, and lagophthalmos is less likely. Recurrence, outcome, and dry eye symptoms are equivalent.

4. **Answer: b.** The inferior oblique arises from the orbital surface of the maxilla, lateral to the lacrimal sac and inserts into the scleral surface. Its primary action is extorsion (external rotation); secondary action is elevation; tertiary action is abduction. The field of maximal inferior oblique elevation is in the adducted position. A superior rectus palsy would present with limitation of upgaze in abduction, and a superior oblique injury would have limited downgaze in adduction. An inferior rectus palsy would limit abducted downgaze.

5. **Answer: a.** Acute tearing is usually self-limited and will resolve within weeks. Prolonged tearing may be due to poor lid position or, rarely, an injured canalicular system. A Jones test evaluates lacrimal outflow by placing fluorescein into the conjunctiva and then testing for it in the inferior nasal meatus.

6. **Answer: a.** A canthoplasty divides the canthus before reinserting it. Both procedures tighten the canthus by suture fixation and are used to correct lid laxity.

7. **Answer: d.** A lateral canthotomy should be done immediately to decrease pressure. Other treatments such as steroids, mannitol, beta blockers, and acetazolamide all take longer to lower pressure and are secondary measures.

8. **Answer: b.** A distraction of the lid from the globe of more than 6 mm is indicative of poor lid tone, and lower blepharoplasty alone will cause ectropion. A canthopexy, canthoplasty, or lateral tarsal strip is needed.

CHAPTER 51 Facelift and Necklift

Gabriele C. Miotto and Foad Nahai

KEY POINTS

- Facial anatomy as it is applied to facial rejuvenation
- Patient evaluation by thorough history, physical examination in the preoperative planning; safety checklist
- Surgical technique selection and different applications
- Postoperative care and patient management
- Common complications and adequate management strategies for good results and patient satisfaction

Facial aging is a multifactorial process involving the skin, soft tissues, and facial skeleton. The major goal of facial rejuvenation is to restore smooth contours and soft transitions between facial units. As the face ages there are predictable surface, volume, and positional changes acting as landmarks for soft tissue manipulation and repositioning. Facial skeleton work is limited in facelift. Soft tissue augmentation with autologous fat transfer can significantly improve structural bony deficiencies and is included frequently to enhance results in facial rejuvenation surgery.[1,2]

ANATOMY

Skin

Intrinsic and extrinsic factors contribute to aging of the skin. Intrinsic factors such as epidermal thinning, dermal elastosis, decreased elasticity, and decreased collagen production are hallmarks of normal aging. Chronic UVA exposure, smoking, radiation, and chronic diseases are extrinsic factors that accelerate skin aging.

Permanent skin wrinkling and dark spots are visual characteristics of photoaging. They are best treated through skin care and resurfacing procedures such as chemical peels and lasers. Skin wrinkling with dynamic movements is best treated with neuromodulators or selective muscle ablation procedures, such as corrugator muscle resection. Facelifting techniques have little effect on skin texture, elasticity, and discoloration, but they improve folds resulting from tissue shifting and descent.

Retaining Ligaments and Fat Compartments

Described by Furnas in 1989, retaining ligaments are fibrous structures in predictable locations of the face connecting bone to the overlying facial skin, crossing all layers of soft tissue. Alghoul and Codner reviewed and clarified the nomenclature of the retaining ligaments of the face by integrating earlier descriptions.[3] Retaining ligaments are landmarks for facial rejuvenation procedures as they separate facial fat compartment, are intimately related to the branches of the facial nerve, and are structural components of facial support and aged appearance (**Figure 51.1**). Laxity of the ligaments and fat compartment deflation create visible surface depressions and creases seen with aging.

The facial fat compartments are pockets of facial adipose tissue confined within a relatively impermeable membrane (the septum). Fat compartments are divided into superficial and deep in relationship to the superficial musculoaponeurotic system (SMAS).[4] They exist in the forehead, periocular, cheek, and perioral areas, and are separated by retaining ligaments and septa that determine the location of the fat compartments.[5] During facelift, the deep and superficial cheek compartments may be repositioned and/or refilled.

Superficial Musculoaponeurotic System and Mimetic Muscles

The term *superficial musculoaponeurotic system* (SMAS) was popularized by Mitz and Peyronie in 1976, describing the SMAS as a superficial fascia investing the face and the superficial mimetic muscles. It is contiguous with the galea aponeurotica, the temporoparietal fascia, parotid masseteric fascia, platysma muscle, and superficial cervical fascia. The SMAS is an important anatomical structure for facial rejuvenation and is often divided into mobile and fixed SMAS. The fixed SMAS is firm and lateral over the parotid gland. The mobile SMAS is softer and medial, over to the zygomatic and masseteric retaining ligaments toward the central face. The mobilization and suspension of the mobile SMAS to the fixed SMAS is an essential step in any SMAS facelift. It lifts and repositions descended facial tissues. The SMAS lies on top of the deep facial fascia, a layer protecting the branches of the facial nerve. Sub-SMAS dissections may result in facial nerve injury if the deep fascia is violated.

The mimetic muscles of the face are arranged in layers according to their origin and insertion. The superficial mimetic muscles include the zygomaticus major and minor, levator labii superioris, risorius, depressor anguli oris, orbicularis oculi, and orbicularis oris. The deeper facial muscles include the buccinator, mentalis, and depressor labii. The most superficial layer of muscles is intimately related to the medial extension of the SMAS. Traction and suspension of the SMAS will also suspend the muscles.

Motor and Sensory Nerves

The facial nerve (seventh cranial nerve) innervates the mimetic muscles and has five main branches: temporal, zygomatic, buccal, mandibular, and cervical. The facial nerve emerges from the stylomastoid foramen and enters the parotid gland where it branches. Within the parotid gland, the branches of the facial nerves are deeply located, deep to the parotid fascia, and they become more superficial at the anterior boarder of the gland. The facial nerve branches transition from the deep superficial fascia through SMAS fusion zones and retaining ligaments. They run as deep as possible until they reach the edge of the muscles they innervate.[6]

The facial nerve usually innervates the superficial mimetic muscles through their deep surfaces (the zygomaticus major and minor, levator labii superioris, risorius, depressor anguli oris, orbicularis oculi, and orbicularis oris) and the deeper facial muscles such as the buccinator, mentalis, and depressor labii, from the superficial surface. Facial nerve injury is rare in facelift surgery with an estimated incidence of below 1%. Permanent loss of function from injury is estimated to be around 0.1% in most cases.

The trigeminal nerve (fifth cranial nerve) is the sensory nerve of the face. The great auricular nerve is a nerve of the cervical plexus (C2, C3) that provides the dominant sensory innervation to the ear (lobule, concha, and posterior auricle). It is also the most common nerve injured in facelift surgery.[7]

These are known as "zones of danger" of the face, where the main nerves are most vulnerable to injury during face and necklift dissections (**Figure 51.2**).[8]

Vascular Supply

The main blood supply to the soft tissues of the face comes from branches of the external carotid artery and internal jugular vein (**Figure 51.3**). The main arterial supply to the central face is the facial artery. The facial artery branches off the external carotid in the neck and crosses over the mandible approximately 3 cm from its angle to

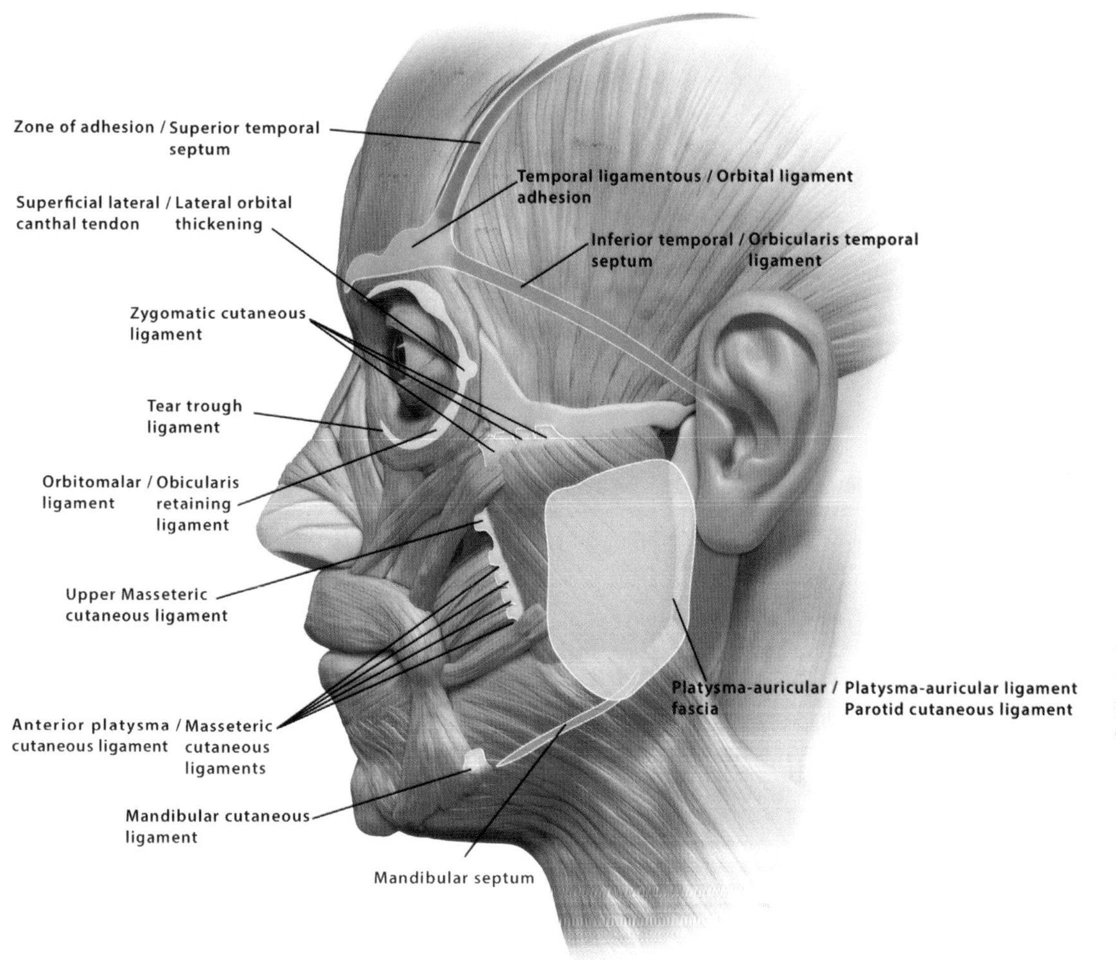

FIGURE 51.1. The retaining ligaments of the face and different nomenclatures since the initial description by Furnas in 1989. (Adapted from Alghoul M, Codner MA. Retaining ligaments of the face: review of anatomy and clinical applications. *Aesthet Surg J*. 2013;33(6):769-782. Reproduced by permission of The American Society for Aesthetic Plastic Surgery, Inc.)

run into the face, deep into the mimetic muscles. Its branches are the submental artery, upper and lower labial arteries, angular artery, and nasal artery. This rich arterial network allows for the elevation of a facelift flap. The infraorbital artery, another branch of the external carotid artery (from the maxillary artery), also supplies the medial cheek and lower lid. The lateral face is supplied by the transverse facial artery. The transverse facial artery branches off the superficial temporal artery at the level of the external auditory meatus and travels anteriorly supplying the lateral face and lateral orbital area. The territories of the facial artery and transverse facial artery overlap in the cheek. The superficial temporal artery provides blood supply to the lateral forehead and scalp.

The facial vein provides the main venous drainage of the face. It runs parallel to and behind the facial artery and flows into the internal jugular vein.

The internal carotid artery and vein also contribute to the vascular supply of the face, mainly in the periocular area and forehead through the supratrochlear and supraorbital vessels.

PATIENT EVALUATION

Good results in facial surgery rely on facial analysis and understanding of the patient's anatomy, including morphology and the extent of aging. Aesthetic analysis is done by dividing the face into horizontal thirds and vertical fifths (Figure 51.4). It includes assessment of the skin surface, facial volume, and position of facial structures. The neck is included in the lower horizontal third of the facial analysis, because neck aging is also addressed with a facial rejuvenation surgery. Differences in width and length of each side of the face should be noted. The volume and position of tissues will define the need for asymmetrical undermining and SMAS elevation, or a combination of a facelift with fat grafting.[9]

Evaluation of the skin includes skin type, pigment changes, wrinkles, elasticity, and thickness. Dyschromias are common concerns for patients looking for facial rejuvenation and the choice of skin resurfacing often depends on the skin type. Poor skin elasticity and severe degree of wrinkling should alert the surgeon that a combination of surgery and resurfacing procedures would provide the best results.

The Fitzpatrick classification is a useful guide for planning skin-resurfacing procedures.[10] Patients with Fitzpatrick skin type I–III are generally good candidates for skin resurfacing procedures such as dermabrasion, with lower risk of postinflammatory hyperpigmentation, hypopigmentation, and blotchiness. For patients with skin types IV–VI, the risks are weighed against potential benefits, and other treatments (nonablative laser rejuvenation, microneedling, and superficial chemical peels) may be considered.

Special consideration should be given to certain skin pathologies. Patients diagnosed with cutis laxa, a rare connective tissue disorder that presents with varied degrees of loose hypoelastic skin throughout the body, are candidates for elective aesthetic surgery because there is no underlying issue with wound healing. Patients with genetic connective tissue disorders such as Ehlers-Danlos syndrome, pseudoxanthoma elasticum, elastoderma, progeria, and Werner syndrome have limited and unpredictable wound healing and should not undergo elective procedures.[11]

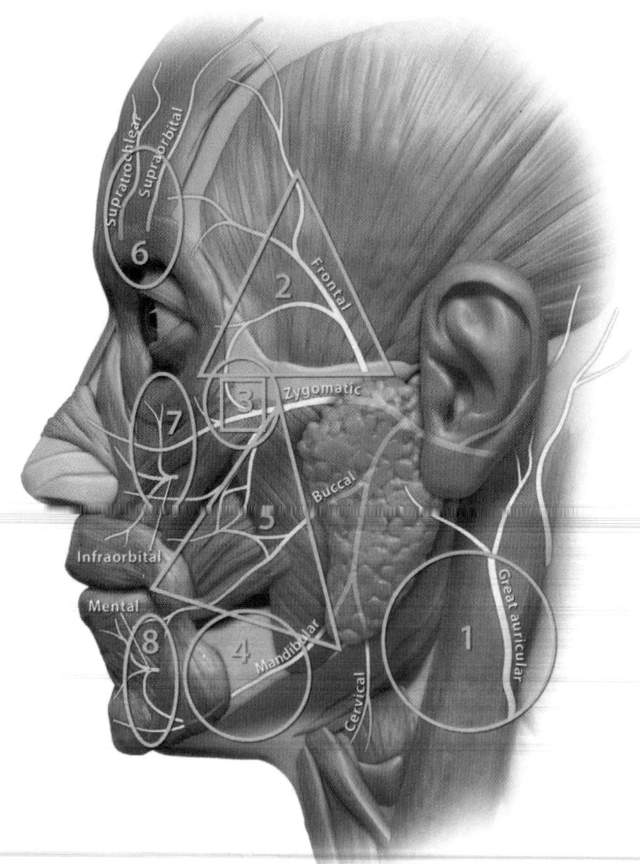

FIGURE 51.2. Zones of danger for nerve injury during face and necklift. The eight zones are indicated and correspond to both sensory and motor nerve danger areas. (1) The frontal branch is vulnerable to injury as it crosses the zygomatic arch 2.5 cm anterior to the external auditory meatus deep into the temporoparietal fascia. (2) The zygomatic branch is vulnerable during the zygomatic retaining ligaments release. (3) The buccal branch is vulnerable during dissection at the anterior edge of the parotid and during buccal fat pad manipulation. (4) The marginal mandibular branch is vulnerable during lateral platysma work and submental dissections as it exits the parotid inferiorly and runs along the mandibular angle. (5) The great auricular nerve branch is vulnerable when dissecting the posterior neck, as it emerges at the posterior border of the sternocleidomastoid muscle, about 6.5 cm inferior to the exterior auditory canal. (6) The supraorbital and supratrochlear nerves are vulnerable during brow lifts and dissections along the supraorbital rim, such as during transpalpebral corrugator resections. (7) The infraorbital nerve is vulnerable during deep dissections of the midface in subperiostal or supraperiostal midfacelift. (8) The mental nerve is vulnerable during deep fat grafting injection in the prejowl sulci and during chin augmentation procedures. (Adapted by permission from Seckel BR. Facial danger zones: avoiding nerve injury in facial plastic surgery. *Can J Plast Surg*. 1994;2(2):59-66. Copyright © 1994 SAGE Publications.)

Anesthesia Evaluation

Preoperative evaluation is performed by a thorough history and physical examination with the assistance of the anesthesia team. According to the American Society of Anesthesiology preoperative evaluation guidelines, preoperative tests should not be ordered routinely but may be required for purposes of guiding or optimizing perioperative management of selected patients.[12] If the patient has chronic medical issues, the preoperative evaluation may include an ECG, clearance from a specialist, X-rays, and adjustment of current medications. Secondary facelift patients are usually older and may require a more extensive preoperative evaluation and management in the postoperative period. Identification of high-risk patients for VTE events is done with the use of a modified Caprini risk assessment scale as proposed by the American Society of Plastic Surgery.[13] Perioperative pneumatic compression pump and early ambulation are useful for all facelift patients. For patients with Caprini scores higher than 7, 40 mg of subcutaneous enoxaparin is used as a single dose 8 to 12 hours postoperatively or extended to a week of treatment according to preoperative clinical evaluation.

FACELIFT TECHNIQUES

Incisions

Facelift and necklift techniques include periauricular skin incisions, varying degrees of skin undermining, and different SMAS manipulation maneuvers. Incisions in front of the ear extend from the base of the ear lobe, into the pretragal or retrotragal area, and then transition along the hairline or into the temporal scalp. Incisions behind the ear are placed just anterior to the retroauricular crease and usually curve posteriorly at the level of the tragus into the hairline or into the occipital scalp (**Figure 51.5**). The term *short-scar facelift* was coined by Baker, referring to a limited incision length around the ear for patients who do not have severe skin laxity in the neck.[14]

Skin-only Lifts

Subcutaneous lifts rely on the undermining of the skin flap only to improve facial aging. They have been used for over a century and have evolved from a limited undermining in the periauricular area to an extensive skin undermining releasing the main retaining ligaments in a superficial plane. Skin traction repositions the facial tissues and follows a superolateral vector of pull. Skin lifts are not universally popular as most surgeons prefer SMAS manipulation because of the tension that is placed adjacent to or in the suture line.[1,2]

SMAS Procedures

Dual-plane Approach

A dual-plane approach includes undermining of the skin flap and the superficial musculoaponeurotic system (SMAS) separately. It facilitates SMAS and the skin modification in different vectors. The soft tissue support of a dual plane approach is at the SMAS level rather than at the skin. The elevation vector of the SMAS is usually superolateral, and the vector of the skin redraping is usually posterolateral. The SMAS can be elevated as a flap (high SMAS technique), can be resected (SMASectomy), or can be plicated with or without tissue stacking (**Figure 51.6**).

In the high SMAS technique, the SMAS flap is elevated at or above the zygomatic arch with medial dissection with at least partial transection of the zygomatic and masseteric-cutaneous ligaments for full mobilization of the cheek and jaw line. The platysma-cutaneous ligaments are preserved for proper elevation and fixation of the SMAS and to prevent the lateral sweep deformity. The subcutaneous undermining accompanies the SMAS undermining and extends anteriorly to include the area of the mandibular ligaments and the neck[15,16] (**Figure 51.7**).

The lateral SMASectomy technique was popularized by Baker and includes resection of a diagonal strip of SMAS from the malar eminence to the angle of the mandible, parallel to the nasolabial fold with posterior SMAS plication. The edges of the fix and mobile SMAS are brought together with sutures for elevation of the jowls and cheek[17] (**Figure 51.8**).

In the SMAS plication technique, there is no flap elevation or resection of SMAS. The edges of the fixed and mobile SMAS are simply plicated together with sutures. The vectors can be diagonally oriented such as in the lateral SMASectomy technique or vertically oriented, such as in the high SMAS technique, depending on the desired outcome. The SMAS stacking procedure proposed by Rohrich includes a limited lateral SMAS dissection and stacking of the SMAS during plication for volume increase in the lateral cheek.

In the minimal access cranial suspension lift (MACS lift) developed by Tonnard, large purse-string suture loops are used to suspend

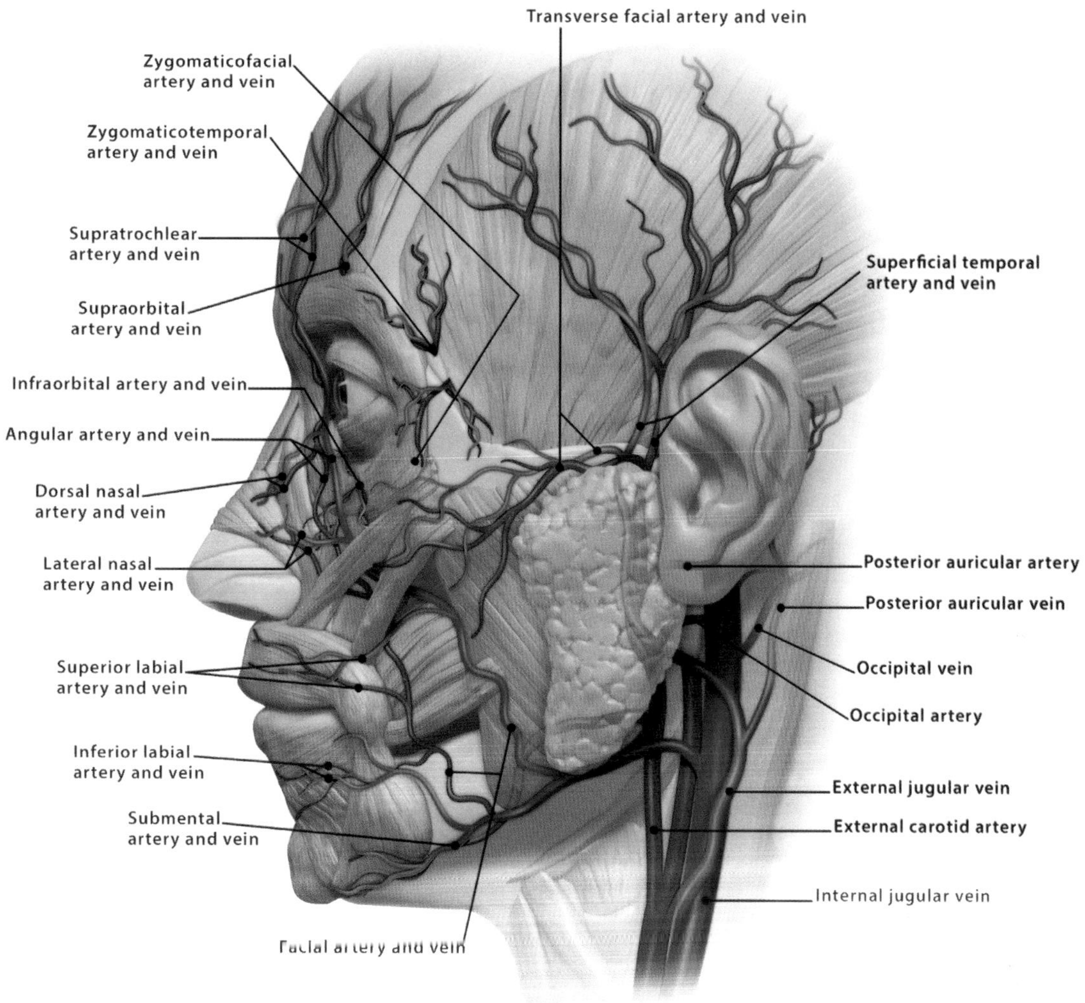

Transverse facial artery and vein
Zygomaticofacial artery and vein
Zygomaticotemporal artery and vein
Supratrochlear artery and vein
Supraorbital artery and vein
Infraorbital artery and vein
Angular artery and vein
Dorsal nasal artery and vein
Lateral nasal artery and vein
Superior labial artery and vein
Inferior labial artery and vein
Submental artery and vein
Facial artery and vein
Superficial temporal artery and vein
Posterior auricular artery
Posterior auricular vein
Occipital vein
Occipital artery
External jugular vein
External carotid artery
Internal jugular vein

FIGURE 51.3. Vascular supply to the face.

Periorbital zone
(upper third)
Perioral zone
(middle third)
Neck zone
(lower third)

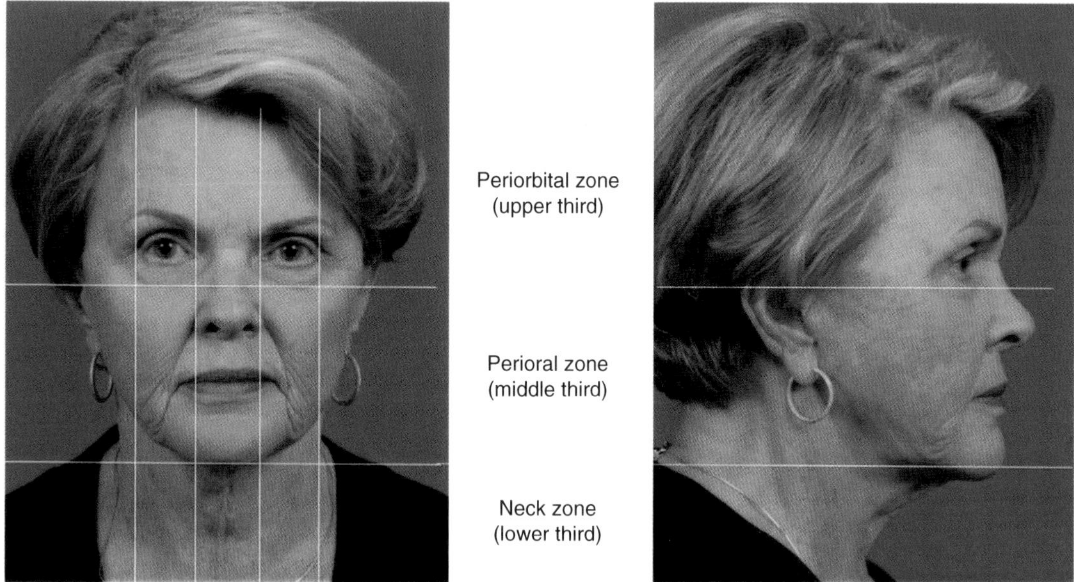

FIGURE 51.4. Upper third (periorbital zone) starts at the hairline (trichion) to mid cheek. Middle third (perioral zone) starts at the mid cheek (line over zygomatic arches) to the chin (mentum). Lower third goes from the mentum to the sternal notch and upper border of the clavicles. Lines crossing the inner and lateral canthus divide the face into vertical fifths.

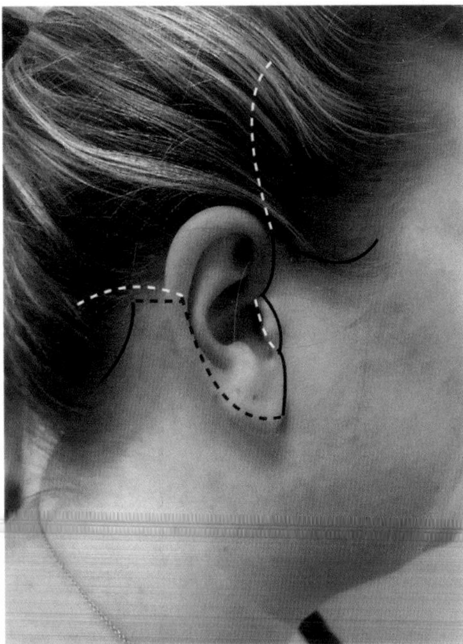

FIGURE 51.5. The most common variations in the preauricular and postauricular scar placement for facelift and necklift surgery.

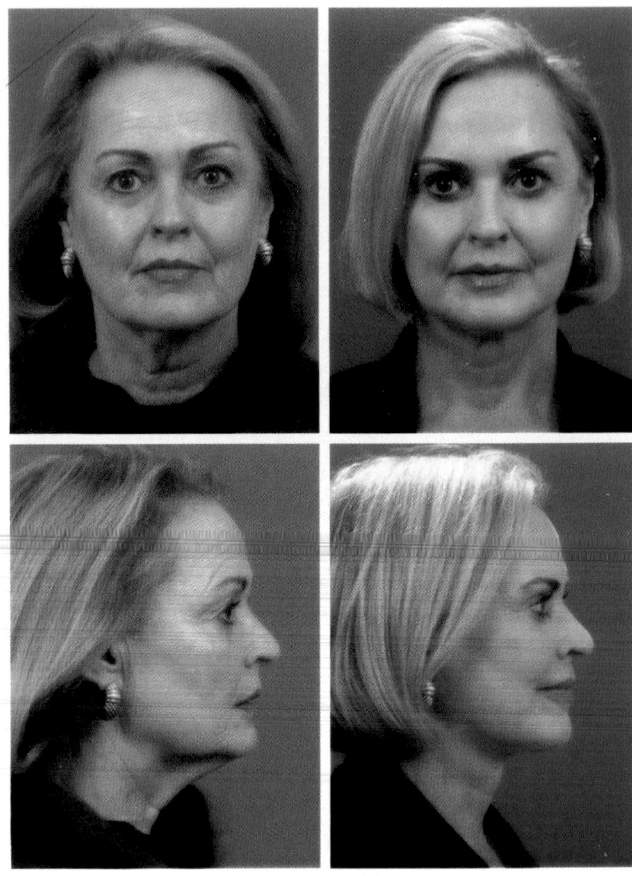

FIGURE 51.7. Preoperative (left) and 3-year follow-up (right) photos of a woman in her 60s who underwent a high SMAS face and necklift with anterior platysmaplasty and partial platysma transection, upper and lower blepharoplasty, and lateral brow lift.

the SMAS platysma in a cranial position instead of using the traditional individual plication sutures placed parallel to the nasolabial fold.[18,19]

Deep Plane (Composite) Approach

The deep plane approach repositions the SMAS and skin as a single unit. The skin flap dissection in front of the ear is limited and there the transition into a skin–SMAS flap starts laterally, over the deep parotid fascia.[20] The skin–SMAS composite flap is suspended as a single structure in a superolateral vector. This composite flap is thick and has robust vascularization, being a good option for patients with potential would healing issues, such as smokers and diabetic patients. The critics of this technique point out that the skin of the neck is

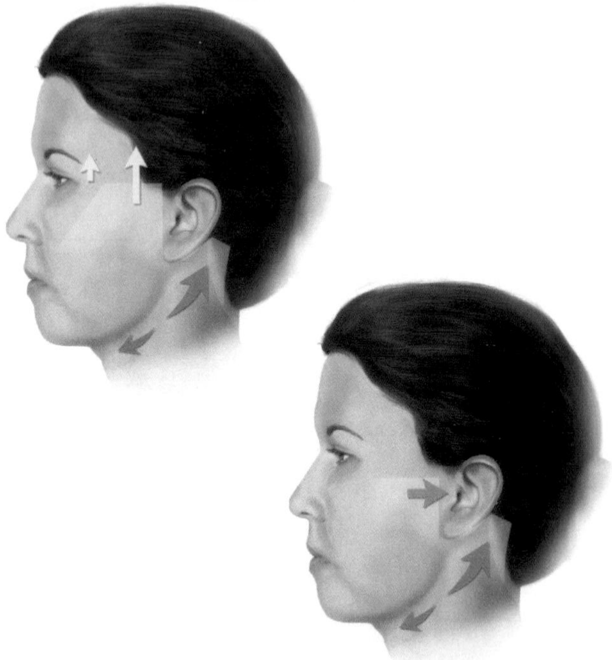

FIGURE 51.6. The different vectors of traction of the SMAS flap during a high-SMAS facelift. Vertical vector is used for elevation of midface, jowls, and neck. Lateral vector can be used for elevation of jowls and neck only.

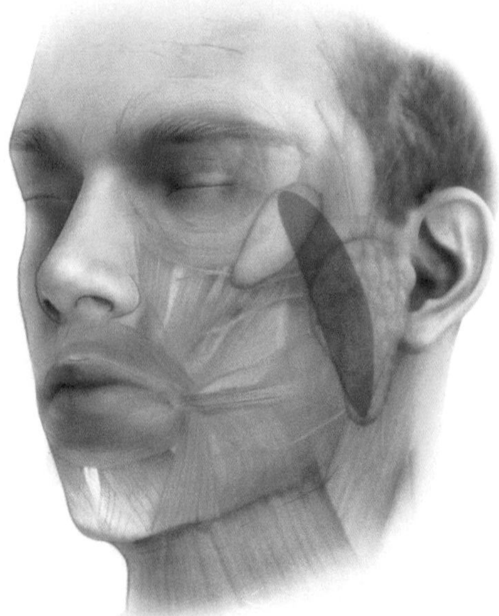

FIGURE 51.8. Location of the lateral SMASectomy, which extends from the tail of the parotid to the lateral canthus.

usually shifted into the facial skin, and adjustments of the skin and SMAS flaps cannot be performed independently and can cause artificial facial contour.

In selected patients, other facial sub-SMAS procedures are needed to adjust facial volume and shape.[8] These include buccal fat pad excision or suspension and trimming of the parotid gland to reshape the face. Buccal fat pad may be approached through the mouth, through the temple, or through the sub-SMAS dissection. There is a close relationship between the buccal fat pad and branches of the facial nerve and the parotid duct.

Fat Grafting

Fat grafting is used to improve facial appearance by volumetric enhancement of deflated areas. Fat integrates well with facial tissues and when used in conjunction with a facelift, it can enhance the overall results. The most common fat injection locations are the midface, temporal fossa, periocular and perioral areas. Facial lines can also be treated with fat injections.

Facial fat grafting should be performed by avoiding bolus injections or the use of large particle sizes. The most common fat grafting techniques and tools were developed by Coleman and Tonnard, and consist of small size harvesting and injection cannulas. Harvesting cannulas vary from 2.1 to 2.4 mm in diameter, and injection cannulas vary from 1.2 to 0.7 mm.[21,22]

Microfat is a term that was coined by Tonnard and is defined as fat harvested in small particle sizes utilizing tumescent infiltration and small gauge harvesting cannulas (2.0–2.4 mm). Microfat can be used for facial volume restoration and is the preferred method used by the authors for volumization.

Nanofat is a fat grafting derivate from emulsification of microfat. There are no viable fat cells in the nanofat solution. Adipose stromal cells are preserved in nanofat preparations and have been credited for the restorative skin effects seen with the nanofat use. Nanofat should not be used for volume enhancement, but as an adjuvant to skin quality improvement.

Preparation of the fat through decanting, straining, washing, or centrifugation procedures seems to be equally effective for fat survival. Time from harvesting to injection seems to be the crucial point for optimal fat intake. The quicker the fat injected after harvesting the better the result.[24] Exact fat grafting survival is still uncertain, with reported rates of fat grafting survival varying from 40% to 80%. Therefore, overcorrection is necessary for long results. The use of fat grafting can enhance results, but increase operating room time, postoperative bruising, and swelling. Obtaining fat from multiple sites may be needed for thin patients and may help prevent donor site deformities.

NECK CONTOURING TECHNIQUES

Necklifts can be performed in isolation or combined with a facelift, and all facelift procedures will have some effect on the neck (**Table 51.1**). The goal of neck rejuvenation is to modify and improve the submental area and cervicomental angle. Depending on the patient's anatomy and morphology, the surgical options may include single or combined strategies that reduce the fat, remove skin, or modify the muscles and deeper structures of the neck.

TABLE 51.1. DECISION MAKING AND PATIENT SELECTION FOR TREATING THE AGING NECK

Skin	Fat	Platysma Laxity ± Subplatysma Volume	Treatment
Good elasticity	Yes	None	Liposuction
Good elasticity	Yes	Yes	Submental necklift
Laxity	Yes/no	Yes/no	Necklift Anterior neck resection

The most common surgical techniques for neck rejuvenation are liposuction for superficial fat contouring, platysmaplasty for muscle and fascia plication and reshaping, subplatysmal work for treatment of the subplatysmal fat excess, digastric muscles and submandibular glands, lateral skin excision of the neck flap, or direct anterior neck resection.

Liposuction

The neck contains fat in the subcutaneous tissue between the skin and platysma muscle and in the deep plane under the platysma, between the platysma medial borders, and above the digastric muscles. To differentiate between subcutaneous fat and deep fat during the clinical exam, the submental fat is pinched and the patient is asked to grimace to contract the platysma muscle. If the amount of fat does not change with contraction, it indicates that most of the fat is subcutaneous and liposuction is a good option for fat removal. If the fat pinch diminishes upon contraction, most of the fat is subplatysmal requiring an open neck procedure to remove the fat.

The amount of fat in each plane varies according to patient's weight and anatomy and is usually more abundant in the central submental area.

Liposuction can be used to remove superficial fat between the skin and platysma. Used in isolation for neck reshaping, it is ideal for patients who have good skin tone and elasticity. Liposuction is also combined with necklift procedures. All liposuction modalities such as suction assisted liposuction (SAL), power-assisted liposuction (PAL), ultrasound-assisted liposuction (UAL), and laser-assisted liposuction (LAL) can be used. Small cannulas (size 2–3) are recommended to prevent excessive resection of fat and surface irregularities.

Platysmaplasty and Subplatysmal Procedures

The platysma is a pair of superficial muscle of the neck that originates from the pectoralis major muscle fascia and inserts into the mentum and the inferior mandibular border. Its fibers ascend into the lower face connecting to the depressor anguli oris and to the orbicularis oris. It is the extension of the SMAS in the lower face and neck. Within the submental area, the anatomy and the level of midline decussation between the muscles varies greatly from individual to individual. Cardoso de Castro classifies the platysma decussation into Type 1, 2, and 3. Type 1 is the most common (75%) with limited submental decussation. Type 2 (15%) shows decussation from the mandibular symphysis to the thyroid cartilage and Type 3 (10%) shows no decussation.

Stuzin discussed the importance of the platysma retaining ligaments in the aging neck. These ligaments are a series of fibrous bands connecting the mandibular symphysis to the thyroid and once attenuated contribute to platysma descent, band formation, and the oblique cervical angle of the aging neck.

Platysma work is indicated in patients with neck laxity and the presence of platysma bands.

Submental necklifting consists in treatment of the central neck through a submental incision. The submental necklift may be performed in isolation or in combination with a facelift. The submental incision is placed just posterior to the submental crease, with subsequent flap elevation with scissors or electrocautery, liposuction or direct resection of the subcutaneous fat if necessary, and a combination of central platysma plication (anterior platysmaplasty) with or without transection of the medial platysma borders. The extension of the transection usually depends on the thickness and location of the bands and helps with neck reshaping.[20]

Anterior platysmaplasty consists of suturing the medial platysma borders from the submental area to the thyroid cartilage for tightening of the neck. The borders of the muscle can be simply approximated or overlapped with or without transverse partial or complete platysma transection to weaken the platysma bands. Transections usually start centrally at the level of the cricoid cartilage and extends laterally, but this maneuver can also be performed from lateral to medial through the facelift incision. Absorbable and permanent sutures may be used for plication through simple or continuous running sutures.

Other structures that influence the neck shape and aesthetics are located deep into the platysma muscle, such as the subplatysmal fat, the anterior belly of the digastric muscles, and the submandibular glands. The digastric muscles are paired and have an anterior and a posterior belly. The anterior bellies extend from the posterior mandibular symphysis to the lesser cornu of the hyoid bone. The anterior belly and posterior belly of each digastric muscle form two sides of the submental triangles. The submandibular glands are located in the submental triangles and can produce a visible bulge in the lateral neck. The facial artery and vein and the marginal mandibular branch of the facial nerve crosses the gland superficially outside its capsule. The safest approach to the gland is intracapsular resection to avoid neurovascular injury.

To access these deep structures, the surgeon should elevate the central platysma borders. Partial but not complete subplatysmal fat is known to avoid submental depression. When prominent, the anterior belly of the digastric can be partially or totally excised without noticeable loss of function. Enlarged submandibular glands can be visualized laterally to the anterior belly of the digastric muscles. The superficial lobe of the gland is exposed into the operating field by an Allis forceps or a strong suture placement through the gland. The capsule is incised with needle-tip cautery, and the gland excess resected piecemeal until ideal contour of the submandibular area is achieved. Thorough gland hemostasis is important to avoid hematoma in this area and the risk of airway obstruction.

Direct Anterior Neck Resection

Direct resection of the submental skin and fat excess with or without platysmaplasty is an option for neck rejuvenation in selected patients. Good candidates for direct neck resection are usually males or older patients of both genders who tolerate a central and more visible scar, who are not suitable for longer operations or prefer a less extensive procedure. In an anterior neck, the superficial and deep planes of the neck can be resected. Different incision designs have been proposed and straight resections are avoided to prevent banding and scar contraction. Most incision patterns are variations of z-plasty in the midline. Visible scars, hypertrophic scars, and long lasting scar erythema are some of the downsides of this approach.

POSTOPERATIVE MANAGEMENT

The use of drains under the skin flap is a common practice for neck and facelift. Small size Jackson-Pratt drains to bulb suction are usually left on each side of the face for 24 h after surgery. Drains have not shown to prevent hematomas or seromas but are advocated by many authors to help decrease the amount of swelling and bruising after a facelift and help the patient return quickly to social activities.[15]

Facial dressings and head wrapping are commonly used after face and necklifts and removed 24 h after surgery. After this, a compressive, nonbinding chin strap or garment is recommended for a couple of weeks. Head elevation during sleep can help with swelling, as well as low salt intake in the postoperative period.

COMPLICATIONS

Face and necklifts are considered safe procedures with a low overall complication rates. According to a 2016 large prospective cohort study by Gupta et al., the incidence of facelift complications that need hospitalization within 30 days of surgery is 1.8%. Hematoma (1.1%) and infection (0.3%) were most common. The same study found male gender an independent factor for hematoma. Body mass index >= 25 and combined procedures increased the infection risk.[25]

Hematoma is the most common early complication of a face and necklift and it usually occurs in the first 24 to 48 h after surgery. The overall incidence of all (minor-large) postoperative hematoma is variable due to lack of consistent classification, usually reported to be 4% to 8% for men and 1% to 3% for women. Minor hematoma is defined as a collection of blood that does not require surgical evacuation but is amenable to treatment by bedside aspiration, with volumes under 30 cc. An expanding hematoma is a serious complication with an incidence of 1.8% that requires immediate recognition and treatment due to impending risk of skin necrosis, airway obstruction, and death. Minor hematomas can lead to persistent face and neck edema, nerve compression, skin necrosis, and unpleasant aesthetic results.

Several strategies have been proposed to decrease the incidence of post facelift hematoma. Strict blood pressure control in the operating room (SBP < 150 mm Hg) is a widely recognized preventive intervention. Antihypertensive clonidine has been used successfully in the postoperative period to keep SBP under 140 mm Hg. The use of fibrin glue, absence of epinephrine in the local anesthetic solutions, and compressive dressings have been reported to be beneficial but are not completely effective in preventing hematomas. A few recent studies have demonstrated that the use of quilting sutures is a promising strategy in prevention of hematoma in the face by reducing the rate of hematoma to zero in the published series.[26]

Injuries to motor and sensory facial nerves are also acute complications of face and necklift. The great auricular nerve is the most commonly injured nerve and will lead to numbness of the lower part of the ear and earlobe. Its superficial location on the sternocleidomastoid muscle surface places the nerve at risk of transection during the neck flap dissection. Nerve compression by sutures during platysma suspension can also cause numbness and chronic pain.[7]

Injury to the marginal mandibular branch of the facial nerve results in weakness of the ipsilateral lower lip depressors (denervation of the depressor anguli oris). It also affects the ipsilateral mentalis muscle. Neurapraxia is more common than complete nerve transection in this area, and can return within a few days to 3 to 6 months. Another common cause of nerve dysfunction in the immediate postoperative period is temporary paralysis of the facial nerves due to injection of local anesthetic in the dissected areas. It usually takes a few hours for the local anesthetic to wear off.

Smoking can increase the chance of skin necrosis and poor wound healing after cosmetic surgery.[27-29] Rees found that the incidence of skin slough after facelift was 7.5% in smokers compared to 2.5% in nonsmokers. A recent systematic review and meta-analysis by Rohrich shows that at least 4 weeks of abstinence from smoking reduces respiratory and wound-healing complications. Skin necrosis is initially managed with local wound care. They can heal as wide or hypertrophic scars, and further treatments with steroid injections or excision of the scars and flap readvancement are common treatments.

Poor wound healing can be a consequence of poorly planned incisions, too much tension placed on the skin during closure, or poor healing characteristics related to ethnicity (Asians, African Americans).

The "pixie ear" deformity is a known tell-tale sign of previous facelift. It is caused by tethering and forward rotation of the base of the lobule due to excessive tension during wound closure and distortion of natural axis of rotation of the lobule. Other tell-tale signs of previous facelifts are "joker lines", "lateral sweep", postauricular banding, facial deformities related to abnormal SMAS and skin traction, suturing points, or noncorrection of facial deflation.

Secondary facelifts have similar complications to a primary procedure, and the timing for a secondary facelift is in average a decade after the first procedure. Secondary facelift patients are older and usually have thinner tissues. Ancillary procedures such as skin resurfacing and fat grafting are often added to secondary facelifts to improve outcomes. Beale at al proposed the "five Rs" or tenets for performing a sound secondary rhytidectomy: (1) resect skin/scar, (2) release abnormal vectors, (3) refill by fat grafting, (4) reshape with SMAS procedures, and (5) redrape skin.[30]

REFERENCES

1. Mustoe T, Park E. Evidence-based medicine face lift. *Plast Reconstr Surg*. 2014; 133:1206.
2. Wan D, Small KH, Barton FE. Face Lift. *Plast Reconstr Surg*. 2015;136:676e-689e.
3. Alghoul M, Codner MA. Retaining ligaments of the face: review of anatomy and clinical applications. *Aesthet Surg J*. 2013;33(6):769–782.
4. Mitz V, Peyronie M. The superficial musculo-aponeurotic system (SMAS) in the parotid and cheek area. *Plast Reconstr Surg*. 1976;58:80–88.
5. Rohrich R, Pessa J. The retaining system of the face: histologic evaluation of the septal boundaries of the subcutaneous fat compartments. *Plast Reconstr Surg*. 2008;121(5):1804–1809.
6. Roostaeian J, Rohrich RJ, Stuzin JM. Anatomical considerations to prevent facial nerve injury. *Plast Reconstr Surg*. 2015;135(5):1318–1327.
7. Rohrich RJ, Taylor NS, Ahmad J, Lu A, Pessa JE. Great auricular nerve injury, the "subauricular band" phenomenon, and the periauricular adipose compartments. *Plast Reconstr Surg*. 2011;127(2):835–843.
8. Seckel BR. Facial danger zones: avoiding nerve injury in facial plastic surgery. *Can J Plast Surg*. 1994;2(2):59–66.
9. Rohrich RJ, Pessa JE. The fat compartments of the face: anatomy and clinical implications for cosmetic surgery. *Plast Reconstr Surg*. 2007;119(7):2219–2212.
10. Fitzpatrick TB. The validity and practicality of sun-reactive skin types I through VI. *Arch Dermatol*. 1988;124(6):869–871.
11. Nahas FX, Sterman S, Gemperli R, Ferreira MC. The role of plastic surgery in congenital cutis laxa: a 10-year follow-up. *Plast Reconstr Surg*. 1999;104(4):1174–1178; discussion 1179.
12. Practice advisory for preanesthesia evaluation: an updated report by the american society of anesthesiologists task force on preanesthesia evaluation. *Anesthesiology*. 2012;116(3):522–538.
13. Wilkins EG, Pannucci CJ, Bailey SH, et al. Preliminary report on the PSEF Venous Thromboembolism Prevention Study(VTEPS): validation of the Caprini Risk Assessment Model in plastic and reconstructive surgery patients. *Plast Reconstruc Surg*. 2011;126(4):107.
14. Baker DC. Minimal incision rhytidectomy (short scar face lift) with lateral SMASectomy: evolution and application. *Aesthet Surg J*. 2001;21:14–26.
15. Marten TJ. High SMAS facelift: combined single flap lifting of the jawline, cheek and midface. *Clin Plast Surg*. 2008;35(4):569–603.
16. Trussler AP, Stephan P, Hatef D, Schaverien M, Meade R, Barton FE. The frontal branch of the facial nerve across the zygomatic arch: anatomical relevance of the high-SMAS technique. *Plast Reconstr Surg*. 2010;125:1221–1229.
17. Baker DC. Lateral SMASectomy. *Plast Reconstr Surg*. 1997;100:509–513.
18. Saylan Z. The S lift for facial rejuvenation. *Int J Cosmet Surg*. 1999;7:18–23.
19. Tonnard P, Verpaele A, Monstrey S, et al. Minimal access cranial suspension lift: a modified S-lift. *Plast Reconstr Surg*. 2002;109:2074–2086.
20. Stuzin JM, Feldman JJ, Baker DC, Marten TJ. Cervical contouring in face lift. *Aesthet Surg J*. 2002;22(6):541–548.
21. Coleman SR. Structural fat grafting: more than a permanent filler. *Plast Reconstr Surg*. 2006;118(3 suppl):108s–120s.
22. Tonnard P, Verpaele A, Peeters G, et al. Nanofat grafting: basic research and clinical application. *Plast Reconstr Surg*. 2013;132(4):1017–1026.
23. Sinno S, Wilson S, Brownstone N, Levine SM. Current thoughts on fat grafting: using the evidence to determine fact or fiction. *Plast Reconstr Surg*. 2016;137(3):818–824.
24. Rohrich RJ, Ghavami A, Constantine FC, Unger J, Mojallal A. Lift-and-fill face lift: integrating the fat compartments. *Plast Reconstr Surg*. 2014;133:756e-767e.
25. Gupta v, Winocour J, Shi H, Shack RB, Grotting JC, Higdon KK. Preoperative risk factors and complication rates in facelift: analysis of 11,300 patients. *Aesthet Surg J*. 2016;36(1):1–13.
26. Neto JC, Rodriguez DE, Boles FM. Reducing the incidence of hematomas in cervicofacial rhytidectomy: new external quilting sutures and other ancillary procedures. *Aesthet Plast Surg*. 2013;37(5):1034–1039.
27. Krueger JK, Rohrich RJ. Clearing the smoke: the scientific rationale for tobacco abstention with plastic surgery. *Plast Reconstr Surg*. 2001;108:1063-1073; *discussion* 1074–1077.
28. Rees TD, Liverett DM, Guy CL. The effect of cigarette smoking on skin-flap survival in the face lift patient. *Plast Reconstr Surg*. 1984;73(6):911–915.
29. Wong J, Lam DP, Abrishami A, Chan MT, Chung F. Short-term preoperative smoking cessation and postoperative complications: a systematic review and meta-analysis. *Can J Anaesth*. 2012;59(3):268–279.
30. Beale EW, Rasko Y, Rohrich RJ. A 20-year experience with secondary rhytidectomy: a review of technique, longevity, and outcomes. *Plast Reconstr Surg*. 2013;131(3):625-634.

SEMINAL ARTICLES

1. Mitz V, Peyronie M. The superficial musculo-aponeurotic system (SMAS) in the parotid and cheek area.1976. *Plast Reconstr Surg*. 58:80–88. The first detailed anatomic description of the superficial facial fascia. The authors called it the superficial musculo-aponeurotic system, stablishing the acronym SMAS in facial surgery
2. Alghoul M, Codner MA. Retaining ligaments of the face: review of anatomy and clinical applications. *Aesthet Surg J*. 2013;33(6):769–782.Review article that clarifies the anatomy and nomenclature of the retaining ligaments of the face and its importance in facial rejuvenation surgery.
3. Marten TJ. High SMAS facelift: combined single flap lifting of the jawline, cheek and midface. *Clin Plast Surg*. 2008;35(4):569–603. Comprehensive description of the high-SMAS flap surgical anatomy and technique for face and neck rejuvenation.
4. Gupta v, Winocour J, Shi H, Shack RB, Grotting JC, Higdon KK. Preoperative risk factors and complication rates in facelift: analysis of 11,300 patients. *Aesthet Surg J*. 2016;36(1):1–13. Large prospective study with current data evaluating risk factors and complication in face lift patients.
5. Rohrich RJ, Pessa JE. The fat compartments of the face: anatomy and clinical implications for cosmetic surgery. *Plast Reconstr Surg*. 2007;119(7):2219–2212. Facial deflation is an important feature of facial aging. The authors describe the fat compartments of the face and its implications in facial rejuvenation surgery.Aesthetic Surgery

AESTHETIC SURGERY

QUESTIONS

1. **A 62-year-old healthy woman comes to the office for her preoperative visit in preparation for her facelift surgery in 2 weeks. You explain the risks and benefits of the surgery, and she asks what the most common complication of a facelift is. What do you answer?**

   a. Facial nerve injury
   b. Skin necrosis
   c. Seroma
   d. Hematoma
   e. Infection

2. **A 59-year-old woman comes back to the office for follow-up 3 months after surgery. She is pleased with the aesthetic results but refers complete numbness of the left earlobe. Which nerve was most likely injured during the surgical procedure?**

   a. Posterior auricular nerve
   b. Spinal accessory nerve
   c. Cervical branch of the facial nerve
   d. Great auricular nerve
   e Mandibular branch of the facial nerve

3. **During the 2-week follow-up visit of a patient submitted to a high SMAS face and necklift, you noticed a 3 × 4 cm dark patch of skin in the left postrauricular area adjacent the retroauricular suture line. There is no redness or secretion in the area. Which of the following is the most appropriate next step to manage this patient?**

   a. Placement of a negative pressure treatment
   b. Wide debridement
   c. Debridement and full thickness skin graft
   d. Local wound care
   e. Oral antibiotics for a week

4. **Hematoma is a common complication of facelift surgery. Which of the follow options is a known risk factor for this complication?**

   a. Operation performed in an office-based facility
   b. Hyperthyroidism
   c. Loose surgical dressing
   d. History of previous hematoma
   e. Male gender

5. **Six months after a primary facelift with SMASectomy, a 70-year-old man comes back for follow-up. He was overweight and has lost 15 lb since surgery. Now he complains of midface hollowing, depressed temporal area and visible marionette lines. On examination, there is deflation of temples, midface, and perioral area with good tension on the skin. What is an appropriate option for improving this patient's concerns?**

   a. SMAS plication procedure
   b. Chemical peels
   c. Placement of cheek implants
   d. Laser resurfacing
   e. Fat grafting to the face

1. **Answer: d.** The most common complication of a facelift is a hematoma, with an incidence that varies from 1% to 8% in most series. Hematoma that requires surgical evacuation in the operating room has an incidence of 1.8% according to a large prospective study from Gupta et al. Minor hematomas can be drained at the bedside and are likely underreported. Facial nerve injury, skin necrosis, seroma, and infection are not the most common complications of a facelift. Infection is the second most common complication that requires hospital admission within 30 days of surgery.[1,25]

2. **Answer: d.** The overall incidence of nerve injury in facelift surgery is low. Transection of the great auricular nerve is the most frequent nerve injury of facelift surgery, with an estimated incidence of up to 2.6%. Common symptoms associated with great auricular nerve injury are numbness of the earlobe, concha, and posterior auricle or focal pain in case of nerve entrapment from suture placement around the nerve or from neuroma formation. The nerve is located about 6.5 cm inferior to the external auditory canal on the surface of the sternocleidomastoid muscle.[6,7]

3. **Answer: d.** Minor wound issues are known complications of facelifts. The initial treatment is daily local wound care without debridement. In the absence of infection, the eschar will act as a biological dressing and reepithelialization occurs with minor consequences, most commonly wide or hypertrophic scars. Unfavorable scars can be further treated with steroid injections, local resection, or flap readvancement to improve tension upon closure.[1,2]

4. **Answer: e.** According to a 2016 large prospective cohort study by Gupta et al., the incidence of facelift complications that need hospitalization within 30 days of surgery is 1.8%. Hematoma (1.1%) and infection (0.3%) were most common. This same study found male gender an independent factor for hematoma. The same study showed that operations performed in an office-based facility have less risk of hematoma and infection. Surgical dressing, use of drains, and a history of previous hematoma are not risk factors for hematoma after facelift.[1,2,25]

5. **Answer: e.** Facial aging, weight loss, and systemic diseases can cause facial deflation. When there is minimal or no skin laxity associated with facial deflation as in this case, fat grafting is a good option to improve facial deflation by itself. It can be used in combination with a facelift (lift and fill technique). The most common fat injection locations are the midface, the temporal fossa, the periocular, and the perioral areas. Facial lines can also be treated with fat injections. Facial fat grafting should be performed with a proper technique, avoiding bolus injections or the use of large particle sizes. Synthetic fillers such as hyaluronic acid fillers can also be used to improve facial deflation.[5,9,21,22]

CHAPTER 52 Rhinoplasty

Robert H. Gilman and Jeremy Warner

KEY POINTS

- Nasal surgery requires accurate evaluation, assessment, and treatment of both aesthetic and functional components.
- Rhinoplasty surgery can be approached through both open and closed approaches, and there are a number of factors that will direct the surgeon on the most appropriate approach.
- Thorough knowledge of the functional aspects of nasal surgery is critical to prevent postoperative functional airway issues.
- There is a range of technical maneuvers available, from basic to complex, for safe and effective rhinoplasty, septorhinoplasty, and revision rhinoplasty.
- The rhinoplasty surgeon will need to have knowledge of both short-term and long-term facets of the healing process.
- Although rhinoplasty and revision rhinoplasty share many commonalities, there are specific issues with revision rhinoplasty surgery that the surgeon must be aware of.

TERMINOLOGY

Table 52.1 contains terms associated with rhinoplasty.

NASAL ANATOMY (FIGURE 52.1)

- *Skin:* Thicker over the upper and lower third of the nose and thinner over the middle third muscle-osseocartilaginous framework
- *Bones:* Nasal, frontonasal process, and palatal crest of the maxilla, nasal process of the frontal, perpendicular plate of the ethmoid, vomer
- *Cartilage:* Upper lateral and lower lateral, accessory, sesamoid, quadrangular
- *Arterial blood supply* (Figure 52.2)
  - External nose
    - Internal carotid-ophthalmic-anterior ethmoid-external nasal branch of anterior ethmoid
      - Lateral nasal
    - External carotid-facial-angular-lateral nasal
      - Superior labial-columellar
    - External carotid-maxillary-infraorbital
  - Internal nose
    - Internal carotid-ophthalmic-anterior and posterior ethmoid
    - External carotid-sphenopalatine and greater palatine
      - Angular and labial
- *Venous blood supply*
  - Generally follows the arterial supply
  - The nasal veins do not have valves
  - The nasal venous system has direct communication to the cavernous sinus, thus making nasal infections potentially a life-threatening event
- *Nerve supply* (Figure 52.3)
  - Trigeminal-ophthalmic-nasociliary-anterior ethmoid: supplies the anterior half of nasal cavity
  - External branch of the anterior ethmoid: supplies the nasal skin from rhinion to tip
  - Posterior ethmoid: supplies the superior half of nasal cavity
  - Infratrochlear: supplies the nasion and bony dorsum
- *Mucosa*
  - The vestibule is lined by hair-bearing squamous epithelium up to the level of the caudal margin of the alar cartilage, where it transitions to pseudostratified ciliated columnar respiratory epithelium with abundant seromucinous glands

FUNCTIONAL NASAL CONDITIONS

Physiologic: airway obstruction caused by nonanatomic, nonmechanical conditions

- Allergy
- External irritants
- Tobacco
- Medications
- Vasomotor rhinitis
- Rhinitis medicamentosa
- Nasal sinus disease
- Sexual or emotional stimulation
- Hyperthyroidism
- Pregnancy

Anatomic: airway obstruction caused by mechanical or anatomic impingement on the physical airway

- Congenital or acquired nasal septal deviation
- Congenital or acquired nasal bony deviation
- Congenital or acquired nasal cartilage weakness
- Internal valve collapse
- External valve collapse
- Nasal turbinate bone and/or mucosal hypertrophy
- Nasal polyps
- Synechiae

PATIENT HISTORY AND EXAMINATION

Patient Concerns and Goals

- It is very important to determine exactly why patients seek a consultation for potential nasal surgery.
- The patient is asked to look at a mirror and describe exactly what they see, what bothers them, and specifically as possible in what ways they would change their nasal appearance.
- The patient is told that for the purposes of the exam they can assume that anything that they might want changed can be done but they are also told that in reality it may not be possible.
- It is incumbent upon the surgeon to assess that the patient's goals are indeed realistic. A patient with a concern that is disproportionate to the actual degree of deformity that is present should be approached with great caution.[1-3]

Aesthetic Nasal History

- History and nature of any nasal trauma
  - Pretrauma photos when available
  - Emergency department (ED) notes and radiologic exam records when available. Note whether closed reduction or surgical intervention was attempted

TABLE 52.1. TERMINOLOGY ASSOCIATED WITH RHINOPLASTY
Alae/ala: The outer skin of the nostrils from the nostril margin to the skin overlying the alar cartilage making up the lateral surface of the external nose and composed of fibrofatty tissue
Alar groove: The transition between the alae and the lateral nasal sidewalls, defined by a shadow or crease
Anatomic dome: The area of transition between the medial and lateral crura of the alar/lower lateral cartilage. The anatomic dome usually but not always corresponds to the most projecting point of the nasal tip (the clinical dome).
Anterior septal angle: The junction of the caudal septum and the dorsal septum
Anterior: Toward the forward surfaces on lateral view
Cartilage-splitting incision: Intranasal incision within the body of the lower lateral cartilage
Caudal septum: The caudal most portion of the cartilaginous septum
Caudal: Toward the nostrils or the same as inferior when referring to the nose
Cephalic: Toward the root or radix of the nose for the same as superior when referring to the nose
Clinical dome: The apparent point(s) of maximum projection of the tip
Columella: The anatomic columnar structure of the nose that includes the paired lower medial crura of the lower lateral cartilages and its surrounding soft tissues.
Columellar labial angle: Formed by the angle between the columella and the upper lip. This angle is not dependent on the nasal base position, as in the nasolabial angle.
Columellar lobular angle: The angle formed at the junction of the columella and the infratip lobule. The angle is usually 35°–45° in females and 0°–35° in males.
Dorsal aesthetic lines: Imaginary lines starting at the medial edge of the brows and tracing a gentle curve down the lateral side of the dorsum to the tip-defining points.
Dorsal: Along and toward the bridge of the nose, either on anterior-posterior or anterior on a lateral view
External nasal valve: Corresponds to the support of the nostril with deep inspiration. A competent valve will keep the nostril open during deep inspiration
Hemitransfixion incision: An incision along one side of the caudal septum, not going through and through only
Infratip lobule: Transition area between the tip (domes) and the columella
Intercartilaginous incision: Intranasal incision between the upper and lower lateral cartilages
Internal nasal valve: Supportive functional opening within the nasal cavity at the junction of the lower lateral and upper lateral cartilages (scroll area), the angle of which is defined by the septum and the upper lateral cartilage as it diverges from the septum. An angle of less than 15° may contribute to a greater tendency for valvular insufficiency on inspiration.
Keystone area: The area where the bone structures meets the cartilage structures along the dorsum of the nose
Lateral alar crus (crura): Lateral wing of the alar cartilage
Lower lateral cartilages: Paired cartilage structure of the nasal tip also known as the alar cartilage and composed of the medial and lateral crura and dome. It gives support to the nostrils and the external nasal valve and gives rise the tip shape
Marginal incision: An incision caudal to the lower lateral cartilage
Medial alar crus (crura): medial wing of the alar cartilage
Menton: The most inferior point of the mandible/chin as seen on lateral view of a cephalogram
Nasal horizontal facial plane: Corresponds to the Frankfort Horizontal line, the plane defined by a 90° plane from the vertical facial plane, with the line drawn from the inferior portion of the external auditory canal to the bony inferior orbital rim
Nasal pyramid: Corresponds to the bony structure of the upper nose, pyramidal in shape
Nasal septum: The anatomic structure that separates the nasal airway into two separate nasal cavities, with a portion being cartilaginous and a portion being bony
Nasal turbinate: Intranasal mass structures consisting of mucosa, erectile tissue, and thin bone, which helps to humidify and control the flow of air as it passes through the nose. Of the three turbinates located on each side, the inferior turbinate is the most important.
Nasolabial angle: Formed by a line drawn through the anterior and posterior ends of the nostril and vertical facial plane. The angle is usually 95°–100° in females and 90°–95° in males.
Pogonion: The most anterior projection of the mandible as seen on a cephalogram
Pyriform aperture: Area of the bony midface that corresponds to the nasal cavity opening
Radix: The area deepest point of transition of the bony forehead to the bony upper nose
Scroll area: The area where the cephalic edge of the lower lateral cartilage interlocks with the caudal edge of the upper lateral cartilage.
Sesamoid cartilages: Accessory lateral cartilage structures lying between just lateral to the lower lateral cartilages and the pyriform aperture.
Soft triangle/facet: On basal view, the area of transition between the columella and the nostril rim, corresponding to the area just caudal to the domes where there is no cartilaginous structure
Stomion: Midpoint of the oral fissure with the lips closed
Supratip: The area just above the tip or the transition area between the dorsum and tip
Tip: Includes the paired alar cartilages (lower lateral cartilages), tip complex, columella, and nostrils
Tip-defining points: Refers to the light reflex on the outer skin corresponding to the structural paired cartilaginous domes. Ideally, they are paired, symmetrical, and distinct.

TABLE 52.1. TERMINOLOGY ASSOCIATED WITH RHINOPLASTY (Continued)

Tip projection: Refers to how far the nasal tip projects from the face. There are multiple ways to determine tip projection. One of the more common ways is to measure two lines: (A) the length from the nasal base crease to the tip on lateral view and (B) the length of nose on lateral view from radix to nasal tip. Line A should be about 0.67 the length of B (B divided by A = 0.67).
Tip rotation: Refers to the angle of rotation of the nasal tip. There are multiple ways to measure tip rotation. One of the more common ways is to draw a line from the alar base crease to the nasal tip and compare this angle to the vertical facial plane.
Transcolumellar incision: Incision used in an open rhinoplasty approach, along the mid columella, to allow nasal flap elevation. Most surgeons use either a "stairstep" or an "inverted V"
Transfixion incision: A through-and-through incision that is made along both sides of the caudal septum
Upper lateral cartilages: Paired cartilages along the middle third of the structural nose, extending from the septum medially to the pyriform bones laterally and from the cephalic border of the lower lateral cartilage to the nasal bone. The nasal bone overlaps the cephalic edge of the upper lateral cartilage.
Vertical facial plane: Defined by a 90° plane from the Frankfort horizontal

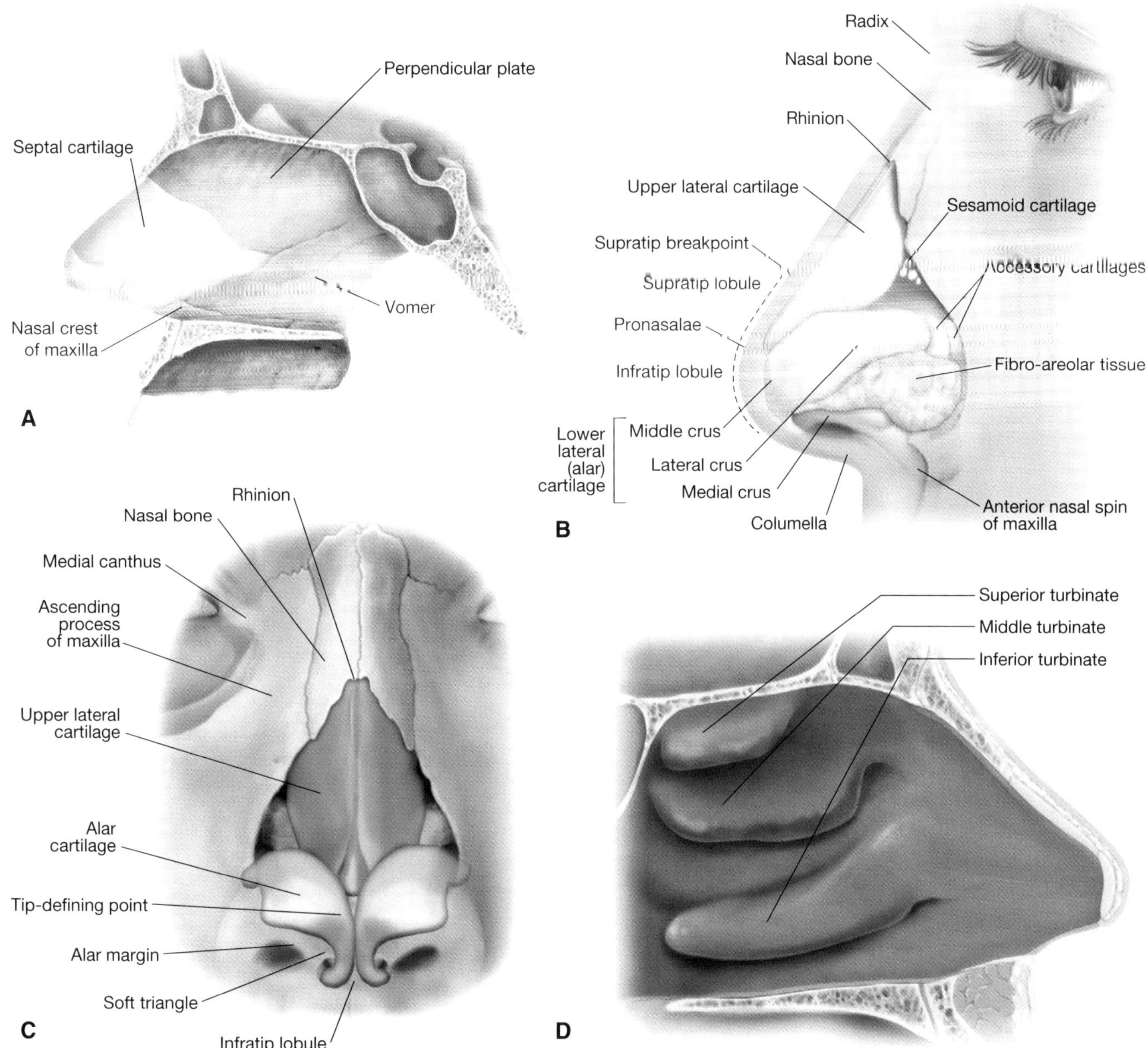

FIGURE 52.1. Nasal anatomy. **A.** Nasal septum. **B.** Lateral view. **C.** Anterior-posterior view. **D.** Internal side wall.

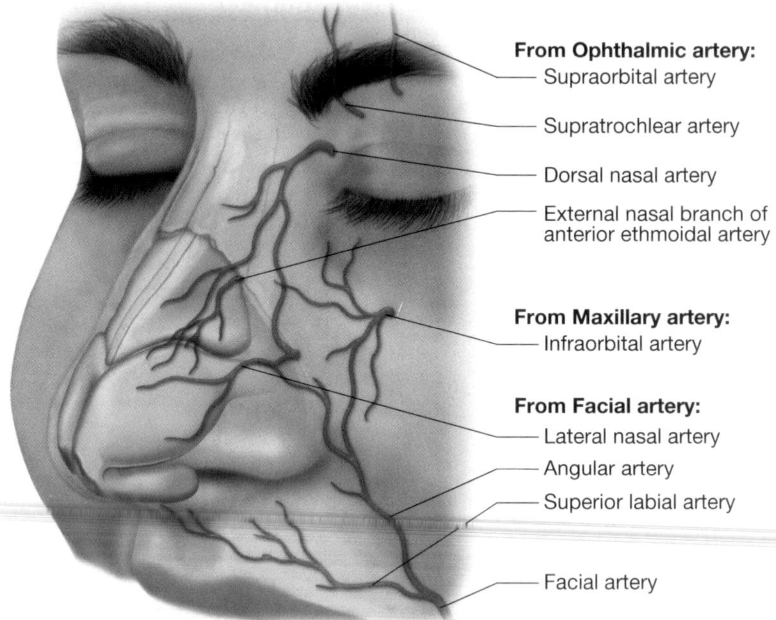

FIGURE 52.2. Nasal arterial supply.

- □ Operative reports when available
- □ Presence of nasal obstructive symptoms related to trauma or disease
  - Constant
  - Intermittent
- □ Epistaxis and or rhinorrhea

History of Previous Nasal Surgery

- Copy of operative notes when available

Psychological History

- Consider psychologic consultation and clearance
- Be aware of body dysmorphic disease

Current Medications

- Medications that can increase nasal obstruction
- Negative medication interactions
- Feedback from prescribing medical doctor regarding medication stops for surgery
- Adequate control of unrelated systemic medical conditions

History of Bleeding Disorders or Difficulties With Previous Surgeries

- Hematology consultation when necessary
- Anesthesia consultation when necessary

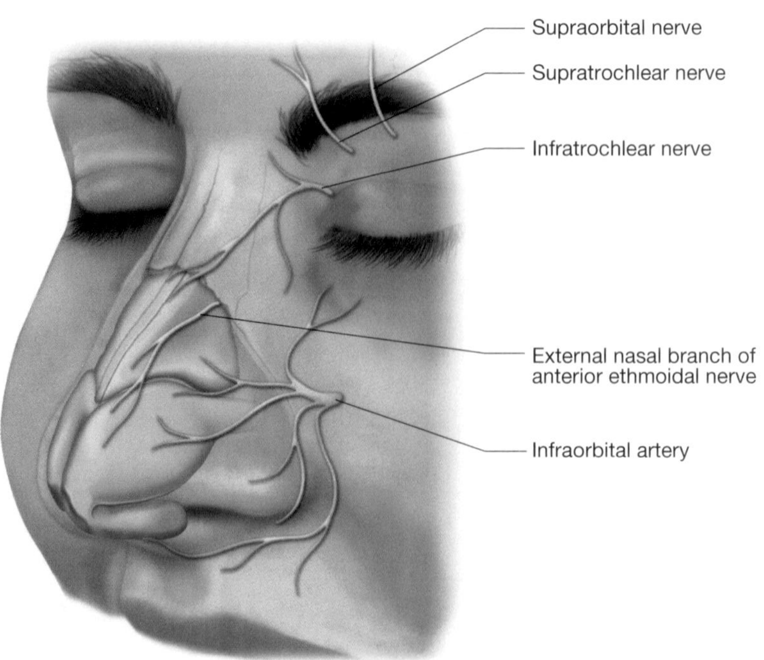

FIGURE 52.3. Nasal nerve supply.

Current Employment

- Need to factor in recovery time off work
- Physical labor versus desk job

Current Physical Activities

- Time away from vigorous exercise, gym, working out, or running

Health History

- Epistaxis
- Rhinorrhea
- Allergies
- Work and home environmental assessment (exposure history)
- Chronicity, seasonality
- Medications
- Previous surgery
- History of cocaine abuse

Physical Examination

- External evaluation
- Cottle testing
- Anterior rhinoscopy before and after vasoconstriction
- Nasoendoscopy (if available)
- Rhinomanometry (if available)

Diagnostic Testing

- CT scanning
- MRI
- Allergy testing

FOCUSED NASAL EXAMINATION

External Examination

- Apparent length and projection of the nose
- Dorsal profile
- Symmetry of the external nose, including deviations
- Width of the alar and bony bases
- Visible and/or palpable bony and/or cartilaginous irregularities
- Condition of the nasal skin and its thickness or thinness
- Presence or absence of nasal scars and skin lesions
- Size, shape, and width of the nostrils
- Presence of prominent medial crural footplates
- Degree of columellar show

Internal Examination

- Cottle tests for both internal and external valve dysfunction first without and then with vasoconstrictor[4]
- Anterior rhinoscopy with evaluation of the nasal mucosa, its moisture, and color
- The presence or absence of discharge
- The presence or absence of nasal polyps
- The shape and alignment of the caudal nasal septum and caudal aspect of the nasal turbinates particularly inferior turbinate
- The presence of any nasal septal perforations
- The presence of scars or scar contracture along with signs of previous nasal surgery
- If the patient has had previous nasal surgery palpation of the nasal septum with a Q-stick can identify whether cartilage has been previously removed. If available, nasoendoscopy can be performed under topical anesthesia to better visualize the posterior aspects of the nasal airway including the posterior septum and turbinates.

Computer Imaging

The use of computer imaging can help to determine the types of changes that can reasonably be made, and it is a visual way of demonstrating the surgeon's concept of the change in the patient's nose directly to that patient. It is important to stress to the patient that computer-imaged results cannot be construed as a guarantee of that exact result. The computer image is a tool that allows the patient and the surgeon to view the same proposed result at the same time.[5,6]

Nasal Analysis

Much has been previously published regarding the ideal nasal aesthetics.[7-9] Byrd analysis looks at idealized relationships between nasal landmarks. Comparison of these idealized measurements with the patient's actual measurements suggests quantifiable changes that can be made in that patient's nose. Computer image analysis uses the surgeon's aesthetic eye to draw the planned change in the patient's nose and then figure what maneuvers are needed to achieve those changes. At this time, the projection or lack thereof of the chin can be analyzed on the lateral photographs by using either Byrd analysis or computer-imaged change. This is one of the few areas where a procedure not directly mentioned by the patient may be legitimately proposed. The use of computer imaging can be very helpful in this situation to demonstrate the change that can be made by genioplasty. General analytic guidelines have limitations based on variability of ideals presented by racial, age, and gender differences.[10-12]

- *The facial thirds* (Figure 52.4A): Transverse lines drawn tangent to the hairline, brow at the level of the supraorbital notch, nasal base, and at the chin (menton) roughly divide the face into thirds. The forehead third shows significant variability because of the differences in forehead height as determined by hairline. The lower third of the face can be subdivided into thirds by adding a horizontal line at the level of the oral commissures (stomion). The upper third defines the upper lip including the Vermillion while the lower two thirds define the lower lip and chin. Attention to these measurements helps the surgeon to assess overall maxillofacial harmony. Underlying facial disharmony should be discussed with patients prior to any facial aesthetic surgery (not just rhinoplasty) to ensure that the patient understands what is beyond the scope of the planned surgery.
- *The facial fifths* (Figure 52.4B yellow lines): Vertical lines are drawn tangential to the periphery of the ears on both sides, the lateral canthi on both sides, and the medial canthi on both sides. Ideally, each segment to the face defined by these vertical lines should be of equal width.
- *Midline facial vertical* (Figure 52.4B, black line): A line drawn from the midglabella to the menton. This line can be used to help determine nasal symmetry in the anterior-posterior view
- *Dorsal aesthetic lines* (Figure 52.5A): These are curved and opposing lines traced from the super orbital ridges curving in toward the keystone area and then flaring slightly as they curve outward toward the tip-defining points.
- *Alar base width* (Figure 52.5B): This distance should be roughly equal to the distance between the medial canthi, as in lines labeled *a*.
- *Bony base width* (Figure 52.5B): This distance should be roughly 80% of the distance between the medial canthi, as in lines labeled *b*.
- *Alar rim orientation* (Figure 52.5C): The alar rims should be symmetrical and flare slightly in it inferolateral direction anterior tip assessment: the supratip break, tip-defining points, and columellar lobular angle are used to define two opposing triangles over the tip of the nose. The intersecting bases of these triangles form a horizontal line through the tip-defining points. These triangles should be roughly symmetrical.
- *Gull wing line* (Figure 52.5D): A line drawn along the superior border of the ala from one side curving around the columellar to the other side should describe a gentle curve similar to the sweep of a seagull in flight.

AESTHETIC SURGERY

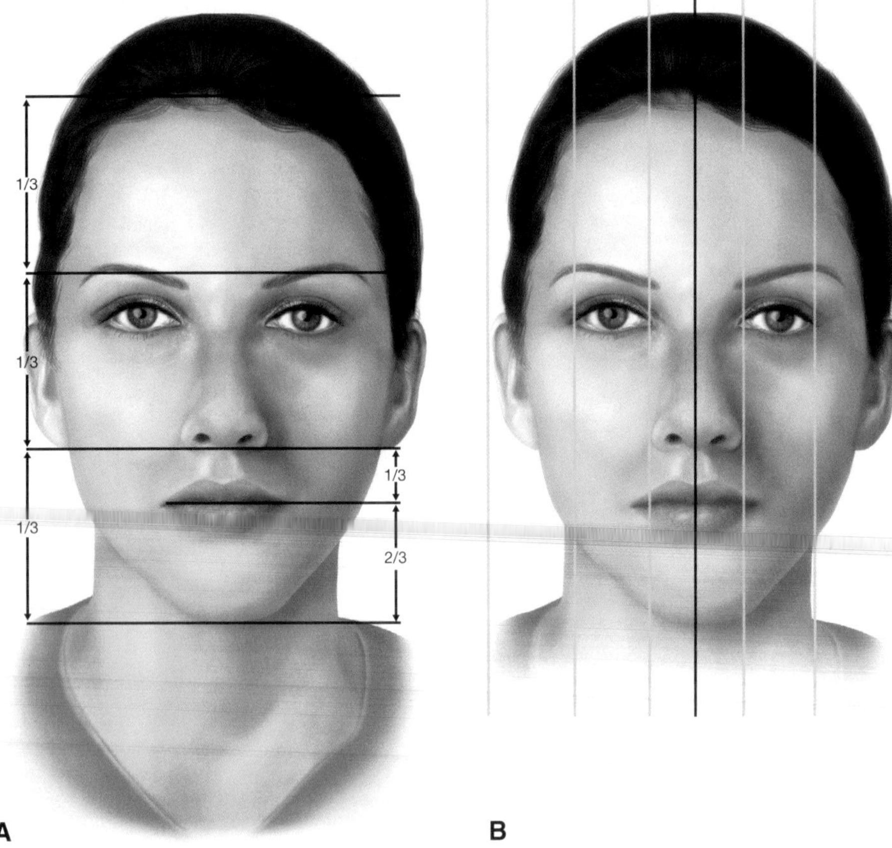

FIGURE 52.4. A. Facial thirds. B. Facial fifths (yellow lines) and midline facial vertical for symmetry (black line).

- *Opposing equilateral triangles* (**Figure 52.5E**): Draw two equilateral triangles with their bases opposed to one another. The corners of the diamond thus formed are the two tip-defining points—the supratip break and the columellar lobular angle. These structures should ideally be symmetrical.
- *Base view triangle* (**Figure 52.6**): In the worm's eye view, a triangle is drawn with its base horizontally through the alar bases and its sides, tangent to the lateral nasal walls. This should form an equilateral triangle.
- *Lobular to nostril ratio* (Figure 52.6): The nostril should be two thirds and the lobule one third of the nasal height in the worm's eye view.
- *Nostril shape* (Figure 52.6): The nostrils should be roughly teardrop shaped with the base wider than the apex and with the axis oriented in a slight medial direction from based apex.
- *Nasal length* (**Figure 52.7**): The apparent length of the nose from radix to tip. This should be approximately the same as the distance from the stomion to the menton.
- *Perceived nasal length:* The apparent length of the nose can be changed by changing the position of the nasal frontal angle or the tip-defining point. Decreasing the rotation of the tip and/or elevating the area of the radix thus moving the nasal frontal angle cephalad will give the perception of a longer nose while increasing tip rotation and/or lowering the radix thus moving the nasal frontal angle caudad will give the appearance of shortening the nose. In addition, a more anterior position of the nasal frontal angle can make the nasal tip look less projecting while a more posterior or deeper position for the nasal frontal angle can make the nasal tip look relatively more projecting.
- *Horizontal ideal chin position* (**Figure 52.8A**): A vertical line can be drawn from a point that is one-half the distance between the radix and the nasal tip and tangent to the anterior most projection of the upper lip. The anterior most projection of the lower lip should be about 2 mm posterior to this line. A parallel line dropped from the anterior most projection of the lower lip should be anterior to the anterior projection of the chin in women and should be tangent to the anterior projection of the chin in men.
- *Nasolabial angle* (**Figure 52.8B**): The angle that is formed between the facial vertical line and the line drawn through the most anterior and posterior edges of the nostril. The degree of rotation of the nasal tip is assessed by evaluating the nasolabial angle. The angle is usually 95° to 100° in women and 90° to 95° in men.
- *Nasofrontal angle* (**Figure 52.8C**): This is determined by the angle of intersection of a line from the tip to the radix corresponding the dorsal plane of the nose and a line along the plane of the brows. Analysis of aesthetically pleasing noses reveals angles ranging from 128° to 140° with the ideal for females being 134° and for males being 130°.
- *Columellar lobular angle* (**Figure 52.8D**): This is the angle formed by the intersection of a line drawn tangential to the columella and to the infratip lobule. This angle is ideally 30° to 45°.
- *Supratip break* (see Figure 52.8C): A pleasing appearance particularly for the female nose is the presence of a supratip break. This is a slightly greater dorsal angulation between the plane of the nasal dorsum and the plane from the cephalic edge of the dome to the tip-defining point.
- *Tip projection* (**Figure 52.9**): The degree to which the nasal tip extends from the face. This can be measured by drawing a line from the alar cheek junction to the nasal tip, and the distance between these two points should be approximately equal to the distance of the alar base width and should be approximately 0.67 times the radix-to-tip distance or the nasal length (Figure 52.9A). Another measure of tip projection states that 50% to 60% of a line drawn from the alar cheek junction to the tip should lie anterior to a line drawn tangent to the most projecting portion of the upper lip (Figure 52.9B). Finally, the tip projection as measured from the alar base should equal the alar base width (Figure 52.9C).
- *The alar-columellar relationship* (**Figure 52.10**): Two lines are drawn, one through the long axis of the nostril and the other from the alar

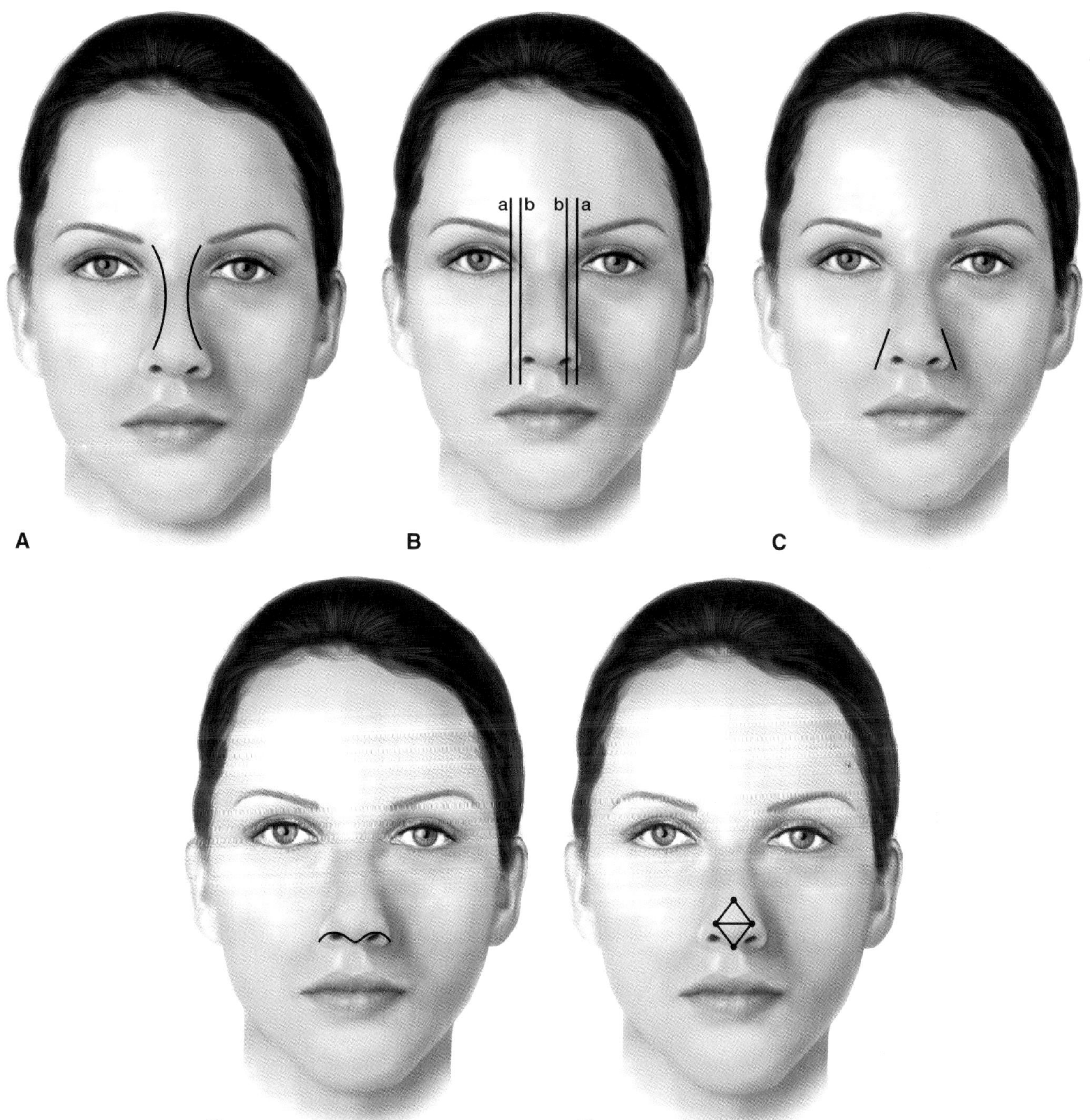

FIGURE 52.5. **A.** Dorsal aesthetic lines. **B.** Alar base width (*a*) and bony base width (*b*). **C.** Alar rim orientation. **D.** Gull wing line. **E.** Opposing equilateral triangles.

rim to the columellar rim at the midpoint of the first line. The distance from the alar rim to the first line should be the same as the distance from the columellar rim to the first line. Increase in either of those distances may represent alar retraction or columellar show.

Regardless of which method one uses to analyze the patient's nose, the idea is to have a specific and detailed operative plan for the procedure prior to entering the operating room.

TREATMENT PLAN

Many nasal surgeries are in fact a combination of procedures for both aesthetic and functional conditions.

Aesthetic rhinoplasty unless traceable to documented trauma is seldom covered by insurance, while functional septorhinoplasty or rhinoplasty performed for correction of deformity secondary to documented trauma or disease may be covered by insurance. Prior approval and contemporaneous records are often required for coverage. The combined case, coding and billing, for the covered aspect of the procedure is often computed by timing the portion of the case that is functional in nature. Most surgeons performing aesthetic rhinoplasty require out-of-pocket payment in full for the procedure in advance of the operation.

Common functional procedures:

- Septoplasty/submucous resection
- Septorhinoplasty

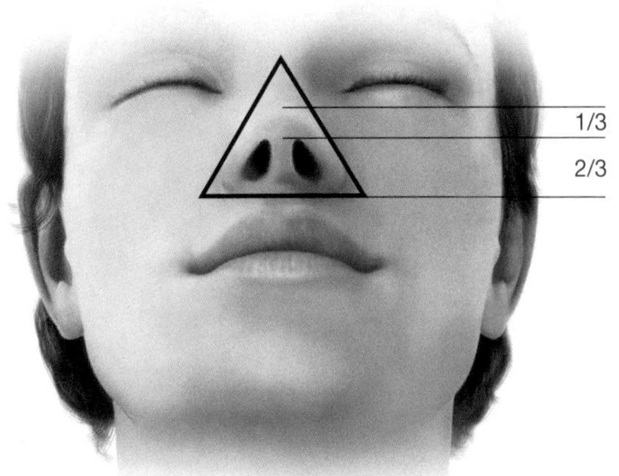

FIGURE 52.6. Base view/worm's eye view showing triangle, lobular to nostril ratio, and nostril shape.

- Reconstruction of the internal nasal valve
- Reconstruction of the external nasal valve
- Nasal turbinate modification
- Anterior turbinectomy
- Submucous resection of the inferior turbinate
- Out fracture of the inferior nasal turbinates
- Bipolar cautery of the inferior nasal turbinates
- Endoscopic polypectomy

Medical Treatment

Medical treatment is used in conjunction with surgical treatment or when mechanical airway obstruction is ruled out and includes the following:

- Systemic antihistamines and decongestants
- Topical vasoconstrictor, steroid, and antihistamine sprays
- Allergic desensitization
- Medication changes; avoidance of medications known to contribute to nasal congestion

Surgical Treatment

Anesthesia

- Managed anesthesia care
    - □ Popular in past years when closed, rapid, and often "cookie-cutter" rhinoplasties were performed
    - □ Requires expertise and experience in sedative of anesthesia by both the anesthesiologist and the surgeon.
    - □ Not recommended *except* for very minor revisions

General

- Allows the surgeon the time needed to perform the individualized operation that each patient requires.
- Ensures that the patient is comfortable throughout the operation

Approach: Considerations

Closed Rhinoplasty

- No external scar
- Limited undermining
- Less postoperative edema
- Faster recovery
- Less operative time
- Difficult to assess and visualize anatomic variations and therefore make an appropriate operative plan
- More difficult to teach this technique because it does not allow simultaneous visualization by the surgeon and residents or students

Open Rhinoplasty

- Three-dimensional binocular visualization
- Simultaneous visualization by the surgeon, residents, and students
- More accurate assessment of anatomic variations
- Requires wider dissection
- More postoperative edema particularly at the tip
- Exposure takes more time
- Possible longer recovery time
- Columellar scar

Operative Order

The question for operative order is tip then nose versus nose then tip.

In closed rhinoplasty, many surgeons would argue that "as goes the tip so goes the nose." This is a reasonable approach in closed rhinoplasty particularly when there is limited tip suturing and/or grafting.

In open rhinoplasty, many surgeons would recommend modification of the tip as the last step in the procedure. Given modern rhinoplasty techniques with multiple tip sutures and grafts, the possibility of disrupting the tip modifications during performance of the remaining portions of the rhinoplasty argues for performing most of the tip modifications later in the procedure.

Localization and Preparation

This can be done prior to washing the face with prep solution. Local anesthesia with epinephrine is ideal to minimize intraoperative

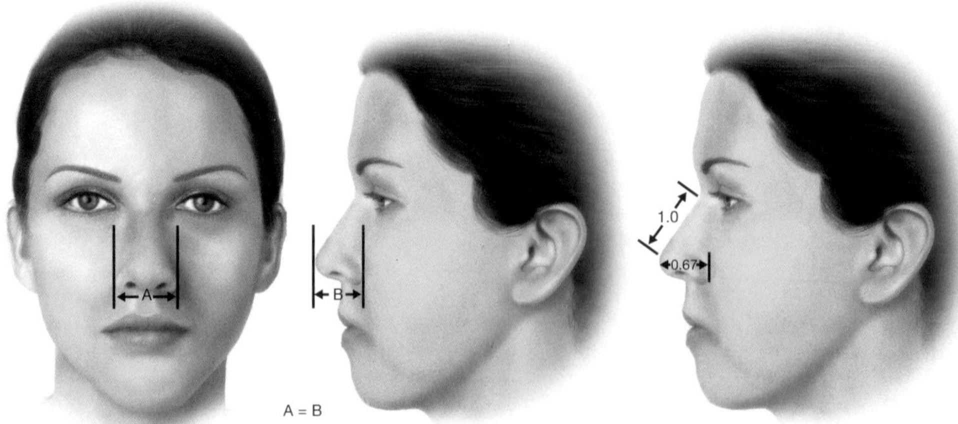

FIGURE 52.7. Nasal length. Ideal nasal length is equivalent to the stomiom-to-menton distance. *A*, ala; *M*, menton; *R*, radix; *S*, stoma; *T*, tip.

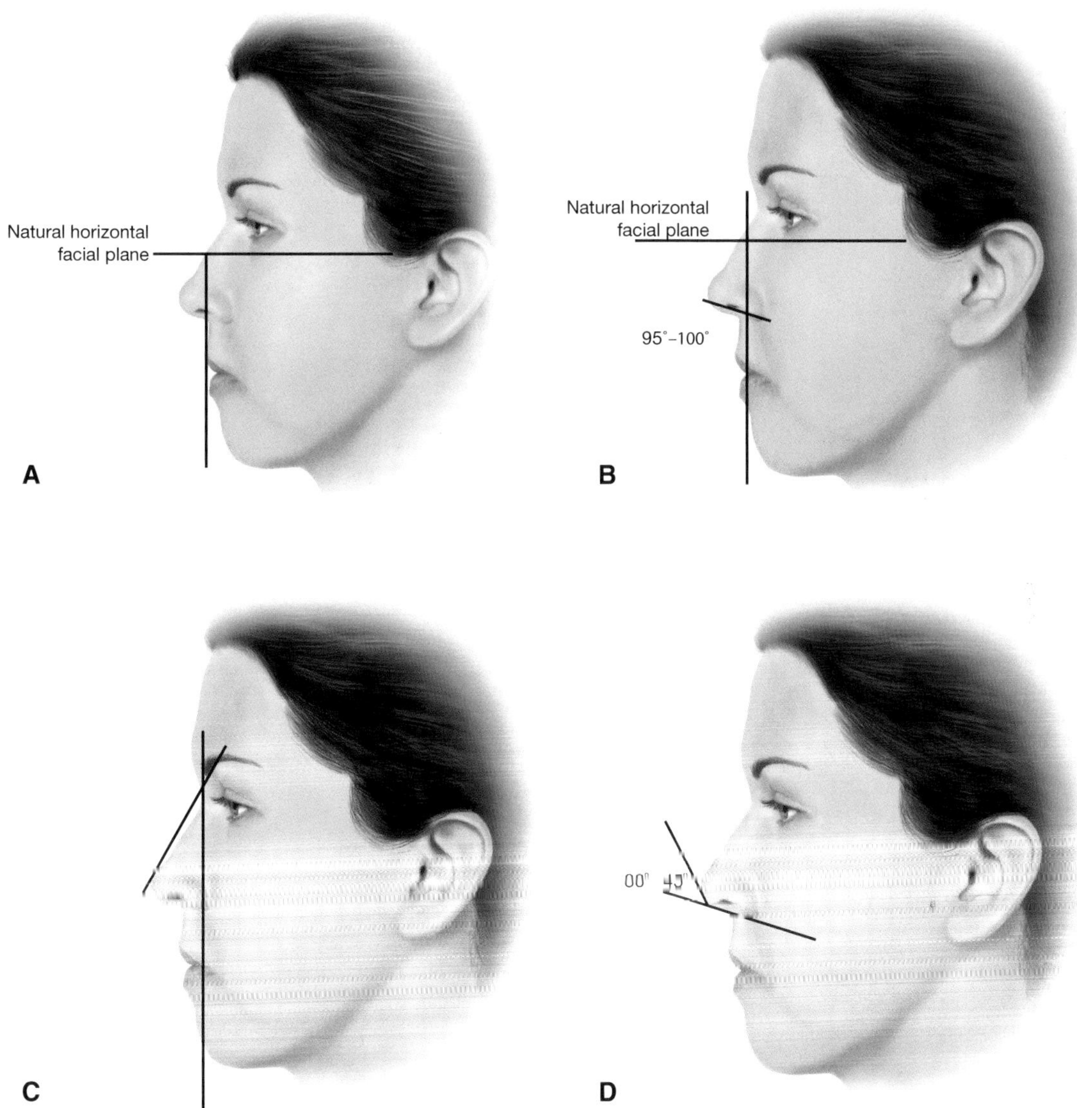

FIGURE 52.8. **A.** Ideal chin position. **B.** Nasolabial angle. **C.** Nasofrontal angle, dorsal line. **D.** Columellar lobular angle.

bleeding. Typically, 1% lidocaine with epinephrine or 1% lidocaine with epinephrine mixed 50/50 with 0.25% Marcaine without epinephrine is used. Intranasal cottonoids soaked in Afrin or epinephrine 1:1000 are used to decrease bleeding and to shrink the turbinates. The face wash should be nontoxic to the eyes.

Incisions and Patient Preparation

Options for incisions (Figure 52.11):

- Transcolumellar stairstep with intranasal marginal incisions: standard for open rhinoplasty
- Cartilage-splitting incision: often used in closed rhinoplasty
- Intercartilaginous incision: often used in combination with marginal incision to "deliver" cartilage in closed rhinoplasty

Marking

Outline the proposed transcolumellar incision using methylene blue pen (Figure 52.12). Methylene blue tattoos strategically placed on either side of the proposed incisions can aid in the closure at the end of the case.

Optional: Outline the nasal anatomy, including the outline of the upper lateral cartilages, the lower lateral cartilages, and the nasal bones as well as outline the planned incisions and any proposed nasal dorsal reduction, proposed placement of grafts, and proposed modification of the lower lateral cartilages, as well as the location of any planned osteotomies.

Trim the nasal vibrissae.

Use the local solution described above in a 10-cc syringe with a 25 gauge 1.5 inch needle to inject the nose in the intended plane of dissection. When injecting the nasal septum, use a 3-cc syringe with a 20 gauge 1.5-inch needle thus providing better hydraulic advantage and making it easier to dissect the septal mucoperichondrial flap from the cartilage.

Place Afrin-soaked cottonoids along the floor of the nose and in the middle meatus and against the roof of the nose to constrict the mucosal vessels and reduce the size of the turbinates. In the past, cocaine in a 4% solution was commonly used because of it being both a vasoconstrictor and a topical anesthetic. It is not necessary nor indicated to use cocaine when performing this operation under general anesthesia.

Prep and drape the patient's face consistent with your institution's approved method.

BASIC OPEN RHINOPLASTY

Opening

Mark a transcolumellar stair-step incision (or an inverted V) across the narrowest portion of the columella. We suggest that the stairs

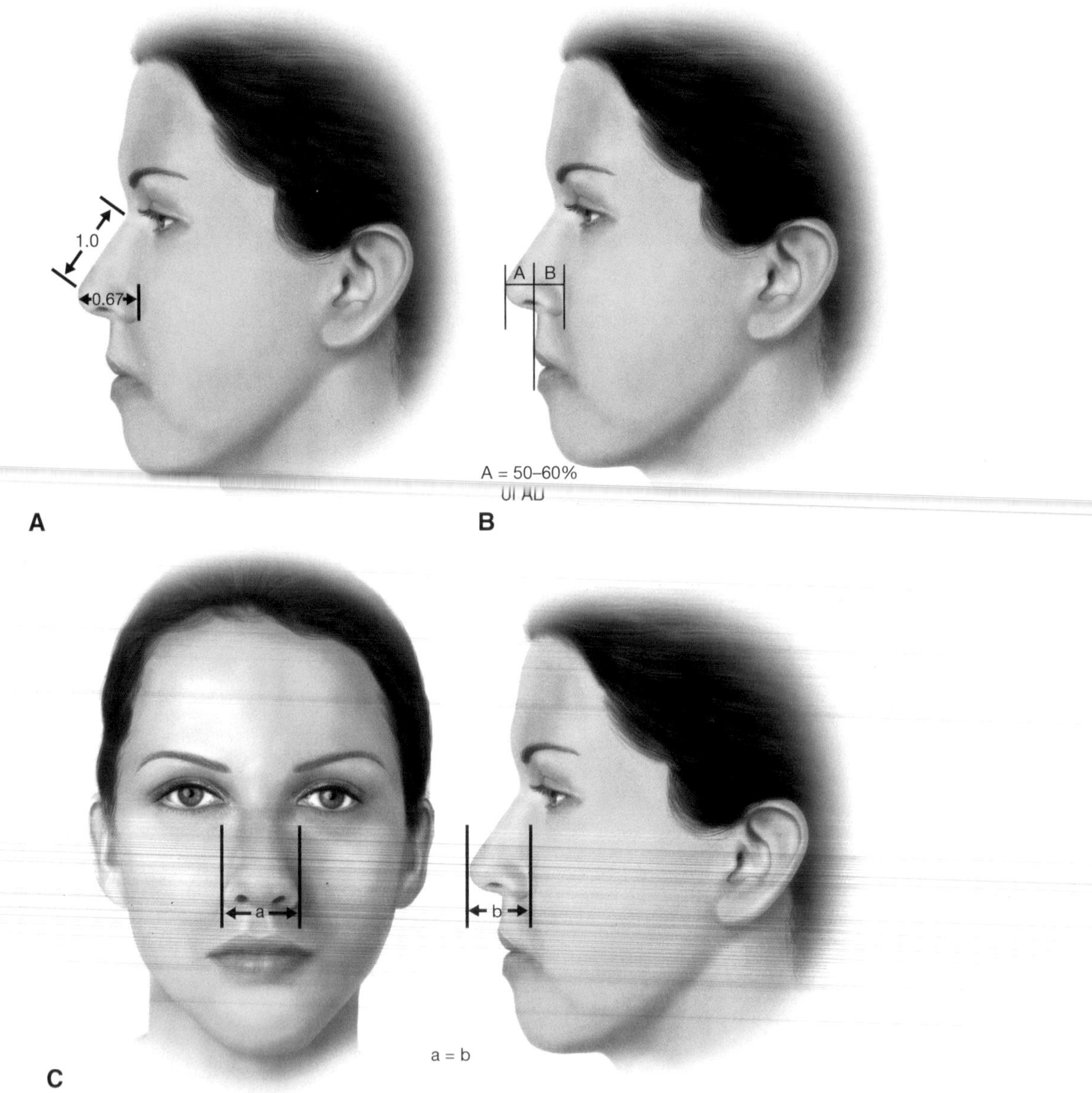

FIGURE 52.9. **A.** Tip-to-length ratio. **B.** Tip projection. **C.** Tip projection to alar base width.

step "down" from the operator's side of the table as it is a little easier to see the opposite nares when making and elevating that portion of the columella flap. Use the tip of a no. 11 scalpel blade to describe the central stair-step right angles. Use the flat of the blade to make the remaining horizontal incision over the medial crura being careful to stay superficial so as not to injure the cartilage, which is immediately under the skin. This incision will intersect at a right angle with a superficial vertical incision that can be made with a no. 15 scalpel blade and that is located just cephalic to the caudal roll of the medial crura. Again, this should be very superficial as this incision overlies the medial crura. The columellar elevation begins in the midline using a no. 4 angled Converse scissors. The elevation continues carefully over the medial crura, dissected as far toward the domes as possible. Everting the left alar rim with a double hook and your middle finger identify the caudal border of the lateral crus and make an incision from just medial to the pyriform up over the dome with care not to violate the soft triangle and joined this incision with the previously made columellar vertical incision. The double hook will have to be moved toward the dome straddling the area of the dome and pushing with the middle finger to see the caudal margin of the alar cartilage. With the assistant retracting the caudal edge of the now exposed lateral crus, use the Converse no. 4 scissors to identify the plane immediately above the perichondrium. In a primary rhinoplasty, you should now be able to use a Q-stick to continue the dissection in this plane with gentle pushing action exposing all of the lateral crus up to and including the domes. Any remaining attachments of the columella flap overlying the dome can be severed with the scissors. Repeating this on the opposite side should allow the dorsal flap to be completely elevated to the level of the upper lateral cartilages. A Q-stick to be used to continue the dissection in this plane over the dorsum of the nose to approximately the level of the nasal bones. The dissection can be completed using a curved Joseph-Peck scissors spreading and elevating just enough to insert an Aufricht retractor. It is important to only elevate enough to allow whatever modifications are planned but not so much as to decrease tissue attachments to the bone thus making it potentially unstable after osteotomies. Staying in this relatively avascular plane immediately above the cartilage and bone will give you good exposure with minimal bleeding (**Figure 52.13**). At this time, any individual bleeding vessels can be cauterized.

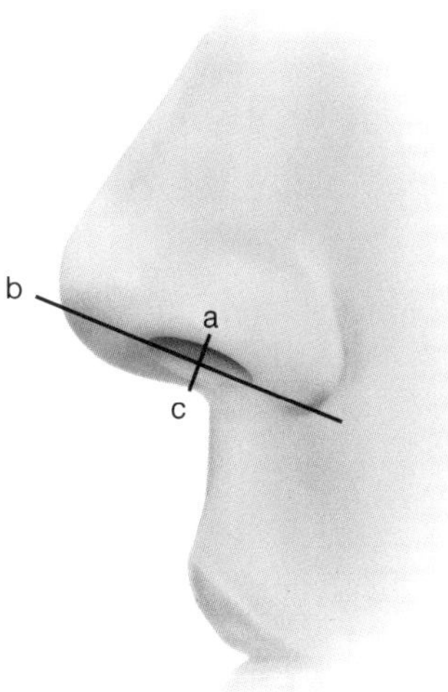

FIGURE 52.10. Alar-columellar relationship.

Modifying the Dorsum

In this case, we will modify the bony dorsum followed by modification of the cartilaginous dorsum. After elevating the periosteum from the nasal bones using a Joseph elevator, a pull rasp is used to take the dorsum down to the desired height. Incremental reduction and frequent checking with the skin redraped and a wet index finger will help to avoid overcorrection. Orientation of the rasp head in exactly the right plane both horizontal and vertical by stabilization through the skin with the operator's nondominant hand will ensure even takedown of the nasal bones. When proper bony height is achieved, attention is turned to separate the dorsal septum from the medial aspect of the paired upper lateral cartilages.

The cartilaginous reduction is begun by exposure of the junction of the upper lateral cartilages with the dorsal nasal septum by means of the creation of a superior Cottle tunnel. The caudal septal angle is exposed with scissors and a mucoperichondrial elevation is begun on one side of the dorsal septum (**Figure 52.14**). Care is taken to be directly on the glistening bluish cartilage. A mucoperichondrium flap is elevated along the dorsum of the nasal septum using a Cottle elevator. This tunnel is dissected in the cephalic direction at the junction of the septum with the upper lateral cartilage to and just beyond the junction of the perpendicular plate of the ethmoid bone with the undersurface of the nasal bone. By sweeping the mucoperichondrium laterally using the Cottle elevator, the junction of the dorsal septum and medial upper lateral cartilage is defined (**Figure 52.15**). If a no. 15 scalpel can be placed within the tunnel with its flat surface on the [illegible] dorsal septum and with the blade oriented dorsally and with the skin protected by the Aufricht retractor, then the upper lateral cartilage can be sharply separated from the dorsal septum from the junction with the nasal bone to its most caudal attachment. Repeating this process on the opposite side will now expose the dorsal septum as well as the medial aspect of the right and left upper lateral cartilages. Each of these structures can be independently trimmed or manipulated at this time. If carefully done, the mucoperichondrium

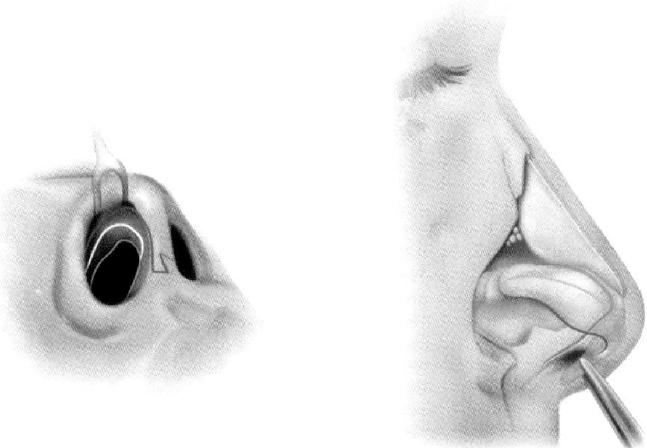

FIGURE 52.11. Incisions. The transcolumellar stairstep with intranasal marginal incisions (shown in red) is standard for open rhinoplasty. The cartilage-splitting incision (shown in yellow) is often used in closed rhinoplasty. The intercartilaginous incision (shown in green) is often used in combination with marginal incision to "deliver" cartilage in closed rhinoplasty.

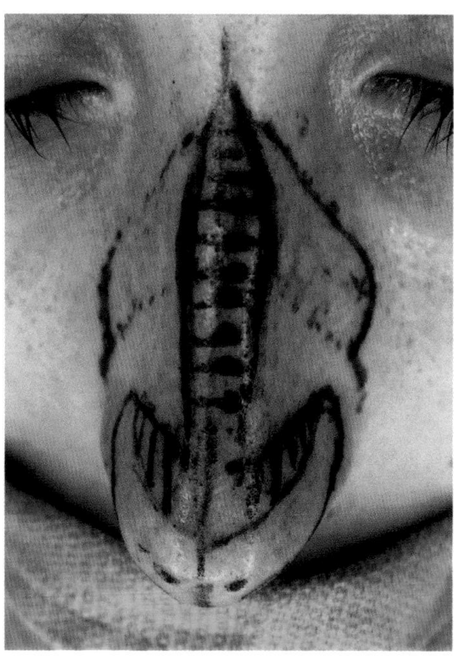

FIGURE 52.12. Nasal anatomy and general operative plan outlined on skin.

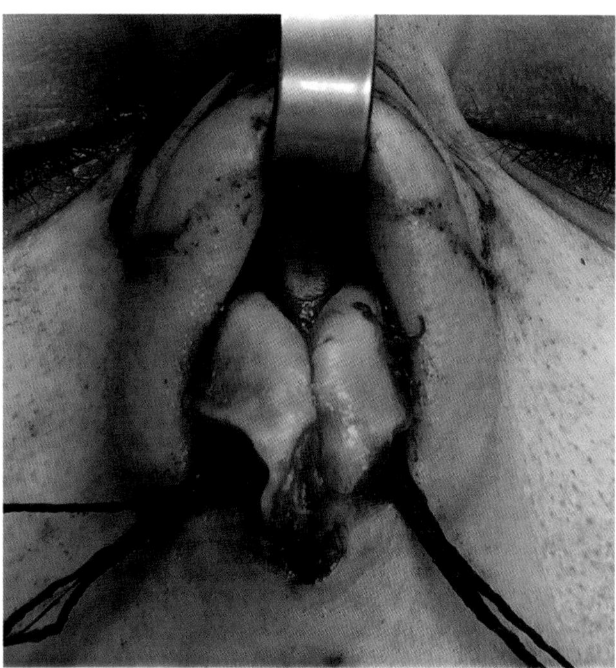

FIGURE 52.13. Skin elevated.

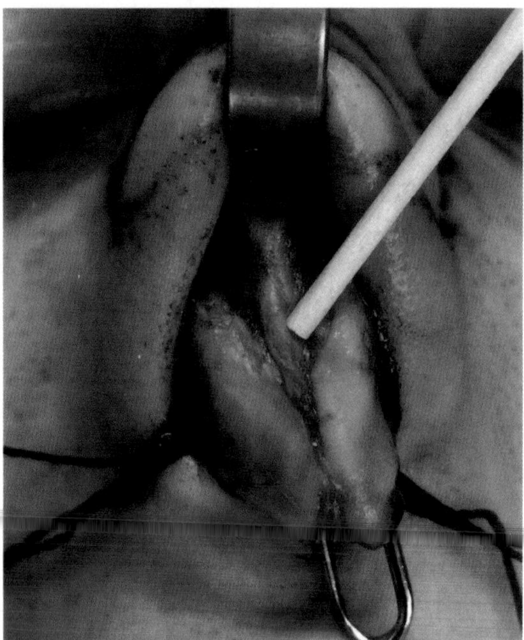

FIGURE 52.14. Anterior superior septal angle.

remains intact without communication to the nasal cavity. The dorsal septum can be lowered using angled scissors or a scalpel. The upper lateral cartilages can be trimmed as well or scored and enfolded on themselves to make auto spreader flaps or maintained for resuturing to the dorsal septum. Note that the cartilaginous dorsum can be lowered first followed by lowering the dorsal bone en bloc using an osteotome.

Septoplasty, Caudal Septal Modification, or Septal Cartilage Harvesting

If the caudal septum is to be modified to shorten the nose or modify the columella labial angle, mucoperichondrium will need to be elevated from that portion that is to be resected beginning dorsally at the septal angle where previous superior Cottle tunnels were made. At this point, it is a good idea to again inject local anesthetic into the plane of dissection on both sides of the septum. Once exposed on both sides, the caudal septum can be modified with scissors or scalpel. If there is a need for septal cartilage grafting or there is deviation of the quadrangular cartilage that is to be corrected, a complete mucoperichondrial elevation on one side is necessary. In general, the first side to be elevated is that side opposite the operator. The elevation can be done with a Cottle or a Freer elevator being careful to be in the relatively avascular plane directly over the cartilage. If only a small piece of cartilage is necessary, then a limited elevation can be performed. If there is need for more graft material, complete elevation is necessary. At this point, it is important to ensure that a minimum of 1 cm of dorsal and caudal septum is preserved as an L-shaped strut to support the nasal structure. The more that can be left, the stronger the nasal structure. If the continuity of this L-shaped strut is accidentally interrupted, it must be repaired and reinforced with cartilage or polydioxanone suture plate gussets. The cartilage to be harvested or removed can be outlined on the surface of the quadrangular cartilage in methyl and blue pen. A curved septal knife can then be used to incise along the outlined cartilage dorsally and caudally. A Cottle elevator can then be used to carefully elevate the opposite side through these incisions only elevating the opposite side over the cartilage that is to be removed. Once the opposite side is elevated, the remaining incisions can be completed with scissors, scalpel, Ballenger swivel knife, and elevator without perforating the mucoperichondrium. It is important to remember the shape of the quadrangular cartilage particularly where it abuts the junction of the vomer and the perpendicular plate of the ethmoid. There is usually a significant tongue of cartilage in this area that can provide important additional material for grafting. At this point, any additional deviation of either the perpendicular plate of the ethmoid, the vomer or the maxillary crest can be dealt with using a Jantzen-Middleton rongeur. The airway should now be assessed for patency, and when indicated out-fracture of the inferior turbinate, Dennis bipolar cautery of the inferior turbinate or anterior turbinectomy can be done. The flap should be inspected for perforations but unless they are large and/or they communicate with a perforation on the opposite flap at the same level repair is not necessary.

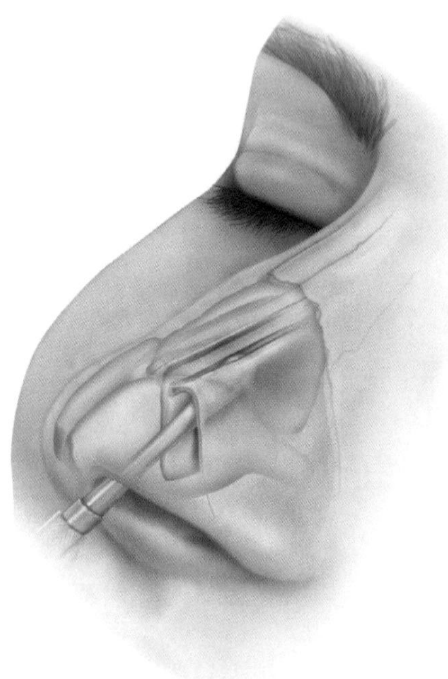

FIGURE 52.15. Elevating superior Cottle tunnels.

Spreader Grafts and Flaps

Spreader grafts or flaps are useful to prophylactically maintain or to widen the internal valve area when a narrow valve angle is contributing to obstructive symptoms[13,14] (**Figure 52.16**). Grafts are generally made from harvested septum but may also be made from rib or auricular cartilage. They can also be used to strengthen the dorsal septum as well as to help straighten dorsal septal deviations. They can be stabilized with 30 gauge needles to allow them to be sutured in place flush with the dorsal septum with 5-0 PDS. Excess medial upper lateral cartilage can be folded on itself and sutured in a similar manner.

Open rhinoplasty allows you to see the nasal tip as it sits in vivo. It is beyond the scope of this chapter to provide a comprehensive compendium of all potential tip modifications.[7-9,15,16] The most common tip modifications involve some form of cephalic lateral alar crural resection, intradome and interdome suturing, and/or the placement of a columellar strut. In principle, as much supporting structure of the alar cartilages as possible should be left in place. The alar cartilages should be assessed for their thickness and strength. If the alar cartilages are of sufficient thickness and strength, a cephalic resection leaving an uninterrupted 6 to 8 mm caudal strip of cartilage can be removed (**Figure 52.17**). If there is unwanted cephalic fullness but the cartilages of questionable strength than the removed cephalic segment can be slid into a pocket made between the nasal mucosa and the remaining caudal cartilage and sutured into position to bolster the lateral alar crus. If there is too much convexity in the segment, the cephalic cartilage can be inverted before being sewn into place thus counteracting the tendency for convexity). If the domes are widely

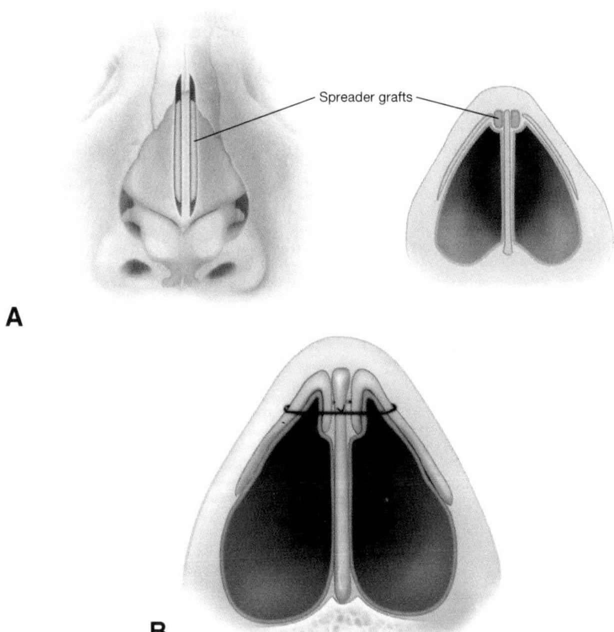

FIGURE 52.16. **A.** Spreader grafts. **B.** Spreader flaps.

separated or are of unequal height, they can be adjusted by interdomal mattress sutures of 5-0 PDS (**Figure 52.18A**). The individual domes can be narrowed and accentuated with intradomal (transdomal) mattress sutures of 5-0 PDS (**Figure 52.18B**). Combination interdomal and intradomal/transdomal sutures can be used to both narrow the individual domes and as well as the interdome distance (**Figure 52.18C**). Further strengthening of the medial crura for maintenance of projection or to increase projection can be accomplished by the insertion of a columellar strut (**Figure 52.19**). This can be fashioned from harvested septum and trimmed to be 0.5 cm in width and up to 3 cm or more in length. A tunnel is made with scissors between the medial crura and extending to the nasal spine. The pocket should be made as close to the width of the strut as possible. The strut can be placed in the pocket against the nasal spine and while the assistant holds the domes at the appropriate level the strut can be sewn in a through-and-through fashion to the medial crura with 5-0 PDS mattress sutures with the knot placed internally between the crura. After each maneuver, the skin should be redraped and the contours carefully inspected and palpated with a wet gloved index finger.

Osteotomies

Generally, osteotomies are performed at this time for closing the open roof that is to say the gap between the nasal bones created when the bony dorsum is reduced.[17] The path that the osteotomies will take will depend upon the degree and length of the open roof as well as the desired change in the width of the base of the nasal bones. Medial oblique osteotomies are first performed by insertion of a curve-guarded osteotome at the junction of the septum and nasal bones at the most cephalic aspect of the open roof (**Figure 52.20**). The osteotomy line is carried in oblique fashion away from the Keystone area for about 5 to 10 mm. This helps to control the position of the osteotomies preventing injury to the Keystone area or the creation of a rocker deformity. Lateral osteotomies can be performed intranasally using a curve-guarded osteotome after elevation of the periosteum overlying the nasal bone-cheek junction or using a 2 mm osteotome through an external percutaneous approach. The osteotomy is begun slightly higher on the pyriform lip preserving a triangle of bone along the pyriform, the Webster triangle, where the lateral most aspect of the alar cartilage anchor and provide stability to the nasal valve. If the bony bases are to be narrowed, the osteotomies are carried from this position staying low on the nasal bones (low to low) to the level of the previously made medial oblique osteotomy. Gentle inward digital pressure will green stick fracture the remaining bridge of nasal bone between the end of the medial oblique and lateral osteotomies. If narrowing of the nasal bony base is not indicated, then the osteotomy can curve in a more dorsal direction, low to high, joining and closing the open roof directly (**Figure 52.21**). Lateral osteotomies can also be performed using a percutaneous 2-mm osteotome. A small puncture is made through the skin in the natural skin tension line, and then the osteotomy is made along the same lines as described for the intranasal curved osteotome by walking the 2-mm osteotome along its desired path with gentle taps from the mallet. An advantage of the 2-mm osteotome is that the periosteum is not elevated and therefore remains intact on both the nasal and the facial side of the bone adding stability to that bony segment.

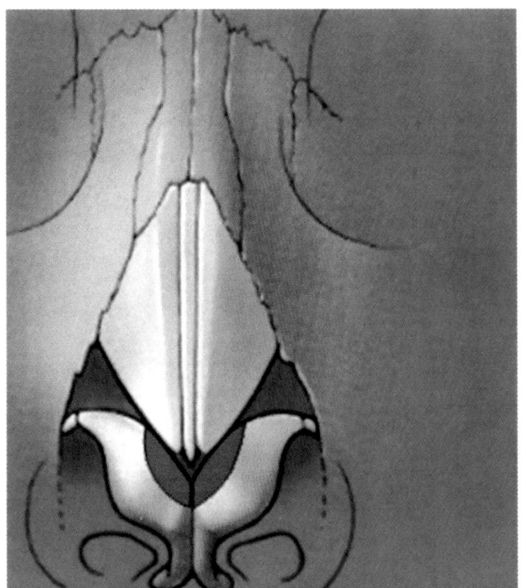

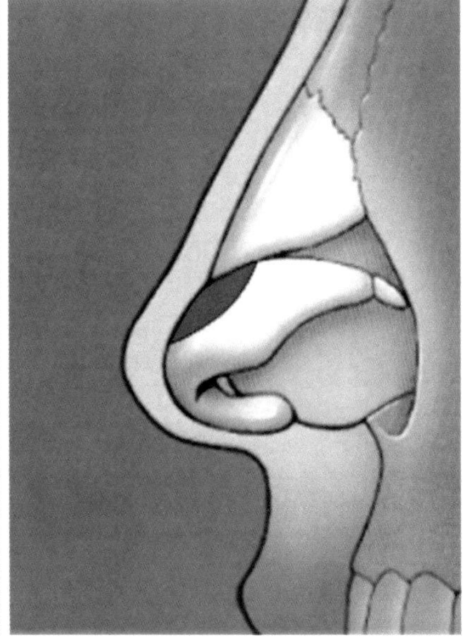

FIGURE 52.17. Cephalic lateral crural resection.

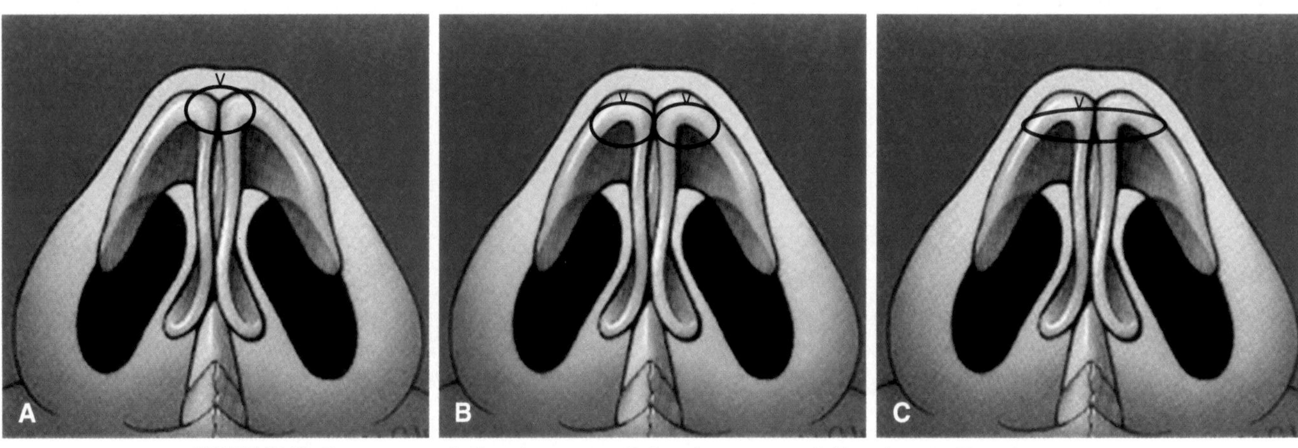

FIGURE 52.18. Dome sutures. **A.** Transdome suture. **B.** Intradome sutures. **C.** Transdome and intradome suture.

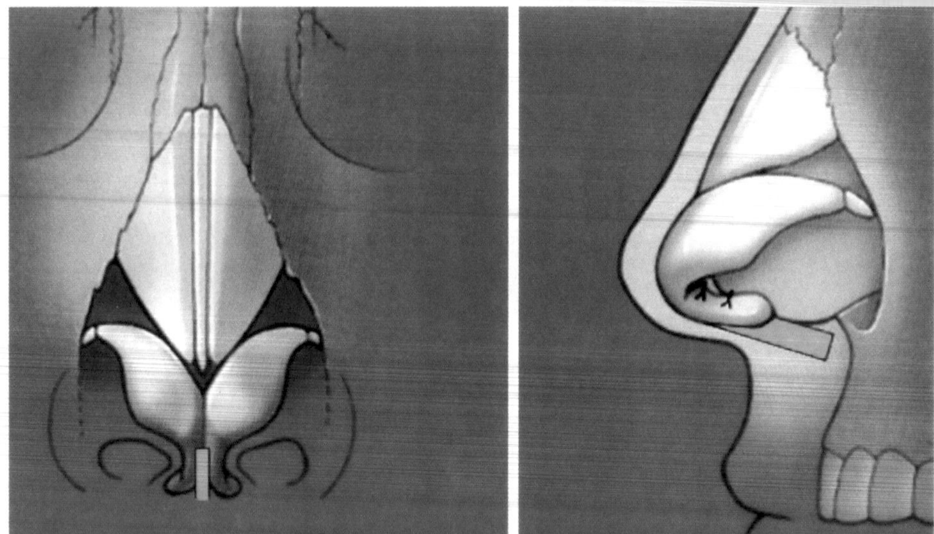
FIGURE 52.19. Columellar strut.

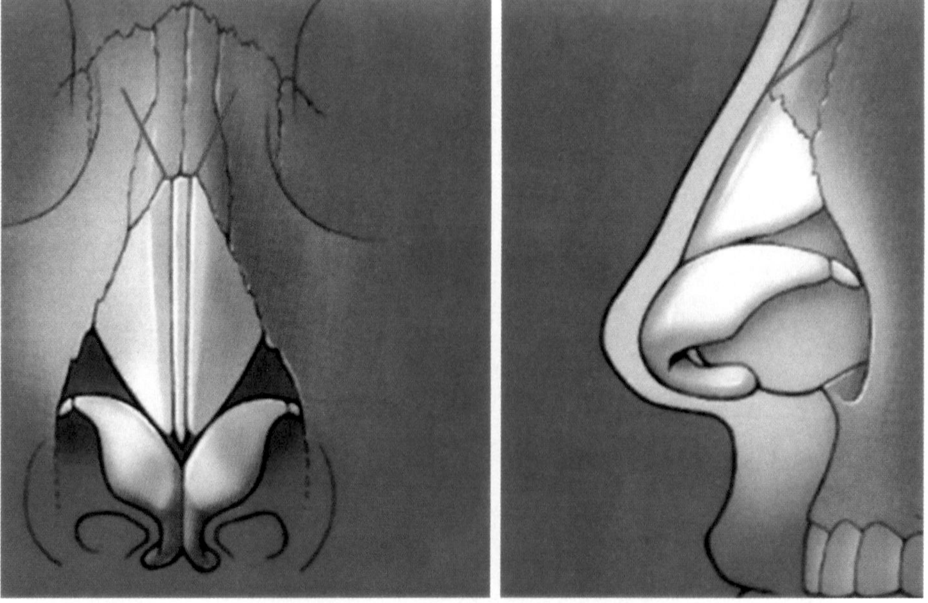
FIGURE 52.20. Medial oblique osteotomies.

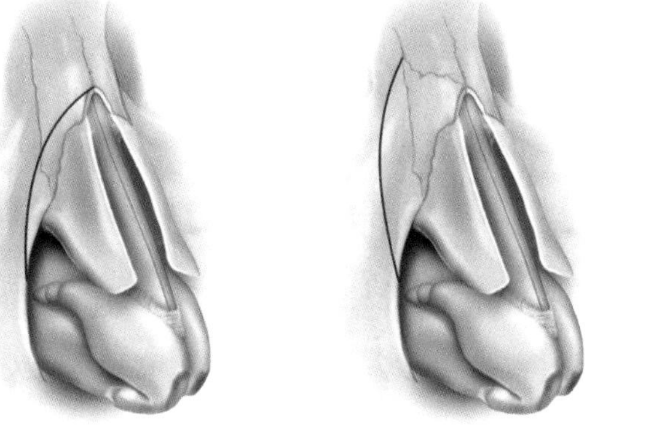

A B

FIGURE 52.21. Osteotomies and the Webster triangle (blue). **A.** Low to high. **B.** Low to low.

The disadvantage is the necessity for an external puncture though experience has shown that these punctures are virtually invisible once healed.

Final Inspection and Closure

Throughout the procedure, the nose should be assessed by observation and comparison to the operative plan. Palpation of the nose using a wet gloved index finger slid along the dorsum should reveal smooth contours without defects. Any residual bony defects should be treated with further rasping using a diamond rasp, while any cartilaginous irregularities should be smooth with a scalpel. Further options for dealing with and "fine tuning" remaining problem areas will be dealt with later in this chapter.

Prior to closing the incisions, the nasal septal flaps are quilted using a 4-0 plain catgut suture passing it back and forth from one side to the other through and through from the caudal septum as far posteriorly as possible in several rows. This is the best way to prevent septal hematoma.

Intranasal incisions are closed with interrupted 5-0 chromic in the same way as in the closed rhinoplasty. The transcolumellar incision is closed very carefully with interrupted 6-0 fast absorbing plain catgut suture, which is then reinforced with skin glue. A careful and meticulous closure of the transcolumellar incision should result in a virtually invisible scar once fully healed. If alar base modifications are planned, they can be performed once the nasal incisions have been closed completely. Alar base modifications include alar base narrowing, nostril size adjustments, alar flare reduction, alar hooding reduction, and alar margin grafting to adjust the position of the alar position on both anterior-posterior and lateral views.[12,18]

When both nasal septal surgery and turbinate modification are done, a Doyle septal splint is placed in each nostril and suture to the membranous columella with a 3-0 Prolene through-and-through suture. The purpose of this splint is not to prevent septal hematoma but rather to provide insulation preventing the formation of synechiae between the septum and the inferior turbinate. Finally, the nose is taped, and a thermoplastic splint is applied (Figure 52.22).

BASIC CLOSED RHINOPLASTY

Tip Delivery Method

A combination of a marginal incision along the caudal border of the lateral alar crus and an intercartilaginous incision at the junction of the cephalic alar crus and the upper lateral cartilages and continued with a transfixion incision at the caudal and cephalic margin of the medial alar crus will allow the total delivery of the dome and lateral alar crura into the nostril for subsequent manipulation. This maneuver is repeated on both sides and allows for increased visualization of the alar cartilages. The bucket handle dissection of the cartilages can be stabilized for manipulation or trimming by passing the handle of a Neivert double ball retractor beneath. The exposure of the domes can allow for moderate manipulation in this area as well

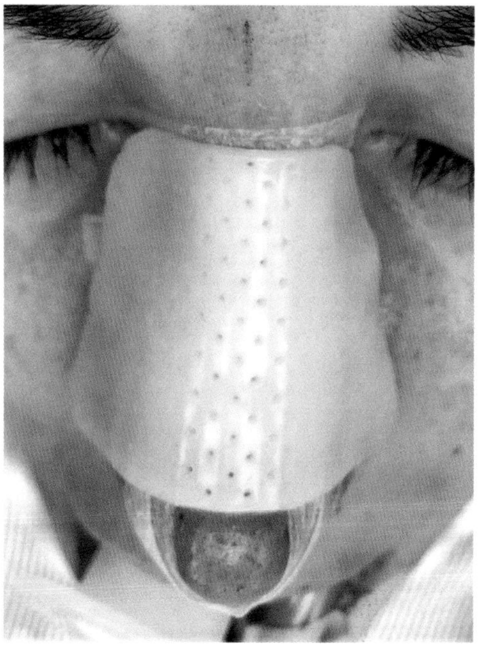

FIGURE 52.22. Thermoplastic splint.

Tip Cartilage-Splitting Method

An intracartilaginous incision is made at the point where the planned cephalic resection of the lateral alar crus begins. It is carried through the nasal vestibular skin and through the cartilage. The vestibular skin can then be dissected from the nasal side of the cephalic alar cartilage, which can then be separated from its attachment to the upper lateral cartilage and removed.

Dorsal Elevation and Reduction

Once the tip is modified, a curved Joseph-Peck scissors can then be used to elevate the nasal dorsum over the cartilage and bone. The plane of dissection should be immediately superficial to the perichondrium and periosteum. Care to stay in this plane will result in a relatively bloodless dissection. The dissection should be wide enough to allow the insertion of a Aufricht retractor for visualization of the dorsum but should be limited to only that needed to make the planned dorsal modifications. A Joseph elevator can then be used to elevate the periosteum over the nasal bones to allow reduction by rasp or osteotome. If the rasp is to be used the bony modification is done at this point followed by reduction of the cartilaginous dorsum. If an osteotome is to be used to lower the bony dorsum, then modification of the cartilaginous dorsum is done first. Many surgeons prefer the rasp, because it allows a more incremental reduction of the dorsum and is less likely to result in accidental overcorrection. The cartilaginous reduction is begun by exposure of the junction of the upper lateral cartilages with the dorsal nasal septum by means of the creation of a superior Cottle tunnel. Through the previously made transfixion incision at the junction of the caudal septum and medial alar crura a mucoperichondrium flap is elevated along the dorsum of the nasal septum using a Cottle elevator. This tunnel is dissected in his cephalic direction at the junction of the septum with the upper lateral cartilage to and just beyond the junction of the perpendicular plate of the ethmoid bone with the undersurface of the nasal bone. By sweeping the mucoperichondrium laterally using the Cottle elevator, the junction point is defined. A no. 15 scalpel can then be placed within the tunnel with its flat surface on the exposed dorsal septum and with the blade oriented dorsally and with the skin protected by the Aufricht retractor, the upper lateral cartilage can be sharply separated from the dorsal septum from the junction with the nasal bone to its most caudal attachment. Repeating this process on the opposite side will now expose the dorsal septum as well as the medial aspect of the right and left upper lateral cartilages. Each of these structures can be independently trimmed or manipulated at this time. If carefully done, the mucoperichondrium remains intact without communication to the nasal cavity. The dorsal septum can be lowered using angled scissors or a scalpel. The upper lateral cartilages can be trimmed or left in place for later use as auto spreader flaps.

Septoplasty

If correction of septal deviations or harvesting of septal cartilage to use for grafting is indicated, then this should be done at this time after the dorsal profile has been set. Using the previously made transfixion incision, a mucopericondrial flap is elevated in the same manner as described for open rhinoplasty. In closed rhinoplasty, where visualization is more difficult, an inferior Cottle tunnel can aid in the elevation of the mucoperichondrial flap along the junction of the quadrangular cartilage and the Vomer. A Freer or McKenty elevator is used to elevate the periosteum along the medial surface of the floor of the nose and the lateral surface of the Vomer up to the attachments at the cartilage-Vomer junction. Scissors can then be used to cut the attachments between the cartilage and the vomer from caudal to cephalic under direct vision therefore minimizing the risk of flap perforation. Once exposed on one side, the modifications can proceed as described for open rhinoplasty.

Spreader Grafts and Flaps

These can be placed in a manner similar to that described in the open rhinoplasty section. Exposure is more limited, and placement and fixation are more difficult in the closed rhinoplasty.

Tip Modification

Tip modifications are considerably more difficult in the closed rhinoplasty though virtually any modification done in the open setting can be done in the closed rhinoplasty. The authors encourage using the open approach until the surgeon has gained considerable experience.

Osteotomies

Osteotomies are also performed as described for open rhinoplasty.

Final Inspection and Closure

The intranasal incisions are now closed with interrupted 5-0 chromic suture. The nasal dorsum is cleansed with saline, dried, and then treated with Mastisol, and then Steri-Strips are placed in such a way as to try to eliminate any dead space between the skin and the refined cartilage and bone. Finally, a thermoplastic splint is applied. Routine nasal packing is not necessary.[19,20] A Doyle internal splint may be desirable when both septoplasty and anterior turbinectomy are performed to prevent synechia.

ADVANCED MANEUVERS

Advanced rhinoplasty maneuvers include the following:

- Septal extension grafts
- Onlay grafts
- Rim grafts
- Tip grafts
  - Dome grafts
  - Shield graft/infratip grafts
  - Supratip graft
  - Lateral crural strut grafts
  - Lateral crural spreader grafts
  - Tip diverging grafts
  - Tip width-control grafts
- Lateral crural shaping sutures to increase external convexity or concavity
- Through-and-through suturing to narrow the columellar base with or without footplate resection
- Columella to septum anchoring sutures
- Alar base excisions to decrease flare or narrow the base

REVISION RHINOPLASTY

The principles for approaching revision rhinoplasty are the same as those for primary rhinoplasty: careful analysis, diagnosis of the problem, and application of appropriate surgical maneuvers. Revision surgery often involves reconstructive principles because the presenting anatomy is no longer standard. There will be scar tissue encountered during dissection and distorted, missing, and possibly extra nasal tissue or alloplastic implants discovered. Additional cartilage sources, including rib or ear cartilage and bone sources including outer table of the calvarium may be necessary. The guiding principle of revision surgery is that regardless of the deformity encountered, the revision surgeon must be prepared to use all tools available to make the anatomical structures as normal as possible to achieve satisfactory appearance and function. Revision rhinoplasty patients also require greater attention to the psychological aspects involved, as these patients tend to be more anxious about repeating another surgery and risking another disappointing outcome. It is important to obtain the operative records of previous surgeries whenever possible. Bear in mind that not all operative reports are entirely accurate. Preoperative CT scans and office-based nasoendoscopy when available can be helpful as can endoscopy in the OR just prior to the procedure.

Common presenting deformities in revision rhinoplasty include a residual dorsal hump, an overprojected nose, a crooked dorsum, a crooked and asymmetric tip, and an overdone "pinched" tip. Other common problems encountered are an overresected dorsum (saddle nose deformity), alar retraction, dorsal asymmetry, visual or palpable irregularities, and a widened dorsum. In addition, one may encounter functional nasal obstruction that is either new or was not optimally dealt with in previous surgery. Given the numerous possible deformities, addressing every problem is beyond the scope of this chapter. The goal is to use whatever tools necessary to fix the problem and create a "normal" structural appearance and normal function. Often, structures need to be reconstructed using strong normal cartilage, which can include residual septal cartilage, previously placed grafts that have been removed during the revisional surgery, rib cartilage, or ear cartilage. Variously prepared allograft materials have also found their way into complex nasal revisional surgery. Extra care is needed in dissecting the skin flap from the underlying skeleton as tenacious scar tissue may be encountered the dissection through which can lead to accidental perforation of the skin flap. Dorsal humps may need to be shaved down using rasps or power burrs if necessary. Repeat osteotomies can create better symmetry in nasal bones but may also lead to comminution and instability. Crooked dorsal septal cartilage may need to be straightened and reinforced using strong cartilage batten grafts applied to one or both sides. The tip can be reconstructed using a variety of means, including grafts to reinforce or replace the lower lateral cartilages and tip grafts to create a more normal looking symmetric tip. Suture can be used to achieve these goals and can also be used to narrow a wide middle third (with care taken not to create a functional problem in the internal nasal valve). Revision septoplasty, anterior turbinate reduction, turbinate cautery, turbinate out-fracture, and internal nasal valve reconstruction using spreader grafts and/or lateral crural strut grafts may be necessary to reconstruct functional airway problems.

COMPLICATIONS

- Bleeding
- Septal hematoma
- Infection
- New or persistent obstruction
- Scarring/skin loss
- Aesthetic irregularities

PATIENT OUTCOMES

Patient outcomes are critically important with any surgery. Measuring individual outcomes quality depends on close and thorough follow-up for at least 1 year if not longer, asking patients questions about their satisfaction with their results, excellent standardized photography at every patient visit, and surgeon dedication to reviewing preoperative photographs and 1 year follow-up photographs in conjunction with the surgical operative report to determine if the operative plan and postoperative treatment were appropriate.[5,21] Many variables affect the result of rhinoplasty surgery, and it is incumbent upon the surgeon to critically analyze his or her results and patient satisfaction to obtain the most optimal outcomes. Objective patient-related outcome (PRO) scales have been developed; however, the perfect qualitative validated scale remains elusive. PRO scales with acronyms such as SCHNOS, NOSE, SNOT, RHINO, and Face-Q are available to the rhinoplasty surgeon but vary in their usefulness. An ideal PRO scale should be validated, reproducible, and easy to administer.[22-27]

REFERENCES

1. Constantian MB. Four common anatomic variants that predispose to unfavorable rhinoplasty results: a study based on 150 consecutive secondary rhinoplasties. *Plast Reconstr Surg*. 2000;105:316.
2. Constantian MB, Lin CP. Why some patients are unhappy. Part 1. Relationship of preoperative nasal deformity to number of operations and a history of abuse or neglect. *Plast Reconstr Surg*. 2014;134(4):823-835.
3. Constantian MB, Lin CP. Why some patients are unhappy. Part 2. Relationship of nasal shape and trauma history to surgical success. *Plast Reconstr Surg*. 2014;134(4):836-851.
   References 2 and 3 are paired articles by Constantian and Lin that provide insight into the recognition of the body dysmorphic patient. They should be read by anyone interested in rhinoplasty.
4. Heinberg CE, Kern EB. The Cottle sign: an aid in the physical diagnosis of nasal airflow disturbances. *Rhinology*. 1973;11:89-94.
5. Guyuron B. Precision rhinoplasty. Part I: the role of life-size photographs and soft-tissue cephalometric analysis. *Plast Reconstr Surg*. 1988;81:489-499.
   First in a set of two articles showing the methodology used by Guyuron as a master rhinoplastic surgeon to obtain consistently good results,
6. Mehta U, Mazhar K, Frankel AS. Accuracy of preoperative computer imaging in rhinoplasty. *Arch Facial Plast Surg*. 2010;12(6):394-398.
7. Daniel RK. Rhinoplasty: creating an aesthetic tip. *Plast Reconstr Surg*. 1987; 80:775.
8. Rohrich RJ, Adams WP Jr, Deuber MA. Graduated approach to tip refinement and projection. In: Gunter JP, Rohrich R, Adams, eds. *Dallas Rhinoplasty: Nasal Surgery by the Masters*. St Louis, MO: Quality Medical Publishing; 2002:333.
9. Toriumi D. New concepts in nasal tip contouring. *Arch Facial Plast Surg*. 2006;8:156-185.
10. Byrd HS, Hobar PC. Rhinoplasty: a practical guide for surgical planning. *Plast Reconstr Surg*. 1993;91:642-654.
    Describes Byrd's method for mathematically analyzing nasal anatomic relationships based on measurements of a particular population judged as having attractive noses.
11. Chauhan N, Alexander AJ, Sepehr A, Adamson PA. Patient complaints with primary versus revision rhinoplasty: analysis and practice implications. *Aesthet Surg J*. 2011;31:775.
12. Gunter JP, Hackney FL. Clinical assessment and facial analysis. In: Gunter JP, Rohrich RJ, Adams WP Jr, eds. *Dallas Rhinoplasty: Nasal Surgery by the Masters*. St Louis, MO: Quality Medical Publishing; 2002:53.
13. Rohrich RJ, Hollier LH. Use of spreader grafts in the external approach to rhinoplasty. *Clin Plast Surg*. 1996;23(2):255-262.
14. Sheen JH. Spreader graft: a method of reconstructing the roof of the middle nasal vault following rhinoplasty. *Plast Reconstr Surg*. 1984;73(2):230-239.
    An early presentation of spreader grafts by their inventor.
15. Adamson PA, Funk E. Nasal tip dynamics. *Facial Plast Surg Clin North Am*. 2009;17:29-40.
16. Hewell TS, Tardy ME. Nasal tip refinement. *Facial Plast Surg*. 1984;1:87.
17. Sullivan PK, Harshbarger RJ, Oneal RM. Nasal osteotomies. In: Gunter JP, Rohrich RJ, Adams WP Jr, eds. *Dallas Rhinoplasty: Nasal Surgery by the Masters*. St Louis, MO: Quality Medical Publishing; 2002:595.
18. Gunter JP, Rohrich RJ, Friedman RM, et al. Importance of the alar-columellar relationship. In: Gunter JP, Rohrich RJ, Adams WP Jr, eds. *Dallas Rhinoplasty: Nasal Surgery by the Masters*. St Louis, MO: Quality Medical Publishing; 2002:105.
19. Guyuron B. Is packing after septorhinoplasty necessary? A randomized study. *Plast Reconstr Surg*. 1989;84(1):41-44.
20. Mansfield CJ, Peterson MB. Toxic shock syndrome: associated with nasal packing. *Clin Pediatr (Phila)*. 1989;28:443-445.
21. Guyuron B. Precision rhinoplasty. Part II: prediction. *Plast Reconstr Surg*. 1988;81:500-505.
    Second in a set of two articles showing the methodology used by Guyuron as a master rhinoplastic surgeon to obtain consistently good results,
22. Klassen AF, Cano SJ, East CA, et al. Development and psychometric evaluation of the FACE-Q scales for patients undergoing rhinoplasty. *JAMA Facial Plast Surg*. 2016;18(1):27-35.
23. Kosowski TR, McCarthy C, Reavey PL, et al. A systematic review of patient-reported outcome measures after facial cosmetic surgery and/or nonsurgical facial rejuvenation. *Plast Reconstr Surg*. 2009;123(6):1819-1827.
24. Menger DJ, Richard W, Swart KM, et al. Does functional septorhinoplasty provide improvement of the nasal passage in validated patient-reported outcome measures? *ORL J Otorhinolaryngol Relat Spec*. 2015;77(3):123-131.
25. Rhee JS, Sullivan CD, Frank DO, et al. A systemic review of patient-reported nasal obstruction scores: defining normative and symptomatic ranges in surgical patients. *JAMA Facial Plast Surg*. 2014;16(3):219-225.
26. Schwitzer JA, Sher SR, Fan KL, et al. Assessing patient reported satisfaction with appearance and quality of life following rhinoplasty using the FACE-Q appraisal scales. *Plast Reconstr Surg*. 2015;135(5):830e-837e.
27. Stewart MG, Witsell DL, Smith TL, et al. Development and validation of the Nasal Obstruction Symptom Evaluation (NOSE) scale. *Otolaryngol Head Neck Surg*. 2004;130(2):157-163.
    One of the first validated patient-reported outcome measured instruments for functional septorhinoplasty.

QUESTIONS

The patient is a 27-year-old man who presents to you with two complaints concerning his nose: dislike for the appearance of his nose and nearly complete obstruction of his left nasal airway. He states that he has broken his nose at least two times playing collegiate rugby. He was seen the first time in the ED where a closed reduction was attempted after X-rays confirmed a fracture. He states that his nose has been crooked ever since and that his nasal breathing, though problematic his whole life has been much worse since that trauma. He did not seek medical attention after his second nasal trauma. He denies any known inhalant allergies, takes no medication, denies using nasal sprays or having had any previous nasal surgery other than the attempted reduction in the ED. When asked to be specific about his nasal appearance, he states that he does not like the crookedness of his nose, nor is he happy with the prominent dorsal hump. He is fine with the appearance of the tip of the nose. His family history is unremarkable, as is his review of systems.

Focused nasal exam reveals a moderately large and projecting nose with a prominent nasal dorsal bony and cartilaginous hump. The nose shows a significant C-shaped deformity concave to the right. He has a narrow supratip and a wide and boxy tip. His skin is intermediate in thickness. His caudal septum presents in his left nostril. He has marked septal deviation to the left with near total obstruction of the left nasal airway. There is a significant spur of the junction of the quadrangular septal cartilage and the vomer extending into the right nasal airway. He has significant enlargement of the right nasal turbinate and moderate enlargement of the left. He has a sharply positive Cottle test on the right and minimal improvement on the left. You devise a treatment plan, which you go over at length and in detail with the patient.

1. You propose an open septorhinoplasty to be done in the hospital under a general anesthetic as an outpatient. Which of the following statements is most accurate regarding the osteotomies in your surgical plan?

a. He will require osteotomies to straighten his nose and correct the incompetent internal nasal valve.
b. He will require osteotomies to close an open roof deformity and straighten the nose.
c. He will require osteotomies to narrow the nasal bases and straighten the nose.
d. He will require oseotomies to close an open roof deformity and straighten the nasal septum.
e. Low to high osteotomies would be ideal to correct the bony asymmetry.

2. You perform the septorhinoplasty using an open approach, transcolumellar stair-step incision. To surgically treat the exam finding of a positive Cottle test, which of the following would you perform?

a. Quadrangular septal cartilage and bony septum excision
b. Bilateral inferior turbinate submucosal resection and outfracture
c. Cartilage spreader graft placement between the septum and upper lateral cartilage on the right side
d. Cartilage spreader graft placement between the septum and upper lateral cartilage on the left side
e. Cartilage lateral crural strut graft placement under each lower lateral crura

3. You perform the septorhinoplasty using an open approach, transcolumellar stair-step incision. Given the marked septal deviation preoperatively, dissection around the deviation was difficult and fractures within the septum from previous trauma presented difficulty in elevating the septal mucoperichondrial flaps. Following completion of septal cartilaginous and bony resection, you note perforations in the septal flaps on both sides. You decide that suture repair of the perforations are not necessary for which of the following reasons?

a. Septal perforations always heal on their own and close secondarily.
b. The opposing perforations are anterior.
c. The opposing perforations are posterior.
d. The perforations will close with spreader graft placement.
e. The perforations on each side are not opposing.

4. The patient you just treated was happy with the results of his rhinoplasty and refers his 22-year-old sister to you for revision rhinoplasty. She has no functional nasal concerns and her nasal history and exam are unremarkable for any breathing disturbance. Her concern is a residual prominent nasal dorsal hump, and she feels that her tip is still too projecting and too bulbous. Her primary rhinoplasty surgery was 3 years ago. You receive a copy of her original operative report, and there is no mention of septal cartilage harvest. You do a nasofacial analysis and find that her tip projection is 70% of her radix-to-tip length and her nasolabial angle is 100°. Your operative plan and consent process should include which of the following?

a. Reduction of the bony and cartilaginous nasal dorsum and tip suturing to better define the domes with no change to the nasal labial angle, tip deprojection, and septal cartilage harvest for columellar strut grafting
b. Reduction of the bony and cartilaginous nasal dorsum and tip suturing to better define the domes, increasing the nasal labial angle, tip deprojection
c. Reduction of the bony and cartilaginous nasal dorsum and tip suturing to better define the domes with no change to the nasal labial angle, tip deprojection, septal cartilage harvest for columellar strut grafting, and possible ear or rib cartilage graft harvest
d. Reduction of the bony and cartilaginous nasal dorsum and tip grafting to better define the domes with no change to the nasal labial angle, tip deprojection, and septal cartilage harvest for columellar strut grafting
e. Reduction of the bony and cartilaginous nasal dorsum and tip grafting to better define the domes with no change to the nasal labial angle, tip deprojection, septal cartilage harvest for columellar strut grafting, and possible ear or rib cartilage graft harvest

5. You perform revision rhinoplasty on the 22-year-old woman in the previous question in the operating room under general anesthesia. Which of the following is not accurate regarding optimal patient outcome assessment?

a. The patient should be followed for 1 year after surgery to assess the final result.
b. Standard photographs should be taken at only at the 1-year postoperative visit for comparison.
c. Functional assessment should be made at each postoperative visit.
d. The patient should be asked directly about satisfaction with the procedure at each postoperative visit.
e. Given the reproducible validity of objective patient reported outcomes scales, it is critically important to use them with every patient.

1. **Answer: b.** Two indications for performing osteotomies are to straighten the nose and to close and open roof deformity after the bony hump is rasped. As he has a C-shaped deformity and crooked nose from his trauma, and because the plan would include rasping of the dorsal bony hump to correct his dissatisfaction cosmetically, answer #2 would be most accurate. Osteotomies are not performed to correct incompetent nasal valves or to straighten the septum. Low-to-high osteotomies are used to prevent further narrowing of the nasal bone bases, not to correct nasal bone asymmetry.

2. **Answer: c.** A positive Cottle test reveals incompetent unilateral internal nasal valve or bilateral internal nasal valves. In this case, the patient had relief of Cottle test on the right side only. Spreader graft placement on the right side is indicated to open the angle of the internal nasal valve on the affected side. Surgery on the septum or turbinates will not treat the internal valve problem. Lateral crural strut grafts are used to treat external nasal valve incompetence.

3. **Answer: e.** Perforation of one or both sides of the septal mucoperichondrium may occur during septoplasty, especially when dissection is exceptionally difficult. Unilateral perforations do not require suture closure. Perforations that are nonopposing will not heal with a persistent open perforation. Tears in the mucosa that are opposing must be closed with suture on each side to prevent a persistent open perforation that can lead to bleeding, crusting, whistling, and functional airflow issues.

4. **Answer: c.** The patient's concerns are residual hump deformity and an overprojected bulbous nasal tip. The plan should include bony and cartilaginous hump reduction, tip suturing to better define the domes of the tip and reduce bulbosity, and deprojection of the tip. Deprojection of the tip will require columellar strut grafting to resupport the new position of the tip. A columellar strut graft can be fashioned from septal, rib, or ear cartilage. Even though the previous operative report does not mention previous septal cartilage harvest, operative reports are not always accurate. Therefore, the operative plan and informed consent for all revision rhinoplasty patients should include the possibility of ear or rib cartilage harvest.

5. **Answer: b.** Patients should be followed postoperatively for at least 1 year after rhinoplasty surgery. Standard photographs should be taken at each postoperative visit throughout the year to track and document the patient's progress. Asking the patient about their satisfaction at all time points, as well as surgeon assessment of both functional and aesthetic outcomes, is critical to evaluate the overall results. Objective patient reported outcome scales can sometimes be useful in the postoperative setting, but the scales available today may be difficult to administer and the perfect validated scale remains elusive.

CHAPTER 53 Otoplasty

Arin K. Greene

KEY POINTS

- Ear anomalies can be characterized by having excess structures, deficient parts, or adequate components that need to be rearranged.
- Ear molding may correct some anomalies during the neonatal period.
- Most otoplasty procedures are best performed ≥3 years old when most ear growth is completed.
- Otoplasty should aim to achieve symmetry on frontal view.
- Simple otoplasty techniques are considered before more complicated reconstructive procedures.

About 50% of newborns have an auricular deformity that persists in 33% by 1 month old[1]; as many as 84% of deformities continue to improve over the first year of life.[2] An exception is prominent ears, which increase from birth to 1 year old, suggesting that postnatal deformation can contribute to this condition (e.g., infant sleep position may push the ear outward).[1,2] Half of children have a bilateral deformity, and when deformity is unilateral, the right and left sides are affected equally.[1] No difference in the prevalence or type of ear deformity exists among males and females.[1] A helical anomaly/constricted ear is the most common disorder at birth (15%).[1] Vaginal delivery and increased birth weight increase the risk of ear anomalies, likely due to forces on the ear causing deformations.[1]

Otoplasty is used to reconstruct several types of ear abnormalities. The primary morbidity of an ear deformity is psychosocial. Ear anomalies do not affect hearing and thus insurance companies often do not cover the procedure. Correction of some deformities (e.g., cryptotia) can facilitate the use of eyeglasses. In the pediatric population, ear anomalies can be particularly worrisome for families because they often have to pay for the procedure, and they are subjecting their child to general anesthesia for a "cosmetic" problem. Consequently, surgeons treating ear anomalies should be well trained on the subject and ensure that patients and families have reasonable expectations.

The ears are particularly tolerant of asymmetry because of their lateral position over the temporal bones. The full appearance of the ears cannot be appreciated on frontal view. To compare the ears, an individual must look at one ear first and then change positions to see the contralateral side. Consequently, it is most important to have the ears as symmetrical as possible on frontal view. Because most ear anomalies cause a "cosmetic" problem, patients and families can be focused on minor asymmetries. It is important that families understand that asymmetries between the ears are common in the general population[3,4] and that there will be some asymmetry following the procedure.

DIAGNOSIS

Diagnosis of an ear anomaly is made by physical examination. Ear abnormalities can be broadly separated into malformations (absence of part of the ear) or deformations (fully developed ear but misshapen). The surgeon should be able to identify the abnormality and list reconstructive options. I approach the management of ear anomalies by dividing them into three categories:

- Excess components—treated by excision
- Deficient parts—managed by addition of tissues
- Adequate structures that are malformed—treated by rearrangement of tissues

The surgeon must understand normal ear anatomy and can use the contralateral ear, if normal, as a guide (**Figure 53.1**). The axis of the ear is angled approximately 20° more posterior than a vertical line. The top of the helix is at the level of the eyebrow and the lobule is at the base of the columella. The height of the ear is 6.5 (±1) cm,

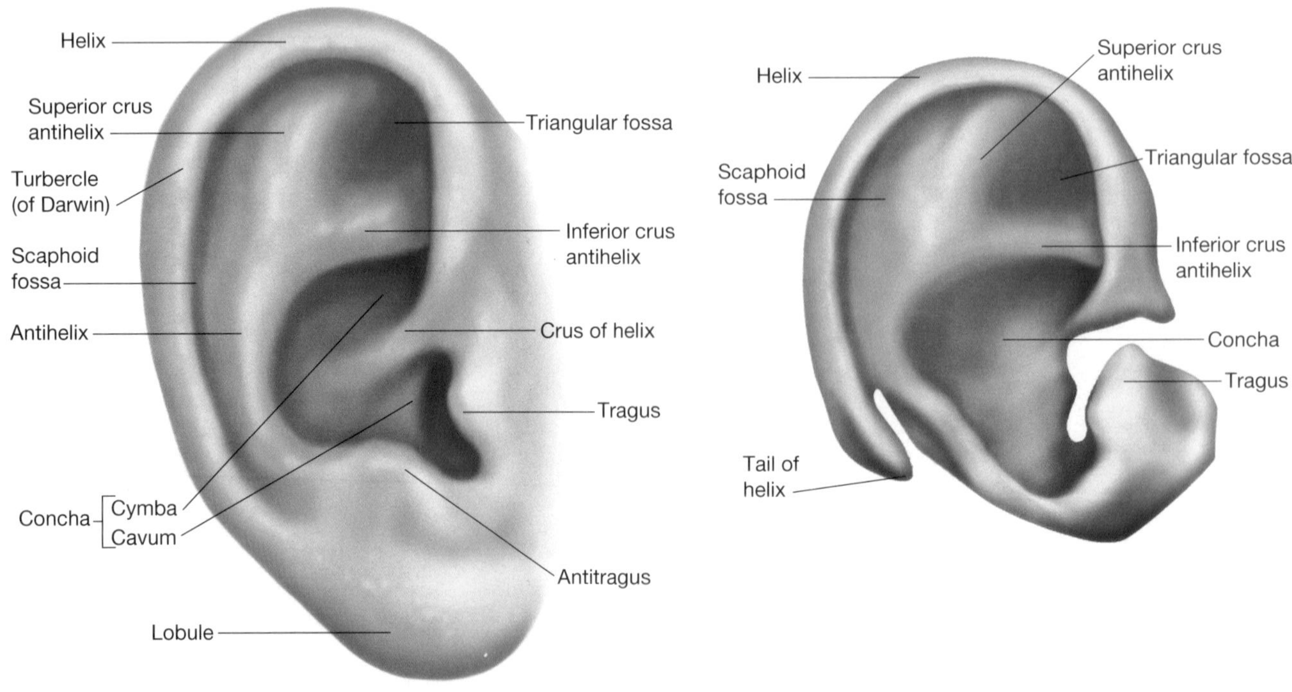

FIGURE 53.1. Ear anatomy.

and its width is 4.0 (±0.5 cm).[5,6] It is located one ear length (6–7 cm) posterior to the lateral canthus. Although several measurements for abnormal protrusion from the mastoid have been described, I use greater than 18 mm at the top of the helix and 21 mm at the midhelix.[3]

NONOPERATIVE TREATMENT

A window exists during the neonatal period when the ear can be molded.[7] Because some anomalies improve during the first week of life, molding should not be initiated until at least 1 week old to allow for possible spontaneous correction.[8] Ideally, molding is started between 1 and 3 weeks old when maternal estrogens in the child facilitate cartilage manipulation. The ear can be molded using wire and tape or a commercially available system (Figure 53.2).[8,9] Unfortunately, patients often are referred after the window to mold their ears has passed. At 6 weeks old, estrogens in the child equal that of an adult and if ear molding is initiated after this time, patients are likely to have a poor response.[9] If the mother is breast-feeding, initiation of ear molding can be attempted up to 8 to 10 weeks old. After 12 weeks old, ear molding is not effective.[9] The ear deformity that is most amenable to molding is a prominent ear. The antihelical fold is recreated to set back the ear. A mildly constricted ear with overhanging helical cartilage can be improved by lifting the helical cartilage into better alignment. A Stahl deformity can be corrected by flattening the abnormal crus.

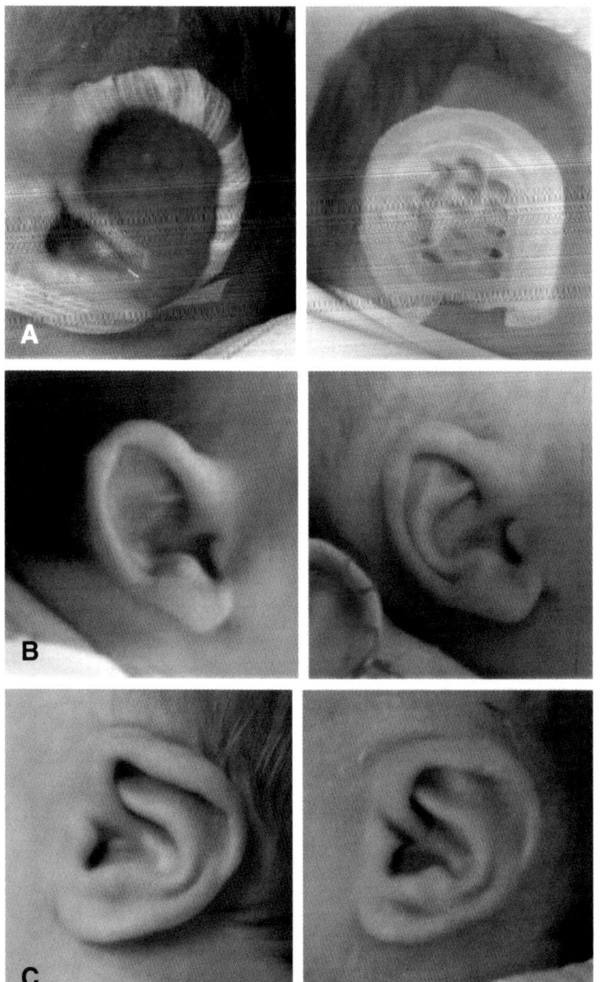

FIGURE 53.2. Ear molding. **A.** Two methods of ear molding. Wire and tape (left) and a commercially available system (right). **B.** Before (left) and after (right) molding of a prominent ear deformity. **C.** Before (left) and after (right) molding of a mildly constricted ear.

TIMING OF OPERATIVE TREATMENT

The primary indication for otoplasty is to improve the patient's self-esteem. Cryptotia and moderate/severe constricted ears can inhibit the ability to wear eyeglasses. Timing of intervention falls into three categories: infancy, 3 to 4 years old, and late childhood or adolescence. Simple excisions of excess structures can be performed during infancy with local anesthesia. Parents having children with preauricular cartilage remnants usually are eager to remove them as soon as possible. Most are small and able to be excised using local anesthesia in the office, as early as 4 to 6 weeks old. After 12 months old, however, it is difficult to restrain an awake child and I will perform the procedure in the operating room with sedation or wait until the child is old enough to cooperate in the clinic. If a child has an ear deformity that cannot be corrected simply using local anesthesia, then I prefer general anesthesia.

Because long-term memory and self-esteem begin to form at approximately 4 year old, many parents decide to correct an ear anomaly when the child is between 3 and 4 years old. At this time, the ear has achieved 85% of its size and the risk of scar limiting ear growth is reduced.[6,10] Most ear growth is completed by 6 years old.[6,10] Although data have shown that operating on ears before 3 years old does not inhibit growth,[11] I prefer to wait until at least 3 years old because (1) the ear is larger to facilitate the procedure and (2) it is not urgent to intervene before this time because memory and self-esteem have not yet formed. An advantage of early intervention is that children tolerate the procedure more favorably than older patients who are more anxious about the operation and are busier with activities such as sports and school.

If an individual has a mild deformity that he/she may not want to have improved, then it is prudent to wait until they are older to determine if they become bothered by it. Some families choose to wait to correct a significant ear anomaly until the child is old enough to participate in the decision to have the procedure. Children between 5 and 8 years old typically are bothered by a deformity, but fear of the operation outweighs their desire to improve their appearance. At 9 to 10 years old, the child's interest in correcting the anomaly begins to outweigh the anxiety about the operation. Girls typically present later than boys, because they are better able to camouflage their deformity with hair. Males often will grow their hair long to hide their ear.

PROMINENT EAR

Approximately 5% of the population has a prominent ear caused by an absent or weak antihelical fold and/or overgrown concha (Figure 53.3).[1,2] Most patients will require recreation of the antihelical fold and setback of the concha. Rarely, a patient will have a normal antihelix and only require a procedure on the concha. Similarly, an individual may have a normal concha and only require formation of the antihelical fold. The prominence of the auricle can be evaluated by considering the upper, middle, and lower thirds of the ear. Although all patients will need to have the upper and/or middle third of the ear setback, 25% of patients in my practice will benefit from having their lobule setback as well. Three-fourths of patients in my experience undergo bilateral setback otoplasty, whereas one-fourth of individuals have prominence of only one ear.

Although setback otoplasty is a clean case, I give one dose of intraoperative antibiotics because I am placing permanent foreign bodies (merseline sutures) and exposing cartilage. I do not prescribe postoperative antibiotics. After the patient is under general anesthesia, I measure the distance of the ears to the mastoid from the most prominent part of the superior helix and from the midhelix at the level of the root. I favor measurements because it improves the likelihood of symmetry between the ears and also reduces the risk of overcorrection. The ear is folded and the position of the antihelical

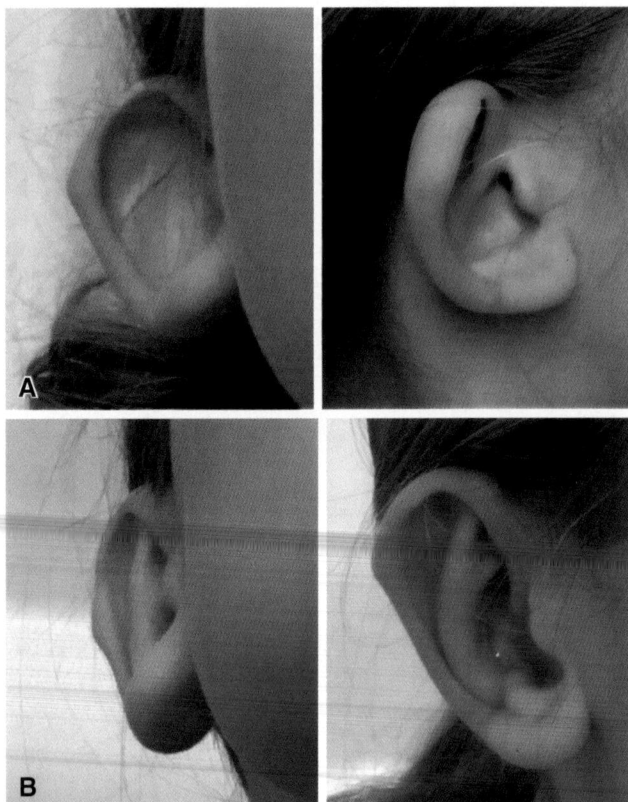

FIGURE 53.3. Otoplasty for a prominent ear. **A.** Preoperative view illustrating the absence of the antihelical fold and overgrown conchal bowl. **B.** Postoperative appearance.

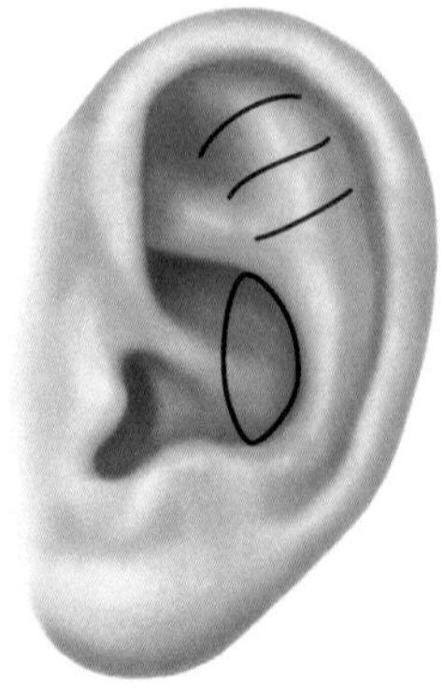

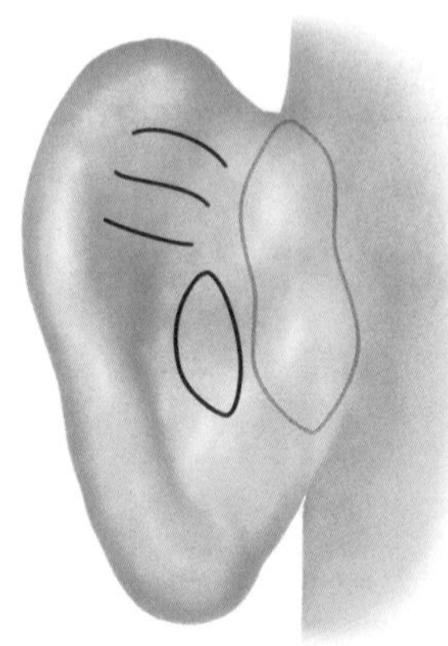

FIGURE 53.4. Illustration of operative methods to reduce the prominence of an ear. Anterior **(A)** and posterior **(B)** views showing the position of scapha-concha sutures to strengthen the antihelical fold and set-back the superior 1/3 of the ear (3 lines) as well as concha excision to reduce the prominence of the middle 1/3 of the ear (black ovals). The outline at the junction of the ear and mastoid on the posterior view represents the skin excision performed to access the ear cartilage.

fold is marked. Local anesthetic with epinephrine is infiltrated to hydrodissect the skin off the cartilage to facilitate suture placement. A posterior skin excision is performed at the junction of the ear and mastoid skin. The incision in this location is hidden in the natural crease. I perform a skin excision because it facilitates the procedure by enhancing exposure, and once the ear is set back, there is sufficient skin to reapproximate.

Superior Third

Techniques to set back the superior third of the ear require strengthening or recreation of the antihelical fold by (1) placement of scapha-concha sutures (Mustarde technique),[12] or (2) cartilage scoring (Stenstrom technique)[13] (**Figure 53.4**). I prefer scapha-concha sutures because it gives greater control and more predictability compared to scoring the cartilage. In addition, scoring the cartilage can cause damage to the cartilage and contour abnormalities. In an adult with very stiff cartilage, scoring may be considered as an adjunct to weaken the cartilage to facilitate its bending during the placement of sutures. The ear is folded, and the position of the antihelical fold is marked. Intraoperatively, a 27 gauge needle is used to transpose the position of the antihelical fold to the posterior cartilage. I typically place three or four 4-0 Mersilene mattress sutures to recreate the fold. It is important not to pull the sutures too tight that can cause the ear to be positioned too close to the mastoid and create an unnatural sharp antihelical fold. On front view, the antihelix should have a gentle curve and the helix should be visible behind the antihelix. I measure the distance from the most superior point of the helix to the mastoid and achieve a distance of 15 mm (±3 mm). Occasionally, the superior third remains prominent despite scapha-concha sutures. In this situation, one or two sutures can be placed from the scapha to the temporal fascia or conchal cartilage. Alternatively, scapha and helical cartilage can be excised.[14]

Middle Third

Options to set back the middle third of the ear include excision of concha or concha-mastoid sutures (Furnas technique).[15,16] I prefer a cartilage excision because it reduces the risk of recurrence and weakens the area to facilitate the antihelix contour provided by the scapha-concha sutures.[16] I have found that suturing the hard cartilage to the weak mastoid fascia/periosteum has an increased risk of recurrence of prominence because of suture dehiscence and/or stretching of tissue. I measure the distance from the midhelix at the level of the root to the mastoid and attempt to achieve a distance 18 (±3 mm).

An approximately 2.0 to 2.5 cm long piece of superior conchal cartilage is removed just below the scapha-concha sutures. Depending on the amount of prominence, the width of the area can be 2 to 7 mm. The cartilage defect is repaired with interrupted 4-0 PDS suture. A line of excess skin may be present anteriorly, but this flattens over time. If more than a 7 mm width of cartilage is removed, then it is possible that the excess skin anteriorly might be bothersome to the patient and require excision. Care must be taken to not overcorrect the middle third of the ear to prevent a telephone deformity.

Lower Third

Lobule prominence is present in approximately one-fourth of patients and is often not appreciated preoperatively.[17] If the lobule remains prominent after setting back the superior and middle third of the ear, I first place a Mersilene suture through the area of the tail of the helix to the base of the conchal bowl. Another option is to extend the conchal cartilage excision inferiorly. A posterior lobule skin excision also can be performed.[16,18] Finally, a suture can be placed from the posterior lobule to the conchal cartilage.[18,19] The goal is to prevent the appearance of a hockey stick appearance of the ear.

Closure

Before closing the incision, I ensure that the helix has a straight contour, a telephone deformity is not present, and the superior helix is visible beyond the antihelix. I also perform repeat measurements; the superior distance of the helix to the mastoid must be 15 (±3 mm) and the middle distance 18 (±3 mm). These measurements should have a difference of ≤2 mm between the ears to ensure adequate symmetry. It is important that the ear is not approximated too close to the mastoid that can cause a deformity. The incision is closed using interrupted 5-0 Vicryl suture followed by a running 6-0 Chromic suture. Cyanoacrylate glue and a Steri-Strip are placed.

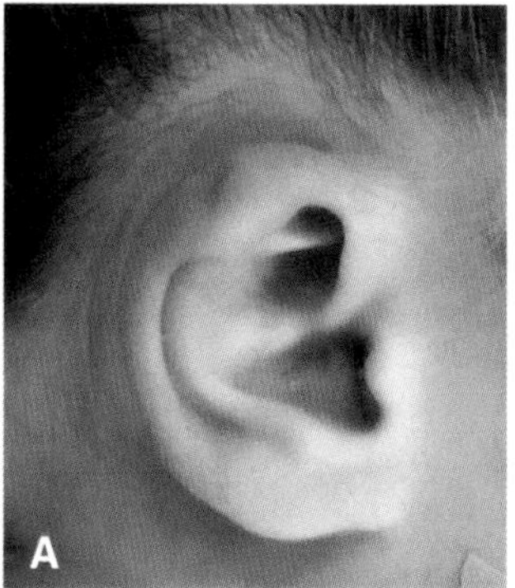

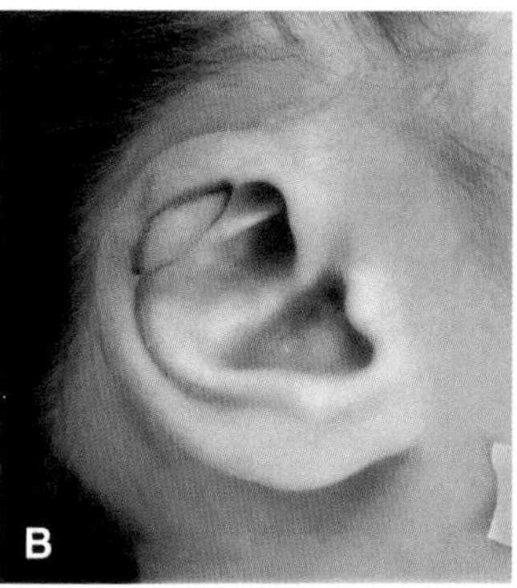

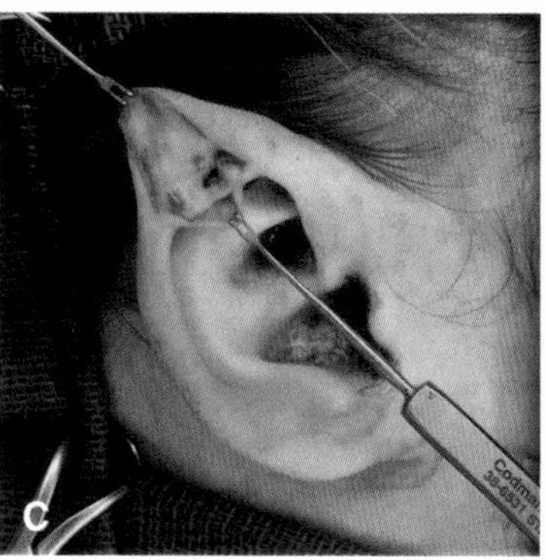

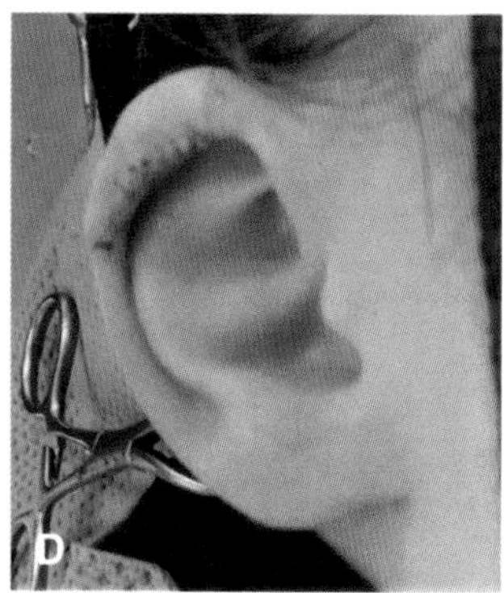

FIGURE 53.5. Correction of a mildly constricted ear. **A.** Preoperative image shows abnormal helix covering a portion of the superior crus of the antihelix. **B.** Outline for soft-tissue and cartilage excision. **C.** Intraoperative view following removal of cartilage. **D.** Immediate postoperative appearance.

Postoperative Care

I place a head-wrap (large piece of cotton over the ear followed by a gauze wrap) that is worn for up to 1 week until the first clinic appointment. I do not attempt to place pressure on the ear with bolster sutures or pieces of cotton soaked in mineral oil. Patients then are instructed to wear a soft head band at night for 6 weeks postoperatively to prevent accidental anterior displacement of the ear that could dehisce the antihelical sutures causing recurrent prominence. Six weeks postoperatively scar tissue is strong enough to maintain the shape of the ear.

CONSTRICTED EAR

A wide spectrum of constricted (e.g., lop, cup) ear anomalies exist. They range from minor helical problems to a variant of microtia and consist of (1) lidding of the helix, (2) prominence, and/or (3) reduced size from deficient structures. If possible, I prefer to manage these deformities as low on the reconstructive ladder as possible before considering cartilage grafts and retroauricular flaps. Minor deformities of the helix can be improved with simple excisions (Figure 53.5). Moderately constricted ears that contain a sufficient amount of structures may be improved using techniques employed for prominent ear deformities (Figure 53.6). Generally, the primary morbidity of a constricted ear is that it is prominent. If the ear is set back by strengthening the antihelical fold and placing sutures from the cartilage to the mastoid and temporal fascia to lengthen the vertical dimension of ear, the appearance of the child can be significantly improved. Severely constricted ears that approximate conchal-type microtia require partial or total auricular construction using cartilage grafts (Figure 53.7).

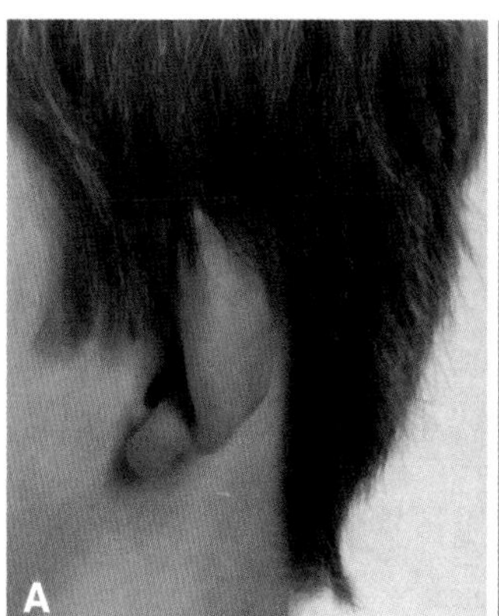

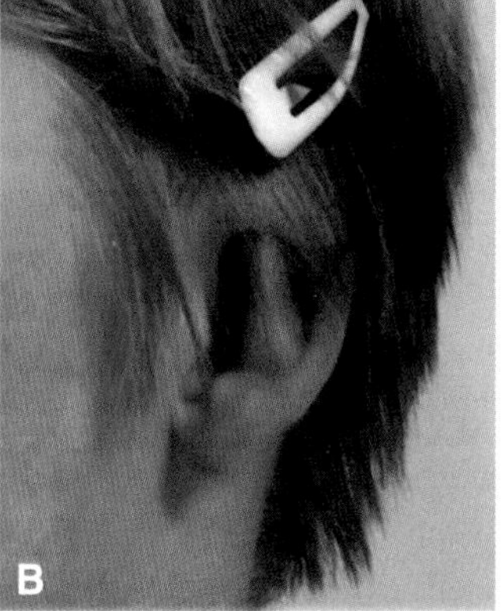

FIGURE 53.6. Treatment of a moderately constricted ear. **A.** Preoperative image shows a cupped ear with reduced vertical height and deficient helix and antihelix. **B.** Postoperative view after placement of scapha-concha, concha-mastoid, and scapha-temporal sutures.

CRYPTOTIA

Patients with cryptotia have a superior helix that is attached to the postauricular skin without a sulcus. In addition to causing a deformity, patients have difficulty wearing eyeglasses. Many techniques have been described to reconstruct the anomaly, including local flaps, skin grafts, and tissue expansion. I prefer using a one-stage V-Y advancement flap from the scalp to recreate the retroauricular sulcus.[20] This leaves a hidden scar behind the ear and in the hairline (Figure 53.8). Occasionally, the helical cartilage may be significantly deformed and require scoring, sutures, and/or grafts to improve its shape.

STAHL DEFORMITY

This abnormality describes the presence of a third crus of the antihelix that can cause the helix to have a pointed appearance. Usually, the anomaly is minor and does not cause psychosocial morbidity. Operative intervention may be indicated to treat a severe deformity. The anomaly is improved surgically through an anterior incision at the junction of the helix and scapha. The anterior skin is elevated, and the abnormal crus is resected (Figure 53.9).[21] If the superior crus of the antihelix is missing, then the excised crus can be grafted or rotated to reconstruct this structure. Occasionally, patients may have a prominent ear deformity as well requiring setback otoplasty techniques.

ACCESSORY CARTILAGE

Accessory cartilage in the preauricular area is the most common ear anomaly. I prefer to remove the tissue during the neonatal period using local anesthesia in the office to obviate general anesthesia. If an infant has a large lesion with a wide cartilage base that cannot be easily excised and closed, the procedure is performed in the operating room. Patients who present after 12 months old as well are managed in the operating room because it is difficult to restrain the child in the clinic.

LOBULE ABNORMALITIES

Split Ear Lobe

This deformity results from an earring being pulled through the lobule. The cleft is rapidly epithelialized preventing the edges from reapproximating. Split ear lobes in older children and adolescents can be repaired with local anesthesia; young children require general anesthesia. The cleft is de-epithelialized and approximated using absorbable sutures in a straight line. The end of the cleft is closed with

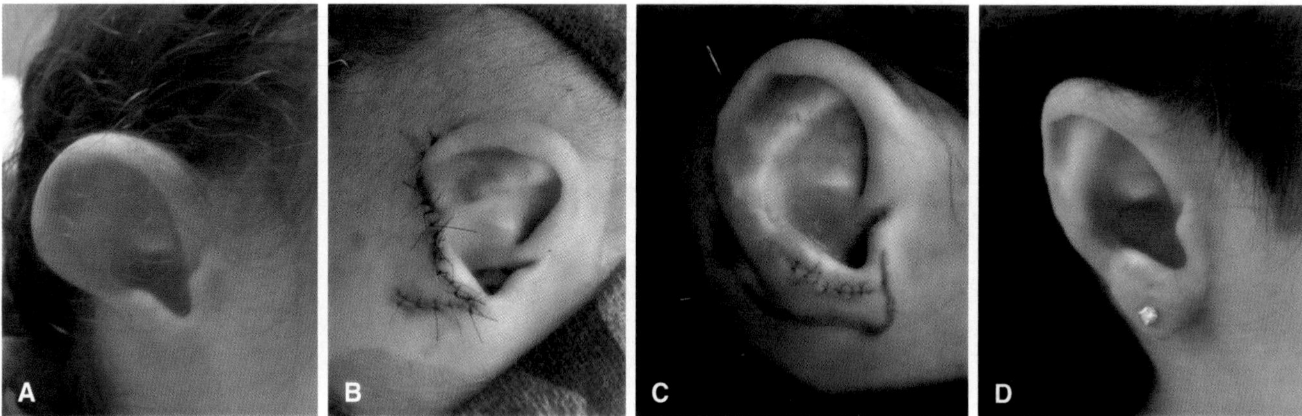

FIGURE 53.7. Reconstruction of a severely constricted ear with the absence of the lobule and part of the helix, concha, and antihelix. **A.** Preoperative appearance. **B.** Following first-stage advancement of a retroauricular flap to add soft tissue to the middle and lower one-third of the ear. The upper one-third of the ear was set back using scapha-concha sutures to recreate the antihelical fold. **C.** Appearance after staged placement of a conchal cartilage graft harvested from the contralateral ear. The outline of the graft is illustrated by the blue marking. **D.** Appearance after completing the reconstruction. The lower third of the ear containing the cartilage graft was separated from the retroauricular area using local flaps.

a mattress suture for eversion to prevent a notch from scar contraction. The scar can be repierced 3 months later when it has achieved its maximal strength. The advantages of repiercing along the scar are that the scar is camouflaged and if the earring pulls through again, a second scar is not formed. The disadvantage of piercing the scar is that it is not as strong as the adjacent lobule and thus has a higher risk of pulling through again.

Keloid

The ear lobe has a greater risk of forming keloid scars from piercings, compared to other parts of the ear. Keloids are managed with pressure, corticosteroid injection, and/or resection. Small lesions can be treated with pressure only. Patients are advised to wear a clip-on earring or purchase a pressure earring designed for keloids.

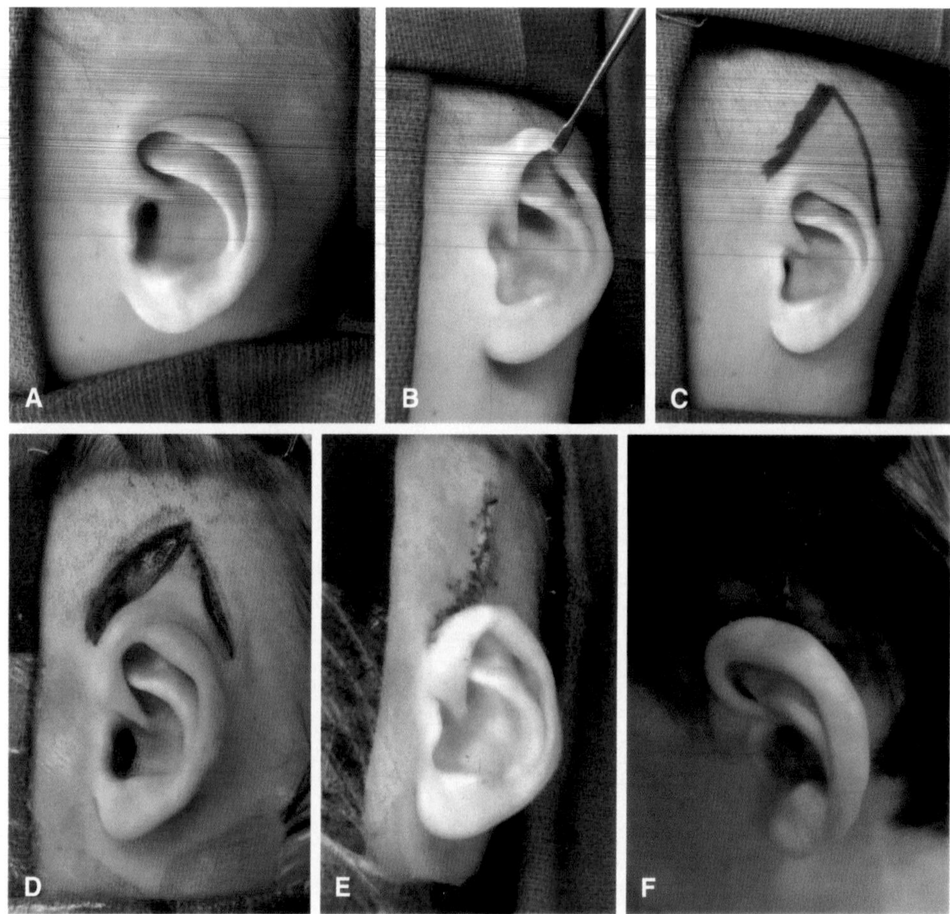

FIGURE 53.8. Correction of cryptotia. **A.** Preoperative appearance. **B.** The normal components of the helix are identified by pulling the ear outward. **C.** Outline of the V-Y advancement flap to recreate the retroauricular sulcus. **D.** Flap raised. **E.** After advancement of the flap and closure of the donor site. **F.** Postoperative view.

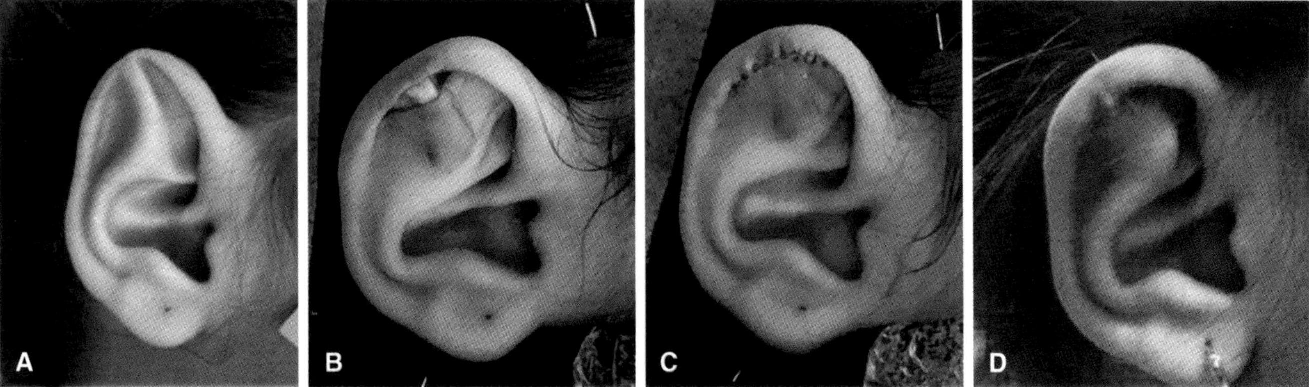

FIGURE 53.9. Correction of a Stahl deformity. **A.** Preoperative view illustrating the abnormal one third crus of the antihelix and a pointed appearance of the helix. **B.** Intraoperative image of the incision along the junction of the helix and scaphoid fossa exposing the abnormal crus. **C.** Following resection of the abnormal cartilage. **D.** Postoperative appearance illustrates improved contour of the helix and scaphoid fossa.

The pressure device is worn at night when sleeping. A pressure earring is a good first-line intervention for minor keloids in young children who are less tolerant of undergoing a corticosteroid injection in the clinic. Older children can be managed with serial triamcinolone injections in addition to the pressure earring. Large keloids are best managed with resection because pressure/injections will only give minimal improvement and the patient will continue to have a significant deformity. Families are educated that resection is exponentially more traumatic to the ear than the piercing that caused the keloid. Consequently, without close follow-up and the use of postoperative compression and corticosteroid injections, the keloid will return and can be worse. After resecting the keloid, the patient wears a pressure earring beginning 2 weeks following the procedure at night. Four weeks postoperatively, the patient returns for monthly evaluations and possible corticosteroid injections. After 6 months, the patient follows up as needed. Although radiation has been described as a treatment for keloids, I have not had a patient require this intervention.

Congenital Deficiency

The most common lobule deficiency is a cleft that causes a deformity and obviates the ability to place earrings. The cleft is deepithelialized and corrected by advancing the tissue to form a lobule (**Figure 53.10**). Rarely, a patient can have an absent lobule on the spectrum of microtia. The lobule can be constructed using staged skin flaps from the adjacent neck, or by placing a conchal cartilage graft. I have found that using cartilage gives the most favorable outcome (see Figure 53.7).

COMPLICATIONS

Rarely, a skin abrasion or full-thickness wound can occur with ear molding; molding is discontinued until the area has healed. The most common problem is an unfavorable "cosmetic" outcome. Infection, hematoma, extrusion of sutures, or wound dehiscence is uncommon. Before reconstructing an ear, patients/parents must have reasonable expectations. The ears are tolerant to asymmetry, and the primary goal is to improve their appearance on frontal view.

SUMMARY

Otoplasty is based on principles. The surgeon must be able to identify the deformity and determine if there are excess structures, deficient structures, or adequate structures that need to be rearranged. Although many options often exist to improve a specific type of ear deformity, the simplest technique often is preferred.

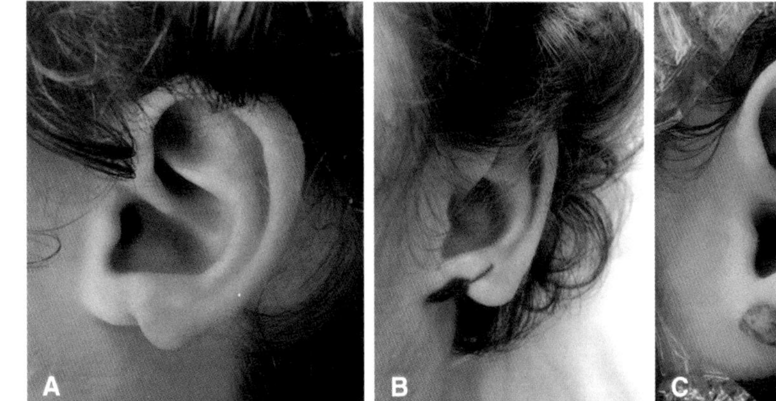

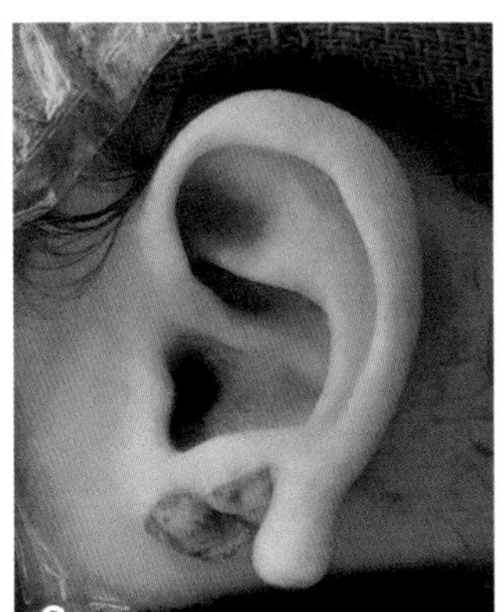

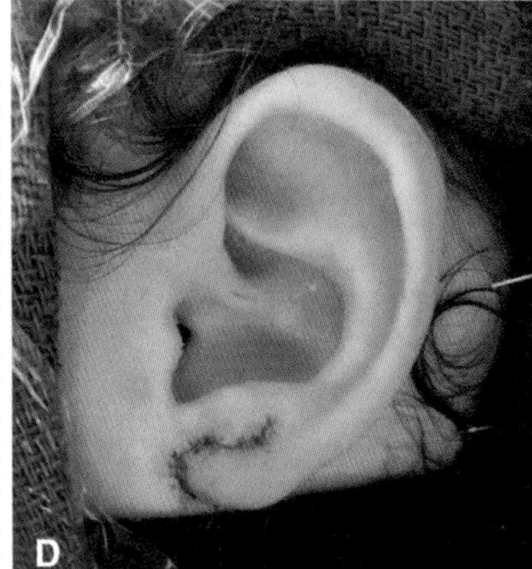

FIGURE 53.10. Congenital lobule deficiency. **A.** Preoperative view. **B.** Outline of flap and area of de-epithelialization. **C.** Prior to flap advancement. **D.** Following inset of the flap.

REFERENCES

1. Zhao H, Ma L, Qi X, et al. A morphometric study of the newborn ear and an analysis of factors related to congenital auricular deformities. *Plast Reconstr Surg.* 2017;140(1):147-155.
   This was a prospective study of 1500 newborns performed at 7 and 30 days of life. Ear anomalies and risk factors were documented as well as the maturation of ear deformities over time. The investigation provided epidemiological data about the incidence and natural history of ear anomalies.
2. Matsuo K, Hayashi R, Kiyono M, et al. Nonsurgical correction of congenital auricular deformities. *Clin Plast Surg.* 1990;17(2):383-395.
3. Driessen JP, Borgstein JA, Vuyk HD. Defining the protruding ear. *J Craniofac Surg.* 2011;22:2102-2108.
4. Shokrollahi K, Manning S, Sadri A, et al. The prominent antihelix and helix—the myth of the 'overcorrected' ear in otoplasty. *Ann Plast Surg.* 2015;74(suppl 4):S259-S263.
5. Tolleth H. Artistic anatomy, dimensions, and proportions of the external ear. *Clin Plast Surg.* 1978;5(3):337-345.
6. Bauer BS. Nonmicrotia. In: Bentz M, Bauer BS, Zucker , eds. *Principles and Practice of Pediatric Plastic Surgery*. New York, NY: Thieme; 2016.
7. Matsuo K, Hirose T, Tomono T, et al. Nonsurgical correction of congenital auricular deformities in the early neonate: a preliminary report. *Plast Reconstr Surg.* 1984;73(1):38-51.
   This was the first report for ear molding of auricular anomalies in newborns. This observation lead to the development of commercially produced ear-molding devices and decreased the need for operative otoplasty in children.
8. Byrd HS, Langevin CJ, Ghidoni LA. Ear molding in newborn infants with auricular deformities. *Plast Reconstr Surg.* 2010;126:1191-1200.
9. Tan ST, Abramson DL, MacDonald DM, Mulliken JB. Molding therapy for infants with deformational auricular anomalies. *Ann Plast Surg.* 1997;38:263-268.
10. Adamson JE, Horton CE, Crawford HH. The growth pattern of the external ear. *Plast Reconstr Surg.* 1965;36(4):466-470.
11. Gosain AK, Kumar A, Huang G. Prominent ears in children younger than 4 years of age: what is the appropriate timing for otoplasty? *Plast Reconstr Surg.* 2004;114(5):1042-1054.
    This study prospectively studied 12 patients who underwent otoplasty for prominent ears between 9 months and 3 years old. The length of the surgically corrected and the normal contralateral ears were the same at follow-up (range 2–7 years). This investigation showed that otoplasty can be performed in early childhood without inhibiting ear growth.
12. Mustarde JC. Correction of prominent ears using buried mattress sutures. *Clin Plast Surg.* 1978;5:459-464.
13. Stenstrom SJ, Heftner J. The Stenstrom otoplasty. *Clin Plast Surg.* 1978;5:465-470.
14. Sinno S, Chang JB, Thorne CH. Precision in otoplasty: combining reduction otoplasty with traditional otoplasty. *Plast Reconstr Surg.* 2015;135(5):1342-1348.
15. Furnas DW. Correction of prominent ears by conchamastoid sutures. *Plast Reconstr Surg.* 1968;42(3):189-193.
16. Bauer BS, Song DH, Aitken ME. Combined otoplasty technique: chondrocutaneous conchal resection as the cornerstone to correction of the prominent ear. *Plast Reconstr Surg.* 2002;110(4):1033-1040.
    The authors present a surgical technique that is a fundamental component of many otoplasty procedures. They describe the resection of conchal cartilage that enables the setback of the middle third of the ear as well as facilitates the formation of the antihelical fold with scapha-concha sutures.
17. Ungarelli LF, de Andrade CZ, Marques EG, et al. Diagnosis and prevalence of prominent lobules in otoplasty: analysis of 120 patients with prominent ears. *Aesthet Plast Surg.* 2016;40(5):645-651.
18. Thorne CH, Wilkes G. Ear deformities, otoplasty, and ear reconstruction. *Plast Reconstr Surg.* 2012;129:701e-716e.
19. Gosain AK, Recinos RF. A novel approach to correction of the prominent lobule during otoplasty. *Plast Reconstr Surg.* 2003;112(2):575-583.
20. Cho BC, Han KH. Surgical correction of cryptotia with V-Y advancement of a temporal triangular flap. *Plast Reconstr Surg.* 2005;115(6):1570-1581.
    The authors present a technique for the correction of cryptotia that uses a one-stage V-Y advancement flap from the postauricular area. This procedure obviates the need for skin grafts or tissue expansion to recreate the sulcus.
21. Kaplan H, Hudson D. A novel surgical method of repair for Stahl's ear: a case report and review of current treatments modalities. *Plast Reconstr Surg.* 1999;103:566-569.

QUESTIONS

1. A 5-year-old girl has an ear anomaly showing poor definition of the superior helix without a retroauricular sulcus. Which of the following is the most likely diagnosis?
   a. Microtia
   b. Prominent ear
   c. Stahl ear
   d. Cryptotia
   e. Constricted ear

2. A 5-year-old boy has an ear anomaly showing a pointed helix and a third crus of the antihelix. Which of the following is the most likely diagnosis?
   a. Microtia
   b. Prominent ear
   c. Stahl ear
   d. Cryptotia
   e. Constricted ear

3. Which of the following is the most ideal time to initiate non-surgical molding to correct a prominent ear deformity?
   a. 1 month
   b. 3 months
   c. 6 months
   d. 12 months
   e. 24 months

4. Which operative technique is used to recreate the antihelical fold in a patient with a prominent ear?
   a. Cartilage graft
   b. Cartilage excision
   c. Mustarde sutures
   d. Furnas sutures
   e. Postauricular flap

5. Which operative technique is used to set back the middle third of the ear in a patient with a prominent ear?
   a. Cartilage graft
   b. Cartilage excision
   c. Mustarde sutures
   d. Stenstrom technique
   e. Postauricular flap

1. **Answer: d.** The patient has cryptotia because the superior helix of the ear is buried underneath the scalp skin.

2. **Answer: c.** The patient's anomaly described is a Stahl deformity.

3. **Answer: a.** Circulating maternal estrogens in newborns allows the molding of ear cartilage. Moreover, 1 to 3 weeks is the ideal time to initiate ear molding because the younger the patient, the more malleable the ear and the more likely the patient will have a favorable outcome. Ear molding cannot be started at 3 months old or later.

4. **Answer: c.** Mustarde sutures (also known as scapha-concha sutures) are used to recreate the antihelical fold. Another method to establish the antihelix is to abrade the anterior aspect of the cartilage (Stenstrom technique). A cartilage graft commonly is used to reconstruct deficient areas of the helix. Cartilage excision minimizes the prominence of the middle third of the ear by reducing the size of the concha. Furnas sutures also decrease the prominence of the concha by suturing the concha to the mastoid fascia and periosteum. A postauricular flap is used to cover exposed areas of helical cartilage.

5. **Answer: b.** Cartilage excision minimizes the prominence of the middle third of the ear by reducing the size of the concha. Mustarde sutures (also known as scapha-concha sutures) are used to recreate the antihelical fold. Another method to establish the antihelix is to abrade the anterior aspect of the cartilage (Stenstrom technique). A cartilage graft commonly is used to reconstruct deficient areas of the helix. Stenstrom technique is the scoring of cartilage to make it bend and is a technique used to strengthen the antihelical fold and set back the superior third of the ear. A postauricular flap is used to cover exposed areas of helical cartilage.

CHAPTER 54 Facial Skeletal Augmentation With Implants and Osseous Genioplasty

Paul D. Durand, Christopher C. Surek, and James E. Zins

KEY POINTS

- Proper preoperative assessment and planning are crucial prior to attempting any modification of the facial skeleton.
- The subperiosteal plane is typically preferred for implant placement.
- Incisions should be planned away from the implant pocket.
- Two most commonly used materials for facial skeletal augmentation are solid silicone and porous polyethylene.
- Rigid fixation minimizes implant malposition and reduces risk of infection.
- Skeletal augmentation should not be viewed as a substitute for soft tissue suspension.
- Horizontal osteotomies should be placed at least 5 mm caudal to the canines to avoid tooth root injury as well as to reduce risk of mental nerve injury.
- Mental nerve exits the mandible through the mental foramen, which is located between the first and second premolars.
- Placement of intraoral incision should be 1 cm anterior to the gingivolabial sulcus, allowing for proper wound closure.
- Using a submental incision for alloplastic augmentation genioplasty may reduce risk of infection, wound dehiscence, and implant migration.

FACIAL SKELETAL AUGMENTATION WITH IMPLANTS

Preoperative Evaluation

As in any preoperative assessment, a thorough physical examination is of paramount importance. Aesthetic concerns and expectations should then be discussed. Reviewing photos of the patient's front, oblique, and profile proves to be particularly useful for both the surgeon and patient. The facial skeleton should be assessed for asymmetry and dysmorphology. Minor modifications of the facial skeleton can significantly accentuate areas of mild asymmetry.

Established anthropometric measurements of balanced faces can provide the surgeon with some objective basis that can be used in deciding what areas need to be augmented or reduced and to what extent.[1]

Recent advances in preoperative evaluation including 3D CT scanning, stereolithographic modeling, 3D printing, and a variety of other software programs are available. Nevertheless, posteroanterior and lateral cephalometric radiographs and panoramic x-rays can be particularly useful when planning augmentation of the chin and mandible. Skeletal dimensions in relation to soft-tissue thickness can be assessed.

Alloplastic Materials

Aesthetic facial skeletal augmentation is generally performed with alloplastic implants. An ideal implant material is one that is biocompatible and has minimal interaction with the surrounding tissues, such that its morphology is maintained after placement. In contrast, skeletal augmentation with autogenous bone can remodel, in time affecting its size and shape.[2,3]

The host tissue response includes some level of capsule formation around the implant being placed. The most important determinant of the degree of this response is the material in the outer surface of the implant. Porous implants typically result in less robust capsule formation compared to smooth implants. Implant migration and adjacent bone erosion also tend to be lower in porous implants.[4,5] Solid silicone implants offer several advantages over other materials—they can be effortlessly carved to achieve a desired shape and size, as well as be easily fixated with screws or sutures. Incidence of infection, although low regardless of the implant type, has been reported to be lower when silicone implants are used.[6]

Positioning and Immobilization

Implant placement is described in both supraperiosteal and subperiosteal planes (**Figure 54.1**). The subperiosteal pocket dissection is preferred as it involves a plane of dissection that is bloodless and safe relative to surrounding neurovascular structures. Regardless of the area being augmented and the type of implant used, proper immobilization of the device can provide a more accurate, reproducible result. A major advantage of screw fixation over the other methods (e.g., sutures) relates to more accurate final contour because gaps between host bone and the implant are eliminated.

Midface Augmentation

Most aesthetic facial augmentation occurs in the middle and lower thirds of the face. Augmentation of the midface can be divided in four major areas: malar, submalar, paranasal, and infraorbital rim.

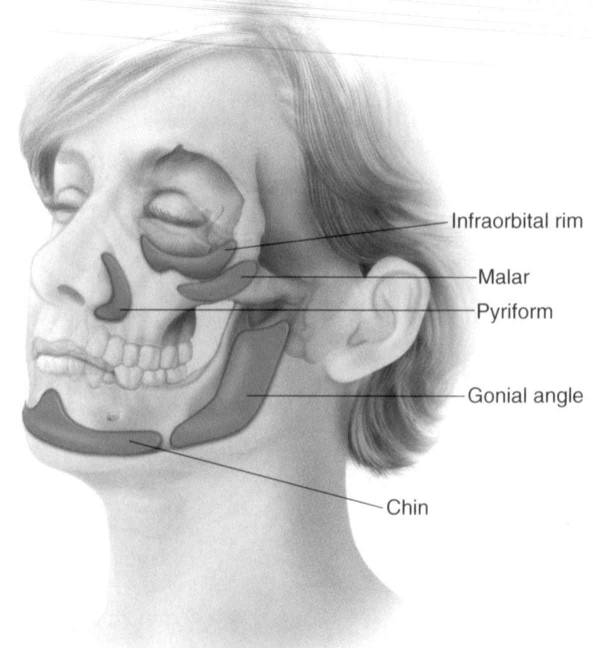

FIGURE 54.1. Location of various facial implants for skeletal augmentation.

Malar

The malar area is a frequent area of alloplastic augmentation. Full cheeks and prominent malar bones are associated with youth and attractiveness. Patients seeking augmentation of this area can either have normal anatomy or a true skeletal deficiency of the midface such as congenital deformities.[7] Such distinction is important, as in the latter case; malar augmentation alone can be insufficient to address the aesthetic issue at hand. Finally, skeletal augmentation should not be seen as equivalent to soft-tissue augmentation and resuspension; these are two separate entities that when used appropriately can have a synergistic effect.

Incision placement for insertion of malar implants can vary and include the intraoral, coronal, or eyelid routes, all of which have been described.[7] An intraoral approach is preferred as it provides good exposure and avoids any external scars. When performing an upper sulcus incision, sufficient labial tissue should be left on either side to allow for a secure, two layered watertight closure. After careful identification of the infraorbital nerve, dissection is carried out in the subperiosteal plane over the malar eminence and onto the zygomatic arch. The pocket size can be tailored to the implant being used and its desired aesthetic outcome. Screw fixation provides for more freedom in pocket dissection and thus greater exposure at the time of implant insertion. Careful carving of the implant on its posterior surface and rigid fixation minimize visibility and malposition.

Paranasal

Deficiency of midface projection can either be congenital or acquired. It is present in individuals who have undergone cleft surgery, traumatic facial fractures, or due to developmental deformities. In patients with a relatively normal occlusion, deficient midface projection can be corrected with facial implants. By increasing nasal base projection, paranasal augmentation serves to open the nasolabial angle and effaces the depth of the nasolabial fold. When properly placed, paranasal implants can simulate the visual effect of LeFort I advancement.[8]

Paranasal augmentation is done intraorally. To avoid placing incisions directly over the implant, the upper gingival buccal sulcus incision is made just lateral to the piriform aperture. As with malar augmentation, dissection is carried out subperiosteally, while the nearby infraorbital nerve is identified and protected. Screw fixation minimizes asymmetries and malposition. When screw fixation is employed, care should be taken to avoid the root of the canine. Compromise of the nasal airway can occur if implants are positioned over the piriform aperture.[8,9]

Infraorbital Rim

The morphology of the infraorbital rim skeleton plays a crucial role in supporting soft tissue of the lower eyelids and cheeks. Lack of projection of this skeletal component can be responsible for premature descent of such structures and result in early facial aging. A characteristic "negative" vector, in which the most anterior projection of the globe lies anterior to the lower lid and malar eminence, is commonly noted in these individuals (**Figure 54.2**). This finding is associated with significant risk of lower eyelid malposition after blepharoplasty. Augmentation of the infraorbital rim can decrease the incidence of lower lid malposition by reversing the "negative" vector.[10,11]

Various types of incision can be used for insertion of infraorbital rim implants, including subciliary skin and skin-muscle flap incisions. If a transconjunctival incision is used, it can be lengthened with a lateral canthotomy. Better exposure of the midface skeleton can be obtained by incorporating an intraoral sulcus incision.

Dissection is carried out in a subperiosteal plane. Infraorbital rim implants can be carved to tailor lateral and medial extension depending on the specific area to be augmented. Screw fixation is beneficial in this area to avoid implant malposition. Prior to closure, malar soft tissue should be resuspended over the secured implant.[11]

Temporal Augmentation

The deepest portion of the temporal fossa is the anterior inferior fossa, which is the sphenoid bone contribution.[12] Facial aging, trauma including previous surgery, weight change, and a variety of other causes can lead to soft-tissue deficiency of muscle and fat in the temporal fossa. Yaremchuk used polymethylmethacrylate (PMMA) to fill up temporal depressions. If a previous reconstructive surgery was performed in the temporal area, access is gained through the old scar and the PMMA is placed over the deficient muscle. To prevent implant motion, titanium screws are secured along the lateral orbital rim. If patients have not had surgery or have had the temple used as a remote access to other regions of the face (i.e., subperiosteal facelift), then the implant is placed beneath the temporalis muscle though an incision in the temporal hair-bearing scalp.[12,13]

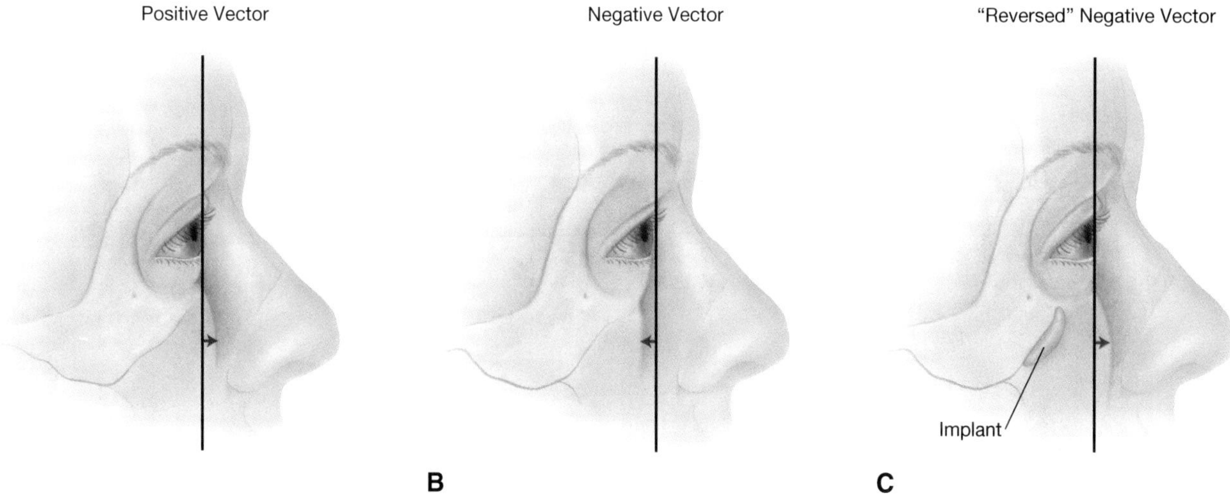

FIGURE 54.2. Globe-orbital rim relationships have been categorized by placing a line or "vector" between the most anterior projection of the globe and the malar eminence and lid margin. **A.** Positive vector relationship. In a youthful face with normal globe-to-skeletal rim relations, the cheek mass supported by the infraorbital rim lies anterior to the surface of the cornea. The position of the cheek prominence beyond the anterior surface of the cornea is termed a positive vector. **B.** Negative vector relationship. In patients with maxillary hypoplasia, the cheek mass lies posterior to the surface of the cornea. The position of the cheek prominence beyond the anterior surface of the cornea is termed a negative vector. **C.** "Reversed" negative vector relationship. Alloplastic augmentation of the infraorbital rim can reverse the negative vector.

Mandibular Augmentation

Chin

Augmentation of the chin area can have a profound effect on the facial profile. In an ideal face, the upper lip should be projecting 2 mm beyond the lower lip, whereas the lower lip should be projecting the same distance beyond the chin.[14] Riedel's line is a rapid means of assessing the adequacy of chin projection. A line is drawn tangential to the upper lip and lower lip and the chin should fall on this line (**Figure 54.3**). Men tend to have larger, more projected chins compared to women. Placing too large of an implant in a woman can have an unattractive masculinizing effect and should be avoided.[14–16]

An ideal chin implant is one that augments the mentum while merging laterally with the anterior aspect of the mandibular body. As with skeletal augmentation of other facial areas, implant materials used are either porous or smooth (see Alloplastic Materials section). Extended porous implants have limited flexibility and are typically designed in two pieces to allow placement through a reduced incision.[16]

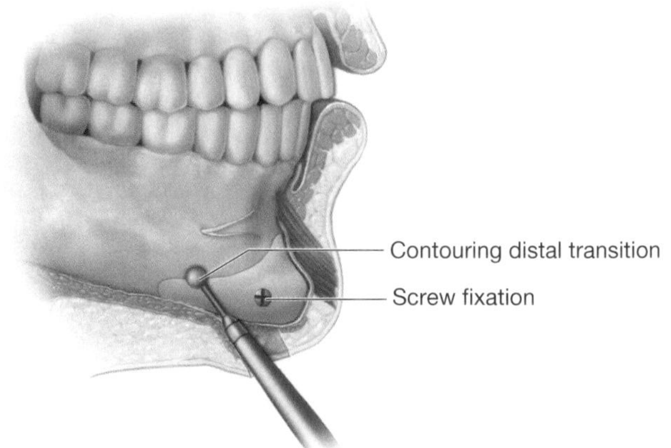

FIGURE 54.4. Representation of a preferred technique for chin augmentation. Through a submental approach, a two-piece porous polyethylene implant is fixed to the skeleton with titanium screws. This maneuver immobilizes the implant and obliterates any gaps between the implant and the underlying bone. The implant is being contoured to provide an imperceptible implant-native mandible transition.

Chin implant insertion can be performed through a submental or an intraoral incision (**Figure 54.4**). However, we use the submental incision exclusively. The intraoral incision avoids an external scar but provides limited exposure of the anterior mandible. In addition, the intraoral incision is associated with superior malposition of the implant and soft-tissue ptosis, and in our opinion it should be avoided.[16] This is usually secondary to improper mentalis muscle repair at the time of wound closure and results in a witch's chin deformity.[17] Regardless of the incision being used, care should be taken to identify and protect the mental nerves during subperiosteal dissection.

Other (Body/Angle/Ramus)

Although chin augmentation remains the most popular type of mandibular augmentation, certain patient populations may benefit from augmentation of other areas. Yaremchuk identifies two main groups of patients who usually seek such enhancement. The first group includes individuals who display normal mandibular dimensions in relation to other facial thirds. They perceive a wider lower face as more attractive and want to emulate the more angular lower face seen in models and actors. The other group includes those who have an actual deficiency of the mandibular skeleton. They may have a normal occlusion or may have had malocclusion previously corrected by orthodontics alone. In these patients, mandibular augmentation of the ramus and body is often paired with an extended chin implant to address poor mental projection.[18]

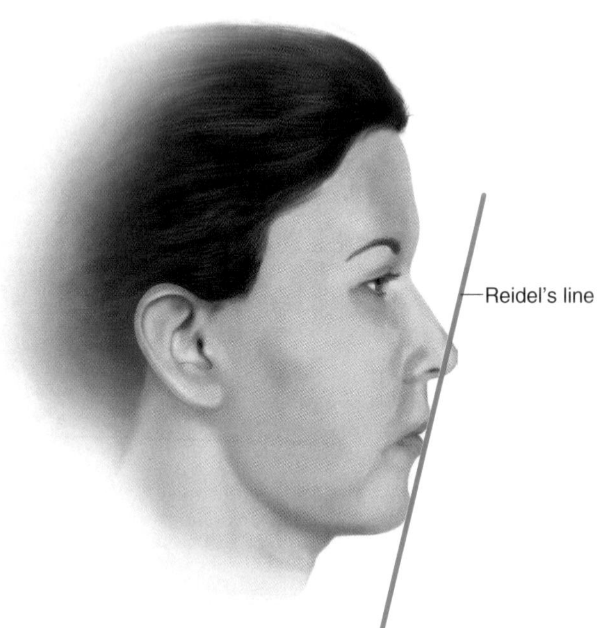

FIGURE 54.3. Riedel line.

An intraoral mucosal incision provides adequate exposure of the mandibular ramus and body in the subperiosteal plane. It can be extended anteriorly if concomitant chin augmentation is being performed. Care must be taken to identify and visualize the mental foramen. Screw fixation of the implants can either be done intraorally or through a percutaneous incision for trocar placement (**Figures 54.5 and 54.6**). A suction drain is usually placed in the operative site which exits through the postauricular area.[18]

Complications in Alloplastic (Implant) Augmentation

Alloplastic implant complications include infection, migration, malposition, and asymmetry. Serious complications after alloplastic augmentation of the facial skeleton are rare. Bone resorption of adjacent areas has been reported and is associated with solid implants. Bone resorption is significantly less likely with porous implants.[19] In his series of 162 patients, Yaremchuk reported an acute infection rate for implants of 2%. The total reoperation rate was 10% and mostly due to implant malposition, asymmetry, or displeasing contours. If implant infection does occur, antibiotic treatment alone is usually not sufficient. In such cases, implant removal is recommended along with an antibiotic regimen. Implants can be replaced at 12 months after infection cessation.[19]

OSSEOUS GENIOPLASTY

The horizontal genioplasty remains as the second most commonly performed osteotomy of the facial skeleton, next to rhinoplasty.[20] Compared to prosthetic chin implants, osseous genioplasty allows for a more powerful and versatile alteration of chin morphology and shape. This includes not only correction of sagittal deficiency, but also can include vertical lengthening, reduction, and correction of asymmetries.

Anatomy

To ensure a safe and predictable result in osseous genioplasty, knowledge of muscle attachments and adjacent neurovascular structures is important. The three muscles that attach to the anterior plane of the chin include: mentalis, depressor angularis, and depressor labii inferioris. Equally important are muscle attachments on the lingual aspect of the chin, which include mylohyoid, geniohyoid,

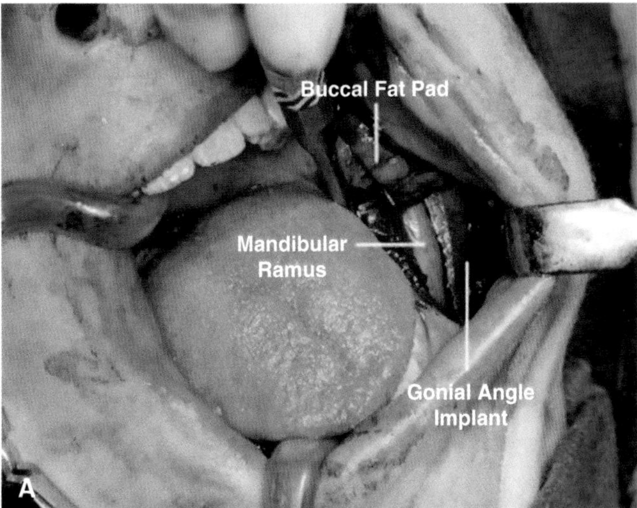

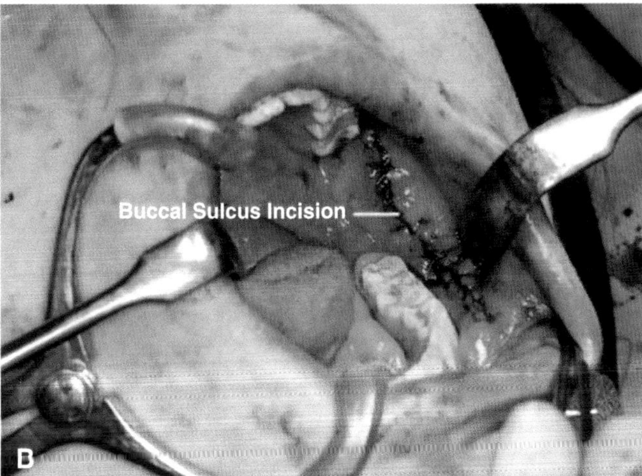

FIGURE 54.5. **A.** Intraoperative photograph following placement of polyethylene gonial angle implant through an intraoral buccal sulcus incision. The periosteum is stripped and the implant is contoured to the appropriate shape and taper. The implant was fixed in place using two screws flush with bone by two titanium screws, one into the gonial angle and the other cephalic in the mandibular ramus. **B.** An intraoperative photograph demonstrating the location of the buccal sulcus incision that was utilized to perform gonial angle implant placement. It is important to leave an adequate mucosal cuff on the lingual side of the incision in order to get a good watertight closure. This photo is taken at the end of the operation demonstrating a multilayered closure.

and genioglossus. It is the latter group that contains the perforating branches responsible for maintaining blood supply of the caudal chin segment following elevation of the anterior periosteum and horizontal osteotomy.

An important structure that is vulnerable to injury during soft-tissue dissection and osteotomy is the mental nerve. A continuation of the inferior alveolar nerve, it exits the mandible via the mental foramen. The latter is located in the vertical plane between the first and second mandibular premolars. To avoid injury to the mental nerve, the horizontal osteotomy should be planned at least 5 mm caudal to the foramen in a caudal-oblique angle. The mental nerve makes a gentle curve as it approaches the mental foramen. Therefore it lies caudal to the foramen distally and can be injured if a bone cut is made just below the foramen.[21,22]

Limitations of Alloplastic (Implant) Augmentation

Those favoring alloplastic augmentation over osseous genioplasty cite several theoretical advantages including: technical ease, less pain, and a relatively low complication risk. Conversely, the horizontal genioplasty offers potential correction in multiple planes, anterior, posterior, and vertical. Alloplastic augmentation with chin implants can be effective in correcting mild to moderate volume deficiencies in the sagittal plane. Major limitations of alloplastic methods occur when trying to correct vertical excess or any asymmetries of the anterior mandible. Furthermore, osseous genioplasty is more amenable to surgical revision if such a condition is indicated. In the latter, soft tissue of the chin has not been degloved and there is no scar capsule formation to address.[16,23]

Preoperative Evaluation and Indications

It is important to note that genioplasty is performed solely to address chin disharmony and should not be seen as a replacement to orthognathic surgery. Proper preoperative evaluation should include a complete history and physical examination with special attention to the occlusion. Specific complaints and cosmetic objectives need to be discussed with the patient. The surgeon should also inquire about previous orthodontic treatments or prior orthognathic surgery. Comorbid conditions and anesthetic contraindications are to be weighed in the decision to perform surgery.

Physical Examination

Physical examination should include appreciation of chin projection, symmetry, and vertical length. In assessing the vertical dimension of the chin, the lower third of the face should be subdivided using a line passing through the stomion (Figure 54.7). The distance from the stomion to the menton should be twice the length of the distance between the subnasale and the stomion.

Chin projection is better assessed in the profile view using Riedel's plane. In the latter, a line is drawn tangential to the upper and lower lip (see Figure 54.3). In a balanced face, this line should touch the most prominent anterior portion of the pogonion. Chin position in relation to Riedel's plane dictates the amount of horizontal microgenia or macrogenia present.[20,24] The lower lip, and not the other structures in the mid and upper face, determines the extent to which the chin should be advanced.[20] In the sagittal dimension, it is always preferable to undercorrect than overcorrect, resulting in an aesthetically displeasing outcome. When advancing the chin, the ratio of soft tissue to skeletal displacement is generally 3:2. Conversely, the response of soft tissue to a posteriorly repositioned chin is less predictable and typically 0.5:1.[20,24]

Labiomental groove depth should also be evaluated when determining if a patient is a good candidate for osseous genioplasty; it should measure 4 mm in women and 6 mm in men. Sagittal advancement or vertical shortening of the symphyseal segment would result in deepening of the labiomental groove. Conversely, vertical lengthening softens the labiomental crease (Figure 54.8). In the setting of a long lower face and a deep labiomental fold, correction should include orthognathic surgery rather than osseous genioplasty alone.[20]

An intraoral examination should be performed to evaluate occlusion and presence of any significant periodontal disease. The majority of individuals requesting aesthetic enlargement of the chin have class II malocclusion secondary to mandibular retrognathia. Although prior orthodontic treatment can convert class II malocclusion into type I, it corrects the underlying skeletal problems.[20] Routine workup includes a lateral cephalometric and panoramic x-ray and frontal, profile, and oblique photographs at a minimum.

Surgical Technique

Operative Approach

Although osseous genioplasty can be performed under local anesthesia with intravenous sedation, general anesthesia with either orotracheal or nasotracheal intubation is recommended. Prior to incision, the chin is infiltrated using xylocaine with epinephrine

AESTHETIC SURGERY

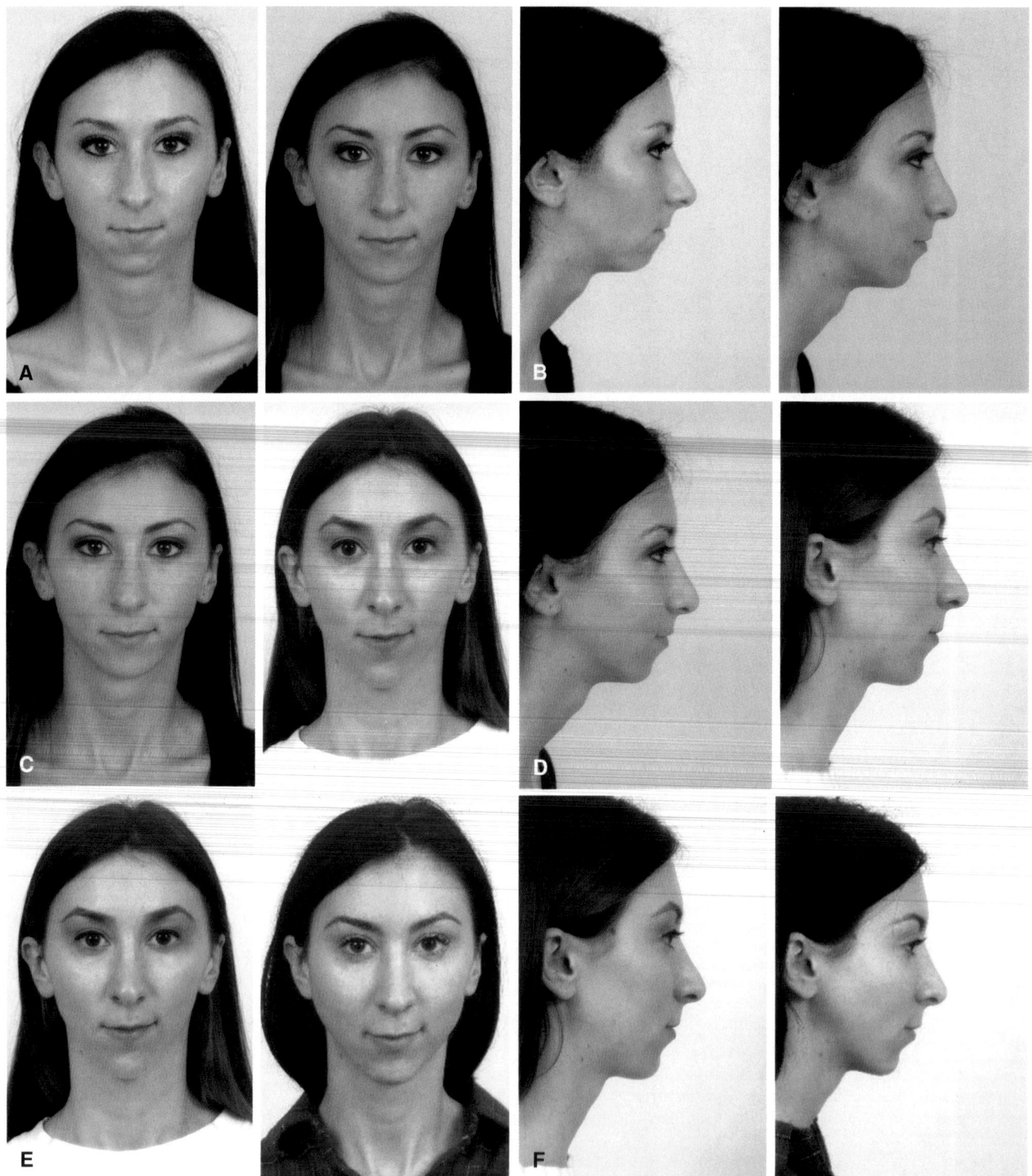

FIGURE 54.6. A, B. An 18-year-old female had a chin implant placed for sagittal microgenia by another surgeon: preprocedure (*left*) and 4 months postprocedure (*right*) photographs. **C, D.** At age 22, the patient was not satisfied with the aesthetic result, so the chin implant was removed and horizontal advancement genioplasty for sagittal and vertical microgenia was performed: preprocedure (*left*) and 11 months postprocedure (*right*) photographs. **E, F.** At 23, the patient underwent gonial angle implant placement and mandibular fat grafting for jawline contour augmentation: preprocedure (*left*) and postprocedure (*right*) photographs. The postprocedure photo is 7 months following the gonial angle implant placement and 4 months following mandibular fat grafting.

solution. An incision is planned at least 1 cm away from the mandibular buccal sulcus and is 2 to 4 cm in length. The mentalis muscle is exposed after incising the mucosa and submucosa. Maintaining a 1 cm cuff of mucosa and mentalis in the gingival side of incision will facilitate later muscle repair and incision closure. After muscle division, subperiosteal dissection of the anterior mandibular symphysis is performed. Inferior dissection is performed only far enough for sufficient exposure to performing the osteotomy and subsequent fixation. Complete degloving of the symphysis is not preferred as reattachment of soft tissues can be unpredictable, increasing the risk for a witch's chin deformity.[17] Exposure is carried laterally until both mental nerves are visualized and posteriorly to the inferior border of the mandible, but not further.

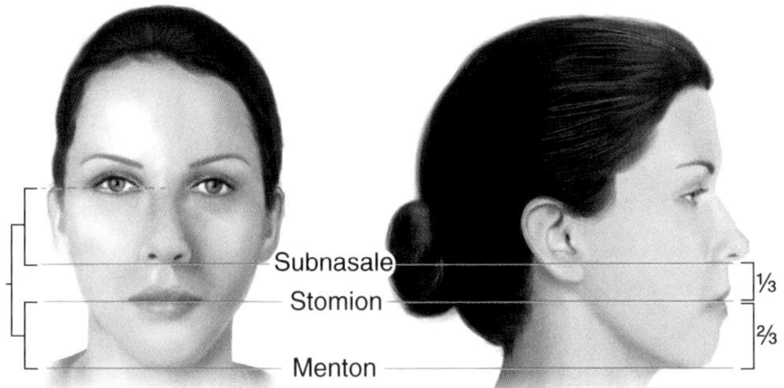

FIGURE 54.7. Lower facial third division.

Prior to performing any osteotomies, the chin midline is marked with a bone bur for proper positioning of symphyseal bone segments at the time of fixation. Horizontal osteotomy should be performed using a reciprocating saw at least 4 mm below the mental foramina to avoid nerve injury. Retractors can be used to protect the nerves. The osteotomy is then carried as far posteriorly as possible to prevent excessive visibility of step-offs in the inferior mandible border. If extensive anterior movement of the chin segment is anticipated, it might be necessary to detach the anterior belly of the digastric muscles from the lingual surface. After proper mobilization is achieved, fixation of the bone segment is performed with either plate and screws or wires (**Figure 54.9**).[22,23] A temporary drill hole and wire through the anterior surface of the mobilized segment allows easy handling of the osteotomy.

Osteotomy patterns vary depending on the type of chin deformity to be corrected (**Figure 54.10**). For vertical shortening of the chin, two parallel horizontal osteotomies with removal of the intervening bone segment are used. The inferior cut is always made first for ease of handling. Conversely, if vertical elongation is needed, interposing blocks of bone substitute can be inserted into the osteotomy gap previously created.[22,23] A gap of less than 5 mm needs no interposition implant.

After appropriate bony fixation is obtained, the wound is irrigated with either dilute povidone-iodine solution or antibiotic irrigation. Mentalis muscle is then reattached using interrupted sutures, a crucial step in preventing soft-tissue ptosis and a witch's chin deformity.[17] Mucosa is then repaired using chromic sutures until watertight closure is achieved.

Complications in Osseous Genioplasty

Wound dehiscence and infection are rare after osseous genioplasty. In the setting of a dehiscence without infection and with no loose or exposed hardware, most resolve without intervention. If infection is suspected and bone fixation is not loose, localized debridement and irrigation followed by antibiotics serve to avoid unnecessary removal of hardware. Because this is a vascularized osteotomy, the bone is not at risk. Hematomas should be promptly evacuated to prevent abscess formation.

More than half of all patients undergoing osseous genioplasty will have some degree of temporary neurosensory loss. Most of these are due to traction and should return days to weeks after the operation. If the nerve is cut during surgery, it should be repaired.

Dental complications can also occur. Root exposure can occur if incision is placed too close to the gingiva and is most likely in patients with gingival resorption. It presents as a caudal retraction of gingival tissue and results in exposure of the sensitive portion of teeth. Gingival grafting might be needed to treat such a complication. Tooth devitalization is probably one of the most serious complications after osseous genioplasty and can be avoided by placing the osteotomy at least 30 mm caudal to the occlusal edge of the mandibular canines.[22]

Soft-tissue ptosis is usually secondary to improper mentalis muscle repair at the time of wound closure and results in a witch chin's deformity. It can be corrected by excising soft tissue through an elliptical incision in the submental area. Lower lip retraction resulting in increased lower incisor show can also occur secondary to improper mentalis muscle repair. Correction can be achieved through an intraoral incision and cephalically suspending anterior periosteum.[17,25]

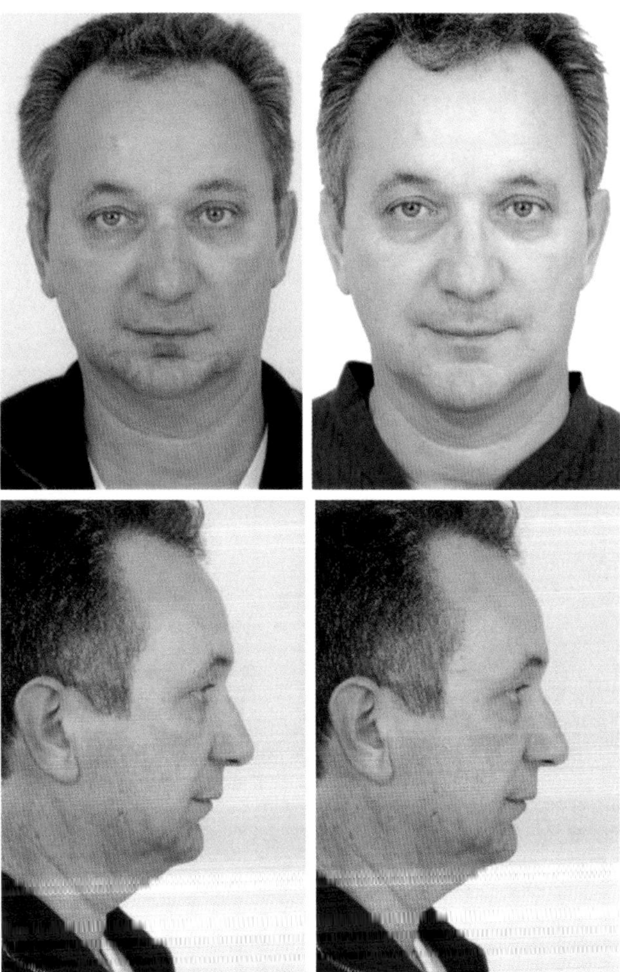

FIGURE 54.8. Preprocedure (*left*) and postprocedure (*right*) photographs of a 55-year-old man who underwent vertical lengthening genioplasty. Note the improvement in lower vertical faical height and softening of the labiomental crease. The postprocedure photo is 2.5 years after the operation.

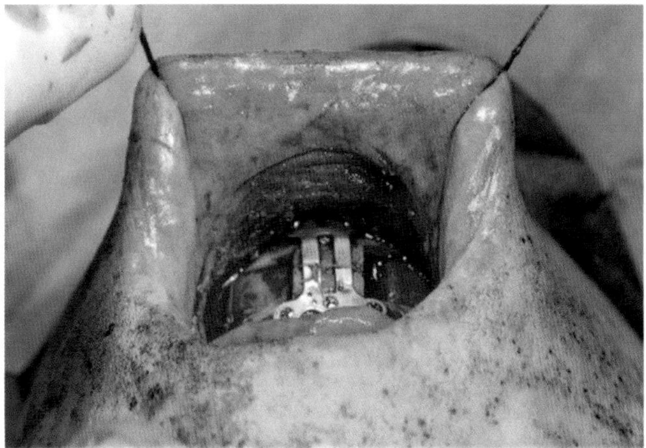

FIGURE 54.9. Intraoperative photograph demonstrating screw and plate fixation of a horizontal advancement genioplasty.

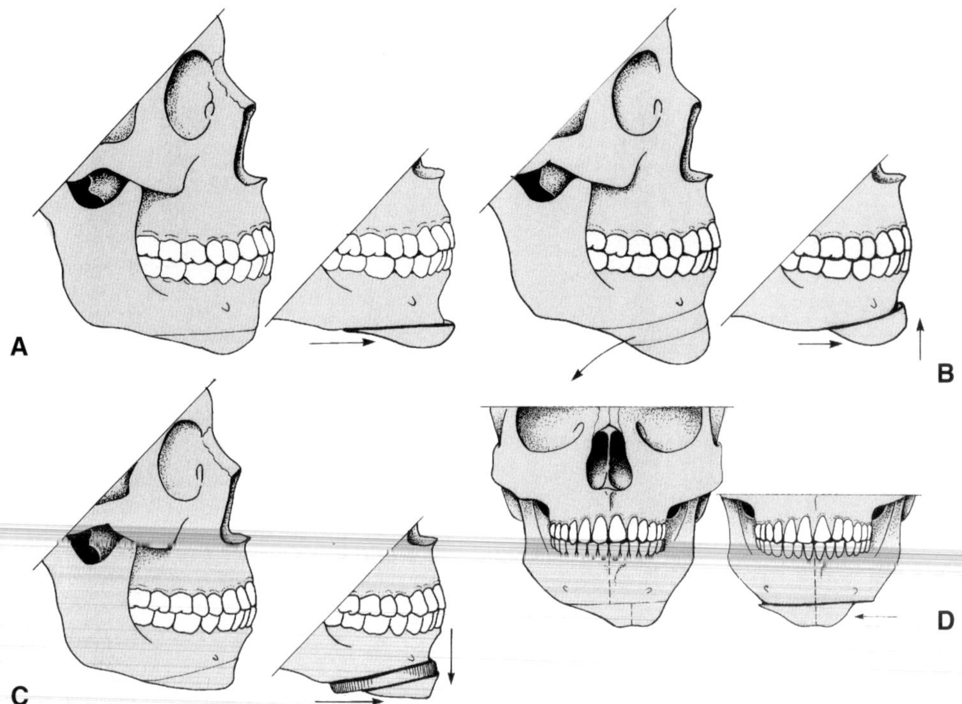

FIGURE 54.10. A. Standard location and orientation of the advancement osseous genioplasty. Note that the osteotomy is placed well below the mental foramina to avoid injury to the inferior alveolar nerve. The osteotomy extends well posterior to the vicinity of the molar teeth. The angulation of this osteotomy allows forward advancement of the chin without any vertical changes. **B.** Simultaneous advancement and vertical reduction of the chin. Note that the two parallel osteotomies are performed with an intervening ostectomy. **C.** Simultaneous advancement and vertical elongation of the chin. The interpositional material typically employed includes blocks of porous hydroxyapatite. **D.** Lateral shifting of the symphyseal segment to restore lower face symmetry.

REFERENCES

1. Farkas LG, Kolar JC. Anthropometrics and art in the aesthetics of women's faces. *Clin Plast Surg.* 1987;14:599.
   Classic article exploring the importance of anthropometric dimensions in female face aesthetics.
2. Chen NT, Glowacki J, Bucky LP, et al. The roles of revascularization and resorption on endurance of craniofacial onlay bone grafts in the rabbit. *Plast Reconstr Surg.* 1994;93:714.
3. Saulacic N, Bosshardt DD, Jensen SS, et al. Impact of bone graft harvesting techniques on bone formation and graft resorption: a histomorphometric study in the mandibles of minipigs. *Clin Oral Implants Res.* 2015;26(4):383-391.
4. Maas CS, Merwin GE, Wilson J, et al. Comparison of biomaterials for facial bone augmentation. *Arch Otolaryngol Head Neck Surg.* 1990;116:551-556.
5. Yaremchuk MJ, Chen YC. Enlarging the deficient mandible. *Aesth Surg J.* 2007;27(5):539-550.
6. Carboni A, Gasparini G, Perugini M, et al. Evaluation of homologous bone graft versus biomaterials in the aesthetic restoration of the middle third of the face. *Minerva Chir.* 2002;57(3):283-287.
7. Whitaker LA. Aesthetic augmentation of the malar midface structures. *Plast Reconstr Surg.* 1987;80:337.
   Another classic article that reviews various preoperative and technical aspects of facial aesthetic augmentation with a focus on the midface.
8. Yaremchuk MJ, Israeli D. Paranasal implants—correct midface concavity. *Plast Reconstr Surg.* 1998;102:1676-1684.
9. Yaremchuk MJ. Secondary malar implant surgery. *Plast Reconstr Surg.* 2008;121:620.
   Offers a complete examination of how to deal with implant-related complications of the malar area, with a focus on secondary revision surgery.
10. Jelks GW, Jelks EB. The influence of orbital and eyelid anatomy on the palpebral aperture. *Clin Plast Surg.* 1991;18:193.
11. Yaremchuk MJ. Infraorbital rim augmentation. *Plast Reconstr Surg.* 2001;107:1585.
12. Vaca EE, Purnell CA, Gosain AK, Alghoul MS. Postoperative temporal hollowing: is there a surgical approach that prevents this complication? A systematic review and anatomic illustration. *J Plast Reconstr Aesthet Surg.* 2017:70(3):401-415.
13. Gordon CR, Yaremchuk MJ. Temporal augmentation with methyl methacrylate? *Aesthet Surg J.* 2011;31(7):827-833.
14. McCarthy JG, Ruff GL. The chin. *Clin Plast Surg.* 1988;15:125.
15. Flowers RS. Alloplastic augmentation of the anterior mandible. *Clin Plast Surg.* 1991:18:107-137.
16. Yaremchuk MJ. Improving aesthetic outcomes after alloplastic chin augmentation. *Plast Reconstr Surg.* 2003:112(5):1422-1432.
17. Zide BM. The mentalis muscle: an essential component of chin and lower lip position. *Plast Reconstr Surg.* 1989;83:413.
   Emphasizes the importance of properly repairing the mentalis muscle when using an intraoral approach. Describes technique and potential pitfalls.
18. Yaremchuk MJ. Mandibular augmentation. *Plast Reconstr Surg.* 2000;106:697.
19. Yaremchuk MJ. Facial skeletal reconstruction using porous polyethylene implants. *Plast Reconstr Surg.* 2003;111(6):1818-1827.
   Extensive single surgeon experience of 162 patients undergoing facial skeletal augmentation. An excellent review of potential complications and their management.
20. Rosen HM. Aesthetic guidelines in genioplasty: the role of facial disproportion. *Plast Reconstr Surg.* 1995;95:463.
21. Hwang K, Lee W, Song Y, Chung I. Vulnerability of the inferior alveolar nerve and mental nerve during genioplasty: an anatomic study. *J Craniofac Surg.* 2005;16(1):10-14.
22. Ousterhout D. Sliding genioplasty: avoiding mental nerve injuries. *J Craniofac Surg.* 1996:7(4):297-298.
23. Sawkat S, Havlik RJ. An evidence-based approach to genioplasty. *Plast Reconstr Surg.* 2011:127(2):898-904.
24. Michelow B, Guyuron B. The chin: skeletal and soft-tissue components. *Plast Reconstr Surg.* 1995;95(3):473-478.
25. Chashu G, Blinder D, Taicher S, Chaushu S. The effect of precise reattachment of the mentalis muscle on the soft tissue response to genioplasty. *J Oral Maxillofac Surg.* 2001;59(5):510-516.

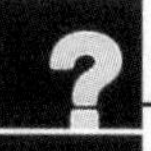

QUESTIONS

1. **Riedel's plane corresponds with a line connecting the most projected points of the upper and lower lip to what structure?**
   a. Nasal tip
   b. Labiomental crease
   c. Pogonion
   d. Base of nasal ala

2. **Inadequate reapproximation of the mentalis muscle following genioplasty surgery can lead to what deformity?**
   a. Inability to depress the oral commissure
   b. Inability to pucker lips
   c. "Witch's chin" abnormality
   d. Decreased ability to suck from a straw

3. **Which of the following tooth root apexes is at greatest risk for damage during osteotomy at the time of sliding genioplasty?**
   a. Bicuspid
   b. Central incisor
   c. Lateral incisor
   d. Canine
   e. First molar

4. **A 22-year-old man is evaluated for lower facial asymmetry. He is scheduled to undergo sliding genioplasty. At the time of osteotomy, the nerve more likely to be injured exits mandible adjacent to what landmark?**
   a. Canines
   b. Between lateral and central incisors
   c. Between second and third molar
   d. Between first and second premolars
   e. Between lateral incisors and canines

5. **A 34-year-old woman with class I occlusion comes for orthognathic evaluation. She is displeased with her lower face profile. On examination, isolated retrogenia and moderate vertical mandibular excess are noted. Which is the most appropriate genioplasty for this particular patient?**
   a. Advancement with horizontal osteotomy only
   b. Advancement with inferiorly angled osteotomy
   c. Alloplastic augmentation, extraoral approach
   d. Alloplastic augmentation, intraoral approach
   e. Advancement with horizontal osteotomy and downgrafting

1. **Answer: c.** Riedel's line is a rapid means of assessing the adequacy of chin projection. A line is drawn tangential to the upper lip and lower lip and the chin should fall on this line (see Figure 54.3).

2. **Answer: c.** During wound closure in genioplasty, the mentalis muscle is then reattached using interrupted sutures; this is a crucial step in preventing soft-tissue ptosis and a witch's chin deformity. If this deformity occurs, it can be corrected by excising soft tissue through an elliptical incision in the submental area.

3. **Answer: d.** The canine tooth root is the longest tooth root and therefore is at risk during sliding genioplasty. Tooth devitalization is probably one of the most serious complications after osseous genioplasty and can be avoided by placing the osteotomy at least 30 mm caudal to the occlusal edge of the mandibular canines.

4. **Answer: d.** The mental foramen is located between the first and second premolars. Note that the mental nerve makes a gentle curve as it approaches the mental foramen. Therefore, it lies caudal to the foramen distally and can be injured if a bone cut is made just below the foramen. Horizontal osteotomy should be performed using a reciprocating saw at least 4 mm below the mental foramina in order to avoid nerve injury.

5. **Answer: b.** This patient has microgenia and therefore needs horizontal advancement. Given that she has vertical excess of the mandible, an angled osteotomy, and possible wedge excision can be performed to help normalize vertical height of the mandible. Patients with retrogenia and vertical mandibular deficiency would be best suited for genioplasty and downgrafting to increase vertical mandibular height (answer e). Patients with normal mandible vertical height and isolated microgenia would receive a horizontal advancement without vertical height manipulation.

CHAPTER 55 Augmentation Mammoplasty, Mastopexy, and Mastopexy-Augmentation

Ali A. Qureshi and Terence M. Myckatyn

KEY POINTS

- Breast augmentation can be performed with implants in the subglandular, subfascial, and submuscular planes with the primary goal to increase the size of the breast. Fat grafting can be used alone or as an adjunct procedure for breast augmentation.
- Breast implants can be saline or silicone, smooth or textured, round or anatomic. These devices can rupture or form capsules that lead to capsule contracture and distortion of the breast.
- Mastopexy aims to change the shape of a breast that has become ptotic or involuted as result of age, hormonal changes, or weight loss by altering the skin and parenchyma of the breast.
- Management of capsular contracture or rupture of a prosthetic device can present a unique set of challenges and often requires operative intervention. A new pocket may need to be created or adjunct materials like acellular dermal matrices may be helpful.
- Mastopexy-augmentation can be performed as a single-stage procedure to alter both the size and shape of the breast at the same operation and presents a unique set of challenges.

AUGMENTATION MAMMOPLASTY

Augmentation mammoplasty or breast augmentation (BA) continues to be one of the most commonly performed aesthetic breast procedures in the United States.[1] The primary goal of the surgery is to increase the size of the breast, but there are simultaneous changes to the shape of the gland and nipple-areola complex (NAC) position. Thoughtful planning and use of devices individualized for the patient help the surgeon to achieve a patient's goals. Although historically BA has been performed with a prosthetic device, advances in flap design and fat grafting have led to a paradigm shift where now BA can be performed almost exclusively with a patient's own tissue if desired.

Preoperative Assessment

The consultation for BA, like that for any aesthetic procedure, is an art and a science. It requires a thoughtful assessment and understanding of a woman's goals for the size and shape of her breasts. This must be complemented by the surgeon's evaluation of objective parameters of anatomy and tissue dynamics. Together, the subjective assessment of expectations and objective physical examination creates an individualized plan for a patient seeking BA. The astute surgeon is aware, and communicates to the patient, that not only will BA affect the size of the breast, but also the overall gland shape and position of the NAC. After any aesthetic breast procedure, the breast will continue to age and patients should be warned that further procedures may be necessary in the future if they desire restoration of a youthful breast.

Patient's seeking BA have often invested a large amount of time in thinking about their ideal breast size and shape. They have researched implants, planes of implant placement, and incisions, and have explored the experiences of friends, family, and internet bloggers before seeing a plastic surgeon in consultation. It is not uncommon for a BA candidate to have met with other plastic surgeons in consultation and continue to search until she finds the "right" surgeon who has the skill, results, reputation, or price point that fits with her expectations. The artful history taker will be able to elicit this and tailor a unique surgical plan using all the information available. Clinical intuition and experience of the surgeon cannot be underestimated. Unrealistic expectations or indications of psychologic instability should raise a red flag to the provider; surgeons should have a low threshold for a second or even third consultation prior to offering surgery, if at all.

The main goal is to increase the volume of the breast and centralize the nipple on the breast mound. The breast mound should reside completely or largely above the inframammary fold (IMF) although this can vary with age. Upper pole fullness and specifically superomedial fullness is generally desired. Asking a patient to bring photographs of augmented breasts that she finds desirable and undesirable can help the surgeon understand the patient's aesthetic expectation for her own breasts. When a potential BA candidate mentions a "natural look," it is important to inquire further and clarify what characteristics of the breast create a "natural look" in the eyes of the patient. Often, but not always, it is equated with a sloped upper pole that transition to the curve of the lower two-thirds of the breast. Some women may desire a convex upper pole and have an "augmented" look that is "natural" to them. Clear communication of expectations of outcomes in and out of clothes is also important.

A thorough medical and surgical history should be obtained. Candidates should be asked about their current bra size and desired cup size. Patients with a history of prior BA and complications necessitating a revision are different than those seeking a primary BA. For example, it would be useful to know if a patient has had a previous breast reduction surgery or radiation because of breast cancer. Additionally, it is important for a surgeon to understand a patient's hobbies and interests. Patients who are highly athletic and perform weight training or yoga for example may be less amenable to submuscular placement of an implant because of animation deformity or changes to the pectoralis muscle.

Physical examination before BA should be systematic and include an assessment of the chest wall. The chest wall is the foundation upon which a prosthetic device will sit, and chest wall asymmetries or abnormalities recognized preoperatively can allow for better operative correction. This is especially true in women who have a history of congenital chest wall abnormalities or scoliosis. Standard measurements before BA include base width (BW), sternal notch to nipple distance (SN-N), nipple to inframammary fold (N-IMF), NAC diameter, and internipple distance (Figure 55.1). Base width

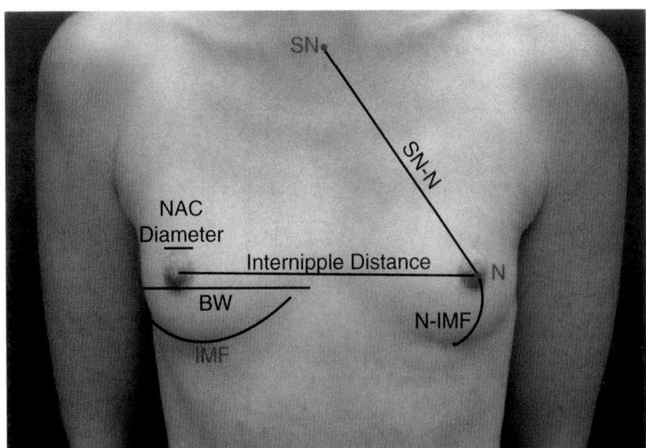

FIGURE 55.1. Key landmarks and measurements for breast augmentation and mastopexy. For both breasts, the sternal notch (SN), nipple (N), and inframammary fold (IMF) are marked. The sternal notch to nipple (SN-N) distance and the nipple to inframammary fold (N-IMF), and internipple distance are key metrics for analyzing nipple position and assessing symmetry between sides. The BW is a key measure for determining the appropriate transverse dimension of a breast implant and chest wall diameter. The nipple-areola complex (NAC) dimensions can affect incision design, particularly for a periareolar or circumvertical mastopexy and may contribute to asymmetry between sides.

can be measured from the medial aspect of the breast footprint to the anterior axillary fold. Tissue quality should also be assessed. This can be done by measuring the pinch thickness of the breast, particularly in the upper pole where involution can be easily appreciated. Generally, 2 cm of pinch thickness is considered the minimum necessary for placement of an implant in the subglandular or subfacial plane. Patients with less than 2 cm of pinch thickness may be better candidates for implant placement behind the pectoralis muscle. The interface between the skin and the breast parenchyma should also be evaluated, as postpartum women or patients with poor dermis due to massive weight loss may have skin that very easily glides over the underlying breast parenchyma. The lower pole of the breast can be constricted in patients with micromastia or mild tuberous breast deformity. Lowering of the IMF and recruitment of upper abdominal skin may be warranted in these patients and should be considered during the evaluation. An assessment of the width of the sternum is a nuance that can help the surgeon talk to a patient about expected superomedial fullness and interbreast distance that will likely persist after augmentation. This distance can be decreased and even lead to symmastia when the implant is placed subglandularly, but is less likely with submuscular placement because the medial pectoralis muscle attachments are left intact and prevent medial migration.

According to current epidemiologic studies, one in eight women will get breast cancer. Women with augmented breasts are at no increased risk of breast cancer compared to women with nonaugmented breasts. There is no difference in breast cancer survival rates among women with and without augmented breasts.[2] Women with a history of breast augmentation undergo screening mammography with special implant-displaced or Eklund views to better assess the tissue anterior to the implant.[3] The sensitivity is increased with ultrasound (US) or magnetic resonance imaging (MRI). When silicone implants were reintroduced into the market in 2006, the Food and Drug Administration (FDA) recommended screening with MRI for silent ruptures 3 years after placement and then every 2 years thereafter. For women desiring breast augmentation, routine mammographic screening should be performed or reviewed if indicated preoperatively using the US Preventative Services Task Force guidelines based on age over 40 and risk.[4]

Assessment of the NAC relative to the IMF is a common way to assess breast ptosis (**Figure 55.2**). In general, patients who have visible breast skin below the NAC (pseudoptosis or grade I and II ptosis) on a frontal view may be candidates for BA alone. Patients who seek BA who have no visible breast skin below the NAC on a frontal view (grade III ptosis) likely need a mastopexy as well to reposition the NAC on the breast mound.

The location of the breast and its footprint on the chest should be evaluated preoperatively during the consultation. There are several ways to make this assessment. Hall-Findlay describes that a patient can be "high" or "low" breasted based on the location of the breast on the chest wall relative to the clavicle and/or humerus.[5] For example, a patient with an IMF at the junction of the middle and distal thirds of the humerus may be considered "low" breasted whereas another with the IMF at the middle of the humerus may be considered "high" breasted.

The location of the pectoralis muscle relative to the breast mound and the IMF should also be assessed. In some women, the pectoralis major muscle and anterior axillary fold are well defined. The pectoralis major's inferior attachments can be above or below the NAC and at or above the IMF. This can be particularly meaningful when thinking about how a prosthetic device will affect the upper breast border if the implant is placed submuscularly versus subglandularly. For example, a low breasted patient with a pectoralis major muscle attachment that is higher than the NAC may not benefit from subpectoral placement of the breast because the implant will ride high behind the pectoral muscle whereas the NAC will remain in a lower position and not be centered on the implant and augmented breast mound.

Patients being evaluated for BA with fat alone or composite BA with fat and an implant should be evaluated for potential donor sites for fat grafting. Common areas include the abdomen, flanks and medial thighs. Finding suitable donor sites and adequate fat can be challenging in women with a low body mass index (BMI) who also have micromastia.

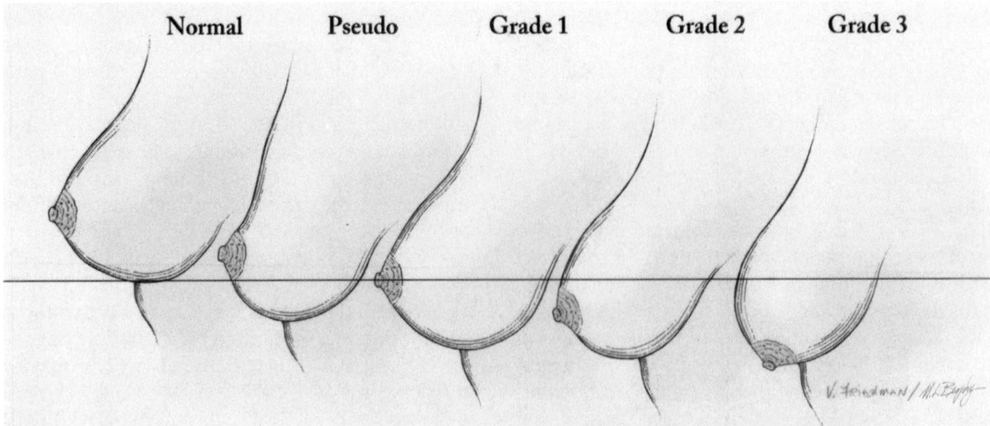

FIGURE 55.2. Grades of breast ptosis based on the position of the gland and nipple relative to the inframammary fold. (From Qureshi AA, Myckatyn TM, Tenenbaum MM. Madtopexy and mastopexy-augmentation. *Aesthet Surg J*. 2018;38:374-384.)

Standardized preoperative photographs should be obtained as a way to document and review anatomy and asymmetries with the patient. Many times, differences between breasts that are not visible to the patient in the mirror can be more apparent in a photograph. Asymmetries noted preoperatively may require correction, can persist, or become more noticeable after a BA. The impact of asymmetries on the operative plan should be discussed with the patient. Three-dimensional imaging has emerged as a newer technology that can also aid with educating patients.[6] Newer virtual reality simulation technologies have also enhanced the preoperative consultation.

Augmentation With Implants

Breast implants for augmentation vary in composition, shape, and shell texturing. Implants are filled with either saline or silicone. However, even saline filled implants have a silicone outer shell. During the FDA moratorium on silicone implants in the 1990s, saline implants were the only implants available for use. This was reversed in 2002 when silicone implants again became available for use in BA and breast reconstruction largely from combine efforts of plastic surgeons and industry. Silicone implants are considered "off label" when used in women less than 22 years old per the FDA.

Just how different saline and silicone implants feel is subjective. A major difference besides cost and feel is that saline and silicone implants differ in how a device rupture is detected. Regardless of type or manufacturer, implant rupture is inevitable. Detection of a rupture in saline implants is fairly straightforward as deflation of the implant and an obvious decrease in an augmented breast indicates a rupture. Silicone implants, including the modern fifth generation cohesive gel implants, differ from the first silicone implants in the 1960s in that the amount of cross-linking of the silicone has increased. First and second generation silicone ruptures led to free floating silicone in the pocket leading to inflammation and silicone granuloma formation. Ruptures of the current fifth generation implants are very different. Silicone ruptures with cohesive gel implants can be detected on mammogram but more often require MRI to confirm a suspected rupture. Often delayed capsular contracture can be due to a silent rupture of a highly cohesive gel implant.

Implants can be anatomically shaped or round devices. Different manufacturers have implants of both types with variable dimensions including height, width, projection, and volume. For a round device, height and width will be the same. Therefore, for a given base width with a round device, an implant can vary in volume and projection. Anatomic implants will have variable height, width, volume, and projection and hence, they have many more permutations. This variability and plethora of implant options help the plastic surgeon to customize the BA and even choose different devices for each breast to correct asymmetries.

Whether shaped or round implants have a different look is controversial. Some studies have shown that it is not possible to accurately detect a shaped versus round implant in the submuscular plan intraoperatively.[7] Proponents of each type of implant may argue that a round implant has a more round superomedial curve whereas an anatomic implant has a more teardrop look when placed in the subglandular or subfascial plan. Additionally, anatomic implants have been argued to have unique uses in breast reconstruction and tuberous breast deformity, though this is debated.

The outer shell of an implant can be either smooth or textured. Textured devices offered by the various implant manufacturers are differentiated by the proprietary methods used to texture the device and surface texture characteristics. Macrotextured devices are characterized by heterogeneously arranged pores with a diameter of 600 to 800 μm and a depth of 150 to 200 μm. Microtextured devices possess a more uniform pore distribution whose diameters range from 70 to 150 μm with a depth of 40 to 100 μm. Pore size and distribution of other textured implant brands run intermediate to the micro- and macrotextured devices. Surface area, pore size, and distribution may play a role in soft tissue integration with the breast implant surface, the organization of myofibroblasts and matrix proteins, and potential for accumulation of bacterial biofilms.[8-10] Textured devices increase friction between the implant and the surrounding tissues that encompass an implant. Anytime a foreign body is placed into a cavity, whether a prosthetic hip in a hip joint or a chin implant in the face, a capsule forms around the device and it happens in the breast around a breast implant. Textured devices have lower rates of capsular contracture, or the formation of a capsule that leads to deformity and/or pain in the breast following BA. This is particularly true when a textured implant is placed in a subglandular or subfascial plane. Textured devices are thought to be less likely to migrate beyond the dissected pocket, but recent data with anatomic, textured devices have demonstrated that even these implants can have rotation and malposition necessitating reoperation.[11] Currently, anatomic implants are all textured devices. Round devices can come as either textured or smooth.

Incisions and Planes for Implant Placement

The implant in BA can be placed in different planes using a number of incisions for exposure. Options for planes of implant placement include subglandular, subfascial, submuscular, and dual-plane (Figure 55.3). The subglandular plane is below the breast parenchyma but above the fascia of the pectoralis major muscle. The subfascial plane is below the fascia of the pectoralis muscle and above the muscle itself and is the same plane used by the breast surgeons when they perform mastectomies. The submuscular plane is below the pectoralis muscle superiorly and inferiorly below the pectoralis muscle fascia as it interdigitates with the rectus muscle fascia

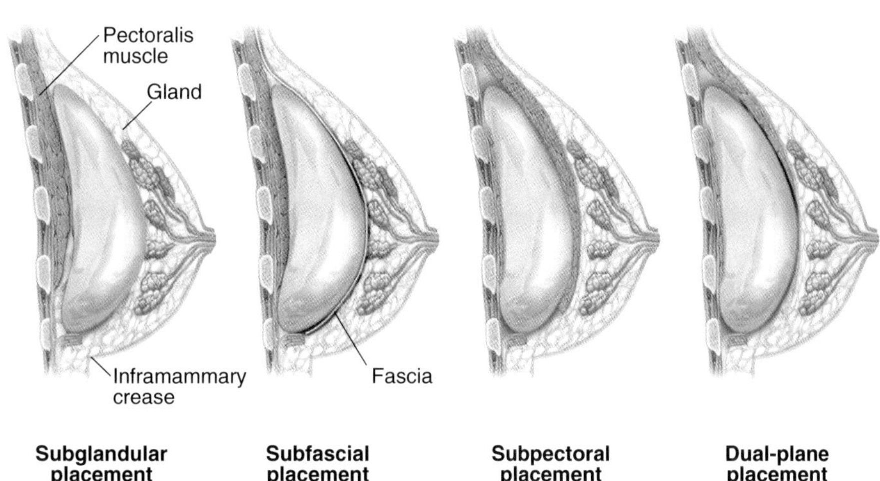

FIGURE 55.3. Options for planes of placement of the breast implant include subglandular, subfascial, subpectoral, and dual-plane.

BREAST

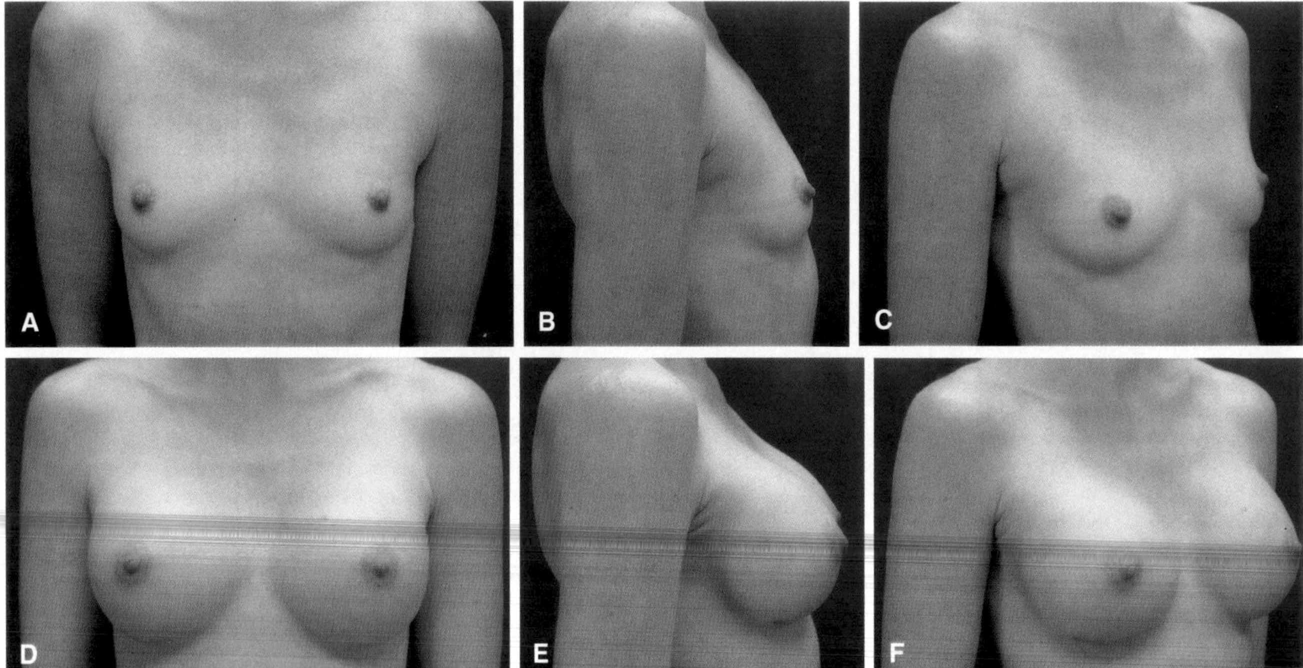

FIGURE 55.4. **A–C.** Preoperative photographs of a 29-year-old woman with micromastia, and minimal asymmetry in good health for breast augmentation. Three-dimensional image simulation in addition to tissue-based planning was performed to facilitate implant selection. Bilateral 330 cc moderate profile smooth round silicone breast implants were placed using a submuscular approach with inferior release of the pectoralis muscle but fascial preservation. **D–F.** Two-year postoperative results.

(Figure 55.4). This is also sometimes referred to as a retropectoral pocket. Dual-plane breast augmentations take advantage of having superior pole coverage with muscle with variable lower pole coverage with breast parenchyma. Dual-plane breast augmentations, as graded I, II, and III, vary by the amount of pectoralis muscle release inferiorly and subsequent amount of contact between the implant and breast parenchyma inferiorly.

Incision options for BA include IMF, periareolar, and transaxillary approaches. The IMF incision is placed in the desired IMF crease, which may be below the native IMF if the IMF is going to be lowered in a BA. Periareolar incisions are made along the junction of the areola and the breast skin. Transaxillary incisions are made in the hair-bearing region of the axilla.

Complications

Delayed seromas with or without an associated mass should raise suspicion for breast implant-associated anaplastic large cell lymphoma (BIA-ALCL). In line with current National Comprehensive Cancer Network Guidelines, suspicious fluid should be sent with fine needle aspiration and tested as BIA-ALCL fluid is CD30 positive and anaplastic large cell lymphoma kinase (ALK) negative prior to surgical intervention.[12] A PET-CT scan is recommended to visualize a suspicious seroma or mass. Treatment always requires complete capsulectomy, and depending on stage of disease, it may also need adjuvant chemotherapy or immunotherapy. This is a rare disease process, and the understanding of its etiology is rapidly evolving.

Revisions rates for BA are largely surgeon dependent. The threshold to perform a revision because of patient complaints or dissatisfaction varies by surgeon. Database studies of complications after BA have shown rates of less than 1% to 2% for hematoma and less than 1% for infection and deep vein thrombosis/pulmonary embolism (DVT/PE).[13] Capsular contracture rates from long-term studies demonstrate variability based on implant manufacturer.

Capsular Contracture

Capsule formation around an implant in any part of the body is a reaction to a foreign body. When the body forms a capsule that distorts the breast and/or causes pain in the breast following BA, this is known as capsular contracture. The Baker classification system is a routine method of categorizing capsular contracture in patients with BA (**Table 55.1**). It relies on physical examination to assess how soft the augmented breast and whether or not the patient reports pain. Applanation tonometry, adopted for measuring intramammary compliance, and ultrasound elastography represent more modern and quantitative, but less widely adopted techniques for assessing capsular contracture.[14,15]

The etiology of capsular contracture is multifactorial and may differ based on whether capsule contracture occurs early or late. Capsular contractures can occur "early" within 1 year of placement or in a delayed fashion several years later. Historically, smooth devices placed in the subglandular plane have had the highest rates of capsular contracture.

Patients with grade III or IV capsular contracture with or without concomitant silicone rupture or silicone granulomas, and those with asymmetry requesting a revision procedure will require operative management. Treatment involves either open capsulectomy or capsulotomy. These can be challenging operations due to silicone rupture, scar formation, thin tissues, and highly vascularized tissue from chronic inflammation. Depending on the plane of the BA, removal of the capsule off the breast parenchyma and/or chest wall can be difficult and techniques including tumescence of the capsule can aid in identifying the correct plane of dissection. Posterior capsulectomy or removal of the capsule of the chest wall should be done with caution

TABLE 55.1. BAKER CLASSIFICATION SYSTEM FOR CAPSULAR CONTRACTURE

Baker Grade	Physical Examination	Patient Report of Pain
I	Soft	No pain
II	Palpable, minimal firmness	No pain
III	Easily palpable, moderate firmness	Pain
IV	Firm, distorted	Painful

as the tissue can be thin and can lead to inadvertent penetration into the thoracic cavity leading to a pneumothorax. Some advocate partial removal or curettage of the posterior capsule for this reason. Closed capsulotomy that involved external, manual compression to break through the capsule is no longer recommended due to risk of implant rupture or possible hematoma formation and incomplete management of the problematic capsule. Medical therapy with leukotriene inhibitors has shown some benefit in preventing and improving capsular contracture.[16] Intraluminal steroids and pocket irrigation with steroids were once performed, but no longer are common practice due to risk of implant rupture, wound dehiscence, and atrophy of tissues. Recurrent capsular contracture often requires placement in an alternative plane or neosubpectoral pocket after a capsulectomy.[17] Acellular dermal matrices (ADM) have also been used in recalcitrant cases of capsular contracture to create an interface between implant and breast tissue.[18]

Implant Rupture

Implant rupture can occur regardless of implant fill material. Saline rupture can easily be identified by unilateral deflation and breast asymmetry that occurs suddenly. This can sometimes be preceded by trauma. Silicone rupture can present with the presence of silicone granulomas or can be silent and diagnosed on mammography or MRI. Rupture can be intracapsular or extracapsular. Treatment of rupture often requires removal of one or both implants and any ruptured material in the case of silicone rupture with or without capsulectomy or capsulotomy. This is can be followed by replacement with a new implant.

Augmentation With Fat and Flaps

BA can be performed with fat grafting or autologous tissue. Fat grafting alone can be used to augment a breast. However, with unpredictable rates of long term fat graft survival, it may be difficult to reliably augment a breast to a desired cup size. More than one surgery or round of fat grafting may be required to achieve a patient's goals. Composite BA is a procedure in which implant-based BA is combined with fat grafting, often placed in the superior pole to blunt the transition between native tissue and the implant. Fat can be placed laterally and inferiorly when the soft tissue envelope is thin to reduce visible rippling or mask implant palpability. Autologous BA with flaps are common in patients who have had a massive weight loss because they have a paucity of breast tissue, which is often atrophic because of major fluctuations in weight. A number of perforator flaps based on intercostals have been used for this purpose.

MASTOPEXY

Mastopexy focuses on changing the shape of the breast to one that appears youthful and beautiful; it also addresses descent of the NAC relative to the IMF.[19] Aging, hormonal changes associated with pregnancy, and weight loss can all affect the skin envelope and breast parenchyma. By addressing the outer lamella of the breast (the skin) and/or the inner lamella of the breast (the parenchyma), the discrepancy between the skin and breast tissue can be reduced. Similar to BA, mastopexy is a very common aesthetic breast surgery and can often be combined with augmentation as a single or two-staged procedure. One of the most litigated plastic surgery operations, mastopexy-augmentation, has increasingly become safer and more acceptable to well-informed patients.

Preoperative Assessment

Analysis of the breasts and chest wall for mastopexy is similar to that described earlier for BA. An assessment and documentation of breast ptosis is essential. The density of the breasts and superior pole involution should be assessed. Additionally, the interaction between skin and breast parenchyma must be critically evaluated as this may help the surgeon counsel the patient on whether mastopexy alone will help achieve the patient's results or whether the addition of an implant will also help restore shape, structure, and volume to the breast.

If the planned procedure is a secondary mastopexy or mastopexy-augmentation, an attempt to obtain previous operative reports should be made. Scars and examination can provide a roadmap, but operative notes can help provide information to reduce the risk of complications from compromised blood supply to the NAC or parenchyma.

Surgical Approaches

Three major categories of surgical approaches for mastopexy have been described: periareolar, vertical, and Wise pattern.[19] A paradigm shift in mastopexy took place when Benelli demonstrated that skin only mastopexies were not as durable as mastopexies that address the skin and parenchyma by redistributing the parenchyma.[20] Plastic surgeons now understand that by addressing both the outer lamella (skin) and inner lamella (parenchyma), more durable and predictable changes can be achieved in the ptotic, involuted breast.

Periareolar mastopexies can be used in patients who have grade I or II ptosis, nipple asymmetry, or widened areola (Figure 55.5). This technique can be used to elevate the nipple no more than 2 cm with an eccentrically designed oval. A variation of the periareolar mastopexy is the crescentic mastopexy in which a crescent is designed only superior to the existing areola. The periareolar mastopexy hides the scar along the areolar-breast junction. Removing skin in a concentric pattern can, however, flatten and reduce breast projection. Scar widening and eventual widening of the areola can occur, but some have advocated the use of a barbed or permanent suture to control this. If there is circumferential full thickness violation of the dermis, decreased nipple sensitivity may occur.

Vertical mastopexies have evolved from reduction mammoplasty techniques described by Lassus, Peixoto, Pitanguy, and Lejour to mention a few.[19] The underlying premise of vertical techniques is to both incorporate ptosis correction with excision of glandular material using a periareolar approach with a vertical component in line with the breast meridian (Figure 55.6). This technique can be used for all grades of breast ptosis. The short-scar periareolar inferior-pedicle

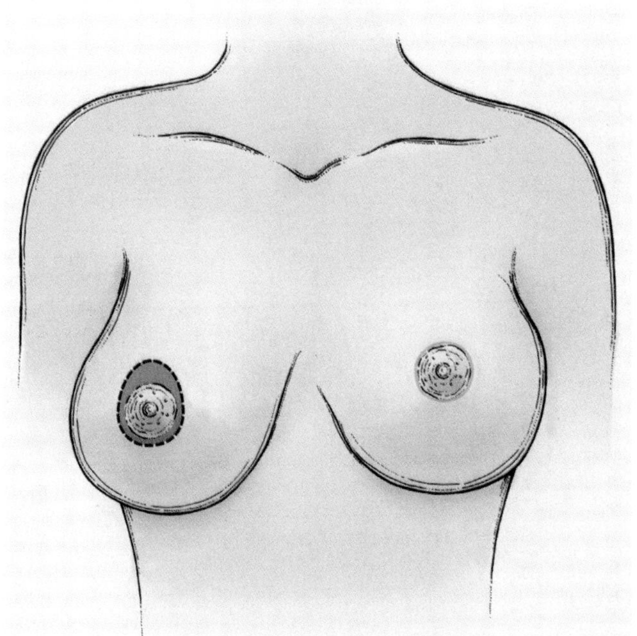

FIGURE 55.5. Periareolar mastopexy incision placement and final scar location. (From Qureshi AA, Myckatyn TM, Tenenbaum MM. Madtopexy and mastopexy-augmentation. *Aesthet Surg J.* 2018;38:374-384.)

BREAST

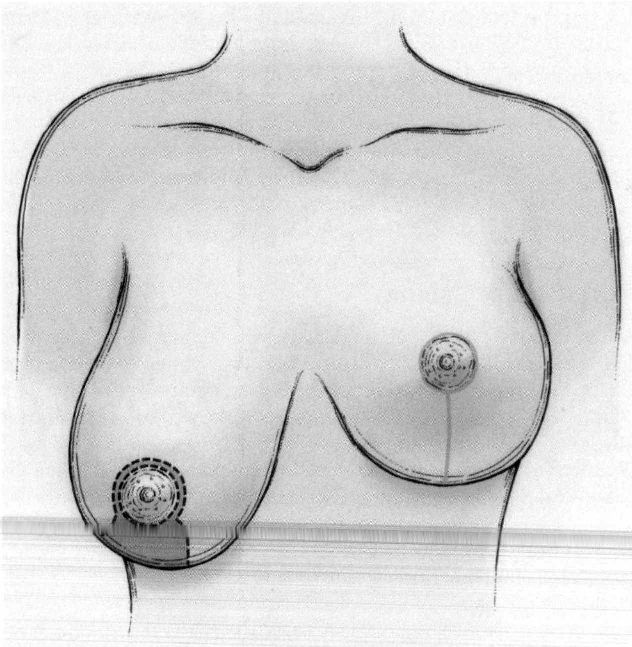

FIGURE 55.6. Vertical mastopexy incision placement and final scar location. (From Qureshi AA, Myckatyn TM, Tenenbaum MM. Madtopexy and mastopexy-augmentation. *Aesthet Surg J*. 2018;38:374-384.)

reduction (SPAIR) and Hall-Findlay mastopexy techniques are the two vertical mastopexies with the highest surgeon satisfaction.[21]

Hammond popularized the SPAIR mastopexy that relies on the fourth intercostal perforator or inferior pedicle for blood supply to the nipple.[22] It involves a periareolar closure in a pin-wheel or interlocking pattern, sometimes with a permanent suture. Suspension sutures to the pectoralis fascia can be used to elevate the breast onto a higher position on the chest wall, though the durability of such techniques is hotly debated. The redundant skin inferiorly can be excised in a "J" or "T" pattern. Because weight remains in the inferior portion of the breast, bottoming out remains a shortcoming. The periareolar closure can widen or have pleating that persists. This technique is not typically complemented with implant placement.

The Hall-Findlay vertical mastopexy most commonly uses the superomedial or medial pedicles for the NAC based on the second and third intercostal perforators, respectively (Figure 55.7).[23] Different from the SPAIR technique that preserves the inferior pedicle, the inferior pole of breast tissue is excised in the Hall-Findlay technique. The medial and lateral pillars are then sutured together, and this provides structural support and buttresses the elevated NAC. By removing weight from the inferior pole of the breast, less gravitational pull will be exerted on the raised NAC and breast. Similar to the SPAIR technique, inferior skin redundancy can be excised as a "J" or "T." An implant can be placed in the subglandular, subfascial or submuscular planes without concern for blood supply to the NAC as the second and/or third intercoastal perforators travel superficially in the gland and remain undisturbed by an augmentation.

In general, vertical mastopexies create an inverted breast shape at the end of the procedure with exaggerated upper pole fullness and a sloped inferior pole. Patients should be counseled that it can take weeks to months for the breast and/or implant to settle and for the breast to take on its final appearance.

The Wise-pattern or inverted-T mastopexy has been a powerful, traditional method for reducing the discrepancy between skin and breast parenchyma. It can be used for all types of ptosis but carries a large scar burden. It was first described in the 1950s by Wise when he developed templates for a skin only mastopexy. Since that time, the technique has evolved to include parenchymal redistribution and can be used with practically any pedicle for blood supply to the NAC. This versatility makes it popular among surgeons, as it is easily adapted from traditional Wise-pattern inferior pedicle reduction mammoplasty techniques. Final scars are along the areola, the vertical meridian of the breast, and along the IMF ending

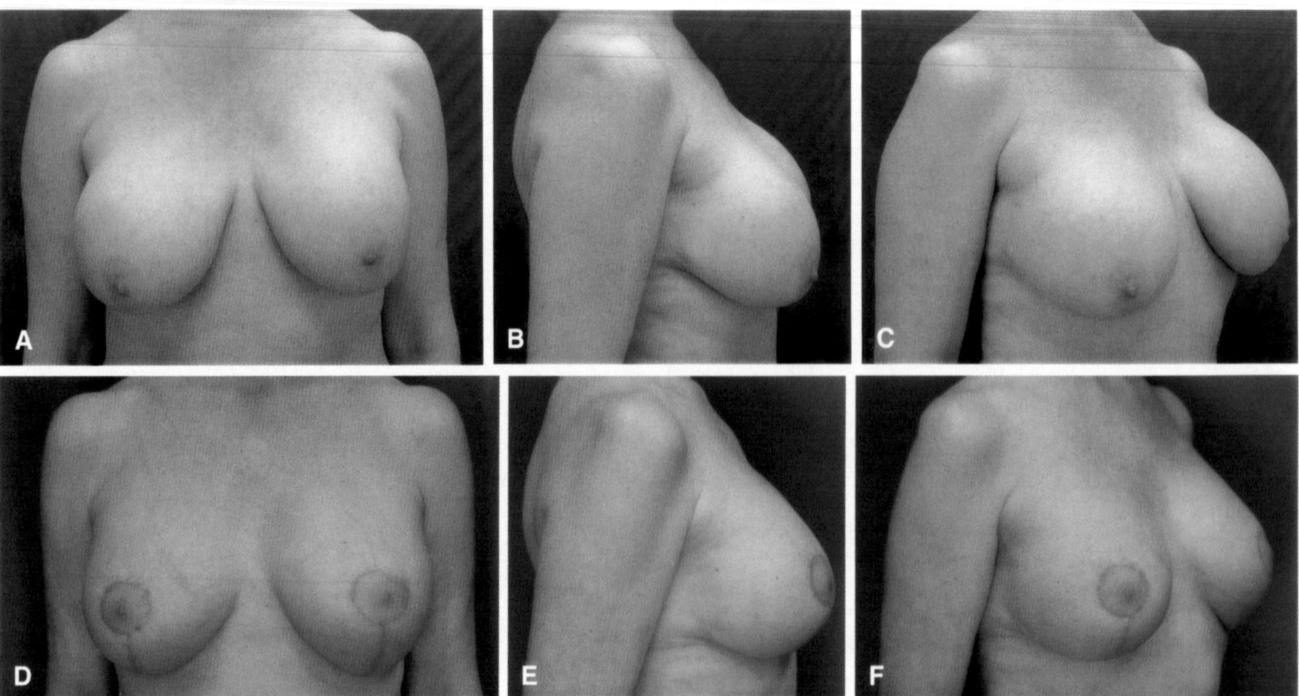

FIGURE 55.7. **A–C.** Preoperative photographs of a nonsmoking, healthy 51-year-old woman with ptosis and moderate asymmetry in which the right breast was more ptotic, had a lower inframammary fold, and was slightly larger than the left. She was interested in improving breast symmetry, shape, and nipple-areolar positioning. A Hall-Findlay vertical mastopexy was performed with a slight parenchymal reduction and more aggressive nipple-areolar elevation on the right. **D–F.** Six-month postoperative results.

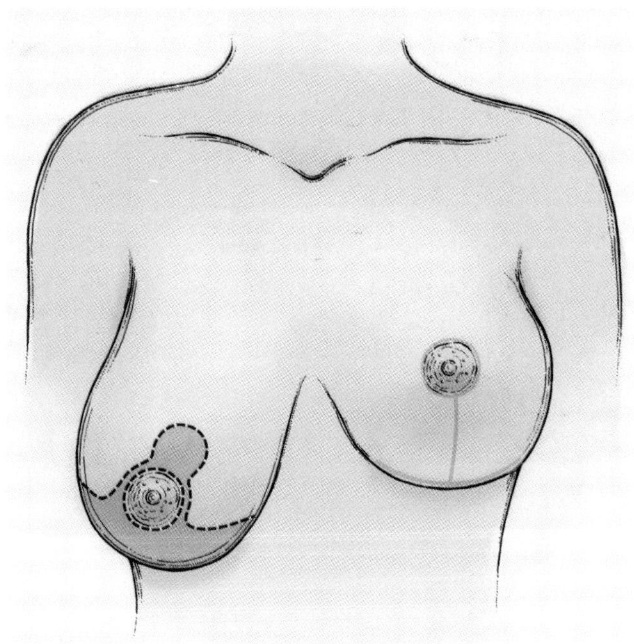

FIGURE 55.8. Wise-pattern or inverted-T mastopexy incision placement and final scar location. (From Qureshi AA, Myckatyn TM, Tenenbaum MM. Madtopexy and mastopexy-augmentation. *Aesthet Surg J*. 2018;38:374-384.)

up as an inverted-T or anchor pattern (Figure 55.8). This technique has the largest scar burden of any mastopexy method and can experience bottoming out when combined with an inferior pedicle.[21] An implant can be placed in the subglandular, subfascial, or submuscular plane depending on where the blood supply to the NAC is coming from.

Complications

Complications in mastopexy have been found to be around 1% in large database studies, with less than 1% rates for hematoma, infection, and DVT/PE.[13] Survey studies of plastic surgeons reporting complications found suture spitting, excess scarring, and bottoming out to be the most commonly reported complications.[21] Specifically, excess scarring was noted with the periareolar technique, suture spitting with the SPAIR technique, persistent asymmetry with the vertical technique, and bottoming out with the inverted-T or Wise-pattern mastopexy. Revision rates have been reported to be as high as 50% in periareolar approaches.

MASTOPEXY-AUGMENTATION

Single or two-staged mastopexy-augmentation is a powerful way to reshape and add volume to a breast (Figure 55.9). The surgeon must be mindful that there are competing forces at play during this procedure. Mastopexy addresses the skin envelope and shape and often requires removal of skin and parenchyma. In an augmentation, volume is being added or redistributed either with autologous breast tissue, implants, or fat. Caution and planning must be applied as the surgeon keeps in mind the blood supply to the NAC and plane of augmentation. Tension-free closure increases the likelihood of a well-appearing scar.

Single-stage mastopexy-augmentation with implants was once considered a controversial and risky procedure, highlighted in 2003 when Spear published "Augmentation/Mastopexy: Surgeon, Beware." Although first described in the 1970s, the safety of single-stage mastopexy-augmentation gained traction with large experiences by Stevens and Calobrace et al. who reported revision rates between 8.6% and 23.2%, which was less than the 100% two-operation rate when mastopexy-augmentation was not performed as a single-stage procedure.[24,25] Other studies demonstrated the safety of blood supply and perfusion to the NAC when mastopexy-augmentation was

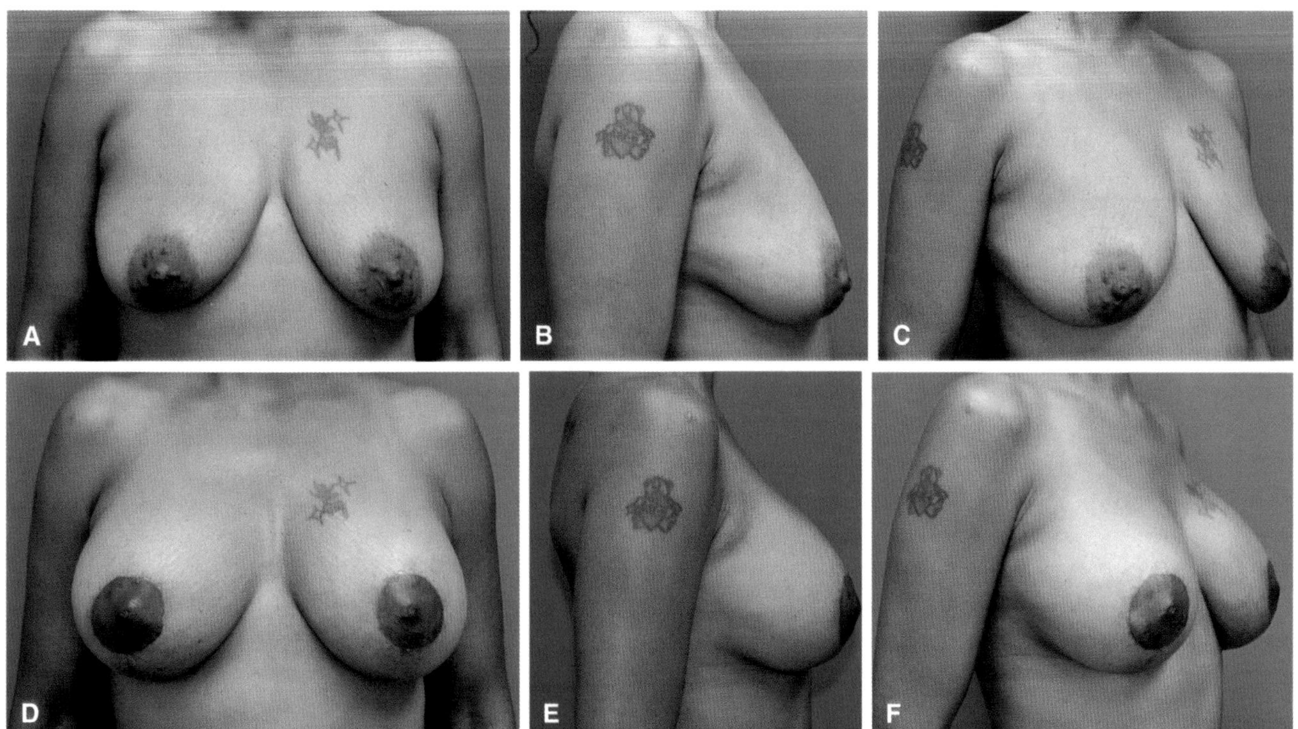

FIGURE 55.9. **A–C.** Preoperative photographs of a nonsmoking, healthy 43-year-old woman with grade 1 ptosis who desired increased upper pole fullness, overall breast volume, and elevation of the nipple-areola complex. The patient had reasonable expectations and understood that simultaneous breast augmentation-mastopexy is associated with a higher revision rate than when either procedure is performed alone. She underwent a simultaneous augmentation-mastopexy with bilateral 385 cc moderate profile round textured breast implants placed using a type 2 biplanar approach. **D–F.** One-year postoperative results.

performed with an implant.[26] Meta-analyses of reports of single-stage mastopexy-augmentation have found an overall complication rate of 13% with a reoperation rate of 11%.[27]

Two-stage mastopexy-augmentation can also be performed. Some surgeons prefer this method because it allows them to address one issue in the first stage, namely shape or volume and then address the other at a second operation, if even necessary. However, a staged approach commits a patient to two operations and recoveries. There is no consensus of whether augmentation or mastopexy should be performed in a two-staged plan.

Mastopexy-augmentation has been found to have a complication rate of less than 2% in large database studies with rates of less than 1% for hematoma, infection, and DVT/PE.[28]

ACKNOWLEDGMENTS

The authors thank Drs. W. Grant Stevens, Andrea E. Van Pelt, and Adrian M. Przybyla, who wrote the chapter on mastopexy and mastopexy-augmentation and Dr. Steven A. Teitelbaum who wrote the chapter on breast augmentation in the 7th edition of this book.

REFERENCES

1. American Society of Plastic Surgeons. *Cosmetic Surgery National Data Bank Statistics*. 2016:1-26.
2. Bryant H, Brasher P. Breast implants and breast cancer—reanalysis of a linkage study. *N Engl J Med*. 1995;332(23):1535-1539.
3. Eklund GW, Busby RC, Miller SH, Job JS. Improved imaging of the augmented breast. *AJR Am J Roentgenol* 1988;151(3):469-473.
4. Siu AL; US Preventive Services Task Force. Screening for breast cancer: U.S. Preventive Services Task force recommendation statement. *Ann Intern Med*. 2016;164(4):279-296.
5. Hall-Findlay EJ. The three breast dimensions: analysis and effecting change. *Plast Reconstr Surg*. 2010;125(6):1632-1642.
This is an important article on understanding the dimensions of the breast. It describes whether different parameters of the breast can be changed and how.
6. Overschmidt B, Qureshi A, Parikh RP, et al. A prospective evaluation of three dimensional image simulation: patient-reported outcomes and mammometrics in primary breast augmentation. *Plast Reconstr Surg*. 2018;142(2):133e-144e.
7. Hidalgo DA, Weinstein AL. Intraoperative comparison of anatomical versus round implants in breast augmentation: a randomized controlled trial. *Plast Reconstr Surg*. 2017;139(3):587-596.
8. Wolfram D, Rainer C, Niederegger H, et al. Cellular and molecular composition of fibrous capsules formed around silicone breast implants with special focus on local immune reactions. *J Autoimmun*. 2004;23(1):81-91.
9. Maxwell GP, Scheflan M, Spear S, et al. Benefits and limitations of macrotextured breast implants and consensus recommendations for optimizing their effectiveness. *Aesthet Surg J*. 2014;34(6):876-881.
10. Brown T. Breast implant-associated anaplastic large cell lymphoma in Australia and New Zealand: high-surface-area textured implants are associated with increased risk. *Plast Reconstr Surg*. 2018;141(1):176e-177e.
11. Sieber DA, Stark RY, Chase S, et al. Clinical evaluation of shaped gel breast implant rotation using high-resolution ultrasound. *Aesthet Surg J*. 2017;37(3):290-296.
12. Clemens MW, Horwitz SM. NCCN Consensus Guidelines for the diagnosis and management of breast implant-associated anaplastic large cell lymphoma. *Aesthet Surg J*. 2017;37(3):285-289.
13. Gupta V, Yeslev M, Winocour J, et al. Aesthetic breast surgery and concomitant procedures: incidence and risk factors for major complications in 73,608 cases. *Aesthet Surg J*. 2017;37(5):515-527.
This large database study provides invaluable information about complications in aesthetic breast surgery.
14. Prantl L, Englbrecht MA, Schoeneich M, et al. Semiquantitative measurements of capsular contracture with elastography: first results in correlation to Baker Score. *Clin Hemorheol Microcirc*. 2014;58(4):521-528.
15. Moore JR. Applanation tonometry of breasts. *Plast Reconstr Surg*. 1979;63(1):9-12.
16. Graf R, Ascenco AS, Freitas Rda S, et al. Prevention of capsular contracture using leukotriene antagonists. *Plast Reconstr Surg*. 2015;136(5):592e-596e.
17. Maxwell GP, Gabriel A. The neopectoral pocket in revisionary breast surgery. *Aesthet Surg J*. 2008;28(4):463-467.
This is a seminal article for understanding operative management of capsular contracture and/or implant rupture. It describes a reproducible technique of managing the diseased capsular and creation of a new pocket for implant replacement.
18. Maxwell GP, Gabriel A. Acellular dermal matrix for reoperative breast augmentation. *Plast Reconstr Surg*. 2014;134(5):932-938.
19. Qureshi AA, Myckatyn TM, Tenenbaum MM. Mastopexy and mastopexy-augmentation. *Aesthet Surg J*. 2018;38(4):374-384.
This recent [illegible] types and approaches for mastopexy and mastopexy-augmentation.
20. Benelli L. A new periareolar mammoplasty: the "round block" technique. *Aesthet Plast Surg*. 1990;14(2):93-100.
21. Rohrich RJ, Gosman AA, Brown SA, Reisch J. Mastopexy preferences: a survey of board-certified plastic surgeons. *Plast Reconstr Surg*. 2006;118(7):1631-1638.
22. Hammond DC. Short scar periareolar inferior pedicle reduction (SPAIR) mammoplasty. *Plast Reconstr Surg*. 1999;103(3):890-901.
This landmark article describes the technique of Hammond in the SPAIR procedure.
23. Hall-Findlay EJ. Pedicles in vertical breast reduction and mastopexy. *Clin Plast Surg*. 2002;29(3):379-391.
This seminal article describes various pedicles and the technique used in a vertical mastopexy by Hall-Findlay.
24. Stevens WG, Macias LH, Spring M, et al. One-stage augmentation mastopexy: a review of 1192 simultaneous breast augmentation and mastopexy procedures in 615 consecutive patients. *Aesthet Surg J*. 2014;34(5):723-732.
This article describes a large series of single-stage mastopexy-augmentation and describes complications and safety profiles.
25. Calobrace MB, Herdt DR, Cothron KJ. Simultaneous augmentation/mastopexy: a retrospective 5-year review of 332 consecutive cases. *Plast Reconstr Surg*. 2013;131(1):145-156.
This article describes a large series of single stage mastopexy-augmentation and describes complications and safety profiles.
26. Swanson E. Safety of vertical augmentation-mastopexy: prospective evaluation of breast perfusion using laser fluorescence imaging. *Aesthet Surg J*. 2015;35(8):938-949.
27. Khavanin N, Jordan SW, Rambachan A, Kim JY. A systematic review of single-stage augmentation-mastopexy. *Plast Reconstr Surg*. 2014;134(5):922-931.
28. Winocour J, Gupta V, Kaoutzanis C, et al. Venous thromboembolism in the cosmetic patient: analysis of 129,007 patients. *Aesthet Surg J*. 2017;37(3):337-349.

QUESTIONS

1. A 45-year-old woman with whom had a gastric bypass performed 3 years ago has lost 125 lb and currently has a BMI of 29, which has been stable for a year. She is bothered by her grade III ptosis and involuted breasts. She presented for single-stage mastopexy-augmentation and a decision is made to perform a Wise-pattern mastopexy with retropectoral placement of a smooth, round silicone device. Which of the following is the most likely sequela of the procedure?
   a. Complete nipple necrosis
   b. Delayed seroma
   c. Implant rupture and silicone leak
   d. Lateral malpositioning of the implant
   e. Symmastia

2. A 33-year-old woman presents for evaluation of nipple asymmetry. She is bothered by the discrepancy between her NAC as the right is 4 cm and the left is 6 cm in width. The left nipple is also 1 cm lower than the right. Which of the following techniques is most suited to correct her asymmetry?
   a. Breast augmentation with implants
   b. Circumvertical mastopexy
   c. Free nipple grafting
   d. Inverted T-mastopexy
   e. Periareolar mastopexy

3. A 25-year-old woman presents for evaluation of bilateral breast augmentation. She is interested in a smooth, silicone round device and wants the implant to be placed underneath the breast but not the muscle. Which of the following is she at greatest risk based on the implant type and plane of placement?
   a. Animation deformity from the pectoralis muscle
   b. Capsular contracture
   c. Deflation and subsequent loss of volume
   d. Superior implant migration
   e. Widening of the areola

4. A 39-year-old woman with a history of bilateral breast augmentation with textured, silicone anatomic implants 7 years ago presents with asymmetric breast swelling of the left breast with no antecedent trauma. Ultrasound demonstrates a capsule with fluid in the periprosthetic space. Which of the following is the next appropriate step in management?
   a. Observation
   b. MRI study of both breasts
   c. Compression garment with repeat evaluation in 2 weeks
   d. Ultrasound guided aspiration of fluid and cytology tests for ALK and CD30
   e. Surgical exploration with explant and capsulectomy

5. A 62-year-old woman is dissatisfied with the appearance of the size and shape of her breasts. She currently wears a 32B bra and has grade III ptosis. A decision is made to perform a single-stage mastopexy-augmentation. Which of the following is the most likely complication after single-stage mastopexy-augmentation?
   a. Asymmetry
   b. Capsular contracture
   c. Poor scarring
   d. Recurrent ptosis
   e. Seroma

6. Which of the following best represents the existing Food and Drug Administration recommendation on screening for silent ruptures in silicone implants used for breast augmentation and/or reconstruction?
   a. MRI annually after placement
   b. MRI 2 years after placement and then every 2 years thereafter
   c. MRI 3 years after placement and then every 2 years thereafter
   d. MRI at 5 years and then as needed
   e. MRI only if palpable changes in silicone

1. **Answer: d.** Lateral malposition is a common problem seen in mastopexy-augmentation in the massive weight loss patient population. These patients have attenuated tissues and with placement under the muscle the implant can migrate laterally. Some have advocated the use of acellular dermal matrix or mesh support of the lateral buttress of the augmented breast. Complete nipple necrosis is a devastating and exceedingly rare complication. Delayed seroma can occur but its less likely than implant malposition. Implant rupture and silicone leaks can also occur but it is not higher in massive weight loss patients. Symmastia is unlikely with retropectoral implant placement because the medial pectoralis muscle fibers prevent medial migration of the implants.

2. **Answer: e.** This is a young woman with NAC asymmetry with regards to diameter as well as nipple position. A periareolar mastopexy can correct the NAC diameter discrepancy and also help elevate a nipple up to 2 cm. Breast augmentation is unlikely to address the underlying problem. The other mastopexy techniques can also correct the nipple asymmetry but are likely to carry a larger scar burden and alter the shape of the breast. Free nipple grafting involves completely removing the NAC and is not appropriate for correction of isolated nipple asymmetry.

3. **Answer: b.** Subglandularly placed smooth devices are at greatest risk for capsular contracture. This rate can be decreased by using a textured device or placing the implant partially or completely behind the muscle as in a dual-plane or retropectoral augmentation. Animation deformity can occur after placement of an implant placement behind, not in front of, the pectoralis muscle. Deflation is possible and common with saline not silicone implants. Superior implant migration is not a common complication. Areola can widen after an augmentation but that is not the greatest risk associated with this augmentation.

4. **Answer: d.** A delayed seroma after placement of a texture implant should raise suspicion for BIA-ALCL. The fluid should be aspirated and sent specifically for ALK and CD30 as the fluid will be ALK negative and CD30 positive. This is the first test that is done in the diagnostic work-up of BIA-ALCL and precedes surgical intervention. If a diagnosis of BIA-ALCL is made (CD30+/ALK-), then a PET-CT scan of the chest is indicated to further characterize the mass and fluid collection associated with the implant capsule and breast tissue. The case should be reported to the PROFILE Registry, sponsored by the Plastic Surgery Foundation, which tracks BIA-ALCL cases. Treatment will be dictated based on staging thereafter and will require surgical exploration with explant and complete capsulectomy. The capsule should be sent for pathology. Observation, further imaging, and compression garment placement are not appropriate next steps.

5. **Answer: d.** In a meta-analysis by Khavinin et al., pooled complication rates in aesthetic breast surgery were examined. Recurrent ptosis was the most commonly encountered complication after single stage mastopexy augmentation at 5.2%. This was followed by poor scarring (3.74%), capsular contracture (2.97%), asymmetry (2.94%), and seroma (1.42%).

6. **Answer: c.** The current FDA recommendation is for an MRI to be performed 3 years after placement and then every 2 years thereafter. The purpose of this is to identify silent ruptures of the implant that would otherwise go unnoticed.

CHAPTER 56 Breast Reduction

Paul H. Izenberg and Nicholas L. Berlin

KEY POINTS

- Integrate anatomic, functional, and aesthetic principles of plastic surgery.
- Perform thorough physical examination and document findings related to macromastia.
- Each technique has its own indications and limitations.
- Preoperative markings and planned resection are essential to achieve consistently good results.
- Appreciate the desired three-dimensional shape of the breast and underlying neurovascular structures throughout the operation.
- Counsel patients regarding risks for short-term and long-term complications.
- Address acute postoperative issues promptly to avoid long-term sequela.

The breast reduction procedure demands that the surgeon integrates anatomic, functional, and aesthetic principles into the design and execution of the operation. This chapter will emphasize principles and techniques for surgeons to achieve aesthetically and functionally pleasing results on a routine basis. There have been numerous techniques for breast reduction described in the literature over the past decades, each adding improvements in the reliability, perioperative risk reduction, and the enhancement of the final appearance. This chapter will not attempt to review all of the previously published data. Instead, we will emphasize techniques that have worked well for the senior author in the majority of clinical cases over 40 years of practicing plastic surgery.

RELEVANT ANATOMY AND PHYSIOLOGY

The breast is a subcutaneous structure with the strongest attachments to the chest wall medially along the sternum and at the inframammary (IM) fold. The primary blood supply originates from the internal mammary system and its arteries perforate the breast from deep to superficial. The venous drainage is located more superficially. Pedicle design should be based on dominant blood vessels for each specific technique for perfusion and sensation to the nipple-areolar complex (NAC) without compromising the intended shape and underlying breast parenchyma. The superior pedicle approach relies on internal mammary perforators from the second rib intercostal space, whereas the blood supply to the superomedial pedicle originates from both the second and third rib intercostal space. The blood supply to the inferior pedicle is based upon the fourth rib intercostal space. All skin and subcutaneous flaps rely on a network of subdermal venous drainage.

Lymphatic pathways parallel the venous drainage and include cutaneous, internal mammary, posterior intercostal, and axillary routes.

The lateral branches of the fourth, fifth, and sixth intercostal nerve supply the primary sensation to the NAC.[1,2] Deep and superficial sensory nerve branches allow any full thickness pedicle described to supply sensibility to the NAC without much impact, provided there is careful dissection, limited undermining, and the muscle fascia remains intact.

PATIENT HISTORY

The surgeon must carefully document any symptoms associated with enlarged breasts and attempted nonsurgical approaches to resolve these issues (physical therapy, pain medications, weight loss). Some findings that have been associated with macromastia include occipital headaches, neck pain, shoulder pain, midback and lower back issues, shoulder grooving, intertrigo or skin rashes, sensory changes including upper extremity paresthesias, difficulty participating in recreational activities, work, sleep, ill-fitting clothes, and anything else that may be attributed to breast hypertrophy. In addition, changes in breast size, as well as previous breast surgery, biopsies, scars, and asymmetries as noted by the patient should be recognized. Document skin lesions, changes with pregnancy, and a personal or family history of cancer (particularly if the family history includes members with breast, colon, prostate cancer or melanoma). If there is any concern for a genetic predisposition for breast cancer, it is recommended that the patient obtain a genetic consultation preoperatively. Consider the potential role of medications that may increase breast size (e.g., hormones, oral contraceptives, and steroids). Additionally, some systemic diseases may affect wound healing, especially related to skin vascularity (e.g., scleroderma, lupus, Raynaud disease, or other connective tissue disorders).

Preoperative mammography is not necessary for elective breast reduction before the age at which screening mammography is generally recommended. Unless there are concerning aspects of the patient's history or examination that call for further investigation, patients should follow the existing clinical practice guidelines that recommend annual screening for patients of certain age groups.[3]

PHYSICAL EXAMINATION

There are multiple aspects of the physical examination that need to be documented for patient selection and surgical planning (Figure 56.1). Furthermore, specific findings in the physical examination may anticipate potential limitations of the procedure in achieving the desired aesthetic result. Therefore, it can be helpful to integrate a standardized checklist into the clinical encounter.

- *Stature:* Height and weight are used to calculate total body surface area, which determines the amount of tissue that must be resected based on the Schnur or other scales required for insurance coverage.[4]
- *Shoulder grooving and hyperpigmentation:* These findings are typically minimal in younger patients with excellent skin.
- *Scoliosis and chest wall asymmetries:* These findings may disguise breast volume or width differences that become more apparent postoperatively and should be discussed with the patient in the preoperative setting.
- *Manubrial projection, pectus excavatum, and pectus carinatum:* Breast reduction will not change these abnormalities and may even make them more apparent postoperatively.
- *Soft tissue fullness of the anterior axillary folds and lateral chest:* Suction-assisted lipectomy (SAL) may reshape these areas. The effects may be limited in obese patients, especially in those patients with fullness extending posteriorly.
- *Deficient cephalic and medial breast:* Emphasize the challenges involved in filling these areas and limit the resection of breast parenchyma in these areas if already deficient.
- *Skin quality:* Document scars, skin lesions, striae, or dimpling with motion. Youthful and elastic skin appears to have a greater risk for hypertrophic scarring postoperatively. A vertical approach may reduce this risk.
- *IM fold asymmetries:* These may become more apparent to the patient once volume is removed.
- *Intertrigo:* Document open wounds, acne, hidradenitis suppurativa, or hyperpigmentation.

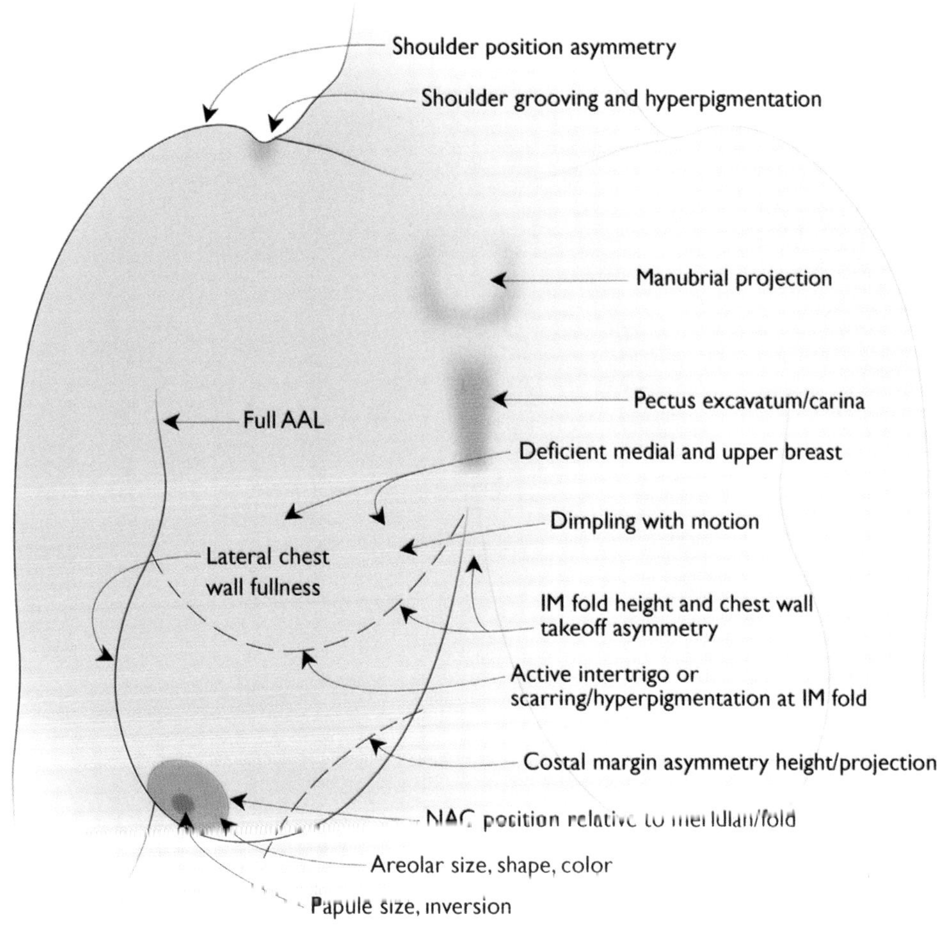

FIGURE 56.1. Key aspects of the physical examination for patients with macromastia. AAL, anterior axillary line; IM, inframammary; NAC, nipple-areolar complex.

- *NAC position:* Wide, narrow, or asymmetric nipple positioning can be corrected to a limited degree. Note the position of the NAC relative to:
  - The breast mound
  - The IM fold
  - Current and intended breast meridian
  - Sternal notch
  - Contralateral NAC
- *Papule:* Note the size and shape of the papule, including continuous or episodic inversion. It may not improve postoperatively. Complete nipple inversion may be dealt with at the time of the breast reduction if needed.
- *Areola:* Document abnormal size, shape, color, and symmetry relative to the contralateral side.
- *Costal margins:* Note any abnormal projection and asymmetries, because this may become more noticeable postoperatively.
- *Breast parenchyma:* Estimate any volume discrepancies, density (e.g., fatty versus fibrous), estimated volume to be removed, and presence or absence of masses.

PREOPERATIVE PHOTOGRAPHY

Standardized photography of women considering breast reduction is essential for insurance approval, for operative planning, and to identify preoperative asymmetries that may affect the final result (Figure 56.2).

- Anterior views with arms elevated and at the sides
- Lateral views with arms elevated and at the sides
- Optional: oblique views
- Posterior view (useful for documenting the presence of scoliosis, shoulder grooving, and chest wall asymmetries)

PREOPERATIVE MARKINGS

Each breast reduction technique is unique and requires variations in markings. We will review a general approach to initial markings. Surgeons generally have two decisions to make: the pedicle type and the pattern of skin resection.

Preoperative markings for keyhole pattern technique:

1. Ask patient to stand with arms at her sides.
2. Mark the IM fold and extend this marking medially to a point that is still hidden in the fold. In the midline (at a point corresponding approximately to the breast meridian that will be marked in the next step), make a small peak or upswing of about 1 cm, which may take some tension off the flaps (Figure 56.3). Curve the medial marking cephalically, as this incision tends to straighten postoperatively potentially resulting in visible scarring. Extend the IM fold markings laterally to a point that corresponds with the anterior axillary line, approximately where the breast ends. Avoid extending this mark toward the back chasing skin folds laterally.

BREAST

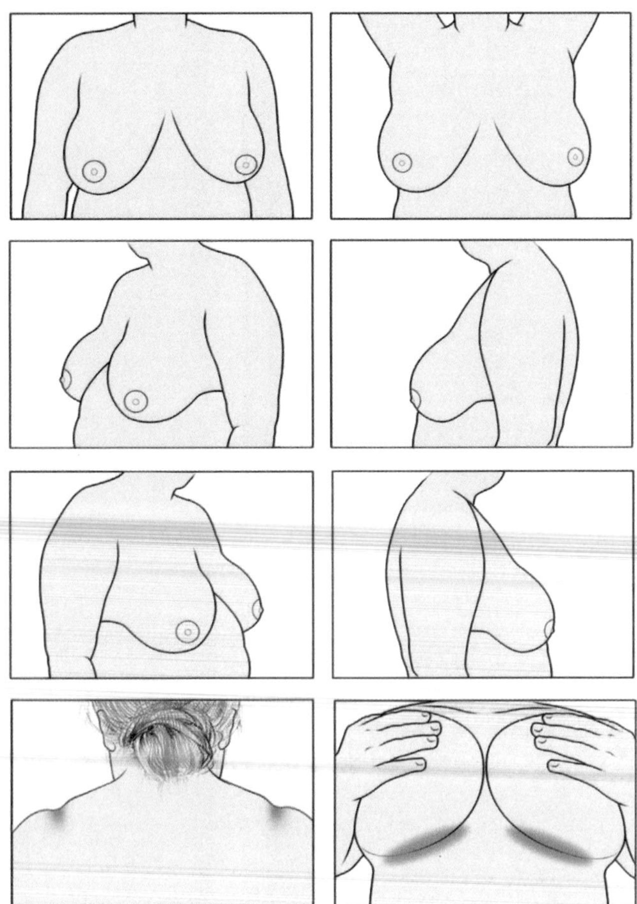

FIGURE 56.2. Suggested preoperative photography.

3. With a measuring tape hung around the neck or using the mid-clavicle, mark out the intended breast meridian bilaterally (this may not align with the current nipple position) (Figure 56.4). Carry this line down under the breast crossing the IM fold at the central peak.

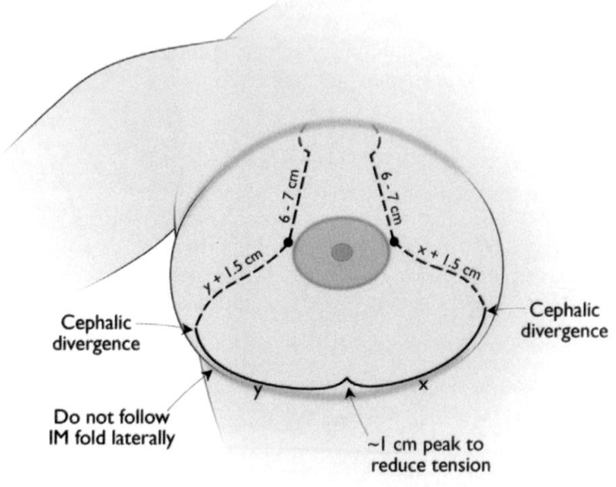

FIGURE 56.3. How to mark the inframammary (IM) fold and determine lengths of upper flap incisions. Extend mark medially and laterally to points that are still hidden in fold and curve cephalically. At the breast meridian, make a small peak of about 1 cm to reduce tension on the final closure. Measure the length of the medial and lateral limbs of the IM fold. Add 1 to 1.5 cm to each distance and transpose to the corresponding inferior margins of the upper flaps, 8 to 9 cm below the new papule position.

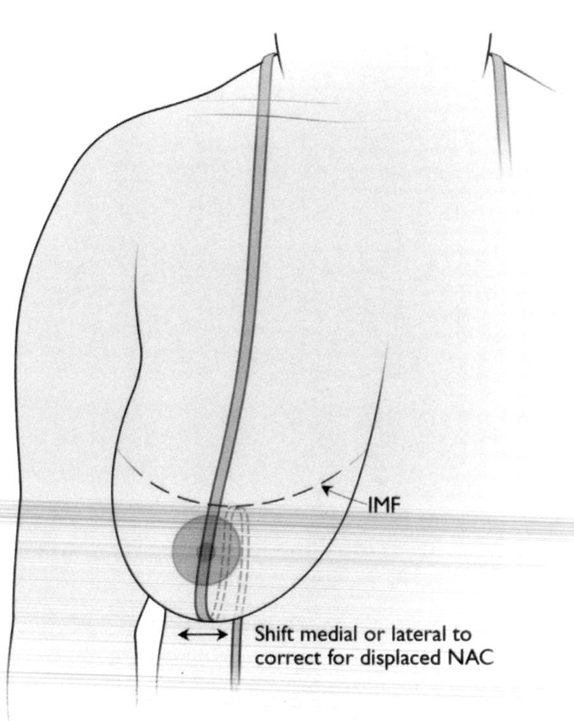

FIGURE 56.4. How to find the intended breast meridian with a measuring tape hung around the neck. IMF, inframammary fold; NAC, nipple-areolar complex.

4. Mark the new nipple position: This is critical and can be done using a number of techniques (Figure 56.5). The distance from the sternal notch to nipple can vary with height, but an example is that a 5′6″ woman who is a 34/36 C will be about 23 to 24 cm (**Table 56.1**). This mark should be very close to a hypothetical line that connects laterally to ~2 cm below the midpoint of the upper arm. And finally, it should be ~2 cm above the projected IM fold onto the anterior breast. Be sure to compensate modestly for skin elasticity which can cause some postoperative retraction cephalically. All three marks should be very close, and most importantly, the appearance of the final NAC position should appear reasonable.
5. Measure the length of the medial and lateral limbs of the IM fold from the midline peak. Add 1 to 1.5 cm to each distance and transpose this point to the planned corresponding inferior margins of the upper flaps, ~8 to 9 cm below the new papule position (see Figure 56.3). Adding this horizontal length to the upper flaps reduces tension and may help to avoid wound healing issues at the trifurcation.
6. With a flexible wire keyhole template, place the areolar opening over the new nipple position and open to the previously marked upper flap lengths. Draw the new NAC position and the vertical limbs. The limbs will be ~5 cm for a small breast and ~6 to 7 cm for a larger final breast. Extend the upper flap incisions from these points to join the IM fold incision medially and laterally with a gentle *S-shaped* curve.
7. Finally, mark topographically areas for planned liposuction as needed (lateral chest, anterior axillary fold) and estimate the amount to be removed with suction.

INFERIOR PEDICLE TECHNIQUE

This technique may be considered for breasts in which the NAC falls significantly below the triangle formed by the planned vertical flaps. It can be done in very large breasts, but size can be a limiting factor and the amputation/free nipple graft technique may be considered.

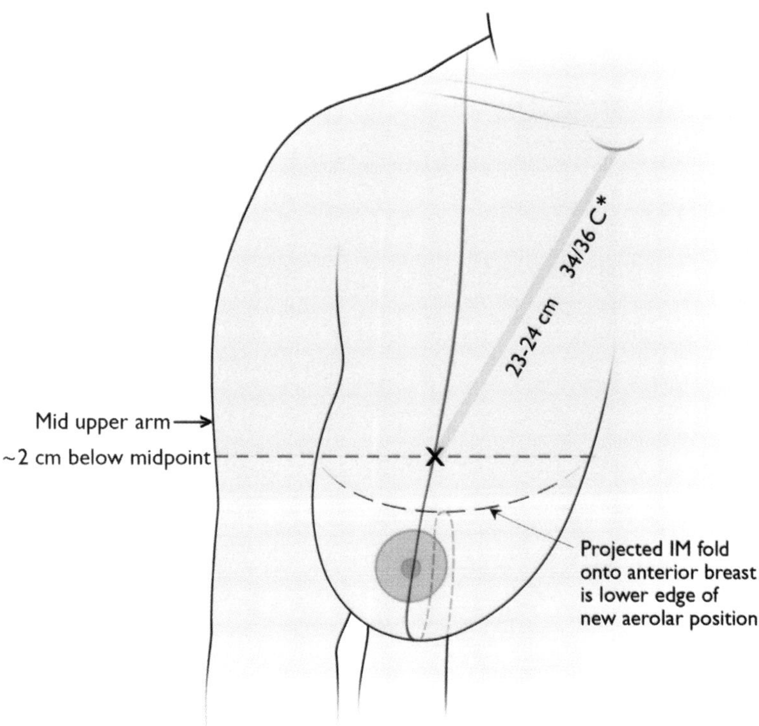

FIGURE 56.5. Three approaches to marking the new papule location. (1) Mark about 2 cm below the midpoint of the upper arm on the meridian. (2) Mark about 2 cm above the transposed position of the inframammary (IM) fold. (3) Refer to Table 56.1 for example sternal notch-to-nipple distances based on desired brassiere size. Remember to compensate for skin elasticity.

After prepping and draping the patient in the usual manner, reinforce your markings at the IM fold. Mark out the new areolar size (3.0–5.0 cm depending on final breast size) with the breast under some mild tension. Design the inferior pedicle from about 1 cm above and around the NAC and flare down toward the IM fold medially and laterally. This pedicle base is generally ~8 to 10 cm or wider. Remeasure and then join the vertical flap incisions in the center of the planned location of the NAC, not fully committing to the final NAC location (Figure 56.6). Tattoo key points for closure with a needle and marking ink including NAC orientation to avoid inadvertent rotation during insetting.

If planning to perform SAL laterally, infiltrate with tumescent solution in the intended areas at this time. Placing the breast base under tension, make all planned incisions and deepithelialize the inferior pedicle with knife or scissors. Proceed with the SAL.

Some surgeons prefer to elevate the upper flaps first. We have found that elevating the inferior pedicle initially works best for us. Make the dermal incisions medially and laterally on the IM fold carrying them about about halfway up the pedicle. Flare this dissection at the IM fold away from the pedicle to leave some added volume and to preserve NAC sensation. Now complete the incision around

TABLE 56.1. NORMATIVE VALUES OF COMMON PREOPERATIVE BREAST MEASUREMENTS [REPORTED IN INCHES (CENTIMETERS)]

	32			34			36			38		
Measurement	B	C	D	B	C	D	B	C	D	B	C	D
Sternal notch to nipple (left)	7.8 (19.9)	8.2 (20.8)	9.6 (24.4)	8.3 (21.0)	8.8 (22.4)	9.9 (25.1)	8.7 (22.1)	9.4 (24.0)	10.2 (25.9)	9.1 (23.1)	10.1 (25.6)	10.5 (26.6)
Sternal notch to nipple (right)	8.1 (20.4)	8.3 (21.1)	9.5 (24.1)	8.3 (21.1)	8.9 (22.5)	9.8 (25.0)	8.6 (21.8)	9.4 (23.9)	10.2 (25.9)	9.1 (22.5)	9.9 (25.2)	10.6 (26.8)
Nipple to nipple	7.9 (20.0)	8.0 (20.3)	8.4 (21.4)	8.1 (20.7)	8.3 (21.0)	8.6 (21.8)	8.4 (21.3)	8.6 (21.7)	8.7 (22.2)	8.6 (21.9)	8.8 (22.4)	8.9 (22.5)
IMF to nipple	3.3 (8.4)	3.8 (9.7)	4.0 (10.2)	3.5 (8.9)	4.0 (10.2)	4.3 (10.9)	3.8 (9.7)	4.3 (10.9)	4.5 (11.4)	4.0 (10.2)	4.5 (11.4)	4.8 (12.2)
Areolar width	1.8 (4.6)	2.0 (5.2)	2.1 (5.3)	1.9 (4.7)	2.0 (5.3)	2.1 (5.3)	1.9 (4.9)	2.0 (5.1)	2.1 (5.3)	2.0 (5.0)	2.1 (5.2)	2.1 (5.4)
Breast width	5.8 (14.7)	5.8 (14.7)	6.2 (15.7)	5.9 (15.0)	6.0 (15.2)	6.4 (16.3)	5.9 (15.0)	6.2 (15.7)	6.6 (16.8)	6.0 (15.2)	6.4 (16.3)	6.8 (17.3)

Values obtained from a study of 30 women for each breast size by Robert Oneal, MD, Denis Lee, and Art Rathjen.

IMF, inframammary fold.

BREAST

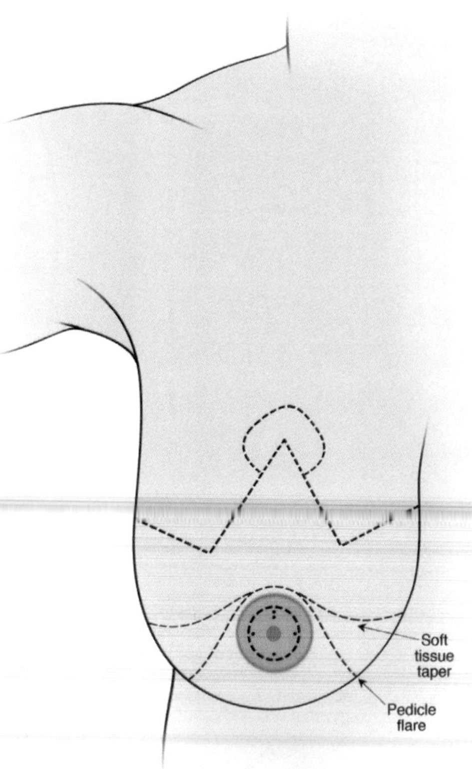

FIGURE 56.6. The preoperative markings for an inferior pedicle technique with a keyhole pattern skin resection. Note the anticipated flaring of the pedicle shape and tapering of the soft tissues.

top of the pedicle and dissect toward the chest wall following natural tissue planes of the breast parenchyma (*Wuringer's Planes*) and avoiding larger vessels at the pedicle base.[5,6] Carry this dissection to the chest wall without injury to the muscle fascia.

Proceed to elevate the medial and lateral flaps. Incise down to the breast capsule along the flap margins, and at the flap corners, tack the capsule to the dermis to assist in avoiding stripping the soft tissues from the overlying dermis, thus protecting blood supply to the skin edges (Figure 56.7). Trim and taper the flaps as needed for shaping the breast and removing the needed volume. Try to limit the resection from the medial flap, as this area is frequently already deficient. Once the flaps are elevated, remove the breast from the chest wall en bloc leaving the pectoralis fascia intact and avoiding injury to the blood supply of the pedicle. Weigh the specimen. Consider dividing and labeling as *central, medial, and lateral* so as to be able to help localize any pathology if inadvertently found.

Divide the dermis at the base of the inferior pedicle to assist in closure. After hemostasis, staple the flaps into position, sit the patient up, and if available, hold a sterilized bra of the planned postoperative breast cup size in position to assess the size and to determine asymmetries (Figure 56.8). Return the patient to supine position, and if necessary, release staples and resect additional tissue as indicated. Once both sides are symmetric volumes, restaple, sit up, and mark the new NAC position measuring from the sternal notch with a suture with patient as vertical as possible. They should be symmetric. Modify the NAC position if needed. Excise the skin for the new NAC position, bring the NAC to the skin surface, and confirm that the NAC is not rotated. You can remove some additional volume from the NAC defect if needed. Drains are placed prior to closure for 24 hours *only* if large amounts of tumescent fluid were used for lateral SAL or if a large potential *dead* space persists. This is usually not necessary.

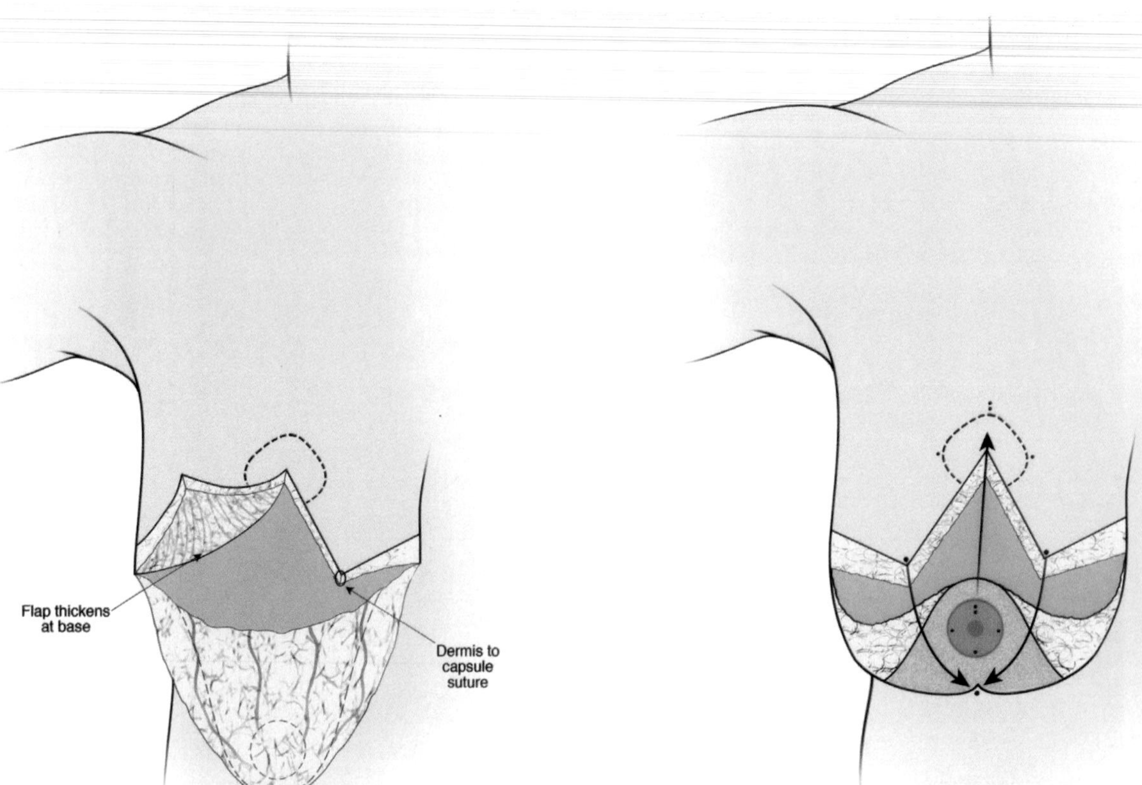

FIGURE 56.7. Elevation of the upper flaps and suturing the breast capsule to the dermis at the corners to prevent stripping the soft tissues from the overlying dermis.

FIGURE 56.8. The inferior pedicle is then brought into position and the upper flaps are brought down and stapled at the meridian. Confirm the correct orientation of the nipple-areolar complex based upon preoperative markings.

SUPEROMEDIAL PEDICLE TECHNIQUE

This technique (popularized by Hall-Findley and others)[7] has increased in popularity over the last two to three decades and continues to be a primary approach for many surgeons in moderate-size breasts. Adapting from the more classic inferior pedicle approach is not an easy transition but well worth the effort. It does require a substantially different three-dimensional understanding and visualization of the planned tissue rearrangement. The resection in the superior and superomedial pedicle approach is mostly from the lower and lateral poles where many volumetric issues exist with breast hypertrophy. The final breast shape can be additionally controlled with some deeper breast pillar sutures to assist in coning the tissues.

The marking of these patients is similar to the inferior pedicle approach using a keyhole pattern. Theoretically, using this technique reduces the risk for bottoming out over time as more lower and lateral pole tissues are resected. There is minimal resection of upper and medial breast tissue, which, along with rotation of the pedicle cephalically, may help to increase upper breast fullness.

After prepping and draping the patient, reinforce the markings at the IM fold and sweep up about 1 cm at the breast meridian (to reduce tension at the T-junction). Staple the inferior corners of the new NAC position together to mark the areola because it is incised initially. Mark out the new areola size with the breast on mild tension at the base. Release the staples and design a superomedial pedicle from just below the 3-o'clock position on the right (9-o'clock on the left) and extending the pedicle around the NAC inferiorly and laterally with ~1 cm margins. If necessary, the lower portion of the pedicle extends a bit beyond the tip of the medial flap to maintain a wider pedicle base (Figure 56.9). This base is ~8 to 10 cm in diameter. Mark key points for closure including the orientation of the areola. Note that the NAC will eventually rotate ~90°.

Infiltrate for SAL, if indicated. With the breast base under tension, perform all planned incisions including the new NAC position, and deepithelialize the superomedial pedicle. Proceed with SAL. Make incisions along the caudal border of the medial flap directly down to chest wall, leaving the pectoralis fascia intact. Continue incisions around the superomedial pedicle up to the new NAC position by avoiding any undermining of the pedicle. The pedicle should rotate easily.

Incise along the medial and lateral thirds of the IM fold directly down to chest wall, but in the central third bevel cephalically to allow some soft tissue to remain to fill potential *dead* space that may persist after superomedial pedicle rotation. Dissect around the new NAC position ~1.5 to 2 cm into the breast tissue and then bevel caudally to create a *platform* for the rotated NAC to rest on. Incise along the vertical and horizontal aspects of the lateral flap, leaving at least 3 cm of thickness to the flap at the tip. Taper the dissection cephalically along the lateral flap (Figure 56.10). This resection is important for reduction of lateral fullness and achieving coning. Resect the specimen from the chest wall en bloc, leaving the pectoralis fascia intact. Weigh the specimen. Divide into medial, central, and lateral aspects for pathology. Carefully incise the dermis at the base of the pedicle for ease of rotation into the new NAC position.

Place pillar sutures (2-0 absorbable) in the deep tissues of the vertical limbs of the tips of the medial and lateral flaps. These are placed ~2 to 3 cm below the flap corners and should assist in coning the breast when tied without skin distortion (Figure 56.11). A second pillar suture can be placed slightly more superficially. Approximate the skin edges with staples, advancing the upper flaps on the IM fold to avoid *dog-ears* medially and laterally. Staple the vertical incision. In the sitting position check for symmetry, volume, and position on the chest wall. Modify as necessary. The NAC position has already been determined and can only be minimally changed. After confirming that the NAC is oriented correctly, staple it into position.

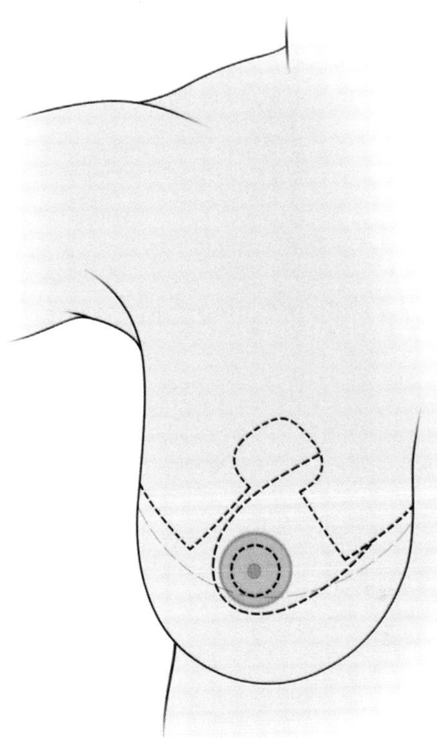

FIGURE 56.9. The preoperative markings for a superomedial pedicle technique with a keyhole pattern skin resection. Note that the position of the nipple-areolar complex is generally within or just below the vertical limbs of the keyhole pattern.

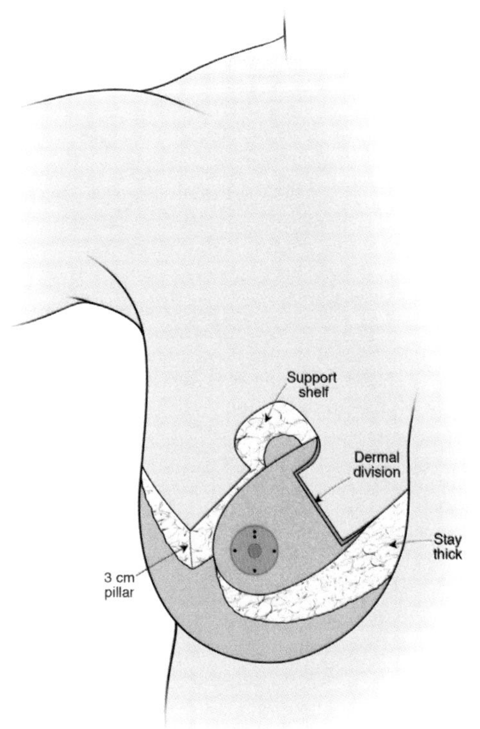

FIGURE 56.10. The relative thicknesses of the dissection of the superomedial pedicle and upper flaps, leaving a support shelf of breast tissue below the new nipple-areolar complex position for projection.

BREAST

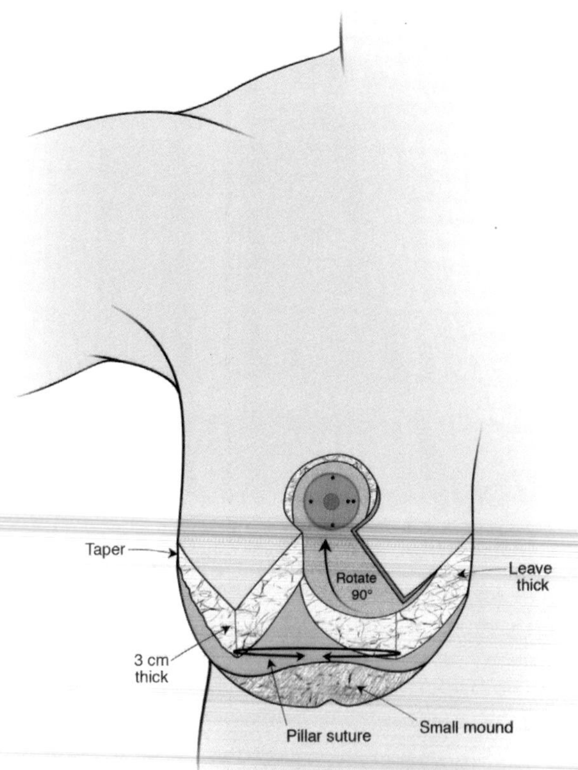

FIGURE 56.11. The upper flaps are then sutured together with pillar sutures and the superomedial pedicle is rotated about 90°. Confirm the correct orientation of the new nipple areolar complex position with the preoperative markings.

SUPEROMEDIAL PEDICLE WITH VERTICAL SKIN RESECTION

In patients with good skin elasticity, small to moderate amounts of planned tissue resection, and a reasonable distance between the papule and IM fold, a vertical skin resection approach may be used that will eliminate the transverse IM incisions. This approach relies upon lower pole skin contraction after elevating thin flaps down to the IM fold. Resection of breast tissue under the skin flaps is identical to the resection of breast tissue performed for the superomedial pedicle with a keyhole pattern. The vertical approach can significantly decrease the risk for hypertrophic scarring medially and laterally. A full understanding of the superomedial pedicle keyhole approach allows transitioning to this technique more easily. If the NAC is positioned high in the superior aspect of the keyhole pattern, the surgeon may want to consider using a superior pedicle.[8]

Preoperative Markings

The surgeon must be familiar with the key differences in the surgical markings for the vertical approach. Mark the breast in a similar manner to the standard superomedial pedicle reduction with a keyhole pattern, except just dot the transverse incisions at the IM fold and the medial and lateral flaps. These marks create a reference on the surface where the resection will be performed underneath the thin skin flaps (also called *ghost areas*). Extend down the vertical limbs beyond the transition point to the medial and lateral flaps of the keyhole pattern. The vertical limbs will continue caudally to ~3 to 4 cm above the IM fold and join in a gentle curve. The breast tissue will be resected caudally to this point to level of the IM fold. The scar will shorten as the tissues heal and the breast will drop down to a new higher IM fold, leaving just a vertical scar below the NAC.

Operative Technique

Once on the table, reinforce and remeasure the lines previously described. The superomedial pedicle and the new position and size of the NAC will be marked. The key points will be tattooed as in previous markings. The incisions are made by avoiding the dotted transverse and IM incisions of the previously described keyhole pattern. Deepithelialize the superomedial pedicle as usual and then begin by undermining the ghost areas between the dotted lines down to the IM fold (Figure 56.12). The skin flaps should be thin with minimal fat, but avoiding injury to the dermis. In patients with very thin subcutaneous tissue overlying the breast, dissection may proceed directly on the breast capsule. Once the undermining is completed under the *ghost areas*, the breast resection is identical to the instructions in the previously described technique for the superomedial pedicle, but with less skin resection.

After the resection of breast tissue, place the pillar sutures in the usual location in the upper flaps and rotate the NAC into position. The vertical incision is closed in either a single or a double layer. Do not attempt to shorten the incision during the closure for the first 2 cm below the NAC. This will place the 6-o'clock position of the NAC under tension caudally and distort its shape. Shorten the incision with a cinching closure beginning about 2 cm below the NAC (Figure 56.13). Barbed sutures may be helpful. It may also be beneficial to hold the skin at the inferior apex of the vertical limbs with a hook retractor during the closure. The final resulting caudal fullness that persists in many cases can be purse stringed or just closed. This redundant tissue can be dressed with a small temporary bolster of Vaseline gauze held by tape for 7 to 10 days.

There is the possibility of this residual redundancy needing some eventual resection transversely under local anesthesia, but the surgeon should wait at least 4 to 6 months as it frequently resolves on its own.

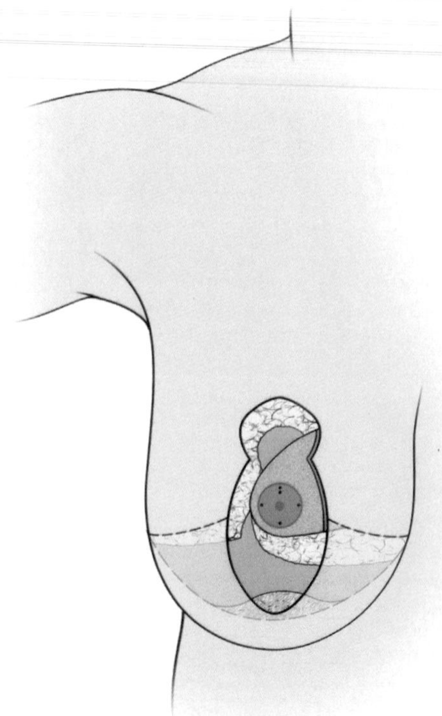

FIGURE 56.12. The intended resection of tissues and the *ghost areas* above the medial and lateral areas of breast tissue resection.

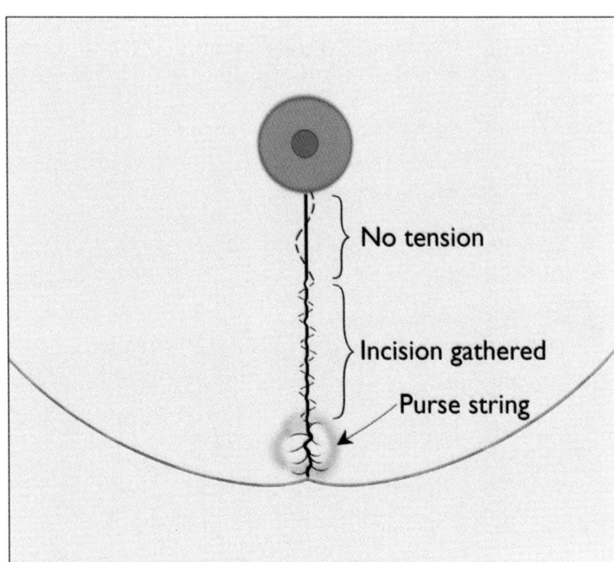

FIGURE 56.13. Distribute the redundant tissue during the closure of the vertical approach inferiorly to avoid distorting the shape of the nipple-areolar complex postoperatively.

AMPUTATION/FREE NIPPLE GRAFT

If the anticipated length of the inferior pedicle or superomedial pedicle raises concern of potential vascular compromise of the NAC, consider an amputation/free nipple graft technique.[9] This approach is generally ideal for patients with macromastia of excessive proportions that may limit pedicle viability, final aesthetics, and planned reduction goals. Generally, this refers to patients with a nipple to IM fold distance >20 cm. This technique may also be appropriate if there are breast scars that cross planned skin flaps or pedicles. This approach may also be preferred in the setting of a history of previous reduction mammoplasty of known or unknown technique, a history of radiation or for patients with systemic vascular issues due to connective tissue disorders, with an extensive smoking history, or autoimmune disorders. This technique allows the surgeon to achieve an excellent result with some projection and volume. Counsel the patient regarding the loss of NAC sensation and the risks of NAC graft failure. Even with these limitations, it is important for plastic surgeons to be able to utilize this technique.

Preoperative Markings

The preoperative markings are identical to the standard keyhole pattern described earlier (Figure 56.14). Because this technique is usually performed in the setting of very heavy breasts, remember to correct for the elasticity of the upper skin by lowering the final nipple position markings as needed. The major difference from previously described markings is that the width of the vertical portions of the keyhole may change once the resection is completed. The length of these vertical limbs should be 6 to 7 cm depending on the final size considered. Also, plan to leave a mound of lower breast tissue at the IM fold, which improves final projection.

Operative Technique

With the breast under mild tension, remove the NAC as full-thickness graft. It may be easier to keep the NAC thin to reduce the time needed to perform defatting. Also consider amputation of the tip of the nipple papule in circumstances where the length of the papule exceeds 1 cm to help it to survive as a full-thickness graft. Place it on a *labeled* moist sponge on the back table to prevent operating room staff from accidentally discarding it.

Deepithelialize a small lower flap along the IM fold (Figure 56.15). Incise down to the chest at the IM fold tapering cephalically over this small mound. The upper flap is incised along the caudal edge directly down to the chest wall, avoiding any undermining.

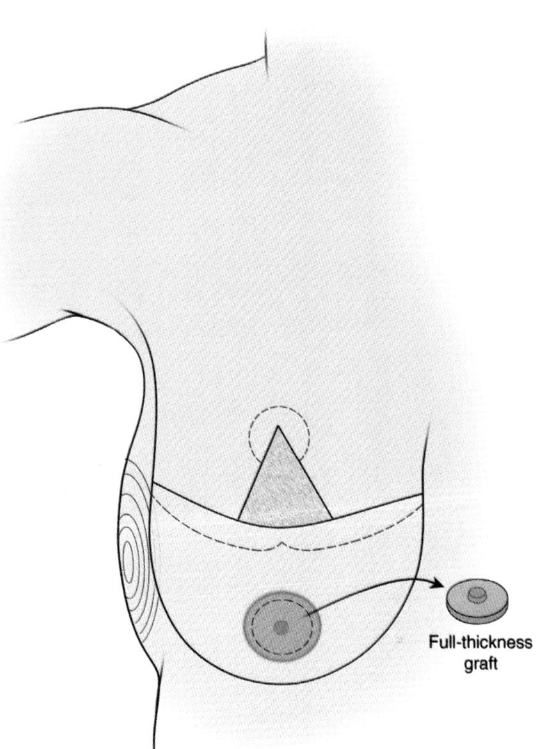

FIGURE 56.14. Preoperative markings for amputation/free nipple graft with suction assisted lipectomy and depiction of the nipple-areolar complex harvested as a full-thickness graft.

The breast tissue that was amputated will then be resected and weighed. Staple the upper incision to the lower advancing from the medial and lateral corners of the upper flaps centrally. The flaps should come together at the planned vertical marks but, depending on the size of the remaining breast, this triangle may need to be enlarged

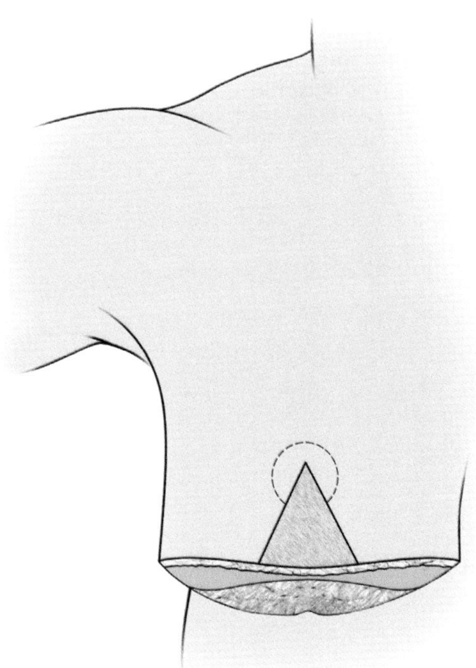

FIGURE 56.15. Following resection of breast tissue and deepithelialization of a central triangle. The new nipple-areolar complex position should then be confirmed and prepared for the full-thickness skin graft and bolster.

BREAST

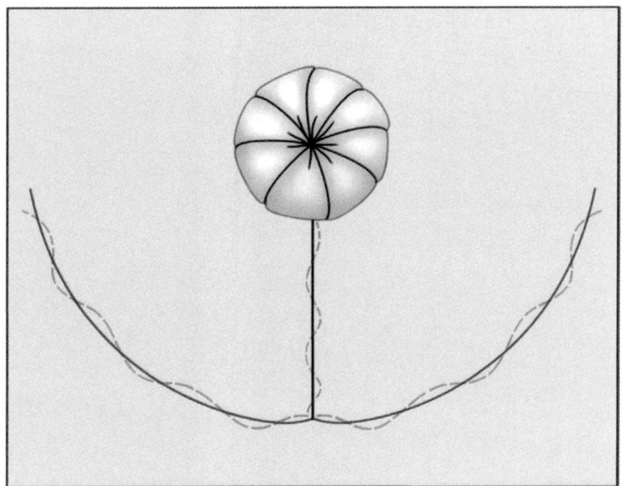

FIGURE 56.16. Final closure with a tie-over bolster for the amputation/free nipple graft technique.

or reduced to achieve good approximation of the skin edges. Staple the *vertical limbs* together and assess the new breast size and shape. Mark out the new vertical limbs as needed, remove staples, and now deepithelialize the triangle.

Restaple the skin edges together again, and in the sitting position, mark the new NAC positions symmetrically and very thinly deepithelialize this area. After closing the horizontal and vertical incisions, secure the NAC grafts to their new positions with tie-over bolsters (Figure 56.16). Drains are not necessary. SAL laterally can help contour as needed.

SUCTION-ASSISTED LIPECTOMY

This technique is helpful ideally for treating limited macromastia in circumstances when the breast tissue contains a high proportion of fatty tissue, the planned reduction would not require significant excision of overlying skin, and the skin has good elasticity.[10] For more dense breasts, modified suction equipment (i.e., ultrasonic, reciprocating, laser assisted) may be more helpful. We consider this for limited asymmetries, small reductions, and previous reductions with asymmetry needing additional volume removal, or for patients who have undergone previous reductions of unknown techniques and are not candidates for amputation with free nipple grafts. This procedure may be performed in a single or a staged manner that may include mastopexy after successful SAL.

POSTOPERATIVE COMPLICATIONS (FIGURE 56.17)

Acute Complications

Hematoma

Estimated to occur in up to 4% of cases.[11] It is important to recognize a hematoma early as it may result in vascular compromise to the NAC. Although surgical drains may initiate an earlier diagnosis, they will not prevent a hematoma from occurring. A small, localized hematoma can be directly drained or allowed to liquefy and then evacuated with a large bore needle or fat harvesting cannula in 1 to 2 weeks postoperatively.

Delayed Wound Healing

Estimated to occur in 10% of cases. Usually occurs at the lower skin trifurcation (*T-junction*), but may also occur along any incision lines. It may be due to the flaps closed too tightly over the remaining mound or in patients with any history of scars, or active smoking. It is not uncommon for mild epidermolysis to occur, which is treated with conservative wound care. To prevent wound healing complications, consider tacking the dermis to the breast capsule at the flap corners with absorbable sutures to avoid stripping the underlying blood supply.

Seroma

Leaving a small mound of breast tissue at the midline along the IM fold in the superomedial pedicle breast reduction approach helps to avoid this complication. If significant SAL of the lateral breast is performed, consider leaving a surgical drain overnight which helps remove residual tumescent fluid.

Vascular Compromise

If the breast reduction is designed and executed correctly, this is a rare complication involving the NAC and hopefully only temporary after the pedicle elevation, positioning, and rotation. It can be difficult to evaluate if local anesthetic with epinephrine was used during the case. Try to identify the underlying cause for vascular compromise and release sutures as needed to avoid necrosis and loss of the NAC. Assess the NAC for proper rotation or consider additional reduction of breast to decrease intrinsic pressure. Vascular compromise also can result in fat necrosis and fibrosis, thus potentially leading to the need for future biopsies or operative interventions. Removal of the NAC as a full-thickness graft and regrafting can be done but has limited results. History of radiation therapy, Raynaud disease, scleroderma, and smoking increases risk for vascular compromise.

Long-term Complications

Asymmetry

Identify and point out asymmetries to the patient preoperatively, including chest wall, costal margins, manubrium, IM folds, or anticipated discrepancies in the amount of breast volume that will be resected. Furthermore, try to predict the volume discrepancies between the breasts preoperatively. Intraoperatively, sit the patient up to determine symmetry by visual inspection and palpation. Use of a sterile bra in the operating room helps to recognize volume differences. Preoperative breast asymmetries will be more obvious after a symmetrical resection. Small to medium differences may be treated postoperatively with SAL.

Fibrosis and Fat Necrosis

Fibrosis may resolve with time and massage and generally is not visible. This finding may cause anxiety for the patient and lead to unnecessary testing or breast biopsies. Fibrosis and fat necrosis may also affect future mammography. Occasionally an area of firmness may be an inclusion cyst, which is a result of inadequate deepithelialization of the pedicle.

Inability to Breastfeed

The impact of breast reduction on ability to breastfeed postoperatively appears largely related to preservation of the subareolar parenchyma. Rates of successful breastfeeding range from <5% for techniques with no preservation of subareolar parenchyma such as an amputation/free nipple graft to 75% to 100% for techniques with full preservation of the subareolar parenchyma.[12]

Inverted Nipples

If the patient has a history of periodic nipple inversion, inform them that it might worsen postoperatively. This may improve with time and scar massage, but might require future surgical correction. Nipples that are always inverted will usually remain that way postoperatively.

Loss of Nipple Areolar Sensation

This rare complication tends to be a transient, and some patients may even experience hypersensitivity that resolves eventually. Be sure to counsel the patient preoperatively regarding this potential complication. To prevent loss of nipple sensation, avoid injury to the pectoralis fascia and if possible, leave small amounts of soft tissue over the muscle, design a wider inferior pedicle base, and avoid undermining the

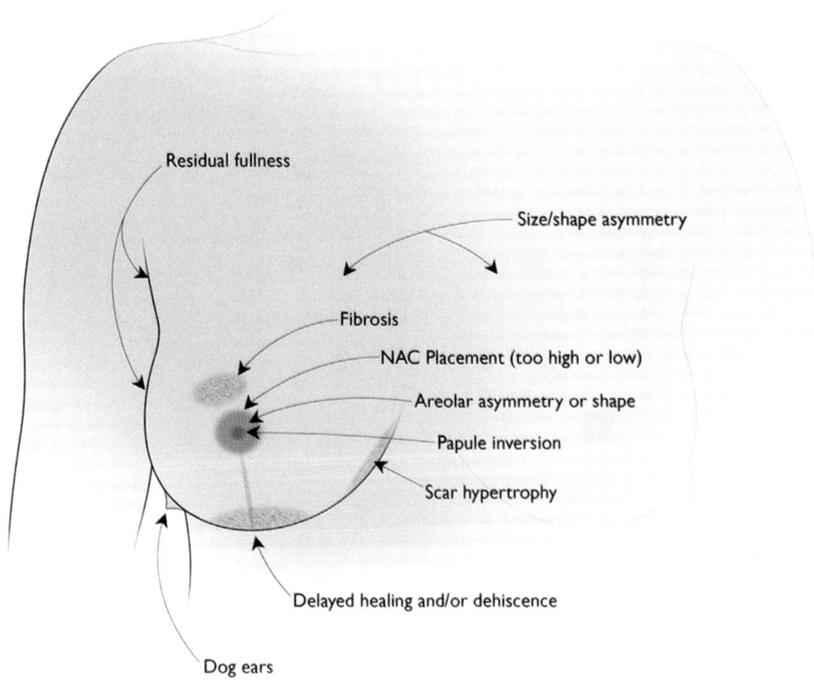

FIGURE 56.17. Potential complications following breast reduction.

superomedial pedicle. Ask patients preoperatively about their nipple sensation, because not infrequently women with macromastia have some reduced sensation at baseline.

Hypertrophic Scarring

This complication is more likely to occur in patients with a propensity for developing these scars, if there is increased tension on the closures, and also in situations with delayed wound healing. It may help to assess other scars on the patient. A vertical approach avoids the lateral and medial IM incisions, which, in the senior author's experience, are more likely to develop hypertrophic scarring. Potential interventions to address hypertrophic scarring include silicone sheeting, steroid injections, fractional CO_2 laser resurfacing, and scar revision. In our experience, true keloid scarring is a rare complication in breast surgery.

High NAC Position

This complication is extremely difficult to correct without significant additional scarring. It is best to avoid this issue by properly planning NAC position and anticipating additional elevation of the new NAC due to weight reduction and the overlying skin elasticity. Undercorrection of the final NAC height can be revised with a small mastopexy or crescentic excision at a later date.[13] The final NAC position of the inferior pedicle and amputation/free nipple graft techniques can be adjusted to a small degree intraoperatively at the initial procedure. In the superomedial pedicle technique, the NAC position is typically determined prior to the incisions because it is integral to the design of the pedicle and resection. Finally, if the NAC position is too high, consider a lower concentric skin excision at the IM fold to reduce the distance of the nipple to IM fold or further reducing the overall breast size.

Discovery of Breast Cancer

Although not a true complication (unless missed on a mammogram or exam), this finding will affect the planned treatment by the surgical oncology team. Preoperative mammograms are important, and age 40 years has been suggested for screening depending on family history.[14] All specimens go to pathology and by dividing the specimen into medial, central, and lateral components, the patient may not need to undergo additional surgery if the location and extent of the carcinoma resection can be determined.

REFERENCES

1. Jaspars JJ, Posma AN, van Immerseel AA, Gittenberger-de Groot AC. The cutaneous innervation of th[illegible] breast and nipple-areola complex: implications for surgery. *Br J Plast Surg*. 1997;50(4):249-259.
2. Sarhadi NS, Shaw Dunn J, Lee FD, Soutar DS. An anatomical study of the nerve supply of the breast, including the nipple and areola. *Br J Plast Surg*. 1996;49(3):156-164.
3. Available athttp://www.choosingwisely.org/wp-content/uploads/2015/02/ASPS-Choosing-Wisely-List.pdf. Accessed June 4, 2018.
4. Schnur PL, Schnur DP, Petty PM, et al. Reduction mammaplasty: an outcome study. *Plast Reconstr Surg*. 1997;100(4):875-883.
5. Wuringer E, Mader N, Posch E, Holle J. Nerve and vessel supplying ligamentous suspension of the mammary gland. *Plast Reconstr Surg*. 1998;101(6):1486-1493.
6. Hamdi M, Van Landuyt K, Tonnard P, et al. Septum-based mammaplasty: a surgical technique based on Wuringer's septum for breast reduction. *Plast Reconstr Surg*. 2009;123(2):443-454.
7. Hall-Findlay EJ. A simplified vertical reduction mammaplasty: shortening the learning curve. *Plast Reconstr Surg*. 1999;104(3):748-759.
This landmark article discusses modifications to the standard vertical reduction mammoplasty technique in a series of 400 breasts. The author made this technique easier and more reliable through a medial dermoglandular pedicle, avoiding undermining of skin, and not using pectoralis fascia sutures.
8. Lejour M, Abboud M, Declety A, Kertesz P. Reduction of mammaplasty scars: from a short inframammary scar to a vertical scar. *Ann Chir Plast Esthet*. 1990;35(5):369-379.
Although not the initial description of the vertical skin resection for breast reduction, this study provided the foundation for procedural advances in breast reduction such as the superomedial pedicle with a vertical skin resection by Hall-Findlay in the 1990s.
9. Oneal RM, Goldstein JA, Rohrich R, et al. Reduction mammoplasty with free-nipple transplantation: indications and technical refinements. *Ann Plast Surg*. 1991;26(2):117-121.
10. Gray LN. Update on experience with liposuction breast reduction. *Plast Reconstr Surg*. 2001;108(4):1006-1010.
11. Cunningham BL, Gear AJ, Kerrigan CL, Collins ED. Analysis of breast reduction complications derived from the BRAVO study. *Plast Reconstr Surg*. 2005;115(6):1597-1604.
12. Kraut RY, Brown E, Korownyk C, et al. The impact of breast reduction surgery on breastfeeding: systematic review of observational studies. *PLoS One*. 2017;12(10).
13. Spear SL, Albino FP. Management of the high-riding nipple after breast reduction. *Clin Plast Surg*. 2016;43(2):395-401.
14. Greco R, Noone B. Evidence-based medicine: reduction mammaplasty. *Plast Reconstr Surg*. 2017;139(1):230e-239e.
15. Mistry RM, MacLennan SE, Hall-Findlay EJ. Principles of breast re-reduction: a reappraisal. *Plast Reconstr Surg*. 2017;139(6):1313-1322.
16. Pannucci CJ, Wachtman CF, Dreszer G, et al. The effect of postoperative enoxaparin on risk for reoperative hematoma. *Plast Reconstr Surg*. 2012;129(1):160-168.
17. Nahabedian MY, Mofid MM. Viability and sensation of the nipple-areolar complex after reduction mammaplasty. *Ann Plast Surg*. 2002;49(1):24-31.

QUESTIONS

1. **What are the reported rates for the following complications:**

   I. Delayed wound healing
   II. Hematoma[16]
   III. Seroma
   IV. Nipple areola loss
   V. Loss of nipple sensation[17]

2. **A 43-year-old woman is seeking a plastic surgery consultation for symptoms associated with macromastia. She reports shoulder grooving, shoulder and back pain, recurrent intertrigo in her IM folds, and difficulty exercising because of her large breasts. She has large, grade III ptotic breasts, with sternal notch to nipple and nipple to IM fold distances of 30 and 25 cm, respectively. Which operation is most appropriate to achieve breast reduction in this patient?**

   a. Inferior pedicle with keyhole pattern skin resection
   b. Superomedial pedicle with keyhole pattern skin resection
   c. Amputation and free nipple graft
   d. SAL and mastopexy

3. **A 32-year-old woman presents for a consultation about breast reduction procedures. She underwent breast reduction 10 years ago by an unknown technique and the operative reports are no longer available. Since that time, she has gained 50 pounds and her breasts have increased in size as well. On examination, she has well-healed scars from a previous keyhole pattern skin resection. She has grade II ptotic breasts with sternal notch to nipple and nipple to IM fold distances of 24 and 12 cm, respectively. Which approach is most appropriate and safe for this patient?**

   a. Superomedial pedicle
   b. Inferior pedicle
   c. Resection of inferior wedge of breast tissue
   d. Amputation/free nipple graft[15]
   e. SAL and mastopexy

1. **Answer:** 10%, 4%, 10-15%, 1%, and 2%.

2. **Answer: c.** When the nipple to IM fold distance is greater than 20 cm, that the surgeon should consider using an amputation/free nipple graft technique to reduce the risk for postoperative vascular issues to the NAC. Often, this technique is also needed for women of much larger body habitus with associated comorbidities and the resulting need to limit anesthesia time for patient safety.

3. **Answer: c.** It is important to know that breast rereduction can be performed safely, even when the previous technique is unknown. The surgeon should appreciate that there is minimal amount of skin excision in this rereduction described by the clinical scenario and thus a vertical or horizontal pattern skin resection would be appropriate to achieve the desired result. In an outcome study of rereduction by Mistry et al., a resection of a small wedge of breast tissue in the lower pole was performed safely in most cases.[15] The NAC then relies on a random pattern blood supply. In circumstances of a much larger breast, the amputation/free nipple graft technique may be the safest option. However, in this case that technique would likely leave the patient described here with breasts that are much smaller than she desires. There is no need to reelevate pedicles such as the superomedial or inferior pedicles in this situation.

CHAPTER 57 Gynecomastia

Ashley N. Amalfi and Nicole Z. Sommer

KEY POINTS

- Gynecomastia is physiologically normal and transient during the neonatal period, puberty, and in old age.
- Persistent or asymmetric gynecomastia should be evaluated by thorough history and physical exam, assessing for systemic or exogenous pathology as the cause of breast enlargement.
- Gynecomastia is the result of an imbalance of hormone levels. Alterations in the ratio of estrogens to androgens caused by systemic illness, neoplasm, pharmacologic agents, or other idiopathic factors may contribute.
- Gynecomastia can have significant social, emotional, and psychological impacts on adolescents, and practitioners should screen patients accordingly and provide appropriate resources and care.
- The plastic surgeon should evaluate the excess stromal tissue, adipose tissue, skin redundancy, degree of ptosis, and size and location of the nipple areolar complex to formulate an individualized surgical plan.
- Ideal proportions in the male breast are quite different compared to the female breast, as to create a masculine appearing chest contour postoperatively.
- Each patient should be approached as an individual to evaluate the patient's desired aesthetics. Sometimes, a staged approach is necessary to achieve an ideal result.

Gynecomastia is the benign enlargement of glandular breast tissue in males. It is the most common breast condition in males.[1] At various stages of development, male breast growth is a normal and transient physiologic response to the balance of androgens and estrogens in the body. Persistent or asymmetric gynecomastia should be evaluated by a thorough history and physical exam, looking for systemic or exogenous pathology as the cause of breast enlargement. This often requires the cooperation of a multidisciplinary team that includes plastic surgery, primary care, endocrinology, and psychiatry.

NATURAL HISTORY

Physiologic breast growth is hormonally driven, and the trimodal distribution of gynecomastia is testament to this. We see normal breast development in males during the neonatal period, puberty, and in aging men. Neonatal mastauxe, or breast enlargement of the newborn, is directly correlated to circulating maternal estrogens, and is seen in almost 70% of infants. A small breast bud of 1 to 2 cm is often palpable in the newborn. As maternal estrogen levels fall, some neonates experience a surge of prolactin, which may cause the temporary secretion of milk. Within the first month of life, hormones normalize, and these self-limiting symptoms dissipate.[2]

The second peak in gynecomastia is seen during puberty, and can last for a period of months to years. Up to 65% of adolescent boys experience transient gynecomastia during this period of development.[3] An elevated ratio of circulating estradiol to testosterone during puberty is thought to be causative, with an onset between the ages of 10 and 13 years. Approximately 4% of males will have persistent gynecomastia beyond this period, defined by breast bud enlargement of greater than 4 cm.

Senile gynecomastia is attributed to decreases in testosterone and an increase in adipose tissue, leading to the peripheral conversion of androgens to estrogens. Once again, this imbalance of hormones leads to breast enlargement that affects up to 65% of men.[4]

PATHOPHYSIOLOGY

Various pathologies that disrupt the delicate hormone balance and result in androgen deficiency, or estrogen excess, can lead to the development of gynecomastia. Systemic disease, neoplasm, pharmacologic agents, or other idiopathic factors may be the causative agents (Table 57.1). Thorough workup by plastic surgeon, primary care physicians, and endocrinologists may be necessary to evaluate the underlying illness or agents that cause male breast enlargement.

Medications and illicit drugs are the most common causes of gynecomastia in men (Table 57.2). Antiandrogens, steroids, antipsychotics, and antiretrovirals are some of the more common classes of medications implicated. Illicit drugs including marijuana, alcohol,

TABLE 57.1. PATHOLOGIC CAUSES OF GYNECOMASTIA

Endocrine
Testicular
Hypogonadism
Klinefelter syndrome (XXY)
Adrenal
Congenital adrenal hyperplasia
Cushing syndrome
Thyroid
Hyperthyroidism
Hypothyroidism
Disorders of sexual differentiation
Androgen insensitivity syndrome
17-B-hydroxysteroid dehydrogenase deficiency
Aromatase excess syndrome
Systemic
Chronic liver disease
Chronic kidney disease
Refeeding syndrome
Malnutrition
Neoplasms
Breast carcinoma
Testicular tumors
Leydig cell
Sertoli cell
Adrenal cortical carcinoma
Lung carcinoma
Liver carcinoma
hCG-secreting tumors
Infectious
HIV
Other
Obesity

TABLE 57.2. PHARMACOLOGIC CAUSES OF GYNECOMASTIA

Illicit Drugs of Abuse
Marijuana
Anabolic steroids
Alcohol
Opiates
Amphetamines
Hormone and Hormone Modulators
Testosterone
Estrogen
Flutamide
Bicalutamide
Leuprolide
Finasteride
Gn-RH analogs
Prednisone
Cardiovascular Medications
Calcium channel blockers
Spironolactone
Digoxin
ACE inhibitors
Amiodarone
Psychiatric Medications
Benzodiazepines
Phenothiazines
Tricyclic antidepressants
Olanzapine
Haloperidol
Risperidone
Antimicrobials and Antiretrovirals
Ketoconazole
Metronidazole
Isoniazid
Protease inhibitors
Nucleoside reverse transcriptase inhibitors
Chemotherapeutics
Methotrexate
Imatinib
Cyclophosphamide
Alkylating agents
Vinca alkaloids
Antireflux Medications
Cimetidine
Omeprazole
Ranitidine

and heroine, as well as anabolic steroids are well-documented causes of gynecomastia. When possible, offending agents should be discontinued to evaluate for resolution of symptoms. A softening and dissipation of the glandular breast enlargement should be seen within 1 month of discontinuation of the offending agent.

PATIENT EVALUATION

Thorough evaluation by the treating provider is necessary to look for underlying pathology as the cause of gynecomastia. In an adolescent with suspected disorders of sexual differentiation and hormone differences, referral to a pediatric endocrinologist is warranted. Often, no true etiology is found and the gynecomastia is thought to be idiopathic. In a review by Cordova et al., 102 of 123 patients had idiopathic gynecomastia without an identifiable cause.[5]

All patients with gynecomastia require thorough history and physical examination. A full record of previous and current medications, including supplements as well as illicit drugs, should be obtained. For pediatric patients, it is often wise to examine them privately, so that they feel comfortable sharing any illegal consumption without the retribution of a parent present.

Physical exam should begin with the palpation of the breast for any discernible masses. The breast bud beneath the nipple areolar complex should be palpated, and is often tender to the patient with idiopathic gynecomastia. Glandular breast tissue should be differentiated from diffuse fatty enlargement of the male breast, often termed pseudogynecomastia. Asymmetries of the breasts and chest wall should be noted. The nipple areolar complex should be evaluated for size, shape, and location. A thyroid and testicular exam should be performed to thoroughly evaluate for underlying systemic pathology.

Less than 1% of all breast malignancies develop in males. Although rare, breast cancer must always remain on the differential diagnosis when examining breast enlargement in male patients. One should specifically palpate for discernible masses located outside of the nipple areolar complex and evaluate for significant asymmetry. Skin dimpling, nipple retraction, nipple discharge, and bleeding are all symptoms suggestive of malignancy.[6] If there is concern based on physical exam, further workup is necessary with an ultrasound or mammogram. In patients with Klinefelter syndrome, their risk of developing breast cancer is almost 60 times greater than the general male population, and excisional surgical techniques are preferred in this high-risk population.

A variety of classification schemes exist to further describe the degree of deformity. Despite their differences, all of these classification systems focus on the degree of breast enlargement as well as the skin redundancy and nipple ptosis seen with these deformities. Simon's classification is a historic and well-referenced system used to evaluate gynecomastia, and includes these basic variables (**Table 57.3**).[7] Other factors to be evaluated include skin elasticity, and the size and shape of the nipple areolar complex, which are not accounted for in this classification system.

Psychological implications of gynecomastia in adolescents are well documented. Nuzzi et al. reported a significant impact on adolescent social functioning, mental health, and self-esteem, regardless of the severity or grade of the gynecomastia.[8] These patients often exhibit anxieties and social phobias, with many teenagers refusing to participate in physical education or sports. The treating physician should consider referral for counseling or psychiatric treatment as an adjunct to medical and surgical management for these patients.[9] Due to these psychological effects, gynecomastia in adolescents is sometimes considered medically necessary by some insurance companies. If gynecomastia is adversely affecting a patient's mental health and wellbeing, it is reasonable to ask for prior authorization for coverage of surgical correction in the appropriate patient.

NONOPERATIVE MANAGEMENT

Nonsurgical management of gynecomastia should be explored first. Any offending agents should be discontinued to allow for resolution of symptoms. Underlying disease processes should be controlled and treated, and their effect noted. For those with pseudogynecomastia, weight loss is an effective strategy to reduce the amount of adipose tissue and help improve the contour of the chest.

In most instances, no causative agent or illness is identified, and the gynecomastia is considered idiopathic. Many small-scale clinical

TABLE 57.3. SIMON GYNECOMASTIA CLASSIFICATION SYSTEM

Grade	Breast Enlargement	Skin Excess
1	Small	None
2a	Moderate	None
2b	Moderate	Skin redundancy
3	Marked	Skin redundancy

trials have evaluated the efficacy of tamoxifen, a selective estrogen receptor modulator, on the treatment of gynecomastia. Khan et al. reported complete resolution of gynecomastia in 83.3% of their patients treated with tamoxifen, with noted decrease in breast tenderness for 84% of men during treatment.[10] Despite multiple randomized and nonrandomized trials in the literature, tamoxifen is not yet approved by the Food and Drug Administration as a treatment for gynecomastia. Clomiphene citrate has also been trialed in small studies, with minimal improvement in the adolescent population.[11]

Patients with prostate cancer treated with bicalutamide monotherapy commonly experience gynecomastia and mastodynia. These patients may receive off-label prophylactic or therapeutic treatment with tamoxifen or anastrazole, an aromatase inhibitor, with varying levels of efficacy. Tamoxifen, when taken as a prophylactic measure at 10 to 20 mg daily, is shown to be most effective in these patients. Prophylactic radiotherapy has also been found to be effective at mitigating approximately one third of the gynecomastia and mastodynia seen with bicalutamide therapy.[12]

SURGICAL MANAGEMENT

If exogenous causes are controlled and the patient's gynecomastia persists for at least 1 year, surgical treatment is warranted. Surgical treatment options vary depending on the severity of the gynecomastia. The goal of surgical management is to achieve a more masculine appearing chest while managing realistic patient expectations. Operative procedures are designed to remove the excess glandular and fatty tissue, reduce the diameter of the nipple areolar complex, relocate the nipple to the appropriate position on the chest wall, and achieve symmetry.

All patients should be marked preoperatively in the sitting or standing position. The sternal notch, midline, and inframammary fold are marked. The nipple areolar complex is also marked and measured. Areas of glandular and fatty excess are delineated. The border of the pectoralis major muscle is palpated and transposed onto the skin (Figure 57.1).

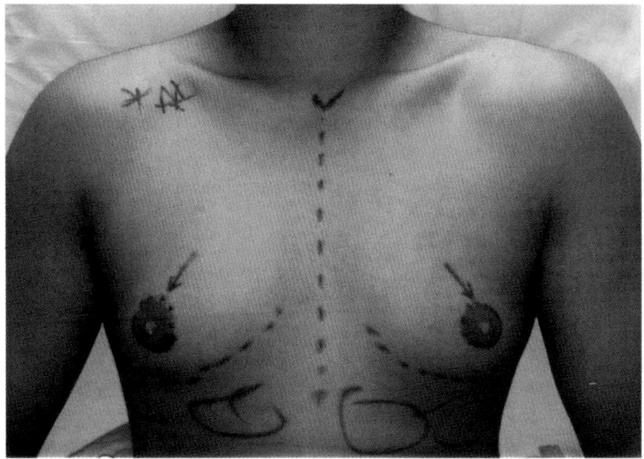

FIGURE 57.1. Preoperative markings for gynecomastia correction show the sternal notch and midline marked, as well as the inferior periareolar incision. The arrow delineates the superior medial pedicle that will be used to preserve nipple viability. The inframammary fold is marked and will be disrupted via liposuction, along with fatty deposits on the inferior chest, which have been circled.

Suction-assisted lipectomy is an excellent option for patients with minimal to moderate tissue and skin excess. If the breast enlargement is predominantly adipose tissue, liposuction is an ideal method to remove the unwanted fat and create a more pleasing contour (Figure 57.2). The use of ultrasound-assisted liposuction has broadened the indications for liposuction, as it is able to address the firmer glandular breast tissue under the nipple areolar complex. The ultrasound-assisted device uses a process of fat emulsification via cavitation, which is highly effective at disrupting dense, glandular tissue. This

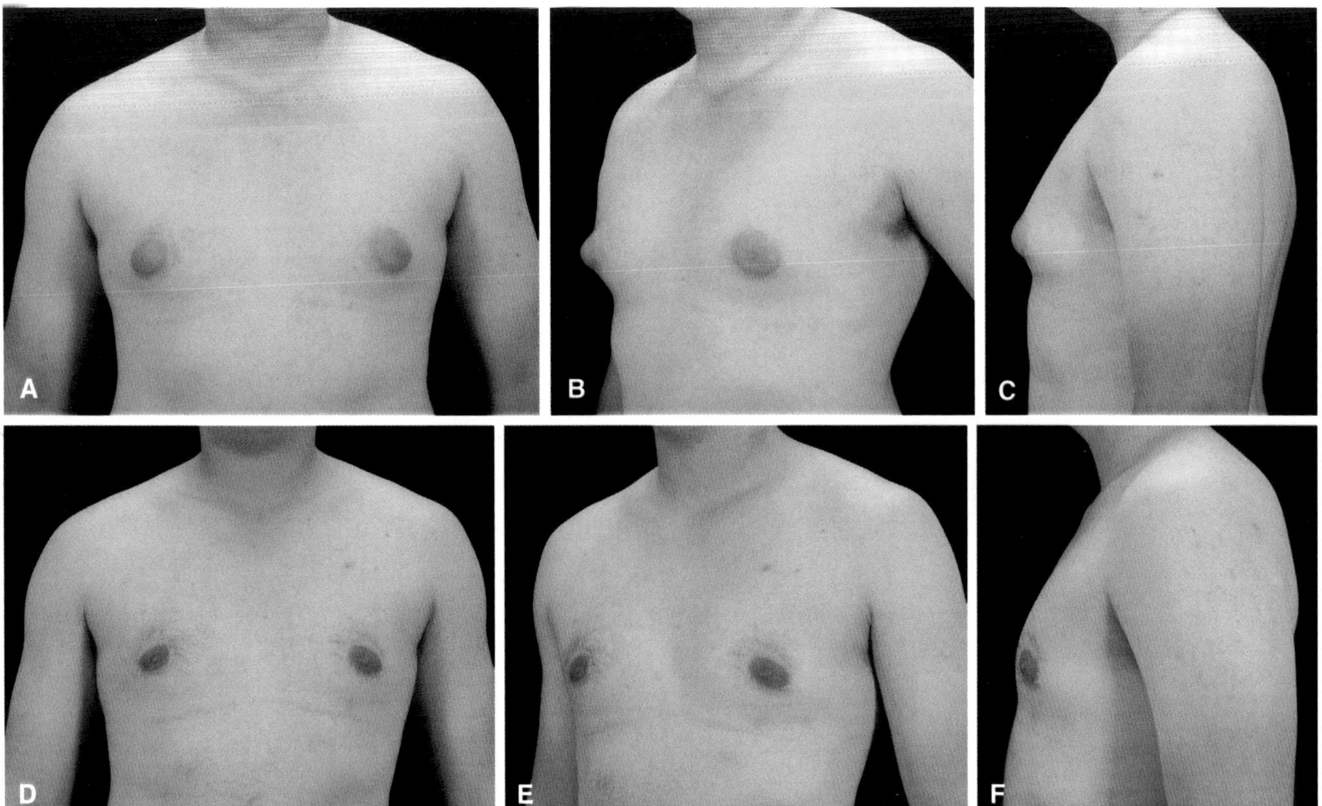

FIGURE 57.2. This patient with minimal fatty gynecomastia without skin excess underwent liposuction correction of gynecomastia. **A–C.** Preoperative photographs. **D–F.** Postoperative photographs.

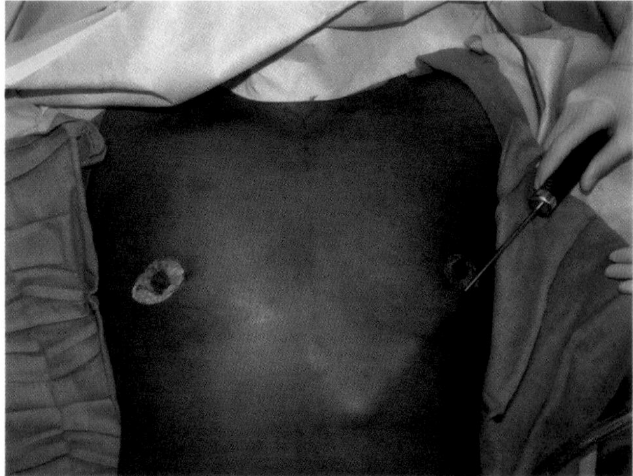

FIGURE 57.3. Intraoperative photo of a liposuction technique to efface the inframammary fold and create a more masculine lower pole contour.

technique also offers skin tightening as an additional benefit when performed in a more superficial plane. Rohrich et al. discussed their technique of tumescence and ultrasound-assisted liposuction followed by traditional liposuction to achieve excellent cosmetic results in their gynecomastia patients.[13] With any of the various types of liposuction, it is important that fanning liposuction of the entire chest be performed to create a smooth and pleasing contour. The surgeon should intentionally disrupt the inframammary fold, because such dermoglandular attachment is feminizing (Figure 57.3). Instead, the lower pole may be contoured via liposuction to emphasize the inferior border of the pectoralis major muscle and create more masculine definition.

In patients with moderate glandular excess as well as moderate skin excess, it is advisable to stage skin excision by performing liposuction or direct glandular excision first. If there is good skin elasticity, the loose skin envelope will contract following surgery. In older individuals or those with poor elasticity, a second procedure may be necessary to trim the excess skin and improve shape. A period of at least 6 to 12 months postoperatively allows the tissue to retract, and the decision to pursue further skin excision can then be made. Most patients will exhibit adequate skin retraction, and do not elect further surgery. For those that require skin excision, incisions are often limited, and the amount of skin removed is far less than if it had been completed at the initial surgery. It is important to manage patient expectations related to skin and nipple appearance, and the potential need for staged procedures.

For patients with minimal to moderate excess that is predominantly glandular, a direct excision technique is preferred. A limited periareolar incision offers access to the parenchyma for direct excision and creates a well-concealed scar. Placing the incision along the inferior lateral aspect of the areola further shadows the incision and leads to a minimally perceptible scar. Another technique involves a transareolar incision hiding the scar in the pigmented areola in a transverse manner (Figure 57.4). Using a pull-through technique, the dense breast parenchyma is delivered through the limited incision and removed in piecemeal fashion using a pair of sharp scissors or electric cautery. In larger patients, this periareolar incision may be extended laterally onto the breast skin in an omega pattern to gain better access to the breast. With direct excision techniques, the surgeon has better visualization and more control of the resection. A mastectomy is performed through this approach to remove the entire glandular breast. It is imperative that a mound of at least 1.5 cm of gland be left below the nipple areolar complex to prevent over resection and a concavity below the nipple. The flaps are created with some subcutaneous tissue to prevent a concave postoperative appearance of the male chest. It is preferred to leave too much tissue here, as it can be further trimmed to improve the contour at the end

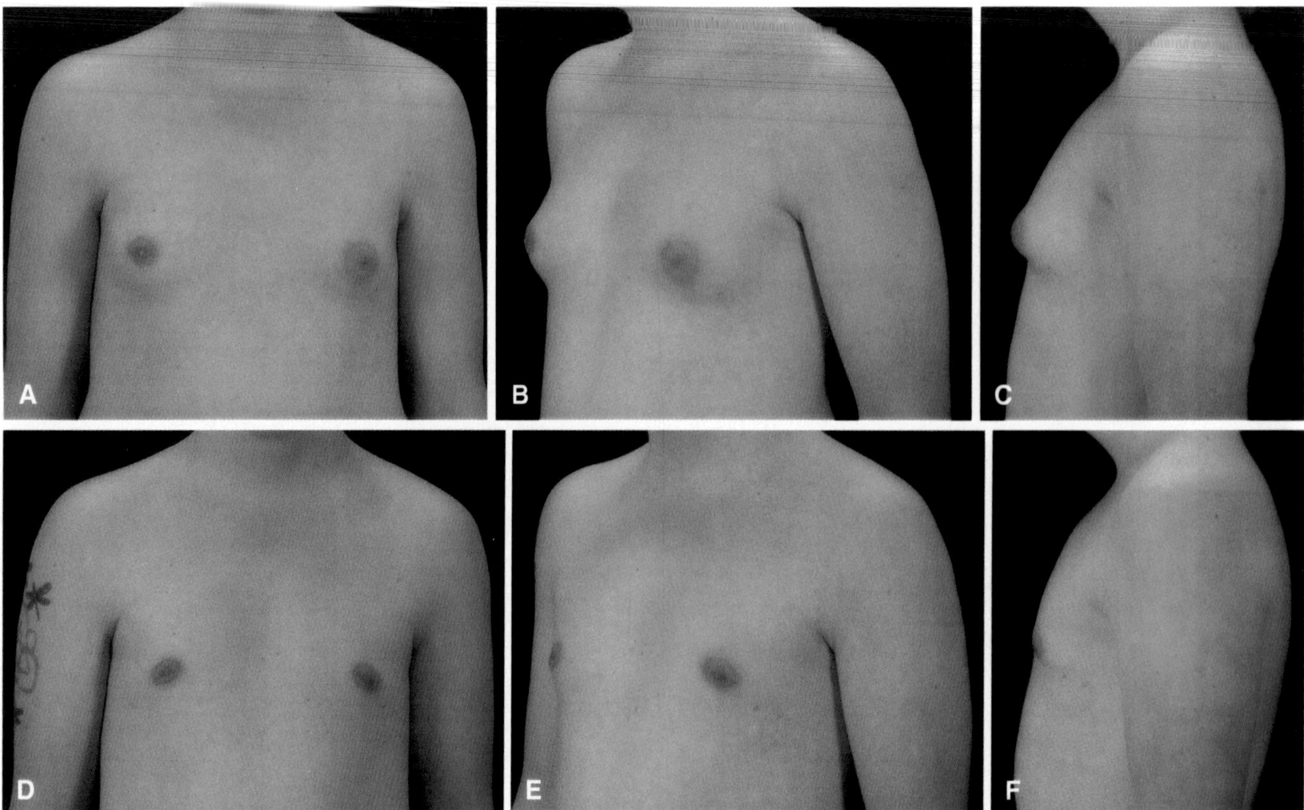

FIGURE 57.4. This patient with moderate glandular gynecomastia without skin excess underwent direct excision via transareolar approach for correction of gynecomastia. **A–C.** Preoperative photographs. **D–F.** Postoperative photographs.

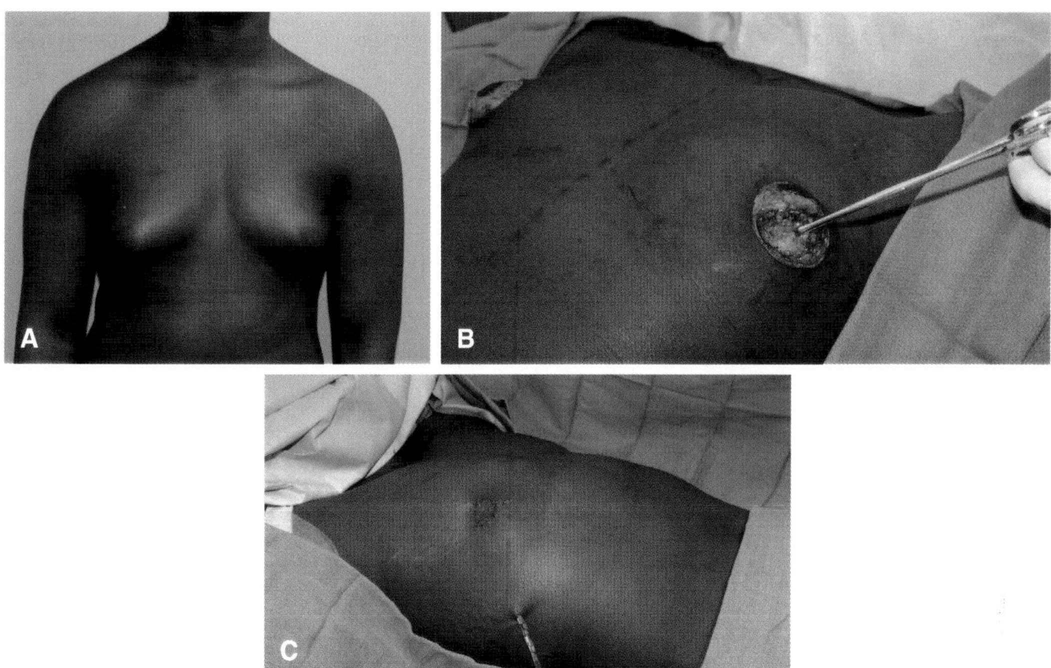

FIGURE 57.5. **A.** Preoperative AP view of patient with moderate glandular gynecomastia and enlarged areolas. **B.** Intraoperative photo after deepithelialization of excess areola and a pull-through technique demonstrating the dense glandular bud of tissue beneath the nipple areolar complex. **C.** Immediate postoperative result showing improved chest contour and areolar diameter.

of the procedure. Liposuction may be used as an adjunct to a direct excisional technique, and fanning is performed to optimize contour.

Gynecomastia is often accompanied by an increased diameter of the nipple areolar complex, contributing to the feminine appearance of the chest. After liposuction or direct excision, some retraction in the size of the nipple areolar complex is expected. However, if the areolar diameter is very large, or the skin has poor elasticity, reduction of the diameter of the areola should be considered at the time of the initial surgery. A circumareolar mastopexy pattern may be performed with deepithelialization to reduce the diameter of the areola and possibly skin envelope (Figure 57.5). Some puckering of the tissue occurs initially, but this settles out postoperatively. This could also be performed in a staged manner if retraction in the areolar diameter does not occur postoperatively.

Patients with moderate to severe enlargement and skin excess require excisional techniques that address both the glandular and skin redundancy. If the nipple lies at or slightly below the fold, a periareolar excision may be sufficient to remove the skin excess. When the nipple is more ptotic and there is marked tissue excess, a reduction mammoplasty approach is necessary. The skin is excised in a vertical pattern, wise pattern, or in a total amputation technique with an inframammary scar only. The nipple may be left on a glandular pedicle to preserve vascularity and sensation. This is sometimes difficult in larger breasted males, as a glandular pedicle requires that significant breast tissue be preserved, often leaving the male breast larger than is cosmetically desirable. The nipple can also be preserved on a dermal pedicle to reduce bulk; however, the blood supply is less reliable with such a technique. Alternatively, a direct amputation technique with free nipple grafting may be indicated (Figure 57.6). Patients should be well informed of the consequences of free nipple grafting, including graft loss, sensory changes, pigment loss, and asymmetry.

Relocating the nipple in these patients is one of the most challenging aspects of gynecomastia surgery. Unlike the female breast, the nipple should be placed inferior and lateral at the level of the inferior border of the pectoralis muscle. A variety of complex mathematical formulas have been postulated to help with nipple placement. Beckenstein et al. studied normal male subjects and determined an ideal sternal notch to nipple distance to be 20 cm, with 21 cm between each nipple. The average diameter of a male nipple in their study is 2.8 cm.[14] Shulman et al. extrapolated on the data, creating a three point mathematical ratio based upon the patient's own height and chest circumference to determine the ideal nipple position. Using these simple measurements, the new nipple should be located at 0.722 of the patient's height. At that level, chest circumference is then measured, and the distance between the nipple areolar complexes should be 0.213 of the circumference. Finally, the patient's height is multiplied by 0.104, which should correlate to the distance between the sternal notch and new nipple location.[15]

Special Patient Populations

Certain patient populations deserve specific attention and evaluation to help with comprehensive surgical planning.[16] In the postbariatric patients, skin elasticity should be evaluated. The entire chest wall should be examined for redundant, loose tissue extending from the breast to the lateral axilla. Due to volume loss and tissue redundancy, these patients often require the direct excision of skin in both the vertical and horizontal direction. Hurwitz described a successful technique with a boomerang-patterned excision in these patients.[17] With this approach, the ptotic nipple areolar complex is relocated, while simultaneously excising breast and torso laxity in the patient. This pattern may then be extended laterally to remove lateral tissue excess on the male chest and axilla.

Bodybuilders are another population specifically affected by gynecomastia. The cause of the breast enlargement in this population may be anabolic steroid use, or related to the hormones in over the counter supplements used to maintain their muscular habitus. The breast enlargement often persists in these patients with low body fat, despite cessation of the offending agents.[18] Persistent stromal and periductal tissue becomes fibrotic with time, and this tissue is unlikely to dissipate if longstanding. In bodybuilders, the gynecomastia is usually glandular and fibrotic, as these patients have a paucity of body fat. Surgical intervention should be planned according to the pathology, and minimally invasive techniques such as liposuction are less effective in these patients. Direct excision of the enlarged gland via a pull-through technique is often indicated.

Pseudogynecomastia refers to enlargement of the male breast in the morbidly obese. In this population there is significant

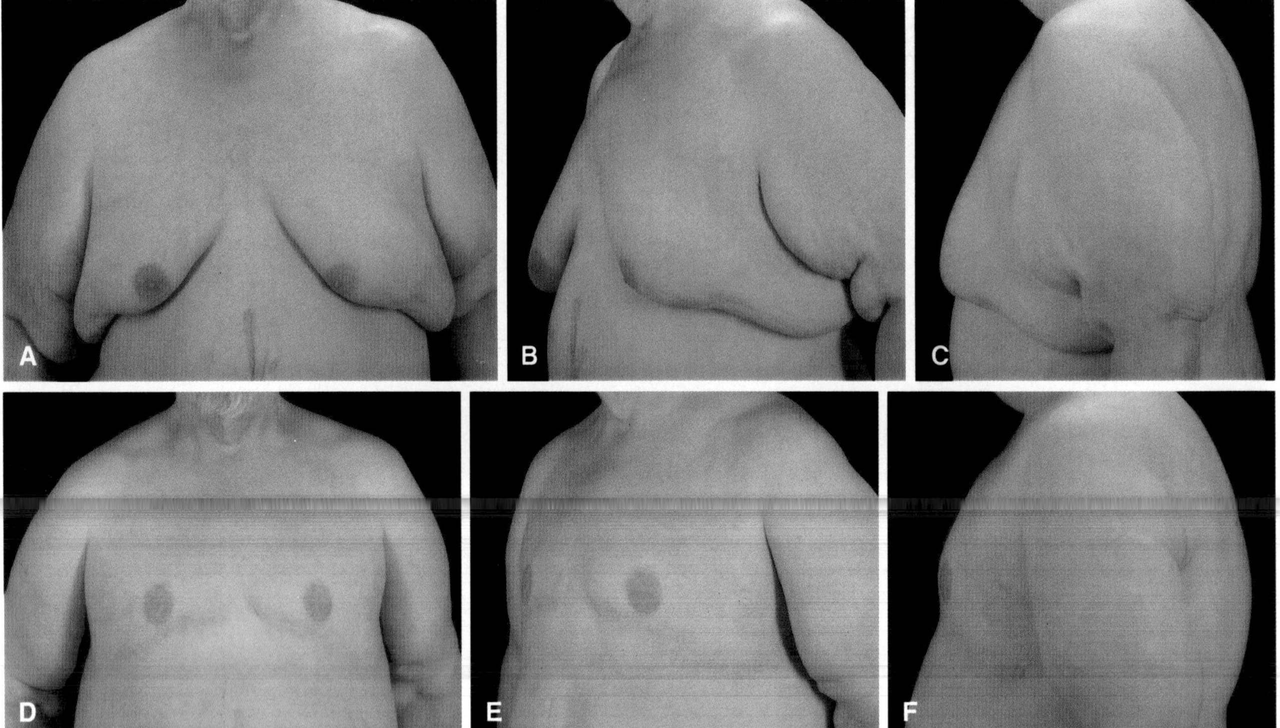

FIGURE 57.6. This patient with marked glandular excess and significant skin redundancy underwent IMF amputation with free nipple grafting. **A–C.** Preoperative photographs. **D–F.** Postoperative photographs.

adiposity in all areas of the body, and the breast is not spared. Due to excess skin and adipose tissue, an open approach with skin excision is often necessary. The treating physician should always counsel these patients on preoperative weight loss to decrease risk of major surgical complications and to achieve a desired cosmetic result.

POSTOPERATIVE MANAGEMENT

Following all types of surgical intervention, postoperative compliance with compression is essential to achieve an optimal cosmetic result. Suction drains should be considered in patients after direct excision, or when there is significant dead space present. Compression should be applied with specialized garments or compression wraps to allow the tissue to heal down to the chest wall and prevent seroma formation. The patients should continue compression for up to 3 months postoperatively throughout the healing process to reduce postoperative edema and ensure a flat contour.

Complications of surgical intervention include under resection, over resection, contour irregularity, and asymmetry. Patients may also experience hematomas, seromas, scarring, and infection. Patients with direct excision via a limited incision are the most likely to experience hematoma, as the visibility with this technique may be poor, leading to postoperative bleeding complications. When ultrasound-assisted liposuction is used, contact burns may occur, especially at the port entry site when moist towels are not used to protect the skin. In patients with skin excess and relocation of the nipple, partial or complete nipple loss and sensory changes may occur.

Most patients are quite satisfied with their outcomes after surgical correction of gynecomastia. They report confidence with their new appearance, and consistently report improved quality of life in all aspects, especially social functioning regardless of the stage of the gynecomastia treated.[19]

REFERENCES

1. Guss CE, Divasta AM. Adolescent gynecomastia. *Pediatr Endocrinol Rev.* 2017;14(4):371-377.
This article discusses the pathophysiology of gynecomastia. The medical workup is fully explained to help with management of these patients. Medical management and nonsurgical options are also discussed.
2. Raveenthiran V. Nenotal mastauxe (breast enlargement of the newborn). *J Neonatal Surg.* 2013;2(3):31.
3. Rohrich R, Ha RY, Kenkel RY, Adams WP Jr. Classification and management of gynecomastia: defining the role of ultrasound-assisted liposuction. *Plast Reconstr Surg.* 2003;111(2):909-923.
This landmark article discusses the use of ultrasound-assisted liposuction for the treatment of gynecomastia. The authors explain the role of skin tightening this therapy has on the gynecomastia patients, and note safe and reproducible results using ultrasound-assisted liposuction to treat gynecomastia. Their experience and surgical technique are highlighted.
4. Cuhaci N, Polat SB, Evranos B, et al. Gynecomastia: clinical evaluation and management. *Indian J Endocrinol Metab.* 2014;18(2):150-158.
5. Cordova A, Moschella F. Algorithm for clinical evaluation and surgical treatment of gynaecomastia. *J Plast Reconstr Aesthet Surg.* 2008;61:41-49.
6. Braunstein GD. Gynecomastia. *N Engl J Med.* 2007;357:1229-1237.
This is a comprehensive review article on the topic of Gynecomastia. The author discusses the pathophysiology of the disease and early patient management and workup. Evaluation and treatment are also discussed with equal attention to nonsurgical and surgical options. Useful algorithms for patient management are also presented.
7. Simon BE, Hoffman S, Kahn S. Classification and surgical correction of gynecomastia. *Plast Reconstr Surg.* 1973;51:48-52.
8. Nuzzi L, Cerrato FE, Erickson CR, et al. Psychosocial impact of adolescent gynecomastia: a prospective case-control study. *Plast Reconstr Surg.* 2013;131:890-896.
9. Kinsella C Jr, Landfair A, Rottgers SA, et al. The psychological burden of idiopathic adolescent gynecomastia. *Plast Reconstr Surg.* 2012;129:1-7.
Gynecomastia is a significant psychological burden for teenage boys, and patients often site social concerns during their consultation. This study used psychological interviews to measure anxiety, depression, and social phobias in this population. They determined that gynecomastia in adolescents placed them at high risk for issues with self-esteem and sexual identity.
10. Khan HN, Rampaul R, Blamey RW. Management of physiological gynaecomastia with tamoxifen. *Breast.* 2004;13(1):61-65.
11. Plourde PV, Kulin HE, Santner SJ. Clomiphene in the treatment of adolescent gynecomastia. *Am J Dis Child.* 1983;137(11):1080-1082.
12. Fagerlund A, Cormio L. Gynecomastia in patients with prostate cancer: a systemic review. *PLoS One.* 2015:1-11.

13. Rohrich RJ, Beran SJ, Kenkel JM, et al. Extending the role of liposuction in body contouring with ultrasound-assisted liposuction. *Plast Reconstr Surg*. 1998;101(4):1090-1102.
14. Beckenstein MS, Windle BH, Stroup RT. Anatomical parameters for nipple position and areolar diameter in males. *Ann Plast Surg*. 1996;36(1):33-36.
15. Shulman A, Badani E, Wolf Y, Hauben DJ. Appropriate location of the nipple-areola complex in males. *Plast Reconstr Surg*. 2001;108(2):348-351.
16. Waltho D, Hatchell A, Thoma A. Gynecomastia classification for surgical management: a systematic review and novel classification system. *Plast Reconstr Surg*. 2016;139(3):638-648.
17. Hurwitz D. Boomerang pattern correction of gynecomastia. *Plast Reconstr Surg*. 2015;135:433.
This technique article discusses an optimal technique for body contouring patients after massive weight loss, who are dissatisfied with their gynecomastia. Dr. Hurwitz presents a safe and effective combination of a torsoplasty with gynecomastia correction to address both the vertical and horizontal tissue excess in this patient population.
18. Blau M, Hazani R. Correction of gynecomastia in body builders and patients with good physique. *Plast Reconstr Surg*. 2015;135:42.
The authors discuss their technique for addressing subareolar glandular excess in bodybuilders and those with minimal body fat. Using a direct glandular excision, they are able to safely achieve a desired cosmetic outcome for these patients.
19. Kasielska-Trojan A, Antoszewski B. Gynecomastia surgery: impact on life quality. *Ann Plast Surg*. 2017;78(3):263-268.

QUESTIONS

1. A 20-year-old male presents with complaints of painful enlargement of breasts bilaterally. He notes that his breast enlargement began about 4 years earlier and has not dissipated. He is embarrassed to take off his shirt in the summer to swim and refuses to participate in organized sports. History, physical examination, and workup should include all of the following *except*:
   - **a.** History of illicit drug use
   - **b.** Testicular exam
   - **c.** Mammography
   - **d.** Medication history

2. A 53-year-old man is referred to your plastic surgery office for gynecomastia. On examination, he has a painless, firm mass of 2 cm located lateral to the nipple areolar complex in the left breast. He first experienced bloody nipple discharge about 6 months ago, and then discovered the breast enlargement. The right breast appears to be normal, and the remainder of his physical exam is unremarkable. Which of the following is the next step in the workup of this patient?
   - **a.** Mammography
   - **b.** Referral to Endocrinology
   - **c.** Observation and follow-up in 3 months
   - **d.** Observation and follow-up in 1 year

3. Which of the following grouping contains a medication or drugs NOT associated with gynecomastia?
   - **a.** Amphetamines, anabolic steroids, marijuana
   - **b.** Digoxin, ACE inhibitors, spironolactone
   - **c.** Benzodiazepines, risperidone, haloperidol
   - **d.** Cephalosporins, metronidazole, isoniazid

4. A healthy 32-year-old man with a BMI of 23.5 comes to your office for evaluation of asymptomatic gynecomastia that has been present for 15 years. He does not have any medical problems, take any medications, or use illicit drugs. On evaluation, he has firm, rubbery tissue below the nipple areolar complex bilaterally. The nipple areolar complex is located at the inferior border of the pectoralis major muscle and is 28 mm in diameter. The remainder of his physical exam is normal. Which of the following is the appropriate recommendation for this patient?
   - **a.** Limited periareolar incision with a pull-through direct excision technique
   - **b.** Suction-assisted lipectomy with disruption of the inframammary fold
   - **c.** Wise pattern reduction mammoplasty with inferior dermoglandular pedicle
   - **d.** Breast amputation technique with free nipple grafting

5. A 13-year-old boy comes to the office accompanied by his mother. For the last [illegible] years, the patient has had progressive increase in size of his breasts. The boy refuses to participate in physical education, and is suffering from failing grades due to his unwillingness to participate. On physical exam, he has marked bilateral breast development with well-defined inframammary folds. No true masses are identified. The patient has underdeveloped testes, and his body habitus and overall appearance is quite feminine. Following your examination, what is the most appropriate next step?
   - **a.** Ultrasound-assisted liposuction technique
   - **b.** Mammography
   - **c.** Referral to pediatric endocrinology
   - **d.** Breast amputation with free nipple grafting

1. **Answer: c.** A thorough history and physical examination are necessary to evaluate patients with gynecomastia. Illicit drugs including heroin, marijuana, and the abuse of anabolic steroids can cause gynecomastia. Similarly, a number of pharmacologic agents have been linked to gynecomastia. These include, but are not limited to, digoxin, cimetidine, spironolactone, verapamil, phenytoin, diazepam, and amphetamines. Neoplastic causes of gynecomastia include a variety of testicular tumors, and therefore physical examination should include a scrotal and testicular exam to rule out such pathology. Mammography is not needed in evaluation of routine adolescent bilateral gynecomastia. Imaging only needs to be obtained if there is concern for malignancy, such as in a unilateral presentation or in men with karyotype anomalies such as Klinefelter syndrome.

2. **Answer: a.** Breast malignancy must always remain on the differential diagnosis for a patient presenting with gynecomastia. Signs of malignancy include a nontender mass located outside of the nipple areolar complex. Asymmetry, skin dimpling, nipple retraction, nipple discharge, and bleeding are all symptoms suggestive of pathology. When these symptoms are present, the patient should have imaging with mammography or ultrasound to evaluate for breast carcinoma. Referrals for further workup should wait until the patient has been evaluated for malignancy.

3. **Answer: d.** Multiple classes of medications are linked to the development of gynecomastia. Illicit drugs, including marijuana, anabolic steroids, alcohol, opiates, and amphetamines, have been linked to gynecomastia. Cardiovascular medications including calcium channel blockers, spironolactone, digoxin, ACE inhibitors, amiodarone, and antipsychotics including benzodiazepines, phenothiazines, tricyclic antidepressants, olanzapine, haloperidol, and risperidone are well-documented causes. Metronidazole and isoniazid are linked to gynecomastia; however, cephalosporin antibiotics have not been associated with the development of gynecomastia.

4. **Answer: a.** Glandular gynecomastia is best treated with a pull-through technique and direct excision. This firm tissue is often difficult to remove with traditional liposuction techniques. Only patients with moderate to marked skin excess should undergo skin reduction procedures with wise pattern reduction mammoplasty or amputation techniques with free nipple grafting.

5. **Answer: c.** Adolescents with feminizing features and significant gynecomastia should be evaluated by pediatric endocrinologists for disorders of sexual differentiation and Klinefelter syndrome (XXY). Surgical intervention should not be planned before underlying pathology and system illness have been ruled out as the cause of gynecomastia. Mammography is not indicated in the workup of bilateral gynecomastia, unless there is clinical suspicion of malignancy with asymmetry, a palpated mass, skin dimpling, nipple retraction, or nipple discharge.

CHAPTER 58 Breast Cancer: Current Trends in Screening, Patient Evaluation, and Treatment

Alvin C. Kwok and Christopher J. Pannucci

KEY POINTS

- In the United States, a woman born today has about a 1 in 8 chance of being diagnosed with breast cancer during her life.
- The American Cancer Society guidelines from 2015 recommend that women at the age of 55 years or older with average risk should have biennial screening mammography.
- Indications for postmastectomy radiation therapy include patients with large tumors (>5 cm), four or more involved lymph nodes, positive or close margins, and those with locally advanced breast cancer.
- The 2014 American Society of Clinical Oncology guidelines recommend axillary lymph node dissection for patients who have three or more metastatic sentinel lymph nodes on sentinel lymph node biopsy (SLNB) or who have one or two metastatic lymph nodes on SLNB but who do not desire whole-breast irradiation.
- Oncologic factors suggestive of suitable cases for nipple-sparing mastectomies include tumors >2 cm from the nipple and no clinical involvement of the skin or nipple.
- In breast cancer patients who have undergone mastectomy, there is no difference in survival in patients receiving chemotherapy within 4 to 8 weeks of surgery.

INTRODUCTION

Breast cancer is the most common malignancy diagnosed worldwide; currently, it is the leading cause of cancer-related death in women.[1] It is estimated that in 2017 there were 252,710 Americans diagnosed with invasive breast cancer and 40,610 died of the disease. The lifetime risk of women developing breast cancer is approximately 12.4%, or 1 in 8 women. Over the last 10 years, the incidence of new female breast cancer cases has been relatively stable. Most women are diagnosed between 55 and 64 years old. The average 5-year survival rate is 89.7% and patients with higher disease stage have decreased 5-year survival. Death rates have been falling at an average rate of 1.8% per year.[2]

The Women's Health and Cancer Rights Act of 1998 increased access to reconstructive services for women with breast cancer. Since that time, an increased proportion of women have undergone reconstructive procedures by plastic surgeons. In the United States, there has been a nearly 20% increase in rates of reconstruction from 1998 to 2007. During the same time period, there was an increasing proportion of implant-based breast reconstruction compared with autologous-based breast reconstruction and higher rates of bilateral mastectomy.[3,4]

RISK FACTORS

Although the etiology of most breast cancer is unknown, risk factors have been clearly defined. These include female gender, increasing patient age, family history of breast cancer at a young age, early menarche, late menopause, older age at first live childbirth, prolonged hormone replacement therapy, previous exposure to therapeutic chest wall irradiation, benign proliferative breast disease, increased mammographic density, and genetic mutations. Aside from gender, increasing age and genetic mutations are the only substantial risk factors.

The National Cancer Institute (NCI) and National Surgical Adjuvant Breast and Bowel Project (NSABP) have developed the Breast Cancer Risk Assessment Tool that can help women to estimate their risk of developing invasive breast cancer (https://www.cancer.gov/bcrisktool/). This tool is also known as the Gail Model. The model uses a women's history of prior breast malignancy, gene mutations, age, age to menarche, age at the time of her first live birth of child, family history, history of breast biopsy, and race/ethnicity to calculate 5 year and lifetime risk of developing breast cancer. The Gail Model has only been validated for women in the United States who are screened regularly for breast cancer.

Hereditary breast cancer accounts for up to 20% of breast cancer cases. More common syndromic breast cancer susceptibility genes include BRCA 1 and 2, TP53 (Li-Fraumeni syndrome), PTEN (Cowden syndrome), CDH1 (hereditary diffuse gastric cancer syndrome) STK11 (Peutz-Jeghers syndrome), mismatch repair genes (Lynch syndrome), and NF1 (Neurofibromatosis 1). More common nonsyndromic breast cancer susceptibility genes include PALB2, CHEK2, and ATM. Genetic testing should be performed if a patient has a known mutation in a breast cancer susceptibility gene, if there are two or more primary breast cancers on the same side of the family (in the same person or two separate individuals), if there is one or more ovarian cancers on the same side of the family, if there is a first- or second-degree relative who was diagnosed with breast cancer before the age of 45 years, or male breast cancer.[5] Patients with strong family history of breast cancer or known genetic predisposition should always be seen in coordination with a certified genetic counselor.

The BRCA1 and BRCA2 genes are autosomal dominant tumor suppressor genes that help to repair damaged DNA. BRCA 1 and 2 gene mutations account for 20% to 40% of the hereditary breast cancers. Women with the BRCA1 mutation have a 55% to 65% risk of developing breast cancer and a 39% chance of developing ovarian cancer by age 70 years. In contrast, women with the BRCA2 mutation have a slightly lower risk of 45% for developing breast cancer and 11% to 17% chance of developing ovarian cancer by age 70 years. In addition to breast and ovarian cancers, patients with the BRCA gene mutation are also at higher risk for fallopian tube, peritoneal, prostate, and pancreatic cancer. Although tests are helpful for identifying known genetic risk factors, those who have significant family history may have genetic mutations that have not yet been formally identified.[6,7]

TYPES OF BREAST CANCER

The most common types of breast cancer include ductal carcinoma in situ (DCIS), invasive ductal carcinoma, and invasive lobular carcinoma. In situ, or noninvasive, cancers increase a patient's risk for developing invasive cancer. DCIS can transform into invasive cancer. Lobular carcinoma in situ (LCIS) does not transform into invasive disease but instead increases one's risk by 7 to 12 times for developing invasive cancer in either breast.[8,9] Other less common types of breast cancer include inflammatory breast cancer, Paget disease, Phyllodes tumor, and angiosarcoma.

SCREENING

The updated American Cancer Society guidelines of 2015 recommend that women with an average risk of breast cancer should undergo regular screening mammography starting at age 45 years. Women between the ages of 45 and 54 years are recommended to have annual screening mammography whereas women at the age of 55 years and older are recommended to have biennial screening mammography. Screening mammography is recommended to continue for as long as the patient has a life expectancy of 10 years or longer. In contrary to previous guidelines, no regular clinical breast examinations for breast cancer are recommended for average-risk women at any age.[10] Mammography is the standard imaging technique for breast cancer screening. Other screening modalities such as MRI are only indicated for patients with higher-than-average risk of developing breast cancer.

STAGING

Tumor classification using the TNM staging system outlined by the American Joint Committee on Cancer (AJCC) is used to assist in prognosis and treatment of breast cancer. This system is built upon the extent of disease for the tumor (T), status of the regional lymph nodes (N), and presence of distant metastases (M). More recently, the AJCC has also added tumor grade, HER2, estrogen receptor (ER), progesterone receptor (PR), and genomic assays as part of the breast cancer staging system.[11] Early-stage breast cancer (stages I–II) is disease that is confined to the breast without extension to the chest wall or locoregional lymph nodes. Early-stage breast cancer is usually treated surgically and in selected patients with radiotherapy. Breast cancers that are stage III and above require locoregional control usually consisting of surgery and adjuvant systemic therapy.[12] Surveillance, Epidemiology, and End Results Program data from 2007 to 2013 showed that women with stage 0 or stage 1 breast cancer have a 5-year relative survival rate of nearly 100%. Women with stage II breast cancer have a 5-year relative survival rate of approximately 93%. Women with stage III and stage IV breast cancers have poorer prognoses with 5-year relative survival rates of 72% and 22%, respectively.[13]

WORK-UP

An abnormal palpable breast mass or new mammographic finding is usually followed by an ultrasonic examination that can differentiate between solid and cystic breast masses. Ultrasound can also be used to detect lymph nodes that are suspicious for axillary metastases. The primary tumor is then evaluated by an image guided biopsy that, if found to be positive for malignancy, is treated with surgery. Although breast MRIs are generally more sensitive than mammography or ultrasonography, they have not been found to improve overall survival outcomes or improve locoregional recurrence rates.[14-17]

SURGICAL TREATMENT

Improved local control is causally associated with improved breast cancer survival.[18] The surgical treatment of breast cancer has evolved. The first surgical treatment of breast cancer was the radical mastectomy that was popularized by William Halstead at the end of the nineteenth century. Since then, there has been a trend toward increasingly less invasive surgical management of breast cancer. Since the introduction of the radical mastectomy, other techniques, such as the modified radical mastectomy, partial mastectomy, skin-sparing mastectomy (SSM), and nipple-sparing mastectomy (NSM), have been developed. Although traditional surgical management has been used to treat the breast affected by cancer, there has also been an increasing trend toward risk reducing procedures such as contralateral prophylactic mastectomies.

BREAST CONSERVATION THERAPY

Breast conservation therapy (BCT) couples surgical excision of the tumor with local radiotherapy. BCT is appropriate for early stage breast cancer and has been shown to provide equivalent overall survival rates compared to total mastectomy while still preserving the breast.[18] Despite similar survival rates, BCT has a reported positive margin incidence rate of 20% to 70%. Several techniques have been developed to decrease the positive margin rates including ultrasound needle localization, stereotactic needle localization, bracketing, or taking additional margins.[19]

NEOADJUVANT SYSTEMIC THERAPY

Neoadjuvant systemic therapy is indicated for patients with inoperable tumors or if BCT is desired and the tumor size would have otherwise required a mastectomy. Cytotoxic, hormonal, and/or trastuzumab therapy can be used to reduce the amount of tumor burden in the breast and axilla without compromising survival. Although the entire initial tumor bed does not need to be removed, any residual palpable or radiographic lesions should be excised. For those who have complete clinical response, surgical excision is still indicated.[18] Decisions regarding radiation therapy should be based upon maximal stage from prechemotherapy tumor characteristics and/or pathologic stage regardless of the tumor's response to adjuvant systemic therapy.[20]

MASTECTOMY

The goal of a mastectomy is to remove all breast tissue thus decreasing the risk for cancer recurrence. The anatomic borders of the breast are defined by the midline medially, the latissimus dorsi muscle laterally, the clavicle superiorly, and the insertion of the rectus abdominus muscle inferiorly. Contemporary techniques such as the SSM and the NSM can improve aesthetic outcome.[21]

The SSM was first described in June 1991 by Toth and Lappert. This technique is defined by removal of breast tissue with modified minimal incisions leaving as much skin as possible. Contraindications for SSM are inflammatory carcinomas, locally advanced carcinomas, and smoking (relative contraindication). Local recurrence rates after SSM are similar to other forms of mastectomy.[22]

The NSM was a natural evolution from the SSM. It is performed by removal of all breast tissue without excision of skin and the nipple-areolar complex. Oncologic contraindications for NSM include a tumor to nipple distance of <2 cm or clinical involvement of the skin and/or nipple. The NSM is generally performed with a frozen section from the posterior nipple margin to confirm no cancer invasion. If this frozen section is positive, the NSM is converted into a SSM. Partial or full nipple necrosis has been reported in 2% to 20% of NSMs. Overall survival, disease-free survival, or local recurrence has been shown to be similar between NSM, SSM, and modified radical mastectomy.[21]

CONTRALATERAL MASTECTOMY

Rates of contralateral prophylactic mastectomy are increasing without evidence of substantial improvement of overall survival. The National Comprehensive Cancer Network currently recommends that women with breast cancer who are 35 years or younger, premenopausal, and carriers of a known BRCA gene mutation should only consider additional risk-reduction strategies with appropriate counseling. Except for the populations outlined earlier, risk-reduction prophylactic mastectomies of the breast contralateral to the known unilateral breast cancer are discouraged. It is important to discuss with those considering contralateral risk-reduction prophylactic mastectomy that these procedures are not without their own risk of minor and major complications, and that symmetry procedures match the native breast to the reconstructed side.[20]

TIMING OF CANCER THERAPIES BEFORE AND AFTER SURGERY

Patients who do not receive neoadjuvant chemotherapy and who undergo surgery within 60 days of their diagnosis have improved overall survival.[23] For patients requiring neoadjuvant chemotherapy, overall survival, 5-year recurrence-free survival, and locoregional recurrence-free survival are equivalent when undergoing surgery within 8 weeks of completion of their neoadjuvant chemotherapy.[24] After a mastectomy for patients with estrogen receptor, progesterone receptor, or HER-2/neu-positive breast cancer, adjuvant systemic therapy has been shown to have similar outcomes on overall survival if initiated within 4 to 8 weeks of surgery. Patients with triple negative breast cancer (estrogen receptor, progesterone receptor, and HER-2/neu-negative breast cancers) have been shown to have an overall survival benefit if adjuvant chemotherapy is initiated within 30 days of their surgery.[25] Postmastectomy radiation therapy is associated with improved outcomes when performed within 6 to 8 weeks of surgery.[26-29]

MANAGEMENT OF THE AXILLA

Removal of axillary lymph nodes both provides pathologic staging data and helps with local control. Unfortunately, removal of lymph nodes also results in significant morbidity. An axillary lymph node dissection (ALND) has a 16% risk of the development of lymphedema at 5 years. Although a sentinel lymph node biopsy (SLNB) is minimally invasive, it is still associated with a 5% rate of the development of lymphedema at 5 years. In addition to lymphedema, there can be arm stiffness, pain, and paresthesia. In the 1980s, two large studies (NSABP-B04 and the King's-Cambridge trials) compared ALND and radiation therapy with no treatment to the axilla in clinically node-negative patients. Each study demonstrated that treating the axilla significantly decreased the recurrence rate but did not improve survival rates in early stage breast cancer patients. With the development of lymphatic mapping techniques, SLNB became established as the new standard for staging the axilla. The SLNB was first described in 1994. The orderly manner with which lymph nodes drained allowed surgeons to use blue dye and/or radioactive technetium to biopsy the first 1 to 4 nodes that took up the technetium or blue dye to evaluate for metastases to the nodes.[30] SLNBs have been shown to have significantly less morbidity than an ALND. Patients who undergo SLNB have improved arm volume, sensibility, and ROM compared to those who undergo ALND.[31] In 2011, the American College of Surgeons Z0011 study was a prospective multicenter randomized trial that showed that for clinical T1-T2 invasive breast cancer patients with clinically negative lymph nodes that a SLNB with one to two positive SLNs was not inferior to a complete ALND for regional control of the axilla. Patients with clinically positive nodes at the time of diagnosis confirmed by fine needle aspiration (FNA) or core biopsy or patients who had no sentinel nodes identified (e.g., a failure of the sentinel lymph node mapping procedure) are recommended to have an ALND.[21,32,20,33]

SYSTEMIC THERAPY

Systemic therapy has become increasingly precise. Chemotherapeutic regimens are becoming largely based on the pathologic analysis of one's tumor. In addition to a tumor's molecular profile, indications for chemotherapy include large tumor size (>2 cm), positive lymph nodes, ER-negative and PR-negative tumors, HER-2/neu-positive tumors, and inflammatory breast cancer. Anthracycline-based systemic therapies have been shown to improve survival compared to methotrexate-based regimens but they also have more substantial side effects. Anthracyclines can have associated cardiotoxicity and thus should be used carefully or avoided when treating elderly patients and those with previous cardiac disease. Taxanes in combination with chemotherapy have also been shown to be more effective and thus have become used as standard treatment.[5]

RADIATION THERAPY

Radiotherapy is an important component of local regional disease control. Whole-breast radiation therapy with or without boost to tumor bed is required as a part of BCT and occurs after lumpectomy. Current guidelines also recommend chest wall radiation after mastectomy if tumors are >5 cm, if pathology margins are positive, or if there are positive ALNs. Accelerated partial breast irradiation (APBI) is a technique that provides a more focused field of radiation after complete surgical excision of in-breast disease but is still considered investigational and should be used within the confines of clinical trials. The benefit of APBI is that it can be administered over a 1 to 2 week period as compared to the typical 6 to 7 week period for whole-breast radiation. APBI commonly combines brachytherapy with external-beam photon therapy to the tumor bed.[20]

HORMONAL BLOCKADE AND BIOLOGIC THERAPIES

The relationship between breast cancer and hormone receptors has been well established since the 1950s. Since them, endocrine therapies such as tamoxifen have been used to treat breast cancer. Selective estrogen receptor modulators (SERMs), such as tamoxifen, block estrogen receptors in the breast, and effectively block estrogen activity in breast tissue. Tumors that are progesterone receptor positive often respond similarly to SERMs as ER-positive tumors. Hormonal blockade therapies are not without adverse events. Tamoxifen, while reasonably well tolerated, has been shown to be associated with hot flushes, headaches, menstrual abnormalities, a higher risk for endometrial cancer (cumulative risk 3.1% versus 1.6%), and a twofold increase in the incidence of pulmonary embolism. Current recommendations call for at least 5 years of treatment with a longer course of 10 years having been shown to further reduce recurrence and increase survival.

Aromatase inhibitors, such as anastrozole, have been demonstrated to increase disease-free survival, increase time to recurrence, and decrease rates of distant metastases and contralateral breast cancer with fewer adverse side effects compared to tamoxifen in ER-positive postmenopausal women.[5,34-36]

Targeted biologic therapies are used to treat patients with HER-2/neu receptor positivity. HER-2/neu receptor positive tumors are known to have a poorer prognosis with high rates of recurrence, relative resistance to hormonal therapy, and resistance to some chemotherapeutics. The monoclonal antibody against HER-2/neu, trastuzumab, has been shown to significantly improve outcomes in HER-2-positive cancers. Current guidelines recommend the use of trastuzumab in patients with HER-2/neu-positive tumors for 1 year.[5]

REFERENCES

1. Network NCC. NCCN Guidelines Version 3.2017 Breast Cancer. https://www.nccn.org/professionals/physician_gls/pdf/breast.pdf. Accessed November 11, 2017.
2. Surveillance E, and End Results Program. Cancer Stat Facts: Female Breast Cancer. https://seer.cancer.gov/statfacts/html/breast.html. Accessed November 11, 2017.
3. Jagsi R, Jiang J, Momoh AO, et al. Trends and variation in use of breast reconstruction in patients with breast cancer undergoing mastectomy in the United States. *J Clin Oncol*. 2014;32(9):919-926.
4. Kwok AC, Goodwin IA, Ying J, Agarwal JP. National trends and complication rates after bilateral mastectomy and immediate breast reconstruction from 2005 to 2012. *Am J Surg*. 2015;210(3):512-516.
5. Matsen CB, Neumayer LA. Breast cancer: a review for the general surgeon. *JAMA Surgery*. 2013;148(10):971-980.
6. NIH NCI. *BRCA1 and BRCA2: Cancer Risk and Genetic Testing*; 2017.

BREAST

7. Frey JD, Salibian AA, Schnabel FR, Choi M, Karp NS. Non-BRCA1/2 breast cancer susceptibility genes: a new frontier with clinical consequences for plastic surgeons. *Plast Reconstr Surg Glob Open*. 2017;5(11):e1564.
8. Society AC. *Lobular Carcinoma In Situ (LCIS)*; 2017.
9. Society AC. *Types of Breast Cancer*; 2017.
10. Oeffinger KC, Fontham ET, Etzioni R, et al. Breast cancer screening for women at average risk: 2015 guideline update from the American Cancer Society. *JAMA*. 2015;314(15):1599-1614.
11. Cancer AJCo. *Breast cancer. AJCC Cancer Staging Manual*. 8th ed.; 2017.
12. Teven CM, Schmid DB, Sisco M, Ward J, Howard MA. Systemic therapy for early-stage breast cancer: what the plastic surgeon should know. *Eplasty*. 2017;17:e7.
13. Society AC. *Breast Cancer Survival Rates*; 2017.
14. Turnbull L, Brown S, Harvey I, et al. Comparative effectiveness of MRI in breast cancer (COMICE) trial: a randomised controlled trial. *Lancet*. 2010;375(9714):563-571.
15. Morris EA. Should we dispense with preoperative breast MRI? *Lancet*. 2010;375(9714):528-530.
16. Shin H-C, Han W, Moon H-G, et al. Limited value and utility of breast MRI in patients undergoing breast-conserving cancer surgery. *Ann Surg Oncol*. 2012;19(8):2572-2579.
17. Weber JJ, Bellin LS, Milbourn DE, Verbanac KM, Wong JH. Selective preoperative magnetic resonance imaging in women with breast cancer: no reduction in the reoperation rate. *Arch Surg*. 2012;147(9):834-839.
18. Kaufmann M, Morrow M, von Minckwitz G, Harris JR. Locoregional treatment of primary breast cancer. *Cancer*. 2010;116(5):1184-1191.
19. [illegible], [illegible] IM, Wengrofsky AJ, et al. Identifying factors and techniques to decrease the positive margin rate in partial mastectomies: have we missed the mark? *Breast J*. 2016;22(3):303-309.
20. Gradishar WJ, Anderson BO, Balassanian R, et al. Invasive breast cancer version 1.2016, NCCN clinical practice guidelines in oncology. *J Natl Compr Cancer Netw*. 2016;14(3):324-354.
21. Cil TD, McCready D. Modern approaches to the surgical management of malignant breast disease: the role of breast conservation, complete mastectomy, skin- and nipple-sparing mastectomy. *Clin Plastic Surgery*. 2018;45(1):1-11.
22. González EG, Rancati AO. Skin-sparing mastectomy. *Gland Surg*. 2015;4(6):541.
23. Bleicher RJ, Ruth K, Sigurdson ER, et al. Time to surgery and breast cancer survival in the United States. *JAMA Oncol*. 2016;2(3):330-339.
24. Sanford RA, Lei X, Barcenas CH, et al. Impact of time from completion of neoadjuvant chemotherapy to surgery on survival outcomes in breast cancer patients. *Ann Surg Oncol*. 2016;23(5):1515-1521.
25. Gagliato Dde M, Gonzalez-Angulo AM, Lei X, et al. Clinical impact of delaying initiation of adjuvant chemotherapy in patients with breast cancer. *J Clin Oncol*. 2014;32(8):735-744.
26. Whelan TJ. Use of conventional radiation therapy as part of breast-conserving treatment. *J Clin Oncol*. 2005;23(8):1718-1725.
27. Buchholz TA. Radiation therapy for early-stage breast cancer after breast-conserving surgery. *New Engl J Med*. 2009;360(1):63-70.
28. Punglia RS, Saito AM, Neville BA, Earle CC, Weeks JC. Impact of interval from breast conserving surgery to radiotherapy on local recurrence in older women with breast cancer: retrospective cohort analysis. *BMJ*. 2010;340:c845.
29. Silva SB, Pereira AAL, Marta GN, et al. Clinical impact of adjuvant radiation therapy delay after neoadjuvant chemotherapy in locally advanced breast cancer. *Breast*. 2018;38:39-44.
30. Rao R, Euhus D, Mayo HG, Balch C. Axillary node interventions in breast cancer: a systematic review. *JAMA*. 2013;310(13):1385-1394.
31. Madsen AH, Haugaard K, Soerensen J, et al. Arm morbidity following sentinel lymph node biopsy or axillary lymph node dissection: a study from the Danish Breast Cancer Cooperative Group. *Breast*. 2008;17(2):138-147.
32. Ozmen T, Vinyard AH, Avisar E. Management of the positive axilla in 2017. *Cureus*. 2017;9(5).
33. Giuliano AE, Hunt KK, Ballman KV, et al. Axillary dissection vs no axillary dissection in women with invasive breast cancer and sentinel node metastasis: a randomized clinical trial. *JAMA*. 2011;305(6):569-575.
34. Burstein HJ, Temin S, Anderson H, et al. Adjuvant endocrine therapy for women with hormone receptor–positive breast cancer: American Society of Clinical Oncology Clinical Practice Guideline focused update. *J Clin Oncol*. 2014;32(21):2255-2269.
35. Shagufta, Ahmad I. Tamoxifen a pioneering drug: an update on the therapeutic potential of tamoxifen derivatives. *Eur J Med Chem*. 2018;143:515-531.
36. Cuzick J, Forbes JF, Sestak I, et al. Long-term results of tamoxifen prophylaxis for breast cancer—96-month follow-up of the randomized IBIS-I trial. *J Natl Cancer Inst*. 2007;99(4):272-282.

KEY REFERENCES

1. Network NCC. NCCN Guidelines Version 3.2017 Breast Cancer. https://www.nccn.org/professionals/physician_gls/pdf/breast.pdf. Accessed November 11, 2017.
   These are peer reviewed national guidelines for the work-up and treatment of breast cancer.
2. Matsen CB, Neumayer LA. Breast cancer: a review for the general surgeon. *JAMA Surg*. 2013;148(10):971-980.
   This is a concise review of screening, work-up, and treatment of breast cancer with a focus on pertinent information for a surgeon.
3. Oeffinger KC, Fontham ET, Etzioni R, et al. Breast cancer screening for women at average risk: 2015 guideline update from the American Cancer Society. *JAMA*. 2015;314(15):1599-1614.
   These paper outlines the most recent American Cancer Society guidelines for breast cancer screen for women at average risk.
4. Gagliato Dde M, Gonzalez-Angulo AM, Lei X, et al. Clinical impact of delaying initiation of adjuvant chemotherapy in patients with breast cancer. *J Clin Oncol*. 2014;32(8):735-744.
   This paper examines the risks of delaying adjuvant chemotherapy.
5. Giuliano AE, Hunt KK, Ballman KV, et al. Axillary dissection vs no axillary dissection in women with invasive breast cancer and sentinel node metastasis: a randomized clinical trial. *JAMA*. 2011;305(6):569-575.
   This is also known as the American College of Surgeons Z0011 study. The results of this paper set the standard for how surgeons decide on whether or not to perform an ALND.

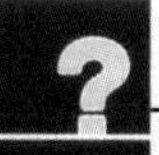

QUESTIONS

1. **A 62-year-old female presents with stage II invasive ductal carcinoma. The tumor measures 2.8 cm and is positioned 1.3 cm from her nipple. Clinically, she has no involvement of her axillary lymph nodes. She desires to undergo a NSM. What are her oncologic contraindications to undergoing a NSM?**

   a. Tumor is within 2 cm of her nipple
   b. Tumor is >2.5 cm in size
   c. Tumor is consistent with invasive ductal carcinoma
   d. Patient is older than 60 years of age
   e. Patient has stage II breast cancer

2. **A 53-year-old female presents with stage III, ER/PR-positive, and Her-2/neu-positive right breast cancer. She undergoes a right SSM with placement of a prepectoral tissue expander. Her oncologist has recommended chemotherapy and would like to initiate it as soon as possible. How long after her mastectomy can you delay chemotherapy without impacting her overall survival?**

   a. 8 weeks
   b. 9 weeks
   c. 10 weeks
   d. 12 weeks
   e. 14 weeks

3. **A 56-year-old female comes to your clinic to be evaluated for bilateral mastopexy. She appears to be a good candidate for a mastopexy. She has no personal or family history of breast cancer and denies any new masses in her breasts. Her last mammogram was performed 14 months ago, and there was no evidence of malignancy. How frequently should she have screening mammography?**

   a. Annually
   b. Every 5 years
   c. Biennially
   d. No need for screening mammogram giving her low risk profile
   e. Every 6 months

4. **A 43-year-old female with an extensive family history of breast cancer was recently diagnosed with stage IIA left breast cancer. Her mother was diagnosed with breast cancer at age 46 and her sister was diagnosed at age 42. Genetic testing was performed, and she has no known genetic predisposing for breast cancer. She presents for a NSM with SLNB with a submuscular tissue expander placement. She had no clinically positive nodes preoperatively. Her SLNB demonstrated three positive lymph nodes, and she undergoes an ALND. What are her indications for the ALND?**

   a. Stage IIA breast cancer
   b. Preoperative history of clinically negative nodes
   c. Family history of breast cancer
   d. Greater than 2 positive sentinel lymph nodes
   e. NSM

5. **Patients with the BRCA gene mutations are at increased risk of developing breast and ovarian cancer as well as which of the other cancers listed below?**

   a. Lung cancer
   b. Pancreatic cancer
   c. Basal cell carcinoma
   d. Lymphoma
   e. Glioblastoma

1. **Answer: a.** NSM is becoming more popular technique. The overall rate of occult nipple malignancy is 11.5%. Characteristics of the primary tumor that increase the risk for occult nipple malignancy include tumor-nipple distance <2 cm, tumor stage >2, lymph node metastasis, lymphovascular invasion, human epidermal growth receptor-2-positive, estrogen receptor/progesterone receptor-negative, tumor size >5 cm, retroareolar/central location, and multicentric tumors.

Reference:

Mallon P, Feron JG, Couturaud B, et al. The role of nipple-sparing mastectomy in breast cancer: a comprehensive review of the literature. *Plast Reconstr Surg*. 2013;131(5):969-984.

2. **Answer: a.** There is no difference in overall survival when comparing initiation of adjuvant chemotherapy within 4 weeks or within 8 weeks after surgery for patients who have estrogen receptor, progesterone receptor, or HER-2/neu-positive breast cancers. In patients with triple negative breast cancers, initiation of adjuvant chemotherapy within 4 weeks of surgery has been shown to improve overall survival.

Reference:

Gagliato Dde M, Gonzalez-Angulo AM, Lei Xet al. Clinical impact of delaying initiation of adjuvant chemotherapy in patients with breast cancer. *J Clin Oncol*. 2014;32(8):735-744.

3. **Answer: c.** The updated American Cancer Society guidelines of 2015 recommend that women with an average risk of breast cancer should undergo regular screening mammography starting at the age of 45 years. Women between the ages of 45 and 54 years are recommended to have annual screening mammography while women at the age of 55 years and older are recommended to have biennial screening mammography. Screening mammography is recommended to continue for as long as the patient has a life expectancy of 10 years or longer.

Reference:

Oeffinger KC, Fontham ET, Etzioni R, et al. Breast cancer screening for women at average risk: 2015 guideline update from the American Cancer Society. *JAMA*. 2015;314(15):1599-1614.

4. **Answer: d.** In 2011, the American College of Surgeons Z0011 study was a prospective multicenter randomized trial that showed that for clinical T1–T2 invasive breast cancer patients with clinically negative lymph nodes that a SLNB with one to two positive SLNs was not inferior to a complete ALND for regional control of the axilla. Patients with clinically positive nodes at the time of diagnosis confirmed by FNA or core biopsy or patients who had no sentinel nodes identified (e.g., a failure of the sentinel lymph node mapping procedure) are recommended to have an ALND.

Reference:

Giuliano AE, Hunt KK, Ballman KV, et al. Axillary dissection vs no axillary dissection in women with invasive breast cancer and sentinel node metastasis: a randomized clinical trial. *JAMA*. 2011;305(6):569-575.

5. **Answer: b.** The BRCA1 and BRCA2 genes are autosomal dominant tumor suppressor genes that help to repair damaged DNA. BRCA 1 and 2 gene mutations account for 20% to 40% of the hereditary breast cancers. Women with the BRCA1 mutation have a 55% to 65% risk of developing breast cancer and a 39% chance of developing ovarian cancer by the age of 70 years. In contrast, women with the BRCA2 mutation have a slightly lower risk of 45% for developing breast cancer and 11% to 17% chance of developing ovarian cancer by the age of 70 years. In addition to breast and ovarian cancers, patients with the BRCA gene mutation are also at higher risk for fallopian tube, peritoneal, prostate, and pancreatic cancer.

Reference:

https://www.cancer.gov/about-cancer/causes-prevention/genetics/brca-fact-sheet.

CHAPTER 59 Breast Reconstruction: Prosthetic Techniques

Peter W. Thompson and Grant W. Carlson

KEY POINTS

- Implant-based reconstruction is the most common method of breast reconstruction employed by plastic surgeons.
- Advantages of implant-based reconstruction include decreased operative time, no donor site morbidity, and faster patient recovery.
- Disadvantages include implant-related complications such as infection, capsular contracture, and implant malposition.
- Prosthetic reconstruction may be performed in an immediate or delayed fashion, in one or two stages. Healthy patients with smaller breasts, early stage breast cancer, and healthy mastectomy skin flaps are the best candidates for immediate and single-stage reconstruction.
- Acellular dermal matrix in implant-based reconstruction is a useful adjunct to provide total implant coverage while defining and maintaining implant position.
- Adjuvant radiation therapy significantly increases the rate of complications and reconstructive failure following implant-based reconstruction while decreasing patient-reported aesthetic outcomes and quality-of-life measures.
- Acute complications such as hematoma, infection, and mastectomy skin flap necrosis must be treated quickly and aggressively to avoid implant loss and suboptimal aesthetic outcome.

The primary technical goal of breast reconstruction is to recreate a breast mound in the postmastectomy patient. Prosthetic breast reconstruction techniques use tissue expanders and breast implants to accomplish this goal.

In 2002, breast reconstruction using prosthetic techniques became the most popular method of immediate breast reconstruction, outpacing autologous methods. According to a survey of the Nationwide Inpatient Sample database, the rate of immediate prosthetic breast reconstructions increased by 11% per year over a period of time from 1998 to 2008, whereas the rate of autologous reconstruction remained stable.[1] The reasons for this trend are likely multifactorial, including the increased prevalence of contralateral prophylactic mastectomy, a favorable operative morbidity profile for prosthetic reconstruction, and changes in patterns of reimbursement for breast reconstruction procedures.[2] In 2016, 81% of breast reconstructive procedures used prosthetic techniques.[3]

Prosthetic breast reconstruction techniques, also called implant-based reconstructions, hold certain widely accepted advantages over autologous methods (**Table 59.1**). First, prosthetic techniques minimize operative and donor site morbidity. The time required to perform placement of an implant or tissue expander is significantly shorter (around 1–1.5 hours) than that required for an autologous flap, which can extend beyond 6 hours of operative time. No dissection of donor site tissue, tunneling into the mastectomy defect or dissection of recipient vessels, is necessary with prosthetic techniques. Prosthetic techniques preserve autologous methods of reconstruction as options for future procedures, should patient preference or necessity determine the need for conversion. Hospital length of stay and patient recovery are generally shorter with prosthetic techniques compared to autologous reconstruction.

Prosthetic reconstruction techniques also have several disadvantages compared to autologous methods (see **Table 59.1**). First, it can be more difficult to match the appearance of an implant reconstruction to a contralateral native breast in the setting of unilateral reconstruction, making symmetry harder to achieve. Second, breast implants and tissue expanders can experience device-related complications including implant infection or exposure, capsular contracture, implant malposition, implant visibility or rippling, and implant rupture. Third, an implant does not behave like normal breast tissue or autologous tissue in look, feel, and development of ptosis over time.

For properly selected patients undergoing breast reconstruction, prosthetic techniques have the potential to create an attractive breast mound that can help improve a patient's psychosocial, physical, and sexual well-being following mastectomy.[4] In this chapter, we highlight some of the different viewpoints concerning timing, technique, and patient selection for implant-based reconstruction.

PATIENT SELECTION FOR PROSTHETIC TECHNIQUES

Successful prosthetic breast reconstruction begins with proper patient selection. Careful attention to patient and oncologic factors in the planning stages of breast reconstruction will ensure an optimal aesthetic outcome with an acceptable complication profile. Risk factors for complications in implant reconstruction include the following:

- Smoking
- Obesity (BMI >30)
- Large breasts
- Diabetes (Hgb A1C >6.5%)

The patient selection process begins with a thorough discussion of patient expectations. One important consideration is the desired postoperative breast volume. Maintaining premastectomy breast volume after reconstruction in a patient with macromastia may be difficult or impossible using prosthetic reconstruction techniques if an appropriately sized implant is not available; in addition, large mastectomy specimen weight was found to be an independent risk factor for implant loss in prosthetic reconstruction.[5]

Certain patient comorbidities make the rate of complications following prosthetic reconstruction unacceptably high. It is accepted that smokers have an increased rate of overall complications, tissue necrosis, and need

TABLE 59.1. ADVANTAGES AND DISADVANTAGES OF IMPLANT-BASED RECONSTRUCTION

Advantages
■ Shorter operative time ■ Shorter hospital stay ■ Shorter recovery ■ No donor tissue or recipient vessel dissection necessary
Disadvantages
■ Implant-related complications (implant infection, capsular contracture, implant malposition, rippling, rupture) ■ Less natural feel compared to autologous tissue ■ Difficult to achieve symmetry in unilateral reconstruction

for reoperation in general following plastic surgical procedures[6]; there is also ample evidence that smoking increases the rate of complications specifically following prosthetic breast reconstruction. An analysis of ACS-NSQIP data demonstrated that active smokers have an odds ratio of four for early tissue expander loss compared to nonsmokers.[7] Two studies from the Memorial Sloan-Kettering Cancer Center demonstrated that smoking more doubles the rate of mastectomy skin flap necrosis, infection, and reconstructive failure in patients undergoing implant-based reconstruction (Figure 59.1).[8,9] The authors also demonstrated a dose-response effect for tobacco use, with the incidence of complications increasing with the number of packs per day smoked.[8] Interestingly, although some surgeons recommend smoking cessation for at least a month prior to surgery, there is some evidence that the rate of complications in *former smokers*, those who stopped smoking 1 month or more before surgery, is similar to the rate of complications in active smokers.[8,9] Patients should be thoroughly educated about the detrimental effects of tobacco, and if active smoking continues, serious consideration should be given to delaying reconstruction.

Diabetes has been associated with an increased risk of wound healing complications in a variety of surgical procedures, and breast reconstruction is no exception. NSQIP database analysis suggests that diabetes increases the overall 30-day complication rate and the rate of wound healing complications in expander/implant-based reconstruction.[10] In addition, data from Hart et al. suggest that even well-controlled diabetes (average preoperative blood glucose 137 mg/dL) increases the 1-year rate of wound healing problems following prosthetic but not autologous reconstruction.[11] In patients with poorly controlled diabetes, referral to diabetic educators and endocrine specialists may be appropriate before consideration of reconstruction. A team-based approach to perioperative glucose management should be undertaken with the goal of preoperative Hgb A1C <6.5%, and perioperative glucose levels under 200 mg/dL.[12]

Obesity is also associated with worse outcomes following breast reconstruction. Using the MarketScan database, Huo et al. demonstrated that the 1-year rate of infectious and wound complications in patients undergoing expander/implant reconstruction was significantly higher in patients with BMI >30.[13] Similarly, McCarthy et al. demonstrated that patients with BMI >30 were almost seven times more likely to experience reconstructive failure following prosthetic reconstruction than their nonobese counterparts.[9] In addition, device projection may be severely limited in patients with overly thick mastectomy flaps; therefore, obese patients should be counseled that preoperative weight loss will not only decrease their risk of postoperative complications, but also potentially improve the appearance of the final result.

Successful patient selection for prosthetic breast reconstruction must also consider oncologic factors. Close communication with the ablative surgeon is extremely important during the planning phase of breast reconstruction to avoid complications and optimize outcomes. The size of the tumor and lymph node status are crucial pieces of information for the reconstructive surgeon; clinical staging helps determine the likely need for adjuvant radiotherapy, which can greatly affect complication rates following implant-based reconstruction. Other important factors to discuss with the ablative surgeon that may influence the choice to pursue implant-based reconstruction include the plan for unilateral versus bilateral mastectomy, and whether a nipple-sparing mastectomy approach is appropriate.

A thorough physical exam can help determine if a patient is an appropriate candidate for prosthetic reconstruction. The preoperative breast size must be taken into account; macromastia is not a contraindication to implant-based reconstruction, but does require attention to tailoring of the skin envelope, such as with skin-reducing mastectomy methods (Figure 59.2).[14] Examination of potential donor sites is important, as a lack of adequate tissue or volume will immediately disqualify patients from undergoing reconstruction with autologous techniques.

TIMING OF PROSTHETIC RECONSTRUCTION

The plastic surgeon undertaking an implant-based breast reconstruction must decide whether to perform the reconstruction in an immediate fashion (at the time of mastectomy) or delayed fashion (as a staged procedure following recovery from mastectomy and/or adjuvant therapy). Each approach has distinct advantages and disadvantages (**Table 59.2**). Immediate breast reconstruction, by preserving the original skin envelope and native breast borders, has been purported to optimize aesthetic outcomes and patient satisfaction,[15] while minimizing the negative psychological impact of mastectomy on a patient's self-image.[16] In addition, immediate reconstruction potentially minimizes the number of trips to the operating room and recovery downtime. Proponents of delayed prosthetic reconstruction have argued that this approach results in a lower rate of complications including mastectomy skin flap necrosis, capsular contracture, and need for device removal.[17,18] The decision to perform a prosthetic reconstruction in an immediate or delayed fashion should be based on patient factors, oncologic factors, and technical aspects of the mastectomy itself. In general, immediate reconstruction will achieve

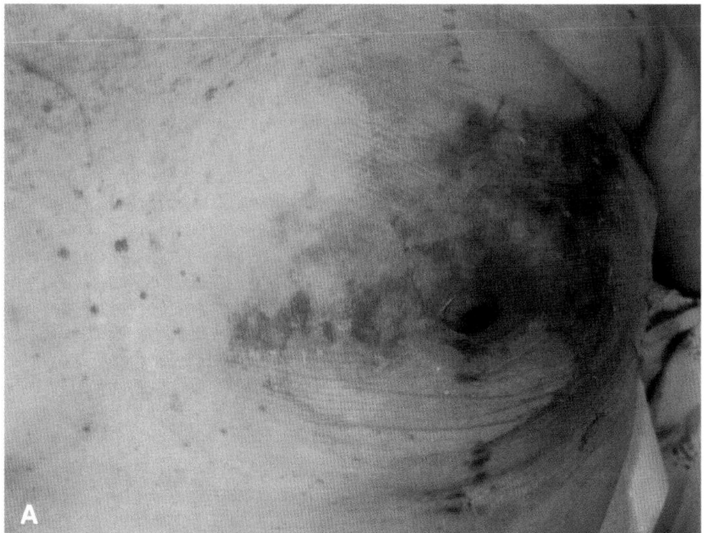

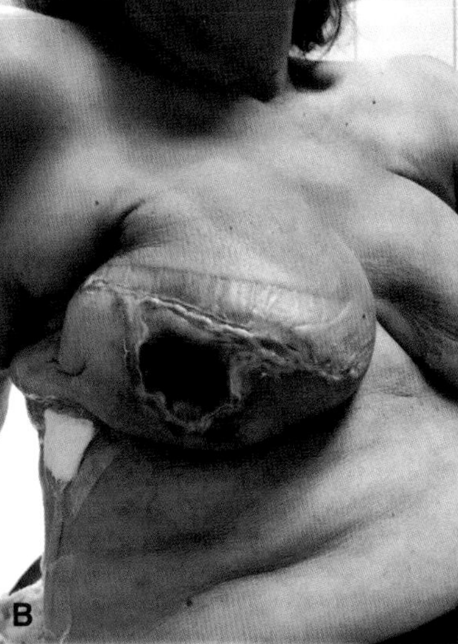

FIGURE 59.1. Mastectomy skin flap necrosis. Partial-thickness **(A)** and full-thickness **(B)** mastectomy skin flap necrosis following implant-based reconstruction in patients with history of smoking.

BREAST

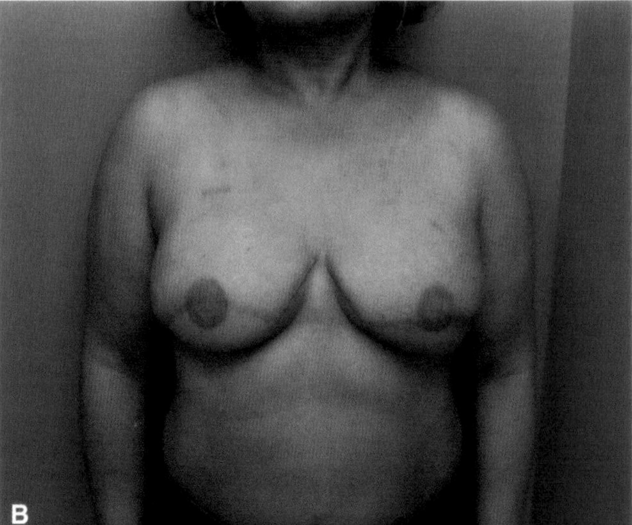

FIGURE 59.2. Skin-reducing mastectomy. Preoperative **(A)** and postoperative **(B)** views following skin-reducing mastectomy with implant reconstruction and nipple-areola reconstruction.

optimal results in patients with a lower preoperative risk profile (nonsmoker, nonobese) and early stage cancers. Delayed reconstruction is more appropriate in patients with advanced stage cancers in whom close tumor surveillance is needed or adjuvant therapy is likely; in addition, if there is concern about the viability of the mastectomy skin flaps and adequate tissue for device coverage at the time of mastectomy, an intraoperative decision to delay reconstruction may be appropriate (Figure 59.3).[19]

TECHNICAL CONSIDERATIONS IN IMPLANT-BASED RECONSTRUCTION

Single- Versus Two-Stage Reconstruction

As previously mentioned, prosthetic breast reconstruction may be completed with either a two-stage (placement of tissue expander followed by exchange for permanent implant) or single-stage (direct placement of permanent implant after mastectomy) approach. A *direct-to-implant* approach has the obvious advantage of eliminating (1) multiple office visits for device expansion, (2) risk of infection related to expander filling access and manipulation, and (3) second-stage surgery for expander-to-implant exchange. Single-stage implant breast reconstruction can achieve excellent outcomes with acceptable revision rates in properly selected patients, but is technically demanding, requiring precise implant selection and positioning following an often unpredictable extirpative procedure. A quality mastectomy is a major determinant of the success of direct-to-implant reconstruction; a skin-sparing or nipple-sparing mastectomy with appropriate skin flap thickness and viability that preserves the inframammary fold will help avoid the complications of implant malposition, skin flap necrosis and device exposure.

TABLE 59.2. ADVANTAGES OF IMMEDIATE AND DELAYED PROSTHETIC RECONSTRUCTION

Immediate
■ Preserves native skin envelope and breast borders ■ Minimizes trips to the operating room ■ Improved psychological and emotional outcome
Delayed
■ Decreased risk of complications in setting of patient comorbidities or need for adjuvant radiation ■ Decreased risk of mastectomy skin flap necrosis

Adjuncts such as indocyanine green angiography can provide an objective assessment of skin flap perfusion, and acellular dermal matrix (discussed later) is a useful tool for providing total implant coverage and securing implant position. Patient comorbidities such as diabetes and smoking, need for adjuvant radiation, and increasing premastectomy breast size have all been found to be risk factors for postoperative complications following single-stage reconstruction.[20,21] Few individual studies have demonstrated any significant difference in complication rates between single- and two-stage prosthetic reconstruction; however, in a recent systematic review and head-to-head meta-analysis, Basta et al. found a significantly increased risk of skin flap necrosis, need for reoperation, and reconstructive failure in patients undergoing direct-to-implant reconstruction (OR 1.43, 1.25, and 1.87, respectively). The overall absolute rate of implant loss was 14.4% for single- and 8.7% for two-stage reconstruction.[22]

Acellular Dermal Matrix

Acellular dermal matrix (ADM) exists in various forms as human or animal cadaveric, decellularized dermis. It is useful as an adjunct to prosthetic breast reconstruction for its ability to better define the mastectomy space and provide support to soft tissues, essentially acting as a hammock to stabilize the implant or expander device. When used in single- or two-stage reconstruction, ADM can help maintain the device in the optimal position on the chest wall, add definition to the inframammary fold and lateral breast border, and improve lower pole projection (Figure 59.4). In several studies, these advantages have translated into improved aesthetic outcomes as determined by independent observer subjective review,[23] compared to prosthetic reconstruction without ADM or even compared to total submuscular coverage.[24] In the setting of two-stage prosthetic reconstruction, the use of ADM was associated with a higher intraoperative fill volume and shorter time to optimal expansion.[25] There are data suggesting that ADM is useful in both the primary prevention and secondary treatment of capsular contracture. Compared to an expected 5-year capsular contracture rate of between 10% and 30%, multiple series in the recent literature have demonstrated a much lower rate (between 0% and 4%) when ADM is used as an adjunct to prosthetic reconstruction.[23,26,27] Several of the patients in these studies had breast irradiation before or after surgery, suggesting that the use of ADM may ameliorate some of the negative sequelae associated with radiation treatment. These benefits may come at the expense of a higher complication rate; multiple retrospective reviews have demonstrated a higher incidence of acute postoperative complications including infection, seroma, skin

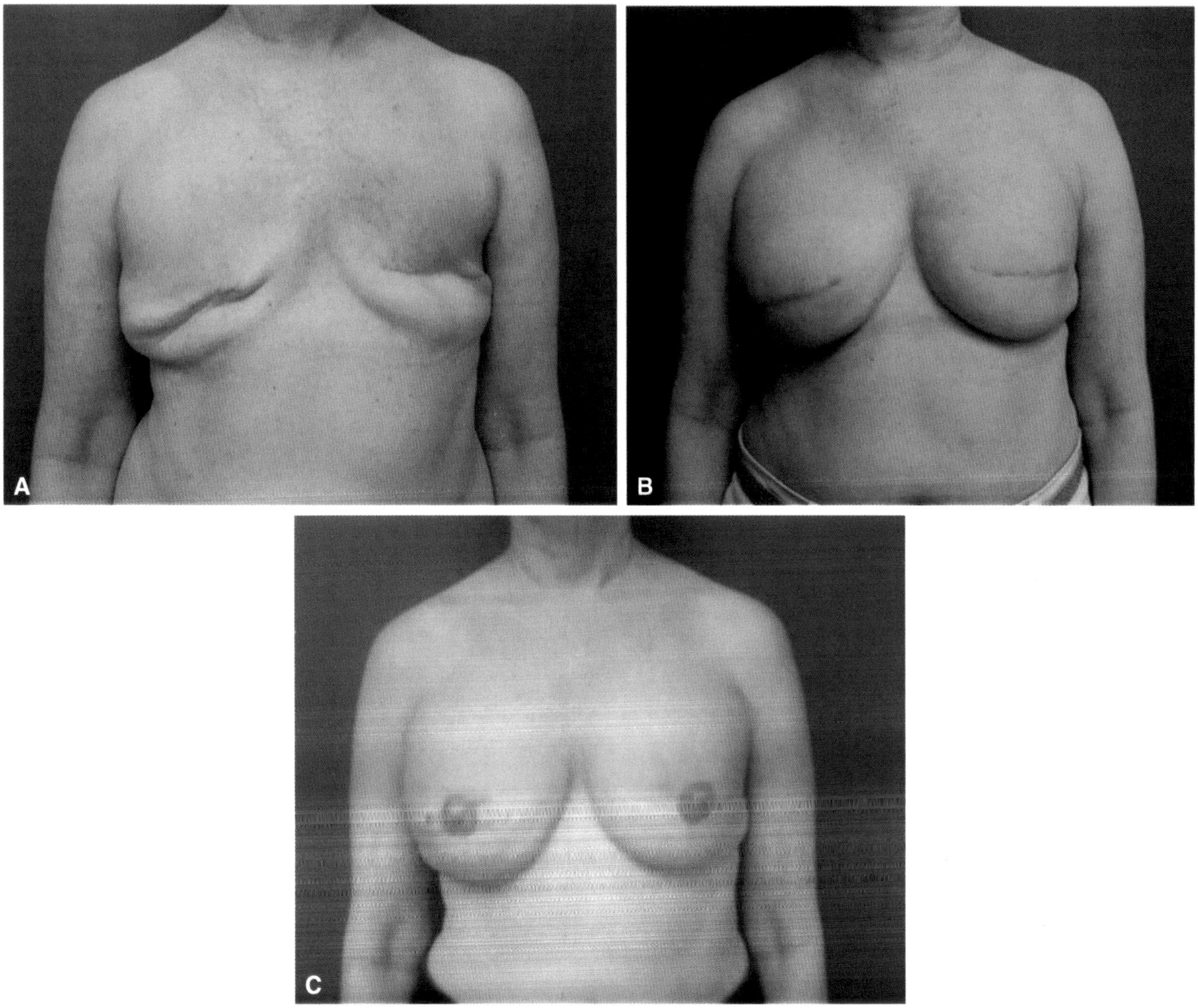

FIGURE 59.3. Delayed placement of tissue expander in breast reconstruction. **A.** Preoperative view following bilateral mastectomy. **B.** Following delayed placement of tissue expander and inflation. **C.** Following exchange for permanent implant and nipple-areola reconstruction.

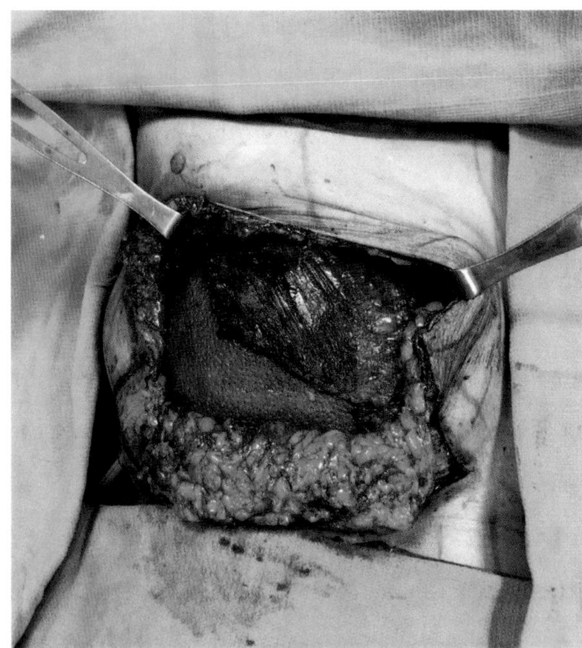

FIGURE 59.4. Submuscular placement of tissue expander with acellular dermal matrix for lower pole support and coverage.

flap necrosis, and reconstructive failure in prosthetic reconstructions employing ADM.[28-30] The strength of this data is diminished by selection bias and confounders such as morbid obesity, which is also known to contribute to higher seroma rates. Taken together, most surgeons feel that, in properly selected patients (i.e., normal BMI, nonsmokers), the benefits of ADM use likely outweigh the potential drawbacks.

Implant Selection

Choice of device is an important component of planning both expander-based and direct-to-implant reconstruction. There are many options for size, shape, and texture of both expanders and permanent implants.

There is a more limited range of options in choice of tissue expanders. Most commercially available tissue expanders designed for use in breast reconstruction use a textured surface, a relative anatomic shape for differential filling of the lower pole, and a magnetic port for filling with saline. Expanders are available in different height, projection, capacity, and base width. Among these, base width is the most important parameter for intraoperative device selection; matching the device base width to the width of the breast footprint on the chest wall eliminates dead space and skin redundancy while optimizing the final expansion pocket. Expander capacity is less important, as many expander devices may be filled well beyond their stated maximum volumes.[31]

Permanent implants are available in an ever-increasing variety of sizes, shapes, textures, fills, and cohesivity. In general, there are several decisions that must be made when selecting a permanent implant. Most available data directly comparing different types of implant exist in the breast augmentation literature, and must be extrapolated to breast reconstruction.

Saline Versus Silicone

Both saline and silicone have distinct advantages and disadvantages from both the patient and surgeon perspective. It is easier to detect a saline implant rupture. Saline implants require a less rigorous surveillance protocol, but likely have higher rates of implant visibility and rippling. Silicone implants more closely resemble the look and feel of the native breast tissue, but silicone leak or implant rupture may be harder to detect and can lead to capsular contracture; in contrast, saline is physiologically inert and is simply absorbed if there is a leak. Available data suggest that rates of rupture and capsular contracture may be slightly higher in silicone implants than in saline at 10 years following implantation.[32-34] There is also some evidence that patients have improved overall satisfaction as well as self-assessed psychological and sexual function after receiving silicone versus saline implants in breast reconstruction.[35] There is no evidence to support the idea that patients with silicone implants are more likely to develop rare neurologic or connective tissue diseases.[36]

Smooth Versus Textured

Textured implants were developed in an attempt to reproduce lower rates of capsular contracture obtained historically with placement of polyurethane-coated devices. In general, rates of capsular contracture do appear to be lower with textured devices, though this difference appears less significant when implants are placed in the submuscular position.[37,38] Again, these data are extrapolated from literature specific to breast augmentation. Another benefit of textured implants includes a more stable position within the pocket, which theoretically decreases lower pole stretch over time. There appears to be a small increase in risk of breast-implant-associated anaplastic large-cell lymphoma (BIA-ALCL) with use of textured devices. This effect may be greatest with macrotextured implants. The overall incidence of this complication is still low (~1/30,000), but discussion of BIA-ALCL is an important part of the informed consent process.[39]

Round Versus Anatomic

Anatomic-shaped implants have been in use for several years and are preferred by some plastic surgeons in breast reconstruction for their ability to better match the device to the original breast footprint following mastectomy. Shaped implants may result in improved upper pole shape and volume, especially in reconstruction of breasts that are taller than they are wide. Placing an anatomic implant is more technically challenging, because without precise pocket control, implant rotation may result. Patients may also report a somewhat firmer feel compared to a softer, round silicone implant. In practice, there has been little detectable difference in patient satisfaction, aesthetic outcome, or complication rates between shaped and round implants in breast reconstruction. Interestingly, blinded expert observers in one study were not routinely able to differentiate which type of implant a patient had received.[40] All currently available anatomic-shaped implants are also textured to limit unwanted implant movement/rotation; therefore, all of the risks and benefits of textured devices also apply to shaped devices.

Standard Technique for Submuscular, Two-Stage Implant-Based Reconstruction With Acellular Dermal Matrix

Procedure begins with assessment of mastectomy cavity, including evaluation of mastectomy skin flap thickness/regularity, hemostasis, and preservation of native breast footprint (i.e., violation of inframammary fold). The breast base width may be measured, and expander size selection is made. Note is made of the mastectomy specimen weight. Indocyanine green angiography may be performed as an adjunct to evaluate mastectomy skin flap viability. If viability or skin quality is a concern, placement of a device is relatively contraindicated and may be deferred to a later time. If native breast borders have been violated, recreation of these natural landmarks such as the lateral breast border and inframammary fold may be accomplished with placement of absorbable sutures.

The lateral border of the pectoralis muscle is identified and raised; the submuscular plane is defined superiorly and medially to the sternal origin of the muscle. A lighted retractor or headlamp, long cautery tip, and muscle paralysis help with this step. After the submuscular plane is developed, the inferior origins of the pectoralis muscle along the inframammary fold are divided and released to the level of the sternum. Additional muscle origin along the most inferior portions of the sternum may be divided further if increased lower pole projection is needed or desired. Care is taken to maintain perfect hemostasis when large intercostal and internal mammary artery perforators are encountered.

A rectangular or contoured piece of ADM is brought onto the field. Usually, a piece 8 × 16 cm in size is more than sufficient. The ADM is anchored medially at the junction of the muscle and chest wall, and then anchored with interrupted absorbable sutures to the thick fascial attachments of the inframammary fold. Laterally, the ADM is sutured to the chest wall to reapproximate the lateral breast border. Excess ADM is trimmed away, leaving a curvilinear sling along the lower and lateral aspects of the mastectomy cavity.

At this point, the cavity is irrigated with antibiotic solution and hemostasis confirmed once again in both the subcutaneous and submuscular space. The previously selected tissue expander is brought onto the field and all air removed from the device. The expander is then inserted into the submuscular space and anchored medially and laterally to the chest wall using the suture tabs on the device (if available).

The inferior border of the pectoralis muscle is sutured to the superior border of the ADM sling to prevent *window-shading* of the muscle. Excess ADM is removed to set the appropriate muscle tension. The device should now be completely covered by the combination of muscle in the upper pole and ADM in the lower pole. Drains are placed in the subcutaneous space and brought out below the lateral aspect of the inframammary fold. One or two drains may be used depending on the amount of dead space. The tissue expander port may now be accessed and the expander filled as desired. After filling the expander, the mastectomy incision may be tailor tacked and a final indocyanine green perfusion assessment performed. If there is a worsening in the appearance of the flaps with the expander in place, volume may be removed from the device, as appropriate, to take pressure off of the skin flaps. The mastectomy incision is meticulously closed in two layers with absorbable monofilament suture. A surgical dressing is applied and the patient is placed in a surgical bra or chest binder. Overnight admission for pain control is standard at our institution.

IMPLANT-BASED RECONSTRUCTION IN THE SETTING OF ADJUVANT THERAPY

The need for adjuvant or neoadjuvant therapy can complicate the decision to employ prosthetic techniques in breast reconstruction, negatively impacting the ability of the reconstructive surgeon to create an aesthetic and natural appearing breast mound (**Figure 59.5**). Radiation of a prosthetic device can lead to increased rates of early complications such as infection, seroma, and mastectomy flap necrosis, as well as delayed complications such as capsular contracture, poor aesthetic outcome, and reconstructive failure. The odds ratio of developing any complication following radiation of an implant-based reconstruction is approximately 4.2 compared to no radiation,[41] and the rate of reconstructive failure is generally accepted to be around 20% compared to 3% in those not receiving adjuvant radiotherapy.[42]

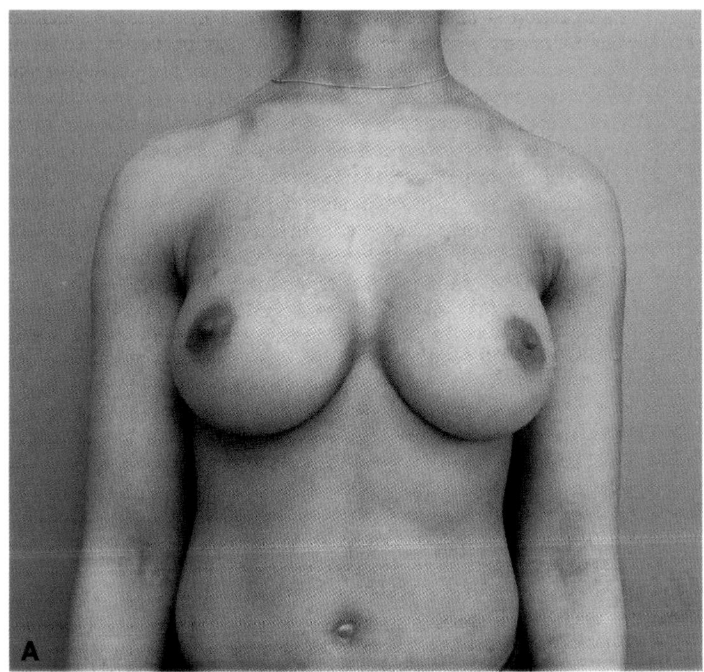

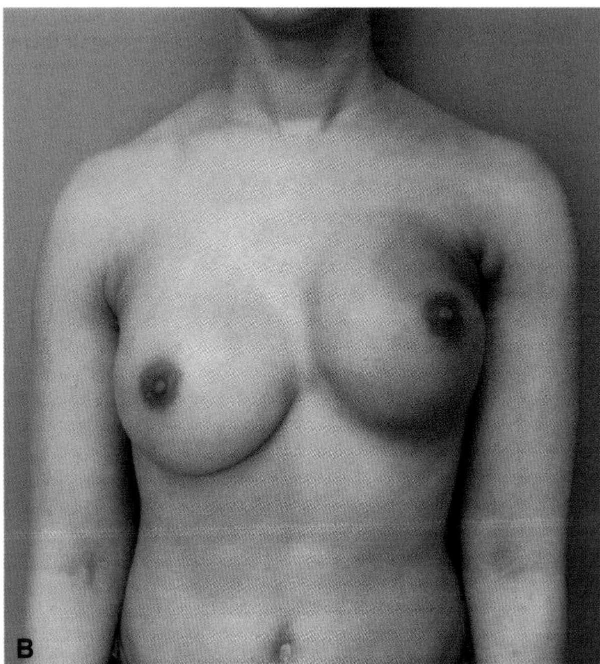

FIGURE 59.5. Effect of radiation on appearance of reconstructed breast. Preradiation **(A)** and postradiation **(B)** views of implant reconstruction, demonstrating skin color change, contraction of skin envelope, and nipple-areola malposition.

Compared to radiation of an autologous reconstruction, patients undergoing postmastectomy radiation therapy following implant reconstruction have been shown to have higher rates of overall complications and significantly lower patient-reported quality-of-life scores as determined by the BREAST Q.[43] However, patient desire for implant-based reconstruction, a shortage of autologous options or unplanned need for adjuvant therapy may still result in the need to radiate a prosthetic reconstruction. Considerable effort has been devoted to determining the optimal timing and protocol for radiation therapy to minimize complication rate while maximizing aesthetic outcome and patient quality of life.

When breast reconstruction is undertaken in the setting of adjuvant radiation therapy, the plastic surgeon's goal of creating an aesthetic, symmetric, and natural appearing breast mound must not overshadow the oncologic goals of local and systemic eradication of breast cancer cells. Further complicating reconstructive planning, the indications for radiotherapy in breast cancer appear to be expanding. In general, postmastectomy radiation is considered in any clinical scenario with an elevated risk of locoregional recurrence. The indications for radiation therapy as outlined by the National Comprehensive Cancer Network (NCCN) are as follows[44]:

Radiation indicated

- Following breast conservation therapy
- Inflammatory breast cancer (may also be considered as neoadjuvant therapy)
- Any T4 tumor
- Four or more positive axillary lymph nodes
- Local or regional recurrence (if radiation not previously administered)

Radiation should be strongly considered

- Tumor >5 cm
- Between one and three positive axillary lymph nodes
- Positive margins

Radiation may be considered

- Close margins (<1 mm)
- High-risk features (central or medially located tumor, tumor >2 cm in young patient or with pathologic extensive lymphovascular invasion)

Timing of Adjuvant Radiation Therapy

Following two-stage prosthetic reconstruction (placement of a tissue expander followed by second-stage replacement with a permanent implant), the treatment team must decide whether to administer radiation before or after exchange of the expander for a permanent implant. Multiple studies have addressed the question of timing, comparing outcomes in patients who have received radiation to the expander versus radiation to the permanent implant. Some studies have found an increased rate of reconstructive failure (complication necessitating device removal) when the permanent implant undergoes radiation,[45,46] but others have found no significant difference in the rate of any complication including reconstructive failure.[47] In a 2015 study by Cordeiro et al., radiation of the permanent implant was associated with a higher rate of capsular contracture and subsequently worse aesthetic outcomes.[46] In this same study, however, patient-reported quality-of-life measures were no different between radiation of the expander versus the permanent implant. In the setting of radiation of the tissue expander, increasing the interval of time between completion of radiation and exchange to permanent implant appears to improve outcomes, with intervals ranging from 3 to 8 months.[48,49]

Technical Aspects of Radiation Delivery

Other factors that may influence prosthetic reconstructive outcome include the dose and fractionation of radiation delivery, as well as whether treatment is delivered to a fully expanded, partially expanded or fully deflated tissue expander. A full discussion of the data supporting different radiation doses, targets, and delivery methods is beyond the scope of this chapter, except to say that there is significant variability in practice patterns in both the United States and abroad.[50] It is possible that these factors may affect reconstruction success and complication rates in a given practice, and it is important to be familiar with the protocol used in a given institution when evaluating published results. With regard to radiation of tissue expanders, some controversy exists regarding the optimal inflation status at the time of radiation delivery. Some authors argue that attempting to radiate a fully or even partially inflated expander may result in alteration of the dose delivered to the chest wall and internal mammary nodes, and that complete deflation of the expander followed by reexpansion at completion of radiation is preferable.[51] However, with modern techniques and modeling, more recent data seem to suggest that radiation of even a fully inflated expander or permanent implant is safe, does not result in decreased radiation dose administration, and may result in a lower rate of complications compared to radiation of a deflated device.[52] Again, the importance of a team approach is emphasized; detailed discussion and close coordination of care between the plastic surgeon, breast surgeon, and radiation oncologist will help to optimize the patient experience and reconstructive outcome.

Implant Reconstruction in the Setting of Previous Radiation Treatment

Another common clinical scenario is the patient who requires salvage mastectomy following previous breast conservation therapy with local recurrence. In these patients, reported complication rates in patients undergoing breast reconstruction with prosthetic techniques vary widely. One systematic review reported the rate of major complications associated with prosthetic reconstructions of previously irradiated breasts at 49%.[53] The rates of early complications such as infection, seroma, and mastectomy skin flap necrosis are significantly higher in previously radiated patients undergoing prosthetic reconstruction compared to nonirradiated patients.[53-56] In addition, late complications such as capsular contracture and reconstructive failure appear to be two to three times more likely in previously irradiated patients.[57] The well-known chronic tissue effects of radiation such as fibrosis and decreased vascularity are likely to blame for the increased complication rate; the soft tissue envelope of the breast simply does not respond as well to stress or expansion following radiation. Compared to postmastectomy radiation, prosthetic reconstruction of the previously irradiated breast appears to have a similar or slightly worse risk profile.[53,56] Sbitany et al. demonstrated that compared to patients who underwent preoperative radiation, patients with postmastectomy radiation exposure had lower rates of wound breakdown and infections requiring procedures for resolution.[56] Despite the complication rate, in their systematic review, Momoh et al. conclude that the rate of successful completion of prosthetic reconstruction in previously irradiated breasts was 83%.[53] This supports the conclusions of multiple authors that despite a higher rate of complications, prosthetic reconstruction can be effectively accomplished in the previously irradiated breast.[54-56] Attempts to maximize the safety of this approach include a careful clinical assessment of the skin for discoloration, quality and elasticity, as well as the location of previous scars, which may necessitate removal of prohibitive amounts of skin. Interestingly, the use of ADM in previously irradiated patients is not protective against reconstructive failure and may increase the rate of skin flap and infectious complications, perhaps due to its inability to incorporate into a poorly vascularized, irradiated mastectomy flap.[56] Although increasing the time interval between previous irradiation and salvage mastectomy beyond 1 year does not appear to improve the rate of complications, performing the reconstruction in a delayed rather than immediate fashion may result in a lower rate of reconstructive failure.[57] All things considered, undertaking a prosthetic reconstruction in a previously irradiated breast can be done effectively and with acceptable aesthetic outcomes. Patient education should include a frank discussion of the possible postoperative course and a realistic appraisal of expectations. Reconstructive failure and need for conversion to an autologous reconstruction is a realistic potential outcome.

Effect of Systemic Therapy on Prosthetic Reconstruction

Neoadjuvant or adjuvant systemic therapies used in the treatment of breast cancer include chemotherapeutic regimens and hormonal therapies. Chemotherapeutics have varying degrees of myelosuppressive potential, resulting in thrombocytopenia, anemia, and neutropenia. These adverse effects raised concerns about the safety of breast reconstruction in patients receiving chemotherapy either before or after expander or implant placement. Several experimental studies demonstrated an increased rate of wound healing complications in animals receiving specific chemotherapeutic agents,[58,59] however similar results in clinical trials have not been reliably reproduced. On the balance, there is no clear evidence that either neoadjuvant or adjuvant chemotherapy increases complication rates in patients undergoing prosthetic reconstruction,[60-62] but these studies varied in the timing, dose, and regimen of chemotherapy administered. Similarly, there is no evidence that hormonal therapies such as tamoxifen or aromatase inhibitors increase complication rates in prosthetic reconstructions.[63] Many patients who require adjuvant systemic therapy for advanced stage breast cancer will also require radiation therapy; as expected, patients who receive both chemotherapy and radiation also experience radiation-related complication profiles.

COMPLICATIONS IN IMPLANT-BASED RECONSTRUCTION

Hematoma

Hematoma is estimated to occur in 2% to 3% of implant-based reconstructions.[23] Acute hematoma is most likely to occur in the first 24 to 48 hours after surgery, and the telltale swelling and ecchymosis are often clinically obvious (Figure 59.6). Surgical drains are not useful for evacuation of blood clots; most hematomas require return to the operating room for evacuation, though finding a single bleeding source at the time of reexploration is rare. Left untreated, even small hematomas can increase the risk of mastectomy skin flap necrosis, capsular contracture, and poor aesthetic outcome.

Infection

The overall rate of infection following implant-based reconstruction was estimated at 7.6% in a recent meta-analysis.[64] Surgical site infections present in a spectrum of severity, from cellulitis involving the incision to frank abscess in the implant pocket with whole breast erythema, swelling and purulent output from the incision and drain (Figure 59.7). Minimal cellulitis may often be managed with empiric outpatient antibiotic therapy, whereas pocket infections often require admission for IV antibiotics, surgical exploration, and

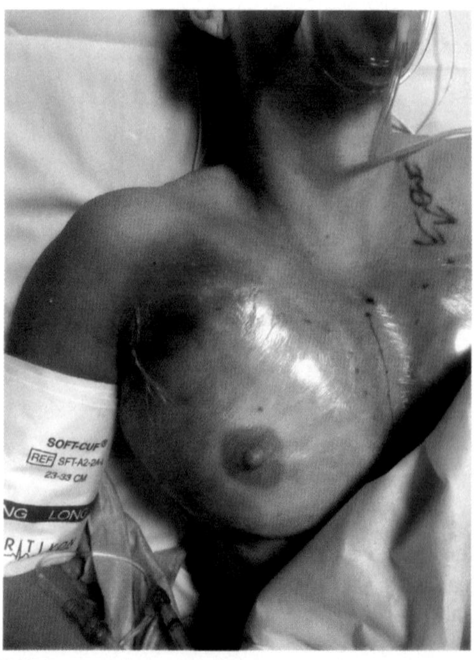

FIGURE 59.6. Acute hematoma following nipple-sparing mastectomy.

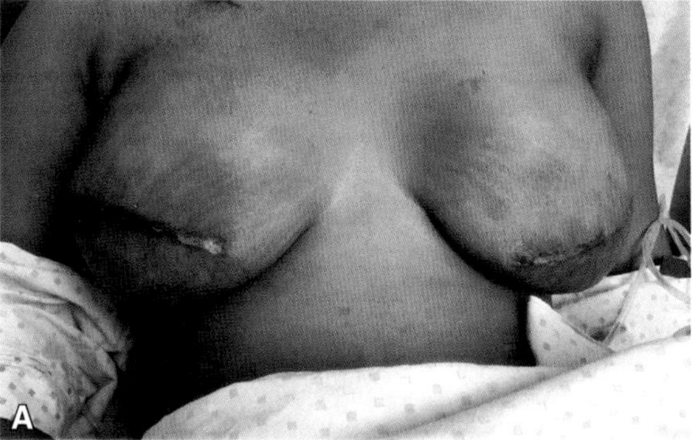

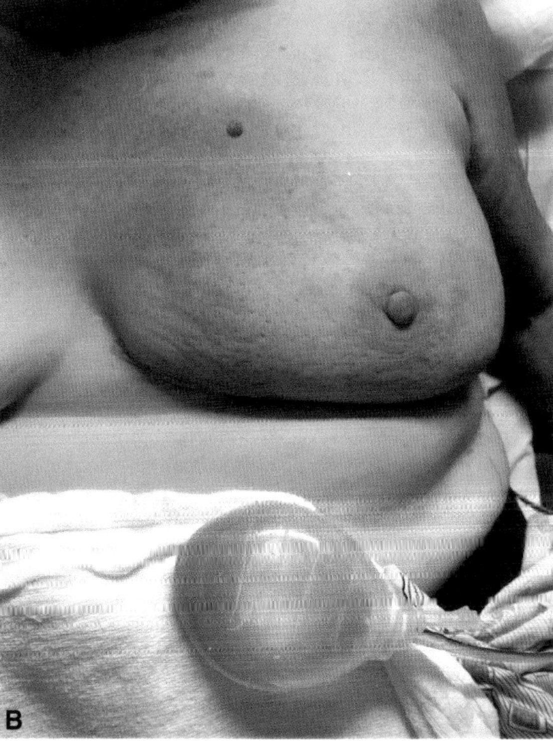

FIGURE 59.7. Infection following implant-based reconstruction. Incisional erythema **(A)** and whole breast erythema **(B)** with purulent drain output approximately 3 to 4 weeks following mastectomy and placement of tissue expander.

implant removal. Implant salvage may be considered in properly selected cases; a recent retrospective review by Reish et al. identified elevated white blood cell count at admission and methicillin-resistant *S. aureus* (MRSA) infection as predictors of salvage failure.[65] Gram-positive bacteria such as *Staphylococcus, Streptococcus,* and *Propionibacteria* are the most common pathogenic organisms in implant-associated infection.[66]

Capsular Contracture

Capsular contracture is a pathologic process thought to result from chronic inflammation of the periprosthetic capsule, resulting in thickening of the capsule and tightening around the implant (Figure 59.8). The Baker Scale is used to grade severity of capsular contracture: grade 1 is a normal, soft breast; grade 2 is a minimally firm breast; grade 3 capsular contracture results in a visible distortion of the breast, and grade 4 capsular contracture causes a painful breast with severe distortion. Rates of capsular contracture following implant-based reconstruction at 3 years are estimated at between 10% and 13% in core studies from Mentor and Allergan. Hematoma, radiation, silicone rupture, and biofilm formation are all considered to increase the incidence of capsular contracture. Techniques for prevention of capsular contracture attempt to target these risk factors (meticulous sterile technique, hemostasis, and pocket irrigation), but an evidence-based approach to treatment of capsular contracture is lacking. A good summary of the current evidence for capsular contracture management was published by Wan and Rohrich; in general, effective surgical techniques require capsulectomy, implant exchange, change of implant position, and use of ADM.[67]

Implant Malposition or Asymmetry

Breast symmetry can be difficult to achieve, particularly in patients with significant premorbid breast asymmetry with respect to both breast size and shape. It is important to point out to the patient any notable asymmetries preoperatively because these may become more apparent after reconstruction. In unilateral reconstruction, contralateral procedures such as breast reduction or mastopexy may be needed to achieve better symmetry. It is important to discuss the likelihood of needing secondary procedures to achieve the best overall result.

Implant malposition is a common complication that may result from overdissection of the mastectomy pocket, expansion in an inappropriate vector, poor implant choice, or capsular contracture. Attention to maintaining or recreating the native breast landmarks at the first stage of reconstruction, in particular the inframammary

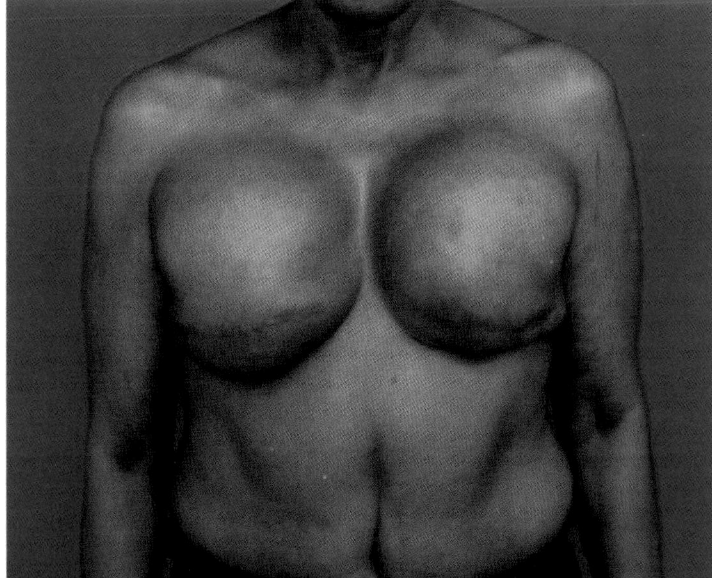

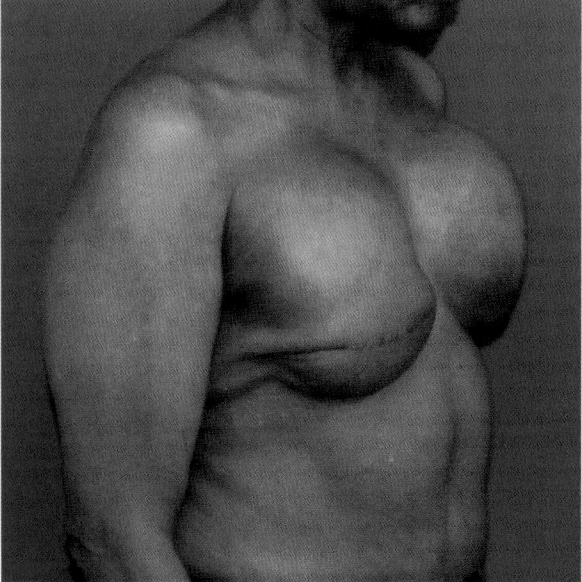

FIGURE 59.8. Severe capsular contracture several years following implant-based reconstruction resulting in pain and implant malposition.

fold and lateral breast border, can help prevent this complication. At the second stage of reconstruction, capsulorrhaphy may be needed to reestablish the optimal implant pocket.

POSTOPERATIVE CARE

Drains

Drains are considered a standard though inconvenient part of implant-based reconstruction. Practice patterns vary considerably, but in our practice one or two closed-suction drains are left in the subcutaneous space until output is less than 30 cc over a 24-hour period. Typical drain duration is 1 to 2 weeks. Persistent high output from a drain can sometimes be improved by partially inflating the tissue expander to decrease the amount of dead space.

Antibiotics

The data supporting antibiotic use in implant-based reconstruction are mixed, and practice patterns vary significantly. Whereas some surgeons treat patients with a preoperative dose of antibiotics only, others prefer to treat with oral outpatient therapy until surgical drains are removed. A recent review by Phillips and Halvorson noted that although data seem to support preoperative antibiotic dosing in decreasing the risk of infectious complications, there was insufficient evidence to recommend continuing antibiotics on an outpatient basis.[68]

REFERENCES

1. Albornoz CR, Bach PB, Mehrara BJ, et al. A paradigm shift in U.S. breast reconstruction: increasing implant rates. *Plast Reconstr Surg*. 2013;131(1):15-23.
2. Farhangkhoee H, Matros E, Disa J. Trends and concepts in post-mastectomy breast reconstruction. *J Surg Oncol*. 2016;113(8):891-894.
3. *2017 plastic surgery statistics report*. Procedural Statistics from the American Society of Plastic Surgeons. 2017. Available from http://www.plasticsurgery.org. Accessed July 19, 2017.
4. Pirro O, Mestak O, Vindigni V, et al. Comparison of patient-reported outcomes after implant versus autologous tissue breast reconstruction using the BREAST-Q. *Plast Reconstr Surg Glob Open*. 2017;5(1):e1217.
5. Woerdeman LA, Hage JJ, Hofland MM, Rutgers EJ. A prospective assessment of surgical risk factors in 400 cases of skin-sparing mastectomy and immediate breast reconstruction with implants to establish selection criteria. *Plast Reconstr Surg*. 2007;119(2):455-463.
6. Coon D, Tuffaha S, Christensen J, Bonawitz SC. Plastic surgery and smoking: a prospective analysis of incidence, compliance, and complications. *Plast Reconstr Surg*. 2013;131(2):385-391.
7. Fischer JP, Nelson JA, Serletti JM, Wu LC. Perioperative risk factors associated with early tissue expander (TE) loss following immediate breast reconstruction (IBR): a review of 9305 patients from the 2005-2010 ACS-NSQIP datasets. *J Plast Reconstr Aesthet Surg*. 2013;66(11):1504-1512.
8. Goodwin SJ, McCarthy CM, Pusic AL, et al. Complications in smokers after postmastectomy tissue expander/implant breast reconstruction. *Ann Plast Surg*. 2005;55(1):16-19.
9. McCarthy CM, Mehrara BJ, Riedel E, et al. Predicting complications following expander/implant breast reconstruction: an outcomes analysis based on preoperative clinical risk. *Plast Reconstr Surg*. 2008;121(6):1886-1892.
   A large retrospective review examining the impact of individual clinical risk factors on outcomes in implant-based reconstruction.
10. Ibrahim AM, Shuster M, Koolen PG, et al. Analysis of the National Surgical Quality Improvement Program database in 19,100 patients undergoing implant-based breast reconstruction: complication rates with acellular dermal matrix. *Plast Reconstr Surg*. 2013;132(5):1057-1066.
11. Hart A, Funderburk CD, Chu CK, et al. The impact of diabetes mellitus on wound healing in breast reconstruction. *Ann Plast Surg*. 2017;78(3):260-263.
12. Endara M, Masden D, Goldstein J, et al. The role of chronic and perioperative glucose management in high-risk surgical closures: a case for tighter glycemic control. *Plast Reconstr Surg*. 2013;132(4):996-1004.
13. Huo J, Smith BD, Giordano SH, et al. A comparison of patient-centered economic and clinical outcomes of post-mastectomy breast reconstruction between obese and non-obese patients. *Breast*. 2016;30:118-124.
14. Dietz J, Lundgren P, Veeramani A, et al. Autologous inferior dermal sling (autoderm) with concomitant skin-envelope reduction mastectomy: an excellent surgical choice for women with macromastia and clinically significant ptosis. *Ann Surg Oncol*. 2012;19(10):3282-3288.
15. Drucker-Zertuche M, Robles-Vidal C. A 7 year experience with immediate breast reconstruction after skin sparing mastectomy for cancer. *Eur J Surg Oncol*. 2007;33(2):140-146.
16. Al-Ghazal SK, Sully L, Fallowfield L, Blamey RW. The psychological impact of immediate rather than delayed breast reconstruction. *Eur J Surg Oncol*. 2000;26(1):17-19.
17. Sullivan SR, Fletcher DR, Isom CD, Isik FF. True incidence of all complications following immediate and delayed breast reconstruction. *Plast Reconstr Surg*. 2008;122(1):19-28.
18. Seth AK, Silver HR, Hirsch EM, et al. Comparison of delayed and immediate tissue expander breast reconstruction in the setting of postmastectomy radiation therapy. *Ann Plast Surg*. 2015;75(5):503-507.
19. Nahabedian MY. Implant-based breast reconstruction: strategies to achieve optimal outcomes and minimize complications. *J Surg Oncol*. 2016;113(8):895-905.
20. Colwell AS, Damjanovic B, Zahedi B, et al. Retrospective review of 331 consecutive immediate single-stage implant reconstructions with acellular dermal matrix: indications, complications, trends, and costs. *Plast Reconstr Surg*. 2011;128(6):1170-1178.
21. Gdalevitch P, Ho A, Genoway K, et al. Direct-to-implant single-stage immediate breast reconstruction with acellular dermal matrix: predictors of failure. *Plast Reconstr Surg*. 2014;133(6):738e-747e.
22. Basta MN, Gerety PA, Serletti JM, et al. A systematic review and head-to-head meta-analysis of outcomes following direct-to-implant versus conventional two-stage implant reconstruction. *Plast Reconstr Surg*. 2015;136(6):1135-1144.
   A meta-analysis of studies comparing single- versus two-stage implant reconstruction complication rates and outcomes.
23. Vardanian AJ, Clayton JL, Roostaeian J, et al. Comparison of implant-based immediate breast reconstruction with and without acellular dermal matrix. *Plast Reconstr Surg*. 2011;128(5):403e-410e.
24. Forsberg CG, Kelly DA, Wood BC, et al. Aesthetic outcomes of acellular dermal matrix in tissue expander/implant-based breast reconstruction. *Ann Plast Surg*. 2014;72(6):S116-S120.
25. Sbitany H, Serletti JM. Acellular dermis-assisted prosthetic breast reconstruction: a systematic and critical review of efficacy and associated morbidity. *Plast Reconstr Surg*. 2011;128(6):1162-1169.
26. Breuing KH, Colwell AS. Inferolateral AlloDerm hammock for implant coverage in breast reconstruction. *Ann Plast Surg*. 2007;59(3):250-255.
27. Salzberg CA, Ashikari AY, Berry C, Hunsicker LM. Acellular dermal matrix-assisted direct-to-implant breast reconstruction and capsular contracture: a 13-year experience. *Plast Reconstr Surg*. 2016;138(2):329-337.
28. Antony AK, McCarthy CM, Cordeiro PG, et al. Acellular human dermis implantation in 153 immediate two-stage tissue expander breast reconstructions: determining the incidence and significant predictors of complications. *Plast Reconstr Surg*. 2010;125(6):1606-1614.
29. Chun YS, Verma K, Rosen H, et al. Implant-based breast reconstruction using acellular dermal matrix and the risk of postoperative complications. *Plast Reconstr Surg*. 2010;125(2):429-436.
30. Lanier ST, Wang ED, Chen JJ, et al. The effect of acellular dermal matrix use on complication rates in tissue expander/implant breast reconstruction. *Ann Plast Surg*. 2010;64(5):674-678.
31. Treiser MD, Lahair T, Carty MJ. Tissue expander overfilling: achieving new dimensions of customization in breast reconstruction. *Plast Reconstr Surg Glob Open*. 2016;4(2):e612.
32. Cunningham BL, Lokeh A, Gutowski KA. Saline-filled breast implant safety and efficacy: a multicenter retrospective review. *Plast Reconstr Surg*. 2000;105(6):2143-2149; discussion 2150–2141.
33. Holmich LR, Friis S, Fryzek JP, et al. Incidence of silicone breast implant rupture. *Arch Surg*. 2003;138(7):801-806.
34. Rohrich RJ, Reece EM. Breast augmentation today: saline versus silicone—what are the facts? *Plast Reconstr Surg*. 2008;121(2):669-672.
35. Macadam SA, Ho AL, Cook EF Jr, et al. Patient satisfaction and health-related quality of life following breast reconstruction: patient-reported outcomes among saline and silicone implant recipients. *Plast Reconstr Surg*. 2010;125(3):761-771.
36. Singh N, Picha GJ, Hardas B, et al. Five-year safety data for more than 55,000 subjects following breast implantation: comparison of rare adverse event rates with silicone implants versus national norms and saline implants. *Plast Reconstr Surg*. 2017;140(4):666-679.
37. Barnsley GP, Sigurdson LJ, Barnsley SE. Textured surface breast implants in the prevention of capsular contracture among breast augmentation patients: a meta-analysis of randomized controlled trials. *Plast Reconstr Surg*. 2006;117(7):2182-2190.
38. Wong CH, Samuel M, Tan BK, Song C. Capsular contracture in subglandular breast augmentation with textured versus smooth breast implants: a systematic review. *Plast Reconstr Surg*. 2006;118(5):1224-1236.
39. Calobrace MB, Schwartz MR, Zeidler KR, et al. Long-term safety of textured and smooth breast implants. *Aesthet Surg J*. 2017;38(1):38-48.
40. Gahm J, Edsander-Nord A, Jurell G, Wickman M. No differences in aesthetic outcome or patient satisfaction between anatomically shaped and round expandable implants in bilateral breast reconstructions: a randomized study. *Plast Reconstr Surg*. 2010;126(5):1419-1427.
41. Barry M, Kell MR. Radiotherapy and breast reconstruction: a meta-analysis. *Breast Cancer Res Treat*. 2011;127(1):15-22.
42. Lam TC, Hsieh F, Boyages J. The effects of postmastectomy adjuvant radiotherapy on immediate two-stage prosthetic breast reconstruction: a systematic review. *Plast Reconstr Surg*. 2013;132(3):511-518.
43. Jagsi R, Momoh AO, Qi J, et al. Impact of radiotherapy on complications and patient-reported outcomes after breast reconstruction. *J Natl Cancer Inst*. 2018;110(2). doi:10.1093/jnci/djx148.

44. National Comprehensive Cancer Network Clinical Practice Guidelines in Oncology: Breast Cancer. Version 2. Published April 26, 2017; Accessed July 19, 2017.
45. Nava MB, Pennati AE, Lozza L, et al. Outcome of different timings of radiotherapy in implant-based breast reconstructions. *Plast Reconstr Surg*. 2011;128(2):353-359.
46. Cordeiro PG, Albornoz CR, McCormick B, et al. What is the optimum timing of postmastectomy radiotherapy in two-stage prosthetic reconstruction: radiation to the tissue expander or permanent implant? *Plast Reconstr Surg*. 2015;135(6):1509-1517.
    Single surgeon experience looking at both surgeon and patient-reported outcomes following radiation of either the tissue expander or the permanent implant in two-stage reconstruction.
47. Santosa KB, Chen X, Qi J, et al. Postmastectomy radiation therapy and two-stage implant-based breast reconstruction: is there a better time to irradiate? *Plast Reconstr Surg*. 2016;138(4):761-769.
48. Peled AW, Foster RD, Esserman LJ, et al. Increasing the time to expander-implant exchange after postmastectomy radiation therapy reduces expander-implant failure. *Plast Reconstr Surg*. 2012;130(3):503-509.
49. Lentz R, Ng R, Higgins SA, et al. Radiation therapy and expander-implant breast reconstruction: an analysis of timing and comparison of complications. *Ann Plast Surg*. 2013;71(3):269-273.
50. Chen SA, Hiley C, Nickleach D, et al. Breast reconstruction and post-mastectomy radiation practice. *Radiat Oncol*. 2013;8:45.
51. Kronowitz SJ, Lam C, Terefe W, et al. A multidisciplinary protocol for planned skin-preserving delayed breast reconstruction for patients with locally advanced breast cancer requiring postmastectomy radiation therapy: 3-year follow-up. *Plast Reconstr Surg*. 2011;127(6):2154-2166.
52. Woo KJ, Paik JM, Bang SI, et al. The impact of expander inflation/deflation status during adjuvant radiotherapy on the complications of immediate two-stage breast reconstruction. *Aesthet Plast Surg*. 2017;41(3):551-559.
53. Momoh AO, Ahmed R, Kelley BP, et al. A systematic review of complications of implant-based breast reconstruction with prereconstruction and postreconstruction radiotherapy. *Ann Surg Oncol*. 2014;21(1):118-124.
54. Persichetti P, Cagli B, Simone P, et al. Implant breast reconstruction after salvage mastectomy in previously irradiated patients. *Ann Plast Surg*. 2009;62(4):350-354.
55. Cordeiro PG, Snell L, Heerdt A, McCarthy C. Immediate tissue expander/implast breast reconstruction after salvage mastectomy for cancer recurrence following lumpectomy/irradiation. *Plast Reconstr Surg*. 2012;129(2):341-350.
56. Sbitany H, Wang F, Peled AW, et al. Immediate implant-based breast reconstruction following total skin-sparing mastectomy: defining the risk of preoperative and postoperative radiation therapy for surgical outcomes. *Plast Reconstr Surg*. 2014;134(3):396-404.
    Retrospective review comparing outcomes of immediate reconstruction in setting of premastectomy or postmastectomy radiation.
57. Lee KT, Mun GH. Prosthetic breast reconstruction in previously irradiated breasts: a meta-analysis. *J Surg Oncol*. 2015;112(5):468-475.
58. Devereux DF, Thibault L, Boretos J, Brennan MF. The quantitative and qualitative impairment of wound healing by adriamycin. *Cancer*. 1979;43(3):932-938.
59. Lawrence WT, Talbot TL, Norton JA. Preoperative or postoperative doxorubicin hydrochloride (adriamycin): which is better for wound healing? *Surgery*. 1986;100(1):9-13.
60. Caffo O, Cazzolli D, Scalet A, et al. Concurrent adjuvant chemotherapy and immediate breast reconstruction with skin expanders after mastectomy for breast cancer. *Breast Cancer Res Treat*. 2000;60(3):267-275.
61. Donker M, Hage JJ, Woerdeman LA, et al. Surgical complications of skin sparing mastectomy and immediate prosthetic reconstruction after neoadjuvant chemotherapy for invasive breast cancer. *Eur J Surg Oncol*. 2012;38(1):25-30.
62. Warren Peled A, Itakura K, Foster RD, et al. Impact of chemotherapy on postoperative complications after mastectomy and immediate breast reconstruction. *Arch Surg*. 2010;145(9):880-885.
63. Wang F, Peled AW, Chin R, et al. The impact of radiation therapy, lymph node dissection, and hormonal therapy on outcomes of tissue expander-implant exchange in prosthetic breast reconstruction. *Plast Reconstr Surg*. 2016;137(1):1-9.
64. Zhao X, Wu X, Dong J, et al. A meta-analysis of postoperative complications of tissue expander/implant breast reconstruction using acellular dermal matrix. *Aesthet Plast Surg*. 2015;39(6):892-901.
65. Reish RG, Damjanovic B, Austen WG Jr, et al. Infection following implant-based reconstruction in 1952 consecutive breast reconstructions: salvage rates and predictors of success. *Plast Reconstr Surg*. 2013;131(6):1223-1230.
66. Washer LL, Gutowski K. Breast implant infections. *Infect Dis Clin North Am*. 2012;26(1):111-125.
67. Wan D, Rohrich RJ. Revisiting the management of capsular contracture in breast augmentation: a systematic review. *Plast Reconstr Surg*. 2016;137(3):826-841.
68. Phillips BT, Halvorson EG. Antibiotic prophylaxis following implant-based breast reconstruction: what is the evidence? *Plast Reconstr Surg*. 2016;138(4):751-757.
69. Hu ES, Pusic AL, Waljee JF, et al. Patient-reported aesthetic satisfaction with breast reconstruction during the long-term survivorship Period. *Plast Reconstr Surg*. 2009;124(1):1-8.

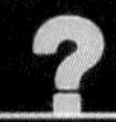

QUESTIONS

1. **A 44-year-old woman undergoes immediate right breast reconstruction with placement of a tissue expander in the partial submuscular position. ADM is used to cover the lower pole of the device. Which of the following is *not* a potential advantage of ADM use in this patient?**

   a. Maintains optimal implant position on the chest wall
   b. Reduced risk of seroma and implant infection
   c. Reduced rate of capsular contracture
   d. Improved definition of inframammary fold and lateral breast border
   e. Improved aesthetic outcome

2. **A 30-year-old fitness instructor comes to clinic to discuss prosthetic breast reconstruction. She would like to know if she is a candidate for single-stage *direct-to-implant* reconstruction. Which of the following patient characteristics is *not* a contraindication to single-stage prosthetic reconstruction?**

   a. BMI >30
   b. Active smoker
   c. Thin mastectomy skin flaps
   d. B-cup breasts prior to mastectomy
   e. Desire for larger postreconstruction breast size

3. **A 38-year-old woman with large breasts comes to clinic to discuss reconstruction after planned mastectomy for a newly diagnosed right breast cancer. Which of the following is *not* considered an advantage of implant-based reconstructions over autologous reconstruction methods?**

   a. Shorter operative time
   b. Easier to achieve symmetry with contralateral breast
   c. Greater long-term patient satisfaction
   d. Improved control over final reconstructed breast volume
   e. Both b and c

4. **A 45-year-old woman who underwent bilateral breast reconstruction with tissue expanders 3 weeks prior comes to clinic with a warm, swollen, red right breast. Her drain output is cloudy. She has a low-grade temperature. Her WBC is 13. She is admitted for IV antibiotic therapy and attempted implant salvage. Which of the following clinical findings is most predictive of failure of implant salvage?**

   a. Diffuse breast erythema
   b. Purulent drain output
   c. Temperature greater than 38.6
   d. WBC greater than 13
   e. Wound cultures growing methicillin-sensitive staphylococcus.

1. **Answer: b.** ADM has become a useful adjunct in implant-based breast reconstruction as a reliable method to maintain the implant pocket, specifically by reconstituting the inframammary fold and lateral breast border, thereby maintaining the device in the optimal position on the chest wall. This has been shown in some studies to translate into improved aesthetic results as graded by both surgeon and patient. Evidence from multiple studies demonstrated decreased risk of capsular contracture when ADM is used at the time of reconstruction. Despite this positive effect, several retrospective reviews have demonstrated an increased risk of other complications including seroma and infection with ADM. A recent meta-analysis of ADM use demonstrated no clear increase in incidence of seroma or infection when ADM was used, but there is no evidence that ADM results in a lower incidence of these complications.[2]

2. **Answer: d.** When considering single-stage implant-based reconstruction following mastectomy, patient selection is key. There are added technical considerations when direct placement of permanent implant is performed that must be considered to obtain the best possible outcome. None of these appears more important than the overall quality and viability of the mastectomy skin flaps. Flaps that are overly thin or that exhibit poor bleeding are more prone to skin necrosis, implant exposure, and reconstructive failure from the added stress of the device, and are therefore a contraindication to single-stage implant reconstruction. Along similar lines, smoking significantly increases the risk of wound complications following direct-to-implant reconstruction, and is a relative contraindication to this technique. Healthy patients without comorbidities such as obesity and diabetes have been shown to have the best outcomes with this technique. The need for revision and complication rates appear to correlate with increasing premastectomy breast size; therefore, patients with small (A or B cup) breasts tend to make the best candidates for a single-stage technique.

3. **Answer: e.** Implant-based reconstruction techniques have several advantages when compared to autologous reconstructions. Implant-based reconstructions can typically be performed in a much shorter period of time, as they do not require dissection of autologous donor tissue or, as in the case of microsurgical reconstruction, the dissection of recipient vessels. Although the volume of an autologous reconstruction is limited by the quantity of donor tissues, the final volume of an implant-based reconstruction can to a certain extent be controlled by the surgeon, both through tissue expansion and final implant selection. One downside of implant-based reconstruction is the ability to obtain symmetry of the reconstructed breast with contralateral native breast tissue. Over time, as the contralateral breast develops ptosis, asymmetry may become even more evident. The difference in the long-term behavior of an implant reconstruction may partially account for differences in long-term patient satisfaction between prosthetic and autologous methods. There are data that though patient satisfaction initially is no different between prosthetic and autologous reconstruction, over time patients tend to become less satisfied with the appearance of an implant reconstruction whereas their satisfaction with an autologous reconstruction remains relatively constant.[69]

4. **Answer: d.** There is a broad range of severity of surgical site infections following implant-based reconstruction. Although erythema isolated to the mastectomy incision may represent a more superficial process that can be managed with outpatient oral antibiotics, infections involving the implant pocket itself may present with whole breast erythema, purulent drain output, and systemic signs such as fever and leukocytosis. Even in the setting of more severe infections, implant salvage is possible and can be considered for certain properly selected patients. A recent study of nearly 2000 implant reconstructions identified elevated WBC at admission and intraoperative cultures growing MRSA as independent predictors of salvage failure.[65] Diffuse erythema, character of drain output, fever, and methicillin-sensitive *Staphylococcus aureus* growth were not predictive of need for explantation.

CHAPTER 60 Breast Reconstruction: Autologous Flap Techniques

Shailesh Agarwal and Adeyiza O. Momoh

KEY POINTS

- Autologous flap breast reconstruction is a mainstay in modern day approach to postmastectomy breast reconstruction.
- An understanding of the multidisciplinary aspects and components of cancer care is important when formulating a plan for reconstruction
- Free flap selection is based on surgical history and presence of sufficient tissue at proposed donor site.
- A variety of flap donor options exist including the abdomen, buttocks, and thighs.
- Preoperative imaging may elucidate vessel anatomy, but is not always critical.
- Clinical exam remains the standard for postoperative flap monitoring.

Breast reconstruction is a critical component of the comprehensive management of the breast cancer patient. The primary goal of breast reconstruction is to restore a natural appearing form of the breast, with additional benefits in the quality of life experienced after cancer treatment. Breast reconstruction may be performed using implants or tissue derived from the patient (autologous tissue). A number of studies evaluating national reconstruction trends have reported ratios of implant to autologous breast reconstruction in the range of 2:1 to 9:1.[1-4] That a minority of breast reconstruction patients undergo autologous tissue reconstruction is likely due to patient- and nonpatient-related factors. Patient-related factors include a lack of donor site tissue, comorbidities that preclude use of flaps, desire to avoid recovery from the donor site and patient preference. Operative requirements, such as increased operative time, need for specialized instruments, specialized technical training and skills, and greater resources, comprise nonpatient-related factors that impede the utilization of autologous breast reconstruction.[4-6] However, by using autologous tissue, one may obviate the postoperative risks of morbidity associated with implants including infection, rupture, capsular contracture, and malposition. In addition, autologous tissue is generally preferred in patients expecting to receive radiation therapy, or with a history of radiation therapy including radiation previously delivered as part of breast conservation therapy (BCT).[7-10] Finally, quality of life in patients undergoing autologous tissue reconstructions is maintained at a high level over time after completion of reconstruction.[11]

PREOPERATIVE EVALUATION

Breast Cancer Treatment Plan

The preoperative evaluation of the patient interested in postmastectomy breast reconstruction includes a thorough history and physical examination. The patient's goals, including desired breast size, should be discussed in the context of the utility and limitations of the reconstructive options. The oncologic plan should also be reviewed including the possibility of chemotherapy, radiation therapy, and contralateral prophylactic mastectomy (CPM). Tamoxifen increases the likelihood of thrombotic complications.[12] A history of radiation or plan for future radiation delivery may make autologous breast reconstruction more desirable given greater morbidity with radiation and implant reconstruction.[7-10] Often, patients presenting for mastectomy have previously been treated for breast cancer with BCT, which includes whole breast radiation (Figure 60.1). These variables should be considered in decisions made for immediate or delayed breast reconstruction and on the type of reconstruction recommended.

Timing of Breast Reconstruction

When possible immediate breast reconstruction tends to be preferred by a majority of patients undergoing mastectomies. The decision on immediate or delayed reconstruction in general is influenced by cancer staging, with delayed reconstruction favored in advanced stage cancers that require postmastectomy radiation therapy (PMRT) or close surveillance. Some patients may also opt to wait on reconstruction if the combined process of oncologic treatment and reconstruction seems overwhelming. The need for PMRT, though not an absolute contraindication to immediate reconstruction, tends to be the predominant reason to consider delayed reconstruction. Delayed reconstruction is typically advocated for multiple reasons including

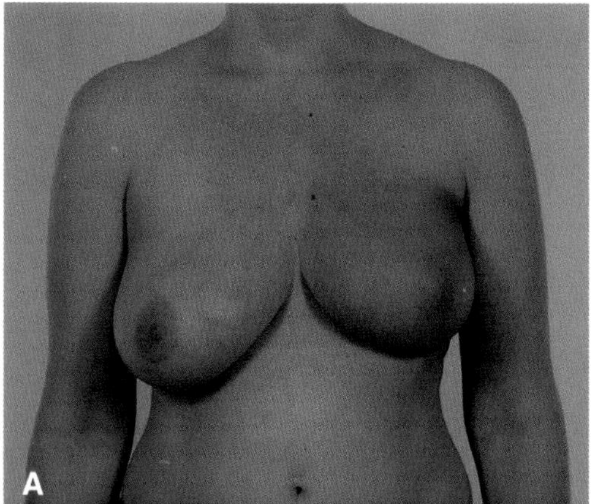

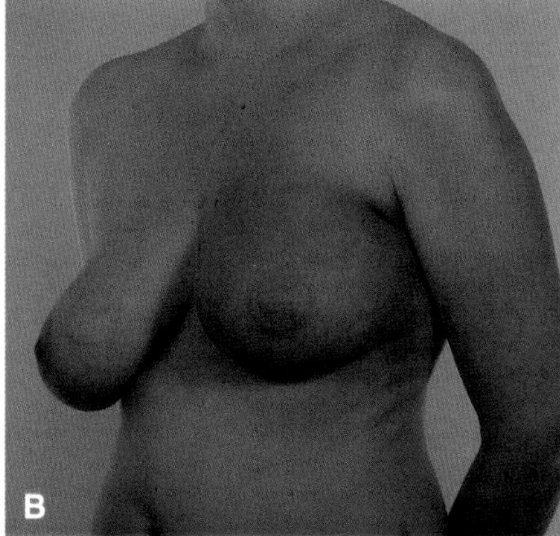

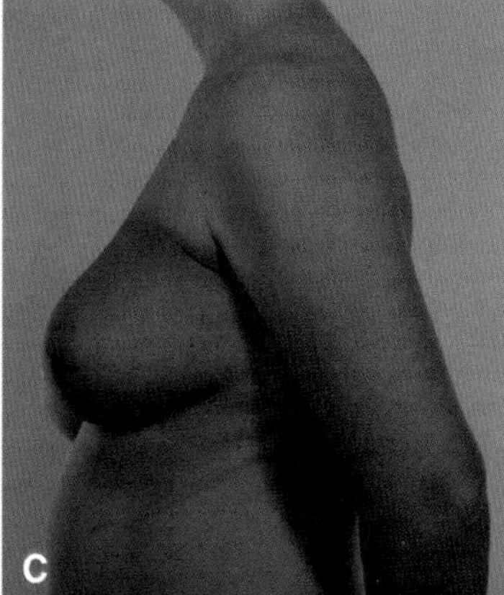

FIGURE 60.1. A patient with a left invasive breast cancer who has undergone breast conservation therapy (BCT—lumpectomy, adjuvant chemotherapy, and radiation) with gross changes to the left breast seen on AP **(A)**, oblique **(B)** and lateral **(C)** views.

the avoidance of untoward effects of radiation on the results of an immediate reconstruction and the potential for delaying oncologic treatment because of complications from reconstruction.

History and Exam

Obtaining an accurate medical and surgical history is critical when evaluating patients for autologous reconstruction. Because autologous operations often require longer operative times, it is imperative to ensure that the patient is medically appropriate for a longer operation from cardiac and pulmonary perspectives. In addition, a history of previous surgeries may impact the use of specific donor sites for autologous breast reconstruction. For instance, previous abdominal operations that compromise abdominal soft tissue blood supply may preclude use of the abdomen as a donor site for reconstruction. A known history of hypercoagulable conditions would be a contraindication to performing a free tissue transfer with an increased risk for vessel thrombosis; pedicled flap options would be possible in this context. Active smoking would be a relative contraindication for performing any autologous flap procedure with increased risk for wound dehiscence and delayed wound healing. Patients are typically counseled to quit smoking for a minimum of 4 weeks before surgery and often preoperatively evaluated with a urine cotinine test.

Patient preferences for postreconstruction breast size is also important for operative planning. For example, thin patients with a paucity of abdominal tissue who desire CPM may not be candidates for bilateral breast reconstruction using abdominal tissue alone. In some patients, use of the entire lower abdominal soft tissue in the form of bipedicled or stacked flaps may be required to attain unilateral breast reconstruction of sufficient size. Alternative donor sites such as the buttocks (superior gluteal artery perforator flap), medial thigh (transverse upper gracilis flap), or posterior thigh (profunda artery perforator flap) may also be options for patients with insufficient abdominal tissue. All potential donor sites should be examined for the presence of adequate skin laxity and adipose tissue by inspection for scars, palpation, and pinch testing.

Perforator and Pedicle Evaluation

Although useful for preoperative planning, imaging is not absolutely needed in patients without a surgical history that raises concerns about pedicle compromise. Scans may be necessary to evaluate the thoracodorsal (TD) vessels in patients desiring latissimus dorsi reconstruction who have undergone axillary lymph node dissections, where the status of the TD vessels is unclear. Similar concerns exist and may prompt imaging to confirm an intact pedicle in patients with low and lateral abdominal incisions in patients considered for abdominal free flaps. Computed tomography angiography (CTA) provides information regarding perforator distribution and pedicle course (Figure 60.2). Studies have shown that CTA may reduce

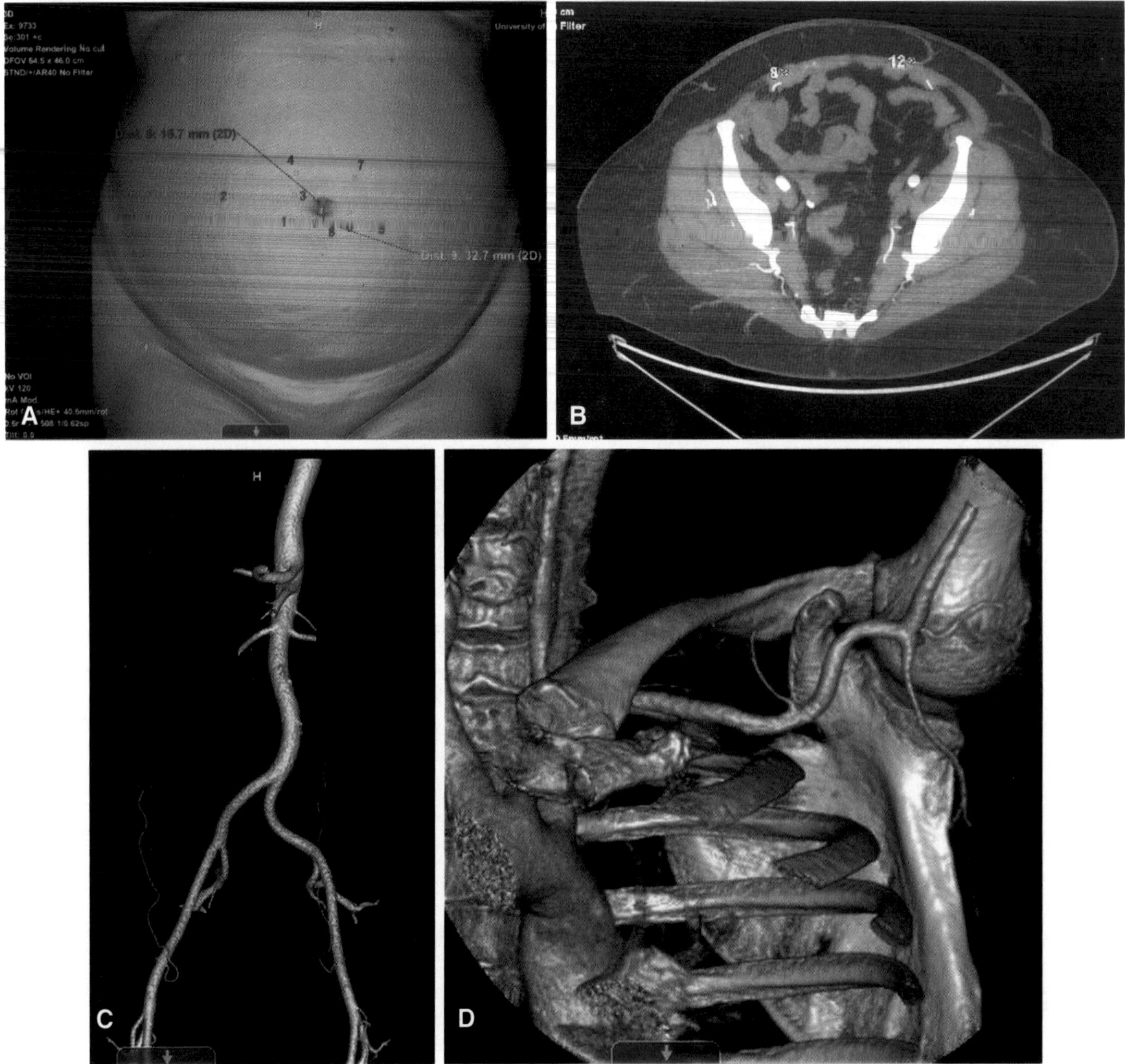

FIGURE 60.2. Preoperative CT angiogram of the abdomen **(A)**, identifying perforators **(B)** and outlining the branching pattern **(C)** of the abdominal vascular pedicle. Also, valuable in evaluating thoracodorsal vessel patency **(D)** with a history of axillary lymph node dissection.

operative time for abdominal-based reconstruction, ostensibly by aiding in perforator identification/selection and deep inferior epigastric artery dissection; however, CTA may also lead to increased healthcare costs.[13-19] Alternative imaging techniques have also been studied including duplex ultrasound and MR angiography, although to a lesser extent. Many surgeons who do not implement preoperative imaging may instead use the pencil Doppler to simply confirm perforator location on the abdominal wall. Still others may choose not to perform any initial perforator or pedicle evaluation, but rather begin flap elevation knowing that the abdomen has reliable perforator anatomy.

PEDICLED FLAPS

Latissimus Dorsi Flap

The latissimus dorsi (LD) myocutaneous flap is a well-established pedicled flap option for breast reconstruction. The LD flap is based on the thoracodorsal vessels, which arises from the subscapular vessels that branch off of the axillary vessels (Figure 60.3). Within the latissimus the thoracodorsal branches into a medial or transverse and a lateral or descending branch, which allow for muscle-sparing procedures with use of part of the LD for reconstruction. The LD flap is a broad muscle that covers a large surface area and can be used with or without a skin paddle for reconstruction. However, the muscle harvested with a skin paddle typically does not provide sufficient volume for breast reconstruction. To achieve a desired breast volume the LD flap is often used in combination with a prosthesis (Figure 60.4). The LD may also be used in setting of salvage procedures to replace compromised mastectomy skin flaps over implants or in cases of failed free-flap breast reconstructions.

Pedicled Transverse Rectus Abdominis Myocutaneous (TRAM) Flap

The pedicled TRAM flap takes advantage of lower abdominal soft tissue adiposity that is present in many patients and is based on the superior epigastric artery, a continuation of the internal mammary artery (IMA). The pedicled TRAM is elevated with the ipsilateral rectus muscle and tunneled into the mastectomy defect site through the inframammary fold.[20-22] Flap harvest includes fascia overlying the rectus muscle and often requires mesh placement for closure of the donor site. The use of the rectus muscle contributes to weakened abdominal wall strength and an increased risk for abdominal bulge.[23-25] Because the deep inferior epigastric artery system is the more dominant blood supply to the abdominal skin and fat, maneuvers to improve the blood supply (from the superior vasculature) to the flap are sometimes employed. One such maneuver is a delay procedure, which is often performed 2 or 3 weeks before the pedicled TRAM procedure, when the ipsilateral deep inferior epigastric artery is ligated to facilitate the recruitment of choke vessels with perfusion from the superior epigastric vessels.[26] Efforts to avoid donor site morbidity while taking advantage of the more dominant deep inferior epigastric system encouraged the evolution of free tissue transfer options described later.

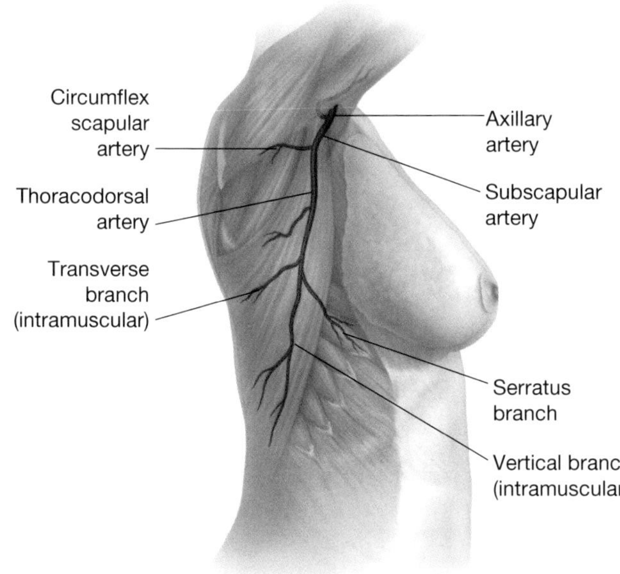

FIGURE 60.3. Thoracodorsal vascular anatomy. (Reproduced with permission from Kung TA, Momoh AO. Recipient vessel exposure: internal mammary and thoracodorsal. In: Chung KC, ed. *Operative Techniques in Plastic Surgery*. Philadelphia, PA: Wolters Kluwer; 2019. Part 4, Figure 24-1.)

FREE FLAPS

Abdomen-Based Flaps

Abdomen-based breast reconstruction is the mainstay of autologous microvascular breast reconstruction. The benefits of this well-described reconstructive technique include reliable vascular anatomy, extensive reported clinical experience, reduced donor site morbidity with muscle-sparing/perforator flap options, a long pedicle with similar caliber to recipient vessels, and typically, the presence of sufficient soft tissue for reconstruction.

Flap types include the free transverse rectus abdominis musculocutaneous (TRAM), free muscle-sparing TRAM (MS-TRAM), deep inferior epigastric perforator (DIEP), and the superficial inferior epigastric artery (SIEA) perforator flaps. The free TRAM, free MS-TRAM, and DIEP flaps are based on the deep inferior epigastric vessels, which are branches from the external iliac vessels. Perforating vessels from the deep inferior epigastric system perfuse varying aspects or zones of the abdominal wall skin and adipose tissue. The SIEA flap is based on the superficial inferior epigastric vessels, which are branches from the femoral vessels, run superficial to the abdominal wall fascia, and perfuse the abdominal soft tissue in parallel to the deep inferior epigastric system (Figure 60.5); violation of the anterior rectus fascia is avoided with this flap. A small percentage of flaps (less than 10%) are reported to be superficially dominant.[27]

The operation is performed with the patient in the supine position. For patients who are undergoing immediate breast reconstruction, flap elevation may be performed while the breast surgery team performs the mastectomy. A lenticular design is employed with tissue based around and inferior to the umbilicus (Figure 60.6). Consideration is given for SIEA flap reconstruction whenever possible. Early in the abdominal flap elevation, along the inferior aspect of the designed abdominal flap, generally superficial to the Scarpa fascia and within 5 to 10 cm lateral from the midline, is explored for the SIEA and SIEV (Figure 60.7).[28] SIEA/V vessels that can be used are reported to be present in 30% of patients.[29] In flaps with vessels that are present and of appropriate size (1.5 mm diameter SIEA at the inferior edge of the flap) dissection of the SIEA and SIEV are carried to the femoral vessels.[29] Once adequate perfusion based on the superficial vessels is confirmed, all other perforators from the deep inferior epigastric system are divided. Perfusion of flaps based on the SIEA/SIEV is not reliable across the midline.

Most of the perforators required for DIEP flap elevation are located within a 10 cm radius from the umbilicus.[30] These perforators perfuse predictable zones of the lower abdominal soft tissue, with perfusion zones initially described by Hartrampf for TRAM flaps and subsequently modified by Holm for DIEP flaps[22,31] (see Figure 60.8). Zones of perfusion have since been shown to be

BREAST

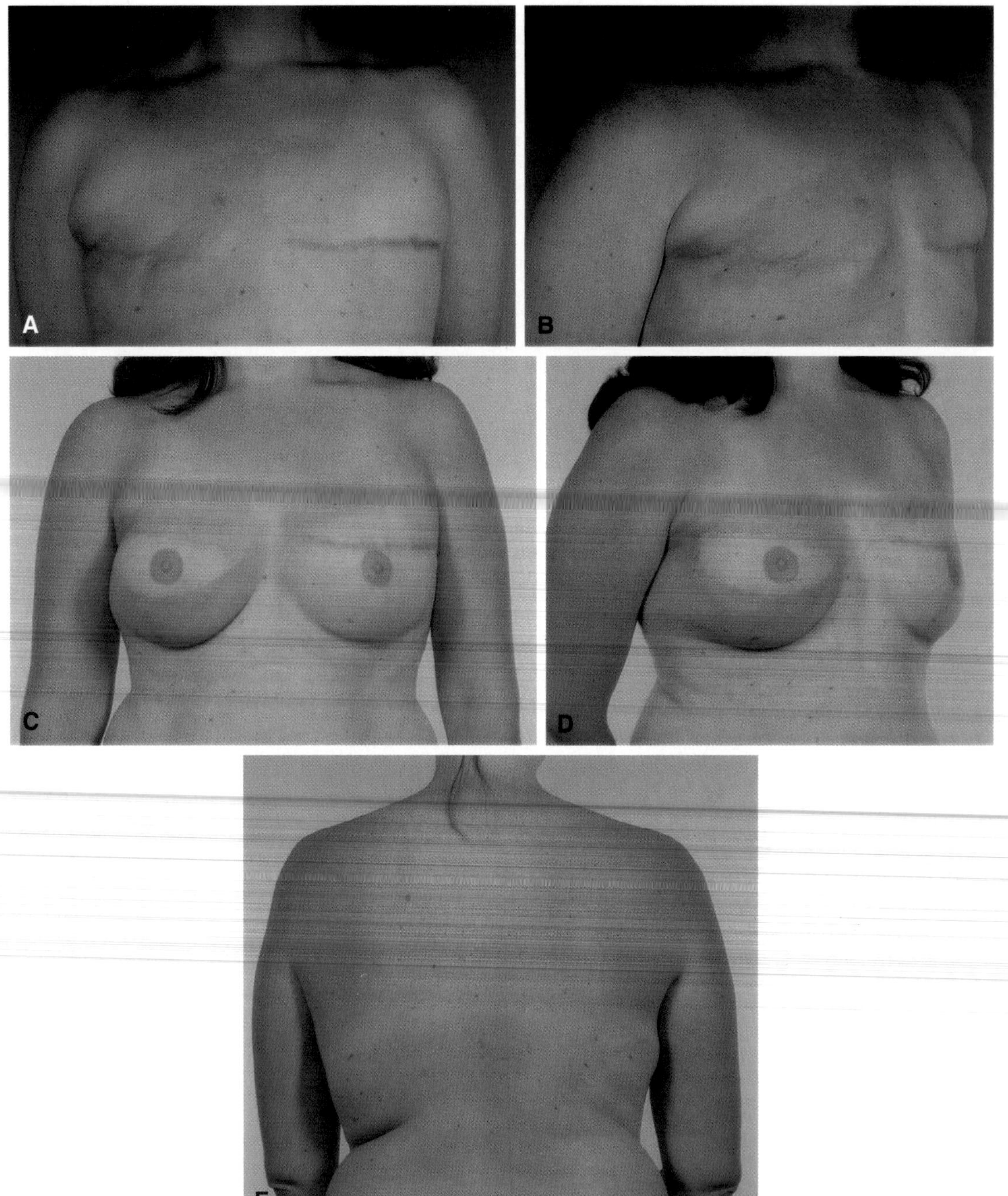

FIGURE 60.4. **A, B.** A patient with a history of invasive right breast cancer who has undergone bilateral mastectomies with right chest wall radiation. **C, D.** Postoperative result after completion of delayed bilateral breast reconstruction with a latissimus dorsi myocutaneous flap and implant on the right and an implant alone on the left. **E.** Obliquely oriented donor site scar on the right back.

varying depending on the row of perforators (medial or lateral) selected (Figure 60.8).[30] When reconstructing a single breast, the midline may be crossed to include the zone immediately adjacent to the midline to provide sufficient tissue for symmetry with the contralateral side; for bilateral breast reconstruction, the abdominal tissue is bisected down the midline. The superior abdominal flap is elevated from the superior incision for closure with the inferior incision, which is not undermined. The umbilicus is transposed and delivered through the superior abdominal flap. At the inferior aspect of the flap, even in cases where the SIEA is absent or too small to rely upon, the SIEV if present is dissected out to a length (5–7 cm) for potential use as an alternate flap outflow option.

Suprafascial identification of lateral and medial row perforators (over the rectus abdominis muscle) is performed and an ideal perforator or group of perforators are selected. With use of a preoperative CT scans, identification of perforators may be simplified.

Perforator row selection may be based on a combination of factors including perforator size, location (central or peripheral) and branching pattern within the adipose tissue of the flap. In addition, perforators considered for exclusion may be clamped temporarily with assessment of flap perfusion by assessing color and capillary refill; perfusion with select perforators clamped may also be assessed with indocyanine green perfusion imaging. Once perforators are selected, the anterior rectus fascia is incised and careful intramuscular dissection of the selected perforators through the

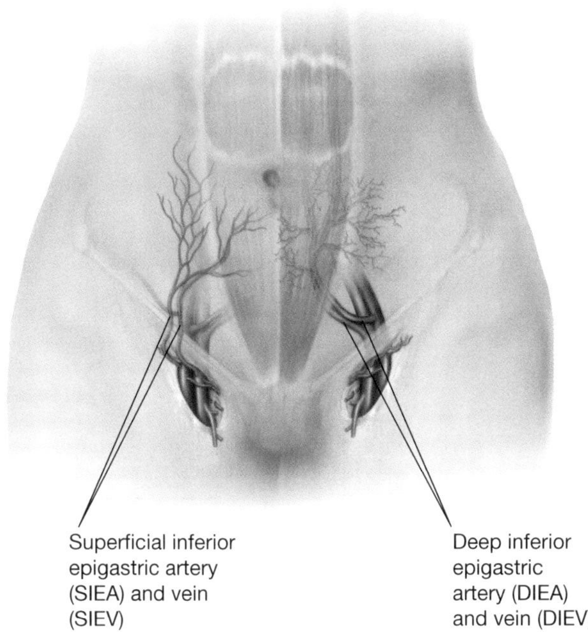

FIGURE 60.5. Superficial inferior epigastric and deep inferior epigastric vascular anatomy.

rectus muscle is performed down to the deep inferior epigastric vessels (Figure 60.9). If perforators from separate rows (e.g., medial and lateral row) are to be included to improve tissue perfusion, the intervening segment of muscle between the two rows may be harvested with the flap as a muscle-sparing TRAM flap, obviating perforator dissection through the muscle. Complete transection of a segment of the rectus muscle that includes perforators without preserving continuity of any aspects of the rectus muscle constitutes a free TRAM flap. In all three described flaps, the pedicle is traced proximally toward its takeoff from the external iliac vessels. The pedicle, typically consisting of two veins and one artery, is ligated distal to the takeoff from the external iliac vessels. The pedicle is ligated to ensure sufficient vessel length and caliber for anastomosis with the internal mammary vessels. In the repair of abdominal fascial defects after flap harvest, primary closure without mesh is often possible with DIEP flap and free ms-TRAM flap harvests. Free TRAM harvests tend to include wide sections of anterior rectus fascia and may require mesh placement, particularly in cases with bilateral flaps.

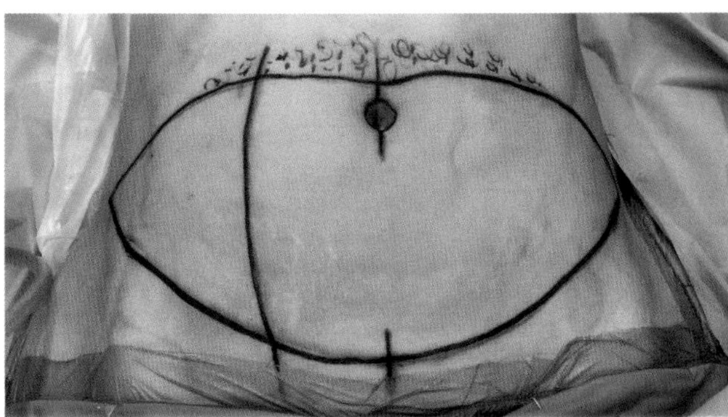

FIGURE 60.6. Preoperative markings for abdominal based flap breast reconstruction. The flap is designed to capture perforators typical localized around the umbilicus (superior marking just above the umbilicus and extending laterally toward the anterior superior iliac spines). Consideration is given for primary closure of the donor site, which determines the position of the lower marking above the pubis.

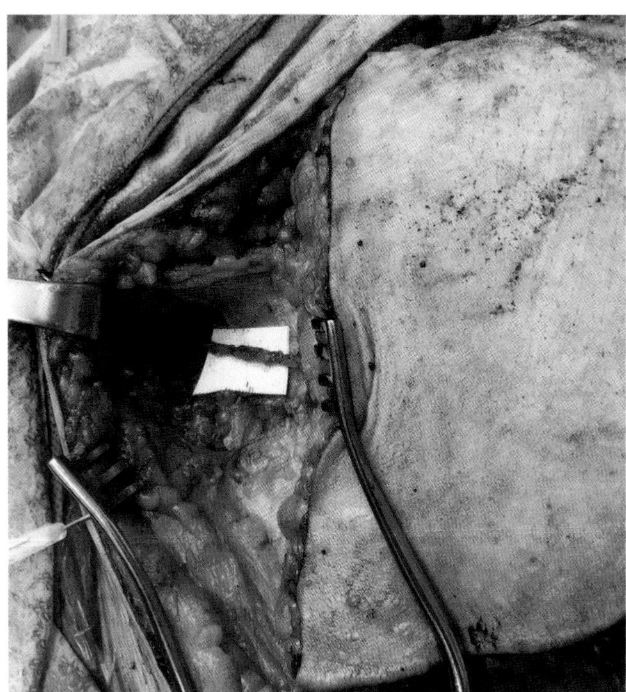

FIGURE 60.7. Superficial inferior epigastric artery and vein, at the inferior border of abdominal flap dissected toward the femoral vessels.

On completion of the microvascular anastomoses, with perfusion reestablished, flaps are shaped on the chest wall to achieve the contour of a breast mound. Varying amounts of skin and adipose tissue are utilized based on existing deficiencies as is encountered in cases of immediate and delayed breast reconstruction (Figures 60.10 and 60.11).

Medial Thigh Flaps

Medial thigh flaps incorporating the gracilis muscle provide another option for breast reconstruction in patients who have had previous abdominoplasty or abdominal flaps, or insufficient abdominal tissue.[32] The medial circumflex femoral artery, a branch of the profunda femoris artery, serves as the pedicle to the gracilis muscle to support the overlying fat and skin (Figure 60.12). The pedicle is identified in the interval between the gracilis and adductor longus muscles and is traced proximally (Figure 60.13). The skin may be oriented transversely (transverse upper gracilis (TUG) flap), vertically (vertical upper gracilis (VUG) flap) or designed as a combination of both with a bipedicled skin paddle.[32] Although the TUG does not provide as much skin or fat as the VUG, it may provide a more reliable skin paddle. The transverse upper thigh scar is better hidden than the vertical scar; however, excessive tension from closure of the transverse skin paddle donor site may cause labial spreading. Medial thigh flaps are ideal for patients with small- to moderate-sized breast who desire similar-sized reconstruction. The overall availability of sufficient tissue for breast reconstruction is one drawback of medial thigh flaps. In a retrospective study, Park et al. reported a mean weight of 342 g among VUGs and 268 g among TUGs[32]; however, use of bilateral stacked flaps (bilateral upper gracilis (BUG) flap) may address this concern for patients undergoing unilateral breast reconstruction.[32] One advantage of this form of reconstruction is that flap harvest and breast reconstruction can be performed in one position with the patient supine and the hip externally rotated (thigh frog legged) for flap harvest. However, the length of the vascular pedicle is relatively short, measuring approximately 7 cm and the flap artery is often smaller than recipient arteries used for breast reconstruction (e.g., internal mammary or thoracodorsal vessels).[33]

Lateral row perfusion Medial row perfusion

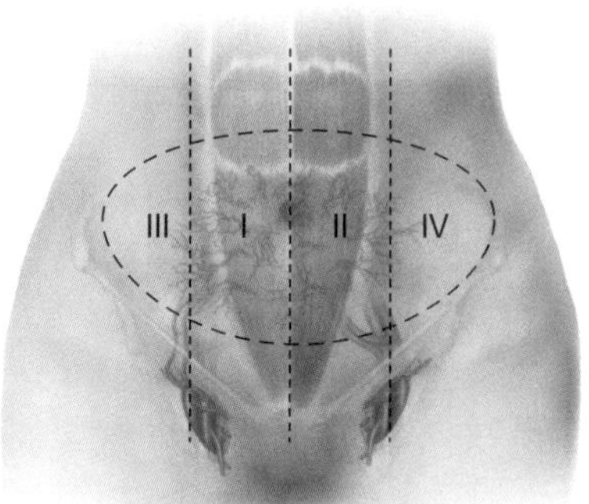

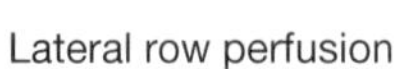

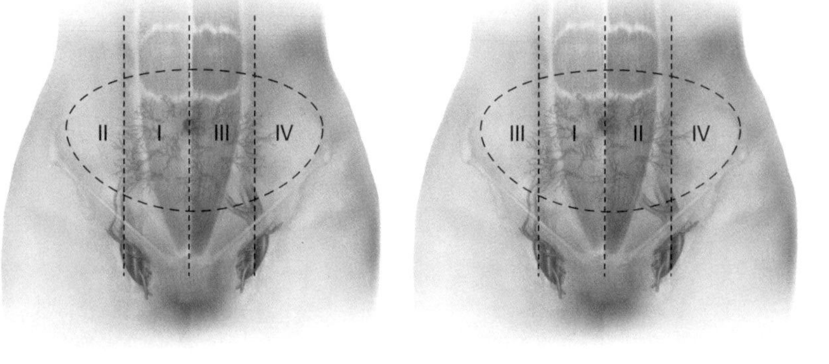

FIGURE 60.8. DIEP flap zones of perfusion.

Posterior Thigh Flaps

The profunda artery perforator (PAP) flap uses posterior thigh skin and adipose tissue as an option for breast reconstruction[34] (Figure 60.14). The consistent presence and length of the pedicle—reported to average 10.6 cm—allows for the internal mammary or thoracodorsal vessels to serve as recipient vessels.[35,36] Perforators from the pedicle are located roughly 5 to 6 cm below the gluteal crease, both medial and lateral to the midline of the posterior thigh.[36,37] The flap is designed as a horizontal ellipse with superior incision at or immediately below the gluteal crease; the perforator travels through the adductor magnus. Flap elevation can be performed in the prone position; however, to avoid intraoperative position change and to facilitate a two-team approach, the flap may also be elevated in a lithotomy or frog-leg position (Figure 60.15). Although it has been reported that the horizontally designed PAP flap offers mean weight of 220 g, larger flaps are possible with the PAP designed as a fleur-de-lis (range 340–735 g).[38]

Gluteal Artery Perforator Flaps

The superior or inferior gluteal artery perforator (SGAP or IGAP) flaps are autologous alternatives to abdominal-based flaps for patients who do not have reliable abdominal vascular anatomy due to previous surgery, or who do not have sufficient abdominal tissue to reconstruct breasts of sufficient size. The superior gluteal artery exits the pelvis superior to the piriformis muscle at approximately the point marking the junction of the upper and middle third of a line drawn from the posterior superior iliac spine (PSIS) to the greater trochanter. The inferior gluteal artery exits the pelvis inferior to the piriformis muscle, at approximately the point marking the junction of the upper and middle third of a line drawn from the PSIS to the ischial tuberosity.[39] Perforators are identified preoperatively using CT angiogram and/or Doppler probe. Patients are either positioned lateral or prone and might need position changes for flap elevation and for transfer of the flap to the breast. A skin paddle is designed over anticipated perforators and an adipocutaneous flap is elevated intramuscular perforator dissection (Figure 60.16). One perforator is many times sufficient to support the GAP flap. One advantage provided by use of this flap is the presence of a good amount of adipose tissue for reconstruction even in patients with lower BMIs. However, the length of the vascular pedicle for this flap is relatively short, measuring 5.6 cm on average.[40]

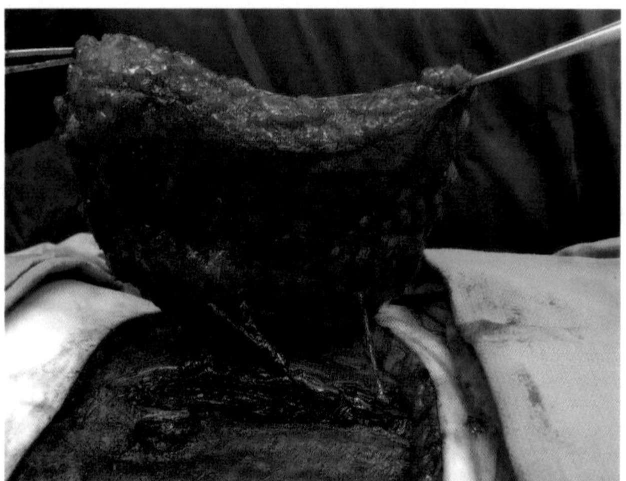

FIGURE 60.9. DIEP flap with three medial row perforators dissected through the rectus muscle and inclusion of a zone across the midline.

RECIPIENT VESSELS

The IMA and internal mammary vein (IMV) are the more commonly utilized recipient vessels for free flap breast reconstruction; alternatives are the thoracodorsal artery and vein. The IMA arises from the subclavian artery, run 1 to 2 cm lateral to the sternum, deep to the intercostal muscles and ribs, and are in continuity with the superior epigastric vessels. The internal mammary vessels can be accessed by removal of the third or fourth rib cartilage; the rib level is determined by ease of access and size of the flap pedicle to avoid a significant vessel size mismatch. At the level of the third rib, the IMA generally lies lateral to the IMV. The right and left IMAs are of similar diameter (1.9–2.1 mm) at third and fourth intercostal spaces. The left IMV bifurcates at a higher level than the right IMV (third rib on the left vs. fourth rib on the right). At the level of the third intercostal space, the left IMV is on average smaller than the right (2.5 mm vs. 3 mm).

Branches of the IMA and IMV are ligated using clips under Loupe magnification, and further under the microscope if necessary. Alternatively, a rib-sparing approach may be performed if the interspace width is adequate to perform anastomoses. This approach limits vessel exposure and introduces greater technical challenge. Here, the intercostal muscles are elevated to access the internal mammary vessels. Care is taken during internal mammary vessel exposure to avoid injury to the pleura, deep to the vessels, which could result in a pneumothorax.

The thoracodorsal vessels arise from the axillary artery and travel along the lateral thoracic wall and into the latissimus dorsi muscle. The vessels are typically identified at the lateral border of a mastectomy defect on the deep surface of the latissimus muscle.

Microvascular Anastomosis

Once flap harvest and recipient vessel exposure is complete, flap vessels are divided rendering the flap ischemic. End-to-end arterial and venous anastomoses are performed either under loupe magnification or using an operating microscope. Arteries are typically hand sewn with fine sutures (8-0 to 10-0 nylon sutures) and veins coupled with a coupling device (Figure 60.17).

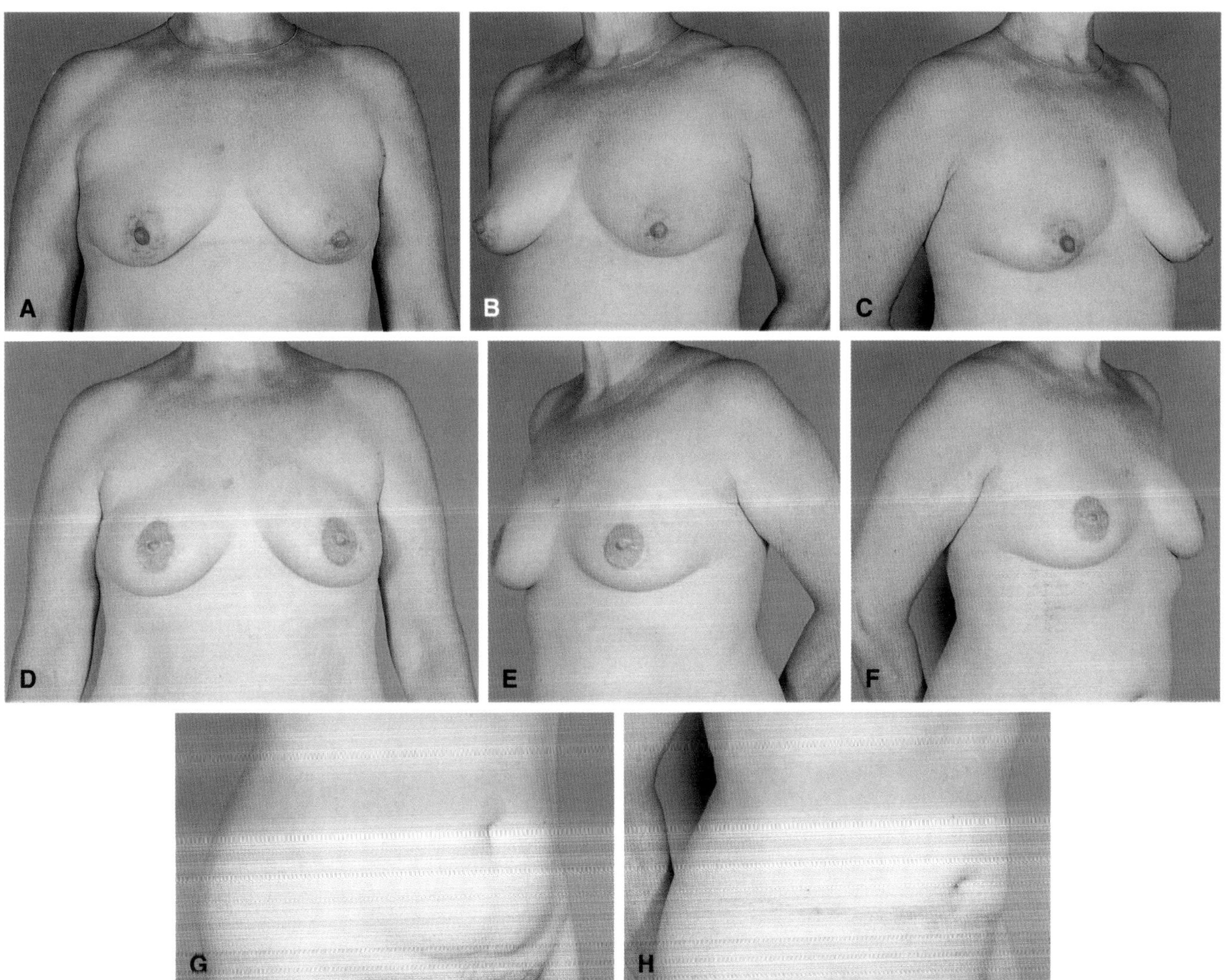

FIGURE 60.10. **A–C.** Preoperative views of a patient with a right invasive breast cancer considering bilateral mastectomy and immediate reconstruction. **D–F.** Postoperative results after immediate bilateral DIEP flap breast reconstruction, with nipple reconstruction and tattooing. **G, H.** Abdominal donor site before and after reconstruction.

After completion of the arterial and venous anastomoses, assessment of perfusion can be determined by confirming capillary refill time (~2–3 seconds), warmth, and flap edges with bright red bleeding. Hand-held Doppler ultrasound may be used to confirm a signal over perforators within the flap and on the external surface of the flap. The external site can then be marked with a suture to facilitate postoperative monitoring as well. Venous outflow can be confirmed based on appearance of the flap—a congested flap typically appears dark and has dark red blood from the edges. The identification of venous congestion without obvious mechanical obstructions within the pedicle and perforators may lead the surgeon to consider augmenting venous outflow through use of the superficial inferior epigastric vein (SIEV).

POSTOPERATIVE FREE FLAP CARE AND MONITORING

Postoperatively, flaps are kept warm with either a blanket with forced warm air over the flap or with control of the room temperature. Flaps are evaluated often, typically every hour for the first 24 hours. Postoperative flap monitoring consists of clinical exam including capillary refill (~2–3 seconds), color, warmth, and hand-held Doppler signals. Adjuncts to the clinical exam that are often implemented include near-infrared tissue oximetry, implantable arterial Doppler, or venous flow coupler. Tissue oximetry reflects a combination of arterial inflow and venous outflow. The implantable arterial Doppler provides real-time audible information regarding arterial inflow. The venous flow coupler provides real-time audible information regarding venous outflow. Anticoagulation with an antiplatelet agent (Aspirin) and venous thromboembolism (VTE) prophylaxis (subcutaneous heparin or enoxaparin) is typical.

FLAP AND DONOR SITE COMPLICATIONS

During the first 24 to 48 hours, vascular compromise may occur due to occlusion of the artery or vein due to thrombus, compression caused by hematoma, or positioning of the vessels (e.g., kinking). Vascular compromise can be identified on the basis of postoperative monitoring techniques described earlier; the rule of thumb is that early vascular compromise necessitates reoperation for salvage. Beyond the early postoperative vascular compromise other flap-related complications include fat necrosis, partial flap loss, wound dehiscence, infections, hematomas, and seromas.

Donor site complications also occur and include infection, hematoma, seroma, wound dehiscence, skin flap necrosis, umbilical necrosis, abdominal wall hernias and bulges, medial thigh lymphatic leaks, and unfavorable scars.

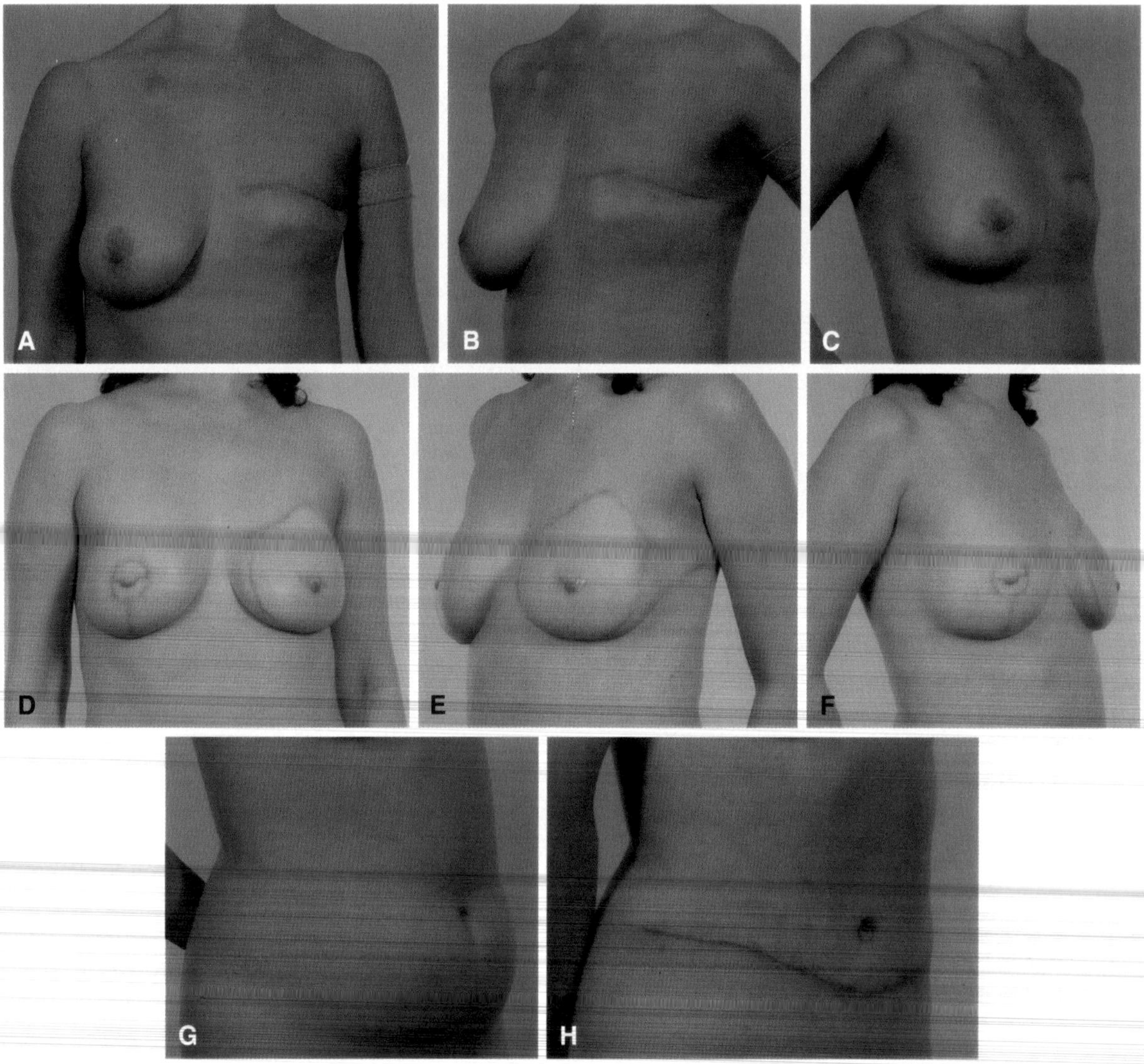

FIGURE 60.11. **A–C.** Preoperative views of a patient with a left invasive breast cancer who has undergone a left mastectomy with postmastectomy radiation therapy. She plans on a right contralateral prophylactic mastectomy with bilateral breast reconstruction. **D–F.** Postoperative results after immediate right and delayed left breast reconstructions. **G, H.** Abdominal donor site before and after reconstruction.

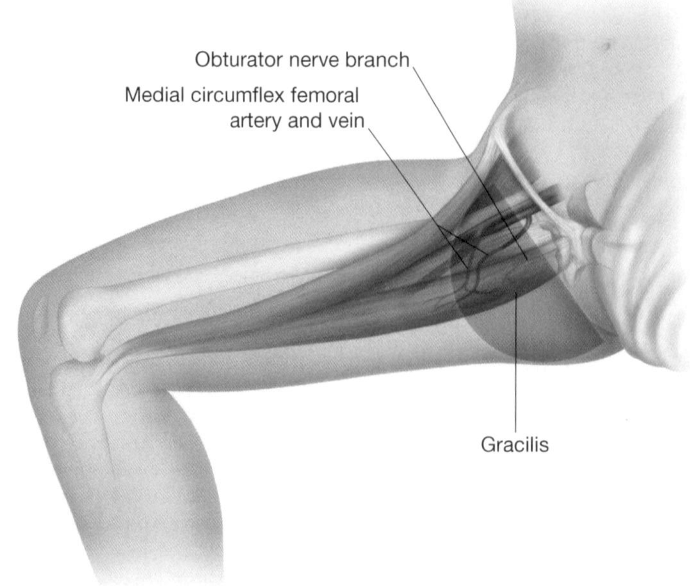

FIGURE 60.12. Medial circumflex femoral artery and vein anatomy with transversely oriented skin paddle for medial thigh flap. (Reproduced with permission from Momoh AO. Transverse upper gracilis flap for breast reconstruction. In: Chung KC, ed. *Operative Techniques in Plastic Surgery*. Philadelphia, PA: Wolters Kluwer; 2019. Part 4, Figure 28-2.)

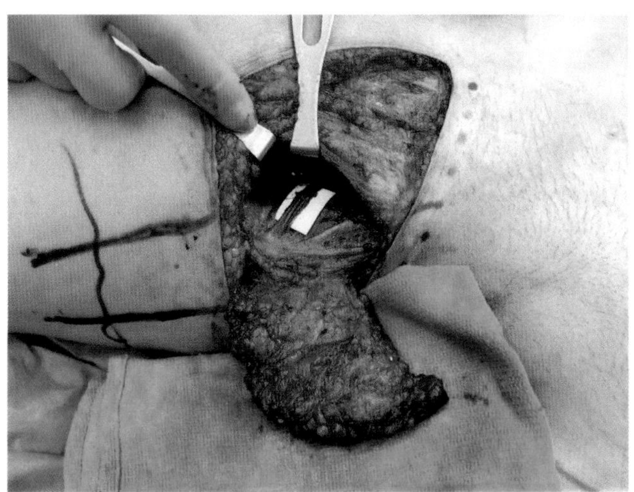

FIGURE 60.13. Medial circumflex femoral vessels extending from the medial border of the gracilis. Vessels are dissected underneath the adductor longus muscle (retracted) to the profunda femoris.

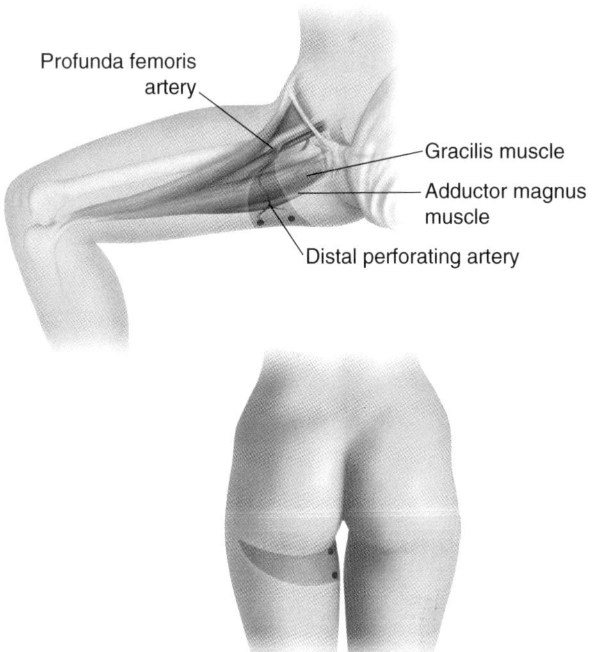

FIGURE 60.14. Profunda artery perforator vascular anatomy with transversely oriented skin paddle for a posterior/medial thigh-based flap.

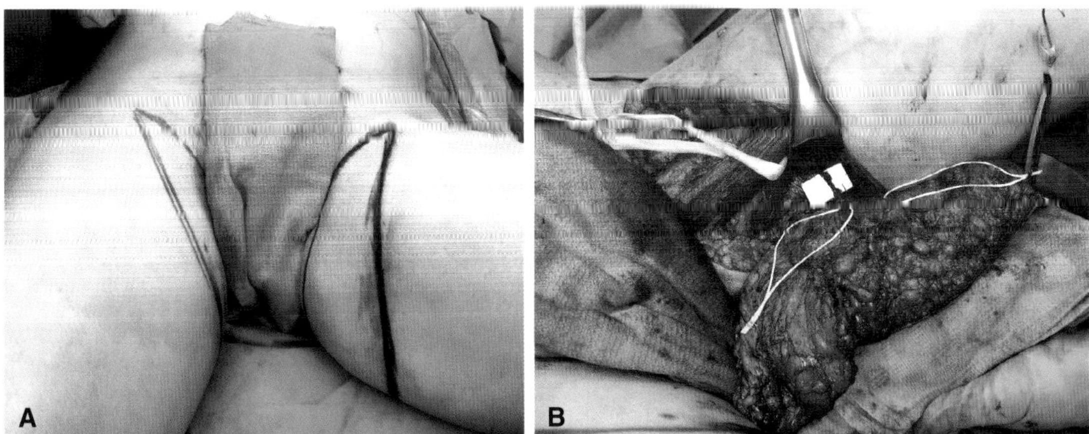

FIGURE 60.15. **A.** Supine position with medial thigh marking of flap visible. **B.** Two perforators dissected underneath the gracilis and thrugh the adductor magnus muscle (both retracted), towards the profunda femoris.

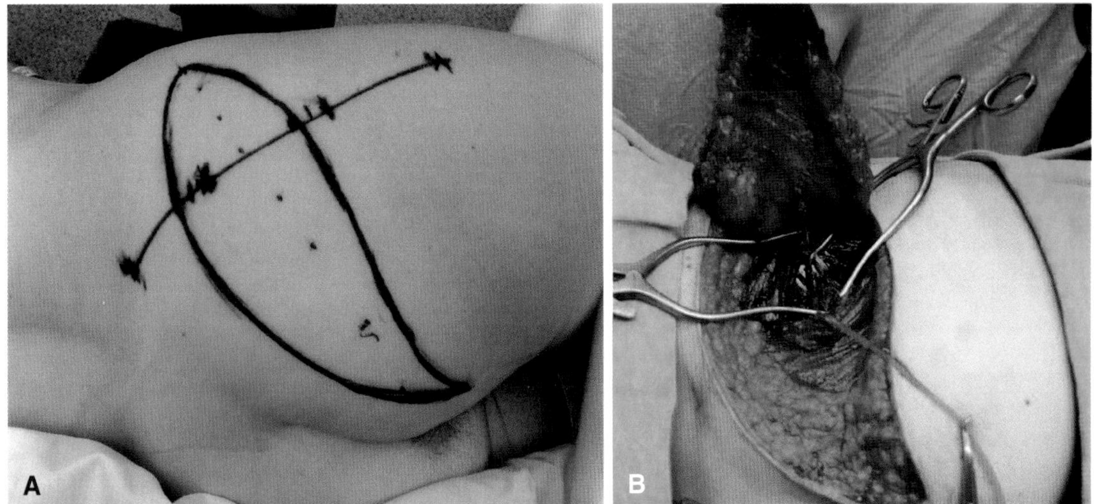

FIGURE 60.16. **A.** Lateral positioning for SGAP flap harvest with flap centered over the upper to middle third of axis from PSIS to greater trochanter. **B.** Single perforator dissected between gluteal muscle fibers.

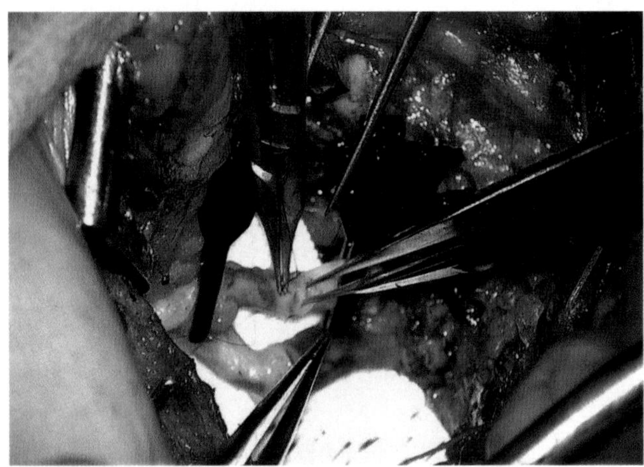

FIGURE 60.17. Hand-sewn arterial anastomosis to the IMA. Coupled veins in the background.

REFERENCES

1. Albornoz CR, Bach PB, Mehrara BJ, et al. A paradigm shift in U.S. breast reconstruction: increasing implant rates. *Plast Reconstr Surg*. 2013;131:15-23.
   Cross-sectional study of immediate breast reconstruction trends in a national patient sample. One of the better known contemporary studies that demonstrates rising reconstruction rates following the Women Health and Cancer Rights Act of 1998. Also, a key study that shows a rise in implant use in the United States.
2. Panchal H, Matros E. Current trends in postmastectomy breast reconstruction. *Plast Reconstr Surg*. 2017;140:7S-13S.
3. Barnow A, Canfield T, Liao R, et al. Breast reconstruction among commercially insured women with breast cancer in the United States. *Ann Plast Surg*. 2018;81:220-227.
4. Sheckter CC, Panchal HJ, Razdan SN, et al. The influence of physician payments on the method of breast reconstruction: a national claims analysis. *Plast Reconstr Surg*. 2018;142(4):434e-442e.
5. Billig JI, Lu Y, Momoh AO, Chung KC. A nationwide analysis of cost variation for autologous free flap breast reconstruction. *JAMA Surg*. 2017;152:1039-1047.
6. Sheckter CC, Yi D, Panchal HJ, et al. Trends in physician payments for breast reconstruction. *Plast Reconstr Surg*. 2018;141:493e-499e.
7. Jagsi R, Momoh AO, Qi J, et al. Impact of radiotherapy on complications and patient-reported outcomes after breast reconstruction. *J Natl Cancer Inst*. 2018;110(2):157-165.
   A multicenter observational study from the Mastectomy Reconstruction Outcomes Consortium (MROC) focusing on postoperative morbidity and patient reported outcomes (PROs) in radiated and nonradiated patients undergoing breast reconstruction. Findings of superior PROs and lower risk of complications with autologous reconstruction in patients receiving postmastecomy radiation therapy.
8. Billig J, Jagsi R, Qi J, et al. Should immediate autologous breast reconstruction be considered in women who require postmastectomy radiation therapy? A Prospective analysis of outcomes. *Plast Reconstr Surg*. 2017;139:1279-1288.
9. Aliu O, Zhong L, Chetta MD, et al. Comparing health care resource use between implant and autologous reconstruction of the irradiated breast: a national claims-based assessment. *Plast Reconstr Surg*. 2017;139:1224e-1231e.
10. Chetta MD, Aliu O, Zhong L, et al. Reconstruction of the irradiated breast: a national claims-based assessment of postoperative morbidity. *Plast Reconstr Surg*. 2017;139:783-792.
11. Santosa KB, Qi J, Kim HM, et al. Long-term patient-reported outcomes in postmastectomy breast reconstruction. *JAMA Surg*. 2018;153(10):891-899.
    A multicenter observational study from the Mastectomy Reconstruction Outcomes Consortium (MROC) evaluating long-term patient reported outcomes in patients undergoing implant or autologous breast reconstruction. Patients undergoing autologous breast reconstruction (relative to implant reconstructions) were found to be more satisfied with their breasts, in addition to other specific quality of life measures, 2 years after reconstruction.
12. Kelley BP, Valero V, Yi M, Kronowitz SJ. Tamoxifen increases the risk of microvascular flap complications in patients undergoing microvascular breast reconstruction. *Plast Reconstr Surg*. 2012;129:305-314.
13. Agarwal S, Talia J, Liu PS, et al. Determining the cost of incidental findings for patients undergoing preoperative planning for abdominally based perforator free flap breast reconstruction with computed tomographic angiography. *Plast Reconstr Surg*. 2016;138:804e-810e.
14. Rozen WM, Ashton MW, Grinsell D, et al. Establishing the case for CT angiography in the preoperative imaging of abdominal wall perforators. *Microsurgery*. 2008;28:306-313.
15. Rozen WM, Phillips TJ, Ashton MW, et al. Preoperative imaging for DIEA perforator flaps: a comparative study of computed tomographic angiography and Doppler ultrasound. *Plast Reconstr Surg*. 2008;121:1-8.
16. Malhotra A, Chhaya N, Nsiah-Sarbeng P, Mosahebi A. CT-guided deep inferior epigastric perforator (DIEP) flap localization—better for the patient, the surgeon, and the hospital. *Clin Radiol*. 2013;68:131-138.
17. Teunis T, Heerma van Voss MR, Kon M, van Maurik JF. CT-angiography prior to DIEP flap breast reconstruction: a systematic review and meta-analysis. *Microsurgery*. 2013;33:496-502.
18. Klasson S, Svensson H, Malm K, et al. Preoperative CT angiography versus Doppler ultrasound mapping of abdominal perforator in DIEP breast reconstructions: a randomized prospective study. *J Plast Reconstr Aesthet Surg*. 2015;68:782-786.
19. Offodile AC II, Chatterjee A, Vallejo S, Fisher CS, Tchou JC, Guo L. A cost-utility analysis of the use of preoperative computed tomographic angiography in abdomen-based perforator flap breast reconstruction. *Plast Reconstr Surg*. 2015;135:662e-669e.
20. Alderman AK, Kuzon WM Jr, Wilkins EG. A two-year prospective analysis of trunk function in TRAM breast reconstructions. *Plast Reconstr Surg*. 2006;117:2131-2138.
21. Wilkins EG, August DA, Kuzon WM Jr, et al. Immediate transverse rectus abdominis musculocutaneous flap reconstruction after mastectomy. *J Am Coll Surg*. 1995;180:177-183.
22. Hartrampf CR, Scheflan M, Black PW. Breast reconstruction with a transverse abdominal island flap. *Plast Reconstr Surg*. 1982;69:216-225.
    A classic article and one of the earlier descriptions of the the pedicled TRAM flap and its vascular anatomy for breast reconstruction.
23. Vyas RM, Dickinson BP, Fastekjian JH, et al. Risk factors for abdominal donor-site morbidity in free flap breast reconstruction. *Plast Reconstr Surg*. 2008;121:1519-1526.
24. Nahabedian MY, Dooley W, Singh N, Manson PN. Contour abnormalities of the abdomen after breast reconstruction with abdominal flaps: the role of muscle preservation. *Plast Reconstr Surg*. 2002;109:91-101.
25. Nahabedian MY, Manson PN. Contour abnormalities of the abdomen after transverse rectus abdominis muscle flap breast reconstruction: a multifactorial analysis. *Plast Reconstr Surg*. 2002;109:81-87.
26. Atisha D, Alderman AK, Janiga T, et al. The efficacy of the surgical delay procedure in pedicle TRAM breast reconstruction. *Ann Plast Surg*. 2009;63:383-388.
27. Sbitany H, Mirzabeigi MN, Kovach SJ, et al. Strategies for recognizing and managing intraoperative venous congestion in abdominally based autologous breast reconstruction. *Plast Reconstr Surg*. 2012;129:809-815.
28. Reardon CM, O'Ceallaigh S, O'Sullivan ST. An anatomical study of the superficial inferior epigastric vessels in humans. *Br J Plast Surg*. 2004;57:515-519.
29. Spiegel AJ, Khan FN. An Intraoperative algorithm for use of the SIEA flap for breast reconstruction. *Plast Reconstr Surg*. 2007;120:1450-1459.
30. Schaverien M, Saint-Cyr M, Arbique G, Brown SA. Arterial and venous anatomies of the deep inferior epigastric perforator and superficial inferior epigastric artery flaps. *Plast Reconstr Surg*. 2008;121:1909-1919.
    Contemporary cadaver studies of DIEP and SIEA flap zones of perfusion that demonstrate similar perfusion pattens for lateral row perforators and SIEA vascular pedicles, consistent with Holm's Zones of perfusion. Medial row perforators were found to perfuse in a pattern similar to Zones described by Hartrampf.
31. Holm C, Mayr M, Hofter E, Ninkovic M. Perfusion zones of the DIEP flap revisited: a clinical study. *Plast Reconstr Surg*. 2006;117:37-43.
    An evaluation of DIEP flap zones of perfusion using laser-induced fluorescence that redefined the zones of perfusion as described earlier by Hartrampf.
32. Park JE, Alkureishi LW, Song DH. TUGs into VUGs and friendly BUGs: transforming the gracilis territory into the best secondary breast reconstructive option. *Plast Reconstr Surg*. 2015;136:447-454.
33. Arnez ZM, Pogorelec D, Planinsek F, Ahcan U. Breast reconstruction by the free transverse gracilis (TUG) flap. *Br J Plast Surg*. 2004;57:20-26.
34. Allen RJ, Haddock NT, Ahn CY, Sadeghi A. Breast reconstruction with the profunda artery perforator flap. *Plast Reconstr Surg*. 2012;129:16e-23e.
35. Saad A, Sadeghi A, Allen RJ. The anatomic basis of the profunda femoris artery perforator flap: a new option for autologous breast reconstruction—a cadaveric and computer tomography angiogram study. *J Reconstr Microsurg*. 2012;28:381-386.
36. DeLong MR, Hughes DB, Bond JE, et al. A detailed evaluation of the anatomical variations of the profunda artery perforator flap using computed tomographic angiograms. *Plast Reconstr Surg*. 2014;134:186e-192e.
37. Haddock NT, Greaney P, Otterburn D, et al. Predicting perforator location on preoperative imaging for the profunda artery perforator flap. *Microsurgery*. 2012;32:507-511.
38. Hunsinger V, Lhuaire M, Haddad K, et al. Medium- and large-sized autologous breast reconstruction using a fleur-de-lys profunda femoris artery perforator flap design: a report comparing results with the horizontal profunda femoris artery perforator flap. *J Reconstr Microsurg*. 2019;35(1):8-14.
39. LoTempio MM, Allen RJ. Breast reconstruction with SGAP and IGAP flaps. *Plast Reconstr Surg*. 2010;126:393-401.
40. Rad AN, Flores JI, Prucz RB, et al. Clinical experience with the lateral septocutaneous superior gluteal artery perforator flap for autologous breast reconstruction. *Microsurgery*. 2010;30:339-347.

QUESTIONS

1. **You plan to perform a pedicled TRAM flap for breast reconstruction and would like to physiologically augment blood flow to the flap through the intended pedicle. What can you do to achieve this?**

   a. Ligate the superior epigastric artery 3 weeks before the TRAM procedure
   b. Ligate the deep inferior epigastric artery 3 weeks before the TRAM procedure
   c. Ligate the intercostal arteries 3 weeks before the TRAM procedure
   d. Elevate the entire TRAM flap and then replace it on the abdomen
   e. Perform an additional microvascular anastomosis

2. **A 45-year-old patient with a history of right-sided breast cancer treated with BCT 5 years ago comes to your clinic to discuss reconstructive options to restore size and symmetry. She has a history of abdominoplasty at the age of 35 years. On examination, her left breast is approximately a B-cup bra-size. Her BMI is 30 kg/m^2. Which of the following reconstructive options would be most appropriate for her?**

   a. Ipsilateral breast reconstruction with DIEP flap
   b. Ipsilateral breast reconstruction with latissimus dorsi musculocutaneous flap
   c. Contralateral breast reduction
   d. Ipsilateral breast reconstruction with PAP flap
   e. Silicone implant placement

3. **In preparation for microvascular reconstruction of the left breast with a DIEP flap (pedicle: 2.5 mm artery/3.0 mm vein), exposure of the IMA/IMV is planned with a rib cartilage resection. Which rib is the most appropriate to resect?**

   a. Rib 1
   b. Rib 2
   c. Rib 3
   d. Rib 4
   e. Rib 5

4. **A 37-year-old woman with a genetic predisposition for breast cancer undergoes bilateral nipple-sparing prophylactic mastectomies with immediate microvascular breast reconstructions. The flaps are buried and without skin paddles. Which of the following offers you the ability for postoperative monitoring of the flap?**

   a. Transcutaneous tissue oximetry
   b. Pencil Doppler
   c. Exam (warmth, color)
   d. Venous coupler
   e. Arterial Doppler probe

5. **You are in the operating room and performing autologous breast reconstruction with a DIEP flap. Immediately on completion of the arterial and venous anastomoses, you note that both anastomoses are patent, but you also see dark red blood from the edges of the flap. What is the next appropriate action to take?**

   a. Begin intraoperative leeches
   b. Perform additional venous anastomosis with SIEV from the flap to the retrograde IMV
   c. Give the flap 5 to 10 minutes to allow for old venous blood to clear
   d. Take down and redo the venous anastomosis with the IMV
   e. Initiate an intravenous heparin drip

1. **Answer: b.** Ligating the deep inferior epigastric artery several weeks before the TRAM flap is performed is known as a TRAM delay procedure. Studies have shown that this improves flap survival and augments blood flow through the superior epigastric artery. The pedicled TRAM flap is based on the superior epigastric artery. Ligating this artery would render the flap unuseable. Ligating the intercostal arteries would risk causing abdominal necrosis superior and lateral to the TRAM donor site. It would not be reasonable to elevate the entire TRAM flap and then replace it on the abdomen. In addition, this would not augment flow through the superior epigastric artery. Additional microvascular anastomosis can be performed if the superior epigastric artery is injured during flap elevation. In that setting, the DIEA, if left long enough can be used to augment flow. However, this would not augment flow through the pedicle (superior epigastric artery).

2. **Answer: d.** The PAP flap provides a reasonable alternative to abdominal-based free flaps in patients with a prior history of abdominal surgery, which would place abdominal-based flaps at risk. In this patient with a history of abdominoplasty, an abdominal-based free flap would not be a viable reconstructive strategy. The PAP flap can provide sufficient tissue in patients with B or C-cup breasts. The DIEP flap is no longer an option in patients who have had an abdominoplasty. The latissimus dorsi musculocutaneous flap is not likely to provide sufficient tissue to reconstruct B-cup breasts in this patient. A contralateral breast reduction is unlikely to restore size, one of the concerns for this patient. In many patients, breast reduction is also unlikely to yield symmetry unless additional operations are performed on the ipsilateral side. A silicone implant would be inadvisable in a patient with a history of radiation on the ipsilateral side, which is a part of the BCT protocol.

3. **Answer: c.** The IMA and particularly the IMV have sufficient size on the left side to match the flap pedicle diameters at rib 3. In addition, if the vessel is injured during exposure, there is an opportunity to obtain sufficient exposure to anastomose proximal on the vessels. On the right side, the veins are slightly larger than they are at the same rib level on the left and as such should be of reasonable size for the described flap at either rib 3 or 4. Rib 1 sits just below the clavicle and resection of this rib would not be appropriate for anastomosis. Rib 2 is still located too far superior for anastomosis between the IMA/IMV and DIEA/DIEV. In addition, if any difficulty is encountered during exposure of the IMA/IMV, use of the second rib does not allow sufficient operative exposure superiorly to perform anastomosis. IMV on the left side can be substantially smaller at ribs 4 and 5.

4. **Answer: e.** The arterial Doppler probe, or Cook arterial Doppler, is a probe that wraps around the artery distal to the anastomosis and provides audible feedback. If the Doppler no longer provides a signal, the reasons can include thrombosis of the artery or in some circumstances, dislodgement of the probe. Transcutaneous tissue oximetry, pencil Doppler, and physical examination all require exposed skin paddle on the flap to be useful. The venous coupler facilitates the anastomosis and has been shown to reduce operative time. However, it alone does not provide monitoring. However, modifications of the venous coupler include the implantable venous flow coupler with Doppler, which allows for venous monitoring.

5. **Answer: c.** Giving the flap 5 to 10 minutes to allow for blood inflow through the DIEA-IMA anastomosis will help determine whether the observed dark blood is a symptom of true venous congestion or of stagnant blood in the flap that remained from the flap harvest. If venous congestion persists despite an intact DIEV-IMV anastomosis, additional anastomosis with the SIEV

to the retrograde IMV can be performed. Leeches would be typically used postoperatively. However, in the setting of free-flap breast reconstruction, postoperative venous congestion should be treated with operative exploration. Additional SIEV anastomosis to the retrograde IMV would be appropriate if the flap exhibits congestion for a prolonged period of time in the operating room despite a patent DIEV-IMV anastomosis. This would not be the next action to take, however. The DIEV-IMV anastomosis is patent based on the question stem. Therefore, it would not be appropriate to redo the anastomosis at this time. There is no evidence of thrombosis and as such anticoagulation in response to the clinical finding would not be indicated.

CHAPTER 61 Reconstruction of the Nipple-Areolar Complex

Anne C. O'Neill and Toni Zhong

KEY POINTS

- Reconstruction of the nipple-areolar complex (NAC) is the final step in the breast restoration process and should only be performed when optimal breast symmetry has been achieved.
- The nipple and areola are reconstructed separately.
- A number of local flaps have been described for reconstruction of the nipple. Maintaining nipple projection is one of the greatest challenges in NAC reconstruction.
- Areolar reconstruction can be achieved with pigmented skin grafts or tattooing.
- Nonsurgical options are also available and can achieve satisfactory reconstitution of the NAC.

Reconstruction of the nipple-areolar complex (NAC) is most commonly performed as a component of breast reconstruction following mastectomy for the treatment of cancer. Other indications for NAC reconstruction may include trauma, burns, nipple loss following reduction mammoplasty, or congenital absence of the NAC (athelia) or breast (amastia). Reconstruction of the NAC was first described by Adams in 1944 and was followed by a steady evolution of techniques up to the early 2000s.[1,2] In recent years, however, there has been increasing acceptance of nipple sparing mastectomies, and the demand for NAC reconstruction has consequently declined.[3] Reconstruction of the NAC is usually the final stage in breast reconstruction and so for many women marks the completion of their breast cancer treatment. Although reconstruction of the NAC is a relatively simple procedure, it can make a significant contribution to patient satisfaction and psychosexual well-being.[4,5]

PREOPERATIVE PLANNING

The nipple is an elevated structure that projects approximately 5 to 10 mm and arises in pigmented skin known as the areola, which is on average 4.2 to 4.5 cm in diameter. The NAC is a critical landmark of the breast. Other aesthetic components of the breast such as the inframammary fold (IMF), breast meridian, and parenchymal position are frequently assessed in terms of their relationship to the NAC. The NAC is generally situated at the prominence of the breast mound, but there is considerable variation in position, size, color, and texture in individual patients. The ideal NAC position is variably described as 22 to 24 cm from the sternal notch or the level of the midhumerus. In unilateral cases, the size and position of the reconstructed NAC is designed to match the contralateral side. In bilateral cases, the optimal position must be carefully selected, and the breast prominence, the breast meridian, the IMF, and the midline of the chest must be considered. Although some surgeons advocate simultaneous reconstruction of the breast and NAC, most would agree that NAC reconstruction should be performed 3 to 6 months later.[6-8] This enables the reconstructed breast to settle into its final position and allows the surgeon to consider any contralateral balancing procedures that may be required.

For the purposes of reconstruction, the nipple and the surrounding areola are generally considered separately.

NIPPLE RECONSTRUCTION

Grafts

The nipple share technique was introduced by Millard in 1972 and remains a popular technique in selected patients.[9] A segment of the contralateral natural nipple is harvested and transferred to the reconstructed breast as a composite graft. This technique is most effective in patients with a large contralateral nipple where projection exceeds 5 to 6 mm. It has been reported that composite nipple grafting can provide sensation and erectile function in the reconstructed nipple in some cases.[10] However, many patients are reluctant to have surgery on the normal nipple. The risk of reduced sensation and impaired erectile function at the donor site has limited the popularity of this technique. In an effort to avoid contralateral surgery, banking of the affected nipple at the time of mastectomy has been proposed. However, cryopreservation of the nipple results in tissue damage and loss of pigmentation that adversely affects aesthetic outcomes.[11]

The desire to avoid surgery on the contralateral nipple has resulted in a number of alternative donor sites for nipple grafts including labia, earlobe, toe pulp, and skin from the postauricular area, medial thigh, and axilla.[12,13] Although most of these areas provide hyperpigmented skin, they usually fade over time and are a poor match for the contralateral nipple. The popularity of grafting has waned with the advent of a multitude of local flap techniques that eliminate the need for a secondary donor site and the risk of associated morbidity. Grafting remains a favorable option in patients who have thin skin and subcutaneous tissues following alloplastic breast reconstruction.

Local Flaps

The first description of nipple reconstruction using local skin flaps was by Berson in 1946.[14] A recent review by Sisti et al identified 30 subsequently described flap designs that have contributed to the evolution of nipple reconstruction in the intervening 70 years.[15] Nimboriboonporn and Chuthapisith proposed a simple classification system for these techniques that divided them into (1) centrally based flaps, (2) subdermal pedicle local flaps with single pedicle, and (3) subdermal pedicle local flaps with double pedicle.[16]

Description of all the described local flap options for nipple reconstruction is beyond the scope of this chapter. The commonest techniques currently in use (skate flap, star flap, and C-V flap) consist of two larger lateral flaps that are approximated to create the circumference of the nipple and a smaller central flap that forms the tip of the nipple (Figure 61.1). Although several more complicated techniques have been described, most surgeons favor modifications of these classic flap designs because of their relative simplicity and the fact that complex designs with multiple incisions may be more prone to complications including contracture and loss of projection.

The skate flap was among the first simple and effective techniques described and is named for its similarity to a skate fish.[17] It consists of two lateral *wing* flaps and a central *head* flap. It incorporates a superior deepithelialized area, which, together with the flap donor areas, accommodates application of a skin graft for reconstruction of the areola. The star flap described by Anton in 1991 is simpler in design than the skate flap and allows primary closure of the donor site.[18]

The C-V flap represents a further simplification and has become a popular choice among surgeons with many minor modifications of the design described in the literature.[19-21]

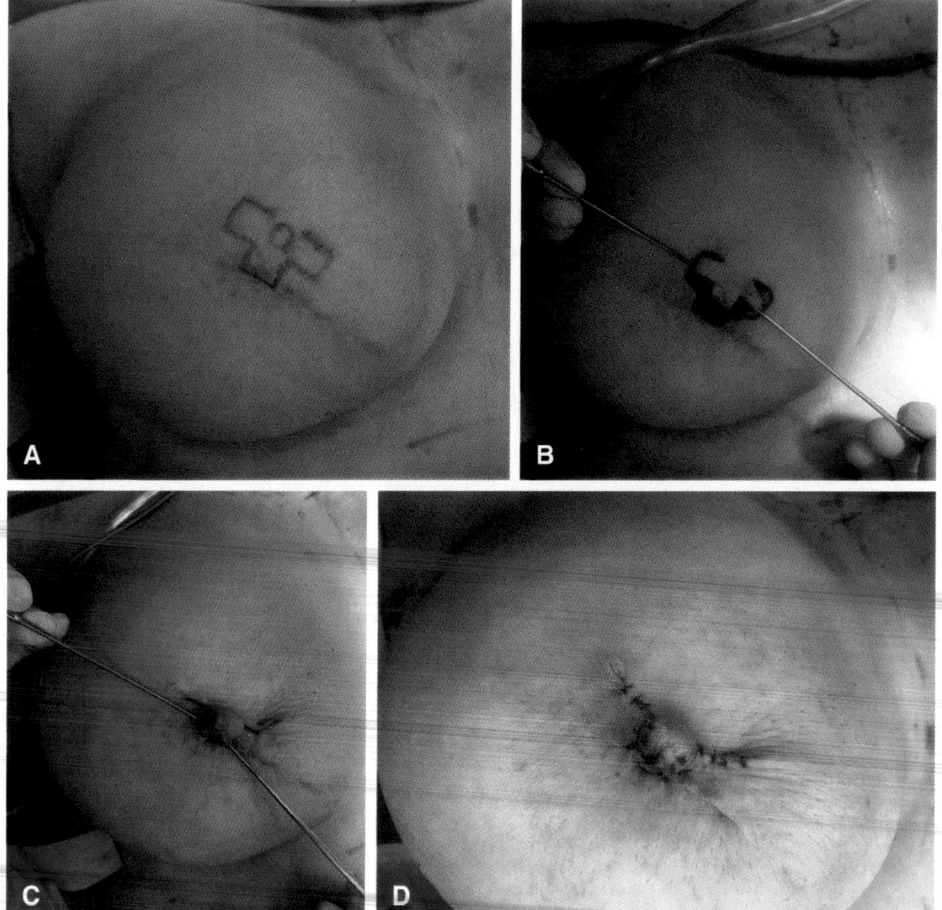

FIGURE 61.1. **A.** Preoperative marking of a C-V flap for nipple reconstruction on a breast mound. Note that the base of the C-V flap does not cross the mastectomy incision. **B.** C-V flaps incised and raised. **C.** The wings of the C-V flap and the cap of the C-V flap are closed. **D.** Final C-V flap closure.

Nipple Projection

One of the greatest challenges in nipple reconstruction is achieving sustained projection.[22] Both graft and flap techniques retract over time, with long-term loss of nipple projection reported to be between 40% and 70%.[15] Studies suggest that the reconstructed nipple loses projection in the first 2 years postoperatively, after which time the height remains relatively stable. A good flap design can help minimize contracture of the nipple by providing well-vascularized tissue and reducing the number of incisions and subsequent scars that are subject to contractile forces. Although there have been few studies that directly compare flap techniques, it is though designs that include double wide-based flaps that preserve rich subdermal vascularity may limit postoperative contracture.[16] Incorporation of subcutaneous fat or de-epithelialized dermis into the lateral flaps may increase the bulk of the reconstructed nipple.[20,23] Centrally based flaps such as the quadrapod flap are subject to the highest degree of postoperative retraction.[24] Flap design must anticipate long-term loss of projection, and surgeons should aim to create a nipple that is at least 50% larger than required. Protective dressings or padding is frequently used to prevent local trauma and compression of the nipple in the early postoperative period.

Augmentation techniques have been described in an effort to improve nipple projection. The addition of autologous auricular cartilage was advocated in the 1970s.[25] With the advent of microvascular breast reconstruction, costal cartilage was identified as a more accessible autologous material because it could be harvested and banked at the time of the initial breast reconstruction and eliminated the need for additional donor sites.[26] Although cartilage can help maintain projection, its use is associated with relatively high complication rates. Pressure necrosis can lead to ischemia of the flaps with exposure and loss of the cartilage graft. In more recent years, there has been increasing interest in the use of fat as an alternative autologous material. The soft consistency of fat grafts may reduce the risk of flap necrosis, but the impact on long-term nipple projection has yet to be established.[27] Acellular dermal matrix and prefabricated collagen tubes can also be used to support local flap reconstruction, but studies still report significant loss of projection over time.[28,29] Several alloplastic augmentation techniques have also been described including calcium hydroxylapatite, silicone, hyaluronic acid, and polytetrafluoroethylene.[30-32] Alloplastic materials carry the risk of infection and extrusion, making them less attractive than autologous options.

AREOLA RECONSTRUCTION

Skin-Grafting Techniques

Skin grafts are commonly used for reconstruction of the areola, as they recreate natural variation in pigmentation and texture that can mimic Montgomery tubercles. The contralateral areola is the ideal source of donor skin but is rarely used unless the patient is undergoing a concomitant balancing breast reduction. Skin is more commonly harvested from areas of increased pigmentation such as the inner thigh, groin, or axilla. Grafting of the areola usually occurs at the same time as nipple reconstruction. An area of deepithelialization can be incorporated into the nipple flap design to accommodate the skin graft. Fading of pigmented skin grafts commonly occurs over time.

Tattooing

Intradermal tattooing has become a popular method of areola reconstruction.[33] It eliminates the need for additional donor sites and allows customization of areolar pigmentation, which optimizes aesthetic outcomes. Tattoo pigments, consisting of iron and titanium oxides, are deposited into the dermis using a dermabrasion technique. One of the commonest problems is fading of the pigment over time and the need for touch-up procedures.[34] The initial tattoo should be darker than required in anticipation of this. Deposition of pigment at the correct dermal level is also important because if it is too superficial, it will slough off in the early postoperative period, but if it is too deep, it will be degraded by macrophage activity. Tattooing is generally performed 6 to 8 weeks after reconstruction of the nipple. It can be challenging to achieve homogenous deposition of pigment in scarred tissues. In an effort to avoid this, some surgeons advocate tattooing of the areola prior to nipple reconstruction.[35]

Recent years have seen significant advances in tattoo techniques. Using color shading, a very convincing NAC can be recreated without the need for flaps or grafts. The tattoo simulates the nipple projection through color contrasts and also mimics the texture of a natural areola.[36] Three-dimensional tattooing is generally performed by specialized medical tattoo artists and requires several sessions to achieve the end result.

Prosthetics

Nipple prostheses are an attractive option for patients who wish to avoid further surgery on the reconstructed breast. They may also be recommended in cases where NAC reconstruction might be considered high risk. The prostheses are made of soft silicone and are attached to the breasts using adhesives. They can be customized for color, shape, and texture to provide an exact match to the contralateral NAC.

PITFALLS AND COMPLICATIONS

Although NAC reconstruction is relatively simple, it can be associated with significant complications including infection and flap or graft failure. Overall complication rates are lower with flap reconstruction of the nipple and tattooing of the areola, but selection of the optimal reconstruction technique in each individual patient is critical.[15] Particular caution is necessary in patients who have had alloplastic reconstruction with thin skin flaps and those who have had prior radiation. Local flap failure may be more common in these patients, resulting in dehiscence and, in severe cases, exposure of the underlying implant.

Malposition of the NAC can compromise the overall aesthetic outcome of breast reconstruction and can be very difficult to correct. Repositioning of the reconstructed NAC usually requires local transposition flaps, which result in additional unfavorable scarring on the breast. Careful initial planning of NAC position and appropriate timing of reconstruction is essential.

The commonest complications are loss of projection and fading of pigmentation over time. As these are almost inevitable with all current techniques, they must be anticipated and adjustments should be made to the reconstructive design to accommodate them.

REFERENCES

1. Adams W. Free transplantation of the nipples and areola. *Surgery*. 1944;15:186-189.
2. Farhadi J, Maksvytyte GK, Schaefer DJ, et al. Reconstruction of the nipple-areola complex: an update. *J Plast Reconstr Aesthet Surg*. 2006;59(1):40-53.
3. Peled AW, Wang F, Foster RD, et al. Expanding the indications for total skin-sparing mastectomy: is it safe for patients with locally advanced disease? *Ann Surg Oncol*. 2016;23(1):87-91.
4. Momoh AO, Colakoglu S, de Blacam C, et al. The impact of nipple reconstruction on patient satisfaction in breast reconstruction. *Ann Plast Surg*. 2012;69(4):389-393.
   This article demonstrates the effect of nipple-areolar complex reconstruction on overall satisfaction and aesthetic scores in a large series of breast reconstruction patients.
5. Wellisch DK, Schain WS, Noone RB, Little JW III. The psychological contribution of nipple addition in breast reconstruction. *Plast Reconstr Surg*. 1987;80(5):699-704.
6. Delay E, Mojallal A, Vasseur C, Delaporte T. Immediate nipple reconstruction during immediate autologous latissimus breast reconstruction. *Plast Reconstr Surg*. 2006;118(6):1303-1312.
7. Losken A, Duggal CS, Desai KA, et al. Time to completion of nipple reconstruction: what factors are involved? *Ann Plast Surg*. 2013;70(5):530-532.
8. El Amm CA, Sung JS, Sawan KT, et al. Immediate nipple reconstruction using the everted umbilicus. *Plast Reconstr Surg*. 2011;128(2):91e-92e.
9. Millard DR Jr. Nipple and areola reconstruction by split-skin graft from the normal side. *Plast Reconstr Surg*. 1972;50(4):350-353.
10. Zenn MR, Garofalo JA. Unilateral nipple reconstruction with nipple sharing: time for a second look. *Plast Reconstr Surg*. 2009;123(6):1648-1653.
    This article discusses the benefits of the nipple share technique in selected patients and demonstrates that this is an excellent option particularly following alloplastic reconstruction or post radiation where local flaps may have high complication rates.
11. Nakagawa T, Yano K, Hosokawa K. Cryopreserved autologous nipple-areola complex transfer to the reconstructed breast. *Plast Reconstr Surg*. 2003;111(1):141-147; discussion 8-9.
12. Adams WM. Labial transplant for correction of loss of the nipple. *Plast Reconstr Surg*. 1949;4(3):295-298.
13. Klatsky SA, Manson PN. Toe pulp free grafts in nipple reconstruction. *Plast Reconstr Surg*. 1981;68(2):245-248.
14. Berson MI. Construction of pseudoareola. *Surgery*. 1946;20(6):808.
15. Sisti A, Grimaldi L, Tassinari J, et al. Nipple-areola complex reconstruction techniques: a literature review. *Eur J Surg Oncol*. 2016;42(4):441-465.
    The authors provide a detailed review of the many nipple-areolar reconstruction techniques that have been described and the associated risks and benefits. This is the most comprehensive review in the current literature.
16. Nimboriboonporn A, Chuthapisith S. Nipple-areola complex reconstruction. *Gland Surg*. 2014;3(1):35-42.
    This article provides an excellent review of nipple-areolar reconstruction and presents a useful classification system for flap techniques. It also provides important insights into the mechanism of retraction in the reconstructed nipple.
17. Little JW, Spear SL. The finishing touches in nipple-areolar reconstruction. *Perspect Plast Surg*. 1988;2:1-22.
18. Anton LE, Hartrampf CR. Nipple reconstruction with local flaps: star and wrap flaps. *Perspect Plast Surg*. 1991;5(1):67-78.
19. Losken A, Mackay GJ, Bostwick J III. Nipple reconstruction using the C-V flap technique: a long-term evaluation. *Plast Reconstr Surg*. 2001;108(2):361-369.
20. [illegible], Yesiloglu N, Sirinoglu H, Sarici M. A new modification of C-V flap technique in nipple reconstruction: rolled triangular dermal-fat flaps. *Aesthet Plast Surg*. 2015;39(1):172-175.
21. Witt P, Dujon DG. The V-V flap—a simple modification of the C-V flap for nipple reconstruction. *J Plast Reconstr Aesthet Surg*. 2013;66(7):1009-1010.
22. Zhong T, Antony A, Cordeiro P. Surgical outcomes and nipple projection using the modified skate flap for nipple-areolar reconstruction in a series of 422 implant reconstructions. *Ann Plast Surg*. 2009;62(5):591-595.
    This article provides a detailed long-term evaluation of outcomes following nipple-areolar reconstruction using a single technique in a large series of patients.
23. Jamnadas-Khoda B, Thomas R, Heppell S. The 'cigar roll' flap for nipple areola complex reconstruction: a novel technique. *J Plast Reconstr Aesthet Surg*. 2011;64(8):e218-e220.
24. Little JW 3rd, Munasifi T, McCulloch DT. One-stage reconstruction of a projecting nipple: the quadrapod flap. *Plast Reconstr Surg*. 1983;71(1):126-133.
25. Brent B, Bostwick J. Nipple-areola reconstruction with auricular tissues. *Plast Reconstr Surg*. 1977;60(3):353-361.
26. Mori H, Uemura N, Okazaki M. Nipple reconstruction with banked costal cartilage after vertical-type skin-sparing mastectomy and deep inferior epigastric artery perforator flap. *Breast Cancer*. 2015;22(1):95-97.
27. Bernard RW, Beran SJ. Autologous fat graft in nipple reconstruction. *Plast Reconstr Surg*. 2003;112(4):964-968.
28. Garramone CE, Lam B. Use of AlloDerm in primary nipple reconstruction to improve long-term nipple projection. *Plast Reconstr Surg*. 2007;119(6):1663-1668.
29. Tierney BP, Hodde JP, Changkuon DI. Biologic collagen cylinder with skate flap technique for nipple reconstruction. *Plast Surg Int*. 2014;2014:194087.
30. Evans KK, Rasko Y, Lenert J, Olding M. The use of calcium hydroxylapatite for nipple projection after failed nipple-areolar reconstruction: early results. *Ann Plast Surg*. 2005;55(1):25-29.
31. Lennox K, Beer KR. Nipple contouring with hyaluronics postmastectomy. *J Drugs Dermatol*. 2007;6(10):1030-1033.
32. Wong RK, Wichterman L, Parson SD. Skin sparing nipple reconstruction with polytetrafluoroethylene implant. *Ann Plast Surg*. 2008;61(3):256-258.
33. Spear SL, Convit R, Little JW III. Intradermal tattoo as an adjunct to nipple-areola reconstruction. *Plast Reconstr Surg*. 1989;83(5):907-911.
34. Spear SL, Arias J. Long-term experience with nipple-areola tattooing. *Ann Plast Surg*. 1995;35(3):232-236.
35. White CP, Gdalevitch P, Strazar R, et al. Surgical tips: areolar tattoo prior to nipple reconstruction. *J Plast Reconstr Aesthet Surg*. 2011;64(12):1724-1726.
36. Halvorson EG, Cormican M, West ME, Myers V. Three-dimensional nipple-areola tattooing: a new technique with superior results. *Plast Reconstr Surg*. 2014;133(5):1073-1075.

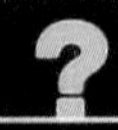

QUESTIONS

1. **A 59-year-old woman is planning to undergo a delayed right breast reconstruction with a free deep inferior epigastric perforator (DIEP) flap. She will require a left-sided balancing mastopexy for symmetry. When is the optimal time to perform NAC reconstruction?**
   - a. At the time of DIEP breast reconstruction
   - b. 3 months after DIEP breast reconstruction
   - c. At the time of balancing mastopexy
   - d. 3 months after balancing mastopexy

2. **All the following materials have been used to augment nipple projection in a reconstructed NAC *except*:**
   - a. Silicone
   - b. Calcium hydroxylapatite
   - c. Hyaluronic acid
   - d. Polyurethane
   - e. Acellular dermal matrix

3. **Possible complications following nipple-areolar reconstruction include the following *except*:**
   - a. Nipple malposition
   - b. Loss of projection
   - c. Increase in pigmentation
   - d. Decrease in pigmentation
   - e. Partial or complete nipple necrosis

4. **What is the safest method of NAC reconstruction in a patient with a radiated implant-reconstructed breast?**
   - a. 3D NAC tattooing
   - b. Labial graft
   - c. Nipple share
   - d. C-V flap
   - e. Skate flap with skin graft

5. **The following landmarks should be taken into consideration for placement of the NAC reconstruction on the reconstructed breast mound *except*:**
   - a. Position of the opposite native NAC
   - b. IMF
   - c. Midhumeral point
   - d. Breast meridian
   - e. Midclavicular point

1. **Answer: d.** NAC reconstruction should be the final step in the reconstructive process. Although it is possible to reconstruct the nipple at the time of DIEP, it is difficult to predict the final position especially in delayed breast reconstruction when the flap would be expected to develop increased ptosis over time. Correct positioning of the reconstructed NAC is essential, and both the position of the NAC on the reconstructed breast and its relationship to the contralateral natural NAC must be considered. It is therefore important to perform the mastopexy prior to NAC reconstruction and to allow some time to determine the final position of the natural NAC following the balancing procedure. Nipple malposition can have a significant adverse effect on the final outcome of breast reconstruction. Correction of nipple malposition is difficult and results in additional scarring on the reconstructed breast.

2. **Answer: d.** Several alloplastic augmentation techniques have also been described including calcium hydroxylapatite, silicone, hyaluronic acid, and polytetrafluoroethylene. Acellular dermal matrix has been inserted as well to increase nipple projection. Polyurethanes are in the class of compounds called reaction polymers, which include epoxies, unsaturated polyesters, and phenolics. They are not safe for placing into human tissues.

3. **Answer: c.** A common complication after nipple reconstruction is fading of nipple-areolar pigmentation over time, rather than increase in pigmentation. The decrease in NAC tattoo pigment can occur months to years after the procedure, and this is more commonly observed in patients with fair skin.

4. **Answer: a.** The safest method of NAC reconstruction in a patient with radiated breast implant reconstruction is 3D tattooing. In all the other methods of NAC reconstruction, incisions have to be placed, a flap has to be recreated, or a recipient bed has to be made to accept the flap or skin graft. In radiated breast tissue, vascularity is compromised, and all the techniques of grafts or flaps that rely on blood supply may be complicated by wound healing problems. Therefore, noninvasive procedures such as 3D tattooing may be the safest choice.

5. **Answer: e.** In a patient undergoing unilateral NAC reconstruction, the opposite or native position of the NAC must be taken into consideration when designing the placement of the NAC. In a patient undergoing bilateral NAC reconstruction, the caudal-cephalic position of the NAC needs to take into account the mid-humeral point, the IMF, and the sternal notch to reconstructed NAC distance. The medial to lateral position of the NAC needs to be placed along the meridian of the breast mound.

CHAPTER 62 Congenital Anomalies of the Breast: Tuberous Breasts, Poland Syndrome, and Asymmetry

Kenneth L. Fan and Maurice Y. Nahabedian

KEY POINTS

- Broadly speaking, pediatric breast disorders may be categorized into hypoplastic, hyperplastic, and deformational.
- Key moves in correction of tuberous breast deformity are periareolar approach to the breast, with radial scoring of constriction bands to the deep dermal plane as necessary, as well as partial subpectoral implant placement and circumareolar reduction of areola and herniated breast tissue.
- Classically, Poland syndrome has been treated with a pedicled latissimus flap and implants. In such a scenario, tissue expansion has been undertaken in the first stage to expand deficient breast tissue. A pedicled latissimus flap with implant placement is performed in a second stage. Increasing implant volume can provide an adjunct to camouflage chest wall deformities. Some authors have had success with multiple stages of lipofilling and free flap reconstruction.
- Gynecomastia requires complete medical workup for concomitant abnormalities in conjunction with medical physicians. At onset during adolescence, 1 year of observation is required as spontaneous regression may occur. Treatment involves liposuction with or without subglandular resection.

Congenital breast deformities represent a source of significant anxiety and distress to the pediatric patient and their families. Broadly categorized, pediatric breast disorders can be thought of as hypoplastic, hyperplastic, or deformational as a framework for discussion among plastic surgeons. The first two are discussed in this chapter. The timing of surgical correction is critical as the operative plans must balance growth-related factors in light of the psychological trauma that may result from a persistent deformity. As a result, treatment goals rely on accurate diagnosis, timing, and technique selection in order to provide the best aesthetic result while addressing psychosocial needs.

EMBRYOLOGY

The breast is a modified apocrine sweat gland that commences development at around 6 weeks of life. Paired, proliferating epidermal cells migrate into mesenchymal tissue and form primitive mammary ridges, or milk line that extends ventrally along the embryo, from the axilla to the groin roughly lateral to the midclavicular line (Figure 62.1). Failure of development within this time results in complete absence of the breast.[1] Portions atrophy, except at the fourth intercostal space, which set the foundation for the primary mammary bud. Incomplete regression gives rise to ectopic breast tissue (polymastia) or supernumerary nipples (polythelia). Breast growth consists of ectodermal plaques branching into underlying mesenchyme, which proliferate and canalize to form lactiferous tissue by 8 weeks.[1] The lactiferous ducts open into the surrounding ectoderm, which develops into the areola at 5 months. By 6 months of gestational age, the basic framework and tubular architecture of the breast can be seen. With circulating estrogen and progesterone from the placenta, the lactiferous tissue continues branching into 2 years of life. The normal gland remains quiescent from 2 years until puberty.

At birth, the neonatal mammary tissue is functional. Seventy percent may secrete colostrum because of rise in prolactin. The nipples evert soon after birth because of proliferation of the underlying mesoderm. However, inverted nipples that remain until puberty is not uncommon. By 2 years of age, breast tissue grows at the same rate in the body, so long as estrogen levels are low. Sex hormones heavily influence the development of the breast in morphological stages as described by Tanner.[2] During Tanner stage 1, the breast is prepubertal, without appreciable breast parenchyma and slight nipple elevation. Tanner stage 2 begins with thelarche, around 9.7 years, as the nipple-areolar complex (NAC) widens and the breast and nipple become a small mound. Stage 3 is heralded with a further enlargement, as the breast extends beyond the borders of the areola. The NAC elevates above the breast contour as a secondary mound in stage 4. In stage 5, the breast achieves the final mature size and form.

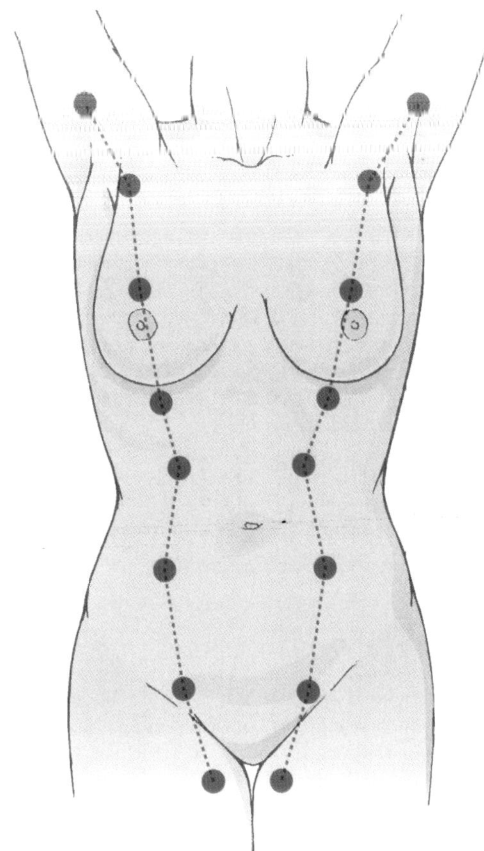

FIGURE 62.1. Embryonic mammary ridges. (Reproduced with permission from Weber JR, Kelley JH. Assessing breasts and lymphatic system. In: Weber JR, Kelley JH, eds. *Health Assessment in Nursing*. 5th ed. Philadelphia, PA: Wolters Kluwer Health/Lippincott Williams & Wilkins; 2014:396-415. Figure 19-3.)

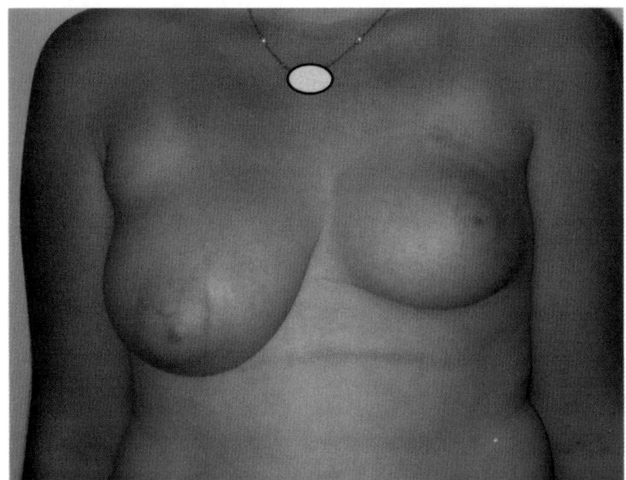

FIGURE 62.2. Typical appearance of breast hypoplasia.

HYPOPLASTIC DISORDERS

Breast hypoplasia presents in a wide spectrum of phenotypes reflecting their underlying disease (Figure 62.2). Amazia, the absence of the breast without nipple absence, may occur unilaterally or bilaterally, in isolation or in conjunction with pectoralis hypoplasia. Athelia describes the absence of the NAC. Amastia is the complete absence of the breast unit, including the gland and nipple. Although these terminologies suggest otherwise, these abnormalities often occur together: athelia often occurs in conjunction with amazia.

Accordingly, Trier et al. broadly categorized observed patterns of amastia and its suspected mode of inheritance into three groups: bilateral absence of the breast associated with congenital ectodermal defects, unilateral absence of the breast, and bilateral absence of the breast.[3] In congenital ectodermal defect, a sex-linked recessive disorder, additional abnormalities with the skin and its appendages, the teeth, and nails are present. Unilateral absence of the breast, when combined with pectoralis aplasia or hypoplasia, is considered a variant of Poland syndrome. Genetically inherited bilateral absence of the breast has been described.[1]

Management of the hypoplastic/aplastic breasts requires consideration of the patient's growth and contralateral breast size. Optimal timing is contingent on the deformity and the psychological and physical manifestations. Tissue expanders may be placed in the breast should the deformity cause profound psychosocial effects while the child is growing or if the skin envelope requires expansion. Implants, myocutaneous flaps, and autologous fat transfer are viable methods of reconstruction. Careful consideration of familial breast cancer history is mandatory when employing fat transfer techniques. Usually, nipple-areolar reconstruction is undertaken after a breast mound is created. Techniques include local flaps, skin grafts, cartilage grafts, acellular dermal matrices (ADMs), and/or NAC tattooing.[4]

TUBEROUS BREAST

First described by Rees and Aston in 1976, the tuberous breast (e.g., tubular breast, herniated areola complex, snoopy breast, constricted breast, lower pole hypoplastic breast, narrow-based breast, domed nipple, and nipple breast) abnormality represents a spectrum of abnormal breast shape (Figure 62.3).[5-7] The term *tuberous* refers to the similarity in shape to root tubers.[6] Rearing its phenotype only during puberty, the tuberous breast is characterized by[6]:

- Constricted skin envelope in the vertical and horizontal dimensions
- Deficiency in the base diameter (breast footprint)
- Elevated inframammary fold (IMF)
- Short nipple-to-IMF distance (*high, tight fold*)
- Herniation of the breast parenchyma through the areola resulting in enlarged diameter of the NAC. NAC involvement is present in about 50% of cases[8]
- Parenchymal hypoplasia
- Asymmetry

Grolleau proposed the most widely used classification scheme based on the initial work by Von Heimburg[7] (Figure 62.4):

Type I Deformity: Only the medial quadrant is absent, the lower medial edge is shaped like an *italic S*, and the lateral breast is larger in comparison.
Type II Deformity: Both lower quadrants are deficient, the areola points down, and the lower pole is constricted.
Type III Deformity: All quadrants are deficient, the breast base is constricted both horizontally and vertically, and the breast is shaped like a tubercle.

Kolker and Collins further described the three tiers with additional pathologic findings (**Table 62.1**).[9]

Several etiologies have been proposed. Grolleau et al. postulated that anomalies in the superficial fascia in the lower pole of the breast lead to strong adherence between the dermis and the muscular plane.[7] During breast development, the growth of the breast cannot overcome this adherence. The peripheral expansion of the breast is restricted, resulting in preferential development forward. When the connective and muscular structure of the areola is weak, as seen in the severe variants, the gland herniates through the NAC.

Mandrekas expanded on this with a *ring theory* by histologically demonstrating a dense *constricting ring* spanning from the periphery of the NAC to the lower part of the breast representing a thickening of the superficial fascia.[10] He postulated that this condensation of fascia may be caused by the joining of the deep and outer layers of the superficial fascia, which collectively envelope the breast, at a higher level, or a thickening of penetrating suspensory ligaments in the area. The constricting ring prevents normal breast expansion and development, and the breast tissue is forced through the outer layer of the superficial fascia resulting in vertical breast development herniating through the areola.

The true incidence of tuberous breast deformity is variable and somewhat unknown. DeLuca-Pytell et al. reported 73% of females presenting for breast augmentation were found to have tuberous breast deformity, with the 60% of breasts having the most severe phenotype

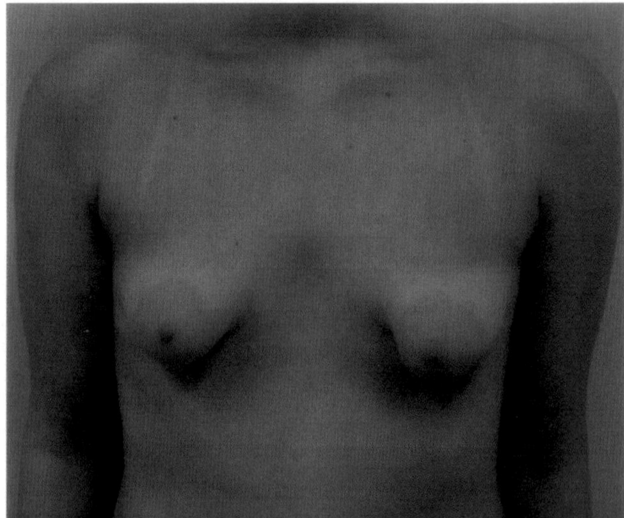

FIGURE 62.3. Bilateral type III tuberous breast. Both sides suffer from constricted envelope, deficiency of the base diameter, elevation of the inframammary fold with short nipple to inframammary fold distance, parenchymal hypoplasia, and asymmetry. The left side has more areolar herniation than the right.

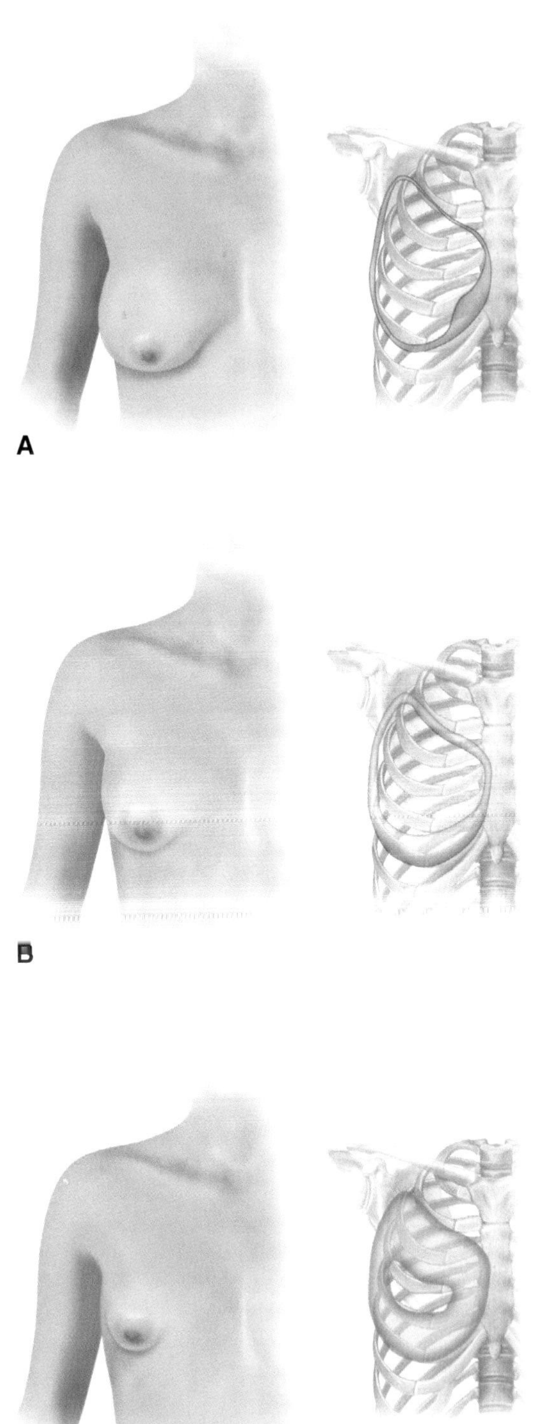

FIGURE 62.4. Grolleau classification of tuberous breast deformity. *Blue* on the right represents missing tissue. **A.** Type I: Medial quadrant absent. Lateral breast is large in comparison. **B.** Type II: Both lower quadrants are absent. The areola points down, and the lower pole is constricted. **C.** Type III: All quadrants are absent. The breast is constricted both in the horizontal and vertical dimension.

(Type III).[8] Ninety-eight percent of the patients with tuberous breasts were asymmetrical in size as well. However, such high incidence is debated, particularly by Zambacos and Mandrekas who report a 7% incidence among those who present for mammoplasty.[11] This discrepancy represents a diagnostic dilemma in tuberous deformity, as milder forms are commonly underappreciated and underdiagnosed.[9]

Surgical Correction of Tuberous Breast Deformity

- Surgical management of tuberous deformity requires close counseling and management of patient expectations. Although patients have semblance of breast deformity, few fully understand the anatomic deficits present and the challenge of restoration to a near normal appearance. Without proper education, many patients expect outcomes seen with primary breast augmentation. These principles of surgical treatment in tuberous breast deformity are adapted from Brown and Somogyi[12]:
  - Release of the constricted base in both the vertical and horizontal plane from the tethering fibrous attachments and/or bands between the breast parenchyma and deep fascia and pectoralis muscle[6]
  - Restoration of a normal nipple-to-IMF distance through expansion and/or mastopexy and lowering of the IMF
  - Obliteration of the old IMF to avoid a double-bubble deformity
  - Reduction of herniated tissue
  - Correction of areola hypertrophy
  - Restoration of breast volume
  - Correction of breast asymmetry

Critical analysis of deficiencies helps formulate a surgical plan. Simply placing an implant will fall short in correcting the tuberous breast (Figure 62.5). Kolker and Collins recently published an algorithm that should be helpful in approaching the tuberous breast deformity (Figure 62.6).[9] In most cases, when the soft tissues are distensible and the size goals are attainable, correction can be performed in a single stage. Two-stage procedures with expanders are reserved for the most severe cases when the lower pole skin is severely deficient, the base/IMF is severely constricted, and/or the patient desires a fuller size. In Kolker and Collins' series, 8% of total or 30% of Groleau type III tuberous breast required expansion.[9]

Approach

The periareolar incision has become the most widely used as it provides access for the reduction of the areola, to the lower pole subglandular plane, and for radial division of the constriction ring.[4,9,13] It is important to avoid reduction of the areola until the implant is placed or tissue rearrangement is performed because the skin envelope is deficient: what may seem to be excess initially may ultimately not be. The alternative approach to the breast tissue is through an inframammary incision.

Radial Scoring and Internal Tissue Rearrangement

Release of the glandular and breast base constriction with radial scoring is an essential component of surgical correction. Rees and Aston first described radial scoring on the undersurface of the breast for expansion.[5] However, their description did not call for scoring to the deep dermis. For adequate release, bands at the base of the breast parenchyma and along the IMF are radially dissected from deep to the superficial until the deep dermis to the point visual and palpable release of the lower pole (Figure 62.7).[9]

Several methods of internal tissue rearrangements have been described. Dinner and Dowden advocated full-thickness skin and glandular incisions with transposition flaps, as they considered the skin itself to be constricting.[14] The addition of internal gland reshaping allowed for release of the constricting base and redistribution of tissue without external scars or contour abnormalities.[12] Puckett and Concannon[15] as well as Riberio et al.[16] described horizontal transection of the gland with folded-down internal flaps based on the subareolar tissue or posterior chest wall, respectively, to reconstitute the lower pole. Mandrekas and Zambacos utilized a periareolar incision to exteriorize the lower half of the breast.[10] A radial six o'clock incision was made to release the constricting ring, creating pillars to redrape and reconstitute the lower pole.

Abbate, Fan, and Nahabedian described a new technique for correction of a tuberous breast with sufficient volume using a central mound mastopexy via an inverted-T incision.[17] The undersurface of

TABLE 62.1. KOLKER AND COLLINS' ADDITIONS TO THE MODIFIED GROLLEAU CLASSIFICATION

Type	Base	Inframammary Fold	Skin Envelope	Breast Volume	Ptosis	Areola
I	Minor constriction	Normal laterally, minor elevation medially	Sufficient	Minimal deficiency, no deficiency, or hypertrophy	Mild, moderate, or severe	Enlargement
II	Moderate constriction	Medial and lateral elevation	Inferior insufficiency	Moderate deficiency	None or mild	Normal, mild, or moderate herniation
III	Severe constriction	Elevation of the entire fold, or fold absence	Global insufficiency	Severe deficiency	Mild ormoderate	Severe herniation

(From Kolker AR, Collins MS. Tuberous breast deformity: classification and treatment strategy for improving consistency in aesthetic correction. *Plast Reconstr Surg*. 2015;135(1):73-86.)

the breast was scored to correct the base constriction without violating the central mound perfusion. The parenchymal herniation through the NAC was managed by de-epithelizing the central mound followed by imbrication sutures to create a tight dermal base and minimize the risk for future herniation. The success of these internal rearrangement techniques is contingent on the presence of enough tissue to augment the hypoplastic lower pole. In severe cases, these techniques may be less successful because of the paucity of breast tissue, thus necessitating the use of an implant.

Implants

Volume correction is often required because of the prevalence of asymmetries. Selection of the appropriate implant requires biodimensional planning that includes breast height, width, and tissue compliance.[12] Devices of various projections can be utilized to augment deficiency in the lower pole and maintain expansion of the released constricted base. The use of anatomical implants for tuberous breast can be considered to increase the volume in the lower pole and for tailoring of height, width, and projection.[12]

Careful attention needs to be given to the IMF. Extending beyond the intended footprint of the breast during dissection may be difficult to correct. Some surgeons avoid lowering the IMF whenever possible owing to the possibility of implant malposition.[12,18] In patients with less severe tuberous deformities, the IMF is well defined, and further lowering the IMF may be counterproductive. In patients with severe tuberous breasts, correction is mandated because of a short nipple-to-IMF distance. In such situations, effacement of the existing IMF is necessary to avoid the double-bubble deformity by lysing fascial connections between the dermis and superficial fascia.[19] Extending radial scoring to the deep dermis may assist in this endeavor. Algorithms, such as ones borrowed from the breast augmentation literature by Tebbett based on implant volume,[20] Mallucci and Brandford ICE principle,[21] and Per Heden's Akademikliniken method,[22] can assist in planning the final IMF location. The surgeon may also use cues from the contralateral IMF or the ridges made by the patient's ideal bra to roughly determine where the IMF will sit. Working backwards from the aforementioned IMF algorithms can help in selecting an implant preoperatively. Correction of asymmetry may be adjusted by varying implant sizes, although some authors remove excess gland from the deepest aspect of the subareolar gland to keep the implant size similar and prevent future herniation.[9]

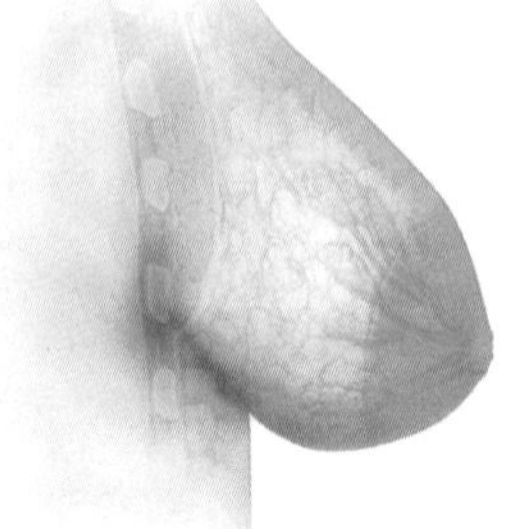
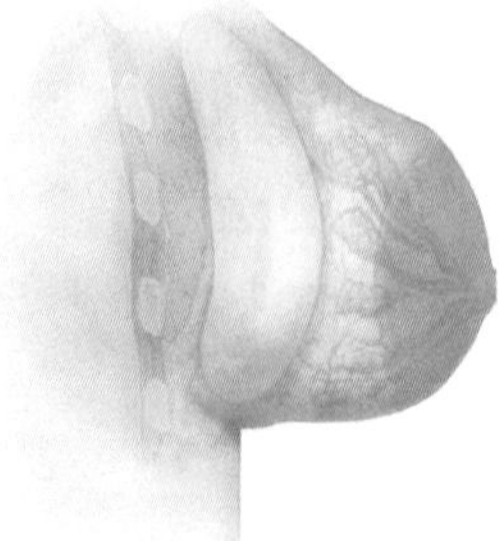

FIGURE 62.5. A standard augmentation mammoplasty will fall short in correcting the tuberous breast deformity.

The ideal plane for implant placement is somewhat controversial. The initial descriptions for correction of tuberous breast demonstrated that implant placement should be in the subglandular plane for the prosthesis to shape and expand the constricted breast without tethering of the pectoralis muscle.[9,12] However, subglandular implants have been associated with increased rates of capsular contracture with visible implant margins and rippling in patients because of a paucity of parenchyma. The use of anatomic implants can mitigate these effects, especially when placed in a dual-plane position. In patients with a tuberous breast deformity, a dual-plane III, which is defined as prepectoral undermining to the upper edge of the NAC, is usually performed to redrape the gland over the implant, and expand the parenchymal malposition and the short lower pole skin.

Mastopexy

Following placement of the permanent implant, final determination on the extent of areolar correction is judged. The periareolar incision may be converted to circumareolar mastopexy with an interlocking purse-string suture technique to reduce areolar dimensions.[9,23] When a patient presents with severe ptosis and a less severe tuberous deformity, a circumvertical mastopexy can be performed as needed using a tailor-tack approach. Complications seen in tuberous breast deformity are similar to that observed in mastopexy. Implant insertion with the additional complications from implant malposition and persistence of the fold produces a double-bubble contour. Management of these complications is further discussed in the cited articles.[12,19,24]

POLAND SYNDROME

Poland syndrome, described by Alfred Poland in 1851, is a rare congenital malformation with an incidence of 1 in 7000 to 100,000.[4] Generally cases are unilateral, but bilateral anomalies have been described. Sporadic cases are hallmarked by 2 to 3:1 higher incidence in males, with 60% to 75% affecting the right side (Figure 62.8).[25] Familial cases have equal incidence in sexes and laterality. Classically, Poland syndrome was defined as the absences of the pectoralis major and ipsilateral hand abnormality (Figure 62.9). Hypoplasia or absence of the sternocostal head of the pectoralis major results in the absence of the anterior axillary fold, subclavicular hollowing, and a pathognomonic groove at the junction of the superior anterior axillary line and chest wall.[13] However, current thought is that Poland syndrome comprises hypoplasia/absence of the pectoralis major with at least two of these minor criteria[4,25,26]:

- Hypoplasia or absence of the breast
- Absence of the nipple
- Absence of axillary hair
- Absence of adjacent muscles (e.g., latissimus dorsi, serratus anterior, external oblique, deltoid, infraspinatus, supraspinatus, and pectoralis minor)
- Absence of costal cartilage and anterior ribs
- Absent subcutaneous tissue
- Axillary webbing
- Ipsilateral brachydactyly, brachysyndactyly, or amelia

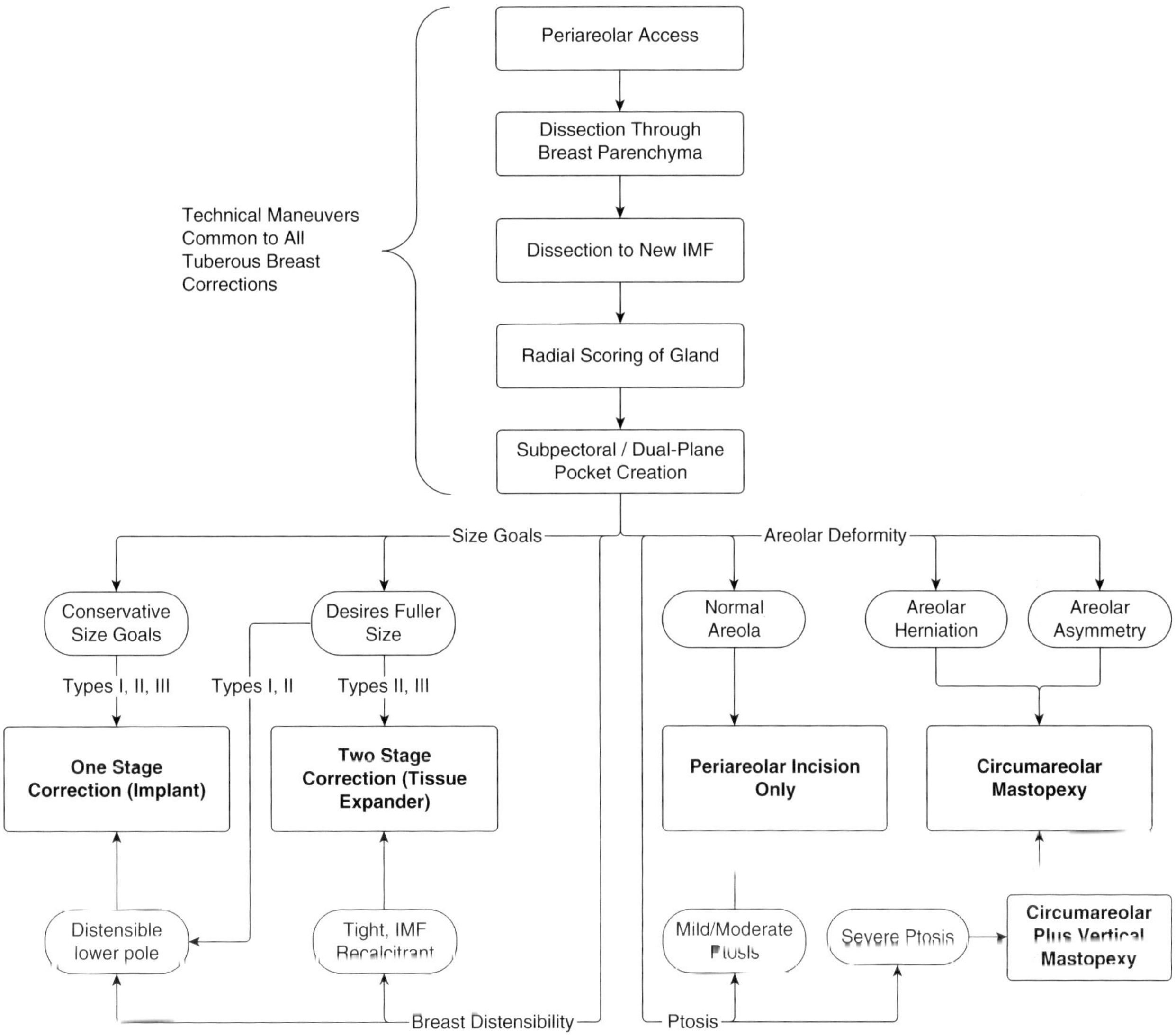

Technical Maneuvers Common to All Tuberous Breast Corrections
Periareolar Access
Dissection Through Breast Parenchyma
Dissection to New IMF
Radial Scoring of Gland
Subpectoral / Dual-Plane Pocket Creation
Size Goals
Areolar Deformity
Conservative Size Goals
Desires Fuller Size
Normal Areola
Areolar Herniation
Areolar Asymmetry
Types I, II, III
Types I, II
Types II, III
One Stage Correction (Implant)
Two Stage Correction (Tissue Expander)
Periareolar Incision Only
Circumareolar Mastopexy
Distensible lower pole
Tight, IMF Recalcitrant
Mild/Moderate Ptosis
Severe Ptosis
Circumareolar Plus Vertical Mastopexy
Breast Distensibility
Ptosis

FIGURE 62.6. Treatment algorithm for tuberous breast deformity. (From Kolker AR, Collins MS. Tuberous breast deformity: classification and treatment strategy for improving consistency in aesthetic correction. *Plast Reconstr Surg*. 2015;135(1):73-86.)

Pectoralis major muscle
Circumareolar incisions
Areolar margin
Old IMF
Radial scoring of gland
Proposed IMF

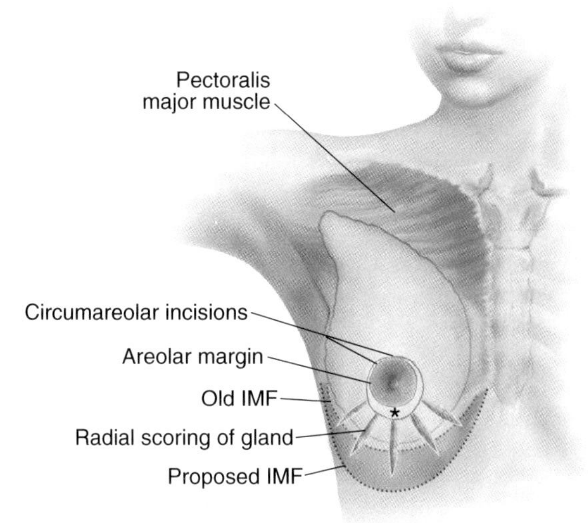

FIGURE 62.7. Radial scoring for release of the glandular and native inframammary fold constriction. (From Kolker AR, Collins MS. Tuberous breast deformity: classification and treatment strategy for improving consistency in aesthetic correction. *Plast Reconstr Surg*. 2015;135(1):73-86.)

Comprehensive clinical classification is difficult because of the diversity in presentation. The general classification used was introduced by Foucras et al. and categorized the severity of disease to mild, moderate, and severe, as summarized in **Table 62.2**.[4,6,27]

Breast anomalies among females are variable and range from mild hypoplasia to amastia.[25] Poland syndrome is involved in 14% of breast aplasia.[6] In the mild form, structural abnormalities may only be appreciated radiographically.[28] These patients may be referred to the plastic surgeon for mild asymmetry, without a formal diagnosis.[29] The mild variant of Poland syndrome is more common than the classic full presentation with an incidence of 1 in 16,500 live births.[25] The moderate variant of Poland syndrome represents the *classic* form and is characterized by hypoplasia of breast parenchyma, high IMF, and an underdeveloped and superiorly displaced NAC, with the absence of the anterior axillary fold. The severe variant of Poland syndrome represents the most challenging to reconstruct and is characterized with a marked deformity of the chest wall with tight chest skin and axillary webbing.[28] Ribiero and colleagues suggested obtaining CT scans to evaluate the structural abnormalities.[29] Cases have been reported in which a prominent posterior fold was evident on clinical examination with compensatory hypertrophy of the teres major that simulated the normal contraction of the latissimus dorsi muscle.[30]

The frequency of hand abnormalities with Poland syndrome is 13.5% to 56%; in turn, 10% of syndactyly is a result of Poland syndrome.[25] The spectrum may range from webbing of the fingers, fusion

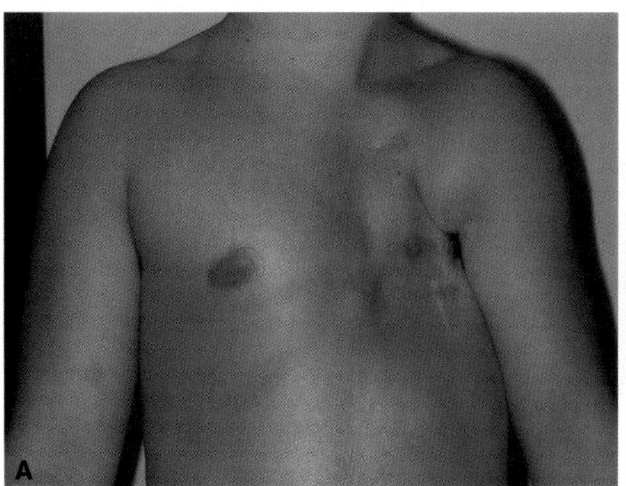

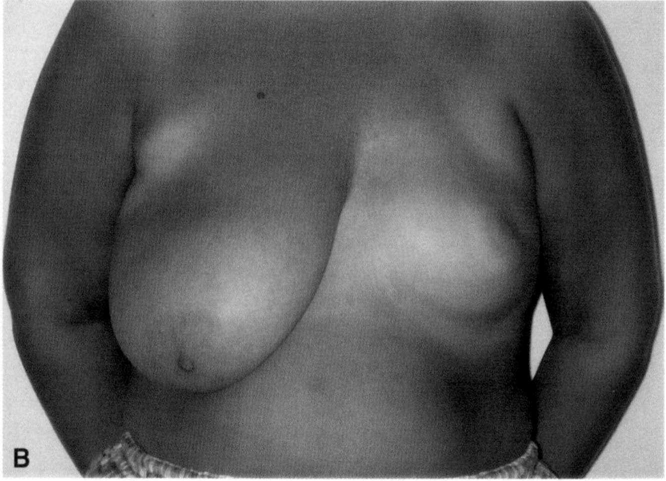

FIGURE 62.8. **A.** Moderate to severe Poland syndrome in a male patient. Note the lack of anterior axillary fold and sunken chest. **B.** Moderate Poland deformity in the female patient. Note the lack of anterior axillary fold and subclavicular hollowing. The breast is characterized by hypoplasia, elevated inframammary fold, and superiorly displaced and underdeveloped nipple-areolar complex.

of the carpal bones, absence of phalanges, and syndactyly to shortened forearm and/or upper arms. Aplasia of the ribs and cartilage involving rib segments two to five often leads to severe chest depression in 11% to 25% of patients. Eight percent of patients may have lung herniation. Dextrocardia is present in 5.6% of patients, which rises to 9.6% when the deformity was on the left side.

Poland syndrome can be associated with Mobius and Klippel-Feil syndrome.[25] Termed acro-pectoral-renal defect, an association with aplasia of the pectoralis major exists with renal anomalies (e.g., unilateral renal agenesis or duplication of the urinary collecting system).[5] Renal ultrasounds are recommended for all patients with aplasia of the pectoralis. Certain cancers are known to exist with Poland syndrome owing to suppression of homeobox and tumor suppression genes; leukemia, non-Hodgkin lymphoma, cervical cancer, leiomyosarcoma, and lung cancer. Despite being hypoplastic, breast cancer has been reported to occur in patients with Poland syndrome and therefore standard monitoring is required.

FIGURE 62.9. Anatomic representations of the classic Poland syndrome.

The etiology of Poland syndrome remains unclear; however, the leading theory suggests by the sixth week of gestation, when the limb bud is adjacent to the chest wall, interruption of the embryonic blood supply results in hypoplasia of the subclavian artery or its branches.[25] The severity and location of the flow impairment dictates the structures compromised (i.e., internal thoracic artery leading to absence of the sternocostal head of the pectoralis major; brachial artery leading to hand anomalies; and suprascapular artery leading to elevation or winging of the scapula, Sprengel deformity).

Surgical Correction of Poland Syndrome

Skeletal deformities should be addressed before breast reconstruction.[13] Significant chest wall depression, inadequate protection of the mediastinum, and paradoxical movement of the chest wall are indications for chest wall reconstruction.[6] When residual chest wall defects persist, custom silicone implants can be considered. Owing to the lack of a pectoralis major as an interposing muscle, placement of a chest wall prosthesis will result in implant-to-implant contact that may increase the likelihood of reconstructive failure.[31] Seyfer et al. reported a 100% complication rate using this technique and eventually abandoned it because of local complications that included migration, contour irregularities, and discomfort.[32] An alternative for the simple chest deformity included using the latissimus dorsi muscle to contour the chest wall followed by placement of a thin mammary prosthesis to correct the subclavicular hollow and to provide a more tolerable feel and appearance.

The timing of breast reconstruction for patients with Poland syndrome is another important consideration. It is commonly delayed until late adolescence or adulthood when breast development is complete, with the pedicle latissimus dorsi flap most commonly used. Patients who have completed breast reconstruction during their later years have been shown to have body image disorders that are unalleviated by reconstructive efforts.[33] Therefore, there is a trend toward less invasive modalities such as fat grafting and tissue expander placement at earlier ages to relieve psychosocial morbidity. The breast of the Poland syndrome patient presents several challenges: deficient subcutaneous tissue, contracted skin envelope, deficient subcutaneous tissue, NAC malposition or absence, high IMF, and caliber of recipient vessels if free flap reconstruction is necessary.[6] Combination of modalities as listed below is often necessary for optimal reconstruction in severe cases.

Fat Grafting

The use of lipofilling to correct contour abnormalities has become a cornerstone in treatment of mild Poland deformity. Lipofilling can

TABLE 62.2. EXPANDED CLASSIFICATION OF POLAND SYNDROME[27,29]

Type	Breast	Nipple Areola	Pectoralis Major	Thoracic Skeleton
Mild	Hypoplasia, asymmetry	Small, elevated	Hypoplasia	None
Moderate	Significant hypoplasia, aplasia, asymmetry	Hypoplastic, absent	Absent sternocostal head	Moderate
Severe	Complete aplasia	Hypoplastic, absent	Complete absence (including surrounding musculature)	Severe

be used primarily or secondarily with other procedures. Fat grafting has made the correction of mild to moderate contour abnormalities, such as improvement of the subclavicular hollow and absence of the anterior axillary fold, possible in short procedures.[34] Lipofilling can also be used to camouflage chest abnormalities and may obviate the need for custom silicone devices. The low morbidity of this procedure has permitted its safe use in adolescent females at the onset of puberty. Transfers may be staged at 4- to 6-month intervals to simulate natural breast growth.[35] Fat grafting techniques have also been used in patients with a history of breast cancer with long-term follow-up demonstrating oncologic safety.[36] Although radiographic distortions are possible with fat grafting, modern imaging modalities are able to differentiate between microcalcification due to fat grafting and malignancy.

Expander and Implant Reconstruction

Patients with less severe phenotypes (grade I or mild II) may be managed with prosthetic reconstruction alone. A prerequisite to direct to implant reconstruction is adequate soft-tissue coverage. When there is a soft-tissue deficiency and the IMF is high and tight, placement of tissue expanders can be beneficial. The expansion of the breast lower pole may bring down a superiorly malpositioned NAC. A contralateral symmetry procedure, such as a mastopexy or augmentation, may be required.

The primary complication arising from the placement of an implant alone is capsular contracture and is most likely increased because ofsubcutaneous placement. Seyfer's series treated 15 patients with implants alone, and 6 (40%) required open capsulotomy.[32] In the event of prosthetic failure, autologous tissue may be added to improve outcomes. In a series by Gautam et al., there were 12 cases in which a perforator flap was used in patients with Poland syndrome who had prior implant failure.[37] Although our understanding of prepectoral implant placement using ADMs has improved in patients following mastectomy, there have been no descriptions of use of ADM to secure the implant and to reduce the incidence of capsular contracture in Poland syndrome.

Autologous Tissue

The pedicled latissimus dorsi flap in combination with a prosthetic device has been the most common form of reconstruction in women with Poland syndrome. This can be performed simultaneously or in stages. The staged approach often begins with tissue expansion followed by a latissimus dorsi flap.[13] Seyfer et al. reported a 0% revision rate of patients treated with this technique. The transfer of the latissimus dorsi flap facilitated the creation of an anterior axillary fold and also camouflaged the subclavicular hollow. The latissimus muscle may be reinserted anteriorly on the humerus, simulating the pectoralis major insertion. Although 66% of patients required a contralateral symmetry procedure, the latissimus transfers were well tolerated without upper extremity weakness.

The correction of Poland deformity with free tissue transfer is another option when pedicled options are not available. Longaker et al. described their experience using free flaps (eight TRAMs, two SGAPs, one IGAP, and one contralateral TRAM) in nine patients with Poland syndrome.[38] Complications included one flap loss because of venous outflow anomalies in the subscapular system. Gautam et al. described a series of 12 perforator flaps to reduce donor site morbidity.[37] The recipient vessels in all patients were the internal mammary vessels. Success was excellent with no take-backs or flap failures.

Dos Santos Costa et al. described using a laparoscopically harvested pedicled omentum flap based completely on the right gastroepiploic artery and tunneled subcutaneously through the IMF.[39] Four to six months are required for volume equalization of the omentum. Eighty percent of patients required additional implants. Huemer utilized myocutaneous gracilis flaps to approach reconstructions.[40] When correction of the infraclavicular territory was necessary, an ipsilateral free gracilis flap was anastomosed to the thoracodorsal vessels. When correcting for breast volume, the free gracilis flap was placed in a retroglandular position and anastomosed to the internal mammary vessels.

Because of the incidence of vascular anomalies in the recipient vessels, preoperative angiography should be strongly considered when proceeding with free tissue transfer options.[30] A secondary implant or lipofilling can be considered as needed for additional volume.

ANTERIOR THORACIC HYPOPLASIA

Anterior thoracic hypoplasia was described by Spear et al. and represents a distinct entity separate from Poland syndrome.[31] Although Poland syndrome has a hallmark of hypoplasia or aplasia of the pectoralis major, anterior thoracic hypoplasia presents with hypoplasia of the ipsilateral breast, superior displacement of the NAC, and posterior displacement of the ribs with sunken chest wall but a *normal* pectoralis major and sternum position. All patients in his series were treated with a partial submuscular anatomical implant.

HYPERPLASTIC DISORDERS

Virginal Mammary Hypertrophy

Virginal hypertrophy (e.g., juvenile hypertrophy, gigantomastia) of the breast is a rare condition characterized by rapid, excessive, and unyielding proliferation of one or both breasts in the adolescent years for at least 6 months (Figure 62.10). Reports have demonstrated that breasts may grow as large as 13 to 23 kg.[41] Virginal hypertrophy, which occurs after a few months after puberty, is differentiated from prepubertal hypertrophy, which is before puberty and usually bilateral. Associated symptoms include shoulder and neck pain, bra strap grooving, and rashes. The parenchyma is often tender, with thin skin and dilated veins. Although there is no consensus on exact etiology, the leading theories include excess local estrogen production and estrogen end-organ sensitivity.[6] The differential diagnosis includes but is not limited to fibroadenoma, phyllodes tumor, lymphedema, endocrine conditions, rheumatologic diseases, and lymphoma.[42] Optimal management usually requires a team approach with pediatric and medical disciplines involved in making the diagnosis.

There has been a myriad of medical options for management that have included dydrogesterone, bromocriptine, and medroxyprogesterone; however, tamoxifen administration for 4 months has been shown to be the most effective in retarding or arresting breast growth. Its use is limited by the side effects in the pediatric population, which includes hot flashes, venous thrombosis, osteoporosis, and endometrial hyperplasia. The ultimate treatment, however, remains surgical and most

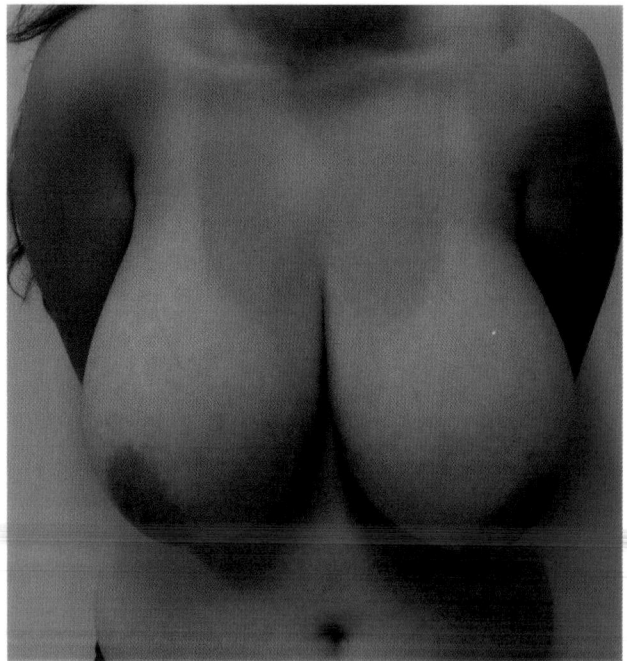

FIGURE 62.10. Bilateral virginal hypertrophy in a 16-year-old girl.

commonly includes reduction mammaplasty and in some cases, mastectomy. Hoppe et al., in the largest systematic review of virginal hypertrophy, demonstrated that recurrence of breast growth is sevenfold higher following a reduction mammaplasty compared with mastectomy.[47] To preserve lactation and aesthetic outcome, most physicians recommend reduction mammaplasty with preservation of the NAC on a vascularized pedicle to avoid the psychologic sequela of a mastectomy in the pediatric patient. It is best to defer reduction mammaplasty until the later years of adolescence to reduce the risk of recurrence and revision surgery.[41,43] In severe cases, early identification is important to minimize the extent of surgery and associated morbidity.[4,42]

It is important to have in-depth discussions with patients preoperatively to set expectations and review sequela, especially relating to breast feeding. With careful preservation of the subareolar gland, most studies have indicated the rates of breast feeding in patients with breast hypertrophy with and without reduction mammaplasty to be equivalent (~60%).[44] In both control and operated groups, 34% to 39% of these patients required supplementation of breast milk. Although this was not studied directly in virginal hypertrophy, these statistics are helpful in counseling.

Giant Fibroadenoma

During adolescence, 75% to 95% of breast lesions are fibroadenomas.[41] Generally, they are well-circumscribed, painless, rubbery, and mobile masses of benign connective tissue and epithelial proliferation. Giant fibroadenoma refers to when the tumor is larger than 5 cm in diameter and/or weighs more than 500 g (Figure 62.11). At this point, skin changes, venous dilation, and in severe instances, skin ulceration of overlying tissue may occur. Ultrasound may reveal a well-circumscribed avascular mass. Although the diagnosis is clinical, confirmation may be obtained with a fine-needle aspiration.[41] Timing is dictated by rate of growth. However, earlier intervention may be necessary to prevent distortion of existing tissue. Treatment involves removing the lesion in the well-demarcated plane. To fill in large cavities, tissue rearrangement techniques are required with consideration to the pedicle and nipple perfusion. Pathologically, fibroadenoma is difficult to distinguish from phyllodes tumor, which has an incidence of less than 1.3%.[6,41] Should a diagnosis of malignant phyllodes tumor be made, consultation with surgical oncology or pediatric surgery is appropriate.

Polythelia and Polymastia

Polythelia is relatively common and occurs in up to 5.6% of male and female patients along the milk lines.[45] These cases are generally sporadic; however, cases of familial inheritance patterns have been reported. They may be associated with nephrourologic abnormalities and therefore a urinalysis and renal ultrasound is necessary. Excision is typically performed before puberty begins with an elliptical excision. Delay of treatment, especially in females, may require a wider incisional pattern as glandular tissue may become involved.

Polymastia, with or without the NAC, may also occur along the embryonic mammary ridges, most commonly in the axilla with a prevalence of 1% to 2%.[46] Although sporadic, familial cases and associated renal abnormalities have been identified. Polymastia differs from ectopic breast tissue, as ectopic breast tissue is outside the mammary ridges. Unlike polythelia, polymastia is usually not identified until after puberty, pregnancy or lactation, and when hormonal influences enlarge the breast tissue. These lesions generally present with discomfort during certain points of the menstrual cycle. This accessory breast tissue may be excised and closed primarily over a drain as needed. If excision is forgone, then screening for malignancy is necessary because breast cancer can occur with the accessory tissue at an equal rate to the natural breast.

Gynecomastia

Gynecomastia is the most common form of breast hypertrophy in men with an overall incidence of 32% to 36% and up to 65% in adolescent males (Figure 62.12).[47] Bilateral disease occurs in 25% to 75% of individuals. Although most cases of gynecomastia during adolescents are idiopathic, the most common cause in those >40 years old is most often drug induced. Idiopathic or physiologic gynecomastia is typically a reflection of the hormonal milieu, with a relative predominance of estrogen. Such times occur with neonates because of circulating maternal estrogen, puberty when there is an excess amount of estradiol versus testosterone, and in the elderly (>65) when both a decline in androgen and aromatization peripherally of testosterone to estrogen occur.

Workup of gynecomastia begins with a detailed history and physical examination as outlined by Rohrich.[47] It is necessary to identify pathologic causes that include testicular cancer, pituitary tumors, adrenal tumors, liver disease, paraneoplastic syndrome, Klinefelter syndrome, thyroid disease, renal failure, myotonic dystrophy, human immunodeficiency virus, marijuana use, alcohol, anabolic steroids, and medications (Figure 62.13).[47] Physical examination will help distinguish pseudogynecomastia, for which enlargement is due to fat deposition in light of obesity without glandular hypertrophy.

Various staging classifications have been described. Simon and Kahn described a classification system based on skin and tissue excess: Grade 1: slight breast enlargement without redundancy, Grade

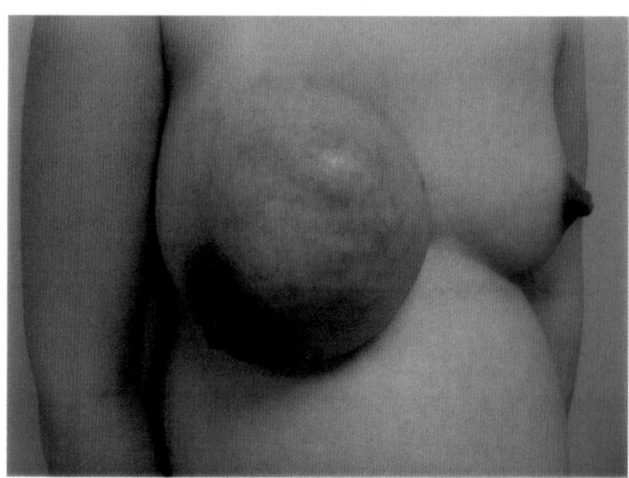

FIGURE 62.11. Giant fibroadenoma.

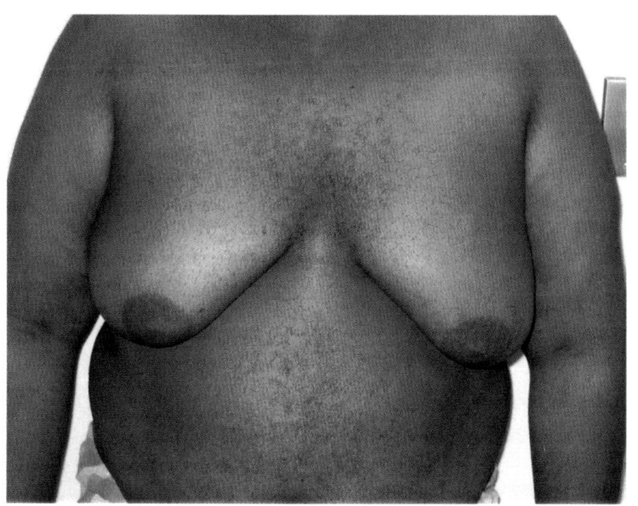

FIGURE 62.12. Bilateral gynecomastia.

2A: moderate breast enlargement without skin redundancy, Grade 2B: moderate breast enlargement with marked skin redundancy, and Grade 3: marked breast enlargement and skin redundancy.[48] Webster described a classification based on tissue type[49]:

Type I: Presence of glandular tissue
Type II: Presence of fatty and glandular mix
Type III: Presence of simple fatty tissue

Rohrich described the most utilitarian method for classifying gynecomastia, based on the amount and character of breast hypertrophy and degree of ptosis (**Table 62.3**).[47]

The onset of gynecomastia is characterized by fibroblastic stromal and ductal proliferation, which may resolve spontaneously. However, when persisting beyond a year, these tissues rarely regress, as stromal fibrosis and hyalinization occur with minimal ductal proliferation. Should a pathologic cause be present, treatment of such agents or disease is required in conjunction with a medical doctor. The risk of breast cancer in patients with gynecomastia remains equivalent when compared with the normal male population. The incidence of breast cancer is 60 times higher in patients with gynecomastia associated

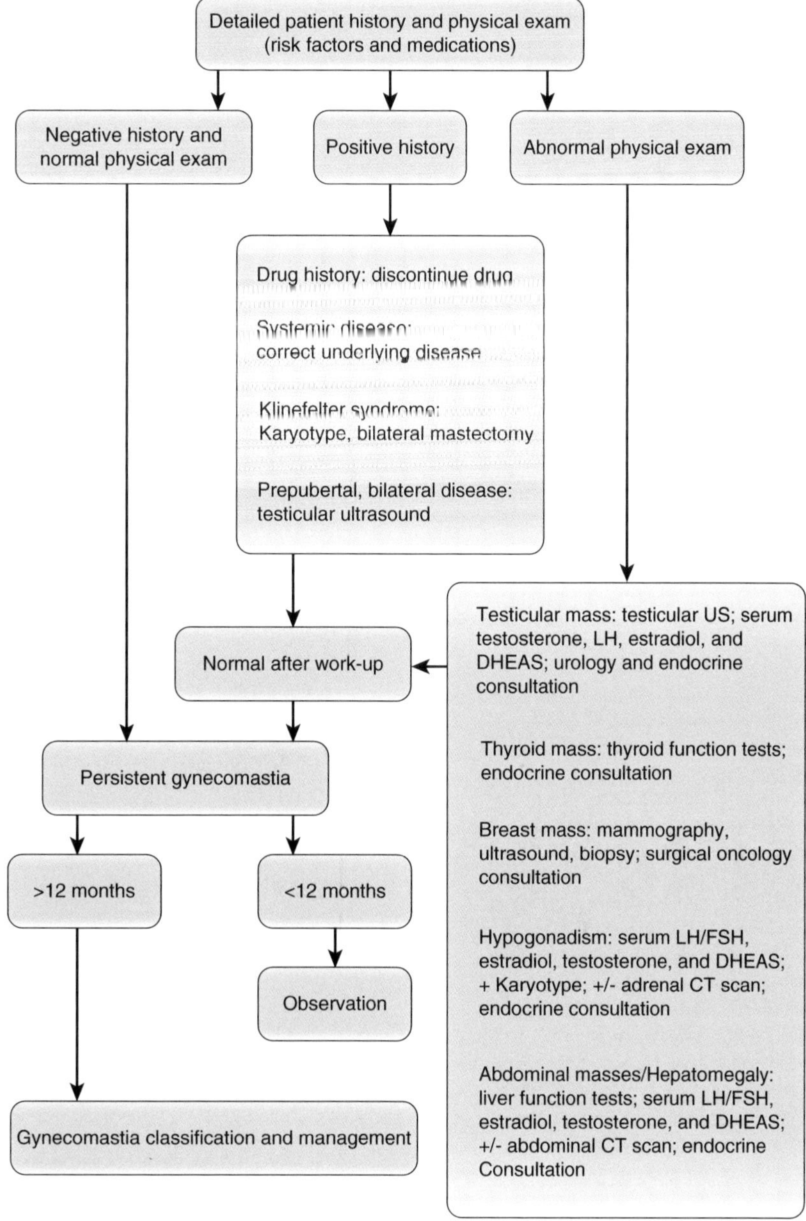

FIGURE 62.13. Preoperative algorithm for gynecomastia. (From Rohrich RJ, Ha RY, Kenkel JM, Adams WPJr. Classification and management of gynecomastia: defining the role of ultrasound-assisted liposuction. *Plast Reconstr Surg.* 2003;111(2):909-923.)

TABLE 62.3. CLASSIFICATION AND MANAGEMENT OF GYNECOMASTIA

Classification	Description	Management
Grade I	Minimal hypertrophy (<250 g of breast tissue) without ptosis	
IA	Primarily glandular	Ultrasound-assisted liposuction or suction-assisted lipectomy
IB	Primarily fibrous	Ultrasound-assisted liposuction
Grade II	Moderate hypertrophy (250–500 g of breast tissue) without ptosis	
IIA	Primarily glandular	Ultrasound-assisted liposuction or suction-assisted lipectomy
IIB	Primarily fibrous	Ultrasound-assisted liposuction
Grade III	Severe hypertrophy (>500 g of breast tissue with grade I ptosis Glandular or fibrous	Ultrasound-assisted liposuction with or without staged excision
Grade IV	Severe hypertrophy with grade II or III ptosis Glandular or fibrous	Ultrasound-assisted liposuction with or without staged excision

(From Rohrich RJ, Ha RY, Kenkel JM, Adams WPJr. Classification and management of gynecomastia: defining the role of ultrasound-assisted liposuction. *Plast Reconstr Surg*. 2003;111(2):909-923.)

with Klinefelter syndrome when compared with the general population and thus necessitates mastectomy.[47] Tamoxifen has been successful in the treatment of glandular gynecomastia in which there is a palpable nodule under the areola.[50] Other medications such as testosterone, danazol, and clomiphene have had limited success.

Surgical management is considered for persistent breast enlargement after 1 to 2 years. Techniques have evolved from the classic open approach to the minimally invasive approaches. Liposuction presented a breakthrough when it was introduced as a primary modality over surgical excision, reducing the incidence of postsurgical contour abnormalities and asymmetry. Rohrich advocates use of ultrasound assisted liposuction as a first-line treatment, arguing that the emulsification of the fat, connective tissue, and skin retraction is advantageous when compared with traditional liposuction.[47] In addition to suctioning in the intermediate fat layer, the subdermal and subareolar regions are suctioned for maximal skin retraction and disruption of the fibroconnective tissues (Figure 62.14). In this study, 87% of men were treated with traditional or ultrasound-assisted liposuction alone. In 13%, 6 to 9 months were allowed to elapse for maximal skin retraction before secondary excision was performed.

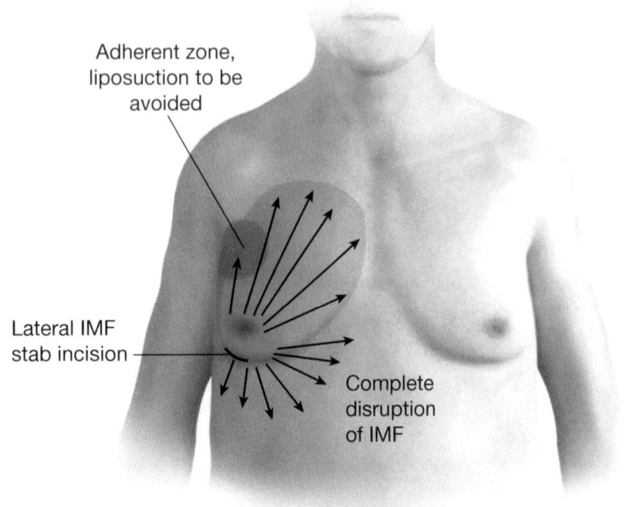

FIGURE 62.14. Pattern of ultrasound-assisted liposuction. Liposuction ports are made in the lateral inframammary fold crease. Adherent zones in the upper outer quadrants (*red*), in proximity to the axillary tissue, should be suctioned with caution. (From Stranix JT, Hazen A. Gynecomastia. In: Chung KC, ed. *Operative Techniques in Plastic Surgery*. Philadelphia, PA: Wolters Kluwer Health; 2019.)

Most practitioners perform a single-stage correction, with liposuction and the excision of the subglandular tissue through a partial periareolar approach. Overzealous subareolar resection may lead to a saucer-type deformity under the areola. It is therefore advisable to leave a layer of fibrous tissue under the areola for a smooth contour to avoid this complication. An alternative to excision is to use an arthroscopic shaver to treat the excess subareolar tissue, obviating the need for an incision.[51] In patients with severe gynecomastia, there are several methods by which the excess skin and gland can be managed. These include circumareolar de-epithelialization and gland resection through an inferior transdermic approach, circumvertical reduction pattern, or free nipple graft.[52,53] Postoperatively, compression garments are worn for at least 6 weeks, and heavy exercise should be avoided for 1 month.

CONCLUSION

Congenital anomalies of the breast represent a rare and diverse set of disorders requiring application of various principles of breast reconstruction with consideration of growth and psychosocial impact. Careful determination of all the deformities present is crucial, and surgeons need to have a frank discussion of goals and the potential impact correction has to the aesthetic and functional (e.g., breast feeding) outcomes. It has become commonplace for early identification of hyperplastic disorders and intervention to limit the extent of surgery and body image disorders, as well as to preserve lactation and optimize aesthetic outcomes.[42] Although correction of hypoplastic breast deformity has traditionally been postponed until late adolescence after growth completed, studies now demonstrate improved psychosocial benefit with the early minimally invasive techniques.[33]

REFERENCES

1. Lin KY, Nguyen DB, Williams RM. Complete breast absence revisited. *Plast Reconstr Surg*. 2000;106(1):98-101.
2. Marshall WA, Tanner JM. Variations in pattern of pubertal changes in girls. *Arch Dis Child*. 1969;44(235):291-303.
3. Trier WC. Complete breast absence: case report and review of the literature. *Plast Reconstr Surg*. 1965;36(4):431-439.
4. Egro FM, Davison EH, Namnoum JD, Shestak KC. Congenital breast deformities. In: Neligan P, ed. *Plastic Surgery*. Vol 2. Philadelphia, PA: Elsevier; 2017.
5. Rees TD, Aston SJ. The tuberous breast. *Clin Plast Surg*. 1976;3(2):339-347.
   The authors describe the tuberous breast deformity for the first time and postulate reconstruction efforts that now serve the basis of modern techniques.
6. Shestak KC, Rottgers SA, Grunwaldt L, et al. Congenital anomalies of the breast: tuberous breasts, Poland's syndrome, and asymmetry. In: Thorne C, ed. *Grabb and Smith's Plastic Surgery*. 7th ed. Philadelphia, PA: Lippincott Williams & Wilkins; 2014:668-677.

7. Grolleau JL, Lanfrey E, Lavigne B, et al. Breast base anomalies: treatment strategy for tuberous breasts, minor deformities, and asymmetry. *Plast Reconstr Surg.* 1999;104(7):2040-2048.
8. DeLuca-Pytell DM, Piazza RC, Holding JC, et al. The incidence of tuberous breast deformity in asymmetric and symmetric mammaplasty patients. *Plast Reconstr Surg.* 2005;116(7):1894-1899.
9. Kolker AR, Collins MS. Tuberous breast deformity: classification and treatment strategy for improving consistency in aesthetic correction. *Plast Reconstr Surg.* 2015;135(1):73-86.
This recent article demonstrates a large series (n = 51) on correction of tuberous breast. The authors comprehensively discuss their classification system, their algorithm for correction, and their results.
10. Mandrekas AD, Zambacos GJ. Aesthetic reconstruction of the tuberous breast deformity: a 10-year experience. *Aesthet Surg J.* 2010;30(5):680-692.
11. Zambacos GJ, Mandrekas AD. The incidence of tuberous breast deformity in asymmetric and symmetric mammaplasty patients. *Plast Reconstr Surg.* 2006;118(7):1667.
12. Brown MH, Somogyi RB. Surgical strategies in the correction of the tuberous breast. *Clin Plast Surg.* 2015;42(4):531-549.
13. Nahabedian MY. Breast deformities and mastopexy. *Plast Reconstr Surg.* 2011;127(4):91e-102e.
14. Dinner MI, Dowden RV. The tubular/tuberous breast syndrome. *Ann Plast Surg.* 1987;19(5):414-420.
15. Puckett CL, Concannon MJ. Augmenting the narrow-based breast: the unfurling technique to prevent the double-bubble deformity. *Aesthet Plast Surg.* 1990;14(1):15-19.
16. Ribeiro L, Canzi W, Buss A Jr, Accorsi A Jr. Tuberous breast: a new approach. *Plast Reconstr Surg.* 1998;101(1):42-50.
17. Abbate OA, Fan KL, Nahabedian MY. Central mound mastopexy for the correction of tuberous/tubular breast deformity. *Plast Reconstr Surg Glob Open.* 2017;5(11):e1545.
18. Swanson E. Can we really control the inframammary fold (IMF) in breast augmentation? *Aesthet Surg J.* 2016;36(10):NP313-NP314.
19. Handel N. The double-bubble deformity: cause, prevention, and treatment. *Plast Reconstr Surg.* 2013;132(6):1434-1443.
This in-depth article reviews the double-bubble deformity in the context of the inframammary fold. The authors describe the pathologic and clinical basis of the IMF, a commonly poorly understood and complicated structure.
20. Tebbetts JB, Adams WP. Five critical decisions in breast augmentation using five measurements in 5 minutes: the high five decision support process. *Plast Reconstr Surg.* 2005;116(7):2005-2016.
21. Mallucci P, Branford OA. Design for natural breast augmentation: the ICE principle. *Plast Reconstr Surg.* 2016;137(6):1728-1737.
22. Heden P, Jernbeck J, Hober M. Breast augmentation with anatomical cohesive gel implants: the world's largest current experience. *Clin Plast Surg.* 2001;28(3):531-552.
23. Hammond DC, Khuthaila DK, Kim J. The interlocking Gore-Tex suture for control of areolar diameter and shape. *Plast Reconstr Surg.* 2007;119(3):804-809.
24. Brown MH, Somogyi RB, Aggarwal S. Secondary breast augmentation. *Plast Reconstr Surg.* 2016;138(1):119e-135e.
25. Fokin AA, Robicsek F. Poland's syndrome revisited. *Ann Thorac Surg.* 2002;74(6):2218-2225.
This article is the most comprehensive review on the clinical findings and chest reconstruction associated with Poland syndrome.
26. Yiyit N. Definition of the inclusion criteria of Poland's syndrome. *Ann Thorac Surg.* 2014;98(5):1886.
27. Foucras L, Grolleau-Raoux JL, Chavoin JP. [Poland's syndrome: clinic series and thoraco-mammary reconstruction: report of 27 cases]. *Ann Chir Plast Esthet.* 2003;48(2):54-66.
28. Namnoum JD. Breast Reconstruction in patients with Poland syndrome. In: Spear SL, ed. *Surgery of the Breast: Principles and Art.* 3rd ed. Philadelphia, PA: Lippincott Williams & Wilkins; 2011:1416-1424.
29. Ribeiro RC, Saltz R, Mangles MG, Koch H. Clinical and radiographic Poland syndrome classification: a proposal. *Aesthet Surg J.* 2009;29(6):494-504.
30. Beer GM, Kompatscher P, Hergan K. Poland's syndrome and vascular malformations. *Br J Plast Surg.* 1996;49(7):482-484.
31. Spear SL, Pelletiere CV, Lee ES, Grotting JC. Anterior thoracic hypoplasia: a separate entity from Poland syndrome. *Plast Reconstr Surg.* 2004;113(1):69-77.
32. Seyfer AE, Fox JP, Hamilton CG. Poland syndrome: evaluation and treatment of the chest wall in 63 patients. *Plast Reconstr Surg.* 2010;126(3):902-911.
The authors describe their method of correction in 63 patients with Poland syndrome. They outline their methods of correction for each deformity.
33. Baldelli I, Santi P, Dova L, et al. Body image disorders and surgical timing in patients affected by Poland syndrome: data analysis of 58 case studies. *Plast Reconstr Surg.* 2016;137(4):1273-1282.
34. Pinsolle V, Chichery A, Grolleau JL, Chavoin JP. Autologous fat injection in Poland's syndrome. *J Plast Reconstr Aesthet Surg.* 2008;61(7):784-791.
35. Delay E, Sinna R, Chekaroua K, et al. Lipomodeling of Poland's syndrome: a new treatment of the thoracic deformity. *Aesthet Plast Surg.* 2010;34(2):218-225.
36. Cohen O, Lam G, Karp N, Choi M. Determining the oncologic safety of autologous fat grafting as a reconstructive modality: an institutional review of breast cancer recurrence rates and surgical outcomes. *Plast Reconstr Surg.* 2017;140(3):382e-392e.
37. Gautam AK, Allen RJ Jr, LoTempio MM, et al. Congenital breast deformity reconstruction using perforator flaps. *Ann Plast Surg.* 2007;58(4):353-358.
38. Longaker MT, Glat PM, Colen LB, Siebert JW. Reconstruction of breast asymmetry in Poland's chest-wall deformity using microvascular free flaps. *Plast Reconstr Surg.* 1997;99(2):429-436.
39. dos Santos Costa S, Blotta RM, Mariano MB, et al. Aesthetic improvements in Poland's syndrome treatment with omentum flap. *Aesthet Plast Surg.* 2010;34(5):634-639.
40. Huemer GM, Puelzl P, Schoeller T. Breast and chest wall reconstruction with the transverse musculocutaneous gracilis flap in Poland syndrome. *Plast Reconstr Surg.* 2012;130(4):779-783.
41. Chang DS, McGrath MH. Management of benign tumors of the adolescent breast. *Plast Reconstr Surg.* 2007;120(1):13e-19e.
42. Hoppe IC, Patel PP, Singer-Granick CJ, Granick MS. Virginal mammary hypertrophy: a meta-analysis and treatment algorithm. *Plast Reconstr Surg.* 2011;127(6):2224-2231.
43. van Aalst JA, Phillips JD, Sadove AM. Pediatric chest wall and breast deformities. *Plast Reconstr Surg.* 2009;124(suppl 1):38e-49e.
44. Cruz NI, Korchin L. Lactational performance after breast reduction with different pedicles. *Plast Reconstr Surg.* 2007;120(1):35-40.
45. Schmidt H. Supernumerary nipples: prevalence, size, sex and side predilection—a prospective clinical study. *Eur J Pediatr.* 1998;157(10):821-823.
46. Grossl NA. Supernumerary breast tissue: historical perspectives and clinical features. *South Med J.* 2000;93(1):29-32.
47. Rohrich RJ, Ha RY, Kenkel JM, Adams WP Jr. Classification and management of gynecomastia: defining the role of ultrasound-assisted liposuction. *Plast Reconstr Surg.* 2003;111(2):909-923.
In this landmark article, the authors classify gynecomastia, review historical correction, describe algorithm of workup, present treatment plan, and review results. They make a strong case for the use of ultrasound assisted liposuction in the correction of gynecomastia.
48. Simon BE, Hoffman S, Kahn S. Classification and surgical correction of gynecomastia. *Plast Reconstr Surg.* 1973;51(1):48-52.
49. Webster JP. Mastectomy for gynecomastia through a semicircular intra-areolar incision. *Ann Surg.* 1946;124:557-575.
50. Khan HN, Rampaul R, Blamey RW. Management of physiological gynaecomastia with tamoxifen. *Breast.* 2004;13(1):61-65.
51. Petty PM, Solomon M, Buchel EW, Tran NV. Gynecomastia: evolving paradigm of management and comparison of techniques. *Plast Reconstr Surg.* 2010;125(5):1301-1308.
52. Persichetti P, Berloco M, Casadei RM, et al. Gynecomastia and the complete circumareolar approach in the surgical management of skin redundancy. *Plast Reconstr Surg.* 2001;107(4):948-954.
53. Hammond DC. Surgical correction of gynecomastia. *Plast Reconstr Surg.* 2009;124(suppl 1):61e-68e.

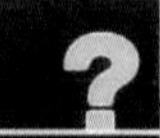

QUESTIONS

1. **What is the key pathological feature of Poland syndrome?**
   a. Hand abnormalities
   b. Chest depression
   c. Hypoplasia or absence of the pectoralis major
   d. Hypoplastic or absent breast
   e. Absence of the latissimus dorsi

2. **Where is the most common site for polymastia to occur?**
   a. Axillary region
   b. Underneath the breast
   c. Near the groin
   d. On the abdomen

3. **An 18-year-old female with a history of tuberous breast deformity comes into your clinic requesting evaluation for unsatisfactory aesthetic appearance. She has had a previous partial submuscular breast augmentation performed by another surgeon. On examination, she appears to have a double-bubble deformity. What key maneuver was missed in the initial operation?**
   a. Complete release of the pectoralis major
   b. Ablation of the old IMF
   c. Placement of the implant's partial submuscular plane
   d. Radial scoring of the undersurface of the breast

4. **A 13-year-old boy with a BMI of 22 presents with bilateral fibrofatty tissue underneath his nipples recalcitrant to exercise regimens for the past 3 months. The lesions have caused him significant distress at the gym and when swimming. A full workup has elicited no pathologic cause. What is the most appropriate next step in management?**
   a. Surgical excision
   b. Selective estrogen receptor modulators
   c. Continued weight loss
   d. Observation and follow-up for 6 to 8 months

5. **What tumor is most clinically difficult to distinguish from fibroadenoma?**
   a. Phyllodes tumor
   b. Intraductal carcinoma
   c. Fibrocystic lesion
   d. Intraductal papilloma

1. **Answer: c.** Poland syndrome represents a highly variable constellation of syndromes revolving around structures supplied by the subclavian vessels. Hypoplasia or absence of the pectoralis major represents the central pathologic finding of Poland syndrome. Additional abnormalities that may be seen include hypoplasia or absence of the breast, absence of the nipple, absence of the axillary hair, absence of adjacent muscles (e.g., latissimus dorsi, serratus anterior, external oblique, deltoid, infraspinatus, supraspinatus, and pectoralis minor), absence of costal cartilage and anterior ribs leading to chest wall abnormality, and upper limb malformations.

2. **Answer: a.** The most common location of the polymastia is the axillary region.[46] These lesions typically present with pain that may coincide with menstrual cycles or lactation separate from the breast tissue itself. Excision requires preservation of the intercostobrachial and associated nerves. The rate of malignancy is equal, and pathologic examination of the sampling is necessary.

3. **Answer: b.** Ablation of the old IMF is the key maneuver to eliminate double-bubble deformity. In an excellent review of the topic by Handel, he demonstrates the double-bubble deformity is not caused by disruption of an IMF ligament but by failure to fully detach the superficial fascial system from the dermis.[19] The IMF is created by attachment from the superficial fascial system to the dermis. In routine breast augmentations without manipulation of the fold, the implant lies beneath the pectoralis fascia, and the superficial fascia relationships are undisturbed. In the more severe cases of tuberous deformity, owing to the short nipple-to-IMF distance, inferior dissection and displacing the fold to a caudal location is typically necessary. Dissection is continued in a plane underneath the superficial fascia. The superficial fascia and dermis attachments from the old IMF persist with inadequate ablation, resulting in double-bubble deformity.

4. **Answer: d.** The patient likely suffers from benign pubertal gynecomastia, which may respond spontaneously. Therefore, observation is prudent. Beyond 1 year, the tissue rarely regresses as stromal fibrosis and hyalinization set in. At this point, surgical therapy is indicated. While weight loss is encouraged, suggesting continued weight loss would resolve gynecomastia is inappropriate.

5. **Answer: a.** Fibroadenoma can be clinically difficult to distinguish from phyllodes tumor. Making such diagnosis may require pathological examination.[41] Histologically, phyllodes tumor shows more stromal proliferation. However, malignant phyllodes tumor has the ability to metastasize and recur locally. These lesions are hallmarked by obvious sarcomatous elements. In adults, surgical treatment requires a 1 cm surgical margin to reduce recurrence rates. There are some who believe the adolescent phyllodes tumor is less aggressive and therefore can be excised with a small rim for a surgical margin.

CHAPTER 63 Principles of Plastic Surgery After Massive Weight Loss

Omar E. Beidas, Jeffrey A. Gusenoff, and Ernest K. Manders

KEY POINTS

- Massive weight loss patients require comprehensive preoperative evaluation and management of expectations.
- Optimization of patients preoperatively is paramount to minimizing or avoiding complications.
- Multiple procedures can be performed simultaneously depending on patient priorities and degree of deformities.
- Staging procedures can minimize operative time and avoid opposite vectors of tension.
- Although complications following body contouring for the massive weight loss patient are common, most are minor and managed as an outpatient basis.

The obesity epidemic in the United States and subsequent popularity in weight loss, whether by means of bariatric surgery or diet and exercise, echeloned a new subspecialty of plastic surgery. Massive weight loss (MWL), commonly defined as a loss of greater than 50% of excess weight above ideal body weight (IBW), has caused an explosion of patients seeking removal of excess skin and fat. This population deserves special consideration, as MWL has been found to be a predictor for wound complications in those undergoing body contouring surgery.[1] A comprehensive evaluation must take a multitude of factors into account to safely and effectively care for the patient. Every patient presents an interesting and unique challenge; therefore, approaches must be tailored to the individual. Attention to detail keeps both surgeon and patient out of trouble. This chapter focuses on the overall assessment and management of the weight loss patient, with procedural details described in Chapters 64–66.

PREOPERATIVE PLANNING

MWL leads to various deformities in all regions of the body, resulting in excess loose skin and fat. Although many medical diseases are improved or even cured by means of weight loss, the redundant skin is a constant reminder of the patient's former self when looking in the mirror. Common complaints from patients include inability to properly fit in clothing, buildup of moisture in skin folds leading to intertriginous rashes and recurrent infections, and social stigma. Regardless of the weight loss method, patients should be congratulated on their tremendous achievement and reminded that their visit with the plastic surgeon ushers the beginning of the end of their journey. It is imperative that the surgeon performs a careful assessment of any patient who presents for body contouring after MWL to optimize the patient and minimize complications.

Weight Loss Method

Most patients undergo weight loss surgery, some achieve weight loss via diet and exercise, whereas a few resort to medication-induced methods of weight loss. If surgery was performed, it is important to note the type of procedure, whether laparoscopic or open, need for revisions or adjustments, and presence of a subcutaneous port. Weight loss by pharmacologic methods can be risky and unpredictable given the lack of long-term data. Dietary supplements or drugs may not have Food and Drug Administration approval and can have serious untoward effects. Similarly, fad diets do not have enough evidence to substantiate them. Interestingly, complications from body contouring in this population are similar independent of weight loss method.[2]

Weight History

History should include the timeline of weight gain and subsequent loss, with particular attention paid to the method of weight loss. Bariatric surgery typically causes a precipitous drop in weight for the first year, thereafter a slow decline. A patient often reaches a nadir then climbs to within 10% of this value before plateauing at this new level. Additional information to obtain at the initial visit is maximum, minimum, and current weights. MWL patients have an almost three-fold increased risk of wound healing complications compared to non-MWL patients, and the risk is highest in those who have lost over 100 pounds.[1]

Before enlisting a patient for body contouring after weight loss, weight should remain stable—within 5 kg—for at least 3 months.[3] If a patient is still actively losing weight, or intends to, then he or she should be reevaluated at 3 to 6 month intervals until down to the desired weight. Ideally, patients should be at or close to their goal weight, as results are significantly improved when weight is shed before surgery rather than after.

Nutritional Assessment

Because most patients presenting to the plastic surgeon for body contouring achieve MWL by means of bariatric surgery, it is vital to perform a comprehensive nutritional assessment as part of the evaluation. Diet, including daily protein and liquid intake, should be documented. The American Dietetic Association (ADA) recommends a daily protein intake of 1 to 1.5 g/kg of IBW, or approximately 60 to 80 g for most adults. ADA guidelines suggest 2 L (8 cups, or 64 ounces) of fluid intake per day. It is best that patients eat a healthy-balanced diet and exercise regularly.

Given that the stress of surgery can increase energy expenditure up to 25%,[4] patients should be accordingly counseled to increase their daily protein consumption to 75 to 100 g in the perioperative period. This increased protein intake should be maintained for at least 2 weeks preoperatively and 4 weeks postoperatively.

Symptoms of chronic malnutrition range in form and severity, including but not limited to fatigue, muscle aches, and peripheral neuropathy. A history of dumping syndrome should be elicited, characterized by postprandial symptoms of abdominal pain, nausea, emesis, and diarrhea. Dumping syndrome is seen mostly in gastric bypass patients and is caused by a rapid emptying of stomach contents into the small intestine. Generally, the solution is to avoid foods with a high sugar content as these are not well-tolerated by the postbariatric surgery patient. If any concerns arise from the patient or physician perspective, the patient should be referred to their bariatric team to address these issues before proceeding with body contouring.

As many as 50% of postbariatric surgery patients have at least one elemental or nutritional deficiency as a result, with a greater risk after procedures with a malabsorptive component such as Roux-en-Y gastric bypass surgery.[5-7] Many of these nutrients and vitamins are necessary cofactors for general metabolism and wound healing.[8] Patients who achieved weight loss by surgical means often require supplementation.[9] Therefore, nutritional assessment should include screening of iron, albumin, and vitamins A, B, and D. Iron-deficiency anemia is the most common perioperative deficiency found in the MWL population[10] and is most prevalent in women of childbearing age.[11] Referral to a hematologist to optimize hemoglobin before surgery can avoid need for perioperative transfusion. Not only are low albumin levels associated with poor wound healing, but also levels below 2.1 g/dL are predictive of increased mortality rates postoperatively.[12,13] Vitamin B (thiamin) deficiency should be suspected in any patient with intractable emesis, as late recognition can lead to serious consequences[14,15] (**Table 63.1**).

Medical Comorbidities

It is important to document a patient's medical comorbidities before and after weight loss, as many conditions will improve if not resolved after achieving a more IBW. Medical diseases such as diabetes, hypertension, hyperlipidemia, gastroesophageal reflux disease, and obstructive sleep apnea, among others, are improved or possibly entirely eliminated. However, these and others may be present and must be optimized before any operative procedure. Principles outlined in Chapter 16 should guide management options, and referrals to specialists made accordingly. It is recommended that a complete blood count be obtained on all patients who have experienced MWL.

Although all patients will experience some degree of amelioration in medical conditions, not all will be completely alleviated. Therefore, surgeons treating these patients should be familiar with common disease states with which they may present. The three most common diseases patients present with after MWL are depression (53%), arthritis (41%), and anxiety (27%).[10]

Body Mass Index

A crucial factor in determining a patient's suitability for surgery is body mass index (BMI). Although no threshold exists, BMI should be under or as close to 30 kg/m² preoperatively, because there is an increased risk of complications in patients who have a BMI above this threshold. Specifically, in the body contouring population, higher BMI at time of presentation is associated with increased complications.[17] Deformities can vary after weight loss so distribution of residual obesity is best evaluated on an individual basis. An example could be performing a patient with a BMI above 40 kg/m² who has difficulty ambulating secondary to a heavy, hanging panniculus that ulcerates and makes exercise difficult. Patients such as these should be optimized and offered a panniculectomy to motivate further weight loss. Such procedures should be focused and expedited to minimize complications in this patient population.

Medical, Surgical, and Social History

The surgeon must be conscientious that body contouring after weight loss is elective and should remind the patient as such. Even though surgery may be life-changing, it will likely never be life-saving as

TABLE 63.1. COMMON VITAMINS AND ELEMENTS THAT REQUIRE SUPPLEMENTATION AFTER BARIATRIC SURGERY[a]

Vitamin/ Mineral	Deficient Patients (%)[10,16-19]	Etiology of Malabsorption	Symptoms/Complications of Deficiency	Supplementation Recommendations[b]
Calcium	40%-50%	Absorption sites (duodenum and jejunum) bypassed	■ Muscle weakness/tetany ■ Osteoporosis	Calcium citrate 1500 mg PO daily
Iron (Fe)	25%-50%	Decreased gastric acid	■ Microcytic anemia ■ Fatigue ■ Generalized weakness	Iron sulfate 325 mg PO daily
Vitamin B_1 (thiamin)	20%-30%	Decreased oral intake; persistent nausea/vomiting	■ Neurologic manifestations ■ Wernicke encephalopathy ■ Beriberi	12 mg PO daily
Vitamin B_9 (folate)	30%-50%	Poor dietary intake	■ Thrombocytopenia ■ Changes in pigmentation or ulceration of skin or mucosa	500 μg PO daily
Vitamin B_{12}	10%-15%	Decreased intrinsic factor (produced in antrum of stomach) required for absorption in terminal ileum	■ Megaloblastic anemia ■ Peripheral neuropathy	PO: 500 μg daily IM or SQ: 1000 μg injection monthly
Vitamin D	20%-40%	Poor sun exposure	■ Osteoporosis ■ Increased risk of infection, chronic disease	Ergocalciferol (D_2) or cholecalciferol (D_3) 3000 IU PO daily
Zinc	20%-40%	Absorption sites (duodenum and jejunum) bypassed	■ Decrease immune system function ■ Poor wound healing ■ Hair loss ■ Folate deficiency	10 mg PO daily

[a]Signs of deficiency should be screened for at any visit to allow for correction before serious complications arise.

[b]These are recommendations for supplementation in a person with already-established normal levels of micronutrients based on the American Society for Metabolic Surgery.[20] In a patient with lower than reference range levels, patients require larger doses and closer monitoring. Recommendations for women attempting to get pregnant or currently pregnant are generally higher. This table is not all-encompassing, and there are several other doses and routes of administration for many of these supplements.

IM, intramuscular; IU, international units; PO, per os (oral); SQ, subcutaneous.

these patients are unlikely to suffer a mortality if they do not undergo surgery. With that in mind, modifiable risk factors should be maximally optimized before signing a patient up for these operations.

Use of nicotine products, as discussed in Chapter 16, is the single most easily modifiable risk factor. It is not advisable to operate on patients actively using any form of nicotine product as these procedures often have lengthy incisions that are at high risk for wound dehiscence or delayed healing.

History of previous surgeries should be elicited, and scars in the anatomical region of the procedure should be sought to avoid complications secondary to vascular compromise. Planned surgery on the abdomen should include a thorough examination of the abdominal wall and any potential hernias. Patients who have undergone adjustable gastric band (AGB) procedures should have a subcutaneous port on the abdominal wall, and this may need to be relocated intraoperatively.

Given that many of these procedures have a significant scar burden, patients must be willing to accept a trade-off of aesthetic result for a scar. Patients need to understand that there is a delicate balance between scar burden and aesthetic outcome, but certain deformities can only be corrected with a greater scar load.

Medications

Guidelines for management of medications for the body contouring patient in the perioperative period is akin to most patients, and is covered in Chapter 16. Additional care should be taken if patients are actively taking weight-loss drugs. Surgeons must ask about birth control or other hormone medications, as this is pertinent for calculating a Caprini score.

The surgeon must be aware of restrictions on postoperative medications in bariatric surgery patients. Patients who have undergone AGB must take oral medications in crushed, liquid, chewable, suspension, or sublingual forms. In those who have had Roux-en-Y gastric bypass, nonsteroidal antiinflammatory drugs are contraindicated due to the perceived risk of ulceration,[illegible] although this has not been studied.

Staging

Patients presenting after MWL usually have many areas in need of body contouring. It is best to have the patient prioritize the regions they desire corrected and, together with the surgeon, create a plan. Variables that may influence the timing and staging include the number of surgeons, procedure setting, regional laws, and the patient's financial resources. Procedures may have to be staged to minimize operative time and avoid opposite vectors of skin tightening. Some procedures may be combined safely, whereas certain procedures should not be combined in the same operative setting.[22,23] Given that many of these procedures are not covered by health insurance carriers, patients may space surgeries due to financial implications. Staging may not be a bad option, however, because it allows for minor revisions and corrections of areas previously operated on. Finally, patients generally desire new areas contoured after initial stages and may return to have other body regions corrected.[24]

For global body contouring, including procedures on the chest or breast, trunk, upper and lower extremities in a healthy patient without financial constraints, a two-stage approach may be used. A common two-stage practice involves a circumferential trunk procedure and upper body procedure such as either mastopexy or brachioplasty, followed later by the second stage to encompass the other upper body procedure and thigh lift. Unless extraordinary circumstances dictate a more accelerated timeline, surgeries should be spaced with a minimum of 3 months in between to allow for the tissues to heal, assessment of skin relaxation, and improved patient recovery.

Markings

Preoperative markings serve for surgeons either as an estimate that is verified intraoperatively or as the final cutting guide. Therefore, it is critical that the patient understand the markings and final scar placement. An easy approach is to mark the patient in clinic the day before surgery in front of a mirror and show the patient the expected scar location. This allows ample time for marking without interruptions, is less invasive and more comfortable for the patient than the holding area, and provides time for questions.

Special Considerations

Despite being already covered in Chapter 16, perhaps in no other patient is attention to certain perioperative factors as important as the MWL patient, namely venous thromboembolism (VTE) prophylaxis and intraoperative body temperature. For truncal reshaping procedures, some surgeons prefer to prep the patient while in the standing position, then have him or her move onto a sterile draped operating room table. Extremities should be prepped circumferentially for easy movement and access to all areas, permitting liposuction of other regions of the extremity or the excision site itself.

VTE Prophylaxis

Worthy of mention in the patient population is proper management of VTE prophylaxis. Risk of VTE in the post-MWL patient is around 3%, and the risk in those with a BMI over 35 kg/m^2 triples to approximately 9%.[25] Although no consensus guidelines exist for the post-MWL patient, the 2005 Caprini score should be used as a reference. At a minimum, either compression stockings or intermittent pneumatic compression devices should be applied throughout the patient's stay, and patient should be encouraged to ambulate on the evening of surgery.

Body Temperature

Given that hypothermia can increase complications postoperatively and body-contouring procedures often require exposure of a large body surface area, it is critical to take all possible precautions to avoid hypothermia.[illegible] Hypothermia is easier to treat before rather than after it sets in, so appropriate measures should be in place to prevent its occurrence. In addition to the methods described in Chapter 16, certain techniques can be employed in the MWL patient to decrease the risk. One technique involves making a sterile warming blanket sandwich, using a forced air heating pad interposed between two sterile drapes. In this manner, the entire surgical region may be prepped, but any areas not actively being operated on may be covered and warmed without interrupting the flow of the procedure.

COMPLICATIONS

Even though postoperative complications in the MWL population can be quite frequent, fortunately they are usually minor and amenable to treatment on an outpatient basis. Most commonly observed are delayed wound healing and wound dehiscence, underscoring the importance of preoperative nutrition optimization. Wound breakdown should be presumed to be a result of nutritional deficiency until proven otherwise. Another common complication is seroma, which can be decreased with drain use. If drain output continues to preclude removal of drains, chemical sclerosis can be performed. If drains were not used or a seroma appears after drain removal, percutaneous needle aspiration can be done up to three times, after which time placement of a seroma catheter is recommended. Rarely, the patient may require reoperation to excise the seroma cavity.

Systemic complications tend to be more serious and can range from VTE to death. Early serious surgical site complications that may require intervention include hematoma, which may require operative drainage; surgical site infection, necessitating oral or intravenous antibiotics; nerve injuries, possibly needing exploration in the operating room. Late surgical site complications include scar widening or hypertrophy, as well as chronic draining wounds or sinus tracts. Surgery on the extremities can lead to lymphedema, with the lower extremities more commonly affected.

Postoperative numbness of the surgical site is normally transient and resolves with time. If a nerve injury is identified intraoperatively, it should be repaired. If a patient complains of numbness postoperatively, it is expected to resolve with time, sometimes taking up to a year. However, if a patient reports numbness in a nerve outside of the zone of operation, such as an ulnar nerve neuropathy during abdominoplasty, this is more likely to be related to improper positioning or padding of the nerve intraoperatively. These nerve symptoms generally resolve spontaneously, although patients require reassurance throughout this period.

The most feared complication of body contouring surgery is resecting so much tissue that closure becomes impossible with the tissue left behind. This is prevented by use of judicious measuring and resection of tissue. The best practice to avoid this complication is by verifying the marks several times, and by committing to only one margin of resection and raising flaps toward the opposite margin until these edges can be brought together without undue tension.

OUTCOMES

Studies have shown that, overall, patients who have body contouring after weight loss have better quality of life (QoL) outcome measures as compared to weight loss patients who do not undergo plastic surgery. Body contouring after MWL provides patients with improved self-esteem, social life, work ability, and sexual and physical activity.[28] Specifically, after lower body lift, patients have higher levels of self-esteem and self-confidence and feel more attractive.[29] These improved QoL measures persisted for years after plastic surgery.

REFERENCES

1. Constantine RS, Davis KE, Kenkel JM. The effect of massive weight loss status, amount of weight loss, and method of weight loss on body contouring outcomes. *Aesthet Surg J*. 2014;34(4):578-583.
   This study examined the differences in complication rates between MWL and non-MWL patients undergoing the same procedures. Results from 450 patients showed that those who lost more than 100 lb of weight were in the highest risk category.
2. Chetta MD, Aliu O, Tran BA, et al. Complications in body contouring stratified according to weight loss method. *Plast Surg (Oakv)*. 2016;24(2):103-106.
3. Bond DS, Phelan S, Leahey TM, et al. Weight-loss maintenance in successful weight losers: surgical vs non-surgical methods. *Int J Obes (Lond)*. 2009;33(1):173-180.
4. Van Way CW III. Nutritional support in the injured patient. *Surg Clin North Am*. 1991;71(3):537-548.
5. Halverson JD. Metabolic risk of obesity surgery and long-term follow-up. *Am J Clin Nutr*. 1992;55(2 suppl):602S-605S.
6. van der Beek ES, Monpellier VM, Eland I, et al. Nutritional deficiencies in gastric bypass patients; incidence, time of occurrence and implications for postoperative surveillance. *Obes Surg*. 2015;25(5):818-823.
7. Stein J, Stier C, Raab H, Weiner R. The nutritional and pharmacological consequences of obesity surgery. *Aliment Pharmacol Ther*. 2014;40(6):582-609.
8. Agha-Mohammadi S, Hurwitz DJ. Potential impacts of nutritional deficiency of postbariatric patients on body contouring surgery. *Plast Reconstr Surg*. 2008;122(6):1901-1914.
9. Austin RE, Lista F, Khan A, Ahmad J. The impact of protein nutritional supplementation for massive weight loss patients undergoing abdominoplasty. *Aesthet Surg J*. 2016;36:204-210.
10. Naghshineh N, O'Brien Coon D, McTigue K, et al. Nutritional assessment of bariatric surgery patients presenting for plastic surgery: a prospective analysis. *Plast Reconstr Surg*. 2010;126(2):602-610.
    A prospective study examining nutritional status of 100 consecutive patients presenting for plastic surgery after bariatric surgery. Eighty percent of patients had inadequate protein intake. The most common deficiency was iron deficiency anemia, with almost 40% of patients.
11. Zimmermann MB, Hurrell RF. Nutritional iron deficiency. *Lancet*. 2007;370:511-520.
12. Gibbs J, Cull W, Henderson W, et al. Preoperative serum albumin level as a predictor of operative mortality and morbidity: results from the National VA Surgical Risk Study. *Arch Surg*. 1999;134(1):36-42.
13. Correia MI, Waitzberg DL. The impact of malnutrition on morbidity, mortality, length of hospital stay and costs evaluated through a multivariate model analysis. *Clin Nutr*. 2003;22(3):235-239.
14. Sebastian JL, V JM, Tang LW, Rubin JP. Thiamine deficiency in a gastric bypass patient leading to acute neurologic compromise after plastic surgery. *Surg Obes Relat Dis*. 2010;6:105-106.
15. Gardiner S, Hartzell T. Thiamine deficiency: a cause of profound hypotension and hypothermia after plastic surgery. *Aesthet Surg J*. 2015;35(1):NP1-NP3.
16. Carlin AM, Rao DS, Meslemani AM, et al. Prevalence of vitamin D depletion among morbidly obese patients seeking gastric bypass surgery. *Surg Obes Relat Dis*. 2006;2:98-103.
17. Coon D, Gusenoff JA, Kannan N, et al. Body mass and surgical complications in the postbariatric reconstructive patient: analysis of 511 cases. *Ann Surg*. [illegible]
    A study examining differences between body contouring patients undergoing single versus multiple operations in a single setting. 449 patients were included, and complications were correlated with current and maximum BMIs in the single procedure group, but with change in BMI in the multiple procedure group.
18. Gletsu-Miller N, Wright BN. Mineral malnutrition following bariatric surgery. *Adv Nutr*. 2013;4(5):506-517.
19. Clements RH, Yellumahanthi K, Wesley M, et al. Hyperparathyroidism and vitamin D deficiency after laparoscopic gastric bypass. *Am Surg*. 2008;74(6):469-474.
20. Parrott J, Frank L, Rabena R, et al. American Society for Metabolic and Bariatric Surgery Integrated Health Nutritional Guidelines for the surgical weight loss patient 2016 update: micronutrients. *Surg Obes Relat Dis*. 2017;13(5):727-741.
21. Mechanick JI, Kushner RF, Sugerman HJ, et al. American Association of Clinical Endocrinologists, The Obesity Society, and American Society for Metabolic & Bariatric Surgery medical guidelines for clinical practice for the perioperative nutritional, metabolic, and nonsurgical support of the bariatric surgery patient. *Surg Obes Relat Dis*. 2008;4(5 suppl):S109-S184.
22. Coon D, Michaels J IV, Gusenoff JA, et al. Multiple procedures and staging in the massive weight loss population. *Plast Reconstr Surg*. 2010;125(2):691-698.
    Looking at 609 patients undergoing body contouring after MWL, the authors showed that the per-procedure complication rate was the same whether performing one or many procedures in the same stage.
23. Pascal JF, Le Louarn C. Remodeling bodylift with high lateral tension. *Aesthetic Plast Surg*. 2002;26(3):223-230.
24. Song AY, Rubin JP, Thomas V, et al. Body image and quality of life in post massive weight loss body contouring patients. *Obesity (Silver Spring)*. 2006;14(9):1626-1636.
25. Shermak MA, Chang DC, Heller J. Factors impacting thromboembolism after bariatric body contouring surgery. *Plast Reconstr Surg*. 2007;119(5):1590-1596.
    The authors looked at their 10-year experience with 129 patients having body contouring after MWL. BMI was the leading risk factor, and recommendations for prophylaxis are discussed.
26. Kurz A, Sessler DI, Lenhardt R. Perioperative normothermia to reduce the incidence of surgical-wound infection and shorten hospitalization: study of wound infection and temperature group. *N Engl J Med*. 1996;334(19):1209-1215.
27. Coon D, Michaels J IV, Gusenoff JA, et al. Hypothermia and complications in postbariatric body contouring. *Plast Reconstr Surg*. 2012;130(2):443-448.
28. Modarressi A, Balagué N, Huber O, et al. Plastic surgery after gastric bypass improves long-term quality of life. *Obes Surg*. 2013;23(1):24-30.
29. Vierhapper MF, Pittermann A, Hacker S, Kitzinger HB. Patient satisfaction, body image, and quality of life after lower body lift: a prospective pre- and postoperative long-term survey. *Surg Obes Relat Dis*. 2017;13(5):882-887.

QUESTIONS

1. **A 45-year-old woman presents for abdominoplasty. She has two children delivered via C-section and desires improved abdominal contour. She smokes half a pack of cigarettes a day but is otherwise healthy. Which of the following is the best approach to her operative management?**
   a. Ask her to quit and proceed with surgery next week
   b. Deny her surgery for her smoking habit
   c. Proceed with surgery since half a pack of cigarettes a day is not detrimental
   d. Refer her to another physician willing to operate on smokers
   e. Wait until she has stopped smoking for 4 weeks and check her urine cotinine before proceeding with surgery

2. **A 37-year-old woman presents to your clinic desiring correction of breast ptosis and abdominal skin laxity. She underwent laparoscopic Roux-en-Y gastric bypass surgery 6 months ago and reports her weight has been stable for the past month. Her BMI in your office is 33 kg/m². She has no other significant medical problems and she would like both procedures at the same stage. What is the best management of this patient?**
   a. Defer surgery until her weight has been stable for a minimum of 3 months
   b. Defer surgery until she is 1-year postbariatric surgery
   c. Perform the abdominoplasty first to promote further weight loss, then the mastopexy in a second stage
   d. Proceed with surgery as soon as possible

3. **A 41-year-old man presents after losing 50 kg through diet and exercise. He has gynecomastia as depicted in Figure 63.1. On physical examination, there is significant fibrous tissue in the retroareolar region. What is the best treatment option for this patient?**
   a. Inframammary fold excision with free nipple graft
   b. Liposuction only
   c. Periareolar incision, direct excision
   d. Wise-pattern reduction

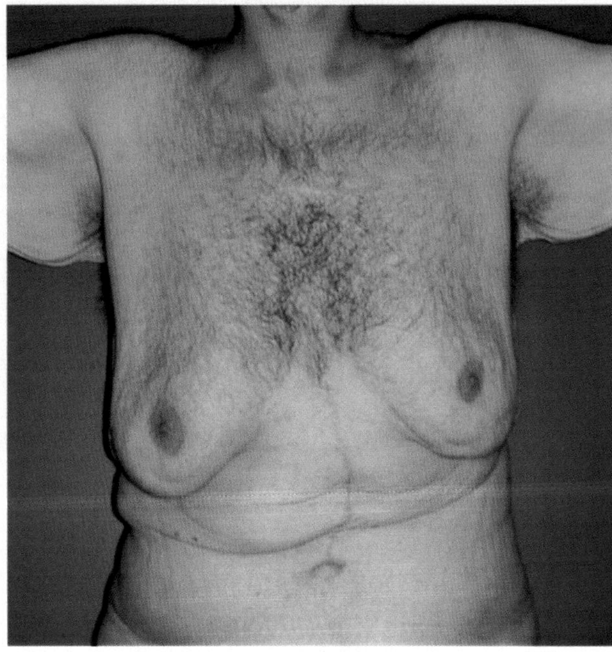

FIGURE 63.1.

4. **What is the appropriate antibiotic and dose for preoperative prophylaxis in a 50-year-old man who has no known drug allergies and weighs 128 kg?**
   a. Cefazolin 2 g
   b. Cefazolin 3 g
   c. Clindamycin 600 mg
   d. Clindamycin 900 mg
   e. Vancomycin 1500 mg

1. **Answer: e.** Smoking is a modifiable risk factor that can reduce complications after surgery. Nicotine can lead to vasoconstriction and reduced oxygenation of healing tissues, leading to increases in wound healing problems and infection. The best option is to counsel the patient to stop and check her urine for smoking 2 weeks before surgery. Urine cotinine tests can take up to 10 days to get the results, so it should not be used close to the surgical date. Many surgeons advise smoking cessation for 4 weeks before and after surgery. Having a smoking policy in place can avoid postoperative complications.

2. **Answer: a.** Patients who present after MWL, regardless of weight method, should have a stable weight for at least 3 months before undergoing a body contouring procedure. Patients often lose weight and reach plateaus at several points in their weight loss cycle then go on to lose again; therefore, a one-month period is of insufficient length to deem stable. In addition, further weight loss will surely improve this patient's BMI, perhaps even bringing it below 30 kg/m², reducing her risk substantially.

3. **Answer: a.** In a patient with excess bulk and a long nipple to inframammary fold distance such as the one pictured, a direct excision with free nipple graft is needed to remove the tissue and move the nipple-areola complex (NAC) to the proper location on the chest wall. Liposuction only or direct excision would be insufficient to treat the excess tissue or move the NAC to the correct location, or both. A pedicled reduction would be too bulky to fit the pedicle under the skin envelope.

4. **Answer: b.** The correct dosing for a patient who has no allergy to penicillin or cephalosporins is 2 g in patients under 120 kg of weight and 3 g in patients over 120 kg of weight. Clindamycin 600 mg is no longer recommended, and the standard dose for patients with a true cephalosporin allergy is 900 mg. In special circumstances, including a history of methicillin-resistant *Staphylococcus aureus* infection, vancomycin 1500 mg should be used.

CHAPTER 64 Liposuction, Abdominoplasty, and Belt Lipectomy

Terri A. Zomerlei and Jeffrey E. Janis

KEY POINTS

- Selection of the correct body contouring procedure—liposuction versus skin resection technique—is essential to optimize outcomes.
- Obtain a thorough personal and family medical history to appropriately calculate the patient's venous thromboembolism risk and plan mechanical and chemoprophylaxis for prevention of VTE.
- Perform anatomic based markings to keep incisions in cosmetically acceptable locations.
- Be mindful of zones of adherence.
- Decrease potential complications by proper positioning and padding and preventing hypothermia, calculating local anesthetic dosing, and respecting blood supply and previous scars.

Selection of the appropriate body contouring procedure(s) is based on the presence and degree of skin and adipose excess. Body contouring procedures are not strictly for weight reduction and patients should be counseled in this regard.

LIPOSUCTION

Liposuction, the surgical aspiration of fat from the subcutaneous plane, is one of the most popular procedures performed by plastic surgeons. The first description of surgically removing fat for body contouring is from the 1920s. Dr. Dujarrier, an obstetrician and surgeon, utilized a uterine curette to remove fat from the knees of a ballerina resulting in catastrophic complications and eventual leg amputation. Modern liposuction became popularized in the 1970s by Drs. Illouz, Fournier, and Otteni. The key advancements and contributions by these surgeons were the use of a wetting solution, blunt cannulas, and negative pressure evacuation. This greatly improved the safety of the procedure.[1]

Patient Selection and Evaluation

Suction-assisted lipectomy, or liposuction, is indicated for removal of localized excess adipose tissue or *lipodystrophy* ideally in areas with good overlying skin quality and minimal excess skin. The patient's motivation and surgical expectations should be garnered early in the consultation process to sort out those with unrealistic expectations or mental disorders such as body dysmorphic disorder.

A thorough medical history should be obtained on all patients. Nonessential supplements and vitamins should be discontinued 3 weeks prior to surgery. Medications that could interfere with lidocaine metabolism (such as psychotropics) should be noted.[2] Patients with a history of nicotine use or poorly controlled diabetes should be counseled on the increased risk of wound healing complications, and strong consideration should be given to deferring their procedures until they have had nicotine cessation for 4 weeks prior to the proposed elective operation (compliance can be tested with a urine cotinine test) and an A1C of less than 7.5.[3,4] In those patients who will be receiving large-volume liposuction (defined as aspiration of greater than 5 L), a complete blood count should be performed preoperatively. In addition, assessing personal and family history of bleeding problems, blood clots, and miscarriages is important. The practitioner should obtain labs and/or hematology consultation as appropriate so that venous thromboembolism (VTE) prevention is optimized.

Liposuction should not be offered as a treatment for global obesity or cellulite, and ideally patients should be within 30% or their ideal body weight.[5] Women typically have a gynoid pattern of fat distribution with accumulation in the lower trunk, hips, upper thighs, and buttocks. Men often exhibit an android fat accumulation pattern with increased abdominal girth, thickened torso, and upper abdomen. During examination of the abdomen, particular attention should be paid to any surgical scars that can affect blood supply and also signal possible hernias.[4] A Valsalva maneuver or having the patient perform a small *sit-up* should reveal the presence of any hernias. Obtain a computed tomography (CT) scan, if needed. During the examination, the presence and extent of a diastasis recti should also be evaluated in addition to assessing the degree of visceral versus external fat. Location of adipose deposits and asymmetries should also be noted and discussed with the patient. Skin quality and quantity should also be assessed noting that those with good skin quality will have more optimal results.

Pertinent Anatomy

Thorough understanding of the pertinent anatomy is essential for effective liposuction treatment. The subcutaneous adipose tissue is supported and separated into compartments and layers by a fibrous network called the superficial fascial system.[6,7] The adipose tissue in a given region can roughly be divided into two layers:

- *Superficial layer:* Dense fat, contained within tight septae and adherent to the dermis. This layer is most susceptible to contour irregularities.
- *Deep layer:* Loose fat and less compact. This is the safest layer to suction.

Zones of adherence are recognized regions in which the subcutaneous tissues are securely adherent to the deep fascia. Liposuction should be avoided or used with extreme caution in these areas as the risk of contour irregularities is high[5] (Figure 64.1):

- Gluteal crease
- Lateral gluteal depression
- Middle medial thigh
- Distal iliotibial tract
- Distal posterior thigh

Marking, Positioning, and Safety

Patients should be marked in the standing position with an indelible marker. Areas to be suctioned are marked with concentric circles in a topographical pattern, typically with an X at the most protuberant point. Zones of adherence are noted and are marked with straight parallel lines or hash marks. Natural creases should be noted, as these will be optimal areas to perform the incisions for liposuction to minimize visibility[5] (see Figure 64.1).

Safety is of utmost importance in surgery, and several precautions should be taken with liposuction procedures.[8] With large areas of the body usually exposed for the liposuction procedure, care should be taken to avoid intraoperative hypothermia. Intravenous fluids (IVFs)

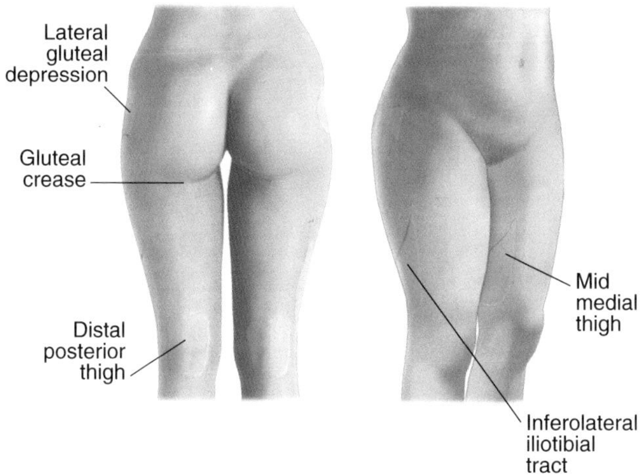

FIGURE 64.1. In addition to surrounding the superficial fat layer, the superficial fascial system sends components through the deep fat compartment attaching to the investing fascia of the underlying musculature. These extensions, where the superficial subcutaneous plane is adherent to the underlying muscle fascia, are collectively called zones of adherence. These zones, which include the lateral gluteal depression, the gluteal crease, the distal posterior thigh, middle medial thigh, and inferolateral iliotibial tract, are much more susceptible to contour irregularities.

and wetting solutions should be warmed. Forced warm air blankets should be placed over areas not being suctioned, and the ambient room temperature can be raised. Pressure points should be appropriately padded, as improper pressure on the neurovascular structures in the body can lead to short- or long-term disability. Padding and flexion of the arm and elbow less than 90 degrees and use of an axillary roll in the lateral decubitus position reduces the risk of upper extremity nerve compression. The surgeon should work closely with the anesthesia provider to ensure that the patient's eyes are protected, the head is supported, and the neck is in a neutral position. In the prone position, a soft hip roll placed beneath the iliac crests aids in elevating treatment areas off the operative table. If the patient will be repositioned during the procedure, close attention should be paid to careful choreography of all details.

Body contouring operations such as liposuction and abdominoplasty have a higher incidence of venous thrombotic complications than other plastic surgery procedures. In 2011, the American Society of Plastic Surgeons Venous Thromboembolism Task Force recommended a stepwise approach for plastic surgery patients that includes:[9]

- Preoperative risk stratification
- Prevention with mechanical and/or chemoprophylaxis
- Patient education

At minimum, patients undergoing liposuction should have pneumatic compression stockings in place (if the leg is not being treated). The use of chemoprophylaxis will depend on the preoperative risk stratification.

Wetting Solution and Fluid Management

First introduced by Illouz, the advent of the use of wetting solution has greatly improved the safety of liposuction.[1] Wetting solutions can be a variable composition but usually include saline or lactated Ringer's, lidocaine, epinephrine, and sometimes sodium bicarbonate. The wetting solution has multiple functions and aids with anesthesia, hemostasis, and emulsification of adipocytes. There has been an evolution of wetting solution techniques that have helped decrease blood loss (**Table 64.1**).[10-12] The desired wetting solution composition and amount is instilled into the treatment area via a fine infiltration cannula through a small stab incision that will also function as the liposuction port. Ideally, the fluid resides at least

TABLE 64.1. COMMONLY USED WETTING SOLUTION TECHNIQUES[a]

Technique	Infiltrate Volume	Estimated Blood Loss (as % of Aspirate Volume) (%)
Dry	No infiltrate	~20–40
Wet	200–300 mL/area	~25
Superwet	1 mL infiltrate: 1 mL aspirate	~1–4
Tumescent	To skin turgor 2–3 mL infiltrate: 1 mL aspirate	~1

[a]The essential difference among these techniques centers on the amount of solution infused into the tissue and the resultant blood loss with aspiration.

7 to 10 minutes in the tissue for optimal vasoconstrictive effect. High lidocaine doses can result in severe systemic complications. Traditionally, maximal lidocaine dosing is 7 mg/kg. In wetting solution, however, much higher doses, up to 35 mg/kg, have been reported as safe. The maximal safe dose of lidocaine should be calculated for each patient.[12-14]

Intraoperatively, appropriate fluid administration and balance is critical.[15] This will include IVF administration to replace preoperative deficit and to provide appropriate maintenance fluids, which can vary depending on whether the patient is undergoing large-volume liposuction. Clear communication with anesthesia staff is essential.

Treatment Types

Once the patient has been deemed an appropriate candidate for adipose reduction, technique selection is the next step. Current options for traditional liposuction include suction-assisted liposuction (SAL), power-assisted liposuction (PAL), ultrasound-assisted liposuction (UAL), and laser-assisted liposuction (LAL). SAL is the most frequently utilized modality among plastic surgeons.

Traditional Liposuction

SAL is a two-stage technique that requires infiltration of wetting solution followed by suction evacuation. This technique is popular because of its lower cost of equipment investment, ease of use, and reliability. However, SAL is more labor-intensive and does not perform as well on areas with fibrous fat.

PAL is a technique that uses a variable- speed motor that provides oscillation in a reciprocating motion at rates of 4000 to 6000 cycles per minute. Because PAL can break up fibrous fat more readily, this modality can significantly cut down on physician fatigue due to shorter procedure times and employing less physical labor to use.

UAL applies ultrasonic energy to break down fat and facilitate suction aspiration. UAL works to emulsify the fat by three mechanisms:[16,17]

- *Mechanical*: direct tissue effects by the ultrasound wave; this is the primary mechanism
- *Cavitation*: tissue fragments based on the formation and collapse of intracellular microbubbles
- *Thermal*: absorption of the ultrasound waves produces heat

Treatment with UAL involves three stages:

1. Infiltration of wetting solution
2. Emulsification with ultrasound treatment
3. Evacuation of emulsified fat and final contouring

With the use of smaller cannulas and conservative ultrasound application times, the frequently cited complications of UAL (contour deformities and thermal injury) can be avoided.

LAL uses a small laser fiber to emulsify fat and tighten skin. A four-step technique is used:

1. Infiltration
2. Application of energy to the tissue
3. Evacuation
4. Subdermal skin stimulation

This treatment modality is purported to have the benefit of skin tightening. However, several well-designed studies have failed to show a significant benefit over SAL.[18]

Peer-reviewed studies failed to show consistent evidence-based benefits for the use of UAL and LAL over SAL. The aesthetic outcomes, patient satisfaction, and incidences of long-term complications appear to be more related to technique and not technology. As a result, SAL/PAL remains the leading techniques employed.[18]

Surgical endpoints for liposuction can be divided into primary and secondary endpoints and depend on the treatment modality used:

Primary endpoints

- SAL/PAL: contour, symmetrical pinch test, and presence of bloody aspirate
- UAL: loss of tissue resistance, contour, and presence of bloody aspirate

Secondary endpoints

- SAL/PAL/UAL: treatment time and volume

Cryolipolysis

In select patients who prefer to avoid surgery for adipose reduction, treatment with cryolipolysis may be employed. Cryolipolysis is a noninvasive technique to destroy adipose cells through administration of controlled thermal reduction via a specialized machine.[19,20] Because of their susceptibility, exposure of adipose cells to below normal temperatures (+5° to −5°C) results in apoptosis-mediated cell death with preservation of overlying skin integrity. The subsequent inflammatory cascade results in removal of the damaged cells over the course of 3 months. The most common complication following cryolipolysis is hypoesthesia of the treatment area that usually resolves over several months. Other less common complications include surface contour irregularities, chronic pain, and rarely, paradoxical adipose hyperplasia.[21]

Technique

Once the wetting solution has been instilled and allowed sufficient time for effect, the liposuction cannula is introduced. The cannula is inserted into the access incision(s) and using even strokes, the cannula is moved in a fanlike pattern. The deep plane is suctioned first, with the dominant hand guiding the liposuction cannula and the nondominant hand overlying the treatment area, providing stereotactic feedback on the cannula location and depth.

To mitigate the most frequently cited liposuction complication, contour irregularities, careful attention to technique is important. *Cross-hatching* or *cross-tunneling* is the method of using the liposuction cannula via multiple access sites to create intersecting sets of parallel lines over the treated area. This helps to ensure the tissue is suctioned more symmetrically and evenly.

In 2016, Wall proposed a multistep process for nonthermal comprehensive fat management that focuses on minimizing tissue injury and prevention of contour irregularities.[22] The SAFE (separation-aspiration-fat equalization) liposuction technique is based on the following principles:

- Optimize fat removal
- Provide comprehensive means of body contouring
- Preserve vascular integrity
- Maximize skin retraction
- Minimize potential for complications/revisions

Briefly, the separation step uses an exploded-tip (basket-tip) cannula with no suction to separate and mechanically emulsify the fat. This step comprises 40% of the operating time and addresses both the superficial and deep fat compartments. Aspiration is then performed with less aggressive cannulas. This step should take approximately another 40% of the procedural time. The last step, fat equalization, again uses an exploded tip without suction. During this step, the fat layer evens out the thicker and thinner areas that may exist.

An extension of the SAFE liposuction technique utilizes the aspirated fat to perform expansion vibration liposuction of the gluteal area.[23] This technique utilizes exploded liposuction tip and other nondisposable existing instrumentation. Close attention is given to patient safety and avoiding critical structures when lipofilling.

Large-Volume Liposuction

The ASPS Patient Safety Committee has recommended, when the anticipated lipoaspirate amount is expected to be greater than 5 L, several precautions should be taken. For safety reasons, the procedure should be performed in a hospital setting as opposed to an ambulatory surgical center. In addition, fluid shifts with large-volume liposuction can be significant, and thus specific fluid replacements should be performed.

Maintenance IVF should be administered up to 5 L. Every 1 mL of aspirate beyond 5 L should be replaced with 0.25 mL of IVF. Overnight monitoring of fluid balance (based on vital signs and urinary output) should be considered.[24]

Treatment Areas

Many areas of the body can be treated with liposuction. The practitioner should keep in mind ideal aesthetic contours based on gender.

Arms

The upper arm can be contoured with liposuction alone or with concomitant brachioplasty to resect excess skin (see Chapter 65).[25] Liposuction of the tissues that will be excised can facilitate direction of the tissues. Adiposity is usually focused at the posterior third of the arm and can be addressed through access points on the distal radial side of the arm. The ulnar nerve can be superficial near the elbow and could be inadvertently injured during the procedure. In addition, the medial antebrachial nerve pierces the fascia of the arm approximately 14 cm proximal to the medial epicondyle and is susceptible to injury in this area. The ideal aesthetic arm is lean with merging deltoid and biceps convexities.

Back

The back anatomy is characterized by a thick dermis and fibrous, dense fat. Lipodystrophy of the back tends to result in folds, especially inferior to the *bra line*. Improved contour can be obtained when the fibrous attachments creating the folds are disrupted. The *buffalo hump* is an enlargement of the dorsocervical fat pad and can be present because of genetics, certain medical conditions, or medication use. In appropriate candidates, this area can be successfully liposuctioned. Because of the dense nature of this fat, UAL is a commonly employed technique for this area.

Abdomen

Lipodystrophy in the abdomen is predominantly in the infraumbilical region. Care must be taken to ensure no hernias are present. In cases of significant excess skin or poor overlying skin quality with poor elasticity, skin resection techniques are indicated. Ideal abdominal contour is gender-dependent, with the female aesthetic having an hourglass figure defined by the flanks and a slight supraumbilical concavity and infraumbilical convexity. Men should have no flare at the iliac crest and the infraumbilical area should be flat.

In a leaner patient, improved body contour can be achieved with high definition liposuction or etching. With this method, the fat in the superficial plane is liposuctioned to improve or provide the appearance of muscular definition. This technique can be used in conjunction with focused fat transfer. This technique should be used only by the trained practitioner as there is a high risk for contour irregularities.[26]

Hips/Flanks

These areas are treated most often in the prone or lateral decubitus positions. There are gender aesthetic differences and fat distribution tendencies that must be taken into consideration when treating this area. In women, the adipose deposits are commonly in the hip overlying the iliac crest and extending down to the lateral thigh zone of adherence. In contrast, the men tend to have adiposity in the *flank* or lateral lumbar area.

Buttocks/Thigh

There are also gender differences in the ideal gluteal region aesthetic. Women desire a rounded more protuberant buttock without ptosis that merges with lateral thigh. Male gluteal area aesthetic is flatter and angular with a squared off lateral contour. The fat in the gluteal area is denser and fibrous. The thigh is a difficult area for liposuction because of the circumferential approach that is usually required. In addition, zones of adherence and natural creases (gluteal crease) need to be recognized and appreciated. Overzealous suctioning in the buttock can result in ptosis and in the thigh can lead to unflattering skin redundancy. For this reason, liposuction in these areas should be approached with caution.

Postoperative Care

Following a liposuction procedure, massage excess wetting solution out of access incisions and either close primarily with suture or leave open, if small enough. Absorbent dressings are applied along with a compression garment. The dressing can be changed as needed for drainage and the compression garment should be worn at all times except during showering. Various lengths of time have been proposed for length of time to wear compression garments but most advocate a duration of 2 to 4 weeks.

Complications

Postoperative complications following liposuction can roughly be divided into *early* and *late* complications. Patients should be aware that postoperative edema and ecchymosis are an *expected* side effect of the procedure and occur to varying degrees in all patients.

Early Complications

- Inadequate fluid resuscitation: communication with anesthesia team is vital
- Sinus tachycardia: can develop after administration of wetting solution because of the epinephrine effect
- Injury to solid organs, bowel, or blood vessels: always be aware of the plane the cannula is in
- Hypothermia: use warming techniques
- Skin slough: local wound care
- VTE: the most common cause of death following liposuction. Risk for this complication increases with large-volume aspirate (>5 L), increased wetting solution infiltration
- LAST (local anesthetic system toxicity): begins with symptoms of central nervous system excitation such as perioral numbness, lightheaded, and dizziness. Can progress with seizures and cardiac arrest. Calculate safe lidocaine dosing prior to procedure. Treat with ABCs of resuscitation and lipid emulsion infusion.[27]

Late Complications

- Neurapraxia: motor weakness or sensory disturbance (numbness/pain) after liposuction. Should observe and reassure the patient. Should resolve within 3 to 4 months.
- Contour irregularities: this is the most common postoperative complication and can occur in up to 20% of patients. Techniques to help prevent include use of small cannulas, multiple access incisions, and cross-tunneling. Treatment of irregularities requires secondary fat equalization and fat grafting to oversuctioned regions, if needed.

Conclusion

Liposuction is artistry as well as surgery. It entails a practical application of anatomic knowledge with precision and craftsmanship and is a skill that can be attained and refined with clinical experience.

ABDOMINOPLASTY

Abdominoplasty is a procedure that removes excess skin and fat and, in most cases, restores the rectus muscle to a more anatomical position, creating an abdominal profile that is smoother and firmer. Abdominoplasty outcomes can be optimized and complication reduced with a strong understanding of the anatomy.

Pertinent Anatomy

The abdominal wall is composed of seven layers:

- Skin
- Subcutaneous fat (superficial layer of fat—thicker and dense)
- Scarpa fascia (superficial fascial system)
- Subscarpal layer (deep layer of fat—less dense)
- Anterior rectus sheath
- Muscle
- Posterior rectus sheath

There are four paired muscle groups that comprise the abdominal wall:

- Rectus abdominis
- External oblique
- Internal oblique
- Transversus abdominis

The aponeurotic portion of the oblique muscles and the transversus abdominis envelope the rectus muscles forming the anterior and posterior rectus sheaths. The composition of the anterior and posterior sheaths varies in relation to the arcuate line. The sheaths meet in the midline forming the linea alba. Pregnancy and weight gain can result in a separation of the rectus muscles in the midline termed a diastasis rectus.

The vascular perfusion of the abdomen is supplied by the deep epigastric arcade, the superficial epigastric arcade, and contributions of the intercostal and subcostal vessels bilaterally. The regional blood supply to the abdomen is defined by three zones, first elucidated by Huger[28]:

- Zone I is the midabdomen, supplied by deep superficial and deep inferior epigastric arcades.
- Zone II is the lower abdomen and is supplied by the superficial and deep circumflex arteries.
- Zone III is the lateral abdomen and is supplied by the intercostal, subcostal, and lumbar arteries.

Prior to abdominoplasty, the major blood supply to the abdomen is from zone I. Following abdominoplasty, zone I blood supply is lost and the abdominoplasty flap is predominantly supplied via zone III segmental perforators with minor collateral flow from zone II.

There are several sensory nerves that supply the abdominal wall (**Table 64.2**). In abdominoplasty, the lateral femoral cutaneous nerve emerges into the superficial plane approximately 2 cm medial to the anterior superior iliac spine (ASIS), and therefore, dissection in this area should be superficial to reduce the risk of meralgia paresthetica, a syndrome characterized by tingling, burning, and numbness in the lateral thigh.

TABLE 64.2. NERVES AT RISK FOR INJURY DURING AN ABDOMINOPLASTY

Nerve	Danger Zone	Symptoms of Injury
Lateral femoral cutaneous	Passes through inguinal ligament 1 cm medial to ASIS	Numbness/pain along anterolateral thigh
Iliohypogastric	Lateral aspect of low horizontal incision near inguinal ligament	Numbness/pain along the inguinal crease and lateral gluteal region
Ilioinguinal	Lateral aspect of low horizontal incision near inguinal ligament	Numbness along the medial thigh and scrotum/labia
Intercostal	Plane between the internal oblique and transversus abdominis. Lateral branches penetrate fascia at midaxillary line and travel in subcutaneous tissues	Numbness in abdominal/flank dermatome

ASIS, anterior superior iliac spine.

The umbilicus is located at or near the midline at the level of the iliac crests. The umbilicus is the central focus of the abdomen. The ideal umbilicus has superior hooding, round or oval shape, is shallow, and has inferior retraction. The blood supply is based on the subdermal plexus, the ligamentum teres remnant, and perforators from the deep inferior epigastric system.

Patient Selection and Evaluation

Pertinent history to obtain from patients seeking abdominoplasty include gravidity and parity history, previous abdominal surgeries (including cesarean sections), history of weight loss/gain, gastrointestinal or respiratory ailments, and tobacco abuse. Patients should be nicotine free for a minimum of 4 weeks prior to and after an abdominoplasty to minimize postoperative complications. Compliance can be tested with a urine cotinine test.[3,4]

On examination, assess for the presence of hernias (order a CT if needed) and take note of the excess fat and skin, skin tone and appearance, and the presence of scars.[29,30] Small hernias may be addressed at the time of abdominoplasty depending on the surgeon's comfort level. The amount and location of excess fat and skin will aid in determining the best technique to address the abdomen. Patients with striae, which represents a thinning or rupture of the dermal layer, must be counseled that an abdominoplasty will remove stria located inferior to the umbilicus but those located supraumbilically may be made worse by the procedure. Scars may limit the movement of the abdominal skin flap and a subcostal scar has potential to compromise the vascular supply to the skin flap. Examination of the patient should also include assessment of myofascial laxity via a diver's test (worsening lower abdominal fullness with flexion at the waist) and a pinch test (assessing abdominal fullness with the abdomen both relaxed and tensed). When the patient is supine, tensing of the abdominal muscles with a small *sit-up* should reveal a diastasis rectus if present.

Marking, Positioning, and Safety

Patients should wear an undergarment or swim bottom of choice to their operation so that the incision can be planned with minimal exposure. Anatomical points should be marked including the xiphoid, midline, ASIS, and pubic bone. Previous scars should be marked. The lower excision should be at least 5 to 7 cm above the vulvar commissure and should be below any cesarean scar if possible. The upper marking is made based on pinch test of the abdomen both centrally and laterally. This marking should come down inferior to the ASIS to minimize visibility.

Prior to entering the operating room, the operative table should be checked that it is able to flex. The patient should be padded appropriately, and previously described measures to minimize hypothermia should be employed. Sequential compression stocking should be applied. Data accrued by the American Association for Accreditation of Ambulatory Surgery Facilities (AAAASF) from 2001 to 2006 indicate abdominoplasty is the procedure with the highest frequency of death due to pulmonary embolism (PE). All patients undergoing abdominoplasty should be carefully risk stratified and at minimal receive sequential compression stockings.[9,31] Any excessive hair can be clipped and the patient is prepped with a wide field ensuring that the umbilicus is free from debris.

Operative Options and Techniques

There are a variety of abdominoplasty techniques that can be employed to improve the contour of the abdomen. Selecting the correct procedure is based upon the examination of the amount and distribution of excess fat and skin, assessment of skin tone and quality, and the presence of a diastasis (Table 64.2).

Traditional Abdominoplasty

In a traditional abdominoplasty, the umbilicus is transposed and the rectus muscles are plicated. A circumumbilical incision is made and dissection is carried down to the rectus sheath. An orientation suture placed in the umbilicus will aid in prevention of twisting at inset. The lower incision is incised and dissection is carried up to the xiphoid, minimizing extensive lateral dissection to preserve blood supply and taking care to keep the disinserted umbilicus intact to the abdominal wall (Figure 64.2A). A marking pen or methylene blue is used to outline the medial edge of the rectus bilaterally. The rectus sheath is then plicated (Figure 64.2B). The bed is flexed at the waist, and the amount of abdominal wall skin that can be safely excised while maintaining a tension-free closure is marked (this may be slightly different than the preoperative estimation). The surgeon can determine where the area of greatest tension will be on the closure based on the patient's needs. The upper incision is made, the abdomen irrigated, and meticulous hemostasis achieved. To minimize dead space and tension at the closure, a surgical assistant can aid in advancing the abdominal skin flap and progressive tension sutures can be placed.[32] Drains can then be placed; however, some studies have found foregoing drains with the use of progressive tension sutures is safe and without increased risk of seroma formation.[33] The neoumbilicus spot is located on the abdominal skin flap based on the umbilical location on the abdominal wall. A small circular or ovoid opening is made and the umbilicus is reintroduced into the skin flap and secured with several suture layers, keeping in mind ideal umbilical aesthetics and the patient's body habitus and preference. The closure of the abdomen is performed in multiple layers with sutures in the Scarpa layer, deep dermis, and subcuticular space.

Miniabdominoplasty

In the miniabdominoplasty, also referred to as a *short-scar abdominoplasty*, the surgical goal is to remove a small amount of skin and subcutaneous tissue from the lower abdomen only. The scar is limited and the position of the umbilicus remains unchanged. Usually no plication of the rectus muscles is performed. The option of a short scar can be appealing to younger patients, but dog-ears can be problematic because of the shorter incision. Careful patient selection is crucial for patient satisfaction.

High Lateral Tension

Popularized by Lockwood, the high lateral tension abdominoplasty endorses an oblique vector of pull of the abdominal skin flap.[34] The oblique vector aids in reducing the horizontal epigastric laxity. In this technique, more skin is excised from the abdominal skin flap laterally than centrally. The tension at the line of closure is borne by meticulous closure of the superficial fascial system (Scarpa fascia).[7]

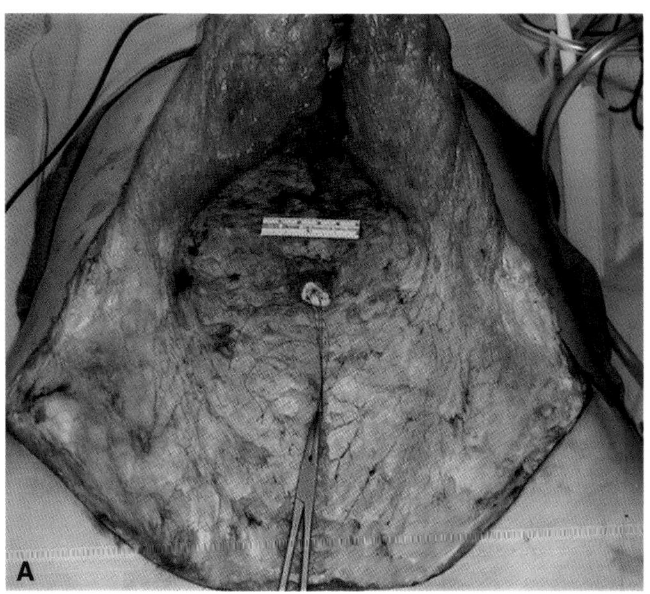

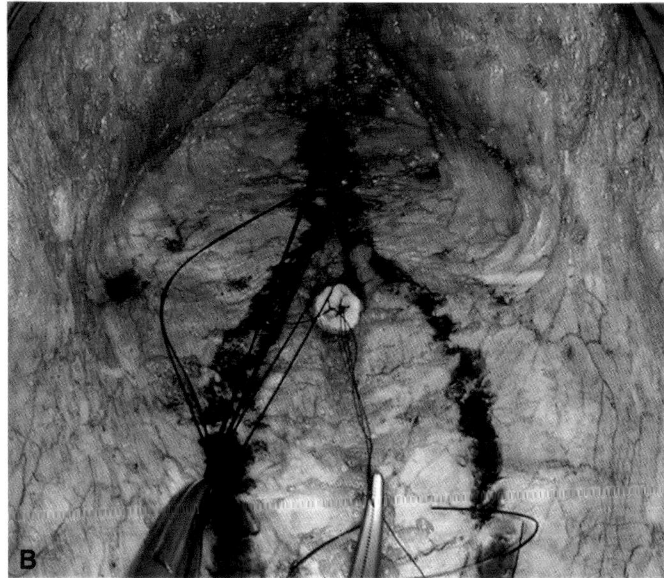

FIGURE 64.2. **A.** The abdominal flap is dissected up to the xiphoid, minimizing excessive lateral dissection. A stitch in the umbilicus helps with orientation when it is delivered through the new opening in the abdominal flap. **B.** The edges of the rectus are outlined and plication is performed to restore the muscles to their anatomic position abutting each other on the midline.

Fleur-de-lis

With the fleur-de-lis technique, the standard low horizontal incision is combined with excision of a vertical ellipse of abdominal tissue (Figure 64.3). This procedure is best for a patient who has both horizontal and vertical skin and tissue excess that is commonly the case in a weight loss patient.[35] First described by Dellon, the procedure seeks to restore a more aesthetic abdominal contour.[36] The major disadvantage of this procedure is an additional scar that is on the vertical midline. Care must be taken to only undermine to the degree necessary for skin resection. The addition of liposuction to the lateral abdomen will result in a discontinuous undermining that will aid in increasing excursion of the abdominal skin flap laterally without increasing the risk of vascular compromise to the skin flap.

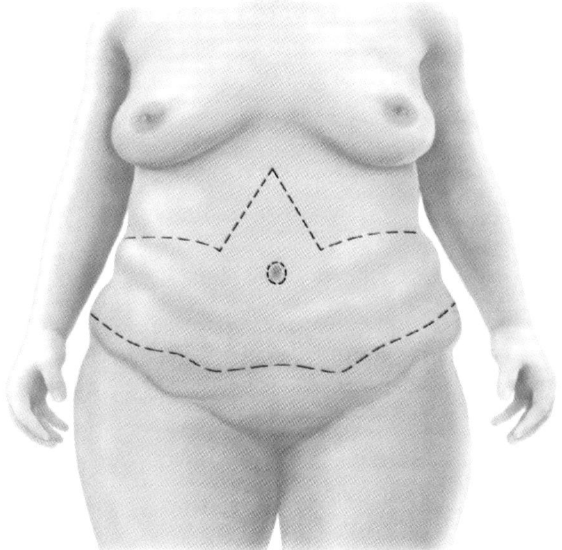

FIGURE 64.3. In the fleur-de-lis abdominoplasty technique, a horizontal and vertical wedge of tissue is excised in order to address excess tissue in both directions.

Lipoabdominoplasty

Popularized by Saldanha, this abdominoplasty technique substitutes liposuction of the abdominal skin flap in lieu of wide lateral undermining in an effort to preserve perforating vessels and thus the blood supply to the skin.[37] Undermining of the skin flap is limited to the area that will be plicated, and the liposuction with a superwet technique is performed in the areas lateral to the rectus.[38] Liposuctioning of the undermined regions of the flap could result in skin flap necrosis and must be avoided or performed with extreme caution.

Postoperative Care

At the conclusion of the abdominoplasty procedure, the patient will be flexed at the waist. To minimize tension at the closure, the patient should be transferred to a stretcher/bed that is likewise flexed at the waist with the knees elevated (beach-chair position). Most would recommend that the patient maintain a semiflexed position at the waist, even when ambulating, for several weeks duration to minimize tension at the closure. If drains are utilized, the patient and/or a caregiver must be educated on proper drain care.[39] A compression garment is worn by the patient for several weeks duration. The patient should avoid heavy lifting and vigorous activity for up to 6 weeks postoperatively.

As described previously, abdominoplasty carries an increased risk of VTE, and thus patients should be encouraged to ambulate early. Low molecular weight heparin or other anticoagulant should be given to those patients deemed to be at higher risk when performing risk stratification.[31]

Scar Management

Scars, especially those that are widened or hypertrophic, can be troublesome to patients. Intraoperatively, wound eversion and minimization of excess tension have been proven to improve scar appearance. In addition, the use of dermal sutures with a self-adherent mesh and octyl-2-cyanoacrylate (PRINEO, Ethicon, Raleigh, NC) has been shown to provide equivalent scar results as dermal sutures, and a subcuticular stitch and is more than four times faster to perform.[40] In the presence of hypertrophic scars, there is evidence that the use of pressure garments, scar massage, and pulsed-dye lasers can improve the appearance.[41]

Complications

The surgeon's efforts both preoperatively and intraoperatively should be focused on mitigating any potential complications through careful preparation and technique.

Complications of abdominoplasty, however, do occur but are usually minor and may include small areas of wound healing problems, poor scars, and lateral dog-ears. Small areas of wound dehiscence, suture abscess, etc. can frequently be treated with local wound care. Those with widened scars or dog-ears can be treated with minor revisional procedures, usually performed in an office setting several months later.

More significant complications can include persistent seroma, areas of flap ischemia, and larger areas of wound dehiscence. Seroma is a common problem with abdominoplasty because of the larger area that is usually undermined. As described previously, the use of progressive tension sutures or quilting sutures has been shown to reduce *dead space* and in turn lessen the frequency of seroma formation.[32,33] The use of drains and compression garments may also reduce the incidence of seroma.[42] Should the patient develop a seroma, it can frequently be aspirated in an office setting using sterile technique so as not to introduce an infectious nidus to the seroma. Larger areas of wound dehiscence can be allowed to heal via secondary intention and be revised at a later date, or a delayed primary closure may be an option. Vascular compromise of the abdominal skin flap can usually be avoided by minimizing large area of undermining. If necrosis does occur, the wound is treated conservatively and allowed to heal by secondary intention with revision at a later date.

The most worrisome complications are those that could prove life-threatening or severely compromise the final aesthetic results. These include VTE and PE, large hematomas, infection, and large areas of flap necrosis. As described previously, abdominoplasty carries with it a relatively high risk of VTE thought to be attributable to the tightening of the abdominal wall, which may increase intra-abdominal pressure. Therefore, *all* patients should undergo a thorough risk assessment, and mechanical and chemoprophylaxis should be utilized.[31] Patients with any symptoms related VTE or PE such as extremity pain and swelling or shortness of breath should be worked up immediately. Large hematomas should be treated via surgical drainage and meticulous hemostasis. Infection is not a frequent abdominoplasty complication. Areas of cellulitis can be treated expectantly with oral antibiotics. More concerning infections may warrant surgical exploration. Larger areas of skin necrosis should be treated with local wound care and subsequent debridements.

Conclusion

Abdominoplasty is a powerful body contouring technique and requires understanding of the relevant anatomy. A thorough physical examination helps the practitioner tailor the procedure to meet patient's specific needs. Complications can occur with any surgical procedure. Fortunately, with good patient and procedure selection and meticulous planning and surgical technique many potential complications can be avoided.

BELT LIPECTOMY

Body contouring procedures address the soft tissue redundancy after weight loss. The popularity of these procedures has increased in conjunction with the number of patients undergoing weight loss procedures. In patients with generalized laxity of the truncal tissues, belt lipectomy is a high yield surgery because it is a circumferential procedure that addressed multiple anatomic areas including the abdomen, back, flanks, and thighs.

Pertinent Anatomy

The surgeon should be familiar with the anatomy of the abdomen (see Abdominoplasty section) and regional blood supply when performing body contouring of the trunk. Zones of fascial adherence are five fixed points that serve as important anatomical landmarks (see T 1). Commonly, in the weight loss patient, zones of adherence as well as a midabdominal fascial thickening are preserved.

Patient Selection and Evaluation

A full history and physical should be performed on all body contouring patients. The medical interview should include questions about the patient's motivation for surgery and their expectations to identify those who may have body dysmorphic disorder. Other questions include the method of weight loss (i.e., diet and exercise vs. a weight loss surgery). The specific type of weight loss surgery (restrictive vs. malabsorptive) should also be obtained as those with malabsorptive surgeries have specific nutritional needs (see Chapter 63). Weight loss before surgery should be stable for a minimum of 3 months prior to surgical interventions.[43] The patient should be questioned about VTE risk factors so that they can be properly risk stratified, and appropriate mechanical and chemoprophylaxis can be anticipated.[31] Many times, weight loss or bariatric patients have a history of several medical comorbidities. All these should be assessed and specialists should be engaged when appropriate to assess surgical risk and assist with medical optimization.

On examination, the skin should be examined for rash, intertrigo, previous incisions, and striae. The thickness and distribution of excess skin and subcutaneous tissue should be evaluated. The abdomen should be examined for the presence of hernias. A CT scan can be ordered if needed. There are a variety of names to describe body contouring procedures. As described by Aly, the belt lipectomy addresses the lower truncal area by removing a wedge of tissue to improve the abdominal contour and create definition between the lumbar area and the buttock.[44] However, with this procedure, the fascial zones of the trunk and lower extremity are not markedly disrupted. This limits the ability of this procedure to substantially address the thighs, and patients with concerns in this area may be better served with a lower body lift (see Chapter 65).[45] The goals of the belt lipectomy are to eliminate the ptotic panniculus to define the waist, eliminate lower back rolls, and elevate the lateral thighs and mons pubis. Proper patient selection is the most important preventative measure available to the surgeon to mitigate the risk of postoperative complications in the body contouring patient; thus a thorough preoperative assessment is crucial.

Marking, Positioning, and Safety

The patient is marked in the standing position. Anatomic landmarks including the anterior and posterior midlines, the suprapubic crease, and the iliac crests are marked. Based on pinch test and anatomic landmarks, the upper and lower incisions are all marked with the anterior superior marking being similar to that for an abdominoplasty and the midline posterior having the narrowest resection width. The posterior markings should be based on pinch test both in the erect and flexed at the waist positions to ensure the area is not overresected. The proposed line of closure is then marked by ensuring that it is at or above the ASIS so the scar can be hidden with undergarments (Figure 64.4). Vertical hash marks through the horizontal markings will assist with realigning the tissues after tissue excision. The markings will be cursory as intraoperative adjustments may need to be made.

Based on surgeon preference, patients undergoing belt lipectomy will be repositioned a minimum of twice. Because of intraoperative positioning changes, padding of extremities to prevent neurapraxias is of utmost importance. The operative table should be tested to ensure it is in good working order and the operative team should be well versed in optimizing patient safety through use of padding, positioning, warming, and VTE prevention techniques.[46]

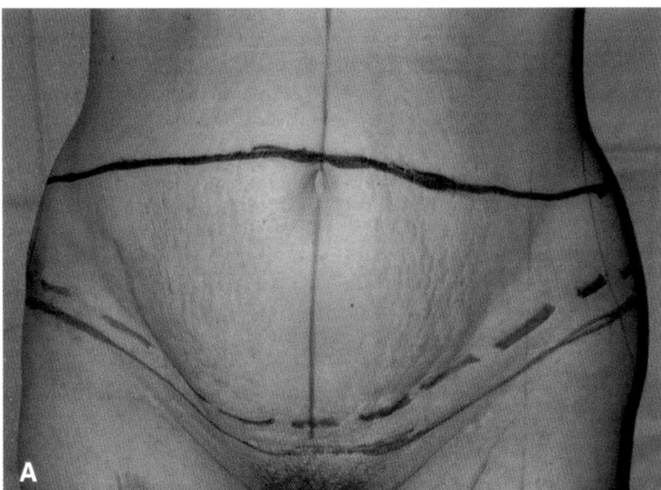

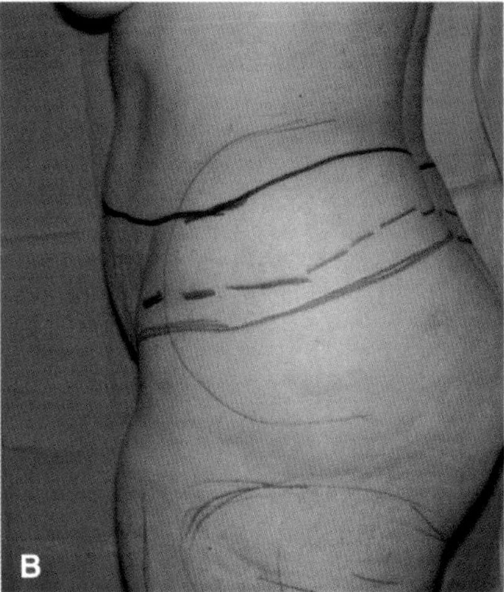

FIGURE 64.4. **A.** Anterior view of the markings for a belt lipectomy. The red line marks the inferior incision. The black mark indicates the proposed superior incision. The green dashed line is a visual indicator of the eventual scar location. **B.** Lateral view of the marking for a belt lipectomy. Black line marks the upper incision, red indicates the inferior incision, and the green is to visually indicate the eventual scar location.

Technique

The surgeon should have well-laid plans for their operative approach to minimize operative time. The patient position changes (supine to prone or lateral-lateral-supine) should be anticipated and communicated with the operative team who should be sufficiently equipped to facilitate safe patient turns. Starting in the supine position, the trunk is widely prepped and draped. The umbilicus is incised and freed from the abdominal tissues and the lower abdominal incision is made. The dissection is carried up to the xiphoid similar to that with abdominoplasty with the exception that the lateral area is undermined to a greater degree. Any rectus diastasis is repaired and the abdominal flap is redraped. Progressive tension sutures can be used if desired and/or closed suction drains are placed. The new umbilical location is anatomically determined and the umbilicus is delivered and sutured into place. The anterior abdomen is sutured closed in the standard fashion working some of the excess abdominal tissues laterally. These lateral dog-ears are stapled closed provisionally and the patient is repositioned into the prone or lateral position and appropriately positioned, padded, prepped, and redraped. The posterior incisions are made based on tailor-tacking and a *cut as you go* technique, if that is the surgeon preference to prevent overresection. The dissection is carried down to the musculofascia. Little to no undermining of the superior or inferior skin flaps is performed. To optimize the superior excursion of the lateral thigh and minimize contour irregularities, this area is liposuctioned in a discontinuous manner to partially disrupt the pelvic rim zone of adherence. The lateral areas and the posterior resection areas are closed over drains. The patient is then repositioned from the prone or lateral position back to the supine *beach chair* position for extubation and application of compression garments.

Complications

With a proper preoperative assessment and close attention to detail in the operative room, efforts can be made to reduce complications by selecting appropriate patients, avoiding hypothermia, correct positioning, and appropriate VTE prophylaxis.[47-49] In addition, controlling for overresection can minimize tension and wound dehiscence. This is performed by committing to only one incision and the undermining the skin resection estimated by pinch test. Prior to making the resection incision, the skin flap is transposed under the first incision to estimate the safe amount of tissue resection.

Despite the surgeon's best efforts, complications can occur.[49] The outcome can still be controlled with early recognition and prompt steps to remedy concerns. Superficial wound healing problems and minor wound dehiscence are the most common complications that occur with circumferential body contouring procedures such as the belt lipectomy because of the competing tensions of the anterior and posterior incisions. These can almost universally be treated with attentive local wound care. Seromas can also be a troublesome postsurgical complication. Seroma formation can be minimized by only undermining the tissues to the degree necessary for excision and closure. Other measures such as sharp dissection, closed suction drains, and quilting or progressive tension sutures are also proven to reduce seroma rates.[42] If a seroma does occur, it can commonly be treated with serial aspirations in the office or placement of a seroma catheter. Untreated seromas can lead to infections, so these should be treated aggressively. Because of the large tissue surface area, bleeding and hematomas can be a potential complication. Large hematomas should be evacuated. Small hematomas that are not expanding and well drained can be treated expectantly. Skin flap necrosis can also occur in the belt lipectomy patient and this is usually due to excessive tension, previous incisions that compromise regional blood flow, and aggressive liposuction. If this occurs, the area is treated with local wound care and allowed to heal secondarily. A revisional procedure can be performed at a later date. The complication with the most potential for mortality is VTE. Procedures that tighten the abdominal wall, such as recuts plication, are theorized to increase intra-abdominal pressure, which affects the compression susceptible venous system. Risk stratification and assertive use of mechanical and chemoprophylaxis is critical.[9,31] Patients should be counseled on the signs and symptoms of VTE so that they can obtain prompt evaluation should they experience these.

Belt lipectomy is a circumferential procedure performed following massive weight loss that improves the abdominal contour and laxity, back rolls and buttock, and lateral thigh ptosis. Proper patient selection and optimization is essential to maximize outcomes and prevent complications.

REFERENCES

1. Illouz YG. Body contouring by lipolysis: a 5-year experience with over 3000 cases. *Plast Reconstr Surg*. 1983;72:591.
   Illouz's technique of using a wetting solution, blunt cannulas, and negative pressure aspiration improved the safety of lipolysis and is the foundation of how liposuction is performed today. Illouz also recognized over the course of his experience represented in this paper that deeper liposuction tunnels allowed for a smoother contour and less skin excess.
2. Broughton G, Crosby MA, Coleman J, Rohrich RJ. Use of herbal supplements and vitamins in plastic surgery: a practical review. *Plast Reconstr Surg*. 2007;119(3):48e.
3. Harrison B, Khans I, Janis JE. Evidence-based strategies to reduce postoperative complications in plastic surgery. *Plast Reconstr Surg*. 2016;138:51S.

4. Rinker B. The evils of nicotine: an evidence-based guide to smoking and plastic surgery. *Ann Plast Surg*. 2013;70:599.
5. Chia CT, Neinstein RM, Theodorou SJ. Evidence-based medicine: liposuction. *Plast Reconstr Surg*. 2017;139(1):267e.
6. Markman B, Barton FE. Anatomy of the subcutaneous tissue of the trunk and lower extremity. *Plast Reconstr Surg*. 1987:80:248.
7. Lockwood TE. Superficial fascial system (SFS) of the trunk and extremities: a new concept. *Plast Reconstr Surg*. 1991;87:1009.
8. Haeck PC, Swanson JA, Gutowski KA, et al. Evidence-based patient safety advisory: liposuction. *Plast Reconstr Surg*. 2009;124(suppl 4):28S.
9. Murphy RX, Alderman A, Gutowski KA, et al. Evidence-based practices for thromboembolism prevention: summary of the ASPS Venous Thromboembolism Task Force Report. *Plast Reconstr Surg*. 2012;130(1):168e-175e.
10. Klein JA. The tumescent technique for liposuction surgery. *Am J Cosmet Surg*. 1987;4:263.
11. Rohrich RJ, Kenkel JM, Janis JE, et al. An update on the role of subcutaneous tissue infiltration in suction-assisted lipoplasty. *Plast Reconstr Surg*. 2003;111:926.
12. Gutowski KA. Tumescent analgesia in plastic surgery. *Plast Reconstr Surg*. 2014;134(4 suppl 2):50S-57S.
13. Klein JA. Tumescent technique for regional anesthesia permits lidocaine doses of 35 mg/kg for liposuction. *J Dermatol Surg Oncol*. 1990;16:248.
14. Swanson E. Prospective study of lidocaine, bupivacaine and epinephrine and blood loss in patients undergoing liposuction and abdominoplasty. *Plast Reconstr Surg*. 2012;130:702.
15. Rohrich RJ, Leedy JE, Swamy R, et al. Fluid [illegible]ution in liposuction: a retrospective review of 89 consecutive patients. *Plast Reconstr Surg*. 2006;117:431.
16. Kenkel JM, Robinson J, Beran SJ, et al. The tissue effects of ultrasound assisted lipoplasty. *Plast Reconstr Surg*. 1998;102:213.
17. Zocchi ML. Ultrasonic assisted liposuction: technical refinements and clinical evaluations. *Clin Plast Surg*. 1996;23;575.
18. Prado A, Andrades P, Danilla S, et al. A prospective, randomized, double-blinded, control clinical trila comparing laser-assisted lipoplasty with suction assisted lipoplasty. *Plast Reconstr Surg*. 2006;118:1032.
19. Ingargiola MJ, Motakef S, Chung MT, et al. Cryolipolysis for fat reduction and body contouring: safety and efficacy of current treatment paradigms. *Plast Reconstr Surg*. 2015;136(6):1581.
20. Derrick CO, Shridharani SM, Broyles JM. The safety and efficacy of cryolypolysis: a systematic review of available literature. *Aesthet Surg J*. 2015;35:83.
21. Stroumza N, Gauhier N, Senet P, et al. Paradoxical adipose hyperplasia (PAH) after cryolipolysis. *Aesthet Surg J*. 2018;38(4):411.
22. Wall SH Jr, Lee MR. Separation, aspiration, and fat equalization: SAFE liposuction concepts for comprehensive body contouring. *Plast Reconstr Surg*. 2016;138(6):1192.
    This article proposes a comprehensive multistep process toward body contouring aimed at reducing complications and fulfilling aesthetic ideals. Wall and Lee describe detailed steps of the process and a retrospective 5-year review of their liposuction results on 129 patients.
23. Del Vecchio D, Wall S Jr. Expansion vibration lipofilling: a new technique in large-volume fat transplantation. *Plast Reconstr Surg*. 2018;141(5):639.
24. Horton BJ, Reece EM, Boughton G, et al. Patient safety in the office based setting. *Plast Reconst Surg*. 2006;117(4):61e.
25. Appelt EA, Janis JE, Rohrich RJ. An algorithmic approach to upper arm contouring. *Plast Reconstr Surg*. 2006;118(1):237.
26. Steinbrech DS, Sinno S. Utilizing the power of fat grafting to obtain a naturally-appearing muscular "6-pack" abdomen. *Aesthet Surg J*. 2016;36(9):1085.
27. Weinberg GL. Lipid emulsion infusion: resuscitation for local anesthetic and other drug overdose. *Anesthesiology*. 2012;117:180.
28. Huger WE Jr. The anatomic rationale for abdominal lipectomy. *Am Surg*. 1979;45:612.
    This anatomic study introduced a simple and reliable regional vascular map of the abdomen. The map is divided into three zones based on regional anatomy. Lipectomy *or abdominoplasty alters the normal anatomic blood supply to the superficial abdominal wall. These postsurgical anatomic changes explain tissue survival following the surgery.*
29. Buck DW II, Mustoe TA. An evidence-based approach to abdominoplasties. *Plast Reconstr Surg*. 2010;126:2189.
30. Gutowski KA. Evidence-based medicine: abdominoplasty. *Plast Reconstr Surg*. 2018;141:286e.
31. Pannucci CJ. Evidence-based recipes for venous thromboembolism: a practical safety guide. *Plast Reconstr Surg*. 2017;139:520e.
32. Pollock H, Pollock T. Progressive tension sutures: a technique to reduce local complications in abdominoplasty. *Plast Reconstr Surg*. 2000;105:258.
33. Macias LH, Kwon E, Gould DJ, et al. Decrease in seroma rate after adopting progressive tension sutures without drains: a single surgery center experience of 451 abdominoplasties over 7 years. *Aesthet Surg J*. 2016;36:1029.
34. Lockwood T. High-lateral tension abdominoplasty with superficial fascial system suspension. *Plast Reconstr Surg*. 1995;96:603.
    In this article, Lockwood introduces his belief that the circumferential trunk is a subunit and provides evidence against two commonly held abdominoplasty principles of that time. Firstly, he challenged the principle that wide undermining of the abdominal flap to the costal margin was necessary by achieving excellent results with widespread liposuction and less flap undermining. Secondly, Lockwood drew attention to the previously neglected lateral abdominal wall tissues and resected excess tissue in this area transferring the tension of closure to the superficial fascial system.
35. Friedman T, O'Brien Coon D, Michaels J, et al. Fleur-de-lis abdominoplasty: a safe alternative to traditional abdominoplasty for the massive weight loss patient. *Plast Reconstr Surg*. 2010;125:1535.
36. Dellon AL. Fleur-de-lis abdominoplasty. *Aesthet Plast Surg*. 1985;9:27.
    This is the first description of this technique. The author emphasizes the advantages of using both a horizontal and a vertical resection in order to restore a favorable contour to the abdomen.
37. Saldanha OR, Federisco R, Daher PF, et al. Lipoabdominoplasty. *Plast Reconstr Surg*. 2009;124(3):934.
38. Matarasso A. Liposuction as an adjunct to a full abdominoplasty. *Plast Reconstr Surg*. 1995;92:1112.
39. Khansa I, Khansa L, Meyerson J, Janis JE. Optimal use of surgical drains: evidence-based strategies. *Plast Reconstr Surg*. 2018;141(6):1542-1549.
40. Richter D, Stroff A, Ramakrishnan V, et al. A comparison of a new skin closure device and intradermal sutures in the closure of full-thickness surgical incisions. *Plast Reconstr Surg*. 2012:130(4):843.
41. Khansa I, Harrison B, Janis JE. Evidence-based scar management: how to improve results with technique and technology. *Plast Reconstr Surg*. 2016;138(3):165S.
42. Janis JE, Khansa I, Khansa L. Strategies for postoperative seroma prevention: a systematic review. *Plast Reconst Surg*. 2016;138(1):240.
43. Rubin JP, Nguyen V, Schwentker A. Perioperative management of the post-gastric-bypass patient presenting for body contouring. *Clin Plast Surg*. 2004;31:601.
44. Aly AS, Cram AE, Chao M, et al. Belt lipectomy for circumferential truncal excess: the University of Iowa experience. *Plast Reconstr Surg*. 2003;111:398.
45. Lockwood TE. Lower body lift. *Aesthet Surg*. 2001;21:355.
46. Colwell AS, Borud LJ. Optimization of patient safety in post-bariatric body contouring: a current review. *Aesthet Surg J*. 2008;28;437.
47. Almutairi K, Gusenoff JA, Rubin JP. Body contouring. *Plast Reconstr Surg*. 2016;137:586e.
48. Hunstad JP. Body contouring in the obese patient. *Clin Plast Surg*. 1996;23:647.
49. Fischer JP, Wes AM, Serletti JM, Kovach SJ. Complications in body contouring procedures: an analysis of 1797 patients from the 2005-2010 American College of Surgeons National Surgical Quality Improvement Program database. *Plast Reconstr Surg*. 2013;132(6):1411-1420.

QUESTIONS

1. Several weeks following an abdominoplasty, your patient presents for follow-up and informs you that she was recently evaluated by her primary care physician because of complaints of outer thigh discomfort. She was diagnosed with meralgia paresthetica. Which structure was likely injured during her procedure?

a. Iliohypogastric nerve
b. Ilioinguinal ligament
c. Genitofemoral nerve
d. Lateral femoral cutaneous nerve
e. Pectineus muscle

2. Following large-volume flank and abdominal liposuction, your patient is taken to the recovery room. While the patient is being transferred to the overnight observation unit, they begin to complain of perioral numbness, develop hypotension, and start seizing. What medication should be administered?

a. Phenobarbital
b. Dantrolene
c. Lipid emulsion
d. Phentolamine
e. Epinephrine

3. You are performing large-volume liposuction at a local hospital. Which of the following is not an endpoint for liposuction aspiration?

a. Pinch test
b. Skin laxity
c. Aspirate volume
d. Skin turgor
e. Length of operative time

4. When assessing a patient during consultation for an abdominoplasty, what is the clinical significance of a positive diver's test?

a. The patient has an incisional hernia.
b. The patient has excess lower abdominal fat.
c. The patient has excess lower abdominal skin.
d. The patient has myofascial laxity.
e. The patient has a diastasis rectus.

5. Which of the following is true regarding belt lipectomy?

a. The postoperative scar is at the same level as with a lower body lift.
b. All zones of adherence are left intact.
c. More than one patient position on the operative table is necessary.
d. The superficial fascial system is not approximated at closure.
e. Belt lipectomy has minimal effect on the waist contour.

1. **Answer: d.** The lateral femoral cutaneous nerve is the most frequently injured nerve during abdominoplasty. Injury to this nerve causes meralgia paresthetica, which is characterized by anterolateral thigh burning, tingling, and numbness. It emerges close to the ASIS, and keeping some fat overlying the musculofascia in this area may prevent nerve injury. The iliohypogastric nerve innervates the suprapubic region. The genitofemoral nerve travels deep into the abdominal wall and originates from L1 to L2. The ilioinguinal ligament is a band that originates from the ASIS and inserts on the pubic tubercle. It is formed by the external oblique aponeurosis and is continuous with the fascia lata of the thigh. The pectineus muscle is a flat, quadrangular muscle on the anteromedial thigh.

2. **Answer: c.** This patient is suffering from lidocaine toxicity or LAST (local anesthetic systemic toxicity). With large-volume aspirates, lidocaine dosage must be carefully calculated and kept below 35 mg/kg. Lidocaine toxicity is best treated with 20% lipid emulsion. The current agreed hypothesis for intravenous lipid emulsion efficacy in treating cardiotoxicity and the effects of lidocaine toxicity is the formation of a ***lipid sink***, that is, an expanded intravascular lipid phase that acts to absorb the offending circulating lipophilic lidocaine toxin, hence reducing the unbound free toxin available to bind to the myocardium. LAST treatment consists of the following steps:

1. Infuse 20% lipid emulsion. (Upper limit is approximately 10–12 mL/kg over the first 30 minutes.)
2. Bolus at 1.5 mL/kg (lean body mass) intravenously over 1 minute.
3. Provide continuous infusion at 0.25 mL/kg per minute.
4. For persistent cardiovascular collapse, repeat bolus up to two times.
5. Double the infusion to 0.5 mL/kg per minute, if remains hypotensive.
6. Continue infusion for at least 10 minutes after circulatory stability is achieved.

Phenobarbital is a barbiturate that acts as a nonselective central nervous system depressant and that is used primarily as a sedative hypnotic and also as an anticonvulsant in certain populations. It is not used for adult status epilepticus. Dantrolene is a postsynaptic muscle relaxant that lessens excitation-contraction coupling in muscle cells. It acts by inhibiting Ca^{2+} ions release from sarcoplasmic reticulum stores by antagonizing ryanodine receptors. It is the primary drug used for the treatment and prevention of malignant hyperthermia, a rare, life-threatening disorder triggered by general anesthesia. Phentolamine is an alpha-1 agonist and results in vasodilation. It can be used to reverse the effects of local anesthetics containing epinephrine. Epinephrine is a direct-acting sympathomimetic drug that acts as an agonist at alpha- and beta-adrenergic receptors. It produces vasoconstriction to counteract the vasodilation and resulting hypotension associated with anaphylaxis and other conditions.

3. **Answer: a.** When performing liposuction, endpoints include contour, pinch test (pinching the operative area between the thumb and index finger to assure evenness of liposuction), and bloody aspirate. The tone of the skin does not dictate an endpoint for liposuction. Skin turgor and the ***fountain sign*** (escape of wetting solution when the infiltration cannula is withdrawn) are endpoints for infiltration of wetting solution. The practice advisory on liposuction released by the ASPS acknowledges that there are no scientific data available to support a specific volume maximum at which point liposuction is no longer safe; with that said, it is important for the surgeon and patient to know that the risk of complications is unavoidably higher as the volume of aspirate and the number of anatomic sites treated increase. Assuming that the patient is tolerating anesthesia and the procedure well, operative length is not an endpoint for liposuction, but should be kept to a reasonable minimum. Close attention to prevent hypothermia, to position and pad the patient appropriately, and to use appropriate deep vein thrombosis prophylaxis will minimize adverse outcomes from a prolonged procedure.

BODY CONTOURING

4. Answer: d. To perform a diver's test, the patient flexes at the waist from a standing position. Presence of a lower abdominal protuberance with flexion that is not present in the erect position indicates laxity of the myofascial system that is most commonly a result of pregnancy. Myofascial laxity can be improved with plication of the rectus muscles.

5. Answer: b. The resultant scar from a belt lipectomy is generally located more superior than that of a lower body lift. With the wedge of tissue being removed located more superior encompassing the abdomen, flanks, and lower back, there is a greater effect on the waist contour. Because of the circumferential nature of the procedure, a minimum of two position changes is necessary during the surgery in order to adequately address the abdomen, back, and lateral flank/thigh area. To obtain maximal lift from the belt lipectomy, the zones of adherence of the lateral thighs are discontinuously disrupted with liposuction.

CHAPTER 65 Lower Body Lift and Thighplasty

Omar E. Beidas and J. Peter Rubin

KEY POINTS

- The lower body lift is a powerful procedure that reshapes the hips, buttocks, and lateral thighs.
- Because the lower body lift does not address the medial thighs, a medial thighplasty is required to treat the thigh deformity.
- Together, these two operations contour the lower trunk and thigh in a single stage or in separate stages.

The massive weight loss (MWL) patient is left with deformities of varying degrees, with somewhat predictable patterns of excess skin and fat. The lower trunk and thighs can be dramatically improved by combining a lower body lift (LBL) and thighplasty. Although many variations of each of these procedures have been described in the literature, key principles are applied according to each patient's anatomy and preferences. Importantly, patients must be accepting of long scars in exchange for improved contour, especially for the medial thighs where a vertical scar is necessary to correct the circumferential excess of skin.[1,2]

Not every patient presenting after MWL needs an excisional procedure; each patient is assessed individually and an operative plan is created based on the nature of the deformity and the patient's goals. Moreover, patients who have plateaued at a high BMI or require optimization of medical comorbidities may not be ready for major elective surgery. The Pittsburgh Rating Scale[3] is a useful tool to grade a patient's deformities and can assist the surgeon with operative planning. Patients with low-grade deformities have excess adipose tissue with adequate skin tone and may be treated with liposuction alone. Patients with high-grade deformities require skin and subcutaneous tissue resection with or without liposuction.

APPROACHES TO THIGH AND BUTTOCK CONTOURING

The LBL was introduced over 25 years ago to treat the ptotic, wrinkled skin and subcutaneous tissue of the abdomen, hips, back, and buttocks.[4] With the understanding of the relevant vectors, Lockwood combined procedures that were typically carried out in multiple stages into a single stage. He introduced the concept of suspending the superficial fascia system (SFS)[5] to anchor the incision and achieve a circumferential correction of the lower trunk. Lockwood referred to this initial technique as the lower body lift #1 (LBL #1)—a combination of abdominoplasty and medial thighplasty—and later developed the lower body lift #2 (LBL #2)—a combination of high-lateral-tension abdominoplasty, lateral thigh lift, and buttock lift. LBL #1 is best suited for patients with minimal abdominal laxity and is infrequently applied to the MWL population as many require a significant abdominal resection. However, the LBL #1 may be useful for patients who had a prior abdominoplasty. The LBL #2 is applied for patients with abdominal skin laxity, and this circumferential approach is the most common and familiar variant in current practice. Both variants exert a significant upward lifting effect on the lateral thighs. The actual vector, though primarily vertical, also causes a mild lateral and vertical rotation (outward spiral motion) of the medial thigh tissues. The correction of medial thigh skin laxity from an LBL is small in magnitude, and patients with significant laxity of the medial thigh skin will require a medial thighplasty procedure.

The medial thigh lift was introduced in 1957,[6] but not widely adopted; over 20 years elapsed before another specific article about thigh lift was described.[7] Complications associated with the original description included vulvar distortion due to scar migration and early recurrence of ptosis. It was not until Lockwood wrote about anchoring the SFS of the thigh to Colles fascia that thighplasty gained popularity.[8]

Thighplasty requires resection of skin and subcutaneous tissue in a longitudinal, transverse, or combined axis. Various incision patterns are described, including a longitudinal medial incision, a longitudinal lateral incision, or a transverse incision in or near the groin crease.[9–11] The transverse thigh lift is also known as a proximal thigh lift, generally reserved for patients with minor deformities.[12] The transverse thigh lift is not the procedure of choice in MWL patients because it can only treat the proximal third of the thigh deformity. It is important to recognize that transverse-only excisions have low power to correct thigh deformities and the force of pull is not transmitted past the proximal third of the thigh. Overly aggressive transverse resection in an attempt to obtain a greater correction of skin laxity can result in labial spreading. The medial vertical thigh lift is better suited for the MWL patient whose excess tissue can be treated along the entire length of the thigh. Lateral vertical thigh excisions are rarely used, but have a role in cases of severe deformities in which both medial and lateral excisions may be of benefit.

LOWER BODY LIFT

Multiple variations of the LBL exist based on the patient's deformity and desired outcome. An LBL generally needs a more inferior resection, and a belt lipectomy resection is located more superiorly, at the level of the waistline. A belt lipectomy (Chapter 63) tends to emphasize waist shape, directly excising central adiposity of the flanks, and is therefore well suited for the typical android body fat distribution. The more inferior resection pattern of an LBL enables more control of lateral thigh and buttock shape and is better for patients with a gynecoid body type whose excess adiposity is in the hips and thighs. Although the higher incisions of a belt lipectomy give the surgeon better control over the contour of the waist and flank, the lower incisions of the LBL exert a more powerful and direct lifting effect of the lateral thighs for gluteal autoaugmentation with autologous flaps. The more caudal the incision, the more buttock autoaugmentation tissue can be incorporated into the dermoglandular flap. Matching the variant of the procedure to individual body types is the key to optimizing outcomes.

Patient Evaluation

Patients almost never present requesting an LBL. Generally, they highlight their dissatisfaction with the appearance of their abdomen, lateral thighs, and/or buttocks. Many do not realize the LBL is an option until brought up by the surgeon. The first determination that must be made is the lower truncal procedure that will best address the patient's deformities and meet their goals; both anterior and posterior deformities must be considered. Candidates for LBL are those with circumferential skin laxity when an anterior approach alone will not treat the 360° nature of the deformity.

The anterior assessment requires a thorough physical examination of the abdomen. The surgeon must evaluate the patient's skin quality, excess skin, subcutaneous versus intraabdominal fat distribution, rectus diastasis, hernias, and existing scars. It is vital to pay attention to the location of previous scars when deciding on any areas that may need liposuction or undermining. Patients who have undergone adjustable gastric banding surgery will have a subcutaneous port along the abdominal wall; it is important to note its location as it may be encountered intraoperatively. Posteriorly, the physical examination focuses on the lower back and buttocks. MWL patients have a characteristic appearance of the buttocks, with loss of adiposity, decreased projection, and ptosis, in addition to lengthening of the infragluteal fold.

Depending on patient and surgical factors, patients may need clearance from other medical specialists. Although these issues are covered in both Chapters 16 and 63, they are worth repeating as MWL patients and body contouring procedures are independent risk factors for complications.[13-15] Please refer to the two chapters referenced above for appropriate venous thromboembolism prophylaxis, pre- and postoperative antibiotic dosing, intraoperative positioning, maintenance of body temperature, and fluid balance. Figures 65.1 and 65.2 depict a patient of each gender who underwent LBL.

Surgical Technique

Markings

Markings begin posteriorly by identifying the midline. The patient and surgeon together decide on the optimal scar placement that is in an acceptable location to the patient to address their chief complaint. The superior line—the stable anchor posteriorly—is marked. Vertical lines are drawn at consistent intervals to align the superior and inferior lines. Next, the width of resection is estimated by means of pulling the caudal tissue in a cephalad direction until the skin is taut in appearance. This marks the inferior line of resection. The posterior resection has the appearance of a bow tie, tapered centrally given the strong zone of adherence and flaring laterally where tissue is more lax. To preserve the sacral dimple, the scar should come together in a "V" at the midline. Maximum buttock projection is most aesthetic when located at the transposed horizontal level of the pubic symphysis; therefore, surgical planning should take this into account. If gluteal autoaugmentation is planned, the resection width is adjusted to accommodate the anticipated additional volume. Male and female markings sometimes differ based on the area to be resected, as shown in Figure 65.3.

Once the posterior markings are complete, they are extended anteriorly, where the inferior line is now the stable anchor. At the midline, the marking is made 7 cm superior to the labial commissure. The marking is carried laterally over the thigh superior to the inguinal ligament to avoid disrupting lymphatic drainage. The superior

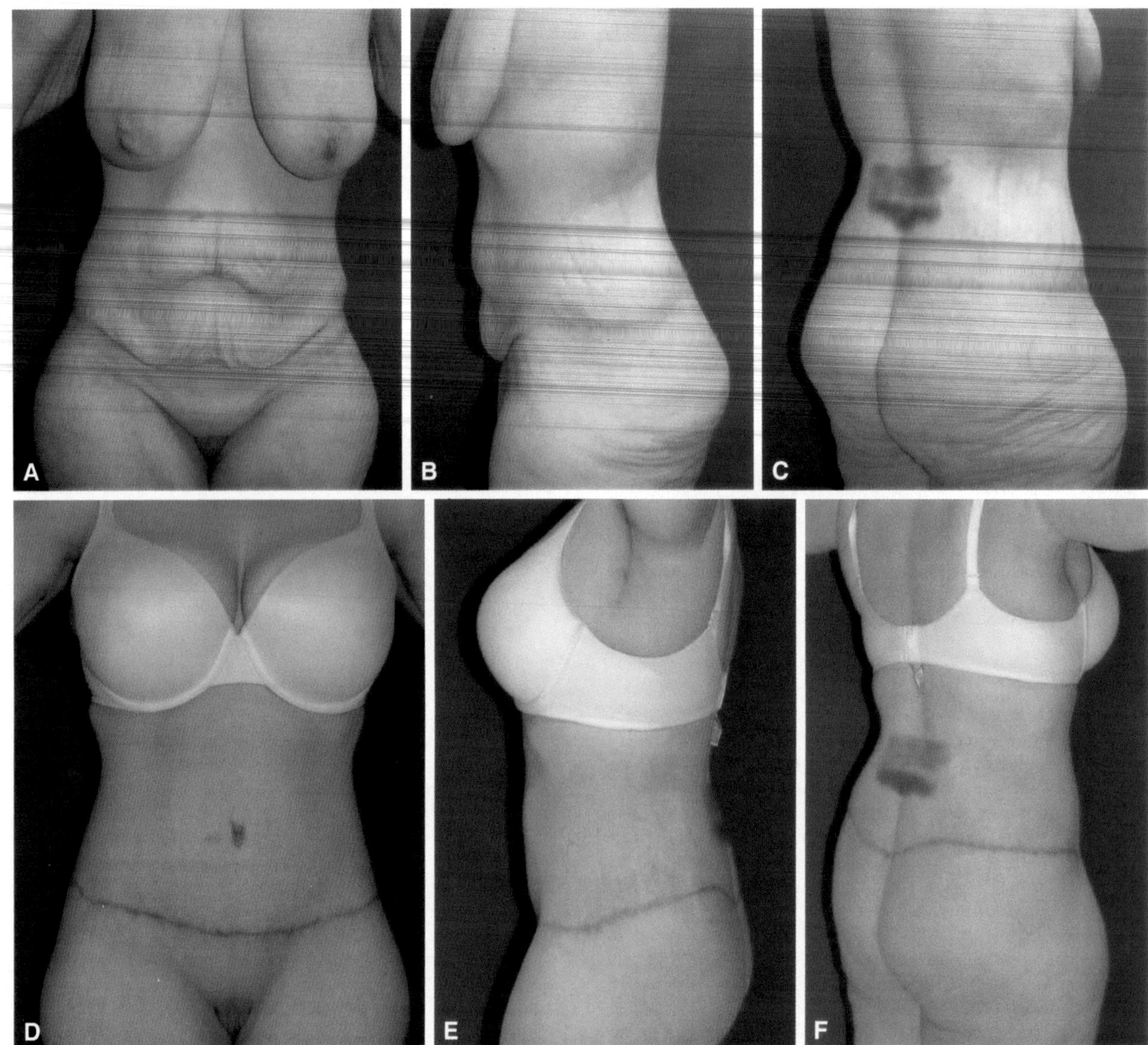

FIGURE 65.1. **A–C.** This 35-year-old woman lost 150 lb after gastric bypass surgery and desired body contouring of multiple areas. She underwent a staged approach with lower body lift and brachioplasty followed 3 months later by dermal suspension parenchymal reshaping mastopexy and thighplasty. **D–F.** Three months postoperative photographs show the first stage of her lower body lift.

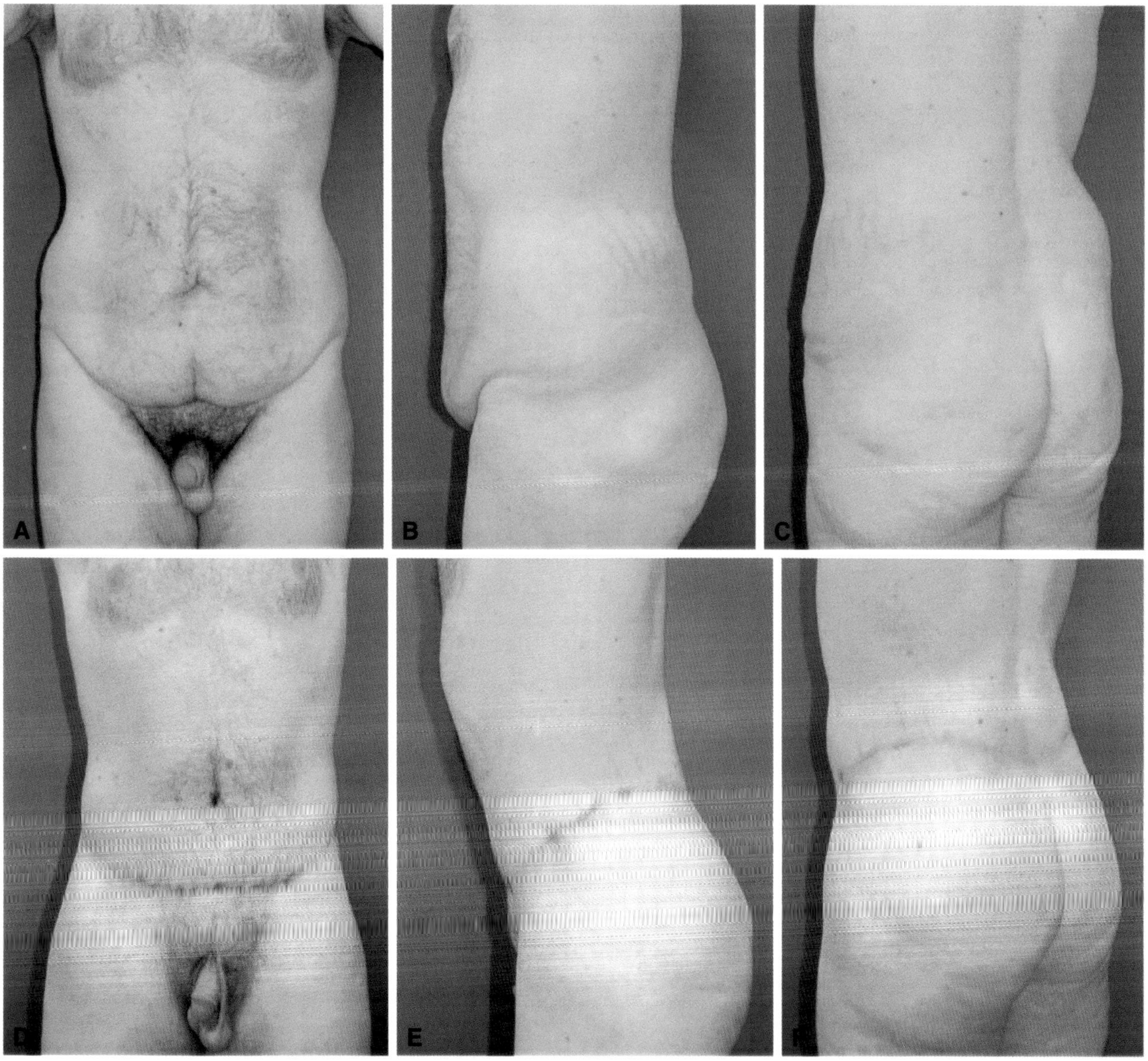

FIGURE 65.2. **A–C.** A 48-year-old male fitness trainer who lost 100 lb through diet and exercise and desired abdominal contouring. **D–F.** One year after lower body lift.

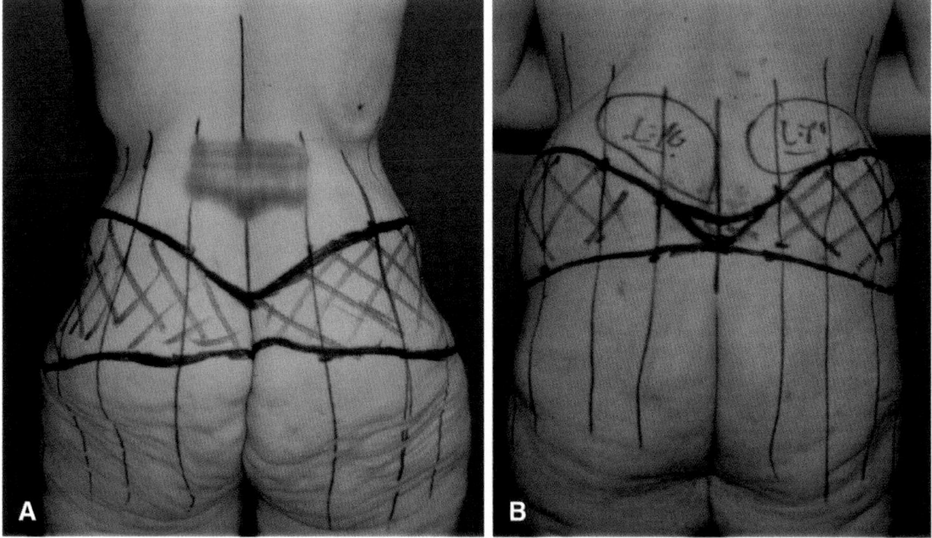

FIGURE 65.3. Side-by-side pictures to demonstrate the sometimes necessary difference in marking a female versus male for lower body lift (LBL) procedure. **A.** The woman in Figure 65.1 marked for her LBL. **B.** The man in Figure 65.2 marked for his LBL with a more cephelad pattern of resection best suited for his specific body type.

line anteriorly need not be drawn as it is determined intraoperatively. Areas of liposuction are marked using different color ink.

Intraoperative Steps

Several different techniques have been described for the LBL. At a minimum, 1 intraoperative patient position change is required to access the torso circumferentially, whereas some prefer 2 position changes. If the procedure is to begin in the lateral or prone position, the patient is intubated and a Foley catheter placed while on the stretcher, then the patient is flipped onto the operating room table. The patient is positioned appropriately, all bony prominences are padded, and the head and neck are placed in neutral alignment. All visible lower truncal surfaces are prepped and draped in typical sterile fashion. Alternatively, some surgeons prefer to prep the patient while standing before moving onto a sterile drape on the operating room table.

The patient's trunk is prepped down to the operating room table along with the thighs circumferentially. As previously described, an additional arm board can be placed adjacent to each thigh to be able to abduct them and decrease tension during the posterior closure.[16] A solution of 1:100,000 of epinephrine in normal saline is injected subcutaneously along the markings. The width of resection is verified with a single towel clamp placed across both incisions, as the LBL is one of the few procedures where the surgeon commits to the entire width simultaneously. After waiting approximately 10 minutes, the incision through the dermis is made. The resection is tailored to the patient, and as is often said in a breast reduction, the tissue left behind is more important than the tissue removed. Preservation of gluteal fat pads to ensure adequate gluteal projection is vital to avoid flattening of the buttock shape.

THIGHPLASTY

Both short and long scar versions of this operation exist, and the incision length is determined according to the patient's preference and soft tissue deformity. In the long scar version, the incision stays medial to the patella before curving inferiorly in a lateral direction. Combined with LBL, thighplasty completely reshapes the lower trunk and thigh circumferentially.

Patient Evaluation

Most patients present in consultation requesting a solution to excess skin in the medial upper thigh that causes chaffing, moisture buildup, and difficulty fitting into clothes. The thigh is assessed in a circumferential fashion to decide on the optimal approach that will address the patient's excess tissue and meet their expectations. Often, vertical thigh lift is combined with liposuction of the lateral thigh and medial knee to debulk tissue that is not treated by the excision. This is discussed with the patient at the preoperative visit. Before and after pictures are shown in Figure 65.4.

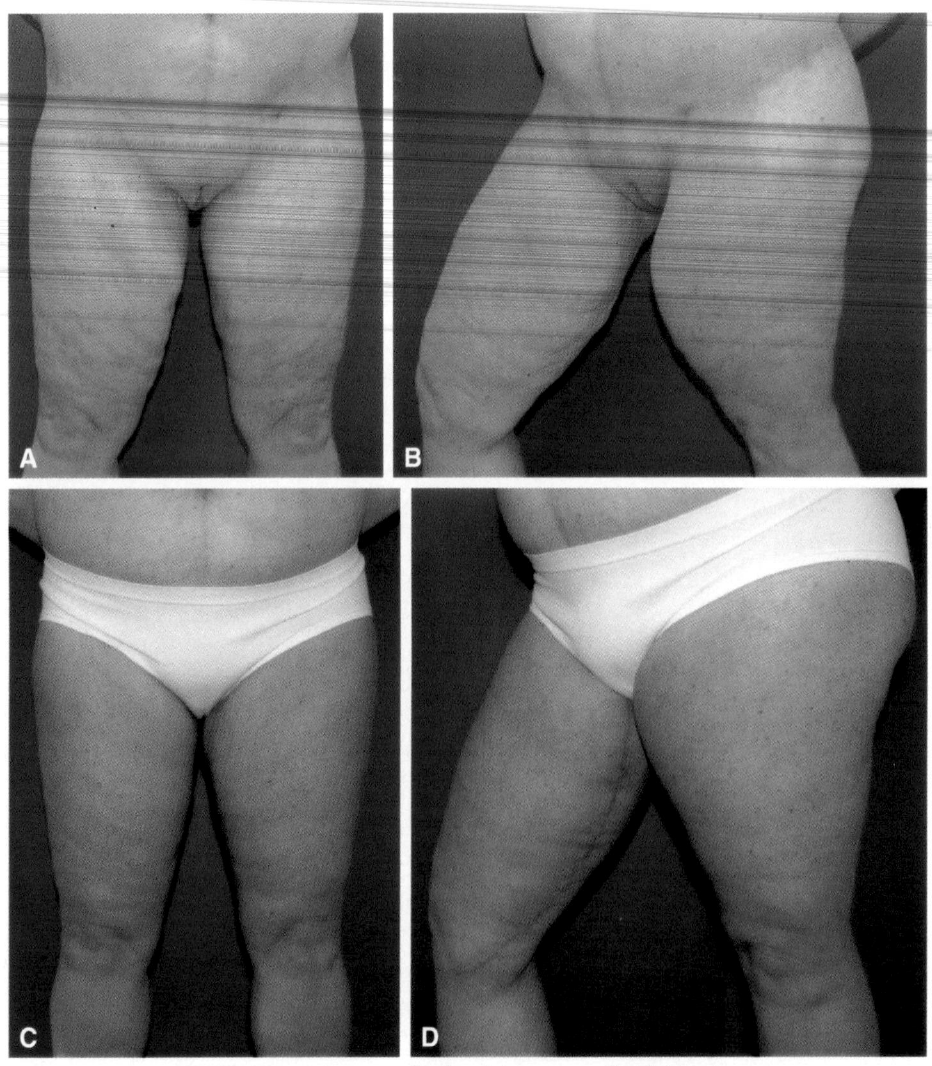

FIGURE 65.4. Preoperative **(A,B)** and postoperative **(C,D)** thighplasty.

Surgical Technique

Markings

The patient is marked with the patient on a bed, in the supine position, with thighs abducted in frog leg position. The first mark is made 4 cm away from the midline at the level of the mons pubis. In the area of the mons, the incision should stay in or near the proximal thigh crease to avoid scar migration and labial widening. This is then extended within the groin crease to mark the natural line that exists in this region. Next, the adductor longus is marked along its course from groin to knee. A pinch or distraction test is used to determine the estimated width of tissue that will be removed. If significant vertical excess is present, a horizontal incision may have to be incorporated; this is done by means of sliding tissue along the adductor longus superiorly and marking the estimated height of resection. Hatch marks are made for easy reapproximation, and symmetry is verified. Representative markings are shown in Figure 65.5.

Intraoperative Steps

The thigh is prepped circumferentially for access to all areas. This permits liposuction of the excision site as well as other regions, if needed (see Alternate Approach: Excision-Site Liposuction section). The procedure begins with subdermal injection of a 1:100,000 epinephrine solution. Alternatively, the epinephrine can be injected after the patient is intubated to allow for maximum effect and minimize wasted time once the procedure has started. After waiting an appropriate amount of time for the epinephrine to take effect, the anterior incision is made along its length. Dissection proceeds in a plan immediately superficial to the muscular fascia toward the posterior marking. Care must be taken during this step to avoid injury to the saphenous vein, which courses superficially, or lymphatic structures of the groin. The dissection must not proceed past the maximum width of resection or risk raising a flap of tissue that will have to be sewed back down. The preoperative markings are guides and therefore the width of resection may differ from the anticipated width. As the surgeon approaches the posterior margin, the ability to close the elevated tissue is intermittently verified.

Once the limit of dissection is reached, the margin of resection is verified by pulling the edges together with a pair of forceps or towel clamp. Perpendicular hash marks are then made to simplify closure, and the posterior incision is infiltrated with epinephrine prior to completing the resection. The wound is irrigated and hemostasis is assured. The SFS of the thigh flap is secured to the Colles fascia using 2-0 absorbable suture to prevent labial distortion. A drain is placed at the base of the wound, exiting lateral to the mons area, and the incision is temporarily closed with staples to mitigate edema. The deep SFS layer is closed with 2-0 absorbable suture and the deep dermis is closed with 3-0 absorbable suture. The skin is closed with 3-0

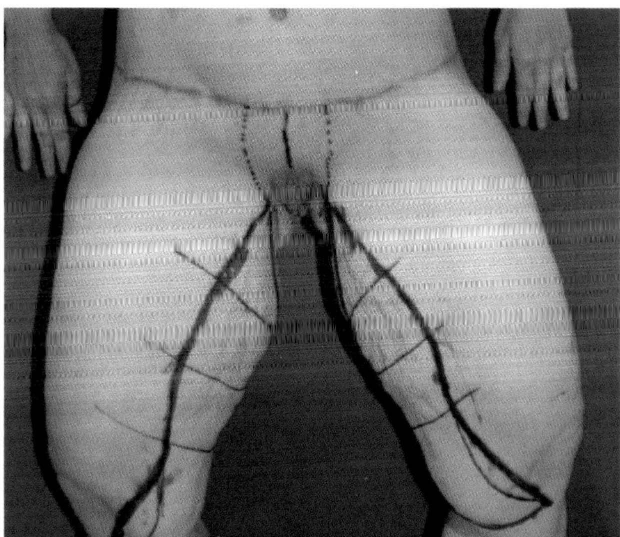

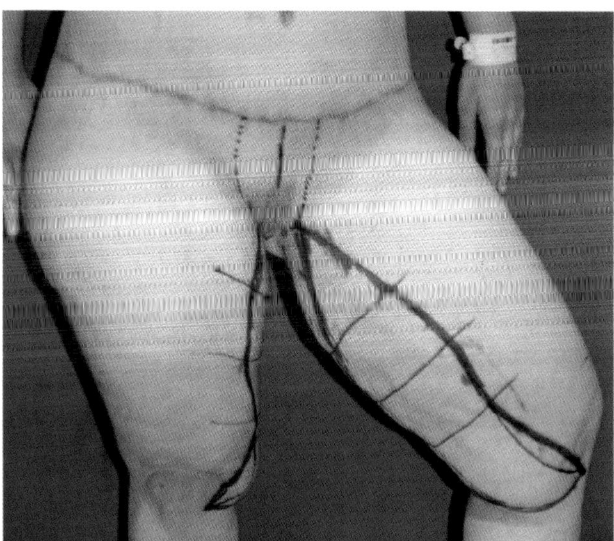

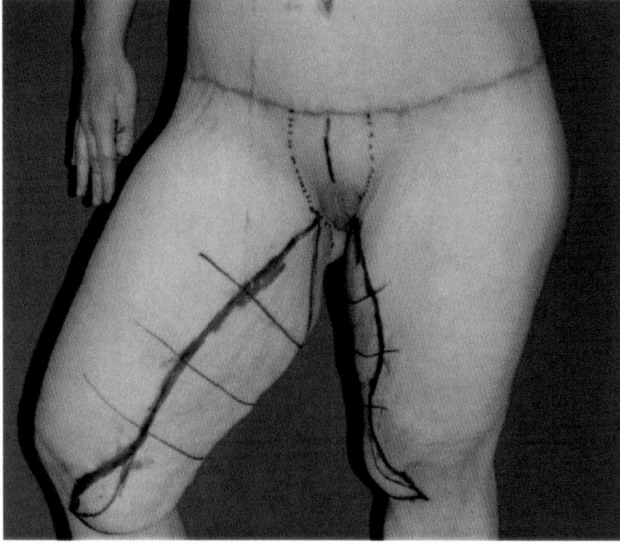

FIGURE 65.5. The same patient at her second stage, with markings performed prior to vertical medial thighplasty. **A.** Anterior and **(B, C)** oblique views of markings.

absorbable suture in the subcuticular layer, and cyanoacrylate glue is used to seal the incision. Lower extremities are wrapped from foot to thigh with a compression bandage.

Alternate Approach: Excision-Site Liposuction

Resection site liposuction as described by Drs. Pascal and Louarn[17] can be applied to thighplasty with comparable results. However, new adopters of this technique should be careful as it requires a commitment to the estimated width of resection and therefore can lead to over-resection. Tumescent solution is infiltrated into the excision site and this area is aggressively lipoaspirated. Alternatively, conservative tumescent followed by liposuction can be performed in an anterior to posterior direction to ensure that the margins of resection can be closed. As much as is feasible, liposuction access sites should be within the safe margin of resection to avoid additional small scars.

Postoperative Care

Patients generally spend one to two nights in the hospital, depending on the concurrent procedure performed. All patients are encouraged to ambulate with assistance on the evening of surgery. While hospitalized, venous thromboembolism prophylaxis is based on a patient's 2005 Caprini score, a validated tool for use in plastic and reconstructive surgery.[18] A Foley catheter is left in place for one evening until the patient can ambulate and use the bathroom. Showering may begin 24 to 48 hours postoperatively. The morning after surgery, dressings are unwrapped and surgical sites examined for signs of bleeding before discharge from the facility. Perioperative antibiotic use and drain placement is left to the discretion of the surgeon.

The patient is seen in clinic within 1 week of surgery for a first postoperative visit. The postoperative dressing is removed to examine the surgical sites. If drains were placed, they are discontinued based on output. Patients are seen weekly until all drains are removed. Compression is maintained for 6 weeks. Patients may use the postoperative medical wrapping or transition to a store-bought compression garment of choice. Lifting is restricted to 5 kg during this same period.

COMPLICATIONS

Common complications with truncal or extremity contouring procedures are usually minor and easily managed on an outpatient basis. Those seen most often are delayed wound healing or wound dehiscence. Another commonly seen complication is a seroma. More serious complications that could require a return to the operating room are hematoma, surgical site infection, and nerve injuries during extremity surgery. Some complications may necessitate revisions, such as scar widening or hypertrophy and chronic wounds or sinus tracts. Recurrent skin laxity is a source of dissatisfaction for the patient and is an unpredictable complication. Systemic complications are generally more worrisome, including but not limited to deep venous thrombosis and pulmonary embolism, which could be fatal. For management of these postoperative problems, refer to Chapter 63.

SUMMARY

Careful planning is the key to successful outcomes in LBL and thigh lift in the MWL population. The surgeon must choose the optimal procedure for the patient's unique deformity rather than stick to one technique and apply it to all comers. Understanding and being able to manage complications is paramount in the care of these patients.

REFERENCES

1. Lockwood T. High-lateral-tension abdominoplasty with superficial fascial system suspension. *Plast Reconstr Surg*. 1995;96(3):603-615.
2. Cormenzana P, Samprón NM. Circumferential approach to contouring of the trunk. *Aesthet Surg J*. 2004;24(1):13-23.
3. Song AY, Jean RD, Hurwitz DJ, et al. A classification of contour deformities after bariatric weight loss: the Pittsburgh Rating Scale. *Plast Reconstr Surg*. 2005;116(5):1535-1544.
   A classification system designed to grade the deformities of 10 anatomical areas after massive weight loss. The Pittsburgh Rating Scale is a validated measure of contour deformities in MWL patients.
4. Lockwood T. Lower body lift with superficial fascial system suspension. *Plast Reconstr Surg*. 1993;92(6):1112-1122.
5. Lockwood TE. Superficial fascial system (SFS) of the trunk and thigh: a new concept. *Plast Reconstr Surg*. 1991;87(6):1009-1018.
6. Lewis JR. The thigh lift. *J Int Coll Surg*. 1957;27:330-334.
7. Schultz RC, Feinberg LA. Medial thigh lift. *Ann Plast Surg*. 1979;2(5):404-410.
8. Lockwood TE. Fascial anchoring technique in medial thigh lifts. *Plast Reconstr Surg*. 1988;82(2):299-304.
   An important article by Ted Lockwood describing the high-lateral tension abdominoplasty with SFS suspension. Fifty patients underwent this technique with excellent lifting of the inguinal and anterior thigh areas.
9. Spirito D. Medial thigh lift and DE.C.LI.VE. *Aesthetic Plast Surg*. 1998;22(4):298-300.
10. Le Louarn C, Pascal JF. The concentric medial thigh lift. *Aesthetic Plast Surg*. 2004;28(1):20-23.
11. Sozer SO, Agullo FJ, Palladino H. Spiral lift: medial and lateral thigh lift with buttock lift and augmentation. *Aesthetic Plast Surg*. 2008;32(1):120-125.
12. Shermak MA, Mallalieu J, Chang D. Does thighplasty for upper thigh laxity after massive weight loss require a vertical incision? *Aesthet Surg J*. 2009;29(6):513-522.
13. Shermak MA, Chang DC, Heller J. Factors impacting thromboembolism after bariatric body contouring surgery. *Plast Reconstr Surg*. 2007;119(5):1590-1596.
14. Kurz A, Sessler DI, Lenhardt R. Perioperative normothermia to reduce the incidence of surgical-wound infection and shorten hospitalization: Study of Wound Infection and Temperature Group. *N Engl J Med*. 1996;334(19):1209-1215.
15. Coon D, Michaels JV, Gusenoff JA, et al. Hypothermia and complications in postbariatric body contouring. *Plast Reconstr Surg*. 2012;130(2):443-448.
   An article examining effects of intraoperative hypothermia in patients undergoing plastic surgery after bariatric surgery. Results demonstrated that hypothermia is associated with an increased risk of seroma formation and bleeding requiring transfusion.
16. Hurwitz DJ, Rubin JP, Risin M, et al. Correcting the saddlebag deformity in the massive weight loss patient. *Plast Reconstr Surg*. 2004;114(5):1313-1325.
17. Pascal JF, Le Louarn C. Brachioplasty. *Aesthetic Plast Surg*. 2005;29:423-429.
18. Caprini JA. Thrombosis risk assessment as a guide to quality patient care. *Dis Mon*. 2005;51(2-3):70-78.
   A landmark article by Caprini wherein the first VTE risk-assessment tool was introduced. This study was later validated in the plastic surgery literature by Panucci et al. and is currently the basis for stratifying outpatient plastic surgery procedures.
19. Shermak MA. Hernia repair and abdominoplasty in gastric bypass patients. *Plast Reconstr Surg*. 2006;117(4):1145-1150.
20. Moreno-Egea A, Campillo-Soto Á, Morales-Cuenca G. Does abdominoplasty add morbidity to incisional hernia repair? A randomized controlled trial. *Surg Innov*. 2016;23(5):474-480.
21. Hughes KC, Weider L, Fischer J, et al. Ventral hernia repair with simultaneous panniculectomy. *Am Surg*. 1996;62(8):678-681.

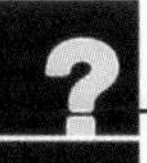

QUESTIONS

1. **A 56-year-old woman presents to clinic after being referred by her bariatric surgeon. She underwent laparoscopic Roux-en-Y 2 years ago. What is the procedure that will best address the deformity shown in Figure 65.6?**

   a. Abdominoplasty
   b. Lateral thighplasty
   c. Liposuction
   d. LBL
   e. Panniculectomy

2. **A 28-year-old man comes to your office after 60-kg weight loss secondary to gastric bypass surgery. He has no major comorbidities and is otherwise healthy. He has an incisional hernia from previous abdominal surgery and is interested in panniculectomy and simultaneous hernia repair. He asks your opinion about a concurrent hernia repair and panniculectomy. What is the appropriate response?**

   a. Both procedures can be safely performed in one operative setting.
   b. It is best to fix the hernia at a first stage then perform the panniculectomy at a second stage.
   c. The risk of complications is less when performed together than individually.
   d. The risk of complications is too high to perform both procedures simultaneously.

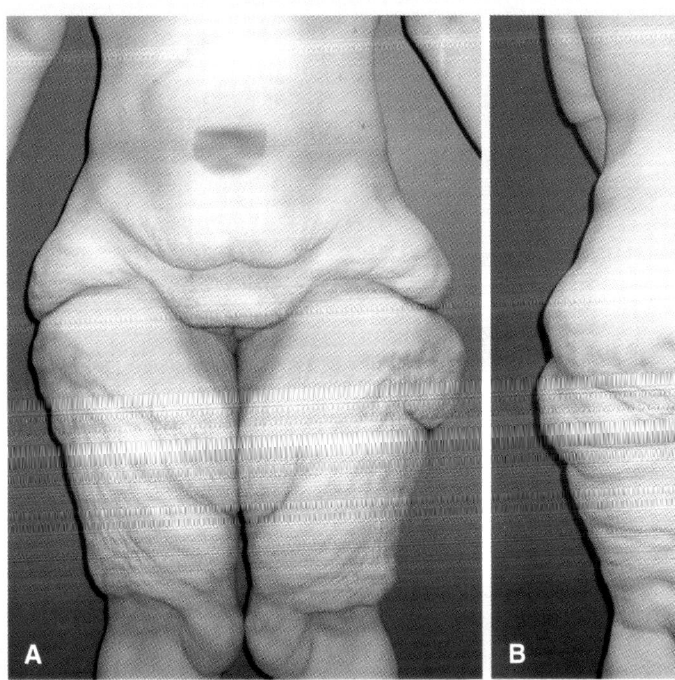

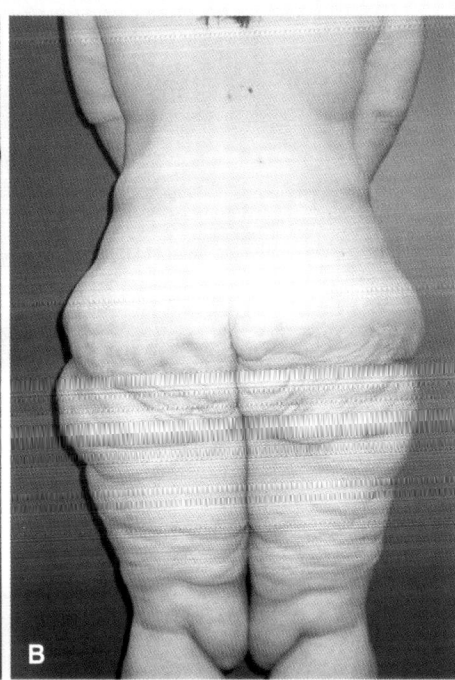

FIGURE 65.6. **A.** Anterior and **(B)** posterior view of patient in question 1.

3. **What is the best treatment option for the patient in Figure 65.7 who has lost 100 lb and presents desiring correction of excess thigh laxity?**

   a. Lateral thighplasty
   b. Liposuction
   c. Short scar vertical thighplasty
   d. Transverse thighplasty
   e. Vertical thighplasty

4. **Which procedure has the highest risk of recurrent skin laxity?**

   a. Abdominoplasty
   b. Brachioplasty
   c. Dermal suspension, parenchymal reshaping mastopexy
   d. LBL
   e. Thighplasty

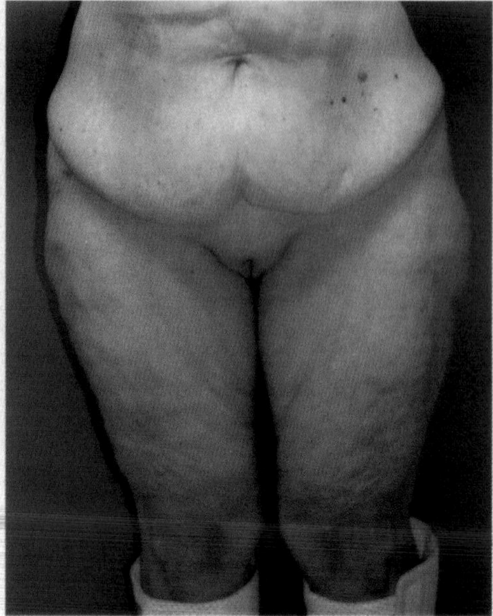

FIGURE 65.7. Anterior view of patient in question 3.

1. **Answer: d.** LBL is the only procedure among the choices that will address the lateral thigh laxity present in the patient depicted. None of the other choices alone would address the circumferential deformity present, which is only treated by means of an LBL.

2. **Answer: a.** Multiple studies have shown the safety of simultaneous panniculectomy or abdominoplasty combined with ventral hernia repair in all patient types (including MWL patients).[19-21] As with all procedures, patient selection and optimization is key, and these operations should not be performed on smokers or poorly controlled diabetics.

3. **Answer: e.** The best treatment for MWL patients for treatment of excess skin and fat of the thigh is a medial vertical thighplasty. Contouring surgery requires a shaping of the thigh in a cylindrical fashion, which can only be obtained via a longitudinal incision on the extremity. Lateral thighplasty may be performed but would place a more visible scar on the outside aspect of the thigh. Liposuction alone would not treat the excess skin present in this patient. A short scar vertical thighplasty would not address the full-length deformity that is present at the knee region. Finally, transverse thighplasty is incorrect as it is a transverse incision that will inadequately treat the distal thigh and is prone to recurrence of laxity.

4. **Answer: e.** Of all the procedures for massive weight loss patients, thighplasty is the one that is most likely to result in recurrent skin laxity. Unfortunately, this is neither avoidable nor predictable by the surgeon preoperatively.

CHAPTER 66 Brachioplasty and Upper Trunk Contouring

Amy S. Colwell and Nicole A. Phillips

KEY POINTS

- Brachioplasty and upper trunk contouring are increasingly performed for patients with redundant skin following massive weight loss.
- The goals of surgery are to remove redundant skin and restore more normal or enhanced contour.
- Patient selection centers on optimizing medical conditions and nutrition while accepting realistic expectations of outcomes.
- Brachioplasty procedures successfully remove redundant skin and fatty tissue from the upper arm. The most common technique leaves a visible scar along the inner aspect of the arm. The patient needs to decide if the benefits of improved contour outweigh the presence of scar.
- The breast deformity is typically characterized by deflated, ptotic breasts. The surgical procedure of choice is related to the current and desired volume of the breasts and includes breast reduction, mastopexy, augmentation-mastopexy, and less commonly autologous augmentation using intercostal artery perforator (ICAP) flaps.
- Upper body contouring includes removal of an axillary roll and back skin to tighten the entire upper torso. This is commonly known as a bra-line lift and may be combined with breast and arm contouring.

Management of excess skin and fat following massive weight loss (MWL) is an area of growing interest and consumer demand. Given the steady rise in popularity of bariatric procedures, it is not surprising that patients are seeking out body contouring procedures at increasing rates. The American Society for Metabolic and Bariatric Surgery reported 216,000 bariatric procedures in 2016, compared with 158,000 procedures just 5 years earlier.[1]

Today's plastic surgeon should be comfortable with the surgical approaches and perioperative care requirements for patients requesting body contouring procedures. The focus of this chapter, brachioplasty and upper body contouring, highlights the upward trend of patient interest in these procedures. According to data from the American Society for Aesthetic Plastic Surgery, breast lift and brachioplasty have shown the most dramatic increase in cosmetic procedures performed since the society began collecting data nearly 20 years ago. More than 24,000 brachioplasty procedures were reported in 2016, representing an 879% increase since 1997. Breast lift was the fourth most commonly performed procedure in 2016 with over 161,000 procedures performed. The popularity of this surgery has increased 712% compared with 1997 rates.[2]

For patients who have successfully lost weight following bariatric surgery or through diet and exercise routines, satisfaction with results can be severely limited by the excess skin and deflated tissue that remains. Although the health benefits of weight loss are undisputed, the psychosocial benefits may lag behind as patients struggle with intertriginous rashes, skin breakdown, difficulty with clothing fit, poor self-image, and functional impairment. The goals of surgery are to restore a more normal contour, achieving improved appearance and function; however, expectations must be frankly discussed with patients prior to surgery, as soft tissues that have been subject to significant weight gain/loss will never recover their pre–weight-gain elasticity and appearance. Patients must fully understand that lengthy scars are the trade-off for improved contour, and that minor complications such as wound dehiscence and seromas are not uncommon. Patients with unreasonable expectations or who are unwilling to accept these risks are not good candidates for body contouring procedures.[3]

At the initial evaluation, special attention should be paid to certain elements of the patient history. The maximum body mass index (BMI) prior to weight loss should be recorded along with the current BMI. Higher BMI at both time points has been associated with higher complication rates after surgery.[4,5] Timing of body contouring procedures should allow at least 12 months after bariatric surgery and 6 months at a stable weight for patients to achieve metabolic and nutritional homeostasis. If patients have experienced a plateau of weight loss at higher-than-expected BMI, or are suffering from significant nausea, vomiting, or nutritional derangement, referral back to the bariatric surgeon for reevaluation is recommended.[4]

Patients with a history of obesity also demonstrate high rates of significant medical comorbidities including cardiac disease, insulin resistance, and obstructive sleep apnea. Risk factors for the aforementioned should be carefully examined, and medical management optimized prior to any planned surgical intervention. Furthermore, if a patient is on chronic anticoagulation, a decision must be made on the safety of being off the medication for the perioperative time period. Finally, the patient's psychological status and social support network should be ascertained. MWL and outcomes after body contouring procedures can precipitate tremendous changes in self esteem, image perception, and interpersonal relationships. Ensuring the safety and stability of the patient from a psychological and social perspective should not be overlooked.[4]

BRACHIOPLASTY

Introduced by Iturraspe and Fernandez in 1954,[6] brachioplasty was designed to tighten and lift the upper arm. Weight fluctuations, aging, and heredity contribute to sagging skin and a droopy appearance of upper arms (Figure 66.1). This excess skin is troubling to patients and has functional consequences including chafing, rashes, and difficulty with clothing fit. No amount of physical exercise will correct an excess of loose skin, and localized adipose deposits can likewise be difficult to target. For these patients, a number of arm contouring procedures have been described, with significant modifications in technique since the original description.[7]

Classification schemes are not widely used in clinical practice; however, knowledge of basic systems may facilitate procedure choices and discussions. The first classification of the upper arm deformity, described by Teimourian and Malekzadeh in 1998, divided upper arm findings into four categories[8]:

- Group 1: Patients with minimal to moderate subcutaneous fat and minimal skin laxity
- Group 2: Patients with generalized accumulation of subcutaneous fat and moderate skin laxity. The authors suggested management of these patients with liposuction, with the possible addition of a small axillary skin excision
- Group 3: Patients with excess fat and extensive skin laxity requiring combined liposuction and direct soft-tissue excision
- Group 4: Patients with minimal excess adiposity but significant skin laxity, requiring brachioplasty without adjunctive liposuction

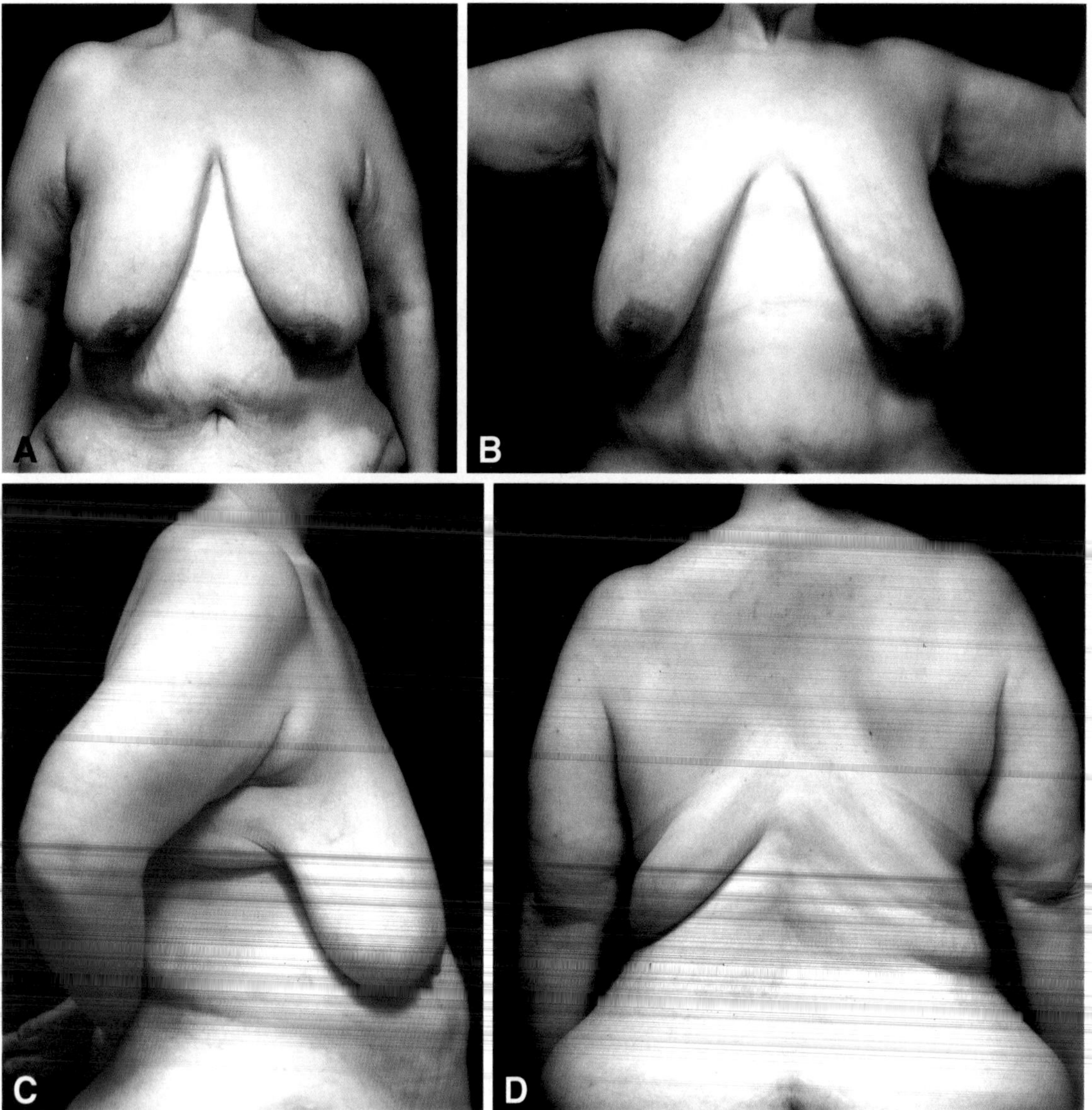

FIGURE 66.1. Massive weight loss upper torso deformity. **A.** The breast deformity is characterized by breast ptosis, lowering of the inframammary fold, upper pole volume loss, and often medialization of the nipples. **B.** The arm deformity consists of variable amounts of excess skin and adipose tissue. **C, D.** The axillary and midback deformity likewise contains excess skin, with or without excess fatty tissue deposits.

Later classification systems built on and refined this concept. In addition to the degree of skin and fat excess, the algorithmic system introduced by Appelt et al. in 2006 added the variable of location of skin excess[9]:

- Type I: Patients with relative excess of adipose tissue but good skin quality and tone, for whom liposuction alone was recommended
- Type II: Patients with minimal to moderate adipose tissue and moderate skin laxity. Excisional brachioplasty techniques were endorsed for this patient population, with a further subdivision into type IIA, IIB, and IIC based on the location of skin excess and the related skin excision pattern
- Type III: Patients with both significant lipodystrophy and redundant skin laxity fall into three categories:
    - Continued weight loss prior to surgery
    - Staged treatment with initial liposuction followed by excisional brachioplasty
    - Combined liposuction-excisional brachioplasty

Type III patients were again subdivided based on location of skin excess, which determines the skin excision pattern for any brachioplasty procedure performed.

Another widely accepted classification system described by El Khatib appeared in the literature the following year with five stages of brachial ptosis and management according to adipose deposits and skin laxity.[10]

Related Anatomy

The fascial systems of the upper arms provide important landmarks for the surgeon performing liposuction or excisional contouring procedures. The superficial fascial system is found between the superficial and deep layers of subcutaneous fat. Loosening of this layer with age or significant weight fluctuations can contribute to upper arm ptosis; as such, some authors advocate plication of this layer during the closing portion of the procedure.[11] The deep fascial system envelops the musculature, and all major neurovascular structures of the arm lie deep to this layer. Care should be taken to avoid violation of this layer during all aspects of the procedure.

Two sensory nerves travel superficial to the deep fascial layer and are thus at risk during brachioplasty procedures: the medial brachial cutaneous nerve and the medial antebrachial cutaneous (MABC) nerve (Figure 66.2). Damage to these nerves results in sensory dysfunction, a well-recognized possible complication of this procedure.

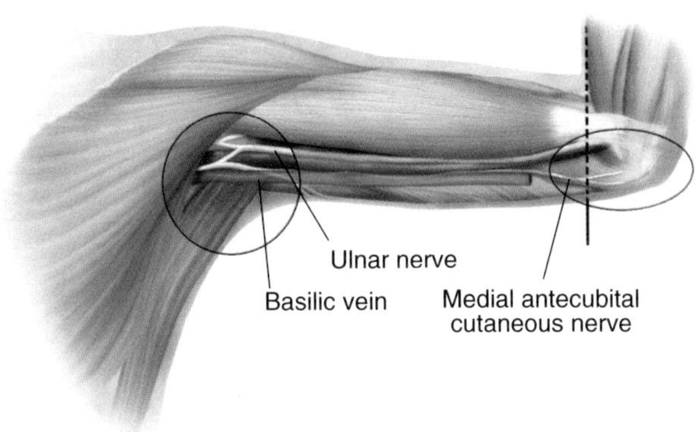

FIGURE 66.2. Upper arm anatomy. During upper arm contouring, knowledge of the relevant anatomy is essential. The shaded areas highlight the axilla and posteromedial elbow, which are approached cautiously secondary to the brachial plexus in the axilla and the superficial path of the ulnar nerve distally. The medial antebrachial cutaneous nerve travels with the basilic vein and should be preserved.

Both nerves arise from the medial cord of the brachial plexus. The MABC nerve, which is the more frequently involved of the two, pierces the deep fascia an average of 14 cm proximal to the medial epicondyle and travels with the basilic vein in the superficial plane of the distal half to third of the upper arm. To prevent damage to these sensory nerves, at least 1 cm of fat should be left on the deep brachial fascia of the upper arm if possible. Adjunctive liposuction can also be employed to facilitate atraumatic dissection and lymphatic preservation of lymphatics to decrease seroma formation. To prevent ulnar nerve injury, liposuction access incisions should be avoided at the posteromedial elbow, and caution should be exercised with the liposuction cannula tip in this same region.

Preoperative Evaluation, Planning, and Marking

A thorough history and physical examination must be conducted at the time of the initial evaluation, with special attention paid to weight loss/gain, stability of current weight, tobacco use, medical comorbidities, and nutritional status. Physical examination should include full motor and sensory examinations of the bilateral upper extremities, in addition to assessment of skin quality and tone. Evaluation of the degree of excess skin and adipose tissue forms the basis for operative planning. Importantly, patients must be willing to accept potentially unfavorable scarring in exchange for improved contour.

To best determine the degree of excess skin, fat, and ptosis, the patient is asked to stand with the shoulder abducted to 90° and the elbow flexed at 90°. Details of marking and surgical technique specific to each approach are highlighted in the relevant sections.

Liposuction

For patients with minimal skin laxity and a mild to moderate amount of adipose deposits in the upper extremity, liposuction can be performed as a stand-alone technique for upper extremity recontouring. It can also be performed as a staged procedure or as an adjunct to traditional excisional brachioplasty procedures. Traditional, mechanical, and/or ultrasound-assisted liposuction may be employed according to the surgeon's preference.

The patient should stand in the position described above, with shoulders abducted and elbows flexed. Pockets of adipose tissue are marked out and access incisions planned by avoiding areas that must be treated with caution while performing liposuction: the axilla, to avoid damage to branches of the brachial plexus, and the posteromedial elbow, to avoid damage to the ulnar nerve (see Figure 66.2).

The operation is performed under local, monitored, or general anesthesia with the patient in the supine position. Arms should be supported on single arm boards, abducted to approximately 80°. Following standard procedures for prepping and draping, tumescent fluid is infiltrated into each arm prior to suction lipectomy. Care should be taken to remain above the deep brachial fascia with the liposuction cannula, leaving a layer of fat over this deep fascial layer to preserve lymphatics and avoid significant contour irregularities. Long, uniform strokes are also recommended to improve outcomes. Liposuction to the bicipital groove is avoided to minimize contour irregularity in this region, which is known anatomically to be relatively devoid of fat.[7,9,12]

Minibrachioplasty (Limited Medial Incision Brachioplasty)

For patients with good skin quality but a moderate excess of skin and adipose tissue limited to the proximal one-half to one-third of the upper arm, the minibrachioplasty is a reasonable option to consider. This procedure has little to no benefit for the MWL patient.

Preoperative planning should begin with the patient standing in the upright position, with arms resting at his or her sides. The anterior and posterior borders of the axillary skin crease are marked, signaling the boundaries of the planned incision (Figure 66.3). The patient is then asked to stand with the arm raised, shoulder abducted, and elbow flexed. The two points are connected along the axillary fold; this line now defines the planned medial incision. A pinch test is performed to determine the extent of resection, which is generally limited to 3 to 5 cm at its widest point. A vertical dart can be added as needed to correct residual horizontal excess. Hatch marks are placed to assist with realignment at the conclusion of the procedure.

The procedure is performed under local, monitored, or general anesthesia. Setup and liposuction should proceed as described in the previous section. The axillary elliptical incisions are made using a scalpel, and then electrocautery is used to raise the tissue in a subcutaneous plane. The medial and lateral skin flaps may be undermined to facilitate closure, but this is typically not necessary. A transverse extension at the midpoint of the incision can be designed to correct a dog-ear or correct for ongoing skin laxity.[7,13]

Extended Brachioplasty

An extended brachioplasty is the procedure of choice for patients with significant skin laxity that cannot be corrected by the methods described earlier. Most MWL patients require this technique

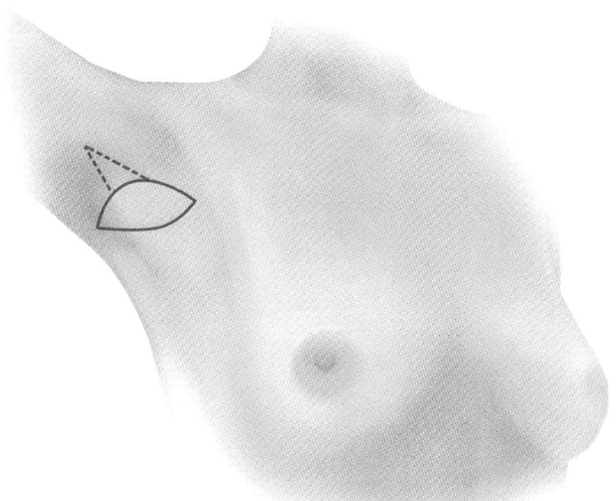

FIGURE 66.3. Minibrachioplasty. For patients with small degrees of skin laxity, with or without excess adiposity, an elliptical incision can be designed in the axilla for skin tightening. This incision may contain a vertical dart (*dashed lines*) for dog-ear removal or to excise more redundant upper arm skin.

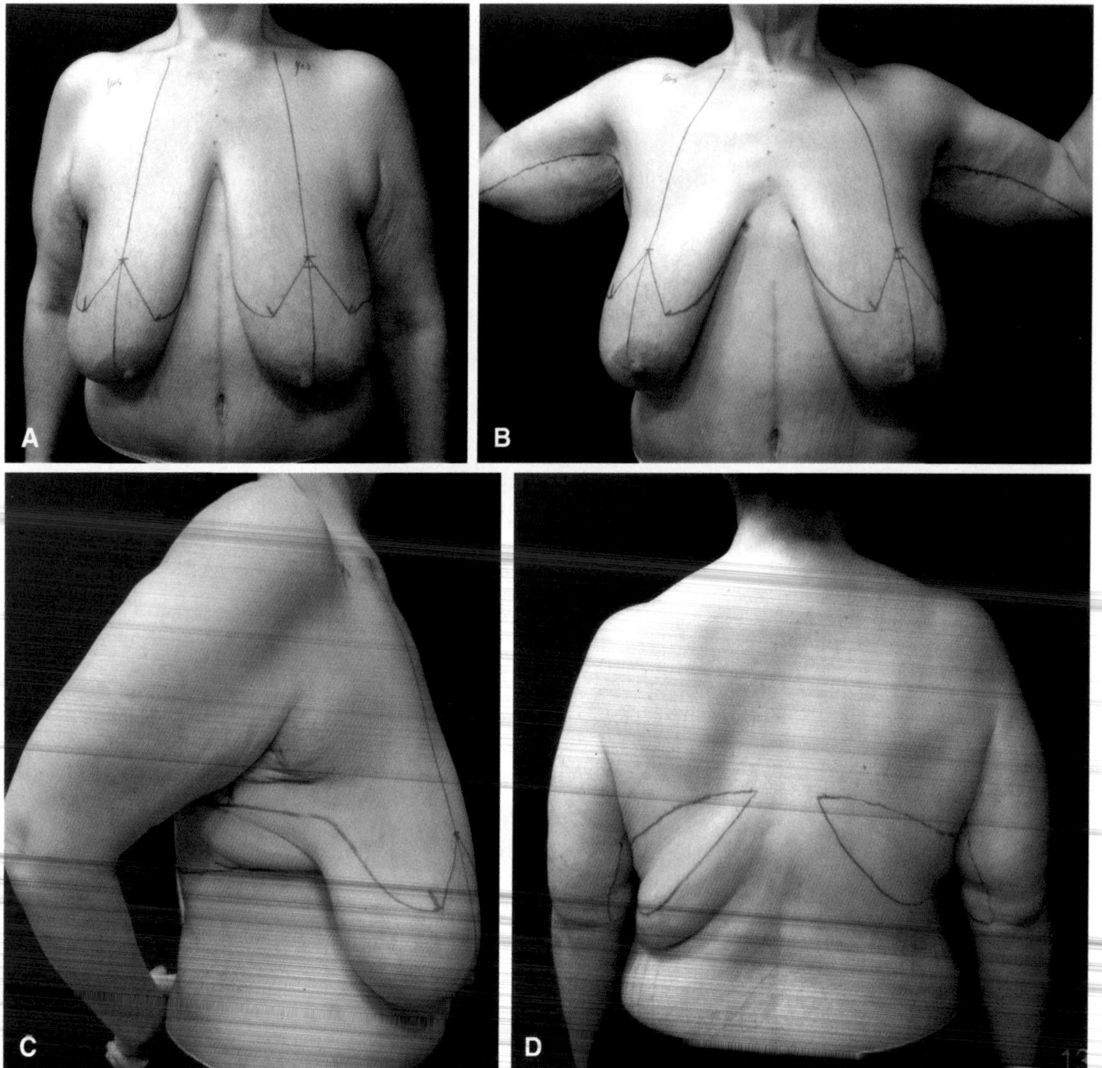

FIGURE 66.4. Markings for upper body lift. This patient had massive weight loss and desired an improvement in her contour. **A.** Markings for Wise pattern mastopexy. **B.** Markings for Wise pattern mastopexy and brachioplasty. **C.** Side view showing continuity of breast and back markings. **D.** Bra-line excision of axilla and back.

if they desire improved arm contour. The superior incision is marked approximately one fingerbreadth above the bicipital groove (Figure 66.4). The inferior incision is then determined with the assistance of a pinch test, often resulting in mark placement just posterior to the inferior-most extent of hanging skin. The final inferior mark is rechecked after skin undermining. An extension to the chest wall is often added and is known as an L-brachioplasty with the superior L-point in or near the deltopectoral groove along the anterior axillary line. The distal extension is planned based on the expected amount of tissue resection and confirmed with a pinch test. Care is taken to avoid overresection and prevent breast lateralization.

The operation is performed under monitored or general anesthesia with the patient in the supine position. Arms should be supported on single arm boards, abducted to approximately 80°. Following standard procedures for prepping and draping, tumescent fluid is infiltrated into each arm if liposuction is going to be used to facilitate the dissection. The amount of tumescent fluid should be minimized, so as to avoid large-volume swelling that may ultimately inhibit the degree of resection. Liposuction is then performed through access incisions placed within the planned area of resection. Liposuction beyond the borders of the planned resection is intentionally limited, as aggressive liposuction of these areas may compromise the remaining soft tissue and lead to postprocedure skin loosening when swelling resolves.

The anterior incision is then made, and dissection of the skin flap from anterior to posterior is performed in the honeycomb plane that has been defined by the previous liposuction (Figure 66.5A). Intermittent pinch tests are performed to ensure the accuracy of the preoperative markings and the ability to close the skin once the inferior incision has been made. The final excision of the skin flap and resultant contour are guided by tailor tacking and either segmental resection or alternatively by committing to the entire inferior incision at once (Figure 66.5B). The longitudinal resection of the upper arm tissue is achieved first, and then adjustments are made to the axillary/chest wall component as needed. Three-layer closure of the wound is also performed using absorbable sutures in a sequential fashion, over a drain (Figure 66.5C). Reapproximation of the superficial fascial system importantly helps maintain contour and prevents scar puckering.[14]

Postoperative Management, Outcomes, and Complications

All patients should be placed into compressive dressings at the end of the procedure, regardless of the selected technique. These compression garments should be worn day and night for at least 6 weeks postoperatively. Drains placed for brachioplasty procedures offload stress on the incisions early and can be removed at the first postoperative visit.

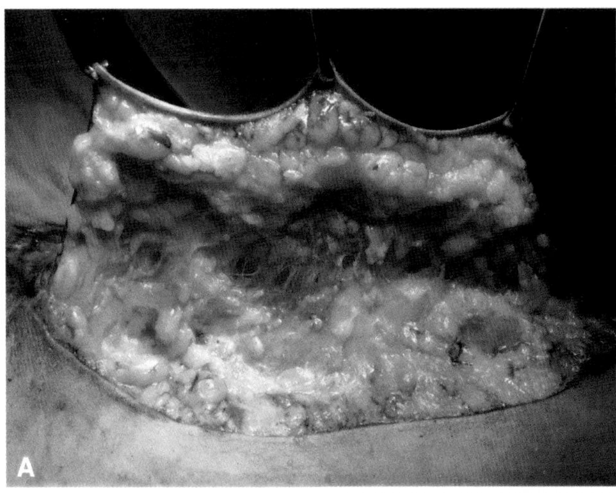

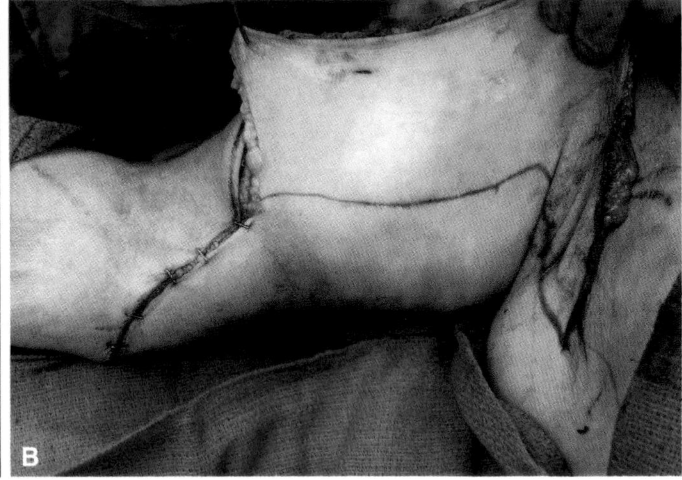

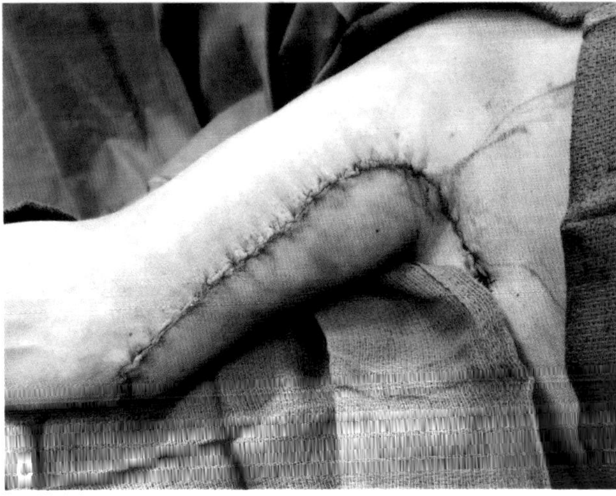

FIGURE 66.5. Extended brachioplasty technique. **A.** Liposuction facilitates the dissection plane and leaves fat down on the deep fascia, thus helping to preserve nerves and lymphatics. **B.** A segmental [illegible] skin excision without risking the ability to close. **C.** The incisions are closed in three layers to avoid indentation and scar puckering.

Recent studies have demonstrated intact sensory and lymphatic function following brachioplasty employing liposuction for atraumatic dissection of tissue planes.[15] This technique helps preserve the layer of fat above the deep brachial fascia harboring the sensory nerves and lymphatics.

Reported complications of the procedure include seroma, hematoma, infection, wound breakdown, slight asymmetries between sides, paresthesias, lymphedema, and unsightly scarring. Risk factors that may increase the chance of overall complications, hematoma, or infection include male gender, BMI >30, and combined procedures.[16] Thoughtful preoperative discussions with patients regarding these risks are critical to ensuring a positive outcome. Patients must be willing to accept these risks to achieve improved contour with decreased volume of the upper arms.

Ongoing debate remains over optimal scar placement. An anterior scar placed just below the bicipital groove of the upper arm is well hidden on both anterior and posterior views with the arms at the side. If the incision is instead placed posteriorly, it will be visible when the patient has his or her arm by the side, but it may have the advantage of avoiding the arm sensory nerves with tissue removal. For thick or heavy scarring, which may occur despite optimal scar placement and technique, regular application of silicone sheeting or scar massage may improve scar appearance.[17]

With careful planning, thorough preoperative discussions, and careful execution, brachioplasty procedures can achieve significant cosmetic and functional improvements for patients. Risk profiles should be carefully considered prior to proceeding; however, with the right patient and operative technique, satisfactory outcomes should be obtainable (Figure 66.6).

BREAST CONTOURING

Related Anatomy

The medial and lateral borders of the breast are defined by the sternocostal junction and the midaxillary line, respectively. The second intercostal space marks the superior boundary. The inframammary fold (IMF) delineates the inferior border of the breast and is formed by the fusion of the deep and superficial fascia with the dermis. Composed of multiple interconnected subunits, the breast is made of mammary glands and associated adipose tissue, which increases as the glandular component subsides after lactation or during menopause. Each mammary gland consists of a host of secretory lobules, which converge to form lactiferous ducts that drain to the nipple. Layers of deep and superficial fascia support the soft tissues of the breast, as do the suspensory Cooper ligaments. Aging and stretch due to weight loss/gain or breastfeeding can lead to attenuation of these structures, contributing to breast ptosis.

Blood supply to the breast must be vigilantly maintained during all contouring procedures. The subdermal plexus provides blood supply to the skin and nipple-areolar complex (NAC). The parenchyma is supported by vascular inflow from perforating branches of the internal mammary artery, the lateral thoracic artery, the thoracodorsal and thoracoacromial arteries, and multiple intercostal perforators.

Innervation of the breast is derived from anteromedial and anterolateral branches of the thoracic intercostal nerves, with the fourth intercostal nerve considered the major contributor to the NAC. Lymphatic drainage occurs via superficial and deep lymphatic drainage systems. The subareolar and subdermal regions drain via the

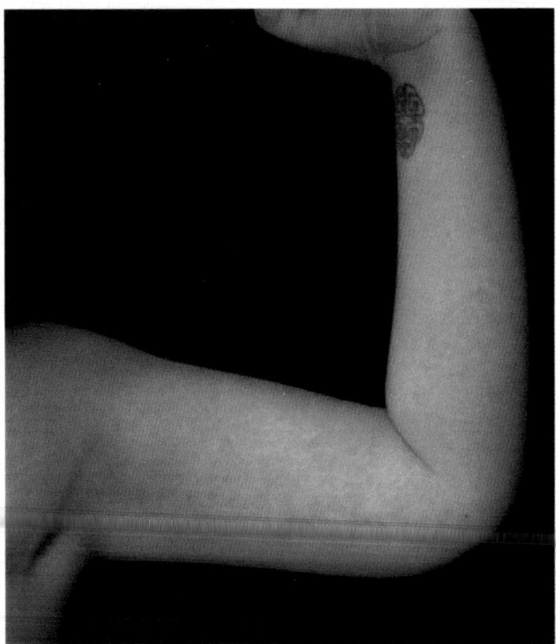

FIGURE 66.6. Brachioplasty result. The scar is located at the level of the bicipital groove and fades over time.

superficial lymphatic system to the axillary basin. The deep lymphatic system drains to the axillary nodes as well, but also exhibits connections with a perforating system that drains to the internal mammary nodes. Other node fields that directly drain the breast include the interpectoral, infraclavicular, supraclavicular, and intercostal nodal basins.[18,19]

Preoperative Evaluation, Planning, and Marking

The loss of volume and attenuation of soft tissue, skin, and ligamentous support associated with MWL results in deflated, ptotic breasts that little resemble the ideal, youthful breast (see Figure 66.1). Given the resultant superior pole deficiency, lack of lateral breast definition, and associated contour deformities of the axilla or posterior trunk, the MWL patient provides the plastic surgeon with a unique set of challenges when attempting to improve breast contour and volume, as traditional techniques may not sufficiently address these concerns.[20] Additionally, the nipple position in MWL patients is frequently located too medial and the IMF too inferior compared with normal breast anatomy, presenting yet other factors to be considered in surgical design and planning.

The breast technique employed largely depends on the current breast volume and desired breast volume[20] (Figure 66.7). Breast ptosis is nearly universal in the weight loss population. If the patient has large breasts and desires smaller breasts, a reduction mammoplasty is performed. If the patient desires to stay the same size, a mastopexy or augmentation mastopexy is offered depending upon the overall size and shape goals. For the patient desiring an increase in breast size, a breast augmentation alone rarely is enough to correct the loose skin and ptosis. Instead, an augmentation mastopexy with implants or autologous tissue is most often chosen. The following breast procedures are covered in separate chapters, but challenges and techniques specific to the MWL population are emphasized in the following sections. As with all patients planned to undergo breast surgery, history of personal or family breast cancer, prior breast procedures, and up-to-date mammography results must be obtained as part of the preoperative workup.

Breast Reduction

For the uncommon MWL patient who retains excess breast volume, standard breast reduction techniques can be employed to provide improved breast shape and position on the chest wall. Although all breast reduction techniques may be considered, the superior safety profile of the inferior pedicle should be taken into account, given the lengthy sternal notch-to-nipple distance typical of weight loss patients. A Wise skin pattern is most commonly chosen to reduce the large skin excess. Dermal suspension techniques and pedicle-shaping sutures as used in mastopexy procedures may improve long-term outcomes and patient satisfaction.[20-22]

Mastopexy

For patients with sufficient volume, standard mastopexy techniques may be employed with the addition of dermal flaps or pedicle-shaping sutures to provide support and maintain breast shape (see Figure 66.4). The

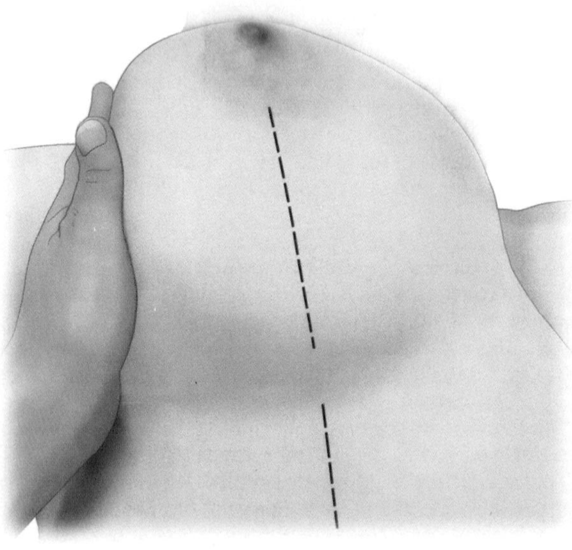

A

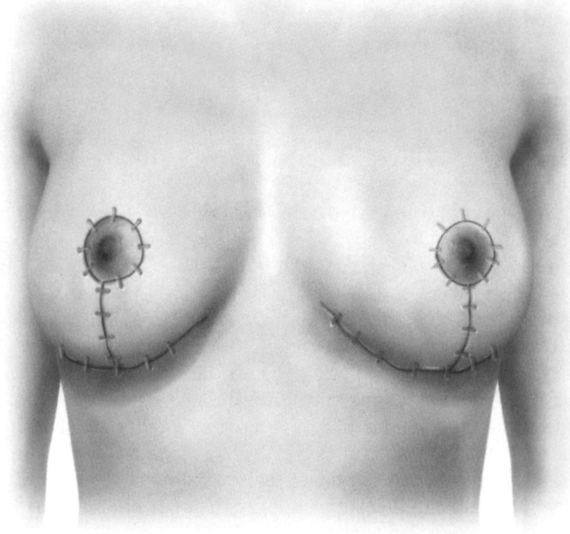

B

FIGURE 66.7. Breast contouring. Options for breast contouring most commonly involve a mastopexy with shaping sutures. A mastopexy with autologous augmentation using an intercostal artery perforator flap can be considered. Augmentation mastopexy is performed in one or two stages. **A.** For a one stage approach, access through a vertical incision preserves lower pole breast support. **B.** Once the implant is placed, the skin is tailor-tacked around the implant for a circumvertical or Wise-pattern mastopexy.

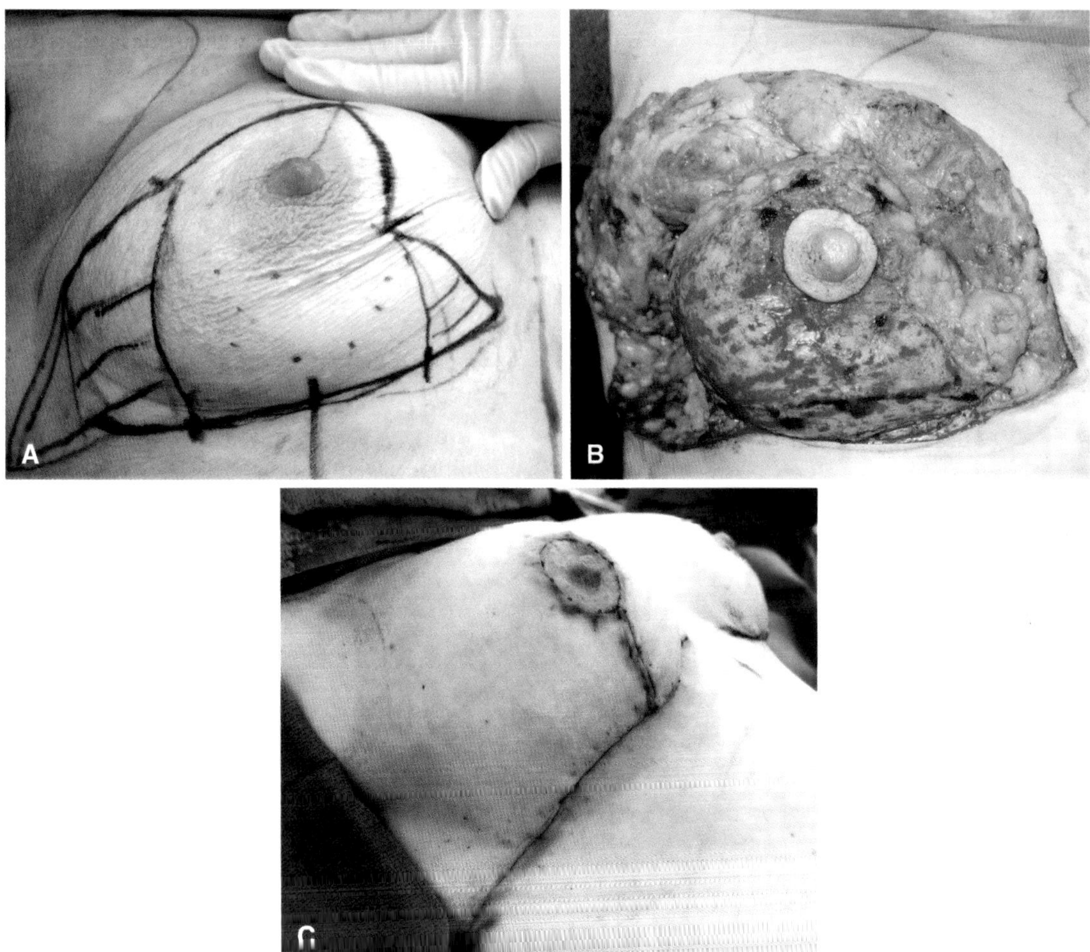

Figure 66.8. Mastopexy with pedicle-shaping sutures. **A**. An 8 to 10 cm inferior and central pedicle is marked around the breast meridian (*dotted area*). **B**. The dermal flap sections are deepithelialized and tacked to the chest wall to support the pedicle shape. **C**. The shaped pedicle resembles the appearance of an implant; however, it descends more than an implant with healing, resulting in less sustained upper pole fullness.

entire Wise pattern is deepithelialized. The lateral most extension of the breast into the axilla may be removed to facilitate a smooth lateral breast border. Skin flaps are then raised approximately 1.5 cm in thickness. The medial and lateral aspects of the deepithelialized breast parenchyma are elevated at the level of the chest wall, maintaining blood supply to the NAC via the preserved 8 to 10 cm inferior and central mound. The inferior pedicle is plicated, leaving 5 to 5.5 cm between the base of the areola and the IMF. Medial, lateral, and superior sections are then tacked to the pectoralis fascia or rib periosteum[20,21] (Figure 66.8).

If the degree of excess skin and ptosis is less severe, a vertical/extended vertical mastopexy with preservation and advancement of the inferior pole tissues can be considered.[23]

Autologous Autoaugmentation

An appealing option for the MWL patient interested in improved breast contour and volume is mastopexy with autologous autoaugmentation using an intercostal artery perforator (ICAP) flap/spiral flap.[20,24-26] This procedure can simultaneously address multiple deformities at once, taking advantage of excess axillary and posterior trunk tissue to provide increased superior pole volume, improved lateral breast definition, and correction of axillary/back irregularities. However, the technical challenges of this technique in achieving adequate mobilization of the flap without injuring the ICAPs have made augmentation using an implant a preferred approach.

For the ICAP flap, patients are marked for a standard inferior-pedicle Wise-pattern mastopexy with extension into the axillary and back regions. Sentinel to this procedure is preservation of the ICAP(s). A Doppler probe is used to confirm perforator location anterior to the anterior axillary line. The flaps are raised from posterior to anterior in the subfascial plane. To obtain adequate rotation of the flap for inset, perforating vessels from the thoracodorsal system must be sacrificed. The skin flaps and inferior pedicle are defined as per routine, and then the mobilized ICAP flap is rotated around the inferior pedicle and secured to the chest wall medially, superiorly, and laterally. Layered closure is performed over a drain. Inadequate mobilization leads to a boxy breast with lateral fullness. Failure to preserve the intercostal arteries leads to fat necrosis.[20,24-26]

Augmentation Mastopexy

For patients who desire more superior fullness, mastopexy with implants is recommended in one or two stages. Owing to the thin, overstretched skin typical of MWL patients, patients are advised to choose a conservative implant size, and two stages may be considered for more predictable results.

In one-stage augmentation mastopexy, the implant pocket is approached through a vertical or IMF incision by preserving the superior and medial blood supplies to the breast. A vertical approach is advantageous for easier exposure compared with an IMF incision because the lateral fold is often anatomically low and for preservation of the inferior breast tissue and fold centrally. The implant is placed subpectorally in a dual plane or in a subglandular position, and a circumvertical or Wise-pattern mastopexy is then tailor-tacked around the implant (Figure 66.9).

In two-stage augmentation mastopexy, the mastopexy is performed first followed by the augmentation procedure 3 to 6 months later. If the inferior blood supply to the nipple is preserved for the

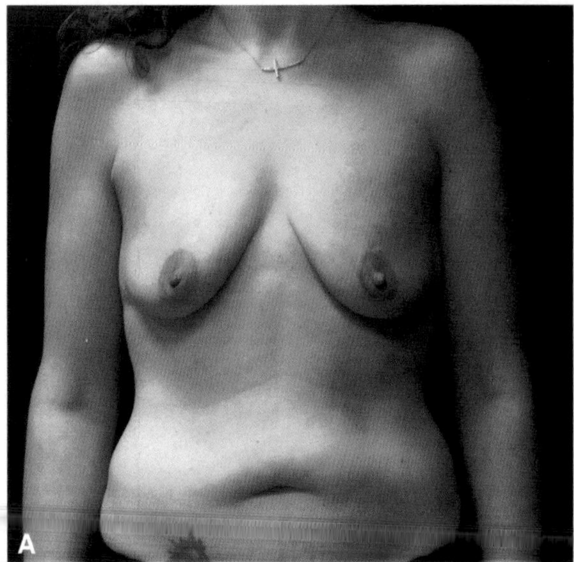

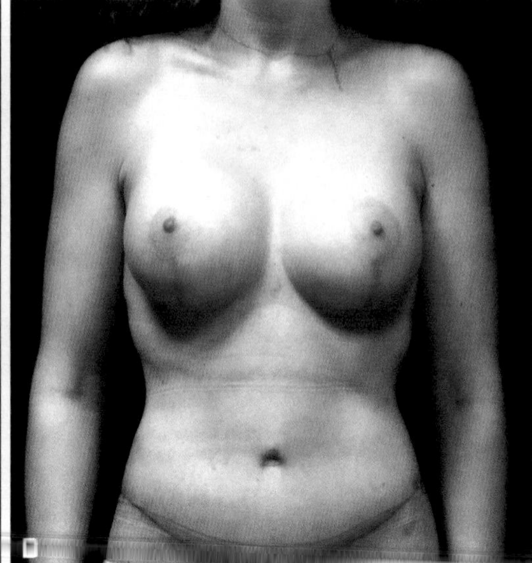

FIGURE 66.9. Augmentation mastopexy with an implant. **A.** This patient had breast ptosis and loss of volume. **B.** She underwent a single-stage augmentation mastopexy with a silicone implant and had a lower body lift at a later date.

mastopexy, care is taken to make a lateral IMF incision for implant placement. If instead the superior/medial blood supply was preserved for the breast lift, the vertical incision may be used to place the implant.

AXILLA AND UPPER/MIDDLE BACK CONTOURING

Excess adiposity and skin laxity of the upper and middle back occurs following MWL or simply as a result of the natural aging process. For patients concerned with the appearance of this region, axillary and back roll excision can be achieved via posterior midback/bra-line lift. This procedure can be performed in conjunction with breast contouring or may be added as a second stage. There are theoretical concerns about opposing vectors if performed at the same time as a belt lipectomy/lower body lift; however, both procedures rely primarily on lifting of the inferior tissues superiorly, so they may be performed together safely and effectively in experienced hands.

Preoperative Evaluation, Planning, and Marking

Evaluation of the degree of excess skin and adipose tissue forms the basis for operative planning. Patients must be willing to accept potentially significant scarring in exchange for improved contour.

According to the Pittsburgh Weight Loss Deformity Scale,[27] the posterior trunk can be evaluated according to a four-point scale:

- Grade 0: Normal contour of the back
- Grade 1: Excess adiposity or a single fat roll
- Grade 2: Multiple skin and fat rolls
- Grade 3: Ptosis of the fat rolls

It is useful for female patients to wear a bra in the initial phase of marking, as this can help determine scar placement—ideally hidden by the posterior bra strap. Once bra strap borders have been marked, the bra is removed. For male patients or patients who do not present with an appropriate undergarment, the ideal placement of the final scar should be set at the level of the planned IMF. The superior incision is designed immediately above the planned final scar; the lower incision can be expected to elevate significantly during closure and is based on a pinch test. The incisions extend from the lateral IMF, along the lateral chest wall, to the posterior chest (see Figure 66.4). The bimanual examination defines how far this excision extends. Severe deformities will require a scar that crosses the midline to avoid a dog-ear. However, for less severe deformity, the central skin of the back is preserved and bilateral wedge excisions are performed. Vertical realignment marks may assist with final closure.

Surgical Technique

The procedure is performed under general anesthesia. The patient is placed in the prone position on gel rolls, with arms flexed at the elbow and extended in the *superman* position. Care is taken to avoid pressure in the axilla. If excess adiposity extends inferior to the planned excision, liposuction is first performed in this area via separate stab incisions. The superior incision is made and carried down through Scarpa fascia using electrocautery (Figure 66.10). The tissue is undermined at the level below Scarpa fascia, leaving fat on the fascia to help prevent seroma. The proposed inferior mark is then rechecked with a pinch test, and the excision is completed. Closure is then performed in three layers over a drain. The wound is dressed with surgical glue

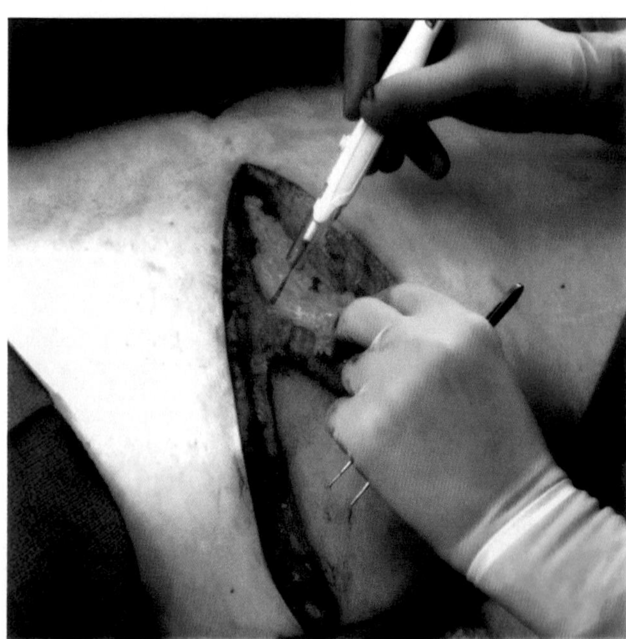

FIGURE 66.10. Bra-line lift. The excess tissue of the back is removed at a level just below Scarpa fascia.

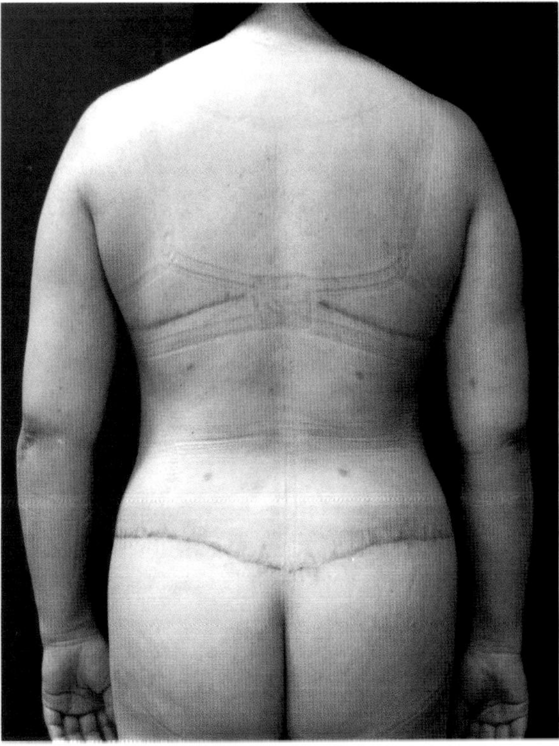

FIGURE 66.11 Bra-line lift result. This 44 year old Asian woman had a bra-line lift combined with a lower body lift and augmentation mastopexy. Liposuction was performed of the midback region and flanks below the bra-line lift. The scar remains covered with a bra.

and steri strips, covered with tegaderm dressings. The patient is then placed supine for completion of the excision or concurrent surgery of the breast and/or arms.

A compression bra, vest, or ace wrap should be placed at the conclusion of surgery. Patients should avoid heavy lifting for 6 weeks postoperatively. Drains are removed at the first postoperative visit. The most common complication reported with this procedure is widening of the scar. Wound healing complications, seroma, hematoma, and infection can also occur.[28-32] A postoperative result is depicted in Figure 66.11.

COMBINED SURGERY

The decision on whether to combine one or more surgical procedures into one operative setting depends upon the age, health, and desire of the patient as well as planned operative time and experience of the surgeon. Upper body contouring procedures are not associated with excessive amounts of blood loss. Therefore, an upper body lift including brachioplasty, excision of axillary and back rolls/bra-line lift, and breast contouring can be combined into one operative procedure in many patients.[5] Upper body contouring can also be combined with lower body contouring procedures; however, a total body lift is typically avoided secondary to excessive operative time, blood loss, and morbidity. There are patient advantages in combined surgeries for time off work and overall costs.[5] However, each patient must be evaluated individually to determine the risk/benefit ratio and to determine the optimal procedure for them.

REFERENCES

1. American Society for Metabolic and Bariatric Surgery. 2016 Statistics. Available at https://asmbs.org/resources/estimate-of-bariatric-surgery-numbers. Accessed March 22, 2018.
2. American Society for Aesthetic Plastic Surgeons. 2016 Statistics. Available at https://www.surgery.org/sites/default/files/ASAPS-Stats2016.pdf. Accessed March 22, 2018.
3. Gusenoff JA, Rubin JP. Plastic surgery after weight loss: current concepts in massive weight loss surgery. *Aesthet Surg J*. 2008;28:452-455.
4. Bossert RP, Rubin JP. Evaluation of the weight loss patient presenting for plastic surgery consultation. *Plast Reconstr Surg*. 2012;130:1361-1369.
Based on years of experience with the massive weight loss population, this paper provides an excellent overview of the complex factors that must be considered in the perioperative period. Medical comorbidities and risk factors associated with obesity are reviewed, as are the psychosocial factors that help determine the patient's candidacy for surgery and chances for a successful outcome.
5. Colwell AS, Borud LJ. Optimization of patient safety in postbariatric body contouring: a current review. *Aesthet Surg J*. 2008;28:437-442.
An extensive literature review was performed to examine and present consensus guidelines for preoperative, intraoperative, and postoperative management of the postbariatric body-contouring patient. This study includes an important discussion of the role of venous thromboembolism prophylaxis among this patient population and provides risk stratification guidelines invaluable for patient counseling and surgical planning.
6. Iturraspe M, Fernandez JC. Brachial dermolipectomy [in Spanish]. *Prensa Med Argent*. 1954;41:2432-2436.
7. Shermak MA. Aesthetic refinements in body contouring in the massive weight loss patient: part 2. Arms. *Plast Reconstr Surg*. 2014;134:726e-735e.
Review article examining evolving trends in brachioplasty classification systems and operative techniques. Succinct overview of relevant anatomy, current practice, and reported outcomes.
8. Teimourian B, Malekzadeh S. Rejuvenation of the upper arm. *Plast Reconstr Surg*. 1998;102:545-551.
9. Appelt EA, Janis JE, Rohrich RJ. An algorithmic approach to upper arm contouring. *Plast Reconstr Surg*. 2006;118:237-246.
10. El Khatib HA. Classification of brachial ptosis: strategy for treatment. *Plast Reconstr Surg*. 2007;119:1337-1342.
11. Ferraro GA, De Francesco F, Razzano S, et al. Modified fish-incision technique in brachioplasty: a surgical approach to correct excess skin and fat of the upper arm (restoring the armpit contour). *Aesthetic Plast Surg*. 2015;39:203-208.
12. de Runz A, Colson T, Minetti C, et al. Liposuction-assisted medial brachioplasty after massive weight loss: an efficient procedure with a high functional benefit. *Plast Reconstr Surg*. 2015;135:74e-84e.
13. Hill S, Small KH, Pezeshk RA, Rohrich RJ. Liposuction-assisted short-scar brachioplasty: technical highlights. *Plast Reconstr Surg*. 2016;138:447e-450e.
Technique article detailing markings and surgical approach for minibrachioplasty/limited medial incision brachioplasty.
14. Hurwitz DJ, Holland SW. The L brachioplasty: an innovative approach to cor- [illegible] 2006;117:403-411.
Technique [illegible] surgical approach, and expected patient outcomes.
15. Gentileschi S, Servillo M, Ferrandina G, Salgarello M. Lymphatic and sensory function of the upper limb after brachioplasty in post-bariatric massive weight loss patients. *Aesthet Surg J*. 2017;37:1022-1031.
16. Nyugen L, Gupta V, Afshari A, et al. Incidence and risk factors of major complications in brachioplasty: anaylsis of 2294 patients. *Aesthet Surg J*. 2016;36:792-803.
17. Meaume S, Le Pillouer-Prost A, Richert B, et al. Management of scars: updated practical guidelines and use of silicones. *Eur J Dermatol*. 2014;24:435-443.
18. Blumgart EI, Uren RF, Nielsen PM, et al. Lymphatic drainage and tumour prevalence in the breast: a statistical analysis of symmetry, gender, and node field independence. *J Anat*. 2011;218:652-659.
19. Manca G, Volterrani D, Mazzarri S, et al. Sentinel lymph node mapping in breast cancer: a critical reappraisal of the internal mammary chain issue. *Q J Nucl Med Mol Imaging*. 2014;58:114-126.
20. Colwell AS, Driscoll D, Breuing KH. Mastopexy techniques after massive weight loss: an algorithmic approach and review of the literature. *Ann Plast Surg*. 2009;63:28-33.
Review article highlighting anatomical changes of the breasts associated with massive weight loss. The authors conduct a literature review examining various techniques for correction of MWL-associated deformities of the breast and offer an algorithmic approach for the management of such.
21. Rubin JP. Mastopexy after massive weight loss: dermal suspension and total parenchymal reshaping. *Aesthet Surg J*. 2006;26:214-222.
The author presents a technique that achieves improved breast contour and volume using the patient's own tissues. This technique has the added advantage of correcting the lateral axillary roll frequently seen in patients following massive weight loss.
22. Colwell AS, Breuing KH. Improving shape and symmetry in mastopexy with autologous or cadaveric dermal slings. *Ann Plast Surg*. 2008;61:138-142.
23. Losken A, Holtz DJ. Versatility of the superomedial pedicle in managing the massive weight loss breast: the rotation-advancement technique. *Plast Reconstr Surg*. 2007;120:1060-1068.
24. Kwei S, Borud SJ, Lee BT. Mastopexy with autologous augmentation after massive weight loss: the intercostal artery perforator (ICAP) flap. *Ann Plast Surg*. 2006;57:361-365.
The authors of this technique paper describe the ICAP flap for autologous autoaugmentation. The article includes detailed information regarding indications for the procedure, surgical planning and execution, and expected outcomes.
25. Hamdi M, Van Landuyt K, Blondeel P, et al. Autologous breast augmentation with the lateral intercostal artery perforator flap in massive weight loss patients. *J Plast Reconstr Aesthet Surg*. 2009;62:65-70.
26. Hamdi M, Van Landuyt K, de Frene B, et al. The versatility of the inter-costal artery perforator (ICAP) flaps. *J Plast Reconstr Aesthet Surg*. 2006;59:644-652.

27. Song AY, Jean RD, Hurwitz DJ, et al. A classification of contour deformities after bariatric weight loss: the Pittsburgh Rating Scale. *Plast Reconstr Surg.* 2005;116:1535-1544.
The authors devise a 10-region, 4-point grading scale for the purpose of providing a validated measure of contour deformities following massive weight loss. This scale can assist with communication between providers, preoperative planning, and patient counseling.
28. Hunstad JP, Repta R. Bra-line back lift. *Plast Reconstr Surg.* 2008;122:1225-1228.
29. Hunstad JP, Khan PD. The bra-line back lift: a simple approach to correcting severe back rolls. *Clin Plast Surg.* 2014;41:715-726.
The authors review relevant anatomy, preoperative markings, and intraoperative technique for the bra-line back lift. The article is accompanied by clear photographs and a concise overview of postoperative care requirements, possible complications, and outcomes.
30. Shermak MA. Management of back rolls. *Aesthet Surg J.* 2008;28:348-356.
31. Soliman S, Rotemberg SC, Pace D, et al. Upper body lift. *Clin Plast Surg.* 2008;35:107-114.
32. Strauch B, Rohde C, Patel MK, Patel S. Back contouring in weight loss patients. *Plast Reconstr Surg.* 2007;120:1692-1696.

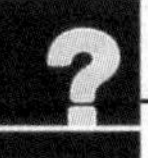

QUESTIONS

1. A 43-year-old woman lost 150 lb through diet and exercise. She had excess skin in her upper arms and underwent a brachioplasty procedure. The patient has persistent numbness in the volar ulnar surface of the forearm. Which nerve was most likely injured during the procedure:

a. Intercostobrachial
b. Lateral antebrachial cutaneous
c. MABC
d. Medial brachial cutaneous

2. A 30-year-old woman who has lost 110 lb after gastric bypass presents for evaluation. She is interested in addressing the excess skin of her upper arms, as this causes her significant distress and difficulty with clothing fit. When counseling the patient about the risks of surgery, which of the following is most likely to lead to dissatisfaction with results and reoperation?

a. Wound dehiscence
b. Hypertrophic scar
c. Seroma
d. Numbness
e. Contour irregularities

3. A 54-year-old woman presents to the office 24 months after gastric bypass surgery. She has lost a total of 170 lb and maintained a stable weight for the past 6 months. Her breasts are characterized by grade 3 nipple ptosis and volume fitting into a C cup bra. She would like to have a more youthful appearance. Which of the following is *least* likely to offer a satisfactory result?

a. Mastopexy
b. Mastopexy with autoaugmentation using an ICAP flap
c. Breast augmentation alone
d. Augmentation mastopexy

4. Which of the following best describes the characteristics most commonly associated with breast appearance following MWL?

a. Deflated superior pole, lateralized NAC position, lowered IMF position
b. Deflated superior pole, medialized NAC position, lowered IMF position
c. Deflated superior pole, medialized NAC, raised IMF position
d. Deflated inferior pole, medialized NAC position, lowered IMF position
e. Deflated inferior pole, lateralized NAC position, raised IMF position

5. A 60-year-old woman presents for consideration of upper body contouring following previous mastopexy. She is primarily concerned about the appearance of her back and posterior trunk. Physical examination is significant for multiple loose, hanging rolls of skin and soft tissue. Which of the following grades best described this deformity, according to the Pittsburgh Weight Loss Deformity Scale?

a. Grade 0
b. Grade 1
c. Grade 2
d. Grade 3

1. **Answer: c.** The MABC nerve is the most commonly cited sensory nerve injury following brachioplasty. The nerve pierces the deep fascia an average of 14 cm proximal to the medial epicondyle and travels with the basilic vein in the superficial plane of the distal half to third of the upper arm. To prevent this complication, at least 1 cm of fat should be left on the deep brachial fascia of the upper arm.

2. **Answer: b.** The most common reason for patient dissatisfaction or reoperation after brachioplasty is unsightly scarring. Patients undergoing this procedure should understand that they are trading improved contour for a significant scar. Because of the tension forces of the upper extremity, thickening or widening of this scar is not uncommon and may require laser treatment, kenalog injections, or revisional surgery to improve scar appearance.

3. **Answer: c.** For patients with MWL, the breast deformity nearly uniformly involves breast ptosis. An implant alone would not be expected to lift the nipple position enough for a satisfactory result. A mastopexy is typically involved, with or without augmentation procedures, or as part of a breast reduction to achieve a good result.

4. **Answer: b.** The loss of volume and attenuation of soft tissue, skin, and ligamentous support associated with MWL results in deflated, ptotic breasts that little resemble the ideal, youthful breast. Characteristic findings include superior pole deficiency, lack of lateral breast definition, medial NAC position, and inferior IMF when compared with normal breast anatomy.

5. **Answer: d.** According to the Pittsburgh Weight Loss Deformity Scale, the posterior trunk can be evaluated according to a four-point scale. A score of "0" indicates a normal contour of the back. Patients with excess adiposity or a single fat roll are classified as grade 1; multiple skin and fat rolls are classified as grade 2. Ptosis of these rolls represents the most severe stage, grade 3. In this patient with multiple loose, hanging rolls of skin and soft tissue, her physical examination findings would qualify as a grade 3 deformity.

PART VIII

HAND

CHAPTER 67 Functional Anatomy and Principles of Upper Extremity Surgery

Robert A. Weber and Wendy L. Czerwinski

KEY POINTS

- The anatomy of the upper extremity follows a form that maximizes its functional output.
- Understanding the relationship between surface landmarks and underlying anatomy facilitates safe and efficient hand surgery.
- A standardized template that identifies functional deficits can facilitate the evaluation of a hand surgery patient to arrive at an accurate diagnosis.
- The restoration of motor and sensory function in the hand is the focus of an upper extremity treatment plan.
- Patient outcomes can be improved by following the principles of Enhanced Recovery After Surgery.

FUNCTIONAL ANATOMY

Form follows function is a particularly useful aphorism when considering the upper extremity. The appearance of the arm is determined by its anatomy, which in turn is a result of the functional demands placed upon it. As such, a way to understand the anatomy of the upper extremity is to think in the following terms: bones, joints, and ligaments function as the *foundation,* muscles and tendons function as *motors*, arteries and veins function as *fuel*, nerves function to *control*, and the skin and subcutaneous tissues function as the *surface interface*.

Bony Foundation

The primary function of the upper extremity skeleton is to provide a stable foundation for purposeful movement. The bones anchor the origin and insertion of musculotendinous units. As such, bone injuries often have concomitant musculotendinous injuries. The bones also resist the compressive and bending forces that these muscles produce, so immobilization must relieve the torque and not create tension in the bone. The joints channel the compressive forces into motion; the configuration of the joints and the constraint of the ligaments determine the degrees of freedom. The majority of functional motion in the arm is flexion and extension in the anterior/posterior plane. The metacarpophalangeal (MP), carpometacarpal (CMC), and wrist joints also allow small amounts of rotation in other axes in order to conform to objects and dissipate forces.

Forearm

The radius and ulna have flat surfaces for multiple muscle origins and insertions. The ulna is constrained to flexion and extension at the elbow, whereas the radius can perform these actions and is also able to rotate longitudinally at the elbow and circumduct around the ulna distally, resulting in proximal translation of the distal radius relative to the distal ulna during pronation. This relative shortening of the radius can cause the distal ulna to impact the lunate or triquetrum (Figure 67.1). The primary stability of the distal radioulnar joint (DRUJ) is provided by the triangular fibrocartilage complex (TFCC) (Figure 67.2); the bony configuration of the sigmoid notch of the radius provides 30% of the DRUJ stability.

Wrist

The radius and ulna articulate distally with the carpus. Because there are no tendinous insertions in any of the carpal bones, the osseous shapes as well as the extrinsic and intrinsic ligaments are vital for functional stability. For the purpose of motion, carpal bone arrangement is usually considered as two arched rows with the lunate as the keystone and the scaphoid extending to both rows. Gilula's arcs represent the curvatures of a ball-within-a-cup configuration of the proximal and distal carpal rows (see Figure 67.1).[1]

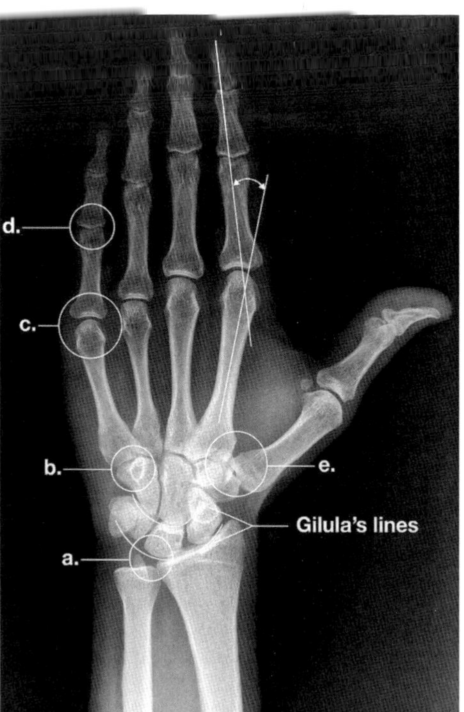

FIGURE 67.1. AP radiograph of the hand. **a.** Location for ulnocarpal impaction due to relative shortening of the radius during pronation. **b.** Hook of the hamate. **c.** Head of the MP demonstrating the recesses where the collateral ligaments insert as well as the ball-and-socket like configuration of the joint. **d.** Bicondylar configuration of the PIP joint adds conformational stability to flexion and extension. **e.** Thumb CMC joint is a saddle joint, which allows flexion and extension in the AP and radioulnar planes (unlike the other CMC joints) and prohibits axial rotation (unlike the MP joints). Note the natural ulnar deviation at the MP joints.

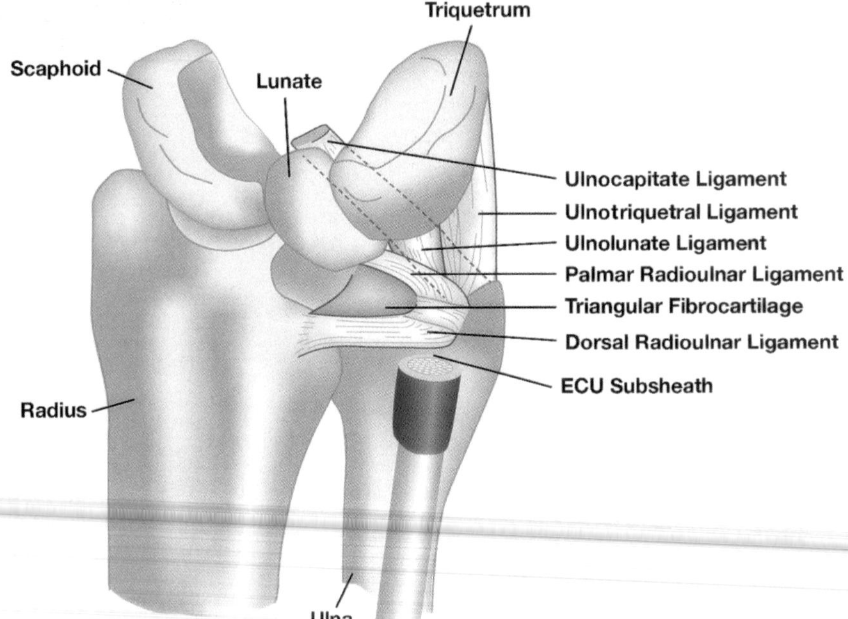

FIGURE 67.2. The TFCC is a complex arrangement of seven soft tissue structures of the ulnar wrist. This includes the TFC proper (a meniscus homologue), the dorsal and volar radioulnar ligaments, the three volar ulnocarpal (UC) ligaments (ulnolunate [UL], ulnocapitate, ulnotriquetral [UT]), and the floor of the extensor carpi ulnaris tendon subsheath. The UC ligament sits volar to the UL and UT ligaments.

The hamate bone has a palpable volar hook that is visible on carpal tunnel view radiographs and represents an attachment of the flexor retinaculum, hypothenar muscles, and pisohamate fascia of the Guyon canal (see Figure 67.1).

The radiocarpal (RC) and the ulnocarpal (UC) joints are restrained by the joint capsule, the volar radioscaphocapitate ligament (the strongest ligament), the long radiolunate ligament, short radiolunate ligament, and the ligament of Testut.[2] The primary dorsal ligaments consist of the dorsal radiocarpal ligament and dorsal intercarpal ligament. A dorsal carpal surgical exposure with a dorsal ligament sparing capsulotomy attempts to preserve the integrity of these structures, thereby improving postoperative stability and mobility.[3] Intrinsic ligaments provide stability between carpal bones within the proximal and distal rows but not between rows and lead to coordinated flexion and extension of these rows. Disruption of intrinsic ligaments can create various instability patterns such as those seen in greater and lesser arc perilunate injuries.[4]

Hand

The metacarpal (MC) bones have a collateral recess radially and ulnarly at their heads for the origin of the proper collateral ligaments (CL) of the metacarpal-phalangeal (MP) joints. These recesses are radiographically visible and serve as excellent insertion points for ideal angulation in placing longitudinal K-wires for fracture fixation (see Figure 67.1). The dorsal convexity of the MC bone results in tension on the dorsal surface with loading, leading to dorsal apex fracture patterns. The MP joints are condyloid in nature, allowing for motion in three planes: flexion/extension, abduction/adduction, and rotation. The volar plate is contiguous with the deep transverse MC ligament, which connects the metacarpal heads and helps maintain the MCs in a slight dorsal arch in the transverse plane. Because the MC head is wider on its volar surface, flexion increases joint stability by tightening the CL and elongating the VP. Thus, the MP joint should be immobilized in flexion to reduce the occurrence of joint contractures. In extension, the MPs are not linear. Instead, there is a 10- to 14-degree natural ulnar deviation, predisposing the finger to ulnar subluxation of the extensor hood and ulnar drift (see Figure 67.1). The carpometacarpal (CMC) joints have limited mobility at the index finger and become progressively more mobile toward the ulnar aspect of the hand, allowing for approximately 30 degrees of flexion/extension at the fourth and fifth with some supination.

The phalangeal heads are bicondylar and form interphalangeal uniaxial hinge joints (see Figure 67.1). The interphalangeal (IP) joints have one axis of rotation in flexion and extension due to their bony configuration as well as a complex arrangement of ligaments, volar plate (VP), joint capsule, and a stout extensor mechanism that resists joint dislocation. Small volar checkrein ligaments arising from the proximal phalanx volar ridges to the VP are thought to contribute to flexion contractures, which can arise at the PIP joints. In contrast to the MP joints, the PIP joints should be splinted in full extension.

The thumb bones are pronated about 90 degrees and volarly abducted about 45 degrees from the plane of the hand. This configuration is what allows the functions of prehension: tip pinch, chuck pinch, key pinch, and grasp. The thumb's MP joint is a shallow ball-and-socket, which permits the thumb phalanges to pronate even more than the metacarpal. Soft tissues are more dominant in creating joint support with the addition of the adductor aponeurosis overlying the ulnar CL. The basilar or carpometacarpal (CMC) joint is a saddle or double ginglymus joint allowing for circumductive motion, and the primary stabilizer is the volar beak/oblique ligament (see Figure 67.1). Laxity of this ligament is considered the origin of first CMC articular changes.

Makers of Movement

The musculotendinous systems of the arm create tension, which is transmitted from the origin to insertion. Working primarily as class 3 levers, longitudinal contraction of the muscle results in rotation around the joint axis. The primary motion is flexion and extension, and the flexors are able to generate more force than the extensors. The primary function of the extensors is to place the hand and fingers in a position to be used optimally. The work of the arm is done by the flexors. Repair or reconstruction of a musculotendinous unit requires that the tension forces be transmitted across the injured site in such a way to minimize adherence to adjacent structures.

Extensors

The musculotendinous system can be differentiated into extrinsic muscles originating in the forearm and intrinsic muscles of the hand including the thenar group. The extrinsic extensors, which are in three groups of three, originate from the dorsal-radial surface of

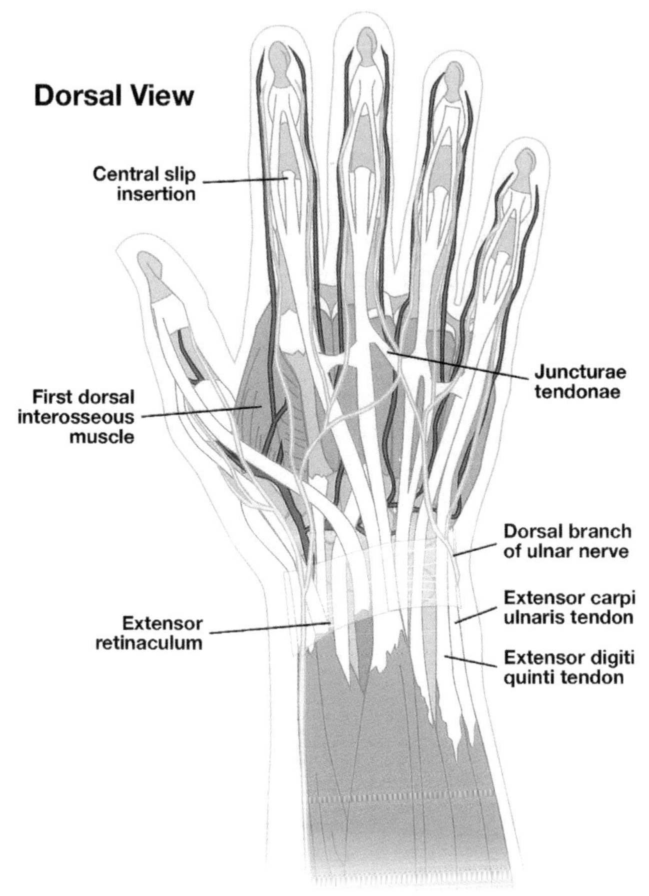

FIGURE 67.3. The extrinsic wrist extensors (extensor carpi radialis longus [ECRL], extensor carpi radialis brevis [ECRB], extensor carpi ulnaris [ECU]), thumb extensors (extensor pollicis longus [EPL], abductor pollicis longus [APL], extensor pollicis brevis [EPB]), and finger extensors (extensor digitorum communis [EDC], extensor indicis proprious [EIP], extensor digiti minimi [EDM]) are organized into 6 compartments with EIP and EDM providing independent extension of the index and small digits and usually lying ulnar to their corresponding EDC slips. The extrinsic tendons continue over the digit stabilized by the extensor hood. The tendinous system continues and becomes a W over the PIP joint. The tendon inserts as the central slip over the middle phalanx with contributions to the lateral bands which extend distally to the terminal triangular ligament over the DIP joint and inserting just proximal to the germinal matrix. The dorsal and volar interossei and lumbricals are intrinsic muscles contributing to the lateral bands running volar to the MP joint axis.

the forearm and serve to extend the wrist, thumb, and remaining digits primarily at the MP level with some contribution to IP extension (Figure 67.3). They are all innervated by the radial nerve. At the wrist, they pass deep to an extensor retinaculum organized into six compartments with extensor indicis proprius (EIP) and extensor digiti minimi providing independent extension of the index and small digits and usually lying ulnar to their corresponding extensor digitorum communis (EDC) counterparts. The EIP is a useful donor motor tendon for functional transfers and can be identified by its muscle belly distal most in the dorsal forearm. The juncturae tendinae, which are interconnections between the extensors over the dorsal hand, can confuse diagnosis of tendon disruptions by the ablility to extend fingers with ruptured tendons to neutral posture through the juncturae tendinae.

The extrinsic tendons continue onto the digit stabilized at the MP joint by the extensor hood/sagittal band (see Figure 67.3). Disruption at this level contributes to improper tendon tracking, and the radial-sided laxity seen in inflammatory joint conditions contributes to ulnar drift. There are no extensor insertions on the proximal phalanx. Instead, the sagittal bands transmit tension to the volar plate to pull the proximal phalanx into extension. At the PIP joint, the intrinsic muscles of the hand join the extensor mechanism (see Figure 67.3). They contribute to the lateral bands, which pass volar to the MP joint axis and thus aid in flexion at that joint. The intrinsic insertions then move dorsal to the axis of the PIP joint and function as the primary IP extensors. The PIP and DIP joints will not extend if the intrinsic muscles do not contract.

Flexors

There are 11 extrinsic flexors, 9 of which pass through the carpal canal (Figure 67.4). The majority of flexors are innervated by the median nerve; the ulnar nerve innervates the flexor carpi ulnaris (FCU) and the flexor digitorum profundus (FDP) to the ring and small digits; however, innervation variability exists in the forearm. The flexor tendon sheath extends from the proximal edge of the A1 pulley to the DIP joint, provides tendon nutrition and facilitates glide. Annular pulleys (A1-A5) are numbered from proximal to distal with three compressible cruciate pulleys intervening from A2 to A5. These prevent bowstringing in order to allow for improved excursion/moment arcs at the corresponding joint levels.

Intrinsic Tendons

In addition to their contributions to MP flexion and IP extension, the interossei are also responsible for digit adduction and abduction. The first dorsal interosseous muscle is the last innervated muscle by the ulnar nerve; thus, wasting and weakness assessed are often first noted here by Froment's test. The adductor pollicis (AdP) is responsible for thumb adduction. The thenar group is innervated by the median nerve, whereas the deep head of FPB and the transverse head of the AdP are innervated by the ulnar nerve. Although this group contributes to precise thumb motion, patients with long-standing carpal tunnel syndrome and thenar wasting are often not aware of any functional deficit.

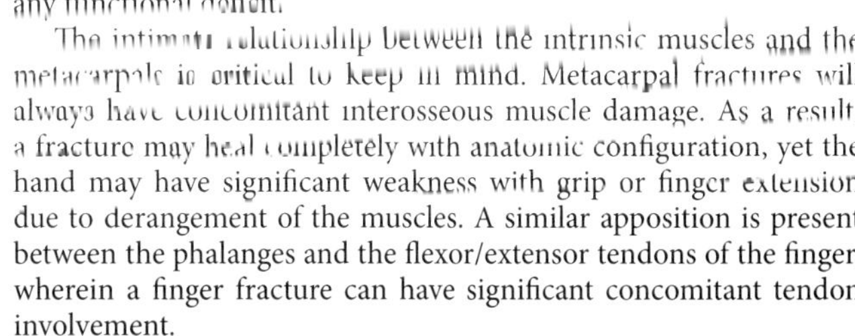

The intimate relationship between the intrinsic muscles and the metacarpals is critical to keep in mind. Metacarpal fractures will always have concomitant interosseous muscle damage. As a result, a fracture may heal completely with anatomic configuration, yet the hand may have significant weakness with grip or finger extension due to derangement of the muscles. A similar apposition is present between the phalanges and the flexor/extensor tendons of the finger, wherein a finger fracture can have significant concomitant tendon involvement.

Fuel and Control

The arteries provide metabolic support for the hand, but the majority of blood flow is used for thermoregulation. Within the arm and hand, the arteries and nerves tend to run parallel within a common sheath, protected from compression by the bones and tendons. The neurovascular structures can tolerate some tension and are able to glide longitudinally within the extremity to accommodate the various positions of the bones and joints. Adhesions that restrict gliding can produce pain and interfere with functionality.

Arteries

The brachial artery at the elbow divides into the radial and ulnar arteries in the antecubital fossa. The radial artery runs in a course toward the radial wrist radial to the FCR. There is a larger dorsal branch that passes through the snuffbox to the deep arch in the palm. The small volar branch contributes to the superficial arch. The ulnar artery runs between the FDS and FDP muscle groups and is palpable radial to the FCU. It continues radial to the ulnar nerve through the Guyon canal; its larger volar branch completes the superficial arch, whereas the smaller dorsal branch completes the deep arch. Vascularity to the carpus arises from the posterior and anterior interosseous arteries as well as from the ulnar and radial arteries at the level of the wrist. The common digital arteries arise from the superficial arch, whereas the princeps pollicis artery to the thumb arises from the radial artery

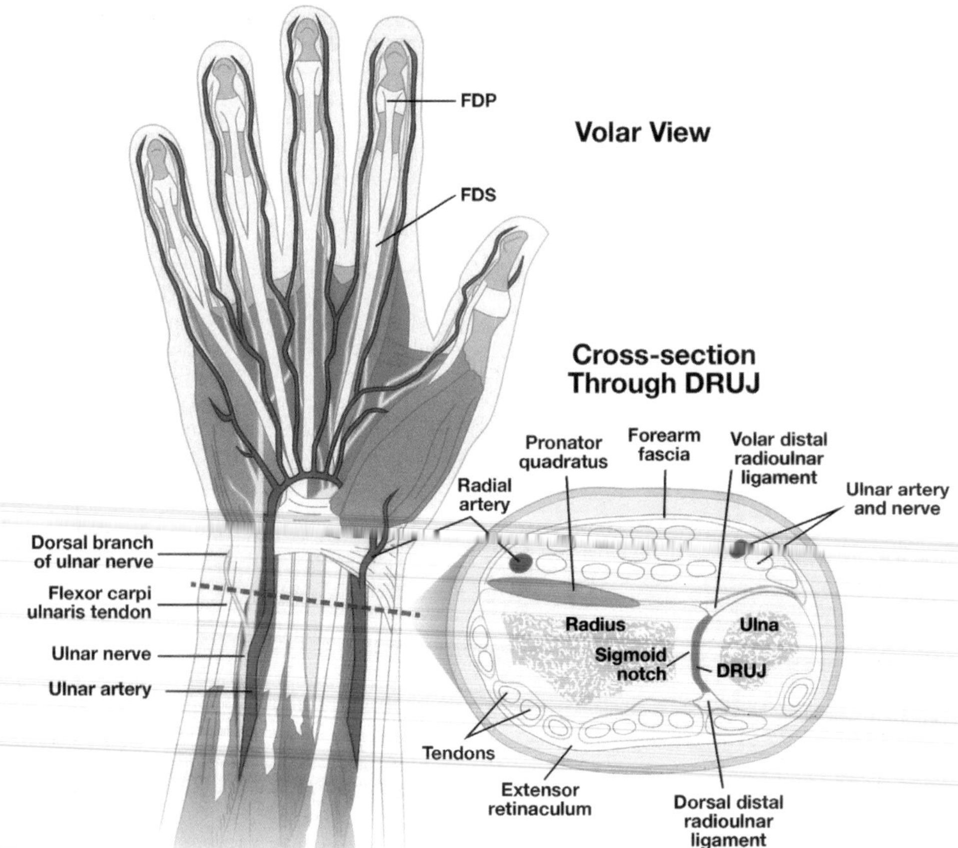

FIGURE 67.4. The FDS runs superficial to FDP and FPL in the carpal tunnel but then has a longitudinal split near its insertion across the PIP joint (Camper's chiasm), which permits FDP to run superficially to reach the distal.

portion of the deep arch. Vascular architecture varies from individual to individual, but within every hand, there are numerous redundant arterial interconnections, so disruption of one artery is unlikely to result in terminal ischemia. Nevertheless, arterial supply to the hand or a digit should be examined before deciding to ligate or not to repair an artery.

Nerves

The peripheral nerves originate from the cervical roots and form the brachial plexus. The median, ulnar, and radial nerve branches that terminate in the hand have fairly consistent anatomic relationships. Cranial to caudal nerve roots correspond to proximal to distal motor control, that is, the shoulder girdle is controlled by C5 nerve roots, and the intrinsic muscles of the hand are innervated from C8/T1 roots. Sensory innervation also follows a cranial to caudal pattern; C5 provides sensation to the radial border of the forearm, T1 provides ulnar forearm sensation.

The internal topography of peripheral nerves has functional implications. For example, some muscles such as the FCR have multiple innervating fascicles, thereby allowing one of the fascicles to be used as motor nerve transfer. Another example of the functional relevance of internal fascicular anatomy is seen in the median and ulnar nerves at the wrist. The motor branches of those nerves are in a predictable location (the median motor is volar radial, and the ulnar motor is dorsal radial), thereby allowing more accurate nerve repairs or nerve transfers.

All the extensors in the arm are innervated by the radial nerve. The elbow flexors are innervated by the musculocutaneous nerve, whereas the wrist and finger flexors are primarily innervated by the median nerve. The ulnar nerve innervates the FCU, the ulnar two FDPs with their associated lumbricals, and all the intrinsics except the thenar muscles. Like the arteries, the location of a peripheral nerve can vary from individual to individual; nevertheless, the ulnar nerve is commonly located adherent to the ulnar artery. The median nerve lies between the superficialis and profundus muscle bellies in the forearm, adherent to the deep surface of the superficialis. This is important to remember when attempting to locate the nerve during trauma exploration. Knowing the functional anatomy of the nerves also allows the surgeon to block the nerves with a local anesthetic for diagnostic and therapeutic purposes.

Surface Anatomy

Understanding how the surface anatomy of the upper extremity (flexion and extension creases, palpable muscle, and bony landmarks) relates to the structures hidden beneath the skin is critical for the management of the hand. The ability to relate what can be seen and palpated to the underlying elements allows effective treatment of those deeper structures with a minimum of damage to the surrounding tissues. Fortunately for the hand surgeon, there are many reliable guides on the surface of the upper extremity.

Forearm

With the elbow flexed at 90 degrees and the wrist in neural pronation, the muscle visible and palpable in the anterolateral portion of the proximal forearm is the brachioradialis (Figure 67.5). The biceps tendon is palpable ulnar to the brachioradialis in the antecubital fossa. The median nerve, anterior interosseous nerve, and the brachial artery are ulnar to the biceps insertion. The extensor wad is dorsal to the brachioradialis.

In the distal volar forearm, flexion of the wrist simultaneous with positioning all the finger tips together reveals the palmaris longus tendon, a source of tendon graft. The palmaris longus (PL), used as both a tendon graft and motor tendon transfer, is absent unilaterally

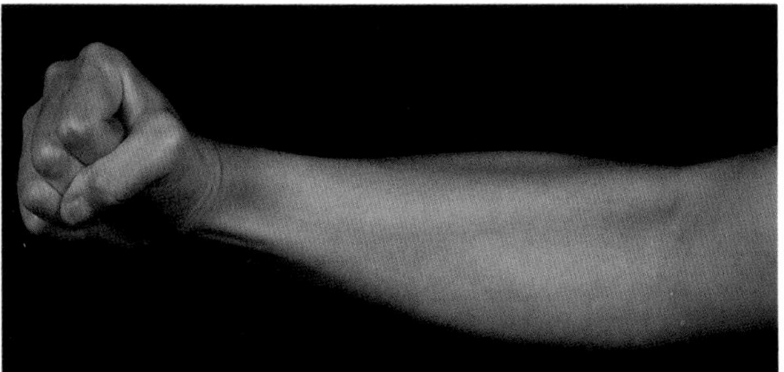

FIGURE 67.5. Right forearm demonstrating the brachioradialis, extensor wad, palmaris longus tendon, and FCR tendon.

in about 15% of the population and bilaterally in 8%. The median nerve is radial to the PL tendon, with the flexor pollicis longus tendon deep to the nerve. All the flexor digitorum superficialis and profundus tendons are ulnar to the PL tendon.

Volar Hand

The volar skin creases provide many landmarks to the musculoskeletal and neurovascular architecture.[5] Figure 67.6 shows the relationship between the major flexion creases and the underlying anatomy. The distal wrist crease lies at the midcarpal joint corresponding to the capitolunate articulation. The distal pole of the scaphoid is distal to the crease. The crease also identifies the proximal edge of the transverse carpal ligament and can be used as a landmark for median nerve blocks. The distal palmar crease overlies the metacarpal necks and is 5 to 8 mm proximal to the metacarpal-phalangeal (MP) joints. This crease should be visible when making volar splints that are intended to immobilize the wrist while allowing MP motion. The misleadingly named MP crease is actually at the same level as the web space and overlies the midportion of the proximal phalanx. The proximal interphalangeal (PIP) and distal interphalangeal (DIP) creases are superficial to the actual joints. They can be used to locate the underlying flexor tendon pulleys. The thenar crease is due to CMC motion and must be visible in any immobilization in which the thumb is allowed to move. The radial digital nerve to the index finger runs deep to the thenar crease. The thumb MP and IP creases overlie the corresponding joints.

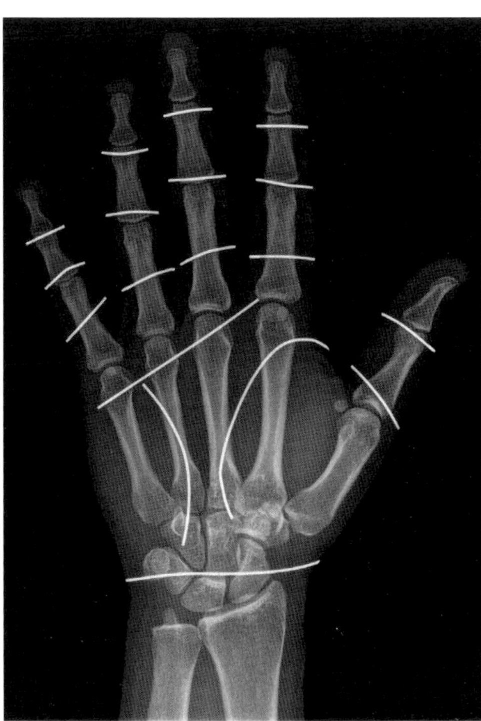

FIGURE 67.6. AP radiograph of the hand with wires on the major hand creases.

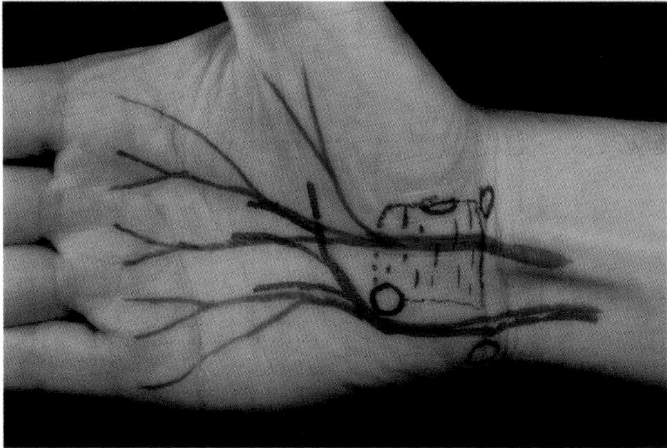

FIGURE 67.7. Volar hand with the palpable pisiform, hook of the hamate, distal pole of the scaphoid, and trapezial ridge identified in *black*. The transverse carpal ligament (*brown*) as well as the relationship of the median and ulnar nerves (*green*) and ulnar artery (*red*) to the palpable bones are drawn. The arterial branches as well as the nerve branches have a more variable location from hand to hand.

Figure 67.7 shows the creases along with the palpable bony landmarks and their relationship to underlying vessels and nerves.[6] The pisiform and hook of the hamate can be used as guides to find the ulnar artery and nerves, and the superficial palmar arch runs transversely across the palm distal to the hamate toward the distal end of the thenar crease. The common digital nerve bifurcates into the digital nerves distal to the distal palmar crease, approximately at the same location where the proper palmar arteries divide.

Dorsal Hand

Lister's tubercle is the key to identifying the important dorsal structures (Figure 67.8).[7] It marks the distal lip of the dorsal radius. Immediately distal to the tubercle is the midportion of the scapholunate ligament, which links the scaphoid and the lunate. The head of the capitate is approximately 1 cm distal to the palpable tubercle. The ulnar surface of the tubercle serves as a pulley for the extensor pollicis longus; the fourth extensor compartment is 1 cm ulnar with its extensor digitorum communis and extensor indicis proprius tendons. The second dorsal extensor compartment with its palpable extensor

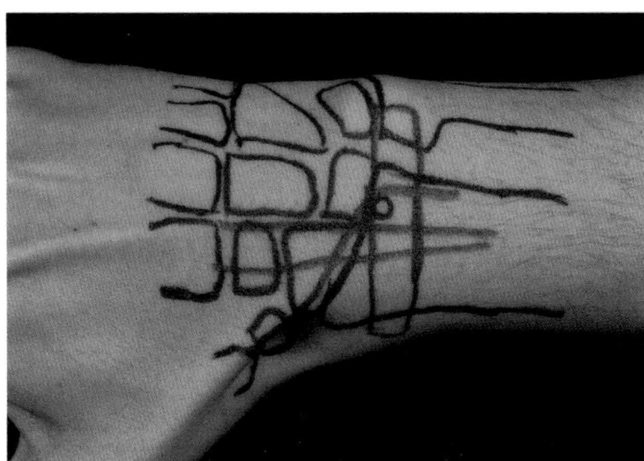

FIGURE 67.8. Dorsal hand with Lister's tubercle identified (*black* circle in center) and the underlying bony anatomy drawn (distal radius and ulna and metacarpal bases in *black*, carpals in *purple*). The ECRL and ECRB in the second compartment and the EPL in the third compartment are drawn in *orange*. The extensor retinaculum is drawn in *brown*.

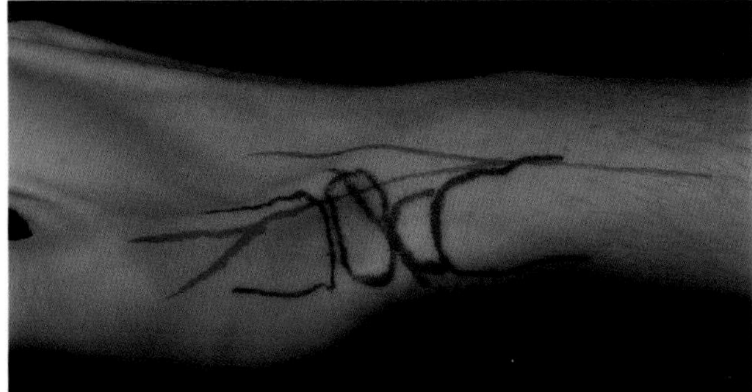

FIGURE 67.9. Radial wrist with the bony anatomy drawn (the radial styloid and metacarpal base in *black*, scaphoid, and trapezium in *purple*). The EPL and EPB/APL ridges are clearly visible. The dorsal branch of the radial artery (in *red*) courses diagonally on the surface of the wrist capsule from volar-proximal to dorsal-distal.

carpi radialis longus and brevis tendons is on the radial border of the tubercle. Proximal to Lister's tubercle is the radial metaphysis, a good source of bone graft.

Radial Hand

The radial styloid, the abductor pollicis longus and extensor pollicis brevis tendons, and the extensor pollicis longus tendon all form the anatomic snuffbox (Figure 67.9).[8] The first dorsal compartment, the artery used in the 1,2 intercarpal radial artery pedicled bone graft, and the sensory branch of the radial nerve all overlie the dorsal radial styloid. The dorsal branch of the radial artery and its venae comitantes are located deep in the snuffbox, easily and reliably identifiable for free flap anastomoses. The thumb CMC joint is the firm bony structure, which creates the distal *lid* of the snuffbox. The bony floor deep is the distal scaphoid and the trapezium.

Ulnar Hand

The palpable ulnar styloid is the origin of the TFCC as well as the border of the sixth dorsal compartment. The bone palpable 1 cm distal to the styloid is the hamate, and the next bony prominence distal is the base of the little finger metacarpal with its concomitant CMC joint. Analogous to the radial snuffbox configuration, the tendon that is palpable dorsal to the styloid and hamate is the extensor carpi ulnaris tendon while the volar border is the flexor carpi ulnaris tendon.

Digit

The junction of the glabrous and nonglabrous skin marks the midlateral line of a finger (Figure 67.10). Points on this line can be found when the PIP and DIP joints are flexed. Incisions in this line are preferable to minimize scar contractures of the joints. The digital neurovascular bundles and flexor tendon sheath are volar to this line, and the bony phalanges are dorsal, a fact to keep in mind when placing percutaneous K-wires.

PRINCIPLES OF UPPER EXTREMITY SURGERY

Assessment

Hand surgery is a discipline in which the practitioner is still a detective. Many patients present with a general concern of pain, stiffness, numbness, weakness, *etc*, and it is incumbent upon the hand surgeon to perform a history and physical sufficient to determine the correct diagnosis. A standard template for asking questions is provided in **Table 67.1**; note the emphasis on functional concerns. There are two particularly important aspects of the patient's narrative that should be elucidated: those circumstances in which the deficit is noted and

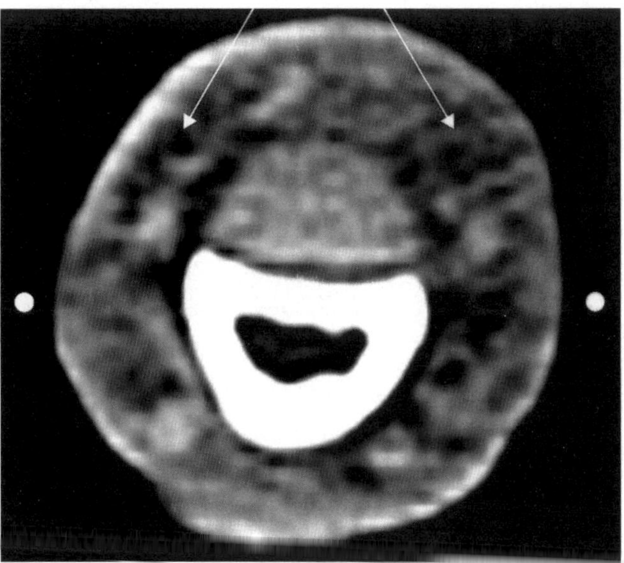

FIGURE 67.10. CT cross-section of the proximal phalanx of the thumb, the volar surface is on the top. The dots are at the junction of the glabrous and nonglabrous skin, which is also the midlateral line. The arrows point to the neurovascular bundles in the 2 o'clock and 10 o'clock positions.

the amount of traumatic energy involved. Symptoms specific to a particular motion or job begin to point the surgeon to the affected anatomy. A fracture from a fall has different accompanying injuries and expected outcomes than a fracture incurred during a high-speed collision.

Having established a differential diagnosis based on the history, the physical exam is used to hone in on the underlying diagnosis;

TABLE 67.1. ELEMENTS OF A HAND HISTORY

History Component	Data Collected
History of present illness	■ Time of onset of symptoms ■ Mechanism of injury or inciting event, or nature of repetitive trauma ■ Type of trauma—blunt, sharp, mechanism, hand position, contamination; estimated amount of force/energy involved ■ Duration of symptoms; continual or intermittent ■ Severity of symptoms ■ Factors that worsen and/or improve the symptoms; cold intolerance ■ History of infection ■ Care to date
General demands on the hand	■ Hand dominance ■ Occupation, hobbies ■ Activity status, walking aids ■ Social status
Medical history	■ Nicotine use ■ Chronic disease—autoimmune, diabetes
Surgical history and prior treatments	■ Prior hand trauma and outcomes ■ Prior surgical interventions and outcomes—remaining hardware
Family history	■ Dupuytren's contracture ■ Lipomas ■ Congenital conditions
Medications/allergies	■ Anticoagulation ■ Immunosuppressants ■ Nonsteroidal anti-inflammatory agents ■ Steroids ■ Opioids

TABLE 67.2. PHYSICAL EXAMINATION OF THE HAND

Physical Examination	Finding
Soft tissue appearance	■ General ■ Gross deformity ■ Cascade ■ Congenital anomalies ■ Wounds—dimension, location, contamination, or presence of foreign body ■ Rashes ■ Nail deformities ■ Masses ■ Contractures versus posturing ■ Symmetry
Vascular	■ Skin color and temperature ■ Atrophic skin changes ■ Allen's test ■ Capillary refill
Motor	■ Flexor and extensor tendon function including forearm musculature ■ Thenar and hypothenar muscle function or atrophy ■ Intrinsic muscle function or atrophy
Sensory	■ Subjective numbness, comparison for symmetry ■ Provocative nerve tests (e.g., Tinel's sign, Phalen's sign) ■ Two-point discrimination
Joint range of motion	■ Arc of rotation: DIP, PIP, MP Wrist, forearm rotation Elbow ■ Joint stability
Bone	■ Angulation/rotational deformity ■ Pain or instability ■ Prominences

again, the focus is on function (**Table 67.2**). It is important to be thorough and examine seemingly uninvolved structures. For example, patients with carpal tunnel syndrome often have thumb CMC arthritis, but unless the arthritic component of their thumb pain is explained prior to surgery, the patient will expect the pain to resolve after carpal tunnel release and be disappointed when it does not. In addition, a thorough functional exam may demonstrate other abnormalities that should be addressed.

Tables 67.1 and **67.2** can also be used to develop a standard history and physical template for use in an electronic medical record. The value of an individually developed standardized evaluation is that repetition allows the clinician to recognize abnormalities and disruptions of patterns better. Subtle diseases are easier to spot in a background of well-understood normal states.

Table 67.3 lists the imaging modalities available to hand surgeons. It is important to choose the proper test for the patient. On one hand, magnetic resonance imaging is overly sensitive and not specific enough to use when a diagnosis is unclear.[9] On the other hand, recent advances in ultrasound make it an excellent investigative and therapeutic tool for multiple conditions involving the soft tissues. Fractures and dislocations are best identified with plain radiographs; palpating a suspected fracture site to make a diagnosis causes pain, tissue damage, and is not diagnostic. The new technology now allows for subtraction of hardware artifact in computerized tomography and has significantly improved resolution.

Treatment

Once a diagnosis has been made, the patient and surgeon collaborate on choosing a treatment plan. Not all hand patients will require surgery. In fact, most patients seen in a hand clinic will be treated nonoperatively with a combination of immobilization, anti-inflammatory medications, therapeutic modalities, and pain management. In patients who have been sent to see a surgeon and are treated without surgery, it is important to make sure the patient understands that the concerns have been taken seriously and are being appropriately addressed.

Preoperative

Patient education and a discussion about expectations are critical in surgical patients. Enhanced Recovery After Surgery (ERAS) is a multidisciplinary and multimodal approach to the care of a surgical patient. Primary elements of ERAS protocols include preoperative patient education, nutritional optimization, early mobilization, and standardized analgesic and anesthetic regimens.[10] Implementation of the ERAS protocol across surgical specialties has demonstrated the decreased average length of stay, complication rates, readmissions, and costs.[11] There has been much research done on improving outcomes in hand surgery patients, and many institutions are utilizing these strategies to decrease costs and improve patient satisfaction. A comprehensive approach to hand surgery utilizing these strategies is outlined below.

Patient education is an important but often overlooked aspect of patient care. A patient's clear understanding of their diagnosis,

TABLE 67.3. IMAGING MODALITIES FOR USE IN THE HAND

Imaging Modality	Evaluation
Plain Radiographs *Most common, most useful, most cost effective imaging modality*	■ Good for assessing fractures, dislocations, arthritic changes ■ Rule of 2's: Two views minimum Joint above and below level of injury Injured and contralateral side Before and after treatment ■ Special views (e.g., carpal tunnel view, scaphoid view) ■ Instability series ■ Evaluation of the image—quality of the radiographs, alignment of the skeleton
CT	■ Provides improved bony detail ■ Good for assessing □ Bone tumors □ Fracture healing □ Carpal or fracture alignment
MRI *Not to be used as a screening test, only order to evaluate a suspected diagnosis*	■ Provides improved soft tissue detail—ligaments, cartilage, muscle ■ Good for assessing possible bony avascular necrosis ■ T1 □ Black = fluid and cartilage □ Gray = tendon and muscle □ White = bone and fat ■ T2 □ Black = bone, tendon, ligament, and cartilage □ White = fluid
Bone scan	■ Three phase assesses vascularity ■ Delayed phase useful for assessing chronic hand pain
Angiography	■ Provides vascular detail for occlusion, aneurysm, ischemia ■ Magnetic resonance angiography is replacing traditional contrast angiography
Ultrasound	■ Identifies and localizes fluid collections (e.g., abscess, ganglion) ■ Localizes radiolucent foreign bodies ■ Identifies ligament and tendon ruptures

perioperative plan, and long-term functional expectations has been shown to improve patient compliance and health outcomes. These are also the key elements of informed consent. Additionally, patient education can benefit the provider by cutting down on unnecessary calls, clinic visits, and medication refills. Providing patients with appropriate educational materials that explain the perioperative course may also reduce patient anxiety and create more reasonable expectations, particularly in the realm of pain control.

Operative

Surgery begins before the patient enters the room. Equipment, positioning, and the anesthetic plan are discussed with operative personnel beforehand and confirmed during the time-out. Surgical site preparation, the operative plan, and subsequent surgical markings should all be performed prior to inflating the tourniquet since the tourniquet time is precious. The *safe* duration of tourniquet-induced ischemia in the upper extremity is 2 hours, but there are few studies other than Wilgis' to confirm this time.[12] His study also suggests that the tourniquet time can be extended by releasing the tourniquet and then reinflating it after the blood supply has had time to circulate to prevent reperfusion injury.[13] Forearm tourniquets may be used in hand cases performed under local anesthesia. These are well tolerated by the patient and provide a bloodless field, but they can encroach on the surgical field.[14]

Details of specific procedures will be provided in the upcoming chapters, but there are several principles that should be followed when operating on the upper extremity.

- *Incisions should be longitudinal.* This minimizes the number of cutaneous nerves that might be transected, allows for wider exposure through simple extension of the incision, and facilitates re-excision of the scar if needed in the future. Transverse incisions at the volar wrist with their attendant stigmata should be avoided.
- *Incisions should not cross flexion creases.* A combination of Bruner and midaxial incisions provides good exposure and can incorporate most traumatic lacerations.
- *Incisions should be long enough to do the job.* A common cause of struggling during surgery is insufficient exposure. The chief goal of hand surgery is restoration of function; patients will trade an additional 2–4 cm of scar for improved use of the hand.
- *Work from normal to abnormal, known to unknown.* Another cause of surgeon distress is the inability to identify structures. The incision should be long enough to expose uninjured, unaffected tissues in order to provide orientation. The temptation to explore a wound through an insufficiently extended traumatic laceration should be resisted.
- *If it does not look right, it will not work right.* Incisions that violate the aesthetics of the hand and closures that produce distortions in hand architecture will result in a wound that may heal, but the functional outcome will be suboptimal.

Postoperative

As noted, optimal postoperative outcomes start with following the principles of ERAS preoperatively. The important points of patient education are reviewed with the patient and his or her support system. Proper dressings, elevation, and activity levels are important and should be described in concert with their concomitant procedures. The key elements of any dressing are edema control, protection of repairs, pain minimization, immobilizing parts of anatomy that must not move, and allowing motion in all other locations.

Pain management in the upper extremity is an important determinant of recovery and overall function. Insufficient pain control in the acute phase increases inflammation and scarring; concerns about opioid dependence are real, but the role of narcotics and nonsteroidal anti-inflammatory medications in the acute phase should be discussed prior to surgery in order to establish expectations. Medication-adverse patients should be reminded that the use of opioids will be limited, and that it is more important to use appropriate pain medication and move the hand than not use pain medication and not move the hand.

One of the most important aspect of postoperative care is the rehabilitation plan. Many hand surgical procedures depend equally on specified hand therapy protocols. The hand surgeon should have an open, well-established line of communication with the hand therapist. The importance of good hand rehabilitation cannot be overstated. In fact, there are numerous procedures in the hand that should not be attempted unless the therapy plan has already been outlined to the patient, compliance has been demonstrated, time off and transportation issues addressed, and insurance coverage for the therapy assured. This last item is important to establish preoperatively because many insurance policies will cover surgery but not rehabilitation.

Since form follows function in the hand, a good hand surgeon should master three areas: functional anatomy, basic surgical techniques, and principles of rehabilitation. Knowing the anatomy allows the surgeon to make a correct diagnosis and construct a plan to restore the anatomy to as close to normal as possible. Because all surgeries are composed of the same basic movements, a good surgeon does not have to memorize a series of specific steps but can apply well-established component steps to create a surgical plan that is tailored to the specific needs of the case at hand. Rehabilitation is the process of returning control of the hand back to the patient. People use their hands in infinite ways; the focus of the hand surgeon is to use all the operative and nonoperative modalities available to return injured or diseased structures to their proper configuration so that the patient can carry on effectively with life.

REFERENCES

1. Linscheid RL, Dobyns JH, Beabout JW, Bryan RS. Traumatic instability of the wrist: diagnosis, classification, and pathomechanics. *J Bone Joint Surg Am.* 1972;54(8):1612-1632.
   This is the sentinel article on wrist biomechanics and instability patterns of traumatic conditions. It reviews the diagnosis, classification, and pathomechanics and relates to radiographic findings of carpal angles.
2. Berger RA, Landsmeer JMF. The palmar radiocarpal ligaments: a study of adult and fetal human wrist joints. *Iowa Orthop J.* 1985;5:32-41.
3. Berger RA, Bishop AT, Bettinger PC. New dorsal capsulotomy for the surgical exposure of the wrist. *Ann Plast Surg.* 1995;35(1):54-59.
4. Mayfield JK. Patterns of injury to carpal ligaments: a spectrum. *Clin Orthop.* 1984;187:36-42.
5. Bugbee WD, Botte MJ. Surface anatomy of the hand: the relationship between palmar skin creases and osseous anatomy. *Clin Orthop Relat Res.* 1993;(296):122-126.
   The volar creases were marked with wires on 50 adult female volunteers. Distance measurements were obtained and analyzed to establish normal anatomic relationships between the creases and radiographic finding.
6. McLean KM, Sacks JM, Kuo YR, et al. Anatomic landmarks to the superficial and deep palmar arches. *Plast Reconstr Surg.* 2008;121(1):181.
7. Ağır I, Aytekin MN, Küçükdurmaz F, et al. Anatomical localization of Lister's tubercle and its clinical and surgical importance. *Open Orthop J.* 2014;8:74-77.
8. Hazani R, Engineer NJ, Elston J, Wilhelmi BJ. Anatomic landmarks for basal joint injections. *Eplasty.* 2012;12:e2.
9. Michelotti BF, Mathews A, Chung KC. Appropriateness of the use of magnetic resonance imaging in the diagnosis and treatment of wrist soft tissue injury. *Plast Reconstr Surg.* 2018;141(2):410-419.
   A retrospective review of 140 patients who had an upper extremity MRI demonstrated that the results only affected treatment recommendations in 28%. The predictor of impact on treatment was the presence of a specific suspected diagnosis.
10. Kehlet H, Wilmore DW. Multimodal strategies to improve surgical outcome. *Am J Surg.* 2002;183(6):630-641.
11. Ljungqvist O, Scott M, Fearon KC. Enhanced recovery after surgery: a review. *JAMA Surg.* 2017;152(3):292-298.
   Enhanced Recovery After Surgery (ERAS) process implementation involves a team consisting of surgeons, anesthetists, an ERAS coordinator (often a nurse or a physician assistant), and staff from units that care for the surgical patient. The care protocol is based on published evidence. The ERAS Society, an international nonprofit professional society that promotes, develops, and implements ERAS programs, publishes updated guidelines for many operations. ERAS protocols have resulted in shorter lengths of hospital stay by 30% to 50% and similar reductions in complications, while readmissions and costs are reduced. The elements of the protocol reduce the stress of the operation to retain anabolic homeostasis. The ERAS Society conducts structured implementation programs that are currently in use in more than 20 countries.
12. Shahryar N, McEwen JA, Kragh JF, et al. Surgical tourniquets in orthopedics. *J Bone Joint Surg Br.* 2009;91(12):2958-2967.
   This article reviews the literature regarding tourniquet use including size, pressure, location, and duration.
13. Wilgis E. Observations on the effects of tourniquet ischemia. *J Bone Joint Surg Am.* 1971;53(7):1343.
14. Cousins GR, Gill SL, Tinning CG, et al. Arm versus forearm tourniquet for carpal tunnel decompression: which is better? A randomized controlled trial. *J Hand Surg Eur.* 2015;40(9):961-965.

QUESTIONS

1. **Surgical exposure of the dorsal carpus should attempt to preserve which of the following anatomic structures?**
   a. Dorsal radiocarpal ligament
   b. TFCC
   c. Gilula's arcs
   d. Dorsal intracarpal ligament
   e. Radioscaphocapitate ligament

2. **Which of the following is correct regarding the bony anatomy of the metacarpal?**
   a. The condyloid nature of the MP joint allows for motion in two planes, flexion/extension and rotation.
   b. The MC head is wider on its volar surface contributing to CL tightening in flexion.
   c. There is a natural radial cant to the MC head of about 10 to 14 degrees.
   d. The volar plate is contiguous with the superficial transverse MC ligament.
   e. The volar convexity of the MC lends to dorsal apex fracture patterns.

3. **Which of the following anatomic relationships is correct?**
   a. Lister's tubercle is just proximal to the lunotriquetral joint.
   b. The palmaris longus is radial to the median nerve.
   c. The distal palmar crease is at the proximal end of the A1 pulley.
   d. The web space is at the proximal portion of the proximal phalanx.
   e. The distal wrist crease is at the level of the DRUJ.

4. **Which of the following anatomic relationships is correct?**
   a. The neurovascular bundle in the proximal phalanx is deep to the midlateral line.
   b. The ulnar artery and nerve are radial to the palpable hook of the hamate.
   c. The trapezoid can be palpated in the depths of the space between the EPL and EPB tendons.
   d. The flexor wad is ulnar to the visible brachioradialis muscle.

5. **Which of the following imaging modalities is best suited to locate a suspected mesquite thorn deep in the thenar eminence?**
   a. Plain film radiograph
   b. Ultrasound
   c. MRI
   d. CT

6. **Which of the following ERAS protocols in hand surgery is *false*?**
   a. Primary elements of protocols include patient education, nutrition optimization, early mobilization, and standardized analgesic and anesthetic regimens.
   b. Implementation of ERAS protocols has demonstrated decreased average length of stay but not complication rates.
   c. ERAS protocols across surgical specialties have been seen to lower readmission rates and hospital costs.
   d. The use of ERAS protocols in hand surgery specifically has not been well established.

1. **Answer: a.** The dorsal ligaments consist of the dorsal radiocarpal ligament and dorsal intercarpal ligament, and a surgical exposure of the dorsal carpal bones, such as a dorsal ligament sparing capsulotomy, attempts to preserve the integrity of these structures, thereby improving postoperative stability and mobility. This is a V-shaped flap elevated from the midpoint between the DRUJ and Lister's tubercle to the tubercle of the Triquetrum and then transversely to the tubercle of the scaphoid. This divides the above to noted ligaments along their midsubstance preserving their integrity. The TFCC is a 7 part soft tissue structure which stabilizes the DRUJ. Gilula's arcs mark the radiographic aspect of the distal and proximal carpal rows. The intracarpal ligaments connect carpal to carpal and are not in the dorsal wrist capsule. The radioscaphocapitate ligament is a volar structure.

2. **Answer: b.** The MP joints are condyloid in nature allowing for motion in three planes: flexion/extension, abduction/adduction, and rotation. Because the MC head is wider on its volar surface, flexion increases joint stability by tightening the CL and elongation of the VP. Thus, the MP joint should be immobilized in flexion to reduce the occurrence of joint contractures. There is a 10- to 14-degree natural ulnar deviation. As a result, the slight ulnar cant to the MP head predisposes to ulnar subluxation of the extensor hood and ulnar drift. The volar plate is contiguous with the deep transverse MC ligament, which connects the metacarpal heads of the index, long, ring, and little fingers and helps maintain the MCs in a slight dorsal arch in the transverse plane. The dorsal convexity to the MC bone results in tension on the dorsal surface with loading, leading to dorsal apex fracture patterns.

3. **Answer: c.** Lister's tubercle is just proximal to the scapholunate ligament and is the radial border of the third dorsal compartment. The palmaris longus is ulnar to the median nerve and serves as a landmark for median nerve blocks. The distal palmar crease is distal to the superficial palmar arch and at the level of the proximal A1 pulleys. The web space is at the mid portion of the proximal phalanx. The distal wrist crease is at the level of the midcarpal joint.

4. **Answer: d.** The neurovascular bundle in the finger is anterior to the midlateral line. The hook of the hamate, which is palpable in the palm, is radial to the ulnar neurovascular structures. The trapezium is palpable in the depths of the anatomic snuffbox. The origin of the flexor wad is the medial epicondyle, which is ulnar to the origin of the brachioradialis on the humerus.

5. **Answer: d.** Like most plant thorns, a mesquite thorn is radiolucent and will not be detected using X-rays. MRI will locate the thorn but is expensive and time consuming. Ultrasound is both sensitive and specific, costs much less than an MRI, and can be used during surgery.

6. **Answer: b.** Primary elements of ERAS protocols include preoperative patient education, nutritional optimization, early mobilization, and standardized analgesic and anesthetic regimens. Implementation of ERAS protocol across surgical specialties has demonstrated decreased average length of stay, complication rates, readmissions, and costs. Although recent research has aimed at improving outcomes in hand surgery, little data are available specific to ERAS protocols.

CHAPTER 68 Hand Infections

Anne Argenta and William W. Dzwierzynski

KEY POINTS

- Obtain a thorough history and physical exam; this will guide treatment.
- Know when urgent surgical intervention is warranted and always be suspicion.
- Persistent symptoms require further review and workup.
- Clearance of infection alone will not always result in a functional hand; stiffness and pain must be addressed.

The hands play a significant role in the way humans communicate and interact with the external environment. Because of this, the hands are particularly vulnerable to infection. Hand infections present in a variety of ways, but they will uniformly have a better outcome when managed expeditiously. When there is suspicion of infection, it is incumbent on the plastic surgeon to be knowledgeable, efficient, and vigilant.

PRESENTATION AND WORKUP

There are two main players during an infectious process: the insulting pathogen and the body's defense mechanism. A thorough workup of each will guide appropriate treatment. Important factors to elicit in the history are the duration and progression of symptoms, history of blunt or penetrating trauma, unusual exposures (animals, water, travel, and sick contacts), alleviating or aggravating factors, and systemic symptoms including fever, nausea, malaise, and altered mental status. Prior treatments and tetanus immunization should be documented.

The same pathogen may present differently in different individuals. Therefore, the patient's comorbidities and risk factors, including occupation, must be identified. Diabetes, obesity, intravenous (IV) drug use, malnutrition, human immunodeficiency virus (HIV/AIDS), autoimmune disease, and use of immunosuppressive medication can predispose patients to infection. Patients with these conditions are more susceptible to opportunistic pathogens and require more aggressive monitoring, with a lower threshold for intervention. Patients who use tobacco should be expected to have slower healing.[1]

On physical exam, the hand should be inspected for swelling, color changes, focal pain, guarding, puncture wounds, lacerations, and active and passive range of motion (ROM). The location of wounds can influence decision-making. For example, a wound over a joint warrants washout and investigation for joint involvement in the setting of a sterile environment, whereas a wound on the dorsum of the hand can usually safely be washed out and explored at the bedside. Similarly, the location of focal swelling should be documented. The compartments of the hand dictate how an infection may spread and, consequentially, influence incision placement during surgery. Signs of progressing infection, such as pain with passive ROM and ascending lymphangitis, should be noted and be treated.

The history and physical exam will guide need for further work up with imaging, cultures, and lab work. Ancillary tests should be used judiciously. Three view X-rays should be done when there is trauma and/or suspicion of foreign body. However, when there are signs of acute rapidly worsening infection, such as with necrotizing fasciitis, imaging will only delay treatment. Computed tomography (CT) and magnetic resonance imaging (MRI) should be reserved for cases where the diagnosis is unclear. A culture or tissue biopsy, if needed, can be taken expeditiously and easily in the emergency department setting before administration of antibiotics, without delaying treatment. Any labs, such as chemistries, complete blood count, and coagulation tests, can be drawn while the physician is examining the patient, thus avoiding treatment delays.

A critical step in the workup of hand infection is determining whether a patient needs hospitalization versus outpatient management. Hospitalization is required in patients with ascending lymphangitis, a failed trial of oral antibiotics, systemic symptoms, elevated white blood cell (WBC) count, a reasonable chance of needing operative intervention, or a high risk of not following-up. When an infection is managed as an outpatient, it is imperative to follow up culture results and adjust antibiotics as appropriate.

GENERAL PRINCIPLES OF TREATMENT

Most hand infections are mild and can be managed in the outpatient setting, but the surgeon should have a low threshold for inpatient care, particularly in rapid onset infections or high-risk patients. Fluctuance, purulent drainage, and worsening pain are all indications for surgical management. Knowledge of anatomy optimizes surgical outcome and minimizes complications.

Antibiotics are the cornerstone of infection management. Cultures of drainage or tissue should ideally be obtained before any antibiotics are given. The most common infections are a result of inoculation of tissues by bacteria normally found on human skin. *Staphylococcus* and *Streptococcus* species are by far the most common and should be covered in initial treatment. A first-generation cephalosporin is usually adequate. Methicillin-resistant *Staph aureus* (MRSA) is becoming more common as both a hospital-acquired and a community-acquired infection. MRSA infections tend to present with more skin necrosis, though cultures should be done to confirm diagnosis. In regions of high MRSA rates and in patients with a history of MRSA or recent hospitalization, empiric coverage with clindamycin, trimethoprim/sulfamethoxazole, a tetracycline (doxycycline or minocycline), or linezolid is indicated.[2] The choice of antibiotic is directed by the patient's community or hospital antibiogram. Immunocompromised patients are more susceptible to fungal, mycobacteria, and other less common pathogens. A high suspicion or an initial lack of response to standard antibiotic regimens may warrant broad-spectrum coverage and tailoring as culture results are obtained. Tissue culture will be more reliable than culture swabs. Confirm with the laboratory proper sampling and storage protocols for adequate testing of fungal and atypical mycobacteria.

Elevation and rest are standard treatment adjuncts for infection and are important components of pain management. Elevation of the hand above the heart level will limit edema. A short period of hand rest for 24 to 48 hours will not have a negative effect on long-term hand function. Hands should be splinted in the position of function (wrist extended 30°, MCP flexed 90°, digits extended) during this rest period. As the acute swelling improves, resumption of ROM exercises is important to limit stiffness and loss of strength.

Hand soaks are commonly used in the acute setting and rehabilitation phase, although their efficacy has not been fully established. Multiple solutions have been advocated. The most important principle is to dilute the betadine or chlorhexidine to a level that is nontoxic to healthy tissue. Soaks are generally performed two or three times a day, 5 to 10 minutes per session. Patients often report better pain control and ability to perform ROM exercises when the hand is submerged in warm solution.

COMMON HAND INFECTIONS

Digits

Paronychia

Paronychias are caused by infection of the skin around the nail fold. Initial violation of the skin barrier is often the result of a hangnail, manicure instruments, or nail biting. Symptoms include swelling, erythema, and pain around the nail plate. Exam should note swelling, discoloration, fluctuance, and drainage. The most common pathogen isolated from culture is *Staph aureus*. If caught early, treatment comprises hand soaks, oral antibiotics, and hand elevation. A first-generation cephalosporin is usually adequate. If an abscess has formed, as indicated by fluctuance and swelling, incision and drainage (I + D) is required. I + D is performed by incising the skin longitudinally with a no. 11 or 15 blade directly over the most prominent area of swelling, bluntly dissecting the cavity with a hemostat, culturing drainage, and copiously irrigating the wound with saline. When the decompressed cavity is large, a gauze wick is placed in the wound for 24 hours to help prevent reaccumulation and early skin closure. A paronychia may extend into the eponychium; in this case, the eponychial fold will need to be elevated. If purulence is noted under the nail plate, part or the entire nail should be removed. All of this can usually safely be performed under a digital block in the emergency room or clinic.

Chronic paronychias present as longstanding induration, pain, erythema along the nail fold, nail plate ridges, elevation of the skin off the nail plate, and occasional drainage. The nail plate may be thickened and discolored due to concomitant onychomycosis. Chronic paronychias are more common in diabetics, immunocompromised patients, women who get manicures, and people who frequently immerse their hand in water (dishwashers, nurses, or swimmers). Antibiotics are less effective and antifungal coverage for *Candida albicans* with nystatin or itraconazole is generally required, along with marsupialization (excision of semilunar patch of eponychial skin and subcutaneous tissue down to the germinal matrix). Topical gentian violet is a historic treatment for chronic paronychia that is gaining popularity again.[1]

Felon

Felons are focal infections within the pulp tissue of the fingertip (Figure 68.1). They are usually initiated by a puncture wound. Because of the extensive septae within the pulp, infection remains localized within a small compartment; this results in abscess formation with throbbing pain, often without visible external swelling until infection is advanced. The most common pathogen is *Staphylococcus aureus*. Very early presentations may resolve with oral antibiotics alone, but usually a focal abscess has formed by the time of presentation. This requires incision and drainage. Incision should be designed longitudinally over the most prominent point of pain, avoiding damage to neurovascular bundles and unnecessarily long incisions over the pulp, as the scars can become hypersensitive. The cavity should be bluntly probed with a hemostat to break up septae and ensure full drainage, and then irrigated. Placing gauze wick in the incision for 24 to 48 hours will help prevent reaccumulation. I + D in the outpatient setting under digital block is generally adequate. Delay in I + D of these abscesses can result in pulp necrosis, osteomyelitis, or extension of infection into the flexor sheath.

Flexor Tenosynovitis

Flexor tenosynovitis presents as an acutely swollen, painful digit (Figure 68.2). Often, there is history of a puncture wound, animal bite, or scrape on the volar surface of digit. When a pathogen, usually *S aureus*, inoculates the flexor tendon region and expands, the flexor sheath guides the infection proximally up the sheath, into the hand and forearm. The four identifying characteristics, known as the Kanaval signs, are as follows:

- Fusiform swelling, or a *sausage-shaped* digit
- Digit resting in flexed position
- Pain with passive extension
- Tenderness to palpation along the flexor tendon sheath into the palm

Untreated infectious tenosynovitis can lead to stiffness, chronic pain, osteomyelitis, and ascending limb-threatening infection. One should have very low threshold for hospitalization and early operative intervention. If caught within 24 to 48 hours with mild or equivocal Kanaval signs, some patients may improve with IV antibiotics, rest, elevation, and inpatient monitoring alone. Broad-spectrum antibiotics should be considered.

Anyone presenting with symptoms longer than 48 hours, Kanaval signs, or worsening symptoms with conservative management should undergo surgical decompression in the operating room (OR). A variety of incisions have been described. Most cases can be treated with two incisions: a standard palmar oblique incision over the A1 pulley (as for trigger finger release), and a midaxial, transverse, or Bruner incision at the distal P2 level. Proximally, blunt dissection with tenotomies will expose the A1 pulley, which is incised longitudinally to view the flexor tendons. A culture should be taken of any fluid in this area. Distally at the midaxial incision, blunt dissection deep to the neurovascular bundle will expose the flexor sheath distally. A small incision in the sheath should be made to inspect the tendons. Any wounds or focal abscesses in the finger should be debrided and cultured. The flexor sheath is then thoroughly irrigated using a 14 to 18 gauge angiocatheter or a no. 5 pediatric feeding tube attached to a syringe of saline and inserted into the tendon sheath through the proximal incision. Saline is pushed though the sheath and drains out the distal incision until the irrigation is clear. The irrigation system can also be inserted into the sheath from the distal incision, if easier but risks pushing the infected fluid proximally into the palm. At least 1 L is irrigated, ensuring that the saline is flowing well through the entire sheath. If there is significant frank

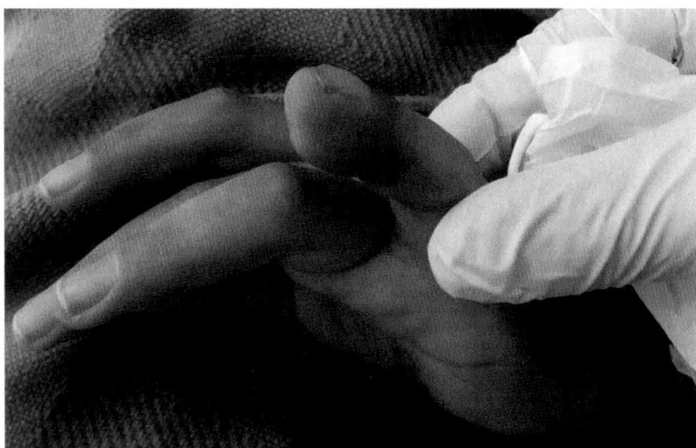

FIGURE 68.1. Felon, presenting in a 12-year-old boy with no recalled history of trauma.

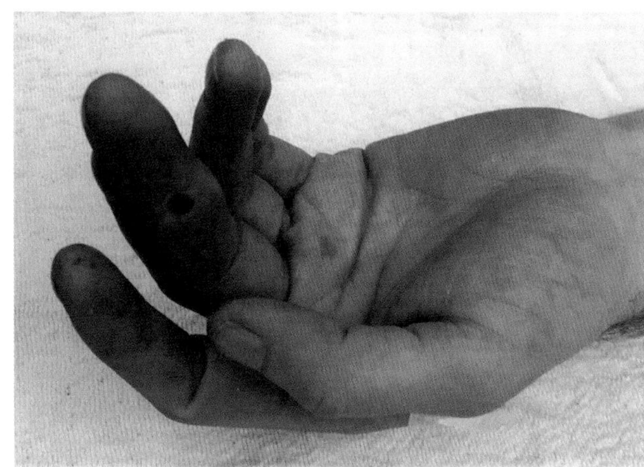

FIGURE 68.2. Flexor tenosynovitis, presenting 3 days after a cat bite to the digit.

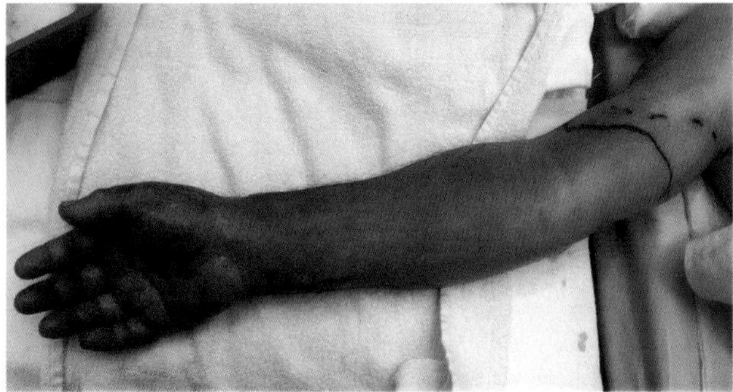

FIGURE 68.3. Cellulitis in a patient with necrotizing fasciitis (dorsal arm view in Figure 68.7).

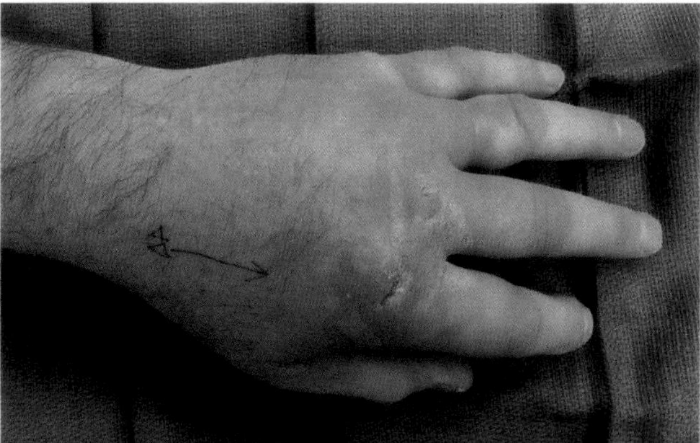

FIGURE 68.4. Fight bite, presenting 3 days after assault.

pus, Bruner incisions may be used to connect the proximal and distal incisions for further exposure. The irrigation system is removed at the end of the case or sutured in place for serial irrigations overnight in the hospital room. Retrospective reviews have not demonstrated that continuous irrigation has better outcomes compared to intraoperative irrigation alone.[4] The palmar and midaxial incisions can be left to close by secondary intention or loosely approximated. Extensive Bruner incisions should be loosely tacked together.

Postoperatively, the hand should be monitored, elevated, and rested for 24 hours in an inpatient setting. If improving, hand therapy can be started 24 to 48 hours after surgery. If pain and swelling persist, return to the OR is necessary. IV antibiotics are generally continued for 5 to 7 days and tailored by the culture results. Subcutaneous purulence and digit ischemia on presentation are indictors of a poor prognosis.[5]

Hand

Cellulitis

Cellulitis is the most common hand infection (Figure 68.3). Patients present with diffuse erythema and nonfocal swelling in the extremity. There may be history of a scratch or insect bite. Exam demonstrates generalize warmth, erythema, stiffness, lymphadenopathy, and edema. Patients rarely have one focal area of pain on exam. *Staph* and *Strep* species are the most common offenders. If the inciting trauma was caused by an animal scratch, additional bacteria may be involved (*Pasturella multocida* in dogs and cats; *Bartonella henselae* in cats). Ascending lymphangitis, elevated WBC, altered mental status, or lack of response to oral antibiotics warrants inpatient admission and IV antibiotics. Erythema should be outlined and dated in permanent marker to monitor progression. High-risk patients should be monitored for septic shock. Surgery is not indicated for cellulitis, but local debridement at the site of inoculation may be necessary if there is tissue necrosis or a localized abscess.

Fight Bites

Fight bites are caused by penetration of a foreign body, usually a tooth, through a joint capsule, resulting in inoculation of sterile joint space with bacteria (Figure 68.4). Patients typically present to the emergency room with a swollen, painful hand 2 or 3 days after punching another person in the face. Exam findings include pain, erythema, swelling over the dorsal metacarpal-phalangeal joint (MCP) region, a benign appearing scab over the dorsal MCP, and pain with axial loading of the joint. X-rays should be performed if there is suspicion of a retained foreign body or fracture.

Fight bites require exploration of the wound to rule out joint-space infection, as the MCP joint is violated in 70% of cases. This is best performed in the OR. The wound should be excised in an elliptical fashion. Because the extensor mechanism glides with ROM, punctures in the extensor mechanism may not directly underlie the skin puncture site. The joint should be fully explored during wound exploration to find violations in the extensor mechanism. If violation is suspected, the extensor should be opened either by longitudinally splitting the tendon or by incising between the extensor and sagittal band. Violation of the underlying joint capsule requires capsulotomy. After cultures are taken of the joint fluid, the patient should be started on broad-spectrum antibiotics covering for *S aureus* and oral flora (*Eikenella corrodens* and *Bacteroides* sp. in human bites) and the joint should be thoroughly irrigated with saline. A small gauze wick is placed in the joint space and the overlying capsule, extensor mechanism, and skin is loosely closed. Postoperative inpatient monitoring is advised. Persistent symptoms require return to the OR. Delay in surgical treatment can result in extensive joint destruction (Figure 68.5).

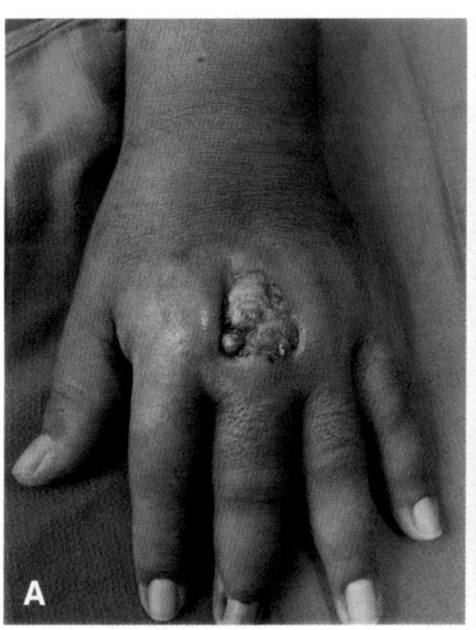

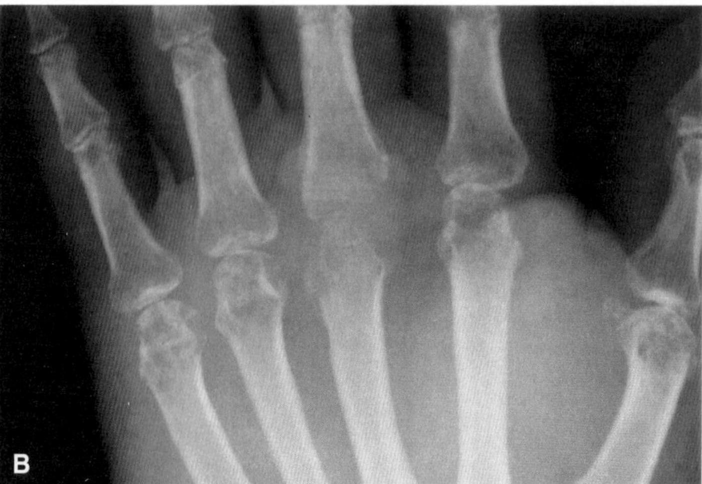

FIGURE 68.5. **A.** Delayed presentation of a fight bite to the left middle finger MCP, 7 months after assault. **B.** X-rays demonstrating joint destruction and osteomyelitis.

Deep-space Infections

Deep-space infections comprise 5% to 15% of all hand infections.[6] Because the hand is compartmentalized by fascial septae, these infections are often naturally confined to predictable locations. A brewing abscess in the thenar region after a puncture wound will be blocked from moving ulnarly toward the small finger by the midpalmar septum. Instead, it travels up flexor pollicis longus into the wrist, where the Parona space allows the infection to cross over to the flexors of the small finger and distally into the ulnar hand, circumventing the mid palm and creating the classic *horseshoe* abscess. A collar button abscess is an infection originating volar webspace and confined distally, because the strong palmar aponeurosis blocks infection from spreading proximally. Instead, the infection spreads dorsally into the dorsal subcutaneous tissues, forming the classic puckering, swelling, and abducted position of the digits.

Patients with deep-space infections will present with pain, swelling, erythema, and increased pain with ROM (Figure 68.6). A CT with contrast, ultrasound, or MRI will help localize and identify the extent of infection when the exam is vague. All deep-space infections require formal I + D and culture, preferably in the OR setting. Care should be taken in designing incisions, ensuring drainage of all areas but avoiding scars over critical structures. Thenar abscesses can be managed with a dorsal incision and dissection between the first dorsal interosseous and adductor pollicis muscles. The midpalmar abscess is accessed with an extended carpal tunnel incision or curved longitudinal incision in the palm. Collar button abscesses generally require volar and dorsal incisions for complete drainage; transverse incisions within the webspace cause adduction contractures and should be avoided. The most commonly isolated pathogens are *S aureus* and group A *Streptococcus*. Gauze wicks should be placed in the wound for continued egress of infection. Inpatient monitoring, broad-spectrum IV antibiotics, and early hand therapy are advised.

Necrotizing Fasciitis

Necrotizing fasciitis is one of the few emergent life- and limb-threatening hand infections. Patients present with cellulitis, discoloration, limited ROM, and rapidly ascending pain. Inciting trauma, if any, is often a minor cut or scrape. Immunocompromised patients (diabetics, chronic steroid use), the elderly, and IV drug abusers are more susceptible to necrotizing fasciitis and have higher mortality rates. There are two types of presentations: type 1, involving multiple anaerobic and aerobic bacteria, and type 2, involving group A *Streptococcus* and *Staphylococcus* sp. More recently, MRSA has been isolated in up to 39% of cases.[7]

Exam reveals erythema, streaking lymphangitis, pain, blistering, and crepitus (Figure 68.7; see Figure 68.3). Signs of hemodynamic instability, such as hypotension, tachycardia, and altered mental status are indicative of septic shock. Stat gram stain should be done without delaying definitive treatment of broad-spectrum IV antibiotics, aggressive resuscitation, and emergent operative debridement. A classic sign of necrotizing fasciitis is cloudy *dishwasher* drainage, due to necrosis of the fascia. Aggressive debridement is vital, as infection spreads rapidly along fascial planes and leads to skin and muscle necrosis. Amputation must be considered in the setting of advanced muscle necrosis and septic shock. Tissue samples should be cultured. Patients should be placed in the intensive care unit if there is any concern of hemodynamic instability. Return to the OR for a second look should occur within 24 to 48 hours. Patients will generally need extensive soft tissue reconstruction once infection is cleared.

Wrist

Septic Arthritis

Similar to a fight bite, septic arthritis of the wrist results from inoculation of the joint with a pathogen. Because joints are avascular *immune privileged* sites, meaning that they do not mount a strong immune response to infection, infection can rapidly progress to permanent cartilage and bone destruction. These infections can arise from a direct penetrating trauma or from hematogenous spread. *S aureus*, *Streptococcus* sp, *Haemophilus influenzae* (in children), and *Neisseria gonorrhoeae* are the most common pathogens. Patients present with gradually worsening pain in the wrist, severe pain with ROM, and swelling. A history of trauma, immunosuppression, autoimmune disease, gout, and sexually transmitted disease should

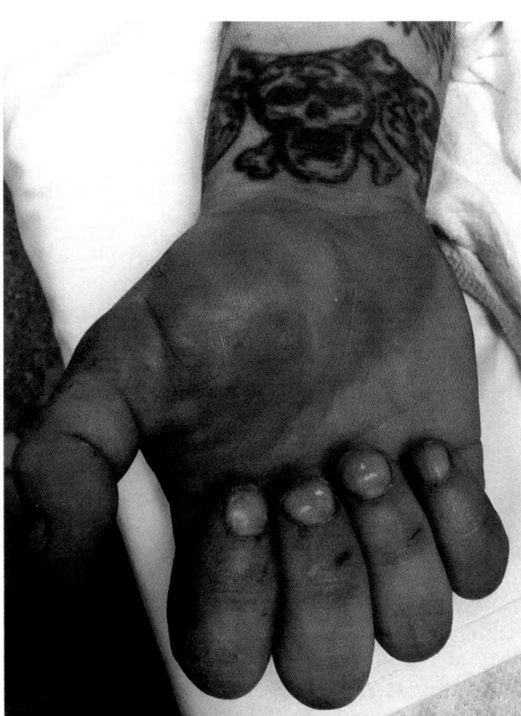

FIGURE 68.6. Thenar deep-space infection in an IV drug user.

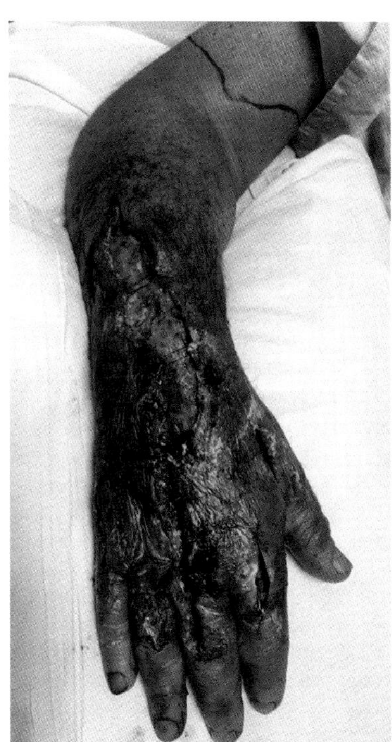

FIGURE 68.7. Necrotizing fasciitis, presenting in a healthy 60-year-old man 4 days after scratching his dorsal hand on a piece of metal (volar arm view in Figure 68.3).

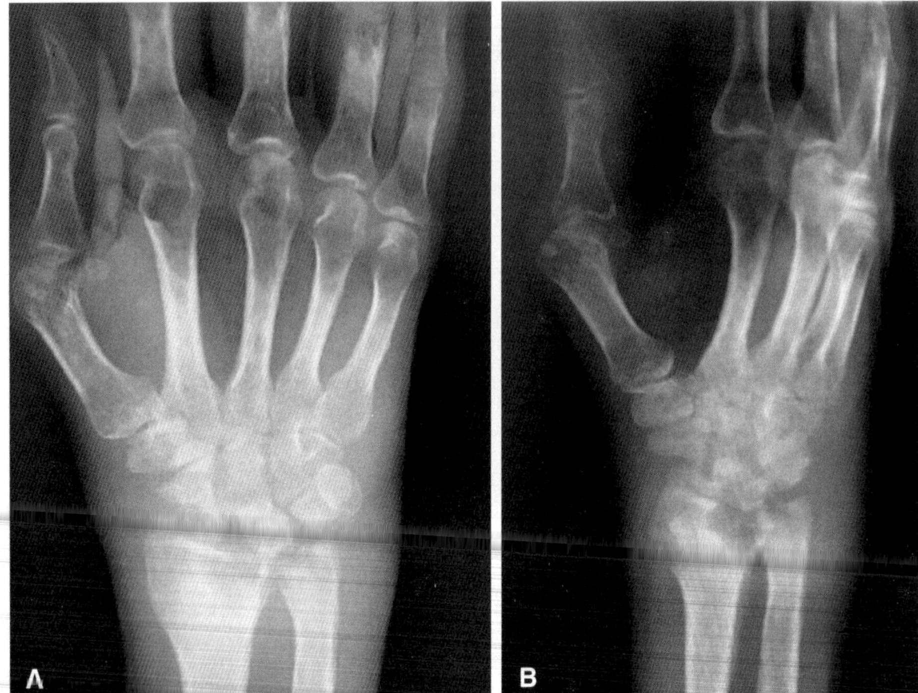

FIGURE 68.8. Advanced septic arthritis and osteomyelitis of the carpus and distal radius in a 50-year-old male with extensive psychiatric history presenting with 7 months of wrist pain. **A.** Anteroposterior radiograph. **B.** Oblique view.

all be noted. Exam reveals pain with wrist ROM and axial loading, swelling, warmth around the joint, and often overlying cellulitis. In delayed presentations, X-rays can identify bony erosion (Figure 68.8).

Septic arthritis of the wrist must be distinguished from simple cellulitis and from acute flares of gout or pseudogout. The history may provide some clues. Prior flares and patchy calcifications of the wrist joint on X-rays would lean toward autoimmune etiology, whereas history of penetrating trauma, fever, erythema, and lymphangitis would be suspicious for infection. A wrist aspiration and joint fluid analysis will confirm diagnosis. This should only be done in the setting of high suspicion, as aspiration risks introduction of pathogen into a joint, creating septic arthritis when it may not have been present initially. To perform a wrist joint aspiration, the 3 to 4 interval on the dorsal wrist is palpated just distal and ulnar to Lister tubercle. The skin is anesthetized, the site sterilized, and the wrist flexed slightly to facilitate entry. A sterile large bore (18–20 gauge) needle is inserted at an angle to avoid the dorsal lip of the distal radius. Ideally, 2 cc of fluid is aspirated. Normal joint fluid is clear or straw colored. The fluid should be sent for crystal analysis and culture, after confirming with the laboratory that the sample is properly packaged for analysis.

Although septic arthritis due to *N gonorrhoeae* can often be treated with IV antibiotics alone, the presence of any other bacterial strain in the joint fluid warrants operative washout and aspiration of frank pus is an indication for urgent surgery. The wrist joint is opened via a longitudinal dorsal skin incision. The wrist capsule can be opened longitudinally or in a ligament-sparing approach to expose the wrist joint. The joint space should be cultured and extensively irrigated with 3 L of saline. Automated pulse lavage is avoided, because the excessive pressure can damage cartilage. The cartilaginous surfaces are inspected. Any frankly necrotic bone is debrided with a rongeur; this is generally only seen in late, advanced cases. The capsule, extensor retinaculum, and skin can be loosely closed, leaving a gauze wick to allow continued egress of bacteria. Arthroscopic wrist washout has been reported to achieve similar results with less postoperative stiffness.[8] Postoperatively, the hand is placed in a wrist splint and elevated for comfort. Patients should be admitted for observation, pain control, and IV antibiotics. One should have a low threshold for a second look in 24 to 48 hours. Once improving, ROM exercises are started while the patient is still admitted.

SPECIAL CASES

Fungal, Mycobacterial, or Viral Infections

The vast majority of hand infections are bacterial in origin. When infections do not respond rapidly to standard antibiotic regimens, one should consider fungal, mycobacterial or viral sources. These pathogens tend to be more indolent. Chronic paronychia, for example, is usually due to candida infection. Mycobacteria are notoriously difficult to culture; suspicion should be raised for mycobacteria when rice bodies are found at time of debridement or granulomas are found on pathology.

Immunocompromised patients and specific patient populations are more susceptible to these less common infections. Hand infections due to *Mycobacterium avium-intracellulare* are increasing in the HIV population. *Mycobacterium marinum* tends to affect fisherman and fish handlers; the infection causes indolent progression of papule clusters on the hand and fingers. Pain is variable. The four other most common pathogens associated with water animal exposure are *Aeromonas* sp., *Edwardsiella tarda*, *Erysipelothrix rhusiopathiae*, and *Vibrio vulnificus*. Sporotrichosis is a fungal infection more common in gardeners who have been pricked by a rose thorn. Coccidioidomycosis in the southwestern United States and histoplasmosis in the midwestern United States are rare fungal causes of synovitis and microabscesses of the hand.

Herpetic whitlow is a viral infection due to the herpes simplex virus, which causes a burning sensation for 1 or 2 days, followed by erythema and blistering around the thumb of fingers (Figure 68.9). It is seen more commonly in children, dentists, and other medical professionals exposed to oral secretions, and in immunocompromised patients. Tzanck smear confirms diagnosis. The infection is self-limited in 2 to 3 weeks; treatment with oral acyclovir or similar antivirals may be used in severe cases or to speed resolution. Aggressive debridement and unroofing of vesicles is ill-advised and can predispose patients to bacterial superinfection.

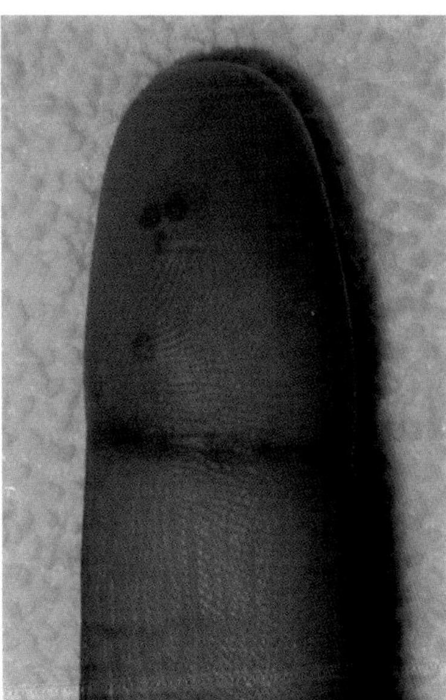

FIGURE 68.9. Herpetic whitlow in a dental hygienist. (Courtesy of Dr James Sanger.)

Osteomyelitis

The ideal time to treat a hand infection is within the first 24 hours. Unfortunately, a lingering infection in the hand, even a simple paronychia, can lead to underlying osteomyelitis if neglected. The standard for diagnosing osteomyelitis is bone biopsy. Any frankly necrotic bone encountered during an I + D should be debrided back to hard, bleeding bone and sent for culture, or it will continue to act as a nidus for further infection. It is prudent to consult an infectious disease (ID) specialist in these cases, to help narrow antibiotics, determine duration, and monitor for any medical [illegible] caused by the antibiotic use. The ID specialists are often more familiar with community antibiotic resistances and cost comparisons of different antibiotics. Patients with osteomyelitis generally require formal hand therapy to limit stiffness and disuse atrophy of the hand during extended treatment. One must consider the pros and cons of amputation over salvage.

Drug Abuse

IV drug use is an unfortunately common cause for hand infections, either by use of a dirty needle, by introduction of skin bacteria by the needle, or by contamination of the substance injected. When the concern is present, patients should be asked directly about drug habits. Particular attention should be paid to track marks along the forearm or antecubital fossa. Puncture marks within the webspace may indicate direct drug injection into the subcutaneous tissues, an increasingly common form of drug delivery known as *skin popping*. A recent history of IV drug use should raise suspicion for both cellulitis and deep-space infections. Mixed flora and anaerobic infections are more common in IV drug use. A drug screen and basic laboratory workup should be performed for anesthesia clearance, if needed. Workup for hepatitis C and HIV should be discussed with these high-risk patients.

Immunocompromised Patients

Immunocompromised patients, including those with diabetes, chronic steroid use, HIV, and malnutrition, require special attention. A higher level of vigilance is needed when monitoring infections in this population. Simple infections can progress rapidly to limb-threatening problems. Because this group has a muted immune response, common presentations such as elevated WBC, fever, erythema, or significant pain may not be present. Inpatient observation and serial exams are recommended.

Problems That Mimic Infection

Several problems can masquerade as an infection. Most commonly, inflammatory arthritis flares, including gout and pseudogout, are confused with septic arthritis of the joints. Proper diagnosis is imperative, as treatments differ dramatically. Factors such as recurrent episodic pain, lack of trauma, elevated blood uric acid levels, and calcium deposits in joints on X-rays may indicate gout or pseudogout, but the presence of crystals on joint aspiration must be confirmed. When in doubt, assume a septic joint until proved otherwise.

Chronic hand wounds that have been maintained on long courses of antibiotics with minimal improvement warrant further investigation. Any wound present for longer than 6 months should be biopsied to rule out cancer, pyogenic granuloma, or pyoderma gangrenosum. Biopsy incisions should be designed longitudinally to allow extension as needed for a wide excision in the future.

OPTIMIZING LONG-TERM OUTCOME

The outcome of hand infections is dependent on rapid diagnosis, efficient treatment, and early rehabilitation. Long after the infection has been treated, the body's inflammatory response may cause residual swelling, stiffness, and pain. As with many other hand conditions, early hand therapy is critical to optimizing function and should, in most cases, be started in the postoperative period while the patient is still in the hospital. When treating hand [illegible], the ultimate goal is not clearance of infection, but the restoration of a functional hand.

REFERENCES

1. Siverstein P. Smoking and wound healing. *Am J Med.* 1992;93(1 suppl A):22S-24S.
2. Liu C, Bayer A, Cosgrove S, et al. Clinical practice guidelines by the infectious diseases society of America for the treatment of methicillin-resistant *Staphylococcus aureus* infections in adults and children. *Clin Infect Dis.* 2011;52:e18-e55.
3. Merritt W. *The Impecunious Treatment for Chronic Paronychia and Ingrown Toenails: Back to the Future.* Presented at American Association of Hand Surgery Annual Meeting; January 21-24; Paradise Island, Bahamas. 2015.
4. Lille S, Hayakawa T, Neumeister M, et al. Continuous postoperative catheter irrigation is not necessary for the treatment of suppurative flexor tenosynovitis. *J Hand Surg Br.* 2000;25(3):304-307.
   This study is a multicenter retrospective review of 75 patients that compares intraoperative and continuous postoperative irrigation (standard of care; n = 55) versus intraoperative flush alone (n = 20) for treatment of suppurative tenosynovitis. Outcomes were not statistically different between the two groups. Intraoperative flush alone simplifies treatment, reduces patient discomfort, and allows for earlier postop range of motion exercises.
5. Pang H, Teoh L, Yam A, et al. Factors affecting the prognosis of pyogenic flexor tenosynovitis. *J Bone Joint Surg.* 2007;89(8):1742-1748.
6. Jebson PJ. Deep subfascial space infections. *Hand Clin.* 1998;14(4):557-566.
7. Lee T, Carrick M, Scott B. Incidence and clinical characteristics of methicillin resistant *Staphlococcus aureus* necrotizing fasciitis in a large urban hospital. *Am J Surg.* 2007;194(6):809-812.
8. Sammer D, Shin A. Comparison of arthroscopic and open treatment of septic arthritis of the wrist. *J Bone Joint Surg Am.* 2009;91A:1387-1393.
   This is a retrospective review out of Mayo clinic that compares open irrigation and debridement (standard of care; n = 19 wrists) versus arthroscopic irrigation and debridement (n = 21 wrists). For isolated septic arthritis of the wrist, arthroscopic treatment resulted in fewer procedures and shorter hospitalization. No differences in procedure number or hospitalization length between the two groups were seen when patients had multiple sites of infection.

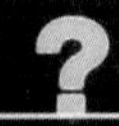

QUESTIONS

1. A 40-year-old homeless diabetic man presents to the emergency room after spontaneous onset of exquisite pain, swelling, and blistering of the dorsal hand 6 hours ago. He is appropriately communicative, tachycardic to the 110s. He has a WBC of 20 and a blood glucose level of 160. On exam, there is blistering and streaking erythema up the forearm and palpable crepitus in the hand and forearm. What is the next step?

   a. X-ray to rule out trauma
   b. MRI to rule out abscess
   c. Emergent surgery
   d. Tissue biopsy

2. A 35-year-old woman with type 1 diabetes presents with worsening pain over the volar index finger after being bitten by her cat yesterday. She has a 2 mm open wound with expressible purulence over the volar surface of the second phalanx. She has full active ROM of the digit with mild pain, no fusiform swelling, and no pain over the volar P1 and palm. Her WBC is 7, her glycosylated hemoglobin is 9.5, and she is afebrile. What is the next step?

   a. X-ray to rule out underlying fracture
   b. I + D of localized abscess and inpatient IV antibiotics
   c. I + D of abscess and discharge with clindamycin
   d. Emergent decompression of the flexor sheath

3. A 75-year-old man with rheumatoid arthritis was referred to you for a persistent infection on the dorsal hand. He reports bumping the hand on a metal railing 10 months ago, resulting in an open, intermittently draining 1 × 1 cm wound overlying the dorsal fifth metacarpal. There is mild cloudy drainage and thickened scar tissue along the wound edges, but no exposed tendon or bone. What is the next step?

   a. Biopsy
   b. IV antibiotics
   c. Formal debridement and closure
   d. Local wound care

1. **Answer: c.** Patient has signs and symptoms of necrotizing fasciitis, which is limb and life threatening. Treatment involves emergent and often serial debridement, broad-spectrum IV, and supportive inpatient care. A tissue sample can be obtained in the OR. Imaging will delay definite treatment.

2. **Answer: b.** Patient is a poorly controlled diabetic with a localized infection that has high risk of developing into flexor tenosynovitis. At present, her wound should be I + Ded and cultured. Monitoring as an outpatient or inpatient can be debated, but clindamycin is not an appropriate antibiotic for *Pasteurella* species, which are most commonly associated with animal bites. At this point, patient does not have flexor tenosynovitis, though she has potential to develop it.

3. **Answer: a.** A biopsy is the necessary next step to rule out skin cancer, which can masquerade as a chronic infection. The other options are appropriate once cancer has been ruled out.

CHAPTER 69

Soft Tissue Reconstruction of the Upper Extremity and Management of Fingertip and Nail Bed Injuries

Sirichai Kamnerdnakta and Kevin C. Chung

KEY POINTS

- The primary goals of soft tissue reconstruction of the hand are restoration of function and appearance.
- As opposed to the historical reconstructive ladder approach, reconstructive elevator approach is more suitable for soft tissue defects of the hand, in which the surgeon selects any procedure that will achieve the desired outcomes.
- Early postoperative mobilization and rehabilitation will achieve maximal functional outcomes.
- A functional hand should possess a stable wrist and at least two opposing, sensate, and painless digits. One finger should be mobile and opposed with another stable finger, with a space between the digits.
- In a mutilated hand injury, pedicle flaps can be used to provide coverage in preparation for a microsurgical procedure, such as a toe transfer or microsurgical bone reconstruction.

An acceptable hand consists of a thumb and at least three fingers that have ample interphalangeal joint motion, adequate length, and preserved sensibility.[1] However, these minimal conditions are sometimes not achievable in extreme reconstruction cases. In such cases, function is prioritized. The minimal functional requirements include a stable wrist and two opposing, sensate, and painless digits. The two fingers should be separated by a gap and should include one mobile finger, along with an opposing, stable finger.[2] Although the functional requirements should be considered during the development of the reconstruction plan, the surgeon should also aim to achieve optimal appearance of the hand.[3] In particular, the surgeon should consider color and texture match, donor/recipient tissue interface, hairiness, and the size and location of the final scar.

PRINCIPLES OF RECONSTRUCTION

One of the fundamental principles of plastic surgery regarding soft tissue reconstruction is the reconstructive ladder, in which surgical decisions are made following a stepwise approach that increases in complexity the higher the ladder goes. The ladder starts with simple primary closure and ends with complex microsurgical free flap surgery. However, modern advancements in plastic surgery suggest a new approach, the reconstructive elevator. With this approach, optimal function and appearance guide the decision that surgeons make regarding reconstruction.[4,5]

Starting with the simplest procedure, definite wound closure should be planned expeditiously. The ultimate goal is to obtain primary wound healing to diminish scar formation and lessen the possibility of contracture and stiffness. However, before any definitive wound coverage is done, wound bed preparation is mandatory before any coverage to ensure proper wound healing of the reconstructed defect. Coverage should be delayed until the wound shows stability and clear demarcation of nonviable tissue, with minimal risk of infection. Although temporary, negative pressure wound therapy (NPWT) provides optimal wound dressing during the serial debridement period because it bridges the gap before definite wound closure and promotes healing. Applying NPWT can reduce exudate, improve local tissue perfusion, and lessen swelling. However, surgeons must exercise caution during prolonged application of NPWT because granulation tissue may form over the wound bed and cause scarring over time.[6] NPWT is often used to promote granulation tissue prior to skin grafting in the lower extremities. However, prolonged use in the hand causes contracture and stiffness. If a patient has vital structures that are exposed, the surgeon must consider an immediate flap coverage. Subsequent debridement and irrigation can be performed to ensure viability of the tissue. Once the wound bed has been prepared adequately, a definitive flap can be performed.

Clinical Consideration

An analysis of a defect is crucial prior to initiating any mode of reconstruction. The surgeon should try to preserve the essential structures as much as possible so that they can maintain their own function. The most effective way to preserve the vital components is to consider early soft tissue coverage as the first step in the management of the severed hand.

In certain scenarios, single-stage reconstructions are not appropriate (e.g., tendon or nerve reconstruction with substantial bony and soft tissue loss) because the formation of scar and fibrotic tissue will hinder functional recovery. Thus, a staged reconstruction is often better than trying to accomplish too much at the onset of the injury. Each defect requires an individualized treatment protocol. While formulating the treatment plan, the surgeon should consider all relevant factors that could affect the success of the reconstruction[7] (**Table 69.1**). Although treatment options vary, all reconstructive procedures of the soft tissue envelope of the hand must follow the basic principles of coverage: replacing like with like, restoring function, and preserving sensibility and mobility. For example, in the effort to reconstruct a mutilated hand that requires secondary reconstruction, surgeons prefer the use of a fasciocutaneous flap over a muscle flap. A fasciocutaneous flap is more pliable and has greater gliding capacity, which facilitates tendon gliding without impairment during motion. On the other hand, a muscle flap can adhere to the wound bed and make a secondary procedure more tedious.

Choosing the optimal flap for each individual defect is an important factor of the hand reconstruction. Choices include a pedicle locoregional flap, a distant flap, and a microsurgical free flap, which all abide by the basic principles of coverage. Depending on the origin site, flaps are defined as the following:

- *Local flap:* Originates from a site directly adjacent to the defect and is typically completed in a single-stage reconstruction (e.g., V-Y advancement flap or Z-plasty)
- *Regional flap:* Originates from areas not adjacent to the defect but is still confined within the ipsilateral limb (e.g., thenar flap, cross-finger flap, radial forearm flap)
- *Distant flap:* Originates from areas that are not from the ipsilateral limb of the defect and almost always requires two stages for harvest and inset (e.g., groin flap)

Surgeons should preferentially consider the use of pedicle locoregional flaps. The defect can be used as a template to simulate the flap design. Pivot point, movement, and length are all factors that should be considered when designing the flap. If a locoregional flap cannot be designed to cover the defect adequately, a distant flap or

TABLE 69.1. INFLUENTIAL FACTORS FOR PERIOPERATIVE CONSIDERATIONS

Factor	Implications
Wound	Size
	Site
	Side (volar/dorsal)
	Amount and type of tissue loss
Donor site	Functional loss
	Scar location
	Morbidity
Flap	Texture
	Color
	Volume
	Hairiness
	Sensibility
Patient	Handiness
	Age
	Sex
	Occupation
	Medical comorbidities
	Preferences
Surgeon	Knowledge
	Technical skill
	Preference

microvascular free flap is needed. A free flap is advantageous because it requires only one procedure, encourages composite reconstruction, allows mobility, and permits earlier rehabilitation.[8] However, the operation is technically demanding and requires advanced microvascular surgery skills. Unstable patients, including those with multiple comorbidities, are normally not the best candidates for free flaps. Additionally, vessel paucity, mutilating hand injuries, or prior history of free flap failure may be indication for a pedicle distant flap.[9] Common scenarios for which the surgeon should consider performing a pedicle distant flap include coverage of digital stump defects in preparation for toe-to-hand transfer, high-voltage electric injuries with diffused thrombosed vessels, and multiple defects.[10-14]

MODES OF RECONSTRUCTION FOR INDIVIDUAL DEFECTS

Partial or Full-Thickness Skin Loss

Skin Grafts

Partial or full-thickness skin defects that do not require additional volume or functional tissue can be covered using a skin graft. Split-thickness skin grafts (STSGs) are more pliable, have an easier "take," conform better on a convoluted surface, and provide more surface coverage than full-thickness skin grafts (FTSGs). However, a FTSG can restore more durability and sensibility, while it can minimize the risk of contracture. Despite their benefits, there are certain contraindications for skin grafting:

- Nonvascularized wound bed such as a bare bone or bare tendon defect
- Exposure of vital structures such as neurovascular bundle
- Defects that are overlying a joint area
- Active infectious status
- Planned secondary reconstruction; tendon graft, nerve graft, implantation, tenolysis, or joint release

The most notable contraindication is that grafts can adhere to the underlying structures, making further reconstruction impossible.

The palmar and dorsal skins of the hand are functionally and anatomically different. The dorsal skin is thin, pliable, and loose, which facilitates smooth tendon gliding and unrestricted movement of the underlying joints. Conversely, the palmar skin is thick, durable, glabrous, and inelastic, which enables to withstand constant external forces and enhance prehensile function through the formation of skin creases and folds. The thick dermal layer of the glabrous skin is rich in exocrine sweat glands, blood vessels, and sensory nerve endings. Therefore, STSGs are typically used for reconstruction of defects of the dorsum of the hand; whereas, volar skin defects almost always require resurfacing by FTSGs. To obtain similarity of the glabrous volar skin, the donor site of FTSGs is harvested from the hypothenar eminence or instep plantar area.

Dermal Substitute

A dermal substitute, in conjunction with an STSG, will provide better quality, thickness, and pliability in comparison to reconstruction with an STSG alone.[15,16] Dermal substitutes are advantageous because they provide a scaffold for growth of neovascularized tissue from the wound bed. Therefore, a dermal substitute can take on tendons devoid of paratenon, cartilage without perichondrium, and bones without the periosteum. Dermal substitutes require a noninfected and well-vascularized wound bed. However, the amount of vascularized tissue necessary for successful incorporation of dermal substitutes is not well defined.[17] Dermal substitutes are used for the reconstruction of acute and chronic burns of the hand, but it lacks evidence-based support to be used over traditional modes of reconstruction in nonburn-related or traumatic wounds.[18-20] Nonetheless, dermal substitutes are a good alternative if the patient cannot tolerate a prolonged operation or needs a shorter period of immobilization. Soft tissue reconstruction using dermal substitutes may deliver acceptable functional and aesthetic outcomes in select situations.[20,21]

However, dermal substitute templates lack many essential components of normal skin, such as hair follicles, sweat glands, or other skin appendages. Furthermore, sensory recovery is unsatisfactory. Injuries that need reconstruction with high sensory demand, such as those in the palm or pulp of the finger, are better suited to be reconstructed with a flap to optimize functional outcomes.

Reconstruction of soft tissue defects via dermal substitutes typically requires STSG. In a two-stage reconstruction, split-thickness skin grafting can be done 2 to 3 weeks after dermal substitute placement. NPWT can be used to bridge the wound before definitive skin graft placement. Full-thickness skin grafting with a dermal substitute is not recommended because there is a high metabolic demand of the FTSG, leading to a risk of ischemia and necrosis of the FTSG.[22]

Fingertip Defect

The goals of reconstructing a fingertip amputation are to restore the padding of the finger to provide maximum tactile gnosis, preserve the length of the finger, keep an intact nail bed, and minimize downtime. Although replantation achieves optimal appearance and functional results, this is not always possible. Surgeons should consider the following factors while formulating the best treatment method: the location of the injury, the dimension of the defect, and any involved structures, such as bone or tendon.

Small fingertip defects that are less than 1 cm^2 with minimal bony exposure or nail matrix involvement should be healed by secondary intention. Secondary intention can restore sensation, appearance of the fingertip, and achieve comparable functionality to skin grafts.[23-25] In cases of defects larger than 1 to 1.5 cm^2, presence of volar oblique injuries, or the exposure of tendon or bone, the mode of surgical closure will be determined.[26] Defects with the largest dimension of less than 1 cm may indicate reconstruction using local tissue coverage, such as V-Y volar or lateral advancement flaps. The V-Y advancement flap is most suitable for coverage of transverse or dorsal oblique fingertip amputations that have exposed bones but sufficient length and bony support of the nail bed. Previous studies have demonstrated near-normal or normal recovery in sensation for most patients after V-Y flap reconstruction.[27-29] However, larger or composite defects will require more soft tissue, suggesting homodigital, heterodigital, locoregional, or free tissue transfers. The location, geometry, and mechanism of the injury will dictate the mode of reconstruction. The indications and contraindications of the available flaps are in **Table 69.2**. Although some locoregional flaps do not require a two-stage reconstruction, cross-finger and thenar flaps do. During a two-stage reconstruction, the affected finger is usually restrained for 2 to 3 weeks before a secondary flap division is performed. This waiting period will delay the onset of rehabilitation, possibly resulting in joint stiffness.

The microvascular toe pulp or the glabrous skin of the foot transfers is an optimal choice for a volar fingertip reconstruction because of the similarity in physical and anatomical factors. Although a free tissue transfer is a prolonged procedure and technically demanding, it should be performed when a locoregional transfer cannot provide adequate soft tissue coverage, the injury affects multiple finger pulp losses, or if the defect of the pulp covers two-thirds of the digital pulp of the first three fingers.[30]

Thumb Fingertip Defect

The thumb is responsible for 40% of total hand function, enabling pinching, grasping, and opposition. Reconstruction of a defect on the thumb should aim to provide adequate length, a nonpainful tip, sensation, mobility, and stability to oppose the other fingers.

The ulnar contact side of the thumb is the most important tactile area on the hand, enabling movements like key pinch and three-point pinch grip. Thus, restoration of the sensory function is vital for normal hand function and grip strength.

A defect without any bony exposure that affects less than half of the finger pulp can heal by secondary intention. Secondary intention results in excellent contour, consistency of the finger pulp, and satisfactory return of sensory function. However, defects that are larger, volar oblique, and leave exposed bones will require flap coverage. The location and size of the defect will influence the flap selection (**Table 69.3**).

Volar or ulnar side defects are best reconstructed by the Moberg flap. A Moberg flap can advance distally by 1.5 to 2 cm without causing flexor contracture (Figure 69.1). A Moberg flap reconstruction can achieve excellent sensory restoration, maintaining contour and suitable fingerprint pattern for friction. However, larger defects that require more than 2 cm of flap advancement are not suitable for reconstruction using the Moberg flap because it requires a more ancillary procedure to diminish flexion contracture of the thumb interphalangeal joint such as division of the proximal skin bridge for additional advancement. Thus, larger defects should be reconstructed with the first dorsal metacarpal artery (DMCA) flap because it provides more soft tissue and can immediately restore sensation by including a branch of the superficial radial nerve (Figure 69.2).[31] If using a first DMCA flap is not possible because of the extent of the injury, an innervated heterodigital island flap from the long or ring finger is an alternative option. However, an innervated heterodigital island flap requires more vascular pedicle dissection into the palm. Furthermore, the use of this flap causes a loss of sensation in the donor finger and a higher rate of venous congestion than with a first DMCA flap.[32,33] Both the first DMCA flap and innervated heterodigital flap will cause dual sensation, requiring cortical reeducation on behalf of the patient to achieve sensory reorientation within a few years.[31,32,34]

Locoregional flaps are not suitable for reconstructing volar or ulnar defects that are accompanied with extensive injuries to the hand. Cases with extreme injury to the hand are an indication for the use of a distant flap or microvascular free tissue transfer. However, the distant flap has some disadvantages including bulky tissue, nonglabrous skin, insensate flap, and prolonged immobilization. Thus, microvascular glabrous skin transfers, such as toe pulp transfers or medial plantar flaps from the foot, are more advantageous than distant flaps.[30,35-38] Toe pulp transfers are preferred over medial plantar flaps because they can provide a sensate flap.[36]

TABLE 69.2. FLAP OPTIONS FOR FINGERTIP RECONSTRUCTION (PIPJ: PROXIMAL INTERPHALANGEAL JOINT)

Flap	Indication	Contraindication
V-Y advancement flap	■ Bony exposure defect from a transverse or dorsal oblique fingertip amputation with adequate length and bony support of the nail bed. ■ Amputation is usually a the midportion of the nail bed.	■ Insufficient tissue on the volar area, such as a volar oblique amputation. ■ Amputation injury proximal to the lanula.
Cross-finger flap	■ Volar soft tissue defects with exposed bone or tendon at the middle or distal phalanx. ■ Defects with exposed bone or tendon at the distal phalanx that cannot be covered with a V-Y advancement flap.	■ Extensive dorsal skin loss and the involvement of the adjacent fingers.
Thenar flap	■ Volar skin avulsion with bony or tendon exposure of the finger pulp of the index, middle, or ring finger. ■ Reconstruction of a near-total or total distal phalangeal pulp loss.	■ Extensive volar and dorsal tissue loss of the finger. ■ Risk of flexion contracture is markedly high when performing this flap in patients who has a concomitant PIPJ injury.
Homodigital island flap	■ Patients with extensive but not complete pulp defects (<2 cm) of the fingers.	■ A negative digital Allen test showing inadequate or nonexistent collateral perfusion. ■ Extensive soft tissue injury of the affected digit. ■ Avulsion injury that affects the digital artery.
Heterodigital island flap	■ A defect with tendon, bone, or neurovascular exposure on the dorsal or volar surface of the finger up to 3.5 cm long.	■ An extensive injury that involves multiple digits of the distal palm in which the pedicle may be injured. ■ Patients with peripheral vascular disease, heavy smoking, or vasculitis that affects the vasculature of the hand. ■ Negative Allen test of the donor finger.
Dorsal metarcarpal artery flap	■ A dorsal defect that affects up to the PIPJ level of a non-thumb digit.	■ Injury to the dorsal carpal circulation. ■ Extensive loss of the dorsal skin.

TABLE 69.3. FLAP OPTIONS FOR THUMB FINGERTIP RECONSTRUCTION

Flap	Indication	Contraindication
Moberg flap	■ Thumb amputation distal to the interphalangeal joint, especially for volar oblique thumb tip defects. ■ Distal volar defects of the thumb, up to 1.5 cm in longitudinal diameter.	■ Extensive soft tissue defects with a lack of volar soft tissue of the thumb.
First dorsal metacarpal artery (DMCA) flap	■ Extensive volar or ulnar defect of the thumb that cannot be treated with a Moberg or digital island flap. ■ Dorsal or radial defect of the thumb with tendon or bony exposure.	■ Injury to the dorsal carpal circulation. ■ Significant loss of the dorsal skin.
Neurovascular heterodigital island flap	■ Extensive volar or ulnar defect of the thumb that cannot be treated with a Moberg or first DMCA flap. ■ Dorsal or radial defect with tendon or bony exposure that is not amendable to first DMCA flap.	■ Injury of the digital artery of the donor or adjacent fingers. ■ Patients with peripheral vascular disease, heavy smoking or vasculitis that affects the vasculature of the finger. ■ Negative Allen test of the donor finger.
Reversed dorsal ulnar or dorsal radial artery flap	■ Dorsal or radial defect of the thumb with tendon or bony exposure.	■ Extensive injury of the dorsal skin over the metacarpophalangeal joint of the thumb. ■ Severe injury that involves the volar and dorsal areas of the thumb that injure the flap pedicle.
Toe pulp transfer	■ Large volar or ulnar pulp defect that is not amenable for an innervated locoregional flap. ■ Multiple finger injuries, in which the transfer of toe pulp allows conservation of the remaining soft tissue coverage. ■ For younger patients who are nonsmokers and are free of vascular disease.	■ Patients medically unfit or unwilling to undergo microvascular surgery. ■ Patients with peripheral vascular disease.

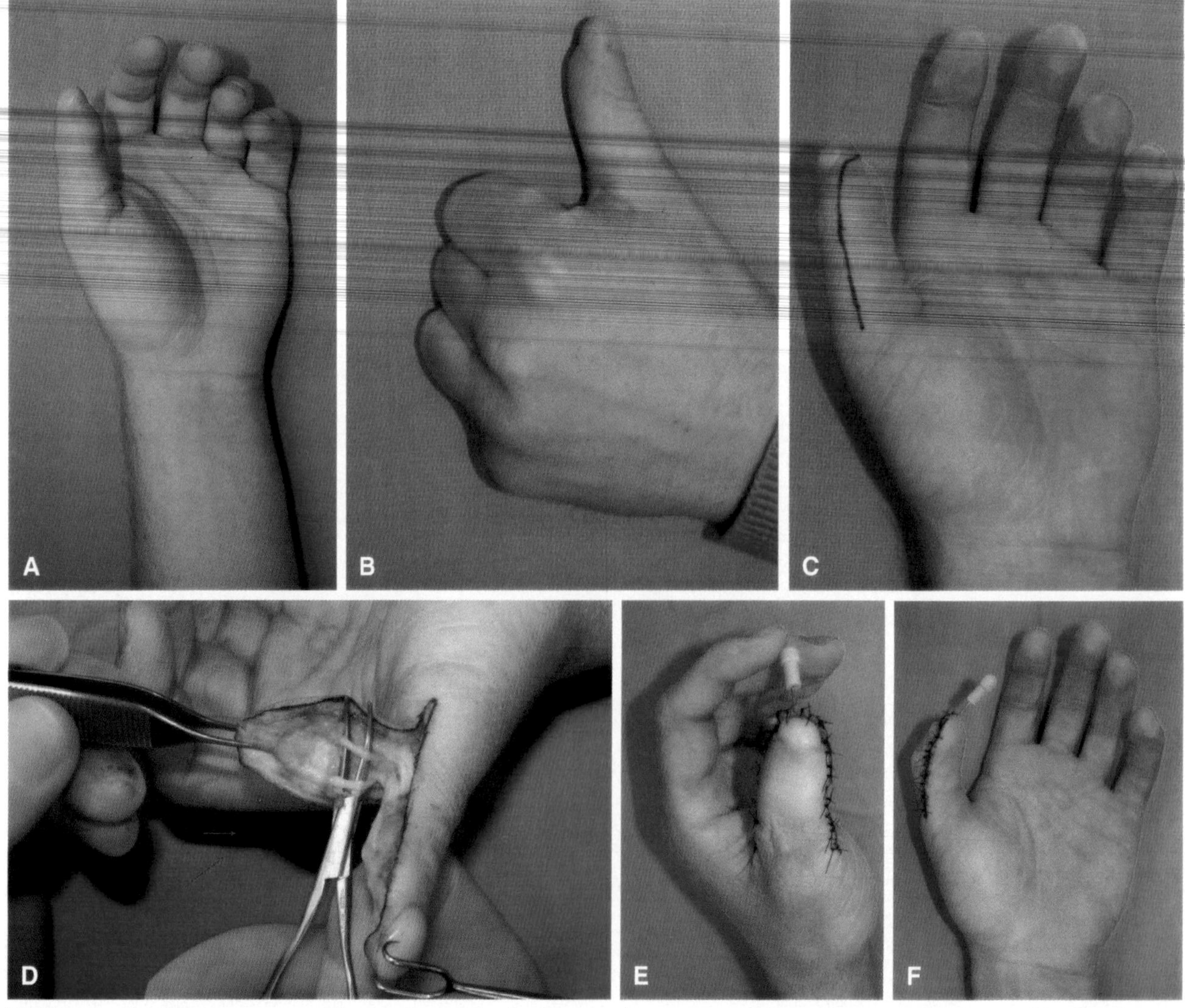

FIGURE 69.1. A volar oblique amputation of the thumb was left to heal by secondary intention. **A, B.** Patient presented with a painful scar and unaccepted thumb appearance. **C.** A Moberg flap is outlined to reconstruct the finger pulp of the thumb. **D.** The bilateral neurovascular bundles were included to provide an innervated finger pulp reconstruction. Note the bilateral proper digital nerves were included with the flap (arrow). **E, F.** A Moberg flap was inset with slight interphalangeal joint flexion of the thumb.

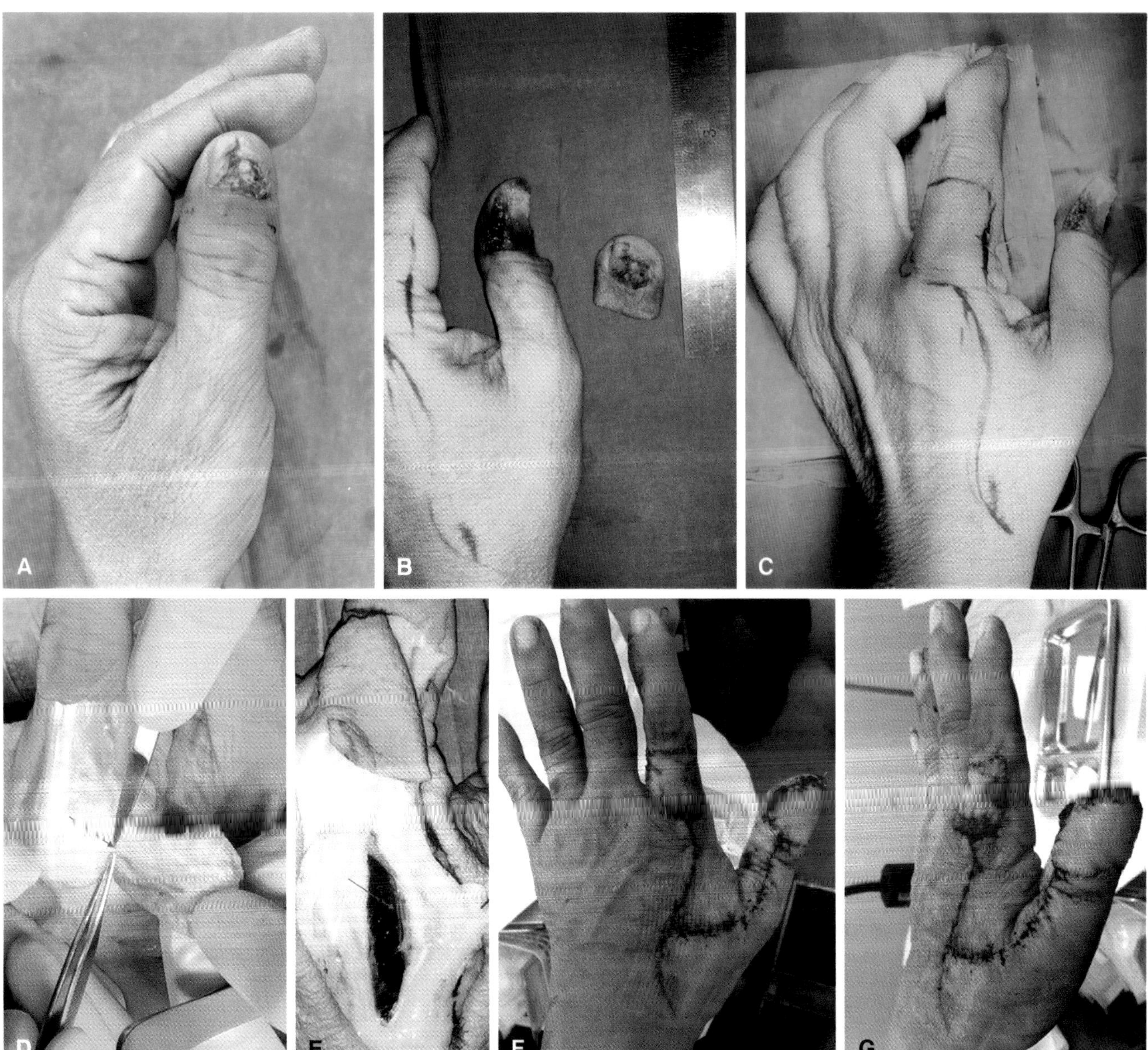

FIGURE 69.2. **A, B.** Post wide excision of the subungual melanoma at the nail bed of the left thumb with sentinel lymph node biopsy. **C.** First dorsal metacarpal artery (DMCA) flap for reconstruction of a bony exposure defect at the dorsal of the distal phalange of the thumb. **D, E.** The pedicle of the first DMCA flap is identified (arrows). Note the pedicle was in the subfascial layer of the first dorsal interosseous muscle. **F, G.** The first DMCA flap was transposed to cover the defect. The flap provided good, pliable, and color-matched skin on the dorsum of the thumb.

In the dorsal or radial areas of the thumb, sensory restoration is not essential. A versatile option for reconstructing defects in these areas is the reverse homodigital dorsal ulnar or dorsal radial flap, except in cases involving crushed or avulsion injuries of the thumb.[39,40] This flap is based either on the dorsal ulnar artery or the dorsal radial artery. The reversed dorsal ulnar artery flap provides soft tissue from the ulnar side of the thumb over the metacarpophalangeal area and first webspace. This flap should only use less than 2 cm of skin.[40] Harvesting a larger flap will use the skin of the first webspace, causing contracture of the webspace. Instead, a reversed dorsal radial artery flap provides a larger skin paddle that can measure up to 4 × 3 cm in dimension.[39]

Dorsal Hand Defect

Reconstructing a dorsal defect of the hand should aim to cover tendinous elements and exposed bone, as well as obtain thin and pliable coverage that facilitates early mobilization. Locoregional fasciocutaneous flaps can reconstruct medium-sized defects that are less than 6 to 7 cm in width. However, locoregional fasciocutaneous flaps can cover larger defects but will require a larger skin paddle from the flap, which will leave a conspicuous skin graft scar. Therefore, free fasciocutaneous flaps are used to reconstruct defects that are larger or more complex and that require more tissue incorporation such as bone, nerve, and tendon.

Medium-sized defects of the hand should be reconstructed using locoregional fasciocutaneous flaps, which include ulnar or radial forearm flaps, posterior interosseous flaps, dorsal ulnar artery flaps, and forearm perforator flaps. Indication for the use of a certain flap depends on the location of the defect (**Table 69.4**). The donor site morbidities of the ulnar or radial forearm flaps are greater than that of the perforator forearm flap, which includes tendon exposure, dysesthesia, and noticeable scarring after skin grafting. Furthermore, the harvesting of ulnar and radial forearm flaps sacrifices one of the major vessels of the hand, making posterior interosseous flaps, dorsal ulnar artery flaps, or forearm perforator flaps more preferable options.

TABLE 69.4. FLAP SELECTIONS FOR THE DORSAL AND VOLAR SURFACE OF THE HAND AND FOREARM

Flap	Indication	Contraindication
Posterior interosseous flap	■ The defect is located at the metacarpophalangeal joint, first webspace and/or the radial palm	■ Severe injury or high-energy fractures of the distal third of the forearm that will affect the competency of the posterior interosseous artery and anterior interosseous artery anastomosis.
Ulnar perforator flap	■ Defect on the dorsal or volar wrist and the dorsum of the distal hand. ■ Defect at the cubital fossa or the distal humerus.	■ Injury to the adjacent perforators that prevent an adequate arc of rotation to cover the defect.
Radial perforator flap	■ A defect of the dorsal or volar surface of the hand that is proximal to the base of the proximal phalanges of the digits ■ The volar or dorsal defect of the distal forearm	■ Significant injury to the distal forearm. ■ A defect that is distal to the metacarpophalangeal joint. ■ Microvascular microangiopathy (extra caution with smokers).
Infraumbilical abdominal-based flap	■ Mutilated hand injuries that require a large area of soft tissue coverage. ■ Complex hand defects in children less than 2 years of age. ■ Soft tissue defects after high-energy injuries or electrical injuries with damage to one of the major vessels of the hand. ■ Soft tissue reconstruction prior to microvascular free tissue transfer (e.g., coverage of digital stump defects in preparation for toe-to-hand transfers).	■ Severely contaminated wounds or active infected soft tissue that requires wound bed preparation.
Anterolateral thigh flap	■ Defects of the upper extremities that include severe hand and forearm injuries that cannot be reconstructed with a locoregional flap.	■ Previous surgeries or injuries affect the viability of the lateral circumflex femoral artery axis.
Lateral arm flap	■ A severe injury to the hand or forearm that cannot be reconstructed with a locoregional flap.	■ Previous surgeries or injuries on the lateral side of the arm such as plate osteosyntheses of the humerus, which could have destroyed the perforators.
Free thenar flap (glabrous palmar flap)	■ Small palmar defect of the hand that measures up to 2 cm × 10 cm.	■ Take caution in patients with peripheral vascular disease.
The medial plantar flap	■ Medium-sized defects on the palmar area of the hand. The flap can be harvested to a maximum of 8 cm × 6 cm of skin.	■ Patients of advanced age, heavy smokers, and peripheral arterial disease.

If a defect requires composite structural reconstruction, distant pedicle flaps or free fasciocutaneous flaps are used. Distant pedicle flaps, such as groin or abdominal-based flaps, can provide a large amount of soft tissue. However, distant pedicle flaps require more than one surgery, which delays the onset of rehabilitation. Furthermore, distant pedicle flaps are usually bulky, which requires a secondary procedure to remove some of the subcutaneous fat. However, distant pedicle flaps are preferred in mutilated hand injuries, especially in cases involving concomitant vascular injuries of the hand or soft tissue reconstruction, prior to microvascular free tissue transfers (see Table 69.4).

Free fasciocutaneous flaps are a versatile option for reconstruction because they provide thin and pliable soft tissue with composite structural reconstruction. With increasing success rates of free flap surgery, patients can initiate early participation in rehabilitation programs and gain satisfactory hand appearance and function. Free fasciocutaneous flaps include flaps from many locations, such as anterolateral thigh (ALT) flaps, lateral arm flaps, superficial circumflex iliac perforator (SCIP) flaps, and medial sural perforator flaps.[41-44] All of these flaps can be raised by a two-team approach. ALT flaps are advantageous over the other free fasciocutaneous flaps because the length of the pedicle reaches up to 16 cm.[45] ALT flaps provide a large surface area of skin that enables composite tissue reconstruction to include the nerve, tendon, or muscle within the same vascular axis.[46] Harvesting a suprafascial ALT flap will result in a thin, pliable flap. Furthermore, as an advantage to the patient, the donor site of the flap can be hidden with clothes.

Lateral arm flaps are thin and pliable with consistent blood supply and usually match in color with the dorsal side of the hand. If the flap that is harvested is less than 6 to 7 cm in width, the donor site can be closed primarily. The pedicle of the flap is dissected toward the spiral groove, which varies in length by 7 to 11 cm.[47] The lateral arm flap is a versatile flap that can provide a vascularized nerve graft of the posterior brachial cutaneous of the forearm. Furthermore, the posterior radial collateral artery extends branches to supply the lateral epicondyle of the humerus and the tricep tendon. Thus, the lateral arm flap can be used for composite reconstruction of the bone and tendons.

SCIP flaps and medial sural artery perforator flaps are not used as frequently as the other free fasciocutaneous flaps. The major disadvantage of the SCIP flap is its short pedicle length, which is around 5 cm.[48] Additionally, medial sural artery flaps have limited amount of skin, which makes the flap only suitable for small-to-medium-sized defects.[41,42]

Free or pedicle fascial flaps with skin grafting is another option for reconstructing a dorsal defect of the hand. One main advantage of fascial flaps is not having to use a skin graft to cover the donor area, which often leaves a discernible scar. Furthermore, previous literature has demonstrated that it is unusual that there will be late scar contracture over the fascial flap after skin grafting on the dorsum of the hand.[49,50]

Palmar Hand Defect

Reconstruction of palmar hand defects aims to create high resistance and durability of the reconstructed tissue, achieve optimal sensory restoration, and provide supple soft tissue for adequate range of motion. To achieve these goals, palmar skin defects should be reconstructed with glabrous skin. The locoregional glabrous skins are usually in the zone of injury. Therefore, complicated microvascular free glabrous skin transfers from the contralateral hand have been described, such as thenar flaps or instep free flaps from the foot. Free thenar flaps can be raised up to 2 cm in width and 10 cm in length. Thenar flaps can be a sensate flap by including a small cutaneous nerve originating from the palmar cutaneous branch of the median nerve.[51] Medial plantar flaps can provide glabrous skin up to 8 cm × 6 cm in dimension with minimal donor site morbidity.[52-54] These flaps can be harvested as a sensate flap by including the medial plantar nerve with the flap. However, in larger defects, there is no supple glabrous skin flap that can provide adequate soft tissue for reconstruction, so nonglabrous skin flaps are used instead.

Posterior interosseous artery (PIA) flaps are considered as the work-horse flap for reconstruction of defects on the dorsum and volar area of the first webspace and the radial palm. PIA flaps provide reliable and pliable soft tissue that facilitates thumb mobility (Figure 69.3). In contrast with the dorsum of the hand, it is not necessary to use a very thin flap. However, for easier tendon gliding, fasciocutaneous flaps are preferred. Furthermore, using fascial flaps and skin grafts are not suitable in the palmar area because scar contracture is likely to occur.

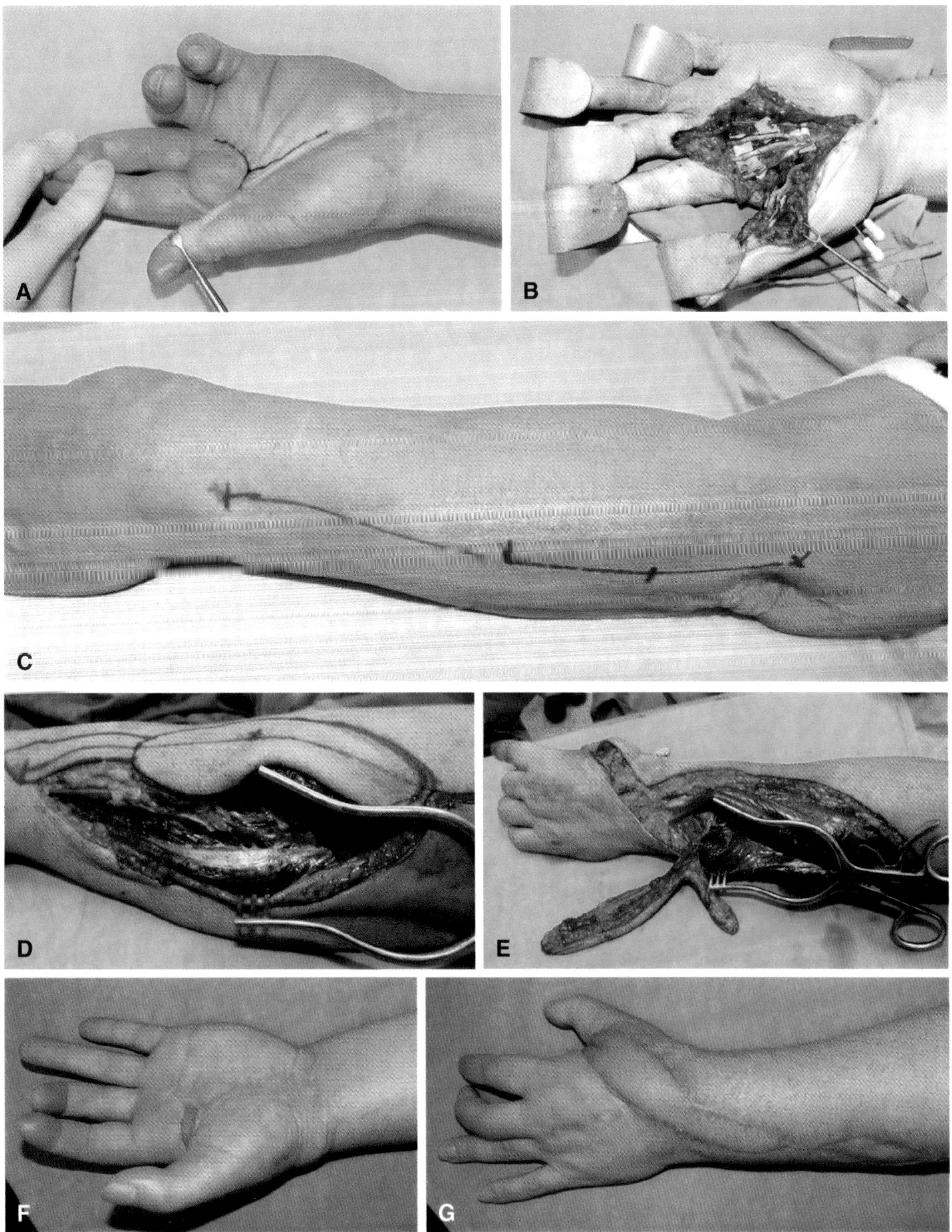

FIGURE 69.3. **A.** Contracted scar at the first webspace on the left hand. **B.** The scar was released and the digital nerve reconstruction was performed. **C.** A reversed posterior interosseous flap was outlined. The axis of the flap was designed by the line from the lateral epicondyle of the humerus and the distal ulnar head in full pronation of the forearm. **D.** The perforators of the posterior interosseous artery were identified in the intermuscular septum between the extensor carpi ulnaris and extensor digiti minimi. **E.** The pivot point was located 3 cm proximal to the distal radioulnar joint. **F, G.** A reversed posterior interosseous flap was inset into the first webspace, which provided stable soft tissue for a mobile thumb. (From Yang G, Chung KC. Pedicled forearm flap. In: Chung KC, ed. *Operative Techniques: Hand and Wrist Surgery*. 3rd ed. Philadelphia, PA: Elsevier; 2018:695-702.)

MANAGEMENT OF NAIL BED INJURY

The nail is a specialized structure that enhances the sensory perception of the pulp of the finger and facilitates precise movements such as grasping small objects. Furthermore, the nail is one of the most imperative, aesthetic features of the hand. Thus, the lost or deformation of the nail can affect both the appearance and function of the hand.

Anatomy of the Fingernail

- Nail plate
- Paronychium—soft tissue fold on the lateral side of the nail plate
- Eponychium—soft tissue that is dorsal to the nail plate that is a continuation of the dorsal skin of the finger. Eponychium creates the matte sheen on the surface of the nail plate
- Hyponychium—keratinous mass that serves as a distal attachment of the nail with the pulp skin.
- Nail bed—lies under the nail plate
    - Lanula—white arc line distal to the eponychium
    - Germinal matrix—nail bed proximal to the lanula, which plays an important role in nail growth.
    - Sterile matrix—nail bed distal to the lanula

Subungual Hematoma

The traumatic conditions that affect the nail bed and cause bleeding under the nail plate are described as subungual hematomas. Subungual hematomas are caused commonly by closed injuries, such as crushing injuries. If the patient is asymptomatic or the hematoma affects less than half of the nail bed, the patient can be treated conservatively, including warm compression and the administration of analgesics. However, if the hematoma affects more than half of the nail bed, it is likely that the nail bed is lacerated and requires repair.[55] In children, if the nail and perionychium are intact, there is no need for an exploration and removal of the nail plate. There are many methods of treatment, such as nail bed exploration and repair, drainage, or conservative treatment. However, the patient's outcome is similar regardless of method.[56,57]

Furthermore, an X-ray will show if there is fracture of the distal phalanx associated with the subungual hematoma. If there is fracture of the distal phalanx, the nail plate should be removed for a more thorough examination of the nail bed and any nail bed laceration can be repaired.

Nail bed Laceration

If the nail plate is not severely disfigured, it can be soaked in betadine solution and reinserted to the nail fold as a stent after initial treatment. Reinserting the nail plate will prevent synechiae of the nail fold to the injured nail bed that will affect the configuration and shining of the nail. If the nail plate is avulsed or partially detached from the nail bed, the nail plate can be removed to permit a thorough examination of the nail bed under anesthesia and tourniquet.

Under magnification, the nail bed is examined carefully. If there seems to be a germinal matrix injury, bilateral incisions on the eponychium are made and the nail fold is elevated to explore the germinal matrix. The nail bed needs to be repaired with 6-0 or 7-0 absorbable monofilament sutures. If there are stellate lacerations to the nail bed, conservative debridement is required to preserve the small pieces of the nail bed as much as possible, followed by a meticulous repair.

Nail bed Avulsion

Nail bed avulsions can result in the detachment of the nail bed from the distal phalangeal periosteum. If the nail bed can be recovered, then it can be sutured with the fine absorbable monofilament suture. However, if the nail bed is partially avulsed from the distal phalanx and it leaves the small defect on the nail bed, the remaining nail bed can be undermined from the periosteum and advanced to close the defect. With severe nail bed avulsion that precludes primary nail bed advancement and repair, a nail bed graft can be harvested from the big toe for reconstruction. After the repair, a nail plate or silicone sheath can be inserted in the nail fold to act as a splint. The nail plate needs to be secured on the hyponychium and paronychium with 5-0 nylon suture, which can be removed 3 to 7 days after surgery.

ACKNOWLEDGMENTS

The work was supported by a Midcareer Investigator Award in Patient-Oriented Research (2 K24-AR053120-06) to Kevin C. Chung. The content is solely the responsibility of the authors and does not necessarily represent the official views of the National Institutes of Health.

REFERENCES

1. del Pinal F. Severe mutilating injuries to the hand: guidelines for organizing the chaos. *J Plast Reconstr Aesthet Surg*. 2007;60(7):816-827.
2. Moran SL, Berger RA. Biomechanics and hand trauma: what you need. *Hand Clin*. 2003;19(1):17-31.
   The authors explain the biomechanics of any anatomical structures of the hand. The effect of each structural loss or disorganization will affect individual function deficit. Any hand injuries are closely scrutinized and determined the reconstructive goals.
3. Rehim SA, Kowalski E, Chung KC. Enhancing aesthetic outcomes of soft-tissue coverage of the hand. *Plast Reconstr Surg*. 2015;135(2):413e-428e.
4. Gottlieb LJ, Krieger LM. From the reconstructive ladder to the reconstructive elevator. *Plast Reconstr Surg*. 1994;93(7):1503-1504.
   The authors of this article initiated the modern concept of the reconstruction. The mode of reconstruction could be acceptable to jump several rungs of the ladder, with the knowledge that some defects require more complex solutions to achieve the functions and appearances.
5. Miller EA, Friedrich J. Soft tissue coverage of the hand and upper extremity: the reconstructive elevator. *J Hand Surg*. 2016;41(7):782-792.
6. Biswas D, Wysocki RW, Fernandez JJ, Cohen MS. Local and regional flaps for hand coverage. *J Hand Surg*. 2014;39(5):992-1004.
7. Rehim SA, Chung KC. Local flaps of the hand. *Hand Clin*. 2014;30(2):137-151, v.
8. Goertz O, Kapalschinski N, Daigeler A, et al. The effectiveness of pedicled groin flaps in the treatment of hand defects: results of 49 patients. *J Hand Surg*. 2012;37(10):2088-2094.
9. Mih AD. Pedicle flaps for coverage of the wrist and hand. *Hand Clin*. 1997;13(2):217-229.
10. Al-Qattan MM, Al-Qattan AM. Defining the indications of pedicled groin and abdominal flaps in hand reconstruction in the current microsurgery era. *J Hand Surg*. 2016;41(9):917-927.
11. Sabapathy SR, Venkatramani H, Bhardwaj P. Reconstruction of the thumb amputation at the carpometacarpal joint level by groin flap and second toe transfer. *Injury*. 2013;44(3):370-375.
12. Wei FC, Seah CS, Chen HC, Chuang CC. Functional and esthetic reconstruction of a mutilated hand using multiple toe transfers and iliac osteocutaneous flap: a case report. *Microsurgery*. 1993;14(6):388-390.
13. Tiwari VK, Sarabahi S, Chauhan S. Preputial flap as an adjunct to groin flap for the coverage of electrical burns in the hand. *Burns*. 2014;40(1):e4-e7.
14. Khandelwal S. An abdominal flap to save the right forearm and the hand, following a high-voltage electric burn in a child: a case report. *J Clin Diagn Res*. 2013;7(7):1473-1475.
15. Janis JE, Kwon RK, Attinger CE. The new reconstructive ladder: modifications to the traditional model. *Plast Reconstr Surg*. 2011;127(suppl 1):205s-212s.
16. Moiemen NS, Vlachou E, Staiano JJ, et al. Reconstructive surgery with Integra dermal regeneration template: histologic study, clinical evaluation, and current practice. *Plast Reconstr Surg*. 2006;117(7 suppl):160s-174s.
17. Iorio ML, Shuck J, Attinger CE. Wound healing in the upper and lower extremities: a systematic review on the use of acellular dermal matrices. *Plast Reconstr Surg*. 2012;130(5 suppl 2):232s-241s.
18. Rehim SA, Singhal M, Chung KC. Dermal skin substitutes for upper limb reconstruction: current status, indications, and contraindications. *Hand Clin*. 2014;30(2):239-252, vii.
19. Dantzer E, Queruel P, Salinier L, et al. Dermal regeneration template for deep hand burns: clinical utility for both early grafting and reconstructive surgery. *Br J Plast Surg*. 2003;56(8):764-774.
20. Cuadra A, Correa G, Roa R, et al. Functional results of burned hands treated with integra. *J Plast Reconstr Aesthet Surg*. 2012;65(2):228-234.
21. Nguyen DQ, Potokar TS, Price P. An objective long-term evaluation of Integra (a dermal skin substitute) and split thickness skin grafts, in acute burns and reconstructive surgery. *Burns*. 2010;36(1):23-28.
22. Rizzo M. The use of Integra in hand and upper extremity surgery. *J Hand Surg*. 2012;37(3):583-586.

23. Soderberg T, Nystrom A, Hallmans G, Hulten J. Treatment of fingertip amputations with bone exposure: a comparative study between surgical and conservative treatment methods. *Scand J Plast Reconstr Surg.* 1983;17(2):147-152.
24. Mennen U, Wiese A. Fingertip injuries management with semi-occlusive dressing. *J Hand Surg (Edinburgh, Scotland).* 1993;18(4):416-422.
25. Lamon RP, Cicero JJ, Frascone RJ, Hass WF. Open treatment of fingertip amputations. *Ann Emerg Med.* 1983;12(6):358-360.
26. Weichman KE, Wilson SC, Samra F, et al. Treatment and outcomes of fingertip injuries at a large metropolitan public hospital. *Plast Reconstr Surg.* 2013;131(1):107-112.
27. Tupper J, Miller G. Sensitivity following volar V-Y plasty for fingertip amputations. *J Hand Surg (Edinburg, Scotland).* 1985;10(2):183-184.
28. Krishnan KG. Sensory recovery after reconstruction of defects of long fingertips using the pedicled V flap. *Br J Plast Surg.* 2001;54(6):523-527.
29. Foucher G, Dallaserra M, Tilquin B, et al. The Hueston flap in reconstruction of fingertip skin loss: results in a series of 41 patients. *J Hand Surg.* 1994;19(3):508-515.
30. Deglise B, Botta Y. Microsurgical free toe pulp transfer for digital reconstruction. *Ann Plast Surg.* 1991;26(4):341-346.
31. Trankle M, Sauerbier M, Heitmann C, Germann G. Restoration of thumb sensibility with the innervated first dorsal metacarpal artery island flap. *J Hand Surg.* 2003;28(5):758-766.
32. Oka Y. Sensory function of the neurovascular island flap in thumb reconstruction: comparison of original and modified procedures. *J Hand Surg.* 2000;25(4):637-643.
33. Krag C, Rasmussen KB. The neurovascular island flap for defective sensibility of the thumb. *J Bone Jt Surg Br.* 1975;57B:495-499.
34. Liu H, Regmi S, He Y, Hou R. Thumb tip defect reconstruction using neurovascular island pedicle flap obtained from long finger. *Aesthet Plast Surg.* 2016;40(5):755-760.
35. Buncke HJ, Rose EH. Free toe-to-fingertip neurovascular flaps. *Plast Reconstr Surg.* 1979;63(5):607-612.
This study demonstrated the results of the reconstruction of pulp defects with a pulp flap from the big toe (hemipulp) and second toe in six patients. The authors emphasized the fundamental of reconstruction, replacing like with like, functional, and sensory restoration.
36. Lin CH, Lin YT, Sassu P, et al. Functional assessment of the reconstructed fingertips after free toe pulp transfer. *Plast Reconstr Surg.* 2007;120(5):1315-1321.
This study was to comprehensively assess the functional outcome of the reconstructed fingertips after free toe pulp transfer. Free toe pulp transfer was the optimal reconstructive option because it could restore the function, sensibility, and durability of the injured fingers.
37. Huang SH, Wu SH, Lai CH, et al. Free medial plantar artery perforator flap for finger pulp reconstruction: report of a series of 10 cases. *Microsurgery.* 2010;30(2):118-124.
38. Koshima I, Urushibara K, Inagawa K, et al. Free medial plantar perforator flaps for the resurfacing of finger and foot defects. *Plast Reconstr Surg.* 2001;107(7):1753-1758.
39. Moschella F, Cordova A. Reverse homodigital dorsal radial flap of the thumb. *Plast Reconstr Surg.* 2006;117(3):920-926.
40. Teran P, Carnero S, Miranda R, et al. Refinements in dorsoulnar flap of the thumb: 15 cases. *J Hand Surg.* 2010;35(8):1356-1359.
41. Lin CH, Lin CH, Lin YT, et al. The medial sural artery perforator flap: a versatile donor site for hand reconstruction. *J Trauma.* 2011;70(3):736-743.
42. Zheng H, Liu J, Dai X, Schilling AF. Free conjoined or chimeric medial sural artery perforator flap for the reconstruction of multiple defects in hand. *J Plast Reconstr Aesthet Surg.* 2015;68(4):565-570.
43. Kuo YR, Jeng SF, Kuo MH, et al. Free anterolateral thigh flap for extremity reconstruction: clinical experience and functional assessment of donor site. *Plast Reconstr Surg.* 2001;107(7):1766-1771.
44. Narushima M, Iida T, Kaji N, et al. Superficial circumflex iliac artery pure skin perforator-based superthin flap for hand and finger reconstruction. *J Plast Reconstr Aesthet Surg.* 2016;69(6):827-834.
45. Lakhiani C, Lee MR, Saint-Cyr M. Vascular anatomy of the anterolateral thigh flap: a systematic review. *Plast Reconstr Surg.* 2012;130(6):1254-1268.
46. Wei FC, Jain V, Celik N, et al. Have we found an ideal soft-tissue flap? An experience with 672 anterolateral thigh flaps. *Plast Reconstr Surg.* 2002;109(7):2219-2226.
This study reviewed the 660 consecutive patients who underwent ALT flap reconstructions. The authors demonstrated the versatility of the ALT flap to reconstruction of various defects and with minimal donor site morbidities.
47. Saint-Cyr M, Wong C, Schaverien M, et al. The perforasome theory: vascular anatomy and clinical implications. *Plast Reconstr Surg.* 2009;124(5):1529-1544.
This vascular anatomic study of the 217 flaps in 40 fresh cadavers demonstrated the direct and indirect linking vessel between the perforator vessels. Implication of the perforasome theory would facilitate the surgeon understand and precisely design the perforator flaps.
48. Goh TL, Park SW, Cho JY, et al. The search for the ideal thin skin flap: superficial circumflex iliac artery perforator flap—a review of 210 cases. *Plast Reconstr Surg.* 2015;135(2):592-601.
49. Carty MJ, Taghinia A, Upton J. Fascial flap reconstruction of the hand: a single surgeon's 30-year experience. *Plast Reconstr Surg.* 2010;125(3):953-962.
50. Taghinia AH, Carty M, Upton J. Fascial flaps for hand reconstruction. *J Hand Surg.* 2010;35(8):1351-1355.
51. Orbay JL, Rosen JG, Khouri RK, Indriago I. The glabrous palmar flap: the new free or reversed pedicled palmar fasciocutaneous flap for volar hand reconstruction. *Techn Hand Upper Extrem Surg.* 2009;13(3):145-150.
52. Zelken JA, Lin CH. An algorithm for forefoot reconstruction with the innervated free medial plantar flap. *Ann Plast Surg.* 2016;76(2):221-226.
53. Acikel C, Celikoz B, Yuksel F, Ergun O. Various applications of the medial plantar flap to cover the defects of the plantar foot, posterior heel, and ankle. *Ann Plast Surg.* 2003;50(5):498-503.
54. Sen SK, Fitzgerald O'Connor E, Tare M. The free instep flap for palmar and digital resurfacing. *J Plast Reconstr Aesthet Surg.* 2015;68(9):1191-1198.
55. Simon RR, Wolgin M. Subungual hematoma: association with occult laceration requiring repair. *Am J Emerg Med.* 1987;5(4):302-304.
56. Roser SE, Gellman H. Comparison of nail bed repair versus nail trephination for subungual hematomas in children. *J Hand Surg.* 1999;24(6):1166-1170.
57. Gellman H. Fingertip-nail bed injuries in children: current concepts and controversies of treatment. *J Craniofac Surg.* 2009;20(4):1033-1035.

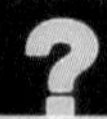

QUESTIONS

1. **According to the volar V-Y flap approach, which one is correct?**
   a. To facilitate flap mobilization, the flap is undermined in the subcutaneous plane until it reaches the distal interphalangeal joint (DIP) joint.
   b. The blood supply perforates the volar digital artery, which lies on both sides of the flap
   c. A volar oblique defect is an ideal injury to use this flap.
   d. To accommodate a large defect of the fingertip, the apex of the triangular flap should extend through the DIP joint crease.
   e. Flap should be inset by loose suturing to the edge of defect, especially to the nail bed, to prevent hook nail deformity.

2. **A patient with a 5 × 12 cm avulsion wound on the dorsum of the forearm with extensor tendon exposure. Wound exploration revealed avulsion of the superficial radial nerve with a 7 cm nerve gap. The surgeon plans to cover the defect with lateral arm free flap with vascularized nerve grafting. Which nerve can be included with the flap to provide a vascularized nerve graft?**
   a. Lateral cutaneous nerve of arm
   b. Lateral cutaneous nerve of forearm
   c. Medial antebrachial cutaneous nerve
   d. Superior lateral brachial cutaneous nerve
   e. Posterior antebrachial cutaneous nerve

3. **A 30-year-old man suffered a crushing injury to his right hand and forearm. The X-rays revealed a comminuted fracture of distal radius and ulna. His thumb was avulsed. What should be the initial method of reconstruction for the avulsion injury of the thumb as shown in Figure 69.4?**
   a. Posterior interosseous flap
   b. Infraumbilical abdominal-based flap
   c. Reversed radial forearm flap
   d. First DMCA flap
   e. Toe-to-hand transfer

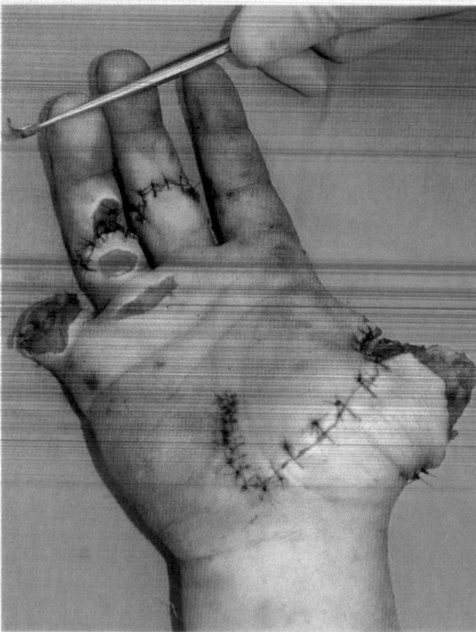
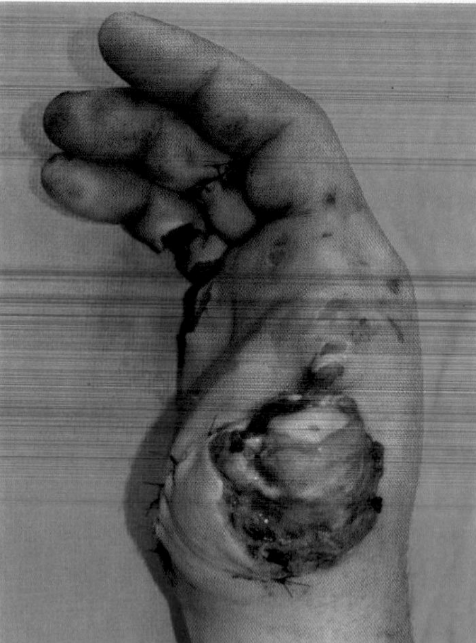

FIGURE 69.4. A crushing injury to the right hand, which underwent wound suturing and revision amputation of the thumb and little finger.

4. **A 40-year-old male had an electrical injury to his right hand. He lost his little finger and the dorsal skin of his middle and ring finger. The injury left the extensor tendon of his middle finger exposed, as well as the bare phalangeal bone (Figure 69.5). A segment of the extensor tendon of the ring finger was also lost. What is the most appropriate choice for reconstructing this defect?**
   a. Radial forearm flap
   b. First DMCA flap
   c. Posterior interosseous flap
   d. Pedicle groin flap
   e. ALT free flap

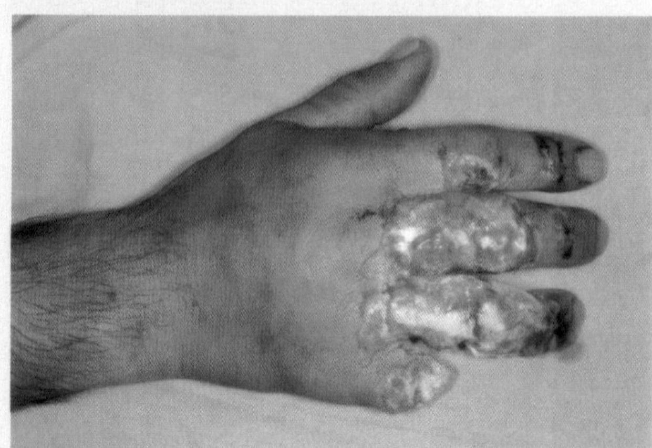

FIGURE 69.5. The postdebridement wounds of an electrical injury to the right hand. After debridement, there was a segmental loss of the extensor tendon of the ring finger and bare phalangeal bone exposure of the middle, ring, and little finger.

5. A 20-year-old man was involved in a motor vehicle crash. He lost the digital pulp of his left thumb, as shown in Figure 69.6. Which flap will provide the best function and sensation for this patient?

a. Visor flap
b. Littler flap
c. Thenar flap
d. Moberg flap
e. Cross-finger flap

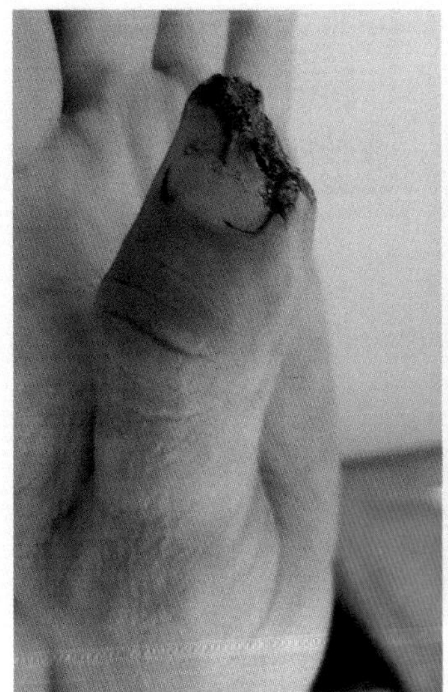
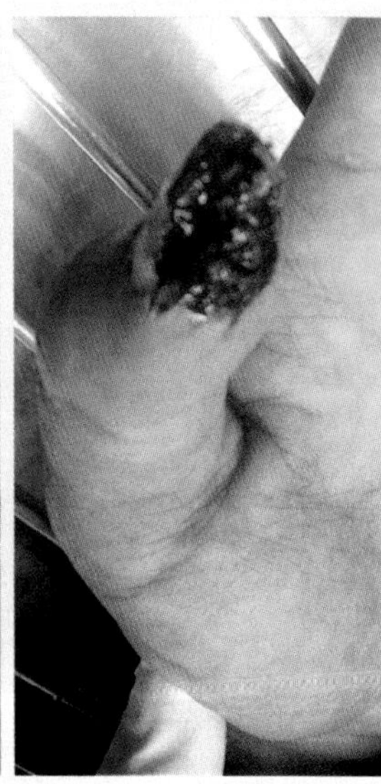

FIGURE 69.6. A 1.5 cm wide traumatic volar oblique soft tissue defect of the thumb tip.

1. **Answer: e.** A volar V-Y advancement flap is best suited for dorsal oblique or transverse fingertip injuries or transverse amputations with a sufficient amount of remaining tissue. The vascular supplies of the flap come from the terminal branches of the digital arteries emerging from the digital transverse arch in the subcutaneous plane. Flap outlines should not extend through the DIP because it will lead to further flexion contracture. To facilitate flap mobilization, the dorsal dissection proceeds proximally on the periosteum until the flexor tendon attachment is seen. Flap should be approximated loosely with the defect, especially to the nail bed to prevent hook nail.

2. **Answer: b.** The posterior cutaneous nerve of the forearm (PCNF) also travels alongside the posterior cutaneous of the arm, within the lateral intermuscular septum. The PCNF runs through the intermuscular septum without any innervation to the skin, but ends with innervation to the posterior forearm skin. The PRCA extends vascular branches to nourish the PCNF. The PCNF can be harvested as a vascularized nerve graft with a lateral arm flap for reconstruction of any nerve defects.

3. **Answer: b.** Reconstructing the thumb is the ultimate goal of reconstruction with avulsion injuries of the thumb. Toe-to-hand transfer will be performed eventually, but preparing the soft tissue to accommodate the neothumb is mandatory. According to the mechanism of the injury, a locoregional flap is located within the zone of the injury. Therefore, a distant pedicle flap is the most appropriate for this patient's case.

4. **Answer: e.** The defect is located distal to the proximal interphalangeal joint and the surface area of the defect is quite large. The defect also needs multiple skin paddles to cover each finger individually. Therefore, the appropriate flap should be large with multiple perforators, which can be divided according to the location of the perforators. The ring finger requires an extensor tendon reconstruction as well. Therefore, an anterior lateral thigh flap can provide a single stage surgery to simultaneously cover the defect while reconstructing the tendon. A locoregional flap cannot provide adequate soft tissue to reconstruct this defect. The pedicle groin flap will need a stage surgery that precludes early rehabilitation.

5. **Answer: d.** A Moberg flap and Littler flap can both provide a sensate, soft tissue reconstruction of the defect. However, the Littler flap requires the patient to retrain the brain to register the sensation in the new area. Therefore, the Moberg flap is a better option. The other flaps cannot provide a sensate flap reconstruction.

CHAPTER 70 Management of Compression Neuropathies of the Upper Extremity

Management of Compression Neuropathies of the Upper Extremity

Loree K. Kalliainen and William B. Ericson, Jr

KEY POINTS

- Peripheral nerve compression occurs at more locations than are classically taught. Symptoms may be vague, and compression can present as motor weakness, deep aching or radiating pain, or numbness, with symptoms where the nerve ends rather than where it is compressed. Detailed knowledge of anatomy is crucial to differentiating potential sites of compression.
- Diagnosis of peripheral nerve compression may often be achieved with history and physical exam alone and without the use of electrodiagnostic or radiologic imaging techniques, including radiographs, MRI, CT scan, and ultrasound.
- Recovery after decompression depends on preoperative duration, severity, and secondary comorbidities such as diabetes, hypertension, hypothyroidism, age, and location(s) of compression.
- There is no single decompression technique at the cubital tunnel that has been shown to be superior.
- Recovery of index and thumb flexion strength is generally rapid following release of the median nerve at the pronator.
- Ulnar nerve compression at the wrist is more likely associated with soft tissue masses, vascular anomalies, and anatomic variations than compression at the elbow.
- Carpal tunnel syndrome is the most commonly recognized peripheral neuropathy of the upper extremity and can be safely and effectively treated surgically under local, regional, or general anesthesia.
- Postoperative splinting is generally unnecessary after nerve decompression.

NERVE DYSFUNCTION RELATED TO CHRONIC NERVE COMPRESSION

Chronic nerve compression causes dysfunction through several mechanisms.[1,2] Enveloping connective tissues become thickened and fibrotic, limiting nerve glide and impairing vascular supply. Edema accumulates in the endoneurium, and because there are no lymphatic channels within it to aid in drainage, microvascular flow is further obstructed.[3] External pressure causes demyelination and axonal degeneration.

Initial symptoms of nerve compression are paresthesia and deep aches. Progression of compression with subsequent loss of axons is associated with a consistent loss of sensation, weakness, and eventually muscle atrophy.[4] If the nerve is decompressed, demyelination can be reversed, and function can improve. Recovery depends upon duration and degree of compression and damage, secondary factors such as hypertension, diabetes, and hypothyroidism, and the presence of multiple sites of compression (the "double crush phenomenon").

DIAGNOSIS

Pathologic compression of a peripheral nerve typically affects a named nerve with paired motor and sensory components, and the combined evaluation of both is critical to determining the source and site(s) of compression. Mild compression of motor nerves causes muscle weakness, and severe, prolonged compression causes atrophy. Compression of sensory nerves causes paresthesias (if the nerve innervates skin) or pain where the nerve ends (e.g., sensory nerve to a joint). The location and timing of symptoms, their severity, and progression are clues as the location and etiology of the nerve compression. Successful treatment requires extensive knowledge of nerve anatomy and physiology, as well as an appreciation for the influence of anatomic and physiologic comorbidities and anatomic variations.

History

Symptoms are defined by location, character, and timing of sensory disturbance, weakness, and/or pain. Numbness as a clinical complaint is clearly related to nerve dysfunction and is often the presenting complaint; it is usually the starting point to establish a differential diagnosis. Paresthesia is painful and clearly nerve-related. Word choice is important, as doctors often use "numbness" and "tingling" interchangeably when examining patients, whereas patients with paresthesia may deny having numbness. Weakness can be caused by compression of motor nerves but can also represent inhibition related to painful processes such as arthritis. Interpreting patient's complaints of pain can be an arduous process. Referred pain, which is pain perceived at a site distant from its origin, is well understood in other compressive neuropathies, such as cervical spondylosis with radiculopathy, but underappreciated in the upper extremity. The examiner must understand not just motor nerve and cutaneous nerve anatomy, but also joint innervation anatomy.

Physical Exam

Accurate testing of motor strength is significantly more complicated than one would assume. The tension of a muscle-tendon unit is created by (1) stretch of the muscle-tendon unit and (2) active contraction of the muscle. To assess muscle weakness related to motor nerve dysfunction, one must test the muscle in a position that eliminates the contribution of tension from stretch. The muscle should be at its "resting length," on the Blix curve, where the sarcomeres are in equilibrium rather than the "position of rest" where the resting tension of the flexors is balanced by the resting tension of the extensors.[5] This principle is used in tendon transfers, where the wrist is placed in extension to gain finger flexion power. If the finger flexors are weak from any cause, actively extending the wrist will increase their tension and apparent strength, potentially masking early weakness related to nerve compression.

Sensory loss is measured subjectively or quantitatively. Semmes-Weinstein monofilaments are used for sensory perception threshold; static and moving two-point discrimination values can be applied to assess nerve continuity and density. Provocative maneuvers such as Tinel, Phalen, manual compression, and scratch-collapse tests can be helpful in supporting a diagnosis if positive.[6] Abnormal deep tendon reflexes are signs of nerve root or spinal cord compression.

Adjunctive Studies

Electrodiagnostic studies remain the primary objective test to assess peripheral nerve dysfunction. Nerve conduction studies quantitate nerve signal velocity, latency, and amplitude and assess myelination. Computer-aided somatosensory measurement devices have higher sensitivity and specificity in quantitating sensory nerve dysfunction but are not in common use. Electromyography assesses muscle innervation integrity via the presence of fibrillations, denervation potentials, and insertional activity. The roles of ultrasound, MRI, and MR neurograms in evaluation of peripheral nerve compression are controversial and are areas of active research.[7,8] Radiographs are frequently used to evaluate complaints of pain in the extremities, and MRIs can show painful conditions that are not apparent on plain radiographs, such as ligament or cartilage tears, and ganglion cysts and other soft tissue processes. Caution is urged when interpreting any diagnostic test: false positives and false negatives exist, and patients can have grossly abnormal tests with no symptoms and significant symptoms with completely normal tests.

Patients who present with abnormalities of multiple peripheral nerves should be evaluated for medical causes of peripheral neuropathy: diabetes, vitamin deficiency, liver disease, and autoimmune disease. Hereditary neuropathy with liability to pressure palsies, related to PMP-22 gene deletion, is an example of a demyelinating polyneuropathy.[9] Acute causes of pain and numbness may rarely be related to other unexpected processes, such as embolic events originating from the heart or aneurysms of the ulnar artery. In those instances, vascular studies such as Doppler, MR angiograms, or CT angiograms may be indicated.[10]

SURGICAL PRINCIPLES

The technique of peripheral nerve decompression is similar at all sites. Patients may often continue taking anticoagulants because expected blood loss is minimal.[11] This shared decision should be made between surgeon, patient, internist, and anesthesiologist. Local anesthesia containing epinephrine is safe and can minimize cutaneous blood loss, optimize visualization, and prolong the duration of anesthesia.[12] The use of a tourniquet is not necessary for the majority of patients, especially if the procedure is being performed under local anesthesia. Hemostasis with bipolar cautery creates less local tissue damage than monopolar cautery, and its use should be considered when operating near nerves.[13] Vascular supply to the nerve should be protected when possible, especially in patients who may already have damage to intrinsic microvasculature. The use of a minimal touch technique, with avoidance of traction, will minimize scar development. Fascial bands around the nerve are exposed and divided. Little evidence exists on operative timing for the less common forms of nerve compression. It is reasonable to use the same guideline used for carpal tunnel syndrome (CTS): persistence of symptoms for 9 to 12 months is a reasonable indication for surgical intervention unless there is rapid deterioration, a diagnosis of tumor, or penetrating trauma.

Routine postoperative splinting is not indicated, and gentle range of motion can be initiated within 1 to 3 days after surgery. Postoperative pain is managed by setting appropriate expectations preoperatively and using rest, ice, elevation, nonsteroidal anti-inflammatory drugs (NSAIDs), and acetaminophen postoperatively (as tolerated by the patient). The prolonged use of opioids should be minimized: up to 10 tablets is acceptable for most operations.[14] For patients on chronic opioids, consultation with their pain physician and the anesthesiologist is recommended to create a plan for multimodal pain management. Intraoperative ketamine is increasingly being used as an adjunct.[15]

Operative risks of nerve decompression include incomplete release, damage to the nerve or surrounding structures, hematoma, infection, devascularization of the nerve, excessive scarring, incomplete recovery, worsened pain, and chronic regional pain syndrome. Risks related to general or sedation anesthesia can be decreased by the use of local anesthesia alone.[16]

MEDIAN NERVE COMPRESSION

Carpal Tunnel Syndrome

Anatomy

CTS is the most commonly recognized compressive neuropathy in the upper extremity, with an incidence of approximately 2.3 cases per 100 person-years.[17] The carpus forms a U-shaped canal, connected anteriorly by the transverse carpal ligament (TCL). The median nerve is protected by the TCL but is subjected to compression by any process that increases the pressure within the tunnel. The tunnel contains nine tendons and the median nerve. The sensory part of the median nerve innervates the volar surfaces of the thumb, index finger, long finger, and the radial half of the ring finger, but not the thenar eminence. The recurrent motor branch of the median nerve innervates the thenar muscles and can be subligamentous, intraligamentous, or extraligamentous.

Etiology

Most cases of CTS are presumed to be idiopathic in origin. CTS is much more common in women than men. Other risk factors include metabolic (obesity, diabetes, pregnancy, hypothyroidism, renal failure, amyloidosis, autoimmune disease), infectious (leprosy), mechanical (trauma, large lumbrical muscles, fibrosis of the tenosynovium), or a combination of factors.[18]

Diagnosis

The diagnosis of CTS is made predominantly by history and physical examination, with adjunctive diagnostic tests when clinically indicated.[18] Early symptoms of CTS include aching pain in the carpal tunnel area, and numbness and/or tingling in the tips of the radial digits, particularly at night or on waking. Numbness on the dorsal hand is inconsistent with the diagnosis. Thenar muscles are examined for strength and bulk (Figure 70.1). Atrophy is a late finding but can also be the result of disuse from thumb carpometacarpal joint arthritis, a common condition in aging women. Provocative maneuvers such as the Phalen test, Tinel sign, Durkan test, and scratch-collapse test are all helpful to some degree to confirm the location of nerve compression. There is no single clinical finding that defines CTS: it involves a constellation of signs and symptoms present over time. Electrodiagnostic studies can be helpful when there is ambiguity or liability involved but they do not add significantly to the decision to operate.[19] Radiographs of the wrist are indicated for evaluation of wrist pain.

For a relatively straightforward anatomic situation, CTS generates considerable controversy regarding diagnostic criteria, the role of diagnostic testing, causality, and treatment. Whether or not CTS is "work-related" remains debatable,[20] but clearly it is much easier to treat strictly as a medical condition rather than a plight of employment.

Nonoperative Treatment

Wrist splints decrease tendon excursion and hold the wrist in a position of decreased tunnel pressure. Hand exercise (tendon excursion under load) tends to aggravate CTS, whereas stretching exercises seem to reduce swelling, and thus pain. Antiinflammatory medications can decrease pain and tenosynovial swelling within the carpal tunnel. Steroid injections can be considered a therapeutic test—if the

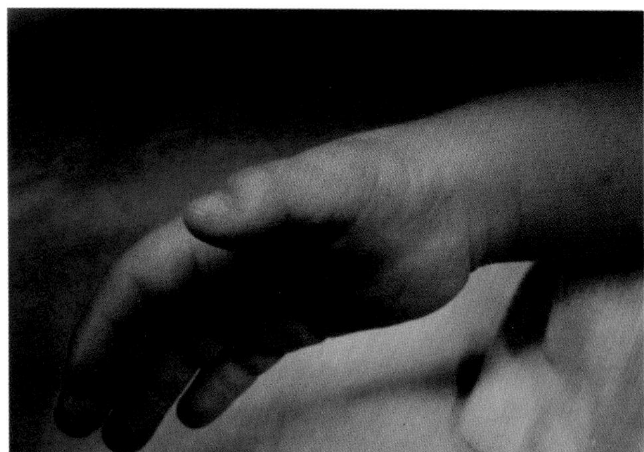

FIGURE 70.1. An 8-year-old patient with dense sensory deficit in median distribution and severe thenar atrophy.

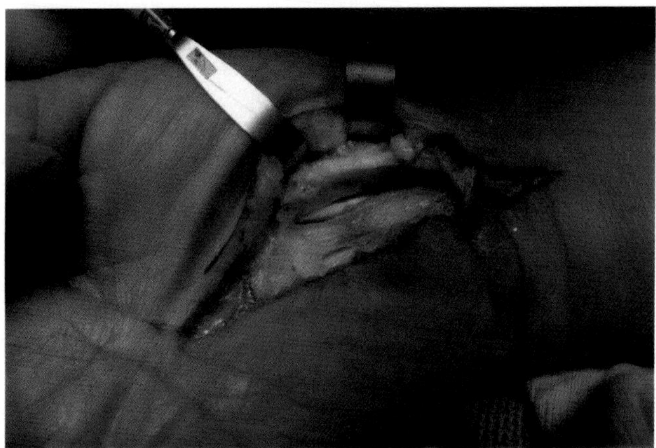

FIGURE 70.2. Severe recurrent carpal tunnel syndrome treated with open carpal tunnel release and internal neurolysis.

symptoms improve then recur after a steroid injection, surgery will generally provide relief. Direct intraneural injections can cause severe, irreversible nerve damage, and ultrasound guidance can help prevent this complication. Diuretics and oral steroids are not indicated. Vitamin supplements such as B6 can be helpful if there is a vitamin deficiency.

Operative Treatment

Operative treatment is reasonable if symptoms progress beyond mild and intermittent despite conservative measures. The TCL and distal antebrachial fascia of the forearm are divided via a palmar incision. Internal neurolysis is not indicated in most cases. Revision surgery or decompression in the setting of rheumatoid arthritis generally calls for an extended incision crossing the wrist crease (Figure 70.2).

The results of surgery are gratifying and consistent, regardless of technique (open versus limited open versus endoscopic), although practitioners are often passionate about their preference. Long-term relief of symptoms is achieved in up to 91% of cases.[21] Postoperative splinting has been found to be unnecessary.[22] Surgical complications are pillar pain (aching of the proximal palm), tendon subluxation over the hook of the hamate, and injury to the ulnar nerve and local median nerve branches.

Recurrence of CTS is rare (it is not less than 53%), and the patient should be questioned about initial postoperative symptom relief.[23] If there was temporary improvement followed by recurrence, scarring should be suspected. If there was minimal to no improvement with surgery, consideration should be given to a diagnosis of incomplete release, permanent uncorrectable intraneural damage, or other sites of nerve compression. Revision carpal tunnel surgery can be performed endoscopically,[24] or open with or without hypothenar fat grafting.

Proximal Median Nerve Entrapment

Pronator syndrome or proximal median nerve entrapment (PMNE) is a subtle diagnosis, also of substantial controversy.[25] It is described as rare in the medical literature but is becoming recognized as being more common than previously thought. Different from CTS, in which pain is at the site of compression, compression of the median nerve at the elbow causes pain in the hand or wrist: there is no spontaneous pain in the region of the pronator. Pain is typically in the palm, wrist, and distal forearm and is exacerbated by activities involving sustained forearm pronation.

Diagnosis

The diagnosis of PMNE is determined predominantly by history and physical exam.[25] Early symptoms include weakness of pinch, dropping things when the wrist is being held in flexion, and vague, intermittent, aching pain in the wrist. Hand weakness involves the flexor pollicis longus (FPL) and flexor digitorum profundus to the index finger (FDP IF). The pronator quadratus (PQ) is the third muscle innervated by the anterior interosseous nerve (AIN), but it is difficult to isolate for strength testing.

The wrist pain is typically diagnosed as "tendonitis" but does not respond to treatment for tendonitis. Numbness with PMNE is a relatively late symptom and typically occurs at night. PMNE is often confused with CTS, and the diagnosis is often only considered after carpal tunnel release fails. The thenar area tends to be involved, distinctly different from CTS. The palmar cutaneous branch of the median nerve exits the median nerve about 5 cm proximal to the wrist and provides cutaneous innervation to the thenar area. Thenar muscles maintain normal strength with PMNE.

Symptoms of hand numbness related to PMNE can be provoked by firm palpation of the median nerve just proximal and distal to the elbow crease and with pronation against resistance. Numbness occurring in less than 60 seconds is considered abnormal.

To assess the strength of the muscles innervated by the AIN, muscles must be tested at their "resting length." The wrist is at neutral position, and the metacarpophalangeal (MCP), proximal interphalangeal (PIP), and distal interphalangeal (DIP) joints are flexed to 90°. The strength of the FDP IF should be similar to that of the FDP of the middle finger. Testing pinch strength of the FPL and FDP IF with the "O" sign is only valid if the wrist is in neutral position and not extended.[5] The FPL is tested with the wrist neutral and the thumb metacarpal in abduction. Weakness of FDP IF and FPL resolves immediately in the recovery room following surgical release.

Patients with preexisting subclinical PMNE are at increased risk for development of AIN palsy with trauma to the forearm, or pressure in the area related to prolonged elbow flexion (as with sling immobilization after shoulder surgery).[26]

Electrodiagnostic studies are not helpful in the diagnosis of PMNE but can exclude other causes of nerve dysfunction. The electromyography should include muscles distal to the area of compression, specifically the FPL, FDP IF, and PQ. The role of ultrasound, MRI, and MR neurograms is not defined.

Nonoperative Treatment

Nonoperative treatment includes avoidance of sustained and/or prolonged pronation and correction of postural issues that magnify other nerve disorders such as thoracic outlet syndrome and cervical spondylosis. Ergonomic modifications such as split keyboards, vertical computer mice, voice-activated software, sit-stand desks, driving with hands on the bottom half of the steering wheel, and modified touring bicycle handlebars may help to reduce symptoms.

Operative Treatment

Operative treatment is an option if the diagnosis is clear by history and examination, if the patient's symptoms are not mild and intermittent, and if they persist or progress in spite of modification of activities. Surgical decompression should address all areas of possible compression of the median nerve around the elbow. From proximal to distal, this includes the fascia of Struthers, the ligament of Struthers (if present), the deep fascia of the proximal pronator teres muscle, the bicipital aponeurosis, the deep fascia of the ulnar origin of the pronator teres muscle, the deep fascia of the humeral origin of the pronator teres muscle, and the fascia of the arch of the superficial flexors. Large incisions are not necessary (Figure 70.3), and there is no indication for postoperative splinting, immobilization, or physical therapy. If wrist pain is the main indication for surgery, release of the bicipital aponeurosis under local anesthesia can be highly effective with a quick recovery.[25]

Anterior Interosseous Nerve Syndrome

The AIN is the most proximal branch of the median nerve in the forearm. There are multiple reported cases of spontaneous AIN palsy, expressed as an acute loss of active flexion of the FPL and the FDP IF and paralysis of the PQ.[27] The cause remains unknown, and treatment is predominantly nonoperative. Weakness is generally self-limited and

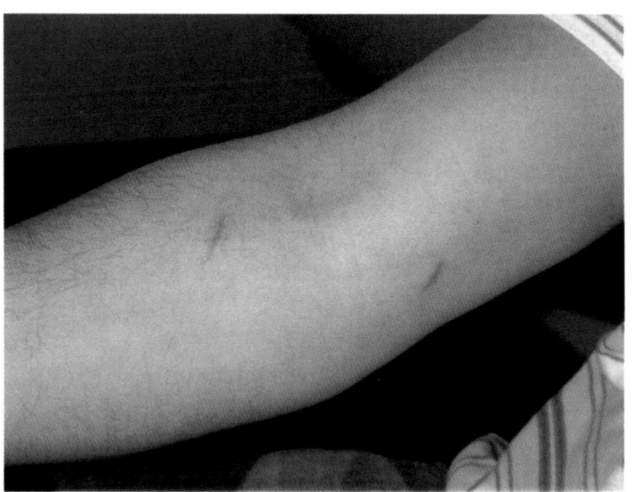

FIGURE 70.3. Typical incisions for decompression of the proximal median nerve.

will often spontaneously resolve. The differential diagnosis includes Parsonage-Turner Syndrome and Kiloh-Nevin Syndrome. Parsonage-Turner is a form of neuralgic amyotrophy thought to be related to the anterior horn cell and preceded by a viral illness. It generally resolves spontaneously.[28] Kiloh-Nevin Syndrome is thought to be focal viral or inflammatory neuritis of the AIN that presents clinically as AIN palsy and that is also expected to recover spontaneously.[29] At least one report, however, demonstrated three cases of prompt return of motor strength following AIN decompression.[30] In one patient, the intraoperative amplitude of the AIN immediately increased from 40 mv to 200 mv after release of the fascia over the AIN.

ULNAR NERVE COMPRESSION

Cubital Tunnel Syndrome

Etiology

Cubital tunnel syndrome is the second most commonly recognized compressive neuropathy in the upper extremity with an incidence of 21 events in 100,000 person-years.[1] It is caused by compression of the ulnar nerve by structures around the elbow. The most common sites of compression are the Arcade of Struthers and intermuscular septum proximal to the elbow, Osborne ligament at the medial epicondyle, and the pronator muscle and flexor fascia distal to the elbow. Other sources of compression are anatomic variations such as the epitrochlearis anconeus muscle, bone spurs, or soft tissue masses in or around the nerve. Risk factors for cubital tunnel syndrome include male gender, performance of heavy manual labor, and tobacco use.[1]

Diagnosis

The diagnosis of cubital tunnel syndrome is made largely by history and physical exam. Early symptoms of cubital tunnel compression include numbness and tingling along the ulnar aspect of the hand, often with proximal radiation of pain along the path of the nerve. Altered sensation of both the dorsal and volar aspects of the ulnar hand distinguishes compression at the level of the elbow from compression at the wrist that causes numbness on the volar surface of the hand. Prolonged compression may lead to complete loss of sensation of the small and ulnar half of the ring fingers and ulnar border of the hand. Ulnar clawing (hyperextension of the MCP with flexion of the PIP and DIP joints), flattening of the palmar arches, and hypothenar atrophy are late findings. Abnormal motor findings include weakness of ulnar-innervated muscles, a positive Froment sign, and loss of ability to concomitantly flex the MCP joints and extend the PIP and DIP joints (the ulnar negative posture). It is important to examine the nerve at both the elbow and hand to determine the level of compression, remembering that compression may be present at both sites. Pain is a variable finding, and patients may use a variety of words to describe the sensations associated with nerve compression.[31]

Intrinsic muscle atrophy combined with sensory loss without a peripheral explanation suggests an unusual underlying neurologic disorder such as Charcot-Marie-Tooth, or syringomyelia. Loss of muscle strength with a normal sensory exam is an early sign of amyotrophic lateral sclerosis.[32]

X-rays of the elbow may be performed if there is a history of trauma or if heterotopic ossification or arthritis is suspected. Electrodiagnostic tests, ultrasound, and MRI have all been used to isolate the level of compression and look for other pathology.[7,8]

Treatment

Nonoperative management with night splinting, physical therapy, and activity and postural modification is indicated for mild disease and has a 50% rate of efficacy.[33] Operative management is indicated when symptoms and signs persist or worsen despite conservative management. Accepted procedures include simple decompression via open or endoscopic approaches, anterior (subcutaneous) transposition, and intra- or submuscular transposition. Although some have advocated a tailored surgical approach, using simple decompression for mild disease and submuscular transposition for severe or recurrent disease, more recent studies suggest that all procedures have high rates of success.[34] The management of the subluxating nerve is still under debate with some surgeons transposing the nerve only if subluxation is noted pre- or intraoperatively. Positive functional and sensory outcomes of cubital tunnel release are high, and have been measured at 77% to 86% at 1 year after surgery.[35,36]

Ulnar Tunnel Syndrome

Anatomy

The ulnar tunnel, also known as Guyon canal, is the site of ulnar nerve compression at the wrist. Distal to the take-off of the dorsal ulnar cutaneous nerve, the ulnar nerve passes between the hamate and pisiform dorsal to the palmar carpal ligament, the palmaris brevis, and fatty tissue and volar to the carpus. It travels ulnar to the ulnar artery and, within the canal, branches into a deep motor branch and a more volar sensory branch. The nerve can be compressed proximal to or within the canal and can involve the motor and/or the sensory branch.

Etiology

Causes of ulnar nerve compression within Guyon canal are more varied than compression at the cubital tunnel and include local fascial bands, ganglion cysts, soft tissue masses, fracture callus, vascular anomalies, aberrant muscles, and tophaceous gout. It is not uncommon to see simultaneous presentation of symptoms of median nerve and ulnar nerve compression at the wrist, and studies have shown improvement in ulnar nerve symptoms after median nerve decompression alone.[37,38]

Diagnosis

Symptoms are similar to those seen in cubital tunnel syndrome but are limited to the hand. A thorough examination of the neck, arm, and hand should be performed to exclude proximal disease. Exams should include palpation, assessment of vascular supply, provocative maneuvers including Tinel, Phalen, and scratch-collapse tests, and evaluation of grip and pinch, and sensory exams. X-ray exams can look for hamate fractures or other bone pathology around the ulnar wrist. Electrodiagnostic tests can assess for muscle involvement. MRI or ultrasound may be useful in looking for anatomic variations and masses within Guyon canal.

Treatment

Splinting and activity modification can be used for mild and intermittent symptoms. If these fail, surgical decompression of the tunnel is reasonable. The incision extends from approximately 4 cm proximal to the wrist crease over the flexor carpi ulnaris (FCU) tendon onto the hypothenar eminence. The FCU is retracted ulnarward, and the nerve is gently dissected free from the ulnar artery and overlying fascia. It is important to identify and release both the motor and sensory branches in the canal as well as the antebrachial fascia in the forearm. The pisohamate ligament should be identified and divided, protecting the nerve at the distal tunnel. Care should be taken to avoid damage to the ulnar artery. Vascular supply to the hypothenar muscles should be preserved if feasible.

The outcomes of ulnar tunnel release have not been examined in the English language literature to the extent of those for cubital tunnel syndrome. Kaiser et al found a 90% rate of subjective and electrodiagnostic improvement in a group of 13 patients.[39]

RADIAL NERVE COMPRESSION

The radial nerve is responsible for extension of the fingers and wrist, and sensation on the dorsal radial hand and radial wrist. Radial nerve entrapment with palsy is relatively rare and presents as loss of finger extension and, if the site of neuropathy is proximal to the posterior interosseous nerve (PIN), loss of wrist extension. The most vulnerable area of the radial nerve is in the spiral groove along the lateral aspect of the distal humerus. "Saturday Night Palsy" refers to temporary paralysis of the motor aspect of the radial nerve from sustained local pressure on this aspect of the upper arm while sleeping or unconscious due to intoxication and generally resolves completely. Radial nerve entrapment at the lateral intermuscular septum causes aching pain distally in the radial tunnel area. Radial nerve palsies associated with distal humerus fractures represent a common therapeutic dilemma as to whether or not the nerve should be explored surgically.[40] If the palsy is from a stretch injury, spontaneous recovery can generally be expected. If the nerve is transected, it should be repaired primarily.

Radial tunnel syndrome (RTS), defined as pain without weakness in the dorsal forearm and wrist provoked by resisted supination, extension of the wrist, or isolated middle finger extension is somewhat controversial. RTS has up to a 41% overlap with lateral epicondylitis, contributing to the debate.[41,42] Electrodiagnostic studies are not helpful for evaluating either condition.

Nonoperative Treatment

Symptoms sometimes resolve spontaneously. Physical therapy can be helpful, particularly with massage and eccentric strengthening. Steroid injections and antiinflammatory medication can give relief, and if so, would imply an inflammatory or edema-related condition. Approximately 25% of patients were observed to improve with conservative care.[41]

Operative Treatment

The approach to the radial tunnel can be anterior, posterior, or between the extensor digitorum communis and the extensor carpi radialis brevis. Dissection using a posterior approach can be tedious because of arborization of the motor nerves to the finger extensors. The anterior approach avoids intramuscular dissection but requires attention to cutaneous nerves and numerous enveloping vessels. Muscular dissection through the extensor carpi radialis brevis may result in a wide scar (Figure 70.4). The fascia of the supinator is released over the PIN (the arcade of Frohse), and a transverse tenotomy of the common extensor fascia is performed.

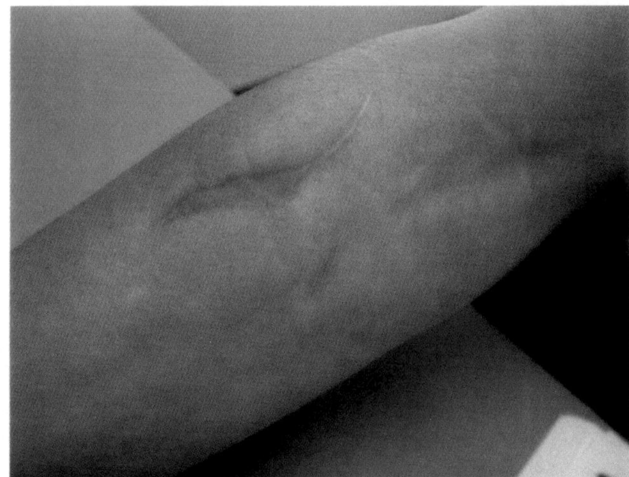

FIGURE 70.4. Widened radial tunnel incision.

Posterior Interosseous Nerve Compression

Compression of the PIN is one of several atraumatic causes of PIN dysfunction, the others being Parsonage-Turner (neuralgic amyotrophy) and spontaneous hourglass deformity of the nerve.[43] Compression can lead to loss of finger extension and radial deviation on extension.[44] If the exam is consistent with PIN palsy, exploration and release of the arcade of Frohse is indicated if there is no recovery after 6 weeks.

Superficial Sensory Branch of the Radial Nerve

Radial sensory nerve entrapment in the distal forearm, also known as Wartenberg Syndrome (WS) or cheiralgia paresthetica, presents with altered sensation and/or pain in the dorsal radial hand, a positive Tinel sign at the site of compression, and provocation of symptoms with ulnar deviation, wrist flexion, or resisted pronation. It is uncommon with a reported incidence of 0.003%, but it may be underdiagnosed.[45] The nerve can be compressed internally by local fascia or more distally and externally by a tight watch or bracelet. Electrodiagnostic testing is not necessary if there is a high degree of suspicion and no proximal symptoms. Ultrasound may demonstrate altered nerve diameter or intraneural masses.

The differential diagnosis of distal radial forearm pain is large, including de Quervain tenosynovitis, thumb carpometacarpal osteoarthritis, lateral antebrachial cutaneous neuritis, intersection syndrome, and proximal nerve compression.[46] Dorsal-radial wrist/hand pain that responds to a nerve block will reliably respond to surgical decompression. WS mimics de Quervain tenosynovitis but does not improve with a steroid injection to the first dorsal extensor compartment, a clue to the diagnosis.

Nonoperative treatments are immobilization with a short thumb spica splint, therapeutic ultrasound or iontophoresis, nerve gliding exercises, or local steroid injections. Conservative therapy has been found to have efficacy of 37% in a small patient sample at 28 months.[47] Surgical treatment is indicated for worsening symptoms or signs of no improvement after a reasonable course of nonoperative treatment. A longitudinal incision is made at the point of maximal tenderness along the radial forearm where the nerve emerges from beneath fascia. Fascia is divided, and the nerve is gently freed from surrounding tissue using tissue scissors and minimal manipulation. In 32 patients who underwent surgical release of the radial sensory nerve, 86% experienced good to excellent outcomes.[47]

CONCLUSION

Upper extremity pain and dysfunction related to nerve compression is likely to be more common than has been historically recognized. Compression of the median nerve at the wrist and ulnar nerve at the elbow and wrist have been the most commonly recognized, but that does not mean that they are the only nerves that *can* be compressed. Success has been reported following decompression of multiple motor and cutaneous nerves, and surgeons should include this category of disorders in evaluation of the upper extremity. Hand surgery is applied anatomy.

REFERENCES

1. Kumar SD, Bourke G. Nerve compression syndromes at the elbow. *Orthop Trauma*. 2016;30(4):355-362.
2. Tapadia M, Mozaffar T, Gupta R. Compressive neuropathies of the upper extremity: pathophysiology, classification, electrodiagnostic findings. *J Hand Surg Am*. 2010;35(4):668-677.
3. Rempel D, Dahlin L, Lundborg G. Pathophysiology of nerve compression syndromes: response of peripheral nerves to loading. *J Bone Jt Surg Am*. 1999;81:1600-1610.
   This broadly quoted article provides an excellent review of nerve anatomy, experimental models of compression, and the effects of compression on the nerve in the acute, short term, and long term. The effects of vibration on nerves, the effect of gliding on the ability of the nerve to glide, and the effects of joint position on extraneural pressure were also measured. The authors concluded that even short periods of nerve compression can have widespread negative effects on structure and function of the nerve.
4. Mackinnon SE. Pathophysiology of nerve compression. *Hand Clin*. 2002;18(2):231-241.
5. Brand PW, Hollister AM. *Clinical Mechanics of the Hand*. 3rd ed. St Louis, MO: Mosby; 1999:17-20.
6. Cheng CJ, Mackinnon-Patterson B, Beck J, Mackinnon SE. Scratch collapse test for evaluation of carpal and cubital tunnel syndrome. *J Hand Surg*. 2008;33(9):1518-1524.
   The authors present a new provocative maneuver, the scratch-collapse test, to provide the surgeon with a rapid, cost-effective, reproducible, objective test for the presence of nerve compression. The study prospectively compared the scratch-collapse test to a Tinel test and a flexion/compression test and found it to be the most sensitive of the three at both the carpal and cubital tunnels.
7. Shen L, Masih S, Patel DB, Matcuk GR Jr. MR anatomy and pathology of the ulnar nerve involving the cubital tunnel and Guyon's canal. *Clin Imag*. 2016;40(2):263-274.
8. Chang KV, Wu WT, Han DS, Ozcakar L. Ulnar nerve cross-sectional area for the diagnosis of cubital tunnel syndrome: a meta-analysis of ultrasonographic measurements. *Arch Phys Med Rehabil*. 2018;99(4):743-757.
9. Farooq MU, Martin JHW, Andary MT. Unusual presentation of hereditary neuropathy with liability to pressure palsies. *J Brachial Plexus Periph Nerve Inj*. 2008;3(1):2.
10. Brinkely DM, Hepper CT. Heart in hand: structural cardiac abnormalities that manifest as acute dysvascularity of the hand. *J Hand Surg*. 2010;35(12):2101-2103.
11. Mckee DE, Lalonde DH, Thoma A, Dickson L. Achieving the optimal epinephrine effect in wide awake hand surgery using local anesthesia without a tourniquet. *Hand*. 2015;10(4):613-615.
12. Lalonde DH, Bell M, Benoit P, et al. A multicenter prospective study of 3,110 consecutive cases of elective epinephrine use in the fingers and hand: the Dalhousie project clinical phase. *J Hand Surg Am*. 2005;30(5):1061-1067.
   This prospective study demonstrated the safety of using local anesthesia containing epinephrine in the hand and fingers. A brief review of the origin of the fallacy that epinephrine causes digital necrosis is provided. This study provides compelling evidence that negates decades of medical school teaching and reminds us to be lifelong students, constantly questioning dogma.
13. Hefermehl LJ, Largo RA, Hermanns T, et al. Lateral temperature spread of monopolar, bipolar and ultrasonic instruments for robot-assisted laparoscopic surgery. *BJU Int*. 2014;114(2):245-252.
14. Stanek JJ, Renslow MA, Kalliainen LK. The effect of an educational program on opioid prescription patterns in hand surgery: a quality improvement program. *J Hand Surg*. 2015;40(2):341-346.
15. Kurdi MS, Theerth KA, Deva RS. Ketamine: current applications in anesthesia, pain, and critical care. *Anesth Essays Res*. 2014;(3):283-290.
16. Hustedt JW, Chung A, Bohl DD, et al. Comparison of postoperative complications associated with anesthetic choice for surgery of the hand. *J Hand Surg*. 2017;42(1):1-8.
17. Dale AM, Harris-Adamson C, Rempel D, et al. Prevalence and incidence of carpal tunnel syndrome in US working populations: pooled analysis of six prospective studies. *Scand J Work Environ Health*. 2013;39(5):495-505.
18. American Academy of Orthopaedic Surgeons. Management of Carpal Tunnel Syndrome: Evidence-Based Clinical Practice Guideline. www.aaos.org/ctsguideline. Published February 29, 2016. Accessed August 1, 2018.
   This high-quality evidence-based clinical practice guideline represents state of the art in diagnosis and treatment of CTS at the time of its production. It is prefaced by a useful summary of graded recommendations and was endorsed by six professional organizations.
19. Graham B. The value added by electrodiagnostic testing in the diagnosis of carpal tunnel syndrome. *J Bone Jt Surg Am*. 2008;90A:2587-2593.
   The CTS-6 model estimates the probability of presence of CTS by asking about six symptoms and signs: numbness predominantly in the distribution of the median nerve, nocturnal numbness, thenar atrophy, positive Phalen test, loss of 2PD, and positive Tinel sign. Point values are assigned to each, and a total of 12 or higher equates with a probability of 80% that CTS is present. Electrodiagnostic tests do not add to the probability of making the correct diagnosis.
20. Andersen JH, Thomsen JF, Overgaard E, et al. Computer use and carpal tunnel syndrome. *JAMA*. 2003;289:2963-2969.
21. Katz JN, Keller RB, Simmons BP, et al. Maine carpal tunnel study: outcomes of operative and nonoperative therapy for carpal tunnel syndrome in a community-based cohort. *J Hand Surg*. 1998;23(4):697-710.
22. Cook AC, Szabo RM, Birkholz, King EF. Early mobilization following carpal tunnel release: a prospective randomized study. *J Hand Surg*. 1995;20(2):228-230.
23. Cobb TK, Amadio PC. Reoperation for carpal tunnel syndrome. *Hand Clin*. 1996;12:313-323.
24. Luria S, Waitayawinyu T, Trumble T. Endoscopic revision of carpal tunnel release. *Plast Reconstr Surg*. 2008;121(6):2029-2034.
25. Hagert E. Clinical diagnosis and wide-awake surgical treatment of proximal median nerve entrapment at the elbow: a prospective study. *Hand*. 2013;8:41-46.
   The author reviews the history of diagnosis and treatment of PMNE and presents her treatment paradigm. Rather than using a large incision, she proposes releasing the lacertus fibrosus with a small proximal forearm incision under local anesthesia. In a prospective study, 44 patients underwent surgery. At the 6-month point, significant improvements were seen in the quick DASH, work DASH, and activity DASH. visual analog scale scores of minimal numbness, almost pain, and high satisfaction were also found.
26. Casey PJ, Moed BR. Fractures of the forearm complicated by palsy of the anterior interosseous nerve caused by a constrictive dressing: a report of four cases. *J Bone Jt Surg Am*. 1997;79A:122-124.
27. Chi Y, Harness NG. Anterior interosseous nerve syndrome. *J Hand Surg*. 2010;35(12):2078-2080.
28. Parsonage MJ, Turner JWA. Neuralgic amyotrophy: the shoulder-girdle syndrome. *Lancet*. 1948;1:973-978.
29. Kiloh LG, Nevin S. Isolated neuritis of the anterior interosseous nerve. *BMJ*. 1952;1:850-851.
30. Garrett JP, Cole DW, Ruch DS. Measurement of intraoperative nerve conduction velocities during anterior interosseous nerve decompression. *Am J Orthop*. 2007;36(12):675-677.
31. Mystakidou K, Parpa E, Tsilika E, et al. Comparison of pain quality descriptors in cancer patients with nociceptive and neuropathic pain. *In Vivo*. 2007;21:93-98.
32. Rowland LP, Shneider NA. Amyotrophic lateral sclerosis. *N Engl J Med*. 2001;344(22):1688-1700.
33. Padua L, Aprile I, Caliandro P, et al. Natural history of ulnar entrapment at elbow. *Clin Neurophysiol*. 2002;113(12):1980-1984.
34. Chimenti PC, Hammert WC. Ulnar neuropathy at the elbow: an evidence-based algorithm. *Hand Clin*. 2013;29:435-442.
35. Malay S, SUN Study Group; Chung KC. The minimal clinically important difference after simple decompression for ulnar neuropathy at the elbow. *J Hand Surg Am*. 2013;38(4):652-659.
36. Jariwala A, Bansal N, Nicol GM, et al. Outcome analysis of cubital tunnel decompression. *Scott Med J*. 2015;60(3):136-140.
37. Bachoura A, Jacoby SM. Ulnar tunnel syndrome. *Orthop Clin North Am*. 2012;43:467-474.
38. Mondelli M, Ginanneschi F, Rossi A. Evidence of improvement in distal conduction of ulnar nerve sensory fibers after carpal tunnel release. *Neurosurgery*. 2009;65(4):696-700.
39. Kaiser R, Houšťava L, Brzezny R, Haninec P. The results of ulnar nerve decompression in Guyon's canal syndrome. *Acta Chir Orthop Traumatol Cech*. 2012;79(3):243-248.
40. Shah A, Jebson PJL. Current treatment of radial nerve palsy following fracture of the humeral shaft. *J Hand Surg*. 2008;33(8):1433-1434.
41. Moradi A, Ebrahimzadeh MH, Jupiter JB. Radial tunnel syndrome, diagnostic and treatment dilemma. *Arch Bone Jt Surg*. 2015;3(3):156-162.
42. Calfee RP, Patel A, DaSilva MF, Akelman E. Management of lateral epicondylitis: current concepts. *J Am Acad Orthop Surg*. 2008;16(1):19-29.
43. Sigamoney KV, Rashid A, Ng CY. Management of atraumatic posterior interosseous nerve palsy. *J Hand Surg*. 2017;42(10):826-830.
44. Spinner M. The arcade of Frohse and its relationship to posterior interosseous nerve paralysis. *J Bone Jt Surg Br*. 1968;50B:809-812.
45. Dang AC, Rodner CM. Unusual compression neuropathies of the forearm. Part 1: radial nerve. *J Hand Surg*. 2009;34(10):1906-1914.
46. Ponnappan RK, Khan M, Matzon JL, et al. Clinical differentiation of upper extremity pain etiologies. *J Am Acad Orthop Surg*. 2015;23(8):492-500.
47. Dellon AL, Mackinnon SE. Radial sensory nerve entrapment in the forearm. *J Hand Surg Am*. 1986;11(2):199-205.

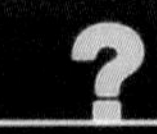

QUESTIONS

1. True or false: The AIN is a pure motor nerve.

 a. True
 b. False

2. A construction worker develops intermittent severe pain in his both carpal tunnels with activities involving sustained pronation of the forearms, associated with awakening with his whole hands numb at night. Over a 10-year period, he has his carpal tunnels released three times on each side. After each operation, he seems to have brief relief of his symptoms but as soon as he goes back to work driving a bulldozer, fully pronated all day long, his wrists hurt, and he is dropping things. He is sent to you by the insurance company for you to perform his seventh carpal tunnel release. Which of the following would be included in successful treatment?

 a. More physical therapy, splinting, NSAIDs
 b. Repeat bilateral carpal tunnel surgery, with internal neurolysis
 c. Psychiatric evaluation for depression
 d. Urine test to assess for drug-seeking behavior
 e. Release of the proximal median nerve

3. Which of the following anatomic structures is associated with cubital tunnel syndrome?

 a. Ligament of Struthers
 b. Arcade of Struthers
 c. Arcade of Frohse
 d. Fascia of Osborne

4. A medical student is injured during an orthopedic case when a heavy drill falls onto the middle of her arm along the radial shaft. She has a large bruise in the midforearm that resolves, but weeks later she has persistent pain in the radial wrist, particularly with combined thumb adduction and ulnar deviation of the wrist. There is no tenderness or swelling at the radial styloid. She has no response to NSAIDs, or steroid injection into the tendon sheath at the wrist. A thumb spica splint helps to prevent the pain but is very uncomfortable to wear and makes it hard for her to perform her duties on the orthopedic service. What would the next step be?

 a. Physical therapy for strengthening exercises
 b. Surgical release of her first dorsal extensor compartment
 c. Cognitive behavioral therapy for disproportionate pain
 d. Blocking of the superficial sensory branch of the radial nerve with local anesthesia

5. A 50-year-old hospital administrator develops swine flu, followed by severe shoulder pain. On recovery, several weeks later, he notes difficulty pulling his zipper up and buttoning his shirt. On exam, he is noted to have no active flexion of this thumb IP joint and index finger DIP joint. What is the diagnosis?

 a. Neuralgic amyotrophy (Parsonage Turner syndrome)
 b. PMNE
 c. Lou Gehrig disease (amyotrophic lateral sclerosis)
 d. Flexor tendon ruptures of the FPL and FDP IF
 e. Stenosing tenosynovitis of the thumb and index finger

1. **Answer: b.** Although there are literally hundreds of descriptions of the AIN as a "pure motor nerve" in medical literature, it is *not* a pure motor nerve. The AIN is a motor nerve to the FPL, FDP IF, and PQ, and terminates in a large sensory nerve to the volar wrist bones. Compression of the AIN branch of the median nerve at the elbow can cause referred pain in the volar wrist/distal volar forearm. Neurectomy of the sensory branch of the AIN is performed to denervate the wrist, useful for painful wrist conditions that are not reconstructable.

2. **Answer: e.** Recurrent or persistent CTSs are rare following carpal tunnel release if the diagnosis is correct and the surgery was performed with proper technique. Wrist pain with sustained pronation in this example is explained by pressure on the sensory branch of the AIN by the deep fascia of the ulnar origin of the pronator teres muscle. Failed carpal tunnel surgery can represent anatomic variation, technical error, excessive scar formation, malingering, somatization, or failure to appreciate a more proximal site of compression that causes very similar symptoms. Electrodiagnostic studies are often ordered to assess patients for PMNE but are rarely helpful.

3. **Answer: d.** Also referred to as the ligament of Osborne, these fascial fibers connect the two heads of the FCU muscle just distal to the interval between the medial epicondyle and the tip of the olecranon, and can flatten the ulnar nerve within the cubital tunnel. The Ligament of Struthers is an anatomic variant that connects the humerus to the medial epicondyle and can cause proximal median nerve compression. The arcade of Frohse is the proximal fascial arch of the supinator, which lies superficial to the PIN in the radial tunnel. The arcade of Struthers is a vascular leash that crosses the median nerve in the upper arm.

4. **Answer: d.** Wartenberg syndrome is a focal neuritis of the superficial sensory branch of the radial nerve, often associated with local trauma. The radial sensory nerve exits between the extensor carpi radialis longus and the brachioradialis as it travels from deep to superficial, and it is particularly vulnerable to blunt trauma along the distal radial shaft, where scar tissue can tether the nerve. The pain from Wartenberg syndrome mimics the pain from de Quervain tenosynovitis.

5. **Answer: a.** This is a classic history for neuralgic amyotrophy (Parsonage Turner syndrome): severe pain following an inciting event such as viral illness, followed by paresis of the upper extremity. PMNE can cause an AIN palsy if there is blunt trauma to or sustained pressure on the proximal medial forearm for several hours. ALS is a fatal motor neuron disease that can present as hand weakness and cramping pain, with muscle twitching and difficulty swallowing. Spontaneous tendon ruptures are rare, but can happen after fluoroquinolone treatment, but tend to be larger tendons, such as the Achilles tendon. Trigger fingers tend to be painful at the site of the stenosing tenosynovitis, and active muscle contraction can be demonstrated even if the tendons are locked.

CHAPTER 71 **Principles and Applications of Nerve Transfers**

Gwendolyn Hoben and Alison K. Snyder-Warwick

KEY POINTS

- Nerve transfers are an evidence-based, reliable, and effective reconstructive tool for both motor and sensory deficits.
- Major indications for nerve transfer include
  - Proximal nerve stump not available (i.e., congenital etiology, root avulsion, hypoplasia, intracranial)
  - Distance to target is prohibitive to recovery (i.e., proximal nerve injury of the upper extremity or late presentation following injury)
- The timeline of muscle atrophy must still be respected with nerve transfers; plan transfers to consider distance of transfer to target and time from injury.
- Donor nerves should be strong, redundant/expendable, modality matched (motor to motor, sensory to sensory), close to target, and preferably synergistic.
- Sensory nerve transfers and tetraplegia transfers (upper motor neuron injury) are exceptions to the timeline used for motor reinnervation.
- When performing a nerve transfer, follow the mantra, *Donor distal, recipient proximal* to guide dissection and transection.

WHY NERVE TRANSFERS?

History

Nerve transfers arose from the natural evolution of inadequate treatment options for patients with nerve injury. Although Ballance published a description of side-to-end nerve transfer of the spinal accessory nerve to the injured facial nerve in 1903, the concept of nerve transfers was accelerated by the injuries seen in World War I. World War I resulted in increased numbers of challenging nerve injuries, particularly gunshot wounds, for which management was inadequate. A German neurophysiologist, self-taught neurosurgeon, and translational neuroscientist, Otfrid Foerster, pushed the envelope of management for his patients with nerve injuries in the quest to achieve better outcomes. He performed three types of nerve transfers[1]:

- End-to-end (he called *copulation*)
- End-to-side (he called *inoculation*) with the inclusion of reverse end-to-side transfers, which we today call *supercharge*
- Partial nerve transfers of up to 30% of the donor nerve diameter (he called *Abspaltung*), analogous to today's fascicular transfers

Foerster reported on over 15 nerve transfers in 1929, emphasized the importance of postoperative rehabilitation and follow-up, and described neural plasticity. Although many of his techniques were forgotten or abandoned for decades, the roots of the recent paradigm shift to nerve transfers for nerve injury management, which has witnessed exponential growth, lie in Foerster's work in the early 1900s.

An Open Door

Nerve transfers have gained popularity due to the shortcomings of previous nerve injury management options. Before nerve transfers, options included primary nerve repair or nerve grafting. Although these options are ideal and preferred for some nerve injuries, multiple clinical scenarios, such as proximal nerve injuries, injuries located distant from their target muscle, and injuries in which no proximal nerve stump is available (e.g., root avulsion, trauma), to name a few, are not amenable to direct repair or nerve grafting. To fulfill this clinical management gap, nerve transfers have come into existence and gained acceptance. Nerve transfers differ substantially from nerve autografts (**Table 71.1**). Nerve transfers have the distinct advantage to provide neural reconstruction in close proximity to the end target muscle, thereby eliminating the need to reenter the zone of injury and promoting faster recovery, which equates to improved functional outcome. Because nerve injuries occur in all body regions, nerve transfers, too, are not limited to any one anatomic area, but may be performed throughout the body.

BASIC PRINCIPLES

The Injured Nerve

Once the decision has been made that a nerve transfer is appropriate, in the case of traumatic proximal injuries, the proximal injury may still be addressed. There are two critical reasons for this: pain control and sensory reconstruction. An unrepaired major nerve injury may result in neuroma formation and potentially debilitating neuropathic pain. Depending on the length of the nerve gap and other reconstructive needs, use of nerve autografts, venous conduits, or acellular nerve allografts are reasonable options to provide a regenerative pathway and prevent neuroma formation. Muscles will atrophy if not reinnervated within 12 to 18 months, but the time frame for sensory regeneration is longer, but not well known. The prognosis for sensory recovery likely declines over time due to mechanisms less well understood than the atrophy of the neuromuscular junction in motor nerves; however, sensory nerve transfers have been successful 20 years after injury and at significant distance to the target.

TABLE 71.1. NERVE GRAFTS VERSUS NERVE TRANSFERS

	Advantages	Disadvantages
Nerve grafts	Reconstruct like with like Little to no motor reeducation Spontaneous, emotional movement (for face)	Requires donor site May be long Involves coaptations Recovery may be less robust
Nerve transfers	Closer to target Avoid additional coaptations Avoid potential graft harvest from distant site May be stronger axonal input Can be use when proximal nerve stump not available Avoid need to reenter zone of injury	Require motor reeducation May involve unwanted movements Movement may not be spontaneous

Indications for Nerve Transfer

Nerve transfers have enabled robust functional recovery in challenging circumstances. Distance and time from injury are the main barriers to functional reconstruction. Nerve transfers enable rapid and successful reinnervation, even when patients present late. They also enable reconstruction when no proximal stump of the injured nerve is available, when a large zone of injury exists, or when the exact location of injury is unknown. Successful reconstructions, like with tendon transfer, require supple joints and careful donor planning. The indications for nerve transfer include

- Injury distant from target
- Proximal nerve stump not available (e.g., intracranial VII, avulsed brachial plexus root)
- Large zone of injury
- Segmental or multiple nerve injuries
- Unknown location of nerve injury
- Partial nerve injuries
- Zone of injury adjacent to critical structures
- Prolonged time from injury

Donor and Recipient Nerve Selection

Similar to tendon transfers, the donor nerve should be selected based on specific characteristics. The criteria for donor nerve selection are as follows:

- Functioning or recovering donor
- Redundant function (expendable)
- Synergistic movement
- Similar power
- Proximity to target muscle
- Reconstruct motor with motor and sensory with sensory

A logical requirement is that the donor nerve be intact and uninjured. There are instances, however, when a recovering nerve may be utilized. In devastating multinerve injuries or cervical spinal cord injuries, it may be reasonable to use a recovering nerve closer to the injury site to transfer to a nerve more distally to reduce the regeneration distance. In the case of tetraplegia, the zone of injury can include lower motor neuron injuries that will recover, and those nerves could be transferred because donor nerves are scarce and may be utilized for a more critical hand function. Clearly, the donor should also be redundant, to avoid functional sacrifice. In contrast to tendon transfers, there are often multiple nerve fascicles going to a single muscle, and transfer of a single fascicle may still retain donor function. Modality specificity (i.e., reconstructing motor with motor and sensory with sensory) is important for improved outcomes. It is intuitive to attempt to match the axonal number in the donor nerve to that of the recipient, similar to the way donor tendons should match the power and excursion of the recipient. There is strong evidence, however, that a definable minimum number of axons will lead to equivalent functional reinnervation. Animal studies indicate regeneration of only 12% to 30% of the native axons leads to motor function equivalent to preinjury function.[2] Schreiber et al. compared outcomes and donor-recipient axon matches in nerve transfers for elbow flexion and found a minimum donor to recipient ratio of 0.7 predictive of good function.[3] Terzis et al. found that donor nerves with over 74% the number of axons in the target nerve led to improved outcomes in cross-facial nerve grafts for facial palsy.[4] In contrast, several examinations of the number of intercostal nerves transferred to the musculocutaneous nerve did not show improving function with additional nerves transferred. Rather, transfers representing roughly two-thirds the number of axons of the musculocutaneous nerve fared no better than those representing one-third the axon number.[5] Maximizing function and reducing donor burden is an ongoing area of research.

Motor retraining must also be considered when choosing the donor nerve. For example, in patients with injury to the musculocutaneous nerve and loss of elbow flexion, described transfers use either a flexor digitorum superficialis (FDS) branch or a fascicle of flexor carpi ulnaris (FCU) to transfer to the biceps. Considering that the biceps is a supinating muscle and that the median nerve controls pronation, this coaptation is antagonistic and retraining is easier with an ulnar fascicle from the FCU. While preferred, this advantage should not limit reconstruction. In pan-plexus injuries, unrelated donors are often the only option and can be successful. For example, during initial retraining following intercostal nerve transfers to the biceps, the patient must learn to inhale to initiate elbow flexion. Over time, however, full voluntary control is possible irrespective of breathing patterns. Excellent cortical plasticity in children often enables motor reeducation of the transferred nerve without learned tricks. Indeed, transfers from the phrenic nerve to the brachial plexus in the setting of birth-related brachial plexus palsy have very good outcomes despite completely disparate prior functions.

Nerve Transfer Coaptations

The general tenants of nerve repair apply to nerve transfers. The coaptation should be tension-free; the donor nerve should be dissected as far distally as possible to maximize length, and the recipient nerve must be divided as proximally as reasonable. We use the mantra, *donor distal, recipient proximal*. It may be intuitive to place the repair distal on the recipient nerve to shorten the distance to the target, but a repair with excessive tension risks poor outcomes. The extremity should be able to move through full range of motion without tension on the coaptation.

Another critical consideration is whether the coaptation should be end-to-end (ETE) or end-to-side (ETS). In ETE repairs, both the recipient and donor nerves are divided and coapted, such that neither the recipient nor donor nerve is left in continuity. When the donor nerve is left in continuity and the recipient end is coapted into the side of the donor nerve, these are classically considered ETS or terminolateral coaptations (Figure 71.1). The most significant advantage of ETS is that donor morbidity is minimized. In this technique, an epineurial window is cut in the donor nerve to facilitate regeneration into the recipient nerve. Many animal studies have confirmed that lateral sprouting from the donor nerve repopulates the recipient nerve without donor morbidity.[6,7] Use of ETS has been studied clinically in facial nerve reconstruction; an intact hypoglossal donor nerve significantly reduces tongue atrophy with excellent facial nerve function.[8] In the upper extremity, there are case reports of M3 elbow function after coapting an avulsed musculocutaneous nerve to the intact median nerve and of reasonable outcomes following digital nerve ETS repairs. ETS is useful when donor nerves are scarce. For this reason, ETS transfers have been increasingly used to reconstruct birth-related brachial plexus injuries.

In contrast, *reverse* ETS or *supercharge* ETS indicates leaving the recipient nerve intact and coapting the proximal end of the donor nerve to the side of the recipient nerve (see Figure 71.1). This technique is particularly advantageous when a large mixed motor and sensory nerve is injured proximally and repaired; preserving continuity of the nerve may allow for sensory regeneration over months to years, whereas the transfer allows motor reinnervation prior to loss of motor endplates. For example, proximal ulnar nerve injuries have a poor prognosis for intrinsic muscle function because the time for regeneration is over 18 months. Sacrifice of the anterior interosseous nerve (AIN) end into the side of the deep ulnar motor branch achieves more rapid intrinsic muscle reinnervation while allowing for sensory regeneration to proceed distally in the ulnar nerve. These reverse or supercharge ETS repairs show augmented regeneration into the recipient nerve in animal models[9] and improved regeneration in clinical application.[10] Current research is examining side-to-side coaptations to harness the advantages of both ETS and reverse/supercharge ETS.[11] A *supercharge* transfer is useful in the scenario of partial nerve injuries. For example, in a partial ulnar injury where electrodiagnostic studies indicate axons in continuity to muscles, but severely reduced in number, the nerve transfer can serve to augment the number of axons supplying those critical muscles and promote a greater functional outcome without sacrificing the axons still in continuity.

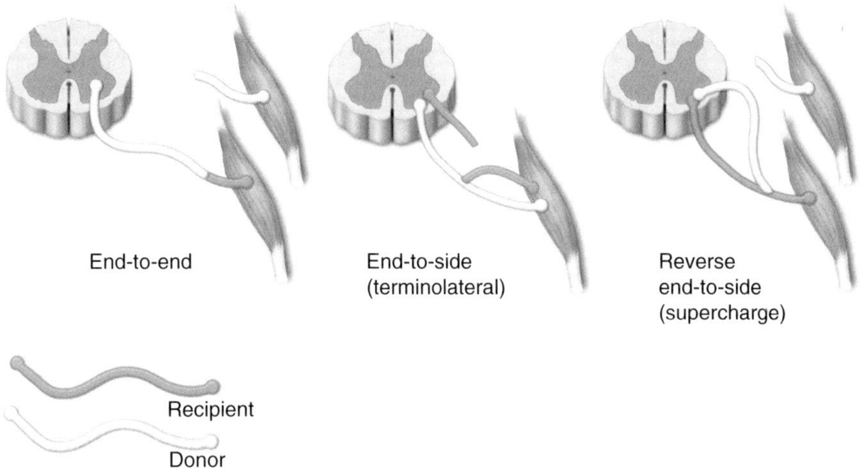

End-to-end
End-to-side (terminolateral)
Reverse end-to-side (supercharge)
Recipient
Donor

FIGURE 71.1. Types of nerve transfer coaptations. Neural coaptation for nerve transfers may be performed via end-to-end (ETE, left), end-to-side (ETS, center), or reverse ETS or supercharge (right) techniques. Both donor and recipient nerves are transected for ETE transfers. Donor nerves remain intact for ETS transfers, and recipient nerves remain in continuity in reverse ETS, or supercharge, transfers.

Confusion exists regarding terminology related to nerve coaptations. As summarized by Dellon et al., describing nerve coaptations in the direction of axonal regeneration may improve clarity.[12] An ETS repair, then, would indicate that the donor nerve is transected and repaired to the side of the injured recipient nerve, which is in actuality a reverse ETS, or supercharge transfer. The term ETS, however, is often used to describe all terminolateral repairs. The classic ETS repair in which the transected end of the recipient nerve is coapted to the side of the donor nerve is in actuality a side-to-end repair. Although we are not able to settle the inconsistencies in terminology reported in the literature, it is important to take detailed note of the scenarios described.

Babysitter Procedures

Babysitter nerve transfers are used to temporarily maintain recipient muscles and may challenge the standard modality matching in donor and recipient nerve selection. This chapter focuses on transfers designed to restore volitional motor control or normal sensation. In these scenarios, the transfers are modality matched: motor to motor and sensory to sensory, and permanent. In scenarios requiring regeneration over very long distances, however, such as cross-facial nerve grafts or extensive brachial plexus grafting, or in cases of delayed treatment, preserving recipient muscle motor endplates is critical to successful eventual regeneration. As first coined in 1984 by Terzis, the first stage of a babysitter procedure for facial palsy involves coapting cross-face nerve grafts to the functional, contralateral facial nerve branches (the distal graft ends were left free). On the injured side of the face, 40% of the hypoglossal nerve is transferred to the critical branches of the nonfunctional facial nerve. In the second stage, 8 to 12 months later, the free ends of the cross-face grafts are connected to the distal stumps of the injured facial nerve and the *mini* hypoglossal nerve transfer is left intact. The intervening hypoglossal transfer preserved the facial mimetic muscle motor endplates, while regeneration proceeded through the cross-facial grafts.[13] Since then, variants on this procedure have evolved, including use of noncritical sensory nerves to maintain muscle mass or to improve axonal regeneration in long nerve grafts. Animal studies have shown that both sensory and motor nerves can be utilized to preserve muscle mass.[14,15] In the scenario of long nerve grafts, sensory nerve transfers are considered to maintain or improve the pathway. For example, Placheta et al. showed that sensory nerve coaptations into the side of long cross-face grafts in rats increased the number of regenerating motor axons and resulted in improved functional outcomes.[16]

APPLICATIONS

Face

Motor

Nerve transfers for reconstruction of facial expression may be performed if conditions are favorable for reinnervation of the native mimetic muscle. Facial muscle differs from skeletal muscle and is thought to have a longer reinnervation window, considered to be up to 12 to 24 months after injury. Each branch of the facial nerve should be assessed for function. Reconstruction may be performed for a specific movement, or more globally for tone or multiple movements. Two of the most integral movements for facial function are eye closure and smile, and these movements should be the focus of reconstruction. The masseteric nerve is likely the most commonly used donor nerve for transfer given its proximity within the ipsilateral cheek, its robust axonal supply,[17,18] and reliable location.[19,20] The advantages of the masseteric nerve include

- Robust axonal supply
- Ability to be transferred without a graft
- Reliable location
- Low donor site morbidity

Postoperatively, there is the challenge of motor reeducation. Use of the masseteric nerve typically results in less spontaneous and emotional movement, although in adults who have had smile movement powered by the masseteric nerve, 85% achieve the ability to smile without biting, with smile spontaneity occurring routinely in 59%.[21] Transfer of the masseteric nerve to the buccal branch of the facial nerve is commonly used for smile reconstruction (Figure 71.2). Reconstruction with the masseteric nerve does not typically reconstruct facial tone well.[22] Use of the hypoglossal nerve has yielded greater results with respect to resting tone. Other donor nerves for transfers to reestablish facial expression include

- The deep temporal nerve[23]
- The platysma motor nerve (for lower lip depression)[24]
- C7
- The phrenic nerve
- The spinal accessory nerve
- The mylohyoid, suprascapular, and long thoracic nerves have been suggested (based on cadaveric studies).

Differential innervation of separate facial movements can decrease unnatural mass movements or unwanted synkinetic movements. Available nerve sources should be inventoried, and the reconstructive plan should be tailored to individual patient needs and preferences.

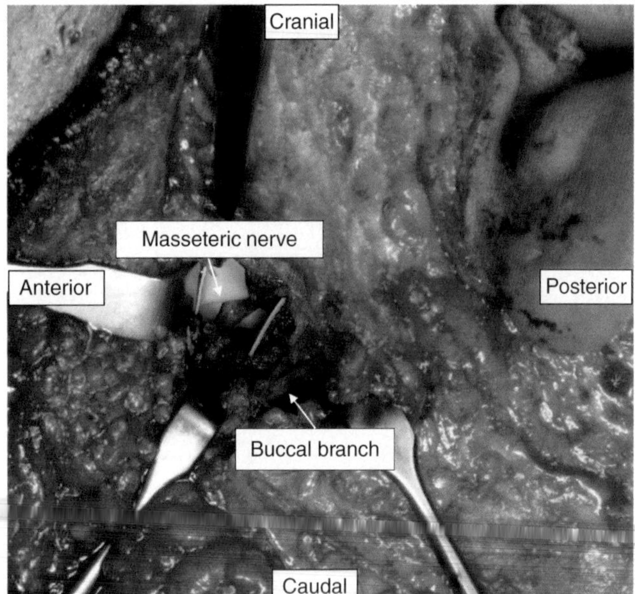

FIGURE 71.2. Masseteric to buccal nerve transfer. The distal end of the buccal branch of the facial nerve can be tunneled through the parotid parenchyma, if needed, to allow direct coaptation without the need for an interposition graft. The masseteric nerve is located on the deep surface of the masseter muscle at a point 3 cm anterior to the tragus and 1 cm inferior to the inferior border of the zygomatic arch. Both nerves are shown here before transection for an end-to-end repair.

Sensory

Concomitant facial paralysis with increased corneal exposure and corneal anesthesia is devastating for corneal health and ultimately leads to ulceration, scarring, and vision loss. Regardless of facial movement, corneal anesthesia can be reconstructed with functional regional sensory nerves. The contralateral supraorbital and supratrochlear nerves are frequently used donors.[25,26] These nerves can be transferred directly or via a nerve graft. After interfascicular dissection of the distal nerve end, fascicles are tunneled in the subtenon plane and grouped three or four locations around the limbus (Figure 71.3). The fascicles are secured and regeneration occurs into the stromal and subbasal layers of the cornea.[27] Preliminary results from patients undergoing a modified technique for corneal neurotization have been promising—most patients regained normal sensation, with all patients achieving protective sensation.[26]

Facial sensory deficits may be reconstructed in a similar manner. Formal sensory mapping confirms functionally intact, nearby nerves that may be used as donors. Branches of the trigeminal nerve can be transferred directly or with a nerve graft to reinnervate important sensory distributions of the face.[28]

Upper Extremity Nerve Transfers

Commonly used upper extremity nerve transfers are listed in **Table 71.2**.

Suprascapular

The suprascapular nerve innervates the supraspinatus and infraspinatus muscles, thus providing shoulder stability and external rotation. A stable shoulder is important for function more distally in the upper extremity. Transfer of the spinal accessory to the suprascapular can be done either through an anterior or posterior approach. The anterior approach combines well with a cervical approach to the brachial plexus. A posterior approach is used to release the suprascapular notch, but does require lateral or prone positioning. In larger patients, this dissection can be quite deep and lighted retractors are necessary. The spinal accessory nerve has multiple branches, and the most robust branch should be used for transfer with care to preserve branches for trapezius function. Transfer of the rhomboid nerve to suprascapular has also been described.[29]

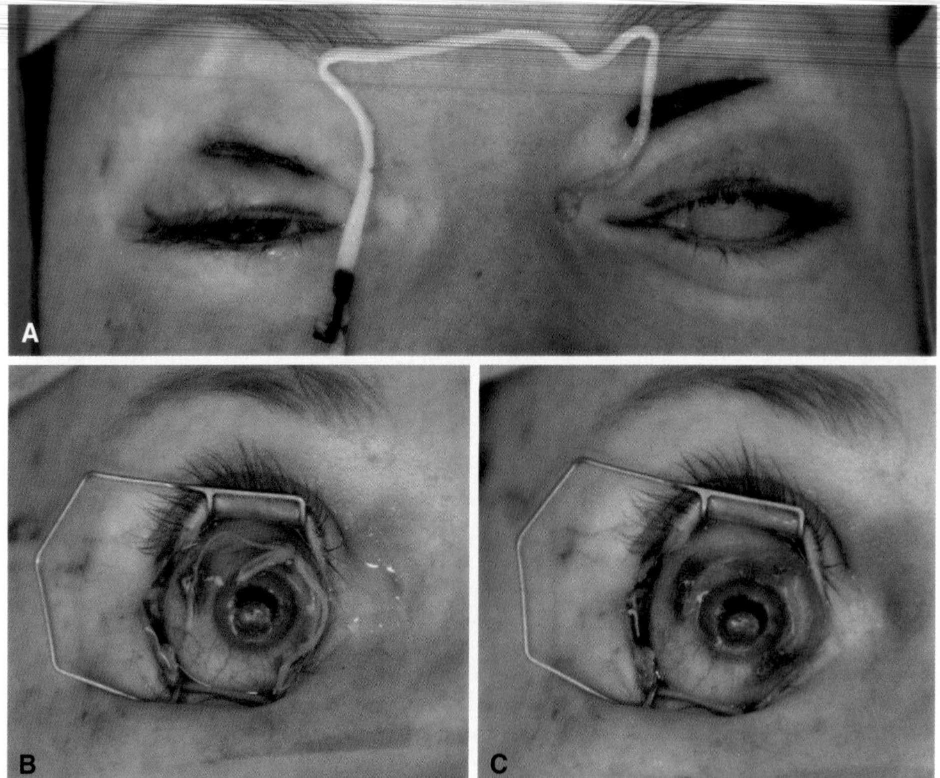

FIGURE 71.3. Corneal neurotization. Corneal anesthesia can be managed by transfer of the contralateral supraorbital or supratrochlear nerve via a sural nerve graft to the cornea. **A.** The nerve graft is tunnelled subcutaneously in the glabellar region via upper lid incisions. **B.** Intraneural fascicular dissection allows placement of the sural fascicles at three locations adjacent to the limbus. **C.** Fascicles are tunnelled in the subtenon layer and dunked into the cornea.

TABLE 71.2. COMMON UPPER EXTREMITY NERVE TRANSFERS

Recipient Nerves and Muscle Targets	Donor Nerves
Suprascapular nerve (C5, 6) Supraspinatus Infraspinatus	Spinal accessory (XI) Dorsal scapular (C3, 4, 5)
Axillary Deltoid (C5, 6)	Radial branch to triceps (C6, 7, 8) Medial pectoral
Musculocutaneous Biceps (C5, 6) Brachialis (C5, 6)	Ulnar branch to FCU (C7, 8, T1) Median branch to FDS/FCR (C6, 7, 8, T1) Thoracodorsal (C6, 7, 8) Medial pectoral (C8, T1)
Radial EPL, EDC (C7, 8) ECRB (C6, 7, 8)	Ulnar branch to FCU (C7, 8, T1) Median branch to FDS/FCR (C6, 7, 8, T1)
Ulnar Intrinsics (C8, T1)	Median branch to pronator quadratus (C7, 8, T1)
Median FPL (C7, 8, T1) FDP (C7, 8, T1) Thenars (C6, 7, 8, T1)	Ulnar branch to FCU (C7, 8, T1) Radial branch to ECRB (C6, 7, 8) Musculocutaneous branch to brachialis (C5, 6) Ulnar to 3rd lumbrical (C8, T1) Ulnar to abductor digiti minimi (C8, T1) Radial to EDQ/ECU (C7, 8)

ECRB, extensor carpi radialis brevis; EDC, extensor digitorum communis; EDQ/ECU, extensor digiti quinti/extensor carpi ulnaris; FCU, flexor carpi ulnaris; FDS/FCR, flexor digitorum superficialis/flexor carpi radialis.

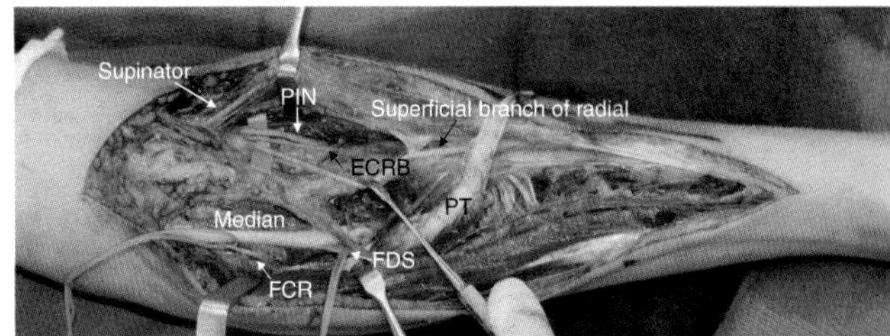

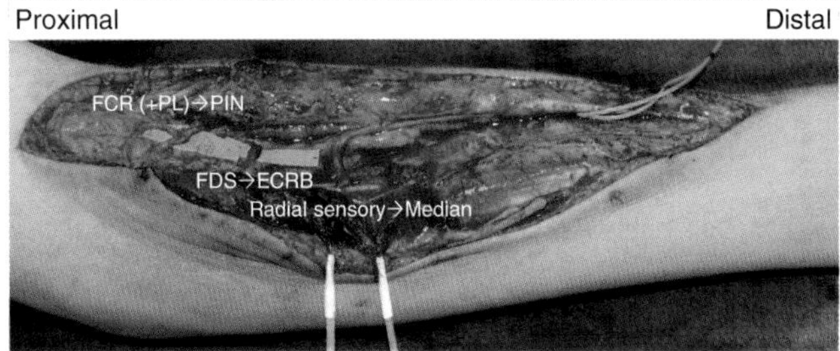

FIGURE 71.4. Median to radial nerve transfers in the forearm. After proximal radial nerve injuries, transfers from the median nerve can restore wrist extension and independent finger extension. A branch to the flexor carpi radialis (FCR), sometimes with the palmaris longus (PL) branch as shown here, is transferred to the posterior interosseous nerve (PIN), and a flexor digitorum superficialis (FDS) nerve branch is transferred to the extensor carpi radialis brevis (ECRB). For sensory reconstruction, the radial sensory nerve is transferred end-to-side (ETS) in the sensory portion of the median nerve. A concomitant pronator teres (PT) to ECRB tendon transfer is included as an internal splint.

Axillary

Deltoid function is the most important deficit with axillary nerve injury. A branch of the radial nerve to the triceps is facile for this transfer, and this procedure is commonly referred to as the Leechavengvong or Somsak procedure. There are three main nerves to triceps: branches to the medial, lateral, and long heads of the muscle. Originally, the branch to the long head of the triceps was favored, but others have argued in favor of the medial branch because it has a longer extramuscular course. This transfer is best done in prone position and can be combined with a spinal accessory to suprascapular nerve transfer. The medial pectoral nerve is another donor. A metaanalysis of grafting versus nerve transfer outcomes for isolated axillary injuries showed no significant differences between the two techniques, and most patients achieve M4 or better shoulder abduction.[30]

Musculocutaneous

Restoration of elbow flexion is a priority in upper trunk injuries as there may be reasonably intact wrist and hand function. There are several options depending on available donors. Transfer of an FCU branch of the ulnar nerve to the motor nerve to biceps, referred to as an Oberlin transfer, is one of the most commonly used and reliable nerve transfers, providing both elbow flexion and supination.[31] An FDS or flexor carpi radialis (FCR) branch of the median nerve can also be transferred to the biceps. The double fascicular transfer, as described by Mackinnon et al., reinnervates two elbow flexors: it combines the Oberlin transfer with transfer of the median FDS/FCR branch to brachialis.[32] This transfer carries a theoretical risk of eliminating both major wrist flexors. In a retrospective review, Carlsen et al. showed that the single versus double nerve transfer resulted in similar elbow flexion strength and disabilities of arm, shoulder, and hand (DASH) scores; the only significant difference was that the double nerve transfer resulted in grip strength 63% of the contralateral side whereas the single nerve transfer resulted in 43% return of grip strength.[33] Other donor options include the thoracodorsal and medial pectoral nerve. In the scenario of complete plexus avulsion injuries, the distal spinal accessory or intercostal nerves can be used with an interpositional nerve graft.

Radial

Elbow extension can be restored via transfer of the nerve branch to FCU to the medial triceps. In the hand, radial nerve function can be restored via median donors—branches to FCR and FDS, and motor branch to pronator quadratus—transferred to posterior interosseous nerve (PIN) and extensor carpi radialis brevis (ECRB) branches (Figure 71.4). Nerve transfer to the PIN is the only method of achieving individual finger extension. If biceps function is intact, the PIN fascicle to supinator should be excluded to maximize reinnervation of the more critical extensors. Although outcome studies are limited, Garcia Lopez et al. reported on six patients who achieved M4 for wrist extension and extensor pollicis longus (EPL) function; two-thirds also achieved M4 metacarpophalangeal extension.[34] The musculocutaneous branch to brachialis is another possible donor. To restore radial hand sensation, lateral antebrachial cutaneous nerve (LABC) to radial sensory can be used. However, because of nerve territory overlap in the hand, the transfer should only be used when necessary.

Ulnar

High ulnar injuries are challenging due to the long distance to the target, the ulnar intrinsic muscles. Transfer of the median AIN branch of pronator quadratus to the motor branch of the ulnar nerve addresses this issue and is likely one of the most commonly used transfers (Figure 71.5). In the presence of an intact pronator teres, there is no donor deficit. Given the challenge of intrinsic recovery, even when the ulnar nerve is in continuity, this transfer may be used in an ETS fashion. Davidge et al. showed that *ulnar supercharge* transfers in the setting of traumatic injuries, severe compression, and traction injuries resulted in M3 or better intrinsic function in 70% of patients.[10] For sensory reconstruction, the median branch to the third webspace can be transferred. The median palmar cutaneous is another possible donor, as is the LABC; however, this transfer usually requires a very lengthy incision, but is of high utility when the median nerve is also damaged. Comparison of grafting versus motor and sensory transfers in proximal ulnar nerve injuries showed significantly improved functional outcomes: 80% were

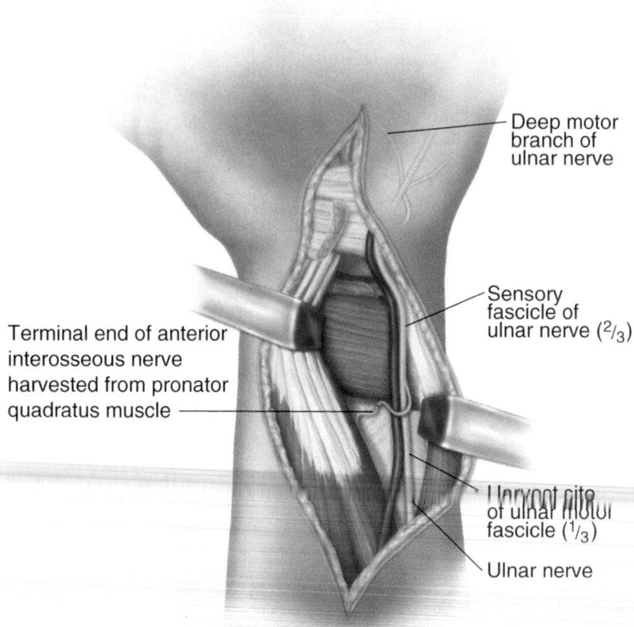

FIGURE 71.5. Anterior interosseous nerve (AIN) transfer to the ulnar deep motor nerve. The terminal AIN to the pronator quadratus can be transferred to the deep motor branch of the ulnar nerve for intrinsic muscle reinnervation. Care must be taken to coapt the AIN to the motor portion of the ulnar nerve and not the sensory region.

at least M3 in the nerve transfer, versus 22% with grafting. Interestingly, sensory outcomes were not significantly different with only 30% to 40% of patients reaching S3 or better at 2 years of follow-up.[34]

Median

The most significant motor deficits in high median nerve injury are flexor pollicis longus (FPL) and flexor digitorum profundus. An ulnar FDS branch, radial branch to ECRB, or musculocutaneous branch to brachialis can be transferred to the AIN branch. Before reinnervation, FPL may lengthen due to unopposed EPL pull and become less effective, thus interphalangeal extension blocking can be a helpful adjunct during reinnervation. The median recurrent motor branch can be restored through an ulnar motor branch to the third lumbrical, nerve to abductor digiti quinti, or a radial PIN branch to extensor digiti quinti and extensor carpi ulnaris. Restoration of sensory function is also crucial in median injuries. Although time is not equal to sensation loss, sensory recovery from grafts in proximal median injuries is typically no better than S3. Transfer of the sensory digital nerve of the 4th webspace end-to-end to the sensory component of the median nerve can be used to restore sensation in the median distribution of the hand. In turn, sensation to the 4th webspace can be returned by coapting the distal end of the 4th webspace sensory branch to the side of the ulnar digital nerve of the small finger.

Flail Arm

In the scenario of a flail arm, there may be no available branches of the brachial plexus for transfer. In these scenarios, donor nerves from the trunk must be judiciously transferred for critical functions. Intercostal (IC) nerve or nerve to rectus transferred to the musculocutaneous nerve, either directly or with an interposition nerve graft, can be used to restore elbow flexion or elbow extension. Given the long distance, this transfer must be done relatively soon after injury. Most publications on IC nerve transfer report transfer of two to four nerves, although up to seven have been reported anecdotally. Kovachevich et al. determined that the number of complications increased significantly when four or more ICs were transferred.[36] It is critical to assess whether the patient has had ipsilateral rib fractures or any respiratory impairment preoperatively, such as phrenic palsy. Prior trauma will increase scarring and has been found to increase the risk of nonviable nerves based on intraoperative stimulation.[36] The risk of iatrogenic pneumothorax in this dissection is 9%.[36] The presence of phrenic palsy has been associated with increased risk of respiratory compromise; however, long-term assessment of patients with combined phrenic and intercostal nerve transfers showed no impact on respiratory function compared to phrenic transfer alone.[37]

Birth-Related Brachial Plexus Palsy

The standard in birth-related brachial plexus palsies (BRBPP) is excision of the neuroma and grafting the intact roots. Distal nerve transfers, however, have several advantages:

- Avoid morbidity of neuroma dissection
- Avoid graft donor site morbidity
- Reduce distance to target muscle (especially advantageous in late presentations)

Moreover, transfers are possible in the scenario of multiple root avulsions when there are minimal donors for grafting. The spinal accessory to suprascapular nerve transfer (Figure 71.6) was accepted early, because the spinal accessory nerve is in the field of the standard cervical approach to the plexus. In a large retrospective study, Tse et al. showed no significant differences in outcomes from grafting C5 to suprascapular versus the spinal accessory transfer. They noted, however, that the transfer was more commonly performed in more severe injuries.[38]

More distal transfers such as the Oberlin transfer and radial to axillary transfers for shoulder abduction have also been utilized in BRBPP. For the Oberlin transfer, retrospective studies have shown

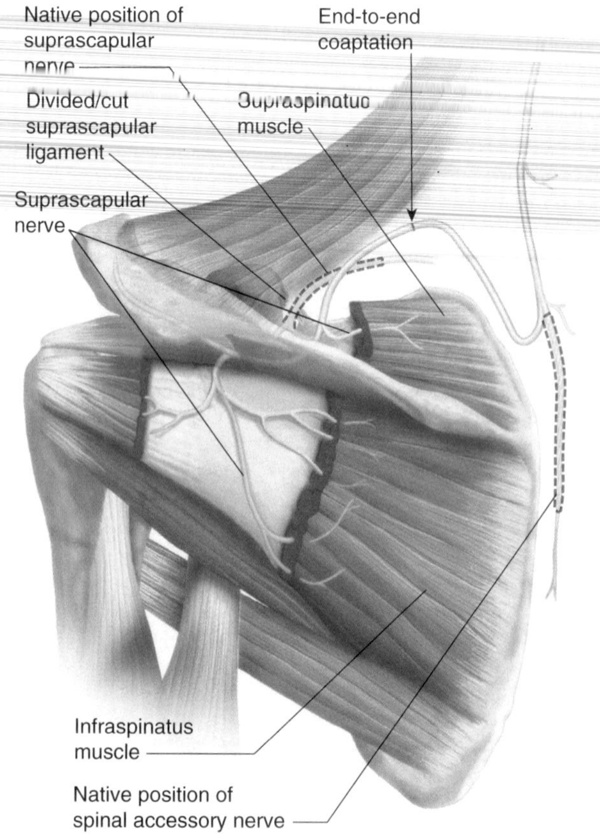

FIGURE 71.6. Spinal accessory nerve to suprascapular nerve transfer for shoulder external rotation. The spinal accessory nerve is in close proximity to the suprascapular nerve. Branches to the superior trapezius muscle can be left intact to minimize donor morbidity. The suprascapular ligament can be divided to decompress the nerve with a posterior surgical approach.

elbow flexion outcomes were similar to grafting at 1 to 2 years follow-up.[39] Chang et al., however, found improved supination with the transfer versus grafting (100 versus 19 degrees), whereas grafting resulted in greater pronation (30 versus 0 degrees).[39] The *triple transfer* of spinal accessory to suprascapular, Oberlin transfer, and radial to axillary shows improved supination and shoulder external rotation compared to grafting.[40,41] Perhaps of greater importance, their group found no donor morbidity with the transfers. Operative time was significantly reduced from more than 8 hours for plexus exploration and grafting to an average of less than 3 hours for the triple transfer, and there was a concomitant drop in length of hospital stay.[40,41] Although there have been no prospective trials of nerve transfers as primary interventions, these results are promising.

The elephant in the room with these studies is the role of neuroma excision and grafting in *sensory outcomes.* Assessments of adults with grafted BRBPP show minimal evidence of chronic pain and remarkably good sensory function, whereas unoperated BRBPP have more mixed outcomes with some reports of chronic pain.[42] Sole utilization of distal transfers for motor function leaves the possibility of sensory recovery through the neuroma, but in cases of severe injury, such as avulsions, lack of proximal reconstruction could prevent sensory recovery. Effects on development of chronic pain are unknown.

Lower Extremity Nerve Transfers

Given the greater regeneration lengths needed in the lower extremity and the excellent outcomes of lower extremity prosthetics, nerve transfers in the lower extremity have not progressed with same rapidity as those in the upper extremity.

Femoral

The femoral nerve most critically supplies the quadriceps and is responsible for knee extension. Unfortunately, this nerve can be injured in common procedures such as total hip arthroplasty. The anterior branch of the obturator, supplying the gracilis, adductor longus, and adductor brevis, can serve as a donor to the femoral branches to rectus femoris and vastus medialis. The rectus femoris provides a straight pull for knee extension whereas the medial pull of the vastus medialis balances the lateral pull of the tensor fascia latae, innervated by the superior gluteal nerve. A case series of two patients demonstrated Medical Research Council (MRC) 4 knee extension and hip flexion, and both patients regained the ability to ambulate normally.[43]

Tibial

Tibial nerve function is a critical decision point for lower extremity amputation. Loss of protective sensation to the plantar foot is linked to failure of limb salvage. The predominant motor role of the tibial nerve is plantar flexion. In proximal tibial nerve injuries, there are multiple redundant femoral branches to the quadriceps muscles that can be used as donors. Branches to the vastus medialis and vastus lateralis can be transferred to the tibial branches of the gastrocnemius to return plantar flexion. This transfer is challenging as the donor and recipient are a significant distance apart. With sufficient neurolysis of the medial gastrocnemius branch, an ETE coaptation can be made with the donor; however, a nerve graft is necessary to connect the vastus lateralis to the lateral gastrocnemius. In two published cases, patients attained MRC 3/3 + gastrocnemius strength.[44] Sensation can be restored with a saphenous to tibial nerve transfer, but the distance between these nerves requires an interposition graft. Transfer of the deep peroneal for plantar sensation has also been successful.[45]

Peroneal

The peroneal branch of the sciatic nerve is unusually superficial and may be involved in knee dislocations and tibial fractures. Peroneal nerve deficits result in foot drop. The tibial nerve branches to flexor digitorum longus or flexor hallucis longus can be used as donors to the anterior tibialis to restore extension. Few case series have been published and they vary in reported outcomes: MRC 4 or better outcomes ranged from 9% to 78%.[46,47] In a case series of 11 patients with average follow-up of 18 months, Giufre et al. reported only one MRC 4 result, notably in a 15-year-old. The remainder of the patients ranged in age from 18 to 59 years, and only three of these reached MRC 3 extension.[46] However, 7 of the 11 no longer required an ankle-foot orthotic. In contrast, Ferris et al. reported seven of nine patients achieving MRC 4 ankle extension by 8 to 26 months postoperatively, with an average follow-up of 30.8 months.[47] Patient age, time from injury, and length of follow-up likely contribute to the discrepancy in outcomes; more studies are necessary before this transfer comes into common use.

POSTOPERATIVE CARE

Postoperative care is important to obtaining successful outcomes after nerve transfer. The surgical dressing frequently includes a splint or bulky soft dressing that is removed at postoperative day 2 or 3. Patients begin working with a therapist who is knowledgeable about motor retraining ideally preoperatively and then beginning at 3 to 4 weeks postoperatively to begin contractions of donor nerve muscles. For sensory transfers, sensory input to the newly reinnervated region is critical for cortical relearning. Cortical remapping is essential for successful outcomes in both motor and sensory nerve transfers.

REFERENCES

1. Gohritz A, Dellon LA, Guggenheim M, et al. Otfrid Foerster (1873–1941)—self-taught neurosurgeon and innovator of reconstructive peripheral nerve surgery. *J Reconstr Microsurg.* 2013;29(1):33-43.
2. Gordon T, Yang JF, Ayer K, et al. Recovery potential of muscle after partial denervation: a comparison between [illegible] and humans. *Brain Res Bull.* 1993;30(3-4):477-482.
3. Schreiber JJ, Byun DJ, Khair MM, et al. Optimal axon counts for brachial plexus nerve transfers to restore elbow flexion. *Plast Reconstr Surg.* 2015;135(1):135e-141e.
4. Terzis JK, Wang W, Zhao Y. Effect of axonal load on the functional and aesthetic outcomes of the cross-facial nerve graft procedure for facial reanimation. *Plast Reconstr Surg.* 2009;124(5):1499-1512.
5. Leland HA, Azadgoli B, Gould DJ, Seruya M. Investigation into the optimal number of intercostal nerve transfers for musculocutaneous nerve reinnervation: a systematic review. *Hand (NY).* 2017;13(6):621-626. doi:10.1177/1558944717744280.
6. Viterbo F, Amr AH, Stipp EJ, Reis FJ. End-to-side neurorrhaphy: past, present, and future. *Plast Reconstr Surg.* 2009;124(6 suppl):e351-358.
7. Cederna PS, Kalliainen LK, Urbanchek MG, et al. "Donor" muscle structure and function after end-to-side neurorrhaphy. *Plast Reconstr Surg.* 2001;107(3):789-796.
8. Slattery WH, Cassis AM, Wilkinson EP, et al. Side-to-end hypoglossal to facial anastomosis with transposition of the intratemporal facial nerve. *Otol Neurotol.* 2014;35(3):509-513.
9. Farber SJ, Glaus SW, Moore AM, Hunter DA, Mackinnon SE, Johnson PJ. Supercharge nerve transfer to enhance motor recovery: a laboratory study. *J Hand Surg Am.* 2013;38(3):466-477.
10. Davidge KM, Yee A, Moore AM, Mackinnon SE. The supercharge end-to-side anterior interosseous-to-ulnar motor nerve transfer for restoring intrinsic function: clinical experience. *Plast Reconstr Surg.* 2015;136(3):344e-352e.
The supercharge technique can be used in scenarios wherein native regeneration is anticipated or some quantity of native axons remain intact. This article reviews the efficacy of supercharge transfers of the AIN branch to pronator quadratus to the ulnar motor branch in injuries ranging from sharp proximal transection to neuritis and chronic radiculopathies. The authors found that there was no donor deficit and over 70% of patients achieved MRC over 3 versus 15% preoperatively. The authors carefully parse out the contributions of the supercharge by assessing the time course of recovery versus what would be expected based on the level of the lesion.
11. Wan H, Zhang L, Li D, et al. Hypoglossal-facial nerve "side"-to-side neurorrhaphy for persistent incomplete facial palsy. *J Neurosurg.* 2014;120(1):263-272.
12. Dellon AL, Ferreira MC, Williams EH, Rosson GD. Which end is up? Terminology for terminolateral (end-to-side) nerve repair: a review. *J Reconstr Microsurg.* 2010;26(5):295-301.
13. Terzis JK, Tzafetta K. The "babysitter" procedure: minihypoglossal to facial nerve transfer and cross-facial nerve grafting. *Plast Reconstr Surg.* 2009;123(3):865-876.
14. Bain JR, Veltri KL, Chamberlain D, Fahnestock M. Improved functional recovery of denervated skeletal muscle after temporary sensory nerve innervation. *Neuroscience.* 2001;103(2):503-510.
15. Zhang F, Lineaweaver WC, Ustüner T, et al. Comparison of muscle mass preservation in denervated muscle and transplanted muscle flaps after motor and sensory reinnervation and neurotization. *Plast Reconstr Surg.* 1997;99(3):803-814.
16. Placheta E, Wood MD, Lafontaine C, et al. Enhancement of facial nerve motoneuron regeneration through cross-face nerve grafts by adding end-to-side sensory axons. *Plast Reconstr Surg.* 2015;135(2):460-471.

17. Snyder-Warwick AK, Fattah AY, et al. The degree of facial movement following microvascular muscle transfer in pediatric facial reanimation depends on donor motor nerve axonal density. *Plast Reconstr Surg.* 2015;135(2):370e-381e.
18. Coombs CJ, Ek EW, Wu T, et al. Masseteric-facial nerve coaptation–an alternative technique for facial nerve reinnervation. *J Plast Reconstr Aesthet Surg.* 2009;62(12):1580-1588.
The masseteric nerve provides a reliable and strong neurotization source for free functional gracilis transfer to the face for dynamic smile reconstruction. In this study, histomorphometric data obtained from masseteric nerve biopsies at the time of gracilis transfer showed an average of 1542 myelinated axons. Based on these data, direct masseteric to buccal branch or facial nerve trunk transfers for facial reanimation were performed in three patients. Outcomes demonstrated improved symmetry at rest and with animation, as well as the possibility for spontaneous expression. No donor morbidity resulted from masseteric nerve use.
19. Borschel GH, Kawamura DH, Kasukurthi R, et al. The motor nerve to the masseter muscle: an anatomic and histomorphometric study to facilitate its use in facial reanimation. *J Reconstr Aesthet Surg.* 2012;65(3):363-366.
This article describes the anatomic landmarks for location of the masseteric nerve. In this cadaver study, the masseteric nerve was consistently located 3.16 cm anterior to the tragus, 1.08 cm inferior to the inferior border of the zygomatic arch, and 1.48 cm deep to the SMAS. The masseteric nerve makes a 50-degree angle with the zygomatic arch and travels 1.33 cm inferior to the arch before branching. The masseteric nerve has an average of 2775 myelinated fibers.
20. Mundschenk MB, Sachanandani NS, Borschel GH, et al. Motor nerve to the masseter: a pediatric anatomic study and the "3:1 rule"Motor nerve to the masseter: a pediatric anatomic study and the "3:1 rule"Motor nerve to the masseter: a pediatric anatomic study and the "3:1 rule". *J Plast Reconstr Aesthet Surg.* 2018;71(1):54-56.
21. Manktelow RT, Tomat LR, Zuker RM, Chang M. Smile reconstruction in adults with free muscle transfer innervated by the masseter motor nerve: effectiveness and cerebral adaptation. *Plast Reconstr Surg.* 2006;118(4):885-899.
22. Chen G, Wang W, Wang W, et al. Symmetry restoration at rest after masseter-to-facial nerve transfer: is it as efficient as smile reanimation? *Plast Reconstr Surg.* 2017;140(4):793-801.
23. Mahan MA, Sivakumar W, Weingarten D, Brown JM. Deep temporal nerve transfer for facial reanimation: anatomic dissections and surgical case report. *Oper Neurosurgery (Hagerstown, Md).* 2017.
24. Rodriguez-Lorenzo A, Jensson D, Weninger WJ, Schmid M, Meng S, Tzou CH. Platysma motor nerve transfer for restoring marginal mandibular nerve function. *Plast Reconstr Surg Glob Open.* 2016;4(12):e1164.
25. Terzis JK, Dryer MM, Bodner BI. Corneal neurotization: a novel solution to neurotrophic keratopathy. *Plast Reconstr Surg.* 2009;123(1):112-120.
26. Elbaz U, Bains R, Zuker RM, et al. Restoration of corneal sensation with regional nerve transfers and nerve grafts: a new approach to a difficult problem. *JAMA Ophthalmol.* 2014;132(11):1289-1295.
Corneal neurotization is a fascinating application of nerve transfers for restoring corneal sensation and preventing blindness resulting from corneal ulcerations and or perforations. This study reviews the outcomes from four corneal neurotization procedures secondary to acquired corneal anesthesia in children. All four patients achieved meaningful corneal sensation using supratrochlear donor nerves and a nerve graft to directly neurotize the cornea.
27. Fung SSM, Catapano J, Elbaz U, et al. In vivo confocal microscopy reveals corneal reinnervation after treatment of neurotrophic keratopathy with corneal neurotization. *Cornea.* 2018;37(1):109-112.
28. Koshima I, Narushima M, Mihara M, et al. Cross-face nerve transfer for established trigeminal branch II palsy. *Ann Plast Surg.* 2009;63(6):621-623.
29. Goubier JN, Teboul F. Rhomboid nerve transfer to the suprascapular nerve for shoulder reanimation in brachial plexus palsy: a clinical report. *Hand Surg Rehabil.* 2016;35(5):363-366.
30. Koshy JC, Agrawal NA, Seruya M. Nerve transfer versus interpositional nerve graft reconstruction for posttraumatic, isolated axillary nerve injuries: a systematic review. *Plast Reconstr Surg.* 2017;140(5):953-960.
31. Oberlin C, Béal D, Leechavengvongs S, et al. Nerve transfer to biceps muscle using a part of ulnar nerve for C5-C6 avulsion of the brachial plexus: anatomical study and report of four cases. *J Hand Surg Am.* 1994;19(2):232-237.
32. Mackinnon SE, Novak CB, Myckatyn TM, Tung TH. Results of reinnervation of the biceps and brachialis muscles with a double fascicular transfer for elbow flexion. *J Hand Surg Am.* 2005;30(5):978-985.
33. Carlsen BT, Kircher MF, Spinner RJ, et al. Comparison of single versus double nerve transfers for elbow flexion after brachial plexus injury. *Plast Reconstr Surg.* 2011;127(1):269-276.
34. García-López A, Navarro R, Martinez F, Rojas A. Nerve transfers from branches to the flexor carpi radialis and pronator teres to reconstruct the radial nerve. *J Hand Surg Am.* 2014;39(1):50-56.
35. Flores LP. Comparative study of nerve grafting versus distal nerve transfer for treatment of proximal injuries of the ulnar nerve. *J Reconstr Microsurg.* 2015;31(9):647-653.
36. Kovachevich R, Kircher MF, Wood CM, et al. Complications of intercostal nerve transfer for brachial plexus reconstruction. *J Hand Surg Am.* 2010;35(12):1995-2000.
37. Zheng MX, Xu WD, Qiu YQ, et al. Phrenic nerve transfer for elbow flexion and intercostal nerve transfer for elbow extension. *J Hand Surg Am.* 2010;35(8):1304-1309.
38. Tse R, Marcus JR, Curtis CG, et al. Suprascapular nerve reconstruction in obstetrical brachial plexus palsy: spinal accessory nerve transfer versus C5 root grafting. *Plast Reconstr Surg.* 2011;127(6):2391-2396.
39. Chang KWC, Wilson TJ, Popadich M, et al. Oberlin transfer compared with nerve grafting for improving early supination in neonatal brachial plexus palsy. *J Neurosurg Pediatr.* 2018;21(2):178-184.
40. Ladak A, Morhart M, O'Grady K, et al. Distal nerve transfers are effective in treating patients with upper trunk obstetrical brachial plexus injuries: an early experience. *Plast Reconstr Surg.* 2013;132(6):985e-992e.
41. O'Grady KM, Power HA, Olson JL, et al. Comparing the efficacy of triple nerve transfers with nerve graft reconstruction in upper trunk obstetric brachial plexus injury. *Plast Reconstr Surg.* 2017;140(4):747-756.
Reconstruction of birth related brachial plexus palsies has evolved significantly over the last several decades. The incorporation of distal nerve transfers into the armamentarium for treating these injuries brings several advantages: reduced operative time, reduced hospital stay, and equivalent to improved outcomes. This article reviews an approach to upper trunk injuries utilizing three different nerve transfers: spinal accessory to suprascapular, radial branch to triceps transfer to axillary, and ulnar branch to FCU transfer to musculocutaneous.
42. Anand P, Birch R. Restoration of sensory function and lack of long-term chronic pain syndromes after brachial plexus injury in human neonates. *Brain.* 2002;125(Pt 1): 113-122.
43. Tung TH, Chao A, Moore AM. Obturator nerve transfer for femoral nerve reconstruction: anatomic study and clinical application. *Plast Reconstr Surg.* 2012;130(5):1066-1074.
44. Moore AM, Krauss EM, Parikh RP, et al. Femoral nerve transfers for restoring tibial nerve function: an anatomical study and clinical correlation: a report of 2 cases. *J Neurosurg.* 2018;129(4):1024-1033.
45. Koshima I, Nanba Y, Tsutsui T, Takahashi Y. Deep peroneal nerve transfer for established plantar sensory loss. *J Reconstr Microsurg.* 2003;19(7):451-454.
46. Giuffre JL, Bishop AT, Spinner RJ, et al. Partial tibial nerve transfer to the tibialis anterior motor branch to treat peroneal nerve injury after knee trauma. *Clin Orthop Relat Res.* 2012;470(3):779-790.
47. Ferris S, Maciburko SJ. Partial tibial nerve transfer to tibialis anterior for traumatic peroneal nerve palsy. *Microsurgery.* 2017;37(6):596-602.
Lower extremity nerve transfers are emerging techniques. Foot drop from common peroneal palsy is debilitating, and outcomes for nerve transfers addressing this problem have had previously relatively poor results in adults. In this prospective series, tibial donors, generally branches to flexor digitorum longus, were used for transfers to tibialis anterior. The series reports 7 of 9 patients achieving MRC better than 4.

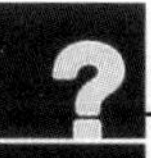

QUESTIONS

1. **A 12-year-old boy presents after falling out of a tree with a right radial nerve avulsion injury proximal to the elbow. The patient is otherwise healthy, is right hand dominant, and enjoys sports and playing the piano. Following an initial washout, the patient returns for definitive reconstruction 3 weeks later. What procedure will give him the best independent finger function?**

   a. Sural nerve grafting to the radial nerve
   b. FCR to extensor digitorum communis tendon transfer
   c. FDS III to extensor digitorum communis III, IV, and V and FDS IV to extensor indicis pollicis tendon transfer
   d. Median branch to FCR nerve transfer to posterior interosseous nerve

2. **A 32-year-old man presents 6 months after a motorcycle accident. He complains of being unable to button his shirt, generalized hand weakness, and weak elbow flexion. An electromyography (EMG) is performed and shows normal motor units in the deltoid and biceps, and there are fibrillations and motor unit potentials in the FCU and the first dorsal interosseous. What intervention will best improve his hand function?**

   a. Transfer of the anterior interosseous branch to pronator quadratus end-to-end to the ulnar motor branch
   b. Transfer of the anterior interosseous branch to pronator quadratus end-to-side (*supercharge*) to the ulnar motor branch
   c. End-to-end Oberlin transfer of the ulnar fascicle to FCU to the musculocutaneous branch to biceps
   d. Continued observation

3. **Twelve months after a knee dislocation injury in a basketball game, a [illegible]-year-old man seeks care for his foot drop. He has reduced sensation along the lateral calf and no anterior tibialis function. What is the most appropriate intervention?**

   a. Posterior tibial tendon transfer to the anterior tibialis tendon
   b. Superficial peroneal nerve decompression
   c. Transfer of the tibial branch to flexor hallucis longus to the deep peroneal branch to tibialis anterior
   d. Transfer of the femoral branch to vastus medialis to the deep peroneal branch to tibialis anterior

4. **A 3-month-old boy presents with a left flail arm and history of shoulder dystocia. At birth, he had a left Horner syndrome that has improved significantly. On examination he has a complete flail arm. Which of the following is correct?**

   a. Excision of the neuroma and nerve root grafting will likely result in near normal function.
   b. The child should be reassessed at 9 months of age with the *cookie test* before determining if an intervention is necessary.
   c. Transfer of the spinal accessory nerve to the suprascapular, intercostal transfer to musculocutaneous, and contralateral C7 transfer for posterior cord will result in the best outcomes.
   d. Transfer of the spinal accessory nerve to the suprascapular, Oberlin transfer and radial branch to triceps to axillary nerve will result in the best outcomes.

5. **A 15-year-old boy presents for evaluation of facial palsy 10 months after resection of a vascular malformation in the brainstem. The patient's facial movement has been unchanged since surgery. On examination, the patient has unilateral complete facial paralysis, and EMG evaluation show no evidence of motor unit potentials on that side of the face. What is the best technique to reconstruct dynamic smile in this patient?**

   a. Segmental sural nerve graft within the ipsilateral buccal branch of the facial nerve
   b. Ipsilateral masseteric nerve transfer to the buccal branch
   c. Cross facial sural nerve graft from the contralateral buccal branch to the affected buccal branch
   d. Free functional muscle transfer to the affected face with neurotization via a cross-facial nerve graft

1. **Answer: d.** In this scenario, the proximal stump of the radial nerve is not available for grafting because it is avulsed. Tendon transfers will result in adequate finger extension, but independent motion will be impossible. The nerve transfer to the PIN will allow for independent finger extension.

2. **Answer: b.** The patient's complaint and EMG are consistent with a pan-plexus injury. However, the presence of motor unit potentials indicates that there is still continuity in the plexus, as is common in traction injuries associated with motorcycle accidents. The generalized hand weakness and weak pinch is indicative of intrinsic loss. Transfer of the anterior interosseous branch to pronator quadratus to the ulnar motor branch has the greatest likelihood of improving hand function given that the injury is quite proximal. As there is still continuity, an end-to-side transfer is most appropriate.

3. **Answer: a.** This patient has a foot drop from an injury to the common peroneal from a knee dislocation. At 12 months after injury and given his age, the best outcome is likely with tendon transfer. Although common peroneal decompression may improve recovery, especially sensory regeneration, the likelihood of regeneration in an older patient that long after injury is very low.

4. **Answer: c.** This infant likely has a complete avulsion injury of C5-T1, and thus there are likely no nerve roots available proximally for grafting. Additionally in the scenario of a flail arm and Horner syndrome, it is recommended that surgery be done prior to 6 months of age. Extraplexal transfers are likely the best option, bearing in mind what proximal donors are available. The Oberlin transfer and triceps to axillary transfer can only be done when C7, C8, and T1 are intact.

5. **Answer: b.** This patient is 10 months out from injury with no clinical or electrodiagnostic evidence of potential for motor recovery. Given the time from injury, the patient's native mimetic musculature is still amenable to reinnervation; therefore free functional muscle transfer is not required. Cross-facial nerve grafting would prolong time to reinnervation, potentially precluding reinnervation within the critical window. A proximal nerve stump is not available; therefore segmental grafting is not possible. Direct transfer of the masseteric nerve to the affected buccal branch provides the most rapid and robust reinnervation for smile.

CHAPTER 72 Management of Brachial Plexus Injuries

Frank Fang and Kevin C. Chung

KEY POINTS

- Brachial plexus injuries are permanently disabling. Even the best results from surgical interventions are only partially restorative of the original functional capacity.
- Surgery is undertaken for closed injuries when physical examination and diagnostic modalities show a plateau or absence of functional recovery (ideally 3–5 months post trauma).
- Surgical interventions can be organized into three broad categories: proximal exploration and reconstruction, distal nerve transfers, and biomechanical restorations.
- Adult and infant brachial plexus injuries are different pathologic entities with varying strategies of surgical intervention.
- There are multiple prevailing philosophies upon management of brachial plexus injuries; rigorous outcomes studies to produce evidence-based conclusions upon best practices are still pending.

Brachial plexus injuries occur in two general categories: adult trauma and obstetric birth trauma. Surgical intervention for these injuries can be categorized into three basic groups—proximal explorations with nerve transfers or nerve grafting, distal (close target) nerve transfers, and biomechanical restorations (tendon transfers and functioning free muscle transplantations). Differing opinions exist regarding the merits and drawbacks of these three groups and their applications. Owing to the atrophy and fibrosis of the neuromuscular junctions that occur approximately 12 to 18 months after denervation, the time elapsed since trauma is the most important factor to consider when determining which surgical intervention is appropriate. The treatment course for these injuries can span a lifetime, and the technical difficulty of many of the involved procedures is high. Permanent functional disability is certain. The severity of the life-changing impairment depends upon the magnitude and foci of the injury. For clarity of presentation within the scope of this chapter, we will first discuss adult brachial plexus followed by coverage of obstetric brachial plexus palsy.

EPIDEMIOLOGY

The mechanism of injury for adult brachial plexus trauma varies by region. The energy of injury differs by the mechanism of injury. For instance, lower-speed moped-associated injuries (accounting for >90% of brachial plexus injuries in regions such as Taiwan, Southeast Asia, and India) generally have a lower energy than high-speed motor vehicle or motorcycle accidents (approximately 84% of cases in Europe and North America).[1,2] Lower-energy mechanisms tend to produce postganglionic nerve ruptures (breakages within the substance of the peripheral nerve, distal to the dorsal root ganglion) as compared with higher-energy mechanisms which tend to produce more preganglionic root avulsions (tearing of the rootlets of the peripheral nerve directly from the spinal cord, proximal to the dorsal root ganglion). Gunshot wounds are typically seen in war zones and also commonly in the United States (17% of brachial plexus injuries), and they can be subdivided into high-velocity (military rifles, hunting rifles, shotguns) versus lower-velocity (handgun) trauma with implications upon prognosis and management.[3–5] Lastly, sharp lacerating injuries of the brachial plexus, such as with knife attacks, account for approximately 10% of presenting cases at a trauma center in the U.S. Despite regional variations in the mechanism of injury, adult brachial plexus trauma mostly affects young males worldwide (>90%).[1]

ANATOMY

The brachial plexus is a confluence of interconnecting nerves that reside in between where the spinal nerves emanate from the spinal cord and ultimately course into the shoulder girdle and upper extremity muscles. Each spinal nerve is formed from rootlets of the ventral and dorsal roots that arise from the spinal cord and unite as the spinal nerve before exiting the dural sac of the spinal cord and running along a groove within the bony vertebra between the anterior and posterior tubercles of the transverse processes of C5 to T1. The dorsal root, which contributes sensory nerves only, is thicker and more resistant to avulsion forces. To note, anatomical variations exist where a prefixed or postfixed brachial plexus has substantive contribution to the innervation of the upper or lower trunk from a C4 or T2 spinal nerve, respectively. These variants may cause a less severe injury deficit than expected for a given injury. The dorsal root ganglion is generally positioned just posterior and medial to the vertebral artery, and it is thus contained within the vertebral bony structure and not visible upon surgical exposure, unless the spinal nerve has been avulsed distally[6] (Figure 72.1). The spinal nerves then coalesce into the upper (C5 and C6), middle (C7), and lower (C8 and T1) trunks which are contained between the anterior and middle scalenic muscles. Each trunk then splits into anterior and posterior divisions within the area deep to the clavicle. To note, the upper trunk's anterior and posterior divisions are also positioned very close to the branch point of the suprascapular nerve, to give the appearance of a trifurcation of nerves near that point. Also notable, the posterior division of lower trunk is quite small. After the divisions emerge inferior to the clavicle, they become the lateral, posterior, and medial cords in the area deep to the pectoralis minor (that inserts upon the useful bony landmark of the coracoid process). At the cord level, the axillary artery is sandwiched between the three cords. From the cords arise the branches that innervate the shoulder girdle and distal upper extremity. The axillary and radial nerve are separable at the region of the posterior cord deep to the lateral border of the pectoralis minor. The musculocutaneous nerve can be located at the proximal arm in the plane between the coracobrachialis and biceps brachialis. The median and ulnar nerves are most easily found in the mid-distal arm deep to the brachial veins as they wrap around the brachial artery (Figure 72.2).

ANATOMIC CLASSIFICATION OF BRACHIAL PLEXUS INJURY

There are multiple systems of anatomic classification of brachial plexus injury that have been popularized by major contributors to surgical advances in brachial plexus injury treatment. We will highlight three classification systems: Terzis' three-level system of root, supraclavicular postganglionic, and infraclavicular injuries[7]; the Alnot classification of preganglionic root, postganglionic root, supraclavicular and retroclavicular, and infraclavicular injuries[8]; and Chuang's level 1 to 4 classification separates injuries into preganglionic (root avulsion), postganglionic, pre- and retroclavicular, and infraclavicular injuries.[9] All three classifications consider the important factors of surgical decision-making: whether spinal root avulsion

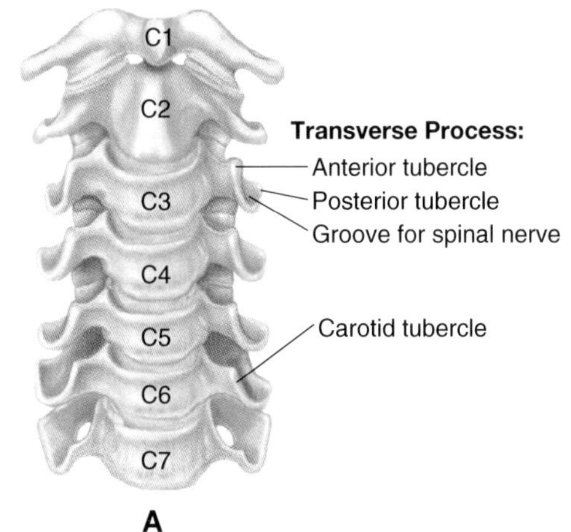

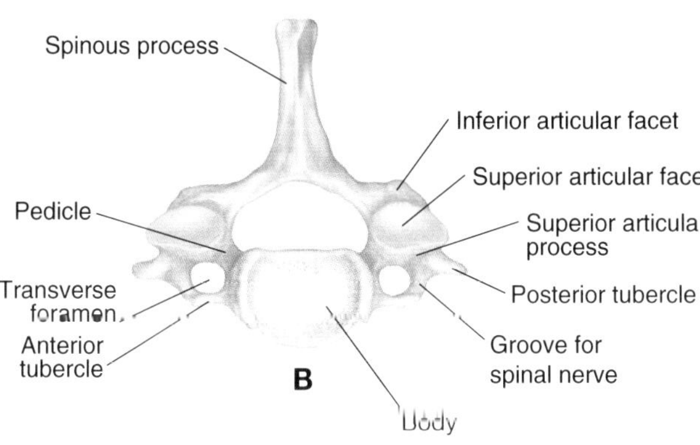

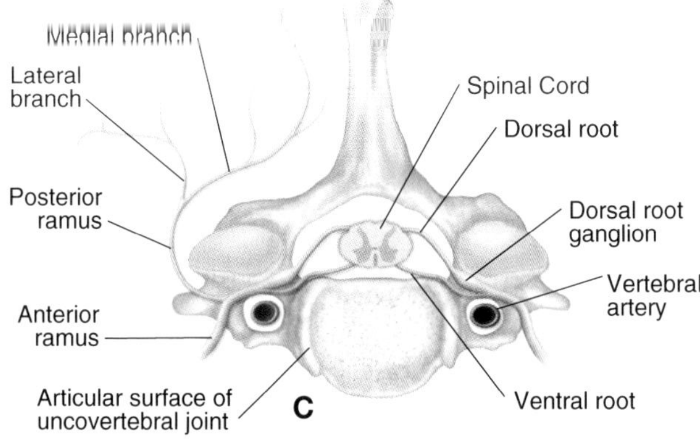

FIGURE 72.1. Spinal nerve and associated anatomy.

has occurred, the location of postganglionic rupture, and the clavicle as an operative landmark and barrier (**Table 72.1**).

Although any combination of spinal nerve rupture or avulsion is theoretically possible with adult trauma, some common injury patterns for closed brachial plexus injury are consistent worldwide with some variability in frequency[3]:

- C5-C6: 15%
- C5-C7: 20%–35%
- C8-T1: 10%
- C5-T1: 50%–70%

The higher frequency of upper trunk pathology with closed injuries may be related to the reflexive terminal position established by a person when encountering impending collision to the head and neck region. The blunt force at the shoulder region in combination with neck flexion to the contralateral side results in sudden caudal force trajectory upon the arm with the greatest energy directed upon the upper and middle trunks (Figure 72.2). Cephalic traction upon the arm with consequent lower trunk injury is much more rarely encountered, and this occurrence can often be attributed to a loss of consciousness prior to the time point of impact.

NERVE INJURY CLASSIFICATION

Classification systems of nerve injury delineate the range of injury from axonotmesis to neurotmesis with progressive involvement of endoneurium, perineurium, and epineurium as injury severity increases[10] (Figure 72.3). Most closed injuries of the brachial plexus are actually mixed in nature (Mackinnon's sixth degree injury). Thus, during the initial period of time (typically at least 3–6 months post trauma), the demyelinated and defunctionalized nerve is in a period where some of the injured elements that meet criteria for Mackinnon's first through third degrees of nerve injury severity will recover spontaneously. Allowing time for the nerve to recover spontaneously is akin to waiting for tissue demarcation as is done after thermal injury to the skin. However, with nerve trauma, it is unclear whether the final severity of the injury is determined by the damage of the initial trauma or if favorable and harmful factors during the initial period of time after trauma can affect the evolution of the final severity of the injury (such as with burn injury).

SURGICAL MANAGEMENT

Timing

Because of the spontaneous recovery that may occur during the initial period after closed brachial plexus trauma, most peripheral nerve surgeons advocate waiting for a period of 3 to 6 months before surgical intervention. Open injuries (e.g., stabbing) where laceration of the nerve is likely warrant exploration within 1 week for direct repair without nerve grafting. Exploration after 2 weeks should be accompanied by preparation for nerve grafting, as the nerve ends will have retracted.

Regarding gunshot wounds, most low-velocity gunshot injuries inflicted by handguns only have a small shock wave and zone of temporary cavitation. They contuse, bruise, and stretch the nerve more often than transecting it. Thus, most civilian gunshot wounds (handguns) are managed conservatively for the first 3 to 5 months in a manner similar to closed injuries. High-velocity gunshot injuries (military style rifles, hunting rifles, and shotguns) cause a large shock wave and permanent cavitation, usually inflicting greater than Mackinnon's fourth degree nerve injury. The prognosis for spontaneous recovery after a high-velocity gunshot wound is poor. Therefore, exploration of these injuries is advisable at 2 to 3 months post injury if clinical and electrodiagnostic evidence of recovery are still absent[4,5,11] (Figure 72.4).

History and Examination

The first visit to the peripheral nerve surgeon is frequently several weeks after the time of trauma, as care for multitrauma or life-threatening conditions will be prioritized. The decision to proceed with surgery is guided by clinical evaluation (history, physical examination, electrodiagnosis, and radiographic imaging [chest X-ray, CT myelography, and magnetic resonance imaging (MRI)]).

Elements of the patient's history can give clues to the type and location of injury to expect. The energy of the injuring mechanism (e.g., high-speed motor vehicle, motorcycle, train, moped at high or low speed, fall from height) is a relevant detail for estimating the severity of nerve injury. Concomitant injuries caused by the injuring mechanism are important to consider. Anterior shoulder dislocation and scapular fracture are associated with posterior cord damage.[12] Spine fractures indicate a more proximal focus of energy

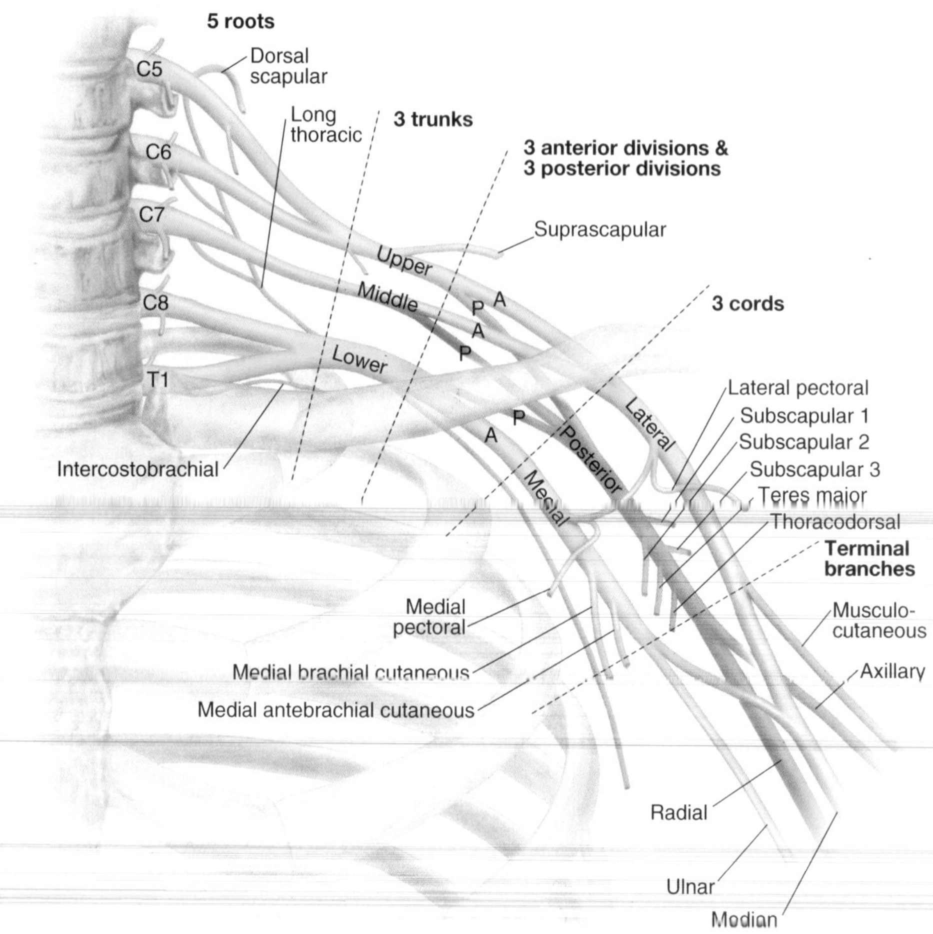

FIGURE 72.2. Brachial plexus anatomy.

from the injury mechanism; thus, the site of nerve rupture or avulsion is likely nearby as well.[13] The position of the patient's head, neck, and arm at the time of impact (if they were conscious) can direct the surgeon to suspect an upper trunk versus lower trunk foci of damage.[14]

The first goal of the physical examination is to determine where upon the brachial plexus the nerve ruptures or avulsions have occurred. To localize the deficit in axonal circuitry, it is helpful to use a chart to systematically examine the dermatomes of sensation and motor function of the shoulder girdle and upper extremity (Figure 72.5). Examination should proceed in a distal to proximal fashion. Deficits in the motor and sensory examination delinate approximately where the zone of injury is. The Hoffmann-Tinel sign is an indicator of regeneration of neurons and is also an indirect indicator of the site of nerve rupture during the early period of time after trauma.[15] Horner syndrome (pupillary miosis, upper eyelid ptosis, and anhidrosis upon the face of the ipsilateral side) indicates disruption of the sympathetic pathways (and a likely presence of a root avulsion involving the lower plexus which is situated just adjacent to the sympathetic plexus).[16] Deafferentation pain (a.k.a. phantom limb pain and sensation) is a sign that root avulsion has occurred. Deafferentation pain is sometimes described as causalgia (pain that is severe, burning in nature, and lancinating).[17] Examination at 1 month intervals from the time of trauma until 3 to 5 months after trauma is an acceptable schedule.

Radiographic imaging is used in conjunction with physical examination. On chest X-ray, diaphragmatic muscle paralysis (hemidiaphragmatic elevation on the injured side) suggests a likely involvement of the upper plexus as the diaphragmatic innervation (C3, C4, and C5) that is involved in the zone of injury is located near the upper trunk. Diaphragmatic function also provides information to the surgeon for consideration about whether the phrenic and intercostal nerves may be used as donor nerves. Some will argue that the phrenic nerve should never be used as a donor nerve because of respiratory morbidity, whereas others believe that using the phrenic donor nerve is safe in lower-BMI patients.[18] Also, some surgeons argue against use of the intercostal nerves for donor innervation if the phrenic nerve on that side is not functional, for fear of respiratory morbidity.[19] MRI and CT myelography can both detect the presence of pseudomeningoceles adjacent to the vertebrae, which develop when the dura tears in conjunction with avulsion spinal nerve roots. MRI can also show

TABLE 72.1. BRACHIAL PLEXUS INJURY CLASSIFICATION SYSTEMS

Alnot	Terzis	Chuang
Preganglionic root	Preganglionic supraclavicular	Preganglionic root (level 1)
Postganglionic root	Postganglionic supraclavicular	Postganglionic spinal nerve (level 2)
Supra-/ retroclavicular	–	Pre-/retroclavicular (level 3)
Infraclavicular	Infraclavicular	Infraclavicular (level 4)

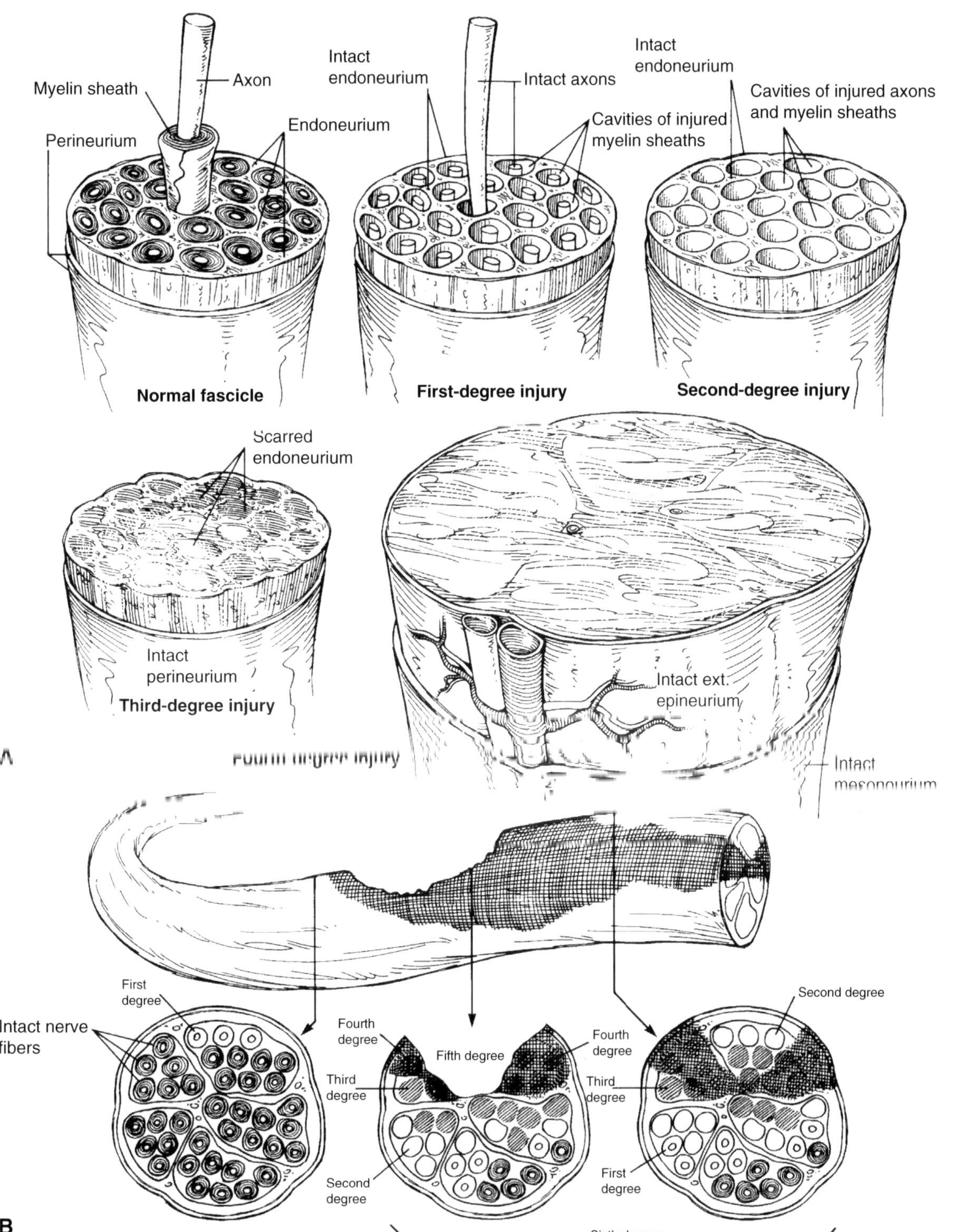

FIGURE 72.3. Classification of nerve injuries. **A.** Uninjured nerve consists of myelinated axons, surrounded by endoneurium, grouped into fascicles surrounded by perineum. The outer layer of the nerve is epineurium. In a first-degree injury, the axons are only demyelinated, whereas in a second-degree injury, the axons are injured and undergo degeneration. A third-degree injury includes damage to the axons, myelin, and endoneurium. A fourth-degree injury is a complete scar block that prevents any regeneration. A fifth-degree injury is a division of the nerve. **B.** The pattern of injury may vary from fascicle to fascicle along the nerve. This mixed pattern of injury is considered a sixth-degree injury.

various signal changes that suggest nerve injury. However, at the current time, MRI has not yet been proven as a reliable modality for delineating nerve rupture or injury within the plexus.[20]

Electrodiagnosis consists of both nerve conduction studies and needle electromyography (EMG). Nerve conduction studies use stimulating and recording electrodes to measure various parameters from both motor and sensory nerves. Needle EMG involves insertion of a needle (intramuscular recording electrode) into a muscle to record insertional, spontaneous, and voluntary electrical activity (useful tips in Table 72.2). The baseline nerve conduction study and EMG should be performed no earlier than 3 to 4 weeks after trauma, as certain acute phase injury changes take that amount of time to become detectable. A

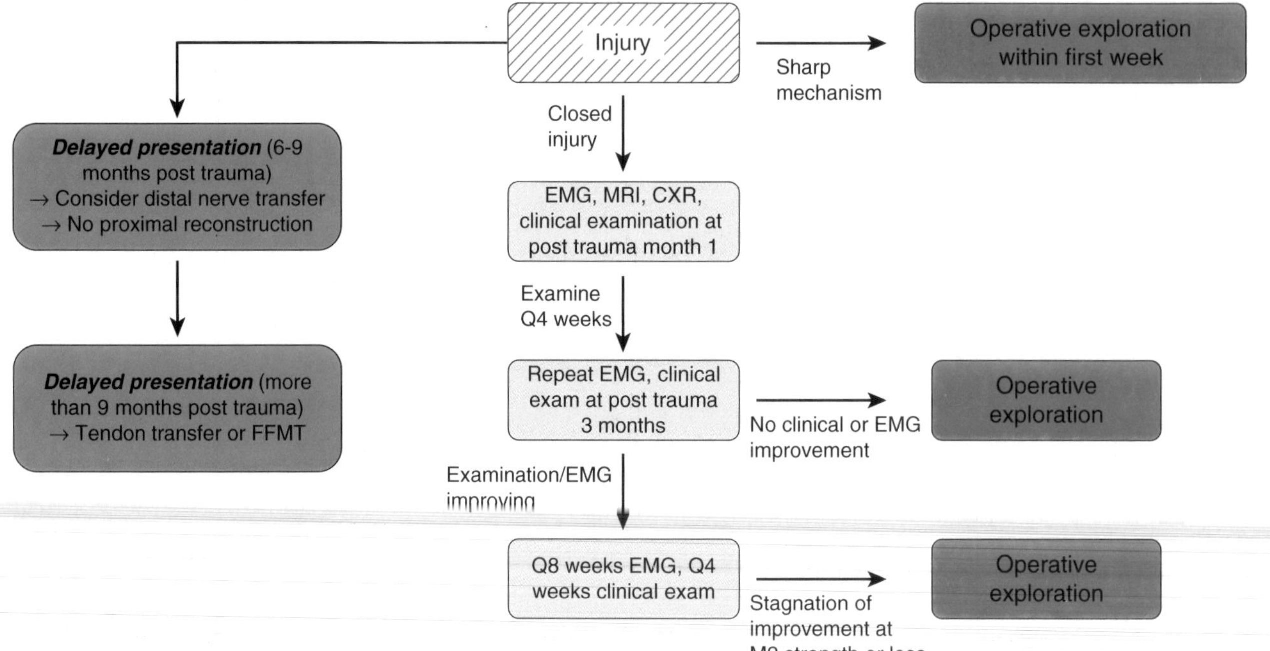

FIGURE 72.4. Approach to brachial plexus injury. *CXR*, chest X-ray; *EMG*, electromyography; *MRI*, magnetic resonance imaging.

follow-up electrodiagnostic study should be repeated at approximately 2-month intervals to monitor for spontaneous recovery versus stable denervation.[21]

A lack of improvement in motor function with progressive examinations combined with electrodiagnostic data consistent with stable denervation points to a state of irrecoverable nerve injury that can only be improved upon by surgical intervention. Contraindications to surgery include traumatic brain or spinal cord injuries that may prevent productive participation in a rehabilitative protocol. Also, medical comorbidities prohibitive of a prolonged general anesthetic session (>6–8 hours) must be considered before committing the patient to a surgical course. Joint contractures also need to be addressed concomitantly if they exist. The surgeon should also take careful consideration of the patient's willingness and ability to comply with postoperative rehabilitation for any patient who has already developed substantial joint contractures during the initial posttrauma time period.

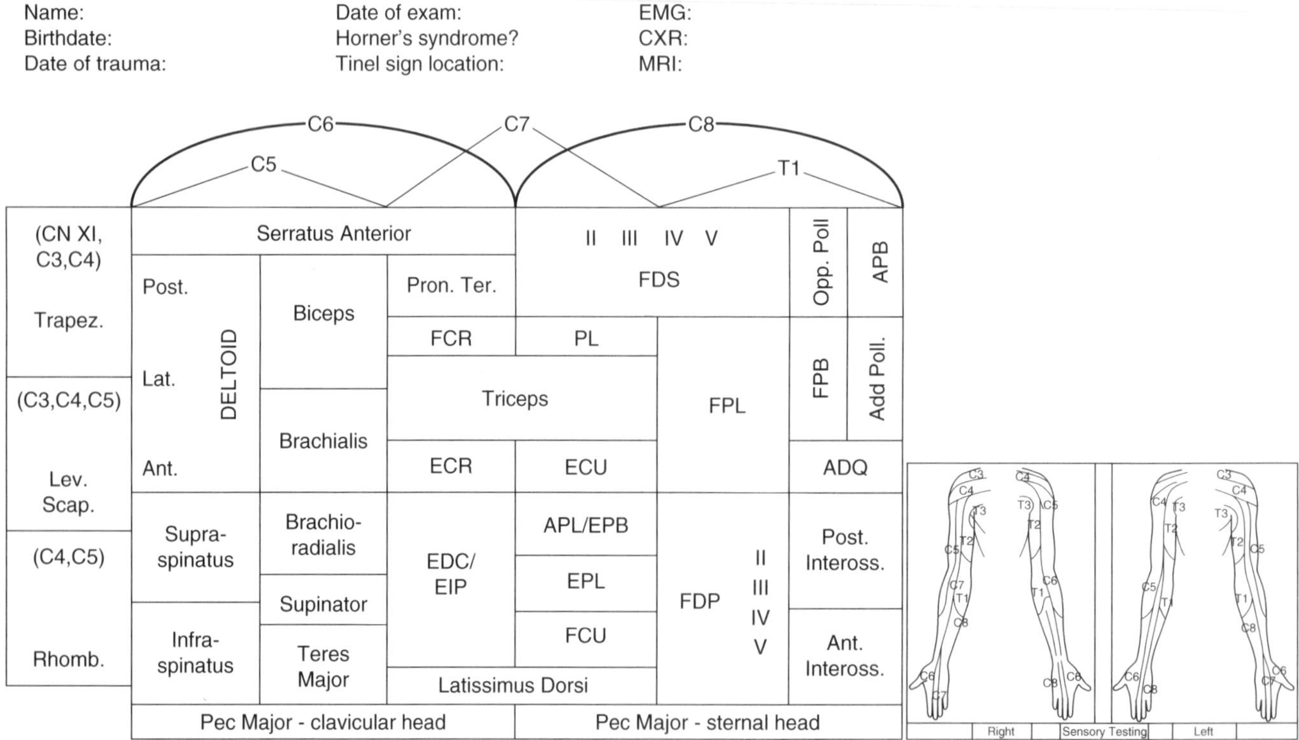

FIGURE 72.5. Worksheet for systematic physical examination of the brachial plexus patient.

TABLE 72.2. TIPS FOR INTERPRETING ELECTRODIAGNOSTIC STUDIES (EDSS)

Basics

Nerve Conduction Studies (NCSs)

- NCSs evaluate larger myelinated nerves.
- SNAP = *sensory nerve action potential* (sensory nerve)—begins to decrease at day 6 after injury and reach nadir at day 10–11.
    - Beware that sensory NCS tends to overestimate severity of injury.
- CMAP = *compound muscle action potential* (motor nerve)—begin to decrease at day 2 or 3 after injury and reach nadir at day 7.
    - CMAP amplitudes are the most useful for quantifying the amount of axon loss (at an early time point *before collateral reinnervation occurs-collateral reinnervation occurs from the remaining nerve fibers when there is an incomplete nerve transection*). Once collateral reinnervation starts to occur, the CMAP amplitude will appear to improve even though the number of degenerated motor nerve fibers is unchanged.
- Amplitude reflects the total number of conducting axons.

Needle Electromyography (EMG)

- MUAP = *(voluntary) motor unit action potential.* (A needle electrode is stuck into the muscle, and the patient voluntarily contracts the muscle; then action potentials are measured). MUAP dropout is proportional to the number of motor axons disrupted; however, MUAP dropout is challenging to quantify and thus less useful for estimating severity.
    - At the late time point (after collateral reinnervation has occurred), MUAP changes (duration and recruitment patterns) are better indicators for motor fiber loss than CMAP changes. However, at least 50% of the motor nerve must be disrupted before these MUAP changes can be discernible.
- The distal stump of a transected nerve can conduct action potentials for ~6 d (motor) and ~10 d (sensory)

Diagnostic Tips

- If muscle is innervated, there are no *spontaneous discharges* (fibrillations and positive sharp waves).
- If EDS shows decreased amplitude (not normal but also not severely decreased), then it suggests that the lesion is *not* a preganglionic avulsion; it is probably a postganglionic rupture and partial rupture of the sensory fibers too.
- PSW (positive sharp waves)—acute phase injury sign (should subside by 1 y post injury).
- Fibrillations—acute phase injury sign (does not appear until 2–3 wk after injury; they should subside by 1 y post injury).
    - Fibrillation potentials tend to overestimate the severity of injury—fibrillations may be quite prominent even when the lesion is minimal.
- Complete denervation (chronically fibrotic muscle will show no spontaneous discharge)—completely reinnervated muscle will also return to the state of no spontaneous discharge.
- Polyphasic waves: if more than five phases occur, the presence of motor unit is likely. Polyphasic waves are a pathologic finding, but the nerve is still alive.
- Fasciculations = *irregular*, normal, or complex MUAP. These can be exercise induced, or they can be indicative of lower motor neuron disorders or peripheral/metabolic neuropathy. (We do not really look at this parameter with acute nerve injury.)
- Voluntary motor units = reflect any presence of motor units (e.g., if empty, then no meaningful recovery, a poor prognostic indicator).
- Recruitment = reflects how many motor unit potentials have survived (e.g., Rare = only a few motor units are surviving, a poor prognostic indicator)
- Velocity will indicate demyelination (large fibers [radial nerve] should normally conduct 50–60 m/s; smaller fibers conduct 25–40 m/s).
- Degeneration of motor fibers is faster than sensory.
- If the EMG suggests no recording at all, then it is probably more accurate than physical examination (in cases where one thinks there may be [illegible] strength on physical examination).
- If motor nerve conduction (amplitude) is absent at 4 months after injury, this as a bad prognostic indicator, and surgical exploration is warranted.

Categories of Surgical Treatment

There are three general categories of surgical management of adult brachial plexus injury:

- Proximal exploration and reconstruction
- Distal (close target) nerve transfers
- Biomechanical restorations (tendon transfers and functioning free muscle transplantations [FFMTs])

Before nerve exploration and repair was possible, there was the biomechanical restorative approach (tendon transfers) that was being done as early as the 1930s with applications to brachial plexus injuries by the 1960s.[22] We have also included the functioning FFMTs that developed in the 1970s in this group.[23] The next approach to surgical intervention for brachial plexus injury was by proximal exploration and visualization of the site of injury directly with concomitant nerve reconstruction (nerve grafting or nerve transfers). Although surgery for the brachial plexus was first attempted in 1900, the field did not see significant advances until the advent of microsurgical techniques in the 1960s.[14] The most recent addition to the toolbox for brachial plexus reconstruction is the distal nerve transfers that utilize intact nerves remote to the zone of injury. With this category of technique developed in the 1990s, a portion of the intact innervation is used to replace the innervation that has been injured.[24] Certain factors affect the selection among these four strategies: time since trauma, surgeon comfort with technique, extent of zone of injury, and availability of donor nerves or musculotendinous units. To note, two or more of these therapeutic categories may be used on the same patient. Furthermore, these surgical categories may be used sequentially in time.

Proximal exploration is performed via a neck incision to gain access to the supraclavicular brachial plexus. The incision can be carried infraclavicularly onto the chest for access to the cords and terminal branches of the brachial plexus. This approach allows for both diagnostic and therapeutic objectives. Typically, nerve ruptures will require cable-grafting between the proximal and distal nerve stumps by using sural, saphenous, median antebrachial cutaneous, or lateral antebrachial cutaneous nerves harvested as nerve grafts. Allografts should not be used in this setting. Occasionally, osteotomy of the clavicle is necessary if the zone of injury terminates retroclavicularly, necessitating coaptation directly behind the clavicle. Root avulsions or spinal nerve ruptures with proximal stumps that are too short to support coaptation can be managed by nerve transfers using intraplexus transfer from proximal stumps of neighboring spinal nerves or from extraplexus donors (e.g., CN XI, contralateral C7, intercostal nerves, phrenic, or cervical motor branches of C3/C4). Proximal exploration is often thought of as the most technically daunting approach to brachial plexus injury because of the need for surgical dissection through the fibrotic scar tissue within the zone of injury. Exploration of the lower trunk can be risky in this regard, as adhesions to the pleural cavity and the proximity to great vessels in this case can sometimes also lead to pneumothorax or vessel injury. Postoperative neck immobilization is crucial, as head-turning can potentially disrupt the delicate nerve coaptations. Proximal exploration with the intent of nerve reconstruction should be done within the posttrauma 3- to 5-month timeframe, to ensure opportunity for reinnervation before the time of motor endplate fibrosis at the neuromuscular junction[9] (**Table 72.3**).

TABLE 72.3. RECONSTRUCTIVE OPTIONS WITH PROXIMAL EXPLORATION

Donor Nerve	Recipient Nerve	Technical Aspects	Functional Objective
CN (cranial nerve) XI (spinal accessory)	Suprascapular/posterior division of C5/C6	Use with phrenic (+/-cervical motor branches [CMBs])	Shoulder abduction
CMBs, (C3, C4)	Suprascapular/posterior division of C5/C6	Use with phrenic and CN XI. (CMBs are too weak to use alone)	Shoulder abduction
Phrenic	Suprascapular/posterior division of C5/C6	(+/-) CN XI and CMB. Phrenic is strong enough to use alone	Shoulder abduction
C5-ruptured proximal stump	Suprascapular/posterior division of C5/C6 versus anterior division upper trunk, median nerve	Will require cable grafting by sural nerve. Pick one target to avoid cross-innervation	Shoulder abduction, elbow flexion, or finger flexion
C6-ruptured proximal stump	Median nerve, C8	Will require cable grafting by sural nerve	Finger flexion
C7-ruptured proximal stump	Median nerve	Will require cable grafting by sural nerve	Finger flexion
Contralateral C7	Suprascapular/posterior division of C5/C6, anterior division upper trunk, median nerve	For five root injuries without other suitable donors. Needs a vascularized nerve graft (ulnar nerve). Pick one target to avoid cross-innervation	Shoulder abduction, elbow flexion, or finger flexion
Intercostal (T3, T4, T5)	Musculocutaneous nerve	Minimum of two intercostals needed. No nerve grafting	Elbow flexion

Distal (close target) nerve transfers are viable options in cases that are within the 3 to 9 month posttrauma timeframe and also with viable donor nerves available that can be used for reinnervating the deficit. The great benefit of this approach is that the operative site is outside of the zone of injury, and thus the surgeon can avoid the difficulty of operating through fibrotic tissue. Furthermore, the time period in which surgical intervention must be performed can be extended by 2 to 3 months (surgery at 6–9 month post trauma is reasonable) because of the much shorter distance that the innervating axons must travel to the target muscle. However, this category of surgical technique is also limited by the severity of injury. For instance, for total root (C5-T1) injuries, only intercostal nerves will be available for use. The disadvantage of distal motor nerve transfer is that it weakens the intact functional portions of the upper extremity in order to restore an incomplete amount of the original function to the injured portion of the upper extremity. Cortical adaptation with postoperative motor reeducation is also required for regaining the use of the reconstructed innervation[24] (**Table 72.4**). A number of accompanying sensory nerve transfers also have been described for restoring sensation (**Table 72.5**).

TABLE 72.4. DISTAL (CLOSE-TARGET) MOTOR NERVE TRANSFER OPTIONS

Deficit	Donor Nerve	Recipient Nerve	Functional Objective
Radial	FDS or FCR/PL fascicles of median nerve	ECRB branch of radial; PIN	Wrist extension, thumb/finger extension
	PT branch of median FCR branch of median	ECRL branch of radial; PIN	Wrist extension, thumb/finger extension
Median	Supinator or ECRB branches of radial nerve	AIN	Finger flexion, thumb flexion
	FCU branch ulnar nerve	AIN	Finger flexion, thumb flexion
	ECRB branch radial nerve/FCU branch ulnar nerve	AIN/PT branch median	Finger flexion, thumb flexion; pronation forearm
	ECRB radial ECRB/supinator radial	PT AIN	Pronation forearm Finger flexion, thumb flexion
	Brachialis branch of musculocutaneous	AIN	Finger flexion, thumb flexion
Distal median	Terminal branch of AIN	Recurrent motor branch median nerve	Thumb opposition
	Third lumbrical branch ulnar	Thenar branch median	Thumb opposition
Ulnar	Terminal branch of AIN	Ulnar motor branch	Ulnar intrinsic muscles
	EDQ/ECU branches of radial nerve	Ulnar motor branch	Ulnar intrinsic muscles
Musculocutaneous	Median and ulnar branches	Musculocutaneous	Elbow flexion
Axillary/suprascapular	Triceps branch of radial CN XI	Anterior branch of axillary nerve; suprascapular nerve	Shoulder abduction, external rotation

AIN, anterior interosseous nerve; *CN*, cranial nerve; *ECU*, extensor carpi ulnaris; *EDQ*, extensor digiti quinti; *ECRB*, extensor carpi radialis brevis; *FCR*, flexor carpi radialis; *FCU*, flexor carpi ulnaris; *FDS*, flexor digitorum superficialis; *PIN*, posterior interosseous nerve; *PL*, palmaris longus; *PT*, pronator teres.

TABLE 72.5. DISTAL SENSORY NERVE TRANSFER OPTIONS

Deficit	Donor Nerve	Recipient Nerve	Sensory Objective
Median	Dorsal cutaneous branch or fourth web space branch ulnar	First web space branch of median	First web space
	Superficial radial	Median nerve	Thumb, index, first web space
	Ulnar digital nerve ring finger	Radial digital nerve index finger	Radial aspect index finger
	Dorsal sensory branch radial	Radial digital nerve index finger	Radial aspect index finger
	Lateral antebrachial cutaneous	Median sensory	Thumb, index, middle fingers
Ulnar	Third web space median	Ulnar sensory branch	Little finger and ulnar aspect of ring
	Third common digital nerve	Ulnar sensory branch	Little finger and ulnar aspect of ring
	Palmar branch median	Ulnar sensory branch	Little finger and ulnar aspect of ring
	Posterior interosseous nerve (PIN)	Ulnar sensory branch	Little finger and ulnar aspect of ring

Biomechanical restoration (tendon transfers and functioning free muscle transplantation) are the third category of reconstruction. This is usually the chosen reconstructive strategy for cases of late presentation (>9 months after the time of injury) that have no opportunity for axonal regrowth within the timeframe before fibrosis of the motor endplates will occur at the neuromuscular junction. The option of tendon transfer or functioning free muscle transplantation is often used as the *lifeboat* for the aforementioned two categories or for augmentation of function after previous reconstruction. To note, conventional tendon transfers are only viable options for incomplete brachial plexus injury, when there are available donor musculotendinous units innervated by uninjured portions of the brachial plexus. Tendon transfers are often paired with arthrodeses (shoulder or wrist) for an enhanced functional result.[25] The gracilis myocutaneous flap is the most popular option for the FFMT for the upper extremity[26] (Tables 72.6 and 72.7).

Complications across these three categories can range from serious to more localized and minor. Proximal exploration can incur lymphatic leak, large vessel injury, or pneumothorax. Distal transfers are typically much safer with a less morbid complication profile with limited exceptions (pneumothorax for intercostal nerve transfer). Tendon transfers have similarly more localized failure consequences (tendon bowstringing, joint posture deviation, etc.). Functioning free muscle transplantations have the complication profile associated with microvascular free flap transfer—vascular pedicle thromboses with partial or total flap loss. Furthermore, the flap donor site can have local complications such as seroma, hematoma, or infection. FFMTs also require a donor nerve for neurotization, which can incur serious complications such as pneumothorax in cases where the intercostal nerves are used.

MULTIDISCIPLINARY APPROACH

Brachial plexus injuries demand a multidisciplinary approach with the involvement of physical medicine and rehabilitation, pain management, and psychiatry teams. From the time of the initial trauma, there is a need for physical therapy and occupational therapy involvement to maintain supple joints; reconstructive intervention is contraindicated if joints are ankylotic. The rehabilitative protocol must be diligently followed for several years after the surgical intervention in order to reap the full benefits of the surgery. Rehabilitative regimens include temperature therapy to aid with dysesthesia and pain, electrical stimulation to minimize atrophy of muscles, and range of motion exercises to maintain supple joints. Orthotic devices may help with shoulder stability and for providing a more natural posture so that the impairment of the injured extremity is less apparent. Involvement of a pain management team is frequently beneficial as the extreme causalgia associated with root avulsion injuries can be debilitating. Pain management therapy will involve pharmacologic agents such as opioid medications,

TABLE 72.6. BIOMECHANICAL RESTORATION: TENDON TRANSFER AND FUNCTIONING FREE MUSCLE TRANSPLANTATION—SHOULDER AND ELBOW

Anatomic Region	Surgical Intervention	Functional Objective	Alternate Intervention
Shoulder	Upper trapezius transfer	Shoulder abduction	Shoulder arthrodesis
	Lower trapezius transfer	External rotation	Shoulder arthrodesis
	Contralateral lower trapezius transfer	External rotation	Shoulder arthrodesis
	Latissimus dorsi transfer	Shoulder abduction, external rotation	Shoulder arthrodesis
Elbow	Biceps to triceps transfer	Elbow extension	
	Brachialis to triceps transfer	Elbow extension	
	Triceps to biceps transfer	Elbow flexion	
	Latissimus dorsi transfer	Elbow flexion	
	Pectoralis major transfer	Elbow flexion	
	Steindler flexorplasty	Elbow flexion	
	Gracilis FFMT (functioning free muscle transplantation)	Elbow flexion	

TABLE 72.7. BIOMECHANICAL RESTORATION: TENDON TRANSFER AND FUNCTIONING FREE MUSCLE TRANSPLANTATION—WRIST AND HAND

Deficit	Anatomic Region	Surgical Intervention	Functional Objective	Alternate Intervention
Radial nerve	Wrist	PT ECRL/ECRB	Wrist extension	Wrist arthrodesis
	Hand	FDS III/IV → EDC	Finger extension	
		FCU → EDC	Finger extension	
		FCR → EDC	Finger extension	
		PL → EPL	Thumb extension	Thumb arthrodesis
		FDS → EPL	Thumb extension	Thumb arthrodesis
Median nerve	Hand	Gracilis FFMT	Finger flexion	
		ECRL → FDP (index/long)	Finger flexion	
		FDP side/side (index/long → ring/small)	Finger flexion	
		BR → FPL	Thumb flexion	
		PL (Camitz)	Thumb opposition	Thumb arthrodesis
		EIP → APB	Thumb opposition	Thumb arthrodesis
		FDS via FCU loop → APB	Thumb opposition	Thumb arthrodesis
		ECRL → APB	Thumb opposition	Thumb arthrodesis
		ADM → APB	Thumb opposition	Thumb arthrodesis
		EDM → APB	Thumb opposition	Thumb arthrodesis
		ECU → EPB	Thumb opposition	Thumb arthrodesis
Ulnar nerve		Fowler wrist tenodesis	Claw correction	
		Zancolli (MCPJ) palmar capsulodesis)	Claw correction	
		EIP/EDM → extensor apparatus	Claw correction	
		FDS III/IV → lateral bands	Claw correction	
		ECRB or ECRL → lateral bands	Claw correction	
		PL → lateral bands	Claw correction	
		ECRB → ADP	Thumb pinch	Thumb arthrodesis
		FDS → ADP	Thumb pinch	Thumb arthrodesis
		EIP → ADP	Thumb pinch	Thumb arthrodesis

ADM, abductor digiti minimi; *ADP*, adductor pollicis; *APB*, abductor pollicis brevis; *BR*, brachioradialis; *ECRB*, extensor carpi radialis brevis; *ECRL*, extensor carpi radialis longus; *ECU*, extensor carpi ulnaris; *EDC*, extensor digitorum communis; *EDM*, extensor digiti minimi; *EIP*, extensor indicis proprius; *EPB*, extensor pollicis brevis; *EPL*, extensor pollicis longus; *FCR*, flexor carpi radialis; *FCU*, flexor carpi ulnaris; *FDP*, flexor digitorum profundus; *FDS*, flexor digitorum superficialis; *FFMT*, functioning free muscle transplantation; *FPL*, flexor pollicis longus; *MCPJ*, metacarpophalangeal joint; *PL*, palmaris longus; *PT*, pronator teres.

anticonvulsants (e.g., gabapentin, pregabalin), or cannabinoids. A high percentage of the brachial plexus–injured population develops chronic pain problems, and there are data suggesting the benefit of pursuing nonopioid therapy instead of narcotic medication. Gabapentin (Neurontin), pregabalin (Lyrica), and cannabinoids have been shown in rat studies to have trophic effects for regenerating neurons after sciatic nerve injury in rats.[27–29] Furthermore, opioids have been shown to have a neurotoxic effect with spinal neuron apoptosis in rats.[30] Psychiatric consultation has been shown to have a beneficial effect in the brachial plexus population (39% of peripheral nerve patients are depressed).[31]

OBSTETRIC BRACHIAL PLEXUS PALSY

Obstetric brachial plexus palsy (OBPP), neonatal brachial plexus palsy, brachial plexus birth palsy, and pediatric brachial plexus injury all refer to the brachial plexus injury incurred during childbirth, most commonly vaginal delivery. Fortunately, owing to better prenatal monitoring with more stringent criteria for conversion to cesarean section delivery, the incidence of birth-related brachial plexus injury in developed countries has continued to decrease in recent years.[32,33] There are numerous risk factors for OBPP (**Table 72.8**). The strongest risk factor is undoubtedly shoulder dystocia (approximately 8.3% chance of sustaining brachial plexus palsy with an occurrence of shoulder dystocia). However, 55% of cases of OBPP had no identifiable risk factor.[33] The most commonly encountered OBPP injury overall (46% of all OBPP) is a classic Erb palsy (C5 and C6 palsy).[34] Fortunately, OBPP has a high frequency of spontaneous resolution (77% to 90%).[32] The most common pattern of injury that necessitates operative exploration is a combination of root avulsions and extraforaminal ruptures of C5, C6, and C7[34,35]. **Table 72.9** describes the other common patterns of OBPP injury presentation. With the greater potential for spontaneous recovery from obstetric-related brachial plexus trauma, it is not surprising that there is much disagreement upon the optimal management of these cases. There are still some practitioners who rarely choose surgical intervention.

Deciphering the clues of the brachial plexus–injured infant is challenging. Rather than a systematic catalog of the presence or absence of each sensory and motor function, the practitioner must use various clever investigative aids to identify deficits and monitor for signs of return of function because the infant is unable to willingly cooperate with a directed examination. The tickle test can

TABLE 72.8. RISK FACTORS AND PROTECTIVE FACTORS ASSOCIATED WITH OBSTETRIC BRACHIAL PLEXUS PALSY (OBPP)[33]

Risk Factors (Odds Ratio)
Shoulder dystocia (113.2)
Birth weight >4.5 kg (26.8)
Excessive fetal weight per gestational week (8.22)
Breech delivery (3.56)
Birth hypoxia (3.08)
Instrumented delivery (3.05)
Protective Factors (Odds Ratio)
Multiple gestation (0.45)
Cesarean delivery (0.16)

elicit upper extremity movement. The towel test is a similar ruse to trigger the baby to move the upper extremity by placing a towel over his or her eyes. There are differing opinions upon the threshold for surgical intervention. Terzis advocated surgical exploration if total palsy with Horner syndrome was present at 2 months of age.[36] Gilbert's threshold was 3 months of age without elbow flexion.[37] Clarke and Curtis described 9 months as the limit for recovery of motor function in response to the "cookie test".[37] Chuang found no difference in the recovery of elbow and shoulder function when surgical intervention was carried out at 2 versus 11 months, but Chuang's threshold for surgical intervention was at 3 months if there was little to no wrist extension and finger flexion. He also determined that a persistent lack or stagnation of improvement in elbow or shoulder function warranted intervention at 6 to 12 months.[illegible] Electrodiagnosis in infants is notoriously unreliable because of its tendency to overestimate the axonal function that is present.[33,38] Surgical intervention within the first year of life involves either proximal exploration with nerve reconstruction or distal nerve transfers in similar fashion as detailed for adult palsy. The notable differences are that the phrenic nerve is generally not used for OBPP, and conventional nerve grafting will frequently involve saphenous, median antebrachial cutaneous , or lateral antebrachial cutaneous nerves in addition to the sural nerves, given the short length of the sural nerve in an infant.

TABLE 72.9. INJURY PATTERNS FOR OBSTETRIC BRACHIAL PLEXUS PALSY (OBPP)

	Cases (n)	Percentage of Cases (n)
Ruptures	**47**	**39%**
UT rupture	17	14%
UT and MT ruptures	24	20%
UT, MT, and LT ruptures	6	5%
Ruptures and Avulsions	72	61%
Single-root avulsion	18	15%
Two-root avulsion	28	24%
Three-root avulsion	17	14%
Four-root avulsion	9	8%

MT, middle trunk; *LT*, lower trunk; *UT*, upper trunk.
Data compiled from David C.C. Chuang's operations from 1994 to 2004.

The hallmark stigmata and primary challenge of OBPP patients later in childhood is aberrant reinnervation manifesting in co-contraction of the muscles of the shoulder girdle and elbow. Several forms exist: Axons of the shoulder abductors may aberrantly reinnervate the shoulder adductors, leading to a limitation of shoulder abduction and eventually causing an adduction contracture of the shoulder girdle. There also is cross-innervation of the elbow flexors (brachialis, biceps) and elbow extensors (triceps) which weakens both elbow flexion and extension movements. There can be cross-innervation between elbow flexors and shoulder abductors (which causes the *trumpet sign*). There can also be cross-innervation of the shoulder abductors and the elbow flexors/finger flexors, leading to involuntary elbow and finger flexion with attempted shoulder abduction. The development of aberrant reinnervation ultimately leads to muscle imbalance that often causes joint deformities.[39]

Interventions for these sequelae of OBPP include biomechanical reconstructions for the shoulder, elbow, and hand and forearm. Shoulder reconstruction involves release of adduction contractures at the shoulder girdle (by releasing both of the hypertrophic pectoralis major and teres major muscles) and performing tendon transfers to augment arm abductors (teres major transferred to infraspinatus).[40–42] Elbow reconstruction should prioritize restoration of elbow extension first, as extension can only be augmented effectively by biceps or brachialis tendon. Biceps to triceps tendon transfer or brachialis to triceps tendon transfers has the two-fold effect of restoring extension at the elbow while concomitantly releasing some of the contracture from the unopposed hypertrophy of the biceps and brachialis. If the preexisting elbow flexion is strong, sacrifice of either the biceps or brachialis can often be tolerated without excessively weakening elbow flexion. However, if necessary, elbow flexion can be augmented by either Steindler flexorplasty or FFMTs.[43–46] To note, prior to undergoing tendon transfer or FFMT reconstruction, the articular integrity of the elbow joint must be excellent. Both shoulder and elbow reconstructions are typically done in the range of 4 to 6 years of age. Hand and forearm function often accommodates surprisingly well. Therefore, waiting until age 6 to 13 years before undertaking hand reconstructive procedures is advisable. Tendon transfers in this regard are highly individualized. Flexors such as PL or FCR may be transferred to the EDC to augment finger extension. A Zancolli procedure might be used for supination contracture. Functioning free muscle transplantation may be required for restoration of finger flexion.[47]

Excellent family participation and investment in the child's postoperative therapy is critical. Surgery without rigorous rehabilitation can render the intervention fruitless, as joint contractures will recur without diligent therapy and continuous lifelong maintenance exercises.

OUTCOMES

Reporting of outcomes in the field of brachial plexus reconstruction currently lacks standardization. This may be attributed to the highly variable combinations of injury circumstances and severity. Most brachial plexus outcomes investigations focus upon motor recovery with little emphasis upon sensory return or quality of life.[48] OBPP outcome evaluation is also confounded by the use of multiple different evaluation systems (e.g., Mallet score,[49] Gilbert and Tassin Muscle Grading System, Clarke and Curtis Active Movement Scale, Narakas' Grading System).[50] Even the MRC grading system may vary substantially among practitioners as it is ultimately a clinical description that is subject to each individual examiner's interpretation. There is currently a focus upon incorporating patient-reported outcome measures (e.g., quality of life, function, pain, satisfaction) into investigations so that we can better understand the effect of brachial plexus injury and reconstruction.

CONCLUSION

Brachial plexus injuries are permanently physically disabling events. Even the best possible therapeutic interventions are only partially restorative, and the therapeutic course often involves multiple surgeries. Future investigations in the field will focus upon comparing the categories of surgical therapy (proximal exploration and reconstruction, distal nerve transfers, and biomechanical restorations by tendon transfers, or FFMTs) by using standardized outcome measures that involve patient-reported outcome measures. Technological advancements in the area of minimally invasive diagnostic techniques are currently poised to transform the field of brachial plexus reconstruction. Da Vinci robot surgery and MRI are both being actively explored for better application to allow early and more accurate diagnosis of brachial plexus injuries. Developing these modalities into reliable tools for early diagnosis can potentially allow earlier surgical intervention to give more time for nerve regeneration before fibrosis of the motor endplates of the neuromuscular junction occurs. Also, emerging technologies in the area of targeted muscle reinnervation and prosthetic replacement that had initially been applied to upper extremity amputees are now being directed to restoration of limb function for the brachial plexus-injury population. Perhaps, we will now begin to see advancements in the field of brachial plexus treatment brought about by technological advances that outpace our efforts to find new surgical techniques to maximize the notoriously limited healing potential of nerves.

ACKNOWLEDGMENTS

The work was supported by a Midcareer Investigator Award in Patient-Oriented Research (2 K24-AR053120-06) to Kevin C. Chung. The content is solely the responsibility of the authors and does not necessarily represent the official views of the National Institutes of Health.

REFERENCES

1. Thatte MR, Babhulkar S, Hiremath A. Brachial plexus injury in adults: diagnosis and surgical treatment strategies. *Ann Indian Acad Neurol*. 2013;16:26-33.
2. Soldado F, Ghizoni MF, Bertelli J. Injury mechanisms in supraclavicular stretch injuries of the brachial plexus. *Hand Surg Rehabil*. 2016;35:51-54.
3. Kim DH, Cho YJ, Tiel RL, Kline DG. Outcomes of surgery in 1019 brachial plexus lesions treated at Louisiana state University Health Sciences Center. *J Neurosurg*. 2003;98:1005-1016.
   Provides a good survey of the range and prevalence of different brachial plexus pathologies that occur at a trauma center in the United States.
4. Kim DH, Murovic JA, Tiel RL, Kline DG. Penetrating injuries due to gunshot wounds involving the brachial plexus. *Neurosurg Focus*. 2004;16:1-6.
5. Secer HI, Solmaz I, Anik I, et al. Surgical outcomes of the brachial plexus lesions caused by gunshot wounds in adults. *J Brachial Plex Peripher Nerve Inj*. 2009;4:11.
6. Groen GJ, Baljet B, Drukker J. Nerves and nerve plexuses of the human vertebral column. *Am J Anat*. 1990;188:282-296.
7. Terzis JK, Vekris MD, Soucacos PN. Outcomes of brachial plexus reconstruction in 204 patients with devastating paralysis. *Plast Reconstr Surg*. 1999;104:1221-1240.
8. Alnot J. Traumatic brachial plexus palsy in the adult: retro-and infraclavicular lesions. *Clin Orthop Relat Res*. 1988;(237):9-16.
9. Chuang DC. Adult brachial plexus reconstruction with the level of injury: review and personal experience. *Plast Reconstr Surg*. 2009;124:E359-E69.
   Excellent overview with tips and insight from the most prolific brachial plexus surgeon currently in practice.
10. Mackinnon SE. New directions in peripheral nerve surgery. *Ann Plast Surg*. 1989;22:257-273.
11. Samardzic MM, Rasulic LG, Grujicic DM. Gunshot injuries to the brachial plexus. *J Trauma*. 1997;43:645-649.
12. Travlos J, Goldberg I, Boome RS. Brachial plexus lesions associated with dislocated shoulders. *J Bone Joint Surg Br*. 1990;72B:68-71.
13. Narakas A. Injuries of the brachial plexus and neighboring peripheral nerves in vertebral fractures and other trauma of the cervical spine. *Orthopade*. 1987;16:81-86.
14. Tung TH, Mackinnon SE. Brachial plexus injuries. *Clin Plast Surg*. 2003;30:269-287.
15. Buck-Gramcko D, Lubahn J. The Hoffmann-Tinel sign. *J Hand Surg Eur Vol*. 1993;18:800-805.
16. Al-Qattan M, Clarke H, Curtis C. The prognostic value of concurrent Horner's syndrome in total obstetric brachial plexus injury. *J Hand Surg*. 2000;25:166-167.
17. Teixeira MJ, Da Paz MG, Bina MT, et al. Neuropathic pain after brachial plexus avulsion-central and peripheral mechanisms. *BMC Neurol*. 2015;15:73.
18. Socolovsky M, Di Masi G, Bonilla G, et al. The phrenic nerve as a donor for brachial plexus injuries: is it safe and effective? Case series and literature analysis. *Acta Neurochir*. 2015;157:1077-1086.
19. Terzis JK, Kostas I, Soucacos PN. Restoration of shoulder function with nerve transfers in traumatic brachial plexus palsy patients. *Microsurgery*. 2006;26:316-324.
20. Fuzari HKB, Dornelas De Andrade A, Vilar CF, et al. Diagnostic accuracy of magnetic resonance imaging in post-traumatic brachial plexus injuries: a systematic review. *Clin Neurol Neurosurg*. 2018;164:5-10.
21. Ferrante MA. Electrodiagnostic assessment of the brachial plexus. *Neurol Clin*. 2012;30:551-580.
22. Granberry WM, Lipscomb PR. Tendon transfers to the hand in brachial palsy. *Am J Surg*. 1964;108:840-844.
23. Ikuta Y, Kubo T, Tsuge K. Free muscle transplantation by microsurgical technique to treat severe Volkmann's contracture. *Plast Reconstr Surg*. 1976;58:407-411.
24. Tung TH, Mackinnon SE. Nerve transfers: indications, techniques, and outcomes. *J Hand Surg Am*. 2010;35:332-341.
    Overview of the "distal nerve transfer" techniques from one of the primary groups that pioneered and popularized this technique.
25. Berger A, Brenner P. Secondary surgery following brachial plexus injuries. *Microsurgery*. 1995;16:43-47.
26. Chuang DC. Nerve transfer with functioning free muscle transplantation. *Hand Clin*. 2008;24:377-388.
    Description of the application of FFMTs to brachial plexus pathology with a comprehensive description of options for neurotization.
27. Camara CC, Araujo CV, De Sousa KKO, et al. Gabapentin attenuates neuropathic pain and improves nerve myelination after chronic sciatic constriction in rats. *Neurosci Lett*. 2015;607:52-58.
28. Celik M, Kose A, Kose D, et al. The double-edged sword: effects of pregabalin on experimentally induced sciatic nerve transection and crush injury in rats. *Int J Neurosci*. 2015;125:845-854.
29. Perez M, Benitez SU, Cartarozzi LP, et al. Neuroprotection and reduction of glial reaction by cannabidiol treatment after sciatic nerve transection in neonatal rats. *Eur J Neurosci*. 2013;38:3424-3434.
30. Mao J, Sung B, Ji RR, Lim G. Neuronal apoptosis associated with morphine tolerance: evidence for an opioid-induced neurotoxic mechanism. *J Neurosci*. 2002;22:7650-7661.
31. Bailey R, Kaskutas V, Fox I, et al. Effect of upper extremity nerve damage on activity participation, pain, depression, and quality of life. *J Hand Surg Am*. 2009;34:1682-1688.
32. Chauhan SP, Blackwell SB, Ananth CV. Neonatal brachial plexus palsy: incidence, prevalence, and temporal trends. *Semin Perinatol*. 2014;38:210-218.
33. Defrancesco CJ, Shah DK, Rogers BH, Shah AS. The epidemiology of brachial plexus birth palsy in the United States: declining incidence and evolving risk factors. *J Pediatr Orthop*. 2019;39(2):e134-e140.
34. Al-Qattan MM, El-Sayed AA, Al-Zahrani AY, et al. Narakas classification of obstetric brachial plexus palsy revisited. *J Hand Surg Eur Vol*. 2009;34:788-791.
35. Chuang DC, Mardini S, Ma HS. Surgical strategy for infant obstetrical brachial plexus palsy: experiences at Chang Gung Memorial Hospital. *Plast Reconstr Surg*. 2005;116:132-142; discussion 43-44.
36. Terzis JK, Papakonstantinou K. Surgical treatment of obstetrical brachial plexus paralysis: the Norfolk experience. *Semin Plast Surg*. 2004;18:359.
    Comprehensive overview of obstetric brachial plexus palsy from one of the pioneers of the field.
37. Gilbert A. *Brachial Plexus Injuries*. Philadelphia, PA: Taylor & Francis; 2001.
38. Slooff AC. Obstetric brachial plexus lesions and their neurosurgical treatment. *Microsurgery*. 1995;16:30-34.
39. Chuang DC, Ma HS, Wei FC. A new evaluation system to predict the sequelae of late obstetric brachial plexus palsy. *Plast Reconstr Surg*. 1998;101:673-685.
40. Chuang DC, Ma HS, Wei FC. A new strategy of muscle transposition for treatment of shoulder deformity caused by obstetric brachial plexus palsy. *Plast Reconstr Surg*. 1998;101:686-694.
41. Narakas AO. Muscle transpositions in the shoulder and upper arm for sequelae of brachial plexus palsy. *Clin Neurol Neurosurg*. 1993;95(suppl):S89-S91.
42. Price AE, Grossman JA. A management approach for secondary shoulder and forearm deformities following obstetrical brachial plexus injury. *Hand Clin*. 1995;11:607-617.
43. Chuang DC, Epstein MD, Yeh MC, Wei FC. Functional restoration of elbow flexion in brachial plexus injuries: results in 167 patients (excluding obstetric brachial plexus injury). *J Hand Surg Am*. 1993;18:285-291.
44. Chuang DC, Hattori Y, Ma HS, Chen HC. The reconstructive strategy for improving elbow function in late obstetric brachial plexus palsy. *Plast Reconstr Surg*. 2002;109:116-126.
45. Haerle M, Gilbert A. Management of complete obstetric brachial plexus lesions. *J Pediatr Orthop*. 2004;24:194-200.
46. Al-Qattan MM. Elbow flexion reconstruction by Steindler flexorplasty in obstetric brachial plexus palsy. *J Hand Surg Br*. 2005;30:424-427.
47. Chuang DC, Ma HS, Borud LJ, Chen HC. Surgical strategy for improving forearm and hand function in late obstetric brachial plexus palsy. *Plast Reconstr Surg*. 2002;109:1934-1946.
48. Dy CJ, Garg R, Lee SK, et al. A systematic review of outcomes reporting for brachial plexus reconstruction. *J Hand Surg Am*. 2015;40:308-313.
49. Tse R, Kozin SH, Malessy MJ, Clarke HM. International Federation of Societies for Surgery of the Hand Committee Report: the role of nerve transfers in the treatment of neonatal brachial plexus palsy. *J Hand Surg Am*. 2015;40:1246-1259.
50. Pondaag W, Malessy MJ. The evidence for nerve repair in obstetric brachial plexus palsy revisited. *Biomed Res Int*. 2014;2014:434619.

QUESTIONS

1. A 20-year-old male was hit by a train traveling approximately 80 mile per hour. His injuries include subdural hematoma, open pelvic fracture, bilateral hemopneumothoraces, and a suspected brachial plexus injury of his left upper extremity. Three months after the injury, he still has no sensation to the left upper extremity on a C5-T1 dermatomal sensory examination, and there is also no detectable motor function of muscles in the left upper extremity. His electrodiagnostic studies are notable for the results shown in Tables 72.10 and 72.11.

TABLE 72.10. NEEDLE ELECTROMYOGRAPHY (EMG) RESULTS

Muscle (Left Side)	Insertional Activity	Fibrillations	Positive Sharp Waves	Amplitude (mV)	Duration (ms)	Polyphasic Waves
FDP	Absent	2+	2+	Absent	No MUPs	
APB	Absent	2+	2+	Absent	No MUPs	
FCR	Absent	2+	2+	Absent	No MUPs	
Biceps	Absent	2+	2+	Absent	No MUPs	
Triceps	Absent	2+	2+	Absent	No MUPs	
Deltoid	Absent	2+	2+	Absent	No MUPs	
Cervical paraspinal muscles	Decreased	2+	2+	Decreased		

APB, abductor pollicis brevis; *FCR*, flexor carpi radialis; *FCU*, flexor carpi ulnaris; *FDP*, flexor digitorum profundus; *MUPs*, motor unit potentials.

TABLE 72.11. NERVE CONDUCTION STUDY RESULTS

	Left		Right	
Sensory	**Latency**	**Amplitude**	**Latency**	**Amplitude**
Median (index finger)	3.1	18.1	3.0	26.3
Ulnar (small finger)	2.7	16.5		
Superficial radial	2.4	22.8	2.5	20.7
LABC	2.4	7.7	2.5	16.3
Median (thumb)	3.2	9.7	3.2	24.8
MABC	2.5	14.0		
Motor				
Median—APB		Not recorded		
Ulnar—ADM		Not recorded		
Radial—ED		Not recorded		14.9
Axillary—deltoid		Not recorded		12.4
Musculocutaneous—biceps		Not recorded		8.7

ADM, abductor digiti minimi; *APB*, abductor pollicis brevis; *ED*, extensor digitorum; *LABC*, lateral antebrachial cutaneous; *MABC*, median antebrachial cutaneous.

His EMG and nerve conduction studies are most consistent with which of the following?

a. Five root neuropraxia
b. Ruptures of C5 and C6; avulsions of C7, C8, and T1
c. Avulsions of C5 and C6; ruptures of C7, C8, and T1
d. Postganglionic ruptures of C5-T1
e. Root avulsions of C5-T1

2. A 25-year-old gang member presents to the trauma center with severe bleeding after a stab wound to the right shoulder region by a knife. The initial exploration by vascular surgery accomplished repair of the axillary artery laceration. Three days after presentation, the patient is hemodynamically stable and without any further transfusion requirement. The trauma team is preparing to discharge the patient to home. The physical examination shows M0 elbow flexion, M3 finger flexion, and anesthesia to the thumb and index fingers. What is the most appropriate next course of action?

a. Immediate reexploration of the site of nerve injury for primary repair
b. Transfer of intercostal nerves (T3-T5) to musculocutaneous nerve for restoration of elbow flexion
c. Double fascicular transfer of expendable flexor carpi ulnaris (FCU) fascicle of ulnar nerve and expendable motor fascicle of median directly to biceps and brachialis branches of the musculocutaneous nerve, for restoration of elbow flexion
d. Functioning free muscle transplantation of gracilis muscle to arm for restoration of elbow flexion
e. Aggressive physical therapy, occupational therapy, electrostimulation, and follow-up in 1 month to monitor for motor and sensory recovery

3. A 6-month-old girl whose birth weight was 5060 g (11.1 lbs) is being followed at your clinic for obstetric brachial plexus palsy. Her birth was notable for vaginal delivery with shoulder dystocia, and forceps were required to facilitate delivery. Initially at birth, she had no abduction of the arm at the shoulder and very weak flexion at the elbow. Currently, she has some evidence of arm abduction and elbow flexion is improving. There has always been good hand function. Of the following factors, which is the strongest risk factor for OBPP?

a. Birth weight >4.5 kg
b. Shoulder dystocia
c. Instrumented delivery (forceps or vacuum)
d. Breech presentation
e. Hypoxia/fetal distress

4. A 38-year-old man was involved in a roll-over motor vehicle accident as an unrestrained driver with loss of consciousness and lower extremity fracture as well. One month after the trauma, he has M0 strength of abduction of the arm at the shoulder and M0 strength of flexion at the elbow. Sensation is severely diminished in the distribution of C5 and C6. What is most appropriate next course of action?

a. Physical therapy and return visit in 1 month
b. Double fascicular transfer of expendable FCU fascicle of ulnar nerve and expendable motor fascicle of median directly to biceps and brachialis branches of the musculocutaneous nerve, for restoration of elbow flexion
c. Surgical exploration with resection of neuroma and nerve grafting
d. Functioning free muscle transplantation of gracilis muscle to arm for restoration of elbow flexion
e. Steindler flexorplasty

5. A 24-year-old man presents to your clinic with M0 strength of elbow flexion and M0 strength of shoulder abduction. It is now 14 months after he developed these deficits after he had landed upon his shoulder when he fell off a roof. What is the most reasonable management strategy for improving his upper extremity function?

a. Aggressive physical therapy and electrostimulation therapy
b. Double fascicular transfer of expendable FCU fascicle of ulnar nerve and expendable motor fascicle of median directly to biceps and brachialis branches of the musculocutaneous nerve, for restoration of elbow flexion
c. Surgical exploration with resection of neuroma and nerve grafting
d. Upper trapezius tendon transfer to restore abduction at the shoulder with functioning free muscle transplantation of gracilis for elbow flexion
e. Shoulder arthrodesis

1. Answer: e. The complete absence of motor unit action potentials on the needle EMG and undetectable motor nerve conduction in combination with the normal amplitude on the sensory nerve conduction studies reflect that the ventral rootlets of the motor innervation and dorsal rootlets of the sensory innervation have all been disrupted. The dorsal root ganglion is still viable, leading to the detectable sensory nerve conduction and amplitudes. However, there is no connection between the peripheral nerve and the spinal cord, so there is no sensation and no motor function detectable in the patient. These EMG and nerve conduction findings are pathognomonic for the occurrence of a preganglionic root avulsion injury.

2. Answer: a. Sharp lacerations of the brachial plexus should be explored within the first week for direct repair if at all possible. Beyond 2 or 3 weeks after injury in the infraclavicular region, the nerve ends will retract, and nerve grafting will likely be necessary to achieve a tension-free coaptation. Repairing within the first week allows for a direct repair (with only a single coaptation site) which will theoretically minimize the loss of regenerating axons (straying away through the discontinuity of the epineurium at the coaptation sites) and maximize the potential for functional recovery.

3. Answer: b. Shoulder dystocia is the factor with the highest odds ratio (OR = 113.2) for occurrence of OBPP. Birth weight >4.5 kg (OR = 26.8), breech presentation (OR = 3.56), instrumented delivery (OR = 3.05), and hypoxia/fetal distress (OR = 3.08) all have substantially lower correlation with OBPP. Much disagreement exists over the criteria and timing by which surgical exploration and intervention should be performed.

4. Answer: a. Closed injuries of the brachial plexus are monitored for the first 3 months. During this time, it is essential to have excellent physical therapy and occupational therapy to keep joints in the hand and upper extremity supple. A baseline electrodiagnostic study may be obtained at approximately posttrauma week 4 and repeated at approximately posttrauma week 12 to monitor for any nerve regeneration. Until month 3, monitoring for motor and sensory recovery at a monthly interval in the clinic is appropriate.

5. Answer: d. At 14 months after injury, nerve surgeries to restore innervation to the native muscles of the shoulder and arm are not an option due to that fibrosis of the motor endplates of the neuromuscular junction will have occurred by the time that axons have the time to regenerate. Salvage procedures such as upper trapezius tendon transfer and FFMT are the only options for improving motor function. Physical therapy and electrostimulation alone without surgical intervention would not be expected to have any significant positive effect upon function. Shoulder arthrodesis may be considered for less-motivated patients or older patients. Arthrodesis leaves the shoulder with a very limited arc of motion with the remaining scapulothoracic muscles driving movement.

CHAPTER 73 Tetraplegia

Jennifer F. Waljee and Kevin C. Chung

KEY POINTS

- Over half of spinal cord injuries (SCIs) involve the cervical spine, and restoration of upper extremity function is consistently rated a top priority by patients.
- Surgical reconstruction of upper extremity function provides an important opportunity to restore independence with transfers and activities of daily living. Reconstruction is considered among patients with pain-free, supple joints and who are able to meet the demands of postoperative rehabilitation once the SCI has plateaued, which typically occurs within 1 year.
- The International Classification for Surgery of the Hand in Tetraplegia (ICSHT) level describes the number of muscles present below the elbow available for tendon transfer and provides the framework for surgical planning.
- Critical functions to restore among patients with SCIs include elbow extension, forearm pronation, wrist extension, key pinch, digit flexion and extension, and intrinsic balance.

Approximately 17,000 new spinal cord injuries (SCIs) occur in the United States each year and are particularly concentrated among young individuals.[1] Most injuries occur among males from trauma, including motorcycle and motor vehicle collisions. Roughly 2,000,000 individuals in the United States live with SCI, and the rates of injury among the elderly due to falls and underlying spinal degenerative disease is increasing.[2] Patients commonly present with concomitant injuries, and over half will develop complications during their initial hospitalization, such as shock, respiratory compromise, and pneumonia.[3] Fortunately, mortality related to SCI has declined considerably in recent decades. Nonetheless, late complications, such as pressure ulceration, sepsis, and venous thromboembolism, remain important causes of death.[4–6]

Of all SCIs, 56% affect the cervical spine.[1] SCI resulting in tetraplegia is a devastating injury, and optimal upper extremity function is consistently rated as a top priority to achieve independence with activities of daily living.[7–12] Upper extremity reconstruction, which can include both nerve and tendon transfers, offers a viable way to restore some elements of upper extremity motion and strength.[13–15] Multiple studies indicate that upper extremity reconstruction can effectively improve hand pinch and grasp, enabling recipients to better perform activities of daily living.[7,16–19] Yet despite these established benefits, rates of procedures are often lagging.[19–21] In this chapter, we will review the principles of upper extremity reconstruction for SCI and common techniques.

PATHOPHYSIOLOGY OF INJURY

Tetraplegia results from traumatic injuries to the cervical spine causing the loss of upper motor and sensory neurons. SCI results from 2 phases of injury: primary and secondary injury. The peripheral and central nervous systems are discontinuous because of blunt, sharp, crushing, or avulsion forces.[22] Secondary injury includes the physiologic events that occur due to disruption of the vasculature, edema, ischemia, and hemorrhage, which further compounds the injury.[23] Above the level of the injured spinal cord, nerve function is normal. However, nerve function below the level of injury is absent. Hyper-reflexia is common and characteristic of the upper motor nerve injury; nerve function can be elicited at levels below the injury if the lower motor neuron unit is intact.

Level of injury is determined by physical examination of motor and sensory function. Symmetry or skip patterns can occur with certain injury types (central cord syndrome, Brown-Séquard syndrome, anterior cord syndrome). Notably, the manifestations of injury may vary between individuals with the same level of injury, and it is important to perform a full examination of the upper extremity muscle units when planning reconstruction.[24] Within the zone of injury, stabilization of recovery occurs as the edema, ischemia, and hemorrhage resolves. In general, the greatest gains of motor and sensory function occur within 6 to 9 months following SCI, after which neurologic stability typically occurs.[25,26]

CLINICAL EVALUATION

Following SCI, loss of function occurs according to the injured segment, and the pattern of function follows the order of innervation by anterior horn cells from cephalad to caudad (Figure 73.1). The American Spinal Injury Association (ASIA) Impairment Scale classification further describes the spinal cord elements related to upper extremity function, and the most common levels of cervical spine injury are at C5 and C6, marked by a loss of elbow extension, wrist flexion, and finger flexion and extension. In general, patients with upper cervical spine injuries have shoulder motion, but absent wrist and hand function. Individuals with midcervical injury typically have elbow flexion, but may have varying degrees of wrist extension, forearm pronation, and hand motion. Patients with lower cervical spine injuries typically have nearly full function of their shoulder, elbow, and wrist, but without intrinsic muscle function. However, there is often variation in the manifestations of each injury, and a full upper extremity examination is necessary to determine reconstructive options.

MANAGEMENT OF TETRAPLEGIA

The management of patients with tetraplegia is multidisciplinary, including surgical care, neurologists, and physical medicine and rehabilitation specialists. Immediately following injury, prevention of contractures ensures options for later reconstruction. Contractures are common, with over half of SCI patients developing a contracture within 1 year of injury, most commonly of the shoulder 43%, elbow and forearm 33%, and wrist and hand 41%.[27] Contractures arise due to spasticity or pathologically increased muscle tone caused by a loss of upper motor neuron innervation and inhibitory control.[28] Stiffness of the soft tissues is caused by shortening and loss of elasticity occurs and can include the skin, subcutaneous tissue, joint capsule, supporting ligaments, tendon, muscle, and neurovascular structures. Mobilization can prevent contractures by providing tensile stress that incites collagen reorganization. Splinting between mobilization exercises is critical, although compliance is variable.[29] The hand should be splinted in a functional position to maximize the potential for tenodesis, with the digits extended and the metacarpophalangeal (MCP) joints in gentle flexion. In addition, the forearm should be positioned in pronation to avoid supination contractures. Medical therapy can also help with prevention of contractures, including the use of spasmolytics (intrathecal, oral, and injected), motor blocks, and targeted electrical stimulation. For patients with severe, refractory spasticity in a nonfunctional limb without expected recovery, motor neurectomy may be considered.[30]

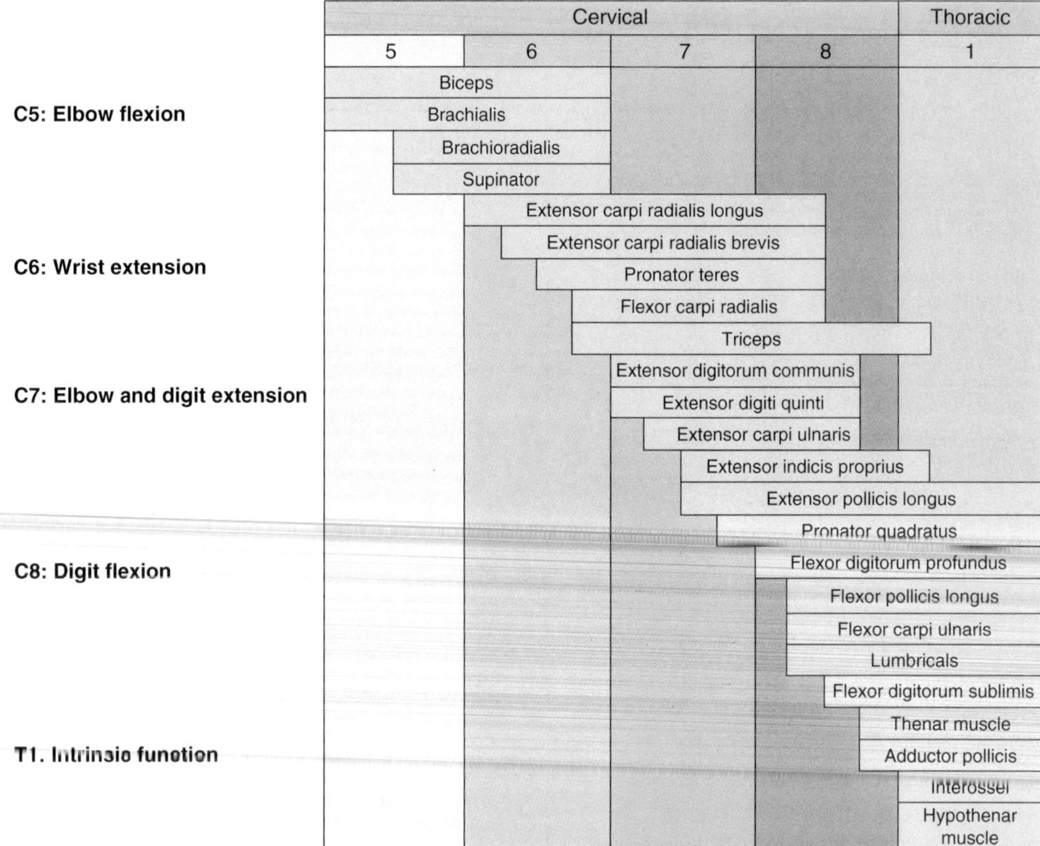

FIGURE 73.1. Spinal cord innervation of upper extremity motor elements and the American Spinal Injury Association (ASIA) Impairment Scale classification.

Reconstructive procedures including tendon transfers, tenodesis procedures, nerve transfers, joint release, and selective arthrodesis can significantly enhance the upper extremity function of patients with tetraplegia. The primary goal of reconstruction is to provide greater independence for SCI patients with activities of daily living. Prior to surgical reconstruction, it is important to ensure that neurologic recovery has plateaued, typically at 1 year after injury, and that the patient has sufficient social support for recovery. In addition, patients should have reasonable expectations for the potential gains provided from reconstructive procedures, demonstrate emotional adjustment to their injury, and have motivation and support to participate in postoperative therapy.[31] Finally, patients should have minimal pain in the upper extremity that may preclude participation in rehabilitation or use of the hand. Traumatic brain injuries commonly occur among patients with SCI, as well as concomitant mood disorders. It is important to ensure that cognition, depression, anxiety, and other mental health conditions are optimized preoperatively.[32]

Prior to any reconstructive procedure, it is essential to ensure that the upper limb is free of contractures, with full passive motion, and in particular the shoulder, elbow, forearm, wrist, MCP, and proximal interphalangeal (PIP) joints. In general, surgical procedures for tendon transfers are delayed for at least 6 to 9 months following injury to establish a baseline for function and identify the motor units that will recover.[26] However, there is no upper limit with respect to timing of tendon transfers from injury for patients who are good candidates. Donor muscles should be strong (M4 or M5 strength) and beyond the zone of injury. Like other tendon transfers, the ideal donor provides synergistic function with a straight line of pull and adequate excursion, and glide through a healthy bed of tissue free of scar.

RECONSTRUCTIVE OPTIONS FOR TETRAPLEGIA

Surgical planning is informed by the patient's International Classification for Surgery of the Hand in Tetraplegia (ICSHT) level, which describes the number of muscles present below the elbow with at least grade 4 strength that are available for tendon transfer (**Table 73.1**). Muscles are listed in the order in which recovery is expected in complete tetraplegia. A muscle is considered functional if the strength is grade 4 or higher based on manual testing (**Table 73.2**). For sensory function, two-point discrimination of 10 mm or less is needed for cutaneous control. Ocular control is needed for patients with wider two-point discrimination. Without adequate sensory input, even the best reconstruction is ineffective because the patient cannot feel or detect how much force is impacted on an object.

The decision for and type of reconstruction planned is then informed by three questions: what muscles are missing, what critical functions are needed, and what donor muscles are available. Critical functions include restoration of elbow extension to facilitate transfer and expand the space around an individual for manipulation of the hand. Other needs are key/lateral pinch, forearm pronation, wrist extension, digit flexion and extension for grasp and release, and hand posture for patients with loss of intrinsic function.[33]

ICSHT Levels

Group 0

Patients with injury levels of C4 and higher are able to elevate their shoulders as the spinal accessory nerve innervating the trapezius muscle is uninjured. However, these individuals are often ventilator

TABLE 73.1. INTERNATIONAL CLASSIFICATION FOR SURGERY OF THE HAND IN TETRAPLEGIA

Sensibility	Level of Injury	Motor Group	Muscles Available for Transfer	Functional Ability	Reconstructive Priorities
O or Cu	C4 and higher	0	No muscle below elbow suitable for transfer		
O or Cu	C5	1	Brachioradialis (BR)	Flexion and supination of the elbow	■ Elbow extension: deltoid to triceps; biceps to triceps ■ Wrist extension: BR to extensor carpi radialis brevis (ECRB) ■ Key pinch: flexor pollicis longus (FPL) tenodesis; Split distal FPL tenodesis
O or Cu	C6	2	Extensor carpi radialis longus (ECRL)	Extension of the wrist	■ Elbow extension: deltoid to triceps; biceps to triceps ■ Key pinch: BR to FPL or FPL tenodesis; Split distal FPL tenodesis ■ Thumb extension: extensor pollicis longus tenodesis ■ Grasp: BR to flexor digitorum profundus (FDP) or ECRL to FDP ■ Release: extensor digitorum communis (EDC) tenodesis
O or Cu	C6	3	ECRB	Extension of the wrist	
O or Cu	C6	4	Pronator teres (PT)	Pronation of the wrist	■ Key pinch: BR to FPL; PT to FPL ■ Split distal FPL tenodesis ■ Grasp: ECRL to FDP; PT to FDP ■ Release: PT to EDC ■ Intrinsic balancing
O or Cu	C7	5	Flexor carpi radialis	Flexion of the wrist	
O or Cu	C7	6	Finger extensors	Extrinsic extension of the fingers	
O or Cu	C7	7	Thumb extensor	Extrinsic extension of the thumb	
O or Cu	C8	8	Partial finger flexors	Extrinsic flexion of the fingers	■ Thumb opposition: ECU to FCU to FPL using flexor digitorum superficialis ■ Intrinsic balancing
O or Cu	C8	9	Lacks intrinsics	Extrinsic flexion of the fingers	
O or Cu		X	Exceptions		

dependent, given the potential injury to the phrenic nerve, and without upper extremity function. Unfortunately, for group 0 patients, there are no muscles below the elbow with sufficient strength for transfer and no options for tendon transfer for upper extremity reconstruction.

Group 1

Patients with C5 injuries (group 1) typically have preservation of elbow flexion and shoulder abduction through the biceps and deltoid. Brachioradialis (BR) is the only muscle below the elbow available to transfer, and critical functions to restore for this group of patients include wrist extension and key pinch. Voluntary active wrist extension and flexion are essential functions for tetraplegia patients as it provides tenodesis that can impart gross grip and lateral pinch with wrist extension, and release with wrist flexion. To accomplish wrist extension, BR is transferred to extensor carpi radialis brevis (ECRB).[34] ECRB is chosen as the recipient because it inserts on the base of the long finger metacarpal and provides centralized wrist extension. BR function is tested by selectively testing the strength of this muscle in a neutral position to avoid the action of biceps and brachialis. The muscle belly is palpated lateral to the biceps tendon at the elbow. The transfer should not be set with excess tension, but should allow the wrist to flex when the elbow is in extension for release with tenodesis. Transfers should also be tensioned to position the wrist in neutral when the elbow is in flexion.

For group 1 patients, flexor pollicis longus (FPL) tenodesis may be performed following BR transfer to restore wrist extension. Key pinch is then accomplished with active wrist extension, with release by passive wrist flexion. To accomplish this, the IP joint of the thumb is stabilized, the A1 pulley around the FPL is released, and the FPL is fixed to the radius. The IP joint of the thumb can either be pinned or fused or a split FPL transfer can be performed (Figure 73.2). In addition, tenodesis of extensor pollicis longus (EPL) and extensor pollicis brevis may be performed to further stabilize the metacarpophalangeal joint.[35] Stabilizing the interphalangeal joint can be accomplished by splitting the FPL tendon and transferring the radial half of the tendon to the EPL. This allows the IP joint to remain straight and stable during attempted key pinch. Alternatively, the EPL tendon may be sutured onto itself in a loop configuration to provide IP joint stability.[36]

TABLE 73.2. MUSCLE GRADING SYSTEM: BRITISH MEDICAL RESEARCH COUNCIL

Grade[a]	Description
0	No contraction
1	Trace contraction
2	Active motion without gravity
3	Active motion against gravity
4	Active motion against gravity and resistance
5	Normal

[a]Only muscles of grade 4 or greater are available for transfer. Tendon transfer results in decline of 1 point due to loss of efficiency.

Groups 2 and 3

Group 2 patients have preservation of extensor carpi radialis longus (ECRL) and group 3 patients preservation of ECRB. Patients with C6 injuries are able to perform wrist extension which affords the benefits of tenodesis for rudimentary grasp and release. Therefore, key pinch is a critical function to restore. Key pinch has three components[37]:

- Allowing FPL to provide active pinch through tenodesis or tendon transfer
- Stabilizing the interphalangeal joint
- Position in the thumb in an effective posture of abduction

Approximately 2.2 kg of strength are needed for effective key pinch, grasp, and release for common activities of daily living such as manipulating adaptive transportation devices and catheter management.

For patients in groups 2 and 3, a one-stage key pinch and release procedure is typically performed, and BR is transferred to FPL (Figure 73.3). Similarly, EPL tenodesis can be performed by creating a loop around the third extensor compartment. The EPL tendon is divided at its musculotendinous junction and sutured to itself distal to the extensor retinaculum and Lister tubercle.[13] Carpometacarpal (CMC) arthrodesis in a position for key pinch is performed to provide stability. To position the thumb, CMC arthrodesis is commonly performed, which may provide greater strength with tendon transfers to actively achieve key pinch, but care is taken not to limit passive and active opening of the hand.[38]

In addition, for groups 1 to 3, pronosupination imbalance can occur due to innervation of the biceps and supinator among patients without function of the pronator teres (PT) or pronator quadratus (groups 1–3).[39–41] Supination deformities impair the ability to position the hand in space for grasp and release and can exacerbate wrist extension contractures due to gravity in the setting of weakened flexors.[37] Reconstruction of pronation provides for more effective tenodesis, grip, and key pinch. Supination contractures often occur in conjunction with elbow flexion contractures, and mild to moderate contractures can be improved with serial casting and splinting. For patients with contracture, correction of a supination deformity can be accomplished by biceps rerouting transfer to the opposite side of the radius with interosseous membrane release as described by Zancolli, which converts the biceps from an active supinator to a pronator.[42,43] Alternatively, derotation osteotomy of the radius can be performed to place the forearm into pronation, and combined with anterior elbow capsule release and fractional lengthening of the biceps and brachialis for patients with elbow flexion contractures.[39]

Groups 4 and 5

Patients in group 4 have preservation of PT and patients in group 5 have preservation of flexor carpi radialis (FCR). Although tenodesis is critical for grasp and release, tenodesis only provides a force around 1 to 2N, and 2N or greater is required to accomplish most activities of daily living.[12] Therefore, in groups 4 and 5, the presence of these additional muscles provides more reconstructive options that can be used to restore the critical functions of finger flexion for grasp and thumb flexion for pinch to hold objects. For these patients, grasp, pinch, and release are accomplished in two phases, an extensor phase (release) and a flexor phase (grasp), and require thumb stability. Reconstruction can be performed in multiple stages in either order (flexion or extension reconstruction) or a single stage depending on surgeon preference and level of injury.[44]

Flexion is restored by transferring ECRL to the flexor digitorum profundus (FDP) tendons, and either BR or PT to the FPL[45] (Figure 73.4). The action of PT is tested by examining the patient's forearm in pronation with resisted supination while palpating the lateral aspect of the forearm distal to the antecubital fossa. ECRL is chosen to restore function to FDP given its greater excursion and strength compared with BR and PT (Figure 73.5). These tendon transfers predictably restore grasp for activities of daily living (Figure 73.6). Extension is accomplished by an extensor digitorum communis (EDC) tenodesis, in which the digit extensors are anchored to the radius. In the forearm, the fourth compartment is exposed, and the periosteum is elevated as a flap. The extensor tendons are sutured together and then anchored to the shaft of the radius. The tension is

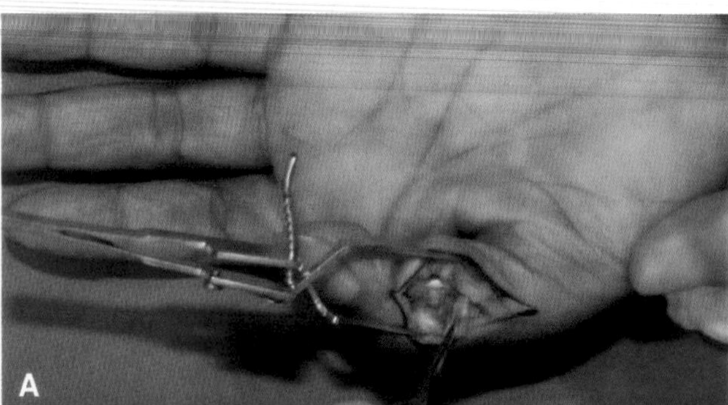

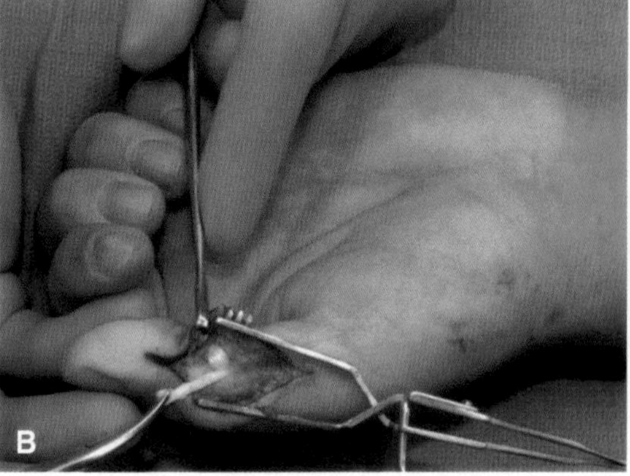

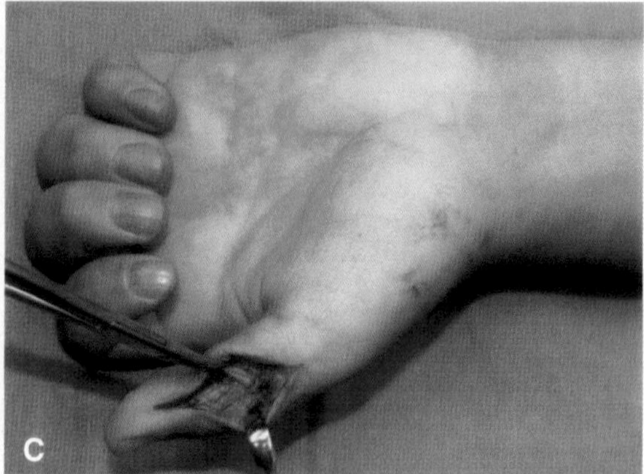

FIGURE 73.2. **A.** Split FPL to EPL tendon transfer to stabilize the thumb interphalangeal joint. **B,C.** Split FPL to EPL tendon transfer to stabilize the thumb interphalangeal joint. *FPL*, flexor pollicis longus; *EPL*, extensor pollicis longus.

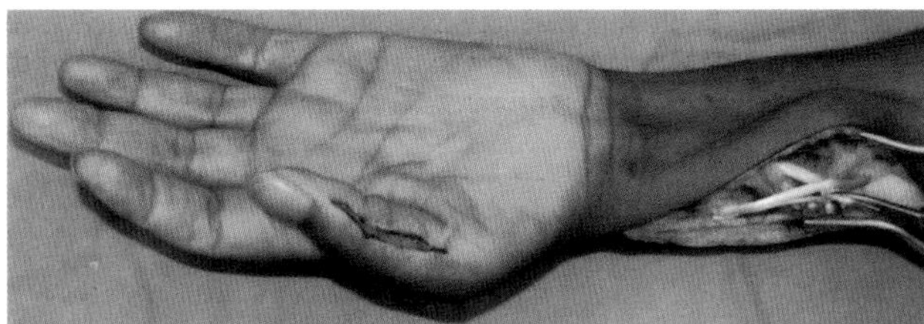

FIGURE 73.3. Brachioradialis to flexor pollicis longus transfer to restore thumb flexion.

set in a reverse cascade, to allow the index finger in the most flexed position for finer pinch, with the MCP joints in extension with the wrist in neutral.[13] The reverse cascade is critical when posturing tendon transfers for patients with SCI as the ulnar digits are less likely to reach the thumb for key pinch. Similar to patients in groups 2 and 3, EPL tenodesis may be performed by constructing a loop around the extensor retinaculum of the third compartment.

The thumb can be stabilized using either an opponensplasty or by performing CMC arthrodesis.[46] Given the limited number of donor tendons, this is performed by transferring PT or BR to the flexor digitorum superficialis (FDS) of the ring finger. The distal aspect of the FDS is then transected at the decussation, routed through a loop of fascia, and transferred to the abductor pollicis brevis insertion at the MCP joint of the thumb.[45] If thumb CMC arthrodesis is performed, the thumb is positioned for lateral pinch in approximately 20° of extension, 45° abduction, and slight pronation.[13] For patients in whom bilateral reconstruction is planned, opponensplasty may be selected for one side and CMC arthroplasty may be selected for the contralateral side, pending on the patient's needs for fine pinch or stronger grip.[46]

Group 6 and 7

For patients in group 6, EDC function is preserved, and patients in group 7 EPL function is preserved. Similar to groups 4 and 5, BR, ECRL, and PT remain available for transfer, and critical functions to restore include restoration of strength for pinch and grasp with finger and thumb flexion. In general, FCR is not used as a donor tendon as its power improves the capacity of the tenodesis effect with the release phase and enhances the ability to power a wheelchair. Grasp and pinch can be reconstructed in one stage to restore the flexor phase, given that the extensors are intact. To do this, ECRL is transferred to FDP to restore finger flexion and BR is transferred to FPL to restore thumb flexion. ECRB is not used as a donor as it provides centralized wrist extension. With respect to the thumb, EPL tenodesis is performed as described above with CMC fusion for patients in group 6. For patients in group 7, EPL is intact, and opponensplasty alone is performed by transferring PT to FDS to the ring finger for power. The FDS tendon to the ring finger is then transferred to the abductor pollicis brevis to provide adduction and opposition.

Group 8

Patients in group 8 have function of digit flexors of the index and middle fingers but lack function of the ring and small fingers. Restoration of full finger flexion is an important reconstructive priority. To do this, side-to-side FDP transfer is performed. In this procedure, the flexor tendons of FDP are anchored together as a single unit to provide finger flexion using either sutures or a free tendon graft.

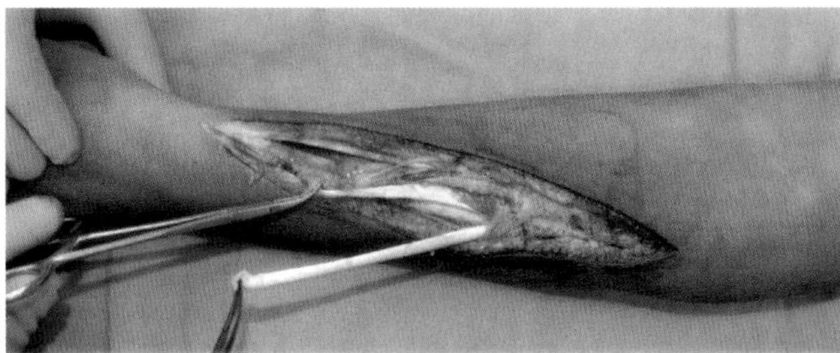

FIGURE 73.4. Brachioradialis and extensor carpi radialis longus tendons for transfer.

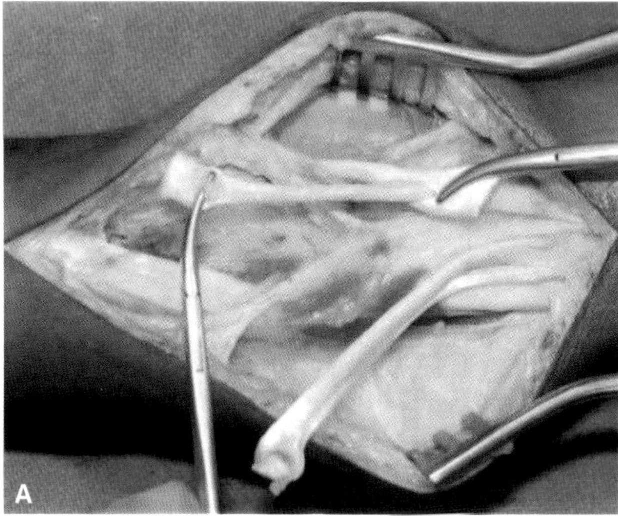

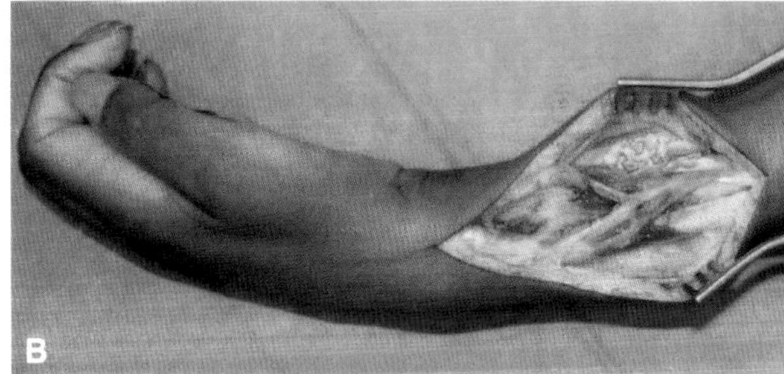

FIGURE 73.5. Extensor carpi radialis longus to flexor digitorum profundus of the index, middle, ring, and small fingers.

Restoration of Elbow Reconstruction

Reconstruction of elbow extension is a top priority to restore the ability to reach, provide stability of hand function, and will augment tendon transfers performed for wrist extension, pinch, and grip. For patients with poor triceps function and injuries at levels of C5 and C6 (typically Groups 1–4), common tendon transfers to achieve elbow extension are the posterior deltoid to triceps transfer, which is achieved with supplemental tendon grafting, and biceps to triceps transfer.[47] It is critical that patients have functional brachialis and supinator muscles to ensure elbow flexion and supination following biceps transfer. The brachialis muscle is palpated during elbow flexion in supination for

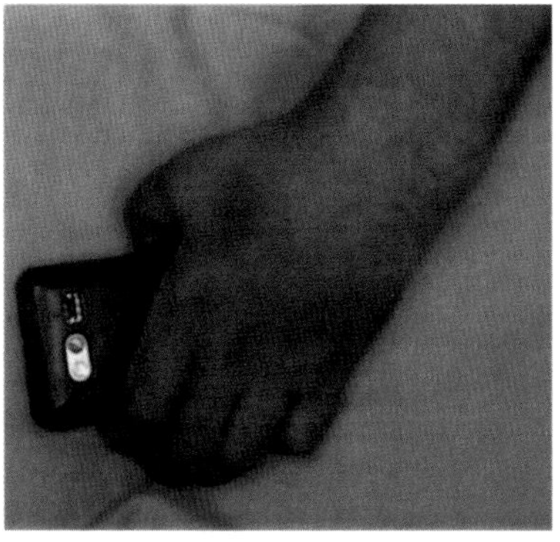

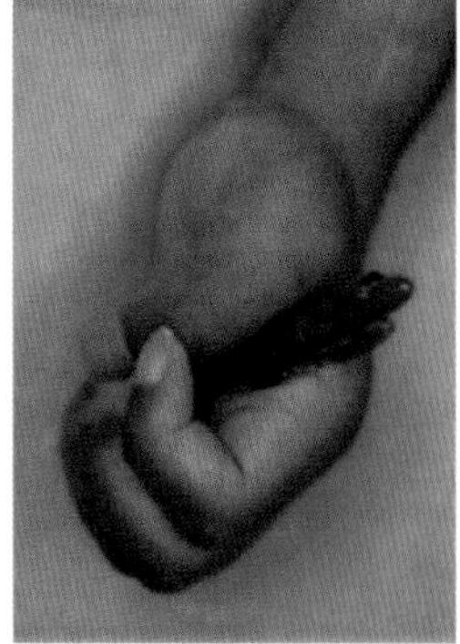

FIGURE 73.6. Grasp following reconstruction of flexion by extensor carpi radialis longus to flexor digitorum profundus transfer.

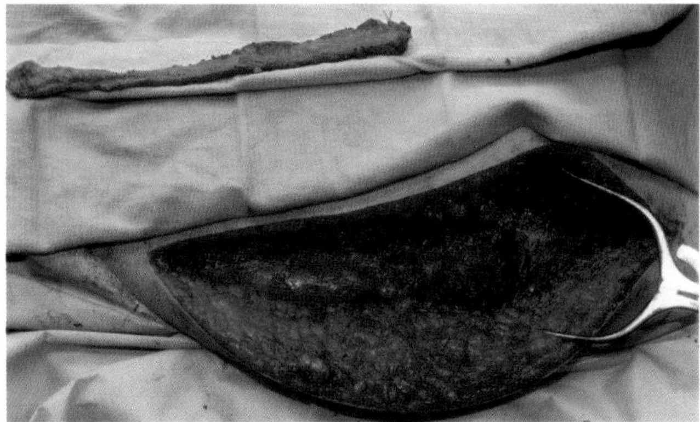

FIGURE 73.7. Harvest of tensor fascia lata graft for posterior deltoid to triceps transfer.

patients without wrist extension. For patients with strong wrist extension, biceps may be used as the level of injury is below the innervation of the brachialis and supinator. Biceps to triceps transfer is performed through a medial approach and routing, rather than posterolaterally, to avoid injury or compression to the radial nerve. The tendon is tunneled in a subcutaneous plane and anchored to the olecranon and/or woven to the triceps tendon.[48] The transfer should accommodate 60° to 90° of elbow flexion passively with tensioning.

Alternatively, the posterior third to half of the deltoid can be transferred to the triceps muscle to provide elbow extension among patients.[49] Typically, an interposition graft of fascia is required (e.g., tensor fascia lata; Figure 73.7). The deltoid is raised distally to proximally, protecting the axillary nerve, and a subcutaneous tunnel or open incision can be used for the interpositional graft. The graft is woven from the distal aspect of the deltoid into the distal aspect of the triceps (Figure 73.8). Overall, biceps to triceps transfers are favored, given the earlier mobilization possible in the rehabilitation period and the potential for stretch of the interposition graft for deltoid to triceps transfer with resultant loss of strength.

Intrinsic Reconstruction

For patients in groups 6 through 9, intrinsic reconstruction can augment hand function by balancing the digit posture in a better position for grasp and release. Patients with intrinsic weakness will have a clawed posture of their hand. The PIP joints are often flexed due to FDS spasticity and hyperextension of the MCP joints due to loss of intrinsic function which provides MCP joint flexion. In addition, an uncoordinated rolling phenomena can occur when grasp is initiated, in which the distal interphalangeal and PIP joints will flex prior to the MCP joint. For the thumb, patients will present with a Froment's sign, in which FPL is flexed with thumb adduction to overcome weakness of the adductor pollicis.

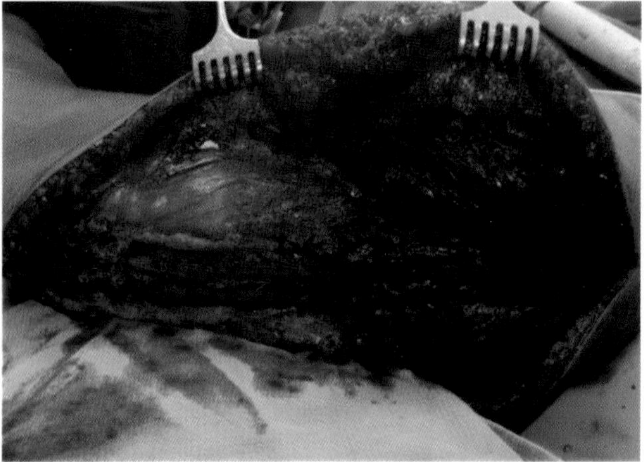

FIGURE 73.8. Posterior deltoid to triceps transfer.

To address intrinsic weakness of the thumb that interferes with key pinch, a portion of the radial aspect of FPL may be transferred to EPL to balance the force across the interphalangeal joint.[50] To create intrinsic balance in the fingers, Zancolli described the creation of a lasso to flex the MCP joints first, followed by the interphalangeal joints, to provide more coordinated movement. To create the lasso, the FDS is released distally and looped onto itself at the A1 pulley to create flexion force at the MCP joint with wrist extension. Alternatively, for patients with central slip deficiencies, free tendon grafts may be used for tenodesis. The integrity of the central slip is identified by the extent to which the digits extend with wrist flexion, and patients with central slip deficiencies will not have digit extension with wrist flexion. Free tendon grafts can be passed around the metacarpal neck volar to the intermetacarpal ligaments and attached to the lateral bands or central slip at the same time. EDC tenodesis is performed to provide extension of the PIP joints with flexion of the MCP joints. Overall, intrinsic reconstruction has been shown to greatly enhance hand function and quality of life among patients with SCI and should be considered among patients with clawing or MCP joint hyperextension after flexor reconstruction due to intrinsic weakness.[51]

FUTURE DIRECTIONS

More recently, nerve transfer procedures have been applied to SCI reconstruction.[52] Nerves that innervate muscles from spinal cord segments above the level of the injury and do not provide essential function can be used as donor nerves for transfer among SCI patients. Nerve transfer procedures may be time dependent, in which the recipient muscle is within the zone of injury, and time independent, in which the recipient muscle is lower than the zone of injury.[52] Nerve conduction studies and electromyography can confirm appropriate recipient and donor nerves.

Nerve transfer procedures have been described to restore elbow extension, wrist extension, finger extension, and finger flexion. Donor nerves to restore elbow extension include branches of the axillary nerve to the teres minor or posterior deltoid transferred to the triceps branches of the radial nerve.[15,52-57] Nerve transfers have also been described to restore finger flexion using branches of the musculocutaneous nerve to the brachialis that are transferred to the anterior interosseous nerve. Additionally, transfer of the branches innervating either BR or ECRB have also been described for transfer to the anterior interosseous nerve to restore finger flexion, achieving up to M4 strength in most patients.[52,58] Although long-term comparative studies of outcomes between nerve transfers and traditional transfers are not yet available, these procedures provide an innovative approach to include in the armamentarium of reconstructive options for SCI.

SUMMARY

Although surgical reconstruction remains underutilized among individuals who suffer cervical SCIs, tendon and nerve transfer procedures can offer substantial gains in upper extremity function and quality of life in properly selected patients (**Table 73.3**). Restoration of upper extremity function is consistently described as a top priority for SCI patients, and integrating surgical care into the multidisciplinary management of these injuries is important to ensure that patients have access to all potential treatment options.

TABLE 73.3. SUMMARY OF RECONSTRUCTION OF UPPER EXTREMITY FUNCTION FOR TETRAPLEGIA

	Available Donors	Reconstructive Priorities	Procedures
Group 1	Brachioradialis (BR)	Wrist extension	BR to extensor carpi radialis brevis (ECRB)
		Pinch	Extensor pollicis longus (EPL) and flexor pollicis longus (FPL) transfer into ECRB, FPL tenodesis, and interphalangeal fusion
Group 2 & 3	BR, extensor carpi radialis longus (ECRL), ECRB	One-stage key pinch and release	BR to FPL EPL tenodesis Carpometacarpal (CMC) fusion
Group 4 & 5	BR, ECRL, ECRB, Pronator teres (PT), Flexor carpi radialis	Two-stage grasp, pinch, release	Flexor phase: BR/PT to FPL ECRL to flexor digitorum profundus Extensor: EPL, extensor digitorum communis tenodesis Thumb: BR or PT to flexor digitorum superficialis (FDS) ring CMC fusion Intrinsic: FDS lasso
Group 6 & 7	BR, ECRL, ECRB, PT, flexor carpi radialis, extensor digitorum communis, EPL	One-stage grasp and pinch	ECRL to flexor digitorum profundus BR/PT to FPL CMC fusion + EPL tenodesis or transfer PT/BR opponensplasty Intrinsics: FDS lasso

ACKNOWLEDGMENTS

The work was supported by a Midcareer Investigator Award in Patient-Oriented Research (2 K24-AR053120-06) to Kevin C. Chung. The content is solely the responsibility of the authors and does not necessarily represent the official views of the National Institutes of Health.

REFERENCES

1. Devivo MJ. Epidemiology of traumatic spinal cord injury: trends and future implications. *Spinal Cord*. 2012;50:365-372.
2. Jain NB, Ayers GD, Peterson EN, et al. Traumatic spinal cord injury in the United States, 1993-2012. *JAMA*. 2015;313:2236-2243.
3. Eckert MJ, Martin MJ. Trauma: spinal cord injury. *Surg Clin North Am*. 2017;97:1031-1045.
4. DeVivo MJ, Black KJ, Stover SL. Causes of death during the first 12 years after spinal cord injury. *Arch Phys Med Rehabil*. 1993;74:248-254.
5. DeVivo MJ. Sir Ludwig Guttmann Lecture: trends in spinal cord injury rehabilitation outcomes from model systems in the United States: 1973-2006. *Spinal Cord*. 2007;45:713-721.
6. Strauss DJ, Devivo MJ, Paculdo DR, Shavelle RM. Trends in life expectancy after spinal cord injury. *Arch Phys Med Rehabil*. 2006;87:1079-1085.
7. Gregersen H, Lybæk M, Lauge Johannesen I, et al. Satisfaction with upper extremity surgery in individuals with tetraplegia. *J Spinal Cord Med*. 2015;38:161-169.
8. Punj V, Curtin C. Understanding and overcoming barriers to upper limb surgical reconstruction after tetraplegia: the need for interdisciplinary collaboration. *Arch Phys Med Rehabil*. 2016;97:S81-S7.
9. Manns PJ, Chad KE. Components of quality of life for persons with a quadriplegic and paraplegic spinal cord injury. *Qual Health Res*. 2001;11:795-811.
10. Manns PJ, Chad KE. Determining the relation between quality of life, handicap, fitness, and physical activity for persons with spinal cord injury. *Arch Phys Med Rehabil*. 1999;80:1566-1571.
11. Putzke JD, Richards JS, Hicken BL, DeVivo MJ. Predictors of life satisfaction: a spinal cord injury cohort study. *Arch Phys Med Rehabil*. 2002;83:555-561.
12. Snoek GJ, Ijzerman MJ, Hermens HJ, et al. Survey of the needs of patients with spinal cord injury: impact and priority for improvement in hand function in tetraplegics. *Spinal Cord*. 2004;42:526-532.
13. Bednar MS. Tendon transfers for tetraplegia. *Hand Clin*. 2016;32:389-396.
14. Freehafer AA. Tendon transfers to improve grasp in patients with cervical spinal cord injury. *Paraplegia*. 1975;13:15-24.
15. Fox IK. Nerve transfers in tetraplegia. *Hand Clin*. 2016;32:227-242.
16. Jaspers Focks-Feenstra JH, Snoek GJ, Bongers-Janssen HM, Nene AV. Long-term patient satisfaction after reconstructive upper extremity surgery to improve arm-hand function in tetraplegia. *Spinal Cord*. 2011;49:903-908.
17. Meiners T, Abel R, Lindel K, Mesecke U. Improvements in activities of daily living following functional hand surgery for treatment of lesions to the cervical spinal cord: self-assessment by patients. *Spinal Cord*. 2002;40:574-580.
18. Wangdell J, Friden J. Satisfaction and performance in patient selected goals after grip reconstruction in tetraplegia. *J Hand Surg Eur Vol*. 2010;35:563-568.
    This study examined patient perspectives of grip reconstruction following spinal cord injury. Using the Canadian Occupational Performance Measure, the authors describe substantial gains in activities of daily living, with an improvement from [illegible]
19. Fox PM, Suarez P, Hentz VR, Curtin CM. Access to surgical upper extremity care for people with tetraplegia: an international perspective. *Spinal Cord*. 2015;53:302-305.
20. Curtin CM, Hayward RA, Kim HM, et al. Physician perceptions of upper extremity reconstruction for the person with tetraplegia. *J Hand Surg*. 2005;30:87-93.
21. Curtin CM, Gater DR, Chung KC. Upper extremity reconstruction in the tetraplegic population, a national epidemiologic study. *J Hand Surg*. 2005;30:94-99.
22. Hachem LD, Ahuja CS, Fehlings MG. Assessment and management of acute spinal cord injury: from point of injury to rehabilitation. *J Spinal Cord Med*. 2017;40:665-675.
23. Tator CH, Fehlings MG. Review of the secondary injury theory of acute spinal cord trauma with emphasis on vascular mechanisms. *J Neurosurg*. 1991;75:15-26.
24. Coulet B, Allieu Y, Chammas M. Injured metamere and functional surgery of the tetraplegic upper limb. *Hand Clin*. 2002;18:399-412.
25. Burns AS, Ditunno JF. Establishing prognosis and maximizing functional outcomes after spinal cord injury: a review of current and future directions in rehabilitation management. *Spine*. 2001;26:S137-S145.
26. Waters RL, Adkins RH, Yakura JS, Sie I. Motor and sensory recovery following complete tetraplegia. *Arch Phys Med Rehabil*. 1993;74:242-247.
    This study prospectively examined the motor and sensory recovery of 61 patients with spinal cord injury. The authors identified that the greatest potential for recovery occurs within the first 6 months, and majority of patients reach plateau of motor recovery between 6 and 9 months following injury.
27. Diong J, Harvey LA, Kwah LK, et al. Incidence and predictors of contracture after spinal cord injury – a prospective cohort study. *Spinal Cord*. 2012;50:579-584.
28. Botte MJ, Nickel VL, Akeson WH. Spasticity and contracture: physiologic aspects of formation. *Clin Orthop Relat Res*. 1988;(233):7-18.
29. Krajnik SR, Bridle MJ. Hand splinting in quadriplegia: current practice. *Am J Occup Ther*. 1992;46:149-156.
30. Strommen JA. Management of spasticity from spinal cord dysfunction. *Neurol Clin*. 2013;31:269-286.
31. Hentz VR. Surgical strategy: matching the patient with the procedure. *Hand Clin*. 2002;18:503-518.
32. Macciocchi S, Seel RT, Warshowsky A, et al. Co-occurring traumatic brain injury and acute spinal cord injury rehabilitation outcomes. *Arch Phys Med Rehabil*. 2012;93:1788-1794.
33. Wangdell J, Friden J. Activity gains after reconstructions of elbow extension in patients with tetraplegia. *J Hand Surg Am*. 2012;37:1003-1010.
34. Johnson DL, Gellman H, Waters RL, Tognella M. Brachioradialis transfer for wrist extension in tetraplegic patients who have fifth-cervical-level neurological function. *J Bone Joint Surg Am*. 1996;78A:1063-1067.

35. Mohindra M, Sangwan SS, Kundu ZS, et al. Surgical rehabilitation of a tetraplegic hand: comparison of various methods of reconstructing an absent pinch and hook. *Hand (NY)*. 2014;9:179-186.
36. Friden J, Reinholdt C, Gohritz A. The extensor pollicis longus-loop-knot (ELK) procedure for dynamic balance of the paralyzed thumb interphalangeal joint. *Tech Hand Up Extrem Surg*. 2013;17:184-186.
37. Friden J, Gohritz A. Tetraplegia management update. *J Hand Surg Am*. 2015;40:2489-2500.
38. Coulet B, Waitzenegger T, Teissier J, et al. Arthrodesis versus carpometacarpal preservation in key-grip procedures in tetraplegic patients: a comparative study of 40 cases. *J Hand Surg Am*. 2018;43:483.
39. Coulet B, Boretto JG, Allieu Y, et al. Pronating osteotomy of the radius for forearm supination contracture in high-level tetraplegic patients: technique and results. *J Bone Joint Surg Br*. 2010;92B:828-834.
40. Friden J, Reinholdt C, Gohritz A, et al. Simultaneous powering of forearm pronation and key pinch in tetraplegia using a single muscle-tendon unit. *J Hand Surg Eur Vol*. 2012;37:323-328.
41. Ward SR, Peace WJ, Friden J, Lieber RL. Dorsal transfer of the brachioradialis to the flexor pollicis longus enables simultaneous powering of key pinch and forearm pronation. *J Hand Surg Am*. 2006;31:993-997.
42. Zancolli EA. Paralytic supination contracture of the forearm. *J Bone Joint Surg Am*. 1967;49A:1275-1284.
43. Gellman H, Kan D, Waters RL, Nicosa A. Rerouting of the biceps brachii for paralytic supination contracture of the forearm in tetraplegia due to trauma. *J Bone Joint Surg Am*. [illegible]
44. Friden J, Reinholdt C, Turcsanyii I, Gohritz A. A single-stage operation for reconstruction of hand flexion, extension, and intrinsic function in tetraplegia: the alphabet procedure. *Tech Hand Up Extrem Surg*. 2011;15:230-235.
45. House JH, Gwathmey FW, Lundsgaard DK. Restoration of strong grasp and lateral pinch in tetraplegia due to cervical spinal cord injury. *J Hand Surg Am*. 1976;1:152-159.
This study describes the reconstruction of grasp and pinch in 7 patients with C6 and C7 level injuries including surgical techniques for the extensor and flexor phase. All patients at follow-up reported gains in activities of daily living, social self-image, and wheelchair use and achieved an average grasp and pinch force of 5.5 and 3.0 kg.
46. House JH, Shannon MA. Restoration of strong grasp and lateral pinch in tetraplegia: a comparison of two methods of thumb control in each patient. *J Hand Surg Am*. 1985;10:22-29.
47. Kozin SH, D'Addesi L, Chafetz RS, et al. Biceps-to-triceps transfer for elbow extension in persons with tetraplegia. *J Hand Surg Am*. 2010;35:968-975.
This retrospective study examined the outcomes of 45 patients who underwent medial biceps to triceps transfer to restore elbow extension. The majority of patients were able to achieve elbow extension against gravity with functional overhead elbow extension.
48. Kuz JE, Van Heest AE, House JH. Biceps-to-triceps transfer in tetraplegic patients: report of the medial routing technique and follow-up of three cases. *J Hand Surg Am*. 1999;24:161-172.
49. Bonds CW, James MA. Posterior deltoid-to-triceps tendon transfer to restore active elbow extension in patients with tetraplegia. *Tech Hand Up Extrem Surg*. 2009;13:94-97.
50. Mohammed KD, Rothwell AG, Sinclair SW, et al. Upper-limb surgery for tetraplegia. *J Bone Joint Surg Br*. 1992;74B:873-879.
The authors review the outcomes of 57 patients undergoing reconstruction for elbow extension, hook grip, and key pinch. This retrospective study highlights the effectiveness of split FPL tenodesis to balance the thumb interphalangeal joint.
51. McCarthy CK, House JH, Van Heest A, et al. Intrinsic balancing in reconstruction of the tetraplegic hand. *J Hand Surg Am*. 1997;22:596-604.

QUESTIONS

1. **A 27-year-old man with a history of SCI from a motor vehicle collision 3 years ago presents for consultation to improve his ability to power his wheelchair. On physical examination, he is able to flex his elbow and extend his wrist. He has M5 strength of biceps, brachialis, BR, extensor carpi radialis longus and brevis, and PT. He is unable to extend his elbow. Which of the following procedures would best enhance his upper extremity function?**
   a. Wrist arthrodesis
   b. Abductor digiti minimi to abductor pollicis brevis transfer
   c. Biceps to triceps transfer
   d. Extensor indicis proprius to EPL transfer
   e. Side-to-side FDP transfer

2. **A 22-year-old woman who suffered a SCI 1 year ago presents for reconstruction to optimize her hand function. She would like to have better hand control to pick up objects. On examination, she has intact elbow flexion and centralized wrist function but is unable to pronate her forearm. She has stiffness with passive motion of her digits and a pressure ulcer across her olecranon. Which of the following options is indicated to optimize her hand function?**
   a. Directed physiotherapy for donor muscle strengthening
   b. Biceps to triceps transfer
   c. BR to FPL transfer
   d. Extensor carpi radialis brevis tenodesis
   e. Directed physiotherapy for range of motion

3. **A 38-year-old man presents for consultation to improve grip approximately 2 years following SCI. On examination, he has intact elbow flexion, wrist extension and flexion, and digit extension. He has weakness with thumb extension and digit flexion. Which of the following procedures would best improve his grasp ability?**
   a. ECRB to FDP transfer
   b. ECRL to FDP transfer
   c. FCR to FDP transfer
   d. BR to FDP transfer
   e. FDS lasso procedure

4. **Which of the following physical examination maneuvers will best assess strength of BR?**
   a. Palpation over the lateral aspect of the mobile wad with the patient abducting the arm in extension
   b. Palpation over the lateral aspect of the mobile wad with the patient flexing the elbow in neutral
   c. Palpation over the lateral aspect of the mobile wad with the patient flexing the elbow in supination
   d. Palpation over the lateral aspect of the mobile wad with the patient flexing the wrist in neutral
   e. Palpation over the lateral aspect of the mobile wad with the patient flexing the wrist in pronation

5. **A 32-year-old patient who suffered a SCI 3 years earlier presents for upper extremity reconstruction. Biceps to triceps transfer to restore elbow extension is planned. The preferred technique for this tendon transfer includes the following:**
   a. Routing the biceps tendon laterally with a supplemental tendon graft (e.g., tensor fasciae latae)
   b. Routing the biceps tendon medially
   c. Routing the biceps tendon medially with a supplemental tendon graft (e.g., tensor fasciae latae)
   d. Routing the biceps tendon laterally
   e. Routing the biceps tendon posteriorly through the triceps muscle

1. **Answer: c.** This individual has intact strength of his PT and is classified in the ICSHT group 1. Critical functions to restore in this group include elbow extension, key pinch, grasp and release, and intrinsic balancing. For this patient, biceps to triceps transfer or posterior deltoid to triceps transfer would provide strength of elbow extension to position the upper extremity in space and facilitate transfer and mobility. Wrist arthrodesis is not performed in SCI patients as it would result in the loss of tenodesis, which is critical for rudimentary key pinch, grasp, and release. Abductor digiti minimi to abductor pollicis brevis insertion at the thumb MCP joint transfer is a commonly used opponensplasty technique for patients with congenital thumb hypoplasia but would not be appropriate or possible for this patient given the level of injury. Extensor indicis proprius transfer is performed for attritional rupture of EPL but is not performed for patients with tetraplegia. Side-to-side FDP transfer is performed among patients with partial innervation of FDP among group 8 patients in whom flexion of the index and long finger is preserved but not of the ring and small finger. However, this option would not be suitable given this patient's level of injury.

2. **Answer: e.** This individual has intact strength of his PT and is classified in the ICSHT group 3, as she is noted to have function of her BR and wrist extensors but does not have recovery of her PT following injury. For this patient, critical functions to restore include elbow extension, forearm pronation, key pinch, and intrinsic balancing. Reconstruction of key pinch could offer this patient a greater ability to pick up objects, including a one-stage key pinch and release procedure including BR transfer to FPL, EPL tenodesis, and CMC arthrodesis. However, this patient has notable stiffness of her hand and a pressure wound across her elbow. Reconstructive options are most appropriate for patients with a pain-free upper extremity without evidence of contracture or neglect. Therefore, physiotherapy to overcome contractures, ensure appropriate pressure offloading, and support and compliance with therapy is indicated first prior to undertaking surgical reconstruction. Biceps to triceps transfer is appropriate for suitable patients to restore elbow extension which can allow patients improved reach for objects. Directed therapy for donor muscle strengthening is an important component of rehabilitation following injury but would not specifically address the wrist contractures or pressure offloading in this patient. ECRB tenodesis would not be recommended as it would reduce the ability of wrist flexion and impair tenodesis, which is critical for release of objects.

3. **Answer: b.** This individual has intact strength of his digital extensors, but not his thumb extensor, and is classified in the ICSHT group 6. For this patient, critical functions to restore include digit flexion and thumb flexion for grasp. BR, ECRL, and PT are available for transfer. Common transfers to restore digit flexion include ERCL to FDP or PT to FDP, and BR to FPL to FPL to restore thumb flexion with EPL tenodesis to provide balance. ECRB is not used as a donor as it provides centralized wrist extension. FCR is not commonly used as a donor tendon as its power facilitates the tenodesis effect and release. The FDS lasso procedure creates a static sling around the A1 pulley to provide improved posture among patients with intrinsic

weakness and place the MCP joints in flexion. Although this procedure can facilitate grip by providing better coordination of interphalangeal joint flexion, it would not specifically address restoration of strength to the digital flexors.

4. Answer: b. BR is innervated by roots C5 and C6 via the radial nerve. It originates along the proximal aspect of the lateral supracondylar ridge of the humerus and the lateral intermuscular septum and inserts on the radial styloid. BR serves to flex the elbow with the forearm in neutral or pronation. It can be palpated lateral to the biceps tendon along the mobile wad. It is best assessed by placing the patient's elbow in 90° and the forearm in neutral and asking the patient to flex the elbow. Maintaining the forearm in pronation or supination is critical to isolate the action of BR from other elbow flexors and supinators including biceps and brachialis.

5. Answer: b. Reconstruction of elbow extension is a top priority following SCI among patients without triceps strength to restore the ability to reach, power assistive devices, and facilitate independence with activities of daily living. Biceps to triceps tendon transfer is commonly performed to accomplish this after action of the brachialis is confirmed to maintain elbow flexion. The biceps tendon is routed medially and anchored to the olecranon and woven to the triceps tendon. Routing the tendon laterally is avoided to prevent injury and compression of the radial nerve. Biceps to triceps tendon transfer typically does not require supplemental tendon grafting but is needed for posterior deltoid to triceps transfer, an alternative procedure to restore elbow extension among SCI patients.

CHAPTER 74 Management of Hand Fractures

Joshua M. Adkinson and Kevin C. Chung

KEY POINTS

- All patients evaluated for a hand fracture should also undergo examination of the skin, tendons, and neurovascular structures.
- Metacarpal fractures typically assume an apex dorsal deformity, whereas proximal phalangeal fractures result in an apex volar deformity. Middle phalanx fracture deformity depends upon the location relative to the flexor digitorum superficialis insertion.
- Operative intervention is indicated for intra-articular incongruity, rotational malalignment, angular deformity, substantial shortening, multiple fractures, and fractures with soft tissue injury or bone loss.
- Select the least invasive method that will achieve satisfactory fracture reduction and stability.
- Prolonged immobilization will invariably lead to stiffness that may be worse than a malunion resulting from no treatment.

Fractures of the hand are common, accounting for 10% of all fractures[1] and 41% of upper extremity fractures.[2] Phalanx fractures occur approximately twice as often as metacarpal fractures[2] and most commonly affect the distal phalanx.[3] The economic impact of hand fractures is substantial, and estimated lost productivity alone exceeds $2 billion per year.[4] Given the individual and societal burden of hand fractures, the ideal treatment is timely, minimizes recovery time, and expedites return to work and other activities. This chapter outlines the most common hand fracture patterns and recommended treatment options.

PRINCIPLES OF MANAGEMENT

A thorough initial history and examination are mandatory. The type of trauma will offer insight into the likelihood of associated injuries as well as any social barriers to effective treatment and an optimal outcome. The time since injury should be determined, as this may influence the timing of surgery. Patient age, hand dominance, occupation, hobbies, comorbidities, and previous hand injuries or surgical procedures should be elicited. Furthermore, the treating physician should discuss patient goals of care and, when possible, ascertain the ability to comply with postoperative instructions and therapy.

The hand is then thoroughly and systematically examined for deformity, tenderness, swelling, open wounds, digital malalignment, tendon integrity, and neurovascular status. Rotational deformity may be subtle, yet clinically significant, and is evaluated through active range of motion or wrist tenodesis; all digits should point to the scaphoid without overlap or rotation (Figure 74.1). Seemingly small amounts of fracture malrotation can result in digital overlap (e.g., 5° of metacarpal rotation leads to 1.5 cm of digital overlap).[5] Range of motion assessment may be facilitated by digital or wrist neuroblockade after sensory evaluation. Three-view (posteroanterior, lateral, oblique) plain radiographs of the hand are mandatory to assess fracture anatomy and any concomitant degenerative, oncological, or rheumatological pathology.[3]

Open fractures of the hand are relatively common and are at an increased risk for infection. Management consists of tetanus administration, antibiotics, irrigation, debridement, and sterile temporary or definitive (e.g., flap) coverage.[6] Definitive fracture treatment is performed when the wound is clean and stable soft tissue coverage can be ensured.

Nearly all closed hand fractures can be initially managed with closed reduction and splinting. Stable, nondisplaced fractures may be definitively treated in this manner. The patient is seen within 7 to 10 days for reexamination and new plain radiographs to confirm stability and to rule out fracture displacement. In general, metacarpal and phalangeal fractures are adequately treated by 3 to 4 weeks of continuous immobilization and judicious use of immobilization beyond this period only for specific activities. There always exists a balance between adequate immobilization to optimize fracture healing and mobilization to counteract the inevitable onset of stiffness. Prolonged immobilization may be worse than no treatment; the duration of immobilization should be as short as possible to allow fracture healing.

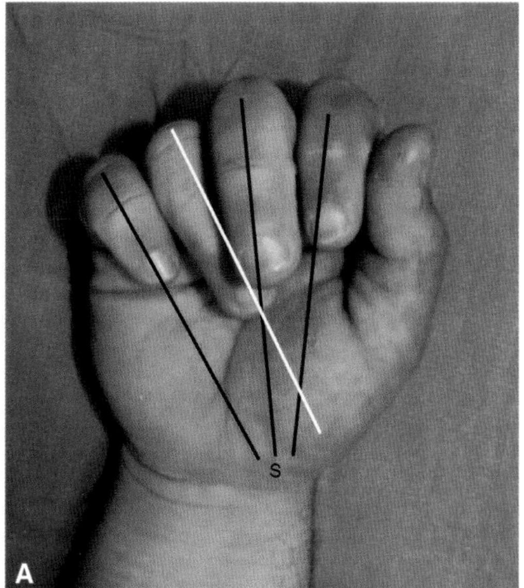

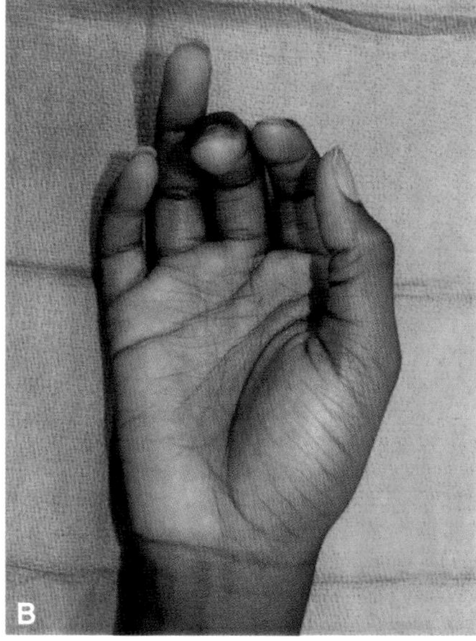

FIGURE 74.1. **A.** Black lines indicate normal alignment of the digits, with the fingertips pointing to scaphoid (S). White line indicates malrotation and digital overlap resulting from a fracture. **B.** Malrotation of ring finger after proximal phalanx fracture.

FRACTURE DEFORMITY

Isolated fractures of the hand lead to a relatively predictable deformity resulting from the muscles and tendons crossing the fracture site. Metacarpal fractures usually lead to an apex dorsal deformity because of intrinsic muscle pull on the metacarpal head. Proximal phalanx fractures typically result in an apex volar deformity because the intrinsic muscles flex the base and the extensor mechanism extends the distal shaft (Figure 74.2). Middle phalanx fracture deformity varies depending on location. Base fractures assume an apex dorsal deformity resulting from the pull of the central slip and the flexion moment imparted by the flexor digitorum superficialis (FDS) insertion. Middle phalanx fractures distal to the FDS insertion assume an apex volar posture because the FDS flexes the shaft and the extensor mechanism extends the distal fragment.

INDICATIONS FOR REPAIR

The primary goals of hand fracture management are to restore anatomic relationships, provide fracture stability with minimal soft tissue injury, and institute early motion. Whereas, most fractures can be managed nonoperatively, surgery may be warranted in the following cases[7]:

- Articular incongruity
- Digital malrotation, shortening, or angulation
- Multiple fractures
- Open fractures
- Fractures with soft tissue injury or bone loss

The amount of tolerable deformity varies by fracture location and pattern of injury.

FRACTURE REPAIR TECHNIQUES

Fracture fixation options are dependent on fracture anatomy, associated injuries, and surgeon preference and experience. In general, fixation options include Kirschner wires (K-wires), interosseous wiring, compression screws, plating, and external fixation[8] (**Table 74.1**).

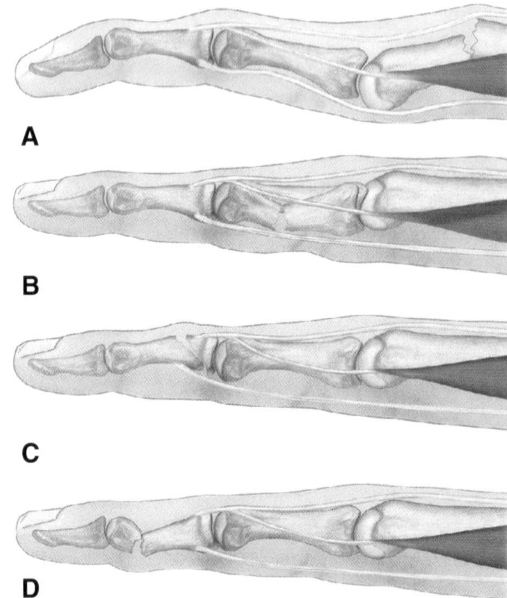

FIGURE 74.2. Fracture site deformity is based on location of the fracture relative to the flexor and extensor tendons. **A.** Metacarpal shaft fracture. **B.** Proximal phalanx fracture. **C.** Middle phalanx fracture proximal to flexor digitorum superficialis insertion. **D.** Middle phalanx fracture distal to flexor digitorum superficialis insertion.

K-Wires

K-wires are a commonly used and versatile fixation method for fractures of the hand. They are inexpensive and relatively easy to apply percutaneously. K-wires alone, however, do not provide rigid fixation or compression across the fracture site.[9] As such, additional immobilization may be necessary to prevent fracture fragment displacement in the postoperative period. Multiple K-wire configurations may be used depending on fracture characteristics. Importantly, a single K-wire does not impart rotational stability, and at least two K-wires should be employed to prevent fracture rotation (Figure 74.3). The crossed K-wire technique is commonly used for treatment of hand fractures. With this technique, two wires cross obliquely in an X configuration. Importantly, the K-wires should never cross at the fracture site, as this will lead to distraction of the fracture fragments and limited fracture stability. Instead, one must ensure that the wires cross proximal or distal to the fracture. Although conceptually simple, optimal application of K-wires can be technically difficult. The wire should be advanced to an appropriate bone entry site under fluoroscopic guidance. Slow, precise entry into the bone allows for trajectory modifications and the wire to gain *purchase* to prevent malposition during advancement.

Tension band wiring is a modification of K-wire fracture fixation that increases construct strength. The tension band concept converts a distraction force (from the flexor tendons) into a compression force at the fracture site. In general, two 0.035- or 0.045-inch K-wires are placed across the fracture site. A 24 gauge (G) or 26G steel wire is then wrapped around the K-wires in a figure-of-eight fashion and secured away from the tendons to prevent attritional injury. This technique can enable immediate motion but requires greater soft tissue exposure than K-wires alone.

Compression Screws

Compression screws may be used for oblique or spiral fractures using the lag principle. This technique is ideal when the fracture length is at least twice the diameter of the bone. Lag screw fixation requires drilling a hole in the near cortex that is the same diameter as the outer diameter of the screw.[10] For example, when applying lag screw fixation for a metacarpal shaft fracture, a 2.0 mm drill bit

TABLE 74.1. COMPARISON OF HAND FRACTURE FIXATION TECHNIQUES

Technique	Advantages	Disadvantages
K-wires	Easily removed, low cost, limited soft tissue damage	Need for additional immobilization, pin tract migration/infection, lack of compression at fracture site
Compression screws	Rigid fixation, limited periosteal stripping needed	Technically demanding
Interosseous wiring	Low profile, provides fracture site compression	Technically demanding, potential wire breakage, requires soft tissue exposure
Plate and screws	Rigid fixation	Technically demanding, requires soft tissue exposure, potentially bulky and/or symptomatic hardware
External fixation	Rapid and easy application, avoids fracture site, allows for soft tissue reconstruction	May not achieve anatomic reduction, pin site infection, requires removal, rarely definitive solution

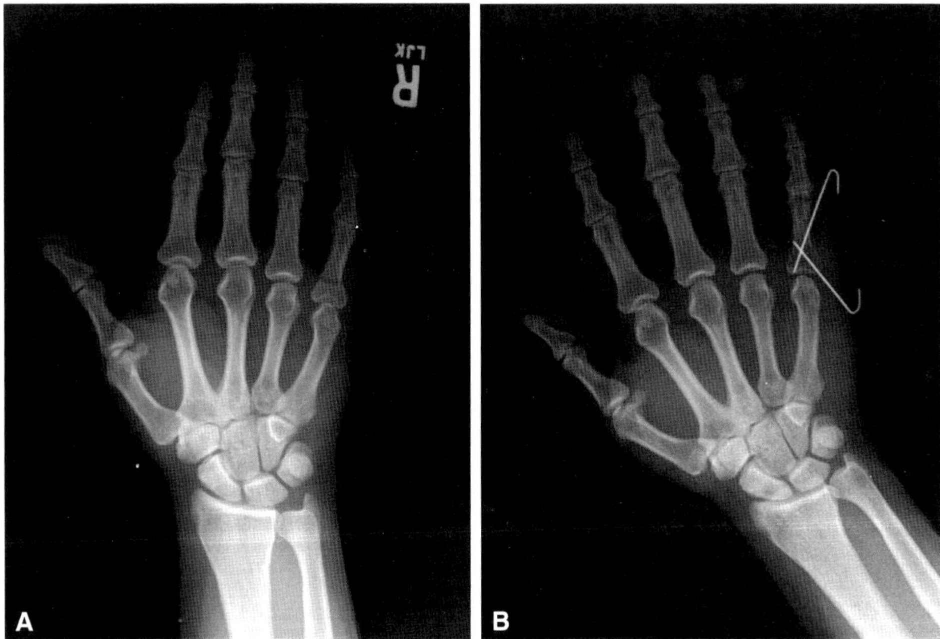

FIGURE 74.3. Right small finger proximal phalanx transverse fracture (Seymour fracture). **A.** X-ray findings. **B.** K-wire fixation.

is used for the near cortex. The far cortex is drilled with a 1.5 mm drill bit. The near cortex acts as a glide hole, whereas the far cortex is captured by the screw threads and leads to compression between the fracture fragments when a 2 mm screw is advanced into the drill hole (Figure 74.4). Prior to screw application, a countersink should be used to prevent screw head prominence. The procedure requires exacting technique and precise fracture reduction. Additional care should be taken when applying lag screws in the softer metaphyseal bone of the metacarpal or phalanges, where aggressive countersinking can lead to the screw head sinking into the medullary canal during tightening. Multiple screws are required to achieve anatomic reduction and impart axial stability of the construct.

Interosseous Wiring

Interosseous wiring is a technically demanding procedure that provides rigid fixation and fracture site compression. It is mainly used for transverse fractures of the phalanges or metacarpals, in joint arthrodesis, or in digital replantation. Typically, a 0.045-inch K-wire is used to create a parallel drill hole in both fracture fragments, dorsal to palmar and radial to ulnar. Alternatively, both wires can be oriented in the dorsal to palmar plane. Through this drill hole, an 18G needle is placed and used a guide for insertion of a 24G or 26G steel wire. The wire is then carefully tightened to prevent breakage.

Plate and Screws

Plate fixation provides a highly stable construct for hand fracture treatment. This technique is most commonly used for metacarpal shaft fractures and for the treatment of nonunion and malunion, where restoring length and stability are essential. Plate fixation is rarely used for phalangeal fractures because of the close relationship of the extensor mechanism to the periosteum of the underlying bone; plate fixation in the phalanges frequently leads to tendon scarring and stiffness. Conversely, the extensor tendons overlying the metacarpals do not sit directly on bone and, as such, are at low risk for adhesions after plate fixation. Dynamic compression style or standard straight plates are available for use in the hand. Compression plate holes are oblong and allow eccentric application of screws. After fixation of one fracture fragment to the plate, the first screw in the adjacent fracture fragment is placed eccentrically away from the fracture; this pulls the fragments into compression as the screw head engages the plate. Subsequent screws are placed in neutral alignment, as no further compression can be achieved with additional screws (Figure 74.5). Compared with other techniques for fracture fixation, plate and screw application requires a relatively large amount of soft tissue dissection and periosteal stripping. Scarring and plate prominence may lead to extensor tendon adhesions and impaired gliding or pain. As a result, tenolysis and/or plate removal may be needed after fracture healing.

External Fixation

External fixation is a relatively simple technique that is useful for fractures with substantial soft tissue injury, marked comminution, bone loss, and/or contamination. It can be rapidly applied, avoids the fracture site, and allows early mobilization. Most commonly, two percutaneous pins are placed proximal and two pins distal to the fracture site. Commercially available external fixator systems connect these pins using a bridging carbon fiber bar. Rarely is external fixation the definitive solution for hand fracture management.

PHALANX FRACTURES

Distal Phalanx

Distal phalangeal fractures are the most common fractures in the hand. They are classified by location as tuft, shaft, and base fractures. Tuft fractures most frequently occur in combination with nail bed injuries and warrant an evaluation of the integrity of the nail plate and nail bed. A concomitant nail bed injury should be washed out and closed with fine absorbable suture. The nail plate may act as a splint for the fracture, although these injuries should be protected with an external splint for approximately 3 to 4 weeks. Tuft fractures often heal with a malunion, but these are rarely symptomatic. Nondisplaced shaft fractures may be managed with immobilization only. Displaced shaft fractures are treated by closed reduction and application of a single longitudinal K-wire. Articular fractures of the dorsal base of the distal phalanx often involve the extensor tendon insertion (i.e., mallet fracture). Most of these injuries may be managed with distal interphalangeal (DIP) joint splinting in full extension for 6 weeks. Dorsal block K-wire fixation is recommended for fractures involving more than one-third of

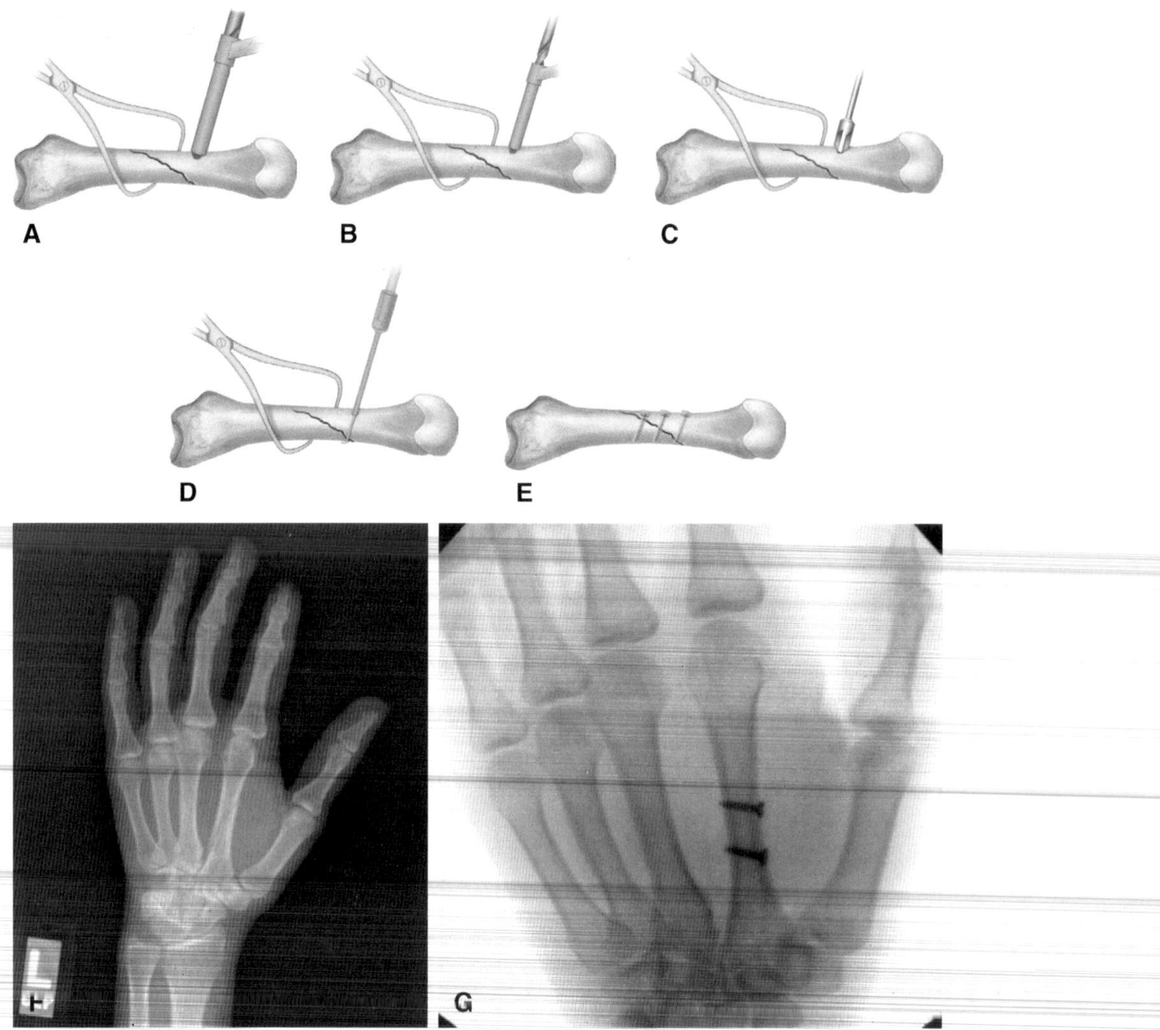

FIGURE 74.4. Technique of lag screw fixation. **A.** Near cortex (gliding hole) is drilled with the larger drill bit. **B.** The smaller drill bit is passed into the same tract and drilled in the same trajectory. **C.** A countersink is used to prevent screw head prominence. **D.** Screw length is determined. **E.** Multiple screws are placed to ensure fracture stability. **F.** A right index finger metacarpal long oblique fracture. **G.** Multiple screws placed using the lag technique.

the articular surface or in the setting of volar subluxation of the distal fragment (Figure 74.6). In children, fractures may occur through the physis and entrap a portion of the nail bed (i.e., Seymour fracture) (Figure 74.7). These fractures should be treated with extraction of the nail bed, irrigation, and K-wire fixation in a timely fashion to prevent infection and subsequent osteomyelitis.

Proximal/Middle Phalanx

Condylar fractures of the proximal and middle phalanges are by definition intra-articular and are associated with development of arthritis. Phalangeal condylar fractures are classified as type I (unicondylar and nondisplaced), type II (unicondylar and displaced), and type III (bicondylar). Nonoperative management may be considered for nondisplaced fractures, but close radiographic follow-up is mandatory to rule out subsequent displacement. Displaced fractures are treated with closed reduction and at least two K-wires or open reduction and screw fixation.[11] Bicondylar fractures may be challenging to manage and are treated by open reduction through the interval between the central slip and lateral band with subsequent screw or K-wire fixation. Extreme care must be exercised when performing open repair of condylar fractures to avoid injury to the vascular supply arising from the attached collateral ligaments. Early motion, when possible, will limit postoperative stiffness and pain.

Phalangeal neck fractures are inherently unstable. As such, the majority of these injuries are treated with K-wire fixation. Nondisplaced shaft fractures may be managed with splinting or buddy tape to an adjacent uninjured digit for 3 to 4 weeks. If malrotated or displaced greater than 10° to 25° in the sagittal plane or 10° to 15° in the coronal plane, reduction and fixation are required. Transverse or short oblique fractures are treated with K-wires or, rarely, plate fixation. Long oblique and spiral fractures are treated with interfragmentary screw fixation (Figure 74.8). The screw diameter should be less than one-third of the length of the fracture. At least two screws are recommended to impart stability to the construct. Nondisplaced phalangeal base fractures are treated with splint immobilization for 3 to 4 weeks. If displaced or associated with malrotation, open reduction and K-wire or screw fixation are warranted. Proximal interphalangeal (PIP) joint fracture-dislocations require special consideration and are discussed elsewhere in more detail. Given the articular incongruity that results from these injuries, patients frequently develop a stiff and painful PIP joint. Treatment options range from dynamic external fixation, K-wire or screw fixation, and dorsal block pinning to more complex volar plate arthroplasty and hemi-hamate reconstruction of the volar base of the middle phalanx.

METACARPAL FRACTURES

Head

Metacarpal head fractures are rare and typically result from an axial load or dorsal fracture-dislocation of the metacarpophalangeal

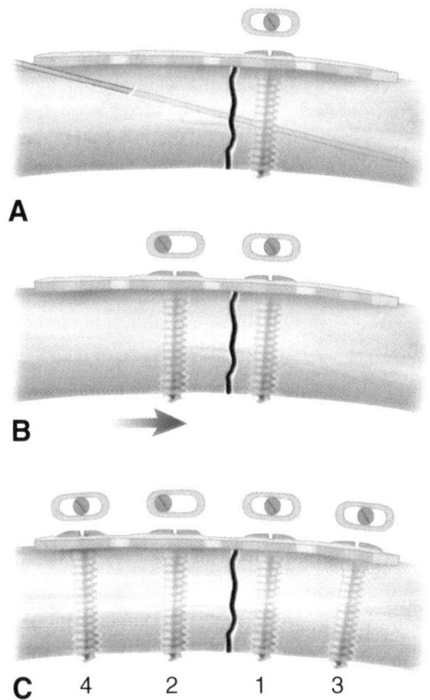

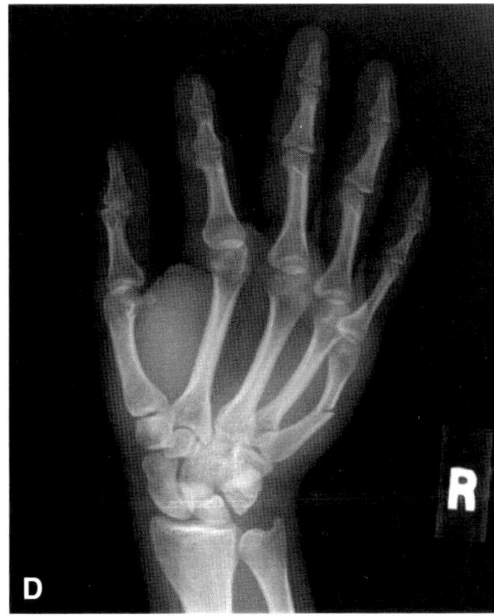

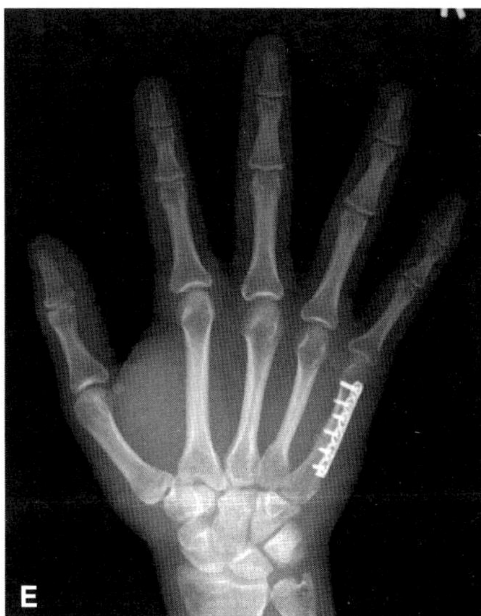

FIGURE 74.5. Technique of compression plate application. **A.** Initial screw is placed in neutral position. **B.** The second screw is placed eccentrically away from the fracture site. **C.** The remaining screws are placed in neutral position as no further compression can occur through the plate. **D.** Right small finger metacarpal shaft fracture. **E.** Compression plate fixation.

(MCP) joint. Computed tomography scan may better visualize the fracture pattern and assist in surgical planning. Nonoperative management is recommended for fractures with less than 25% articular involvement. For fractures with greater articular involvement, >1 mm articular incongruity, or collateral ligament instability, surgery is warranted. Fracture fragments may be small and comminuted, and [illegible] must be taken to avoid stripping the vascular supply arising from the collateral ligaments. Avascular necrosis of the metacarpal head is rare but has been reported.[14] Although headless screw fixation is an optimal choice of fixation for metacarpal head fractures, most injuries are comminuted or associated with joint disruption; these injuries may be best treated by dynamic external fixation or acute arthroplasty.[13]

Neck

Metacarpal neck (i.e., boxer's) fractures are common and typically involve the fifth metacarpal. This injury often results from a punching mechanism in the amateur fighter or someone who strikes a hard object. A relatively large amount of angular deformity is acceptable in the ring and small fingers because of a mobile carpometacarpal (CMC) joint that can accommodate for palmar angulation. As a result, the majority of these injuries are managed nonoperatively. Unreduced metacarpal neck fractures with significant apex dorsal deformity may result in a prominence (metacarpal head) in the palm that is particularly bothersome to athletes and manual laborers. Nonoperatively managed patients should also be [illegible] the loss of the dorsal knuckle prominence.

Closed reduction of a metacarpal neck fracture is accomplished using the Jahss maneuver[14] (Figure 74.9). This is most frequently carried out in the emergency department using a nerve block at the wrist. The MCP and PIP joints are fully flexed, whereas a volar force is directed against the metacarpal shaft, and a dorsal force is applied to the proximal phalanx. This combination of forces is used to lever the metacarpal head into anatomic alignment. The hand is then immobilized in an ulnar gutter splint or cast with the MCP joint in 70° of flexion for 3 weeks, followed by an active range of motion therapy program.

Surgery is recommended in the setting of pseudoclawing (hyperextension of the MCP joint and concomitant PIP joint flexion with attempted digital extension), excessive shortening, and malrotation after attempted closed reduction. Surgical indications for apex dorsal deformity depend upon the involved digit (**Table 74.2**). The amount of tolerated angular deformity is controversial, however, and multiple studies have shown excellent outcomes with substantial angulation (up to 70° in the fifth metacarpal neck). Most commonly, metacarpal neck fractures are managed with percutaneous K-wire fixation and many configurations can be utilized—transverse, retrograde, and antegrade. Buried antegrade intramedullary pin application may be superior because it avoids the extensor mechanism and obviates the risk for pin tract infection (Figure 74.10). Open repair of acute metacarpal neck fractures is reserved for failed percutaneous treatment or an unacceptable closed reduction.

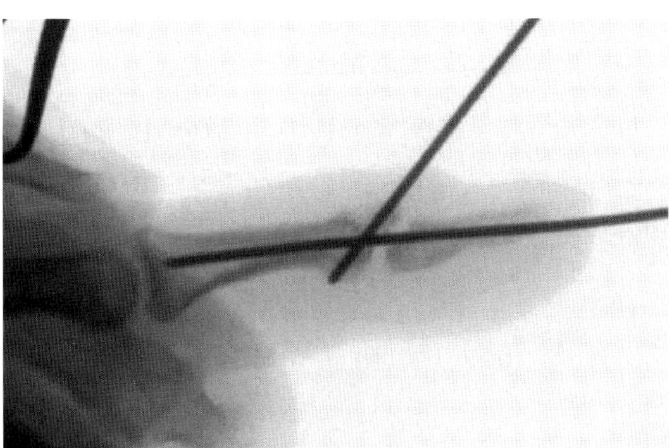

FIGURE 74.6. Dorsal block pinning of a distal phalanx intra-articular fracture.

Shaft

Metacarpal shaft fractures may occur from an axial load, torsion, or crush. Indications for surgical management are similar to metacarpal neck fractures; however, less angular deformity is tolerated in the metacarpal shaft (see Table 74.2). Nondisplaced fractures may be treated with splinting or casting for 4 weeks with

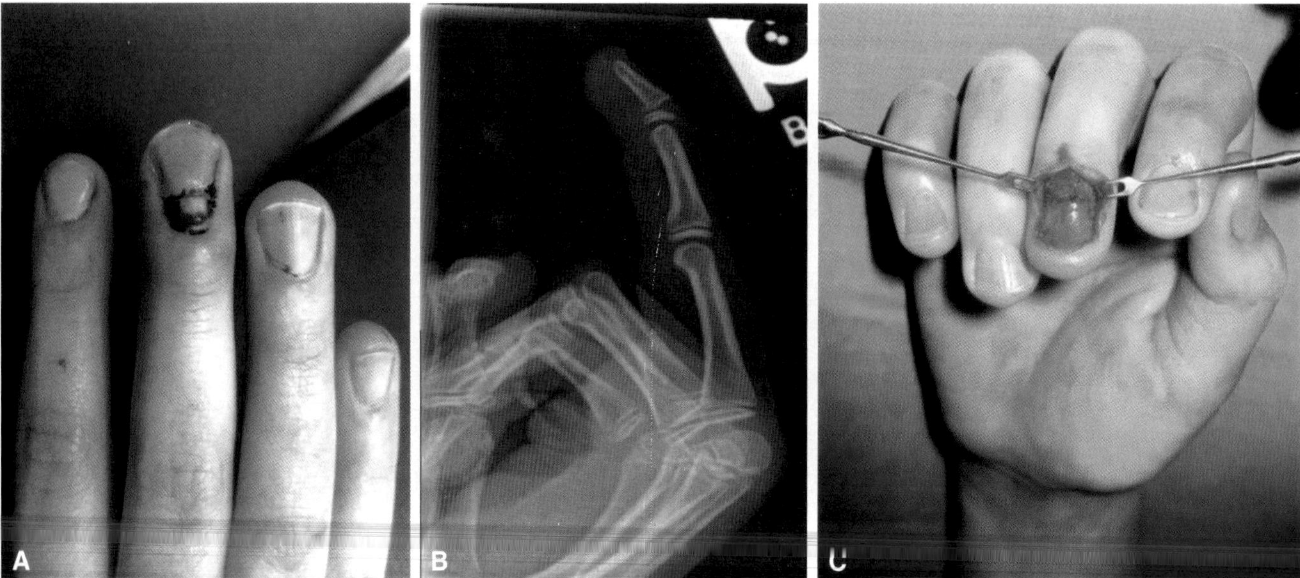

FIGURE 74.7. Seymour fracture. **A.** Clinical findings. **B.** X-ray findings. **C.** Nail bed extracted from fracture site and repaired.

the interphalangeal joints free. Unstable or displaced fractures can be treated with percutaneous pins or open reduction and plate or lag screw fixation. The operative approach is through a dorsal longitudinal incision between the metacarpals. The juncturae may be divided to improve exposure of the fracture. External fixation is reserved for fractures with segmental loss, unstable soft tissue coverage, or contamination. Nondisplaced oblique and spiral fractures are usually unstable and are often best treated with surgery. If nonoperative management is selected, weekly radiographs should be obtained to rule out late displacement. If the fracture is obliquely oriented and the fracture length is at least twice the bone diameter, lag screws may be the best choice, although placement requires exacting technique. Percutaneous pinning may also be used for metacarpal shaft fractures, although this requires longer periods of immobilization and delayed initiation of therapy.

Base

Extra-articular metacarpal base fractures are managed similarly to shaft fractures. Most are nondisplaced and managed with immobilization for 3 to 4 weeks. If displaced or obliquely oriented, closed or open reduction and fixation is recommended. Given the substantial mobility of the thumb CMC joint, a relatively large amount of displacement is well tolerated. Reduction is indicated if the distal fragment is flexed greater than 30°, as this amount of deformity leads to compensatory thumb MCP joint hyperextension.

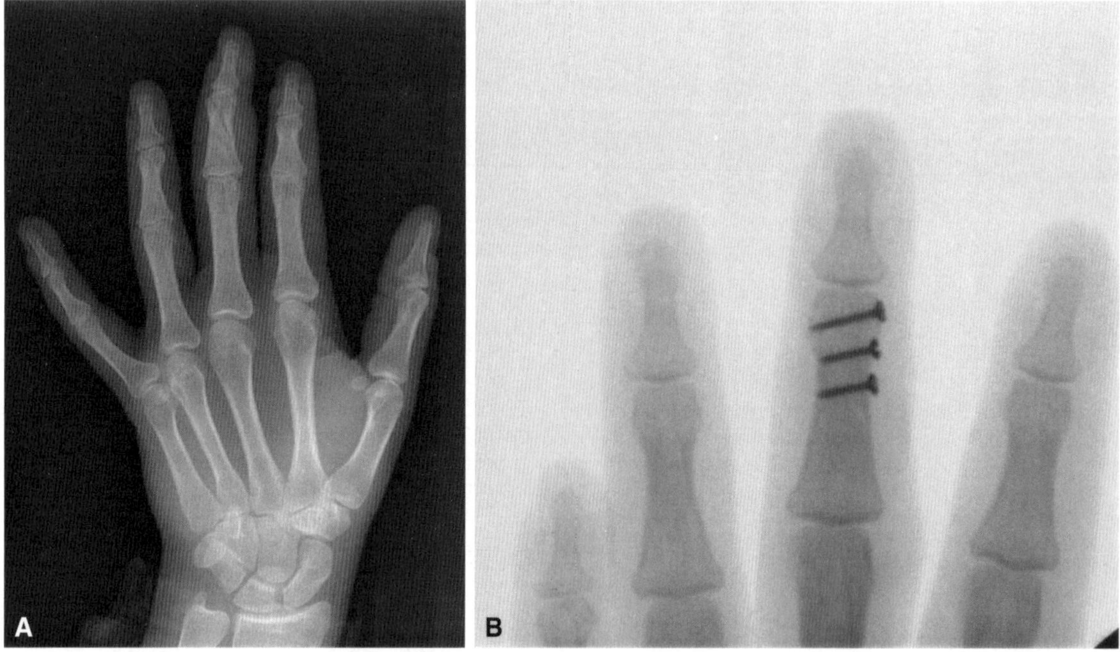

FIGURE 74.8. Left middle finger middle phalanx oblique fracture. **A.** X-ray findings. **B.** After lag screw fixation.

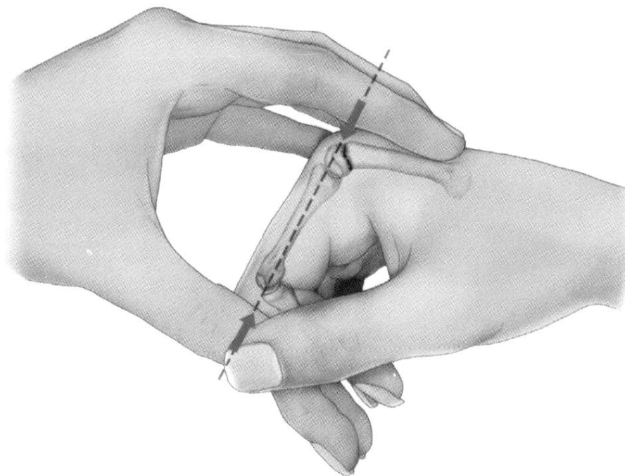

FIGURE 74.9. Jahss maneuver for reducing a metacarpal neck fracture.

TABLE 74.2. ACCEPTABLE ANGULATION FOR METACARPAL FRACTURES

Digit	Angulation (degrees)
Neck	
Index	10
Middle	20
Ring	30–40
Small	50–60
Shaft	
Index	10
Middle	20
Ring	30
Small	40

Thumb (Bennett/Rolando)

A Bennett fracture represents an oblique intra-articular fracture-dislocation of the thumb metacarpal base. The anterior oblique (beak) ligament is the main stabilizer of the thumb CMC joint and is responsible for maintaining the small volar ulnar fragment in anatomic alignment. The metacarpal subluxates proximally, radially, and dorsally secondary to the pull of the abductor pollicis longus, extensor pollicis brevis, and adductor pollicis, respectively (Figure 74.11). Closed reduction is achieved with a combination of thumb axial traction, abduction, and pronation (Figure 74.12). Because the fracture is inherently unstable, percutaneous pinning with K-wires is advocated. A common configuration is to place a K-wire across the articular surface perpendicular to the long access of the metacarpal into the second metacarpal base. An additional wire is placed obliquely across the trapeziometacarpal joint. If an acceptable reduction cannot be achieved with closed reduction, open reduction is performed through an incision overlying the dorsal CMC joint with plate, interfragmentary screw, or pin fixation. A Rolando fracture is similar to a Bennett fracture, except that the fracture is comminuted and characterized by a Y- or T-shaped fracture pattern.

Segmental Loss

Segmental bone loss is common with gunshot wounds to the hand. Self-inflicted injuries typically involve the nondominant hand. Segmental loss is often associated with open and contaminated wounds and is managed with external fixation until the wound is clean and definitive soft tissue coverage can be ensured. On occasion, the distal bone fragment collapses into the void left behind by the bone loss, given the perception of minimal soft tissue loss. However, when the distal fragment is distracted to anatomic length, the soft tissue loss becomes apparent. Bone grafting and rigid fixation is recommended during or after soft tissue reconstruction. Tendon reconstruction is typically delayed because the requisite immobilization needed to ensure bone union will lead to poor tendon glide and an unsatisfactory outcome.

OUTCOMES

The wide variety of hand fracture types and options for management present challenges for outcomes reporting. There is no reference standard objective or subjective outcomes measure for hand

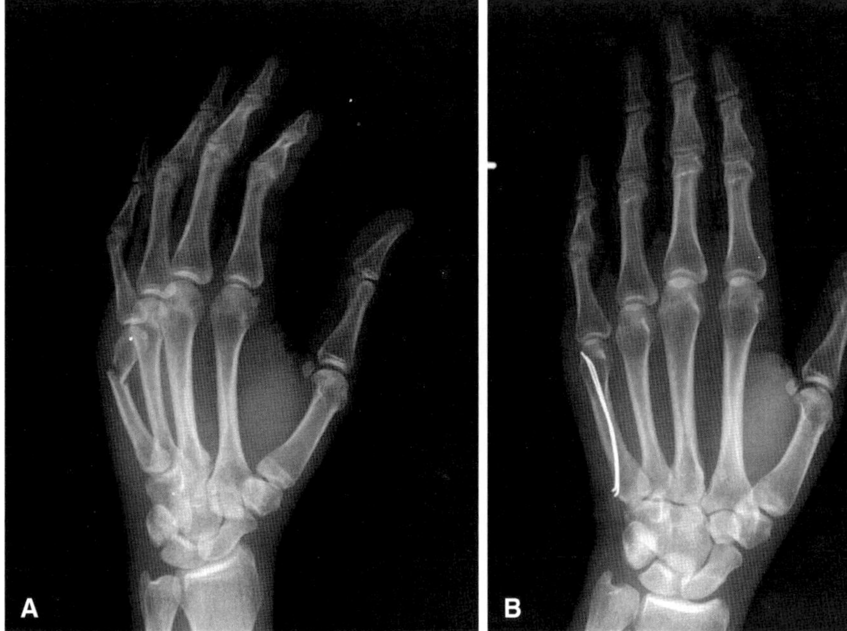

FIGURE 74.10. Left small finger metacarpal neck fracture. **A.** X-ray findings. **B.** After intramedullary pinning with antegrade wires.

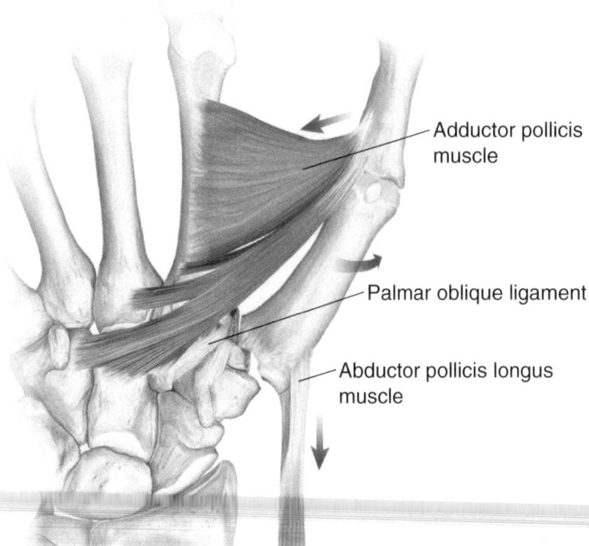

FIGURE 74.11. Deforming forces acting a Bennett fracture.

fracture management. Although radiographic assessments and functional measurements are the classic means by which management options are compared, patient-reported outcome measures have been increasingly used as they provide a greater potential understanding of the patient perception of disability and quality of life. In general, a combination of these measurements provides the clearest picture of function, pain, and disability after treatment. Radiographic outcomes typically include fracture union, residual deformity, hardware complications, or development of arthrosis, whereas functional outcomes include total active motion (**Table 74.3**) and grip/pinch strength. The Jebsen-Taylor Hand Function test is one of the most common functional tests performed to assess outcomes after hand fracture management. The most commonly used patient-reported outcome measures include the Disabilities of the Arm, Shoulder, and Hand, Short Form-36, and Michigan Hand Questionnaire.[15-18]

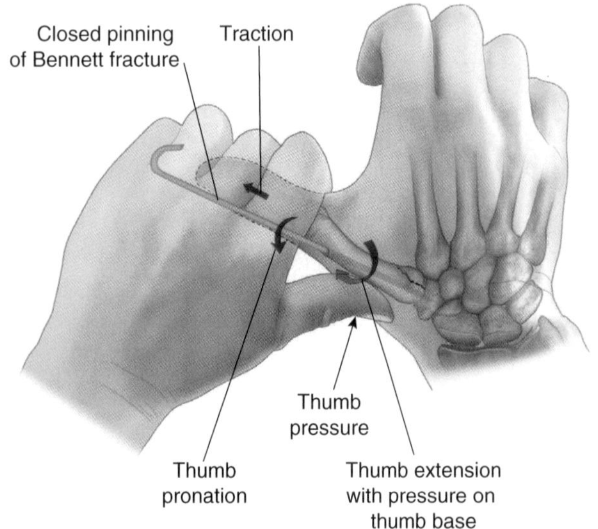

FIGURE 74.12. Reduction maneuver for a Bennett fracture.

TABLE 74.3. TOTAL ACTIVE RANGE OF MOTION

Result	Motion (degrees)
Excellent	>220
Good	180–219
Fair	130–179
Poor	<130

COMPLICATIONS

Complications can and will happen in a busy hand trauma practice, regardless of surgeon skill. Because of the wide range of hand fracture patterns, mechanisms of injury, and available management options, the possible complications after treatment vary widely. In general, complications are more frequent after phalangeal and open fractures than with metacarpal fractures.[19,20] The surgeon should be equipped to identify and treat complications early in an effort to optimize outcomes.

Stiffness is the most common complication after operative or nonoperative hand fracture management.[3] Crush injuries are also a common cause of hand stiffness. Immobilization for greater than 4 weeks increases the likelihood for stiffness and is minimized by initiation of early motion.[7] Stiffness with active and passive motion results from joint contracture, whereas diminished active motion only is often the result of tendon adhesions. Early management is with an intensive rehabilitation program. If there is no improvement after at least 3 months of therapy, capsulotomy and/or tenolysis may be indicated.

Malunion, or the abnormal alignment of a healed fracture, is not always an indication for surgical intervention. The deformity may manifest as shortening, rotation, or angular malalignment. In the immature skeleton, significant intrinsic remodeling ability may result in normal hand function. In older patients, surgery may be required. Depending upon the type of deformity, a variety of osteotomies may be performed to restore anatomic alignment (e.g., step cut, transverse, opening or closing wedge).

Fracture nonunion may be hypertrophic or atrophic. Hypertrophic nonunions require open reduction and stable fixation, typically with a plate and screw construct. These are relatively common in young patients with neglected hand fractures. Atrophic nonunions are more commonly associated with bone loss or infection[21] and are treated with bone grafting and plate fixation.

Infection associated with a hand fracture relates to the extent of trauma and wound contamination. If severe or untreated, a pyogenic infection of the bone (i.e., osteomyelitis) may result. Prompt diagnosis and treatment of osteomyelitis is mandatory to avoid the frequent need for amputation (up to 40% in some studies).[22] In the absence of an abscess, acute osteomyelitis is treated with intravenous antibiotics. If osteomyelitis is chronic or associated with an abscess, intravenous antibiotics and surgical debridement of nonviable soft tissue and bone is recommended. Any unstable hardware should be removed and the fracture site stabilized with external fixation and/or an antibiotic spacer. Once infection clearance has been confirmed, stable fixation is applied with or without bone grafting. K-wire fixation may also lead to infection, many of which are attributable to patient noncompliance.[23] Appropriate pin care and cleaning are required to minimize this risk. Furthermore, if pin duration is anticipated to be greater than 6 weeks, the pins should be buried to decrease the risk for loosening and infection.

Hand fractures may also lead to chronic pain, cold intolerance, and complex regional pain syndrome (CRPS). Acute pain after a hand fracture is to be expected. However, chronic pain is unusual with healed fractures, and other causes of pain (e.g., nerve injury, joint instability, post-traumatic arthritis) should be considered in these cases. Cold intolerance after hand trauma is an unfortunately common occurrence, affecting approximately 38% of patients.[24] Although the pathophysiology of cold intolerance is unclear, it appears to be related to vascular dysfunction and an abnormal rewarming response after hand trauma. CRPS is a chronic, debilitating syndrome characterized by pain, trophic changes, and autonomic dysfunction that can occur after upper extremity trauma or surgery.[25] Patients with suspected CRPS should be promptly referred to a pain specialist for initiation of multimodality treatment, including therapy, antidepressants, anticonvulsants, calcium channel blockers, and adrenergic agents. In rare cases, amputation may be warranted.

CONCLUSION

Hand fracture management is both an art and a science. The surgeon must evaluate not just the fracture *personality* but also the patient socioeconomic situation, social support, risk tolerance, and likelihood for compliance with therapy. Most hand fractures can be treated nonoperatively, yet in certain cases surgery may expedite recovery and avoid the risks of malunion or arthrosis. In general, one should select the least invasive treatment option that will achieve a satisfactory reduction and fracture stability. Early motion is imperative after rigid fixation to combat the inevitable onset of stiffness. The surgeon should be aware of the possible complications after any treatment, including those related to nonoperative management. Appropriate therapy helps to address swelling and stiffness, the most common sequelae of hand fracture management. If managed properly, most hand fractures lead to near normal hand function.

ACKNOWLEDGMENTS

The work was supported by a Midcareer Investigator Award in Patient-Oriented Research (2 K24-AR053120-06) to Kevin C. Chung. The content is solely the responsibility of the authors and does not necessarily represent the official views of the National Institutes of Health.

REFERENCES

1. Bernstein ML, Chung KC. Hand fractures and their management: an international view. *Injury*. 2006;37:1043.
2. Chung KC, Spilson SV. The frequency and epidemiology of hand and forearm fractures in the United States. *J Hand Surg*. 2001;26:908-915.
3. Meals C, Meals R. Hand fractures: a review of current treatment strategies. *J Hand Surg Am*. 2013;38(5):1021-1031.
4. Carpenter S, Rohde RS. Treatment of phalangeal fractures. *Hand Clin*. 2013;29(4):519-534.
5. Diaz-Garcia R, Waljee JF. Current management of metacarpal fractures. *Hand Clin*. 2013;29(4):507-518.
6. Tulipan JE, Ilyas AM. Open fractures of the hand: review of pathogenesis and introduction of a new classification system. *Orthop Clin North Am*. 2016;47(1):245-251.
7. Cheah AE, Yao J. Hand fractures: indications, the tried and true and new innovations. *J Hand Surg Am*. 2016;41(6):712-722.
8. Black D, Mann RJ, Constine R, et al. Comparison of internal fixation techniques in metacarpal fractures. *J Hand Surg Am*. 1985;10(4):466-472.
This biomechanical study compared rigidity and strength in torsion and bending in metacarpal fractures treated by five different types of fixation. The types included dorsal plating, dorsal plating with an interfragmentary lag screw, crossed K-wires, a single intraosseous wire plus a single oblique K-wire, and a single intraosseous wire alone. Plating techniques were superior to wire techniques with regard to dorsal bending and axial torsion. There were no significant differences among the three K-wire methods except in torsion. Plate fixation had higher moments and absorbed more energy than wire fixation.
9. Jones WW. Biomechanics of small bone fixation. *Clin Orthop Rel Res*. 1987;214:11-18.
10. Freeland AE, Roberts TS. Percutaneous screw treatment of spiral oblique finger proximal phalangeal fractures. *Orthopedics*. 1991;14:384-388.
This article describes the genesis of lag screw fixation for phalangeal fractures. The authors sought to balance the risks and benefits of widely used K-wire fixation with the existing plate and screw hardware available at the time. The technique of lag screw fixation was proposed as most suitable for spiral oblique phalangeal fractures in the sagittal plane. They used a 1- to 2-cm mid-axial incision to minimize scar formation and suggested countersinking the screw head to better distribute the forces over a larger area and to avoid screw head prominence.
11. Green DP, Anderson JR. Closed reduction and percutaneous pin fixation of fractured phalanges. *J Bone Joint Surg Am*. 1973;55(8):1651-1654.
This study evaluated 26 displaced proximal phalanx fractures treated by closed reduction, percutaneous pin fixation, and early motion (by means of buddy taping). The proposed advantages were not needed for splinting/casting and earlier return to work. In this series, 18 of 21 patients (26 fractures) regained a full range of motion within 8 weeks following injury.
12. McElfresh EC, Dobyns JH. Intra-articular metacarpal head fractures. *J Hand Surg Am*. 1983;8(4):383-393.
13. Nagle DJ, Ekenstam FW, Lister GD. Immediate silastic arthroplasty for nonsalvageable intraarticular phalangeal fractures. *Scand J Plast Reconstr Surg Hand Surg*. 1989;23(1):47-50.
14. Jahss SA. Fractures of the metacarpals: a new method of reduction and immobilization. *J Bone Joint Surg Am*. 1938;20A:178-186.
This classic article describes what is now known as the Jahss maneuver; reduction of a metacarpal neck fracture by upward or dorsal pressure on the flexed distal fragment, with the metacarpophalangeal and proximal interphalangeal joints of the involved finger held at 90° of flexion. As described in the paper, this position at the metacarpophalangeal joint relaxes the interosseous muscles and at the same time tenses the collateral ligaments, permitting extension (correction of the angulation) of the distal fragment through upward or dorsal pressure on the flexed proximal interphalangeal joint.
15. Baldwin PC, Wolf JM. Outcomes of hand fracture treatments. *Hand Clin*. 2013;29(4):621-630.
16. Davis Sears E, Chung KC. Validity and responsiveness of the Jebsen-Taylor hand function test. *J Hand Surg Am*. 2010;35(1):30-37.
17. Horng YS, Lin MC, Feng CT, et al. Responsiveness of the Michigan hand outcomes questionnaire and the disabilities of the arm, shoulder, and hand questionnaire in patients with hand injury. *J Hand Surg Am*. 2010;35(3):430-436.
18. Chung KC, Pillsbury MS, Walters MR, et al. Reliability and validity testing of the Michigan hand outcomes questionnaire. *J Hand Surg Am*. 1998;23(4):575-587.
19. Page SM, Stern PJ. Complications and range of motion following plate fixation of metacarpal and phalangeal fractures. *J Hand Surg Am*. 1998;23:827-832.
20. Duncan RW, Freeland AE, Jabaley ME, et al. Open hand fractures: an analysis of the recovery of active motion and of complications. *J Hand Surg Am*. 1993;18(3):387-394.
21. Gajendran VK, Gajendran VK, Malone KJ. Management of complications with hand fractures. *Hand Clin*. 2015;31(2):165-177.
22. Reilly KE, Linz JC, Stern PJ, et al. Osteomyelitis of the tubular bones of the hand. *J Hand Surg Am*. 1997;22(4):644-649.
23. Botte MJ, Davis JL, Rose BA, et al. Complications of smooth pin fixation of fractures and dislocations in the hand and wrist. *Clin Orthop Relat Res*. 1992;276:194-201.
This study reviewed the complication rates of pin fixation of fractures and dislocations of the hand or wrist over a 4-year period in 137 patients (422 pins). All pins were unthreaded, measured 0.035 to 0.069 inches (0.9–1.8 mm) in diameter, were placed with a power drill, and were left outside the skin. Mean duration of time that pins were left in place was 6.5 weeks. Minimum follow-up time was 43 days after pin removal. A total of 34 complications occurred in 24 patients, and the overall complication rate was 18%. A total of 45 of the 422 pins were involved (11%). The most common complication was infection (7%), followed by pin loosening (4%), loss of reduction (4%), symptomatic nonunion (4%), impaled flexor tendon (2%), asymptomatic pseudarthrosis (1%), pin migration (1%), median nerve injury (1%), and radial artery injury (1%). Osteomyelitis developed in two of the patients with infections.
24. Nijhuis TH, Smits ES, Jaquet JB, et al. Prevalence and severity of cold intolerance in patients after hand fracture. *J Hand Surg Eur Vol*. 2010;35(4):306-311.
25. Zimmerman RM, Astifidis RP, Katz RD. Modalities for complex regional pain syndrome. *J Hand Surg Am*. 2015;40(7)1469-1472.

QUESTIONS

1. A 25-year-old right-hand-dominant man is seen in the emergency department 1 week after an altercation. He complains of worsening right hand pain and an X-ray confirms a right fifth metacarpal neck fracture (i.e., boxer's fracture; Figure 74.13). What fracture deformity would be predicted based on the location of the fracture?

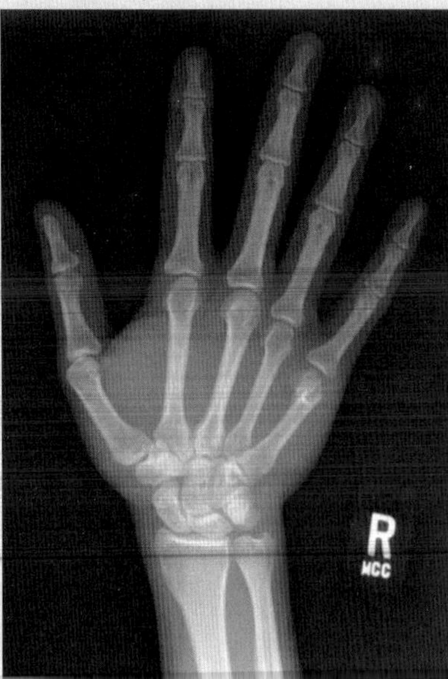

FIGURE 74.13.

   a. Apex ulnar angulation
   b. Apex volar angulation
   c. Apex radial angulation
   d. Apex dorsal angulation
   e. No deformity

2. A 34-year-old right-hand-dominant woman is evaluated in the emergency department after sustaining left hand trauma in a motor vehicle accident. An X-ray confirms a left ring finger proximal phalanx comminuted, extra-articular fracture (Figure 74.14). What finding would be an indication for surgery?

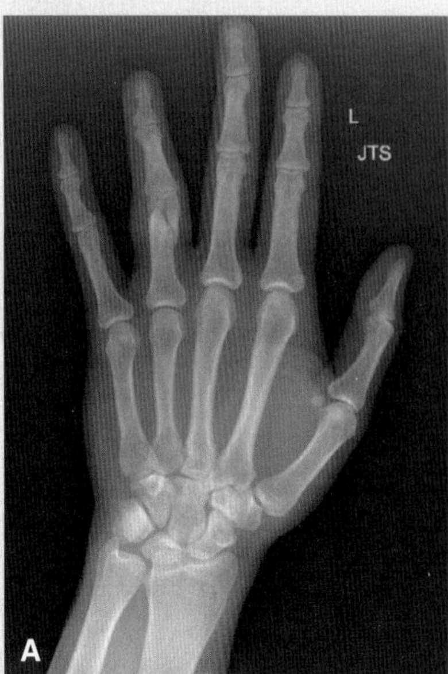

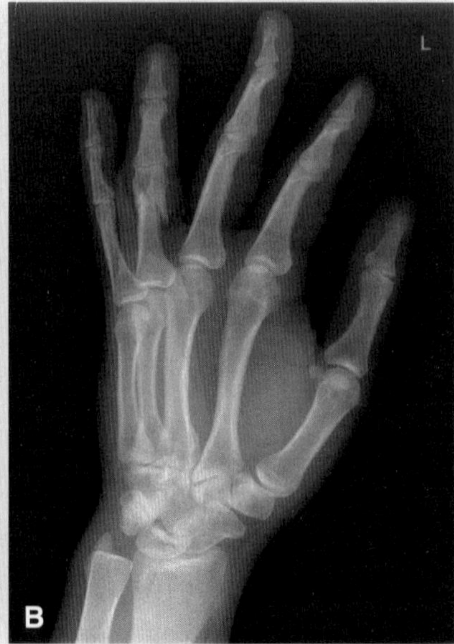

FIGURE 74.14.

   a. 5-degree sagittal plane deformity
   b. Pain at the fracture site
   c. Digital overlap of the ring and small fingers
   d. 5-degree coronal plane deformity
   e. PIP joint intra-articular congruity

3. A 35-year-old right-hand-dominant man is seen in the emergency department 2 hours after sustaining a self-inflicted gunshot wound to his left palm. A 4 × 3 cm open wound is noted on the dorsum of the hand with exposed bone and extensor tendon. An X-ray confirms a comminuted fracture of the left third metacarpal neck with segmental bone loss (Figure 74.15). What would be the most appropriate management of the fracture?

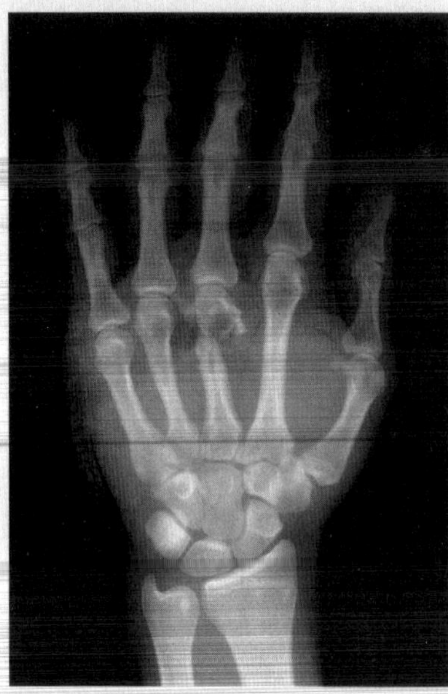

FIGURE 74.15.

   a. Plate and screw fixation of the third metacarpal with interposition bone graft
   b. Synthetic bilaminar skin substitute application to wound bed and delayed bone reconstruction
   c. Wound debridement and application of an external fixator
   d. Immediate third ray amputation
   e. Splint application and delayed fracture fixation

4. **A 35-year-old right-hand-dominant man is referred to the office 3 days after injuring the right ring finger while sliding during a baseball game. He is found to have a flexed resting posture of the ring finger DIP joint without active DIP joint extension. An X-ray shows an intra-articular fracture of the dorsal base of the distal phalanx (50% of the articular surface) with minimal palmar subluxation of the distal phalanx (Figure 74.16). What would be the most appropriate management of this injury?**

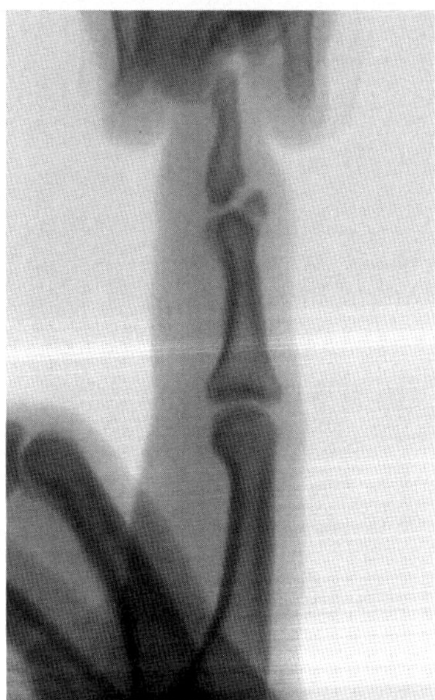

FIGURE 74.16.

a. Open reduction and internal fixation of the fracture
b. Extension block pinning of the fracture
c. Immediate active range of motion exercises
d. 8 to 12 weeks of DIP joint extension splinting
e. Application of an external fixator

5. **A 50-year-old right-hand-dominant man is seen in the office for right thumb pain the day after falling off his bicycle. He is found to have a swelling and pain about the right thumb base with thumb metacarpal adduction. An X-ray shows an intra-articular obliquely oriented fracture of the thumb metacarpal base (i.e., Bennett fracture) with 3 mm of displacement (Figure 74.16). What maneuvers are used to reduce the fracture?**

a. Thumb traction, abduction, and pronation
b. Thumb traction, adduction, and pronation
c. Thumb traction, abduction, and supination
d. Thumb traction, adduction, and supination

1. **Answer: d.** Hand fracture deformities are relatively predictable because of the muscles and tendons crossing the fracture. Metacarpal fractures lead to an apex dorsal deformity due to intrinsic muscle pull on the metacarpal head. Proximal phalanx fractures typically result in an apex volar deformity because the intrinsic muscles flex the base and the extensor mechanisms extend the distal shaft. Middle phalanx base fractures assume an apex dorsal deformity because of the pull of the central slip and the flexion moment imparted by the FDS insertion. Middle phalanx fractures distal to the FDS insertion assume an apex volar posture because the FDS flexes the shaft and the extensor mechanism extends the distal fragment.

2. **Answer: c.** There are multiple indications for reduction of a phalangeal fracture. These include fractures with greater than 10° to 25° of sagittal plane deformity, 10° to 15° of coronal plane deformity, shortening of more than 2 to 4 mm, intra-articular incongruity, multiple open fractures, and fractures with soft tissue injury and/or bone loss. Any rotational deformity leading to digital overlap is poorly tolerated and can impair grip strength and dexterity. Acute fracture site pain is to be expected and is not an indication for surgery.

3. **Answer: c.** Open fractures of the hand are initially treated with washout and debridement. Immediate or delayed definitive reconstruction of composite injuries of the hand is a matter of some controversy. Generally, open fractures with segmental loss combined with substantial soft tissue injury are treated in a staged manner. Temporary skeletal stabilization with wires and an external fixator are appropriate choices until definitive soft tissue coverage can be achieved. Immediate plate and screw fixation with bone grafting is inappropriate in the absence of stable soft tissue coverage. Integra is contraindicated for coverage of open fractures with segmental bone loss. Immediate ray amputation is contraindicated in the setting of a reconstructible bone and soft tissue defect of the hand. Splint application only is an appropriate initial management choice in the absence of significant bone and soft tissue loss. In the setting of segmental bone loss with a soft tissue defect, the goals are to provide fracture stability and maintain length of the digit to prevent shortening of the musculotendinous structures acting on the digit.

4. **Answer: b.** The patient has sustained a mallet fracture. The vast majority of these injuries are managed nonoperatively in the form of extension splinting for 8 to 12 weeks. Indications for surgery include a large, displaced bone fragment (one-third or more of the articular surface), palmar subluxation of the distal phalanx, and loss of DIP joint congruity. Open reduction and internal fixation of this injury is not indicated given that the fracture can be managed with less invasive and technically simpler techniques. Immediate range of motion will prevent fracture healing. An external fixator is unnecessary for a closed distal phalanx fracture without intra-articular comminution. This patient is best managed with extension block pinning.

5. **Answer: a.** A Bennett fracture is an oblique, intra-articular fracture at the base of the thumb metacarpal. The anterior oblique ligament is the main stabilizer of the thumb CMC joint and is responsible for maintaining the small medial fragment in anatomic alignment. The metacarpal, however, subluxates proximally, radially, and dorsally secondary to the pull of the abductor pollicis longus, extensor pollicis brevis, and adductor pollicis. Closed reduction is achieved with a combination of thumb axial traction, abduction, and pronation. Because the fracture is inherently unstable, percutaneous pinning with K-wires is advocated. A common configuration is to place a wire across the articular surface perpendicular to the long access of the metacarpal into the second metacarpal base. An additional wire is placed retrograde across the trapeziometacarpal joint.

CHAPTER 75 Management of Wrist Fractures

Mitchell A. Pet and Warren C. Hammert

KEY POINTS

- Four radiographic measurements describing orientation of the joint surface have been found to correlate with patient outcomes after distal radius fracture. These are radial height, radial inclination, volar tilt, and ulnar variance.
- Development of a treatment plan for a distal radius fracture requires consideration of patient factors, fracture pattern, fracture stability, and associate injuries.
- Initial treatment for most distal radius fractures is closed reduction. This maneuver improves patient comfort, relieves pressure on potentially threatened soft tissues and nerves, and may be the definitive treatment for stable fracture patterns.
- Operative fixation of a distal radius fracture may be achieved using percutaneous pins, volar locking plate, dorsal spanning plate, external fixator, or a combination. Volar locking plates are currently very popular because they offer rigid fixation, which facilitates early rehabilitation and can be safely applied to many fracture patterns.
- Acute scaphoid fractures may be radiographically occult. Clinical suspicion with negative radiographs has historically been followed by immobilization and follow-up radiographic evaluation. However, early advanced imaging in patients with negative plain films has become increasingly popular.
- Operative fixation of a fractured scaphoid is most commonly accomplished using a cannulated headless compression screw. Fracture pattern guides the choice of a dorsal or volar approach.
- The scaphoid has a retrograde blood supply supplied by branches of the radial artery. Because of this unique vascular anatomy, the proximal pole of a fractured scaphoid is particularly prone to avascular necrosis and nonunion.

The diagnosis and treatment of wrist fractures is a constantly evolving field. Development of a safe and effective treatment algorithm requires an understanding of wrist anatomy (Figure 75.1) and biomechanics, adherence to the principles of fracture fixation, and attentive facilitation of prompt rehabilitation.

EVALUATION OF THE PATIENT WITH WRIST TRAUMA

Elements unique to upper extremity injuries history include the timing, mechanism and energy of the injury, occupation/avocation, and prior hand or wrist injuries/surgeries. The injured extremity should be examined beginning at the elbow and moving distally. A displaced distal radius fracture often results in gross deformity of the wrist, but carpal fractures and minimally displaced fractures of the distal radius may not be obvious. Finger, wrist, and forearm motion are assessed, and palpation for focal tenderness with specific attention to the radius, distal radioulnar joint (DRUJ), and carpus helps to determine appropriate imaging studies.

Evaluation of the median, ulnar, and radial sensory nerve function is critical, as injury of each can be associated with an acute wrist fracture. One should be suspicious for acute median nerve dysfunction (carpal tunnel syndrome), and if numbness persists following closed reduction then emergent operative intervention may be indicated.

DISTAL RADIUS FRACTURES

Epidemiology and Cost

Over a half million distal radius fractures occurred in the United States in 2009, with an overall incidence of 16.2 fractures per 10,000 person years. This age distribution of these fractures is bimodal, with the highest rates in persons under 18 and over 65 (30.18 and 25.42 per 10,000 personyears, respectively).[1] In young patients, characteristic injuries occur in men by means of high-energy trauma. In the elderly population, Caucasian women are most at risk. These fractures are often related to osteoporosis and frequently occur after low-energy trauma.

The economic burden of distal radius fractures is difficult to measure because care occurs in varied settings and costs are subject to wide geographic variation. One recent analysis, which stressed exhaustive examination of direct and indirect costs, estimated that operative and nonoperative treatment of a distal radius fracture costs $15,403 and $3,775, respectively. The largest driver of this cost was missed work.[2]

Anatomy

The distal radius is quadrilateral in cross-section with articular surfaces at the radiocarpal joint and DRUJ. The radiocarpal joint surface has distinct scaphoid and lunate facets separated by the interface ridge. On its ulnar side, the cartilage-bearing sigmoid notch articulates with the ulnar head at the DRUJ, which allows pronation and supination of the forearm as the radius rotates and translates around the ulna. The sigmoid notch is a shallow concavity, with a radius of curvature that is about twice that of the ulnar head. Consequently, bony constraints offer little joint stability and the soft tissues supporting this joint are critical. Primary among these is the triangular fibrocartilage complex (TFCC). The TFCC includes the dorsal and volar radioulnar ligaments and has both superficial styloid and deep foveal insertion points.[3]

Volarly the distal radius is concave, with the recessed volar cortex curving anteriorly as it meets the volar lip of the articular surface. The metaphysis is covered by the pronator quadratus. The dorsal distal radius is convex in shape and is intimately related to the extensor tendons. The most palpable dorsal structure is Lister tubercle, which serves as a pulley for the extensor pollicis longus tendon. The dorsal cortex is considerably thinner than the volar cortex, leading to the common occurrence of dorsally comminuted fractures.

Biomechanics of Injury

The three-column theory of the distal radius aids in understanding the biomechanical rationale for treating distal radius fractures. The radial column, composed of the radial styloid and the scaphoid fossa, anchors radiocarpal stability through the styloid's osseous buttress effect and the origin of the volar radiocarpal ligaments. The intermediate column is composed of the lunate fossa and sigmoid notch. The lunate fossa has a volar buttress effect and is the primary load-bearing surface of the radiocarpal joint. The sigmoid notch provides congruity to the DRUJ and tensions its soft tissue attachments. The ulnar column, composed of the distal ulna and TFCC, shares in transmission of the carpal load and serves as a stable pivot point for the rotating radius.

Load distribution across the radiocarpal and ulnar carpal joints is dependent on radial length (ulnar variance). When neutral, 80% of the load is through the radiocarpal joint and 20% through the ulnar carpal joint. As the ulnar variance increases, the load across the radiocarpal joint decreases and ulnar carpal joint increases.

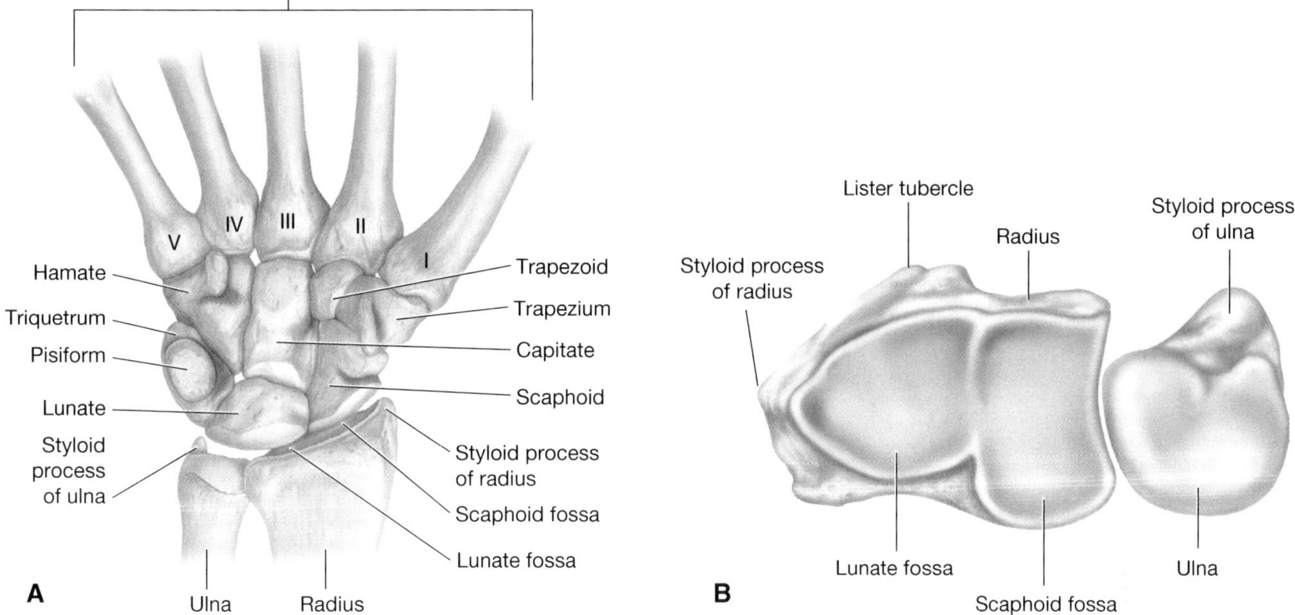

FIGURE 75.1. **A.** The bones of the wrist as seen from the volar surface. **B.** The distal articular surface of the distal radius and ulna and the distal radioulnar joint.

Conversely, as the variance decreases, the load across the ulnar carpal joint decreases and radiocarpal joint increases. This relationship is important because a deranged relationship of the radius and ulna leads to altered load distribution and potentially accelerated arthrosis.

Although distal radius fractures can result from all types of applied forces, the most typical mechanism is hyperextension, often caused by fall on an outstretched hand. The site of fracture is usually at the [illegible] due to its primary composition of weak cancellous bone with a thin dorsal cortex. Given the dorsally and axially directed force of [illegible] comminution are common (Colles fractures with classic *dinner-fork deformity*). However, Pechlaner[4] demonstrated in cadaveric experiments that depending on the energy of the injury, position of the hand during the impact, and on the quality of the bone, widely variable patterns of fracture and soft tissue derangement can occur with hyperextension.

Classification

Several distinct fracture patterns have associated eponyms that are used commonly in the clinical setting (Figure 75.2). In the last 70 years, 15 distinct systems for classifying distal radius fractures have been proposed in the literature. Perhaps the most commonly utilized are the Frykman, Melone, Fernandez, Mayo Clinic, and AO classifications. Unfortunately, no single classification has been able to simultaneously describe fracture characteristics in a simple language, order them into a hierarchy, provide a guide to treatment, and predict outcomes with reliability and reproducibility.[5]

Despite the limited utility of classification systems, we do find that a common nomenclature for the fragments most commonly comprising a complex intraarticular fracture facilitates good clinical communication and treatment planning. These fragments are as follows (Figure 75.3):

- *Radial column:* This is often the largest fragment and bears the insertion of a portion of the brachioradialis tendon.
- *Dorsal ulnar corner:* The fragment may bear a portion of the sigmoid notch and lunate facet.
- *Volar rim/lunate facet:* This fragment supports much of the load transmitted by the carpus and usually maintains a strong radiocarpal ligamentous attachment. For this reason, failure to recognize and stabilize a volar rim fragment can lead to volar subluxation of the carpus.

In more complex fracture patterns, additional dorsal wall and intraarticular fragments may be present. Although every fragment will not necessarily be separate or typical in a given fracture, this framework is useful in considering how derangements of osseous anatomy are reflected radiographically.

Radiographic Evaluation

Initial imaging of wrist [illegible] posteroanterior (PA), lateral, and oblique planes. The PA radiograph is taken with the shoulder in 90° of abduction, the elbow in 90° of flexion, and the wrist and forearm in a neutral position. A standard PA view of the wrist should reveal the extensor carpi ulnaris tendon groove at the level of or radial to the base of the ulnar styloid (Figure 75.4A). For the lateral, the shoulder is adducted and the elbow held in 90° of flexion with the hand positioned in the same plane as the humerus. On a true lateral view, the palmar cortex of the pisiform bone should overlie the central third of the interval between the palmar cortices of the distal scaphoid pole and the capitate head (Figure 75.4B). Careful positioning is important, as small errors at this stage can affect interpretation of critical radiographic parameters.

Four radiographic measurements describing orientation of the joint surface have been found to correlate with patient outcomes.[6] These are radial height, radial inclination, volar tilt, and ulnar variance. *Radial height* is measured on the PA radiograph as the distance between a line perpendicular to the long axis of the radius passing through the distal tip of the sigmoid notch at the distal ulnar articular surface of the radius and a second parallel line at the distal tip of the radial styloid. This measurement averages 10 to 13 mm. *Radial inclination* is also measured on the PA radiograph and represents the angle between one line connecting the radial styloid tip and the ulnar aspect of the distal radial articular surface and a second line perpendicular to the longitudinal axis of the radius. Radial inclination ranges between 21° and 25°. The *volar tilt* of the distal radius is measured on a lateral radiograph. The volar tilt represents the angle between a line along the distal radial articular surface and one perpendicular to the longitudinal axis of the radius at the joint margin. The normal volar tilt averages 11° and has a range of 2° to 20°.[7] *Ulnar variance* refers to the distance between the articular surface of the ulnar head and the ulnar border of the lunate fossa. It is described as neutral when both are at the same level, ulnar positive when the ulna is longer than the radius, and ulnar negative when the

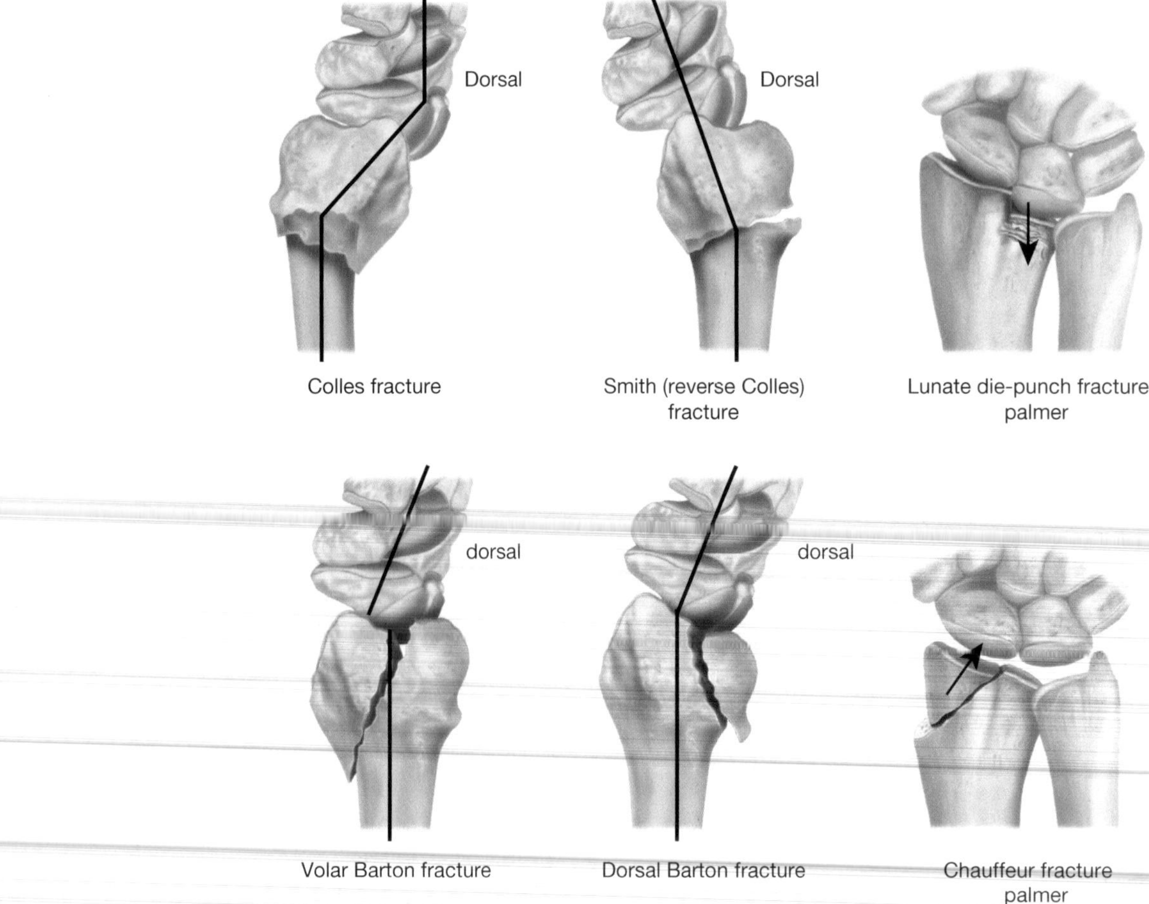

FIGURE 75.2. Eponyms used to describe common patterns of distal radius fracture.

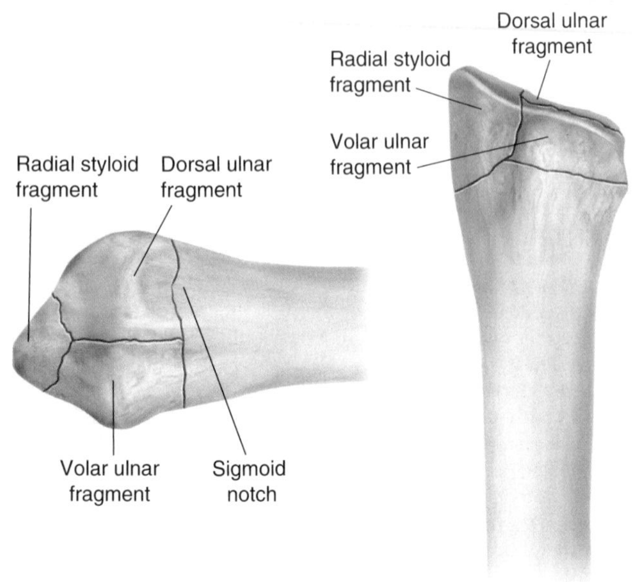

FIGURE 75.3. Many intra-articular distal radius fractures can be described as consisting of radial column, dorsal ulnar corner, and volar rim/lunate facet fragments. Not all fragments are present or typical in every fracture, and additional fragments may be present in complex patterns.

converse is true. Normal ulnar variance can range from 0 ± 2 mm. In cases of distal radius fracture, abnormal ulnar positive variance may indicate loss of radial length due to metaphyseal collapse.[6]

For intraarticular fractures, additional measurements are useful to describe relationships between the articular fragments and the resultant joint (in)congruity. *Step* describes any longitudinal discontinuity in the joint surface. *Gap* refers to transverse separation of articular segments. The teardrop of the distal radius articular surface refers to the U-shaped outline of the volar rim of the lunate facet. The teardrop angle refers to the angle between the central axis of the teardrop and the central axis of the radial shaft, which is normally 70°. A depressed teardrop angle may be the only evidence that the volar rim fragment is incompletely reduced.[6,8] The anteroposterior (AP) distance is measured on the lateral projection from the apices of the dorsal rim and volar lunate facet. Normal AP distance is 17 to 21 mm, and an increased value reflects an unreduced discontinuity between the volar and dorsal lunate facet fragments and potentially a coronal split in the sigmoid notch.[8]

All of the radiographic measurements discussed above are outlined upon a normal radiographic series in Figure 75.5.

Indications for Operative Treatment

A treatment plan for a given distal radius fracture requires consideration of four main factors.

Patient Factors

Patient age and activity level are important patient factors. A 2-mm articular step-off after closed reduction might reasonably prompt

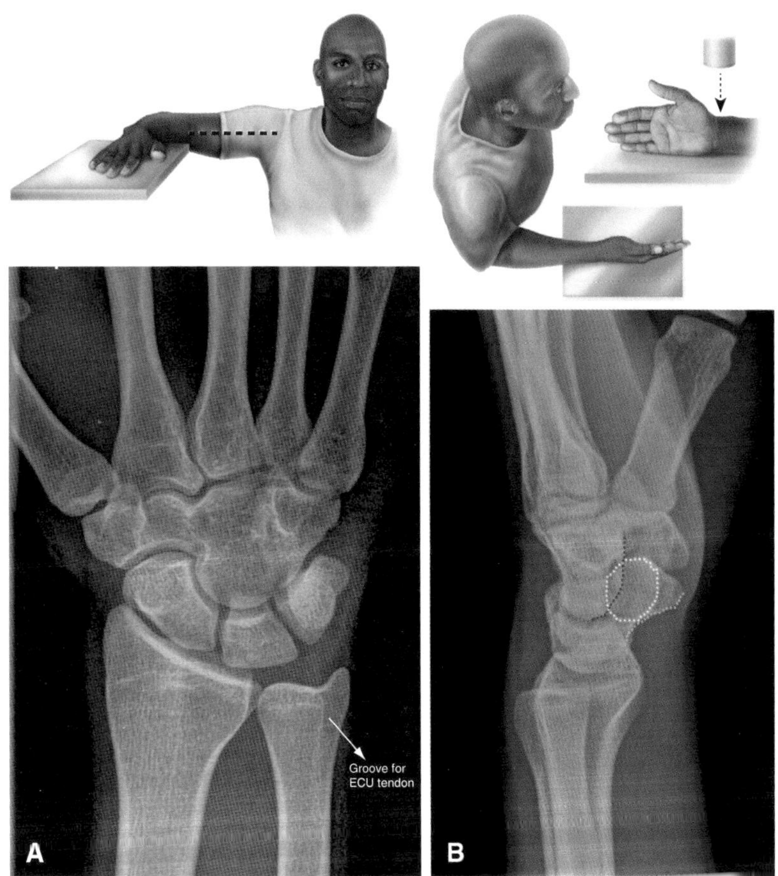

FIGURE 75.4 **A.** Clinical picture (*top*) and a correctly positioned posteroanterior view showing the extensor carpi ulnaris (ECU) groove radial to the ulnar styloid (*bottom*). **B.** Clinical picture (*top*) and a correctly positioned lateral view showing the pisiform (*white line*) overlying the distal scaphoid (*green line*) and the capitate (*red line*) (*bottom*).

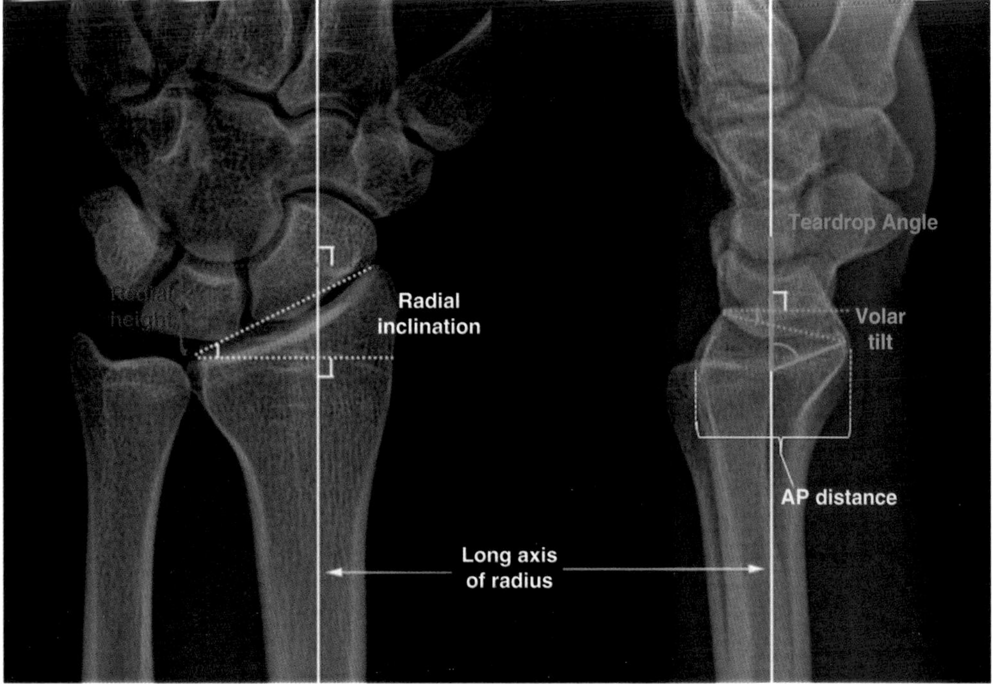

FIGURE 75.5. Measurement of radiographic parameters of the distal end of the radius: radial height (*dotted red lines*), radial inclination (*dotted white lines*), volar tilt (*dotted green lines*), teardrop angle (*solid blue line*), and anteroposterior (AP) distance (*dotted yellow line*).

surgical intervention for a young healthy laborer. However, this same step-off might be acceptable in an 85-year-old high-risk surgical candidate who is already unable to live independently.

Fracture Pattern

Imaging before and after fracture reduction is evaluated to assess adequacy of the reduction. While the definition of acceptable reduction is situational and based upon incomplete evidence, biomechanical and outcomes studies have established some general guidelines.[9]

- Radial inclination greater than or equal to 15°
- Loss of radial length less than 5 mm at the DRUJ (compared to contralateral)
- Volar tilt between 15° dorsal and 20° volar
- Articular step-off of 2 mm or less

Fracture Stability

Fractures for which satisfactory reduction cannot be achieved are unstable, and most require operative treatment. If an acceptable reduction can be obtained, the surgeon must then decide whether it is likely that the reduction can be maintained with cast/splint immobilization. If a fracture is judged to be stable after reduction, then nonoperative management should be considered. If it is unstable, then surgical intervention is usually indicated. Many studies have investigated models for predicting fracture stability. In a classic study, Lafontaine et al concluded that five factors predicted distal radius fracture instability and that the presence of three of them correlated with loss of reduction despite cast immobilization[10]:

- Initial dorsal angulation greater than 20°
- Dorsal comminution
- Radiocarpal intraarticular involvement
- Associated fracture of the ulna
- Age greater than 60 years

In more recent work examining 4000 fractures, Mackenney et al[11] found that the most important predictors of instability and malunion were advanced age, dorsal comminution, and the position of the fracture at presentation.

Associated Injuries

Certain associated injuries may indicate operative treatment of fractures that might otherwise be treated nonoperatively. Contaminated open fractures should be meticulously debrided and fixation may be done in an immediate or interval manner. Compartment syndrome and acute carpal tunnel syndrome require emergent treatment with fasciotomy or carpal tunnel release, respectively, and both are often accompanied by fracture fixation. Finally, patients with multiple injured limbs may benefit from operative fixation of otherwise nonoperative wrist fractures to facilitate earlier weight bearing and rehabilitation.

TABLE 75.1. TECHNIQUE FOR TRACTION-ASSISTED REDUCTION OF DISTAL RADIUS FRACTURE

Step	Details
1. Hematoma block	■ Raise a wheal of 1% lidocaine in the dermis of the dorsal forearm, directly over fracture using a 25 g needle ■ Wait 5 min ■ Enter fracture through dorsal wheal with 18 g needle ■ Feel needle enter fracture, and then withdraw blood from fracture hematoma to confirm position ■ Inject 10 cc of 1% lidocaine
2. Wait 10 min	■ To allow onset of anesthetic
3. Apply finger traps	■ Apply all the way down to the base of index and middle finger. If finger traps slip, apply benzoin
4. Hang arm from IV pole	■ Hang finger traps from an IV pole such that elbow is at 90°
5. Apply weight	■ Tie a length of stockinette into a loop such that it fits loosely around the brachium ■ The stockinette should be spread out to cover much of the brachium to avoid discomfort by distributing pressure ■ Suspend 10–15 pounds of weight from this stockinette
6. Wait 10 min	■ Allow time for deforming muscles to fatigue and fracture to be reduced by ligamentotaxis
7. Fluoroscopy and manual manipulation	■ Use C-arm to visualize reduction ■ If necessary, manually manipulate fragments to improve reduction
8. Splint application	■ While traction is still applied, apply a well-padded plaster splint that is molded to maintain the reduction
9. Removal of traction	■ Remove the weight and finger traps
10. Postreduction radiography	■ C-arm images or formal radiographs are obtained to ensure that reduction has been maintained by the splint

Treatment Modalities

Closed Reduction and Plaster Immobilization

Initial treatment for nearly all fractures is closed reduction. This maneuver improves patient comfort, relieves pressure on potentially threatened soft tissues and nerves, and may be the definitive treatment for stable fracture patterns. Closed reduction is facilitated by ligamentotaxis, whereby intact soft tissue attachments guide the bone fragments into alignment when longitudinal traction is applied.[12]

Our preferred technique for closed reduction of a distal radius fracture is outlined in **Table 75.1** and demonstrated in Figure 75.6. Other variants are acceptable,[13] though we recommend caution when recreating the hyperextension that caused injury, as this can stress the median nerve.

After reduction is achieved, a well-padded plaster splint is applied. Circumferential casting is not recommended in the acute setting because a cast does not accommodate postinjury swelling. For most fractures, a short arm dorsoradial splint out to the level of the metacarpal heads is adequate to immobilize the wrist. Routine use of a sugar-tong splint is common, and Smith fractures and fractures that involve the DRUJ require sugar-tong splinting to control pronosupination. The plaster should be molded and the wrist positioned to oppose the initial pattern of fracture displacement. For a classic Colles fracture, this entails a three-point mold with two points of dorsal pressure proximal and distal to the fracture, and a single point of volar pressure at the level of the fracture. This functions to maintain tension on the intact dorsal periosteal hinge and opposes dorsal displacement. This fracture pattern is immobilized in slight wrist flexion and ulnar deviation. Extremes of flexion/extension and radioulnar deviation should be avoided.

Patients treated initially with closed reduction and plaster immobilization should be followed closely for interval radiographs to ensure that reduction has been maintained. Not infrequently, a fracture of uncertain stability will be treated with initial closed reduction and immobilization and then undergo interval displacement, resulting in conversion to operative treatment. If ongoing closed treatment is planned, the splint should be adapted as the padding compresses and swelling decreases in order to maintain the mold. Transition to a cast is made at 2 weeks and generally continued until 4 weeks postinjury for minimally displaced fractures and 6 weeks for fractures that had initial displacement or comminution. A removable splint is then applied and weaned over the ensuing month.[13]

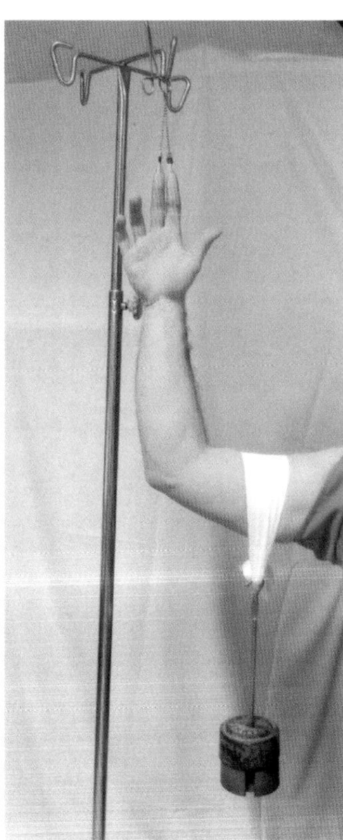

FIGURE 75.6. Distal radius reduction using traction. The patient is seated on a gurney and hung from an IV pole by finger traps applied to the index and small middle fingers. Ten to twenty pounds of weight is suspended from the brachium using stockinette.

Closed Reduction and Percutaneous Pinning

Percutaneous pinning of the distal radius is applicable to extraarticular or simple articular fractures without metaphyseal comminution that are reducible, but unstable after reduction. It is not indicated in severely comminuted or osteoporotic fractures. Pinning is performed in the operating room under fluoroscopic control, usually utilizing 0.062 in Kirschner wires. Several methods of pin fixation have been described—we prefer transradial styloid and Kapandji (intrafocal) pinning.

Transradial styloid pinning simply entails closed reduction of the fracture with or without the use of intraoperative traction. This is followed by placement of one or two retrograde pins beginning in the tip of the radial styloid, directed across the metaphyseal fracture line and into the volar-ulnar cortex of the radius. This may be supplemented by an additional retrograde pin beginning dorsally between the fourth and fifth extensor compartments and directed in a volar-radial direction.

Kapandji (or intrafocal) pinning entails insertion of pins directly into the fracture site from the volar-radial and dorsoulnar aspects. These pins are then levered distally to reduce the fracture and restore radial height/inclination and volar tilt, respectively, before being advanced into the opposite cortex to maintain the reduction.[14]

These techniques have the advantage of low cost and easy removal of all hardware in the office. Concerns of percutaneous pinning include neurovascular injuries during pin placement[15] and pin tract infections. Additionally, pin constructs do not provide rigid fixation, limiting early rehabilitation of the wrist. Required immobilization with closed reduction percutaneous pinning is one reason many surgeons prefer volar locking plate (VLP) fixation, despite some meta-analyses that report similar outcomes with both techniques.[16]

Volar Locking Plate Fixation

Since its introduction by Orbay and Fernandez,[17] VLP fixation has become a popular method for treating distal radius fractures.

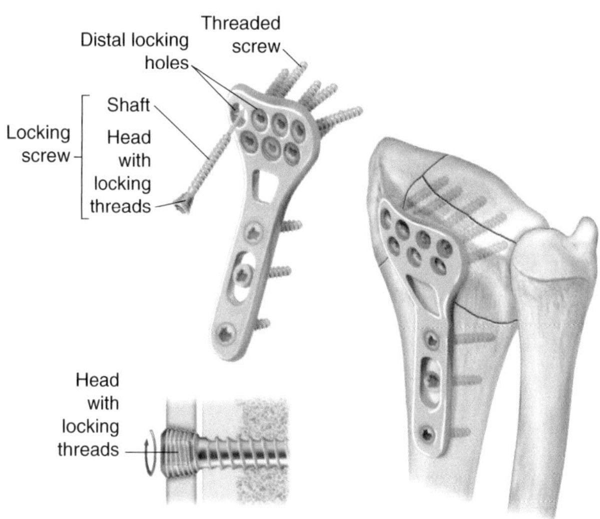

FIGURE 75.7. Anatomy of a volar locking plate.

Even though a wide variety of proprietary devices are available, basic plate design involves a narrow proximal stem that affixes to the radial shaft and a wide distal end, which abuts (and potentially buttresses) the volar aspect of the radial metaphysis with screws or pegs to support articular surface (Figure 75.7). This construct transmits load from the articular surface, via the subchondral locking pegs to the strong volar radial cortex, thereby opposing secondary displacement, even in cases of severe metaphyseal comminution. Subchondral locking pegs provide enough support that bone grafting of dorsal metaphyseal defects is rarely necessary. Fracture fixation using a VLP is demonstrated in [illegible]

Application of a VLP is generally done through a flexor carpi radialis approach. After fracture exposure and mobilization, the fracture may be reduced and the plate is used to stabilize the fracture. The plate must be placed proximal to the *watershed line* to avoid irritation of the flexor tendons,[18] but not so proximal that the locking pegs fail to support the subchondral bone (Figure 75.9).

Advantages of VLP fixation include wide applicability, absence of a need to routinely remove hardware, and a low rate of tendon irritation/rupture. The rigid nonspanning fixation offered by a VLP allows early mobilization and rehabilitation of the injured wrist.[19]

Limitations of the volar approach include poor visualization of dorsal articular surface and centrally impacted fractures. Small but crucial volar or dorsal ulnar corner fragments may be difficult to capture with standard VLP, requiring additional fixation or fragment-specific plates.[20]

Dorsal Plating

Prior to introduction of the VLP, dorsal buttress plating of the distal radius was common. This approach offered easy exposure, facilitated subchondral bone grafting, and allowed effective buttressing of dorsally displaced fractures. Additionally, this approach allowed direct visualization of the articular surface and intercarpal ligament injuries via a dorsal capsulotomy. Unfortunately, dorsal plates were prone to irritate and sometimes rupture the extensor tendons,[21] and hardware removal was frequently required. For this reason, dorsal buttress plating has been supplanted by the VLP as the fixation method of choice for most fracture patterns. Despite this, some fracture patterns are still preferably managed with dorsal plates.

Fragment-Specific Fixation

In some cases, critical articular fracture fragments may be too small to support multiple locking screws/pegs. Furthermore, placing a

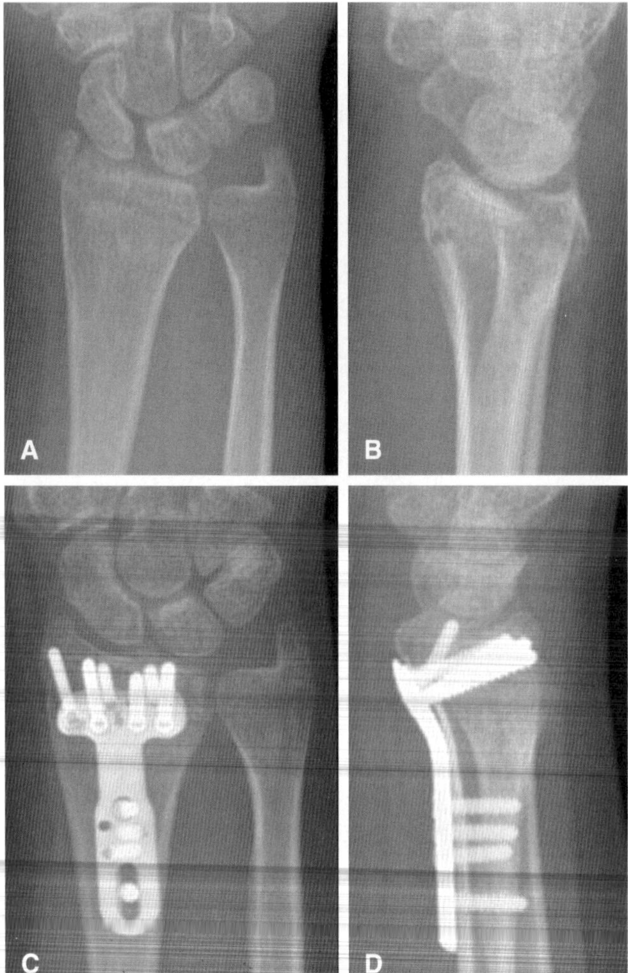

FIGURE 75.8. Preoperative **(A, B)** and postoperative **(C, D)** radiographs demonstrating use of a volar locking plate to stabilize a distal radius fracture.

VLP distal enough to capture small volar rim fragments may cause irritation or rupture of overlying flexor tendons. In these situations, *fragment-specific fixation* can be used. This is a system of ultralow profile miniplates, pin plates, hook plates, and wireforms anatomically designed to fix a single common articular fracture fragment (see *Classification* section above). While this technique often requires both dorsal and volar approaches to the distal radius, each approach can be done with minimal soft tissue dissection owing to the smaller size of the implants (Figure 75.10).

External Fixation and Bridge Plating

External fixation can be used for temporary or definitive treatment of many distal radius fractures, though it is most commonly used in highly comminuted and shortened fracture patterns. Additional indications include situations of excessive edema or substantial soft tissue injury. External fixators maintain length while aligning the joint surface with the radial shaft. The most common configuration is a radiocarpal spanning uniplanar fixator anchored in the radial shaft and second metacarpal. More complex designs including dynamic devices, fixators that do not span the radiocarpal joint, and a device offering multiplanar control are also available.[12]

Advantages of external fixation include the ease of application and avoiding the devascularization of multiple small bony fragments that can occur during open reduction internal fixation. Limitations include the external frame, the risk of pin-related infection, and potential injury to tendons and nerves.

To avoid external pins, dorsal bridge (aka spanning or distraction) plating can be used for similar fracture patterns.[22] A straight plate is affixed to the dorsal radial shaft and proximal second or third

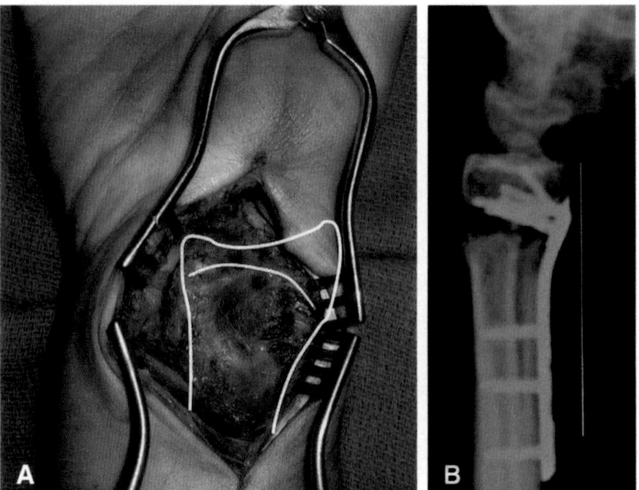

FIGURE 75.9. **A.** The watershed line is a transverse ridge located between the distal border of the pronator quadratus and the origin of the volar extrinsic ligaments of the wrist (*yellow line*). It marks the most prominent portion of the volar distal radius and is thus point of contact for overlying flexor tendons. Volar locking plates should ideally be positioned proximal to the watershed line. **B.** Radiographically, this can be checked by ensuring that the plate does not protrude beyond a tangent line dropped from the most volar portion of the distal radius as visualized on lateral radiograph.

metacarpal, spanning and distracting the fracture to maintain length and axial alignment. This device is mechanically similar to a uniplanar external fixator, in that it provides distraction across the fracture and does not disrupt its vascularity, but the plate sits closer to the fracture and thus provides increased stability. The plate is generally removed at 12 weeks, during which time the wrist should be immobilized to prevent plate breakage.

Because this load-bearing fixation technique allows early weight bearing upon the injured extremity, it is useful in polytrauma patients with multiple injured extremities. A limitation of both external and internal spanning fixations is that ligamentotaxis cannot alone reliably maintain reduction of displaced and impacted articular fragments. For this reason, external and internal spanning fixation is often augmented with other hardware (i.e., K-wires, fragment-specific plates) to maintain articular reduction (Figure 75.11).

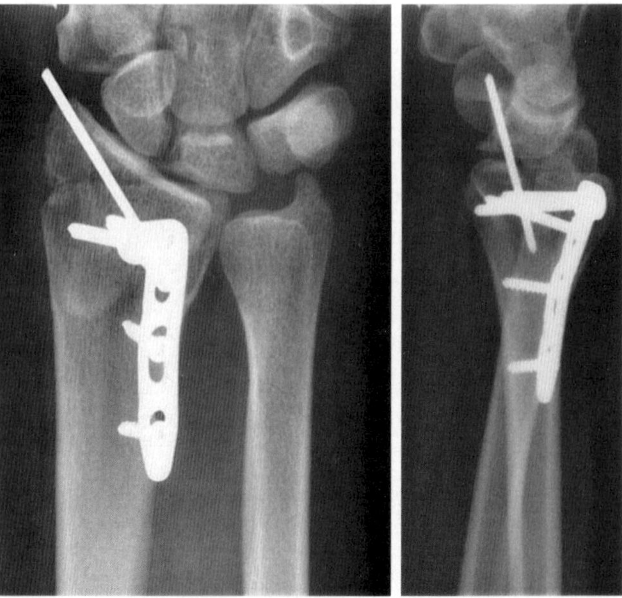

FIGURE 75.10. Posteroanterior **(A)** and lateral **(B)** views of an intra-articular fracture of the distal radius treated with fragment-specific plating of the dorsal ulnar fragment and K-wire fixation of the radial styloid fragment.

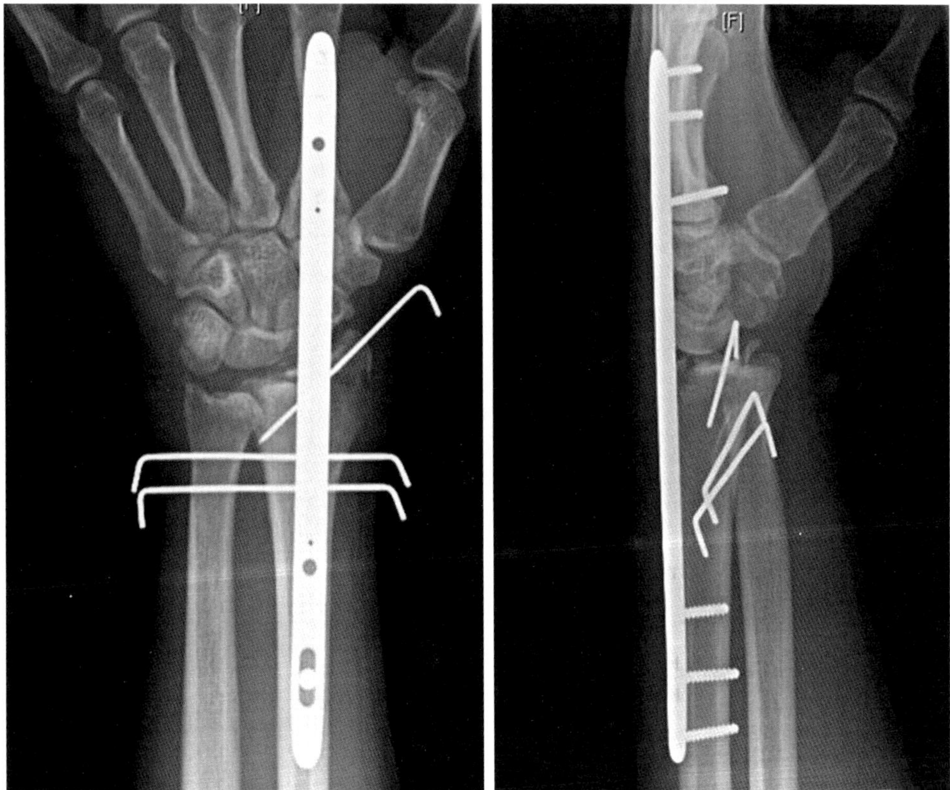

FIGURE 75.11. Posteroanterior **(A)** and lateral **(B)** views of an intraarticular fracture of the distal radius treated with a dorsal bridge plate augmented by a K-wire in the radial styloid. Two radioulnar pins were also used for treatment of traumatic instability of the distal radioulnar joint.

Associated Injuries

Median Nerve Dysfunction

Median nerve dysfunction associated with distal radius fracture is usually due to nerve stretching over a dorsally angulated fracture. Accumulation of hematoma within the carpal tunnel may also irritate and compress the nerve. Median nerve function (two-point discrimination, thenar motor function) should be assessed and documented before and after reduction. If median nerve function worsens or does not improve after reduction, carpal tunnel release (and often surgical treatment of the fracture) is indicated.

Ulnar Styloid Injuries

Ulnar styloid fractures occur commonly with distal radius fractures. They are not independently predictive of outcomes, and the presence of even a large ulnar styloid fragment does not necessarily indicate DRUJ instability.[23] If a large styloid fragment is present in a fracture with DRUJ instability after fixation of the radius, repair of the ulnar styloid is indicated.

Distal Radioulnar Joint Instability

Evaluation of every distal radius fracture should include assessment of DRUJ stability in neutral, supination, and pronation. Following fixation of the radius, the ulna is stabilized in one hand and the radius is *shucked* in an AP direction. Laxity varies among individuals, so suspected instability should always be compared to the uninjured side. If DRUJ instability is detected, this may represent a TFCC disruption.

Treatment for DRUJ instability is based upon fracture pattern and the positions of maintained forearm stability. If a large ulnar styloid fragment is present, this may be fixed with a K-wire, tension band, or screw, thereby reestablishing the TFCC's constraint of the DRUJ. If the DRUJ is stable in supination, postoperative immobilization in this position for 3 weeks and then in neutral for another 3 weeks often allows soft tissue healing to the point that DRUJ stability is restored. If the joint is unstable in supination, TFCC repair or DRUJ pinning is indicated.[24]

Intercarpal Ligament Injuries

Scapholunate and lunotriquetral interosseous ligament tears occur with 16% to 40% and 8.5% to 15% of distal radius fracture respectively.[25] Plain radiographs may suggest the diagnosis, but magnetic resonance imaging (MRI) or arthroscopy can be used to guide treatment. High physical demand patients with static or dynamic carpal instability may benefit from interosseous ligament repair.[25]

Complications

Complications include stiffness, posttraumatic arthrosis of the radiocarpal or distal radioulnar joint, and complex regional pain syndrome (CRPS). CRPS is characterized by pain out of proportion to the injury, edema, vasomotor instability, and stiffness. There is conflicting evidence regarding ascorbic acid reducing the risk of CRPS. In this setting, electrodiagnostic studies to evaluate for peripheral nerve compression are important as missed peripheral nerve compression are easily treatable and can be a cause of CRPS.[26] Early referral to a pain management specialist for initiation of multimodality treatment[27] and to a hand therapist for edema control and joint mobilization are important adjunctive treatments.

Attritional rupture of the extensor pollicis longus after distal radius fracture results from increased pressure within the third extensor compartment and is most often seen in minimally displaced fractures treated nonoperatively. Both flexor and extensor tendon irritation can result from contact with a prominent plate or screw tip.[27] When applying a VLP, this problem can be mitigated by proper implant placement, and choosing distal locking screw/pegs that do not penetrate the dorsal cortex. Biomechanical studies demonstrate support of 75% or articular surface is sufficient to resist displacement.[28] Unexplained pain or crepitus with active range of motion at any interval following plate fixation requires radiographic evaluation, and consideration should be given to removal or exchange of hardware depending on fracture healing.

Rehabilitation of Distal Radius Fractures

Rehabilitation of a distal radius fracture begins promptly after diagnosis. Finger motion is encouraged immediately. The period of strict immobilization following initial fracture treatment will vary based upon the fracture pattern, bone quality, fixation method, patient predisposition, and surgeon preference. Therapeutic concerns and specific protocols for each type of fixation have been described in detail by Slutsky and Herman.[29] In general, the era of rigid VLP fixation has been marked by enthusiasm for early active wrist and forearm motion. After fracture healing, late concerns include scar management and desensitization, strengthening, and restoration of advanced/occupational activities.

Outcomes Assessment

Many level III to IV studies have been published concerning the outcomes of treatment for distal radius fracture. Unfortunately, high-level evidence is still lacking, in part due to the widely varied and incomplete methods of assessment that have been employed. The Distal Radius Outcomes Consortium has recently developed a consensus Unified Approach to Outcomes Assessment for Distal Radius Fractures.[30] In this document, the consortium outlines minimum outcomes to capture after distal radius facture, subdivided into the domains of performance measures, patient reported outcomes, pain, complications, and radiographs. It is their aim that widespread adoption of these measures will provide a deliberate and systematic assessment of both treatment effectiveness and quality that is accessible for review and comparison.

SCAPHOID FRACTURES

Epidemiology

The scaphoid accounts for 60% to 70% of all carpal fractures, and like fractures of the distal radius, it often fractures after falling onto an outstretched hand. Their incidence has been calculated at 12.4 per 100,000 personyears, with a peak occurring in men between the ages of 15 and 19 years.[31]

Anatomy

The scaphoid is the link between the proximal and distal carpal rows, and is described as proximal and distal poles with an intervening waist. The proximal pole articulates with the lunate and the scaphoid fossa of the distal radius, the waist articulates with the capitate, and the distal pole articulates with the trapezium and trapezoid (see Figure 75.1). About 75% to 80% of scaphoid fractures occur at the waist, 10% to 15% occur at the proximal pole, and 5% to 10% occur distally.

Biomechanics of Injury

Scaphoid fractures most commonly occur after fall on an outstretched hand, which causes impaction of the proximal pole upon the dorsal rim of the distal radius. Waist fractures occur around the radioscaphocapitate ligament, which acts as a fulcrum. After scaphoid waist fracture, the distal fragment tends to flex and the proximal fragment tends to extend due to its strong lunate attachment via the scapholunate interosseous ligament. This can be visualized radiographically as an elevated lateral intrascaphoid angle (>35°) and *humpback deformity* on the lateral projection.

Vascularity

The scaphoid is almost entirely covered by articular cartilage; it has a delicate vascular supply with greater than 70% of the scaphoid's intraosseous vascularity from the dorsal scaphoid branches of the radial artery. These vessels enter the dorsal ridge in a retrograde direction, providing the single dominant intraosseous vessel to the proximal pole of the scaphoid. A minor volar contribution comes from the radial artery or its superficial palmar branch.[32] Because of this unique vascular anatomy, the proximal pole of a fractured scaphoid is particularly prone to avascular necrosis and nonunion, especially when the fragment is small.

Classification

At least 13 distinct schemes for classification of acute scaphoid fractures have been proposed based upon assessment by plain radiography. Schemes generally divide fractures by anatomical location, fracture plane orientation, and/or stability and displacement.[33] The most commonly cited classification scheme is the modified Herbert[34] system followed by the Russe[35] system. A summary of the modified Herbert and Russe classifications can be found in **Tables 75.2** and **75.3**.

Radiographic Evaluation

Physical examination has a high sensitivity and low specificity for detecting acute scaphoid fractures, so radiographs including PA, lateral, pronated and supinated oblique, and scaphoid views are utilized. Approximately 20% of patients with negative radiographs have an occult acute fracture. Clinical suspicion with negative radiographs has historically been followed by immobilization in a thumb spica cast and follow-up radiographic examination at 2 weeks. This strategy still fails to detect 9% of scaphoid fractures, results in delayed fracture diagnosis, and unnecessarily immobilizes many patients. For these reasons, early advanced imaging in patients with negative plain films and suspicion for a fracture based upon history or examination findings has become increasingly popular. MRI is the most sensitive and specific imaging modality for diagnosing scaphoid fractures and also allows assessment of osseous blood supply and soft tissue injuries. Computed tomography (CT) scan reformatted in the long axis of the scaphoid is slightly less sensitive and specific for identification of scaphoid fracture, but has the advantage of superior bony detail.[36]

Operative Indications

Operative indications are dependent upon fracture alignment and stability. Nondisplaced fractures may be treated with immobilization. Indications for operative management of the fractured scaphoid include[37]

- Greater than 1 mm of displacement at the waist
- Lateral intrascaphoid angle >35°
- Bone loss or comminution
- Dorsal intercalated segment instability
- Malalignment
- Any proximal pole fracture

Delayed presentation is also a relative indication for surgery, as this population has an increased risk of nonunion with nonoperative treatment. Because of the scaphoid's retrograde vascular supply, distal pole and tubercle fractures have a low incidence of nonunion and can generally be treated nonoperatively.

Less invasive surgical techniques have resulted in an increased operative treatment of nondisplaced scaphoid waist fractures. Proponents cite improvements in union rate and earlier mobilization, but outcomes studies examining operative versus nonoperative management of nondisplaced scaphoid waist are inconclusive.[38]

Nonoperative Treatment

Nonoperative treatment is reserved for nondisplaced scaphoid waist and distal pole fractures. Repeat images at 2 weeks are obtained to verify if alignment has been maintained. Above elbow thumb spica, short arm thumb spica and simple short arm casting have all been advocated,

TABLE 75.2. MODIFIED HERBERT CLASSIFICATION OF SCAPHOID FRACTURES

Type	Description	Depiction	Stability
A1	Tubercle		Stable
A2	Incomplete waist		
B1	Distal oblique		Unstable
B2	Complete waist		
B3	Proximal pole		
B4	Fracture dislocation	Varies, usually waist fracture	
D1	Fibrous union		Nonacute
D2	Pseudoarthrosis		
D3	Sclerotic pseudoarthrosis		

TABLE 75.3. RUSSE CLASSIFICATION OF SCAPHOID FRACTURES

Type	Description	Depiction	Stability
D4	Avascular necrosis		
HO	Horizontal oblique		Most stable
T	Transverse		Intermediate stability
VO	Vertical oblique		Least stable

without conclusive evidence one method is superior. Recently, a randomized trial demonstrated better healing when the thumb is not included.[39]

The duration of immobilization depends upon the patient and the location of the fracture. Distal pole and tubercle fractures generally require only 6 to 8 weeks to heal, whereas scaphoid waist fractures usually require 12 weeks. Immobilization can be discontinued when bony union has been demonstrated. We advocate CT scan to confirm healing between 10 and 12 weeks, when the fracture is no longer visible on plain radiographs.

Open Reduction and Internal Fixation

Until the mid-1980s, most scaphoid fixation was performed using Kirschner wires. In 1984, Herbert and Fisher popularized the use of headless compression screws, revolutionizing the treatment of scaphoid fractures.[40]

The initial screw was not cannulated and required a jig for insertion. Subsequently, a cannulated modification (Herbert-Whipple screw) was developed, allowing insertion over a fluoroscopically targeted guidewire.[41] When there is bone loss or comminution, cancellous or corticocancellous autogenous bone graft from the distal radius can be used to fill the void and aid in healing.

Fracture location often dictates the surgical approach. Because of the volar obliquity of the scaphoid axis, proximal pole fractures are more easily visualized using a dorsal approach, whereas distal pole fractures are amenable to a volar approach. Waist fractures can be addressed from either side, with advantages and drawbacks to each. A volar approach provides wide bony exposure, and facilitates correction of a humpback deformity using structural bone graft to support the collapsed volar cortex. However, the volar margin of the trapezium hinders retrograde screw placement. The dorsal approach to a scaphoid waist fracture provides an unobstructed path for screw placement, but exposure is more limited, and bone grafting for correction of a humpback deformity is more difficult from the dorsal approach. Furthermore, the dorsal location of the dominant blood supply is at risk with distal exposure.

Percutaneous and *mini-open* techniques can be performed from dorsal or volar with minimal soft tissue and vascular disruption.[42] These approaches are best suited for nondisplaced fractures, though displaced fractures can still be treated percutaneously with the aid of joystick manipulation using Kirschner wires and arthroscopic visualization.

Postoperative Management and Rehabilitation

After surgical treatment of a scaphoid fracture, the patient is immobilized in a short arm splint with or without a thumb spica component. Finger motion is initiated immediately and the surgical dressing is changed at 2 weeks to a cast or removable brace. Some surgeons allow intermittent splint removal for light active range of motion exercises at the wrist even before bony union. Assessment of bony union is variable among surgeons, with some relying on CT scans to determine healing. Progressive wrist range of motion and strengthening is initiated following bony union.

Outcomes

Distal pole scaphoid fractures are quite vascular and in the absence of substantial displacement can be treated nonoperatively. Displaced scaphoid waist fractures are treated operatively, and the rate of union is generally thought to be approximately 90%, though this depends upon surgical technique and patient factors. Proximal pole fractures are managed with surgery, with some reports of union at 95%.[43]

Complications

Nonunion is the most important adverse outcome for scaphoid fracture. The overall incidence is approximately 10%, but this rate may be elevated by delayed presentation, fracture comminution, smoking, incomplete immobilization, or errors in surgical technique.[44] Because of the retrograde nature of scaphoid vascularity, proximal pole fractures have an increased incidence of nonunion and avascular necrosis.

The shortening and collapse of the scaphoid is manifested with flexion of the distal fragment and proximal scaphoid extension. When not corrected, a predictable pattern of degenerative changes known as scaphoid nonunion advanced collapse arthritis occurs.

A detailed classification system and complex treatment algorithms have been developed for treatment of scaphoid nonunion.[45] Treatment principles for scaphoid waist nonunion include debridement and reduction of the fracture if necessary, rigid fixation, and bone grafting to restore the native shape and length of the scaphoid and induce osteogenesis. When nonunion is present in the absence of scaphoid flexion, screw fixation and autogenous distal radius cancellous bone grafting can be performed via a dorsal or volar approach (Figure 75.12). When a humpback deformity is present, a volar approach is recommended such that the scaphoid can be extended and then held in alignment with corticocancellous autogenous bone graft.[45]

An alternative to nonvascularized bone grafting is the use of pedicled or free vascularized bone flaps. A variety of these flaps have been applied to nonunions when decreased vascularity of the proximal fragment is suspected, and to those that have been recalcitrant to treatment with nonvascularized autograft. In theory, by bringing new blood supply to the fracture site these flaps can aid in the healing of a hypovascular fracture site. The 1,2 intercompartmental supraretinacular artery (1,2 ICSRA) flap was the first to be described, and several additional pedicled flaps from the dorsal and volar distal radius are available.[46] These are limited by their small size and diminutive vascular pedicles. As an alternative, the medial femoral condyle free flap has been popularized as a robust and reliable source of vascularized bone for treatment of scaphoid waist nonunion.[47]

In cases of proximal pole nonunion with avascular necrosis, the fragment may be too small or sclerotic to allow intercalary bone grafting and fixation of the scaphoid. When this proximal fragment is unsalvageable in a young patient, replacement of the entire proximal pole including the proximal articular surface may be indicated. Options include nonvascularized osteochondral rib graft and a vascularized free medial femoral trochlea osteochondral free flap[48] (Figure 75.13). In patients who are older and have low functional demand and in those who have developed arthritis of the radioscaphoid joint or irreducible flexion of the distal scaphoid fragment, salvage options such as proximal row carpectomy or limited intercarpal fusion are recommended.

OTHER CARPAL FRACTURES

Triquetral Fractures

The triquetrum is the second most common carpal fracture. Dorsal rim fractures result from hyperflexion and radial deviation resulting in avulsion of the dorsal radiocarpal and dorsal intercarpal ligaments with a cortical fragment of the triquetrum. Most injuries can be treated with 3 to 6 weeks of immobilization; however, large fragments may

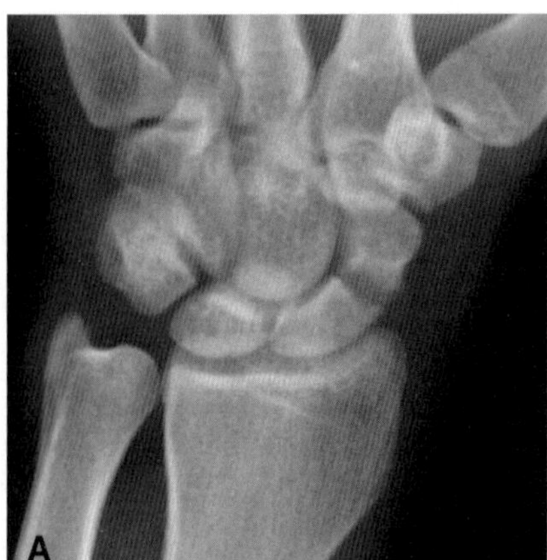

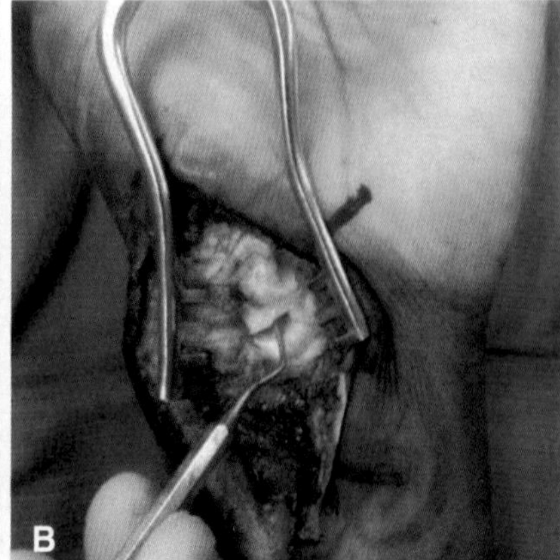

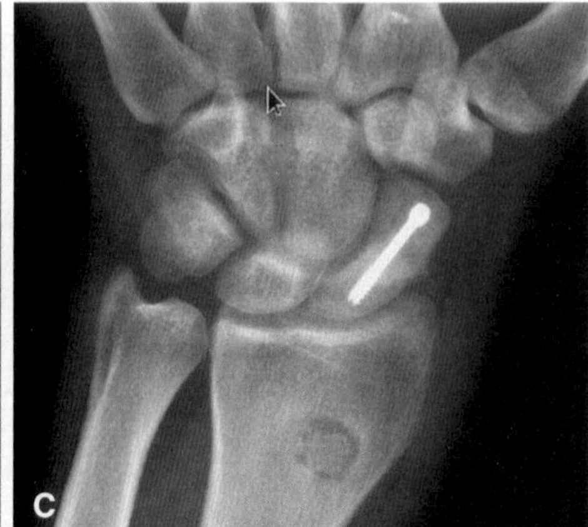

FIGURE 75.12. **A.** This patient presented with subacute wrist pain and radiographs demonstrated a scaphoid waist nonunion. **B, C.** This was treated with debridement of the nonunion, cancellous bone grafting from the distal radius, and stabilization with a headless compression screw via a volar approach.

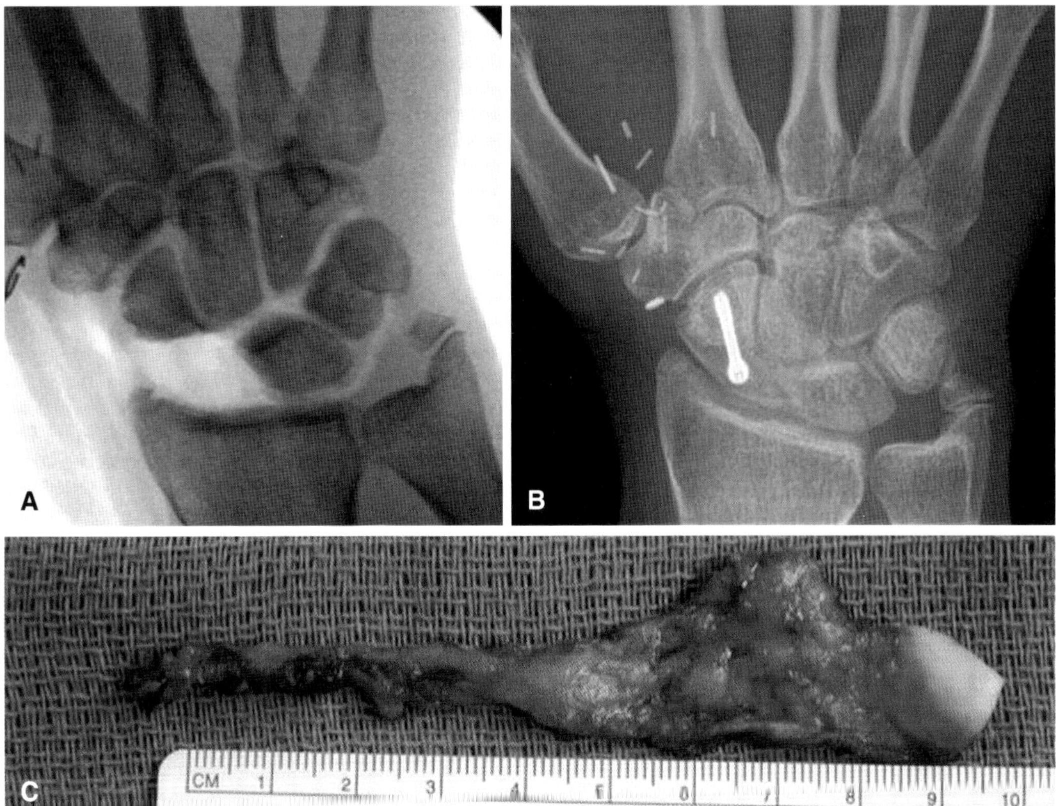

FIGURE 75.13. In cases of proximal pole nonunion with avascular necrosis, the fragment may be too small or sclerotic to allow intercalary bone grafting and fixation of the scaphoid. In this case, the proximal pole can be entirely resected (A), and the scaphoid reconstructed with a medial femoral trochlea osteocartilaginous free flap harvested from the knee (C). Fixation of the osteocartilaginous flap is achieved using a cannulated headless compression screw (B).

require surgical fixation. In dorsal rim fractures with associated lunotriquetral ligament avulsion and resultant instability, the fragment can be ignored and the joint simply pinned.[49] Triquetral body fractures reflect a high energy mechanism and are often associated with other pathology such as a greater arc perilunate dislocation. Displaced body fractures and those associated with carpal instability patterns require surgical treatment.

Hamate Fractures

Hook of Hamate

Two patterns of hamate fracture present with relative frequency: fractures of the hook and hamatometacarpal fracture-dislocations. The hook of the hamate may be injured by compressive trauma during stick-and-ball sports or by avulsion at its attachment to the transverse carpal ligament. This injury may be associated with weak or painful grip due to the hook's role as a pulley for the ring and small flexor digitorum profundus tendons, or with ulnar nerve symptoms due to irritation of the adjacent motor branch. Advanced imaging with CT scan or MRI may be required for diagnosis. Treatment of acute hook fractures is 6 to 12 weeks of immobilization.[49] Established symptomatic nonunions are treated with excision of the hook fragment.

Hamatometacarpal Fracture-Dislocation

An axial load applied to the fourth and fifth metacarpals may result in fracture of metacarpal base, extending through the carpometacarpal joint to include the dorsal hamate. The presence of a hamatometacarpal fracture-dislocation can easily be missed on a standard radiographic series, and clinical suspicion should prompt a pronated oblique film or CT scan. Treatment for these injuries may include closed immobilization, percutaneous pinning of the carpometacarpal joints, or open reduction and internal fixation.[50]

REFERENCES

1. Karl JW, Olson PR, Rosenwasser MP. The epidemiology of upper extremity fractures in the United States, 2009. *J Orthop Trauma*. 2015;29(8):e242-e244.
2. Swart E, Tulipan J, Rosenwasser MP. How should the treatment costs of distal radius fractures be measured? *Am J Orthop*. 2017;46(1):E54-E59.
3. Kleinman WB. Stability of the distal radioulna joint: biomechanics, pathophysiology, physical diagnosis, and restoration of function what we have learned in 25 years. *J Hand Surg Am*. 2007;32(7):1086-1106.
4. Pechlaner S, Kathrein A, Gabl M, et al. Distal radius fractures and concomitant lesions. Experimental studies concerning the pathomechanism. *Handchir Mikrochir Plast Chir*. 2002;34(3):150-157.
5. Shehovych A, Salar O, Meyer C, Ford DJ. Adult distal radius fractures classification systems: essential clinical knowledge or abstract memory testing? *Ann R Coll Surg Engl*. 2016;98(8):525-531.
6. Ng CY, McQueen MM. What are the radiological predictors of functional outcome following fractures of the distal radius? *J Bone Joint Surg Br*. 2011;93(2):145-150.
7. Goldfarb CA, Yin Y, Gilula LA, et al. Wrist fractures: what the clinician wants to know. *Radiology*. 2001;219(1):11-28.
8. Medoff RJ. Essential radiographic evaluation for distal radius fractures. *Hand Clin*. 2005;21(3):279-288.
9. Graham T. Surgical correction of malunited fractures of the distal radius. *J Am Acad Orthop Surg*. 1997;5(5):270-281.
10. Lafontaine M, Hardy D, Delince P. Stability assessment of distal radius fractures. *Injury*. 1989;20(4):208-210.
This study examined 112 distal radius fractures treated with closed reduction and plaster immobilization. Five criteria including dorsal angulation >20, dorsal comminution, intraarticular radiocarpal fracture, associated ulnar fracture, and age exceeding 60 years were found to predict loss of reduction despite immobilization. As a result, the authors recommended close radiological surveillance and possible early fixation of fractures with three or more of these risk factors.
11. Mackenney PJ, McQueen MM, Elton R. Prediction of instability in distal radial fractures. *J Bone Joint Surg Am*. 2006;88A:1944-1951.
Over 4000 distal radial fractures were prospectively assessed for early and late instability. Patient age, metaphyseal comminution of the fracture, and ulnar variance, but not dorsal angluation were identified as the most consistent independent predictors of radiographic outcome. Formulas to predict the radiographic outcome were constructed using these independent predictors, and can be used to inform surgical decision-making.
12. Agee JM. Application of multiplanar ligamentotaxis to external fixation of distal radius fractures. *Iowa Orthop J*. 1994;14:31-37.

13. Fernandez DL. Closed manipulation and casting of distal radius fractures. *Hand Clin*. 2005;21(3):307-316.
14. Trumble TE, Wagner W, Hanel DP, et al. Intrafocal (Kapandji) pinning of distal radius fractures with and without external fixation. *J Hand Surg Am*. 1998;23(3):381-394.
15. Chia B, Catalano LW, Glickel SZ, et al. Percutaneous pinning of distal radius fractures: an anatomic study demonstrating the proximity of K-wires to structures at risk. *J Hand Surg Am*. 2009;34(6):1014-1020.
16. Chaudhry H, Kleinlugtenbelt YV, Mundi R, et al. Are volar locking plates superior to percutaneous k-wires for distal radius fractures? A meta-analysis. *Clin Orthop Relat Res*. 2015;473(9):3017-3027.
This is a metaanalysis of seven randomized controlled trials to determine whether patients treated with volar locking plates achieved better function, wrist motion, radiographic outcomes, or fewer complications patients treated with K-wires for dorsally displaced distal radius fractures. Patients treated with volar locking plates had slightly better early function, fewer superficial wound infections, and similar radiographic outcomes as patient treated with K-wires. The clinical significance of these differences is questionable, and both methods of fixation are still in use.
17. Orbay JL, Fernandez DL. Volar fixation for dorsally displaced fractures of the distal radius: a preliminary report. *J Hand Surg Am*. 2002;27(2):205-215.
This clinical series marks the introduction of volar locking fixation for the treatment of distal radius fractures and is the first documentation of outcomes using this technique. The authors conclude that this is a versatile technique with a favorable complication profile and is applicable to many patterns of distal radius fracture.
18. Soong M, Earp BE, Bishop G, et al. Volar locking plate implant prominence and flexor tendon rupture. *J Bone Joint Surg Am*. 2011;93A:328-335.
This study classified volar locking plates applied to the distal radius according to their degree of volar prominence on the lateral radiograph. The authors conclude that there is an increased risk of flexor tendon rupture when plates are more prominent than the volar rim, corresponding to placement beyond the watershed line.
19. Quadlbauer S, Pezzei C, Jurkowitsch J, et al. Early rehabilitation of distal radius fractures stabilized by volar locking plate: a prospective randomized pilot study. *J Wrist Surg*. 2017;6(2):102-112.
20. Dy CJ, Wolfe SW, Jupiter JB, et al. Distal radius fractures: strategic alternatives to volar plate fixation. *Instr Course Lect*. 2014;63:27-37.
21. Azzi AJ, Aldekhayel S, Boehm KS, Zadeh T. Tendon rupture and tenosynovitis following internal fixation of distal radius fractures. *Plast Reconstr Surg*. 2017;139(3):717e-724e.
22. Hanel DP, Lu TS, Weil WM. Bridge plating of distal radius fractures. *Clin Orthop Relat Res*. 2006;445:91-99.
23. Sammer DM, Chung KC. Management of the distal radioulnar joint and ulnar styloid fracture. *Hand Clin*. 2012;28(2):199-206.
24. Hanel DP, Jones MD, Trumble TE. Wrist fractures. *Orthop Clin North Am*. 2002;33(1):35-57.
25. Desai MJ, Kamal RN, Richard MJ. Management of intercarpal ligament injuries associated with distal radius fractures. *Hand Clin*. 2015;31(3):409-416.
26. Placzek JD, Boyer MI, Gelberman RH, et al. Nerve decompression for complex regional pain syndrome type II following upper extremity surgery. *J Hand Surg Am*. 2005;30(1):69-74.
27. Mathews AL, Chunk KC. Management of complications of distal radius fractures. *Hand Clin*. 2015;31(2):205-215.
28. Wall LB, Brodt MD, Silva MJ, et al. The effects of screw length on stability of simulated osteoporotic distal radius fractures fixed with volar locking plates. *J Hand Surg Am*. 2012;37(3):446-453.
This biomechanical study investigated the effect of screw length upon the stability of distal radius fractures fixed with volar locking fixation. The authors found that locked unicortical distal screws of at least 75% the AP length of the distal radius produce construct stiffness similar to bicortical fixation. They concluded unicortical distal fixation using screws of adequate length does not compromise construct integrity and should be entertained in cases of extraarticular distal radius fracture to avoid extensor tendon injury.
29. Slutsky DJ, Herman M. Rehabilitation of distal radius fractures: a biomechanical guide. *Hand Clin*. 2005;21(3):455-468.
30. Waljee JF, Ladd A, MacDermid JC, et al. A unified approach to outcomes assessment for distal radius fractures. *J Hand Surg Am*. 2016;41(4):565-573.
31. Garala K, Taub NA, Dias JJ. The epidemiology of fractures of the scaphoid: impact of age, gender, deprivation and seasonality. *Bone Joint J*. 2016;98B(5):654-659.
32. Freedman DM, Botte MJ, Gelberman RH. Vascularity of the carpus. *Clin Orthop Relat Res*. 2001;(383):47-59.
33. Berg Ten P, Drijkoningen T, Strackee S, Buijze G. Classifications of acute scaphoid fractures: a systematic literature review. *J Wrist Surg*. 2016;05(02):152-159.
34. Filan SL, Herbert TJ. Herbert screw fixation of scaphoid fractures. *J Bone Joint Surg Br*. 1996;78(4):519-529.
35. Russe O. Fracture of the carpal navicular: diagnosis, nonoperative treatment, and operative treatment. *J Bone Joint Surg Am*. 1960;42A:759-768.
36. Yin ZG, Zhang JB, Gong KT. Cost-effectiveness of diagnostic strategies for suspected scaphoid fractures. *J Orthop Trauma*. 2015;29(8):e245-e252.
37. Cooney WP, Dobyns JH, Linscheid RL. Fractures of the scaphoid: a rational approach to management. *Clin Orthop Relat Res*. 1980;(149):90-97.
38. Ram AN, Chung KC. Evidence-based management of acute nondisplaced scaphoid waist fractures. *J Hand Surg Am*. 2009;34(4):735-738.
39. Buijze GA, Goslings JC, Rhemrev SJ, et al. Cast immobilization with and without immobilization of the thumb for nondisplaced and minimally displaced scaphoid waist fractures: a multicenter, randomized, controlled trial. *J Hand Surg Am*. 2014;39(4):621-627.
40. Herbert TJ, Fisher WE. Management of the fractured scaphoid using a new bone screw. *J Bone Joint Surg Br*. 1984;66B:114-123.
This clinical series marks the introduction of the headless compression screw for the treatment of scaphoid fractures and is the first documentation of outcomes using this technique. The authors document high rates of fracture union in primary and secondary cases and conclude that this device has wide applicability in the treatment of scaphoid fractures. Modern scaphoid (and other) fixation is based upon a cannulated modification of this original headless compression screw.
41. Whipple TL. Stabilization of the fractured scaphoid under arthroscopic control. *Orthop Clin North Am*. 1995;26(4):749-754.
42. Merrell G, Slade J. Technique for percutaneous fixation of displaced and nondisplaced acute scaphoid fractures and select nonunions. *J Hand Surg Am*. 2008;33(6):966-973.
43. Suh N, Grewal R. Controversies and best practices for acute scaphoid fracture management. *J Hand Surg Eur Vol*. 2018;43:4-12.
This review article represents a current and complete collation of the evidence surrounding the diagnosis, management, and outcomes of acute scaphoid fractures. Evidence-based recommendations are included with citation of the supporting literature
44. Pinder RM, Brkljac M, Rix L, et al. Treatment of scaphoid nonunion: a systematic review of the existing evidence. *J Hand Surg Am*. 2015;40(9):1797-1805.
45. Janowski J, Coady C, Catalano LW III. Scaphoid fractures: nonunion and malunion. *J Hand Surg Am*. 2016;41:1087-1092.
46. Rizzo M, Moran SL. Vascularized bone grafts and their applications in the treatment of carpal pathology. *Semin Plast Surg*. 2008;22(3):213-227.
47. Jones DB Jr, Moran SL, Bishop AT, Shin AY. Free-vascularized medial femoral condyle bone transfer in the treatment of scaphoid nonunions. *Plast Reconstr Surg*. 2010;125(4):1176-1184.
48. Higgins J, Burger H. Proximal scaphoid arthroplasty using the medial femoral trochlea flap. *J Wrist Surg*. 2013;2(3):228-233.
49. Pan T, Lögters TT, Windolf J, Kaufmann R. Uncommon carpal fractures. *Eur J Trauma Emerg Surg*. 2016;42(1):15-27.
50. Kim JK. A novel hamatometacarpal fracture-dislocation classification system based on CT scan. *Injury*. 2012;43(7):1112-1117.

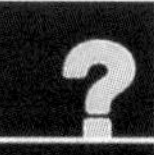

QUESTIONS

1. **A 45-year-old woman presents to the emergency department with snuffbox and distal tubercle tenderness 2 hours after a bicycle accident. She is insistent upon avoiding surgery. A favorable outcome utilizing immobilization without operative intervention is most likely if her X-ray reveals scaphoid fracture of which type?**

   a. Incomplete waist fracture
   b. Nondisplaced proximal pole fracture
   c. Nondisplaced proximal pole fracture with sclerosis
   d. Displaced distal tubercle fracture

2. **Verification that a VLP has been placed upon the distal radius in a position that is unlikely to cause flexor tendon irritation or rupture can be best obtained using which plain radiographic view?**

   a. PA
   b. Lateral
   c. Oblique
   d. Carpal tunnel view

3. **Which clinical factor has *not* been implicated as a risk factor for radius fracture displacement after initial closed reduction and plaster immobilization?**

   a. Dorsal comminution
   b. Age over 60
   c. Associated fracture of the ulna
   d. Volar tilt of 10°

4. **Dorsal bridge plating of a distal radius fracture should be strongly considered for initial management of which patient?**

   a. 35-year-old woman with left closed intraarticular, comminuted distal radius fracture and bilateral operative femur fractures
   b. 95-year-old male with a right intraarticular distal radius fracture characterized by 5° of dorsal angulation, ulnar neutral variance, and 1 mm of articular step-off
   c. 25-year-old male pitcher with depressed fracture of the volar lunate facet
   d. 45-year-old woman with a heavily comminuted metadiaphyseal fracture of the left distal radius and ipsilateral segmental fractures of the second through fifth metacarpals

5. **To what is the high risk of nonunion after treatment of a proximal pole scaphoid fracture attributable?**

   a. The anterograde nature of the primary blood supply to the scaphoid, which enters volarly
   b. The retrograde nature of the scaphoid's blood supply, which enters volarly
   c. The anterograde nature of the scaphoid's blood supply, which enters dorsally
   d. The retrograde nature of the scaphoid's blood supply, which enters dorsally

6. **A 23-year-old woman comes in to the emergency department after falling off her snowboard onto an outstretched left hand. Physical examination demonstrates tenderness in the anatomic snuffbox. Initial PA, lateral, and oblique plain radiographs of the wrist demonstrate no fracture. What additional imaging is most sensitive and specific for detection of an acute scaphoid fracture?**

   a. Immediate MRI
   b. Immediate CT scan
   c. Immobilization and follow-up plain radiography in 2 weeks
   d. Immobilization and follow-up plain radiography in 3 days

1. **Answer: a.** The modified Herbert classification scheme divides scaphoid fractures into three major groups: stable, unstable, and nonacute. Of the types listed above, only incomplete waist is a stable type of fracture. As such, immobilization in a thumb spica cast for up to 12 weeks will likely result in fracture union. Proximal pole fractures are at high risk for nonunion and avascular necrosis, and generally fracture of the proximal pole is considered an indication for operative fixation in order to reduce this risk. Avascular necrosis of the proximal pole occurs with a fracture that is subacute or chronic condition and may be identified following a new acute injury. However, given that acute scaphoid fractures can be easily missed, delayed detection at the time of reinjury symptom exacerbation, or radiographic examination for an unrelated complaint is not uncommon. Nonoperative treatment of a proximal pole nonunion is not recommended. Displaced scaphoid fractures, regardless of the anatomical location, are not amenable to nonoperative treatment.

2. **Answer: b.** A VLP should be placed distal enough that all articular fragments are stabilized by locking screws/pegs supporting the subchondral bone. However, placing the plate too distal leads to volar prominence of the distal edge of the plate putting the flexor tendons at risk for irritation or attritional rupture. As such, when possible, a VLP should be placed be positioned proximal enough that it lies entirely volar to the volar rim of the distal radius. The proximodistal position of the plate and the volar/dorsal relationship between plate and volar rim are best visualized on the lateral projection. Although proximodistal placement of the plate can be assessed to some degree on the PA, oblique views, the volar rim is easily distinguishable only on the lateral. The carpal tunnel view is not applicable to distal radius fractures, but can be used to visualize hook of hamate, pisiform, and trapezium fractures.

3. **Answer: d.** In a landmark [illegible] study, Lafontaine et al demonstrated five clinical/radiographic predictors of distal radius fracture displacement after initial closed reduction and immobilization. These were initial dorsal angulation greater than 20°, dorsal comminution, radiocarpal intraarticular involvement, associated fracture of the ulna, and age greater than 60 years. In a larger 2006 study, Mackenney et al found that the most important predictors of fracture instability were advanced age, dorsal comminution, and the position of the fracture at presentation. Volar tilt of 10° is well within the range of normal and would not be considered a marker of fracture instability.

4. **Answer: a.** A dorsal bridge plate is a long, straight implant which spans the distal radius and is anchored into the radial shaft and second or third metacarpal. By unloading the radiocarpal joint and maintaining distraction across the fracture, dorsal bridge plating can provide rigid stability and maintain some degree of articular reduction via ligamentotaxis. Notably, this technique does not call for direct open manipulation of fracture fragments. For this reason, it is useful for heavily comminuted fractures wherein surgical exposure would result in unacceptable devascularization of the fragments. Additionally, because this bridging technique protects the distal radius from any axial loading, it is relatively indicated in polytraumatized patients who require early upper extremity weight bearing to facilitate lower extremity rehabilitation or transfers.

5. **Answer: d.** Gelberman et al demonstrated that 70% to 80% of the intraosseous vascularity (and the entire proximal pole) comes from the dorsal scaphoid branches of the radial artery, entering through the dorsal ridge. These dorsal vessels enter the scaphoid distally and course in a retrograde direction to supply the proximal pole of the scaphoid. A minor volar contribution

comes from radial artery or its superficial palmar branch, which gives off several volar scaphoid branches at the level of the radioscaphoid joint, entering the bone at its distal tubercle.

6. Answer: a. Approximately 20% of patients with clinical suspicion for a scaphoid fracture and negative initial plain radiographs have an occult fracture. For this reason, patients with negative radiographs have traditionally been immobilized for 2 weeks and then sent for repeat plain radiography seeking interval displacement or resorption. Disadvantages of this strategy include the fact that is unnecessarily immobilizes many of patients and still fails to detect 9% of scaphoid fractures. In an effort to avoid these disadvantages, immediate advanced imaging has gained popularity. MRI is the most sensitive commonly employed modality (97.2%), followed by CT (90.7%).

CHAPTER 76 Flexor Tendon Repair and Reconstruction

Xuan Qiu and Kevin C. Chung

KEY POINTS

- Complete flexor tendon lacerations should be repaired early (preferably within 7 days of injury).
- Flexor tendon undergoes both intrinsic and extrinsic healing after repair.
- At least four-strand core sutures placed 1 cm from the tendon ends should be used to repair flexor tendon lacerations.
- Epitendinous sutures augment flexor tendon repair strength.
- Early protective motion improves the functional outcome of flexor tendon repair.
- Shortening of a single digit flexor digitorum profundus tendon more than 1 cm should be avoided to prevent the quadriga effect.

Finger flexion is powered by the actions of extrinsic and intrinsic muscles of the hand across multiple joints. Flexor tendon injuries result in loss of finger flexion and impair power grip. These injuries are often a result of penetrating trauma to the volar aspect of the fingers, palm, wrist, or forearm. Avulsion of flexor digitorum profundus insertion at the base of the distal phalanx, or degenerative flexor tendon tears in systemic inflammatory conditions such as rheumatoid arthritis, can also result in loss of finger flexion.

Management of flexor tendon injuries can be challenging, especially those within the fibrous digital sheath because of the tendency for restrictive adhesion formation after surgery, which discourages smooth gliding and prevents normal range of motion of the fingers. The evolution of treatment for flexor tendon injuries has exemplified how clinical practice has been driven by our understanding of the molecular biology and biomechanics of tendon healing from basic science and clinical research to ultimately overcome the challenges in managing these conditions. Recent advances in surgical techniques, suture design, and postsurgical rehabilitation protocols have made flexor tendon repair and reconstruction more satisfactory to both the patient and surgeon.

ANATOMY

There are nine flexor tendons in the hand. The flexor pollicis longus (FPL) controls thumb flexion; the flexor digitorum profundus (four FDP) and flexor digitorum superficialis (four FDS) control finger flexions. The flexor tendon muscles originate from the volar proximal to mid forearm, and distally their tendons enter the carpal tunnel before continuing to insert on the palmar aspect of the fingers. The contraction of the flexor tendon muscles leads to flexion of the fingers to make a composite fist; the distal tendon insertions determine the level of flexion (**Table 76.1**).

Unlike the FDP tendons that spread to the fingers in the same coronal plane at the wrist and forearm, the FDS tendons are stacked in two layers, with the more superficial tendons inserting onto the middle and ring fingers, and the deeper tendons inserting onto the index and small fingers, respectively. Additionally, each FDS tendon divides into two slips, radial and ulnar, to wrap around the FDP tendon to continue distally on the dorsal aspect of the FDP tendon. They reunite at the Camper chiasm before dividing again into two slips to insert onto the palmar aspect of the middle phalanx (Figure 76.1).

TABLE 76.1. FLEXOR TENDON MUSCLES

Muscles	Description
Flexor pollicis longus (FPL)	■ Origin: radial shaft and interosseous membrane ■ Insertion: base of the distal phalanx of the thumb ■ Innervation: anterior interosseous branch of the median nerve (AIN) ■ Action: flexion of the interphalangeal (IP) joint of the thumb
Flexor digitorum profundus (FDP)	■ Origin: proximal ulna and the interosseous membrane ■ Insertion: base of the distal phalanx of index, middle, ring, and small fingers ■ Innervation: AIN for the index and middle fingers; ulnar nerve for the ring and small fingers ■ Action: flexion of the distal interphalangeal (DIP) joint
Flexor digitorum superficialis (FDS)	■ Origin: ulnar head from medial humeral epicondyle, the ulnar collateral ligament, and the coronoid process; radial head from proximal radius ■ Insertion: palmar aspect of the middle phalanx ■ Innervation: median nerve ■ Action: flexion of the proximal interphalangeal (PIP) joints

The FDS and FDP tendons within the flexor tendon sheath receive nutritional supply and eliminate wastes by two major routes: vascular perfusion and synovial diffusion. The direct arterial supply to the flexor tendons comes from the well-developed vincular system, which takes off the common digital arteries and continues to the dorsal aspect of the tendon (Figure 76.1). The palmar aspect of the tendon is relatively avascular, and the paratenon promotes material exchange by means of diffusion.[1]

The flexor tendons are covered by a thin layer of fibroblasts known as the epitenon, which is surrounded by a synovial sheath. The membranous inner component of the sheath provides a smooth gliding surface in addition to secreting synovial fluid rich in hyaluronic acid,[2] which provides both lubrication and nutrition. The outer component of the sheath is the retinaculum, which condenses into fibrous bands of tissue that forms a fibro-osseous tunnel on the palmar surface of the fingers to restrain the flexor tendons close to the adjacent bone or joint. These fibrous bands are known as the pulleys (Figure 76.3A). They are named based on the orientation of their fibers, including annular (A)

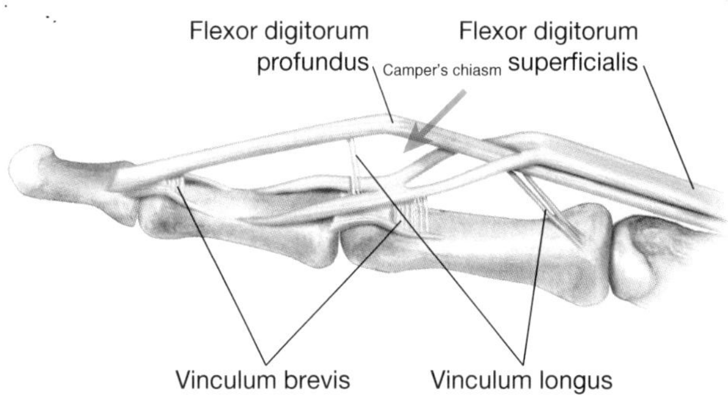

FIGURE 76.1. Anatomy of flexor tendons. (Reproduced with permission from Machol JA IV, Chen NC, Eberlin KR. Acute repair of flexor tendon injuries. In: Chung KC, ed. *Operative Techniques in Plastic Surgery*. Philadelphia, PA: Wolters Kluwer; 2019. Part 6, Figure 37-1a.)

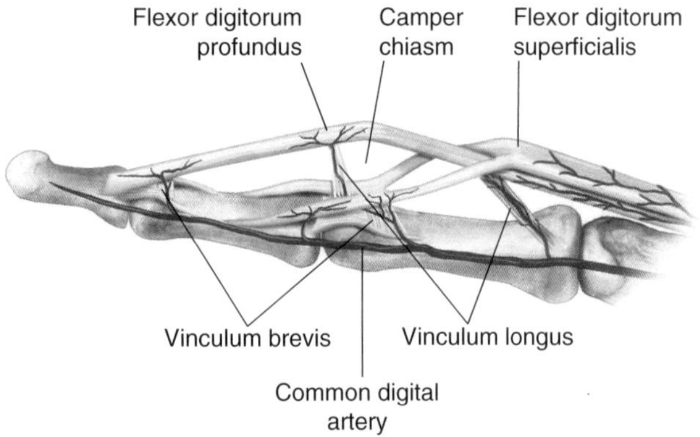

FIGURE 76.2. Vascularity of flexor tendons.

and cruciate (C) pulleys. The thumb has its own pulley system, which includes two annular pulleys, A1 and A2, separated by an oblique pulley which is the most important one in the thumb (Figure 76.3B).[3]

In the fingers, the A pulleys are numbered A1 through A5, and the C pulleys are numbered C1 through C3. The A2 and A4 pulleys originate from the periosteum of the proximal and middle phalanx, respectively. They are the most important pulleys in maintaining grip power and preventing bowstringing of the flexor tendons during active finger flexion. The A1, A3, and A5 pulleys arise from the volar plate of the metacarpophalangeal (MCP), proximal interphalangeal (PIP), and distal interphalangeal (DIP) joints, respectively. They prevent bowstringing of the flexor tendons across these joints during active finger flexion. The A1 pulley is the most commonly affected pulley in trigger fingers and usually divided during trigger finger release. The more flexible cruciate (C1–C3) pulleys are located inbetween the annular pulleys and in close proximity with the joints. They function to accommodate full flexion and extension of the joints without significant collapse or expansion of the adjacent annular pulleys during finger motion.

CLINICAL EVALUATION

Evaluation of patients with possible flexor tendon injuries should begin with a detailed history to determine the mechanism and timing of the injury. The position of the hand and fingers at the time of injury, and the presence of a soft tissue mass on physical examination, can often provide a clue on where the proximal end of the lacerated tendon is located. The location and extent of skin injuries should be carefully assessed. Any notable deformity suggests underlying bone or ligamentous injury, which may require manipulation or reduction. Plain radiographs can help confirm bone or joint abnormalities as well as the presence of a foreign body. Local anesthetics or sedation should be held until after a careful neurovascular examination. Loss of sensation to light touch and two-point discrimination in a digital nerve distribution suggest nerve transection. Delayed capillary refill or an abnormal digital Allen test suggests a digital artery laceration, which can also be confirmed with a Doppler.

Flexor tendon injury can lead to loss of the active finger flexion, normal finger cascade, resting flexor tone resulting in extension posturing, and tenodesis effect. The tenodesis effect is the phenomenon of finger flexion when the wrist is passively extended. Individual fingers should be examined to determine the integrity of the FDS and the FDP tendons. Active finger flexion at the PIP joint while adjacent digits are held down in full extension at the MCP, PIP, and DIP joints indicates that the FDS tendon is intact. Active finger flexion at the DIP joint while the finger is held in full extension at the middle phalanx indicates that the FDP tendon is intact (Figure 76.4). Similarly in the thumb, active flexion at the IP joint indicates that the FPL tendon is intact. Partial tendon injury can manifest as pain with active finger flexion. These injuries are either repaired if the laceration involves more than 50% of the cross-sectional area or debrided if the involvement is less than 50% of the cross-sectional area to minimize catching during finger range of motion.[4]

Flexor tendon injuries are classified into five anatomic zones (zone 1 through zone 5) based on location (Figure 76.5).[5] Zone 1 is the area distal to the insertion of the FDS tendon, i.e., only involving the FDP tendon. Zone 2 describes the area within the flexor tendon sheath distal to the A1 pulley but proximal to the FDS insertion; therefore, injuries within this zone can potentially compromise both the FDS and the FDP tendons. Historically Zone 2 injuries were challenging to manage because of the complex anatomy and the high likelihood of complications after repair, earning Zone 2 the name of *no man's land*.[6] Zone 3 describes the area in the palm distal to the carpal tunnel. Zone 4 is the area within the carpal tunnel. Zone 4 tendon injury is rather uncommon because the overlying trapezium and hamate prominence shield the tendons in this zone from laceration. Zone 5 is the area from the proximal muscle-tendon junction to the carpal tunnel.

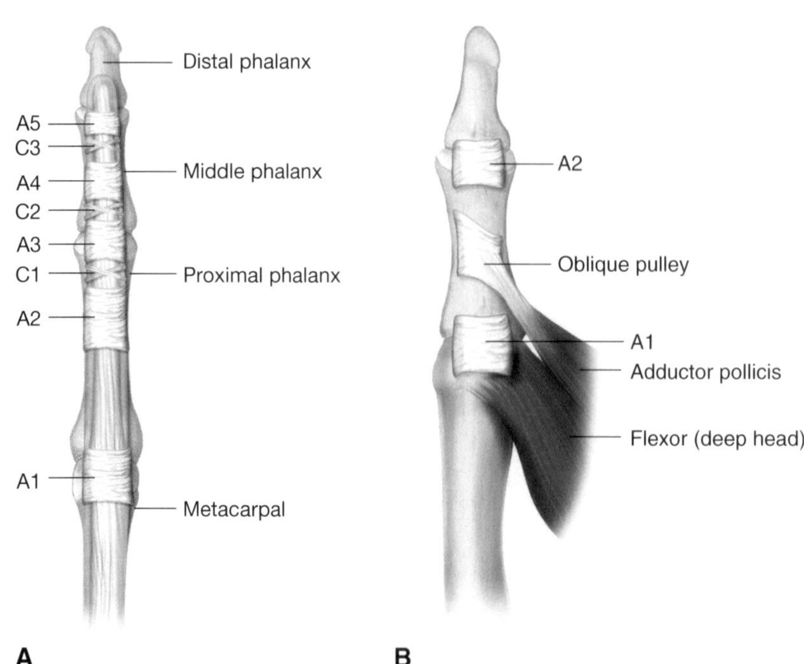

FIGURE 76.3. Pulley systems of the fingers **(A)** and thumb **(B)**. (**A.** Reproduced with permission from Machol JA IV, Chen NC, Eberlin KR. Acute repair of flexor tendon injuries. In: Chung KC, ed. *Operative Techniques in Plastic Surgery*. Philadelphia, PA: Wolters Kluwer; 2019. Part 6, Figure 37-1B.)

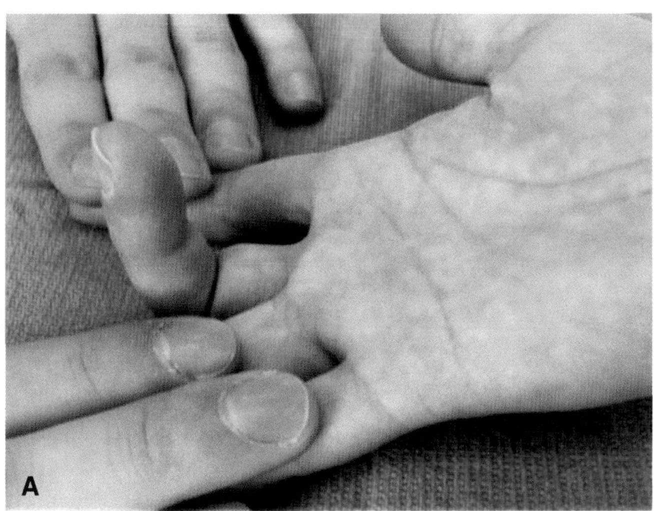

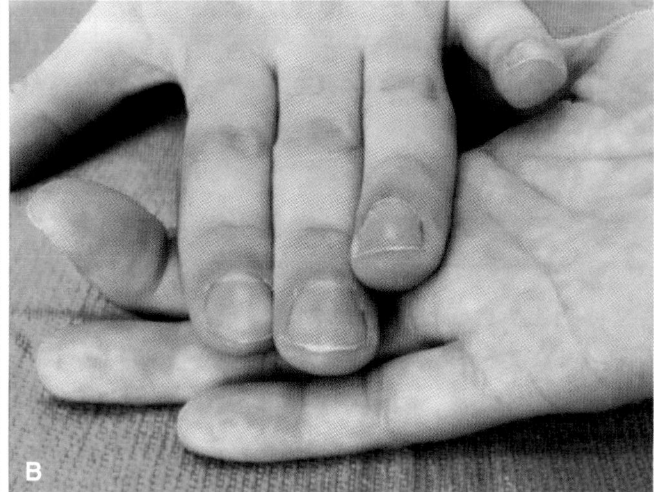

FIGURE 76.4. Physical examination of flexor tendons. **A.** FDS. **B.** FDP.

MANAGEMENT

The treatment goal of a flexor tendon injury is to restore a strong and smooth construct such that a rehabilitation protocol can promote tendon gliding and minimize peritendinous adhesion, and ultimately restore normal motion of the finger. Sometimes this requires partial excision of the FDS tendon to decrease the repair bulk,[7,8] or partial release of the adjacent pulleys.[9] Any fresh open wounds in the hand noted during initial examination should be thoroughly irrigated with sterile saline. A dose of first-generation cephalosporin should be administered if there is no contraindication. Tetanus prophylaxis should also be provided to the patient if not up to date.

In the setting of vascular compromise to the digit with concomitant flexor tendon injury, emergency wound exploration and microvascular repair or reconstruction to restore digital perfusion are indicated, and the lacerated flexor tendons can be repaired at the same time. Otherwise definitive repair of flexor tendon laceration can be scheduled within 7 days of the injury. The injured finger and the wrist should be splinted in slight flexion to prevent further proximal migration of the proximal end of the lacerated tendon. Beyond 6 weeks, the primary repair of flexor tendon is unlikely to succeed because of myostatic contracture of the lacerated tendon and swelling of the tendon ends that do not permit tendons to be retrieved through the pulleys. In the cases of delayed presentation, the surgeon should be prepared for conducting two stage tendon reconstruction or primarily tendon grafting if the wound bed is not too scarred.

Early animal studies suggested that tendon healing required adhesion formation, characterized by infiltration of fibroblasts and capillary buds, which came from the surrounding synovial sheath.[10-12] However, later experiments demonstrated the alternative intrinsic tendon healing without adhesion formation. This was illustrated in an elegant study in which repaired tendon bathed in the synovial fluid of a rabbit knee healed without extrinsic blood supply.[13] This intrinsic tendon healing undergoes three phases of wound healing: inflammation, neovascularization, and remodeling. The earliest stage is characterized by an increase in the inflammatory cells including macrophages[14] and their mediators such as interleukins and matrix metalloproteinases.[15] During tendon healing, neovascularization occurs to bring necessary nutrients for tendon repair and healing,[16] with concomitant early rise of vascular endothelial growth factor[17] and integrin family of cell adhesion receptors.[18] Eventually new collagen formation and reorientation of the collagen fibers restore the tendon morphology and synovial sheath anatomy.[19]

Several factors affect the quality of the flexor tendon repair. Core sutures are those that traverse the main substance of the tendon for coaptation of the repair site. There are different techniques of core suturing, from the classic two-stranded Tajima to the simple four-stranded Strickland and cruciate, and to the more complex multi-stranded Modified Becker/Massachusetts General Hospital (MGH) suture repair (Figure 76.6A–C). Biomechanical studies have shown that increasing the suture caliber can increase the tensile strength at the repair site.[20] Similarly, an increased number of core strands also increases repair strength[21] (**Table 76.2**).[22] Of the two parameters, the core strand number is more important than suture caliber in terms of increasing repair site strength.[23] Based on these data, a nonabsorbable suture, 3-0 to 4-0 depending on the size of the tendon to be repaired, should be placed at 1 cm from the cut edges to provide at least 4-strand core sutures across the repair site to ensure the approximation of the tendon ends for optimal healing.[24] Moreover, locking core suture loops are stronger than grasping loops,[25] and the location of the core suture knot, inside or outside of the repair site, has not been shown to affect the repair site strength.[26]

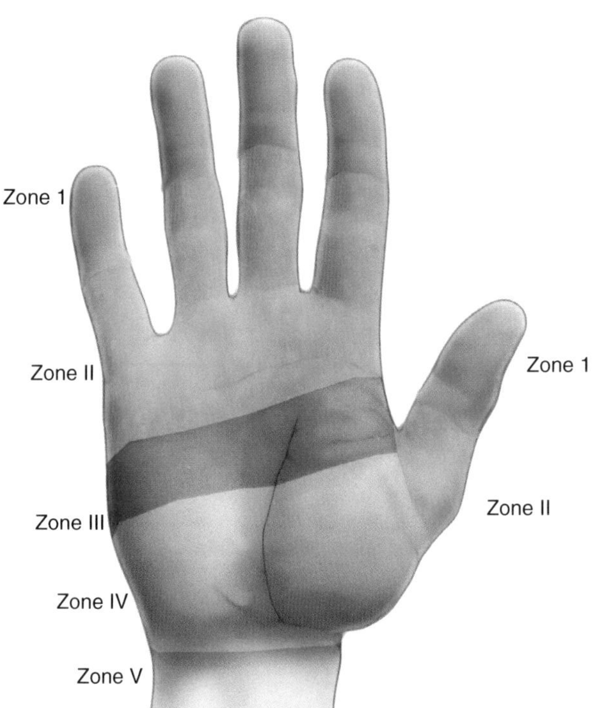

FIGURE 76.5. Flexor tendon zones of injury. (Reproduced with permission from Wiesel SM. Operative Techniques in Orthopaedic Surgery. Philadelphia, PA: Wolters Kluwer Health/Lippincott Williams & Wilkins; 2010. Figure 56-1a.)

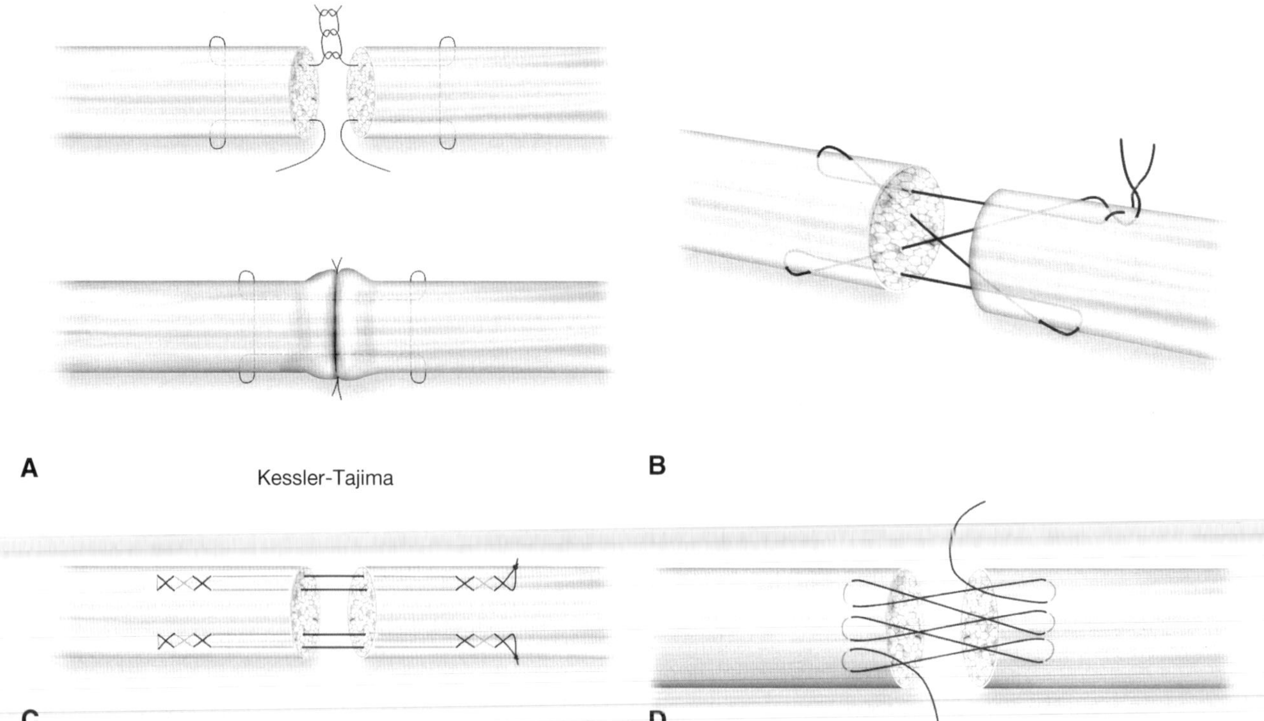

FIGURE 76.6. Flexor tendon repair. Core sutures: Tajima **(A)**, cruciate **(B)**, and modified Becker/MGH **(C)**. **D.** Epitendinous suture. (Reproduced with permission from Machol JA IV, Chen NC, Eberlin KR. Acute repair of flexor tendon injuries. In: Chung KC, ed. *Operative Techniques in Plastic Surgery*. Philadelphia, PA: Wolters Kluwer; 2019. **A.** Part 6, Figure 37-Tech Fig 3. **B.** Part 6, Figure 37-Tech Fig 5. **C.** Part 6, Figure 37-Tech Fig 6. **D.** Part 6, Figure 37-Tech Fig 7a.)

Epitendinous sutures are those that are placed on the superficial aspect of the repair site circumferentially to smoothen the edges for improved gliding and repair site strength (Figure 76.6D). Deeply placed epitendinous sutures provide better repair strength compared to those placed superficially.[27] Epitendinous sutures placed further from the cut edges also improve the tensile strength at the repair site.[28] Therefore, epitendinous sutures for Zone 2 are recommended in addition to the core sutures to augment the repair with a 6-0 nonabsorbable material placed at 2 mm from the cut edges and 2 mm deep. This combination of the core and epitendinous sutures is placed to minimize the gap formation at the repair site, as studies have shown that a gap less than 3 mm is the critical gap to facilitate adequate healing of the tendon and increased repair strength with time.[29]

Shortening of the FDP tendon by more than 1 cm is undesirable because of the *quadriga* effect, when increased tension in the repaired tendon leads to flexion lag and weakened grip in the adjacent fingers, because the FDP tendons share a common muscle belly whose excursion is defined by the shortest tendon. Specific considerations are required for injuries in the different zones. Zone 1 flexor tendon avulsions are further classified into type I through type III by Leddy and Packer (Figure 76.7).[30] In type I avulsion, the FDP tendon retracts into the palm with disruption of the vincular system, and thus needs urgent repair within 2 weeks from the time of injury. In type II avulsion, the FDP tendon retracts to the level of the PIP joint, and can be repaired within 6 weeks from the time of injury, because of preservation of some of the vincular blood supply. Type III injuries usually do not retract proximal to the A4 pulley because of a large bony fragment; these may be repaired with a Kirschner wire or a screw. Pure tendon lacerations in Zone 1, on the other hand, may require tendon-to-bone repair with or without a button if the distal stump is less than 1 cm in length, otherwise it can be repaired primarily. In delayed presentation of Zone 1 injuries outside of the time window for

TABLE 76.2. ESTIMATED REPAIR STRENGTH WITHOUT AN EPITENDINOUS SUTURE

Type of Repair	0 weeks	1 week	3 weeks	6 weeks
Two-strand	1800 g	900 g	1200 g	2200 g
Four-strand	3600 g	1800 g	2400 g	4200 g
Six-strand	5400 g	2700 g	3600 g	6500 g

Reproduced with permission from Strickland JW. Flexor tendon injuries: I. Foundations of treatment. *J Am Acad Orthop Surg*. 1995;3:44-54.

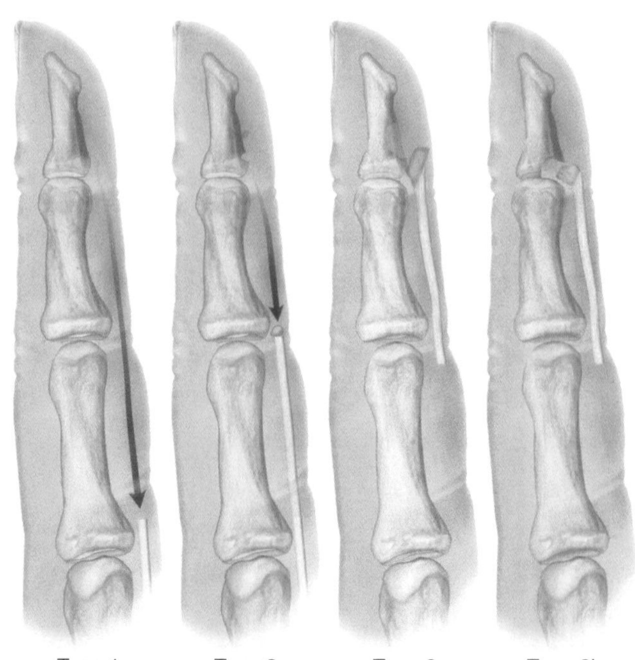

FIGURE 76.7. Leddy classification of Zone 1 flexor tendon injuries.

repair, DIP arthrodesis can be considered in the setting of intact FDS function, understanding that the overall grip strength will be decreased.

Zone 2 flexor tendon injuries are more challenging because of the complex anatomy in this area. Care should be taken to preserve the A2 and the A4 pulleys when the lacerated tendons are passed through them during the repair. The FDP tendon should be carefully pulled through the FDS tendons if it retracts proximal to the chiasm. The proximal end of the FPL laceration in Zone 2 may retract to the thenar musculature or even more proximally, which requires extension of the incision to the thenar eminence, or a separate incision in the carpal tunnel or distal forearm, respectively. Milking the digit from proximal to distal and wrist and MCP flexion can help to deliver the proximal tendon end near the laceration. If the proximal FPL tendon cannot be retrieved readily, we prefer to make an incision at the wrist, radial to the FCR tendon to find the proximal tendon end. A small feeding catheter is threaded into the sheath, taking great care not to create a false path. The proximal tendon is then sutured to the catheter, which is used to guide the tendon through the sheath. After tendon repair, gentle range of motion of the finger can detect repair site gapping or catching at the edge of a pulley.

Flexor tendon injuries in Zones 3, 4, and 5 are repaired with similar techniques as those used in Zone 2 injuries, although epitendinous sutures may not be necessary because there is more room in these zones for tendon excursion, which decreases the intensity of the adhesions. Furthermore, multiple structures are cut in these zones, which require expedient repairs to keep the tourniquet time within 2 hours. Repairs in Zones 3, 4, and 5 have less adhesion formation and better prognosis. Microsurgery may be needed for concomitant nerve or arterial injuries at the time of tendon repair.

REHABILITATION AND OUTCOMES

After successful flexor tendon repair, a dorsal blocking splint is applied to maintain the wrist flexion at 20° to 30°, the MCP joint flexion at 50° to 70°, and PIP and DIP joints in full extension. Animal studies have demonstrated that early protective motion promotes tendon healing.[31] The strength of the repair determines the type of postoperative motion therapy. Studies have concluded that at least four core strands are needed to create a strong enough repair to withstand the strain across the repair site from light active motion (Figure 76.8).[22] Therapy should begin within a week of the surgery under the guidance of an experienced hand therapist. Early motion rehabilitation protocol in the appropriate patients helps to decrease intrasynovial adhesion formation and prevent digital stiffness.

It has been well accepted that 3 to 5 mm of tendon excursion sufficiently prevents adhesion formation in Zone 2 repairs.[32] Within this range, increased tendon excursion does not affect the tensile properties of the repair site.[33] Similarly, increasing the level of applied force during rehabilitation does not affect the ultimate strength of the repaired tendon.[34] A prospective randomized clinical trial demonstrated that the active place-and-hold therapy improved finger active range of motion, compared to passive motion therapy, although functional outcome scores were similar in both groups.[35]

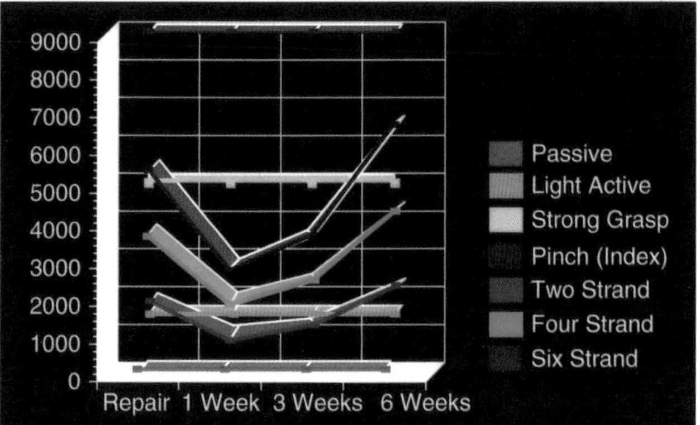

FIGURE 76.8. Estimated strength to failure (in grams) for flexor tendon repairs with epitendinous sutures. (Reproduced with permission from Strickland JW. Flexor tendon injuries: I. Foundations of treatment. *J Am Acad Orthop Surg*. 1995;3:44-54.)

More rigorous active finger range of motion starts at 3 to 4 weeks postoperatively. The protective dorsal splint is eventually discontinued around 6 to 8 weeks postoperatively. Individual digit strengthening is gradually introduced at 10 weeks after surgery, and the patient may return to normal activities at 4 to 6 months after surgery. In pediatric patients and those who are unable to safely participate in an early motion rehabilitation program, cast immobilization for 4 to 6 weeks is used to protect the repair. The cast is applied to maintain the wrist in neutral, MCP joints at 70° of flexion, and IP joints in extension. Careful initiation and progression of range-of-motion exercises with frequent monitoring are critical to achieve a good outcome.

Outcomes of flexor tendon repair surgery depends on multiple factors, including severity of initial injury, timing and quality of the repair, patient's underlying medical conditions that may affect tendon healing, and the quality of postoperative rehabilitation. Majority of Zone 1 and Zone 2 repairs have good to excellent outcomes, almost all Zone 3, 4, and 5 repairs have good to excellent outcomes.

COMPLICATIONS

The most common complication after flexor tendon repairs is finger stiffness, which can be a result of either tendon adhesion or IP joint contractures. Other complications, such as infection, skin flap necrosis, and tendon rupture after repair, can also occur. These complications adversely affect the outcome and should be addressed promptly.

Peritendinous adhesion can happen with crush injuries, inflammatory conditions, fractures, excessive surgical manipulation during primary repair, tendon grafting, poor postoperative rehabilitation, and wound complications. Based on the American Society for Surgery of the Hand guidelines,[36] the postoperative total active motion (TAM) of the digit can be determined using the following formula:

$$TAM = (MCP + PIP + DIP)flexion - extension\,lag$$

A grading system categorizes the functional outcome based on the postsurgical TAM as a percentage of the normal TAM of 260°. An excellent outcome is the recovery of 100% of the normal TAM; a good outcome is the recovery of more than 75% of the normal TAM but less than 100%. A recovery of less than 75% but more than 50% is considered fair, and anything less than 50% is considered poor.

At 4 to 6 months after the flexor tendon repair surgery, if a patient's digit function is no longer improving with occupational therapy and there is still substantial limitation in the active motion but passive motion has been restored, tenolysis followed by immediate mobilization may release the adhesion and help to gain full or near full active range of motion. However, tenolysis is a complicated procedure that can result in neurovascular injury, worsening stiffness, and even tendon rupture; therefore, it should be recommended only for patients with fair or poor outcomes. These risks should be thoroughly discussed with the patient preoperatively. Similarly, IP joint contractures are initially managed with passive stretching exercises and static progressive splinting. Beyond 4 to 6 months after the index procedure, joint releases to correct the contractures can be considered. Rupture within the first 3 weeks of the initial tendon repair warrants an attempt for repeat repair, which has reasonable success. If the rupture occurs more than 3 weeks after the primary repair, tendon reconstruction should be considered.

TENDON RECONSTRUCTION

Single-stage flexor tendon grafting can be used to reconstruct flexor tendon injuries that have significant segmental tendon loss or damage, or those that present late and outside of the time window for primary repair, or ruptures that occur after primary repair but are not amenable to repeat repair. Graft donor sites include the palmaris, plantaris, long toe extensors, extensor indicis proprius and extensor digiti minimi, and toe flexors. Alternatively, the proximal FDS or FDP tendon can be used as a graft depending on which motor source the surgeon chooses to keep to power the tendon graft. Patients with extensive scarring, joint contractures not responsive to aggressive hand therapy, and incompetent pulleys need two-stage reconstruction.

The first stage in the two-stage reconstruction includes the placement of a silicone tendon implant in the flexor tendon sheath, repair and/or reconstruction of the pulley system over the implant, and scar and joint contracture release. This process promotes the formation of a pseudosheath over the silicone implant in the next 3 months. During the second stage of the procedure, a tendon graft is passed through the pseudosheath to replace the implant.

For either single-stage or two-stage flexor tendon grafting, the tendon graft is first repaired to the distal phalanx either directly to the FDP tendon stump, or with a pull-through suture to secure the distal stump in a drill hole in the distal phalanx and the suture tied over a button on top of the nail. After appropriate tensioning, the proximal end of the tendon graft is repaired to the motor unit proximally to the remnant FDS or FDP tendon stump. Early motion rehabilitation under close supervision of an experienced hand therapist can be initiated in a similar fashion as that for primary repair, provided that the graft junctures are strong.

In summary, flexor tendon injuries require early intervention. Understanding the biology of tendon healing and the mechanics of the repair methods can direct treatment to improve functional outcomes. A strong repair of the tendon ends with at least four-strand core sutures and an epitendinous suture minimizes gap formation and creates a coaptation that tolerates early protective motion therapy to promote healing and decrease adhesion formation. Chronic injuries are treated with tendon reconstruction. Appropriately setting tension of the repair or reconstruction prevents the quadriga effect. Modern surgical techniques, suture design, and postsurgical rehabilitation protocols have led to satisfactory outcomes in these otherwise challenging injuries.

ACKNOWLEDGMENTS

The work was supported by a Midcareer Investigator Award in Patient-Oriented Research (2 K24-AR053120-06) to Kevin C. Chung. The content is solely the responsibility of the authors and does not necessarily represent the official views of the National Institutes of Health.

REFERENCES

1. Lundborg G, Myrhage R, Rydevik B. The vascularization of human flexor tendons within the digital synovial sheath region – structural and functional aspects. *J Hand Surg*. 1977;2(6):417-427.
2. Hagberg L, Tengblad A, Gerdin B. Hyaluronic acid in flexor tendon sheath fluid after sheath reconstructions in rabbits: a comparison between tendon sheath transplantation and conventional two stage procedures. *Scand J Plast Reconst Surg Hand Surg*. 1991;25(2):103-107.
3. Doyle JR, Blythe WF. Anatomy of the flexor tendon sheath and pulleys of the thumb. *J Hand Surg*. 1977;2(2):149-151.
4. Chow SP, Yu OD. An experimental study on incompletely cut chicken tendons – a comparison of two methods of management. *J Hand Surg*. 1984;9(2):121-125.
5. Verdan CE. Half a century of flexor-tendon surgery: current status and changing philosophies. *Bone Joint Surg Am*. 1972;54(3):472-491.
6. Bunnell S. *Surgery of the Hand*. 2nd ed. Philadelphia, PA: JB Lippincott; 1948.
7. Tang JB. Flexor tendon repair in zone 2C. *J Hand Surg*. 1994;19(1):72-75.
8. Zhao C, Amadio PC, Zobitz ME, An KN. Resection of the flexor digitorum superficialis reduces gliding resistance after zone II flexor digitorum profundus repair in vitro. *J Hand Surg*. 2002;27(2):316-321.
9. Kwai Ben I, Elliot D. "Venting" or partial lateral release of the A2 and A4 pulleys after repair of zone 2 flexor tendon injuries. *J Hand Surg*. 1998;23(5):649-654.
10. Mason ML, Allen HS. The rate of healing of tendons: an experimental study of tensile strength. *Ann Surg*. 1941;113(3):424-459.
11. Potenza AD. Tendon healing within the flexor digital sheath in the dog. *Bone Joint Surg Am*. 1962;44-A:49-64.
12. Potenza AD. Critical evaluation of flexor-tendon healing and adhesion formation within artificial digital sheaths. *Bone Joint Surg Am*. 1963;45:1217-1233.
13. Lundborg G. Experimental flexor tendon healing without adhesion formation – a new concept of tendon nutrition and intrinsic healing mechanisms: a preliminary report. *Hand*. 1976;8(3):235-238.
Elegant animal study to demonstrate intrinsic healing of tendons.
14. Gelberman RH, Vandeberg JS, Manske PR, Akeson WH. The early stages of flexor tendon healing: a morphologic study of the first fourteen days. *J Hand Surg*. 1985;10(6 Pt 1):776-784.
15. Berglund M, Hart DA, Wiig M. The inflammatory response and hyaluronan synthases in the rabbit flexor tendon and tendon sheath following injury. *J Hand Surg Eur Vol*. 2007;32(5):581-587.
16. Gelberman RH, Khabie V, Cahill CJ. The revascularization of healing flexor tendons in the digital sheath: a vascular injection study in dogs. *Bone Joint Surg Am*. 1991;73(6):868-881.
17. Boyer MI, Watson JT, Lou J, et al. Quantitative variation in vascular endothelial growth factor mRNA expression during early flexor tendon healing: an investigation in a canine model. *J Orthop Res*. 2001;19(5):869-872.
18. Harwood FL, Monosov AZ, Goomer RS, et al. Integrin expression is upregulated during early healing in a canine intrasynovial flexor tendon repair and controlled passive motion. *Connect Tissue Res*. 1998;39(4):309-316.
19. Manske PR, Gelberman RH, Lesker PA. Flexor tendon healing. *Hand Clin*. 1985;1(1):25-34.
20. Taras JS, Raphael JS, Marczyk SC, Bauerle WB. Evaluation of suture caliber in flexor tendon repair. *J Hand Surg*. 2001;26(6):1100-1104.
21. Thurman RT, Trumble TE, Hanel DP, et al. Two-, four-, and six-strand zone II flexor tendon repairs: an in situ biomechanical comparison using a cadaver model. *J Hand Surg*. 1998;23(2):261-265.
Biomechanical study in cadavers to demonstrate increased repair strength with increased number of core sutures.
22. Strickland JW. Flexor tendon injuries: I. Foundations of treatment. *J Am Acad Orthop Surg*. 1995;3(1):44-54.
Classic review on flexor tendon anatomy, biology, biomechanics, and treatment after injuries.
23. Osei DA, Stepan JG, Calfee RP, et al. The effect of suture caliber and number of core suture strands on zone II flexor tendon repair: a study in human cadavers. *J Hand Surg*. 2014;39(2):262-268.
24. Chung KC. *Operative Techniques: Hand and Wrist Surgery*. 3rd ed. Philadelphia, PA: Elsevier; 2018.
25. Hotokezaka S, Manske PR. Differences between locking loops and grasping loops: effects on 2-strand core suture. *J Hand Surg*. 1997;22(6):995-1003.
26. Pruitt DL, Aoki M, Manske PR. Effect of suture knot location on tensile strength after flexor tendon repair. *J Hand Surg*. 1996;21(6):969-973.
27. Lotz JC, Hariharan JS, Diao E. Analytic model to predict the strength of tendon repairs. *J Orthop Res*. 1998;16(4):399-405.
Biomechanical study to establish the added repair strength with an epitendinous suture.
28. Merrell GA, Wolfe SW, Kacena WJ, et al. The effect of increased peripheral suture purchase on the strength of flexor tendon repairs. *J Hand Surg*. 2003;28(3):464-468.
29. Gelberman RH, Boyer MI, Brodt MD, et al. The effect of gap formation at the repair site on the strength and excursion of intrasynovial flexor tendons: an experimental study on the early stages of tendon-healing in dogs. *Bone Joint Surg Am*. 1999;81(7):975-982.
Animal study that established acceptable gap formation for tendon repair.
30. Leddy JP, Packer JW. Avulsion of the profundus tendon insertion in athletes. *J Hand Surg*. 1977;2(1):66-69.
Classification system of Zone 1 flexor tendon injury.
31. Gelberman RH, Manske PR, Akeson WH, et al. Flexor tendon repair. *J Orthop Res*. 1986;4(1):119-128.
32. Duran RJ, Houser RG, Coleman CR, Postlethwait DS. A preliminary report in the use of controlled passive motion following flexor tendon repair in zones II and III. *J Hand Surg*. 1976;1(1):75-83.
Principles for the Duran Protocol after flexor tendon repair.
33. Silva MJ, Brodt MD, Boyer MI, et al. Effects of increased in vivo excursion on digital range of motion and tendon strength following flexor tendon repair. *J Orthop Res*. 1999;17(5):777-783.
34. Boyer MI, Gelberman RH, Burns ME, et al. Intrasynovial flexor tendon repair: an experimental study comparing low and high levels of in vivo force during rehabilitation in canines. *Bone Joint Surg Am*. 2001;83-A(6):891-899.
35. Trumble TE, Vedder NB, Seiler JG III, et al. Zone-II flexor tendon repair: a randomized prospective trial of active place-and-hold therapy compared with passive motion therapy. *Bone Joint Surg Am*. 2010;92(6):1381-1389.
Level I evidence comparing active place-and-hold with passive motion therapy.
36. Kleinert HE, Verdan C. Report of the committee on tendon injuries (International Federation of Societies for Surgery of the Hand). *J Hand Surg*. 1983;8(5 Pt 2):794-798.
American Society for Surgery of the Hand determination of total active motion of the digit.

QUESTIONS

1. A 20-year-old male presents at about 3 weeks after accidentally cutting his right index finger at the distal interphalangeal joint. His clinical photo at presentation and initial radiographs are shown in Figure 76.9. Upon finger exploration the distal tendon stump appeared to be 0.5 cm, and the proximal tendon stump was found within the A4 pulley. Which of the following best describes his injury and the treatment?

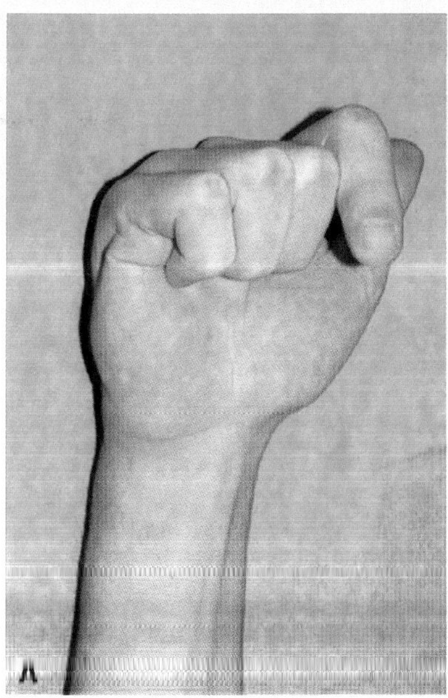

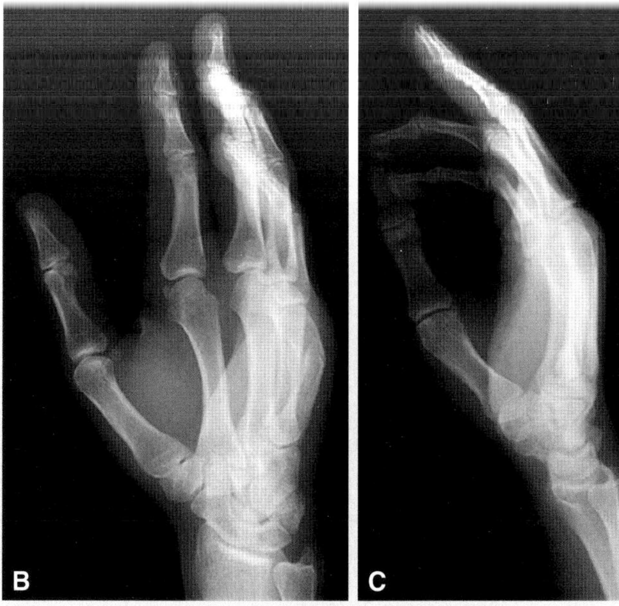

FIGURE 76.9. Clinical photo and radiographs.

a. Zone 1 Leddy type 1 injury, primary repair with four-strand core sutures and an epitendinous suture
b. Zone 1 Leddy type 2 injury, tendon-to-bone repair with nonabsorbable sutures tied over a button
c. Zone 1 Leddy type 3 injury, tendon-to-bone repair with a suture anchor
d. Zone 2 injury, primary repair with four-strand core sutures and an epitendinous suture
e. Zone 2 injury, two-stage reconstruction

2. A 7-year-old girl presents with a laceration to the left index finger that occurred about 5 days previously. Resting hand posture, initial radiographs, and photos from surgical exploration of the finger are shown in Figure 76.10. What is the best treatment for her?

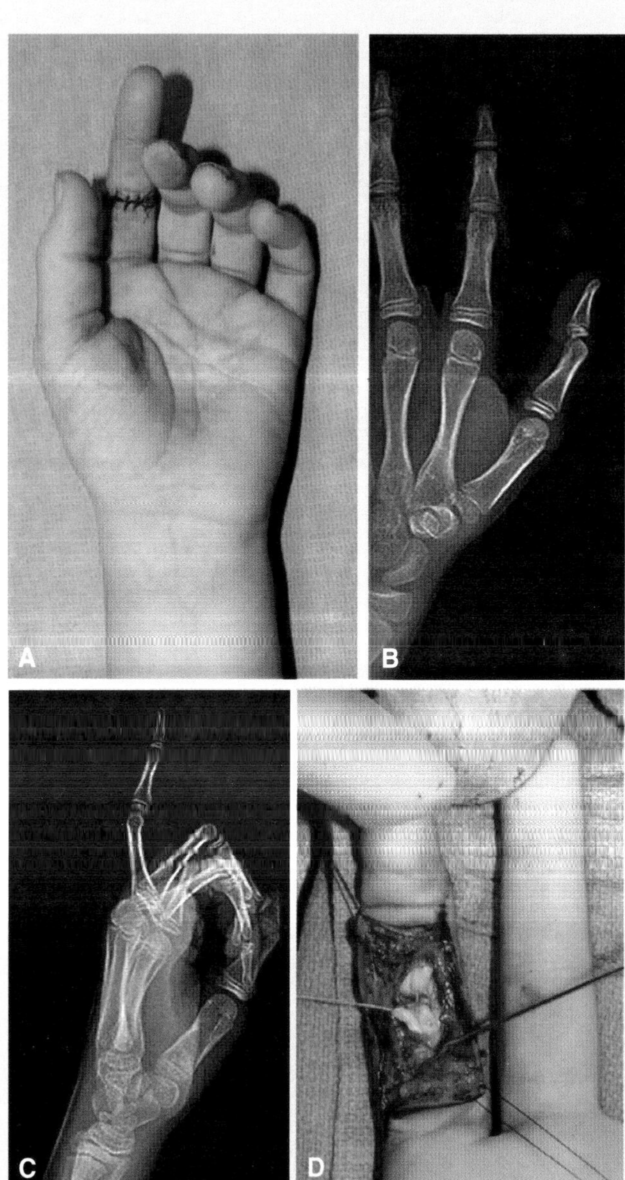

FIGURE 76.10. Clinical and intraoperative photos, and radiographs.

a. Tendon debridement
b. Tendon-to-bone repair with nonabsorbable sutures tied over a button
c. Primary repair with at least four-strand core sutures and an epitendinous suture
d. Single-stage reconstruction with a tendon graft
e. Two-stage reconstruction with a silicone rod followed by a tendon graft

3. **A 32-year-old man presents with a nonfunctioning right small finger from an injury at the proximal interphalangeal joint about 5 months ago. The clinical photo at presentation is shown in Figure 76.11A, and Figure 76.11B–D are pictures from the surgical exploration of the finger, showing the intact and competent tendon sheath. What is the best treatment for him?**

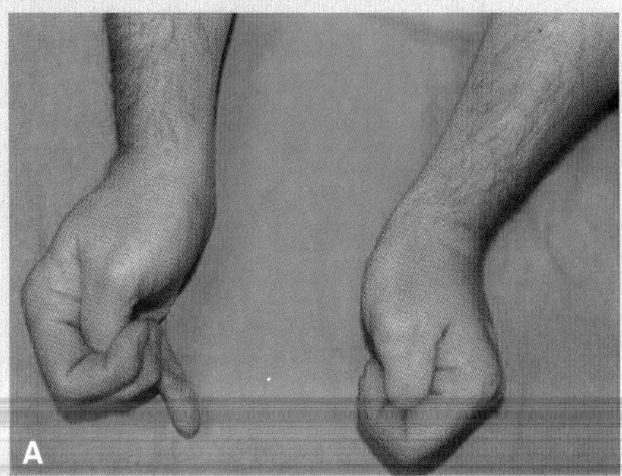

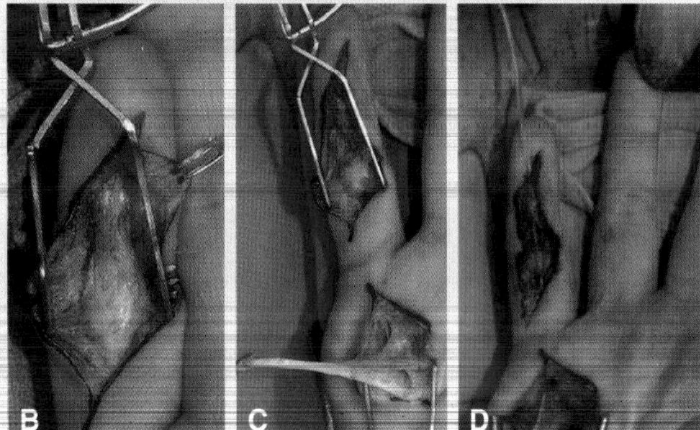

FIGURE 76.11. Clinical and intraoperative photos.

a. Tendon excision
b. Tendon-to-bone repair of the injured tendon using a suture anchor
c. Primary repair with at least four-strand core sutures and an epitendinous suture
d. Single-stage reconstruction with a tendon graft
e. Two-stage reconstruction with a silicone rod followed by a tendon graft

4. **A year after the surgery, the patient in question 3 developed loss of grip in his right small finger. He is able to fully extend the small finger. However, when he attempted to make a fist, the proximal and distal interphalangeal joints of the small finger extend instead. What is the likely cause of this condition and what is the best treatment for him?**

a. Adhesion causing stiffness; hand therapy and progressive static splinting to gain flexion
b. Rupture of the central slip; extension splinting at the proximal interphalangeal joint
c. Attritional rupture of the small finger FDP in the palm; end-to-side repair to the adjacent ring finger FDP tendon
d. Quadriga effect; tendon lengthening
e. Progressive laxity in the tendon graft; lumbrical release

1. **Answer: b.** The clinical history, location of the laceration and proximal tendon stump, and the lack of bony fragment on the radiographs suggest that this was a Zone 1 Leddy type 2 injury of the FDP. The distal tendon stump was too short for primary repair, and therefore the best treatment was a tendon-to-bone repair, which could be achieved with nonabsorbable sutures tied over a button or using a suture anchor.

2. **Answer: c.** The intraoperative photos suggest that this was an acute Zone 2 flexor tendon injury with complete laceration of the FDP tendon, possibly also the FDS tendon. Tendon debridement is only indicated for lacerations less than 50% of the tendon. Tendon-to-bone repair with nonabsorbable sutures tied over a button is usually used to repair a Zone 1 injury. Tendon reconstructions are used for more chronic injuries. This acute flexor tendon injury is best treated by primary repair using at least four-strand core sutures and an epitendinous suture.

3. **Answer: d.** The clinical history and initial clinical photo suggest that this was a Zone 2 flexor tendon injury involving both the FDP and FDS. Tendon excision will not restore finger flexion. Tendon-to-bone repair with a suture anchor is usually used to repair a Zone 1 injury. The chronicity of the injury makes the primary repair not appropriate because of degeneration of the tendon ends, retraction of the proximal tendon stump, and scarring of the soft tissue. The intraoperative photos demonstrate a competent pulley system, so the best treatment option among the choices is a single-stage reconstruction with a tendon graft. Two-stage reconstruction is used when the tendon sheath is so severely scarred that passing of a tendon graft is impossible.

4. **Answer: e.** The clinical scenario describes a ***lumbrical-plus*** finger, characterized by paradoxical extension of the interphalangeal (IP) joints with active finger flexion, likely from progressive lengthening of the tendon graft over time in this case. The lumbricals originate from the profundus tendons and extend the IP joints while flex the metacarpophalangeal joints through pulling the lateral bands. When there is laxity in the FDP tendon, the power of the proximal flexor muscle cannot effectively pull the finger into flexion, and the lumbrical is pulled instead, causing extension of the IP joints. The best treatment therefore is lumbrical release. Adhesions will not result in paradoxical IP joint extension. Central slip rupture causes a Boutonniere deformity characterized by PIP flexion and DIP extension. Attritional rupture of the small finger FDP can lead to a loss of finger flexor; however, it will not result in paradoxical IP joint extension. The quadriga effect is a result of over shortening of the FDP tendon during repair, limiting the ability of the adjacent fingers to fully flex, because the FDP tendons to the long, middle, ring, and small fingers share a common muscle belly and the shortest tendon determines the overall excursion.

CHAPTER 77 Extensor Tendon Repair and Reconstruction

Amir H. Taghinia and A. Samandar Dowlatshahi

KEY POINTS

- The extrinsic extensors of the digits are innervated by branches of the radial nerve and primarily mediate metacarpophalangeal (MP) joint extension.
- The intrinsic extensors of the digits are innervated by the ulnar and median nerves and primarily mediate MP joint flexion and interphalangeal (IP) joint extension.
- At the digit level, minimal tendon excursion translates into substantial change in joint position.
- Redundancies in the extensor system, such as the juncturae tendinae, can initially mask injury.
- Extensor injuries are classified by zones starting at the distal interphalangeal (DIP) joint (zone 1) and sequentially progressing proximally.
- Acute closed injuries of the digital extensor system are best treated with splinting; however, open injuries usually require exploration and repair if the injury is substantial.
- The mainstay of rehabilitation at the digital level (zones 1–4) remains static splinting; however, early motion protocols have shown promising results in more proximal injuries (zones 5–8).

The extensor apparatus is a well-balanced system of interlinking tendons and fibroligamentous bands that orchestrate the fine positional movements of each digit. As opposed to flexor tendons, extensors exhibit minimal excursion, especially in the digits. Seemingly negligible position changes in the extensor mechanism can translate into large degrees of motion in the digits. Thus, even minor disruptions of the delicate balance of these tendons can cause significant functional deficits. Due to the superficial position of extensor tendons, they are vulnerable to injury and exposure. Nevertheless, the phylogenetic evolution of the extensor apparatus has led to interconnections and duplications that allow functional redundancy. This redundancy can compensate for acute injury to one of the parts and lead to misdiagnosis. Once edema has subsided, and secondary support structures have fatigued, clinically significant deformity and functional loss become evident. This combination of factors—redundancy and late manifestation—along with significant anatomic variation in the extensor system makes accurate diagnosis difficult, but crucially important.

After repair, the proximity of the tendons to bone, the high incidence of associated periosteal stripping and capsular injuries, and the limited excursion of the extensors makes repair prone to adherence. Furthermore, the mechanical strength of the repair and status of local soft and hard tissues may not allow early mobilization. The stronger opposing action of the flexor system makes early rehabilitation even more problematic. Although not always preventable, stiffness and adhesions can be minimized with meticulous surgical technique and rational rehabilitation protocols. Associated injuries to the thin soft tissue cover of the dorsum of the hand need to be treated concomitantly because they have a direct impact on functional outcomes.

This chapter will discuss the anatomy and physiology of the extensor mechanism of the hand as well as injury patterns, repair strategies, and rehabilitation protocols. The importance of an in-depth anatomical understanding of this complex system cannot be overstated. Anatomy helps the reader to diagnose injury patterns understand the logic behind repair and rehabilitation.

CLINICAL ANATOMY AND FUNCTION

An appreciation of the fine mechanics and physiology of the extensor apparatus goes well beyond descriptive anatomy. The system is composed of unsheathed extrinsic and intrinsic tendons aided by retinacular structures and stabilized by periarticular constituents. Extension of the fingers follows a slightly different mechanism than the thumb. Full finger extension occurs because of a coordinated proximal to distal contraction of extrinsic and intrinsic muscles that set up an integrated series of tenodesis actions via fibroligamentous interconnections. There is no better way to demonstrate the tenodesis action of these interconnections than to passively flex the wrist. This action relaxes the long digital flexors and stretches the extensors. Performing this passive tenodesis examination in an injured hand is one of the best ways to diagnose an extensor tendon injury, especially proximal to the metacarpophalangeal (MP) joint (Figure 77.1).

Extrinsic System

The extrinsic extensor muscles are so called because they are located outside the anatomic boundaries of the hand. They are innervated by branches of the radial nerve or posterior interosseous nerve (PIN). The radial nerve proper innervates (in order) the brachioradialis (BR), extensor carpi radialis longus (ECRL), and (sometimes) extensor carpi radialis brevis (ECRB) muscles. BR is not a wrist or digital extensor; it flexes the elbow. ECRL and ECRB are both wrist extensors (Table 77.1). BR and ECRL are innervated above the elbow whereas ECRB is innervated below the elbow. Thus, a radial nerve laceration at or below the elbow is likely to maintain wrist extensor function.

All other extrinsic extensor muscles are innervated by the PIN, a branch of the radial nerve. The musculotendinous junctures of these tendons start at the mid to distal forearm. The most distal muscle belly, which occasionally extends beyond the carpus, is the extensor indicis proprius (EIP). This is the last muscle to receive innervation from the PIN, and thus the last to recover after a nerve injury. At the level of the wrist, the tendons are stabilized by a synovial-lined sheath termed the extensor retinaculum. This retinaculum is composed of horizontal fibers that form an overarching system of tunnels spanning the dorsal wrist and acting as a pulley to prevent bowstringing. Vertical, fibrous septae separate the tunnel into six individually numbered compartments (Figure 77.2).

The extensor digitorum communis (EDC) is the shared extensor (with a common muscle belly) for all four fingers. It travels through the fourth extensor compartment along with the EIP, the independent extensor of the index finger. The EIP extends the index finger independently of the other digits, hence inviting its moniker *pointer finger*. The only other independent finger extensor is the extensor digiti minimi (EDM) (also named extensor digiti quinti) that is the sole tendon in the fifth extensor compartment. These two independent tendons provide redundancy of finger extension, thus making them suitable for tendon transfers. They typically lie ulnar to the EDC at the level of the MP joints.

At the distal metacarpal level, the extensors of the fingers are often connected by oblique tendinous connections termed juncturae tendineae (see Figure 77.2). At the MP joint, the extrinsic tendons attach to the sagittal bands, specialized retinacular fibers that encircle the MP joints and insert onto the volar plates (Figure 77.3). These transverse laminar fibers provide radioulnar stability, effectively centralizing the tendon over the convexity of the metacarpal head. The attachments of the extrinsic finger extensors onto these structures make them effective extensors of the

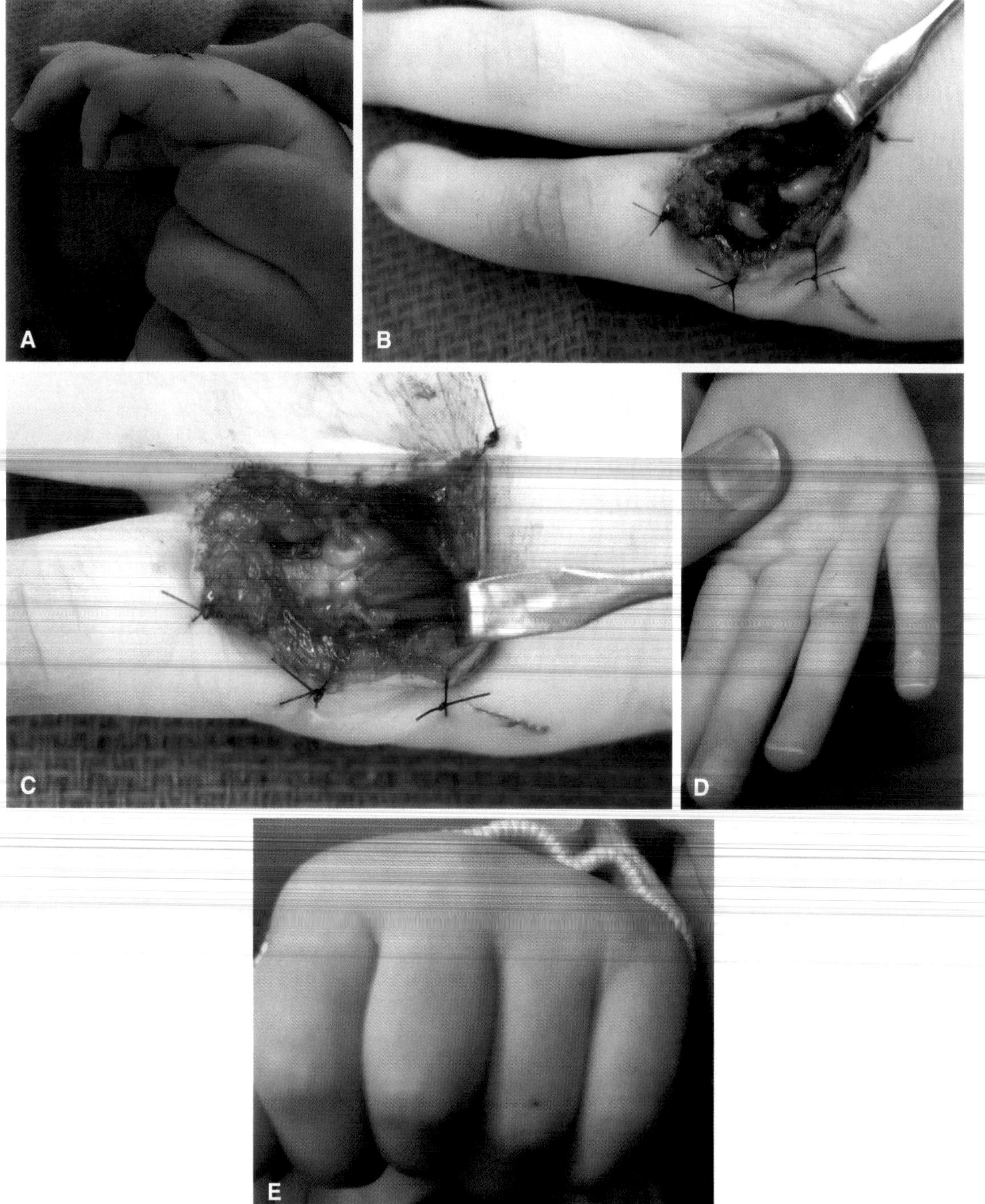

FIGURE 77.1. Wrist tenodesis. This 2-year-old girl sustained a laceration on the dorsum of the small finger MP joint. In this age group, assessing active motion is difficult. Relying on the tenodesis effect, maximal flexion of the wrist demonstrates lack of extensor tone in the small finger **(A)**, and exploration confirms a tendon laceration at zone 5 **(B)**. **C.** Figure-of-eight braided absorbable sutures were used to repair the tendon and the hand was immobilized in a cast for 3 weeks. **D, E.** Full active range of motion is demonstrated 6 months after the repair with minimal hand therapy. Similar injuries in adults can be treated with core and cross-stitch sutures with early mobilization.

MP joints, which are not intuitive, because they do not directly insert onto the proximal phalanges.[1]

Thumb extension is primarily mediated by the extensor pollicis longus (EPL). As it travels through the third extensor compartment, it makes a sharp radial turn around Lister tubercle (a dorsal bony prominence of the radius) and heads towards the thumb. This tendon forms the dorsal boundary of the anatomic snuffbox. It facilitates thumb interphalangeal (IP) joint extension but its most direct action is retropulsion (the act of lifting one's thumb off a table while keeping the palm resting flat) (Figure 77.4). The extensor pollicis brevis (EPB) and abductor pollicis longus (APL) travel through the first dorsal compartment; their action is to extend the thumb MP and carpometacarpal (CMC) joints, respectively.

There is significant variation in extrinsic extensor tendon anatomy. The more common variants and their clinical relevance are outlined in **Table 77.2**.

Intrinsic System

The intrinsic muscles originate and insert within the anatomic boundaries of the hand. For the extensor apparatus, these muscles are the interossei and the lumbricals. There are seven interosseous

TABLE 77.1. EXTRINSIC EXTENSORS OF THE HAND AND WRIST

Muscle	Origin	Insertion	Innervation	Function	Extensor Compartment
Extensor carpi radialis longus (ECRL)	Lateral supracondylar ridge of humerus	Dorsal base of second metacarpal	Radial nerve	Wrist extension and radial deviation	2
Extensor carpi radialis brevis (ECRB)	Lateral epicondyle of humerus	Dorsal base of third metacarpal	Radial nerve	Wrist extension	2
Extensor carpi ulnaris (ECU)	Lateral epicondyle of humerus and posterior border of ulna	Dorsal base of fifth metacarpal	PIN	Wrist extension and ulnar deviation	6
Extensor digitorum communis (EDC)	Lateral epicondyle of humerus	Finger extensor shroud	PIN	Finger MP joint extension	4
Extensor indicis proprius (EIP)	Posterior surfaces and ulna and interosseous membrane	Index finger extensor shroud	PIN	Index finger MP joint extension	4
Extensor digiti minimi (EDM)	Lateral epicondyle of humerus	Small finger extensor shroud	PIN	Small finger MP joint extension	5
Abductor pollicis longus (APL)	Posterior surfaces of ulna, radius, and interosseous membrane	Base of thumb metacarpal	PIN	Thumb abduction, extension at CMC joint	1
Extensor pollicis brevis (EPB)	Posterior surfaces of radius and interosseous membrane	Thumb extensor shroud	PIN	Thumb MP joint extension	1
Extensor pollicis longus (EPL)	Posterior surfaces and ulna and interosseous membrane	Thumb dorsal base of distal phalanx	PIN	Thumb IP joint extension, retropulsion	3

CMC, carpometacarpal; IP, interphalangeal; MP, metacarpophalangeal; PIN, posterior interosseous nerve.

muscles, four dorsal, and three volar. They are all innervated by the deep branch of the ulnar nerve. In addition to abducting (dorsal interossei) and adducting (volar interossei) the fingers, the interossei are the primary flexors of the finger MP joints. They course *dorsal* to the deep transverse metacarpal ligament and insert into the digital lateral bands (see Figure 77.3).

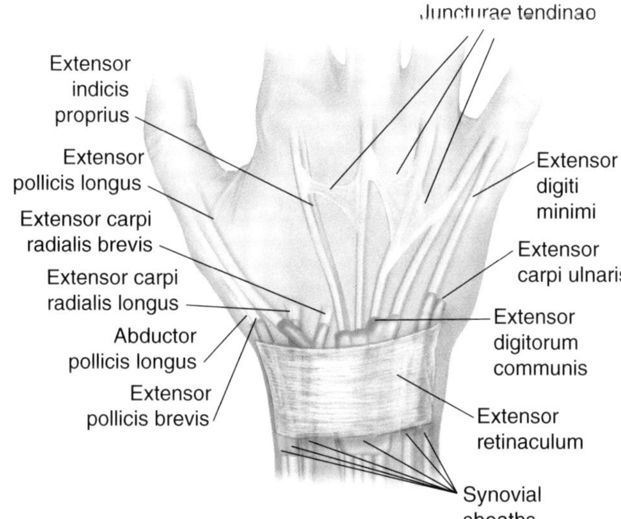

FIGURE 77.2. Illustration of the dorsal extensor system shows the extensor retinaculum covering the extensor tendons at the wrist. Under the retinaculum, the extensors traverse six compartments numbered sequentially: (1) APL and EPB, (2) ECRL and ECRB, (3) EPL, (4) EIP and EDC, (5) EDM, and (6) ECU. The juncturae tendinae connect the finger extensor tendons on the dorsum of the hand; there are no juncturae that link to the thumb extensors. In most cases, the ring finger sends connections to the middle and small fingers; but the connection between the index and middle fingers can be variable. (Reproduced with permission from Shoshana W. Ambani SW, Chung KC. Rheumatoid arthritis of the hand and wrist. In: Chung KC, ed. *Operative Techniques in Plastic Surgery*. Philadelphia, PA: Wolters Kluwer; 2019. Part 6, Figure 24-4.)

The lumbrical muscles are unique in that they originate from the finger profundus flexor tendons. There are four lumbrical muscles in the hand, one for each finger, and they lie on the radial side of the respective flexor tendon. They course *volar* to the deep transverse metacarpal ligament before attaching to the radial lateral band of the respective finger. The median nerve innervates the lumbrical muscles of the index and middle fingers, and the ulnar nerve innervates those of the ring and small fingers.

The intrinsic extensor tendons lie volar to the axis of rotation of the MP joint and dorsal to the axis of rotation of the IP joints. Thus, they cause the MP joints to flex and the IP joints to extend. These musculotendinous units are maximally stretched (taut) when the MP joint is passively extended and the PIP joint is simultaneously flexed. They are maximally lax when the MP joint is passively flexed and the PIP joint is extended (Figure 77.5). Intrinsic muscle action is also responsible for volumetric grip that starts with coordinated MP joint flexion and simultaneous IP joint extension.[2] Patients with combined lower median and ulnar nerve palsy are unable to perform volumetric grip, and instead initiate finger flexion at the IP joints, curling the fingers towards the palm utilizing the extrinsic flexors.

The intrinsic muscles of the thumb are mainly involved in rotational motion. However, both the adductor pollicis (ulnar) and the abductor pollicis brevis (radial) insert onto the EPL tendon at the MP joint level, which along with the EPB, gives them the ability to extend the IP joint of the thumb at least to neutral, thus potentially obscuring an EPL injury.

Digital Extensor System

Just distal to the sagittal bands, the extrinsic extensor system splits into a central slip and two lateral slips (see Figure 77.3).[3] Distal to this trifurcation, there is a crossing of fibers from the lateral bands to the central slip and vice versa. The myriad of crisscrossing fibers create a contiguous coalescence of fibers termed the extensor hood. The central slip then terminates as it inserts onto the dorsal base of the middle phalanx.

The lateral slips pass on either side of the PIP joint and merge with the lateral bands forming the conjoined lateral bands. These bands

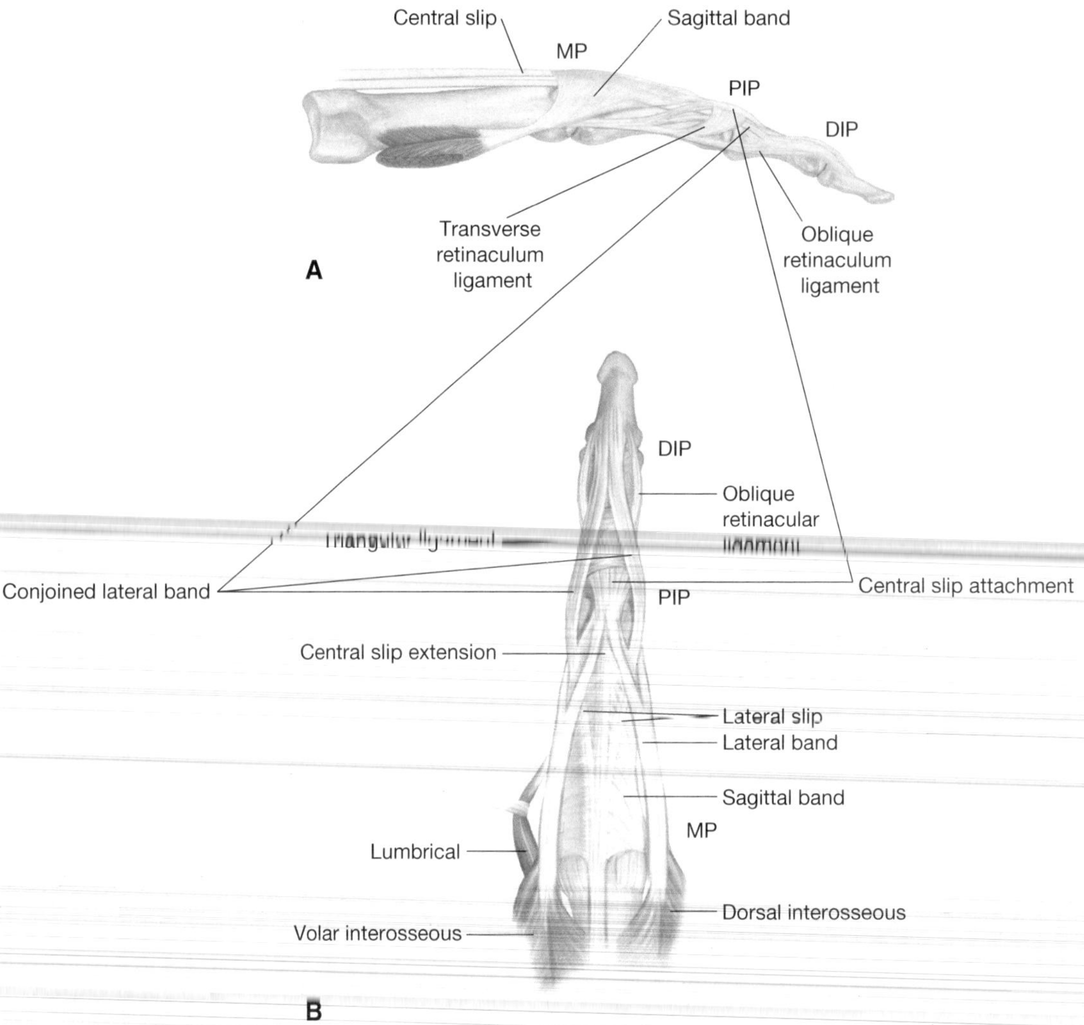

FIGURE 77.3. Finger extensor apparatus. Dorsal (A) and lateral (B) anatomic illustrations of the finger extensor apparatus. (Reproduced with permission from Smith MD, Machol JA IV, Chen NC. Acute repair of extensor tendon injuries in zones I to VI. In: Chung KC, ed. *Operative Techniques in Plastic Surgery*. Philadelphia, PA: Wolters Kluwer; 2019. Part 6, Figure 41-1B and Figure 41-1C.)

then course dorsally and join the triangular ligament on either side, ultimately uniting to form the terminal tendon that inserts onto the dorsal base of the distal phalanx.

At the PIP joint level, the transverse retinacular ligament tethers and stabilizes the extensor mechanism, not dissimilar to the sagittal bands at the MP level. The oblique retinacular ligament (ORL, of Landsmeer) arises from the lateral aspect of the flexor tendon sheath at the neck of the proximal phalanx (A2 pulley) and passes volar to the axis of rotation of the PIP joint, inserting onto the extensor mechanism along the middle phalanx. Although previously thought to link PIP and distal interphalangeal (DIP) motion, the ORL has been found to be variably present and often attenuated—its role remains controversial.[3-5]

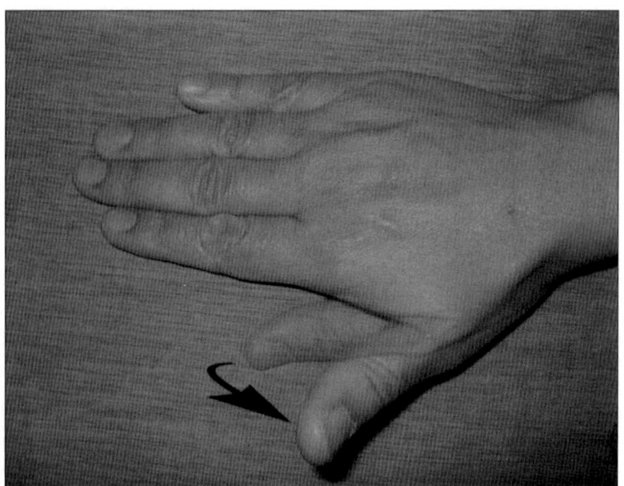

FIGURE 77.4. Retropulsion. The ideal way to test the EPL is by asking the patient to rest the hand, palm down, on a flat surface and lift the thumb.

Extension Function

MP joint extension is primarily mediated by the extrinsic extensor tendons. Historically, it was thought to be mediated by the sagittal bands as they lasso around the base of the proximal phalanx. However, more recent evidence suggests that the extensor continuation to the extensor hood and middle phalanx is the major mediator of MP extension.[6] Interphalangeal joint extension is more complex and requires the interplay of both intrinsic and extrinsic systems (Figure 77.6).

Digital extensor tendon excursion is much wider at the forearm and wrist level than the digit. The excursion of a common extensor proximal to the wrist is approximately 5 cm. The excursion of the extensor mechanism at the PIP joint level is only a few millimeters, despite a PIP joint arc of motion of 100°.[7] Every millimeter of extensor tendon lengthening over the proximal phalanx leads to 12° of extension deficit at the PIP joint.[8] Any small disturbance of this delicate balance causes deformity that can be progressive and difficult to

TABLE 77.2. SURGICALLY RELEVANT ANATOMICAL PEARLS

Anatomical Variant	Surgical Relevance
The first extensor compartment is partially divided by a fibrous septum in 29% of the population, and by a bony septum in 5%. Complete separation has been observed in 8.5% of cases.	During release of the first extensor compartment for de Quervain's syndrome, all subcompartments must be identified and released
An extensor carpi radialis intermedius (ECRI) is present in 12% of limbs, located either radial to ECRL or in between ECRL and ECRB	The ECRI can be used as a tendon graft or in tendon transfers involving the radial wrist extensors
The EIP is absent in 4% of individuals. Its muscle belly extends further distal than other extensor tendons. It is located ulnar and volar to EDC of the index finger.	The EIP is often used for tendon transfers, either after EPL spontaneous rupture or for opponensplasty. Anatomic differences can help more easily localize the tendon.
An extensor medii proprius (EMP) is the middle finger equivalent of the EIP and is present in 10% of individuals.	The EMP, if present, can be used for tendon transfers.
The extensor indicis et medii communis is a variant of EIP that inserts onto the index and middle fingers.	The muscle belly can be hypertrophic to the point where it is mistaken for a ganglion cyst. It can complicate a planned EIP tendon transfer.
The extensor digitorum brevis manus muscle is an anomalous dorsal muscle, present in 3% of hands, which arises distally on the wrist between the index and middle finger metacarpals.	This muscle can be mistaken for a ganglion cyst.
The EDM is doubled in 72% of cases.	This redundancy allows the tendon to be used for tendon grafts or additional tendon transfers.

correct. Similar issues plague the DIP joint where each millimeter of relative terminal tendon lengthening results in 25° of extension lag.[9]

The interlinkages of the extensor mechanism have further pathophysiologic implications. Normal function relies on individual tendons acting about the axis of rotation of multiple joints, and on stabilization of joints between where the axial force is generated and where it is intended to act. If one interlinkage is disrupted, this derangement causes (progressive) reciprocal deformity of adjacent joints. This phenomenon is seen in boutonnière, swan neck, and so called zig zag deformities, where injury/deformity in one joint pathologically alters the position of an adjacent joint.

CLINICAL ASSESSMENT

The clinical assessment of a patient with suspected extensor deficit or derangement requires thorough knowledge of the anatomical and mechanical features of extensor function. Cross-functionality of the extensor mechanism can mask serious injury that may manifest later as recalcitrant chronic deformity. The best way to diagnose injury is to assess function distal to the level of the injury. This is especially relevant in the hand, wrist, and forearm where retraction of the proximal tendon ends may obscure visualization.

In the fingers, accurate diagnosis can be made by exploring an acute wound in the emergency room (ER). Extensors in this area are superficial and will not retract much. However, one needs adequate lighting, retraction, and hemostasis because small wounds with venous bleeding can obscure injury. When in doubt, one should close the wound, apply a splint, and reexamine in a few days.

INJURY PATTERNS, REPAIR, AND REHABILITATION

Extensor tendon injuries are classified based on location. Kleinert and Verdan[10] initially delineated these zones from 1 to 8, and Doyle[11] later added a ninth zone for the muscular area of the mid to proximal forearm. The zones start at the DIP joint and progress proximally. Odd numbers are over joints and even numbers in between. There are separately numbered zones for the thumb (Figure 77.7).

These zones are significant because they require different approaches for repair and rehabilitation. A detailed outline of injury patterns and repair paradigms will follow. However, certain generalizations about rehabilitation are worth mentioning first. Rehabilitation of zone 1 and 2 injuries requires static splinting for 6 weeks followed by night splinting and range of motion exercises. More proximal injuries were traditionally treated by 3 to 4 weeks of static splinting followed by controlled motion. This approach may increase adhesions particularly in those with multiple concomitant injuries that involve bone and other soft tissue, as the tendon forms scars to adjacent structures during healing. Early controlled motion using dynamic splinting has shown promising results for zone 4 to 7 injuries, and may be especially suited for patients who are compliant and have associated bony and soft tissue injuries. The idea is that early controlled gliding of the tendon will break up impending adhesions while minimizing risk of rupture. Dynamic splinting protocols are just as effective as early active motion protocols with less risk of tendon rupture.[15,16] More proximal injuries in zones 8 and 9 carry the least risk of adhesions and can be treated with static splinting for 3 to 4 weeks.

Zone 1

Disruption of the terminal extensor tendon from the base of the distal phalanx results in a mallet finger injury. The mechanism is either an open injury, or more commonly by closed rupture with or without associated fracture of the distal phalanx. Sudden, resisted flexion of the DIP joint is the leading cause. The terminal tendon usually inserts onto a thin area on the dorsal/proximal aspect of the distal phalanx. This area corresponds to the dorsal ledge of the epiphysis prior to skeletal maturity.

The DIP joint is held in a flexed posture with decreased or absent active extension (Figure 77.8). Compensatory hyperextension at the PIP joint (swan-neck deformity) can occur acutely in patients with congenital or traumatic PIP volar plate laxity. Elderly patients with osteoarthritis can present with a mallet deformity that is atraumatic.

Radiographs are necessary to rule out a fracture of the distal phalanx, and need to be appropriately centered on the involved digit. The lateral view is critical, to assess joint congruity and subluxation. Fractures are often missed on the anteroposterior view alone. Injuries presenting within 4 weeks of trauma are considered acute; after 4 weeks, they are chronic. If left untreated, hyperextension of the PIP joint can develop because of proximal and dorsal migration of the lateral bands,[17] creating the swan-neck deformity.

Doyle and others classified mallet finger injuries into four types.[11] **Table 77.3** outlines this classification and the treatment algorithm for each type of injury. Closed injuries without subluxation encompass

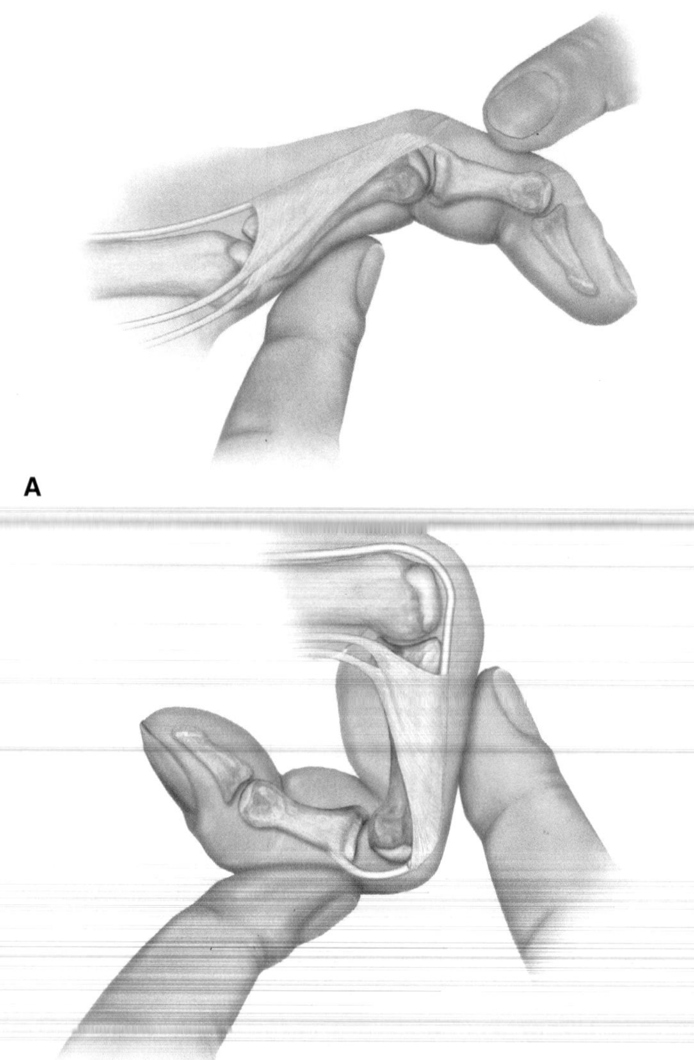

FIGURE 77.5. Intrinsic tightness. The intrinsic muscles flex the MP joints and extend the PIP joints of the fingers. In the passive posture of maximal MP joint flexion and PIP extension, these muscles are fully lax. In contrast, the opposite passive posture of maximal MP joint extension and PIP flexion puts them at peak stretch. When the intrinsic muscles are contracted or tight, achieving this second posture is difficult. **A.** Intrinsic tightness can be demonstrated if the PIP joint cannot be easily flexed when the MP joint is held in extension. **B.** Flexing the MP joint and confirming normal PIP joint flexion rules out a problem with the PIP joint.

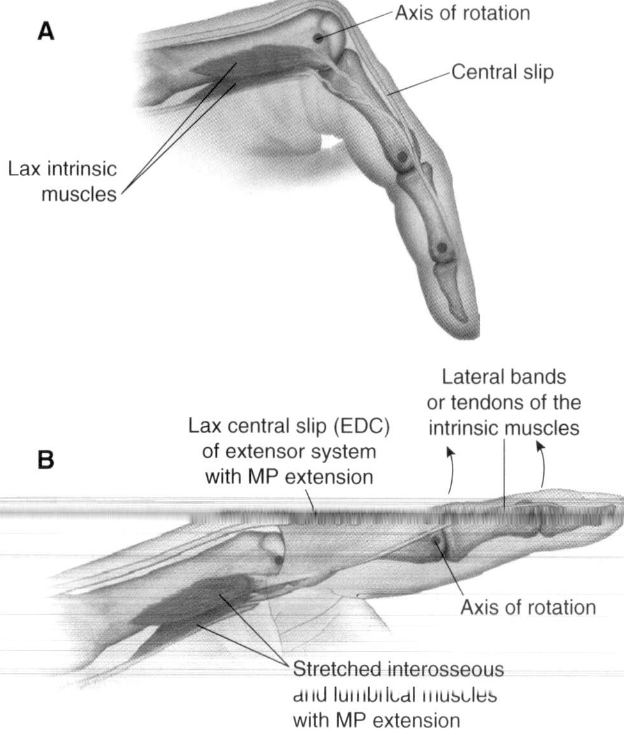

FIGURE 77.6. Coordinating IP joint motion. **A.** When the MP joint is flexed, the extrinsic extensors are rendered tighter while the intrinsic interosseous-lumbrical system is lax and redundant. The lax structures are not able to generate significant force in this situation. Thus, IP joint extension is mediated by the extrinsic system when the MP joint is flexed. In contrast, when the MP joint is extended, the extrinsic system becomes lax and less effective. **B.** Meanwhile, MP joint extension tightens the intrinsic tendons, thus making them better IP joint extensors. In summary, extensor action on the IP joints is mediated by the extrinsic system when the MP joint is flexed and by the intrinsic system when the MP joint is extended.

the great majority of mallet injuries (types I and IVb). These injuries are best treated with continuous splinting of the DIP joint in extension for 6 weeks, followed by 2 weeks of night splinting. Splinting must be continuous. If at any time the patient is to remove the splint (e.g., for hygiene), it must be rested against a flat surface to ensure continuous extension of the DIP joint. Splinting in extreme hyperextension or placing the splint too tightly can cause dorsal skin necrosis. Different types of splints (aluminum foam, premade plastic, or custom-made thermoplastic) placed volar or dorsal have been used in the literature, with comparable outcomes.[18,19] The main predictor of long-term extension lag appears to be compliance with splinting. The authors recommend a dorsal aluminum foam splint with the DIP joint in slight hyperextension. Active PIP joint motion is encouraged.

Residual extensor lag of 5° to 10° is common, despite adequate treatment and patient compliance (Figure 77.9). Erythema and swelling over the dorsal aspect of the DIP joint can last several months.

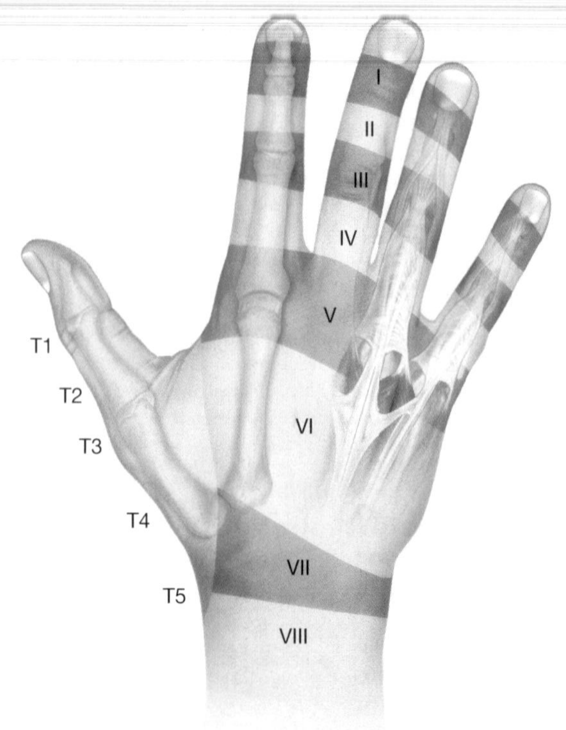

FIGURE 77.7. Zones of extensor muscle and tendon injury. These are numbered from I to IX starting at the DIP joint and progressing proximally. Zone I is over the DIP joint, zone II is over the middle phalanx and so on. Zone IX is located in the forearm proximal to zone VIII (not shown).

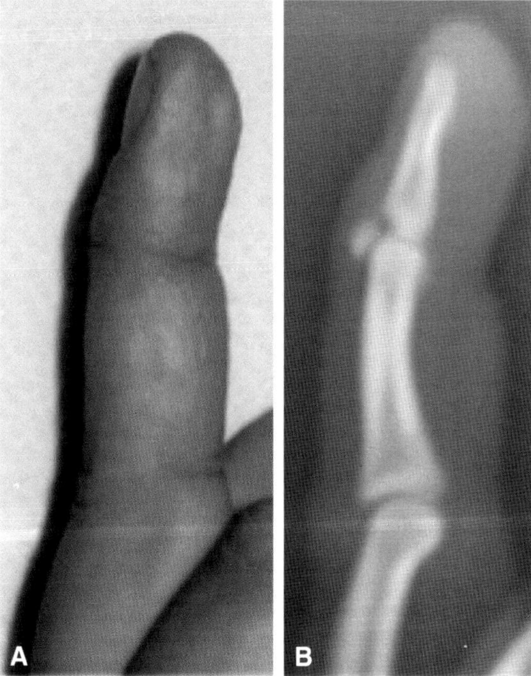

FIGURE 77.8. Type I (closed) bony mallet finger. **A.** Clinical posture of the digit after injury shows extension lag at the DIP joint. **B.** A small bony fragment, still attached to the terminal tendon, has been separated from the distal phalanx. Most mallet injuries present in this way with or without a small avulsion fracture.

Chronic Mallet Injuries

There is no formal time cut off for closed treatment with splinting. Tenderness and inflammation over the DIP extensor surface are considered to be relative indications for closed treatment, even several months after injury. Surgical options include direct tendon repair with or without skin imbrication (tenodermodesis), tendon rebalancing with a central slip tenotomy (Fowler tenotomy), ORL reconstruction, or DIP joint arthrodesis.

- *Technique of skin imbrication/tenodermodesis:* An elliptical wedge of skin and scarred tendon is excised.[20] The closure incorporates both skin and tendon as a single unit. A Kirschner wire maintains the joint in full extension for 6 weeks.
- *Fowler tenotomy/central slip tenotomy:* At least 6 to 12 months are required since injury to allow the terminal tendon to mature. The principle underlying this procedure is a release of the central slip, allowing the now centrally untethered lateral bands to move proximally and reduce the slack within the extensor system distal to the PIP joint, correcting the extensor lag at the DIP joint. A boutonnière deformity is prevented by keeping the triangular ligament intact. The release is performed from underneath the extensor system via a midaxial incision. Passing a freer elevator underneath the lateral bands ensures that any adhesions are released so that they can glide freely.
- *Spiral ORL reconstruction:* This procedure links the position of the PIP joint to that of the DIP joint. Performed with a tendon graft[21,22] or a lateral band,[23] it links the terminal tendon or distal phalanx to the flexor tendon sheath or proximal phalanx, leading to a dynamic tenodesis (Figure 77.10).

Posttraumatic Swan-Neck Deformity

A swan-neck deformity is flexion of the DIP joint with hyperextension of the PIP joint. It occurs after a traumatic (untreated) mallet finger when the PIP volar plate is lax. It is important to ascertain whether the deformity is primarily due to PIP joint laxity or DIP extension lag; this is done by blocking PIP hyperextension and assessing active DIP extension. With PIP hyperextension blocked, if the DIP can be actively extended fully, then the main problem is PIP laxity. Otherwise, the main problem is DIP extension deficit. For PIP joint laxity, one should attempt conservative treatment with figure-of eight splinting. If that is not effective, then volar plate imbrication or FDS tenodesis may work. If the primary issue is DIP extension deficit, then ORL reconstruction or Fowler tenotomy are advocated. Joints should be supple before operative correction is attempted.

TABLE 77.3. DOYLE CLASSIFICATION OF MALLET INJURY

Type	Description	Treatment	Pearls and Pitfalls
I	Closed injury, with or without small dorsal avulsion fracture	8 wk continuous splinting with DIP in full extension, PIP free.	If extensor lag is evident at 8 wk, then resume splinting until extensor lag is resolved.
		After 8 wk, initiate splint weaning and controlled active motion under therapist guidance.	Look for skin maceration and breakdown.
II	Open injury with laceration to the terminal extensor	Surgical tendon repair with running suture incorporating skin and tendon, and transfixation of DIP joint with axial or oblique 0.045 in K wire for 6 wk followed by night time splinting for 4 wk.	Beware of bulky suture material that can become symptomatic and extrude. The DIP joint is invariably open and needs to be washed out.
III	Open injury with loss of skin and/or tendon substance	Primary repair if possible. Positioning of DIP joint in hyperextension is permissible if allows for apposition of tendon ends. May require homodigital or cross-finger flap for coverage with or without tendon graft.	Consider staged reconstruction: soft tissue, then tendon reconstruction.
IV A	Transepiphyseal plate fracture in children (Seymour's fracture)	Requires operative washout, reduction and antibiotic coverage. Longitudinal K wire often necessary.	Dislocated nailplate often present. Untreated Seymour fracture can lead to osteomyelitis.
IV B	Hyperflexion injury with 20%–50% fracture of articular surface	Operative and conservative methods of treatment are acceptable based on current literature, even in the presence of volar subluxation of the distal phalanx. Operative treatment consists of extension block pinning.	Patients are always advised that they may have a permanent dorsal bump with either surgical or nonsurgical treatment.
IV C	Hyperextension injury with >50% fracture of articular surface with early or late volar subluxation of distal phalanx		

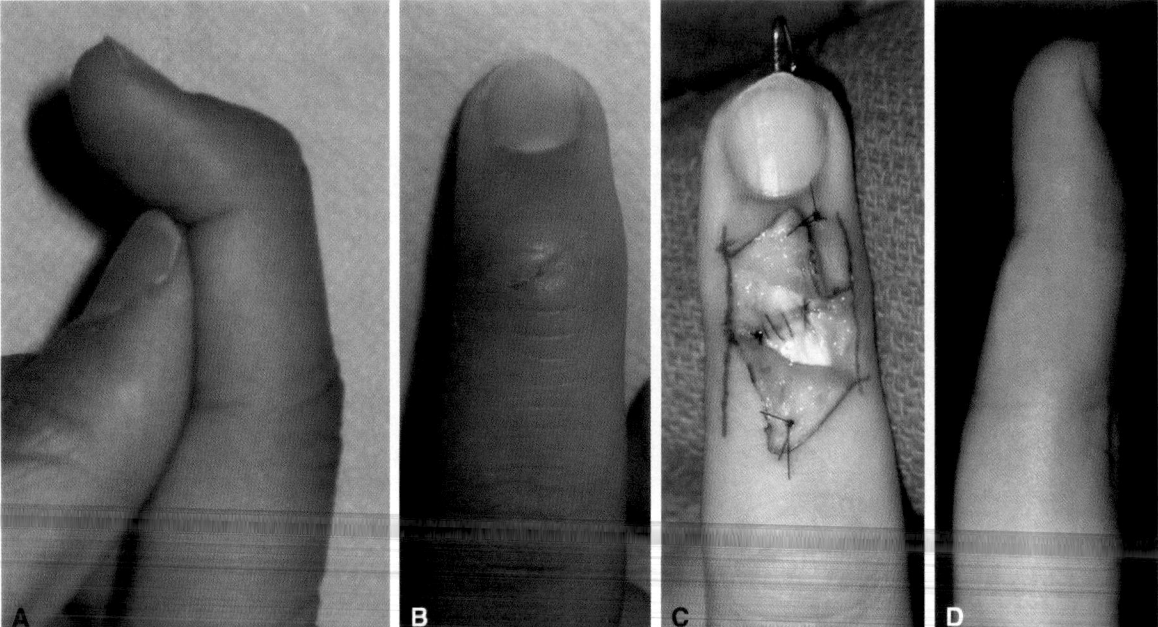

FIGURE 77.9. Type II (open) mallet finger. **A.** Clinical posture of the digit shows a more significant extension lag than typically seen in a closed mallet injury. **B.** Dorsal view demonstrates a healing laceration over the DIP joint. **C.** Repair was performed with a running stitch and protected with a longitudinal pin. **D.** Three months postoperatively, the finger demonstrates mild extension lag as can be seen often in these cases despite timely and adequate repair. Even a miniscule amount of tendon lengthening in this area translates to significant extension lag.

Zone 2

These injuries are located over the middle phalanx and are usually sharp. They can involve the two conjoined lateral bands and the triangular ligament that restrains them in the dorsal midline. Only one lateral band is sufficient to achieve full extension of the DIP joint. If the injury involves less than 50% of the extensor mechanism, then routine wound care and splinting for 7 to 10 days is sufficient treatment, followed by active motion. If greater than 50% of the tendon is cut, then primary repair and a longer period of immobilization is indicated. The extensor system at this level is thin and cannot carry a core suture. A simple running nonabsorbable 5-0 suture can be augmented with a running cross-stitch (e.g., Silfverskiöld; Figure 77.11). PIP motion is permitted postoperatively. The DIP joint is held in extension for 6 weeks after which active motion can commence. Chronic zone 2 injuries can be treated with spiral ORL reconstruction, as in chronic mallet injuries.

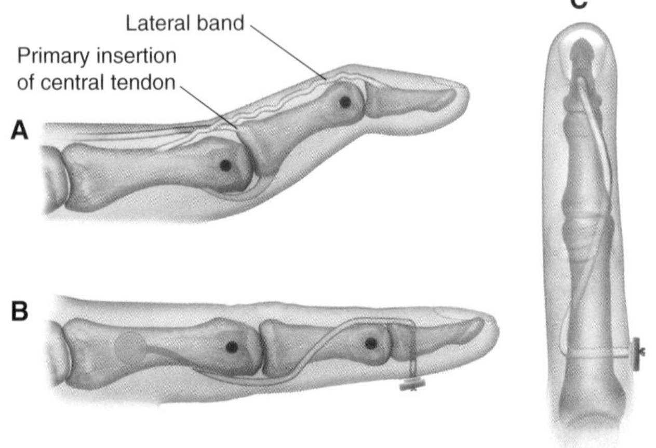

FIGURE 77.10. Spiral oblique retinacular ligament reconstruction. **A.** The swan-neck posture of a mallet deformity is shown with lax lateral bands and PIP volar plate. **B, C.** The tendon graft is secured to the distal phalanx with a pull out suture that is brought volarly and stabilized with a button. It is routed adjacent to the flexor sheath volar to the PIP joint, and then anchored to the side of the proximal phalanx (Thompson) or the flexor sheath (Kleinman and Peterson). Extension of the PIP puts tension on the graft, resulting in extension of the DIP. Flexion of the PIP relaxes the graft and allows flexion of the DIP.

Zone 3

As in mallet injuries, zone 3 injuries can be open lacerations or closed ruptures, the latter with or without avulsion fracture of the middle phalanx. The injury may result in PIP joint extension deficit and DIP joint hyperextension, the so-called boutonnière deformity. In the setting of an isolated (closed) central slip injury, PIP joint extensor lag is usually not present at first. The intact lateral bands and triangular ligament maintain an extension moment on the PIP joint due to their position dorsal to the PIP joint rotation axis. However, the extension torque gets shifted completely to the lateral bands, and over several weeks the restraining triangular ligament stretches out, thereby allowing volar translation and shortening of the lateral bands. This in turn increases direct pull at the terminal extensor tendon, leading to hyperextension of the DIP joint (Figure 77.12), and the boutonnière posture.[24,25] Concomitant injury to adjacent structures may also be necessary to cause a boutonnière deformity.[26]

A more reliable test for central slip disruption was suggested by Elson (Figure 77.13).[27] This test is found to be the most sensitive test for diagnosing acute central slip disruption.[28] In clinical practice, the aforementioned tests are difficult to perform in the acute setting because of pain and swelling. A digital block may be helpful to do a proper Elson test. In suspected cases where the examination is inconsistent or unreliable, the clinician should splint the PIP in extension and reexamine after a week once swelling and pain have subsided.

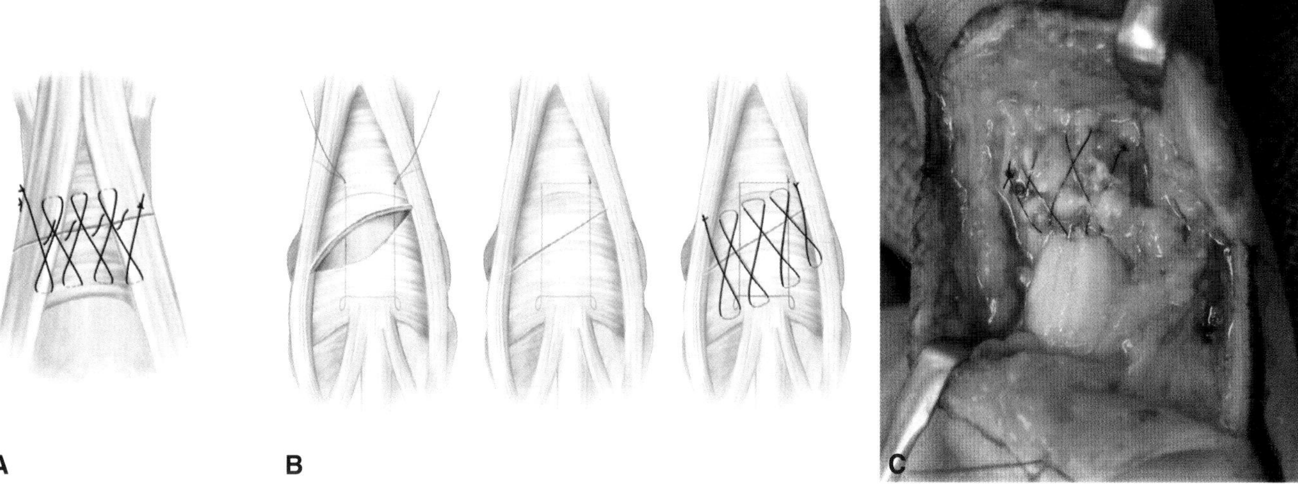

FIGURE 77.11. Extensor tendon repair techniques. **A.** The Silfverskiöld cross-stitch technique is demonstrated for a zone 2 injury. More proximal injuries can be repaired with 2 to 4 core sutures and augmented with the cross-stitch using a finer monofilament suture **(B)**. Repair of a T-2 thumb extensor injury is demonstrated with core Ethibond suture (green) and Silfverskiöld cross-stitch **(C)**.

Closed Central Slip Injury

Treatment of a closed central slip rupture with or without boutonnière deformity consists of splinting or pinning the PIP joint in full extension for 6 weeks, followed by an additional 4 to 6 weeks of protective splinting. The patient performs active DIP flexion and extension exercises to keep the lateral bands gliding. In patients with a boutonnière deformity, active DIP flexion helps to pull the lateral bands back into a more dorsal and central position thus correcting the deformity. When treated early in a compliant patient, the injury will usually respond to this conservative approach.

Closed Central Slip Injury with Associated Avulsion Fracture

Depending on the size of the fracture, these can also be treated closed. Larger fragments can be repaired by Kirschner wire or screw fixation. In the presence of comminution, the fragment(s) can be excised and a tendon-to-bone juncture performed.

Open Zone 3 Injury

A traumatic PIP arthrotomy is usually present and requires joint irrigation. In cases where there is minimal to no distal tendon, a suture anchor is employed or a trough can be created in the middle phalanx for passing a suture. If there is sufficient tendon for repair, a cross-stitch suture with or without a single-core suture is sufficient. A pin protects the repair for 6 weeks. Range of motion exercises can commence after pin removal but night splinting should continue for another 3 weeks.

Posttraumatic Boutonnière Deformity

This deformity refers to DIP joint hyperextension and PIP joint flexion. In addition to trauma discussed earlier, arthritis, burns, and [illegible] of the central slip. The changes occur in three stages: dynamic imbalance (early), established tendon contracture with supple joints (delayed), and fixed contracture (late/chronic). Passively correctable deformities should initially be treated with splinting as even late treatment can allow realignment of the lateral bands.[23]

Surgical treatment of chronic boutonnière deformity is extremely challenging. Supple joints are a necessity before any surgical interventions; thus, fixed chronic cases should be treated with serial splinting and stretching to maximize joint mobility. The distal Fowler tenotomy transversely divides the extensor mechanism at the junction of the middle and proximal thirds of the middle phalanx while

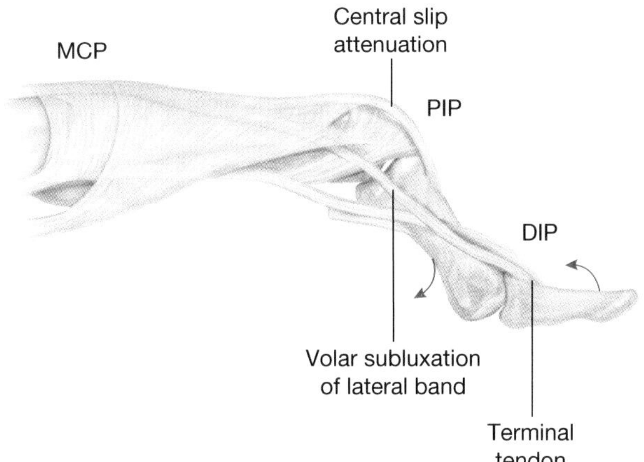

FIGURE 77.12. Development of boutonnière deformity. **A.** The central slip is disrupted from the base of the middle phalanx leading to all extensor forces being concentrated into the lateral bands. **B.** The lateral bands slip volarly and become flexors of the PIP joint and hyperextensors of the DIP joint. (Reproduced with permission from Shoshana W. Ambani SW, Chung KC. Rheumatoid arthritis of the hand and wrist. In: Chung KC, ed. *Operative Techniques in Plastic Surgery*. Philadelphia, PA: Wolters Kluwer; 2019. Part 6, Figure 24-7A.)

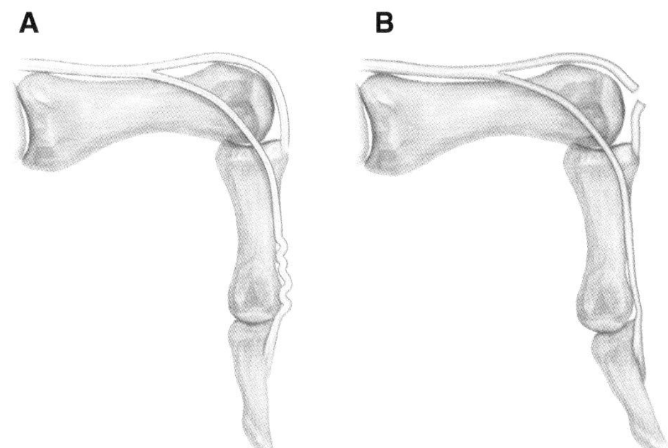

FIGURE 77.13. Elson test. With the finger held at 90° of PIP joint flexion against a right-angled surface (such as the end of a table), active extension is tested. If the central slip is intact, the DIP joint should have very little active extension ability (flail). **A.** This is because an intact central slip will draw the origin of the lateral bands distally. **B.** However, if the central slip is disrupted, the proximal migration of the lateral bands stretches them and allows active DIP joint extension.

preserving the ORL. This effectively creates a surgical mallet finger, decreasing tone at the DIP joint and increasing tension at the PIP by allowing the extensor to slide proximally. A modification of this procedure shifts the lateral bands dorsally and suturing them together over the PIP joint.[29] Lastly, Curtis proposed a four-stage process to correct this deformity with reasonable outcomes.[30] The reconstruction involves tenolysis, sectioning of the transverse retinacular ligament, distal Fowler tenotomy, and advancement and reinsertion of the central tendon.

Zone 4

The extensor mechanism in this zone is broad and the convexity of the proximal phalanx shields the lateral bands, thus most injuries are partial. Surgical exploration is often necessary to diagnose the degree of injury. Injuries that involve less than 50% of the extensor mechanism and/or those in which PIP active extension is spared can be managed conservatively with range of motion exercises after the skin laceration has healed. The choice of repair is variable and includes either figure of eight absorbable sutures or core sutures (2 or 4 of 4-0 or 5-0 nonabsorbable suture) augmented with a cross-stitch on the dorsal surface. Similar to zone 3 injuries, the PIP joint should be splinted in extension for 4 to 6 weeks while the DIP joint is exercised. Dynamic splinting can be considered in this zone.[31,32]

Zone 5

These injuries occur over the MP joint, are almost always open, and should be considered human bite injuries unless proven otherwise. The classic *fight bite* occurs when the fully flexed MP joint forcefully strikes human maxillary incisors. The teeth lacerate the skin, extensor tendon, and joint capsule before inoculating the joint with oral flora. The finger then returns to its natural extended posture, sealing the joint and catalyzing an impending septic arthritis. The clinician should be suspicious for those with innocuous appearing injuries.

Primary tendon repair will be required after thorough joint irrigation. The lacerated tendon is proximal to the area of skin injury. Flexing the joint recreates the multilevel injury tract and wash out all of the inoculated tissues. Once identified, the tendon ends can be repaired with a two- or four-core (e.g., modified Kessler) suture followed by an epitendinous suture. If the sagittal bands are lacerated, they should also be repaired to keep the tendon centralized. Radial sagittal band injuries are particularly prone to subsequent subluxation.[33] The surgeon should obtain wound cultures and commence broad-spectrum antibiotics. If there is frank septic arthritis, the wound and joint need to be opened widely, debrided, irrigated, and left open to allow egress of purulence; and the tendon repaired secondarily once the infection has resolved. Postoperative therapy should be tailored to the patient, mechanism, and extent of injury.

In cases where the injury is not caused by human bite, the layers must be carefully identified and repaired separately. Postoperative rehabilitation with intermittent-controlled active motion and relative motion splinting is particularly useful in reliable, motivated patients (Figure 77.14).

Sagittal Band Injuries

Isolated sagittal band injuries are most often closed injuries resulting from resisted extension of the finger or direct trauma to the dorsum of the MP joint. These are often mistaken for a trigger finger because of the snapping that occurs when the extensor tendon shifts back and forth between its natural position and the intermetacarpal groove. The radial sagittal band is more often affected. Usually, the affected finger cannot be actively extended from a flexed starting position but can be held in the fully extended position. Closed injuries are treated conservatively by relative motion splinting or casting. In late presentations or cases of failed conservative treatment, surgical reconstruction is warranted.

Zone 6

Extensor tendon injuries over the metacarpals may not be readily apparent because the juncturae tendinae can transmit extensor force from adjacent, intact tendons. Although exploration for a suspected tendon laceration may confirm its presence, it should be performed in a controlled setting where visualization is excellent. Venous bleeding in the ER setting can impair visibility and result in misdiagnosis. The ability to hyperextend the MP joint and/or extend against resistance are often better indicators of extensor integrity than direct visualization in the ER. Local anesthesia can be administered before attempting these maneuvers to eliminate the influence of pain.

The tendons in zone 6 are oval-shaped and thick, making them amenable to core suture repair techniques. Injuries that involve greater than 50% of the tendon cross-sectional area may be repaired with 3-0 or 4-0 nonabsorbable core sutures. Various core suture techniques have been proposed; the authors prefer the modified Kessler method. A subsequent circumferential epitendinous suture lends additional strength and smooths the edges of the repair. In injuries not suitable for early mobilization, figure-of-eight absorbable sutures may also be utilized (Figure 77.1). Even if a single slip of the EDC is involved, all fingers should be splinted.

Zone 7

Extensor tendon injuries over the wrist usually damage the extensor retinaculum. Partial release of the retinaculum is often necessary to gain access to the injured tendons. Controversy exists about whether a part of the retinaculum should be excised to minimize adhesions.[34] The surgeon can usually maintain or repair part (about 50% of its length) of the retinaculum to prevent subsequent bowstringing while excising the portion over the repair site to minimize adhesions. The only exception is the EPL tendon (see section on Special Considerations for the Thumb).

The tendons are in close proximity in this zone, thus multiple tendons are usually involved in sharp injuries. Furthermore, retraction is common because there are fewer locally tethering structures. The surgeon must carefully identify all injured structures and make sure that the injured ends match correctly. A four- to six-strand core suture repair is ideal. The close proximity of tendons makes problematic adhesions more likely in this zone. Dynamic splinting or early motion protocols should be considered postoperatively.

Zone 8

Distal forearm extensor tendon injuries are treated similar to zone 7 injuries. Because multiple tendons are often involved, it may be difficult to identify and match ends correctly. A systematic radial to ulnar (or vice versa) survey can be helpful. Independent wrist and thumb motion should be prioritized. Similar to zone 7, core sutures should be used to repair the stout tendons in this area. The extrinsic extensor tendons that have their muscle bellies end most distally in the forearm are the EIP (most distal), EPL, EPB, and APB. The remainder of the extensor musculotendinous junctions is approximately 4 cm proximal to the wrist. Thus, injuries in this zone may present with a mixed picture of lacerations through the tendon substance, at the musculotendinous junction, or the muscle belly. The proximal tendon end may retract into the belly of the muscle. The surgeon should carefully identify as much proximal tendon as possible because tendon-to-tendon repair is much stronger than tendon to muscle. In the forearm, there is no need for Bruner-type zigzag incisions. Linear or curvilinear access incisions look nicer and are less likely to create ischemic skin flaps.

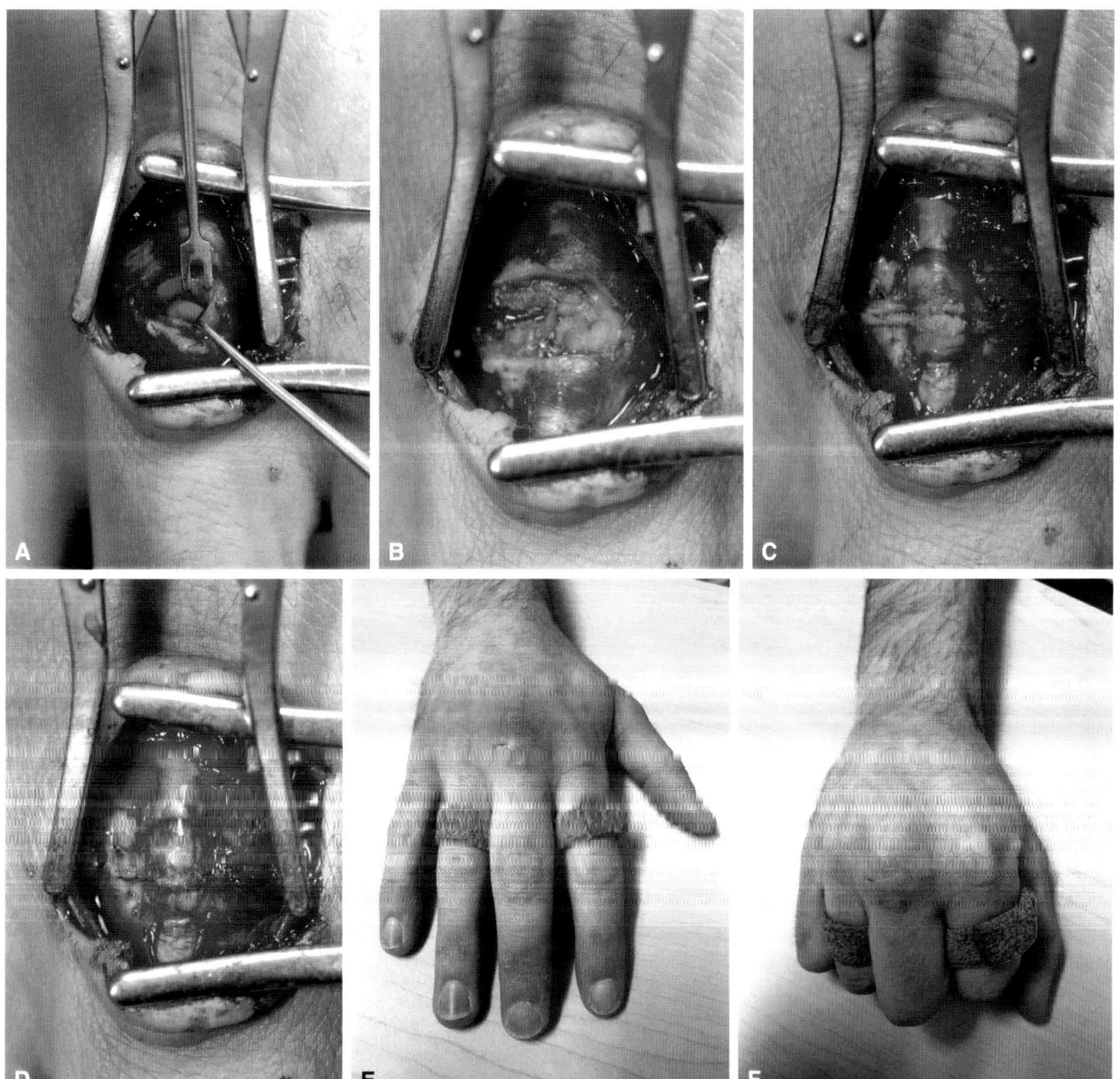

FIGURE 77.14. Zone 5 extensor tendon laceration. This 35-year-old carpenter sustained penetrating trauma to the dorsum of his hand by a screwdriver. Extension deficit was evident preoperatively, but subtle. **A.** Intraoperative exploration revealed a transected EDC tendon as well as injury to the shroud mechanism and traumatic MP joint arthrotomy. **(B)** Repair of the joint capsule with 6-0 absorbable suture. Repair of extensor tendon with 4-0 nonabsorbable core suture (modified Kessler; **C**), augmented with a 6-0 epitendinous suture (locking running; **D**). After repair, the patient is placed in an extension wrist splint and a yoke splint with the affected digit in hyperextension relative to the neighboring digits. **E, F.** Controlled active motion begins immediately with both splints in place. The wrist splint is discontinued at 3 weeks and the yoke splint at 6 weeks, followed by strengthening and passive range of motion. This carpenter returned to work 3 days postoperatively.

Zone 9

In the most proximal zone, penetrating trauma usually causes direct laceration of the muscle bellies. Each can be isolated, identified, and its severed ends carefully matched. The overlying fascia can be repaired either with figure-of-eight absorbable sutures or with barbed sutures. The advantage of barbed sutures is timesavings and knotless repairs that decrease likelihood of muscle strangulation. Given abundant soft tissue, adhesions are unlikely to cause substantial tethering in this zone. Furthermore, repairs are inherently weaker due to closure of the muscle fascia alone without tendon substance. Therefore, these repairs should be protected and immobilized for 3 to 4 weeks before commencing range of motion exercises.

Special Considerations for the Thumb

The treatment of thumb extensor injuries is similar to the finger analog for each of the respective zones of injury T1–T5 (see Figure 77.6) with a few caveats and pearls as outlined herein:

- For zone T5 injuries of the EPL (wrist), the tendon should be displaced out of the third compartment and repaired over the extensor retinaculum. This maneuver should not be replicated with finger extensors that tend to bowstring. The change in EPL tendon routing does not alter its mechanics significantly, but does provide a better soft tissue bed to decrease adhesions.

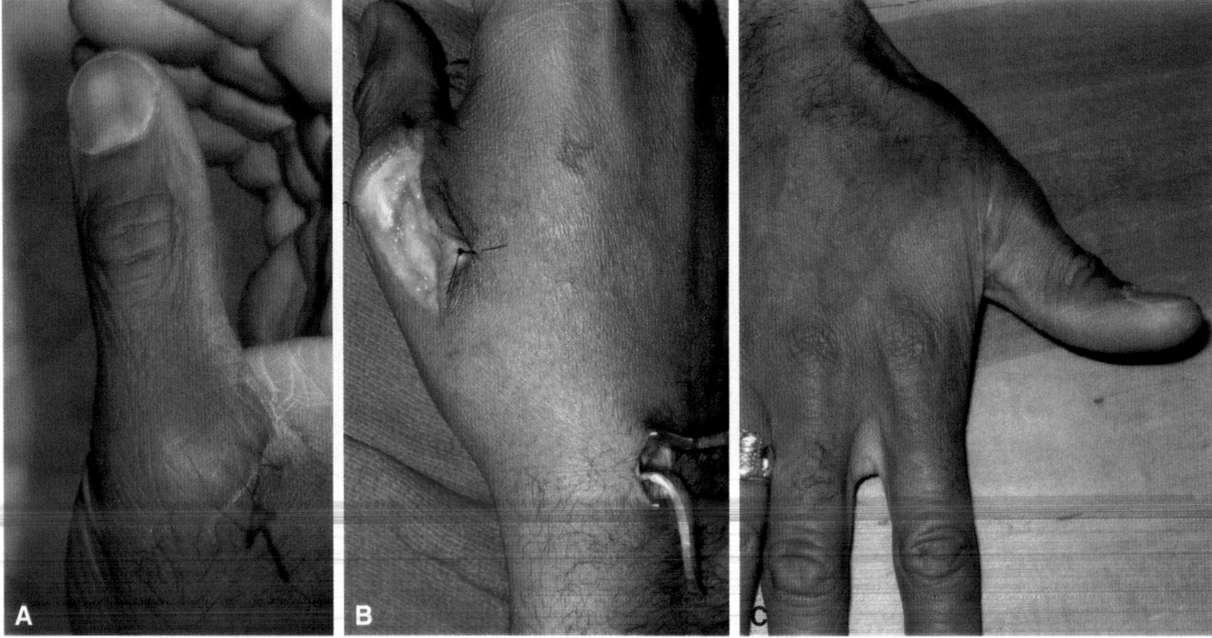

FIGURE 77.15. Proximal EPL laceration. EPL lacerations proximal to the MP joint can retract significantly because there are no tethering linkages such as juncturae tendinae to prevent proximal migration. **A.** This patient sustained such an EPL laceration. Proximal extension of the wound was not enough to uncover the proximal end of the tendon. **B.** Instead, a separate transverse wrist incision exposed the proximal EPL that was then routed to the distal wound. The injury was repaired with nonabsorbable four-core sutures (3-0, modified Kessler) and augmented by an epitendinous cross-stitch. **C.** Three months postoperatively, the patient demonstrates normal thumb retropulsion and IP hyperextension.

- Extensor lacerations just proximal to the MP joint (zones T4 and T5) result in significant recoil of the EPL. It is best to check thumb retropulsion (see Figure 77.3) than to hopelessly explore the wound in the ER. Additional proximal incisions are sometimes needed if the tendon retracts significantly and/or repair is delayed (Figure 77.15).
- An uncommon and unusual tendon injury that occurs in zone T1 is spontaneous rupture of the EPL tendon after distal radius fracture. The rupture usually occurs in closed nondisplaced fractures treated nonoperatively, and it can present weeks to months after the initial fracture. The mechanism is unclear but watershed blood supply and/or extravasation of blood into a tight compartment with subsequent pressure ischemia have been proposed. The best treatment is transfer of the EIP tendon to the EPL tendon.[35] Dividing the EIP proximal to the extensor hood minimizes likelihood of extension lag in the index finger. Patients adjust well to this transfer and start using it naturally soon after rehabilitation. Paradoxically, the majority of patients can still independently extend the index finger.[36] A rarely discussed alternative is EPL reconstruction with a tendon graft that is a closer reconstitution of normal anatomy but requires appropriate tensioning, compensating for a shortened EPL muscle.

REFERENCES

1. Van Sint Jan S, Rooze M, Van Audekerke J, Vico L. The insertion of the extensor digitorum tendon on the proximal phalanx. *J Hand Surg*. 1996;21(1):69-76.
2. Arnet U, Muzykewicz DA, Fridén J, Lieber RL. Intrinsic hand muscle function, part 1: creating a functional grasp. *J Hand Surg*. 2013;38(11):2093-2099.
3. Harris C, Rutledge GL. The functional anatomy of the extensor mechanism of the finger. *J Bone Joint Surg Am*. 1972;54A:713-726.
In this oft-cited classic article, the authors carefully dissect the extension function of the human finger using fresh cadaver specimens. A methodical and precise rendition of the anatomy is provided along with the proposed role of each structure alone and in unison with others.
4. el-Gammal TA, Steyers CM, Blair WF, Maynard JA. Anatomy of the oblique retinacular ligament of the index finger. *J Hand Surg*. 1993;18(4):717-721.
5. Adkinson JM, Johnson SP, Chung KC. The clinical implications of the oblique retinacular ligament. *J Hand Surg*. 2014;39(3):535-541.
The authors review the oblique retinacular ligament, its discovery, functional role, and clinical significance. Although the role of the ligament is now thought to be insignificant, the concept of linking interphalangeal joint motion led to the development of effective surgical interventions for mallet injuries and swan-neck deformities.
6. Marshall TG, Sivakumar B, Smith DJ, Hile MS. Mechanics of metacarpophalangeal joint extension. *J Hand Surg*. 2018;43(7):681e1-681e5.
7. Minamikawa Y, Peimer CA, Yamaguchi T, et al. Wrist position and extensor tendon amplitude following repair. *J Hand Surg*. 1992;17(2):268-271.
8. Vahey JW, Wegner DA, Hastings H. Effect of proximal phalangeal fracture deformity on extensor tendon function. *J Hand Surg*. 1998;23(4):673-681.
9. Schweitzer TP, Rayan GM. The terminal tendon of the digital extensor mechanism. Part II: kinematic study. *J Hand Surg*. 2004;29(5):903-908.
10. Kleinert HE, Verdan C. Report of the committee on tendon injuries (International Federation of Societies for Surgery of the Hand). *J Hand Surg*. 1983;8(5 Pt 2):794-798.
11. Doyle J. Extensor tendons: acute injuries. In: Green D, ed. *Operative Hand Surgery*. 3rd ed. New York, NY: Churchill Livingstone; 1993.
12. Browne EZ, Ribik CA. Early dynamic splinting for extensor tendon injuries. *J Hand Surg*. 1989;14(1):72-76.
13. Mowlavi A, Burns M, Brown RE. Dynamic versus static splinting of simple zone V and zone VI extensor tendon repairs: a prospective, randomized, controlled study. *Plast Reconstr Surg*. 2005;115(2):482-487.
14. Kitis A, Ozcan RH, Bagdatli D, et al. Comparison of static and dynamic splinting regimens for extensor tendon repairs in zones V to VII. *J Plast Surg Hand Surg*. 2012;46(3-4):267-271.
15. Collocott SJ, Kelly E, Ellis RF. Optimal early active mobilisation protocol after extensor tendon repairs in zones V and VI: a systematic review of literature. *Hand Ther*. 2018;23(1):3-18.
16. Neuhaus V, Wong G, Russo KE, Mudgal CS. Dynamic splinting with early motion following zone IV/V and TI to TIII extensor tendon repairs. *J Hand Surg*. 2012;37(5):933-937.
17. Evans D, Weightman B. The Pipflex splint for treatment of mallet finger. *J Hand Surg Edinb Scotl*. 1988;13(2):156-158.
18. Pike J, Mulpuri K, Metzger M, et al. Blinded, prospective, randomized clinical trial comparing volar, dorsal, and custom thermoplastic splinting in treatment of acute mallet finger. *J Hand Surg*. 2010;35(4):580-588.
19. Handoll HHG, Vaghela MV. Interventions for treating mallet finger injuries. *Cochrane Database Syst Rev*. 2004;(3):CD004574.
This Cochrane review assessed four randomized controlled trials for the treatment of acute mallet finger to ascertain effective treatment methods. There was methodological flaws in all of the trials, and there was no comparative advantage seen in different splinting methods or pin fixation. The importance of patient compliance was stressed.
20. Iselin F, Levame J, Godoy J. A simplified technique for treating mallet fingers: tenodermodesis. *J Hand Surg*. 1977;2(2):118-121.

21. Thompson JS, Littler JW, Upton J. The spiral oblique retinacular ligament (SORL). *J Hand Surg*. 1978;3(5):482-487.
22. Kleinman WB, Petersen DP. Oblique retinacular ligament reconstruction for chronic mallet finger deformity. *J Hand Surg*. 1984;9(3):399-404.
23. Oh JY, Kim JS, Lee DC, et al. Comparative study of spiral oblique retinacular ligament reconstruction techniques using either a lateral band or a tendon graft. *Arch Plast Surg*. 2013;40(6):773-778.
24. Hart RG, Uehara DT, Kutz JE. Extensor tendon injuries of the hand. *Emerg Med Clin North Am*. 1993;11(3):637-649.
25. Rockwell WB, Butler PN, Byrne BA. Extensor tendon: anatomy, injury, and reconstruction. *Plast Reconstr Surg*. 2000;106(7):1592-1603, 1673.
26. Grau L, Baydoun H, Chen K, et al. Biomechanics of the acute boutonniere deformity. *J Hand Surg*. 2018;43(1):80e1-80e6.
27. Elson RA. Rupture of the central slip of the extensor hood of the finger. A test for early diagnosis. *J Bone Joint Surg Br*. 1986;68B:229-231.
    Recognizing that closed rupture of the central slip is easily missed until the late appearance of a boutonniere deformity, Elson proposed a new test to assess integrity of the central slip. Absence of extension force at the PIP joint and fixed extension at the DIP joint, when the finger is held in PIP flexion, are signs of complete rupture.
28. Rubin J, Bozentka DJ, Bora FW. Diagnosis of closed central slip injuries: a cadaveric analysis of non-invasive tests. *J Hand Surg Edinb Scotl*. 1996;21(5):614-616.
29. Littler JW, Eaton RG. Redistribution of forces in the correction of boutonniere deformity. *J Bone Joint Surg Am*. 1967;49A:1267-1274.
    The authors describe the pathophysiology of the boutonniere deformity and a method of repair that involves using the lateral bands, where they are detached from the terminal tendon and repaired to the central slip insertion. In this reconstruction for chronic deformity, the new insertion of the bands functions to extend the PIP joint.
30. Curtis RM, Reid RL, Provost JM. A staged technique for the repair of the traumatic boutonniere deformity. *J Hand Surg*. 1983;8(2):167-171.
31. Hung LK, Chan A, Chang J, et al. Early controlled active mobilization with dynamic splintage for treatment of extensor tendon injuries. *J Hand Surg*. 1990;15(2):251-257.
32. Chester DL, Beale S, Beveridge L, et al. A prospective, controlled, randomized trial comparing early active extension with passive extension using a dynamic splint in the rehabilitation of repaired extensor tendons. *J Hand Surg Edinb Scotl*. 2002;27(3):283-288.
33. Koniuch MP, Peimer CA, VanGorder T, Moncada A. Closed crush injury of the metacarpophalangeal joint. *J Hand Surg*. 1987;12(5 Pt 1):750-757.
34. Newport ML, Blair WF, Steyers CM. Long-term results of extensor tendon repair. *J Hand Surg*. 1990;15(6):961-966.
35. De Smet L, Van Loon J, Fabry G. Extensor indicis proprius to extensor pollicis longus transfer: results and complications. *Acta Orthop Belg*. 1997;63(3):178-181.
36. Moore JR, Weiland AJ, Valdata L. Independent index extension after extensor indicis proprius transfer. *J Hand Surg*. 1987;12(2):232-236.

QUESTIONS

1. **A 32-year-old woman with fibromyalgia comes to the office after being seen in the emergency department 3 days prior with a laceration to the dorsal aspect of the right hand caused by broken glass. The laceration was repaired in a single layer in the emergency department. On physical examination, the patient can extend all fingers but cannot hyperextend her long finger beyond the neutral position. The interphalangeal joints can be fully extended actively. What explains the findings?**
   a. There is no tendon injury.
   b. The patient has an accessory extensor tendon to the long finger.
   c. The patient has a partial tendon laceration of less than 50%.
   d. Junctura tendinum and intact intrinsic muscles are extending the finger.
   e. Her inability to fully extend is related to pain and swelling following the laceration.

2. **A 23-year-old right-hand–dominant man presents to clinic after a sprain of the left ring finger sustained while playing flag football. The finger is swollen and bruised. His PIP joint is held in flexion, and is slightly lax to valgus stress. The DIP joint is hyperextended. Which is the most likely diagnosis?**
   a. Avulsion of the superficial flexor tendon
   b. Central slip disruption
   c. Sagittal band rupture
   d. Avulsion of the deep flexor tendon
   e. Swan-neck deformity

3. **A 34-year-old man presents to the office with a mallet deformity of the nondominant index finger sustained 13 years ago. He did not seek treatment at the time. On examination, which of the following deformities is likely to be present?**
   a. Clinodactyly
   b. Hook-nail deformity
   c. Boutonnière
   d. Swan-neck
   e. Camptodactyly

4. **A 37-year-old nurse presents to the emergency department with sudden weakness in his thumb. He fractured his distal radius 3 months previously. This was a nondisplaced fracture. He also has CMC joint laxity, symmetric to the unaffected hand. On exam, thumb retropulsion is absent. Which is the most appropriate treatment?**
   a. Fusion of the CMC joint of the thumb
   b. Fusion of the IP joint of the thumb
   c. Transfer of the anterior interosseous nerve to the recurrent branch of the median nerve
   d. Transfer of the EIP tendon to the abductor pollicis brevis tendon
   e. Transfer of the EIP tendon to the EPL tendon

5. **A 45-year-old man comes to the office because of sudden inability to extend the distal phalanx of the long finger after playing basketball. Physical examination shows that the distal phalanx of the long finger is held in 45° of flexion. The patient has no active extension of the joint. There is only minimal swelling over the DIP joint. X-rays are normal. Which of the following is the most appropriate management?**
   a. Arthrodesis of the DIP joint in 15° of flexion
   b. Exploration and repair of the extensor tendon
   c. Percutaneous pin fixation of the DIP and proximal interphalangeal (PIP) joints
   d. Splinting of the DIP joint at 0°
   e. Observation only

6. **A 17-year-old girl undergoes extensor tendon repair in zone 4 and open treatment of a proximal phalangeal fracture affecting the nondominant fifth finger. At the 6-week postoperative visit, she is unable to actively extend the finger at the DIP and PIP joints. She has been very compliant with splinting. What is the most likely diagnosis?**
   a. An unidentified terminal extensor injury
   b. Rupture of the repaired extensor tendon
   c. Unidentified sagittal band injury
   d. Malingering
   e. Tendon adhesions

1. **Answer: d.** There is redundancy built into the extensor mechanism. Despite complete EDC injury, the neighboring extensor tendons can bypass the site of laceration and exert pull on the distal stump of the extensor via the juncturae tendinae, hereby allowing full digit extension. Suspicion of injury should prompt surgical exploration and repair. Furthermore, the intrinsic system (interossei and lumbricals) inserts onto the extensor hood via the lateral bands and can extend the digit at the IP joints.

2. **Answer: b.** The central slip is ruptured, leading to extension lag at the PIP joint and an acute boutonnière deformity. Although a simple sprain may also cause PIP extension lag, it will not cause simultaneous DIP hyperextension. An abnormal Elson test can confirm the diagnosis. A ruptured superficial flexor tendon is rare and would lead to an inability to flex at the PIP joint with the neighboring digits held in extension. A ruptured deep flexor tendon makes DIP flexion impossible. Sagittal band rupture leads to subluxation of the extensor tendon and weakened extension at the MP joint. Swan-neck deformity results from terminal extensor tendon disruption and inability to actively extend the DIP joint independent of PIP position.

3. **Answer: d.** Flexion deformity of the distal joint seen in mallet finger will lead to secondary hyperextension of the proximal joint. This occurs in a zigzag fashion because of the imbalance of forces. If the terminal tendon is displaced proximally, the conjoined bands will slide proximally and become extensors to the proximal joint. A boutonnière deformity is a flexion deformity of the PIP joint from disruption of the central slip. The lateral slips migrate volarly becoming hyperextensors of the DIP joint clinodactyly is a congenital condition in which there is radial deviation of the fifth finger, usually at the middle phalangeal level. A hook nail results from loss of bone to support the nail, usually after amputation, causing curvature of the nail. Camptodactyly is also a congenital condition in which there is a fixed flexion deformity of the PIP joint of the fifth finger.

4. **Answer: e.** The scenario depicts a classic case of EPL tendon rupture following distal radius fracture. The reported incidence of EPL tendon rupture ranges from 0.2% to 3%. Ruptures can occur after internal or external fixation due to impingement of hardware on the tendon or due to ischemic changes in the tendon within the third dorsal compartment. Reconstruction of the EPL tendon can be accomplished either by tendon grafting, typically palmaris longus interposition between the proximal and distal healthy segments of the EPL tendon, or by transfer of the EIP to the distal segment of EPL tendon. Thumb IP joint fusion may be useful in flexor pollicis longus ruptures that cannot be repaired, but this would not restore thumb retropulsion and is rarely performed in this circumstance. Fusion of the CMC joint can alleviate pain from basal joint arthritis, but would result in further loss of motion of the thumb. Transfer of the EIP to the

abductor pollicis brevis and transfer of the anterior interosseous nerve to the recurrent branch of the median nerve are techniques for restoring thumb palmar abduction/opposition and would not restore retropulsion/extension.

5. **Answer: d.** The physical exam is consistent with an avulsion of the terminal extensor tendon, a mallet injury. In the absence of joint subluxation, conservative nonoperative management with splinting is recommended. This requires splinting the DIP joint in extension or slight hyperextension. One can employ prefabricated stack splints, malleable aluminum splints, or custom-made thermoplastic splints. Outcomes of each of these treatments are similar, but the type of splinting is generally more limited by skin irritation. Pin fixation for the DIP joint is recommended for patients who cannot tolerate splinting or those with special circumstances, such as a surgeon who requires unencumbered use of the hand. Pin fixation should cross the DIP joint only. Arthrodesis is an option for patients with degenerative arthritis of the DIP joint. Surgical mallet treatment is not recommended, unless it is an open injury. Observation is not advised due to the possibility of secondary effects such as a swan-neck deformity.

6. **Answer: e.** Her exam is consistent with adhesions of the repaired extensor tendon at the site of the fracture. This is a common issue, especially when multiple tissues are injured in close proximity. Because the extensor system is stuck at the level of the hood, both the central slip as well as lateral bands are lacking excursion, hence the lack of extension at the PIP and DIP joints. Early motion protocols can be used to minimize adhesions; however, the osteosynthesis and tendon repair should be of sufficient strength to allow early motion. A terminal extensor injury, as in a mallet, would not lead to extension lag at the PIP joint. A rupture of the repaired tendon is a possibility but unlikely in the setting of compliance with postoperative immobilization. A sagittal band injury would influence extension at the MP joint, not the PIP of DIP joints. To rule out malingering, the wrist can be passively flexed and extended (tenodesis) to verify excursion of the extensor system.

CHAPTER 78 Tenosynovitis Disorders of the Upper Extremity

Lydia A. Helliwell and Kyle R. Eberlin

KEY POINTS

- Lateral epicondylitis results from microtears at the origin of the common extensor tendon mass, specifically the extensor carpi radialis brevis tendon, causing mucoid degeneration. It is often a self-limited condition that may take 1 to 2 years to resolve.
- Medial epicondylitis affects the common flexor tendon mass, most often the pronator teres and flexor carpi radialis. Conservative management is the mainstay of medial epicondylitis treatment, and all patients should be assessed for possible ulnar neuropathy.
- De Quervain disease is a stenosing tendiopathy involving the tendons of the first dorsal compartment (abductor pollicis longus and extensor pollicis brevis), resulting in painful wrist and thumb motion. Treatment options include splinting, corticosteroid injections, and operative decompression.
- Intersection syndrome results in pain, swelling and often crepitus over the junction on the first and second extensor compartments, approximately 4 cm proximal to the radiocarpal joint. It often resolves with nonoperative treatment such as therapy and splinting.
- Trigger fingers occur by a combination of thickening of the A1 pulley and nodule formation within the flexor tendon, resulting in pain and locking of the finger. Corticosteroid injections are effective in many patients, but if unsuccessful, surgery may be considered. Diabetics are less likely to respond to nonoperative treatment.

Painful tendinopathy of the elbow, wrist, and hand includes some of the most common issues presenting to upper extremity surgeons. Collectively, these conditions are often described as tenosynovitis disorders; however, this nomenclature can be misleading as the term tenosynovitis implies the existence of an inflammatory process.

In contrast, many common disorders involving the tendons of the upper extremity are the result of degenerative or mechanical stresses, rather than an inflammatory process. These conditions include lateral and medial epicondylitis of the elbow, de Quervain disease, intersection syndrome, and trigger finger. In addition to these common pathologies, there are several less common disorders involving the tendons of the wrist and hand. Almost every tendon in the hand and wrist can cause pain if irritated through mechanical stresses or stenosing forces. Atypical conditions include tendinopathy of the extensor carpi ulnaris (ECU), flexor carpi radialis (FCR), and extensor pollicis longus (EPL) tendons. In addition, there are also inflammatory tendon disorders of the wrist and hand, including rheumatoid arthritis, calcific tendinitis, as well as myriad infections that can affect these areas. The purpose of this chapter is to discuss the common tendinopathies affecting the upper extremity.

Despite the ubiquitous nature of tendon disorders in the upper extremity, treatment controversies remain. Both nonoperative and operative treatments exist and a definitive treatment algorithm remains elusive despite a plethora of studies.

LATERAL EPICONDYLITIS

Lateral epicondylitis is a common cause of lateral elbow pain. First described by Runge in 1873 in a patient unable to write because of pain and tenderness over the lateral epicondyle, it became commonly known as *tennis elbow* after Morris described a similar condition as *lawn tennis arm* in 1882.[1] Despite its common name and association, lateral epicondylitis may be precipitated by any activity that results in forceful repetitive motion of the forearm extensors.[2] It may also develop insidiously without antecedent trauma. The pain can be acute or chronic in nature and typically begins near the lateral epicondyle and radiates distally along the dorsal forearm. Manual activities, particularly lifting loads greater than 20 kg, have been associated with the development of lateral epicondylitis. It has been estimated that approximately 1% to 3% of the population will develop lateral epicondylitis during their lifetime. It is equally common in men and women, and prevalence peaks between the ages of 45 and 54 years.[2]

The lateral epicondyle is the origin for the common extensor tendons that include the tendons of the extensor carpi radialis brevis (ECRB), the extensor digitorum communis (EDC), and the ECU. Although each of these tendons may be involved in the process, the classic finding of lateral epicondylitis includes ECRB tendon pathology. The ECRB is located deep to the extensor carpi radialis longus (ECRL) and EDC and acts as a wrist extensor, inserting distally on the base of the third metacarpal. Changes within the ECRB tendon substance represent the *sine qua non* for lateral epicondylitis.

Although initially believed to be an inflammatory process involving the common origin of the wrist extensors, histopathologic analysis has shown an absence of inflammatory cells and instead has revealed markers of a degenerative process consistent with tendinosis rather than tenosynovitis. The tendons frequently demonstrate repetitive microtrauma, and the body's attempt to repair these microtears results in a number of pathologic findings including hyaline and mucoid degeneration, fibrosis, calcifications, and fibrovascular proliferation. Inflammatory cells, such as macrophages and neutrophils, are lacking.[3] Despite these findings, the true pathogenesis of lateral epicondylitis remains a matter of debate. Many theories have been postulated, with some hypothesizing that repetitive contact between the capitellum and the ECRB tendon may be the causative problem.[4]

Patients often present with pain over the lateral epicondyle and the common extensor tendon origin, immediately distal and anterior to the lateral epicondyle. On exam, resisted wrist extension with the elbow extended and the wrist pronated is a provocative maneuver that may elicit increased pain. A complete elbow examination should be performed to ensure that there is no other source of elbow pain. Other causes of elbow pain, including osteoarthritis, osteochondritis dissecans, occult fracture, lateral ulnar collateral ligament injury, plica, radial tunnel syndrome, and synovitis of the radiohumeral joint should be considered and exonerated.

Imaging studies add limited information in the diagnosis of lateral epicondylitis. Radiographic images of the elbow may be obtained to rule out arthritic changes as a source of pain but have not been found to aid significantly in the diagnosis of lateral epicondylitis. Ultrasound (US) and magnetic resonance imaging (MRI) have both been utilized for diagnosis, to assess disease severity and for purposes of preoperative planning. Ultrasound has been found to have a lower sensitivity for detection of both lateral and medial epicondylitis (64%–82%) and therefore, MRI is often the modality of choice, with a higher sensitivity of 90% to 100%.[5] However, the severity of disease present on MRI does not necessarily correlate with symptoms, and patients with resolved pain may continue to have pathologic findings present on MRI. MRI is often reserved for recalcitrant cases in which the patient fails to improve with 6 months of conservative treatment or when the diagnosis in unclear.[6]

The treatment of lateral epicondylitis remains one of the most controversial subjects in hand and upper extremity surgery. In his paper on tennis elbow published in 1936, Cyriax wrote "the condition usually clears up in eight to twelve months without any treatment except perhaps avoidance of the painful movements."[7] For many surgeons, activity modification continues to be the mainstay of treatment for lateral epicondylitis, with up to 90% of patients improving without intervention in some studies.[8] Other studies, however, suggest that up to 40% of people continue to have discomfort after 1 to 5 years of nonoperative treatment.[9] Modalities for nonoperative management include counterforce bracing, wrist and elbow splinting, physical therapy, iontophoresis, shockwave therapy, laser therapy, nonsteroidal antiinflammatory medications, and a number of different injection therapies (corticosteroids, botulinum toxin, platelet-rich plasma, and autologous blood). Despite numerous randomized controlled studies, none of these interventions has been definitively proven to work better than rest and therapy alone.[8]

Physical and occupational therapy for lateral epicondylitis often includes gentle stretching with progression to more aggressive strengthening. Studies comparing physical therapy to no intervention found patients improved in the short term, but differences in the long term were not significant.[10] Counterforce bracing and wrist splinting are also employed; counterforce bracing appears to work by offloading the common extensor origin by applying pressure to a more distal site on the muscle, which then acts as the new muscle origin. Cock-up wrist splints maintain the wrist in extension, thereby offloading the extensors. Several studies have compared bracing or splinting to physical therapy and to each other with conflicting results.[11]

Injections into and around the lateral epicondyle remain highly controversial. Corticosteroid injection into the site of maximal tenderness is a common intervention performed when pain is not relieved with therapy or splinting alone. Various combinations of dexamethasone, betamethasone, and triamcinolone with or without local anesthesia have been given. Some studies have shown an improvement in pain at 4 to 6 weeks, but this advantage usually is not present at 12 months.[12] The exact mechanism by which steroid injection might improve pain is not well understood as corticosteroids usually counteract inflammation, which as mentioned earlier, is not present in lateral epicondylitis. There is no prospective, randomized trial demonstrating a long-term benefit of steroid injection for lateral epicondylitis. Additionally, complications such as fat atrophy and/or hypopigmentation may occur (Figure 78.1).

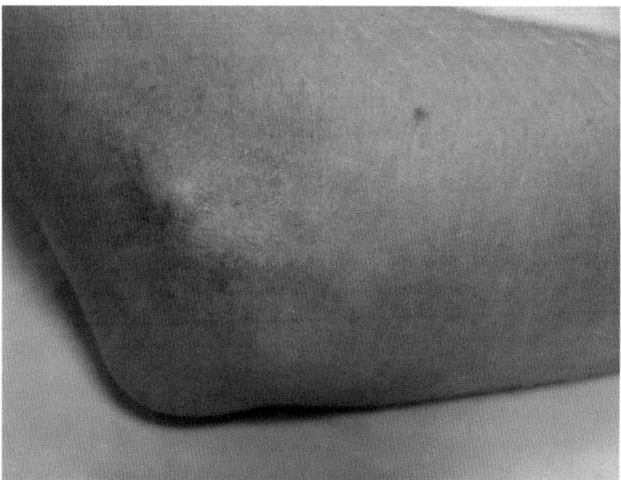

FIGURE 78.1. Atrophy and discoloration after multiple steroid injections for lateral epicondylitis.

Botulinum toxin A has also been used in the treatment of lateral epicondylitis to temporarily paralyze the extensor muscles to reduce further microtrauma and pain. Studies have been variable in their results, with no clear long-term benefit conferred. Transient loss of finger extension is a potential side effect. Platelet-rich plasma and autologous blood are two other injection therapies that have been attempted without demonstrable benefit at long-term follow-up.[12]

Surgical intervention for lateral epicondylitis is usually reserved for the small percentage of patients who fail 6 to 12 months of conservative management and who remain significantly affected by pain. In general, the main surgical tenet includes debridement of the common origin of the wrist extensors at the site of tendinopathy. A number of surgical techniques have been described, including open, percutaneous, and arthroscopic approaches. Many patients will improve with or without surgery, and therefore the decision to proceed with surgical intervention is complicated; the choice of approach is determined by surgeon experience and patient preference.

All surgical procedures for lateral epicondylitis aim to address the pathology associated with the ECRB. Open, percutaneous, or arthroscopic release of the ECRB from the lateral epicondyle, open, or arthroscopic debridement of the ECRB tendinosis, denervation of the lateral epicondyle, and anconeus rotation have all been described with fair to good results. The open approach is performed via a small incision over the common extensor tendon distal to the lateral epicondyle. The interval between the ECRL and EDC is identified and incised. The ECRB is found directly deep to these muscles, and can be divided and the tendonosis debrided. The diseased tissue is usually white-gray in color with a friable, disorganized appearance. The joint can be inspected for plica. Care is taken not to debride the lateral ulnar collateral ligament, as this will lead to elbow instability. A volar wrist splint is usually applied to maintain the wrist in extension and take stress off the common extensor origin until the incision has healed and elbow motion has returned to normal. Outcomes after open treatment have been good to excellent in several studies. Nirschl and Pettrone reported that after 88 open ECRB debridements, 98% of patients improved and 85% were able to return to work.[13]

The arthroscopic approach utilizes the same principles, approaching the diseased ECRB from its medial aspect. This approach has the advantage of visualizing the joint directly and for identifying other pathology, including loose bodies and plicae. Disadvantages include decreased visualization of the ECRB tendon, resulting in potential incomplete debridement of diseased tissues, and greater possibility of radial nerve injury. Studies have shown that the arthroscopic approach has similar results to the open approach at long-term follow-up of 130 months.[14] However, when open, arthroscopic, and percutaneous approaches were compared, no difference in functional outcome, pain intensity, or patient satisfaction was found at 1-year follow-up.[15] Complications from either approach are wound breakdown, infection, injury to the lateral ulnar collateral ligament, neurovascular injury, and incomplete relief of pain with ongoing disability.

Overall, lateral epicondylitis remains a conundrum for upper extremity surgeons, with many available treatment options but no conclusively disease-modifying interventions.

MEDIAL EPICONDYLITIS

Medial epicondylitis, also known as *golfer's elbow*, is a common cause of medial elbow pain. Although less prevalent than lateral epicondylitis (<1% versus 3.4%),[2] it may be more prevalent in patients performing forceful, repetitive manual labor.[16] Similar to lateral epicondylitis, medial epicondylitis is associated with repetitive movements and is often found in patients 40 to 50 years old.[2,16]

On physical exam, point tenderness is usually present over the medial epicondyle and distally over the common flexor tendon. The common flexor tendon is composed of five muscles including the pronator teres (PT), FCR, flexor carpi ulnaris, palmaris longus, and flexor digitorum superficialis. Similar to lateral epicondylitis, microtrauma from repetitive motion, specifically repetitive valgus loads, may result in mucoid degeneration of the tendons resulting in the histopathologic findings of angiofibroblastic hyperplasia, fibrosis, and calcification. The PT and FCR are most frequently affected.

Other sources of medial elbow pain should also be considered including elbow arthritis, osteochondral defects, medial collateral ligament instability, cervical radiculopathy, pronator syndrome, and ulnar neuritis/cubital tunnel syndrome. Ulnar neuritis is especially important as 23% to 61% of patients with medial epicondylitis also have concurrent ulnar neuropathy.[17] Given this high rate of concomitant ulnar neuritis, workup should also evaluate for ulnar nerve pathology.

The diagnosis of medical epicondylitis is most commonly made by physical examination, with point tenderness over the medial epicondyle and pain elicited with resisted forearm pronation and wrist flexion. Ultrasound can be used to assist in the diagnosis, as it has been shown to be both specific and sensitive.[5] MRI may show increased signal on T1 and T2 series, but similar to lateral epicondylitis, the appearance on MRI may not correlate with symptoms. It can be a helpful tool to rule out other causes of elbow pain, including assessing for medial collateral ligament instability.[18]

Treatment of medial epicondylitis is similar to lateral epicondylitis, with nonoperative management the first line therapy for most patients. Activity modification includes avoidance of activities that require repetitive wrist flexion and forearm pronation. Physical therapy, with common flexor mass stretching and strengthening, is recommended for those who do not improve with activity modification alone. Counterforce bracing has shown some success by limiting the maximum forces exerted on the flexor mass. Elbow extension bracing can be useful especially in those with concurrent ulnar nerve symptoms. Corticosteroid injections have been utilized in the treatment of medial epicondylitis with short-term pain relief (6 weeks), although there is no clear benefit over the long term.[19] Overall, in 88% to 96% of cases, nonoperative management and the passage of time has been shown to result in resolution of symptoms.[17]

Surgery for medial epicondylitis should be reserved for patients who do not improve with 6 months or greater of conservative therapy. Open surgical debridement is most commonly used. An incision is made over the common flexor tendon, and the interval between the PT and FCR is developed. The underlying diseased tissue is debrided. Protecting the ulnar nerve, the MCL, and the medial antebrachial cutaneous nerves are all key components of this operation. This open approach has been shown to have good-to-excellent results in up to 97% of patients.[20] Depending on the presence or absence of ulnar neuritis, cubital tunnel release and ulnar nerve transposition may be performed concomitantly. Notably, patients with medial epicondylitis and ulnar neuritis preoperatively have been shown to have increased pain and longer recoveries than those without ulnar neuritis.[17]

DE QUERVAIN DISEASE

De Quervain disease is a stenosing tendiopathy involving the first dorsal extensor compartment. It receives its eponymous name from Fritz de Quervain, a Swiss surgeon, who first described the condition and its treatment in 1895.[21] Patients often present with radial-sided wrist pain exacerbated by ulnar deviation of the wrist and thumb abduction. It is most common in the fifth and sixth decade of life and is up to six times more common in women than men.[22] It is often associated with repetitive motion of the wrist seen in women doing common household chores or other highly repetitive activities, such as typing and lifting.[23] It is also more commonly seen in pregnant and lactating women.[24]

The extensor tendons of the hand and wrist are located within six separate compartments contained within the dorsal carpal ligament. The abductor pollicis longus (APL) and extensor pollicis brevis (EPB) travel together within the first dorsal compartment, which overlies the radial styloid. The APL inserts on the base of the thumb metacarpal, whereas the EPB inserts on the base of the proximal phalanx of the thumb. Both act to abduct the thumb at the carpometacarpal (CMC) joint, and the EPB also helps to extend the thumb at the metacarpophalangeal (MCP) joint. The APL often has several tendinous slips within the compartment and the EPB can travel through its own separate subsheath within the first compartment. Knowledge of this anatomy is particularly relevant to treatment of de Quervain disease, as failure to recognize the presence of this subsheath can lead to incomplete operative treatment.[25]

The frictional forces caused by repetitive motion of the APL and EPB tendons within the tight compartment may lead to swelling and thickening of the retinaculum, causing narrowing of the tunnel and pain with motion. Similar to lateral and medial epicondylitis, histopathologic examination of the tendon sheath in patients with de Quervain disease shows lack of inflammation but myxoid degeneration within a thickened tendon sheath.[26] Patients present with a gradual onset of radial-sided wrist pain and tenderness to palpation over the radial styloid. The Finkelstein test, first described in 1930, is a common physical exam tool used to diagnose de Quervain disease and involves gentle ulnar deviation of the wrist, followed by passive flexion of the thumb into the palm by the examiner.[27] Other common causes of radial-sided wrist pain must be excluded, including CMC joint arthritis of the thumb, scaphotrapezial-trapezoid arthritis, intersection syndrome, scaphoid fracture, and radial sensory nerve pathology.

Similar to other tendinopathies, nonoperative treatment is usually provided first. This may include nonsteroidal antiinflammatory medications along with splint immobilization with or without corticosteroid injection (Figure 78.2). A number of studies demonstrated the high success rate of corticosteroid injections alone or in conjunction with splinting. Harvey et al found in their treatment of 91 wrists in 82 consecutive de Quervain patients, that 80% had complete and lasting relief of symptoms after corticosteroid injection.[28] Splinting alone was observed to be less successful, but when combined with corticosteroids, is likely more successful than injections alone.[22] Corticosteroid injections may cause fat atrophy, skin discoloration, and in rare circumstances, tendon rupture. Patients should be warned of these side effects before injection. Interestingly, patients who fail to improve with corticosteroid injections have been found to have a higher rate of EPB subsheath than the general population.[28]

Surgical release is often performed when symptoms persist despite splinting and/or steroid injection, and is performed by making either a transverse or a longitudinal incision over the first dorsal compartment. The radial sensory nerve is protected, and the first dorsal compartment is sharply divided on its dorsal aspect to prevent volar subluxation of the tendons. The compartment must be closely inspected for the presence of a EPB subsheath. The EPB should be clearly identified and passively tested to ensure thumb metacarpal extension before the surgical release is complete. Studies have shown that a separate subsheath is present in 44% of normal cadavers versus

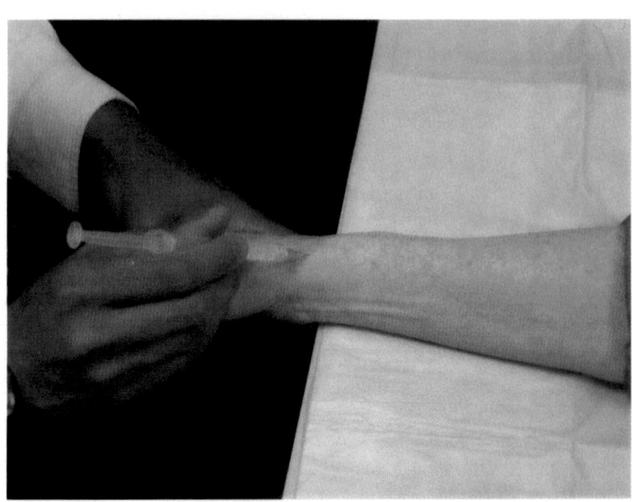

FIGURE 78.2. Site of steroid injection for de Quervain disease.

62% in de Quervain disease patients.[29] Failure to release this subsheath at the time of surgery is a potential cause of failure of surgical release. Other complications include injury to branches of the radial sensory nerve, which can cause symptomatic neuroma and volar subluxation of the APL and EPB tendons after first dorsal compartment release.

INTERSECTION SYNDROME

Intersection syndrome involves the contents of the second dorsal compartment, the ECRL and ECRB as they cross beneath the first compartment muscles (APL and EPB), which occurs approximately 4 to 6 cm proximal to Lister tubercle on the dorsal radial aspect of the forearm. Erythema and crepitation may be present. It can be easily confused with de Quervain disease and should be considered in anyone who presents with both radial-sided wrist and forearm pain. First described by Velpaeu in 1825, intersection syndrome is an uncommon cause of wrist pain, thought to be caused by similar inciting activities as other wrist tendinopathies including activities that cause repetitive wrist, hand, or digital motion.[30] Ulnar and radial deviation of the wrist, as well as thumb abduction and extension are the activities most associated with intersection syndrome. Controversy exists as to whether stenosis of the second compartment sheath alone versus friction between the first and second compartments is the underlying etiology.[31]

Although intersection syndrome is often diagnosed based on physical exam alone, both MRI and ultrasound can be useful modalities for distinguishing between intersection syndrome and other pathologies, such as de Quervain disease.[32] Nonoperative treatment represents the mainstay of care for intersection syndrome. Nonsteroidal antiinflammatory drugs (NSAIDs) combined with splinting of the wrist in 20° of extension for 2 to 3 weeks resolves most cases. Refractory cases can be treated with a corticosteroid injection.[33] For those who fail conservative management, surgical release of the second extensor compartment followed by a short period of immobilization may provide relief.[34]

TRIGGER FINGER

Trigger finger, also known as stenosing tenosynovitis, is one of the most common hand maladies with a lifetime risk of 2.6% in the general population and up to 10% in those with diabetes.[35,36] The flexor tendons pass through tight fibro-osseous canals containing a system of pulleys, which help to maintain the close association of the flexor tendons to the bone and prevent bowstringing of the tendon. The A1 pulley, located at the level of the metacarpal head, is the site of mechanical impingement seen in trigger finger. The thumb's A1 pulley is located near the MCP joint crease and is the site of flexor pollicis longus triggering.

Although the exact etiology of trigger finger is not well understood, it is theorized that repetitive motion of the flexor tendons through the A1 pulley leads to friction within the flexor sheath, causing both thickening of the pulley and nodule formation within the flexor tendon. As these two areas become further hypertrophied, the tendon has difficulty with its normal gliding through the pulley. Motion can become painful, eventually leading to inability of the tendon to pass through the sheath and *locking* of the digit in either flexion or extension. Because of the locking or *popping* sensation noted, it is not uncommon for patients to localize the problem to the proximal interphalangeal (PIP) joint rather than the A1 pulley.

On physical exam, patients frequently have tenderness to palpation directly over the A1 pulley and a nodule within the tendon can sometimes be appreciated. Locking or triggering of the finger may be appreciated (Figure 78.3). Although repetitive motion is thought to be the underlying cause of trigger finger, association with specific occupations has not been found. However, patients with diabetes, hypothyroidism, rheumatoid arthritis, gout, and renal failure develop trigger fingers at higher rates. Similar to other tendinopathies, there is no evidence of inflammation but there is evidence of fibrocartilage metaplasia and upregulation of type 3 collagen.[37]

Nonoperative treatment is used commonly in the initial management approach for idiopathic trigger finger, including splinting and corticosteroid injection. Splinting of the MCP joint has been shown to be successful in up to 66% of cases, with a higher success rate (70%) in digits versus thumbs (50%).[38] The PIP joint can also be splinted, instead of the MCP joint, with similar effect. Splinting is recommended for 6 to 10 weeks both during the day and night, to which some patients can find difficult to adhere.

Corticosteroid has proven effective in treating trigger fingers and can be the first line intervention. Successful resolution of symptoms ranges from 60% to 90% in various studies, and a second injection increases the success rate.[39] Injection with various corticosteroid formulations has been tried without a clear advantage of one formulation over another. Intrasheath injections are not required for effect, and intratendinous injections should be avoided to reduce the risk of tendon rupture.[40] Other risks of corticosteroid injection include pain, infection, fat atrophy, hypopigmentation, and digital nerve injury. Patients with diabetes do not respond as well to steroid injections; some studies advocated for immediate surgical release or only one attempt at injection before surgical intervention is considered.[41] Diabetic patients often experience a transient elevation in blood glucose levels after a corticosteroid injection.[36]

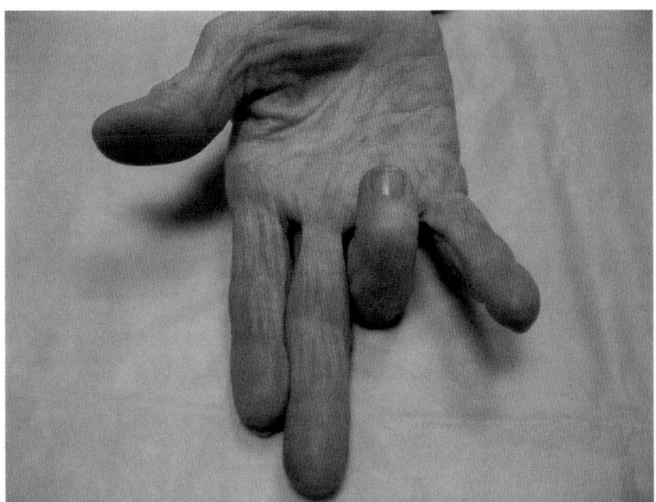

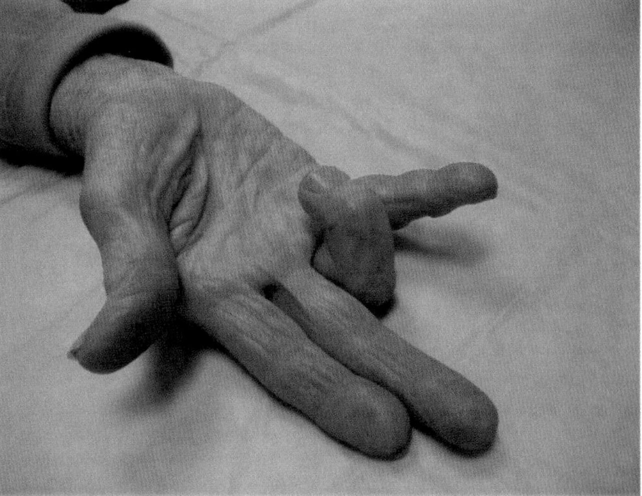

FIGURE 78.3. The ring finger trigger demonstrates active locking. Another view of the locked trigger finger.

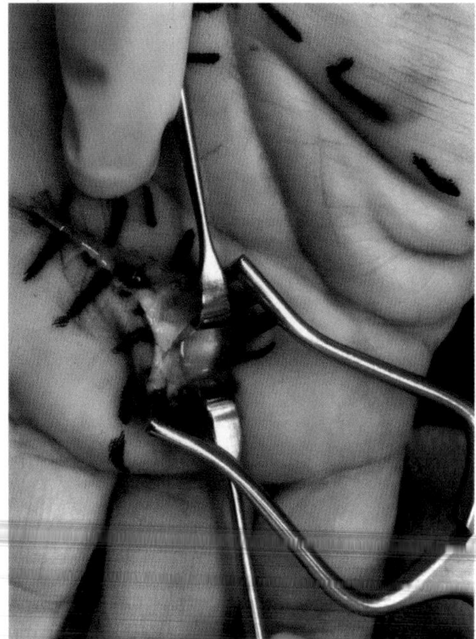

FIGURE 78.4. After surgical release of the trigger finger, a thickening within the flexor tendon is noted.

Both percutaneous and open techniques have been employed successfully for trigger finger. Although the number of injections that should be attempted before proceeding to surgical release has not been established, many surgeons will attempt more than one injection before proceeding with surgical release in patients without comorbidities such as diabetes and hypothyroidism.[42] Percutaneous techniques have been shown to be successful with up to 95% resolution of symptoms.[43] An 18- or 19-gauge needle is inserted into the A1 pulley and moved longitudinally until the *grating* feel of the A1 pulley against the needle disappears and the patient is able to actively flex and extend the digit without recurrent locking. Percutaneous release can be done in the office and has been found to be safe with few complications.[43] However, a study by Guler et al found a statistically significant increase in digital nerve injury with percutaneous release versus open release,[44] which may be most germane to the thumb.

Open surgical release requires an incision over the A1 pulley of either the digit or thumb and opening the pulley completely under direct visualization (Figure 78.4). This protects the neurovascular bundles throughout the procedure and visual confirmation of complete A1 pulley release. Both transverse and longitudinal incisions can be employed to assess the A1 pulley. The proximal edge of the A1 pulley can be successfully localized by measuring the distance from the PIP joint crease to the palmar-digital crease. The leading edge of the A1 pulley can be found at the same distance from the palmar-digital crease.[45] Open surgical release has been shown to be highly effective, with up to 99% of patients achieving successful treatment.[46] However, open surgical release comes with its own risk for complications including chronic pain, infection, iatrogenic digital nerve injury, incomplete release, and bowstringing.

OTHER TENDINOPATHIES OF THE WRIST AND HAND

Although trigger finger and de Quervain disease are the most common tendinopathies of the hand and wrist, most tendons of the wrist or hand can be a source of pain and discomfort. In addition to intersection syndrome, other less common tendinopathies include tendinitis of the EPL, ECU, and FCR. The EPL tendon travels through a tight fibro-osseous tunnel as it passes around Lister tubercle. This area is thought to be a watershed area of decreased blood supply to the tendon. Thus, any swelling in this area can lead to dysvascularity of the tendon.[47] Thus, treatment of EPL tendinitis is often surgical with complete release of the third dorsal compartment, to prevent rupture of the EPL. Patients can present with pain, swelling, and occasionally crepitus and triggering of the EPL tendon.[47]

The floor of the ECU tendon sheath is an important contributor to the triangular fibrocartilage complex, and irritation of the ECU tendon can be difficult to differentiate from other sources of ulnar-sided pain. It is also important to assess for ECU subluxation, which can occur after an acute injury in athletes. Patients often present with point tenderness over the ECU tendon that is worsened with gripping and heavy lifting. Ultrasound and MRI can help differentiate other causes of ulnar-sided wrist pain but is not necessary for diagnosis. Injecting local anesthesia into the ECU subsheath can be a helpful diagnostic tool. Treatment is usually conservative with splinting, NSAIDs, and corticosteroid injections, although surgical release of the ECU subsheath has been shown to be effective in those who do not respond to conservative measures.[48]

The FCR tendon travels through a tight subsheath before inserting onto the base of the second metacarpal. Within this subsheath, it is subject to impingement and irritation from osteophytes from neighboring thumb CMC joint and scaphotrapezial joint degeneration.[49] Patients present with pain and swelling over the FCR tendon at the distal wrist crease, worsened by wrist flexion and radial deviation. Plain radiographs and MRI can assist in the diagnosis and treatment is often conservation, with splinting, steroid injection, and NSAIDs being the first line. Surgical release of the FCR subsheath can be performed in refractory cases.[50]

REFERENCES

1. Cyriax JH. Tennis elbow. *Br Med J*. 1937;1937:559.
2. Shiri R, Viikari-Juntura E, Varonen H, Heliövaara M. Prevalence and determinants of lateral and medial epicondylitis: a population study. *Am J Epidemiol*. 2006;164(11):1065-1074.
   This often-cited population study performed in Finland found a prevalence of lateral epicondylitis of 1.3% and medical epicondylitis of 0.4%, with a higher prevalence seen in patients who are obese and smoke.
3. Khan KM, Cook JL, Bonar F, et al. Histopathology of common tendinopathies: update and implications for clinical management. *Sport Med*. 1999;27(6):393-408.
4. Bunata RE, Brown DS, Capelo R. Anatomic factors related to the cause of tennis elbow. *J Bone Joint Surg Am*. 2007;89A:1955-1963.
5. Miller TT, Shapiro MA, Schultz E, Kalish PE. Comparison of sonography and MRI for diagnosing epicondylitis. *J Clin Ultrasound*. 2002;30(4):193-202.
6. Walton MJ, MacKie K, Fallon M, et al. The reliability and validity of magnetic resonance imaging in the assessment of chronic lateral epicondylitis. *J Hand Surg Am*. 2011;36(3):475-479.
7. Cyriax J. The pathology and treatment of tennis elbow. *J Bone Joint Surg*. 1936;18(4):921-940.
8. Sims SEG, Miller K, Elfar JC, Hammert WC. Non-surgical treatment of lateral epicondylitis: a systematic review of randomized controlled trials. *Hand*. 2014;9(4):419-446.
   Although multiple randomized controlled trials addressing the nonsurgical management of lateral epicondylitis exist, none have provided clear evidence of the superiority of one treatment over another. Lateral epicondylitis is usually self-limited, resolving over 12 to 18 months.
9. Binder AI, Hazleman BL. Lateral humeral epicondylitis—a study of natural history and the effect of conservative therapy. *Br J Rheumatol*. 1983;22(2):73-76.
10. Peterson M, Butler S, Eriksson M, Svrdsudd K. A randomized controlled trial of exercise versus wait-list in chronic tennis elbow (lateral epicondylosis). *Ups J Med Sci*. 2011;116(4):269-279.
11. Garg R, Adamson GJ, Dawson PA, et al. A prospective randomized study comparing a forearm strap brace versus a wrist splint for the treatment of lateral epicondylitis. *J Shoulder Elb Surg*. 2010;19(4):508-512.
12. Coombes BK, Bisset L, Vicenzino B. Efficacy and safety of corticosteroid injections and other injections for management of tendinopathy: a systematic review of randomised controlled trials. *Lancet*. 2010;376(9754):1751-1767.
13. Nirschl RP, Pettrone FA. Tennis elbow. The surgical treatment of lateral epicondylitis. *J Bone Joint Surg Am*. 1979;61A:832-839.
14. Baker CL, Baker CL. Long-term follow-up of arthroscopic treatment of lateral epicondylitis. *Am J Sports Med*. 2008;36(2):254-260.
15. Burn MB, Mitchell RJ, Liberman SR, et al. Open, arthroscopic, and percutaneous surgical treatment of lateral epicondylitis. *Hand*. 2017. doi:10.1177/1558944717701244.
16. Descatha A, Leclerc A, Chastang JF, Roquelaure Y. Medial epicondylitis in occupational settings: prevalence, incidence and associated risk factors. *J Occup Environ Med*. 2003;45(9):993-1001.

17. Gabel GT, Morrey BF. Operative treatment of medical epicondylitis: influence of concomitant ulnar neuropathy at the elbow. *J Bone Joint Surg Am.* 1995;77A:1065-1069.
18. Kijowski R, De Smet AA. Magnetic resonance imaging findings in patients with medial epicondylitis. *Skeletal Radiol.* 2005;34(4):196-202.
19. Stahl S, Kaufman T. The efficacy of an injection of steroids for medial epicondylitis: a prospective study of sixty elbows. *J Bone Joint Surg Am.* 1997;79A:1648-1652.
20. Vangsness CT, Jobe FW. Surgical treatment of medial epicondylitis: results in 35 elbows. *J Bone Joint Surg Br.* 1991;73B:409-411.
21. Ahuja NK, Chung KC. Fritz de Quervain, MD (1868-1940): stenosing tendovaginitis at the radial styloid process. *J Hand Surg Am.* 2004;29(6):1164-1170.
22. Weiss APC, Akelman E, Tabatabai M. Treatment of de Quervain's disease. *J Hand Surg Am.* 1994;19(4):595-598.
 This study comparing splint immobilization versus steroid injection versus a combination of both showed that splint immobilization alone or in combination with injection did not improve outcomes. Additionally, 28 of 42 wrists that ultimately had surgery were found to have a separate EPB subsheath.
23. Moore JS, Steven J. De Quervain's tenosynovitis: stenosing tenosynovitis of the first dorsal compartment. *J Occup Environ Med.* 1997;39(10):990-1002.
24. Avci S, Yilmaz C, Sayli U. Comparison of nonsurgical treatment measures for de Quervain's disease of pregnancy and lactation. *J Hand Surg Am.* 2002;27(2):322-324.
25. Alemohammad AM, Yazaki N, Morris RP, et al. Thumb interphalangeal joint extension by the extensor pollicis brevis: association with a subcompartment and de Quervain's disease. *J Hand Surg Am.* 2009;34(4):719-723.
26. Clarke MT, Lyall HA, Grant JW, Matthewson MH. The histopathology of de Quervain's disease. *J Hand Surg Br.* 1998;23(6):732-734.
27. Finklestein H. Stenosing tendovaginitis at the radial styloid process. *J Bone Joint Surg.* 1930;12A:509-540.
28. Harvey FJ, Harvey PM, Horsley MW. De Quervain's disease: surgical or nonsurgical treatment. *J Hand Surg Am.* 1990;15(1):83-87.
29. Lee ZH, Stranix JT, Anzai L, Sharma S. Surgical anatomy of the first extensor compartment: a systematic review and comparison of normal cadavers vs. De Quervain syndrome patients. *J Plast Reconstr Aesthet Surg.* 2017;70(1):127-131.
30. Thompson AR, Plewes LW, Shaw EG. Peritendinitis crepitans and simple tenosynovitis: a clinical study of 544 cases in industry. *Br J Ind Med.* 1951;8(3):150-160.
31. Luellen JR, Hanlon DP. Intersection syndrome: a case report and review of the literature. *J Emerg Med.* 1999;17(6):969-971.
32. Sato J, Ishii Y, Noguchi H. Clinical and ultrasound features in patients with intersection syndrome or de Quervain's disease. *J Hand Surg Eur Vol.* 2016;41(2):220-225.
33. Chatterjee R, Vyas J. Diagnosis and management of intersection syndrome as a cause of overuse wrist pain. *BMJ Case Rep.* 2016. doi:10.1136/bcr-2016-216900
34. Grundberg AB, Reagan DS. Pathologic anatomy of the [illegible]
 Thirteen patients were treated with decompression of the second dorsal compartment without intervention directed toward that first dorsal compartment and all had resolution of symptoms.
35. Akhtar S, Bradley MJ, Quinton DN, Burke FD. Management and referral for trigger finger/thumb. *BMJ.* 2005;331(7507):30.
36. Stahl S, Kanter Y, Karnielli E. Outcome of trigger finger treatment in diabetes. *J Diabetes Complicat.* 1995;11(5):287-290.
37. Sampson SP, Badalamente MA, Hurst LC, Seidman J. Pathobiology of the human A1 pulley in trigger finger. *J Hand Surg Am.* 1991;16(4):714-721.
38. Patel MR, Bassini L. Trigger fingers and thumb: when to splint, inject, or operate. *J Hand Surg Am.* 1992;17(1):110-113.
39. Peters-Veluthamaningal C, van der Windt D, Winters J, Meyboom-de Jong B. Corticosteroid injection for trigger finger in adults (review). *Cochrane Database Syst Rev.* 2009;(1):CD005617.
40. Kazuki K, Egi T, Okada M, Takaoka K. Clinical outcome of extrasynovial steroid injection for trigger finger. *Hand Surg.* 2006;11:1-4.
41. Luther GA, Murthy P, Blazar PE. Cost of immediate surgery versus non-operative treatment for trigger finger in diabetic patients. *J Hand Surg Am.* 2016;41(11):1056-
42. Kerrigan CL, Stanwix MG. Using evidence to minimize the cost of trigger finger care. *J Hand Surg Am.* 2009;34(6):997-1005.
43. Pope DF, Wolfe SW. Safety and efficacy of percutaneous trigger finger release. *J Hand Surg Am.* 1995;20(2):280-283.
44. Guler F, Kose O, Ercan EC, et al. Open versus percutaneous release for the treatment of trigger thumb. *Orthopedics.* 2013;36(10):e1290-e1294.
45. Wilhelmi BJ, Snyder N, Verbesey JE, et al. Trigger finger release with hand surface landmark ratios: an anatomic and clinical study. *Plast Reconstr Surg.* 2001;108(4):908-915.
 This study identified surface landmarks of the A1 pulley to aid both the open and percutaneous treatment of trigger finger.
46. Sato ES, Gomes dos santos JB, Belloti JC, et al. Treatment of trigger finger: randomized clinical trial comparing the methods of corticosteroid injection, percutaneous release and open surgery. *Rheumatology.* 2012;51(1):93-99.
47. Kardashian G, Vara AD, Miller SJ, et al. Stenosing synovitis of the extensor pollicis longus tendon. *J Hand Surg Am.* 2011;36(6):1035-1038.
 Extensor pollicis longus stenosing tenosynovitis is a rare diagnosis and triggering of the EPL as a result is seen even less frequently. This article presents three cases of cases and reviews pathology and treatment.
48. Kip PC, Peimer CA. Release of the sixth dorsal compartment. *J Hand Surg Am.* 1994;19(4):599-601.
49. Bishop AT, Gabel G, Carmichael SW. Flexor carpi radialis tendinitis. Part I: operative anatomy. *J Bone Joint Surg Am.* 1994;76A:1009-1014
50. Gabel G, Bishop AT, Wood MB. Flexor carpi radialis tendinitis. Part II: [illegible]

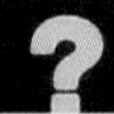

QUESTIONS

1. **A 50-year-old woman presents to your office 6 months after undergoing first dorsal compartment release performed by another surgeon. She reports no improvement in her pain postoperatively. She still has significant discomfort with ulnar deviation of the wrist and a positive Finkelstein test. There is no Tinel sign present at the surgical site, and her axial grind test is negative. She has no history of recent trauma. You decide to bring her back to the operating room for repeat exploration. Intraoperatively, what are you likely to discover at the time of repeat surgery?**

   a. Scaphoid fracture
   b. Injury to the radial dorsal sensory nerve
   c. Radial artery injury
   d. An unreleased subcompartment containing the EPB tendone.
   e. First CMC arthritis

2. **Common tendinopathies in the upper extremity typically have what histopathological feature?**

   a. Acute inflammation with neutrophil and mast cell predominance
   b. Acute inflammation with presence of fibroblasts
   c. Chronic inflammatory changes with predominance of neutrophil infiltration
   d. Chronic inflammatory changes with a T-cell mediated response
   e. Mucoid degeneration and fibrosis

3. **A 55-year-old man presents with pain near the lateral epicondyle, which is exacerbated by activities requiring wrist extension. He does not recall a traumatic injury to this extremity. What is the natural history of most patients with lateral epicondylitis?**

   a. Waxing and waning symptoms, with general progression and worsening of disease over time
   b. Progression to radiocapitellar arthritis and increasing elbow dysfunction
   c. Improvement in symptoms over time without surgical intervention
   d. Requirement for surgical debridement to ameliorate symptoms
   e. Involvement of the radial tunnel with sensory and motor changes in the radial nerve distribution

4. **A 59-year-old nondiabetic patient presents with triggering of her left ring finger. After discussion, she elects to receive a corticosteroid injection near the A1 pulley. The success rate of initial corticosteroid injections for treatment of trigger finger (stenosis tenosynovitis) is closest to:**

   a. 10% to 20%
   b. 20% to 30%
   c. 30% to 40%
   d. 60% to 70%
   e. 90% to 100%

5. **Percutaneous trigger release may have the highest rate of iatrogenic nerve injury in which of the digits?**

   a. Thumb
   b. Index finger
   c. Middle finger
   d. Ring finger
   e. Small finger

1. **Answer: d.** Patients with de Quervain disease have a higher incidence of a subcompartment for the EPB tendon compared with a group of random cadaver wrists. It is important to evaluate for this subcompartment when performing a first dorsal compartment release to ensure adequate EPB release. The multiple slips of APL can be confused for both the EPB and APL.

2. **Answer: d.** The histopathology of most tendinopathies of the upper extremity is one of degenerative change and fibrosis, not inflammatory change. This is a common misconception among many providers and patients. This is particularly true of lateral epicondylitis and de Quervain disease. For this reason, treatment generally should not be directed toward decreasing inflammation alone.

3. **Answer: c.** Lateral epicondylitis is a common cause of lateral arm pain. Many treatments have been described including splinting, injections, and surgery. Lateral epicondylitis appears to be a self-limiting condition in most patients and usually resolves in between 12 and 18 months. Most patients with lateral epicondylitis do not undergo surgery. Radial tunnel syndrome is a distinct pathologic entity with a similar anatomic location of discomfort.

4. **Answer: d.** Steroid injections for trigger finger are a common form of treatment. Injections are typically 60% to 70% effective in improving symptoms but are usually less successful in patients with diabetes. Patients should be counseled about the effectiveness of injection and all other treatment modalities.

5. **Answer: a.** The radial digital nerve of the thumb crosses the MCP flexion crease and is particularly vulnerable to injury during percutaneous trigger release or open surgical release.[43] It is located approximately 2 mm deep to the dermis, and approximately 1 mm volar to the sesamoid bone. Surgeons must understand the pathway of the nerve before proceeding with percutaneous or open release.

CHAPTER 79

Principles and Applications of Tendon Transfers

Michael S. Gart and Jason H. Ko

KEY POINTS

- Before considering tendon transfer surgery, the soft tissue bed must be stabilized; all fractures must be fixated; and passive joint motion should be maximized.
- When possible, protective sensation should be restored prior to tendon transfer.
- An appropriate muscle for transfer is one that is expendable, of appropriate strength and excursion, under volitional control, and preferably synergistic with the recipient muscle's previous function.
- Tendon transfers for radial nerve palsy aim to restore wrist, finger, and thumb extension.
- Tendon transfers for low median nerve injury aim to restore thumb opposition; high median nerve injuries will also lack flexion of the index and long fingers and the thumb interphalangeal (IP) joint.
- Tendon transfers for ulnar nerve injury aim to restore thumb adduction (pinch) and correct clawing for coordinated digital grasp.

Damage to one of the three major peripheral nerves of the upper extremity may result in devastating functional losses and sensory deficits. Tendon transfers can restore many of the functional deficits, albeit without normal strength or coordination. A tendon transfer involves releasing the distal insertion of a functional muscle tendon unit and reinserting it into the tendon of a nonfunctional muscle to recreate its lost action. Owing to the redundant actions of many upper extremity muscles, carefully selected tendon transfers can restore fundamental hand and wrist movements with minimal or no functional sacrifice. It is important to remember, however, that though tendon transfers can reestablish function, they cannot replace a muscle that is damaged or lost; that is, they should not be expected to restore completely normal function and coordination.

Pertinent patient history includes the nature of injury, time from injury, current functional status, and goals of treatment. The time elapsed from injury is critical because this helps to determine the treatment options available to the patient. Nerve transfers are performed with increasing frequency following peripheral nerve injury but are ideally performed within the first 6 months after nerve injury to target muscle reinnervation before motor endplate degeneration at approximately 18 months. Tendon transfers, however, can be performed at any time after a nerve injury. Deciding whether to perform nerve transfers versus tendon transfers depends on the timing, the clinical situation, and the surgeon's discretion. Preoperative planning includes a thorough motor and sensory examination to determine the patient's functional deficits and available muscles for transfer. If the examination is unclear, or if the patient demonstrates variable innervation patterns, electromyography may be useful to determine available donor muscles.

Although many *classic* sets of tendon transfers have been described for specific nerve injuries, a thorough understanding of the principles of tendon transfer surgery will allow the hand surgeon to develop a comprehensive treatment plan for any combination of functional deficits. General indications for tendon transfer include restoring function lost by major central or peripheral nerve injury, posttraumatic reconstruction, and balancing muscle forces in patients affected by neurologic or rheumatologic conditions.[1] Here, we outline the approach to treatment of high and low radial, median, and ulnar nerve palsies, although these same principles can be applied in the posttraumatic, rheumatologic, or neurologic patient.

PRINCIPLES OF TENDON TRANSFERS

The principles of successful tendon transfer surgery have been elucidated over time by some of the pioneers of hand surgery and are briefly outlined here.[2] Strict adherence to these principles will maximize the chances for a successful surgical outcome.

Timing of Surgery

In general, provided the patient's passive range of motion is maintained and available donor muscles are kept strong, tendon transfer surgery is not time dependent. Tendon transfers can broadly be divided into *early* and *late*, depending on the prognosis for spontaneous recovery. Early tendon transfers are performed within weeks of injury, often in combination with nerve exploration or repair, and act as an *internal splint*, whereas the more proximal nerve injury has time to recover. Most often, these are performed in the setting of radial nerve injury to maintain wrist extension and place the hand and fingers into a more functional position. Such transfers can be performed in an end-to-side fashion, substituting for the paralyzed muscle until it is reinnervated. If reinnervation is partial, the transferred tendon can augment its function; if reinnervation fails to occur, the transfer can also act as a permanent solution.

The timing of late tendon transfers varies widely among surgeons and institutions but generally takes place 6 to 18 months following injury. Previous work has established a nerve regeneration rate of approximately 1 mm/day or 1 in/month; therefore, an expected timeframe for functional recovery can be established and used to determine the prognosis for recovery. During this period of observation, it is critical that the therapist utilize orthoses to maintain the limb in a functional position and prevent or treat any soft tissue contractures. Motor endplate degeneration is considered complete and irreversible by 18 months postinjury. Nerve transfers are increasingly being used to treat nerve injuries in the critical time window before motor endplates degenerate; however, this topic is beyond the scope of this chapter and readers are referred to Chapter 71 for further details. Beyond 18 months, tendon transfers remain the only option to restore function.

Protective Sensation

The loss of sensation that accompanies injury to the radial, median, or ulnar nerves cannot be fully restored, but visual input can help to accommodate these sensory losses. Visual feedback, however, is not helpful unless the hand is in the direct line of sight and is lost when searching for an item in a bag or pocket, or in darkness. Therefore, with critical sensory losses, sensation should be restored prior to tendon transfer whenever possible. A minimum goal should be to achieve protective sensation, without which the brain will tend to exclude the insensate limb or digit(s) from functional activities, limiting the utility of the transfer and the functional outcomes of surgery.[3] A number of sensory nerve transfer techniques have been described to restore sensation in the setting of peripheral nerve injury.[4–6] In the case of radial nerve injury, the area of sensory loss is not critical to hand function, so tendon transfers can yield excellent results in the absence of sensory recovery.

Supple Joints

Tendon transfers rely on adequate passive mobility of the joints they act across to effectively exert force. A good rule of thumb is that the active range of motion across a joint following a tendon transfer will never exceed its preoperative passive range of motion. To that end, passive mobility must be maximized prior to tendon transfer. Notably, if a joint contracture that requires surgical release is present, this must be carried out in a staged fashion, separate from any tendon transfers across that joint. The postoperative protocols following contracture release and tendon transfer are diametrically opposed—early, aggressive range of motion is paramount to maintaining the intraoperative gains from joint contracture release, and tendon transfers must be immobilized to allow for sufficient healing. As mentioned above, early involvement of a hand therapist can help to prevent or treat contractures following injury.

Tissue Equilibrium

Tendon transfers should be avoided until all fractures are united and soft tissue equilibrium has been achieved. *Soft tissue equilibrium*, a term coined by Steindler,[7] implies the resolution of any open wounds and tissue induration, supple joints, and scar maturity. Transferred tendons will only glide well if they are routed through a soft tissue bed that is healthy, well vascularized, and free of significant scar burden. If significant scar burden remains or the soft tissues are unstable, local or distant flaps may be necessary to obtain a healthy bed prior to embarking on tendon transfer surgery. In the areas of planned tendon reconstruction or transfer, flaps can be kept slightly thicker to allow passage of the tendons through the subcutaneous fat.[8] In addition, at the time of surgery, atraumatic techniques should be used to minimize the formation of new scar and incisions should be carefully planned such that they do not lie directly over a tenorrhaphy site.[9,10]

One Tendon, One Function

A single transferred tendon should not be used to perform two distinct active functions, or it will preferentially exert a greater force on whatever inset is under greater tension.[11] However, transfers can be inset to multiple tendons that perform the same function (e.g., Flexor carpi radialis [FCR] to the extensor digitorum communis [EDC] of all four fingers) to allow simultaneous movements across multiple joints but without individual control. Similarly, a single tendon transfer can perform one active function combined with different passive functions as in the case of extensor carpi radialis longus (ECRL) transfers to the lateral bands of all four digits, actively flexing the metacarpophalangeal (MCP) joints while passively extending the IP joints.

Straight Line of Pull

A donor muscle-tendon unit should be routed to its recipient tendon in the straightest line possible, as a change in direction of 40° will result in a clinically significant loss of force.[12] Furthermore, the transfer will migrate over time to adapt a straight line of pull, which may result in diminished function. A straight line of pull is more easily accomplished in end-to-end tendon transfers because the recipient tendon is also divided and can be rerouted to *meet* the donor in a more favorable position. In some instances, this is not possible (e.g., flexor digitorum superficialis [FDS] opponensplasty), in which case the transfer must be routed through a smooth and robust pulley which will not migrate over time.

Surgical Considerations for Tendon Transfers

In general, incisions for tendon transfer procedures should be planned such that no incision lies directly over a tenorrhaphy site. When mobilizing muscles for transfer, care must be taken to avoid damage to their neurovascular pedicles. Traditionally, a Pulvertaft weave has been used for tendon transfers, but many alternatives have been described to reduce the bulk of the tenorrhaphy or increase its strength.[13–17] Though some techniques have demonstrated increased strength in biomechanical studies,[14,16] no single one has demonstrated clinical superiority, and surgeon preference varies widely.

SELECTING APPROPRIATE DONOR MUSCLES FOR TRANSFER

There are several principles that guide the selection of appropriate donor muscle-tendon units, all of which aim to maximize functional gains while minimizing donor-site morbidity. Expendable muscles of adequate strength and excursion that are synergistic with the function to be replaced make for optimal donor selections.

Expendable Donor

First and foremost, transfer of a donor muscle must provide more function than it sacrifices. Ideally, donor muscles should not perform essential functions or should have a redundant muscle that performs the same function so that no functional loss is observed following transfer. A general guiding principle is to leave at least one wrist flexor, one wrist extensor, and one extrinsic flexor and extensor to each digit intact.[1]

Adequate Strength and Control

The muscle to be transferred should be free of spasticity with good volitional control and, ideally, an independent function. Good examples of muscles with independent function are the FDS and extensor indicis proprius (EIP). Independent function may simplify the postoperative rehabilitation process from a cortical plasticity standpoint.

The amount of strength necessary in a transferred tendon depends largely on the function it is intended to replace. *Power* transfers require a strong donor muscle to produce significant force (e.g., grasp and pinch), whereas *positional* transfers do not require strength beyond what is necessary to reposition the hand or wrist (e.g., digital extension and opposition). In 1981, Brand published an exhaustive inventory of relative muscle strengths for the purposes of planning tendon transfers in the upper extremity.[18] A donor muscle must be of adequate strength to perform its new function in an altered position but not so strong that it overpowers its new antagonists. Transfer of a muscle to a new location typically results in a loss of one grade of strength on the Medical Research Council (MRC) scale; therefore, muscles that have been previously injured or denervated should only be used if they have recovered normal or near-normal strength. The relative strengths of common donor and recipient muscles in the forearm are presented in **Table 79.1**.

Excursion

The amplitude of excursion of a donor muscle is directly proportional to the length of its individual muscle fibers.[9,19] A practical summary of tendon excursions was proposed by Boyes's 3-5-7 rule.[20] Flexors and extensors of the wrist have an average excursion of approximately 3 cm (33 mm); the extensors of the digits (EDC and extensor pollicis longus [EPL]) have an average of 5 cm; and digital flexors have 7 cm of excursion. The excursion of some muscles can be increased through proximal dissection of the muscle belly, particularly in the case of a brachioradialis (BR) transfer.

In order to restore a full active range of motion, the amplitude of the donor and recipient tendons must be closely matched. When this is not possible (e.g., FCR to EDC transfer), the excursion of the transfer can be increased by 2 to 3 cm through the tenodesis effect of wrist flexion or extension. Because of the reliance on wrist motion for enhancing tendon excursion through tenodesis, wrist fusion should be avoided at all costs in these patients. If wrist fusion is planned, its implications must be fully considered before surgery.

TABLE 79.1. WORK CAPACITY OF DONOR AND RECIPIENT MUSCLES IN THE FOREARM

Muscle	Work Capacity (m-kg)
Donor	
Brachioradialis (BR)	1.9
Pronator teres (PT)	1.2
Flexor carpi radialis (FCR)	0.8
Flexor carpi ulnaris (FCU)	2.0
Palmaris longus (PL)	0.1
Flexor digitorum superficialis (FDS)	4.8
Flexor digitorum profundus (FDP)	4.5
Flexor pollicis longus (FPL)	1.2
Recipient	
Extensor carpi radialis longus (EPL)	0.1
Abductor pollicis longus (APL)	0.1
Extensor pollicis brevis (EPB)	0.1
Extensor digitorum communis (EDC)	1.7
Extensor indicis proprius (EIP)	0.5
Extensor carpi radialis longus (ECRL)	1.1
Extensor carpi radialis brevis (ECRB)	0.9
Extensor carpi ulnaris (ECU)	1.1

Synergy

Synergy in tendon transfer surgery refers to the preferential use of donor muscles that are in phase with their recipient. For example, wrist flexion and digital extension typically occur simultaneously, as do wrist extension and finger flexion. On this basis, it is believed that patients can more easily adapt to transfers that capitalize on these relationships (e.g., wrist flexor for finger extension or wrist extensor for finger flexion). In general, in-phase transfers are preferred but are not always possible. One exception to this is the FDS tendons, which have a high degree of independent cortical control and are easily retrained for a variety of in-phase and out-of-phase movements. Some authors have advocated that synergy is not necessary and that any transfer that performs an advantageous function can be relearned, particularly in young children.[21,22] Standard teaching advocates the use of synergistic muscles when possible.

TENDON TRANSFERS FOR SPECIFIC NERVE PALSIES

Radial Nerve Palsy

Anatomy

As it travels from proximal to distal, the radial nerve innervates the triceps, brachialis, BR, and ECRL before bifurcating into the superficial radial nerve and posterior interosseous nerve (PIN). Innervation to the extensor carpi radialis brevis (ECRB) is variable and can occur proximal to the bifurcation from the main radial nerve or from the PIN distal to the bifurcation. The superficial radial nerve carries sensory fibers only to provide cutaneous innervation over the dorsal and radial aspects of the hand, including the thumb, index, middle, and ring fingers. The PIN is primarily a motor nerve that provides innervation to the supinator, the extensor carpi ulnaris (ECU), the extrinsic extensors of the digits (EIP, EDC, extensor digiti quinti [EDQ]), the extrinsic thumb extensors (EPL and extensor pollicis brevis [EPB]), and the abductor pollicis longus (APL).

Palsies of the radial nerve are classified as high or low, with high palsies occurring above the elbow, proximal to the innervation of the wrist extensors. Depending on the exact location and nature of the injury, the sensory component of the radial nerve may also be lost. However, this is not a critical sensory loss and typically does not require treatment. The functional requirements for a patient with irreparable radial nerve injury include the following:

- Wrist extension (high palsy only)
- MCP joint extension (IP joint extension maintained by intrinsics)
- Thumb extension and palmar abduction

The main clinical distinction between high and low radial nerve palsy is the presence or absence of wrist extension. Patients with high palsy will require active wrist extension to be restored, whereas those with a low palsy will not. Both high and low palsies will require digital extension at the MCP joint and thumb extension/abduction. The intrinsic muscles of the hand will continue to provide extension at the IP joints of the fingers, and supination is maintained by the biceps brachii muscle.

Tendon Transfers for Radial Nerve Palsy

Jones is credited as the main innovator of radial nerve tendon transfers and described two distinct sets of transfers that have become *classic*[23] (**Table 79.2**). The pronator teres (PT) is transferred to the ECRB muscle, which inserts centrally on the base of the third metacarpal, producing wrist extension without radial or ulnar deviation. The flexor carpi ulnaris (FCU) is used to restore digital extension, as wrist flexion and digital extension are synergistic movements. The palmaris longus (PL) is transferred to the EPL, which is rerouted volarly to provide more palmar abduction. If the PL is absent, a slip of the ring finger FDS tendon can be transferred to the EPL. Over time, the use of the PT to restore active wrist extension has become accepted as the standard of care, but much debate has surrounded the best combination of transfers to restore digital extension and thumb extension/abduction.

It should be noted that several modifications of this standard set exist, each bearing the name of the author who described them. In France, Merle d'Aubigné described a slight modification, which includes PT to ECRB, FCU to EDC and EPL, and PL to EPB and APL. Starr originally described use of the FCR instead of the FCU to restore digital extension.[24] Boyes and Brand advocated using the FCR instead of the FCU, arguing that the FCU was more important to wrist flexion, was too strong, and did not provide adequate excursion.[9,20,25] Long-term results, however, have failed to support a functional deficit

TABLE 79.2. COMMON SETS OF TENDON TRANSFERS FOR RADIAL NERVE PALSY

Jones Transfer
■ Pronator teres (PT) to extensor carpi radialis brevis (ECRB)
■ Flexor carpi ulnaris to extensor digitorum communis (EDC)
■ Palmaris longus to extensor pollicis longus (EPL)
Flexor Carpi Radialis (FCR) (Brand, Starr) Transfer
■ PT to ECRB
■ FCR to EDC
■ Palmaris longus to EPL
Superficialis (Boyes) Transfer
■ PT to ECRB and extensor carpi radialis longus
■ FCR to abductor pollicis longus and extensor pollicis brevis
■ Flexor digitorum superficialis of long finger (FDS-III) to EDC
■ Flexor digitorum superficialis of ring finger (FDS-IV) to EPL and extensor indicis proprius

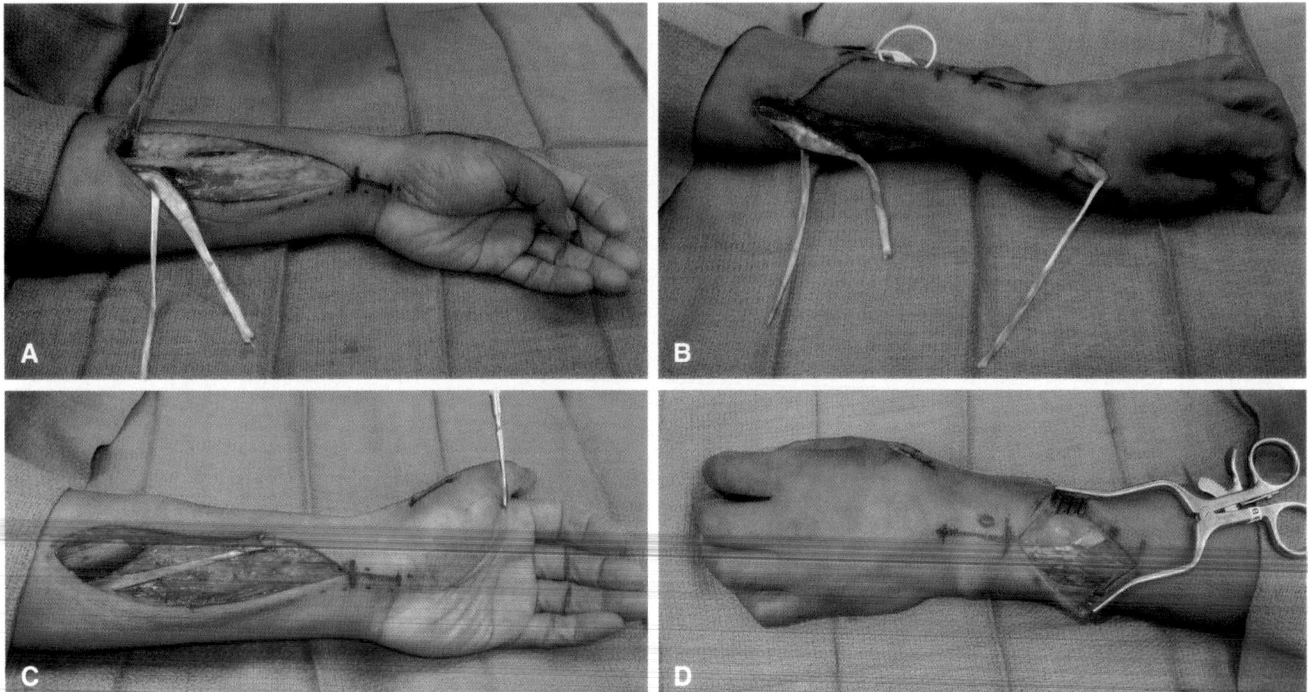

FIGURE 79.1. Median to radial nerve tendon transfers to restore wrist and digit extension. **A.** Pronator teres (PT), flexor carpi radialis (FCR), and palmaris longus (PL) dissected and isolated for transfer. **B.** PT, FCR, PL, and extensor pollicis longus tendons divided before transfer. **C.** PT to extensor carpi radialis brevis and PL to extensor pollicis longus following transfer. **D.** FCR to extensor digitorum communis following transfer.

following FCU transfer[26] (see Table 79.2). One additional argument favoring the FCR is that in radial nerve palsy, the FCU is the only remaining ulnar-sided wrist motor, and its sacrifice eliminates active ulnar deviation (*dart-thrower's* motion), which is increasingly being recognized as an important functional movement. The FCR set of tendon transfers is shown in Figures 79.1 and 79.2.

Boyes later argued that neither wrist flexor was suitable to restore digital extension, as their limited excursion (33 mm) leaves them reliant on tenodesis to fully extend the digits, and simultaneous wrist and finger extension is not possible.[25] Instead, he suggested use of the FDS tendons routed through the interosseous membrane in the Boyes transfer (see Table 79.2).

Each set of radial nerve tendon transfers has been shown in the literature to produce good results, and no head-to-head comparisons exist to suggest the superiority of one over another. The choice of transfers depends largely on surgeon preference and patient specific considerations (i.e., concomitant median or ulnar nerve injury, previous wrist fusion, etc.).

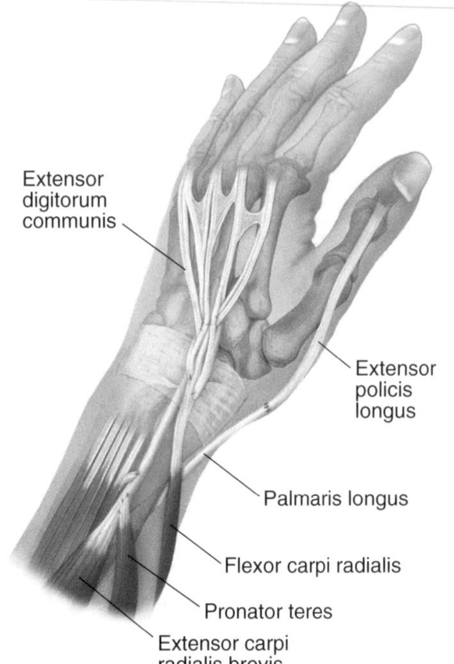

FIGURE 79.2. FCR tendon transfer set consisting of flexor carpi radialis to extensor digitorum communis, pronator teres to extensor carpi radialis brevis, and palmaris longus to extensor pollicis longus.

Median Nerve Palsy

Anatomy

The median nerve enters the forearm between the two heads of the PT, innervating it along with the FDS, FCR, and PL before giving off the anterior interosseous nerve approximately 6 to 8 cm distal to the medial epicondyle. The anterior interosseous nerve is primarily a motor nerve, providing innervation to the flexor pollicis longus (FPL) and flexor digitorum profundus (FDP) to the index and long finger, and terminates as the innervation to the pronator quadratus. The median nerve continues distally and gives off the palmar cutaneous branch, which supplies sensation to the thenar eminence, before entering the carpal tunnel. The median nerve provides sensation to the palmar surfaces of the thumb, index, and long fingers, as well as the radial half of the ring finger. The recurrent motor branch, the distal motor branch of the median nerve, innervates the thenar musculature—the abductor pollicis brevis (APB), the superficial head of the flexor pollicis brevis (FPB), and the opponens pollicis. The motor innervation of the index and long finger lumbricals arises off of their respective common digital nerves.

The functional deficits following median nerve injury depend on the level of the lesion. A high median nerve palsy will manifest with a loss of forearm pronation, index and long finger flexion, thumb IP joint flexion, and thumb opposition. These deficits are due to paralysis of the PT and pronator quadratus, all four FDS muscles, the FDP muscles to the index and long fingers, the FPL, and the thenar intrinsic musculature, respectively. In our experience, FDP function to the long finger is often maintained, presumably by an ulnar nerve contribution. Therefore, the functions that must be restored in median nerve palsy are the following:

- Thumb opposition
- Thumb IP joint flexion (high palsy only)
- Index and long finger DIP and PIP joint flexion (high palsy only)

Thumb opposition is a complex movement which consists of flexion at the MCP joint, palmar abduction, and pronation. Following median nerve injury, MCP joint flexion may be maintained by the ulnar-innervated deep head of the FPB. A patient with a unilateral, nondominant loss of opposition may compensate quite well with MCP joint flexion alone and should be counseled appropriately before attempting surgery to improve function.

In addition to the motor deficits seen with median nerve palsy, the absence of sensation over the thumb, index, long, and radial half of the ring finger is disabling. Bertelli has described sensory transfers in an attempt to restore sensation in high median nerve injuries.[5]

Tendon Transfers for Median Nerve Palsy

Three thenar intrinsic muscles contribute to the complex motion of thumb opposition: the opponens pollicis, the APB, and the FPB. Due to its unique position and mechanical advantages, the APB is the most important muscle in thumb opposition.[27] As such, the ideal vector for an opposition transfer should parallel this muscle, from the pisiform to the insertion of the APB on the abductor tubercle at the base of the thumb proximal phalanx.[27] This insertion site produces the best combination of MCP joint flexion, pronation, and palmar abduction. A pulley is often required to create the proper vector of pull. A variety of pulleys have been described, including loops of the FCU tendon at or near its insertion on the pisiform, the palmar aponeurosis, transverse carpal ligament, and the FCU tendon itself. There are four commonly used, reliable options for restoring opposition (*opponensplasty*), each with advantages and disadvantages (Table 79.3).

Transfer of the PL tendon with an extension of palmar aponeurosis, also known as the Camitz transfer, is often utilized in patients with severe carpal tunnel syndrome and advanced thenar atrophy.[28] The primary advantages of this transfer are the ease of harvest, as it lies in the same surgical field as a carpal tunnel release, and the lack of functional deficit. However, the tendon may be damaged in traumatic median nerve palsy owing to its superficial location; it is a weak muscle; and its vector of pull is not ideal for producing true opposition. It is, however, useful in providing palmar abduction in patients with severe thenar atrophy to aid in grasp.

The FDS opponensplasty was originally described in 1938 by Royle.[29] This transfer typically involves dividing the ring finger FDS tendon distally—in part or whole—and retrieving it through the carpal tunnel before rerouting it to the APB insertion. The original description, which passed the tendon through the sheath of the FPL was later modified by Bunnell, who proposed rerouting the tendon through a pulley created by a strip of FCU tendon to improve its vector of pull.[30] Thompson later advocated tunneling the tendon subcutaneously to reach the thumb.[31] The primary disadvantage of the FDS opponensplasty is that it can only be used when the median nerve injury has occurred distal to the innervation of the FDS.

The abductor digiti minimi (ADM) can be transferred from the hypothenar musculature, providing an excellent vector for opposition and restoring muscular bulk to the thenar eminence (Figure 79.3). This transfer is synergistic to opposition and provides good strength and excursion but has limited ability to produce palmar abduction. This technique, known as the Huber transfer, has been relegated mostly to children with hypoplastic thumb deformity or when other options are not available. The ADM muscle belly provides improved cosmetic appearance of the thenar region in children with hypoplastic thumb deformity, which is one benefit despite its functional limitations.

Lastly, the EIP opponensplasty is an excellent option that can be used in high or low median nerve palsy and, when routed around the ulnar aspect of the wrist, provides an ideal vector for opposition (Figure 79.4). Although the EIP is not a strong muscle, it is sufficient to position the thumb in opposition. This transfer is advantageous

TABLE 79.3. COMMON SETS OF TENDON TRANSFERS FOR MEDIAN NERVE PALSY

Opponensplasty
Palmaris longus transfer (Camitz procedure)
Flexor digitorum superficialis (FDS) ring opponensplasty (Royle-Thompson/Bunnell)
Extensor indicis proprius (EIP) opponensplasty (Zancolli, Burkhalter)
Abductor digiti minimi transfer (Huber transfer)
High Median Nerve Palsy
Smith and Hastings
EIP to abductor pollicis brevis
Brachioradialis (BR) to flexor pollicis longus (FPL) (thumb IP arthrodesis for stability)
Flexor digitorum profundus (FDP) tenodesis (side to side, powered by ulnar)
Burkhalter
EIP to abductor pollicis brevis
BR to FPL
Extensor carpi radialis longus (ECRL) to FDP (index and long)
Boyes
Extensor carpi ulnaris with graft to thumb proximal phalanx
BR to FDP (index and long)
ECRL or extensor carpi radialis brevis to flexor pollicis longus (FPL)
Brand
Extensor carpi ulnaris with graft to thumb proximal phalanx
FDP tenodesis
ECRL to FPL
Flexor carpi ulnaris split to flexor carpi radialis and flexor carpi ulnaris for wrist balance

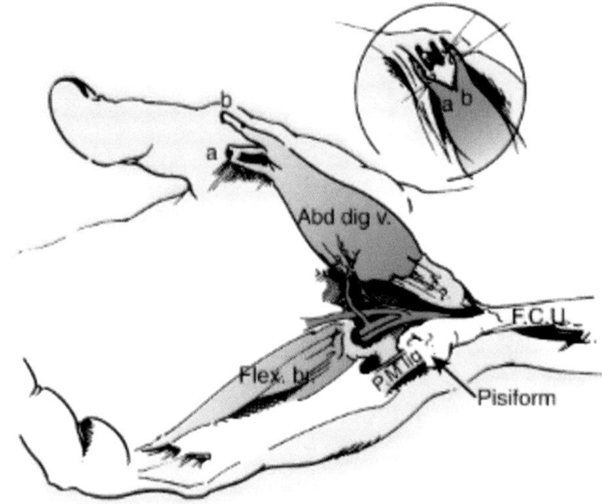

FIGURE 79.3. Huber transfer. The abductor digiti minimi muscle is isolated on its neurovascular pedicle and freed from its attachments to the pisiform and the hypothenar eminence. It is rotated across the palm and tunneled subcutaneously to the abductor tubercle or abductor pollicis brevis tendon.

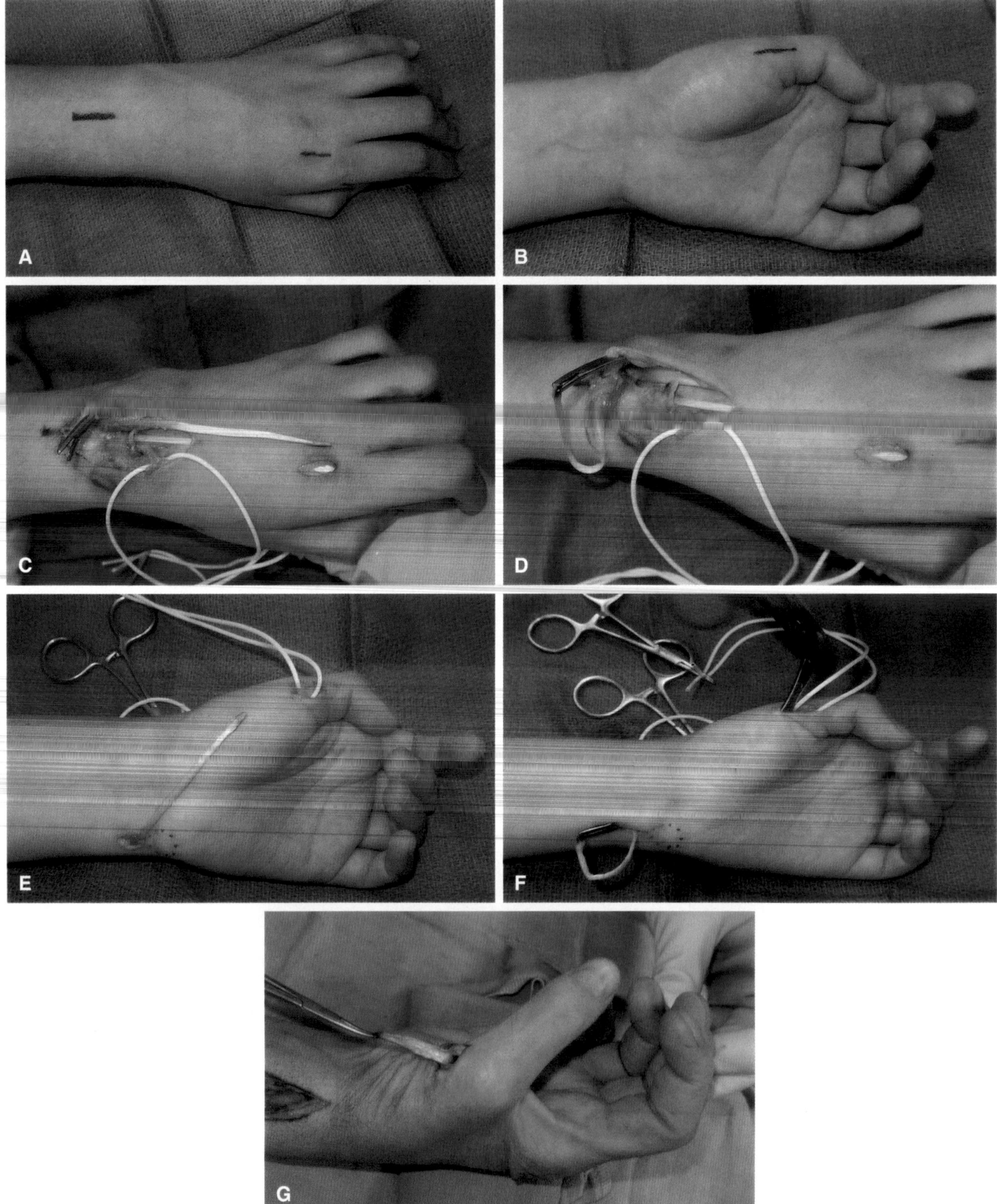

FIGURE 79.4. Extensor indicis proprius (EIP) opponensplasty. **A,B.** Incision markings for harvest of EIP tendon and tenorrhaphy site at the abductor pollicis brevis tendon. **C.** EIP tendon is divided over the metacarpophalangeal joint. **D.** EIP is routed subcutaneously around the ulnar border of the hand. **E.** Planned path of the tendon transfer (note the position of the pisiform marked with dotted line). **F.** Tendon passed subcutaneously to the abductor pollicis brevis tendon using a curved tendon passer. **G.** EIP tendon transferred to the APB to hold the thumb in abduction (photograph of different patient).

due to its ease of harvest, availability in high and low palsies, and minimal functional deficit. In high median nerve palsy, the EIP transfer is most commonly used.

With high median nerve palsy, all of the musculature of the forearm flexor compartment, with the exception of the ulnar-innervated FCU and FDP to the ring and small fingers, are paralyzed. Therefore, many of the *workhorse muscles* for tendon transfer (i.e., FDS, FCR, PL) are unavailable. Only the EIP opponensplasty and Huber transfer are available, and the EIP is typically selected. In addition to restoring opposition, these patients must also regain flexion of the index and long fingers as well as the IP joint of the thumb. In our experience, FDP function to the long finger is often preserved, although may be weak, presumably due to cross-innervation by the ulnar nerve. The only muscles remaining for restoring these functions are the ECU, BR, and ECRL. Some reports of ECU harvest have demonstrated radial deviation wrist deformities in these patients and severe grip weakness.[32] Therefore, the BR is typically selected to restore FPL function, and the ECRL is used for index finger flexion when needed. In most instances, however, adequate index and long finger flexion can be achieved with a side-to-side transfer to the functioning ring and small finger profundus tendons.

The lack of forearm pronation resulting from denervation of the PT and pronator quadratus does not always require treatment, as shoulder abduction can position the forearm in a *pronated* position. If this deficit is a problem, or if shoulder function is abnormal, a biceps rerouting can be performed, which converts the biceps from a supinator into a pronator.[33]

Ulnar Nerve Palsy

Anatomy

Unlike the median and radial nerves, the ulnar nerve has very few motor branches proximal to the hand, innervating only the FCU and the FDP muscles to the ring and small fingers in the proximal forearm. Approximately 7 to 8 cm proximal to the wrist, the ulnar nerve gives off the dorsal sensory branch, providing cutaneous innervation to the dorsal and ulnar hand. The ulnar nerve continues through the Guyon canal at the volar-ulnar wrist, where it again branches into sensory and motor components. At this level, the ulnar nerve provides motor innervation to the hypothenar muscles, palmaris brevis, all of the interosseous muscles, the lumbricals to the small and ring fingers, and the adductor pollicis. Approximately 80% of the time, the ulnar nerve also innervates the deep head of the FPB. Notably, anomalous innervation patterns (i.e., Martin-Gruber and Riche-Cannieu) are not uncommon, and clinical presentations may vary in these patients.[34,35] In such cases, electromyography may be useful to help determine which muscles are available for transfer.

The ulnar nerve is tremendously important to hand function, and a number of clinical manifestations are seen with ulnar nerve palsies (**Table 79.4**). With resisted pinch, weakness of the first dorsal interosseous muscle and adductor pollicis (AP) will result in thumb IP joint flexion as the FPL attempts to substitute for a weak pinch, known as Froment sign. Intrinsic function can also be evaluated by asking the patient to abduct and adduct the fingers, to cross their index and middle fingers, or to perform the Pitres-Testut test—placing the hand flat on a table with the fingers fully abducted and moving the long finger side to side. The small finger may be abnormally abducted, a finding known as Wartenberg sign, which results from third volar interosseous weakness and the unopposed pull of the EDQ muscle.

Clawing of the digits and loss of coordinated digital flexion is the most disabling aspect of ulnar nerve injury and results from intrinsic muscle paralysis in the presence of functioning extrinsic digital flexors and extensors. Loss of the lumbricals and interossei to the ring and small fingers, which normally function to flex the MCP joints and extend the PIP and DIP joints, results in hyperextension at the MCP due to the unopposed pull of the extrinsic digital extensors. Furthermore, the unopposed pull of the FDP tendon produces

TABLE 79.4. DYNAMIC TENDON TRANSFERS FOR CLAW DEFORMITY CAUSED BY ULNAR NERVE PALSY

Technique	Description	Comments
Dynamic tenodesis ■ Wrist tenodesis (Fowler and Tsuge)	■ Free tendon graft attached to central extensor retinaculum and passed from dorsal to palmar, deep to deep transverse metacarpal ligaments (DTMLs) and inserted into lateral bands	■ Tenodesis loosens with time
Extrinsic finger flexors ■ Flexor digitorum superficialis (modified Stiles-Bunnell)	■ Long finger flexor digitorum superficialis split into four slips, routed through lumbrical canal of each finger volar to the DTMLs, sutured to the lateral band of the extensor apparatus	■ Insertions sites modified several times: □ Lateral bands (Stiles,Bunnell) □ Phalangeal insertion (Burkhalter) □ Pulley insertion (Riordan, Zancolli) □ Interosseous insertion (Zancolli, Palande) ■ PIP extensor lag can occur in donor finger
Finger-level extensors ■ Extensor indicis proprius and extensor digiti minimi (Fowler)	■ Extensor indicis proprius and extensor digiti minimi tendons are transferred to lateral bands	■ May produce excessive tension in extensor mechanism (intrinsic-plus deformity) and reverse metacarpal arch ■ Does not add grip strength
Wrist-level motor transfers ■ Dorsal route extensor carpi radialis brevis (Brand)	■ Extensor carpi radialis brevis lengthened by free tendon graft (split into four tails); passed through intermetacarpal spaces, deep to DTMLs, and attached to radial lateral bands long finger, ring finger, small finger, and ulnar lateral band of index finger	■ Uses free tendons for length (adhesions) ■ Does not improve metacarpal arch or grip strength ■ Extensor carpi radialis longus (ECRL) can also be used
■ Flexor carpi radialis (FCR) (Riordan)	■ FCR is augmented with free tendon graft brought dorsally around the forearm and then routed in similar fashion to dorsal Brand transfer	■ Removes FCR, which is a strong wrist flexor
■ Flexor route ECRL (Brand)	■ Free tendon graft is passed through the carpal tunnel (split into four tails), and ECRL is used as the motor and brought around the forearm to the volar side	■ Uses free tendons for length (adhesions) ■ Requires extensive therapy postoperatively ■ Possible crowding of carpal tunnel can occur

flexion at the DIP and PIP joints, which results in the characteristic claw position: MCP joint hyperextension and IP joint flexion of the ring and small fingers.

An additional and functionally devastating complication of intrinsic muscle paralysis is the loss of coordinated finger flexion. A normal grasp begins with MCP flexion, initiated by the lumbricals which arise from the tendons of the FDP, and is followed by IP joint flexion. With clawing, the lumbricals are nonfunctional, and grasp is initiated by the extrinsic digital flexors. As a result, flexion begins distally at the DIP joint and is often coupled with MCP hyperextension (from the radial nerve), which results in objects being *pushed* out of the hand instead of encircled by the digits.

Patients with high ulnar nerve palsy will experience loss of sensation of the dorsal-ulnar hand, loss of FDP function to the ring and small fingers, and FCU paralysis. Paradoxically, clawing is less severe in high ulnar nerve palsy as the FDP paralysis lessens the flexion forces on the PIP and DIP joints of the ring and small fingers. Although sensory nerve transfers have been described for the dorsal-ulnar hand, these are not routine, as the sensory deficit is not as disabling as that seen with median nerve injuries.

The primary functional losses with ulnar nerve palsy are key pinch and grasp, due to both clawing and loss of coordinated finger flexion. Patients with high ulnar nerve palsy will also lack active DIP joint flexion in the ring and small fingers. Wrist flexion is typically preserved through the FCR, and the functional losses from inability to abduct and adduct the digits are minimal. As previously discussed, the FCU paralysis does not result in demonstrable grip weakness.[26] Therefore, the goals of reconstruction in ulnar nerve palsy are as follows:

- DIP joint flexion in ring and small fingers (high palsy only)
- Thumb adduction (*key pinch*)
- Correct clawing/restored digital flexion

With high ulnar nerve palsy, restoring active DIP joint flexion in the ring and small fingers is easily accomplished with a side-to-side tenodesis of these tendons to the functional FDP tendons of the long finger. This extrinsic transfer should typically be performed before correcting clawing to enable the patient to make a strong, full fist after correcting the intrinsic paralysis. It should be noted that this transfer will worsen clawing due to the pull of the FDP tendons until the intrinsic muscle function can be restored with an intrinsic tendon transfer.

Key pinch is a combination of thumb adduction through the AP and index finger abduction through the first dorsal interosseous muscle. Procedures to restore key pinch (*adductorplasty*) only need to restore thumb adduction as the index finger can be stabilized against the adjacent digits, obviating the need for active index finger abduction. Many donor muscles have been described to restore thumb adduction, including wrist flexors, digital flexors and extensors, and the BR. The ECRB[37] and BR are both commonly used to restore thumb adduction; both must be lengthened with free tendon grafts and passed from dorsal to volar in the third intermetacarpal space, using the second metacarpal as a pulley and orienting the vector of pull in a line parallel to the AP (Figure 79.5). The FDS tendons to the long and ring fingers have also been used for adductorplasty.[38] These are divided distally in the digit, retrieved in the palm, and routed in the retroflexor space to reach the AP insertion. Although the FDS tendons have good independent control and excursion, this vector does not mimic that of the AP as well as the ECRB or BR do. Furthermore, the sacrifice of an FDS tendon may weaken grip in these patients who already suffer from a loss of grip strength and can sometimes lead to PIP joint hyperextension. Importantly, the ring finger FDS must never be sacrificed in a patient with high ulnar nerve palsy, as this will leave them without an extrinsic flexor to the ring finger. Digital extensors, including the EIP, EDC-index, and EDQ have also been described as transfers to restore thumb adduction, but these are often weak motors with suboptimal vectors of pull.

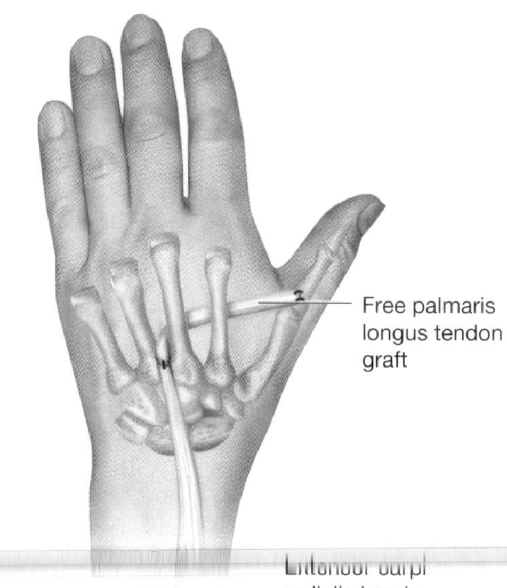

FIGURE 79.5. Extensor carpi radialis brevis adductorplasty. The extensor carpi radialis brevis is extended with a free tendon graft and passed around the third metacarpal (pulley) before inserting into the abductor tubercle or APB tendon.

Physical examination is critical in selecting the appropriate procedure to correct the clawed hand. The Bouvier test involves passively flexing the MCP joints and asking the patient to actively extend the IP joints. If the patient is able to fully extend the IP joints through the extrinsic digital extensors with the MCP joints flexed, the Bouvier test is positive and the clawing is considered simple (static). In these cases, only the MCP joint hyperextension deformity must be corrected. If the extrinsic extensors are unable to extend the IP joints with the MCP joints passively flexed, the Bouvier test is negative and the clawing is considered complex (dynamic). In these cases, the central slip is attenuated, and a tendon transfer must provide IP joint extension in addition to correcting the MCP joint hyperextension deformity.

In the case of simple clawing, several static procedures have demonstrated clinical success in preventing MCP hyperextension, including osseous blocks on the dorsal metacarpal head,[39] volar (Zancolli) MCP joint capsulodesis,[40] and free tendon grafts from the deep intermetacarpal ligament, passed through the lumbrical canal, and secured to the extensor mechanism.[41] Fowler and Tsuge popularized a *dynamic tenodesis* procedure, where a tendon graft is looped through the extensor retinaculum of the wrist, and each end is split in half. The four free ends are then routed along the lumbrical canals and inserted into the lateral bands to provide MCP joint flexion and IP joint extension with wrist flexion[42,43] (Figure 79.6). These procedures are best reserved for patients with a positive Bouvier test (simple clawing).

Transfers of the FDS can be used to correct both simple and complex clawing. In both cases, the tendons are divided distally, retrieved in the palm, and split into four tails that are passed to the fingers via the lumbrical canals (Figure 79.7). If only MCP hyperextension is to be corrected (simple clawing), the transfers can be inserted into the A1 or A2 pulleys[44] or into the proximal phalanx itself[45] (Figure 79.8). If a superficialis transfer must also provide IP joint extension, the modified Stiles-Bunnell procedure describes insertion into the lateral band.[46] It should be noted that in this procedure, sacrifice of the FDS tendon—the primary flexor of the PIP joint—and simultaneous increase in the extension force on the PIP joint by inserting into the lateral bands can increase the risk of PIP

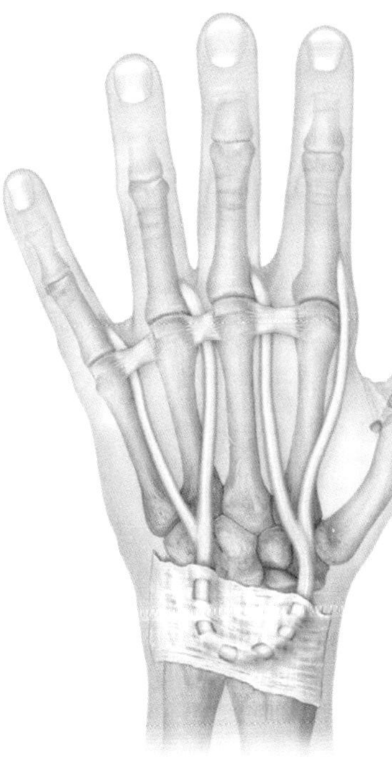

FIGURE 79.6. Dynamic tenodesis for claw hand correction. A free tendon graft is anchored in the extensor retinaculum and each of four slips is passed through the lumbrical canal to insert into the lateral bands.

joint hyperextension and swan neck deformity. This risk can be minimized by suturing one of the distal slips of the FDS remnant across the PIP joint to act as a checkrein to prevent hyperextension or by only performing this procedure in patients with stable joints that cannot be passively hyperextended. The primary drawback to all superficialis transfers is that they may further diminish grip strength.

In an effort to integrate MCP and IP joint flexion while maintaining—or even improving—grip strength, several authors have described transfers utilizing wrist flexors and extensors as donor muscles to correct clawing (Figure 79.9).[47-49] In a similar fashion, these donors are all lengthened with a tendon graft that is split into four tails distally and routed through the lumbrical canals to reach their insertion on the lateral bands. The ECRL, ECRB, FCR, or BR muscles may be used for this transfer, although the wrist extensors provide a higher degree of synergy by coupling wrist extension with grasp. In addition to improving grip strength, the preservation of the FDS tendons in these procedures also minimizes the risk for PIP joint hyperextension deformity.

Tendon Transfers for Combined Palsies and Other Injuries

Patients with combined nerve injuries present a much more difficult problem as the muscles available for transfer become more limited. These patients require an individualized approach that addresses their specific functional priorities. It is often necessary to combine tendon transfers with adjunctive measures, including splinting, tenodesis, nerve transfer, free functional muscle transfer, or selective

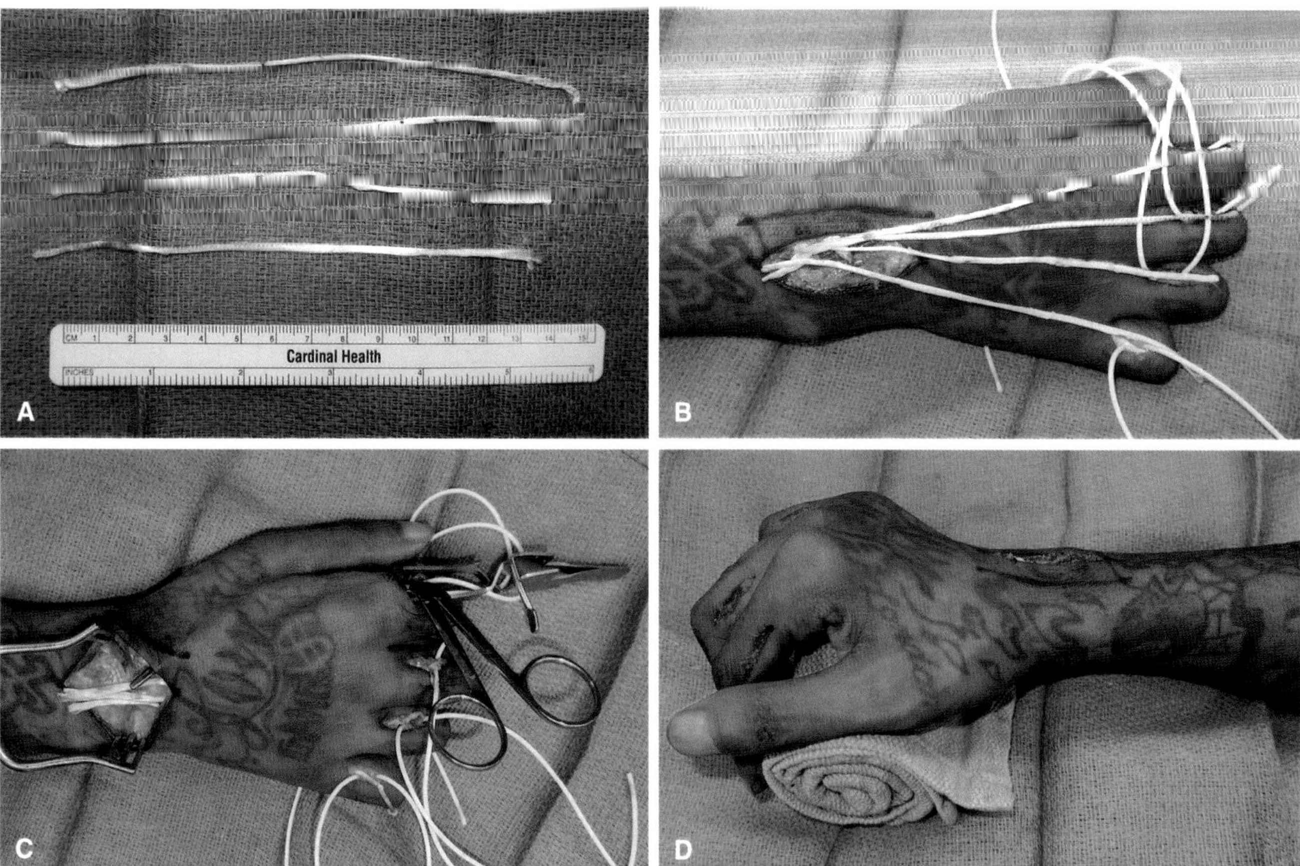

FIGURE 79.7. Brand flexor carpi radialis tendon transfer for ulnar nerve palsy. **A.** A free tendon graft is harvested and divided into four equal slips. **B.** The radial lateral bands are identified and isolated with vessel loops and the free tendon grafts are laid out in the position of the transfer. **C.** A curved tendon passer is used to deliver the tendons through the lumbrical canal of each finger to perform the distal tenorrhaphy first. **D.** The tension of the transfer is set using a rolled towel to simulate a functional grasp position.

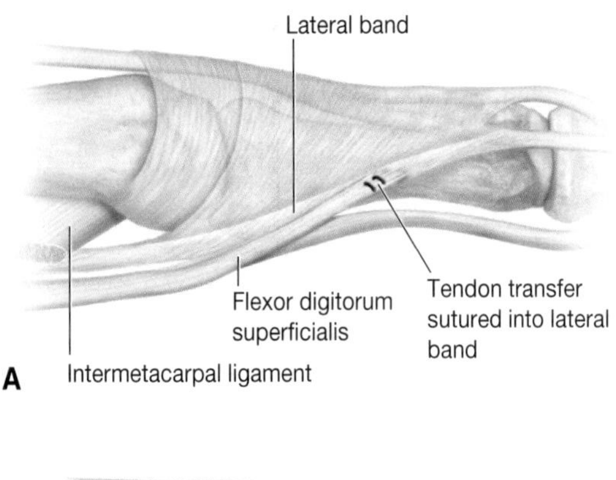

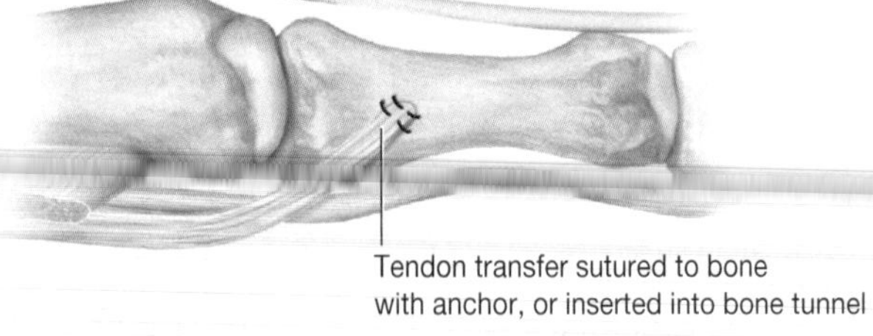

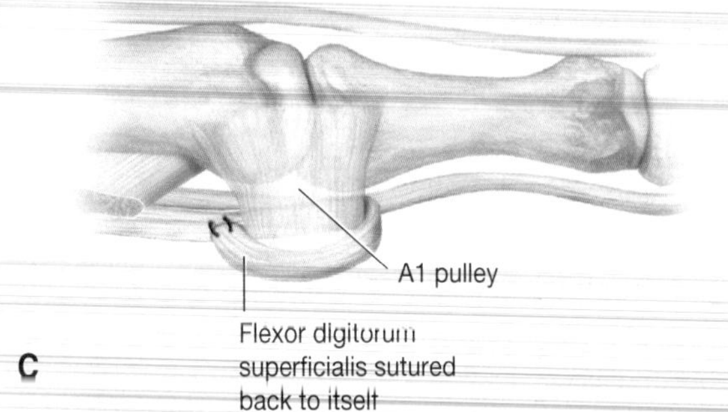

FIGURE 79.8. Classic insertion sites for flexor digitorum superficialis tendon transfers to correct clawing: lateral band **(A)**, proximal phalanx **(B)**, and flexor tendon sheath **(C)**.

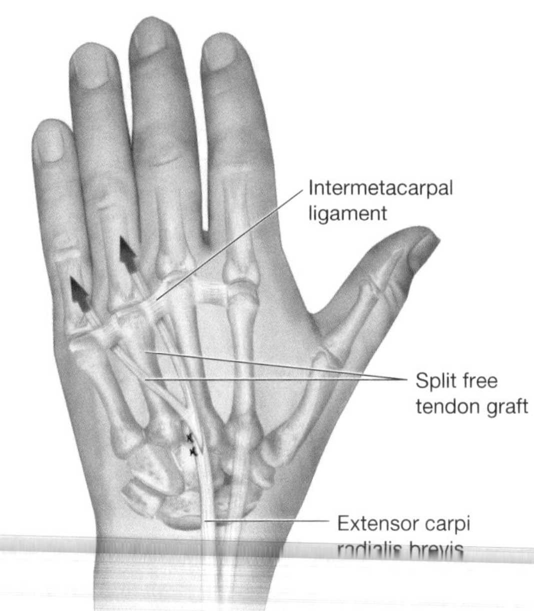

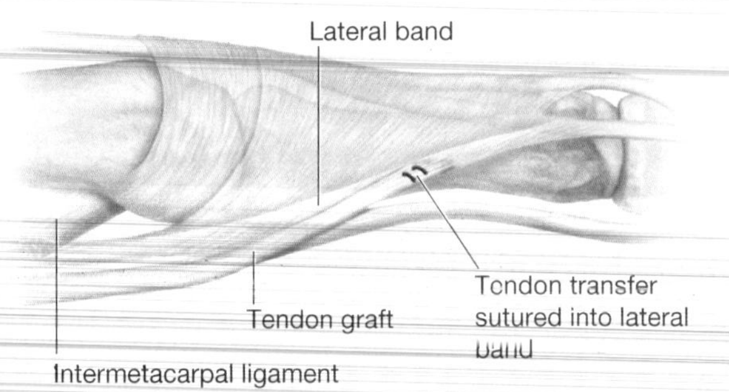

FIGURE 79.9. Transfer of elongated extensor carpi radialis longus to the radial lateral bands of the ring and small fingers for dynamic correction of clawing.

arthrodesis, to improve function in these patients. Tendon transfers can also be used to restore function in patients with brachial plexus injury or tetraplegia, but such procedures are beyond the scope of this chapter. Interested readers are referred to several excellent review articles available on these subjects.[10,50]

POSTOPERATIVE MANAGEMENT

Tendon transfers must be allowed sufficient time to heal before formal therapy can begin. Postoperatively, patients are immobilized in a cast or splint for 4 weeks before transitioning into a removable orthosis, at which time gentle mobilization exercises are initiated. Passive- or active-assisted exercises are continued for an additional 4 weeks, and patients may gradually begin strengthening exercises at 8 weeks postoperative. By 12 weeks, the tendons should be fully healed, and a gradual return to full activity is advocated. The amount of reeducation necessary will depend on several factors, including the timing and nature of injury, age of the patient, specific transfers performed, and patient motivation.

REFERENCES

1. Jones NF, Machado GR. Tendon transfers for radial, median, and ulnar nerve injuries: current surgical techniques. *Clin Plast Surg*. 2011;38(4):621-642.
2. Beasley RW. Principles of tendon transfer. *Orthop Clin North Am*. 1970;1(2):433-438.
3. Wilbur D, Hammert WC. Principles of tendon transfer. *Hand Clin*. 2016;32(3):283-289.
4. Bertelli JA. Distal sensory nerve transfers in lower-type injuries of the brachial plexus. *J Hand Surg*. 2012;37(6):1194-1199.
5. Bertelli JA, Ghizoni MF. Very distal sensory nerve transfers in high median nerve lesions. *J Hand Surg*. 2011;36(3):387-393.
The authors describe the technique of transferring the radial nerve from the dorsal first webspace to restore the thumb and index finger sensation lost in a median nerve injury.
6. Brunelli GA. Sensory nerves transfers. *J Hand Surg (Edinb)*. 2004;29(6):557-562.
7. Steindler A. Reconstruction of the poliomyelitic upper extremity. *Bull Hosp Joint Dis*. 1954;15(1):21-34.
8. Sabapathy SR, Bajantri B. Indications, selection, and use of distant pedicled flap for upper limb reconstruction. *Hand Clin*. 2014;30(2):185-199, vi.
9. Brand PW. Biomechanics of tendon transfer. *Orthop Clin North Am*. 1974;5(2):205-230.
10. Omer GE Jr. Tendon transfers in combined nerve lesions. *Orthop Clin North Am*. 1974;5(2):377-387.
11. Schwarz RJ, Brandsma JW, Giurintano DJ. A review of the biomechanics of intrinsic replacement in ulnar palsy. *J Hand Surg Eur*. 2010;35(2):94-102.

12. Sammer DM, Chung KC. Tendon transfers: part I. Principles of transfer and transfers for radial nerve palsy. *Plast Reconstr Surg*. 2009;123(5):169e-177e.
13. Bidic SM, Varshney A, Ruff MD, Orenstein HH. Biomechanical comparison of lasso, Pulvertaft weave, and side-by-side tendon repairs. *Plast Reconstr Surg*. 2009;124(2):567-571.
14. Brown SH, Hentzen ER, Kwan A, et al. Mechanical strength of the side-to-side versus Pulvertaft weave tendon repair. *J Hand Surg*. 2010;35(4):540-545.
15. Fuchs SP, Walbeehm ET, Hovius SE. Biomechanical evaluation of the Pulvertaft versus the 'wrap around' tendon suture technique. *J Hand Surg Eur*. 2011;36(6):461-466.
16. Rivlin M, Eberlin KR, Kachooei AR, et al. Side-to-side versus pulvertaft extensor tenorrhaphy: a biomechanical study. *J Hand Surg*. 2016;41(11):e393-e397.
17. Vincken NL, Lauwers TM, van der Hulst RR. Biomechanical and dimensional measurements of the Pulvertaft weave versus the cow-hitch technique. *Hand (NY)*. 2017;12(1):78-84.
18. Brand PW, Beach RB, Thompson DE. Relative tension and potential excursion of muscles in the forearm and hand. *J Hand Surg*. 1981;6(3):209-219.
    In this classic article, the authors use cadaveric dissections to quantify the relative strength and excursion of the muscles distal to the elbow. This is the basis for selecting appropriate donor muscles to restore those paralyzed after nerve injury.
19. Wehbe MA, Hunter JM. Flexor tendon gliding in the hand. Part I. In vivo excursions. *J Hand Surg*. 1985;10(4):570-574.
20. Boyes JH. Selection of a donor muscle for tendon transfer. *Bull Hosp Joint Dis*. 1962;23:1-4.
    Boyes presents the 3-5-7 rule for tendon excursion and discusses the need for the tenodesis effect to augment the excursion of some donor muscles.
21. Brand PW. Biomechanics of tendon transfers. *Hand Clin*. 1988;4(2):137-154.
22. Omer GE Jr. Reconstruction of a balanced thumb through tendon transfers. *Clin Orthop Relat Res*. 1985;(195):104-116.
    Omer describes the detailed evaluation of a patient with loss of thumb function due to median or ulnar nerve palsy and the various options available for reconstruction along with their rationale for use.
23. Jones R II. On suture of nerves, and alternative methods of treatment by transplantation of tendon. *BMJ*. 1916;1(2888):641-643.
24. Starr CL. Army experiences with tendon transference. *J Bone Joint Surg*. 1922;4(1):3-21.
25. Chuinard RG, Boyes JH, Stark HH, Ashworth CR. Tendon transfers for radial nerve palsy: use of superficialis tendons for digital extension. *J Hand Surg*. 1978;3(6):560-570.
26. Raskin KB, Wilgis EF. Flexor carpi ulnaris transfer for radial nerve palsy: functional testing of long-term results. *J Hand Surg*. 1995;20(5):737-742.
27. Chadderdon RC, Gaston RG. Low median nerve transfers (opponensplasty). *Hand Clin*. 2016;32(3):349-359.
    A thorough and in-depth discussion of thumb [illegible] and the various options available for opponensplasty.
28. Foucher G, Malizos C, Sammut D, et al. Primary palmaris longus transfer as an opponensplasty in carpal tunnel release: a series of 73 cases. *J Hand Surg (Edinb)*. 1991;16(1):56-60.
29. Royle ND. An operation for paralysis of the intrinsic muscles of the thumb. *JAMA*. 1938;111(7):612-613.
30. Bunnell S. Opposition of the thumb. *J Bone Joint Surg Am*. 1938;20A:269-284.
31. Thompson TC. A modified operation for opponens paralysis. *J Bone Joint Surg Am*. 1942;24A:632-640.
32. Wood VE, Adams J. Complications of opponensplasty with transfer of extensor carpi ulnaris to extensor pollicis brevis. *J Hand Surg*. 1984;9(5):699-704.
33. Zancolli EA. Paralytic supination contracture of the forearm. *J Bone Joint Surg Am*. 1967;49(7):1275-1284.
34. Cliffton EE. Unusual innervation of the intrinsic muscles of the hand by median and ulnar nerve. *Surgery*. 1948;23(1):12-31.
35. Leibovic SJ, Hastings H II. Martin-Gruber revisited. *J Hand Surg*. 1992;17(1):47-53.
36. Ozkan T, Ozer K, Gulgonen A. Restoration of sensibility in irreparable ulnar and median nerve lesions with use of sensory nerve transfer: long-term follow-up of 20 cases. *J Hand Surg*. 2001;26(1):44-51.
37. Smith RJ. Extensor carpi radialis brevis tendon transfer for thumb adduction: a study of power pinch. *J Hand Surg*. 1983;8(1):4-15.
38. Hamlin C, Littler JW. Restoration of power pinch. *J Hand Surg*. 1980;5(4):396-401.
39. Mikhail IK. Bone block operation for clawhand. *Surg Gynecol Obstet*. 1964;118:1077-1079.
40. Zancolli EA. Claw-hand caused by paralysis of the intrinsic muscles: a simple surgical procedure for its correction. *J Bone Joint Surg Am*. 1957;39A:1076-1080.
41. Parkes A. Paralytic claw fingers: a graft tenodesis operation. *Hand*. 1973;5(3):192-199.
42. Riordan DC. Tendon transplantations in median-nerve and ulnar-nerve paralysis. *J Bone Joint Surg Am*. 1953;35A:312-320.
43. Tsuge K. Tendon transfers in median and ulnar nerve paralysis. *Hiroshima J Med Sci*. 1967;16(1):29-48.
44. Hastings H II, McCollam SM. Flexor digitorum superficialis lasso tendon transfer in isolated ulnar nerve palsy: a functional evaluation. *J Hand Surg*. 1994;19(2):275-280.
45. Burkhalter WE, Strait JL. Metacarpophalangeal flexor replacement for intrinsic-muscle paralysis. *J Bone Joint Surg Am*. 1973;55A:1667-1676.
46. Bunnell S. Surgery of the intrinsic muscles of the hand other than those producing opposition of the thumb. *J Bone Joint Surg Am*. 1942;24A:1-31.
47. Burkhalter WE. Restoration of power grip in ulnar nerve paralysis. *Orthop Clin North Am*. 1974;5(2):289-303.
48. Enna CD, Riordan DC. The Fowler procedure for correction of the paralytic claw hand. *Plast Reconstr Surg*. 1973;52(4):352-360.
49. Brand PW. Tendon grafting. *J Bone Joint Surg Br*. 1961;43B:444-453.
50. Bednar MS. Tendon transfers for tetraplegia. *Hand Clin*. 2016;32(3):389-396.

QUESTIONS

1. A patient with high ulnar and median nerve palsy needs an opponensplasty to improve thumb function. The most appropriate tendon transfer is:

   a. EIP
   b. EPL
   c. EDQ
   d. Ring finger FDP
   e. ADM

2. Tendon transfers that attempt to replicate the function of which muscle provides the best thumb opposition?

   a. FPL
   b. Opponens pollicis (OPP)
   c. FPB
   d. APB
   e. AP

3. A patient with known ulnar nerve palsy is unable to actively extend the proximal IP joint of the small finger and exhibits clawing. During physical examination, the MCP joint is stabilized in neutral (0°). The patient is then able to extend the proximal IP joint. What muscle acts alone to extend the proximal IP joint in this circumstance?

   a. Lumbrical
   b. Dorsal interosseous
   c. Volar interosseous
   d. EDC
   e. ADM

4. A 44-year-old man undergoes an elbow arthroscopy and immediately postoperatively, the patient is unable to extend his thumb and fingers. These functions never recover, and tendon transfers are planned. Which of the following tendon transfers would be preferred for this patient?

   a. PT to ECRL, FCR to EDC, PL to EPL
   b. FCR to ECRB, PL to EPL
   c. FCU to ECRB, FCR to EPL
   d. FCR to EDC, PL to EPL
   e. PT to ECU, FCR to EDC, PL to APL

5. Which one of the following muscles has a similar relative strength to the FCU?

   a. BR
   b. ECU
   c. ECRL
   d. APL
   e. FPL

6. Which surgical procedures will improve hand function in a patient with high median nerve palsy?

   a. Ring finger FDS transfer for thumb opposition, BR to the flexor pollicis longus, and FDP of the ring and small fingers side by side to the long and index fingers
   b. EIP to APB for thumb opposition, BR to flexor pollicis longus, and FDP of ring and small fingers side by side to the long and index fingers
   c. Flexor carpi ulnar transfer prolonged with a PL graft for thumb opposition, thumb IP joint arthrodesis, and extensor carpi radialis brevis to the FDP of the index and long fingers
   d. Thumb abduction bone block, transfer of the FCU to the FDP, and BR to flexor pollicis longus
   e. BR transfer prolonged with a PL graft for thumb opposition, extensor carpi radialis brevis to the FDP of index and long fingers, and arthrodesis of the thumb IP joint

1. **Answer: a.** The EIP transfer is appropriate for opponensplasty in patients with a supple hand. The EIP opponensplasty produces good results in restoration of thumb opposition. The EIP is expendable with minimal donor site morbidity, is of sufficient length, and has an optimal line of pull to provide a superior mechanical advantage and a favorable torque when compared with FDS. EPL and EDQ are not suitable for this clinical situation. The remaining alternatives are not available with the high ulnar and median nerve palsies that this patient has.

2. **Answer: d.** Opposition of the thumb results from the abduction, flexion and rotation of the carpometacarpal joint of the thumb and abduction of the MCP joint. The APB, OPP, and superficial head of the FPB produce thumb abduction, and their simultaneous action on both the thumb CMC joint and MCP joint produces thumb opposition. The APB is the primary mover of the thumb as it provides the correct direction of action and proper insertion to produce full thumb opposition. The OPP is an important but less effective muscle in opposition. The FPB is a stronger flexor than the abductor and together they provide for strong key and tip pinch. Based on muscle excursion and tension fraction, the best muscles to use in transfer for thumb opposition are the FDS of the long finger, ECU, FDS of the ring finger and ECRL. A pulley in the area of the pisiform restores the necessary direction of action.

3. **Answer: d.** Bouvier's maneuver is a clinical sign of ulnar nerve dysfunction. It allows the isolation of the components of clawing in a hand with severe intrinsic dysfunction. Patients with a positive test are unable to use their extensor digitorum to extend the PIP joint because of intrinsic weakness and the relative shortening of the length over which the extensor digitorum must act. By stabilizing the MCP joint in neutral to slight flexion, the EDC is then able to extend the PIP joint from its flexed position.

4. **Answer: d.** The patient most likely has a PIN injury distal to the innervation of the ECRB and ECRL, preserving wrist extension. Thus, the primary defects are finger and thumb extension. The best answer for treatment of these deficits includes FCR to EDC and PL to EPL.

5. **Answer: a.** When designing tendon transfers, matching the relative strength of muscles is helpful. Although not always possible, matching a muscle deficit with a muscle transfer of similar relative strength is preferred. The strengths of the muscles in the forearm have been compared to the FCR which was given a relative strength of one. The FCR, ECRL, ECRB, ECU, PT, FPL, FDS, FDP, and APL all have a relative strength of one. The FCU and BR have a relative strength of 2. The strength is related to the cross-sectional area of the muscle.

6. **Answer: b.** This patient has a classic high median nerve lesion. The missing functions that need to be restored are thumb opposition and flexion of the thumb, index, and long fingers. The best set of transfers listed is the rerouted EIP into the APB for thumb opposition, BR to FPL, and FDP side to side of ring/small to index/long finger. When there are enough available transfers to restore the missing function, a tendon transfer is better than an arthrodesis. A thumb abduction block does not provide for thumb opposition, and a transfer for opposition is better. The BR prolonged with a graft would not provide the correct line of pull for thumb opposition unless it were routed more ulnarly through the hand. Option *a* would be reasonable, but it is better to sacrifice a wrist extensor than the superficialis to the ring finger for thumb opposition, especially because the ring profundus is now going to have to provide flexion for the long and index along with the side-to-side transfer.

CHAPTER 80 ▪ Ligament Injuries of the Hand

Aviram M. Giladi and Kevin C. Chung

KEY POINTS

- If a proximal interphalangeal (PIP) fracture/dislocation remains reduced and congruent when splinted at 30° of flexion or less, it is considered stable and can be treated closed.
- Many unstable PIP fracture/dislocation injuries, historically treated with open fixation, are now amenable to treatment with dynamic external fixation, facilitating earlier range of motion and improving long-term outcomes.
- For failed primary treatment of unstable PIP fracture/dislocation injuries with destruction of the volar base of the middle phalanx, or for those that present more than 4 to 6 weeks after injury, the hemihamate arthroplasty is a reliable option for joint reconstruction.
- An acute boutonniere deformity, with DIP extended and PIP flexed, raises concern for a central slip rupture. This can be tested with Elson's test.
- Avoid longitudinal traction when attempting reductions of metacarpophalangeal dislocations—this can entrap the metacarpal head and prevent a successful reduction.
- Maintain suspicion for finger carpometacarpal (CMC) joint dislocation in a patient with trauma, pain, and swelling over the CMC region even if the X-rays are difficult to evaluate. If dislocation is suspected but cannot clearly be seen on X-rays, CT scan may be required to evaluate.

Hand ligament injuries are common and present in a variety of ways. Although some of these injuries are associated with fractures or obvious dislocations, many ligament injuries in the hand are subtle. Appropriate diagnosis and management of these injuries require in-depth knowledge of anatomy and biomechanics, along with thoughtful evaluation and careful examination. In this chapter, we review many of the more common hand ligament injuries, and present the associated anatomy, biomechanics, related pathology, and treatment options for each.

PROXIMAL INTERPHALANGEAL JOINT INJURIES

Proximal interphalangeal joint (PIPJ) injuries are common and fall in to three major categories[1,2]:

- Dislocations
- Avulsions
- Fracture-dislocations

Postinjury stiffness is a substantial problem and is often made worse by improper or prolonged immobilization even within the first 2 weeks after injury. Early treatment is critical.

The PIPJ is a bicondylar hinge with an arc of motion of 110° in a single plane. It accounts for 20% of the total arc of motion of the finger. The major soft tissue contributors to joint stability are the volar plate and the collateral ligaments (Figure 80.1). The collateral ligaments on the ulnar and radial side are composed of two segments, an accessory collateral ligament (more volar) and a proper collateral ligament (more dorsal). The extensor system provides the least amount of support, which makes the joint inherently less stable to dorsal forces. As a result, dorsal dislocations are most common, with the middle phalanx being driven dorsally and then proximally. Lateral and volar dislocations are much less common.

PIPJ Dislocation

Generally, the approach to PIPJ dislocations is as follows:

- Reduction
- Evaluate postreduction for joint congruency through the arc of motion
- Assess stability

If the joint is stable following reduction, nonoperative treatment is generally the best option, and early hand therapy should be used to minimize stiffness. Unstable joints, including those that frankly redisplace after reduction as well as those that do not maintain congruency through the arc of motion, often require operative management.[3,4]

Evaluation

A thorough history will help clarify the mechanism and direction of forces.

Radiographs are done to assess for any associated fractures or avulsion fragments (which may represent ligamentous avulsions) and to see the resting joint congruency:

- True lateral view of the involved finger
- Anteroposterior or posteroanterior (PA) view of the involved finger

If evaluating an acute injury that is in need of reduction:

- Perform a sensory exam.
- Provide a digital block to make the reduction maneuver less painful and more likely to succeed.
- Perform the reduction.
  - □ The reduction maneuver includes hyperextension of the PIPJ following by gentle pressure on the base of the middle phalanx along with axial traction.
  - □ Use fluoroscopic guidance when available.
  - □ Avoid multiple attempts at closed reduction.
    - Irreducible dislocation can be caused by interposed soft tissues, and repeated attempts can create additional tissue and/or articular injury.
    - For dorsal dislocations, the volar plate is most often interposed, although the profundus tendon or part of the extensor mechanism can become entrapped and block reduction.
    - In these cases, open reduction is indicated.

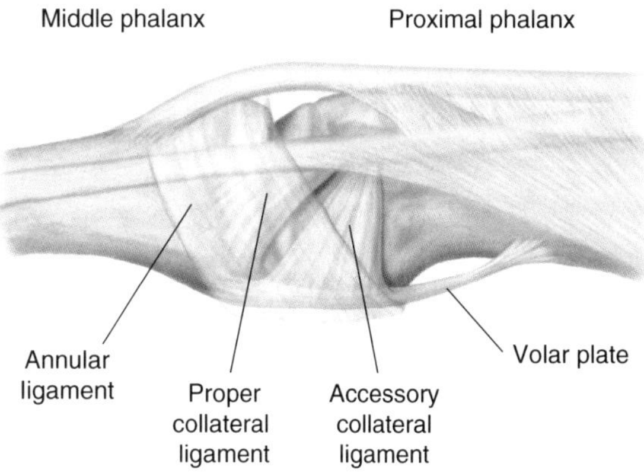

FIGURE 80.1. Anatomy of the PIP joint. Note the volar and lateral stabilizing structures, especially the volar plate and the collateral ligaments. The proper collateral ligament attaches to the middle phalanx and the accessory collateral ligament attaches to the volar plate.

If Closed Reduction Is Successful:

- Assess for tendon function and joint stability.
- Repeat radiographs after reduction to evaluate for congruency and for any subtle fractures that may have been missed.
- Palpate the ligamentous structures to help identify focal areas of pain and potential injury (remember this may be altered by local anesthesia).

It is important to passively stress the joint with radial/ulnar pressure and volar/dorsal translation, as well as to test stability through active motion. Of note, radial/ulnar stressing to test collateral ligament stability should be done with the finger extended to test the accessory collateral, and with the PIPJ at 30° to test the proper collateral. Evaluating joint congruency under fluoroscopy during active motion is the optimal way to test active stability. If the joint is stable after reduction, buddy straps/taping to facilitate early motion with some protection is the optimal treatment, rather than immobilization. If the subluxation or dislocation recurs with active motion, splinting in a position of stability—15° to 30° of flexion—may be required to facilitate ligament healing before allowing motion.

- *Dorsal PIPJ dislocation:* This is the most common PIPJ injury, often occurring because of hyperextension with axial loading (Figure 80.2).
- *Type I (hyperextension):* Hyperextension results in avulsion of the volar plate from the proximal phalanx. However, some contact is usually maintained between the head of the proximal phalanx and the base of the middle phalanx, facilitated by the stable collateral ligaments. This is not a complete dislocation.
- *Type II (dorsal dislocation):* Volar plate avulsion along with separation between the accessory and proper collateral ligaments, allowing complete dorsal dislocation of the middle phalanx that then tends to pull proximally into a bayonet configuration. The proper collateral often remains intact. As long as they can be reduced, type I and II injuries rarely require surgical treatment.
- *Type III (fracture-dislocation):* An additional component of impaction fracture at the volar base of the middle phalanx makes these types of injuries more complicated. Generally, the lip fragment remains attached to the volar plate and collateral ligament, whereas the rest of the middle phalanx dislocates dorsally. Additional X-rays of the finger after reduction can help evaluate subtle bony injuries. Stability of these injuries is largely dependent on the amount of the joint surface that is involved with the fracture, and some mild flexion may be needed to restabilize the joint.
    - Stable fractures tend to involve 30% or less of the articular surface.
    - Some fractures between 30% and 50% will have stability although many will not.

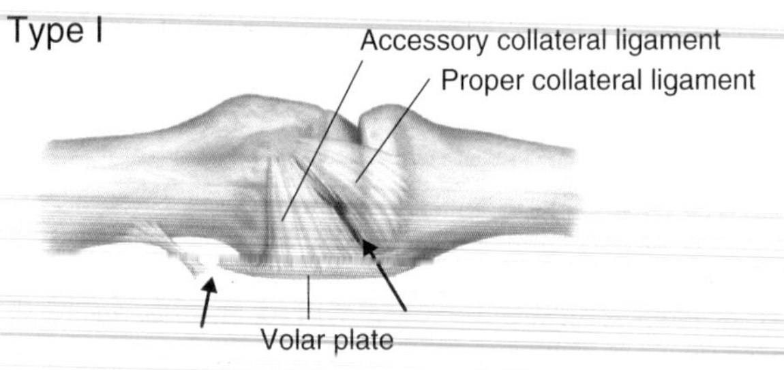

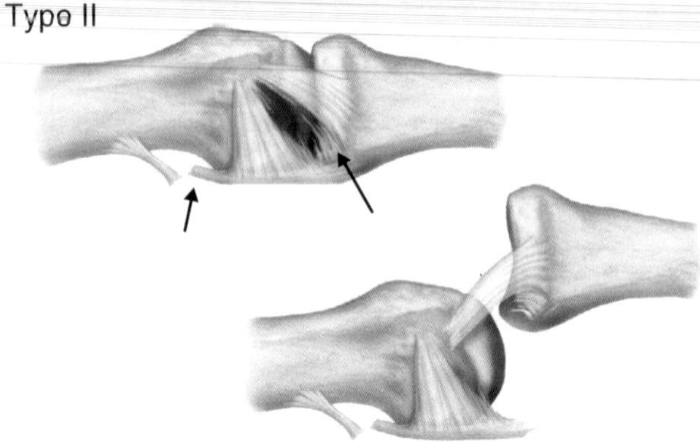

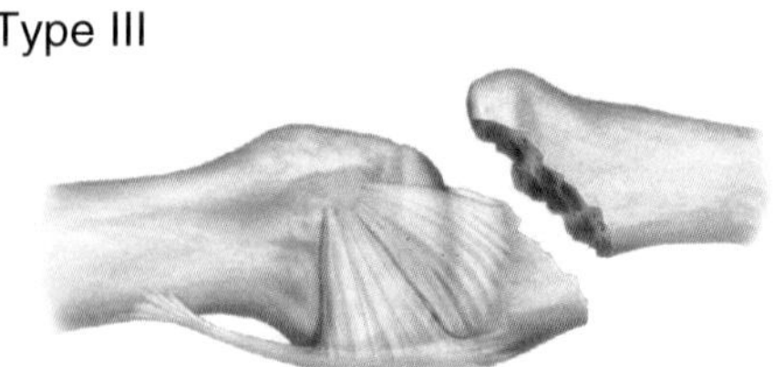

FIGURE 80.2. Dorsal PIP dislocation types (Eaton classification). Type I represents a hyperextension that results in volar plate injury with associated minor tear between the collaterals; however, the joint remains congruent. Type II completely disrupts the volar plate along with a complete tear between the collateral ligaments. The middle phalanx will shift dorsal and the joint is no longer congruent. Type III involves a fracture and dislocation component. The volar plate, as well as accessory and proper collateral ligaments, is damaged, and the volar lip fracture segment stays with these soft tissue elements as the rest of the middle phalanx shifts dorsally and proximally.

The stable fracture-dislocations tend to have the proper collateral on the middle phalanx shaft segment, facilitating postreduction stability, whereas those with more articular surface involvement often have both collateral segments on the broken lip segment, which confers no stability to the reduced middle phalanx. Some of these injuries are obviously unstable after reduction and easily redislocate; however, subtle findings of instability during joint motion—including the *dorsal V sign* (Figure 80.3)—must be evaluated before accepting the reduction as stable. As long as the joint exhibits stability at 30° of flexion or less, it can be considered stable.

Treatment

No matter the treatment, the pain, swelling, and stiffness from these injuries may last for months. The unstable injuries, especially the unstable fracture-dislocations, are prone to long-term stiffness, flexion contracture, and functional limitations. The patient should be counseled about these issues early to help guide expectations.

Stable PIPJ

Almost all type I and II injuries are stable after reduction and can be treated nonoperatively with buddy straps. For patients with stability but substantial discomfort, extension block splinting, preventing full extension of the joint, may be helpful.

- Active motion therapy should begin within 2 or 3 days of injury.
- Beginning this range of motion therapy within the splint maintains reduction while preventing painful full extension.

For stable joints with more structural injury requiring mild flexion to reach full stability, mostly fracture-dislocation injuries of 30% to 40% or less, extension block splinting may be needed for up to 4 weeks.[5]

- Initiate early range of motion within the splint.
- The splint can be set to start at 30° of flexion to provide stability and be adjusted into extension progressively (e.g., 10° per week) so that the patient slowly gets to full extension over 4 weeks while maintaining range of motion in flexion within the splint.
- If the fracture component risks instability with early extension, the splint can be maintained in the flexed position for longer, but no longer than 3 weeks at 20° to 30° to avoid flexion contracture.

In some cases, extension block pinning may be used.[6] This requires passing a Kirschner wire (K-wire) through the proximal phalanx head to structurally block full proximal interphalangeal (PIP) extension. Although this does prevent dorsal translation of the middle phalanx, the downsides are a surgical procedure with complication risks that is not amenable to progressive straightening. Therefore, splinting tends to be a better option if the patient can tolerate it and comply with the protocol.

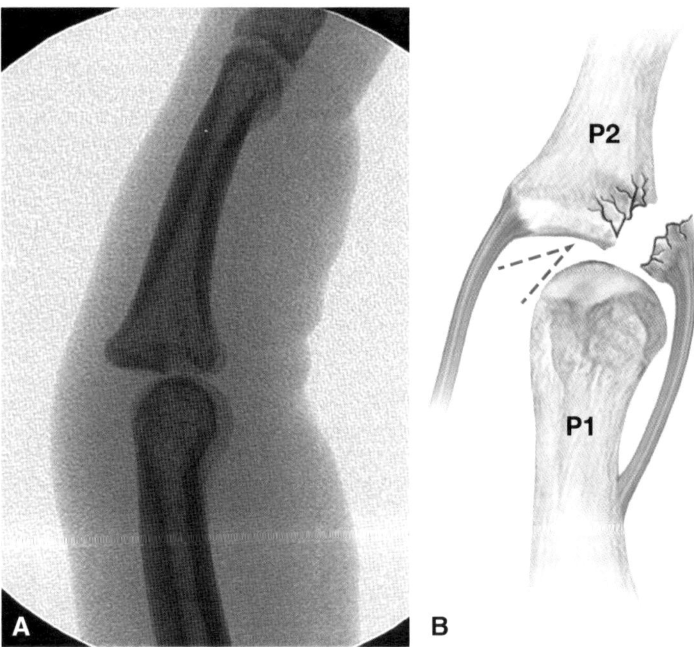

FIGURE 80.3. Dorsal V sign. **A.** X-ray of a *reduced* fracture/dislocation injury demonstrating persistent instability with resultant dorsal V sign. This PIP is hinging, rather than maintaining appropriate congruent alignment and gliding. **B.** Illustration of the dorsal V, indicating persistent PIP instability.

Unstable PIPJ

These injuries—most often fracture dislocations with greater joint surface area involvement—are difficult to treat. Outcomes are often disappointing even with optimal treatment. The goal of treatment is to restore congruity and facilitate early active motion. There are numerous options:

- *Dynamic external fixation/dynamic skeletal traction*[illegible]: The traction from the fixator system creates tension in the soft tissue envelope that helps hold fracture fragments in reduction and stable, and the dynamic component allows for range of motion while traction is maintained (Figure 80.4).
- *Open reduction and internal fixation:* If the volar fragment is not comminuted and is large enough for a screw, it may be amenable to direct repair with a lag screw.
- *K-wire fixation:* A single K-wire is driven across the fracture site and then across the PIPJ with joint at 20° to 30° of flexion. Pin is removed at 3 weeks.

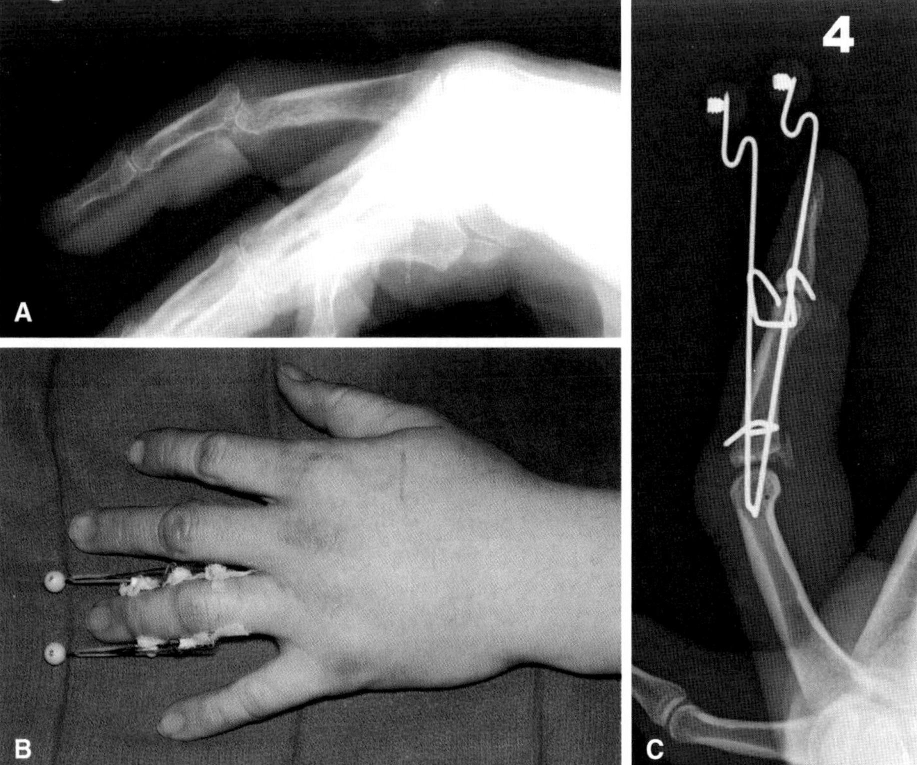

FIGURE 80.4. Dynamic external fixator. **A.** Unstable fracture/dislocation of left ring finger PIP joint. **B.** Dynamic external fixator placed using K-wire and rubber band construct. **C.** Traction via dynamic fixator improves joint alignment and facilitates early motion.

- *Volar plate arthroplasty:* Especially useful when the fracture is comminuted and restoring joint surface is not feasible. This technique uses the volar plate and anchors it in the fracture defect to resurface the middle phalanx base.[10] This holds the PIPJ in mild flexion, and although it does restore stability, the risk of flexion contracture is high.
- *Hemihamate osteochondral arthroplasty:* When the volar base of the middle phalanx is comminuted and unstable, but the dorsal base remains intact, reconstruction of the PIPJ is possible using a nonvascularized osteochondral graft taken from the dorsal distal articular surface of the hamate. This technique can also be useful for fractures that may have been amenable to dynamic external fixation or open reduction and internal fixation (ORIF) but did not present acutely. The articulation between the hamate and the small and ring finger metacarpal bases, notable for having a dorsal central ridge that is an excellent anatomic match to the volar base of the middle phalanx, can be contoured to fit the defect and recapitulate the PIPJ (Figure 80.5). The graft is secured with screws, and range of motion can be started 1 week after surgery. Long-term outcomes of this procedure have an average range of motion between 50° and 75° of PIP flexion, with many patients having a persistent flexion contracture even if active range of motion has improved overall.[11,12]

Volar PIPJ Dislocation and Central Slip Injuries

Volar PIPJ dislocation is rare. If a volar PIPJ dislocation is identified, it is usually facilitated by either rupture of the central slip of the extensor tendon or torsion force causing volar-directed rotatory subluxation of the middle phalanx. A central slip rupture may be associated with an avulsion fracture of the dorsal base of the middle phalanx, but some slip ruptures occur without a fracture and therefore cannot be seen on X-rays.

If the volar PIPJ dislocation was from a rotatory mechanism, only one of the collateral ligaments may be injured, whereas a dislocation after central slip rupture often injures both collateral ligaments. Although a volar dislocation also injures the volar plate and extensor mechanism, closed reduction is usually attainable with longitudinal traction and extension. However, especially with rotatory injuries, the condyle of the proximal phalanx can get interposed between the central slip and the lateral band, making reduction difficult. In this situation, flexing the PIPJ to relax the lateral band (rather than pulling traction) is necessary before recreating the rotational force to facilitate reduction.

Confirm adequate reduction with X-ray. Test active extension to evaluate the integrity of the central slip. An acute boutonniere deformity, with extensor lag at the PIPJ and hyperextension of the distal interphalangeal joint (DIPJ), indicates central slip rupture. Elson's test can be used to evaluate. This is performed by holding the PIP in flexion and having the patient attempt to extend the middle phalanx against resistance—if the DIPJ tightens into extension a central slip rupture has likely occurred. If the DIPJ remains lax, the central slip is intact.

With no central slip injury, these dislocations should be splinted for approximately 2 weeks and then put into buddy straps to facility early motion. In the setting of a central slip rupture, 6 weeks of splinting with the PIPJ in full extension is needed. Even if the central slip rupture is associated with a small avulsion fragment, closed treatment with 6 weeks of splinting is usually adequate. As long as any finger deformity associated with the central slip injury is passively correctable, splinting is often adequate even with a subacute presentation. In the setting of a larger intra-articular fracture fragment that is displaced, ORIF may be required. If the deformity (i.e., boutonniere) is not passively correctable, surgical intervention is needed.[13,14]

Lateral PIPJ Injuries

Forced radial or ulnar deviation of the PIPJ puts stress on the contralateral collateral ligament, which may sustain a partial injury or complete rupture. Often a rupture occurs at the site of the proximal attachment on the proximal phalanx. This creates joint instability, and due to the force of the injury the PIPJ may dislocate. More severe injuries can also disrupt the volar plate. Longitudinal traction is usually adequate for reduction. Once reduced, test for stability through the flexion/extension arc and to lateral stress (as described earlier). If the reduction is stable, splinting in extension for 7 days followed by protected active range of motion with buddy straps is the appropriate treatment.

If reduction cannot be accomplished (often due to interposition of soft tissues), or the joint is persistently unstable, operative intervention is needed. This involves approaching the PIPJ through a midaxial approach, clearing any entrapped tissues, and reconstructing the collateral ligament by attaching it to the phalanx with suture anchors.[15,16]

Outcomes and Complications

PIPJ injuries are notorious for causing some amount of stiffness long term, and it is important to counsel patients about this early. Even for injuries that recover well, the time to recovery can be many months

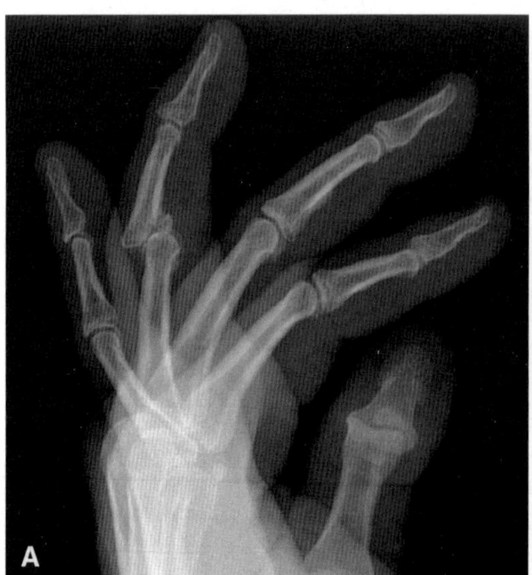

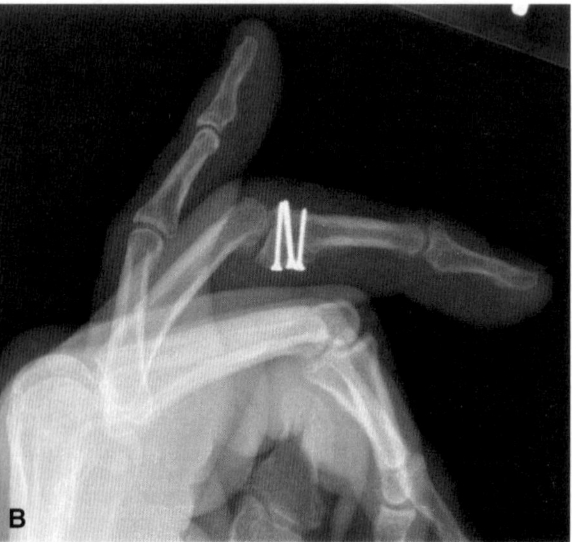

FIGURE 80.5. Hemihamate arthroplasty of the ring finger PIP joint. **A.** Chronic unstable fracture-dislocation of the ring finger PIP joint. **B.** Reconstruction of the volar base of the ring finger middle phalanx using a hemihamate autograft, recreating PIP articular architecture

of edema and pain before resolution. Stiffness and flexion contracture are commonly encountered problems after these injuries, especially the more severe types with fracture components or complete dislocations (and associated soft tissue disruption).[17]

Collateral stiffness is the most common etiology for loss of range of motion as well as flexion contracture. Volar plate stiffness contributes as well. First-line treatment for these findings is early aggressive therapy to restore range of motion. If this is not successful, joint release by releasing the collateral ligaments, and perhaps also the volar plate, may be required. Even after joint release, range of motion does not return to preinjury levels. For PIPJ that remain painful and stiff, conversion to arthroplasty or arthrodesis is then considered.

Long-term instability, although less frequent, can occur due to unrepaired collateral ligament rupture, persistent collateral ligament laxity, persistent central slip injury, or volar plate laxity. Instability from any cause can precipitate early degenerative arthritis. Additionally, chronic hyperextension from volar plate laxity can lead to swan-neck deformity. Unrepaired central slip injuries can result in extensor lag, and if untreated can progress to boutonniere deformity.

FINGER DISTAL INTERPHALANGEAL JOINT/THUMB INTERPHALANGEAL JOINT INJURIES

The DIPJ is similar to the PIPJ in that it is a hinge joint with strong lateral stabilizers. In addition to volar and dorsal support structures seen at the PIPJ (e.g., volar plate), the DIPJ benefits from added volar stability from the insertion of the flexor digitorum profundus (FDP) tendon at the base of the distal phalanx. The thumb interphalangeal joint (IPJ) is structurally similar, with the flexor pollicis longus (FPL) tendon providing the added volar structural stability. Even with the support from the tendon insertion, the finger DIPJ have added hyperextensibility compared to the PIPJ (and IPJ) due to shorter and more laterally positioned checkrein ligaments. DIPJ/IPJ arc of active motion is about 90°, with an additional 10° to 15° of passive hyperextension possible for DIPJ.

DIPJ and thumb IPJ dislocations are rare. Often when these dislocations do occur they are associated with flexor or extensor tendon insertion injuries, which are covered in the flexor and extensor tendon injury sections. If an isolated DIPJ dislocation occurs, it is almost always a dorsal dislocation. Closed dislocations can be reduced with longitudinal traction. If successfully reduced, splint for 1 week and then begin protected active motion in a dorsal blocking splint for an additional 3 weeks. Dorsal dislocations with an associated dorsal laceration are common and should be irrigated thoroughly before reduction and closure. If reducible, the same splinting regimen as reducible closed injuries is the appropriate treatment.

Dorsal DIPJ or thumb IPJ dislocations may be irreducible due to interposition of soft tissue (volar plate, flexor tendon) or sesamoid bones.[18-20] These cases require operative intervention for open reduction but are often stable enough to be treated with splinting after the reduction. If not stable, K-wire pinning may be required. Volar plate arthroplasty is an alternative option, although the potential for flexion contracture is increased with this approach.

Small fractures of the phalangeal base may occur with dislocation or hyperextension injuries of the DIPJ and thumb IPJ. Fractures with small fragments that do not destabilize tendon insertions or joint congruity are generally left alone; however, if the fragment is large and associated with tendon insertion or large part of the articular surface, operative fixation may be required.

Stiffness and even fusion of the DIPJ and thumb IPJ is much better tolerated than at the PIPJ. Most surgical procedures required after a DIPJ or thumb IPJ dislocation, and even reduction and splinting treatments, will result in some stiffness. However, if persistently painful, conversion to a fusion is tolerated well overall and provides pain relief.

FINGER METACARPOPHALANGEAL JOINT INJURIES

The finger metacarpophalangeal joints (MCPJ) is a diarthroidal joint and has a complex stabilization system with contributions from unique bony anatomy, intrinsic components, and extrinsic structures.

The metacarpal head is volarly offset from the shaft. As a result, the arc of rotation moves the articulation further from the shaft as the joint surface progresses volarly (Figure 80.6). This is a cam mechanism. The MCPJ intrinsic stabilizers include a volar plate as well as radial and ulnar accessory and collateral ligaments. Due to the unique bony anatomy of the metacarpal, the collateral ligaments are progressively tightened as the MCPJ flexes and the proximal phalanx base is moved further volarly compared to the ligament attachment on the metacarpal. As a result, the joint is relatively lax in extension, and can glide in abduction and adduction, yet loses much of that lateral gliding as the MCPJ flexes. The MCPJ is therefore more stable, with the collaterals tight, in full flexion. The volar plate is stout distally but much thinner proximally. Different from the PIPJ, there are no checkrein ligaments on the MCPJ volar plate. This facilitates some hyperextension of the MCPJ. The extrinsic stabilizers include flexor tendons, the extensor mechanism, the sagittal bands, and the transverse intermetacarpal ligament that connects across the volar plates.

Because of these stabilizing components around the metacarpal head, major ligamentous injuries and dislocations of finger MCPJ are less common than PIPJ. However, this complex anatomy can contribute to difficulties in management of MCPJ injuries when they do occur.

Sagittal Band Injuries

Sagittal bands contribute to MCPJ and extensor tendon stability. They attach dorsally to the extensor hood and run palmar to insert on the volar plate. They function as the primary lateral stabilizer for the extensor tendon over the MCPJ. Sagittal band rupture results in subluxation or complete dislocation of the extensor tendon during MCPJ flexion and extension. Injury is often identified by subluxation and associated localized pain and edema. The diagnosis is usually made clinically, but ultrasound or MRI can provide confirmation in unclear cases.

For injuries with pain and minimal tendon instability, 4 to 6 weeks of conservative treatment in a splint that holds the affected metacarpophalangeal (MCP) neutral or mildly hyperextended is appropriate. If subluxation or dislocation is identified within 6 weeks of injury, conservative treatment is appropriate first-line treatment for most patients. Even for patients who present with longer delay, a trial of conservative management is often still indicated.[21]

For athletes and very high demand patients who present with complete dislocation, early surgical intervention may be appropriate, as this facilitates primary repair of the sagittal band. For most patients, conservative first-line treatment is appropriate as described

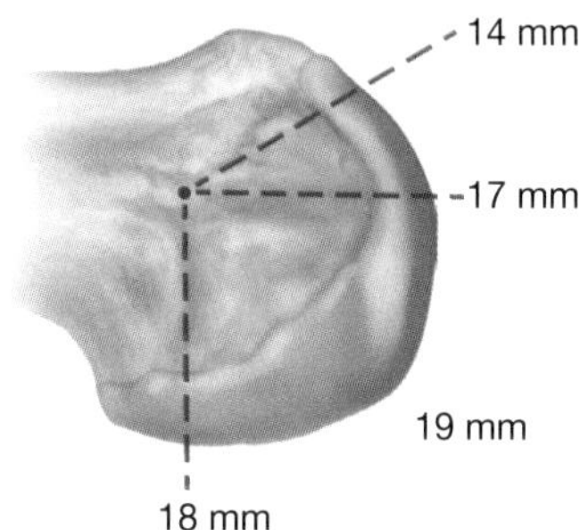

FIGURE 80.6. Anatomy of the metacarpal head, illustrating greater lengths from the center of rotation as the arc progresses volarly.

earlier; however, if painful subluxation or dislocation persists, then sagittal band reconstruction is appropriate to correct the abnormality and decrease pain.[22,23]

Isolated Finger MCPJ Collateral Ligament Injuries

These injuries are rare and when they occur may be associated with a fracture of the base of the proximal phalanx.[24] Appropriate treatment is important, especially for radial-sided injuries, as the radial collateral ligament (RCL) is important to stabilize against pinch forces. Visualizing fractures associated with collateral injuries, especially when they are small avulsion types, can be difficult; a Brewerton view X-ray may be helpful. Physical examination with stress testing is important, similar to collateral testing of the PIPJ. For the MCPJ, flex as far as 60° and then test stability against radial and ulnar stress.

If the joint is stable with a firm end point, 4 weeks of dorsal block splinting in 30° to 60° of flexion with early active motion is appropriate treatment. If the examination identifies a complete tear, or there is an avulsion fracture associated with an unstable joint, surgical repair is often required.

Finger MCPJ Dislocations

Finger MCPJ dislocations, when they occur, are usually dorsal or ulnar. They occur most commonly to the border digits (index or small finger).

Dorsal MCPJ Dislocations

These injuries often occur after forced hyperextension. This results in injury to the volar plate, at the thinner proximal segment. Upon presentation, the degree of deformity can indicate the severity of the injury; however, the more noticeably deformed joints, often with MCPJ held in fixed hyperextension of 60° to 80°, are the result of a *simple* subluxation. The proximal phalanx base remains in continuity with the metacarpal head and, as a result, is amenable to closed reduction. The more inconspicuous *complete dorsal dislocation* may have a subtle presentation, as the proximal phalanx has completely dislocated into a bayonet position atop the metacarpal head, leaving the finger in a relatively straight resting position. This injury is more challenging, and these dislocations can become *complex dislocations* as the torn volar plate can interpose between the phalanx and the metacarpal, blocking reduction.[25] Additionally, the metacarpal head can translate volar and buttonhole between the lumbrical radially and the FDP tendon ulnarly. This can form a noose around the metacarpal neck.

For the simple dislocation, and even the subluxation, traction should be avoided so that the volar plate is kept out of the joint space—undue traction can create a complex dislocation. Additionally, any hyperextension or traction forces used to attempt reduction will make the tendon noose tighter on the metacarpal neck, preventing reduction. Therefore, closed reduction of a dorsal MCPJ injury should be done with PIPJ and wrist flexed (to relax the flexor tendons as much as possible), and with volar- and distal-directed pressure along the base of the proximal phalanx so that it slides over the metacarpal head without losing contact.

Complex dislocations require operative intervention for open reduction. The approach can be volar or dorsal, with different risks and benefits. The volar approach is considered higher risk because the volar displacement of the metacarpal head displaces the neurovascular bundles toward the skin, directly at risk during the surgical approach.[26] However, the volar approach allows for direct visualization of the tendon noose around the metacarpal head and facilitates an A1 pulley release that may be all that is needed to free the metacarpal.[27] The dorsal approach is perceived to be safer and more efficient, and allows direct visualization of the interposed volar plate, but freeing the tendon noose may be more challenging.[28]

After closed or open treatment, radiographically confirm adequate reduction. The patient should then be placed in a dorsal blocking splint for 4 weeks to prevent MCPJ hyperextension while facilitating early active range of motion.

Volar MCPJ Dislocations

Volar MCPJ dislocations are rare, because the volar force required to cause the dislocation is more likely to fracture the proximal phalanx. However, when these injuries occur, they may be amenable to closed reduction under sedation. The reduction can be blocked by soft tissue interposition, as dorsal capsule, distal volar plate, collateral ligament, or junctura can all become entrapped.[29] Open reduction would then be required.

THUMB METACARPOPHALANGEAL JOINT INJURIES

The thumb metacarpophalangeal joint (tMCPJ) has properties of a hinge (ginglymus) joint as well as a condyloid joint, facilitating movement in a flexion-extension arc as well as some elements of rotation and abduction-adduction. Natural anatomic variation in the metacarpal head results in a wide range of *normal* motion in the population. Most of the tMCPJ stability is from soft tissue. These stabilizing structures include collateral ligaments and the volar plate. Additionally, the adductor pollicis inserts into the ulnar sesamoid while the flexor pollicis brevis and abductor pollicis brevis insert into the radial sesamoid. These sesamoid attachments are at the distal margin of the volar plate, and provide volar stability to the tMCPJ. These muscular attachments also have fibrous connections to the extensor mechanism, thereby providing lateral stability as well. Dorsal stability is less stout, provided mostly by the extensor pollicis longus and brevis tendons passing over the joint, along with some strength from the joint capsule itself.

Acute Thumb MCPJ Ulnar Collateral Ligament Injuries

Ulnar collateral ligament (UCL) tear is the most common injury to the tMCPJ.[30-32] It occurs due to hyperabduction and forced radial deviation of the proximal phalanx. Examination will reveal pain and edema along the ulnar border, particularly over the MCPJ. The most common injury type involves avulsion off of the distal attachment on the proximal phalanx. In evaluating these injuries, it is important to discern a partial from a complete tear, identify any fractures, and evaluate for a Stener lesion (described below). Always remember to examine the uninjured thumb as well, as many patients have laxity in these joints/ligaments at baseline.

Partial tears and small avulsion fractures that are stable can be treated conservatively in a thumb spica splint for 4 to 6 weeks.[33] MCP should be ulnarly deviated in the splint, and IPJ can be left free. A complete tear should be repaired. However, it is important to discern if a Stener lesion is present. A Stener lesion occurs when the UCL is torn away from the distal attachment on the proximal phalanx and mobilizes enough to allow the adductor pollicis aponeurosis to interpose between the ligament and the insertion site. Stener lesions can occur with an associated avulsion fracture or with the ligament alone.

Considering all of this, UCL evaluation involves an important series of steps.[34] Collateral ligament testing is similar to as described above for PIPJ injuries, with examination in full extension as well as 30° of joint flexion (Figure 80.7). Pain, as well as adductor pollicis spasm, can make the examination difficult, so a local anesthetic block may be helpful.

- Valgus stress is placed on the joint, evaluate the amount of gapping or angulation that can be created; this is where a comparison to the normal side is important.

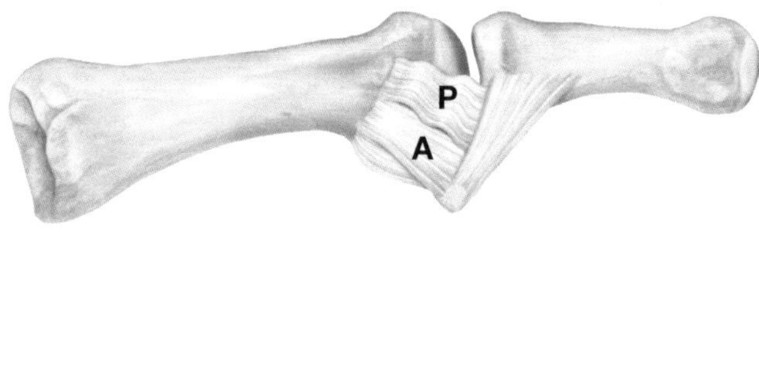

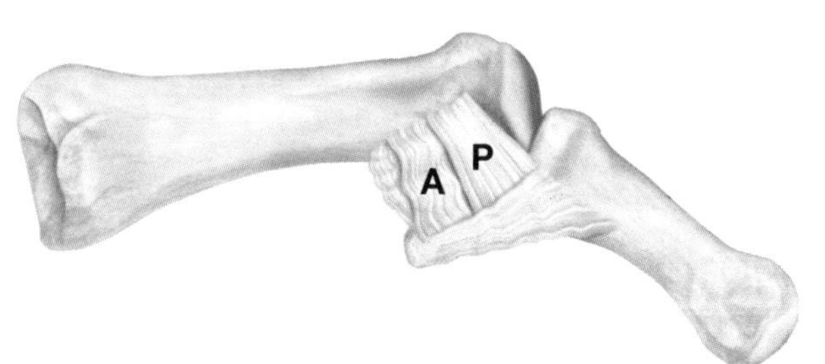

FIGURE 80.7. Thumb MCP anatomy. Note that the proper collateral ligament (*P*) is tight in 30° of flexion, while the accessory collateral (*A*) is tight in full extension. This is why when testing for a collateral ligament injury one must check the joint fully extended and flexed to 30°. This relationship is the same for finger PIP collateral ligaments.

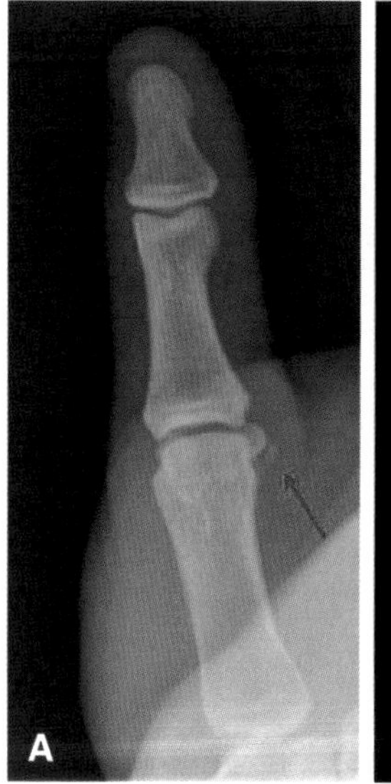

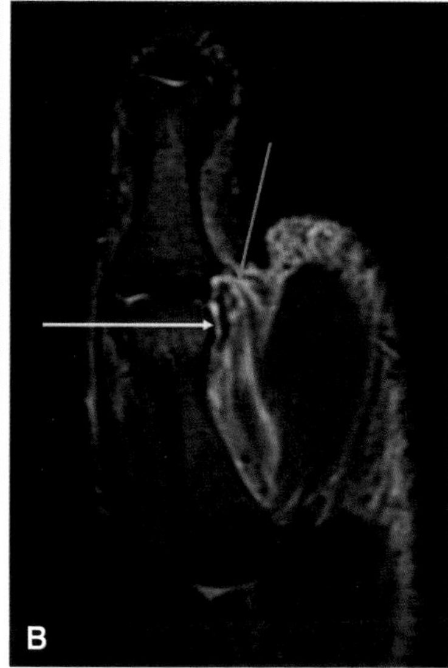

FIGURE 80.8. Stener lesion. **A.** X-ray of a thumb with instability and pain on testing of the ulnar collateral ligament. Note the small fracture fragment proximal to the joint line (*red arrow*). **B.** MRI of the same thumb with avulsed ulnar collateral ligament (*yellow arrow*) retracted proximal to the adductor aponeurosis (*blue arrow*).

- If there is a *firm endpoint*, it is likely a partial tear; if there is no resistance, the ligament is likely completely torn.
  - □ If the joint can be stressed to >35° of angulation, complete ligament tear is likely
    - If this occurs with joint flexed, it is a proper collateral tear
    - If this occurs with joint fully extended, it is an accessory collateral tear
  - □ If the joint can be stressed >15° more than contralateral, a complete tear is likely.
- If a mass is palpable proximal to the tMCPJ, this may indicate a Stener lesion. However, the absence of this finding does not rule it out.
- Evaluate X-rays because avulsion fractures are common.
  - □ Is the avulsion displaced?
    - More than 2 mm of displacement?
    - Is it proximal to the level of the adductor hood? If so, this is likely a bony Stener lesion (Figure 80.8).
  - □ Is 20% or more of the joint surface involved?
  - □ Is the UCL unstable?
- Is advanced imaging necessary?[35]
  - □ Ultrasound
  - □ MRI

If a complete UCL tear is diagnosed (aka Skier's thumb), open repair of the ligament is warranted.[36] These injuries usually involve detachment off of the distal site, but proximal tears and midsubstance tears do occur as well. Small minimally displaced (<2 mm) avulsion fractures can be treated conservatively, similar to partial tears. Larger or displaced fractures likely require open reduction and fixation; however, advanced imaging may be warranted to clarify whether a UCL injury has also occurred, as the examination may not be adequate for diagnosis of the combined bony and ligamentous injury. Stener lesions require operative intervention.

Operative approach is via a lazy-S incision over the ulnar border of the thumb, taking care not to violate the webspace with the incision. Midsubstance tears can be primarily repaired with permanent suture, whereas ligament avulsions are treated with bone anchors. If the distal avulsion donor site is not clear, aim to affix the ligament 3 mm distal to the articular surface and 3 mm dorsal to the volar cortex. If the avulsion is off of the metacarpal, aim to anchor at or dorsal to bony midline. Most surgeons advocate holding the tMCPJ in ulnar deviation and passing a K-wire across the joint to stabilize it during the acute recovery period.

Chronic Thumb MCPJ UCL Injuries (aka Gamekeeper's Thumb)

This injury presents as symptomatic chronic UCL pain and laxity. This can occur due to chronic overuse (i.e., game keepers) or more commonly inadequately treated acute UCL injuries. Confirm that there is no substantial tMCPJ arthritis before attempting to reconstruct the joint—if there is, fusion may be the proper treatment. If there is no arthritis, surgical repair with anchoring of the UCL can be attempted[37]; however, often the ligament is scarred and contracted, and a formal reconstruction is required to stabilize the joint.[38]

- *Static* reconstruction options are most commonly used, involving harvesting a free tendon graft and using it to recreate the ligament via bone tunnels and tenodesis screw fixation.
- *Dynamic* reconstruction options include transfer of adductor pollicis or extensor pollicis brevis insertion to the base of the proximal phalanx to create ulnar pull.

Thumb MCPJ Radial Collateral Ligament Injuries

RCL injuries are more likely to occur from an axial load force and often present later than UCL injuries because RCL instability is not as functionally limiting as UCL instability. Also, in contrast to the UCL, the RCL most commonly ruptures off of the proximal attachment. Additionally, the abductor pollicis brevis inserts more distally on the radial side, covering the RCL and generally preventing a Stener-type lesion.[39,40] One case report presents an exception.[41]

Presentation is similar to UCL injuries, with pain and edema along the radial side of the tMCPJ. The examination should be the same as with UCL injuries, evaluating degree of angulation on joint stressing along with other details reviewed above. Because the radial-sided structures contribute more to dorsal joint stability, also check for palmar subluxation when evaluating RCL injuries, as 3 mm or more of palmar subluxation is an indication of a complete tear.

Partial injuries should be treated conservatively with thumb spica splinting and IP left free. Management of a complete tear is controversial. Because a Stener-type lesion does not occur with RCL injury, some advocate splinting/casting similar to partial injuries. However, concern that thenar muscle ulnar deviation force is too strong to oppose with splinting has led others to advocate surgical repair of complete tears. If surgical repair of an acute tear is pursued, recommendations include fixating the joint in 30° of flexion with a K-wire, so the ligament repair is done on maximal tension and the adductor pollicis pull is prevented. Chronic injuries likely require ligament reconstruction.

Thumb MCPJ Dislocations

Most tMCPJ dislocations are dorsal, often the result of hyperextension that ruptures the volar plate, joint capsule, and at least part of the collateral ligaments.

Dorsal tMCPJ Subluxation

Less severe hyperextension injury can create subluxation injury without complete dislocation. The patient often presents with the joint in hyperextension. Sometimes, the tMCPJ becomes locked and cannot be flexed or extended. This occurs due to entrapment of the radial condyle in a torn segment of the volar plate.

Reduction may be attempted with the assistance of local anesthesia and joint insufflation. Then, apply volar-directed pressure on the proximal phalanx base while twisting on the metacarpal head. Avoid longitudinal traction. If this fails, open reduction may be necessary.

Dorsal tMCPJ Dislocations

Most dorsal dislocations are reducible. As with other MCPJ dislocations, the maneuver should avoid longitudinal traction. Instead, hyperextend and then use volar and distal pressure on the base of the proximal phalanx. This can be aided by local anesthetic block and intra-articular insufflation.

When a dorsal dislocation cannot be reduced, it is usually due to volar plate or FPL interposition. Volar plate obstruction is often made worse by the inclusion of the sesamoid bones, and when this occurs operative intervention is usually required. The FPL can create a noose around the metacarpal head/neck with the displaced thenar muscles, also making the dislocation irreducible.

If open reduction is required, the surgical approach can be dorsal, volar, or lateral. If using a dorsal approach, the goal is to find the interval between the extensor pollicis longus and extensor pollicis brevis tendons to approach the joint capsule. If approaching volar, be cautious about the potential for displaced neurovascular bundles directly under the skin.

Volar tMCPJ Dislocation

Volar tMCPJ dislocations are very rare, and in general are not reducible closed.

THUMB CARPOMETACARPAL JOINT

The articular surfaces of the thumb carpometacarpal joint (tCMC)—connecting the base of the thumb metacarpal with the distal aspect of the trapezium—resemble two opposed saddles. This arrangement facilitates motion in three planes: flexion-extension, pronation-supination, and abduction-adduction. The concavoconvex relationship confers some stability, but a complex ligamentous system and thick joint capsule are the primary sources of tCMC stabilization.[42] The four major ligaments are volar (aka volar oblique, anterior oblique), intermetacarpal, dorsal-radial, and dorsal oblique (aka posterior oblique). Abductor pollicis longus inserts over the dorsal joint, stabilizing the dorsal ligamentous structures. The volar oblique ligament connects the trapezium to the volar beak of the thumb metacarpal, and although there have been recent debates on this issue, the volar oblique ligament is largely believed to provide the major stabilizing force against dorsal metacarpal displacement. This stability is critical in pinch forces.

Thumb CMC Dislocation

These injuries are generally all dorsal dislocations. Although debated, it is generally believed that the dorsal-radial ligament must be torn, along with avulsion of the volar oblique ligament off of the metacarpal beak, to facilitate dislocation of the tCMC.[42,43]

Although a complete dislocation is easier to identify, it is also quite rare. More commonly, these injuries are partial dislocations.

- Evaluate plain radiographs as well as stress radiographs.
  - Standard PA and lateral views
  - Stress view is PA of both thumbs, parallel to the X-ray plate, with distal phalanges pressed together along the radial borders.
- Confirm no associated metacarpal base fracture.

Considering that these injuries are rare, and that partial dislocations/tears are often missed due to the subtle nature of the presentation, the clinical experience with these injuries is limited.[44]

- Closed reduction is often possible, but it is important to confirm that reduction is maintained and that the joint is stable.
  - If stable after reduction, immobilize with plaster.
  - Reexamine in 5 to 7 days, and if still stable treat with casting for a total of 6 weeks.
- If the joint remains unstable, surgical intervention is required.
  - Closed reduction augmented with pin fixation has been attempted, but in limited series this treatment still resulted in long-term instability.
  - Many providers go directly to ligament reconstruction techniques to treat tCMC injuries with persistent instability after initial reduction.

FINGER CARPOMETACARPAL JOINTS

The carpometacarpal joints (CMC) of the index, middle, ring, and small fingers have different degrees of inherent stability and range of motion, with the ring and small finger CMCs being most mobile. As a result, these CMC joints are also most likely to sustain dislocation. The most difficult aspect in managing finger CMC dislocations is identifying these injuries, as the findings are often subtle, and radiographs can be difficult to interpret.

In evaluating X-rays of possible CMC dislocation, any of the following should raise concern[45]:

- Loss of parallel M lines (Figure 80.9)
- Asymmetry of the CMC joint spaces: all should be 1 to 2 mm wide
- Loss of parallel joint lines for each CMC on PA view
- Cortical overlap at the CMC interface
- Indistinct cortical rims of the metacarpals
- Metacarpal axis (on lateral/oblique view) that does not parallel the other metacarpals

If X-rays are inadequate, evaluate under active fluoroscopy if available. CT scan may be needed to assess for dislocation/joint alignment if unable to clearly visualize via X-ray or fluoroscopy.

Once a CMC dislocation is identified, the reduction maneuver is relatively easy compared to other hand joints. Longitudinal traction with associated volarly directed pressure on the dorsal metacarpal base is often adequate.

However, these injuries tend to be unstable and will redislocate, indicating need for operative intervention.

- In isolated dislocations, reduction and K-wire fixation are usually adequate.
- If a fracture component is associated, management can be K-wires or ORIF depending on the extent of injury.

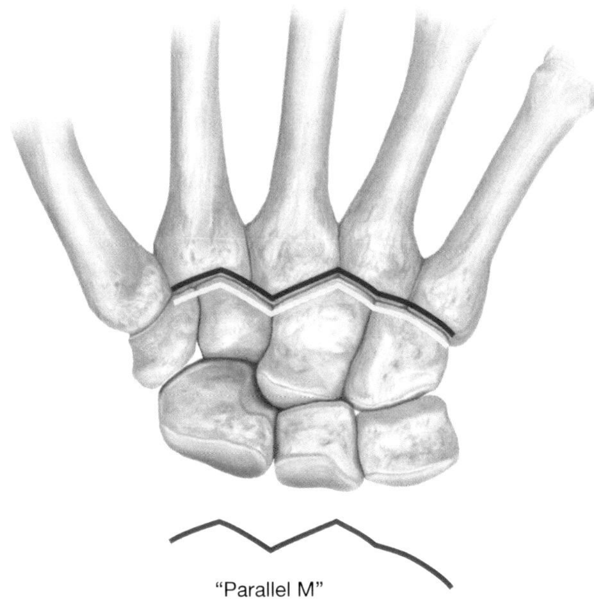

FIGURE 80.9. Parallel M-lines guide the evaluation of finger CMC joint congruency.

Long-term outcomes after dislocation are relatively good with low incidence of long-term pain or instability. Delayed presentation can result in worse outcomes.[46] Fracture-dislocations have mixed long-term outcomes, especially for ring/small finger CMC fracture dislocations, with some patients having persistent pain after initial repair that necessitates conversion to fusion.

ACKNOWLEDGMENTS

This work was supported by a Midcareer Investigator Award in Patient-Oriented Research (2 K24-AR053120 06) to Kevin C. Chung. The content is solely the responsibility of the authors and does not necessarily represent the official views of the National Institutes of Health.

REFERENCES

1. Eaton RG, Littler JW. Joint injuries and their sequelae. *Clin Plast Surg*. 1976;3:85-98.
2. Eaton RG, Glickel SZ, Littler JW. Tendon interposition arthroplasty for degenerative arthritis of the trapeziometacarpal joint of the thumb. *J Hand Surg*. 1985;10A:645-654.
3. Hart DP, Blair WF. Acute dorsal fracture-dislocation of the proximal interphalangeal joint. *J Iowa Med Soc*. 1983;73:359-363.
4. Haase SC, Chung KC. Current concepts in treatment of fracture-dislocations of the proximal interphalangeal joint. *Plast Reconstr Surg*. 2014;134:1246-1257.
   This article provides an excellent comprehensive review of the available techniques and evidence for treating fracture-dislocations of the PIP joint. The approach to these challenging injuries has evolved in recent years, and this article presents a clear review and summary of key studies.
5. McElfresh EC, Dobyns JH, O'Brien ET. Management of fracture-dislocation of the proximal interphalangeal joints by extension-block splinting. *J Bone Joint Surg Am*. 1972;54A:1705-1711.
6. Viegas SF. Extension block pinning for proximal interphalangeal joint fracture dislocations: preliminary report of a new technique. *J Hand Surg Am*. 1992;17A:896-901.
7. Badia A, Riano F, Ravikoff J, et al. Dynamic intradigital external fixation for proximal interphalangeal joint fracture dislocations. *J Hand Surg Am*. 2005;30A:154-160.
8. Ellis SJ, Cheng R, Prokopis P, et al. Treatment of proximal interphalangeal dorsal fracture-dislocation injuries with dynamic external fixation: a pins and rubber band system. *J Hand Surg Am*. 2007;32:1242-1250.
9. Ruland RT, Hogan CJ, Cannon DL, Slade JF. Use of dynamic distraction external fixation for unstable fracture-dislocations of the proximal interphalangeal joint. *J Hand Surg Am*. 2008;33:19-25.
10. Eaton RG, Malerich MM. Volar plate arthroplasty of the proximal interphalangeal joint: a review of ten years' experience. *J Hand Surg*. 1980;5A:260-268.
11. Calfee RP, Kiefhaber TR, Sommerkamp TG, Stern PJ. Hemi-hamate arthroplasty provides functional reconstruction of acute and chronic proximal interphalangeal fracture-dislocations. *J Hand Surg Am*. 2009;34:1232-1241.
   This case series presents 33 patients after hemihamate arthroplasty. Although the study is retrospective, the manuscript nicely reviews the procedure, indications, critical elements of the technique, postoperative management, and comprehensive outcomes. It is one of the more complete representations of this relatively new procedure and helped clarify approach and outcomes expectations as the hemihamate has become more frequently used in PIP reconstruction.
12. Williams RM, Kiefhaber TR, Sommerkamp TG, Stern PJ. Treatment of unstable dorsal proximal interphalangeal fracture/dislocations using a hemi-hamate autograft. *J Hand Surg Am*. 2003;28:856-865.
13. Baugher WH, McCue FC III. Anterior fracture-dislocation of the proximal interphalangeal joint: a case report. *J Bone Joint Surg Am*. 1979;61A:779-788.
14. Rosenstadt BE, Glickel SZ, Lane LB, Kaplan SJ. Palmar fracture dislocation of the proximal interphalangeal joint. *J Hand Surg Am*. 1998;23:811-820.
15. Ali MS. Complete disruption of collateral mechanism of proximal interphalangeal joint of fingers. *J Hand Surg Br*. 1984;9:191-193.
16. McCue FC, Honner R, Johnson MC, Gieck JH. Athletic injuries of the proximal interphalangeal joint requiring surgical treatment. *J Bone Joint Surg Am*. 1970;52:937-956.
17. Kamnerdnakta S, Huetteman HE, Chung KC. Complications of proximal interphalangeal joint injuries: prevention and treatment. *Hand Clin*. 2018;34:267-288.
   This is another review article that should be seen by anyone learning about and treating PIP joint injuries. The authors provide a very clear and thoughtful approach to the development of complications and recovery limitations after PIP injuries, and take a stepwise approach to diagnosing and treating the various complications that can arise after these difficult injuries.
18. Abouzahr MK, Poblete JV. Irreducible dorsal dislocation of the distal interphalangeal joint: case report and literature review. *J Trauma*. 1997;42:743-745.
19. Naito K, Sugiyama Y, Igeta Y, et al. Irreducible dislocation of the thumb interphalangeal joint due to displaced flexor pollicis longus tendon: case report and new reduction technique. *Arch Orthop Trauma Surg*. 2014;134:1175-1178.
20. Kubota R, Nozawa M, Matsuda K, Kim S. Closed irreducible dislocation of the interphalangeal joint of the thumb: report of two cases. *Chir Organi Mov*. 2009;93:85-88.
21. Grandizio LC, Klena JC. Sagittal band, boutonniere, and pulley injuries in the athlete. *Curr Rev Musculoskelet Med*. 2017;10:17-22.
22. Lee JH, Baek JH, Lee JS. A reconstructive stabilization technique for nontraumatic or chronic traumatic extensor tendon subluxation. *J Hand Surg Am*. 2017;42:e61-e65.
23. ElMaraghy AW, Pennings A. Metacarpophalangeal joint extensor tendon subluxation: a reconstructive stabilization technique. *J Hand Surg Am*. 2013;38:578-582.
24. [illegible] joint of a finger. *J Hand Surg Am*. 1988;13:444-448.
25. McLaughlin HL. Complex "locked" dislocation of the metacarpophalangeal joints. *J Trauma*. 1965;5:683-688.
26. Patterson RW, [illegible] joint dislocations. *Orthopedics*. 2008;31:1099.
27. Durakbasa O, Guneri B. The volar surgical approach in complex dorsal metacarpophalangeal dislocations. *Injury*. 2009;40:657-659.
28. Vadala CJ, Ward CM. Dorsal approach decreases operative time for complex metacarpophalangeal dislocations. *J Hand Surg Am*. 2016;41:e259-e262.
29. Renshaw TS, Louis DS. Complex volar dislocation of the metacarpophalangeal joint: a case report. *J Trauma*. 1973;13:1086-1088.
30. Moberg E, Stener B. Injuries to the ligaments of the thumb and fingers: diagnosis, treatment and prognosis. *Acta Chir Scand*. 1953;106:166-186.
31. Frank WE, Dobyns J. Surgical pathology of collateral ligamentous injuries of the thumb. *Clin Orthop Relat Res*. 1972;83:102-114.
32. Smith RJ. Post-traumatic instability of the metacarpophalangeal joint of the thumb. *J Bone Joint Surg Am*. 1977;59A:14-21.
   A classic article that reviews 86 patients with thumb ligamentous and bony injuries. It was one of the earliest comprehensive reviews of the approach to thumb collateral ligament injuries and indications for repair.
33. Carlsen BT, Moran SL. Thumb trauma: Bennett fractures, Rolando fractures, and ulnar collateral ligament injuries. *J Hand Surg Am*. 2009;34:945-952.
34. Pulos N, Shin AY. Treatment of ulnar collateral ligament injuries of the thumb: a critical analysis review. *JBJS Rev*. 2017;5.
35. Mahajan M, Tolman C, Wurth B, Rhemrev SJ. Clinical evaluation vs magnetic resonance imaging of the Skier's thumb: a prospective cohort of 30 patients. *Eur J Radiol*. 2016;85:1750-1756.
36. Wilppula E, Nummi J. Surgical treatment of ruptured ulnar collateral ligament of the metacarpophalangeal joint of the thumb. *Injury*. 1970;2:69-72.
37. Pai S, Smit A, Birch A, Hayton M. Delayed anatomical repair of ruptured ulnar collateral ligament injuries of the thumb using a dissolvable polylactic acid bone anchor. *J Trauma*. 2008;65:1502-1506.
38. Wong TC, Ip FK, Wu WC. Bone-periosteum-bone graft reconstruction for chronic ulnar instability of the metacarpophalangeal joint of the thumb—minimum 5-year follow-up evaluation. *J Hand Surg Am*. 2009;34:304-308.
39. Edelstein DM, Kardashian G, Lee SK. Radial collateral ligament injuries of the thumb. *J Hand Surg Am*. 2008;33:760-770.
40. Melone CP Jr, Beldner S, Basuk RS. Thumb collateral ligament injuries: an anatomic basis for treatment. *Hand Clin*. 2000;16:345-357.
41. Doty JF, Rudd JN, Jemison M. Radial collateral ligament injury of the thumb with a Stener-like lesion. *Orthopedics*. 2010;33:925.
42. Strauch RJ, Behrman MJ, Rosenwasser MP. Acute dislocation of the carpometacarpal joint of the thumb: an anatomic and cadaver study. *J Hand Surg Am*. 1994;19:93-98.

43. Bosmans B, Verhofstad MH, Gosens T. Traumatic thumb carpometacarpal joint dislocations. *J Hand Surg Am*. 2008;33:438-441.

44. Simonian PT, Trumble TE. Traumatic dislocation of the thumb carpometacarpal joint: early ligamentous reconstruction versus closed reduction and pinning. *J Hand Surg Am*. 1996;21:802-806.
A retrospective case series comparing patients treated with two different approaches to a rare condition. Although the manuscript has flaws, due to the uncommon nature of this injury it presents helpful information in the treatment algorithm, favoring early open intervention with ligamentous reconstruction.

45. Fisher MR, Rogers LF, Hendrix RW. Systematic approach to identifying fourth and fifth carpometacarpal joint dislocations. *AJR Am J Roentgenol*. 1983;140:319-324.
An early and very thoughtful review of how to approach these often-missed injuries. The helpful diagnostic and radiographic parameters are reviewed. This article is a high-yield read to help avoid the all too common mistake of missing the CMC dislocation injury.

46. Zhang C, Wang H, Liang C, et al. The effect of timing on the treatment and outcome of combined fourth and fifth carpometacarpal fracture dislocations. *J Hand Surg Am*. 2015;40:2169-2175.

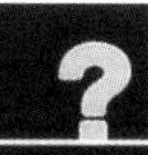

QUESTIONS

1. **An 18-year-old hit his finger on another player's helmet during a football game and felt a pop. He grabbed his finger and pulled it into place. However, he cannot extend the PIP joint beyond 35° of flexion, and his distal phalanx is positioned in notable hyperextension. What soft tissue structure in the finger is most likely injured?**
   - a. Volar plate
   - b. Collateral ligament
   - c. Central slip
   - d. Sagittal band
   - e. Lateral band

2. **A 45-year-old man presents 8 weeks after his left ring finger had been hit with a softball. He noted pain and swelling, as well as difficulty using the finger, but did not seek treatment until now. The patient has 90° of mildly painful active flexion at the PIP joint, and the finger deviates ulnarly during flexion. X-ray reveals destruction of 45% of the volar base of the middle phalanx with dorsal subluxation of the middle phalanx. What treatment should be offered to help preserve range of motion while correcting the deviation and improving pain?**
   - a. PIP fusion
   - b. Buddy straps and therapy
   - c. Volar plate arthroplasty
   - d. Hemihamate arthroplasty
   - e. Dynamic external fixation

3. **A 20-year-old female presents 8 weeks after jamming her long finger. On examination, a passively correctable boutonniere deformity is [illegible]. Active range of motion is preserved at the PIP and DIP joints. X-ray reveals no fracture. What is the best initial treatment?**
   - a. Splinting of the PIP and DIP in extension
   - b. Volar plate arthroplasty
   - c. Splinting of the PIP in extension while allowing active ROM at the DIP
   - d. DIP fusion
   - e. Kirschner wire pinning of the DIP and PIP in full extension

4. **A 48-year-old man presents with thumb pain 3 days after an injury. He has swelling over the thumb MCP joint. He is unable to pinch due to pain, and radial deviation stress of the MCP is painful and unstable. X-ray shows a small fracture off the proximal phalanx base with a displaced fracture fragment seen at the level of the proximal MCP joint. What is the appropriate treatment?**
   - a. Closed reduction and splinting
   - b. Open ligament repair
   - c. Early occupational therapy
   - d. Closed reduction and percutaneous pinning

5. **A 32-year-old police officer presents after feeling a pop in her hand during a training exercise. No soft tissue injuries or lacerations. On examination, she has pain over the dorsum of her hand. No limitations in range of motion. She has notable painful subluxation of the middle finger extensor tendon during range of motion. What is the most likely diagnosis and the best initial treatment?**
   - a. Sagittal band rupture; splinting with middle finger MCP in extension
   - b. Sagittal band rupture; open repair
   - c. Sagittal band rupture; buddy straps and early active range of motion
   - d. Central slip rupture; splinting with PIP joint in extension and DIP active flexion therapy
   - e. Central slip rupture; open repair

1. **Answer: c.** The patient has an acute boutonniere deformity, identified by the fixed position of PIP flexion and DIP hyperextension. This is caused by a rupture of the central slip over the dorsal PIP/middle phalanx. With the central slip detached, the lateral bands (which are held in position in part by their attachments to the central slip) are able to subluxate volarly on the finger, creating the boutonniere deformity.

2. **Answer: d.** The patient has a delayed presentation of fracture/dislocation of the PIP joint with subluxation of the middle phalanx. Although his range of motion is reasonable (the reconstructive PIP options do not reliably restore more than 90° of flexion), he has notable scissoring and discomfort. The hemihamate arthroplasty is the only option on the list that is adequate for such a substantial injury to the PIP and preserves motion. Fusion will leave no motion, buddy straps will not correct the scissoring long term, volar plate arthroplasty is unreliable for a fracture that involves so much of the volar base of P2 especially with a delayed presentation, and the external fixator will only work in the acute setting when the fracture is still malleable.

3. **Answer: c.** With a passively correctable boutonniere deformity due to a central slip injury, even when presenting 8 weeks after injury, splinting the PIP in extension is the best first-line treatment. The extension position provides better continuity for the central slip to heal in appropriate position, while allowing DIP range of motion helps pull the lateral bands more dorsal and prevents unnecessary stiffness. Holding both joints in full extension is unnecessary, and by not allowing DIP flexion may even prevent the deformity from properly correcting. None of the other options will correct the deformity.

4. **Answer: b.** Patient presents with an UCL injury and associated Stener lesion. The fracture fragment represents a distal avulsion of the ligament with displacement preventing successful closed treatment. The appropriate treatment is open repair.

5. **Answer: a.** Sagittal band ruptures can be quite painful without notable functional limitation. Localizing the site of pain and identifying the subluxation of the extensor tendon help confirm the diagnosis. Especially when identified early, most sagittal band ruptures can be treated closed using a reverse yoke splint that keeps the MCP in extension while allowing active range of motion of the finger to prevent stiffness in other joints.

CHAPTER 81 ■ Ligament Injuries of the Wrist

Brett F. Michelotti

KEY POINTS

- Early identification and treatment of wrist ligamentous injury will result in the best clinical outcomes.
- Arthroscopy remains the reference standard for diagnosing wrist ligamentous injuries.
- The type of operation to be performed depends on the chronicity of the injury, the presence of reparable ligament, and presence or absence of wrist arthritis.
- A salvage operation, such as a partial wrist fusion or hemiresection ulna arthroplasty, should be considered when there is clinical and radiographic evidence of wrist arthritis.

The wrist is an extremely complex arrangement of bony and soft-tissue structures. Understanding the normal anatomy and kinematics of the wrist helps identifying and treating the breadth of the pathology. Soft-tissue and ligamentous injury can disrupt normal kinematic processes and lead to inflammation, pain, and joint destruction. Ranging from partial caspuloligamentous tears to complete ligamentous disruption and instability, degree and location of injury, as well as timing of diagnosis can impact the type of intervention and predictability of outcomes. Delayed or missed injuries can result in irreversible joint damage and may require a salvage operation such as a proximal row carpectomy (PRC) or arthrodesis.

ANATOMY AND KINEMATICS

The wrist is the connection between the forearm bones and the hand. It consists of the distal radius and ulna, five metacarpal bases, seven tightly articulated carpal bones, and the pisiform, a sesamoid bone that acts as a lever arm for the flexor carpi ulnaris tendon. The radius and ulna articulate with the proximal carpal row, forming the radiocarpal and ulnocarpal joints. The proximal carpal row is made up of the scaphoid, lunate, and triquetrum. The midcarpal joint is the articulation of the proximal and distal carpal rows. The distal carpal row is formed by the trapezium, trapezoid, capitate, and hamate. These carpal bones articulate with the bases of the five metacarpals.

The stability of the carpus is influenced by bony constraints and intrinsic and extrinsic ligaments. Intrinsic ligaments originate and end within the carpus, otherwise referred to as intercarpal connections. Extrinsic ligaments originate outside the carpus and end within the carpus.

Extrinsic ligaments may be subdivided into three major groups: palmar radiocarpal, palmar ulnocarpal, and dorsal radiocarpal (DRC) ligaments. There are no dorsal ligaments between the ulna and the carpus.

Palmar radiocarpal ligaments consist of the radioscaphoid, radioscaphocapitate (RSC), and long and short radiolunate ligaments. The space of Poirier is the palmar interligamentous space ulnar and proximal to the RSC ligament. This is a weak soft-tissue space through which lunate dislocation occurs.

Arising from the base of the ulnar styloid, the ulnar capitate ligament courses obliquely to attach to the neck of the capitate. The ulnar capitate and RSC ligaments form a V, otherwise known as the arcuate ligament. Originating from the triangular fibrocartilage complex (TFCC) are the ulnar triquetral and ulnar lunate ligaments.

The DRC is a wide, fan-shaped ligament connecting the dorsal edge of the distal radius to the dorsal triquetrum; there are some deeper fibers that connect to the dorsal surfaces of the lunate and scaphoid.

The dorsal intercarpal ligament (DIC) arises from the dorsal triquetrum, traverses along the distal edge of the lunate, and inserts with its fan-shaped terminal extensions on the dorsal rim of the scaphoid, the trapezium, and the trapezoid bones.

Intrinsic ligaments of the proximal carpal row include the scapholunate interosseous ligament (SLIL) and the lunotriquetral interosseous ligament (LTIL). There are many strong ligamentous attachments between the bones of the distal carpal row, named after the bones in which they connect.

There are no tendinous attachments to the bones of the proximal carpal row. With normal wrist mechanics, motion of the proximal carpal row is passive, meaning that it functions as an *intercalated segment* with movement of bones around their articulations dictated by extrinsic ligamentous forces, bony geometry, and interosseous ligamentous connections. The distal carpal row functions as a fixed unit, its articulations held tightly by stout intercarpal ligaments. Movement of the radiocarpal, ulnocarpal, and midcarpal joints is dictated by forces exerted by the tendons crossing the joints.

With radial deviation of the wrist, the scaphoid flexes. This is caused by the forces exerted on the proximal carpal row by the bones of the distal row. A proximally directed force from the hamate into the triquetrum forces the triquetrum to flex. With tight interosseous connections through the lunate (LTIL) to the scaphoid (SLIL), the scaphoid is forced into a flexed position. The opposite is true during ulnar deviation (Figure 81.1). The triquetrum extends, the lunate and scaphoid follow, assuming an extended posture.

Disruption of intercarpal ligaments and secondary stabilizing ligaments leads to carpal instability and altered biomechanics.

CARPAL INSTABILITY

Carpal instability, defined broadly, is abnormal carpal motion that results from injuries to the carpal bones and intrinsic or extrinsic ligaments. Altered kinematics or dyssynchronous motion can occur within bones of the same carpal row or between carpal rows.

- *Carpal instability dissociative (CID):* Instability caused by injury or disease affecting the articulation and motion of bones within the same carpal row. Examples of common dissociative instabilities include scapholunate (SL) dissociation, lunotriquetral dissociation (LT), unstable scaphoid fracture, nonunion or malunion, inflammatory synovitis, and advanced Kienböck disease.
- *Carpal instability nondissociative:* Symptomatic carpal dysfunction between the radius and the proximal row or between the proximal and distal rows, but without disruption of the interosseous ligaments or between the bones of the same row.
- *Carpal instability complex:* Carpal derangement that has features of carpal instability dissociative and carpal instability nondissociative in which there is an altered relationship between the bones of the same row and between rows. These include carpal bone dislocations, such as a perilunate dislocation or carpal bone fracture dislocation, such as a trans-scaphoid perilunate dislocation.
- *Carpal instability adaptive:* Instability within the carpus as a result of a deformity outside of the proximal and distal rows. An example of carpal instability adaptive is a malunited or poorly reduced distal radius fracture that results in altered biomechanics and arthritis of the midcarpal joint. This can be corrected by performing a radial osteotomy, in that the surgical planning is not aimed at the symptomatic midcarpal joint itself.

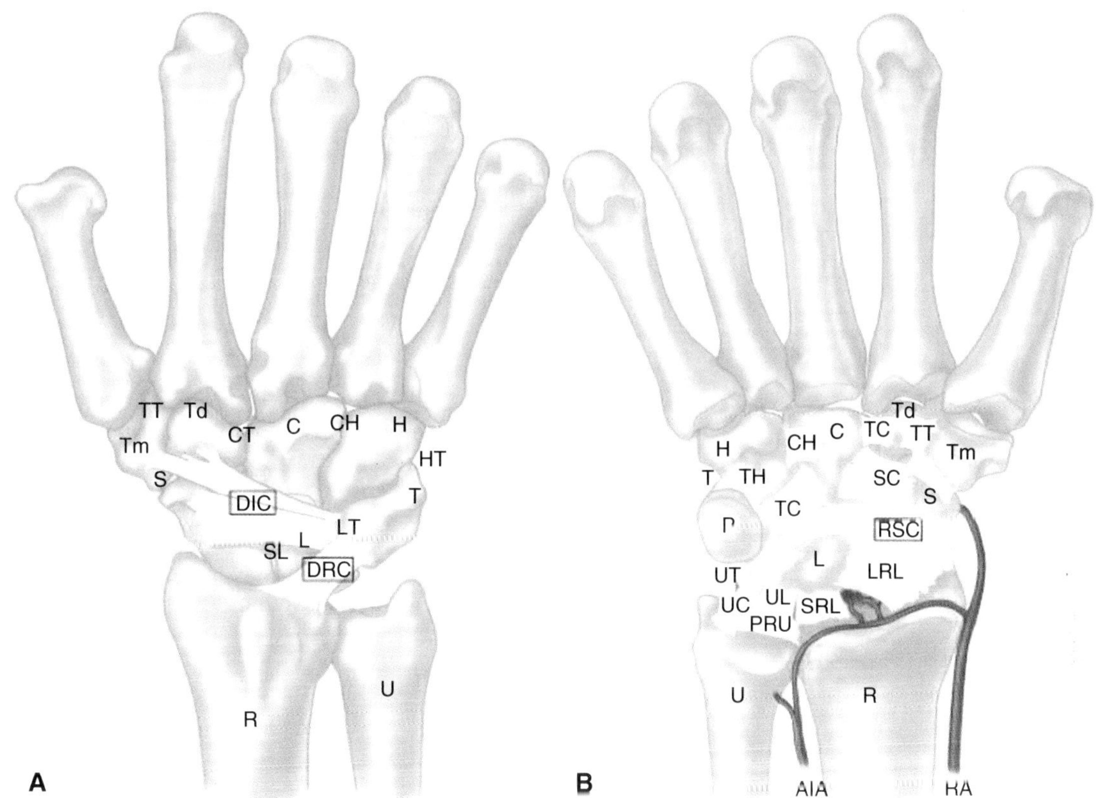

[illegible] Intrinsic ligaments of the wrist. **A.** Dorsal extrinsic and intrinsic ligaments of the wrist. **B.** Volar extrinsic and intrinsic ligaments of the wrist. *AIA*, anterior interosseous artery; *C*, capitate; *CH*, capitohamate; *CT*, capitotrapezoid; *DIC*, dorsal intercarpal ligament; *DRC*, Dorsal radiocarpal ligament; [illegible] *L*, lunate; *LRL*, long radiolunate; *LT*, lunotriquetral; *P*, pisiform; [illegible] *S*, scaphoid; *SC*, scaphocapitate; *SL*, scaphol- [illegible] *T*, triquetrum; *Td*, trapezoid; *Tm*, trapezium; *TC*, triquetrocapitate; *TH*, triquetrohamate; [illegible] ulna; *UC*, ulnocapitate; [illegible] Mayfield JK. Wrist ligamentous anatomy and pathogenesis of carpal instability. *Orthop Clin North Am*. 1984;15(2):209-216. Copyright © 1984 Elsevier. With [illegible])

SCAPHOLUNATE LIGAMENT INJURY

Diagnosis

Early recognition and treatment of SL ligament injury can delay or prevent the onset of arthritis. In a cadaveric study by Lee et al, 35% of cadaveric wrists had some degree of SL tear, and of those wrists with SLIL injury, 29% had evidence of arthrosis.[1]

The SL ligament is a U-shaped soft-tissue structure that has three parts with measurably different biomechanical properties. The strongest part of the ligament runs within the deep portion of the wrist capsule and links the dorsal scaphoid and lunate. The palmar portion of the ligament contains obliquely oriented fibers that are weaker but permit more rotation around the lunate and play less of a role in stability than the stronger dorsal ligament. The proximal membranous portion of the ligament does not play a role in stabilization and often appears perforated in older individuals, but this is not a true indication of SL instability.[2]

Injury to SL ligament occurs during a fall onto an outstretched hand causing wrist hyperextension, ulnar deviation, and midcarpal supination. With complete disruption of all the SL components, the axial load generated by extrinsic forces on the wrist results in flexion of the scaphoid and extension of the lunate—dorsal intercalated segment instability or DISI deformity. Less commonly, SLIL dissociation results from attritional degeneration owing to rheumatoid arthritis, pseudogout, or Kienbock disease.[3–5] SLIL injury should be considered along the spectrum of perilunate dislocation as described by Mayfield[6] (Figure 81.2):

Stage I: SL instability resulting from total disruption of the SLIL and secondary stabilizing ligaments
Stage II: Rupture of the midcarpal joint capsule with dorsal and proximal translation of the capitate over the lunate
Stage III: Lunotriquetral ligament (LT) rupture and tearing of the radio-lunate-triquetral ligaments
Stage IV: Volar lunate dislocation with the remaining carpal bones in line with the radius

SL injury itself can be categorized as predynamic, dynamic, static-reducible, static-irreducible, and scapholunate advanced collapse (SLAC):

- *Predynamic instability* is the result of partial tearing of the ligament that can present as wrist pain, exacerbated by loading or lifting. In this stage of SLIL, X-rays are normal but the diagnosis can be confirmed by wrist arthroscopy.[7]
- *Dynamic instability* can be diagnosed with clenched fist X-rays, which demonstrate widening of the SL interval as the capitate is driven from distal to proximal across the SL articulation.[8]
- *Static instability* results from a complete disruption of the SLIL and tearing or attenuation of the secondary stabilizing ligaments (scaphotrapezio-trapezoid ligament [STT], RSC ligament, and DIC ligament). Gapping between the scaphoid and lunate (normal 1–2 mm, >4 mm with static instability) can be observed with standard radiographs. Reducibility of the scaphoid, or correction of DISI deformity, may signify whether a reconstruction can be performed. If the deformity is not reducible, a salvage operation should be considered, e.g., scaphoidectomy and partial fusion versus PRC.

Long-standing carpal malalignment owing to SL ligament disruption leads to a predictable pattern of wrist arthritis or SLAC. Standard PA X-rays may reveal radial styloid arthritis (stage I), radioscaphoid arthritis (stage II), scaphocapitate arthritis (stage III), or pancarpal arthritis (stage IV). The degree of arthritis and which articular surfaces have been affected or spared become important when deciding which pain-relieving operation to perform. If the

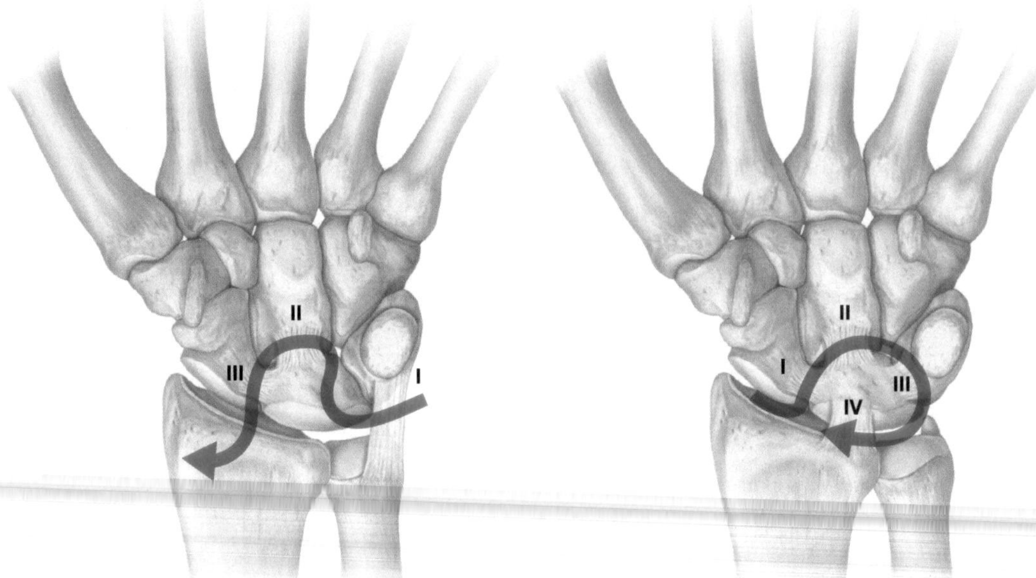

FIGURE 81.2. Stage I is disruption of the scapholunate articulation. Stages II and III are separation of the capitolunate and lunotriquetral joints. Stage IV is a volar lunate dislocation. (From Morris MS, Chung KC. Lunotriquetral ligament reconstruction using a slip of the extensor carpi ulnaris tendon. In: Chung KC, ed. *Operative Techniques in Plastic Surgery*. Philadelphia, PA: Wolters Kluwer; 2019. In press.)

radiolunate or capitolunate joints have been affected, the patient is not a candidate for PRC (Figure 81.3).

Diagnosis of SL injury begins with a focused history and physical examination. History of fall onto an outstretched hand, dorsal wrist pain, and pain that is exacerbated with axial loading should prompt careful examination of the SL interval. Palpation over the SL ligament, just distal to the Lister tubercle and between the EPL and EDQ tendons, may elicit pain. The scaphoid shift test is performed by dorsally directing pressure through the distal scaphoid tubercle while passively moving the wrist from ulnar to radial. With laxity or disruption of the SL ligament, the proximal scaphoid will dislocate dorsally. A clunk is appreciated when the bone is reduced into the scaphoid fossa of the radius. Dislocation in association with pain should prompt further evaluation with adjunctive tests such as noncontrast MRI or wrist arthroscopy.

Standard three-view wrist X-rays may identify widening of the SL interval. More than 4 mm of gapping (Terry Thomas sign) may be static SL instability but it may also be nonpathologic widening of the interval as seen in elderly; therefore, this must be considered in the context of history and physical examination and may be compared with the unaffected side.

A true PA X-ray may reveal the *signet ring* sign, where the distal pole of the scaphoid projects through the proximal pole and appears as a ring. With tearing or attrition of the secondary stabilizing ligaments (STT, DIC, RSC), the scaphoid assumes a flexed position and the lunate extends (DISI deformity). The SL angle is normally between 30° and 60° (mean 47°) but with DISI deformity, the angle exceeds 60° (Figure 81.4).

In the patient with pain but normal X-ray findings (possible predynamic instability) or with evidence of dynamic instability (gapping of the SL interval with wrist loading), arthroscopy may be performed to further characterize the injury pattern. Geissler described an arthroscopic grading system to classify interosseous ligament injury[7]:

Grade I: Attenuation and hemorrhage of interosseous ligament seen from radiocarpal joint, with no step-off present as seen from midcarpal joint

Grade II: Attenuation and hemorrhage of interosseous ligament seen from radiocarpal joint, with step-off seen through midcarpal joint; the probe can be placed between the scaphoid and lunate

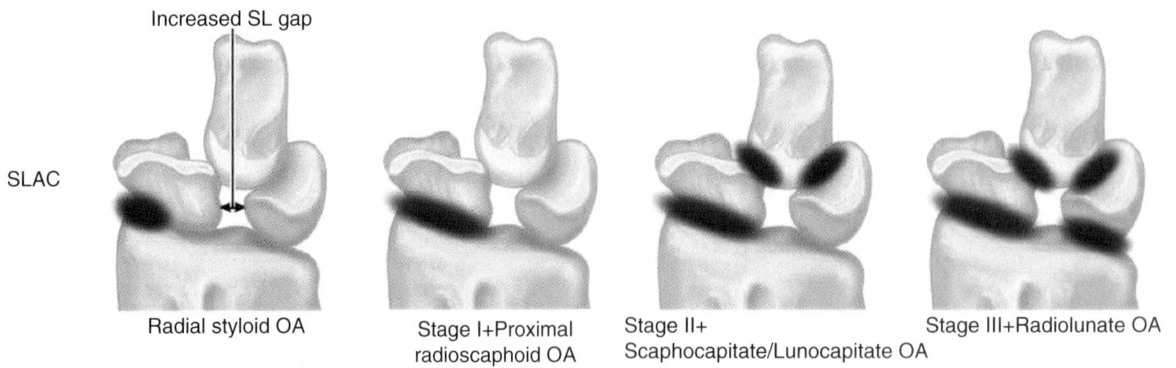

FIGURE 81.3. Scapholunate advanced collapse (SLAC arthritis). (From Michelotti BF, Chung KC. Scaphoid excision and four-corner fusion. In: Chung KC, ed. *Operative Techniques: Hand and Wrist Surgery*. 3rd ed. Philadelphia; PA: Elsevier Saunders; 2017:244; with permission.)

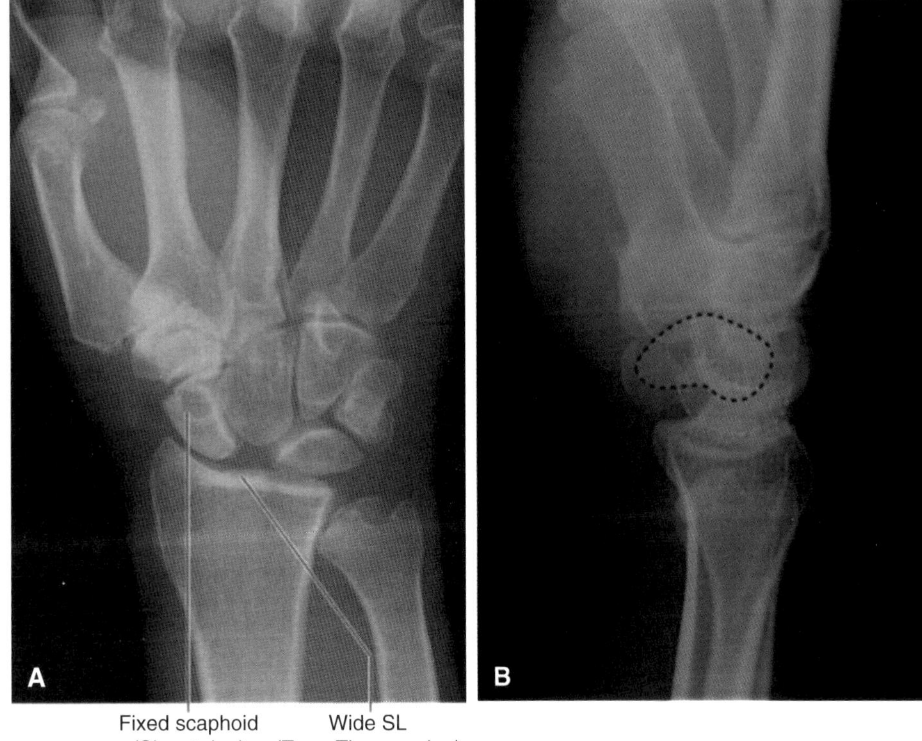

FIGURE 81.4. **A.** Scaphoid ring sign and Terry Thomas sign. **B.** Lateral radiograph demonstrating an increased SL angle. (From Michelotti BF, Chung KC. Scapholunate ligament reconstruction. In: Chung KC, ed. *Operative Techniques: Hand and Wrist Surgery*. 3rd ed. Philadelphia, PA: Elsevier Saunders; 2017.[183]; with permission.)

Grade III Incongruency or step-off is seen between the scaphoid and the lunate from both the radiocarpal and midcarpal portals; the probe can be placed and freely rotated between the scaphoid and lunate

Grade IV Incongruency or step-off is seen between the scaphoid and lunate from both the radiocarpal and midcarpal portals; gross instability is noted, and the 2.7 mm arthroscope may be passed through the gap between the scaphoid and lunate

Grades I to III of the Geissler classification system represent partial injury to the SLIL or *predynamic instability*. Grade IV represents complete disruption of the SLIL and *dynamic instability*.

Treatment

Treatment of SL pathology is dictated by the degree of ligamentous disruption and the chronicity of the injury.

Predynamic Instability

- Arthroscopic debridement and percutaneous pinning of SL interval
- Proprioceptive rehabilitation

Dynamic Instability, Direct Repair Possible

- Dorsal SLIL repair with or without capsulodesis

Dynamic Instability, Direct Repair Not Possible

- Ligamentous reconstruction from DIC and palmaris graft
- Bone-tissue-bone graft
- Three-ligament tenodesis

Static, Reducible Instability

- Three-ligament tenodesis

SLAC

- Scaphoidectomy and partial fusion
- PRC

Predynamic Instability

Initial treatment of suspected predynamic SL should consist of a trial of bracing and nonsteroidal anti-inflammatories. If this fails to reduce pain localizing to the SL interval, Geissler and others suggest that predynamic instability (Geissler grade I to III) can be treated by arthroscopic debridement and/or percutaneous pinning of the SL interval.[7,9,10] Chronic predynamic instability has also been treated with selective proprioceptive rehabilitation, arthroscopic debridement, or capsular shrinkage. Whipple determined that in patients who were treated within 3 months of injury, 83% remained symptom-free and maintained their reduction in up to 7-year follow-up.[9]

Dynamic Instability

Treatment of dynamic instability depends on whether the ligament is repairable. Assuming it has been only 6 weeks from the time of injury (acute), the ligament can either be repaired (midsubstance tear) or anchored to the bone with bone tunnels or suture anchors. Repair of the dorsal portion of the SL ligament is all that is required to restore normal relationships between the carpus.[2,11,12]

When direct repair of the ligament is not possible, a three-ligament tenodesis, or bone-tissue-bone ligament reconstruction may be considered[13–15] (Figure 81.5). Proponents of the bone-tissue-bone construct suggest that bone-to-bone contact may heal more predictably than a bone-tendon interface. However, studies have shown that the tissue portion of the graft may stretch and fail, the bone graft may not unite, and, with static instability, rotatory subluxation of the scaphoid cannot be addressed.

Static, Reducible Instability

When the secondary stabilizing ligaments of the scaphoid fail because of an acute, high-energy injury, or over time with attrition (STT, DIC, RSC), the scaphoid assumes a flexed, pronated posture. It is important to carefully examine the patient for the ability to reduce or correct the DISI deformity and for the absence of articular wear, as both are a contraindication for reconstruction.

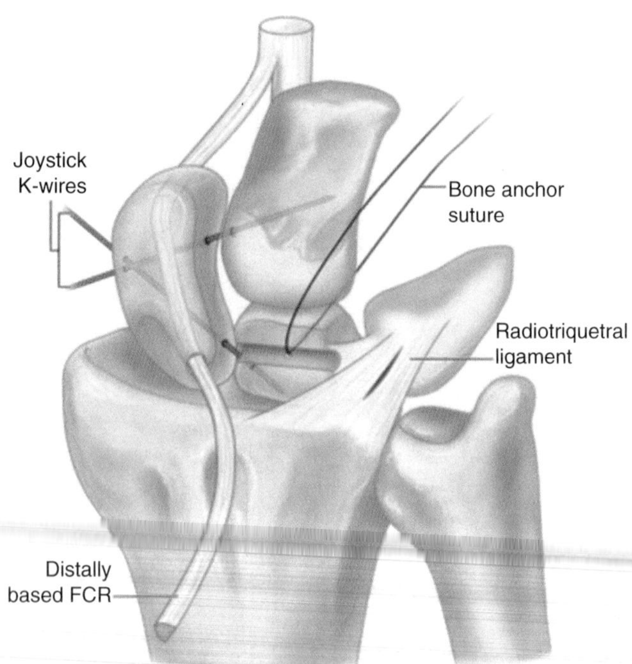

FIGURE 81.5. Tendon reconstruction of the scapholunate interosseous ligament (Brunelli and modifications). *FCR*, flexor carpi radialis. (From Michelotti BF, Chung KC. Scapholunate ligament reconstruction. In: Chung KC, ed. *Operative Techniques. Hand and Wrist Surgery*. 3rd ed. Philadelphia, PA: Elsevier Saunders; 2017:199; with permission.)

The initial three-ligament tenodesis uses a portion of the flexor carpi radialis (FCR) tendon to pass through a bone tunnel in the scaphoid, from palmar to dorsal, to improve the abnormally flexed posture in addition to reconstructing the dorsal portion of the SL ligament. The distal tendon graft is anchored to the radius. This was well tolerated but resulted in average loss in wrist flexion of 45% as compared with the unaffected side.[16] A modified tenodesis addressed the decrease in wrist flexion by anchoring the FCR tendon to the dorsal lunate instead of crossing the radius.[17] In the patient with dynamic or static-reducible instability, long-term data suggest that the modified Brunelli tenodesis is effective at reducing pain, may permit near-normal wrist motion, and will likely improve patient-reported outcome measures. Some patients still develop SLAC arthritis and will need wrist fusion procedures.[18,19]

Static, Irreducible Instability

When the DISI deformity is fixed and cannot be reduced, or there are signs of articular wear, the patient is no longer a candidate for ligamentous reconstruction but should be counseled on salvage procedures for pain relief. Rotatory subluxation of the scaphoid, around the RSC ligament, results in abnormal contact of the scaphoid with the radial styloid and scaphoid fossa of the radius. Over time, this leads to articular wear and a predictable progression of arthritis beginning with the radial styloid, progressing to the radioscaphoid articulation, scaphocapitate and lunocapitate joints, and finally to the lunate fossa. The most common salvage procedures aimed at relieving wrist pain caused by SL or SLAC are scaphoidectomy and intercarpal fusion, and PRC. Recent data suggest that the PRC is more cost-effective.[20]

Rehabilitation and Recovery

Painless motion is the goal of an SL repair or reconstruction. Patients are immobilized in a wrist brace for 8 weeks or until K-wires are removed. Gentle range of motion exercises is initiated and gradually advanced over 3 months. Protecting the reconstruction assures its durability and long-term effectiveness, therefore, a subtle loss in motion is accepted. Patients are counseled to expect loss of motion after any type of wrist surgery.

LUNOTRIQUETRAL LIGAMENT INJURY

Diagnosis

Injury to the LT in isolation is a rare but commonly overlooked diagnosis. This injury may be encountered in a patient with concomitant ulnar-sided wrist pathology and is often seen in athletes who participate in high-energy or impact sports.[21] Lunotriquetral injury can occur after a fall onto an outstretched wrist with a dorsally directed force through a volar-flexed wrist, or as part of the perilunate instability spectrum with pressure directed through the thenar region as the wrist is extended and ulnarly deviated.

The LT is similar to the SL in that it is a U-shaped, interosseous ligament, connecting the lunate to the triquetrum, stabilizing the LT joint. The LT ligament also consists of a dorsal, membranous, and volar portion but differs from the SL ligament in that its volar portion is the strongest. Secondary stabilizers of the LT interval include radiolunotriquetral ligament and the DRC.

The triquetrum is tightly articulated with the hamate, and it is through this interaction that the proximal and distal carpal rows are linked. With radial deviation, the hamate forces the triquetrum to flex, which translates through the LT and SL ligaments resulting in scaphoid flexion. With ulnar deviation, the hamate drives the triquetrum into extension, carrying the lunate and scaphoid into extension as well. With disruption of the LT ligament, and the secondary stabilizing ligaments, in the absence of a concomitant SL tear, the lunate remains tightly articulated with the scaphoid and assumes a flexed position (Figure 81.6). LT injury also exists along an injury spectrum with both dynamic and static instability. With static instability, the SL angle becomes more acute (<30°, normal 30°–60°, mean 47°), known as volar intercalated segment instability.

LT ligament injury can occur with progressive perilunate instability. According to the Mayfield classification system, stage III perilunate instability occurs after a scaphoid fracture or SL tear, dorsal dislocation of the capitolunate joint, and tear of the LT.

Patients often present with ulnar-sided wrist pain, weakness with grip, sensation of instability, and possibly ulnar nerve paresthesias.[22] A systematic examination of the wrist must be performed in an attempt

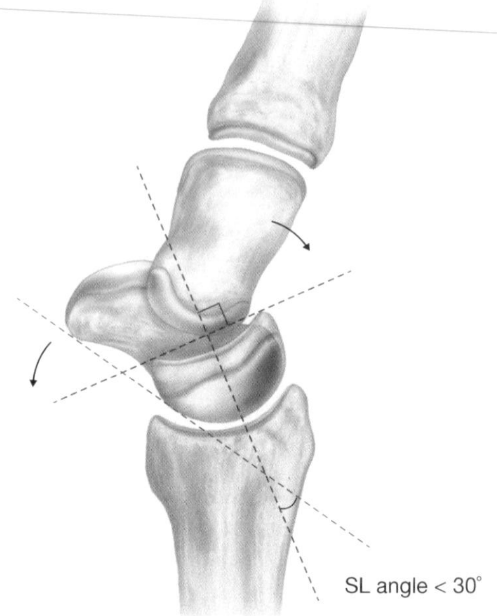

FIGURE 81.6. Radiographic evidence of lunotriquetral ligament dissociation. (From Morris MS, Chung KC. Lunotriquetral ligament reconstruction using a slip of the extensor carpi ulnaris tendon. In: Chung KC, ed. *Operative Techniques in Plastic Surgery*. Philadelphia, PA: Wolters Kluwer; 2019. In press.)

to rule out other sources of ulnar-sided wrist pain. Tenderness with direct palpation of the LT interval, between the fourth and fifth dorsal compartment tendons, should prompt further evaluation for LT injury. The LT ballottement test will result in pain with compression of the lunate and triquetrum.[23] The shear test is the most specific for LT injuries. While supporting the body of the lunate, the examiner compresses the pisotriquetral joint and generates a force across the LT interval. Increased pain during this maneuver may be because of an LT injury.

Standard, three-view wrist X-ray series may reveal gapping of the LT interval or volar intercalated segment instability deformity. Careful examination of static and dynamic X-rays may demonstrate disruption of the Gilula arcs (Figure 81.7), overlap of the lunate and triquetrum, or motion of the scaphoid and lunate independent of the triquetrum.[24] Standard arthrography, MR arthrography, and arthroscopy have been used to detect LT tears.[25-29] Several studies have demonstrated a high rate of membranous LT tears, where there is passage of contrast across the LT interval. A tear in this portion of the LT ligament may not be of biomechanical consequence. Arthroscopy remains the reference standard for diagnosing, classifying, and possibly treating functionally significant LT injury.[29,30]

Treatment

Acute LT Injury

Treatment of LT injuries depends on the degree of instability (dynamic versus static), timing of injury (acute versus chronic), and the presence of articular degeneration as a result of biomechanical alterations. For acute injuries, an initial trial of 6 weeks of nonoperative management with brace or cast immobilization and nonsteroidal anti-inflammatories should be attempted.[31] With failure of nonoperative treatment, as evidenced by continued pain or instability, operative treatment is performed.

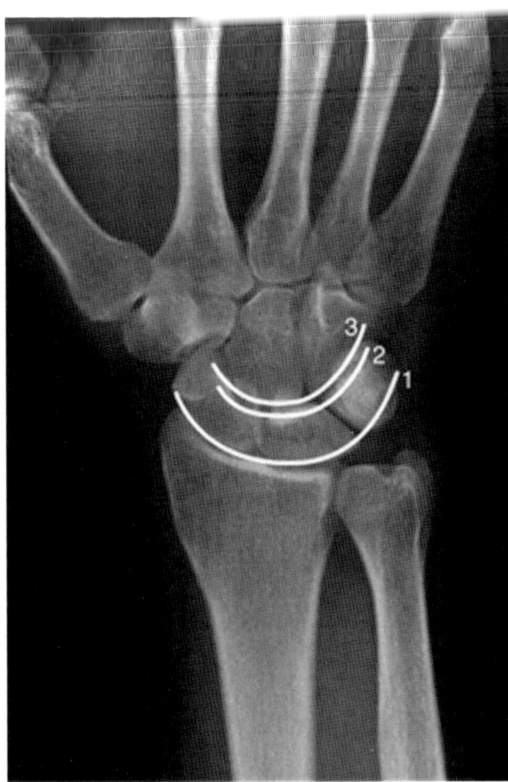

FIGURE 81.7. Gilula arcs. 1. Proximal aspect of proximal carpal row, 2. Distal aspect of proximal carpal row, and 3. Proximal aspect of distal carpal row. (Reproduced with permission from Chhabra AB, Miller CD, Wall L. Imaging. In: Hammert WC, et al, eds. *ASSH Manual of Hand Surgery*. Philadelphia, PA: Wolters Kluwer Health/Lippincott Williams & Wilkins; 2010:7-28.)

Arthroscopy remains the mainstay of diagnosis and treatment in acute, dynamic LT injury. The LT joint is best visualized and interrogated via the midcarpal joint.[32] The joint is normally tightly articulated but gapping may be appreciated when scope is directed between the lunate and triquetrum. Systematic, diagnostic wrist arthroscopy will also permit identification of other wrist pathologies including TFCC injury and articular wear.

Arthroscopic debridement of a fraying LT ligament or synovitis may be performed.[33] Following debridement, reduction of the joint and pin fixation of the LT interval may aid in healing of the ligament. Where Geissler grade IV instability is noted (arthroscope is passed freely between the lunate and triquetrum), direct repair should be performed. A direct approach to the wrist permits identification of the LT interval and reattachment of the ligament to the triquetrum with bone tunnels or suture anchors. A secondary volar approach (through the floor of the carpal tunnel) may be necessary to repair the volar portion of the ligament. Supplemental K-wire fixation is left in place for 8 weeks, at which point the wires are removed and range of motion is initiated. Painless range of motion and prevention of wrist arthrosis can be achieved.[22,34]

Chronic LT Injury

A trial of NSAIDs and brace immobilization should be attempted for 3 months prior to surgical intervention. If this fails, a reconstruction or fusion of the LT interval may be considered. A slip of extensor carpi ulnaris (ECU) tendon can be used to reconstruct the dorsal portion of the LT ligament with good results.[35] Lunotriquetral arthrodesis is less predictable to achieve fusion.[34,36] In patients with concomitant ulnocarpal abutment, an ulnar shortening osteotomy may be beneficial.[34,37]

PERILUNATE DISLOCATION

Diagnosis

Perilunate dislocations are uncommon high-energy soft-tissue injuries (lesser arc injury) and sometimes combined bony and soft-tissue injuries (greater arc injury).[38] As previously discussed in this chapter, perilunate injury progresses as a sequential pattern of ligamentous disruption, starting from the SLIL (Mayfield stage I). As the energy is transmitted around the lunate, the lunocapitate joint is disrupted (Mayfield stage II), followed by tear of the LT (Mayfield stage III), and finally volar dislocation of the lunate from its fossa (Mayfield stage IV). These injuries are most commonly seen in young men as a result of a fall from height, motor vehicle collision, or sports-related accident.

Patients with perilunate injury or dislocation will complain of pain, swelling, and decreased range of motion in the affected extremity. It is important to inquire about median nerve symptoms as acute carpal tunnel syndrome is present in approximately 25% of patients.[39] Patients must be evaluated with a standard three-view X-ray series. With perilunate injuries, there is a disruption of the Gilula arcs and overlapping of the normally tightly articulated carpal bones.

Careful examination of the distal radius, scaphoid, capitate, hamate, and triquetrum must be performed, as there may be associated fractures.[40,41] Radius or carpal bone fractures associated with intercarpal ligamentous disruption around the lunate are described as trans-bony, perilunate injuries. For example, a scaphoid fracture associated with a perilunate dislocation is described as a trans-scaphoid, perilunate dislocation. In stage IV lunate dislocation, the lunate remains attached to the short radiolunate ligament and is seen on the lateral X-ray, displaced volarly, within the carpal tunnel. With a perilunate dislocation, the lunate remains within its fossa on the radius, and the remainder of the carpus is dislocated (Figure 81.8).

Treatment

Careful assessment of the median nerve will guide early treatment. In a stage IV perilunate dislocation (volar lunate dislocation), median nerve symptoms will be present. Reduction of the lunate must be performed in the acute setting. To reduce the lunate with the goal to decrease the pressure over the median nerve before definitive repair, the patient may need to be sedated and traction must be applied. The reduction maneuver involves hyperextending the carpus to recreate the injury, dorsally directing pressure on the lunate to reduce it to the radius and to permit capitate reduction onto the lunate. With volar flexion and continued traction, a palpable clunk and gross correction of the deformity will occur. Postreduction X-rays must be performed to confirm that the lunate has been successfully reduced. If closed reduction fails, the patient should be taken to the operating room for open reduction. This may be the result of interposed soft tissue.[42] If closed reduction and splinting can be performed acutely, the patient must be observed for progression of median nerve symptoms. If the patient has progressively worsening paresthesias and pain (acute carpal tunnel syndrome) despite a successful reduction, he/she must be taken to the operating room for release of the carpal tunnel. Mild paresthesias, without progressing pain, do not require urgent operative decompression.

When closed reduction can be achieved, it is acceptable to delay surgery for up to 2 weeks following the injury. This permits a reduction in swelling that may make the open ligamentous exploration and repair easier. Operative treatment with open repair of injured structures may decrease the rate of subsequent DISI deformity and resulting articular wear as compared with casting or splint immobilization.[43] The interosseous ligaments may be approached from dorsal or by a combined dorsal and volar approach, decompressing the carpal tunnel and repairing the volar capsule and interosseous ligaments.[44–46] Supplemental K-wires are used to immobilize the proximal and distal rows where indicated and removed at 8 weeks following surgery.

Although this is a high-energy injury, many patients return to work and few have permanent disability. Range of motion, grip strength, and presence of arthritis are variable.[43,47,48]

DISTAL RADIOULNAR JOINT AND TRIANGULAR FIBROCARTILAGE COMPLEX INJURY

Diagnosis

The ulna is the fixed unit of the forearm, and muscular forces permit radius rotation (pronation and supination) around the ulna at the level of the distal radioulnar joint (DRUJ). The DRUJ consists of the

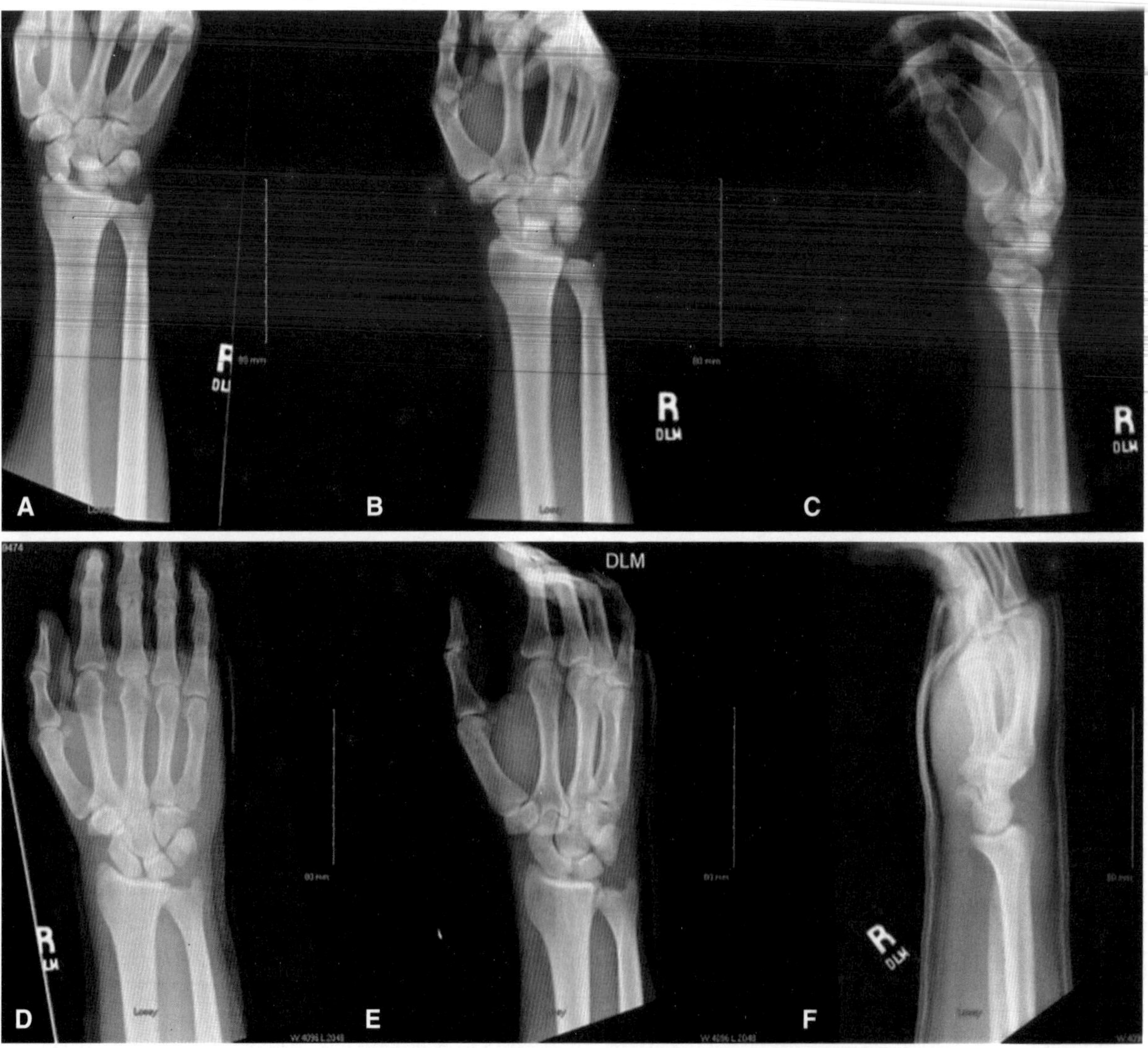

FIGURE 81.8. Transradial styloid perilunate fracture dislocation. A-C. Prereduction X-rays. D-F. Postreduction X-rays.

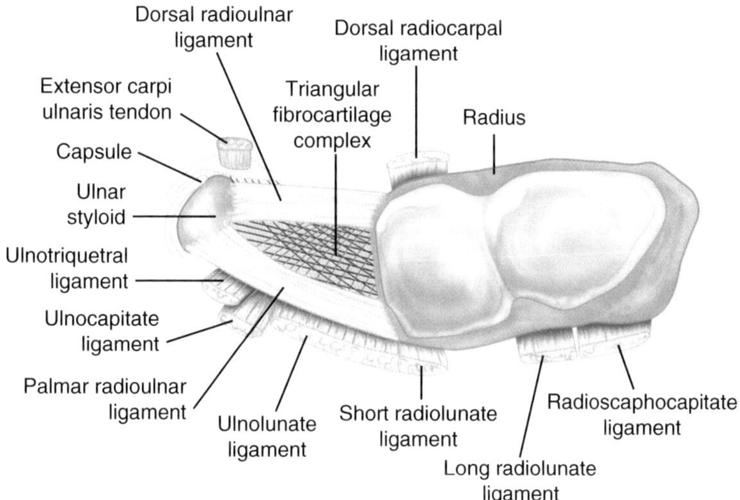

FIGURE 81.9. Triangular fibrocartilage complex and related anatomy. (Reproduced with permission from Dy CJ, Ouellette EA, Makowski AL. Extra-articular reconstructive techniques for the distal radioulnar and ulnocarpal joints. In: Wiesel S, ed. *Operative Techniques in Orthopaedic Surgery*. 2nd ed. Vol 3. Philadelphia, PA: Wolters Kluwer; 2016:3016. Figure 64-10.)

sigmoid notch of the radius and ulnar head. Each of these surfaces is covered by articular cartilage. The curvature of the sigmoid notch is larger than that of the ulnar head, which allows for palmar and dorsal translation of the radius in relation to the ulna.

Soft-tissue constraints of the DRUJ include the TFCC, the palmar and dorsal radioulnar ligaments, the ulnar collateral ligament, the joint capsule, and the interosseous membrane. Muscles that act as dynamic stabilizers include the ECU and pronator quadratus.

The TFCC consists of many soft-tissue structures and acts as both a stabilizer of the DRUJ and shock absorber of loads transmitted through the ulnar side of the wrist. Structures include the dorsal and palmar radioulnar ligaments, the articular disk, the ulnocarpal ligaments, the ECU subsheath, and the meniscus homologue.

Dislocation of the DRUJ may occur as an isolated soft-tissue injury or with a fracture of the radius (distal radius fracture, Galeazzi fracture). Ulnar-sided wrist problems, including TFCC injury, occur up to 37% of the time with an associated distal radius fracture.[49,50] Patients present with swelling, pain, and deformity. TFCC injury with associated fracture may present as ulnar-sided wrist pain, becoming clinically apparent after healing of the radius fracture. Radiographic indicators of DRUJ instability include the following:

- Base of ulnar styloid fracture
- Dislocation of the DRUJ
- Sigmoid notch fracture
- Widening of the DRUJ
- Radial shortening or loss of radial inclination

Treatment

Acute DRUJ Injury

Treatment begins with anatomic reduction of a radius fracture when present. An isolated dislocation should be reduced and the joint assessed for stability in neutral, pronation, and supination. While the joint is stable in supination, the patient is placed in a long-arm splint or cast, in that position, for 4 to 6 weeks. If the joint is unstable in all directions, and an ulnar styloid fracture is present, the fracture should be reduced and fixed. If no ulnar styloid fracture is present, the soft-tissue structures (TFCC) may be repaired, and the reduced DRUJ is pinned for 4 to 6 weeks.

Chronic DRUJ Instability

In patients with clinically apparent instability of the DRUJ (translation of the radius on the ulna at the sigmoid notch with associated pain), and no evidence of arthritis, one should consider a reconstruction. Nonoperative treatment with bracing for 6 to 12 weeks should be attempted prior to operating.

Distal radius or ulnar malunion should be ruled out as a possible cause of instability and corrected where present. If purely ligamentous failure is suspected, a reconstruction is performed using palmaris longus tendon. The goal of reconstructive surgery is to permit a painless arc of forearm motion.

TFCC Injury

Treatment depends on the acuity of the injury. Palmer developed a classification system based on time to presentation and the location of the TFCC tear and/or the presence of cartilage wear[51] (Figure 81.10; Table 81.1).

Initial treatment of TFCC injuries is nonsurgical with bracing or casting, activity modification, NSAIDs, and occupational therapy. If a trial of 6 weeks of conservative therapy fails to improve symptoms, arthroscopic evaluation and/or open treatment is considered. The central portion of the TFCC is often debrided, as this area has less potential to heal. Type 1B, 1C, and 1D injuries may be amenable to arthroscopic or open repair.[52,53]

Degenerative tears may benefit from arthroscopic debridement and/or DRUJ stabilizing, or ulnar shortening procedures when indicated.[54] When DRUJ arthritis exists, the patient may benefit from a salvage operation such as a hemiresection arthroplasty, ulnar head resection, or implant arthroplasty.

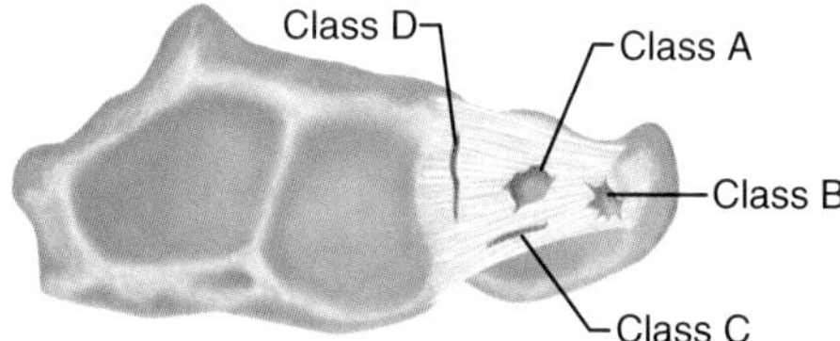

FIGURE 81.10. Palmer classification for acute triangular fibrocartilage complex (TFCC) injuries. A class 1A lesion involves a tear in the central, horizontal portion of the TFCC. A class 1B lesion is a tear of the TFCC from the distal ulna with or without an ulnar styloid fracture. A class 1C lesion is a tear of the TFCC distal attachment to the lunate and triquetrum through the ulnolunate and ulnotriquetral ligaments. A class 1D lesion is a detachment of the TFCC from its insertion on to the radius at the distal sigmoid notch. (Reproduced with permission from Osterman AL. Arthroscopic and open triangular fibrocartilage complex repair. In: Wiesel S, ed. *Operative Techniques in Orthopedic Surgery*. Vol 3. Philadelphia, PA: Wolters Kluwer Health/Lippincott Williams and Wilkins; 2011:2520. Figure 49-2A.)

TABLE 81.1. PALMER CLASSIFICATION OF TRIANGULAR FIBROCARTILAGE COMPLEX (TFCC) TEARS

Type	Description
Type 1	Acute, traumatic
IA	Isolated central TFCC articular disk
IB	Peripheral ulnar-sided TFCC tear (with or without ulnar styloid fracture)
IC	Distal TFCC disruption (disruption from distal ulnocarpal ligaments)
1D	Radial TFCC disruption (with or without sigmoid notch fracture)
Type 2	Degenerative
2A	TFCC wear
2B	TFCC wear with lunate and/or ulnar chondromalacia
2C	TFCC perforation with lunate and/or ulnar chondromalacia
2D	TFCC perforation with lunate and/or ulnar chondromalacia and with lunotriquetral ligament peroration
2E	TFCC perforation with lunate and/or ulnar chondromalacia, lunotriquetral ligament perforation, and ulnocarpal arthritis

CONCLUSION

Wrist ligamentous injuries must be identified and treated early to avoid the sequelae of altered motion, including pain and joint degeneration. Surgical strategies may be employed to repair or reconstruct soft tissues and to restore normal anatomic relationships and kinematics. Salvage operations are considered when there is evidence of articular wear and pain that can be localized to the site of joint destruction.

REFERENCES

1. Lee DH, Dickson KF, Bradley EL. The incidence of wrist interosseous ligament and triangular fibrocartilage articular disc disruptions: a cadaveric study. *J Hand Surg Am.* 2004;29(4):676-684.
2. Berger RA. The ligaments of the wrist: a current overview of anatomy with considerations of their potential functions. *Hand Clin.* 1997;13(1):63-82.
   In this article, the author carefully describes the extrinsic and intrinsic ligaments of the wrist and details the functional implications of injury. This is one of the first comprehensive descriptions of the wrist soft-tissue anatomy and continues to be used as a guide for future publications.
3. Bourne MH, Linscheid RL, Dobyns JH. Concomitant scapholunate dissociation and Kienbock's disease. *J Hand Surg Am.* 1991;16(3):460-464.
4. Chang IY, Mutnal A, Evans PJ, Sundaram M. Kienbock's disease and scapholunate advanced collapse. *Orthopedics.* 2014;37(9):578, 637-579.
5. Muramatsu K, Ihara K, Tanaka H, Kawai S. Carpal instability in rheumatoid wrists. *Rheumatol Int.* 2004;24(1):34-36.
6. Mayfield JK. Wrist ligamentous anatomy and pathogenesis of carpal instability. *Orthop Clin North Am.* 1984;15(2):209-216.
   This is the original publication in which Mayfield describes the progression of bony and ligamentous injury around the lunate. He describes the predictable pattern of instability that usually begins on the radial side of the wrist and progresses to complete lunate dislocation. This seminal work should be appreciated as it remains essential in understanding the spectrum of perilunate pathology.
7. Geissler WB. Arthroscopic management of scapholunate instability. *J Wrist Surg.* 2013;2(2):129-135.
8. Lee SK, Desai H, Silver B, et al. Comparison of radiographic stress views for scapholunate dynamic instability in a cadaver model. *J Hand Surg Am.* 2011;36(7):1149-1157.
9. Whipple TL. The role of arthroscopy in the treatment of wrist injuries in the athlete. *Clin Sports Med.* 1998;17(3):623-634.
10. Whipple TL. The role of arthroscopy in the treatment of scapholunate instability. *Hand Clin.* 1995;11(1):37-40.
11. Linscheid RL, Dobyns JH. Treatment of scapholunate dissociation: rotatory subluxation of the scaphoid. *Hand Clin.* 1992;8(4):645-652.
12. Walsh JJ, Berger RA, Cooney WP. Current status of scapholunate interosseous ligament injuries. *J Am Acad Orthop Surg.* 2002;10(1):32-42.
13. Harvey EJ, Berger RA, Osterman AL, et al. Bone-tissue-bone repairs for scapholunate dissociation. *J Hand Surg Am.* 2007;32(2):256-264.
14. Harvey EJ, Sen M, Martineau P. A vascularized technique for bone-tissue-bone repair in scapholunate dissociation. *Tech Hand Up Extrem Surg.* 2006;10(3):166-172.
15. Shin SS, Moore DC, McGovern RD, Weiss AP. Scapholunate ligament reconstruction using a bone-retinaculum-bone autograft: a biomechanic and histologic study. *J Hand Surg Am.* 1998;23(2):216-221.
16. Brunelli GA, Brunelli GR. A new technique to correct carpal instability with scaphoid rotary subluxation: a preliminary report. *J Hand Surg Am.* 1995;20(3 Pt 2): S82-S85.
   This article covers what has become the reference standard in the reconstruction of SL with associated static deformity. The authors elegantly describe their technique of using the FCR tendon to correct the flexed posture of the scaphoid while simultaneously reconstructing the dorsal SL ligament. This procedure and its associated outcomes has become the benchmark by which all SL reconstructive procedures are compared.
17. Garcia-Elias M, Lluch AL, Stanley JK. Three-ligament tenodesis for the treatment of scapholunate dissociation: indications and surgical technique. *J Hand Surg Am.* 2006;31(1):125-134.
18. Chabas JF, Gay A, Valenti D, et al. Results of the modified Brunelli tenodesis for treatment of scapholunate instability: a retrospective study of 19 patients. *J Hand Surg Am.* 2008;33(9):1469-1477.
19. Nienstedt F. Treatment of static scapholunate instability with modified Brunelli tenodesis: results over 10 years. *J Hand Surg Am.* 2013;38A:887-892.
20. [illegible] Zhong L, Chung KC. A comparative analysis of resource utilization between proximal row carpectomy and partial wrist fusion: a population [illegible]. *J Hand Surg Am.* 2017;42(10):773-780.
21. Linscheid RL, Dobyns JH. Athletic injuries of the wrist. *Clin Orthop Relat Res.* 1985;(198):141-151.
22. Reagan DS, Linscheid RL, Dobyns JH. Lunotriquetral sprains. *J Hand Surg Am.* 1984;9(4):502-514.
23. Kleinman WB. Physical examination of the wrist: useful provocative maneuvers. *J Hand Surg Am.* 2015;40(7):1486-1500
24. Beckenbaugh RD. Accurate evaluation and management of the painful wrist following injury. An approach to carpal instability. *Orthop Clin North Am.* 1984;15(2):[illegible]
25. Mikic ZD. Arthrography of the wrist joint: an experimental study. *J Bone Joint Surg Am.* 1984;66(3):371-378.
26. Trentham DE, Hamm RL, Masi AT. Wrist arthrography: review and comparison of normals, rheumatoid arthritis and gout patients. *Semin Arthritis Rheum.* 1975;5(2):105-120.
27. Viegas SF, Patterson RM, Hokanson JA, Davis J. Wrist anatomy: incidence, distribution, and correlation of anatomic variations, tears, and arthrosis. *J Hand Surg Am.* 1993;18(3):463-475.
28. Cantor RM, Stern PJ, Wyrick JD, Michaels SE. The relevance of ligament tears or perforations in the diagnosis of wrist pain: an arthrographic study. *J Hand Surg Am.* 1994;19A(6):945-953.
29. Weiss LE, Taras JS, Sweet S, Osterman AL. Lunotriquetral injuries in the athlete. *Hand Clin.* 2000;16(3):433-438.
30. Osterman AL, Seidman GD. The role of arthroscopy in the treatment of lunatotriquetral ligament injuries. *Hand Clin.* 1995;11(1):41-50.
31. Gilula LA, Weeks PM. Post-traumatic ligamentous instability of the wrist joint. *Vestn Rentgenol Radiol.* 1993;(2):16-26.
32. Michelotti BF, Chung KC. Diagnostic wrist arthroscopy. *Hand Clin.* 2017;33(4):571-583.
33. Weiss AP, Sachar K, Glowacki KA. Arthroscopic debridement alone for intercarpal ligament tears. *J Hand Surg Am.* 1997;22(2):344-349.
34. Shin AY, Weinstein LP, Berger RA, Bishop AT. Treatment of isolated injuries of the lunotriquetral ligament: a comparison of arthrodesis, ligament reconstruction and ligament repair. *J Bone Joint Surg Br.* 2001;83(7):1023-1028.
35. Shahane SA, Trail IA, Takwale VJ, et al. Tenodesis of the extensor carpi ulnaris for chronic, post-traumatic lunotriquetral instability. *J Bone Joint Surg Br.* 2005;87B:1512-1515.
36. Sennwald GR, Fischer M, Mondi P. Lunotriquetral arthrodesis: a controversial procedure. *J Hand Surg Br.* 1995;20(6):755-760.
37. Wagner ER, Elhassan BT, Rizzo M. Diagnosis and treatment of chronic lunotriquetral ligament injuries. *Hand Clin.* 2015;31(3):477-486.
38. Herzberg G, Comtet JJ, Linscheid RL, et al. Perilunate dislocations and fracture-dislocations: a multicenter study. *J Hand Surg Am.* 1993;18(5):768-779.
39. Trumble T, Verheyden J. Treatment of isolated perilunate and lunate dislocations with combined dorsal and volar approach and intraosseous cerclage wire. *J Hand Surg Am.* 2004;29(3):412-417.
40. Gilula LA. Carpal injuries: analytic approach and case exercises. *Am J Roentgenol.* 1979;133(3):503-517.
41. Gilula LA, Destouet JM, Weeks PM, et al. Roentgenographic diagnosis of the painful wrist. *Clin Orthop Relat Res.* 1984;(187):52-64.
42. Jasmine MS, Packer JW, Edwards GS Jr. Irreducible trans-scaphoid perilunate dislocation. *J Hand Surg Am.* 1988;13(2):212-215.
43. Linscheid RL, Dobyns JH, Beabout JW, Bryan RS. Traumatic instability of the wrist: diagnosis, classification, and pathomechanics. *J Bone Joint Surg Am.* 1972;54(8):1612-1632.
44. Melone CP, Murphy MS, Raskin KB. Perilunate injuries: repair by dual dorsal and volar approaches. *Hand Clin.* 2000;16(3):439.
45. Blazar PE, Murray P. Treatment of perilunate dislocations by combined dorsal and palmar approaches. *Tech Hand Up Extrem Surg.* 2001;5(1):2-7.

46. Sotereanos DG, Mitsionis GJ, Giannakopoulos PN, et al. Perilunate dislocation and fracture dislocation: a critical analysis of the volar-dorsal approach. *J Hand Surg Am*. 1997;22(1):49-56.
47. Hildebrand KA, Ross DC, Patterson SD, et al. Dorsal perilunate dislocations and fracture-dislocations: questionnaire, clinical, and radiographic evaluation. *J Hand Surg Am*. 2000;25:1069-1079.
48. Knoll VD, Allan C, Trumble TE. Trans-scaphoid perilunate fracture dislocations: results of screw fixation of the scaphoid and lunotriquetral repair with a dorsal approach. *J Hand Surg Am*. 2005;30(6):1145-1152.
49. Geissler WB, Fernandez DL, Lamey DM. Distal radioulnar joint injuries associated with fractures of the distal radius. *Clin Orthop Relat Res*. 1996;(327):135-146.
50. Lindau T, Adlercreutz C, Aspenberg P. Peripheral tears of the triangular fibrocartilage complex cause distal radioulnar joint instability after distal radial fractures. *J Hand Surg Am*. 2000;25(3):464-468.
51. Palmer AK. Triangular fibrocartilage complex lesions: a classification. *J Hand Surg Am*. 1989;14(4):594-606.
52. Corso SJ, Savoie FH, Geissler WB, et al. Arthroscopic repair of peripheral avulsions of the triangular fibrocartilage complex of the wrist: a multicenter study. *Arthroscopy*. 1997;13(1):78-84.
53. Anderson ML, Larson AN, Moran SL, et al. Clinical comparison of arthroscopic versus open repair of triangular fibrocartilage complex tears. *J Hand Surg Am*. 2008;33(5):675-682.
54. Seo JB, Kim JP, Yi HS, Park KH. The outcomes of arthroscopic repair versus debridement for chronic unstable triangular fibrocartilage complex tears in patients undergoing ulnar-shortening osteotomy. *J Hand Surg Am*. 2016;41(5):615-623.

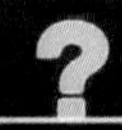

QUESTIONS

1. A 45-year-old roofer presents to the emergency department 45 minutes after he sustained an injury to the right wrist when he fell off a 10-foot ladder. He has extensive swelling of the wrist as well as progressively worsening numbness and pain in the fingers and thumb. Which of the following is the most appropriate management?

a. Elevation of the hand and monitoring of compartment pressures by invasive means
b. Carpal tunnel release only
c. Carpal tunnel release and intercarpal arthrodesis
d. Carpal tunnel release and PRC
e. Carpal tunnel release, relocation of the lunate, and repair of the volar and dorsal extrinsic and intrinsic ligaments

2. A 25-year-old woman fell from a 15-foot ladder and sustained a dorsal perilunate dislocation. The injury was reduced in the emergency department, and she has no clinical evidence of acute carpal tunnel syndrome. Two-week follow-up X-rays demonstrate a widened SL interval (10 mm) and evidence of DISI (SL angle 90°). No bony abnormality is appreciated. What is the most appropriate management?

a. Long-arm cast application for 8 to 12 weeks
b. PRC
c. SL arthrodesis
d. Operative repair of the SL and LT ligaments through a dorsal wrist incision
e. Percutaneous pin fixation of the SL interval

3. A 70-year-old retired steel worker is seen in the clinic complaining of chronic wrist pain and stiffness. He reports a history of falling from a roof onto an outstretched hand in his youth. X-rays are obtained that demonstrate widening of the SL injury, peaking of the radial styloid, narrowing of the radioscaphoid articulation, and preservation of the radiolunate and midcarpal joints. Conservative management has failed, and his pain is interfering with activities of daily living. Which is the most appropriate surgical treatment?

a. Total wrist arthrodesis
b. PRC
c. Scaphoidectomy alone
d. Reconstruction of the SL ligament
e. Radial styloidectomy

4. A 45-year-old woman is seen in the office 3 months after an ice skating injury in which she fell onto an outstretched left wrist. X-rays are obtained which reveal static SL (8 mm SL gap, SL angle 80°). There is no evidence of articular wear or other bony abnormality. All other intercarpal articulations are normal. Which of the following is the best surgical treatment option?

a. Dorsal SL ligament repair
b. SL ligament reconstruction with modified three-ligament tenodesis
c. Scaphoidectomy and partial fusion
d. Distal scaphoid excision
e. Arthroscopic reduction of the SL interval and percutaneous pinning

5. A 35-year-old woman is a restrained driver in a motor vehicle collision in which her left dominant wrist is driven into the steering wheel, resulting in pain and swelling. She is seen in consultation 1 week following the injury and localizes her pain to the ulnar side of her wrist. Examination demonstrates stability of the DRUJ but ulnar foveal tenderness, as compared with the contralateral side. Compression and translation of the lunotriquetral interval do not generate pain. The remainder of the physical examination is normal. X-rays are negative for any bony abnormality, and Gilula arcs are maintained. Which of the structures is most likely to be injured?

a. TFCC
b. ECU tendon
c. Flexor carpi ulnar tendon
d. Occult fracture of the fifth metacarpal base
e. Partial LT tear

1. **Answer: e.** Acute carpal tunnel syndrome is a surgical emergency. If the lunate cannot be reduced by closed means, the patient must be taken to the operating room for reduction and definitive treatment. Casting alone is inferior to open repair of ligamentous structures. Elevation of the hand or carpal tunnel release alone is insufficient. Intercarpal arthrodesis or PRC is not indicated when all joint surfaces are maintained.

2. **Answer: d.** This patient has suffered a lesser arc (soft tissue only) perilunate injury. With dislocation of the lunate, the SL and LT ligaments have been disrupted. Optimal results can be obtained when interosseous wrist ligament injuries are treated within the first 6 weeks. Open repair is superior to pin fixation alone. Long-arm casting results in worse outcomes than open repair of the injured ligaments. PRC and SL arthrodesis are not indicated.

3. **Answer: b.** The patient has evidence of chronic SL injury, time indeterminate, and SLAC. With arthritis of the radial styloid and radioscaphoid articulation, he is not a candidate for SL reconstruction. Scaphoidectomy or removal of radial styloid alone would be insufficient for pain relief. A total wrist arthrodesis is not indicated because the midcarpal and radiolunate joints are preserved. The best answer is PRC, which would remove the pain-generating articulation and preserve 50% of wrist motion when the lunate fossa of the radius articulates with the proximal capitate. This is also more cost-effective than scaphoidectomy and partial wrist fusion.

4. **Answer: b.** The patient has evidence of static SL injury, meaning the SL ligament is incompetent ***and*** the secondary stabilizing ligaments have failed. Repair or reconstruction of the ligament alone is insufficient to durably correct the rotatory subluxation of the scaphoid. Failure will lead to a predictable pattern of wrist arthritis (SLAC). Arthroscopic reduction and pinning is insufficient for correction of a static deformity. At 3 months from the time of injury, with evidence of rotation of the scaphoid, reduction and pinning of the interval will not permit healing of the ligament. Open reduction and reconstruction of the ligamentous complex is required. Because there is no articular wear, scaphoidectomy or distal pole excision is not indicated.

5. **Answer: a.** This patient has sustained an axially directed force through the wrist and is complaining of ulnar-sided wrist pain. Based on the physical examination and standard radiographic assessment, she does not have evidence of an interosseous ligament injury, therefore LT injury is incorrect. The hand and wrist examination is normal except for ulnar foveal tenderness. Pressure in this location suggests injury to the TFCC. All other answers are incorrect based on the pertinent history and physical examination that is presented.

CHAPTER 82 Management of Mutilating Upper Extremity Injuries

Jessica I. Billig and Kevin C. Chung

KEY POINTS

- Owing to the severe nature of these injuries, management begins with Advanced Trauma Life Support.
- Important decision-making regarding limb salvage versus amputation is essential.
- Systematic evaluation of the injury and damaged part facilitates treatment.
- Principles of operative treatment include debridement, possible vascular shunting, skeletal fixation, revascularization, tendon/muscle repair, nerve repair, soft-tissue reconstruction.
- The use of spare parts can deliver a satisfactory functional outcome.

Mutilating trauma to the upper extremity are devastating injuries with complex fracture patterns, substantial soft-tissue deficits, questionable neurovascular viability of the extremity, and possible additional injuries to other parts of the body. Treatment of these injuries is challenging and requires a thorough debridement and often needs creative reconstructive techniques. However, the treating surgeon and physician must adhere to Advanced Trauma Life Support (ATLS) before treatment of these injuries. All patients with mangled upper extremities should be evaluated as trauma patients because they may have additional devastating injuries. Furthermore, major upper extremity injuries may be life threatening, and one must often choose life over limb

Once the patient has been cleared from a trauma standpoint, a thorough evaluation of the upper extremity is essential to catalog all of the injured structures (Figure 82.1). Operative principles include the following:

- Complete debridement
- Restoration of blood flood with possible shunting
- Skeletal fixation
- Muscle and tendon repair
- Arterial and venous repair
- Nerve repair
- Soft-tissue coverage

The surgeons should strive to complete the reconstruction in a one-staged approach if possible, unless the wound is so contaminated that it requires multiple debridements. However, with experience in radical debridement, the surgeon can transform a dirty wound into a relatively clean wound. After the initial debridement, we recommend another debridement within 48 to 72 hours to prepare the wound for coverage at the second operation.

EVALUATION

The principles of ATLS must be strictly followed. Management begins with the primary survey and the ABCs (airway, breathing, circulation). The surgeon must not become distracted by the devastating upper extremity injury and miss other life-threatening injuries. Tourniquets can be used to help control massive hemorrhage and have been shown to improve survival.[1] However, one should also be aware of possible nerve injury with prolonged tourniquet usage, and tourniquets should be released every 2 hours for blood flow to the distal extremity. Blind clamping of vessels is inappropriate, as other surrounding structures may get injured in the process. A secondary survey according to ATLS should be performed quickly and efficiently to uncover any additional injuries. Resuscitation and stabilization of the patient must be performed before treating the mangled upper extremity.

The decision for limb salvage versus amputation is complex. Although difficult to predict, surgeons must determine the functional outcomes of amputation compared with limb salvage. Unlike in the lower extremity where amputation is more tolerable, amputation proximal to the fingers is disabling. The surgeon should always strive for salvage rather than amputation for the upper limb. Patient factors such as age and health status play a critical role in this decision-making process. If the patient is lucid, a thorough history of the incident should be obtained. Important medical information including comorbid medical diseases, occupation, smoking status, hand dominance, and a recount of the injury are beneficial in devising a reconstructive surgical plan. The ultimate decision to attempt limb salvage requires a full evaluation of the patient and the circumstances surrounding the injury. Criteria for considering amputation include the following[2]:

- Open fractures with large soft-tissue defect
- Warm ischemia time longer than 6 hours with muscle involvement
- Proximal major nerve injury (e.g., brachial plexus involvement)
- Unstable patient
- Older patient
- Associated major organ trauma
- Comorbid medical problems with increased risk with prolonged anesthesia (e.g., myocardial infarction, stroke)

When considering limb amputation, current upper extremity prosthetics lack the ability to replicate the functionality and sensibility of the human hand. Even with recent advances in the field, many patients continue to abandon their prosthetics because of limited dexterity[3]; therefore, future prosthetic use must be weighed in the decision for amputation. Furthermore, primary amputation is more beneficial from a functionality standpoint compared with a failed reconstruction attempt. Finally, a surgeon's experience plays a role in the decision to pursue limb salvage or amputation.[4]

Currently, there are no validated scoring systems to predict upper extremity amputations after mutilating injuries. Some surgeons have extrapolated the Mangled Extremity Severity Score, which is used for lower extremity injuries, to guide management of these mutilating upper extremity injuries. However, in the lower extremity, a Mangled Extremity Severity Score of seven or higher has been used as a cutoff to perform amputation, but this has not been validated in the upper extremity.[5] Given the lack of robust data surrounding when to amputate, the surgeon must treat patients and each injury individually.

If amputation in the field has occurred, the appropriate transfer of the amputated part includes wrapping in a protective dressing, such as saline-soaked gauze, and placing the part on ice (Figure 82.2). One should not place the amputated part directly on ice to avoid freezing of the tissues and frostbite injury. Traditionally accepted ischemia time is 6 hours for a warm extremity, 12 hours for a cold extremity, 12 hours for a warm digit, and 24 hours for a cold digit. However, the traditionally accepted digit ischemia times have been challenged by multiple surgeons with successful replantations at longer ischemic intervals.[6,7] As compared with digits, upper extremities

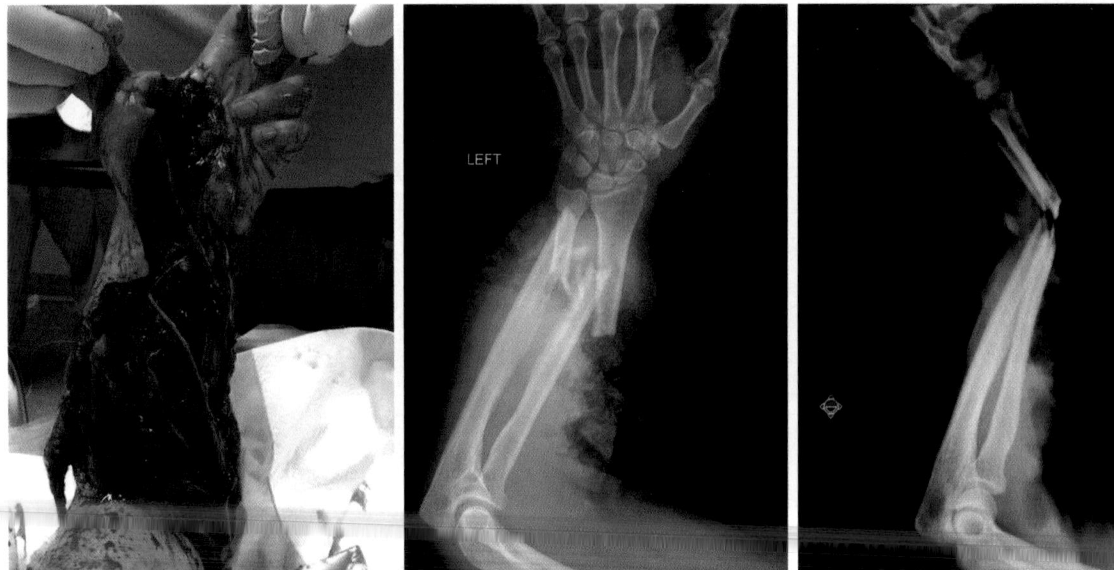

FIGURE 82.1. Initial evaluation in the emergency department of a 63-year-old woman with extensive left forearm crush injury of her forearm and hand after an auger injury.

have shorter ischemia times because of degradation of deoxygenized muscle. In patients with amputations of the upper extremity, functional outcomes are substantially worse than digit replantation. However, transhumeral replantation should be attempted to preserve the elbow, which greatly impacts function and prosthetic use.[8] Additionally, in a study by Atzei et al., the objective long-term results from proximal forearm amputations were poor, but patients found the replanted extremity useful for activities of daily living and were satisfied with their surgical outcome.[9] This highlights the importance of an individualized approach to mutilating upper extremity injuries and amputations.

Prior to going to the operating room, it is preferable to perform a thorough evaluation of the injured extremity. However, this may be impossible in the trauma bay due to pain or other distracting injuries. Nonetheless, the vascularity of the extremity must be assessed immediately, and radiographic examination can easily be performed without wasting time.[10] Splinting of the extremity can be carried out quickly and efficiently. Tetanus prophylaxis should be updated in all patients according to previous immunization status. If the patient presents with an open fracture, early antibiotic administration targeted against gram-negative and gram-positive organisms has been shown to reduce infection rate.[11]

OPERATIVE TREATMENT

Debridement

Adequate wound debridement is the foundation of treatment of mutilating upper extremity injuries. Debridement may be performed in the immediate or delayed setting depending on the stability of the patient and availability of a reconstructive surgeon.[12] If the patient is stable, early aggressive debridement should be performed in the operating room (Figure 82.3). Meticulous debridement using fresh sharp knife blades removes bacteria, foreign bodies, and nonviable tissue. It also facilitates a thorough inspection of the wound and cataloging of all injured entities. We prefer a staged approach to debridement. Early debridement is performed at the time of presentation and then another debridement is performed within a few days in conjunction with definitive reconstruction. The first debridement removes necrotic tissue and infectious burden, permitting adequate time for demarcation of nonviable tissues.[10]

Temporary Shunting

With mutilating upper extremity injuries, the vascular status of the extremity is exceedingly important. Presence of a peripheral pulse

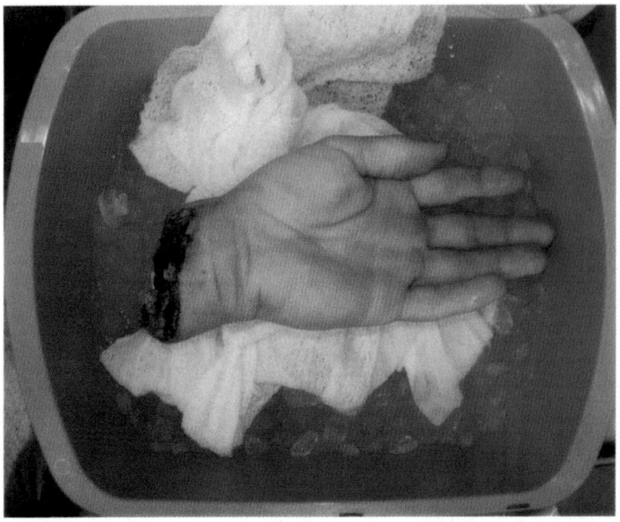

FIGURE 82.2. This 19-year-old suffered a saw amputation at the level of distal third of the forearm. The part was placed in gauze and on ice for transport.

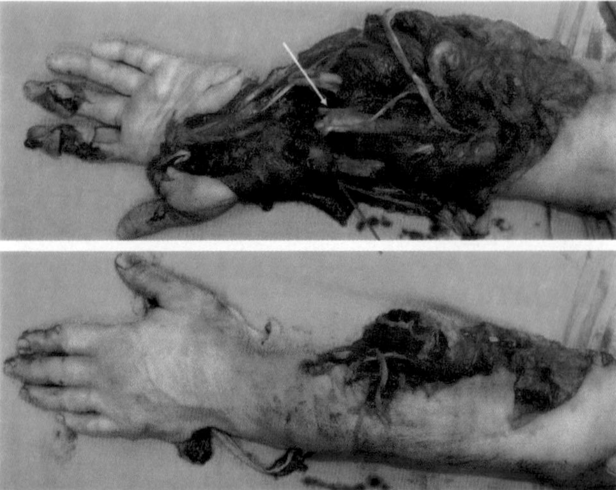

FIGURE 82.3. Operative debridement was performed to remove all nonviable tissue and decrease the infectious burden. The yellow arrow is pointing at the ulna, and the blue arrow indicates the radius.

may not exclude impending arterial compromise. Signs and symptoms of vascular compromise include the following[13]:

Definitive Signs of Vascular Injury

- Pulselessness
- Pallor
- Massive hemorrhage
- Rapidly expanding hematoma
- Palpable thrill/audible bruit

Suggestions of Vascular Injury

- History of bleeding in transit
- Proximity-related injury
- Neurologic injury of known nerve adjacent to a large artery
- Hematoma over a known large artery
- Pain
- Paresthesia
- Paralysis

Doppler ultrasound can be used as an adjunct tool in the trauma bay and has an accuracy of approximately 98% in diagnosing vascular compromise.[13] If the patient is stable, preoperative angiography may provide vital data regarding their vascular status. Criteria for angiography in upper extremity injury include the following[15]:

- Exclusion of vascular injury in absence of clinical signs of definitive vascular injury
- When not evident on physical examination:
  - Determination of level of injury
  - Determination of extent of injury
  - Determination of nature of injury

If there is any concern for vascular compromise, however, delaying surgical intervention with upper extremity angiography is inappropriate because the vascular injury will be apparent upon exploration. When muscles are injured, ischemia time of greater than 6 hours may lead to irreversible myocyte damage and subsequent ischemia reperfusion injury. Ischemia reperfusion injury is associated with decreased viability of the extremity, multiple organ failure syndrome, and acute respiratory distress syndrome.[14]

After debridement, controversy exists regarding the most important next step in surgical management. Most surgeons will perform vascular repair to restore circulation prior to any skeletal fixation. However, some argue that skeletal fixation should be performed prior to vascular repair as it may stabilize the limb and protect the vascular repair.[15] In such cases, temporary shunting is commonly used to minimize the overall ischemia time and reduce postoperative complications. Shunting has been associated with maintenance of tissue viability, thus enhancing the functional outcome of the patient.[16,17] Temporary shunting is commonly performed prior to skeletal fixation and can reestablish arterial flow, mitigating the long-term sequelae of ischemia reperfusion injury.

Skeletal Fixation

Fractures associated with mutilated upper extremity injuries are often comminuted, unstable, and may have bony loss. These fractures are usually open and highly contaminated. Surgeons must decide appropriate fracture fixation with functional recovery in mind. Identification of salvageable components marks the initial step in fracture fixation.[18] This will help determine which type of fixation to use. Treatment of mutilating upper extremity skeletal injuries is technically challenging. The presentation of the injury including degree of displacement and ability to maintain fracture reduction plays a substantial role in surgical management. Duncan et al. investigated complications after open hand fractures and found that final postoperative range of motion was influenced by severity of soft-tissue injury; more extensive soft-tissue injuries were associated with higher infection and amputation rates, thus highlighting the difficulties with providing a good functional outcome in mutilating upper extremity injuries.[19]

Typical fixation used for skeletal stability includes Kirschner wires (K-wires), screw and plate fixation, and external fixators. The most common fixation method in mutilated hand injuries are wires or pins because of the relative ease in placement and universal availability.[20] However, K-wires and pins do not provide strong fracture stability, and patients should not perform early postoperative aggressive range of motion. Many surgeons advocate the use of crossed K-wires to improve rigidity especially in hand injuries.[18] Plate and screw fixation is another method commonly used, specifically in mutilated injuries involving the forearm (Figure 82.4). Plating systems require wide undermining of the periosteum for appropriate exposure and placement, which may compromise the vascular supply to the bone. However, plates and screw provide rigid fixation for earlier mobilization. Finally, in severely comminuted, contaminated, and open fractures, external fixators can be used for immediate fracture stabilization. External fixators are generally applied in severely contaminated wounds, until such time when more definitive fixation can be performed after wound debridement. They can be placed easily with minimal devitalization of bony fragments. No matter what fixation method is chosen, the ultimate goals are initiation of range of motion to provide improved function and minimization of soft tissue stripping to achieve bony healing and union of the fracture.

Tendon and Muscle Repair

Appropriate identification of both proximal and distal musculotendinous units facilitates repair. Given the extensive damage associated with these injuries, it is often impossible to repair all musculotendinous units. In situations with loss of proximal musculotendinous units, Faibisoff et al. advocate repairing the distal tendons to other available tendons/muscles proximally.[21] However, surgeons must consider synergy when performing tendon [illegible] of proximal and distal musculotendinous units. Primary repair of the musculotendinous unit is ideal; however, utilization of tendon grafts or delayed repair with secondary tendon reconstruction may be necessary. Commonly used donors for tendon grafts include palmaris longus, plantaris, toe extensors, or *spare parts* from other tendons in the injured extremity.

Flexor tendon repairs are often challenging and require precise surgical technique. When performing a flexor tendon repair, the strength of the repair will determine early range of motion and the ultimate functional outcome. For optimal flexor tendon repair, multistrand core suture repair techniques should be prioritized to reduce gapping and tendon rupture.[22] In addition to a multistrand core suture repair, the use of an epitendinous suture provides a more robust repair and use of early range of motion protocols.[23] Surgeons should strive to use this technique in all flexor tendon repairs in the mutilated upper extremity to prevent tendon rupture and promote better functional outcomes. However, when there are multiple tendons lacerated in zone 5, the tedious epitendinous sutures are often not performed to expedite the surgical sequence because of the relative lack of restrictive adhesion formation in this zone.

Pulley reconstruction in mutilating upper extremity injuries should be performed if multiple digits are involved.[24] Preservation of A2 and A4 pulleys avoids bowstringing and promotes appropriate tendon gliding. Primary pulley repair should be attempted, but if primary repair cannot be done, reconstruction with tendon grafts wrapped around the phalanx or attached to available remnant pulleys can be performed. Appropriate repair of tendons in these complex injuries will promote optimal function and increased range of motion.

Vascular Repair

Vascular reconstruction involves both the arterial and venous system. When assessing the degree of vascular injury, it is important to debride the artery and vein to outside of the zone of injury. The *ribbon sign* has been used to identify areas of arterial vessel wall avulsion and intimal injury and confers a poor prognosis for replantation.[25] Areas with the ribbon sign should be debrided both proximally and distally,

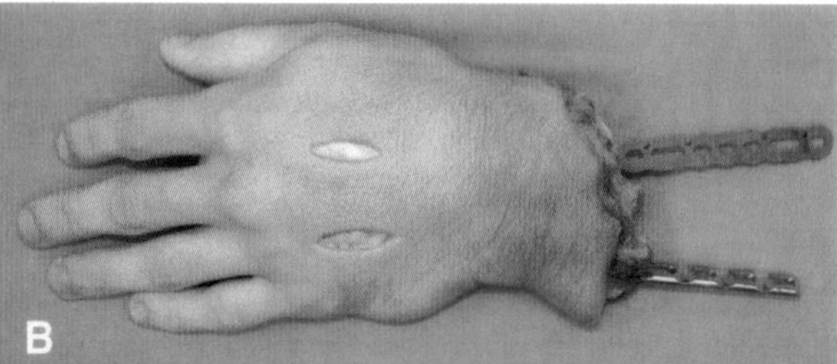

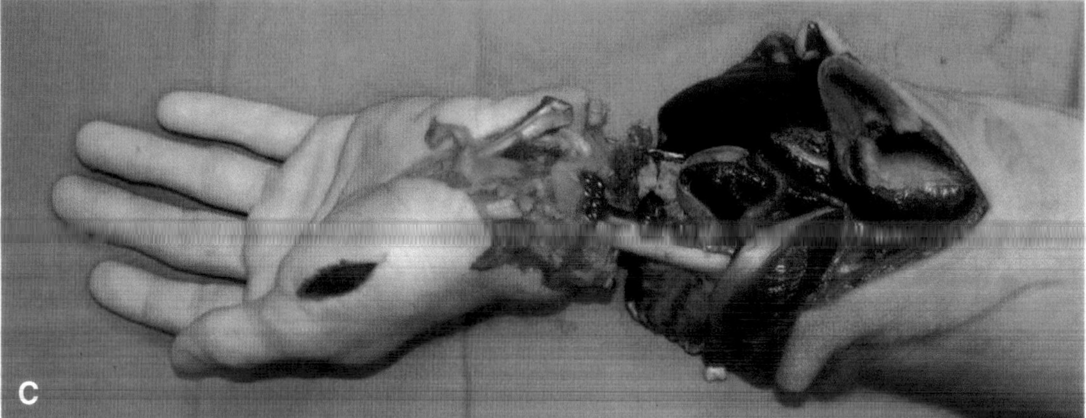

FIGURE 82.4. Same patient as in **Figure 82.2**. **A, B.** Thenar, hypothenar, carpal tunnel, and dorsal fasciotomies of the hand were performed. **C.** The radius and ulna were fixated using plates and screws.

and the gap created should be bridged by a vein graft. Without appropriate debridement, vascular anastomosis will fail. For microsurgical success, Buncke et al. recommended anastomosis of the vessel walls without tension, atraumatic surgical treatment of the vasculature, precise suture placement without trapping the adventitia, and prevention of suture crowding.[26]

If possible, primary anastomosis should be attempted, and in upper extremity injuries, both the radial and ulnar artery should be repaired. If primary anastomosis cannot be accomplished, however, vein grafting should be used to optimize successful repair. Commonly used vein grafts include veins or branches of veins from the dorsal or volar forearm such as the basilic or cephalic vein or the saphenous vein from the lower extremity (used as a reverse saphenous vein graft). Veins from the upper extremity can only be utilized when small segments of graft are required. For more extensive vascular reconstruction, such as the palmar arch, surgeons must use creative and complex reconstructive techniques. To reconstruct the palmar arch, a Y-vein graft from the volar forearm is used to perform end-to-end anastomoses to reconstruct multiple common digital arteries concurrently (Figure 82.5).

With severe crush injuries, revascularization is substantially more difficult. Severely crushed or mangled extremities portend a poorer prognosis with associated vascular compromise.[27] In these injuries, vessels may be damaged beyond the zone of injury and require an extensive debridement. Surgeons must be aware of the degree of vessel injury to optimize successful revascularization.

Venous reconstruction is challenging in the digits, and surgeons should strive for at least one venous repair or more if possible to avoid venous complications. Thrombosis of the repair leads to venous congestion and ultimately replantation and revascularization failure. When faced with venous congestion, surgeons utilize adjunct treatments such as medical leeches and anticoagulation. Every upper extremity surgeon must be equipped with microsurgical skills to optimize vascular repairs and ultimate survival in mutilating upper extremity injuries.

Nerve Repair

In mutilating upper extremity injuries, nerves can be damaged extensively and often have traction or crush injuries. For restoration of sensibility and function, direct end-to-end nerve repair without tension is the primary goal. However, with complex upper extremity trauma, direct repair may not be feasible. Again, surgeons must ensure that an adequate debridement has been performed, and this includes debridement of crushed and avulsed nerves until healthy fascicles are present. This will provide the ideal environment for return of function and sensibility. Additionally, it is preferable to perform the nerve repair outside the zone of injury to ensure success. Once a thorough debridement has been performed, the nerves are aligned according to their fascicular pattern and coapted using an epineural repair using microsurgical techniques.

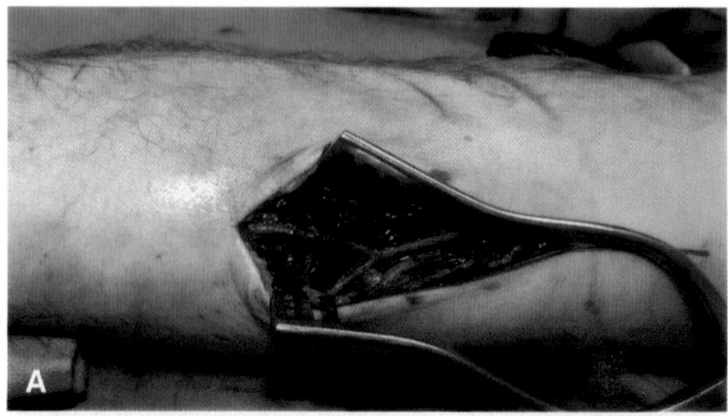

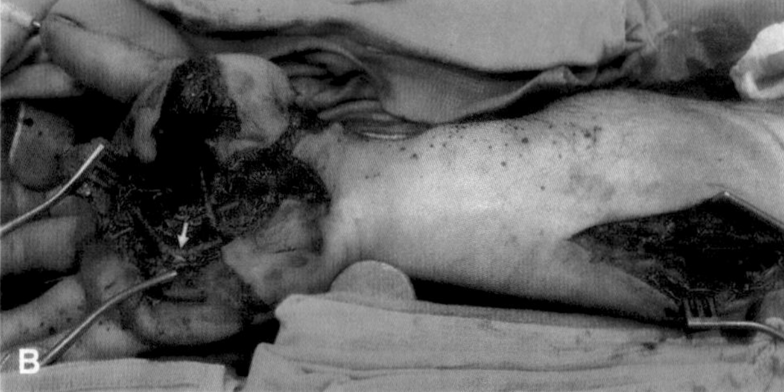

FIGURE 82.5. **A.** A Y-vein graft was used to reconstruct the palmar arch of a 36-year-old man who sustained a crush injury to his right upper extremity. **B.** The arrow indicates the Y-vein graft in situ.

If primary repair has undue tension, surgeons can use interposition autogenous nerve grafts, nerve conduits, or processed nerve allografts to bridge the gap. Primary nerve grafting with interposition autografts from the upper and lower extremity provides viable nerve cells including Schwann cells, which may aid in nerve regeneration.[28,29] Commonly used donor nerves include the medial or lateral antebrachial cutaneous, sural, and posterior interosseous nerve. Cutaneous nerves of the forearm can be easily harvested for grafting. With more extensive injuries, the sural nerve from the lower extremity offers additional grafting material.

Use of autologous nerve grafts is the standard for nerve repairs; however, there are specific instances when nerve conduits or processed nerve allografts are valuable. Given the finite amount of autologous nerve grafts available, in cases with extensive nerve injuries, some surgeons may choose to use conduits or nerve allografts. These nerve substitutes do not require additional donor sites and are available *off the shelf*. Indications for the use of conduits include nerve gaps of less than 3 cm, nerves that are of small diameter, and noncritical, typically sensory nerves.[30,31] Nerve conduits have been shown to provide sensory recovery but are inferior to autologous nerve grafting for motor regeneration.[32]

Processed nerve allografts have shown promise in digital nerve repair and are now commercially available. Rinker et al. showed equivalent sensory outcomes for processed nerve allografts when compared with nerve autografts, and they had superior sensory outcomes when compared with nerve conduits.[33] For motor recovery, there are better motor functional outcomes when 5 to 50 mm processed nerve allografts are used.[34] In specific instances, nerve substitutes such as conduits and processed nerve allografts can aid in nerve recovery.

In proximal injuries, autologous nerve grafting, nerve conduits, and processed nerve allografts may not provide the desired motor and sensory recovery. Certain nerve injuries, specifically those proximal to the elbow, such as the ulnar nerve, will not have a functional recovery because of the long path needed for nerve generation to reach the target muscle. In these instances, surgeons may opt to perform primary nerve transfers or *babysitting* nerve transfers. This promotes continued muscle innervation while the nerve is regenerating, such as the anterior interosseous nerve is transferred in an end-to-side fashion to the ulnar nerve. Surgeons must be well versed in autologous nerve grafting, nerve conduits, processed nerve allografts, and nerve transfers.

Soft-Tissue Coverage

In the mangled upper extremity, there is often extensive soft-tissue and skin loss, requiring complex soft-tissue coverage. When choosing the appropriate soft-tissue coverage, surgeons must provide durable coverage of vital structures. The soft-tissue deficit can be managed with various reconstructive techniques. The *reconstructive ladder*, starting with the simplest surgical technique and moving to more complicated surgical techniques, has been touted as the optimal framework for reconstruction. However, in these complex injuries, the *reconstructive ladder* may get replaced by the *reconstructive elevator*, as simpler reconstructive techniques are not viable with extensive injuries, and surgeons may need to jump to free tissue transfer. In mutilating injuries, skin grafts often cannot be used when there are exposed nerves, vessels, and tendons. However, in skin-only defects, both full thickness and split thickness skin grafts are ideal. Injudicious use of skin grafting delays definitive reconstruction using flaps, which may require more difficult secondary procedures in the future.

Flap-based coverage is often used in mutilating upper extremity injuries and provides ideal durable coverage from both a functional and cosmetic perspective (Figure 82.6). Surgeons must be equipped to use both local flaps and free tissue transfer when treating these complex upper extremity injuries. Because of the extent of the injury, local flap options may not be available; therefore, microsurgical techniques for soft-tissue reconstruction may be needed.[35] However, free tissue transfer may not always be a possibility as the recipient vessels can be damaged, thus rendering microsurgery impossible. Furthermore, there are situations where a trained microsurgeon is unavailable. Therefore, when managing mutilating upper extremity injuries, it is imperative that the surgeon be well versed in all reconstructive techniques to tailor treatment to the individual patient and injury.

For a successful reconstruction, soft-tissue coverage should be taken from outside the zone of injury for adequate healing. Coverage must provide tendon gliding to optimize functional recovery. Timing for flaps reconstruction continues to be controversial. Flaps can be performed as *primary free flap closure* (12–24 hours after injury), *delayed free flap closure* (2–7 days after injury), and *secondary wound closure* (beyond 7 days after injury).[36] We prefer to perform a complete initial debridement at the time of injury and *delayed free flap closure* within 2 to 7 days after the injury. At the second surgery, nonviable tissues will be demarcated and definitive reconstruction can be performed after the second debridement.

Fasciocutaneous flaps are usually the *work horse* flaps for mutilating upper extremity injuries. For optimal color match, local flaps including pedicled radial forearm flap can provide durable coverage with an ideal environment to promote tendon gliding. When the dorsal hand is involved, surgeons may use groin flaps in a two-stage approach. These flaps require an additional operation for flap division. Additionally, there are numerous free flaps that can be used to provide adequate coverage such as the anterior lateral thigh flap. However, in extremely large soft-tissue defects, free muscle flaps, such as the latissimus dorsi, may be used for coverage. Lastly, free functional muscle transfer is often employed to recreate function in addition to coverage. The individual characteristics of the patient and injury should guide the surgeon's choice in flap reconstruction.

Adjunct treatments may aid in successful reconstruction. Negative pressure wound therapy promotes granulation tissue between debridements and definitive reconstruction and is often used as a temporary dressing. Additionally, there has been an increased use of acellular dermal matrix (ADM) in complex upper extremity wounds and burns.[37] ADM replaces the missing dermis prior to placing a skin graft. It promotes granulation tissue over areas lacking paratenon or periosteum that would otherwise desiccate, and ADM can be used to aid in the coverage of exposed vital structures such as nerves, arteries, and tendons. For soft-tissue coverage of mutilating upper extremity injuries, surgeons must use an individualized approach and be able to master all reconstructive techniques from skin grafts to free tissue transfer.

Use of Spare Parts

Spare parts use creative reconstructive techniques to employ presumably unusable tissues that are nonreplantable or unsalvageable. This technique avoids additional donor site morbidity by using parts that would have otherwise been discarded. The spare parts technique affords surgeons the opportunity to match tissue for definitive reconstruction and can be a source of soft tissue, nerves, vessels, tendon, or bones (Figure 82.7). For example, the glabrous skin from a nonreplantable digit is an excellent source of skin for palmar defects. Additionally, bony remnants can be used as a nonvascularized bone graft to provide additional length for an amputated digit. When approaching the mangled upper extremity, the amputated parts should be thoroughly evaluated and not discarded. Preservation of the amputated or mangled entities may provide spare parts that can substantially contribute to the reconstructive treatment plan. The use of spare parts provides additional tools to reconstruct mutilating upper extremity injuries.

Fasciotomy

In upper extremity trauma, patients are at increased risk of compartment syndrome, which if unrecognized can lead to devastating consequences including limb loss and mortality. The clinical diagnosis of compartment syndrome includes pain especially on passive stretch of the muscle, pallor, pulselessness, paresthesias, poikilothermia, and paralysis. However, adjunct measurement of compartment pressures may aid in the diagnosis. In a study by Branco et al., approximately 1%

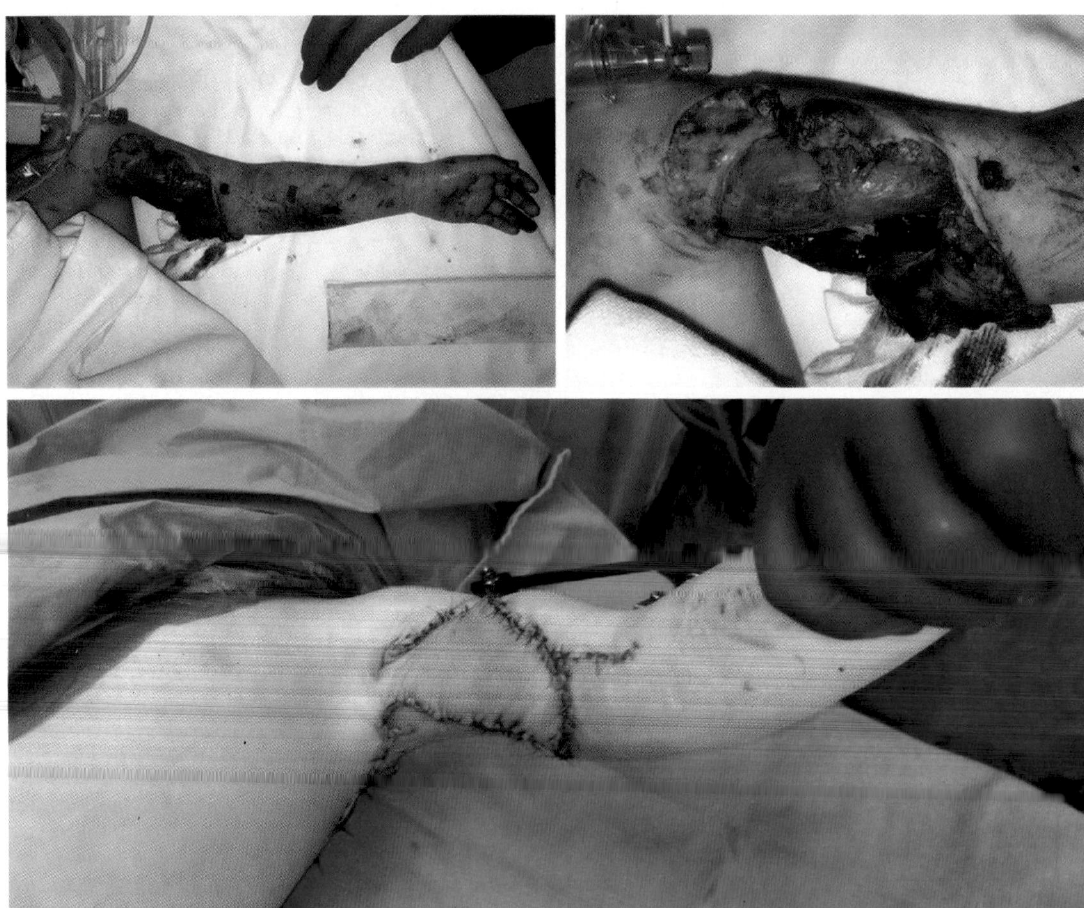

FIGURE 82.6. A 3-year-old boy suffered a left proximal arm avulsion injury from a motor vehicle collision. He underwent debridement, ulnar nerve repair, fasciotomies, and a latissimus dorsi pedicled flap.

of all upper extremity trauma patients will need a fasciotomy, especially in those patients who suffered an arterial and venous injury.[38] Therefore, surgeons must recognize compartment syndrome and have a low threshold to perform fasciotomies. Furthermore, in instances with vascular compromise in the mangled upper extremity, preemptive compartment releases should be performed because of the reperfusion injury and muscle ischemia after the return of blood flow.

All compartments within the hand and forearm must be fully released for adequate decompression. We prefer a two-incision release of the forearm compartments, using two longitudinal incisions—one overlying the flexor muscles on the volar radial aspect of the forearm and another overlying the extensor muscles on the dorsal ulnar aspect of the forearm.[39] This approach can fully release the volar, dorsal, and mobile wad compartments without risking exposure of the median nerve or flexor and extensor tendons. In the hand, a five-incision approach is used. The carpal tunnel, thenar eminence, and hypothenar eminence must be released in the palmar hand. On the dorsum of the hand, we recommend two longitudinal incisions overlying the radial index and ring finger metacarpals. Unrecognized compartment syndrome in the upper extremity can lead to substantial disability and even limb loss and death; thus surgeons must promptly intervene to avoid devastating consequences.

SPECIAL CONSIDERATIONS

Pediatric Injuries

Pediatric mutilating upper extremity injuries are a unique entity because children tend to have better outcomes when compared with adults. Children recover quicker and have increased function with enhanced mobility and sensory return.[40] The mechanisms surrounding these injuries in children substantially differ from adult injuries and can be divided into three categories: accidental, nonaccidental, and self-mutilation.[41] In an epidemiologic study from a regional trauma center, approximately 53% of pediatric amputation injuries occurred without any adult supervision.[42] Common mechanisms of injury include lawn mowers, animal bites, burns, explosives, and injuries from other dangerous household equipment.[40,41,43]

Evaluation of mutilating upper extremity injuries in children poses a unique challenge, as both the parents and child may be anxious and scared. However, similar with adults, ATLS should be followed to assess for other life-threatening injuries. Once the child is cleared from a trauma standpoint and hemodynamically stable, an evaluation of the extremity should be attempted. Children may need anesthetic blocks in the emergency department for examination of the injury. However, a sensory examination should be documented prior to placement of an anesthetic block. As in adults, the operative principles are complete debridement, restoration of blood flood with possible shunting, skeletal fixation, muscle and tendon repair, venous and arterial repair, nerve repair, and soft-tissue coverage. However, in children, epiphyseal plates may still be intact, and bones may continue to grow after the injury or replantation, thus requiring special handling and consideration.[44,45] With any reconstruction, it is important to involve the parents and help them understand the expected outcomes.

In children, postoperative management can be quite difficult. We recommend splinting or casting the patient in an above-elbow fashion for complete immobilization. The operated extremity should remain as inactive as possible to optimize healing. Despite being immobilized for longer periods of time, children recover mobility of the operated extremity much easier than adults.

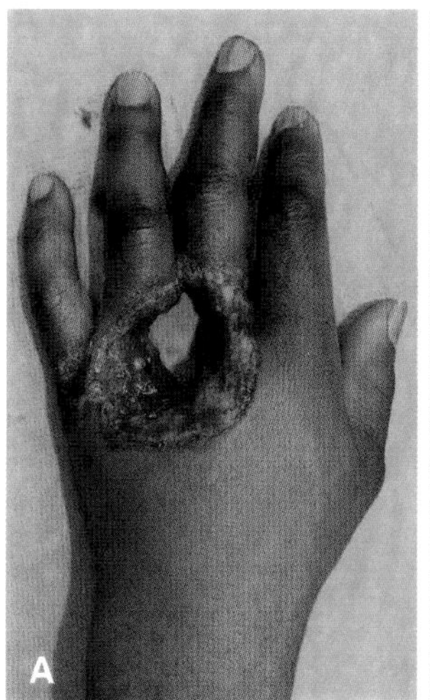

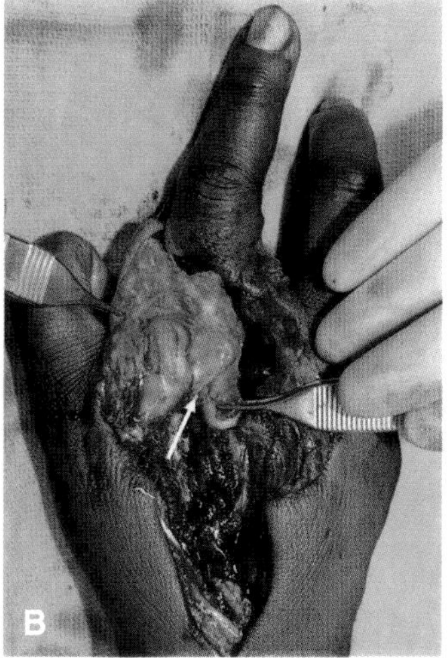

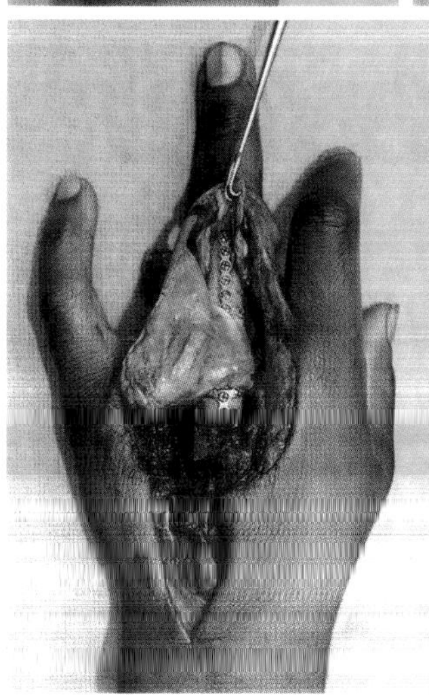

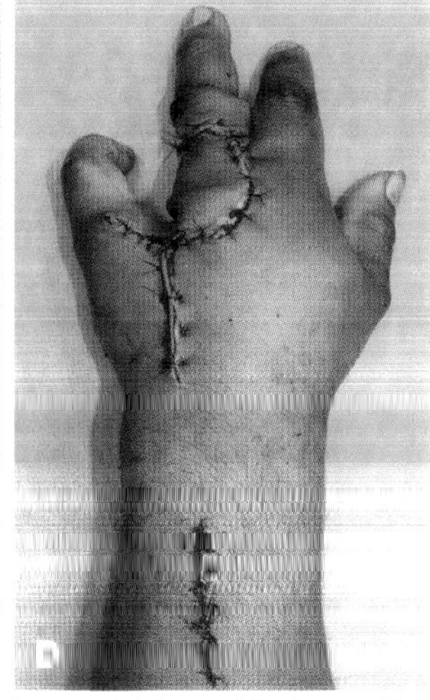

FIGURE 82.7 **A.** This patient suffered a dye punch injury while at work. **B–D.** The spare parts technique was used to transfer his left ring finger proximal interphalangeal joint as a composite pedicled graft to reconstruct the left middle finger metacarpophalangeal joint. The arrow in B indicates the transferred left ring finger proximal interphalangeal joint placed in its new location at the middle finger metacarpophalangeal joint. (Reproduced with permission from Osterman AL. Arthroscopic and open triangular fibrocartilage complex repair. In: Wiesel S, ed. *Operative Techniques in Orthopaedic Surgery*. Vol 3. Philadelphia, PA: Wolters Kluwer Health/Lippincott Williams and Wilkins;2011:2520.Figure 49-2A.)

Treatment of a child with a mutilating upper extremity injury requires participation of the family and can often lead to a functional reconstruction.

Combat Injuries

Mutilating upper extremity injuries during combat are common. War time involves complicating circumstances including limited resources and delayed treatment,[46] which can hinder reconstructive efforts. Management begins with saving the life, then saving the limb, and lastly maintaining function of the upper extremity. In a study by Dougherty et al., there was a 2.3% mortality rate for upper extremity injuries in Operation Iraqi Freedom.[47] Common mechanisms of injury include gunshot wounds and blast injuries from improvised explosive devices or land mines,[48] which can create large segmental mutilating injuries with permanent disability. Additionally, there are substantial late sequelae that combat-wounded service members suffer, subsequently requiring late upper extremity amputation. Krueger et al. determined that loss of wrist and finger motion, neurogenic pain, and heterotopic ossification contribute to delayed upper extremity amputation.[49] Furthermore, revision surgery of upper extremity amputations sustained while in combat are common because of phantom limb pain requiring neuropathic medications.[50] These complications provide barriers to prosthetic use and should be promptly recognized to permit an optimal functional recovery. Combat injuries to the upper extremity create substantial morbidity and mortality and pose unique challenges for the reconstructive surgeon.

CONCLUSION

Treatment of mutilating upper extremity injuries requires creativity and an armamentarium of reconstructive surgical techniques. A thorough primary and secondary survey, in accordance with ATLS, assures that other life-threatening injuries are not missed. Operative treatment should begin with an aggressive debridement and then follow a systematic operative approach. Even with the most meticulous technique, mutilating upper extremity injuries often result in poor motor and sensory recovery. Future research in prosthetics, vascularized composite allotransplantation, and tissue engineering will improve the functional outcomes and make these injuries less devastating.

ACKNOWLEDGMENTS

The work was supported by a Midcareer Investigator Award in Patient-Oriented Research (2 K24-AR053120-06) to Kevin C. Chung. The content is solely the responsibility of the authors and does not necessarily represent the official views of the National Institutes of Health.

REFERENCES

1. Kragh JF Jr, Walters TJ, Baer DG, et al. Survival with emergency tourniquet use to stop bleeding in major limb trauma. *Ann Surg*. 2009;249(1):1-7.
2. Schlickewei W, Kuner EH, Mullaji AB, Götze B. Upper and lower limb fractures with concomitant arterial injury. *J Bone Jt Surg Br*. 1992;74(2):181-188.
3. Pierrie SN, Gaston RG, Loeffler BJ. Current concepts in upper-extremity amputation. *J Hand Surg Am*. 2018;43(7):657-667.
4. Sabapathy SR, Elliot D, Venkatramani H. Pushing the boundaries of salvage in mutilating upper limb injuries: techniques in difficult situations. *Hand Clin*. 2016;32(4):585-597.
5. Prichayudh S, Verananvattna A, Sriussadaporn S, et al. Management of upper extremity vascular injury: outcome related to the mangled extremity severity score. *World J Surg*. 2009;33(4):857-863.
6. Wei FC, Chang YL, Chen HC, Chuang CC. Three successful digital replantations in a patient after 84, 86, and 94 hours of cold ischemia time. *Plast Reconstr Surg*. 1988;82(2):346-350.
7. Chiu HY, Chen MT. Revascularization of digits after thirty-three hours of warm ischemia time: a case report. *J Hand Surg Am*. 1984;9A(1):63-67.
8. Wood MB, Cooney WP III. Above elbow limb replantation: functional results. *J Hand Surg Am*. 1986;11(5):682-687.
9. Atzei A, Pignatti M, Maria Baldrighi C, et al. Long-term results of replantation of the proximal forearm following avulsion amputation. *Microsurgery*. 2005;25(4):293-298.
10. Burkhalter W. Mutilating injuries of the hand. *Hand Clin*. 1986;2(1):45-68.
11. Patzakis MJ, Wilkins J. Factors influencing infection rate in open fracture wounds. *Clin Orthop Relat Res*. 1989;(243):36-40.
12. Ng ZY, Salgado CJ, Moran SL, Chim H. Soft tissue coverage of the mangled upper extremity. *Semin Plast Surg*. 2015;29(1):48-54.
13. Lebowitz C, Matzon JL. Arterial injury in the upper extremity: evaluation, strategies, and anticoagulation management. *Hand Clin*. 2018;34(1):85-95.
14. Gillani S, Cao J, Suzuki T, Hak DJ. The effect of ischemia reperfusion injury on skeletal muscle. *Injury*. 2012;43(6):670-675.
15. Franz RW, Goodwin RB, Hartman JF, Wright ML. Management of upper extremity arterial injuries at an urban level I trauma center. *Ann Vasc Surg*. 2009;23(1):8-16.
16. Weinstein MH, Golding AL. Temporary external shunt bypass in the traumatically amputated upper extremity. *J Trauma*. 1975;15(10):912-915.
17. Nunley JA, Koman LA, Urbaniak JR. Arterial shunting as an adjunct to major limb revascularization. *Ann Surg*. 1981;193(3):271-273.
18. Bhardwaj P, Sankaran A, Sabapathy SR. Skeletal fixation in a mutilated hand. *Hand Clin*. 2016;32(4):505-517.
19. Duncan RW, Freeland AE, Jabaley ME, Meydrech EF. Open hand fractures: an analysis of the recovery of active motion and of complications. *J Hand Surg Am*. 1993;18(3):387-394.
In this study, the authors investigate the long-term functional outcomes after operative fixation of open hand fractures. With more extensive soft-tissue injuries, patients had significantly decreased range of motion. Furthermore, open reduction internal fixation of metacarpal fractures had better range of motion when compared with phalangeal fractures.

20. Henry MH. Fractures of the proximal phalanx and metacarpals in the hand: preferred methods of stabilization. *J Am Acad Orthop Surg*. 2008;16(10):586-595.
21. Faibisoff B, Daniel RK. Management of severe forearm injuries. *Surg Clin North Am*. 1981;61(2):287-301.
22. Osei DA, Stepan JG, Calfee RP, et al. The effect of suture caliber and number of core suture strands on zone II flexor tendon repair: a study in human cadavers. *J Hand Surg Am*. 2014;39(2):262-268.
This is the seminal article that proved the benefit of multistrand core suture repair for flexor tendon injuries in an animal model. An eight-strand repair was approximately 43% stronger than a four-strand repair, highlighting the importance of additional core sutures to strengthen flexor tendon repairs.
23. Fufa DT, Osei DA, Calfee RP, et al. The effect of core and epitendinous suture modifications on repair of intrasynovial flexor tendons in an in vivo canine model. *J Hand Surg Am*. 2012;37(12):2526-2531.
24. Dy CJ, Daluiski A. Flexor pulley reconstruction. *Hand Clin*. 2013;29(2):235-242.
25. Van Beek AL, Kutz JE, Zook EG. Importance of the ribbon sign, indicating unsuitability of the vessel, in replanting a finger. *Plast Reconstr Surg*. 1978;61(1):32-35.
This is the first article to describe the ribbon sign, *which indicates avulsion and crush of an artery. When attempting revascularization, the authors suggest that if the ribbon sign is present, then a thorough debridement of the artery should be performed and a vein graft used to bridge the gap.*
26. Buncke HJ, Alpert B, Shah KG. Microvascular grafting. *Clin Plast Surg*. 1978;5(2):185-194.
27. Cooney WP III. Revascularization and replantation after upper extremity trauma: experiences with interposition artery and vein grafts. *Clin Orthop Relat Res*. 1978(137):227-234.
28. Millesi H. Bridging defects: autologous nerve grafts. *Acta Neurochir Suppl*. 2007;100:37-38.
29. Moore AM, Wagner IJ, Fox IK. Principles of nerve repair in complex wounds of the upper extremity. *Semin Plast Surg*. 2015;29(1):40-47.
30. Moore AM, Kasukurthi R, Magill CK, et al. Limitations of conduits in peripheral nerve repairs. *Hand (NY)*. 2009;4(2):180-186.
31. Mackinnon SE, Dellon AL. Clinical nerve reconstruction with a bioabsorbable polyglycolic acid tube. *Plast Reconstr Surg*. 1990;85(3):419-424.
This is a retrospective study of 15 patients who underwent nerve repair using a bioabsorbable polyglycolic acid nerve conduit. The authors report excellent sensory return with these nerve conduits when used for gaps up to three centimeters. These sensory results were similar to traditional nerve grafts.
32. Safa B, Buncke G. Autograft substitutes: conduits and processed nerve allografts. *Hand Clin*. 2016;32(2):127-140.
33. Rinker BD, Ingari JV, Greenberg JA, et al. Outcomes of short-gap sensory nerve injuries reconstructed with processed nerve allografts from a multicenter registry study. *J Reconstr Microsurg*. 2015;31(5):384-390.
34. Cho MS, Rinker BD, Weber RV, et al. Functional outcome following nerve repair in the upper extremity using processed nerve allograft. *J Hand Surg Am*. 2012;37(11):2340-2349.
35. Lee K, Roh S, Lee D, Kim J. Skin coverage considerations in a mutilating hand injury. *Hand Clin*. 2016;32(4):491-503.
36. Ninkovic M, Mooney EK, Ninkovic M, et al. A new classification for the standardization of nomenclature in free flap wound closure. *Plast Reconstr Surg*. 1999;103(3):903-914.
This is a retrospective review of 68 patients who underwent emergency free tissue transfer. This article classifies free flap reconstruction for traumtic wound closure as three separate entities: primary free flap closure (12–24 hours after the injury), delayed primary free flap closure (2–7 days after the injury), and secondary free flap closure (7 days after the injury). The authors explain that this new nomenclature follows traditional wound-healing biology and chronologic considerations and should be used for uniform communication among surgeons.
37. Ellis CV, Kulber DA. Acellular dermal matrices in hand reconstruction. *Plast Reconstr Surg*. 2012;130(5 suppl 2):256S-269S.
38. Branco BC, Inaba K, Barmparas G, et al. Incidence and predictors for the need for fasciotomy after extremity trauma: a 10-year review in a mature level I trauma centre. *Injury*. 2011;42(10):1157-1163.
39. Giladi AM, Chung KC. Fasciotomy for compartment syndrome of the hand. In: Chung KC, ed. *Operative Techniques: Hand and Wrist Surgery*. New York, NY: Elsevier; 2018. vol. 3:13-22.
40. Buncke GM, Buntic RF, Romeo O. Pediatric mutilating hand injuries. *Hand Clin*. 2003;19(1):121-131.
41. Thirkannad SM. Mutilating hand injuries in children. *Hand Clin*. 2016;32(4):477-489.
42. Trautwein LC, Smith DG, Rivara FP. Pediatric amputation injuries: etiology, cost, and outcome. *J Trauma*. 1996;41(5):831-838.
43. Moore RS Jr, Tan V, Dormans JP, Bozentka DJ. Major pediatric hand trauma associated with fireworks. *J Orthop Trauma*. 2000;14(6):426-428.
44. Demiri E, Bakhach J, Tsakoniatis N, et al. Bone growth after replantation in children. *J Reconstr Microsurg*. 1995;11(2):113-122.
45. Kim JY, Brown RJ, Jones NF. Pediatric upper extremity replantation. *Clin Plast Surg*. 2005;32(1):1-10, vii.
46. Mathieu L, Bertani A, Gaillard C, et al. Surgical management of combat-related upper extremity injuries. *Chir Main*. 2014;33(3):174-182.
47. Dougherty AL, Mohrle CR, Galarneau MR, et al. Battlefield extremity injuries in operation Iraqi freedom. *Injury*. 2009;40(7):772-777.
48. Mathieu L, Bertani A, Gaillard C, et al. Wartime upper extremity injuries: experience from the Kabul International Airport combat support hospital. *Chir Main*. 2014;33(3):183-188.
49. Krueger CA, Wenke JC, Cho MS, Hsu JR. Common factors and outcome in late upper extremity amputations after military injury. *J Orthop Trauma*. 2014;28(4):227-231.
50. Tintle SM, Baechler MF, Nanos GP, et al. Reoperations following combat-related upper-extremity amputations. *J Bone Jt Surg Am*. 2012;94(16):e1191-e1196.

QUESTIONS

1. **A 52-year-old right-hand-dominant farmer is found unconscious in a field next to a haulm topper. He is brought into a community hospital by emergency medical services without access to a hand surgeon. A trauma code is called. Primary survey is performed without any other injuries found except his partially amputated left upper extremity, which has substantial bleeding. What is the next step in management of this patient?**
   a. Place tourniquet on left upper extremity
   b. Intubate the patient
   c. Perform a secondary survey
   d. Go straight to the operating room
   e. Transfer to a more experienced center

2. **A 5-year-old girl was found in her front lawn after suffering a lawn mower injury to her left upper extremity at the level of the forearm. The parents accompany her in the ambulance to a level II trauma center. On examination, her left upper extremity is cool with minimal capillary refill. She has no additional injuries noted on examination. A surgeon is called to the emergency department. What is the next step in management?**
   a. Serial hand examinations
   b. Emergent operative intervention
   c. Transfer to level I trauma center
   d. Place tourniquet on left upper extremity

3. **A 70-year-old left-hand dominant man was using a table saw and amputated his right upper extremity at the midforearm level. A tourniquet is placed in the field, the amputated part is appropriately wrapped and placed on ice, and he is immediately taken to the nearest hospital. There is no hand surgeon on call, so he is transferred to a level I trauma center. By the time he arrives, his upper extremity has been amputated for 6 hours. After evaluation in the emergency department, he is immediately taken to the operating room. Which technique will prevent further systemic injury?**
   a. Skeletal fixation
   b. Microvascular anastomosis with vein grafts
   c. Microsurgical flap reconstruction
   d. Aggressive debridement
   e. Vascularized shunt

4. **A 60-year-old left-hand-dominant man presents to the emergency department after suffering a wood splitter injury to the right hand. There is extensive soft-tissue injury, but the fingers appear to be well perfused with capillary refill less than 2 seconds. He has diminished two-point discrimination in the median nerve distribution. He is taken to the operating room for emergent exploration and debridement. In the operating room, his median nerve is noted to be cut and crushed at the level of the carpal tunnel. What is your next step in the operation?**
   a. Anastomose the cut ends of the median nerve
   b. Use a nerve graft taken from the medial antebrachial cutaneous nerve to bridge the gap
   c. Debride the median nerve back to healthy fascicles
   d. Use a nerve conduit to bridge the gap

5. **A 40-year-old man is found 20 ft from a motor vehicle collision. He is unconscious, and his right upper extremity has a large soft-tissue defect on the dorsum of the hand with gross contamination and debris. He is intubated in the field and taken to the nearest level I trauma center, where a primary and secondary survey is performed. No other injuries are found on examination. X-rays reveal segmental loss of index, middle, and ring metacarpals. He is cleared by anesthesia for operative intervention if necessary. What is the next step in management?**
   a. Serial hand examinations
   b. Wait until he is extubated to perform a more thorough history and physical examination
   c. Obtain consent from his wife and take him to the operating room for debridement and exploration
   d. Obtain consent from his wife and take him to the operating room for debridement and definitive reconstruction with repair of bony loss with bone grafts, nerve conduits, and tendon repairs

1. **Answer: c.** Before transfer to a more experienced trauma center, the patient must be stabilized. According to ATLS, once the primary survey is completed, then the secondary survey commences. Even though the patient is bleeding from the partially amputated left upper extremity, the secondary survey should take less than a few minutes. It is important to not be distracted by the mutilated upper extremity injury. These injuries are often accompanied by injuries to other parts of the body that may be more life-threatening.

2. **Answer: b.** In this scenario, there is concern for vascular compromise. The patient needs to be taken to the operating room for exploration, debridement, and likely vascular repair. There should be a surgeon on call who is capable of treating this injury. Any delay in operative intervention will place the patient at risk for amputation.

3. **Answer: e.** The upper extremity has been amputated for longer than 6 hours, which places the patient at risk for ischemia of the muscle and subsequent ischemia reperfusion injury. This can affect other organ systems such as the kidneys. To avoid this consequence, blood flow should be reestablished to the amputated part as soon as possible; therefore, a vascularized shunt should be used.

4. **Answer: c.** Even though a debridement will create a larger nerve gap, it is necessary to promote healthy nerve regeneration. The first step should be a debridement of the median nerve back to healthy fascicles. Once this has been performed, the nerve gap can be bridged using nerve grafts and an interfascicular repair.

5. **Answer: c.** The injury is grossly contaminated, and the patient needs a debridement to remove nonviable soft tissue and debris. Given the contamination, definitive reconstruction should not be performed in this setting as it will likely lead to infection. Reconstruction should be performed in a delayed fashion with an additional debridement at the time of the secondary surgery. This will allow for demarcation of nonviable tissues and time to develop a reconstructive plan.

CHAPTER 83 Replantation Strategies of the Hand and Upper Extremity

Sang Hyun Woo

KEY POINTS

- Sequences of the operative technique of replantation are variable up to the type of injury and amputation level.
- Postoperative anticoagulation and rehabilitation are important for achieving satisfactory functional restoration.
- Depending on the amputation level and type of amputation, unique characteristics of replantation should be understood.
- Management and prevention of complications of replantation relate to the amputation level

In traumatic amputation of digits, the hand or upper extremities, the decision of whether to perform microsurgical replantation or revision amputation depends on the condition of the amputation stump, the condition of the amputated parts, the level of injury, and the patients' medical condition. By definition, replantation is the reattachment of all structural tissues following complete amputation. The term revascularization is used to refer to the repair of an incomplete amputation where there is some tissue still intact, but without arterial circulation. Malt and McKhann performed the first replantation of an amputated arm at the midhumeral level in 1962. Kleinert reported the first vascular repair in fingers the next year, followed by Tamai reporting replantation of a totally amputated thumb.[1-3]

Since these early developments, microsurgery has become an integral part of the training of plastic surgeons and hand surgeons in most major hospitals. Frequent emergency replantation surgery spontaneously evolves to elective microsurgical free tissue transfer. Even though an emergency replantation surgery as a resident or plastic surgeon can be a laborious job, it should be performed with a sense of responsibility and pride to resurrect amputated dead tissues. Experience of microanastomosis techniques for the replantation of very distal amputation can be developed for supermicrosurgery-related perforator free flaps or lymphatic surgery. Also, emergency replantation of a major limb is sufficient to replace the clinical practice of allotransplantation of the extremities.

With the refinement of microsurgical techniques and development of microscope capabilities, the success rate of replantation has increased dramatically. Most plastic and hand surgeons have tried to perform replantation at all levels and with all types of injury patterns in accordance with the needs of the patients based on cultural background or specific conditions.

INDICATIONS AND CONTRAINDICATIONS

Any patient with any level of amputation from the fingertip to the upper arm is a candidate for replantation. The decision to replant and the outcome of that decision have significant consequences for the patient, the hospital, and the public purse. Before the final decision to proceed with replantation, the following three factors should be considered. The variables in amputation factors are type of injury (guillotine, crush, and avulsion), level of amputation, warm ischemia time, and multiple or bilateral and segmental injuries (Figure 83.1). Patient factors include age, general condition for prolonged anesthesia, preexisting diseases or other combined major injuries, occupation and intelligence for cooperation of postoperative care and rehabilitation, the last factor being a socioeconomic factor which includes relative medical cost per quality-adjusted life-year gained, duration of hospitalization, sick leave, and so on. However, patients' strong demands often override textbook indications for replantation.

The indications for replantation have seen little significant change over the years[4]:

Absolute Indications

- Thumb
- [illegible]
- Transmetacarpal
- Wrist
- Forearm
- Single digit in children
- Individual digit distal to the flexor digitorum superficialis (FDS) tendon insertion

Relative Indications

- Distal to distal interphalangeal joint (DIPJ)
- Single digit proximal to the FDS tendon insertion
- Local crushing or clear avulsion
- Elbow and above elbow, sharply amputated or moderately avulsed
- Patients of advanced age

These indications are not based solely on potential viability but are predicated on the potential for long-term function. In the case of thumb amputation, replantation probably offers the best functional return among any other option for thumb reconstruction. Even with poor motion and sensation, the thumb is useful to the patient as a post for opposition.

Although single-finger replantation is generally not performed, replantation beyond the level of the FDS tendon insertion, and zone 1 in a flexor tendon injury, usually results in satisfactory function. The replantation of a single digit amputated proximal to the insertion of the FDS is more indicative of revision amputation.[5,6] The flexor and extensor tendons can adhere to the healing bone and require secondary tenolysis to improve motion, and the results after tenolysis are often not good. The replanted digit may even interfere with overall hand function. Recent reports, however, demonstrate the justification of replantation of this zone by the benefits of functional and aesthetic improvement in spite of higher cost, longer hospital stay, and sick leave.[7,8] The posttraumatic stress and psychological sequelae of amputation of the single digit should not be underestimated.[9] The severity of consequence of a distal single-digit injury in one patient may be greater than that of a major limb amputation in another individual.

In Asian countries, Confucian moral values and the greater emphasis on maintaining body integrity and appearance give further reason to perform these procedures.[10] Moreover, in situations when amputation of the digit is considered a stigma, when the motivated patient may need all fingers for his or her occupation, when cosmetic considerations are important, or in children, a single-digit amputation may be indicated for replantation.

Replantation of distal digital amputation is becoming more popular in special replantation centers. In the West, the loss of function in the fingertip is perceived to be negligible despite the lack of scientific evidence supporting this.

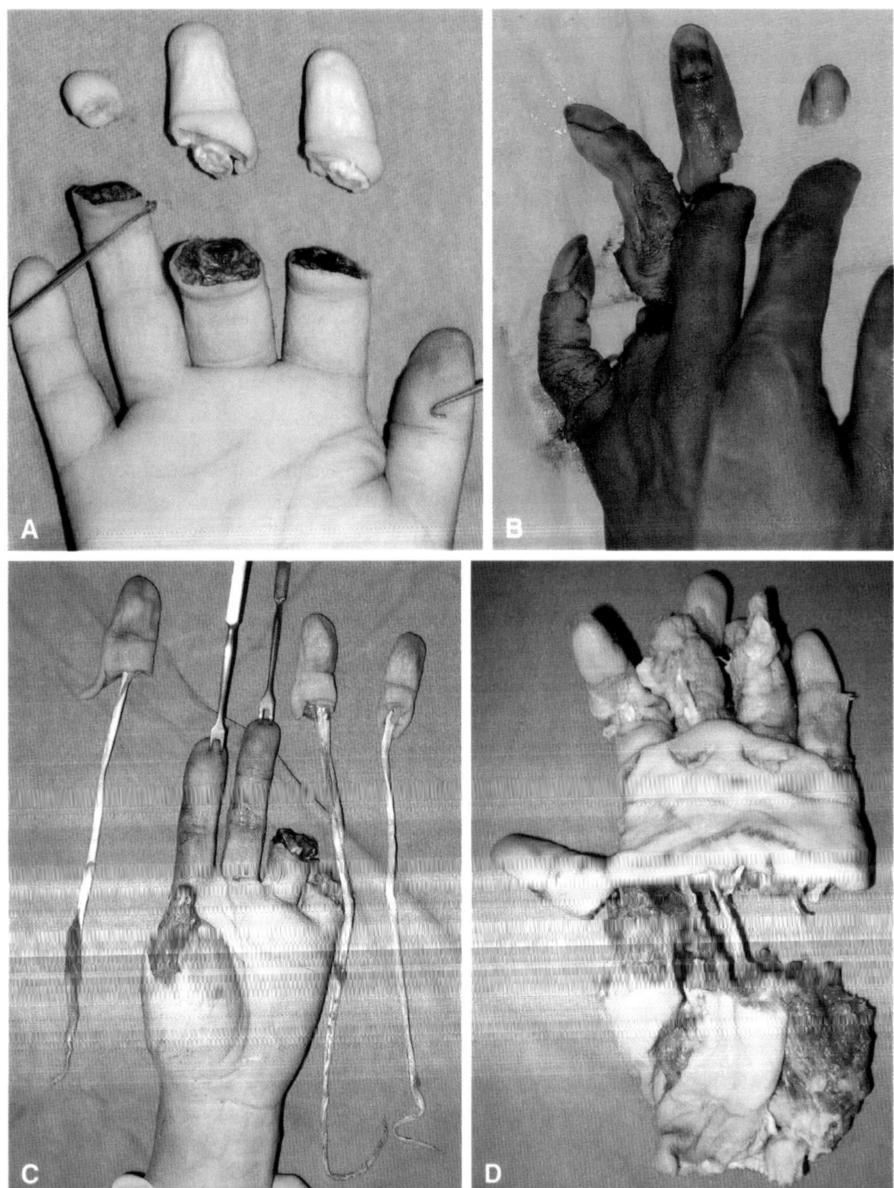

FIGURE 83.1. Different types of amputations. **A.** Guillotine amputation. **B.** Local crushing amputation. **C.** Avulsion amputation. **D.** Combined amputation caused by a combination of crush, avulsion, and segmental injury.

Amputation of digits in children is a clear indication for replantation, no matter whether it is single or multiple-digit or proximal or distal digits involved. Digital replantation in children is no longer a challenging procedure, and survival rates are increasing. With refinement of replantation techniques, the success rate is as high as in adults, and the ultimate functional result is shown to be successful in long-term follow-up studies. Replantation of a single digit is generally indicated in children. Successful replantation provides improved wound healing and nerve regeneration allowing not only improved overall function of the hand but also the child's future potential.

Contraindications to replantation exist when injuries or serious preexisting diseases preclude a prolonged anesthesia:

- Life-threatening-associated injuries
- Psychologically unstable patients
- Systemic illness (e.g., severely arteriosclerotic vessels)
- Severe crushing or avulsion
- Multiple segmental injuries of the amputated part
- Extreme contamination
- Prolonged warm ischemia time in major limb amputation

Suspended or delayed replantation[11] or ectopic transplantation[12] of the digits is another option for patients with acute combined injury or disease and seriously contaminated amputation. Of the factors relating to the injury, amputation level and injury type are not considered as contraindications.

Prolonged warm ischemia time is strongly correlated with contraindication to the replantation of amputation at the proximal forearm or upper arm. Because muscle is the tissue most susceptible to ischemia, in normal ambient temperatures, irreversible changes can develop in muscle within only 2 hours of ischemia.[13] In contrast, digits do not contain muscle and can tolerate much longer ischemic conditions. The recommended ischemic times for reliable success with replantation are 12 hours of warm and 24 hours of cold ischemia for digits, and 6 hours of warm and 12 hours of cold ischemia for major limb replants. Delayed or suspended replantation of the digits even after 48 hours of cold ischemia time can be considered for patients with immediate life-threatening injuries that can be stabilized during the first 24 hours.

In cases of severe crushing or avulsed amputation of the digits, if the patient wants replantation, the decision to go ahead relies on the results of the microscopic exploration of the vessel condition of

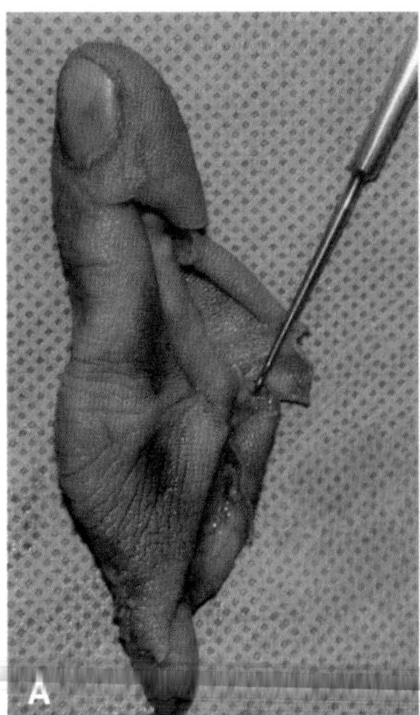
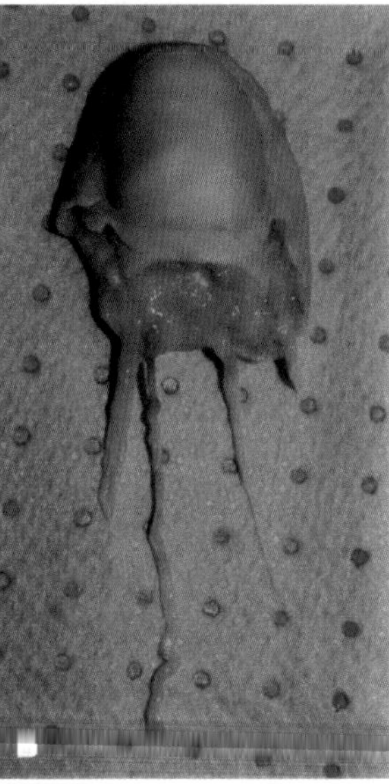

FIGURE 83.2. Clinical signs suggesting injury to the digital arteries. **A.** Red line sign indicating disruption of branches of digital artery. **B.** Ribbon sign indicating avulsion of digital artery.

the amputated part. Severe crushing or avulsion injury shows the *red line sign*, which is a bruised line of the skin along the course of neurovascular bundles (Figure 83.2A). Because of intimal tears and disruption of small branches to the skin, there is no blood flow to the skin even after successful arterial anastomosis. Under loupe magnification, avulsed vessels reveal the *ribbon sign* (Figure 83.2B), demonstrating intimal injury by torsion and stretch on a vessel. The vessel resembles a ribbon like those curled for decoration on a wrapped gift. In these cases, replantation requires vein grafting proximal and distal to this zone of injury.

Even with digit amputation in the elderly, there is no difference in perioperative complications or mortality when comparing replantation patients under 65 years of age and those aged 65 years and above.[14] Advanced age in itself is not a factor for contraindication of replantation. However, extreme contamination or multilevel or segmental amputation of the digit is regarded as a contraindication.

When the patient requests replantation despite one existing contraindication, hand and plastic microsurgeons should try to perform replantation or revascularization surgery at any level of amputation and any type of injury of the digits of patients of any age. Textbook contraindications should not be used as justification for passive surgeons to decline the patients' request for replantation of their amputated tissues under the pretext of failure to achieve functional recovery.

PREPARATION

Transport of Amputated Part to the Replantation Center

The amputated part should be wrapped in saline moistened gauze sponge and placed in a sealed plastic bag, then placed in a container of water and ice at a temperature of 4°C (Figure 83.3). The amputated part should not directly contact the ice and should not be immersed in water. Cold injury directly damages the tissue cells and causes damage to the endothelial lining of small blood vessels with a consequent increase in capillary permeability. Compressive dressing and elevation is sufficient to control bleeding of the amputation stump without clamping. When transferring amputation patients, if necessary, fluid resuscitation, tetanus prophylaxis, and broad-spectrum intravenous antibiotics should be commenced. Upon arrival at the emergency room, it is important that the referring physician inform the patient that they are being transferred for amputation evaluation, not miraculous replantation surgery. An experienced microsurgeon will then determine whether replantation is possible.

Preoperative Evaluation

A physical examination is performed to exclude associated injuries or medical problems. Routine investigations include radiographs, electrocardiogram, complete blood count, and electrolytes. Blood typing and crossmatching are necessary for replantation of a major limb or amputation of two of three digits or more. In this case, a central line should be maintained and Foley insertion implemented for volume monitoring. Protection for pressure point is mandatory to prevent complications.

In the emergency department, discussion surrounding replantation should include the potential need for 5 to 7 days hospitalization, the need for blood transfusion, the potential for emergency re-exploration when the finger becomes ischemic, and the need for revision amputation or local flap coverage when the replantation fails. Intensive care monitoring is necessary for complications caused by massive transfusion as well as for maintaining the patient's general condition. Patients should also be informed that most will require additional surgery in the future to improve the function as well as appearance of the digits.

Anesthesia

Axillary brachial plexus block with long-acting local anesthetics provide satisfactory anesthesia for digital or hand replantation in adults and cooperative adolescents. An axillary nerve block with an infusion mixture of 20 mL 2% lidocaine, 20 mL 0.75% ropivacaine, 10 mL normal saline, and 0.1 mL epinephrine keeps the patient pain free for 6 to 8 hours. If the operation time is prolonged, one more injection is feasible if conditions allow. This offers the additional benefit of decreased postoperative pain and possible vasodilatation. There is another advantage of the regional nerve block in case of amputation with multiple traumas. Intraoperative talk with patients or monitoring of patient's cooperation during the operation is invaluable to assess mental changes, abdominal discomforts, and respiratory difficulty. However, in cases of prolonged anesthesia, patients are frequently uncomfortable after lying supine on the operating table for several hours. Postoperative use of indwelling pain catheters is not recommended because of concerns about hematoma formation secondary to anticoagulation protocols used following replantation.

For proximal amputations above the elbow, younger children, very nervous patients, patients on anticoagulants, and in prolonged surgery such as in multiple-digit or bilateral amputations, general anesthesia is usually preferable.

Preparation of the Amputated Part

The preparation of the amputated part should be started on a back table with sterile drapes before the patient is brought through to the operating room. As for early microsurgical reconstruction, copious irrigation and radical debridement of devitalized and contaminated tissue and foreign materials are the most important steps in promoting neovascularization between the amputated part and stump. Even in very distal replantation, it is as crucial a step as vessel anastomosis as delayed wound healing and inflammation may deteriorate newly established circulation by vessel anastomosis. At the same time, the decision is made whether to proceed with replantation or not depending on the results of the microscopic examination of the vessels. If there are signs of arterial damage, including the telescope, cobweb, and ribbons signs or terminal thrombosis, long segment resection of the injured artery and harvesting of a vein graft is mandatory for successful replantation.

Each finger has a dominant digital artery. The dominant artery of each finger is usually located close to the midline of the hand. In the index finger, the ulnar digital artery is dominant, and in the little finger, the radial digital artery is dominant. In the middle and ring

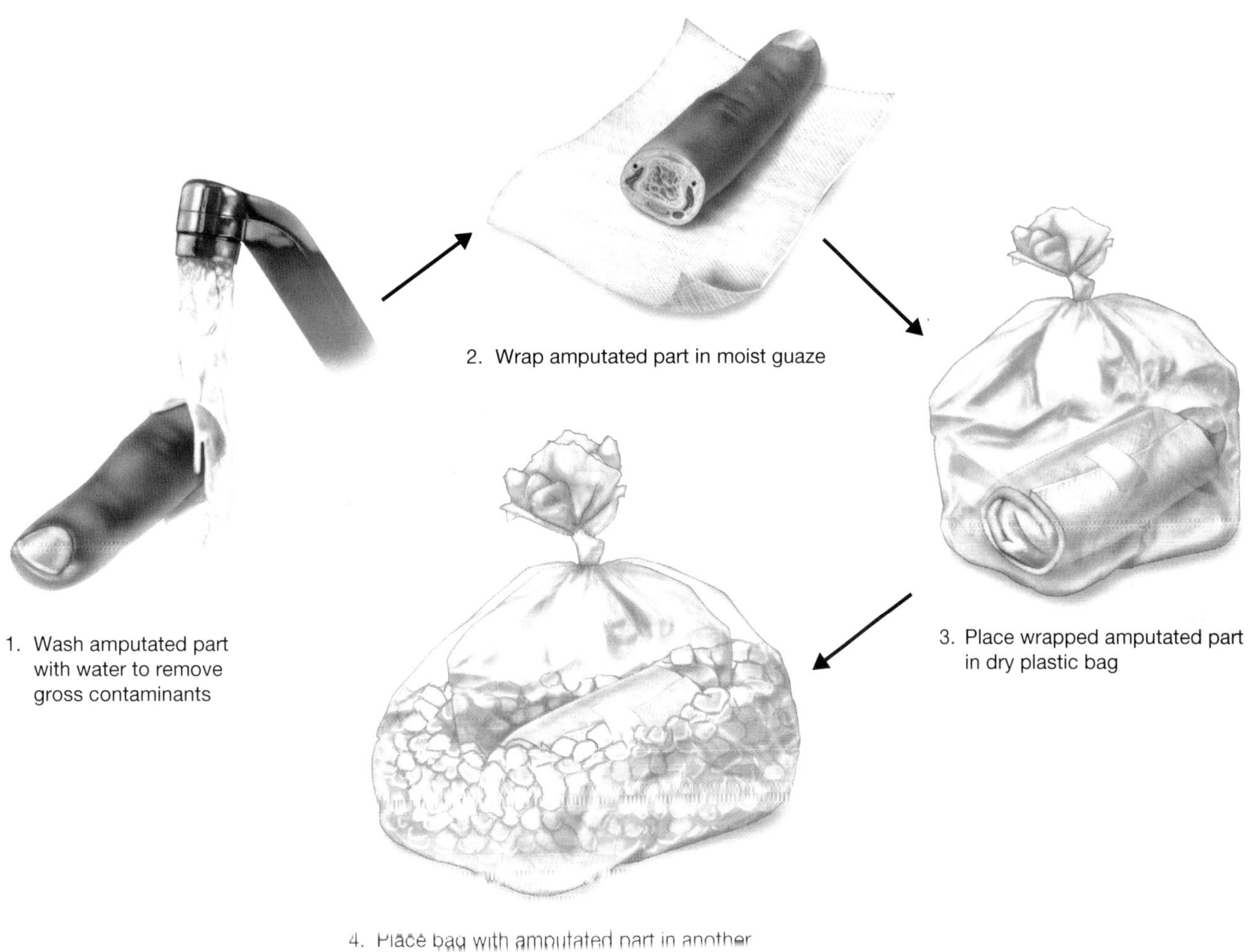
1. Wash amputated part with water to remove gross contaminants
2. Wrap amputated part in moist guaze
3. Place wrapped amputated part in dry plastic bag
4. Place bag with amputated part in another plastic bag with ice

Preservation of the amputated part for transport. **A.** Wash amputated part with water to remove gross contaminants. **B.** Wrap amputated part in moist gauze. **C.** Place wrapped amputated part in water tight plastic bag. **D.** Place bag with amputated part in another plastic bag with ice and water mixture.

fingers, ulnar and radial digital arteries are dominant, respectively, but dominance is less obvious.

The position of the digital nerve can be easily determined by first fully flexing the finger; when the finger is flexed, the most dorsal aspect of both proximal interphalangeal joint (PIPJ) and DIPJ flexion creases should be marked with a dot. Connecting a line between these dots shows the course of the digital nerve (Figure 83.4A). In the thumb, neurovascular bundles are located to both lateral sides of the mid-volar line (Figure 83.4B). The digital artery is always located on the dorsolateral aspect of the digital nerve (Figure 83.5).

A longitudinal mid-lateral incision placed slightly volar to the mid-axial line is made on both sides of the severed digit and extended to the next joint. During elevation of the two dorsal and volar flaps, venous channel should be dissected as a whole and not as separate vein. Skin flap should be preserved at constant thickness to avoid later necrosis. The longitudinal incisions over the vascular pedicles are sometimes difficult to close without compressing the pedicles. Because of this problem, volar zigzag incisions are preferable. It can be left partially open without exposure of vessels to accommodate swelling and can be extended proximally as far as necessary to identify undamaged artery and nerve.

After identification of arteries and nerves, these are then tagged with 6-0 black silk for easy and quick location after later bone fixation and tendon repair. At least 0.5 to 1 cm of intact digital artery and nerve should be dissected free for easy coaptation and placement of vascular or nerve clamp. The ruptured ends of the flexor are easily found at the same level of amputation. The ends of tendons are cut sharply with a scalpel and any ragged or contaminated parts debrided. A core suture with braided nylon is placed into the flexor digitorum profundus (FDP) tendon. This type of incision requires another incision on the dorsum of the digit for dissection of the veins. Tagging of the extensor tendon is not usually necessary.

For rigid fixation, it is advantageous to spend time on the bone shortening procedure as it facilitates primary bone union, direct nerve repair, end-to-end vessel repair, and tension-free closure of the soft tissue without grafts. This reduces the total operation time required for revascularization. Bone shortening of the amputated part is preferred to maintain the maximum stump length if the replantation fails. Acceptable length of the bone shortening is 0.5 to 1 cm of the digits. During the bone shortening, the periosteum on the amputated bone is elevated and preserved for repair after bone fixation. Bone shortening can usually be performed safely with a rongeur and a power saw; the tagged neurovascular structures are gently retracted to avoid injury. If the amputation passes through a joint, primary arthrodesis accomplishes both bony shortening and bony fixation. This is especially indicated in amputations of the DIP joint of the digits, the IP joint or metacarpophalangeal (MCP) joint of the thumb.

Preparation of the Amputation Stump

As described with the amputated part, the same procedures of debridement, identification, and tagging of all structures are performed. Identification of the retracted flexor tendon is time consuming because retrieval of the flexor tendons is not possible at the level of amputation. Additional proximal incision to find and transfix flexor tendon with a 23-gauge needle may be required. A similar core

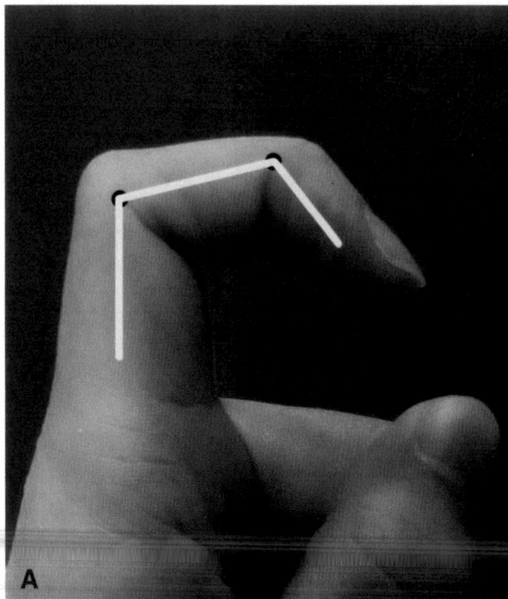

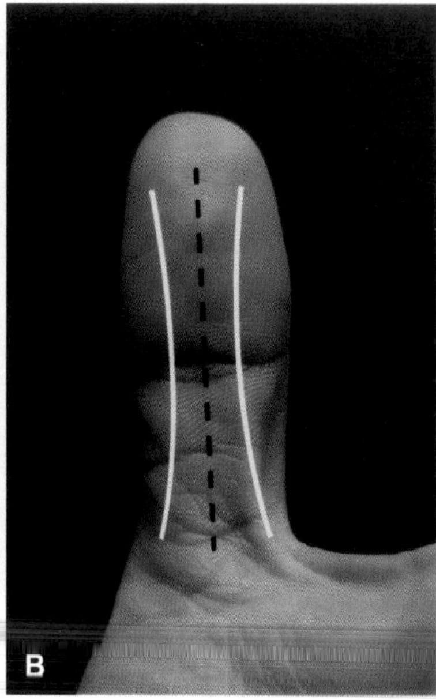

FIGURE 83.4. **A.** Surface anatomy of the neurovascular bundle of the digit. When the finger is flexed, the most dorsal aspect of both proximal interphalangeal and distal interphalangeal joint flexion creases is marked with a black dot. Connecting a yellow line between these dots shows the course of the digital nerve. **B.** In the thumb, the nerves (two yellow lines) are located just lateral to the mid-volar dotted line.

suture of 4-0 braided nylon can be placed into the proximal stump. Spurting of the proximal artery should be checked under deflation of the tourniquet. If the spurt is inadequate, additional shortening of the more proximal vessel is required.

SURGICAL TECHNIQUE OF REPLANTATION

The sequence for repairing the various structures in a finger replant is dependent on the surgeon's preference and the injury. It is probably more logical to perform the bony fixation, extensor tendon repair, and flexor tendon repairs under inflation of the tourniquet, and then after deflation, arterial anastomosis, nerve repairs, venous repair, and skin closure can be carried out. If veins are repaired immediately after extensor tendon repair, it minimizes repositioning of the hand to facilitate venous anastomosis in a bloodless field and may minimize venous congestion. It is also easier to repair the nerve just before repairing the artery.

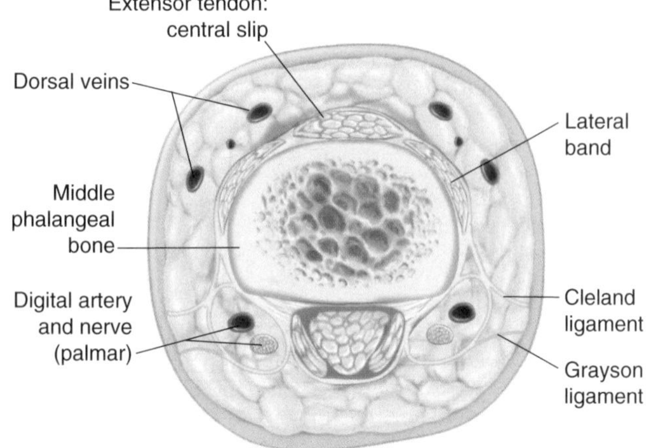

FIGURE 83.5. Cross-section of digit shows the digital artery is always located on the dorsolateral aspect of the digital nerve.

Bone Fixation

The importance of stable bone fixation cannot be emphasized enough, as stability aids in the subsequent steps of replantation and permit early rehabilitation. In guillotine-type injury patterns where the zone of injury is narrow, direct contact between the ends of fractured bone allows easy fixation; however, in most cases, bone shortening is essential as described before.

The method of bone fixation depends on the fracture pattern and level of skeletal injury relative to the joints (Figure 83.6). In the case of phalangeal or metacarpal bone fixation in replantation, it is not necessary to use plates and screws which is an acceptable but time-consuming technique. Bone fixation is usually achieved by using two parallel medullary axial Kirschner (K) wires, and two crossed K-wires or a single axial K-wire with an oblique wire to prevent rotational deformity. Because longitudinal K-wires carry the disadvantage of not offering rigid fixation, not preventing rotation, and of passing through the joint, it should only be used in distal replants and revascularizations where other fixation methods may not be technically feasible. Although cross K-wires are fixed, neurovascular structures need to be protected from spinning or direct injury. The intraosseous 90-90 wiring technique is a quick and secure method of bony fixation for digital replantation and has the lowest nonunion and complication rate irrespective of supplemental fixation with K-wire.[15,16] Three sets of wires, two longitudinal and one radial ulnar, provide as much rigidity as a fixation plate. Even though plate and screw fixation offers secure fixation and compression, it requires more time, wider periosteal stripping, and more extensive soft-tissue exposure resulting in tendon adhesion and increased scarring. Because of lack of adjustability, improper fixation can lead to rotational deformities. A low-profile H-shaped plate may overcome these shortcomings but this is still technically demanding and has the possibility of angulation and malunion for the inexperienced surgeon.

Tendon Repair

Before extensor tendon repair, dorsal periosteum should be sutured with 5-0 absorbable sutures when possible. Repaired periosteum can provide a smooth gliding surface for the tendons and also will cover any exposed wires or metal plates following bone fixation. In zone

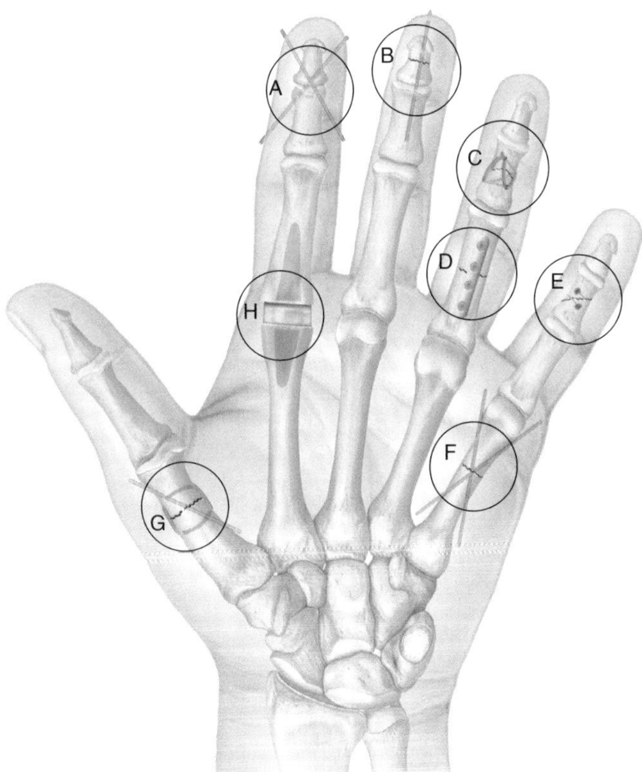

FIGURE 83.6 Various fixation methods of phalangeal bone fractures in digital replantation. **A.** Cross K-wire fixation for arthrodesis of the interphalangeal joint. **B.** Single longitudinal K-wire fixation. **C.** Intraosseous 90-90 wiring technique. **D.** Miniplate fixation with screws. **E.** Double screw fixation. **F.** Cross K-wire fixation. **G.** Intraosseous wiring and additional K-wire fixation. **H.** Implant arthroplasty for [illegible]

1 and zone 2 injuries, extensor repairs are performed with running 5-0 nonabsorbable sutures. For zone 3 or 4 extensor tendon repairs, a modified 4-0 Kessler suture is used with 5-0 or 6-0 running epitendinous suture. A Silfverskiöld cross-stitch epitendinous repair may be useful. In amputations at the proximal phalanx, repair of the lateral bands of the extensor tendon is essential to achieve appropriate extension of the distal joints.

Depending on the surgeon's preference, for flexor tendon repair, a four-strand or more core suture technique with 4-0 nonabsorbable suture is sufficiently strong to provide early rehabilitation. Repairing the proximal FDP to distal FDS tendon is an available option to get flexion in cases of significant injury to the substance of the distal FDP. However, in zone 2 injuries, repair of only the FDP tendon may be undertaken to avoid adhesions between the FDS and FDP tendon suture lines. Currently, repairing the FDS tendon is not mandatory because it simplifies surgery and makes postoperative finger motion easier. Venting the sheath or pulley for a total of 1.5 cm in the areas close to the amputation level should be done to allow smooth gliding of the repaired tendon (Figure 83.7).

Vessel Repair

The order of vessel repair depends on the amputation level, delayed ischemic time, and also the surgeons' preferences. In most digital replantations, performing arterial repair first decreases ischemic time and allows the dorsal veins to fill, aiding in the identification of small and friable veins. Even in cases of more proximal amputation containing more muscle, and in cases where considerable time has passed since amputation, arterial anastomosis should precede vein repair.

Adequate resection of the proximal vessel is verified by checking for blood spurt strength from the cut end. Gentle dilation and irrigation of the cut ends of the artery helps to clear the field of thrombogenic material. Irrigation with heparinized solution at a concentration of 100 units/mL should be under 80 mm Hg of pressure, sufficient to remove clots and avoid damage to the endothelium. Weak spurting and persistent spasm indicates a damaged proximal artery and the artery should be resected back further until pulsatile flow is obtained.

If the digital arteries can be approximated under minimal tension using a microvascular clamp, direct end-to-end anastomosis is performed using interrupted 9-0 or 10-0 nylon sutures or 11-0 sutures for very distal replantation. In [illegible] segmental gap between the proximal and distal ends of the artery, interposition vein graft or shifting artery from the undamaged adjacent artery of the same or another finger is necessary [illegible]. The use of vein grafts is not as time consuming as much as commonly thought and is a straightforward and reliable technique. Rather than struggling to shorten the bones substantially and to repair the vessels under tension, it is more expedient to harvest the vein graft early in the operation and bypass the crushed vessels. Depending on the amputation level, selection of donor sites of the vein graft is important to minimize the discrepancy of diameter between the vein graft and the

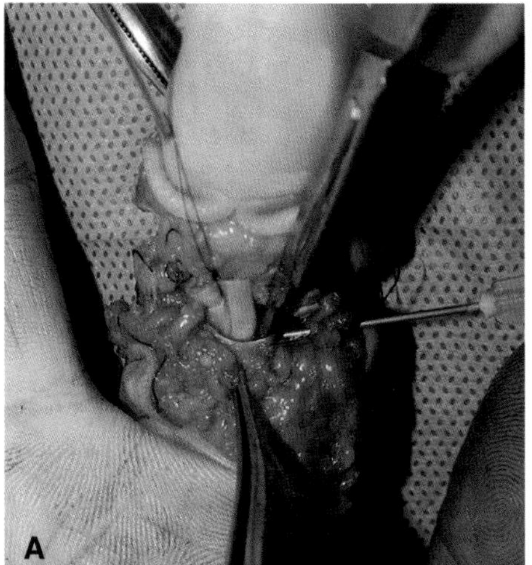

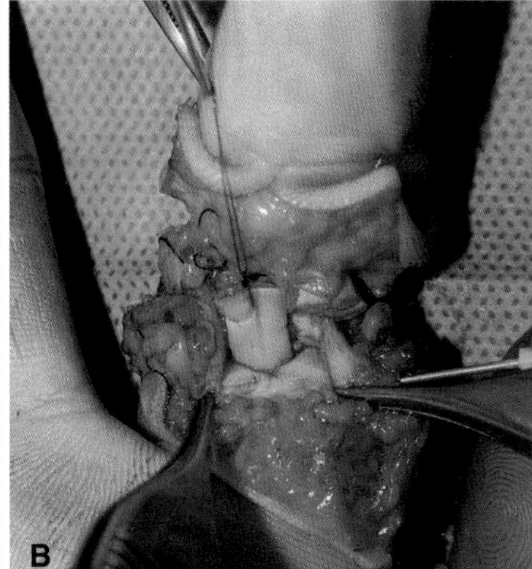

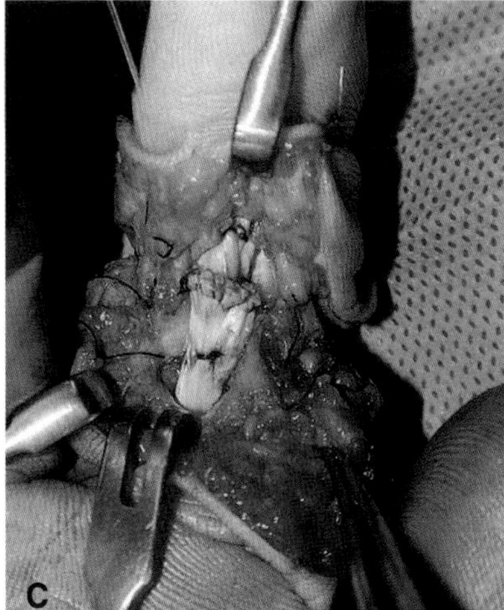

FIGURE 83.7. **A.** After resection of flexor digitorum sublimis, flexor digitorum profundus is retracted with 4-0 Prolene suture. **B.** Distal half of the A2 pulley is vented to allow smooth gliding of the repaired tendon. **C.** Flexor digitorum profundus tendon is repaired with Tang method.

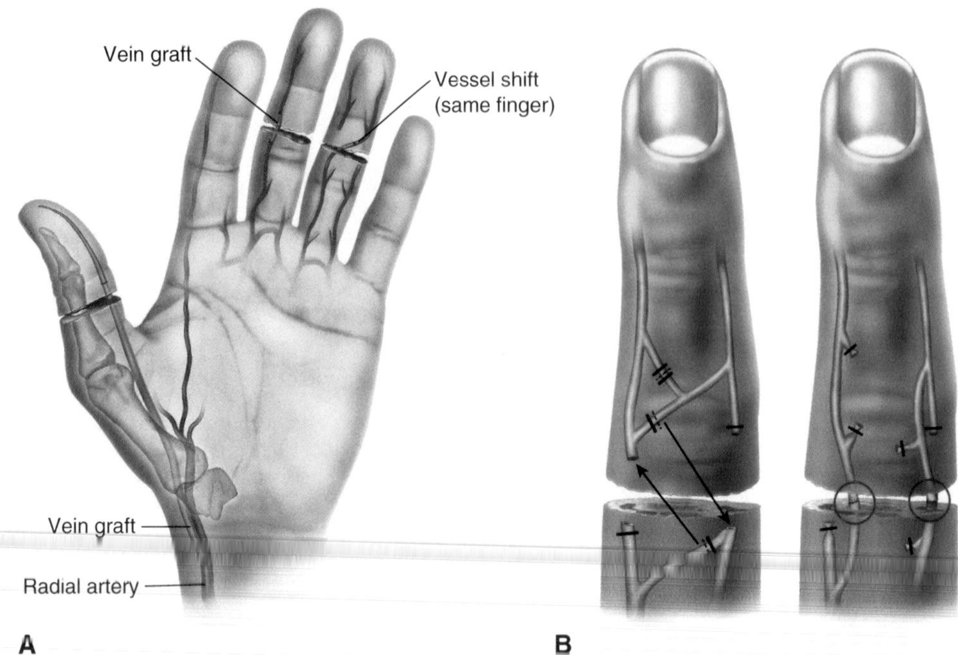

FIGURE 83.8. **A.** Techniques of bridging segmental defects in the digital arteries. **B.** Dividing venous branches will allow mobilization and primary repair of veins (black line, ligation or clipping; dotted line, cut the vein).

artery. Vein grafts can be easily obtained from the volar aspect of the proximal phalanx, thenar area, and the volar wrist (most readily available source) depending on the length and vessel diameter. To match the arterial defect, measuring the length of vein graft in situ before division is probably the best way to avoid making it too short or long.

If the digit or hand does not become pink even after arterial microanastomosis, there are several possible reasons besides technical errors. Arterial thrombosis or spasm is caused by tension on the anastomosis or excessive handling of the intima. Several factors besides vessel condition can affect blood flow to the amputated part including the patient's temperature, the patient's hydration status, systolic blood pressure, and any more proximal arterial injuries.

Maintaining venous drainage is the key to successful replantation because venous insufficiency is the most common cause of replantation failure.[17] It is preferable to repair both digital arteries and as many veins as possible for successful replantation. The vein which is actively draining the most blood should be chosen. In a middle or proximal phalangeal replantation, anastomosis of one artery and two veins is sufficient. If two arteries have been repaired, two or more veins should be repaired. To increase the number of anastomosed veins, it may be necessary to mobilize or harvest adjacent branches of the vein (Figure 83.8B). The digital dorsal venous plexus is conventionally considered as a reliable source for venous repairs. The volar skin of the digit is a useful site for vein repair because it is less likely to be avulsed during injury and in amputations with tissue loss, and the size discrepancy is less for volar veins than for dorsal veins. It also does not require changes in hand position and it is indicated when primary repair of dorsal veins can be difficult due to tightness ensuing from arthrodesis of the underlying joint in flexion.

Nerve Repair

Nerve regeneration is the most important prognostic factor in final functional recovery after replantation. In most replants, nerve repair is not difficult because of the amount of bone shortening. Only two to four epineurial stitches of 9-0 or 10-0 monofilament suture are enough to get approximation of the fascicles.

To prevent neuroma formation in replantation, nerve repair should be performed without tension. A short defect of the nondominant digital nerve is reconstructed with a vein conduit. This is appropriate for defects of less than 1 to 2 cm in length. Nerve conduits consisting of collagen or polyglycolide can also be used. When a nerve graft is required, a terminal branch of the posterior intraosseous nerve or medial antebrachial cutaneous nerve of the forearm is easily harvested from the ipsilateral side. In multiple-digit amputations, nerve grafts may be taken from the discarded digits. In avulsion injuries or digital nerve injuries of different levels, radial to ulnar or reversed cross-pattern digital nerve repair should be considered. In case of long nerve defect or uncertainty regarding the extent of intraneural injury, it is better to delay primary nerve grafting for later reconstruction. The ends of the avulsed or crushed nerve should be marked with 6-0 nylon sutures for easy identification.

Skin Closure

During skin closure, be sure not to create any pressure over the repaired vessels. Just one tight stitch can result in venous congestion. When there is an open wound, small split-thickness skin grafts can be applied, even directly over arterial or venous anastomosis or vein grafts. Soft tissue defect may require a Z-pasty, local flap, or a venous flap to cover tendons as well as the artery or veins. If at any time during skin closure the fingertip loses its pinkish color or becomes dusky, then excessive tension is compromising either arterial inflow or venous outflow. Sutures must be removed and a split-thickness skin graft or artificial skin used to cover the defect. Dressings should be loose and the extremity immobilized in a long-arm splint then elevated.

POSTOPERATIVE MANAGEMENT

Monitoring

Postoperative monitoring of replantation is essential for successful replantation because early recognition of vascular compromise provides the best chance for flap salvage. Patients should be admitted to a warm room and be well hydrated and comfortable to avoid peripheral vasospasm. Circulation status can be assessed by aid of technical devices such as pulse oximeter, implantable venous Doppler probe, digital thermometry, and the laser Doppler. A temperature drop of 1.8 to 3°C or an absolute temperature of less than 30°C mandates immediate re-exploration of the arterial and venous anastomosis.[18] A continuous pulse oximeter can monitor the pulse rate and the oxygen

TABLE 83.1. MONITORING OF CIRCULATION IN REPLANTED DIGIT

	Normal	Arterial Occlusion	Venous Insufficiency
Color	Pink	Pale or white pink	Dark pink or purple
Capillary refilling	Fast	Very slow	Very fast
Temperature	Warm	Cold	Warm-cool
Turgor	Full	Hollow	Swollen
Bleeding	Bright red	Minimal, only serum	Dark red or purple

saturation within the digit. Loss of the pulse rate indicates arterial occlusion, whereas a fall in the oxygen saturation below 90% usually indicates venous occlusion. However, intensive monitoring of capillary refill, temperature, and the color of replanted digits by experienced nursing staff is the most reliable (**Table 83.1**). This should be checked hourly for the first 48 hours, every 2 hours for the next 2 days, and then every 4 hours for the next 3 days because the highest risk of postoperative thrombosis is in the first 72 hours after surgery. Arterial thrombi usually result from platelet aggregation and present on day 1, whereas venous thrombi result from fibrin clotting and usually present by day 2 or 3.

Anticoagulation Therapy

Perioperative anticoagulation therapy varies according to the circumstances of the replant and preference of the surgeons. The most common agents are aspirin, heparin, and low-molecular-weight dextran. Aspirin inhibits the platelet enzyme cyclooxygenase and impedes arachidonic acid breakdown through thromboxane and prostacyclin. Preoperative administration of aspirin decreases microvascular thrombosis formation. Heparin possesses properties of prevention of both platelet-induced arterial thrombi and coagulation induced venous thrombi and vasodilatory effect, but it causes hematoma formation and induces thrombocytopenia. The use of intravenous heparin does not correlate with higher success rates of replantation but it may be indicated in cases of intimal damage by crush and avulsion injuries, intraoperative thrombus, or following successful thrombolysis and arteriosclerotic changes. Dextran 40 is a group of synthesized polysaccharides which interfere with the formation of fibrin clot and to prevent the aggregation of red thrombi. This has a low risk of postoperative bleeding and hematoma formation but in rare cases has the serious consequence of pulmonary edema due to fluid overload.

Regimen of anticoagulation for replantation is recommended as follows.[19] Preoperative loading dose of 1.4 mg/kg (100 mg in the 70-kg adult) of enteric-coated aspirin is started and followed by the same dosage per day for 2 weeks. Before the release of microvascular clamps, heparin bolus of 50 to 100 U/kg is intravenously injected. Intraoperatively, dextran 40 is administered at a dose of 0.4 mL/kg/h, and the dosage is cut in half on postoperative days 3 and 4 and weaned off on postoperative day 5. In cases of suspicious perfusion failure, intravenous bolus injection of heparin of about 100 to 160 U/kg is recommended.

Rehabilitation

Rehabilitation after replantation surgery is unique in that all tendons, bone, joint, and neurovascular structures are involved. An initial period of immobilization is followed by passive and active mobilization with particular emphasis on maintaining the range of motion of the noninjured digits. For an even digital replantation, the splint is applied in a protective position with the wrist neutral, MP joint flexion at 60 to 90 degrees, and IP joint extension. In this position, both tendon systems are protected, the length of the collateral ligament length is preserved, and flexion contracture of the PIP joints can be avoided. A thermoplastic protective splint is fabricated as soon as the anticoagulants are discontinued, usually on the fifth to seventh postoperative day, to allow ease of wound care and exercises in the mobilization phase.

Two stages of supervised exercises, known as early protected motion (EPM), are designed to prevent joint stiffness and to minimize adhesions after digital replantation.[20] EPM I begins at approximately 5 to 14 days after replantation and consists of gentle wrist flexion and simultaneous finger extension by virtue of the tenodesis effect. EPM II begins at 7 to 14 days and consists of the intrinsic minus (hook) and the intrinsic plus (table) position, respectively. The hook position provides the most differential gliding between the FDS and FDP tendons; the table position maintains intrinsic muscle function. After the first 3 weeks, patients are encouraged to participate in a graduated program of active, active-assisted, and protected passive stretching and range-of-motion exercises supplemented by appropriate dynamic and static bracing and splinting. For either digits or thumb replantations, wrist extension beyond neutral, blocking exercises, and tendon gliding exercises are introduced at 4 to 5 weeks. At 5 to 6 weeks, composite motion and functional activities are introduced. Blocking splints and dynamic splints can also be added when the protective splint is discontinued at 6 weeks. Strengthening begins at 6 to 8 weeks.

REPLANTATION FOR SPECIFIC LEVEL OF AMPUTATION

Distal Digital Replantation

Regarding replantation distal to the DIPJ level of amputation, multiple classification systems have been proposed [illegible]. Revision amputation was perceived to be the better choice, given the minimal functional loss and reduced expense compared with replantation. However, systematic review and retrospective studies indicate that high success rates and good functional outcomes and cosmetic results followed distal digital replantation when compared with revision amputation.[23,32] Although it can be technically demanding because of the diminutive size of the distal arteries, successful replantation restores an almost normal appearance and satisfactory sensibility if the digital nerves can be approximated (Figure 83.10). This level of amputation should be included as a formal indication of replantation surgery.[22,23]

This procedure can usually be performed safely and comfortably as outpatient surgery, often under local anesthetic block or under brachial plexus block.[23] It usually takes less than 2 hours for bone fixation with 0.028 or 0.035 K-wires through distal phalangeal bone, one digital artery and/or one vein repair, and where possible two digital nerves and nail plate and skin sutures. Finding a suitable vein at this level is challenging, and venous insufficiency is the most compromising cause of replantation failure. At the DIP joint level, the vein goes distally and the larger vessels are palmar; proximal to the DIP joint, the dorsal veins tend to predominate. At the level of the eponychium, 63% of fingers have a vein of 0.8 mm or larger. Distal venous arch on the lateral nail fold area is reliable to find and to anastomose. This runs around the lateral nail wall and distal pulp forms an arch over the distal phalanx that surrounds the nail proximally. Occasionally after release of the tourniquet, a small vein can be identified dorsally just proximal to the nail fold and a single venous anastomosis performed.

In cases of impossible vein repair, there are suggested methods of salvage procedures with external bleeding with a fish mouth incision or removal of the nail bed, medical leeches, continuous administration of heparinized saline, or creation of an arteriovenous anastomosis between the other distal digital artery and a proximal vein. The external bleeding method for one digit needs blood transfusions of 1.2 to 1.8 units on average and with success rate typically higher than

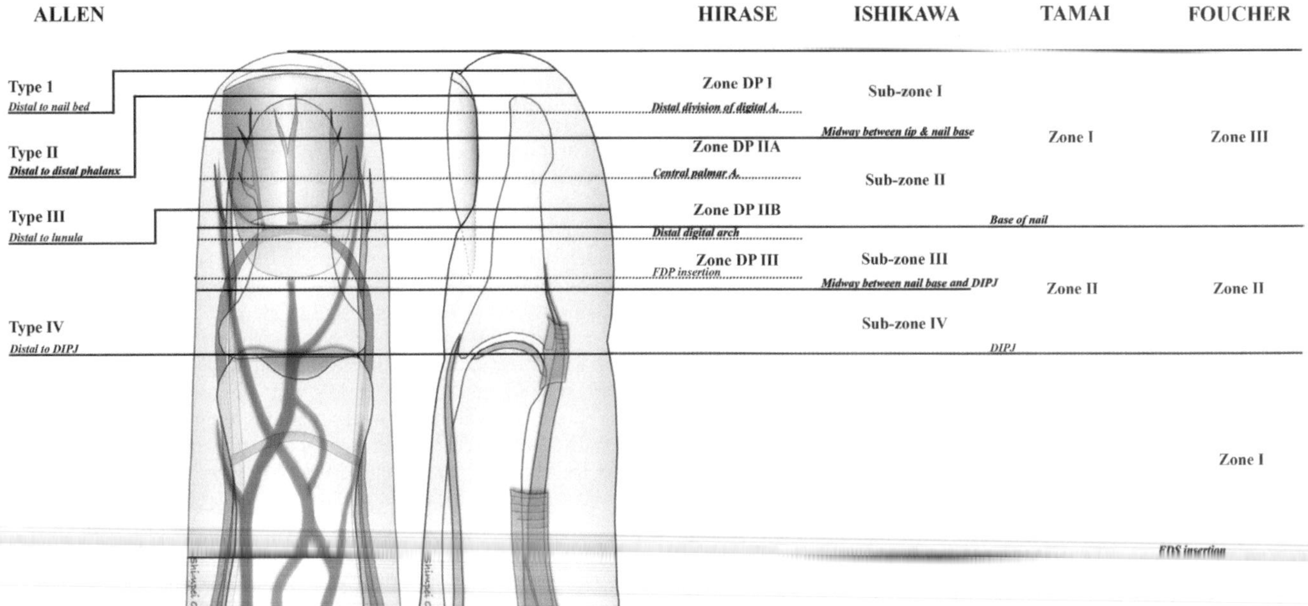

FIGURE 83.9. Amputation level of distal part of digits proposed by Sebastin and Chung, Ishikawa, and Tamai. *DIPJ*, distal interphalangeal joint; *FDP*, flexor digitorum profundus; *FDS*, flexor digitorum sublimus.

85%, including adequate sensory recovery.[24,25] If there is postoperative congestion on the day or days immediately after the primary vascular anastomosis, dilated venules usually become larger and can easily be anastomosed. Delayed venous drainage results in a high success rate in distal phalangeal replantation.[26] To support adequate venous drainage, external bleeding with topical heparinized saline solution with hyperbaric oxygen therapy with venous anastomosis can surely overcome venous congestion.

Leeches are effective at treating venous outflow problems in failing replants (Figure 83.11). The leech saliva contains the effective anticoagulant "hirudin" that acts as a regional anticoagulation of the part. If the venous congestion happens 2 or 3 days after the initial surgery, re-exploration may harm the neovascularization of the replanted parts. When the leech is placed on the failing digit, it bites the digit, then sucks a small amount of blood, and ultimately falls off the digit within 10 to 40 minutes of beginning its meal of blood. Leeches are generally applied on an as-needed basis but can be used up to every 6 hours and are slowly weaned at approximately 5 days until venous circulation should be re-established. The most feared complication of leech use, however, is an infection from the bacterium *Aeromonas hydrophila*. The incidence of this infection ranges from 2.4% to 20%, with clinical presentations ranging from cellulitis or abscess to extensive soft-tissue infections causing tissue loss and systemic sepsis.[27] Routine antimicrobial prophylaxis with a fluoroquinolone should be used for cases of leech therapy.

Pediatric Replantation

Replantation should be considered for all amputated parts in children. Crush by door hinge and avulsion injuries from bicycle chain or mechanical sports equipment are common mechanisms for amputation in children and should not be considered contraindications for replantation. The preponderance of this mechanism of injury results in lower survival rate than in adults. Furthermore, replantation in young children may be more technically demanding because of the small caliber of the vessels and the propensity for vasospasm, but the digit will continue to grow and the results of the tendon and nerve repairs are much better than in an adult. Replantation should consist of minimal bone shortening to preserve epiphyseal plates and simple bone fixation with longitudinal K-wires. Postoperatively, use

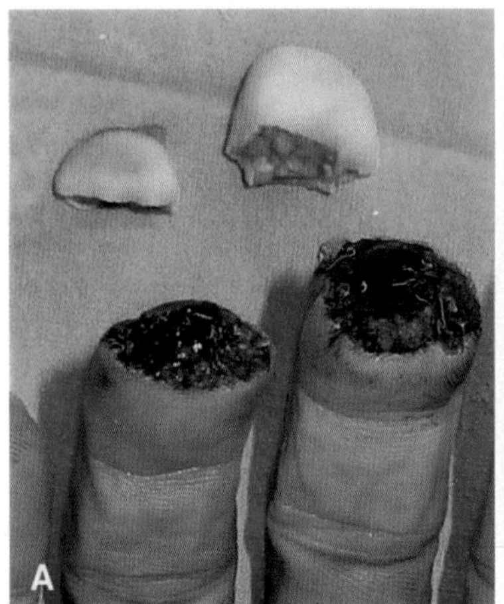

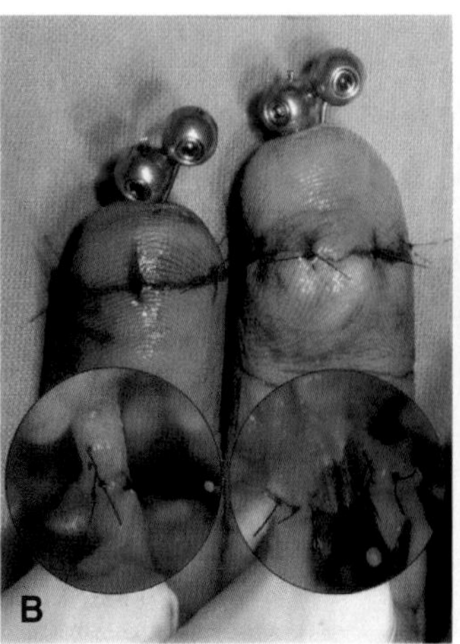

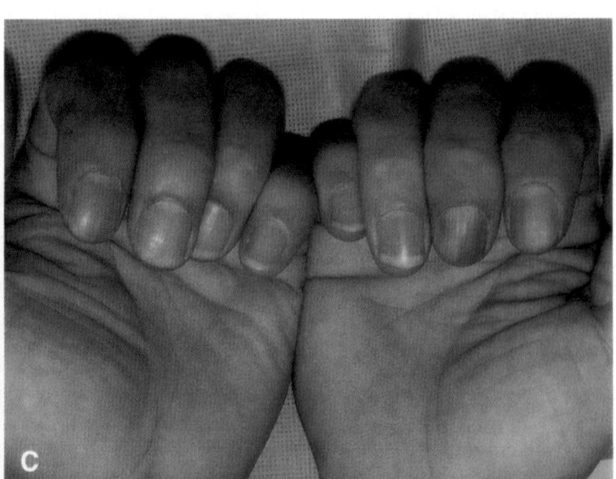

FIGURE 83.10. **A.** Guillotine-type amputation of the long finger at sub-zone II of Ishikawa classification (zone 1A of Sebastin and Chung, zone I of Tamai) and ring finger at sub-zone I by Ishikawa classification. **B.** Anastomosis included two bifurcating central artery repairs at the long finger and one bifurcating artery repair at the ring finger. Immediately after operation. External bleeding with heparin and medical leech application for 5 days. **C.** Twelve months after operation.

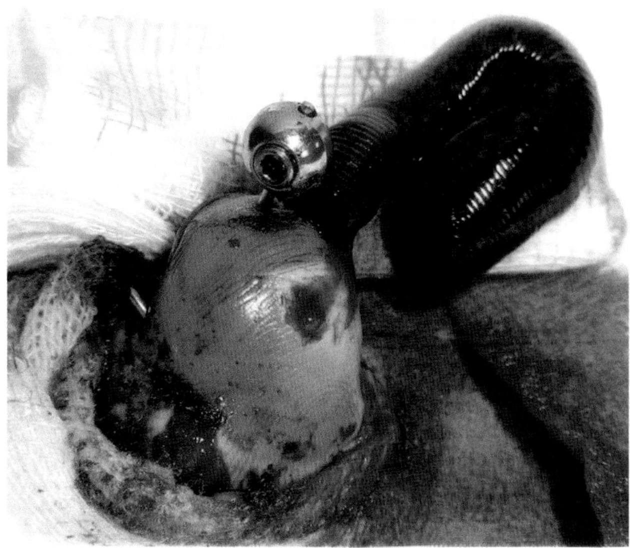

FIGURE 83.11. Medicinal leech on the distal digital replantation. It improves oxygenation and enhanced bleeding in venous congestion.

of sedation to maintain calmness and encourage somnolence can be helpful to prevent vasospasm in children. Recovery of sensibility in the replanted digit is nearly as good as for isolated digital nerve repair. The success rates of pediatric digital replantation have been reported to be as high as 95% to 97%,[28,29] but proximal replantation is less favorable than digital replantation, with a reported success rate of 77% for complete amputations and 80% for revascularization procedures.[30] One long-term study shows that continued skeletal growth occurred and the digit attained 81% to 90% of normal longitudinal length at maturity unless significant damage to the epiphyseal plate is apparent[29] (Figure 83.12). Patient and parent satisfaction is high when replantation is successful, with uniform approval of the extensive effort required.

Thumb Replantation

Thumb replantation should be considered for any traumatically amputated thumb regardless of the type of injury or level of amputation. After successful replantation of the thumb, there is no significant correlation between the level or type of injury and the grip/pinch strength. Compared with the contralateral unaffected hand, grip strength and key pinch strength are 70% to 92% and 68% to 81%, respectively.[31,32] Most patients with traumatic thumb amputation who received replantation are able to return to their previous occupation and are able to perform the activities of daily living. However, a low level of sensory recovery is one of the most critical points which is directly related to crush or avulsion injuries as well as low compliance and insufficient sensory reeducation.

Operative technique of the thumb is a little different from digital replantation. Regarding bone management, shortening of an amputated thumb should be kept to a minimum and an arthrodesis is more generously accepted in cases of amputation around the IP or MCP joint. The thumb with IP fusion can still have useful motion through the MCP joint and carpometacarpal joint without repairing flexor pollicis longus (FPL) and extensor pollicis longus (EPL). Even a thumb with MCP joint fusion maintains the role of post for opposition with digits.

The ulnar digital artery is the dominant artery in the thumb and is most reliable for arterial anastomosis resulting in successful replantation. Proximally, the princeps pollicis artery can provide sufficient

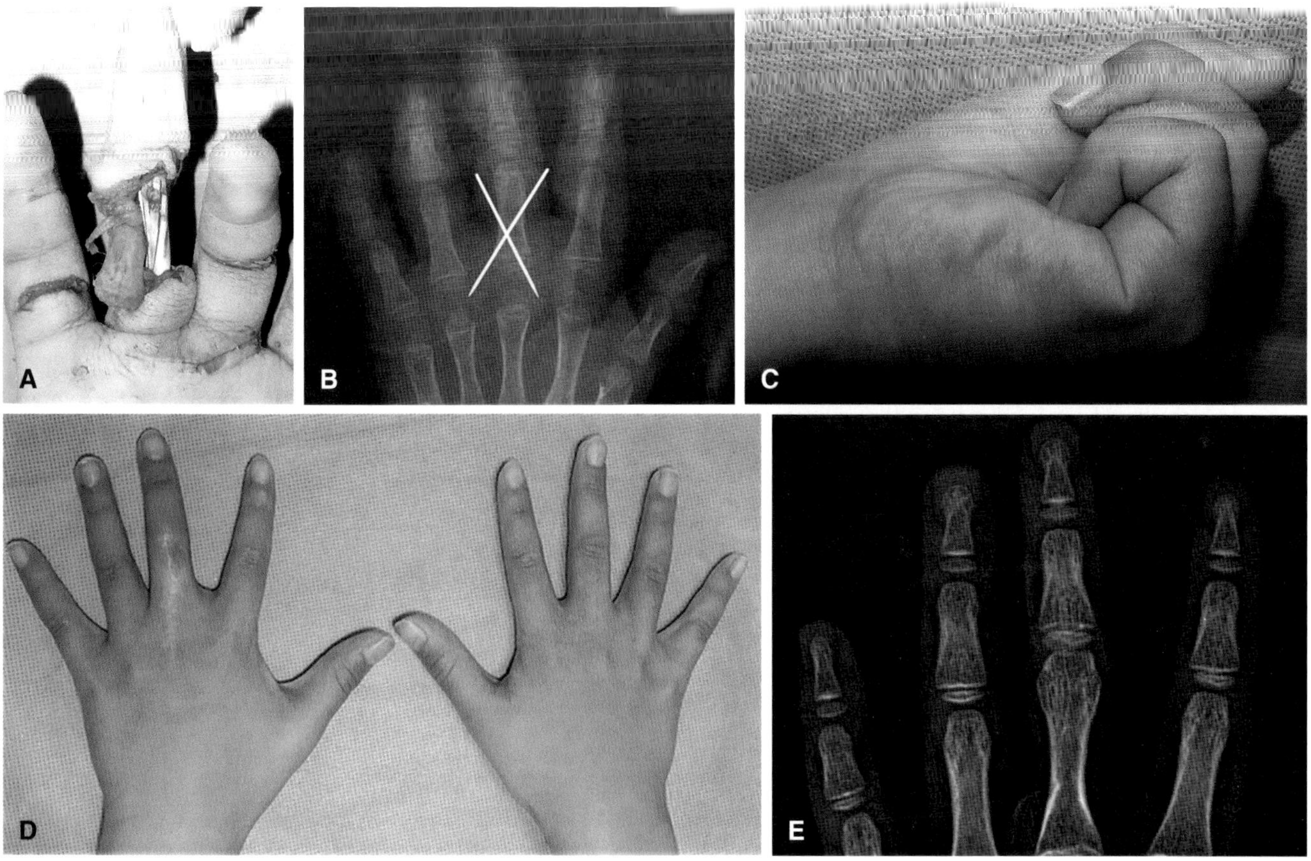

FIGURE 83.12. **A.** In this 40-month-old child, belt injury resulted in incomplete amputation of the left long finger. It was a Salter-Harris type II epiphyseal fracture of the base of proximal phalanx. **B.** Bone fixation with two crossed Kirschner wires. **C, D.** After 6 years of revascularization, the length and joint motion of the replanted digit were found to be nearly normal. **E.** Six years postoperatively.

blood flow from the dorsum if no palmar arteries are suitable for repair. If possible, primary arterial repair is easiest by anastomosis of the severed ends of both digital arteries after bone shortening. If not, interposition of short or long vein grafts is employed from the volar aspect of the wrist or forearm. Microscopic focus on the ulnar artery at different levels is annoying because it requires extreme arm pronation or supination. This can be avoided by either repairing the ulnar digital artery before the bone fixation or using an arterial interposition graft (see Figure 83.8A). It may be easier to anastomose interpositional vein grafts to the terminal branch of the ulnar digital artery and largest vein in a supine position before performing osteosynthesis. The proximal anastomosis can be performed dorsally and proximal to the area of injury.

Thumb avulsions are common industrial injuries by conveyor belt or rotating machines, traditionally by rodeo roping and sports activities like water skiing tow ropes and riding a mechanical bull and team roping. When the FPL and EPL tendons have been avulsed from their musculotendinous junction, treatment options are tendon resection, reattachment to muscle, tendon transfer, side-to-side repair, or insertion of tendon spacer. If these could be reconstructed primarily as a one-stage procedure, the costs would be lower, the patients would return to their work earlier, and the technical difficulties encountered in secondary reconstructions would also be eliminated. Reattachment of the FPL tendon to its muscle belly and direct repair of the EPL is preferred as the most promising technique in the recovery of function (Figure 83.13).

The mean survival of replantation of thumb avulsion injuries is 68% (26% to 100%).[33-35] This variability may in part explain the different success rates in the reports of replantation of the thumb resulting from different causes of avulsion.

Replantation for Ring Avulsion Amputation

A ring avulsion injury is sustained by a sudden and strong traction force as pulling a ring from a finger. These injuries are usually caused by crushing, shearing, and avulsing the soft tissue envelope which results in severe macroscopic and microscopic damage to the digital neurovascular bundle along with tendon rupture, and even bone fractures.[36] Ring avulsion amputation is regarded as a denuded finger necessitating a tubed pedicle flap or primary ray amputation.

Optimal management will vary depending on the pattern of injury, status of the amputated part, and functional requirements and expectation of individual patients. Several classification systems have evolved that are useful to recommend anticipated treatment and to predict possible outcomes (**Table 83.2**).[37-39] Class II injuries are often incorrectly diagnosed as a skin laceration at the emergency room because there is intact tendon and no skeletal injury. If there is inadequate perfusion of the distal digit as evidenced by no capillary refill, poor pulp turgor, coldness, and pallor, immediate care including irrigation and debridement of the wound as well as microsurgical repair of artery or vein and both digital nerves should be performed. Because bone shortening is not available for intact bone, short vein graft is often needed for reconstruction of vessel whether there is damage to the digital arteries, veins, or both. Prognosis of the replanted digits in class II injuries show a better range of motion, sensibility, strength, and appearance when compared with class III injuries which include skeletal injuries.

A class IVd injury is considered as a candidate for replantation, but in patients with an IVp injury, amputation or ray amputation should be considered, as these patients are likely to have poor hand function. Proximal dorsal or volar skin flap of the survived digit tends to be

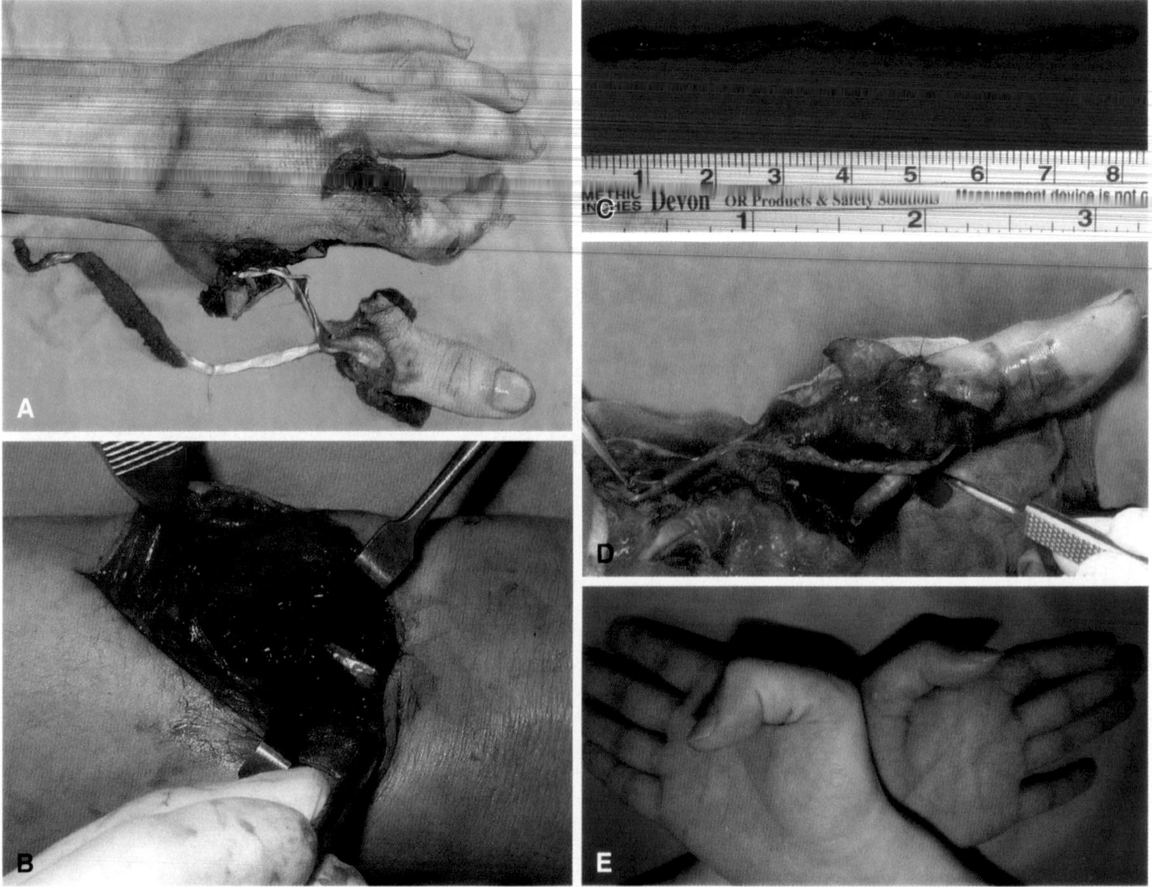

FIGURE 83.13. **A.** Avulsion amputation of the left thumb and incomplete amputation of the index. **B.** After muscle portions of the avulsed flexor and extensor tendons were clearly debrided, both extensor and flexor tendons were reattached to the viable muscle belly by interweaving suture at the dorsal and volar proximal forearm. **C.** Vein graft about 8 cm in length was harvested from the volar aspect of the ipsilateral wrist. **D.** Arterial reconstruction with interpositional vein graft between princeps pollicis artery and ulnar digital artery. **E.** Postoperative appearance about 12 months demonstrating active motion of the interphalangeal joint.

TABLE 83.2. MODIFIED CLASSIFICATION SYSTEM OF FINGER AVULSION INJURY BASED ON URBANIAK CLASSIFICATION

Class	Description
I	Avulsion injuries with adequate circulation
II	Incomplete avulsion injuries with inadequate arterial or venous circulation, without skeletal injury
IIa	Arterial circulation inadequate only
IIv	Venous circulation inadequate only
IIav	Arterial and venous circulation inadequate
III	Incomplete avulsion injuries with inadequate arterial or venous circulation, with fracture or joint injury present
IIIa	Arterial circulation inadequate only
IIIv	Venous circulation inadequate only
IIIav	Arterial and venous circulation inadequate
IV	Avulsion injuries with complete degloving or amputation
IVp	Complete avulsion injuries with amputation proximal to flexor digitorum superficialis insertion
IVd	Complete avulsion injuries with amputation distal to flexor digitorum superficialis insertion

necrosed by direct injury and insufficient circulation. Additional flap coverage is often necessary for the late necrosis (Figure 83.14).

Ring avulsion injuries have traditionally been considered as having low success rate and unsatisfactory functional results. However, systemic review proves the 78% of mean survival rate, protective sensation, and acceptable functional outcomes.[41] Completely amputated ring avulsion injuries with an intact PIP joint and FDS are thus worthwhile replantation procedures.

Multiple-Digit Replantation

Compared with single-digit or double-digit replantation, there are many considerations in replantation operations for three or more digits to avoid systemic or more serious general complications. In terms of prolonged ischemic time, it is preferable to use a digit-by-digit replantation sequence rather than structure-by-structure replantation. However, to reduce operation time, a structure-by-structure sequence is more efficient because prolonged cold ischemic time at this level of amputation does not affect the survival rate and final functional results of the replanted digits.[11] Because of the importance of the pinching and grasping functions of the hand, a good replantation order is the thumb first followed by the middle finger, the ring finger, index finger, and the small finger last. By bone shortening at the phalangeal bone, any graft for vessel or nerve should be avoided. Maintenance of digital length is not a positive factor for the final functional result. However, in cases of guillotine-type injury, direct bone fixation and primary repair of the tendon, nerve, and vessel is possible without any shortening or even any extended incision. A no-incision technique can certainly decrease total operation time as well as improve wound healing and regeneration (Figure 83.15).

However, in case of multiple-digit amputations including nonreplantable thumb, the least damaged digit should be replanted in place of the mutilated thumb (Figure 83.16). Transpositional replantation is aimed to achieve basic pinch, tripod pinch, and even most importantly, opposition grip. Amputated long digit is always used to replace an unreplantable thumb with simultaneous reconstruction of opposition with tendon repair or transfer. In cases of multiple-digit amputations with the thumb intact, the effort is made to replant the digits toward the ulnar side of the hand, so the width of the palm span is preserved and the power grip of the hand can be increased.[40] In cases of bilateral multiple-digit amputations or bilateral multiple-digit and hand amputations, the replantation effort is directed at increasing the dexterity of the dominant hand or restoring basic hand function by transposing digits or hand from relatively less injured part of digits or hand. Cross-hand replantation or cross-arm replantation is aimed to save at least one hand or one limb used for pinch and grasping.

Adequate radical debridement is required to achieve immediate replantation in cases where amputation is combined with extensive soft tissue loss or contamination or where the immediate replantation on the orthotic position seems impossible due to associated severe injuries or with an unstable patient. Even if it performs, it would be functionally or aesthetically inadequate. The amputated part of the upper extremity may be rapidly ectopically banked to the thoracodorsal artery of the axilla or contralateral radial artery of the forearm. This creative and useful concept serves as an important limb-saving technique for the reconstructive hand surgeon in select clinical settings.

Transmetacarpal Replantation

Functional results after this level of replantation have been mainly attributed to poor recovery of intrinsic muscle function, which is due to direct injury to the intrinsic muscle, ischemia, or

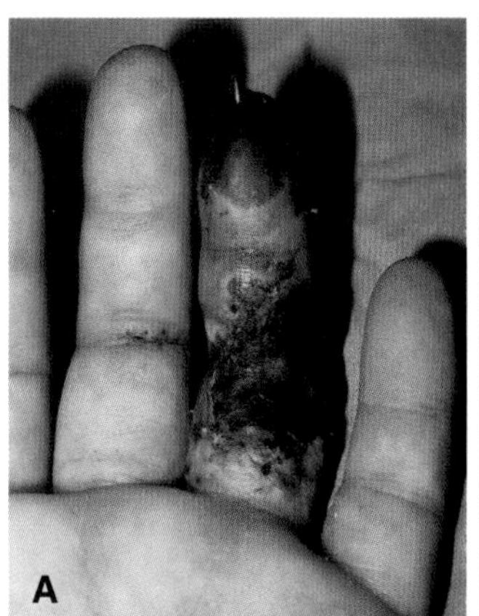

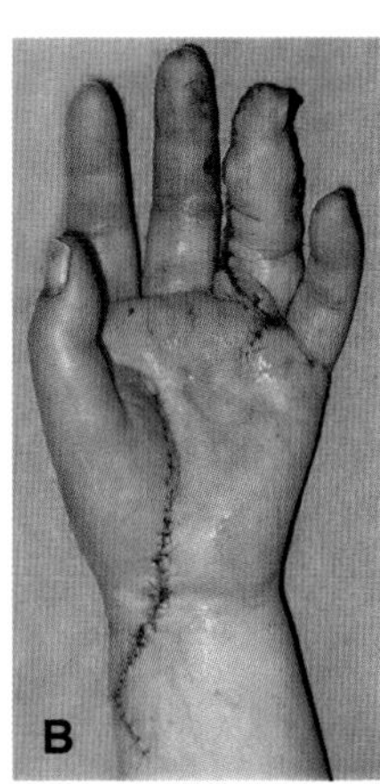

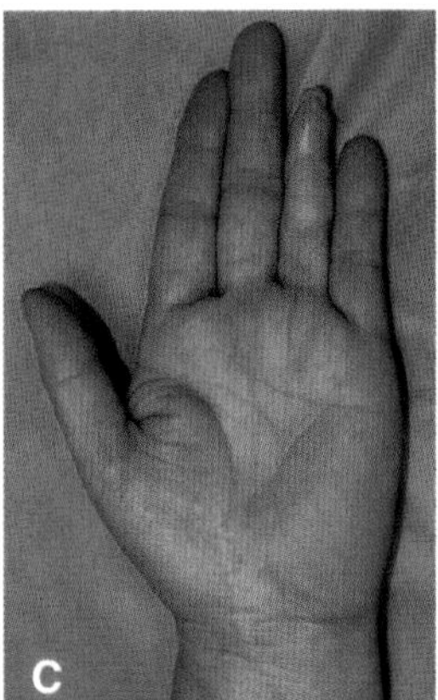

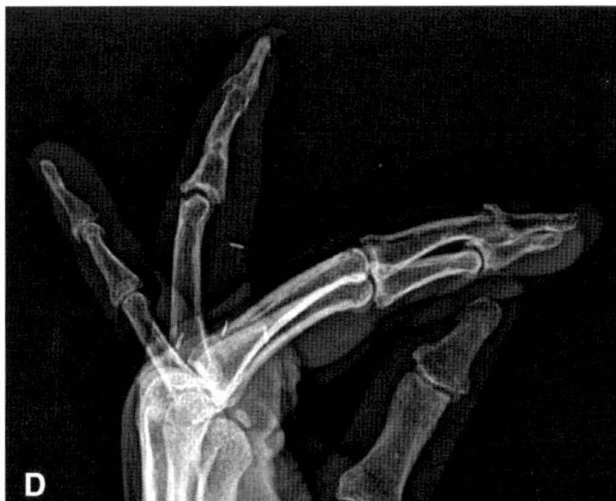

FIGURE 83.14. A 53-year-old woman sustained left ring finger avulsion amputation by henhouse chicken wire. The proximal interphalangeal jointwas intact, but both the digital artery and nerve were avulsed, for class IVd. The ulnar digital artery was anastomosed with vein graft about 1.2 cm from the volar aspect of the proximal interphalangeal joint, and the proximal radial digital nerve was transposed to the distal ulnar digital nerve. **A.** Four weeks after the operation, the volar soft tissue was necrotic. **B.** After debridement of the necrotic tissue, about 7 cm × 3 cm radial artery superficial palmar branch flap is harvested from the ipsilateral thenar area to cover the whole volar aspect of the ring finger. Donor site was closed primarily. **C, D.** Five years postoperatively.

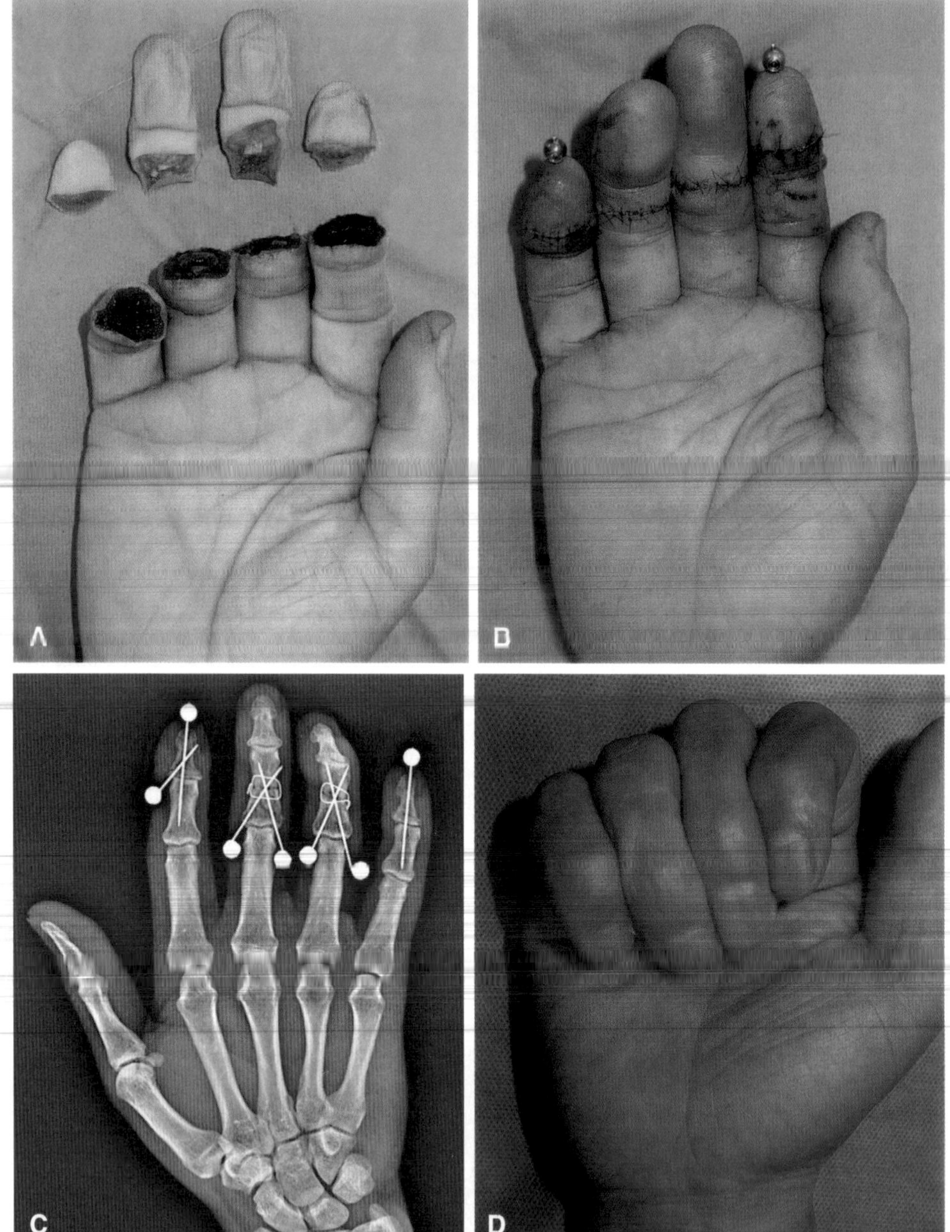

FIGURE 83.15. **A.** A 63-year-old man with a sharp cutting injury on the right hand. The right index and small finger were amputated at the base of distal phalangeal bone, and long and ring finger were amputated at the middle phalanx. **B.** Immediate after replantation by structure-by-structure technique. **C.** Postoperative radiograph. **D.** At 25 months of follow-up, the patient had nearly full flexion of the proximal interphalangeal joint and radiograph.

postoperative scarring.[41] Because replantation at this level is not technically difficult, primary survival rate is reported at a high of 86%.[41]

Regarding operative technique, at least 1 cm of bony shortening is recommended to prevent secondary intrinsic tightness in the fingers. Bone fixation is recommended with longitudinal K-wires in children and minicompression plates in adults. Care must be taken during bony fixation to prevent malrotation of an individual digit because rotation at this level translates into a greater functional deficit than a similar one in the digit. At least three or four dorsal veins should be anastomosed, approximately two veins for each artery. Hemostasis is particularly important at this level where branches of the deep metacarpal arteries may bleed profusely. It should be identified both in the distal amputated part and in the amputation stump and ligated to prevent postoperative hemorrhage causing a hematoma after revascularization is completed. The distal portions of devitalized and denervated interosseous muscles should be completely debrided, which can allow the intrinsic tendons to tenodese in an intrinsic-plus position.

A postoperative protocol should be initiated 72 hours after replantation consisting of early protective active mobilization with anticlaw splinting. This helps prevention of intrinsic minus deformity, provides a more serviceable grasping hand, and improves final functional results.[42] Recovery of sensibility is poor but protective sensory recovery can be expected in most cases; , cold intolerance remains a permanent problem in half of the patients in cold weather areas. Intrinsic muscle function and pinch and grip strengths are weak or absent in most patients (Figure 83.17).

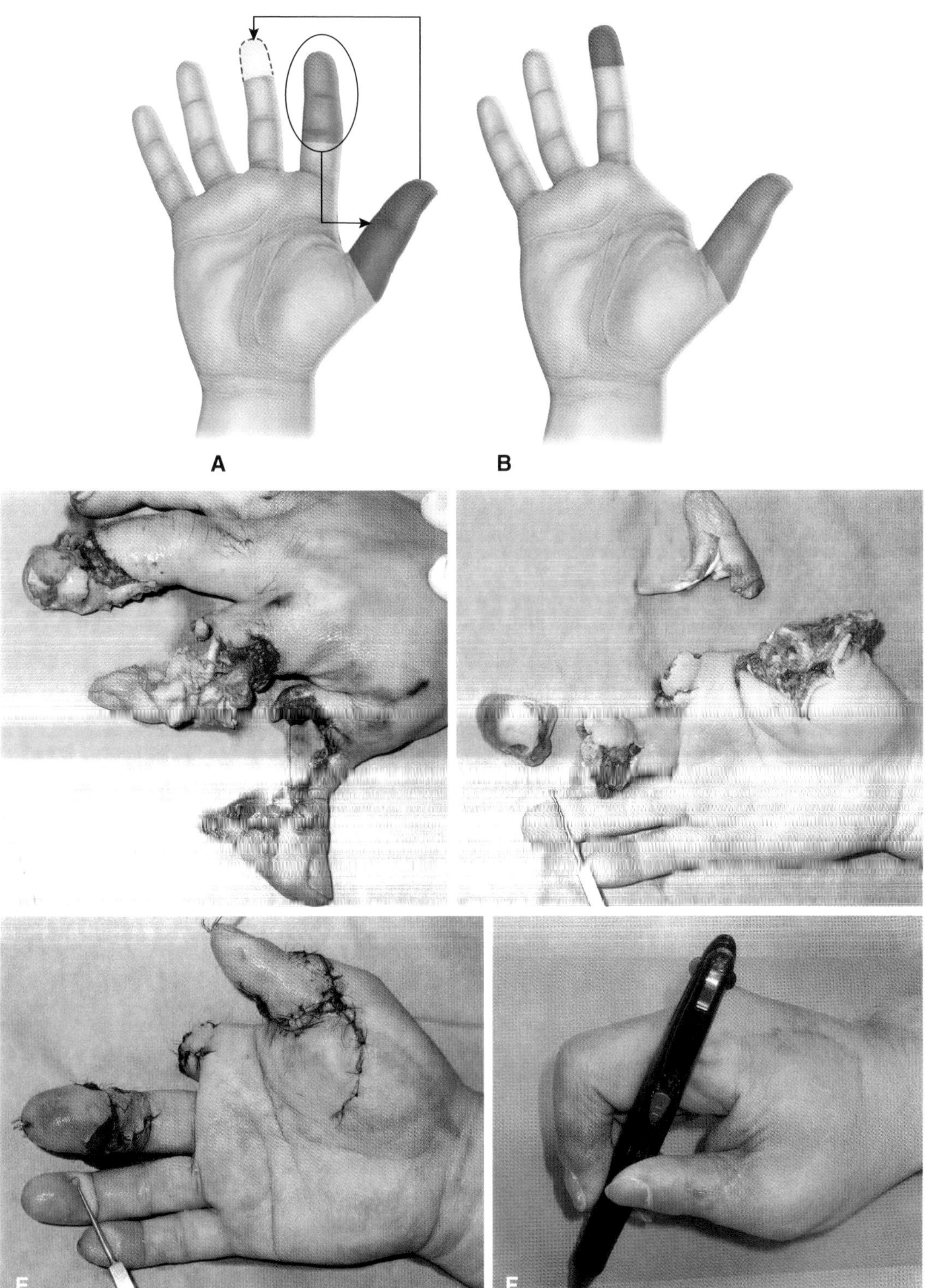

FIGURE 83.16. **A, B.** Illustrations depicting the transposition of the amputated digits. **C.** After a devastating crushed amputation injury by press machine, all three fingers seemed irreplantable. **D.** Amputated part of the right index finger was transposed to the thumb and distal phalanx of the thumb to the long finger. **E.** Immediate postoperative view. **F.** Thirteen months after the second ray amputation.

Major Limb Replantation

Major limb amputations are defined when they occur through or proximal to the radiocarpal joint and include transections at the level of the wrist, forearm, elbow, humerus, or shoulder. In more proximal amputation, there is a high possibility of significant associated injuries such as rib fractures, hemothorax, cervical spine injury, or traction injury of the brachial plexus so the patient should be checked thoroughly by the emergency specialist. These may be life-threatening conditions which may preclude replantation of upper extremity amputation.

There are very different considerations on both preparations and operative techniques compared with digital replantation.[43] First of all, if the total ischemic time extends beyond 8 hours, the operator

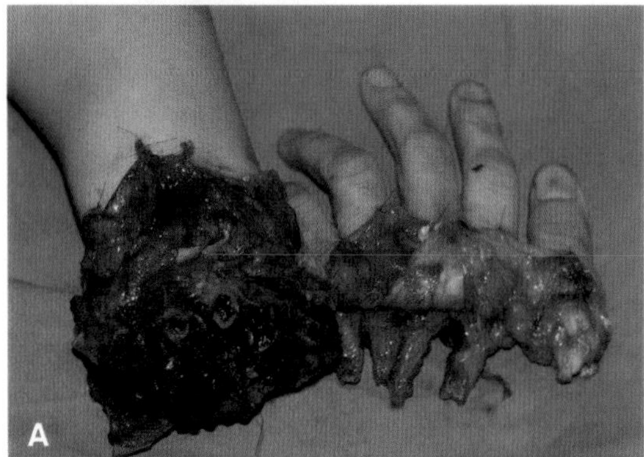

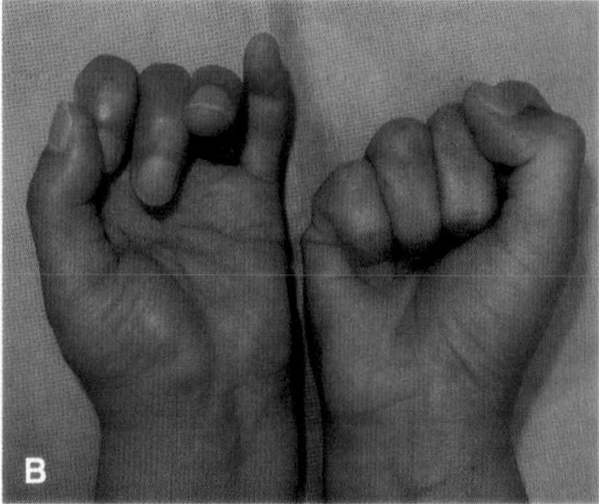

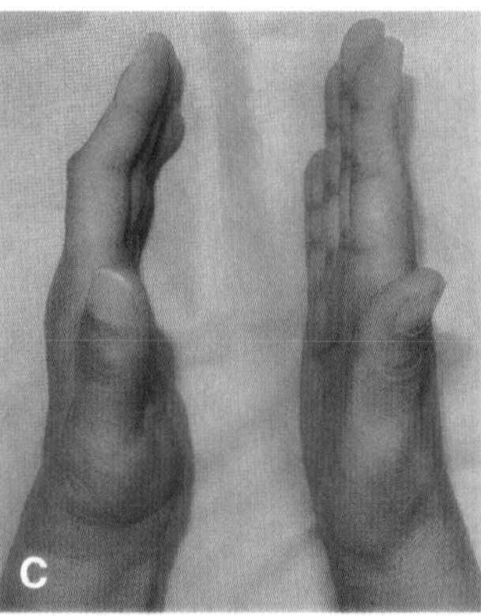

FIGURE 83.17. **A.** A 46-year-old woman sustained a local crushed-type amputation to her nondominant hand. All digits including thumb were amputated through the metacarpal bone. The intrinsic muscles were extensively debrided, and plate and screw fixation of the shortened metacarpals was followed by extensor and flexor tendon repair. Princeps pollicis artery and the second and third common digital arteries were microanatomosed and three dorsal veins were repaired. **B, C.** Fourteen years later.

should think over the replantation attempt once again. From the time of a patient's arrival at the emergency room to restore arterial blood flow to the amputated part, it will take at least 2 hours. Because the most common complication of major limb replantation is infection, debridement is a very critical step in preventing infection and is more radical at the muscles of the distal part. Acutely spreading infection immediately after operation may give rise to ruptured vessels or multiple organ system failure resulting in life-threatening complications. During the whole phase of operation, a hypothermic condition should be maintained by placing the amputated part on ice bags. Temporary vascular stent is used to avoid ischemic risk by connection arterial inflow from the proximal vessel to the amputated part. This can be performed before bone fixation if the duration from amputation to arrival in the operating room is longer than 4 to 6 hours. Hypothermic perfusion with the University of Wisconsin solution may allow longer periods of preservation, which could enable surgeons to take more precise and confirmed preparation procedures before arterial anastomosis.

Replantation at transcarpal and radiocarpal level of amputation is technically much easier but there are different options for joint management. In cases of amputation at the level of the intercarpal joint or radiocarpal joint with intact distal articular surface, proximal row carpectomy is a useful procedure to preserve joint motion of the wrist. An overall shortening effect of 2 to 3 cm by proximal row carpectomy can facilitate radical debridement of the soft tissue as well as direct repair of the vessels and nerves without any graft. Multiple K-wires are used for transarticular fixation for 6 to 8 weeks. The remnant of the joint capsule of the wrist and extensor retinaculum should be robustly repaired. In cases of extensive bone fractures around the radiocarpal joint, partial or total carpectomy and primary arthrodesis of the wrist is recommended. This is indicated especially if the radiocarpal joint is destroyed or in a young, working man. And, if the level of amputation is just proximal to the distal articular surface of the radius, shortening osteotomy of the radius and Darrach resection of the distal ulna are preferred.

At the wrist and proximal forearm, aggressive bone shortening up to 2.5 to 5 cm of both radius and ulna or 6 to 8 cm in length of either of the humeri is essential to make functional restoration possible.[43] The sequence of repair from this point on is from deep to superficial. Motor units of tendons are repaired with braided nonabsorbable sutures using a locking four-strand technique. If no motors are available, the tendons after resection of the muscle portion are left in the floor of the wound.

Regarding vessel repair, two main arteries and their venae comitantes as well as two subcutaneous veins at least should be repaired. Venae comitantes of radial and ulnar artery seem small compared with subcutaneous vein but are capable of draining a significant quantity of blood. Once arterial flow is established, the vein should be allowed to bleed for 5 minutes. Before this critical time, the anesthesiologist should be on standby and supply blood and sufficient fluid to the patient. Acute blood loss may cause transient hypovolemic shock necessitating prompt management. If the ischemic time is over 6 hours and/or there is a considerable muscle mass, the venous blood causes metabolic acidosis, hyperkalemia, cryoglobulinemia, and possibly reperfusion injury. With intensive monitoring of electrocardiogram, sodium bicarbonate is slowly given intravenously over a period of 5 minutes prior to clamp release. Reperfusion injury by reactive oxygen species into systemic circulation causes direct cell damage and produces inflammatory mediators, complements activation, and aids leukocyte adhesion. This cascade increases vascular permeability and can cause cell death despite revascularization. Even to decrease or prevent reperfusion injury, the conditioning maneuvers at the onset of reperfusion are simple, safe, and at least relatively harmless. A postconditioning maneuver should include brief alternative episode or episodes of nonocclusion/reocclusion on the feeding artery. Remote postconditioning is composed with brief alternative episode or episodes of ischemia and reperfusion on one of the nonoperative extremities.

Grouped fascicular primary nerve repair using 9-0 nylon sutures without tension can achieve optimal nerve regeneration which determines final functional results and ultimate use of the hand. Where the nerves are avulsed or segmentally defected, cross nerve suture between proximal radial to distal median repair or proximal ulnar to distal median is an alternative method for providing protective sensation of radial digits. If not, the nerve ends must be tagged with 4-0 nylon sutures at an easily accessible plane for later nerve grafting.

By significant bone shortening, primary skin repair is possible. Skin flap should be placed on the vessel anastomosis sites. If the skin graft is on the repaired vessel, there is a risk of delayed rupture. In cases of large soft-tissue defect possibly exposing vital structures or plate, tentative coverage with artificial skin or thin-split skin graft should be replaced by flap surgery as soon as possible depending on the general condition of the patient.

Major upper extremity replantation is successful in 77% to 93% of cases, depending on the level and mechanism of injury.[44] Better functional outcomes have been reported for distal and sharp injuries.[44] The functional outcomes of proximal amputations often caused by higher energy injury mechanisms are less predictable due to greater tissue damage and longer distances for muscle reinnervation. For improvement of the survived limb replantation, secondary surgical managements of the remaining functional deficits are mandatory. Tenolysis is the most common secondary procedure performed for amputations of the distal forearm to wrist. Free functioning muscle transfer is the most common secondary surgeries for amputations between the elbow and mid-forearm (Figure 83.18) and soft-tissue coverage is the most common secondary procedure in case of upper arm replantation.

Technical innovations and refinement of the indications for major replantation of limb amputations have resulted in a predictably high rate

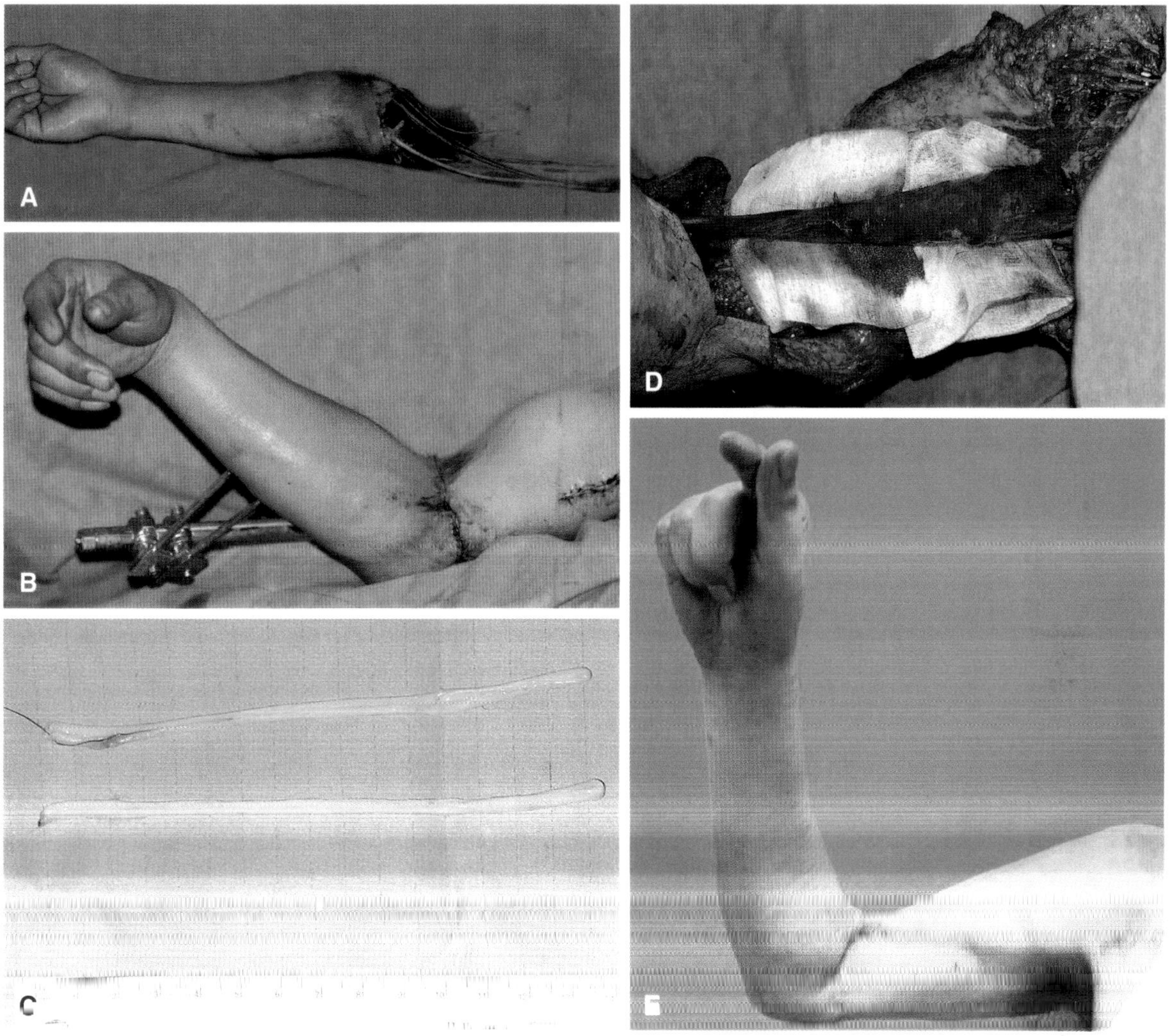

FIGURE 83.18. **A.** A 15 year old man sustained elbow amputation by belt injury. All nerves were avulsed from the upper arm. **B.** Elbow joint was fixed with a temporary K-wire with external fixator. **C.** Six months later, sural nerve grafts were used to reconstruct ulnar and median nerve. **D.** Functioning gracilis muscle was transferred to reconstruct elbow flexion. **E.** Fifteen years after the operation, functional result was grade III by Chen's criteria.

of successful revascularization. Replantation surgery produces superior functional results compared with revision amputation and a prosthesis.[45]

Regarding rehabilitation for more proximal level of replantation at palm, wrist, and forearm, prevention of intrinsic minus deformity, maintaining full passive range of motion at uninjured joints distal to the amputation level, and daily use of the replanted digit is essential to get satisfactory functional restoration. As the intrinsic minus posture is difficult to correct once it becomes fixed, daytime exercise with a dynamic crane outrigger splint with an MP joint extension block and night anticlaw splint are mandatory (Figure 83.19). Even though active motion of the digits is not recovered after replantation, the status of full passive motion of the digits leaves the possibility of functional improvement by later reconstruction with tendon transfer or free functioning muscle transfer.

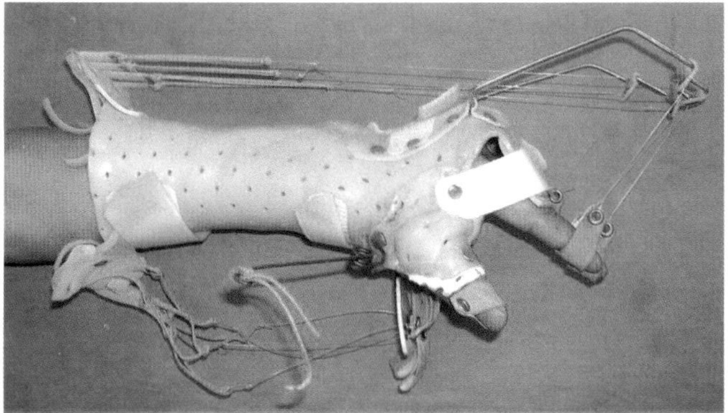

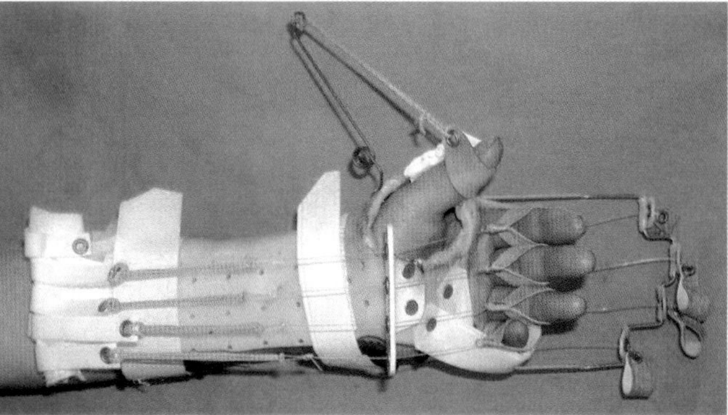

FIGURE 83.19. Active and resisted exercise of the joint with the orthoplast dynamic splint. This can prevent claw deformity of the digits as well as adduction contracture of the thumb.

SECONDARY PROBLEMS AND OUTCOMES

The long-term patency of the microanastomosed digital arteries after successful replantation varies. In spite of successful replantation, the pulsation of Doppler and angiography reveals occlusion of the arteries in 37% of vessels after an average of 15 postoperative days.[46] Therefore, early wound healing of the soft tissue is critical for neovascularization of the replanted finger. In crush amputation cases, neovascularization of the replanted part occurs slowly. In these cases, replantation failures may happen after 1 week to 10 days postoperatively. Radical debridement of the soft tissue, as well as apposition between fresh tissues, is essential upon completion of the case. In cases of soft-tissue defects following replantation, local or free flaps are necessary.

The worst complication in the early postoperative period is replantation failure. Failed distal replants can be allowed to mummify and be left in situ to act as a dressing for the underlying stump. In children, in young women, and in multiple-digit amputation, preservation of middle phalangeal bone length at the time of revision amputation is important to preserve hand competence and prevent objects from slipping through the hand. Later, secondary reconstruction with toe-to-hand transfer is possible only where at least 1 cm of the middle phalangeal bone remains.

In practice, secondary operation after digital replantation is almost a necessity for the improvement of both function and appearance of the digits. About 30% to 50% of replantation cases show problems related to bony healing.[16] Nonunion rates range from 10% to 30% with K-wire fixation having the highest nonunion rates. Malunion rates are about 20% with screw fixation being associated with the highest rates of malunion. Intraosseous wires alone have been found to have the lowest nonunion and complication rates. In cases of rotational deformity or nonunion, secondary revision with corrective osteotomy and internal fixation with or without bone graft are needed.

Stiffness of the MCP, PIP, and DIP joints remains a problem due to edema and swelling in the replanted digit. The surgeon should avoid using longitudinal K-wires to transfix joints. It is important to encourage an active and passive range of motion exercises of the joints of adjacent noninjured digits, otherwise these too can become stiff. To improve joint motion, artificial joint insertion or toe joint transfer is another option depending on the condition of the tissues surrounding the joint.

The indications for flexor or extensor tendon tenolysis of the replanted digits are almost the same as the general indications for tenolysis following isolated flexor tendon injury. These include significant discrepancy between passive and active flexion of the digital joints after a substantial period of more than 6 months. This allows sufficient time for wound healing and maximum rehabilitation therapy. The result of tenolysis after digital replantation is a useful and safe procedure to achieve improvement in the active flexion of the digit. After tenolysis, secondary tendon rupture or subsequent bone fracture may happen due to aggressive rehabilitation. Secondary tenolyses or two-stage flexor tendon grafting may significantly increase the total active range of motion of a replanted digit. In extensor tenolysis, any hardware used in bone fixation should be removed at the same time. An intrinsic reconstruction and dorsal arthrolysis and capsulotomy are worthwhile when active and passive flexions are present. Certain procedures such as tenolysis, capsulotomy, and arthrolysis are performed together because all these procedures need no immobilization.

Factors that influence digital sensibility following replantation include patient's age, level and mechanism of injury, digital blood flow, cold intolerance, and postoperative sensory reeducation. However, there is no significant relationship between the return of sensibility and the length of ischemia time. Thermoregulation following digital replantation is likely to be a complex interaction among vascular, neural, metabolic, and possibly hormonal mechanisms. Cold intolerance after replantation is a significant problem, but the exact mechanism of cold intolerance following digital nerve injury is unknown and clearly, greater than 80% of patients have moderate to severe cold intolerance following digital replantation. In most series, this disabling phenomenon abates somewhat after a period of 2 years but may persist.[6,47] This means that cold intolerance results from a disorder in vasoregulation and not from arterial insufficiency of the digit. Postoperative sensory reeducation and daily use of the replanted digits will continue to improve digital sensibility as well as cold intolerance following replantation. Chen's classic criteria for the evaluation of function after replantation[48] are ideal for assessing multisystem injuries and are general enough to allow comparison of results within complex injury groups. Viable upper extremity replantation without return of sensation does not represent a functional success.

REFERENCES

1. Malt RA, McKhann C. Replantation of a severed arm. *JAMA*. 1964;189:716-722.
2. Kleinert HE, Kasdan ML, Romero JL. Small blood vessel anastomosis for salvage of severely injured upper extremity. *J Bone Jt Surg Am*. 1963;45A:788-796.
3. Komatsu S, Tamai S. Successful replantation of a completely cut off thumb: case report. *Plast Reconstr Surg*. 1968;42:374-377.
4. Chen ZW, Meyer VE, Kleinert HE, et al. Present indications and contraindications for replantation as reflected by long-term functional results. *Orthop Clin North Am*. 1981;12:849-897.
5. Scott FA, Howar JW, Boswick JA Jr. Recovery of function following replantation and revascularization of amputated hand parts. *J Trauma*. 1981;21:204-214.
6. Jones JM, Schenck RR, Chesney RB. Digital replantation and amputation-comparison of function. *J Hand Surg Am*. 1982;7:183-189.
7. El-Diwany M, Odobescu A, Bélanger-Douet M, et al. Replantation vs revision amputation in single digit zone II amputations. *J Plast Reconstr Aesthet Surg*. 2015;68:859-863.
8. Zhu H, Bao B, Zheng X. A comparison of functional outcomes and therapeutic costs: single-digit replantation versus revision amputation. *Plast Reconstr Surg*. 2018;141:244e-249e.
   A retrospective review of 1023 single-digit amputations was performed over a 3-year period. Replantation of thumb, index, long, and ring fingers showed extra benefit compared with revision amputation.
9. Meyer TM. Psychological aspects of mutilating hand injuries. *Hand Clin*. 2003:19:41-49.
10. Nishizuka T, Shauver MJ, Zhong L, et al. A comparative study of attitudes regarding digit replantation in the United States and Japan. *J Hand Surg Am*. 2015;40:1646-1656.
11. Woo SH, Cheon HJ, Kim YW, et al. Delayed and suspended replantation for complete amputation of digits and hands. *J Hand Surg Am*. 2015;40:883-889.
    A retrospective review of 28 cases of delayed and suspended digital replantations was performed. It shows similar survival rates and functional results compared with those involving immediate replantation. This justifies having the option to delay and suspend replantation.
12. Godina M. Early microsurgical reconstruction of complex trauma of the extremities. *Plast Reconstr Surg*. 1986;78:285-292.
13. Nishikawa H, Manek S, Barnett S, et al. Pathology of warm ischemia and reperfusion injury in adipomusculocutaneous flaps. *Int. J. Exp. Pathol.* 1993;74: 35-44.
14. Kwon GD, Ahn BM, Lee JS, et al. The effect of patient age on the success rate of digital replantation. *Plast Reconstr Surg*. 2017;139:420-426.
15. Zimmerman NB, Weiland AJ. Ninety-ninety intraosseous wiring for internal fixation of the digital skeleton. *Orthopedics*. 1989;12:99-103.
16. Whitney TM, Lineaweaver WC, Buncke HJ, et al. Clinical results of bony fixation methods in digital replantation, *J Hand Surg Am*. 1990;15:328-334.
17. Zumiotti A, Ferreira MC. Replantation of digits: factors influencing survival and functional results. *Microsurgery*. 1994;15:18-21.
18. Khouri RK, Shaw WW. Monitoring of free flaps with surface-temperature recordings: is it reliable? *Plast Reconstr Surg*. 1992;89:495-499.
19. Conrad MH, Adams WP. Pharmacologic optimization of microsurgery in the new millennium. *Plast Reconstr Surg*. 2001;108:2088-2096.
20. Silverman PM, Willette-Green V, Petrill J. Early protective motion in digital revascularization and replantation. *J Hand Ther*. 1989;2:84-101.
21. Ishikawa K, Ogawa Y, Soeda H, et al. A new classification of the amputation level for the distal part of the fingers. *J Jpn Soc Microsurg*. 1990;3:54-62.
22. Hattori Y, Doi K, Ikeda K, et al. A retrospective study of functional outcomes after successful replantation versus amputation closure for single fingertip amputations. *J Hand Surg Am*. 2006;31:811-818.
23. Scheker LR, Becker GW. Distal finger replantation. *J Hand Surg Am*. 2011;36:521-528.
24. Buntic RF, Brooks D. Standardized protocol for artery-only fingertip replantation. *J Hand Surg Am*. 2010;35:1491-1496.
25. Erken HY, Takka S, Akmaz I. Artery-only fingertip replantations using a controlled nailbed bleeding protocol. *J Hand Surg Am*. 2013;38:2173-2179.
26. Koshima I, Yamashita S, Sugiyama N, et al. Successful delayed venous drainage in 16 consecutive distal phalangeal replantations. *Plast Reconstr Surg*. 2005;115:149-154.

27. Lineaweaver WC, Hill MK, Buncke GM, et al. *Aeromonas hydrophila* infections following use of medicinal leeches in replantation and flap surgery. *Ann Plast Surg.* 1992;29:238-244.
28. Baker GL1, Kleinert JM. Digit replantation in infants and young children: determinants of survival. *Plast Reconstr Surg.* 1994;94:139-145.
29. Cheng GL, Pan DD, Zhang NP, et al. Digital replantation in children: a long-term follow-up study. *J Hand Surg Am.* 1998;23:635-646.
30. Beris AE, Soucacos PN, Malizos KN, et al. Major limb replantation in children. *Microsurgery.* 1994;15:474-478.
31. Unglaub F, Demir E, Von Reim R, et al. Long-term functional and subjective results of thumb replantation. *Microsurgery.* 2006;26:552-556.
32. Chen HC, Tang YB. Replantation of the thumb, especially avulsion. *Hand Clin.* 2001;17:433-445.
33. Agarwal JP, Trovato MJ, Agarwal S, et al. Selected outcomes of thumb replantation after isolated thumb amputation injury. *J Hand Surg Am.* 2010;35:1485-1490.
34. Bieber E, Wood MB, Cooney WP, et al. Thumb avulsion: results of replantation/revascularization. *J Hand Surg Am.* 1987;12:786-790.
35. Sears ED, Chung KC. Replantation of finger avulsion injuries: a systematic review of survival and functional outcomes. *J Hand Surg Am.* 2011;36:686-694.
A systemic review of ring avulsion amputation was performed. It demonstrates that functional outcomes of sensibility and range of motion after replantation of finger avulsion injuries are better than what is historically cited in the literature.
36. Kupfer DM, Eaton C, Swanson S, et al. Ring avulsion injuries: a biomechanical study. *J Hand Surg Am.* 1999;24:1249-1253.
37. Urbaniak JR, Evans JP, Bright DS. Microvascular management of ring avulsion injuries. *J Hand Surg Am.* 1981,6.25-30.
38. Kay S, Werntz J, Wolff TW. Ring avulsion injuries: classification and prognosis. *J Hand Surg Am.* 1989;14:204-213.
39. Adani R, Pataia E, Tarallo L, et al. Results of replantation of 33 ring avulsion amputations. *J Hand Surg Am.* 2013;38:947-956.
40. Soucacos PN, Beris AE, Malizos KN, et al. Transpositional microsurgery in multiple digital amputations. *Microsurgery.* 1994;15:469-473.
41. Paavilainen P, Nietosvaara Y, Tikkinen KA, et al. Long-term results of transmetacarpal replantation. *J Plast Reconstr Aesthet Surg.* 2007;60:704-709.
42. Scheker LR, Chesher SP, Netscher DT, et al. Functional results of dynamic splinting after transmetacarpal, wrist, and distal forearm replantation. *J Hand Surg Br.* 1995;20:584-590.
43. Sabapathy SR, Venkatramani H, Bharathi RR, et al. Technical considerations and functional outcome of 22 major replantations. *J Hand Surg Eur.* 2007;32:488-501.
Twenty-two consecutive major limb replantations carried out over a 5-year period were assessed. Surgical technique, risk factors, and outcome are discussed. The technical details believed to be important for success are outlined. With decreasing numbers of such injuries in most countries, this paper may help surgeons faced with an occasional patient with a major amputation to make the right decisions.
44. Larson JV, Kung TA, Cederna PS, et al. Clinical factors associated with replantation after traumatic major upper extremity amputation. *Plast Reconstr Surg.* 2013;132:911-919.
45. Pet MA, Morrpetison SD, Mack JS, et al. Comparison of patient-reported outcomes after traumatic upper extremity amputation: replantation versus prosthetic rehabilitation. *Injury.* 2016;47:2783-2788.
46. Lee CH, Han SK, Dhong ES, et al. The fate of microanastomosed digital arteries after successful replantation. *Plast Reconstr Surg.* 2005;116:805-810.
47. Waikakul S, Sakkarnkosol S, Vanadurongwan V, et al. Results of 1018 digital replantations in 552 patients. *Injury.* 2000;31:33-40.
48. Chen CW, Qian YQ, Yu ZJ. Extremity replantation. *World J Surg.* 1978;2:513-524.
The pioneer of replantation surgery in the world discusses traditional surgical techniques and different methods of replantation. Final evaluation of replantation using "Chen's criteria," which are still very useful and reliable, is included.

QUESTIONS

1. Which is mostly related with overnight delay in replantation, with preservation of the amputated part at 4 to 6°C?

a. Correlated with lower overall viability of the replant
b. Resulted in no differences in survival rate
c. Caused hypothermic damage to the replanted finger with later loss
d. Resulted in increased surgeon fatigue

2. Which of the following patients presenting with an amputation would be most appropriate to consider for replantation?

a. A 63-year-old diabetic suffering a crushing amputation of the index finger
b. A 5-year-old boy with a sharp amputation of the little finger
c. A 35-year-old woman with an avulsion amputation of the forearm with 6 hours of warm ischemia
d. A 73-year-old man with an amputation of the arm through the mid humerus

3. What is the appropriate antibiotic prophylaxis against *Aeromonas hydrophila* infection?

a. Penicillin
b. Fluoroquinolone
c. Cefazolin
d. Clindamycin

4. The most common complication of major limb replantation is:

a. bleeding
b. bony nonunion
c. infection
d. adult respiratory distress syndrome

5. A 22-year-old welder with no medical history is brought to the emergency department following a sharp amputation of his dominant right hand following an altercation. Plain film inspection of the hand and amputated part reveals amputation through the distal shaft of the middle phalanx. Physical examination reveals intact FDS. After inspection of the amputated part under the operating microscope, a decision is made to attempt replantation. What is the first step that must be performed in the surgical sequence of replantation?

a. Bone shortening and fixation
b. Flexor tendon repair
c. Arterial anastomosis
d. Venous anastomosis

6. A 15-year-old boy with no medical history is brought to the emergency department following sharp amputation of the dominant right thumb while hunting. What is the best way to preserve the finger until replantation can be attempted?

a. Place the finger directly on ice
b. Allow the finger to soak in a bath of physiologic solution at room temperature
c. Wrap the finger in saline-soaked gauze, place the gauze in a watertight bag, and place the bag on water and ice mixture
d. Place the finger in a dry container and place directly in the tissue freezer

1. Answer: b. The survival rate of digital replantation in the overnight-delayed replantation group was 93.4% and in the immediate replantation group was 91.2%. This difference was not statistically significant.

2. Answer: b. All indications for replantation must take into account the status of the amputated part (sharp amputation versus crush) and the patient (healthy versus systemic illnesses). The degree of tissue injury may argue against replantation, even in the case of a clear indication, such as thumb amputation. Although single-finger replantations are generally not performed, replantation beyond the level of the sublimis tendon insertion (zone 1) usually results in good function. Multiple finger amputations present reconstructive difficulties that may be difficult to correct without replantation of one or all of the amputated digits. Any hand amputation from zone 2 (distally) to zone 4 (proximally) offers the chance of reasonable function after replantation, usually superior to available prostheses. It is generally believed that replantation should be attempted with almost any part in a child. In children, success rates (in terms of viability) are lower, but the functional results are better. Although there have been several reports of successful lower limb replantation, this area remains controversial. The available lower extremity prostheses make amputation less of a functional problem in the leg than in the upper extremity. The leg contains larger masses of muscle (which tolerate ischemia poorly) and without adequate sensory recovery, the foot is at risk for soft-tissue breakdown. Replantation and revascularization of the foot, lower leg, or both in children may give gratifying results, however.

3. Answer: b. If there is total obstruction of venous outflow, near-continuous leeching will be necessary for at least 5 or 6 days, and the patient may suffer significant blood loss (in the 2 to 6 unit range). This blood loss represents the primary potential complication of leech therapy, but they also have the potential to cause infection. ***Aeromonas hydrophila*** is a saprophytic organism in the leech's gut, which, although not a primary pathogen in humans, can cause significant infection. One review article found that infection occurred in 7% to 20% of cases of leech application for venous outflow problems and was associated with a decrease in salvage of the involved tissue. Infection is uncommon in tissue with adequate arterial supply, however, and their use should be avoided if the viability of the tissue is questionable. To minimize the risk of infection, the patient should be covered with appropriate antibiotic therapy during the period of leech application. Studies of leech flora suggest that a fluoroquinolone is appropriate prophylaxis in most cases.

4. Answer: c. Attempting to replant a forearm or arm with a prolonged warm ischemic period can lead to severe metabolic problems and potentially death of the patient. Debridement of nonviable tissue is paramount, and this process leads to the problem of soft-tissue coverage in many of these patients. Although uncommon in digital replantation, infection, and even systemic sepsis, is the number one complication in major limb replants. For this reason, major limb replantation is not to be undertaken without a serious commitment to the endeavor.

5. Answer: a. Identifiable structures should be tagged with suture or microclips. The first step in replantation is bone shortening and fixation. Bone should be shortened enough to take all tension off of the subsequent soft-tissue repairs. In the pediatric population, any bony shortening should take care not to sacrifice the physis. Bony fixation is followed by extensor tendon then flexor tendon repair. Arterial repair should then be undertaken.

6. Answer: c. Transportation of the amputated part is paramount in preserving viability. The most widely utilized and effective method of preservation is wrapping the amputated extremity in gauze moistened with a physiologic solution (normal saline or lactated ringers), placing the wrapped amputated part in a plastic bag, then placing this plastic bag on ice. Alternatively, the part may be immersed in a physiologic solution in one bag which is then placed on ice. Amputated extremity parts should never be placed directly on ice, as this may cause frostbite or other soft-tissue injuries to the amputated part. Such injury may preclude replantation altogether or compromise the achievable functional result of replantation.

CHAPTER 84 Thumb Reconstruction

Patrick L. Reavey and Neil F. Jones

KEY POINTS

- The thumb is responsible for 40% of the overall hand function; therefore, reconstruction of this digit is essential to restore adequate length as well as sensate and durable soft tissue.
- The minimum length for acceptable thumb function is at the interphalangeal joint. Complex injuries at or distal to the IP joint may not require extensive reconstruction.
- Isolated soft tissue defects of the thumb can be reconstructed with either local/regional or microsurgical flaps though selection of sensate flaps is essential.
- Thumbs with inadequate length (proximal to the IP joint) require bony and soft tissue reconstruction and in these cases, microsurgical techniques utilizing a toe-transfer procedure provide superior outcomes.
- In complex hand injuries involving the thumb, replantation of the thumb is an absolute priority; heterotopic replantation and/or pollicization of injured digits should be considered. Secondary reconstruction can be accomplished by conventional techniques of distraction lengthening or pollicization of an injured finger or a normal finger and probably now better by microsurgical toe-to-thumb transfer.

ANATOMY AND BIOMECHANICS

The thumb is unique in humans due to the position of the thumb axis at the trapeziometacarpal (TM) joint, which is pronated and flexed with respect to the other metacarpals. This position allows for circumduction and opposition of the thumb and the versatility of the thumb to participate in prehension. The thumb contributes 40% of hand function but takes on a much more significant role in mutilating trauma when other digits are missing or stiff.[1]

Opposition is necessary for the majority of essential thumb function. Opposition is the result of the abductor pollicis brevis, opponens pollicis, and superficial head of the flexor pollicis brevis flexing and rotating the TM and metacarpophalangeal (MP) joints simultaneously. The abductor pollicis brevis inserts on the radial sesamoid and radial base of the proximal phalanx. It is the main contributor of opposition and every effort should be made to preserve this function during reconstruction. In proximal transmetacarpal thumb injuries, the opponens pollicis, which inserts on the volar-radial aspect of the thumb metacarpal, may still provide some opposition function at the TM joint.[2] However, secondary opposition transfer may be required after reconstruction to maximize thumb function in proximal injuries.

PATIENT EVALUATION

All patients require a comprehensive evaluation. A detailed medical history, including tobacco use, is important as medical comorbidities may preclude long microsurgical procedures in some patients. Handedness, occupation, and any prior injuries or limited function help to determine the goals of reconstruction. Details on the mechanism and timing of injury are crucial in the evaluation of patients presenting at the time of injury or for primary reconstruction. Additional medical records, especially time-of-injury radiologic examinations and prior operative reports, are important for planning in patients presenting for secondary reconstruction.

A complete hand examination should be performed to determine the extent of soft tissue loss, vascular and neurologic status, tendon lacerations, and bone, joint, or ligamentous injuries to the thumb and all digits. In regards to the thumb, specific attention should be paid to the geometry (e.g., dorsal, volar, transverse, oblique) and location of soft tissue loss (e.g., pulp, radial, or ulnar) as well as the quality of remaining tissue adjacent to the injury. The level of amputation or bony injury should be noted relative to soft tissue component and involvement or injury to the first webspace should be noted. Standard anteroposterior and lateral radiographs of the hand or digits should be obtained. Additional views (i.e., Roberts view for evaluation of the TM joint) can be ordered as needed for proximal or carpal injuries. Advanced imaging (computerized axial tomography, magnetic resonance imaging) is not indicated in the evaluation of acute injuries but may be helpful in patients presenting with complicated injuries for secondary reconstruction.

A shared medical-decision making approach is essential to the conversation between the patient and surgeon about the reconstructive options. The patient should be asked what the goals and expectations of reconstruction are. The surgeon should discuss the expected outcomes of any reconstructive options, including details on expected thumb and hand function, the need and extent of postoperative therapy, overall recovery time, donor site morbidity, and the appearance of the reconstructed thumb. Patients may decide to undergo a *suboptimal* functional reconstruction due to the cultural, social, occupational, or financial impact of that option (i.e., choosing not to undergo great toe-transfer due to the inability to wear sandals postoperatively).

RECONSTRUCTIVE GOALS

An optimal thumb reconstruction should restore thumb length, mobility, stability, strength, sensibility, and aesthetics.[3] It is difficult to achieve all of these in every patient so it is important to remember that the overall goal of thumb reconstruction is to maximize *hand function;* this requires that the thumb participates in prehension. The goals of reconstruction can then be simplified into three key objectives: creating a thumb with adequate length, with optimal mobility and/or position for opposition, and with a sensate, painless tip.

Length

The minimum required length for a functional thumb is at the level of the IP joint. An amputation at this level decreases the function of the thumb by 50%; however, the thumb is still able to oppose the other digits and function in prehension. Thumb amputations at or distal to the IP joint do not necessarily require additional length or bony reconstruction. Amputations proximal to the IP joint of the thumb will require a surgical approach that restores a functional length similar to that of a normal thumb or a minimum at the level of the IP joint.

Mobility/Position

The thumb is normally pronated 80° relative to the other digits with additional pronation occurring during opposition to allow tip pinch. In injuries distal to the MP joint, the majority of thumb mobility will be maintained, and the goals of length and sensibility will take precedence. In injuries proximal to the MP joint, the function of any remaining thenar musculature must be assessed and a decrease in thumb mobility is expected. Secondary opposition transfers may be required to maximize the function. Thumb injuries without a functional TM joint require a reconstructive procedure to create a neo-TM joint (e.g., pollicization) or the creation of immobile post that may still serve to restore some hand function. Attention should also be paid to injuries involving the first webspace as contracture in this area will limit thumb opposition and require additional reconstructive procedures.

Sensate and Painless Tip

An optimal thumb has good sensation and preferably stereognosis. At a minimum, the ulnar aspect of the thumb tip/pulp should have sensibility as this is the portion most often involved in pinch and prehension. Additionally, the tip of the thumb should have durable and adequate soft tissue for pain-free use. Restoration of adequate soft tissue and sensibility may be performed in staged procedures; however, the end goal must be to restore as close to normal sensibility as possible.

THUMB REPLANTATION

Replantation of a native thumb will nearly always achieve better outcomes when compared to secondary reconstruction techniques. As such, every effort should be made to replant amputated thumbs including those with relative contraindications to replantation such as crush and avulsion injuries. Distal digital replantations require a supermicrosurgical expertise but have excellent results and survival.[4] Surgeons not facile with these techniques should give consideration to referring distal thumb amputations to a regional center where this care is available prior to performing a revision amputation or planning secondary reconstructive procedures.

Mangled hand injuries involving the thumb are some of the most complicated cases for hand surgeons. A systematic approach is required to achieve optimal outcomes. First priority should be given to the replantation/reconstruction of the thumb. When the amputated thumb is not salvageable, other injured digits should be evaluated for heterotopic replantation to the thumb position. Spare parts from nonsalvageable digits should also be considered for maximizing the outcome of thumb reconstruction in more limited injuries (Figure 84.1).

Severe mutilating hand injuries involving the proximal amputation of all digits, such as in the metacarpal hand, require a thoughtful approach to the initial operation and the plan for secondary procedures. Microsurgical techniques allow for the reconstruction of a hand with a functional thumb or thumb analog and a minimum of a second opposable finger or unit.[5,6]

THUMB RECONSTRUCTION

When replantation is unsuccessful or cannot be performed, thumb reconstruction can still achieve good results. Several classification schemes have been proposed to guide the reconstructive approach to thumb injuries.[1,3,7] We find that a modified version of Lister's scheme is most useful for guiding decision making (**Table 84.1**). This scheme focuses on the two main issues that need to be addressed in reconstructing a thumb—length and soft tissue coverage. The mobility and position of the thumb are often most impacted by the level of the initial injury and proximal injuries may require secondary procedures to maximize function.

Soft Tissue Deficit With Acceptable Length (at or Distal to the IP Joint)

These injuries require only the restoration of a soft tissue envelope to maintain the remaining thumb length. Dorsal soft tissue loss can be adequately covered by any soft tissue procedure because there is no need for normal sensibility in this area. Wounds of the volar pulp

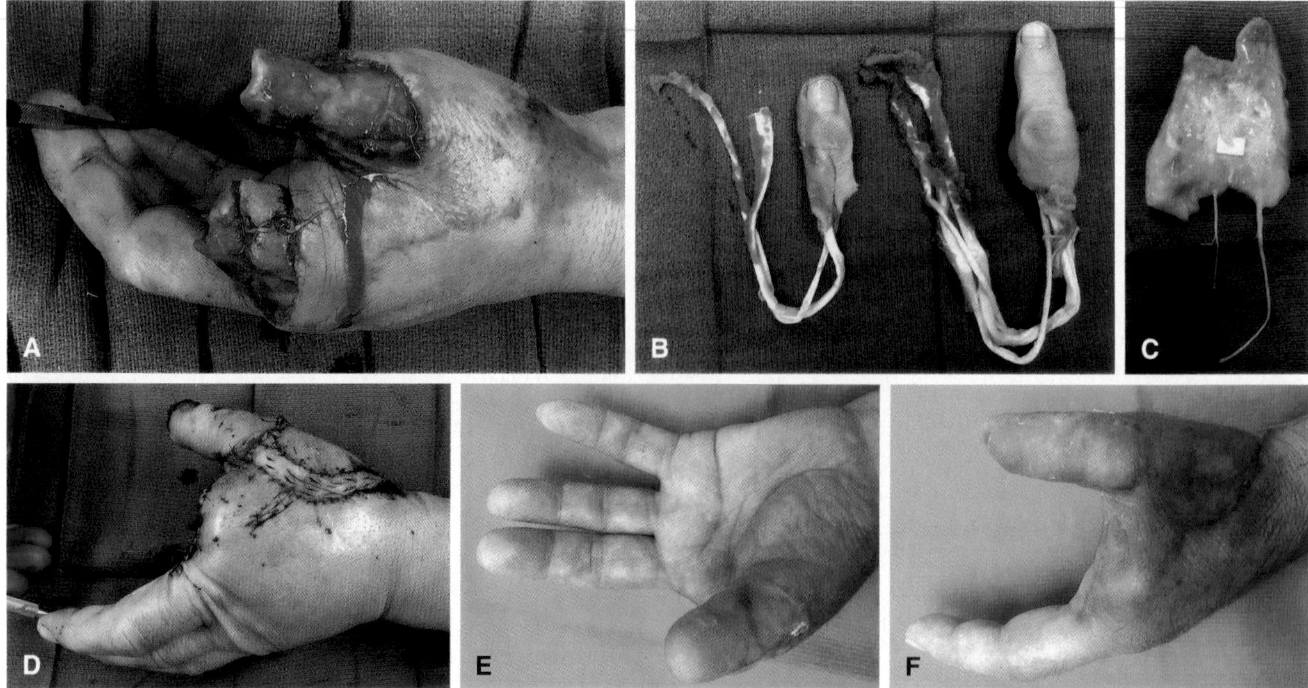

FIGURE 84.1. Avulsion amputation of the index finger and thumb. **A.** The proximal phalanx of the thumb is intact but without soft tissue coverage. **B.** The amputated thumb had a multilevel injury, with better preservation of the index finger. **C, D.** Neurotized fillet of the index finger flap transferred to salvage the remaining thumb. **E, F.** Postoperative outcome at 3 months.

TABLE 84.1. THUMB INJURY CLASSIFICATION AND RECONSTRUCTIVE APPROACH

	Reconstructive Need			
Type of Injury	**Bone**	**Soft Tissue**	**Considerations**	**Options**[a]
Soft-tissue deficit with acceptable length (amputation at or distal to the IP joint)	+/−	+	■ Reconstructive techniques to reestablish the normal thumb length preferred ■ First webspace deepening may improve functional length in distal proximal phalanx injuries	■ Local or regional flaps ■ Osteoplastic reconstruction ■ Free toe-pulp flap ■ Partial trimmed-toe transfer
Amputation distal to the MP joint but inadequate length	+	+	■ Bone and soft tissue reconstruction must restore minimal functional length ■ Reconstructive techniques to reestablish normal thumb length preferred	■ **Great or second toe transfer** ■ **Trimmed toe transfer** ■ **Wrap-around toe-flap** ■ Osteoplastic reconstruction ■ Distraction lengthening.
Amputation proximal to the MP joint but preserved TM joint	++	++	■ Opponens pollicis function on remaining metacarpal should be assessed ■ APB function should be restored if possible ■ First webspace injuries may require additional soft tissue reconstruction	■ **Second toe transfer** ■ Osteoplastic reconstruction ■ Distraction lengthening ■ Pollicization/on-top-plasty
Amputation with destruction of the TM joint	+++	+++	■ Pollicization standard option for the TM joint and thumb reconstruction ■ Creation of stable [illegible] ensure appropriate position ■ First webspace will likely require additional soft tissue reconstruction	■ **Pollicization** ■ Second-toe transfer with TM fusion

[a]Options in bold indicate the first-line reconstructive options when appropriate

with adequate remaining soft tissue and no exposed bone can achieve excellent functional and cosmetic outcomes with good wound care. Significant volar soft tissue loss with exposed bone or tendons require sensate and durable reconstruction. Local, regional, and microvascular flaps can all be considered; the best option is selected after considering the patient's needs.

Local and Regional Flaps

Moberg Flap

The Moberg flap is a bipedicle neurovascular advancement flap from the proximal volar thumb.[8] Because this flap advances in line with the longitudinal neurovascular pedicle, it has a limited range and is only indicated for defects less than 1.5 cm. A proximal transverse incision at the MCP flexion crease, leaving the neurovascular bundles intact, provides greater advancement up to 2 cm but requires a skin graft in the donor site.[9] V-Y or bilateral Z-plasty modifications at the proximal incision yield a similar advancement without the need for a skin graft.[10,11] Although this flap has the advantage of using the native glabrous skin and normal sensibility, IP joint flexion is frequently required to get complete distal coverage and patients may be left with a residual IP joint contracture.

First Dorsal Metacarpal Artery (FDMA) Flap

The FDMA flap (Foucher or kite flap) is a regional flap based on the FDMA supply to the dorsal aspect of the index finger.[12] The flap can include all of the dorsal skin and soft tissue between the MCP and PIP joints of the index finger. The proximal soft tissue pedicle includes dorsal veins and branches of the superficial radial nerve, making it a sensate flap. A key aspect in the flap dissection is to preserve the paratenon over the index finger extensor tendon for a subsequent skin graft to the donor site. After dissecting the pedicle back to the origin of the FDMA, it can then be transposed to the thumb tip either by tunneling under the remaining thumb skin or dividing the bridge during inset. Including a proximal skin paddle in the flap design to inset along the thumb is helpful in avoiding compression of the pedicle (Figure 84.2). This flap is reliable and provides a significant amount of tissue for large defects. The static two-point discrimination (s2PD) of the dorsal index finger is 12 to 15 mm and this sensibility is maintained in the standard flap design.[12-14] Patients may have *double-sensitivity*, experiencing sensation in the dorsal index finger when using the thumb; however, some patients are able to cortically reorient over time.[14,15] An alternative is to divide the radial nerve branches proximally and perform a neurorrhaphy to the proper digital nerves of the thumb to restore normal cortical function and this may improve s2PD to 8 mm.[13] With careful dissection of the pedicle, the flap can be mobilized to reach the tip of the native volar thumb[16]; however, this often requires IP joint flexion or thumb adduction.[13] An additional limitation of this flap is the conspicuous donor site.

Cross-Finger Flap

A cross-finger flap from the dorsal aspect of the index finger is another option for distal thumb coverage. The flap is designed over the proximal phalanx of the index finger and raised in the standard fashion with the donor site covered by a full thickness skin graft.[17] A flap from the dorsal middle phalanx of the index or long finger has also been reported.[18] After the initial inset, the patient is brought back to the operating room for flap division after 2 to 3 weeks. Reported sensory recovery is variable and ranges between poor (>12 mm s2PD) and normal (<6 mm s2PD) sensation, and can take more than a year for the final outcome.[18] Several modifications of the flap to improve sensibility are described; branches of superficial radial nerve can be isolated during proximal flap dissection and pedicled during

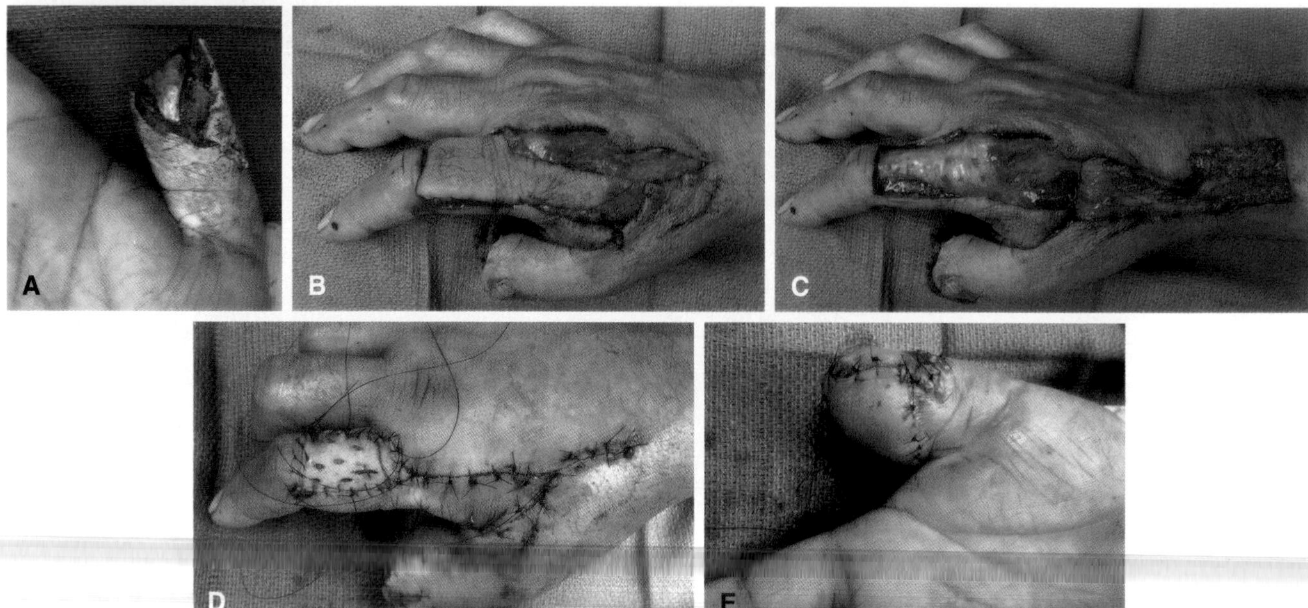

FIGURE 84.2. **A.** Thumb amputation immediately distal to the IP joint. An FDMA flap dissected with proximal skin extension **(B)** and wide soft tissue pedicle preserving paratenon **(C)**. An inset of a flap to tip of thumb without tunneling **(D)** and good tip coverage **(E)**.

flap inset[19] or these nerves can be divided and neurorrhaphy performed to the digital nerves of the thumb.[20] Though this flap has the advantage of being easily executed, the donor site morbidity, need for two operations, and potential index finger and thumb stiffness due to prolonged immobilization[21] limit the routine use of this technique.

Heterodigital Neurovascular Island Pedicle (Littler) Flap

The Littler flap[22] is a flap transferred from the ulnar aspect of the middle finger or radial aspect of the ring finger to the thumb tip. The flap is harvested from the hemipulp of the respective finger and transferred on the neurovascular pedicle after dissection through the palm. The donor site is covered with a skin graft. Due to the inclusion of the donor digital nerve, most patients have s2PD <8 mm but suffer from *double-sensitivity*.[14,23] Cortical reorientation is rare and can take more than 18 months.[23] Division of the nerve and coaptation to the thumb digital nerves result in minimal loss in s2PD (<10 mm) but better cortical integration.[24,25] Due to the issues with donor site morbidity, significant dissection in the palm, and poor cortical reorientation, routine use of this flap should be limited to use in combination with other methods for subtotal thumb reconstruction as discussed later.

Microsurgical Soft Tissue Reconstruction

Microsurgical reconstruction of distal thumb soft tissue defects has the advantage of transferring sensate soft tissue to the thumb while limiting morbidity to the already injured hand. The most common method is the free toe-pulp flap taken from the lateral great toe, though the second toe is an alternative donor site.[26,27] With standard microsurgical techniques, the success of these flaps is greater than 95% and static 2PD <5 mm can be achieved.[27] Partial great and second toe flaps can be customized with skin, skin and bone, and portions of the nail matrix[28] adhering to plastic reconstructive principles of replacing *like-with-like* and maximizing the function and aesthetic appearance of the thumb. Details of flap options anatomy, dissection, and donor site considerations are discussed in the section on toe-transfers.

Amputation Through the Proximal Phalanx With a Preserved MP Joint

Amputations through the proximal phalanx of the thumb can vary widely in their reconstructive requirements. Injuries immediately proximal to the IP joint have a borderline length. They may be salvaged with regional soft tissue coverage techniques to preserve the residual bone and webspace deepening to increase the effective length of the thumb. More proximal injuries require a combination of bony and soft tissue reconstruction for optimal outcomes.

Nonmicrosurgical Techniques

Osteoplastic Reconstruction

Osteoplastic thumb reconstruction is the combination of a bone graft and a skin flap to provide soft tissue coverage over the bone graft. The classic description is an iliac crest bone graft and a pedicled groin flap either in separate (flap followed by graft) or in the same operation.[29,30] These techniques require immobilization for several weeks prior to flap division at the groin. Pedicled flaps from the forearm including the posterior interosseous osteocutaneous and radial forearm osteocutaneous flaps are alternative single stage options. However, this approach does not provide sensibility to the reconstructed thumb and is often augmented with a heterodigital neurovascular island flap at a later operation. Though good functioning of these reconstructions is reported,[31,32] the bulky appearance, bone graft resorption, need for multiple stages, and issues with double sensitivity limit the use of this procedure. One stage sensate osteoplastic reconstruction has been reported[33,34] (Figure 84.3). Though these operations do not require microvascular anastomosis, the complexity of the dissection is significant and provides inferior results compared to microsurgical techniques.[35]

Distraction Lengthening

Matev described distraction lengthening to reconstruct proximal thumb amputations.[36] The technique involves an osteotomy in the metacarpal and placement of an external distractor to lengthen the metacarpal up to 3 cm. The residual defect is left to undergo spontaneous osteogenesis and consolidation or an autologous bone graft can be placed into the defect. A good soft tissue envelope is required at the tip of the thumb to withstand the stress of the process. This technique requires significant patient compliance and can take more than 6 months until a stable construct is complete. Additional soft tissue procedures may be required to provide a durable tip or to deepen the effective webspace.

Microsurgical Reconstruction

Numerous microsurgical options exist for proximal phalanx amputations. Sensate osteocutaneous free flaps such as the radial forearm, lateral arm, or superficial circumflex iliac artery flaps can reconstruct the thumb but may require secondary debulking. As with distal

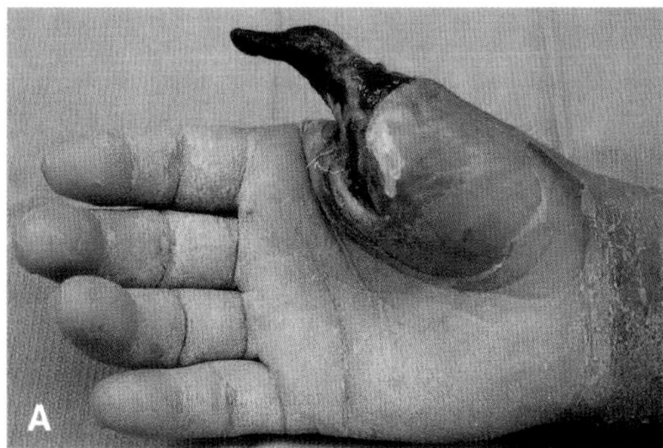

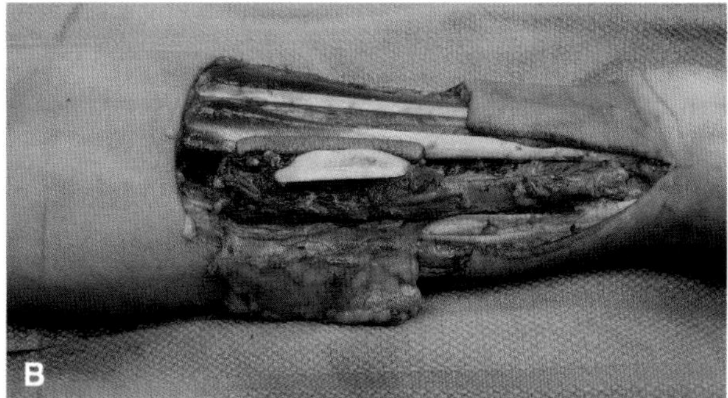

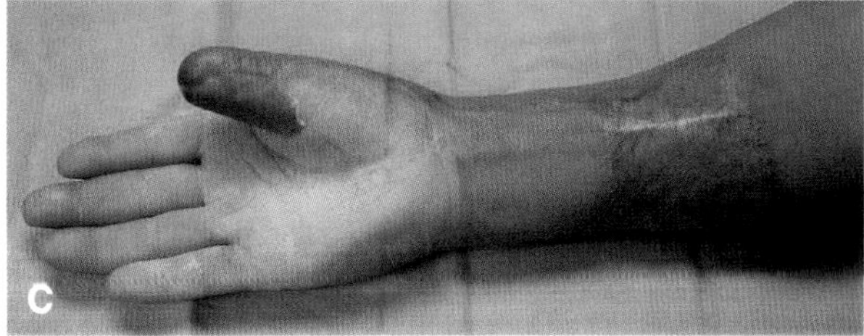

FIGURE 84.3. **A.** Delayed presentation of a ring avulsion of thumb with necrosis of underlying phalanges. **B, C.** Sensate, osteocutaneous radial forearm flap to reconstruct a thumb post.

thumb injuries, toe-to-thumb transfers have the advantage of a single-stage reconstruction and can be tailored to optimally restore a functional and aesthetic thumb. Options from the great and second toe are acceptable. Details of flap options, anatomy, dissection, and donor site considerations are discussed later.

Amputation Through the Metacarpal but With a Preserved TM Joint

These injuries represent a complete loss of the thumb post and require a significant amount of bone and soft tissue. The preserved basilar joint provides stability to the thumb and may provide some degree of abduction and opposition; however, secondary opposition transfers may be required to optimize its function. Additionally, secondary regional flaps or free tissue transfer may be required in injuries that compromise the first webspace.

Nonmicrosurgical Techniques

Osteoplastic reconstruction and distraction lengthening may be options for distal metacarpal amputations, though they will lack an MP joint and serve mostly as a post. Distraction lengthening requires that the majority of the metacarpal remains for placement of the external fixator. Additionally, as the maximum amount of length gained is only 3 cm, it is not likely to adequately create a functional thumb except in the most distal injuries. In proximal metacarpal amputations, osteoplastic reconstruction and distraction lengthening are most successful in combination with other methods such as transfer of an injured index finger ray or microsurgical toe-transfer.

Index Finger On-Top-Plasty

The transfer of an adjacent finger to the thumb position on its intact neurovascular pedicle is called a pollicization (see discussion later). When transferring a partial digit to add length to the reconstructed thumb, the term *on-top-plasty* may be more appropriate. Transfer of an already injured index finger can provide length and sensate soft tissue to reconstruct distal transmetacarpal thumb injuries without the need for microsurgical techniques. With a preexisting injury to the index finger, there may be minimal morbidity to overall hand function; with a fully functioning index finger, loss of grip strength and the resulting three-finger hand provide inferior results when compared to toe-transfer.[37] On-top-plasty may be a suitable option in patients for whom toe-transfer is contraindicated due to comorbidities or the patient's wishes. It may also be a useful adjunct to add length to the proximal thumb in combination with toe-transfer techniques.

Microsurgical Techniques

Toe-to-thumb transfer represents the standard of reconstruction for complete thumb amputations proximal to the MP joint. In distal transmetacarpal injuries, great toe and second toe transfers can provide adequate length and function. However, in more proximal injuries, transfer of the great toe is not an option due to the need to preserve the entire first metatarsal. Transfer of the great toe in these cases will require adjunctive procedures to add metacarpal length in combination with toe-transfer. Details of flap options, anatomy, dissection, and donor site considerations are discussed later.

Amputation With Destruction of the TM Joint

Amputation of the entire thumb metacarpal with loss of the TM joint is a difficult problem with limited reconstructive options. In these cases, special attention to the creation of a stable post with appropriate position relative to the remaining fingers is crucial. These injuries also involve the first webspace and may require regional or free tissue transfer procedures to provide adequate soft tissue for thumb reconstruction and the first webspace.

Pollicization

Pollicization of the index finger (or rarely the long finger) is the best option for reconstruction of these proximal injuries[38] (Figure 84.4). The finger metacarpal is fixed to the scaphoid or the proximal index finger metacarpal base with the MP joint hyperextended to create a TM joint analog. Care to properly position the finger is paramount so it can oppose the remaining fingers. With traumatic thumb amputations, the radial aspect of the index finger is often involved and special consideration must be taken to ensure adequate vascularity to the ulnar aspect of the digit and dorsal veins if microsurgical techniques are to be avoided.[39] Vascularized soft tissue augmentation at the base of the thumb or in the first webspace may be required. Children accommodate extremely well to pollicization in congenital and traumatic cases; however, adults may require a prolonged period of retraining and secondary procedures to optimize the function.

Second-Toe Transfer

Second-toe transfer has been used as an alternative to reconstruct these proximal thumb amputations when pollicization is not an option due to injury to the index finger.[40,41] As much as 5 cm of the second metatarsal may be required to provide adequate length but this has limited donor site morbidity. Motion of the reconstructed

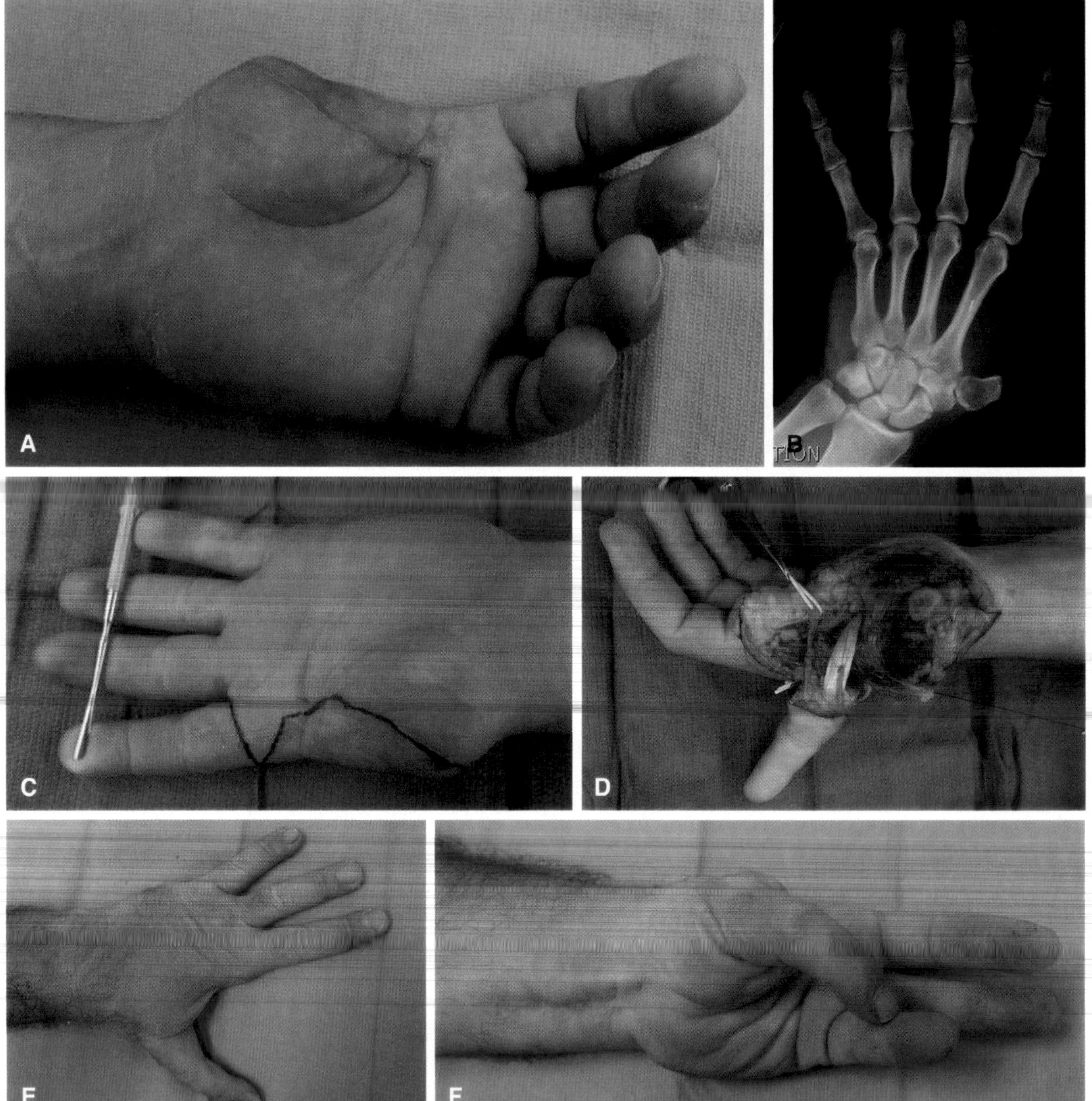

FIGURE 84.4. **A, B.** Amputation of the thumb just distal to the TM joint, with some stiffness of the index finger. **C, D.** Patient elected to undergo pollicization. **E, F.** Postoperative results were excellent.

thumb will be limited to the MTP and IP joints of the thumb, and so special care is needed to properly orient the thumb to oppose the remaining digits. Fixation can be performed to the distal scaphoid or remaining trapezium. Staged reconstruction with a soft tissue flap prior to toe-transfer is usually required to provide coverage for the toe-transfer and new thumb ray.

TOE-TO-THUMB RECONSTRUCTION

The great and second toes provide a multitude of flap options to reconstruct thumb injuries. As discussed previously, this includes isolated thumb pulp soft tissue defects all the way to reconstruction of the entire thumb. All of these flaps are based on the blood supply to the first webspace of the foot, usually from the first dorsal metatarsal artery (FDMtA). There is significant variability in the arterial supply to the first and second toes from the FDMtA and detailed knowledge of this anatomy is crucial to successful transfer.[42] The dominant vascular pedicle can be identified in the first webspace and dissected retrograde without the need for preoperative imaging.[43] One or both of the proper digital nerves and the dorsal nerves are included for neurorrhaphy depending on the flap design. The venous drainage of these flaps is most often the terminal branches of the saphenous vein harvested from the dorsal foot.

Great-Toe Transfer

Great-toe transfer involves isolating the great toe on the FDMtA. Flap harvest is limited to the proximal phalanx of the hallux, preserving at least the entire head of the first metatarsal to avoid uneven plantar weight distribution and unsteady gait. With sacrifice of the great toe, there will be some decrease in push-off strength during ambulation but this is generally well-tolerated. The great toe will appear as a short and broad thumb but has excellent functional outcomes.

Wrap-Around Great-Toe Transfer

The wrap-around toe-transfer is a modification of the great toe flap to preserve all or most of the hallux to avoid donor site morbidity and create a more normal size and contour to the reconstructed thumb. The flap is harvested as an onychocutaneous flap and can include a portion of the distal phalanx. The majority of the toe phalanges and a strip of plantar skin and soft tissue are left behind and the donor site defect reconstructed with a skin graft. The flap is then *wrapped around* a degloved thumb or a bone graft as in traditional osteoplastic techniques.

Trimmed Great-Toe Transfer

The trimmed great-toe transfer is another modification of the standard great-toe transfer designed to improve the appearance of the reconstructed thumb. In this case, the medial skin and dissected off the trimmed-toe flap and a longitudinal osteotomy were performed to remove 2 to 4 mm of the medial phalanges and 4 to 6 mm of the medial prominence at the IP joint. The remaining skin flap is then trimmed and draped over the remaining bone prior to transfer.[44] This technique allows the surgeon to most closely replicate the natural size of the thumb (Figure 84.5). However, due to the longitudinal osteotomy through the IP joint there is some loss of range of motion.

Second-Toe Transfer

The second-toe transfer is an alternative to the great-toe transfer with several advantages. The second toe donor site decreases morbidity to the foot relative to sacrifice of the hallux. The second-toe transfer can also include the majority of the second metatarsal allowing for reconstruction of transmetacarpal thumb amputations. However, the second toe will least resemble a normal thumb in terms of its size and shape. Additionally, the second toe is prone to clawing with hyperextension of the MP joint and flexion of the IP joint and may require capsular procedures to maximize function.[26]

Twisted-Toe Transfer

The twisted-toe transfer is a flap combining tissue from both the great and second toes based on the common FDMtA pedicle. An osteoonychocutaneous flap similar to a trimmed toe is harvested from the lateral great toe and a cutaneous flap is harvested from the medial second toe. The second toe flap is then *twisted* on its pedicle to cover the exposed medial aspect of the great toe flap.[45,46] The advantages of this flap are the creation of a more normal sized thumb and the donor site closure can *recreate* a neo-hallux to minimize donor site morbidity.

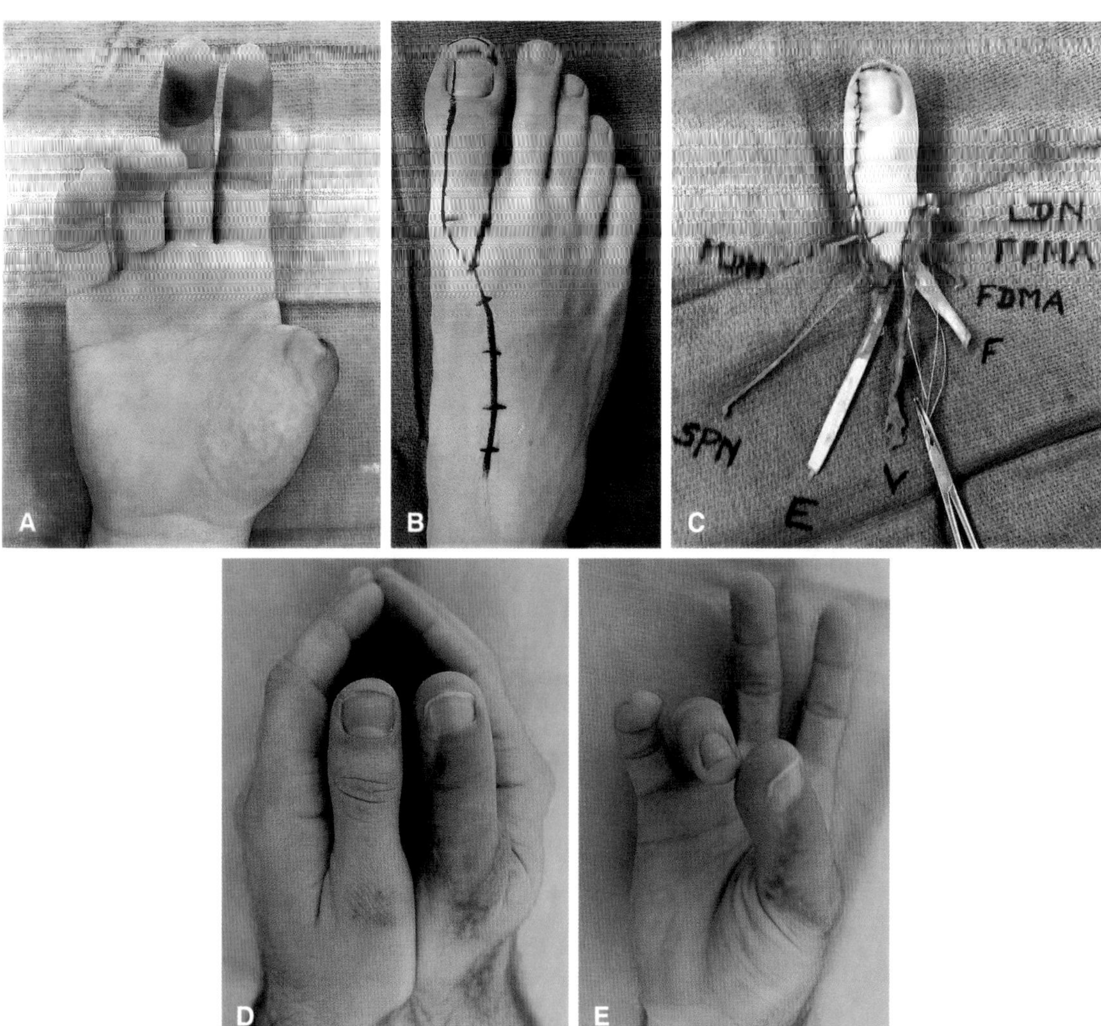

FIGURE 84.5. **A.** Amputation of the thumb distal to the MP joint. **B, C.** The patient underwent trimmed toe-transfer for reconstruction. **D, E.** Postoperative appearance and function were excellent.

Toe Pulp and Distal Trimmed Toe-Transfer

Sensate cutaneous flaps can be harvested from the great and second toes to reconstruct isolated thumb pulp defects. Most often the lateral great toe pulp and medial second toe are selected.[27] These flaps can include portions of the distal phalanx and or nail matrix in a customized fashion to directly reconstruct partial tip amputations, providing optimal aesthetic and functional results.[28,45] Donor sites can be closed primarily, with a skin graft, or amputation of the distal phalanx of the toe. Because of the preservation of most of the donor toes, morbidity is minimal (Figure 84.6).

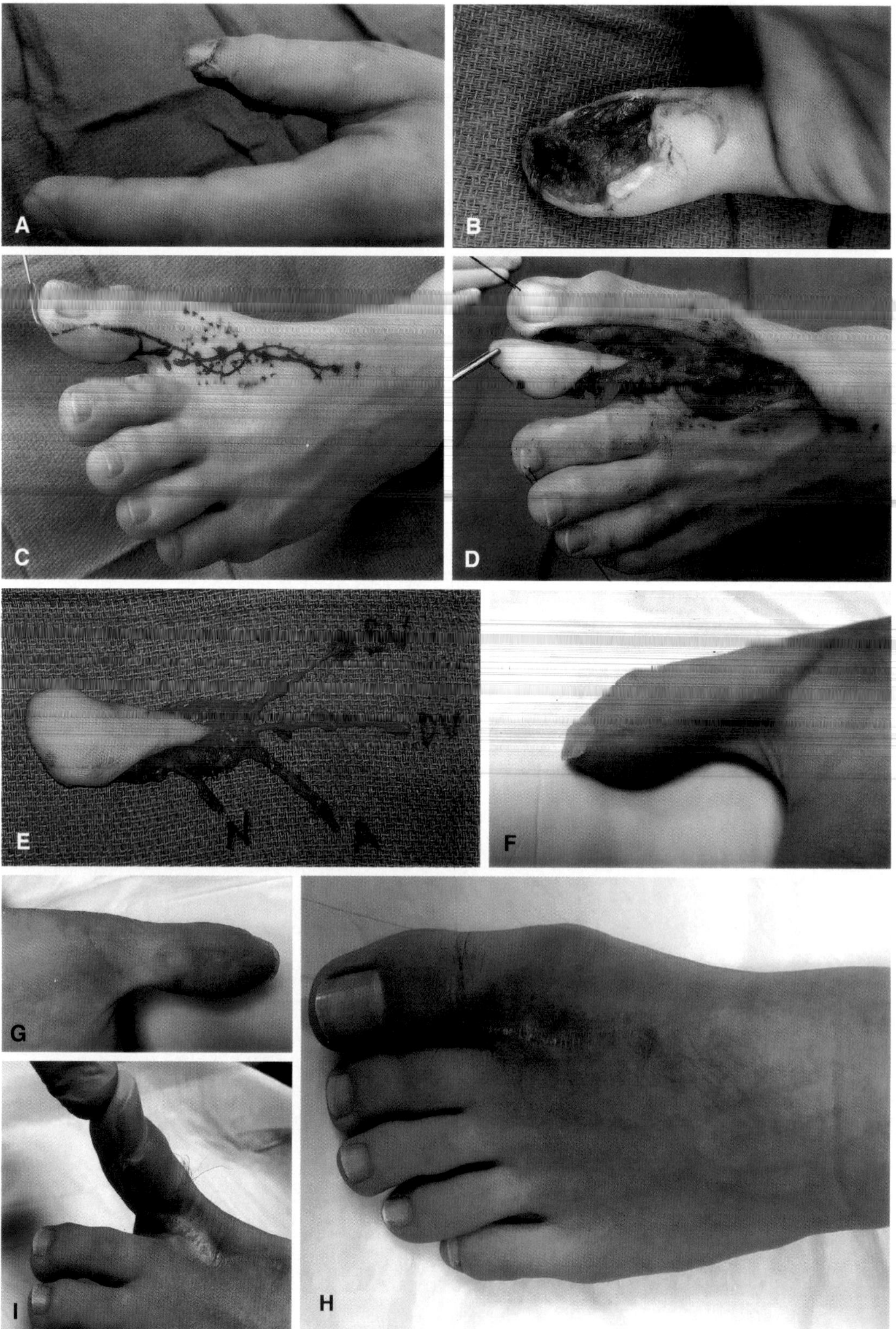

FIGURE 84.6. **A, B.** Partial thumb fingertip amputation with loss of the ulnar pulp. **C–E.** The patient underwent reconstruction with toe-pulp transfer from the ipsilateral great toe. **F, G.** The postoperative appearance is satisfactory at 3 months with slight contracture of the IP joint but return of protective sensation. **H, I.** Minimal donor site morbidity after delayed healing of first webspace incision.

Toe-Transfer Donor Site Morbidity and Outcomes

Donor site complications from toe transfers are common. As much as 35% of patients will have some degree of incisional dehiscence or delayed wound healing. Preservation of the head of the first metatarsal is mandatory to avoid irregular plantar pressure and wear. When the MP joint of the hallux is preserved, both great and second toe transfers have some degree of gait changes, though this is well tolerated in the majority of patients. Additionally, patients with great-toe wrap around transfers have demonstrable changes in gait.[47] Considering this, the major disadvantage of the great-toe transfer relative to the second-toe transfer, with regards to the donor site morbidity, is the change in appearance of the foot and the effect on future footwear (e.g., inability to wear sandals). The twisted-toe technique may minimize these donor site issues.

The survival of toe-transfer techniques is greater than 95% in most series. However, patients must accept the potential loss of the toe-transfer prior to proceeding with this invasive surgery. Functional outcomes of toe-transfer techniques are excellent with good ROM, 70% to 85% grip strength relative to the contralateral side and static 2PD averaging 10 mm. The standard teaching is that the great-toe transfer will result in a stronger and more stable thumb relative to second toe. However, when amputations distal to the MP joint are compared, there are no statistically significant differences between techniques.[48] The decrease in strength seen in some series of second toe transfers may be due to the loss of thenar musculature in proximal amputations where the second toe is required.

In selecting the best option for toe-transfer in thumb amputations, there are several important factors for the surgeon to consider. For injuries in the proximal metacarpal, the second toe is the best option due to the need for additional bony length. The second toe is also preferred in the middle and distal metacarpal amputations; however, these may be salvaged with a great-toe transfer in combination with another method to lengthen the metacarpal. The second important factor is the surgeon's comfort level with the various techniques. The great-toe wrap around, trimmed, and twisted-toe techniques add another layer of complexity onto an already difficult operation. Finally, the surgeon should discuss the donor site morbidity, foot appearance, and the appearance of the reconstructed thumb (Figure 84.7) with the patient and help the patient decide on the best option.

CONCLUSION

Thumb reconstruction is a challenging area of hand surgery due to the functional and aesthetic requirements. However, the rewards for both the patient and surgeon after restoring function to an injured hand are far greater. The evolution of thumb reconstruction since the 19th century demonstrates the ingenuity of surgeons who advanced medical knowledge and technology in hand and plastic surgery, all with the goal to *make a thumb*.[30] Many of the early techniques are still relevant today. However, with increasing experience in microsurgical reconstruction, toe-to-thumb transfer is now the gold-standard as it provides optimal aesthetic and functional outcomes.

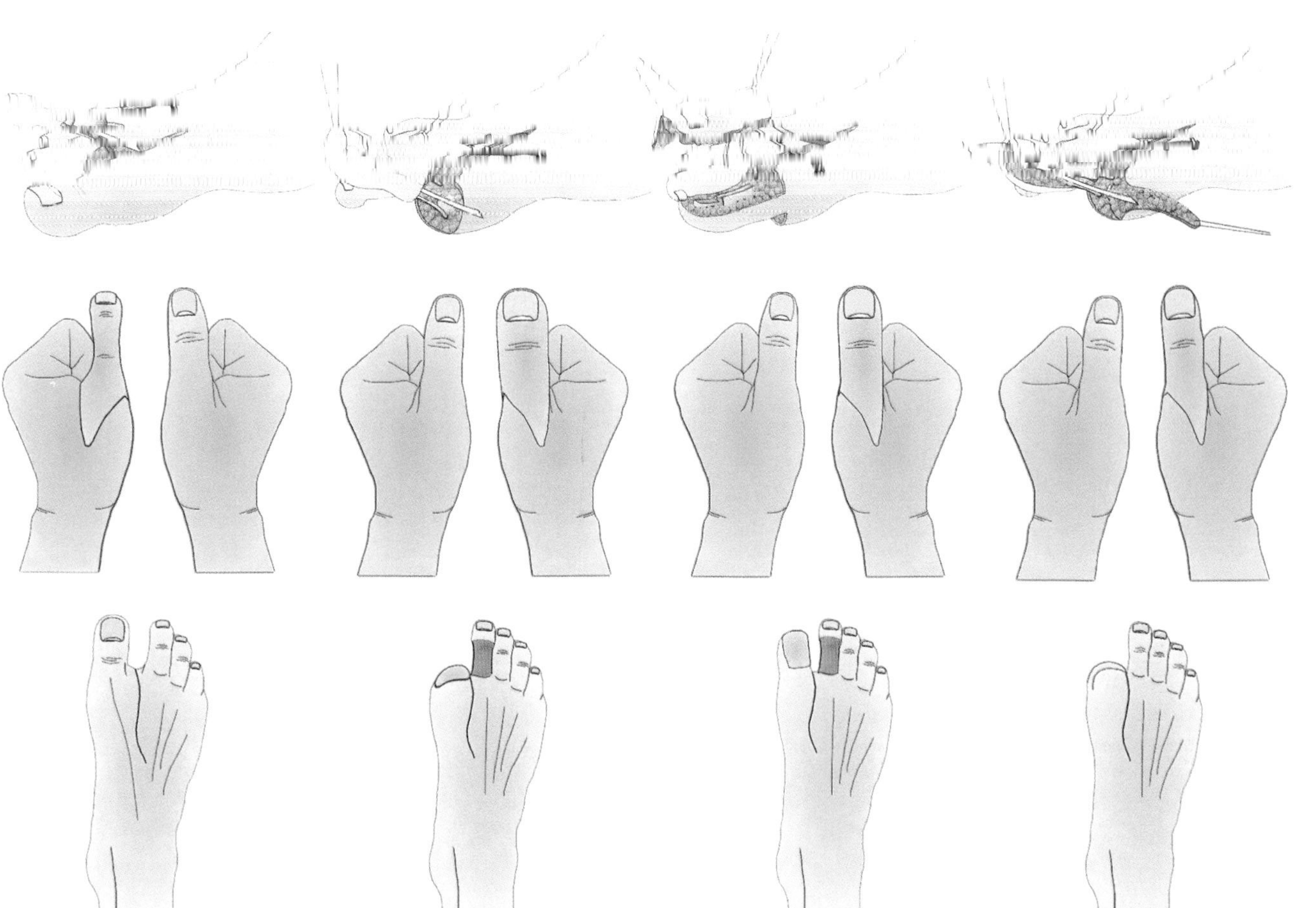

FIGURE 84.7. Diagram depicting the thumb and donor site appearance after great and second toe transfers. (From Lin PY, Sebastin SJ, Ono S, et al. A systematic review of outcomes of toe-to-thumb transfers for isolated traumatic thumb amputation. *Hand*. 2011;6(3):235-243. Copyright © American Association for Hand Surgery.)

REFERENCES

1. Moran SL, Berger RA. Biomechanics and hand trauma: what you need. *Hand Clin.* 2003;19(1):17-31.
   This article provides a detailed and exhaustive review of hand biomechanics as related to trauma. Key points of altered biomechanics that may dictate reconstructive options are discussed.
2. Gupta S, Michelsen-Jost H. Anatomy and function of the thenar muscles. *Hand Clin.* 2012;28(1):1-7.
3. Lister G. The choice of procedure following thumb amputation. *Clin Orthop Rel Res.* 1985;195:45-51.
4. Sebastin SJ, Chung KC. A Systematic review of the outcomes of replantation of distal digital amputation. *Plast Reconstr Surg.* 2011;128(3):723-737.
5. Wei FC, Al Deek NF, Lin YT, et al. Metacarpal-like hand. *Plast Reconstr Surg.* 2018;141(1):128-135.
6. del Piñal F. Severe mutilating injuries to the hand: guidelines for organizing the chaos. *J Plast Reconstr Aesthet Surg.* 2007;60(7):816-827.
   This article presents a simple and thoughtful approach to reconstructing the mangled hand both in the acute and secondary periods.
7. Pet MA, Ko JH, Vedder NB. Reconstruction of the traumatized thumb. *Plast Reconstr Surg.* 2014;134(6):1235-1245.
8. Moberg E. Aspects of sensation in reconstructive surgery of the upper extremity. *J Bone Joint Surg.* 1964;46A(4):1-9.
9. O'Brien B. Neurovascular island pedicle flaps for terminal amputations and digital scars. *Br J Plast Surg.* 1968;21:258-261.
10. Foucher G, Delaere O, Citron N, Molderez A. Long-term outcome of neurovascular palmar advancement flaps for distal thumb injuries. *Br J Plast Surg.* 1999;52:64-68.
11. Baumeister S, Menke H, Wittemann M, Germann G. Functional outcome after the Moberg advancement flap in the thumb. *J Hand Surg.* 2002;27(1):105-114.
12. Foucher G, Braun J-B. A New island flap transfer from the dorsum of the index to the thumb. *Plast Reconstr Surg.* 1979;63(3):344-349.
13. Zhang X, Shao X, Ren C, et al. Reconstruction of thumb pulp defects using a modified kite flap. *J Hand Surg.* 2011;36(10):1597-1603.
14. Delikonstantinou IP, Gravvanis AI, Dimitriou V, et al. Foucher first dorsal metacarpal artery flap versus littler heterodigital neurovascular flap in resurfacing thumb pulp loss defects. *Ann Plast Surg.* 2011;67(2):119-122.
15. Tränkle M, Sauerbier M, Heitmann C, Germann G. Restoration of thumb sensibility with the innervated first dorsal metacarpal artery island flap. *J Hand Surg.* 2003;28(5):758-766.
16. Ratcliffe RJ, Regan PJ, Scerri GV. First dorsal metacarpal artery flap cover for extensive pulp defects in the normal length thumb. *Br J Plast Surg.* 1992;45:544-546.
17. Kleinert HE, McAllister CG, MacDonald CJ, Kutz JE. A critical evaluation of cross finger flaps. *J Trauma.* 1974;14(9):756-763.
18. Woon CY, Lee JY, Teoh LC. Resurfacing hemipulp losses of the thumb: the cross finger flap revisited. *Ann Plast Surg.* 2008;61(4):385-391.
19. Gaul JS. Radial-innervated cross-finger flap from index to provide sensory pulp to injured thumb. *J Bone Joint Surg Am.* 1969;51A(7):1257-1263.
20. Hastings H. Dual innervated index to thumb cross finger or island flap reconstruction. *Microsurgery.* 1987;(8):168-172.
21. Koch H, Kielnhofer A, Hubmer M, Scharnagl E. Donor site morbidity in cross finger flaps. *Br J Plast Surg.* 2005;58(8):1131-1135.
22. Littler JW. The neurovascular pedicle method of digital transposition of the thumb. *Plast Reconstr Surg.* 1953;12(5):303-319.
23. Murray JF, Ord J, Gavlein GE. The neurovascular island pedicle flap. *J Bone Joint Surg Am.* 2006;49A(7):1285-1297.
24. Adani R, Pancaldi C, Castagnetti S, et al. Neurovascular island flap by the disconnecting-reconnecting technique. *J Hand Surg Br.* 1990;15B(1):62-65.
25. Oka Y. Sensory function of the neurovascular island flap in thumb reconstruction: comparison of original and modified procedures. *J Hand Surg.* 2000;25(4):637-643.
26. Foucher G, Binhammer P. Plea to save the great toe in total thumb reconstruction. *Microsurgery.* 1995;16:373-376.
27. Gu JX, Pan JB, Liu HJ, et al. Aesthetic and sensory reconstruction of finger pulp defects using free toe flaps. *Aesth Plast Surg.* 2014;38(1):156-163.
28. Cheng G, Fang G, Hou S, et al. Aesthetic reconstruction of thumb or finger partial defect with trimmed toe-flap transfer. *Microsurgery.* 2007;27(2):74-83.
   A case series of partial trimmed toe flaps to reconstruct small defects of the thumb and fingertips. The clinical cases exemplify the superiority of toe-transfer techniques to maximize form and function in distal thumb injuries.
29. Parmaksizoglu F, Beyzadeoglu T. Composite osteocutaneous groin flap combined with neurovascular island flap for thumb reconstruction. *J Hand Surg Eur Vol.* 2003;28B(5):399-404.
30. Littler JW. On making a thumb: one hundred years of surgical effort. *J Hand Surg.* 1976;1(1):35-51.
   Littler's review of the history of thumb reconstruction discusses the innovative techniques that have evolved into today's gold standards. An essential read for any hand and/or plastic surgeon.
31. Cheema TA, Miller S. One-stage osteoplastic reconstruction of the thumb. *Tech Hand Upper Extrem Surg.* 2009;13(3):130-133.
32. Sabapathy SR, Venkatramani H, Bharathi RR. Functional evaluation of a great toe transfer and the osteoplastic technique for thumb reconstruction in the same individual. *J Hand Surg Eur Vol.* 2003;28B(5):405-408.
33. Yajima H, Tamai S, Yamauchi T. Osteocutaneous radial forearm flap for hand reconstruction. *J Hand Surg.* 1999;24A(3):594-603.
34. Zhang X, Shao X, Ren C, et al. Use of the second dorsal metacarpal artery-based bilobed island flap for thumb reconstruction. *J Reconstr Microsurg.* 2011;28(02):125-132.
35. Lin CH, Mardini S, Lin YT, et al. Osteoplastic thumb ray restoration with or without secondary toe transfer for reconstruction of opposable basic hand function. *Plast Reconstr Surg.* 2008;121(4):1288-1297.
36. Matev IB. Thumb reconstruction through metacarpal bone lengthening. *J Hand Surg.* 1980;5(5):482-487.
37. Michon J, Merle M, Bouchon Y, Foucher G. Functional comparison between pollicization and toe-to-hand transfer for thumb reconstruction. *J Reconstr Microsurg.* 2008;1(2):1-8.
38. Tanzer RC, Littler JW. Reconstruction of the thumb by transposition of an adjacent digit. *Plast Reconstr Surg.* 1948;3(5):533-547.
39. Stern PJ, Lister GD. Pollicization after traumatic amputation of the thumb. *Clin Orthop Rel Res.* 1981;155:85-94.
40. Sabapathy SR, Venkatramani H, Bhardwaj P. Reconstruction of the thumb amputation at the carpometacarpal joint level by groin flap and second toe transfer. *Injury.* 2013;44(3):370-375.
41. Tsai T-M, McCabe S, Beatty ME. Second toe transfer for thumb reconstruction in multiple digit amputations including thumb and basal joint. *Microsurgery.* 1987;8:146-153.
42. Hou Z, Zou J, Wang Z, Zhong S. Anatomical classification of the first dorsal metatarsal artery and its clinical application. *Plast Reconstr Surg.* 2013;132(6):1028e-1039e.
   A detailed discussion of the FDMtA anatomy including important clinical variations. Knowledge of this anatomy is essential prior to undertaking any toe transfer.
43. Wei FC, Silverman RT, Hsu WM. Retrograde dissection of the vascular pedicle in toe harvest. *Plast Reconstr Surg.* 1995;96(5):1211-1214.
   Wei's description of retrograde pedicle dissection in the first webspace is a safe and reliable way to approach toe-transfer without the need for preoperative imaging.
44. Wei FC, Chen HC, Chuang CC, Noordhoff MS. Reconstruction of the thumb with a trimmed-toe transfer technique. *Plast Reconstr Surg.* 1988;82(3):506-513.
45. Foucher G, Merle M, Maneaud M, Michon J. Microsurgical free partial toe transfer in hand reconstruction: a report of 12 cases. *Plast Reconstr Surg.* 1980;65(5):616-626.
46. Kempny T, Paroulek J, Marik V, et al. Further developments in the twisted-toe technique for isolated thumb reconstruction. *Plast Reconstr Surg.* 2013;131(6):871e-879e.
47. Sosin M, Lin C-H, Steinberg J, et al. Functional donor site morbidity after vascularized toe transfer procedures. *Ann Plast Surg.* 2016;76(6):735-742.
   This systematic review compares donor site morbidity after various toe-transfer procedures. The outcomes are important for the physician to understand and discuss with patients prior to choosing the best toe-transfer technique for that patient.
48. Lin P-Y, Sebastin SJ, Ono S, et al. A systematic review of outcomes of toe-to-thumb transfers for isolated traumatic thumb amputation. *Hand.* 2011;6(3):235-243.
   This systematic review compares outcomes of toe-transfer procedures for amputations distal to the MP joint. In general, outcomes for all toe-transfer techniques are excellent. The surgeon must be aware of these outcomes when discussing options with patients.

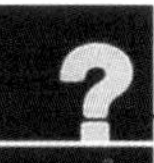

QUESTIONS

1. **A 34-year-old right hand dominant mechanic presents to clinic to discuss options for hand reconstruction. One year earlier he had a significant injury to his right hand from fireworks that resulted in the amputation of his thumb and index finger. On examination, he has functional thenar musculature and approximately 2 cm of thumb metacarpal remaining and a mobile trapeziometacarpal joint. What is the best option to reconstruct his thumb?**
   - **a.** Distraction lengthening
   - **b.** Great-toe transfer
   - **c.** Second-toe transfer
   - **d.** Wrap-around toe-transfer

2. **A 65-year-old right hand dominant man presents with a volar oblique amputation of the distal thumb pulp. The distal phalanx and FPL insertion are exposed within a 2 × 2 cm wound. A Moberg flap is planned. What is the most likely outcome of this reconstructive technique?**
   - **a.** Interphalangeal joint flexion contracture
   - **b.** Lack of functional sensibility
   - **c.** Unaesthetic appearance of the reconstructed thumb
   - **d.** Flap failure

3. **A 32-year-old left hand dominant pianist presents to clinic 3 months after a distal thumb amputation that was treated with a composite graft from the amputated part during the initial ER visit. In clinic, she is noted to be missing 1 cm of the distal phalanx with the proximal portion covered by a [illegible] of glabrous skin graft adherent to bone. There is 4 mm of an intact nail and nail plate dorsally with a hook nail deformity. She would like thumb reconstruction to restore the appearance and function of her thumb. What is the best reconstructive option to achieve these goals?**
   - **a.** Moberg advancement flap
   - **b.** Germinal matrix ablation and first dorsal metacarpal artery flap
   - **c.** Onychoosteocutaneous trimmed toe flap
   - **d.** Second toe pulp flap

4. **A 48-year-old right hand dominant construction worker presents to the ER 1 hour after a saw injury to his left hand. The thumb and index finger were amputated through the proximal phalanges, and the amputated parts were not found. The middle finger is devascularized and has a complex intra-articular fracture through the PIP joint with significant proximal phalanx comminution and only a 4 mm dorsal skin bridge remaining intact. The ring and small finger are devascularized with volar lacerations at the level of the PIP joint but no fractures. What is the best acute operative plan?**
   - **a.** Revascularization of the middle finger, ring, and small fingers; revision amputation of the index and thumb
   - **b.** Revascularization of the middle, ring, and small fingers; revision amputation of the index and FDMA flap to cover the remaining thumb
   - **c.** Revascularization of the ring and small fingers; revision amputation of the index and middle fingers, and a skin graft from amputated parts to cover the thumb tip.
   - **d.** Revascularization of the ring and small fingers; amputation and heterotopic replantation of the middle finger to the thumb; revision amputation of the index finger.

5. **A 40-year-old right-hand-dominant postal worker suffered a severe crush injury to his right hand 2 years earlier. He required amputation of the thumb and index finger and closure of the wound with a groin flap. He now presents for thumb reconstruction. He has normal motion of remaining fingers and a soft, redundant soft tissue flap on the radial aspect of the hand. He has 1.5 cm of the thumb metacarpal remaining and some motion with attempted abduction. The patient elects to undergo second-toe transfer for reconstruction. What secondary procedure will the patient most likely require to maximize hand function after toe-transfer?**
   - **a.** First webspace deepening
   - **b.** Debulking of the thumb
   - **c.** Opponensplasty
   - **d.** Distraction lengthening of the reconstructed thumb

1. **Answer: c.** Due to the significant loss of length in the patient's thumb, adequate reconstruction will require significant bone and soft tissue. Distraction lengthening will not be able to achieve this. Out of the remaining microsurgical options, the second-toe transfer is the only option that can provide the necessary bony length. During harvest of the second toe, a significant portion of the metatarsal can be taken without increased donor site morbidity. However, with great toe transfers, the first metatarsal head must be preserved to prevent destabilization of the foot and gait. Wrap-around toe-transfer would not provide the necessary bone required for optimal reconstruction.

2. **Answer: a.** The Moberg flap is a bipedicle advancement flap of the proximal volar thumb skin. It is very reliable, and because it uses native thumb tissue, it provides near normal sensibility and appearance to the thumb. However, the maximum distance that it can be advanced is 2 cm and this often requires IP joint flexion during inset and may result in a flexion contracture.

3. **Answer: c.** A trimmed great toe flap including portions of the distal phalanx, nail matrix, and skin with its neurovascular pedicle can restore this patient's thumb to near normal appearance and function. The Moberg flap will require significant advancement and result in possible IP joint contracture. The FDMA flap and germinal matrix ablation will provide soft tissue to the tip of the thumb and correct the hook nail deformity but result in an abnormal appearing thumb without a nail. A second toe pulp flap would create durable and sensate soft tissue to the tip but would not restore length to the thumb or the nail.

4. **Answer: d.** In multiple digit amputation and mangled hand injuries involving the thumb, reconstruction of the thumb takes top priority. In this case, the amputated thumb and index finger are not available for replantation. The thumb is amputated through the proximal phalanx which will require a reconstructive procedure to restore function. Revision amputation should not be considered for the thumb. An FDMA flap is not an option given the amputation of the index finger, and a skin graft will provide an inadequate reconstruction. The middle finger has a severe injury with a destroyed proximal phalanx and PIP joint. Revascularization of this finger will not result in a ***functional*** digit. However, the finger can be amputated and the distal portion heterotopically replanted onto the remaining thumb to restore a normal length and near normal function.

5. **Answer: c.** In thumb amputations in the mid-to-proximal metacarpal, there is loss of the thenar muscle insertions and function most importantly the abductor pollicis brevis. The opponens pollicis may provide some motion to proximal metacarpal amputations but will not likely provide adequate strength and abduction. Opponensplasty may be required to maximize this. The first webspace will not likely require deepening given the loss of the index finger and presence of durable soft tissue from a prior groin flap. The second toe does not require debulking to improve appearance or function. The second-toe transfer provides adequate length even in proximal amputations and would not require distraction lengthening.

CHAPTER 85 Dupuytren Disease

Steven C. Haase

KEY POINTS

- Dupuytren disease is a chronic condition without a cure.
- Disease aggressiveness can be predicted by defined risk factors.
- Treatment is indicated for significant contractures and/or disability.
- A detailed knowledge of the disease anatomy can mitigate the risk of surgery.
- Multiple treatment options are available—treatment decisions should be based on available evidence, individual patient characteristics, and the surgeon's clinical experience.
- More aggressive (invasive) treatment options may reduce rate of recurrence, but may be accompanied by increased risk.

Dupuytren disease (DD) is a fibroproliferative disorder affecting the palmar fascia of the hand. In this disease, new tissue is deposited that deforms normal fascial structures (*bands*) into pathologic *cords*. These cords may contract, causing variable contractures of the fingers and/or palm. Many interventions have been described to alleviate the disability associated with these contractures, but there is no cure for this chronic disorder.

HISTORICAL PERSPECTIVE

Medical history enthusiasts continue to discuss who might have been the first to describe the entity we commonly refer to as *Dupuytren disease*. In 1614, Felix Plater of Basel described the case of a stone mason with ridging of the palmar skin that drew the ring and small fingers down into the palm. Whether Plater correctly identified the pathologic cause of the condition is still debated—his exact thoughts may be lost in translation.[1,2]

Many credit Henry Cline, Sr., with first describing this condition in 1777; when in the course of lecturing on anatomy, he dissected two hands to reveal contractures of the palmar fascia. Shortly thereafter, around 1787, he proposed an operative cure by means of palmar fasciotomy, though he had not performed the procedure on a patient at that time. Cline's apprentice, Astley Cooper, ultimately went on to join Cline in practice and publish *A Treatise on Dislocations and Fractures of the Joints*, in which he eloquently describes treating these contractures by means of a small incision to divide the implicated cords—a procedure that sounds much like some of the minimally invasive options used in modern times to treat this condition.[1] Importantly, in this era before the development of anesthesia and antisepsis, very few hand surgeries were performed for nonemergent conditions.

Baron Guillaume Dupuytren, who eventually secured the eponym for this disease, was a prominent Parisian surgeon in the early 19th century. As was perhaps typical of a surgeon in his time and place, he was known for being hard working, but also abrasive. In a famous lecture demonstration in 1831, he recounted his own surgical success with treatment of palmar contractures and then performed his surgical procedure on a patient to illustrate the technique. During the lecture, he gave little credit to Cline and Cooper for their earlier work, and in fact may have misquoted Cooper as stating the disease was incurable. This lecture was reproduced verbatim in the press, and from that point forward, the eponym has persisted.[3,4]

EPIDEMIOLOGY

DD has been described in nearly every ethnicity, but it is certainly most prevalent in persons of Caucasian descent. Studies of DD prevalence may be flawed by difficulty defining the exact study population, or by variability in making the diagnosis of DD.[5] Therefore, prevalence reports tend to vary widely between studies. For example, a 2014 meta-analysis of DD prevalence in Western countries found a range from 0.6% to 31.6%.[6] A population-based US study found that the estimate of prevalence varied between 0.5% and 10.9%, depending on the definition of the disease used.[7] Men are affected more often than women, with increased prevalence between two- and five-fold.[8] Onset is most common in the sixth decade of life; beyond the eighth decade, the incidence of DD in men and women becomes nearly identical.[9] Reports of DD in infants and children are very rare.[10,11]

Nature Versus Nurture

Similar to many other pathologies, DD has both a genetic and an environmental component. Evidence of the genetic influence was nicely demonstrated in a large study of Danish twins, which found that the concordance of DD in monozygotic pairs far exceeded that in dizygotic pairs, meaning genetic factors must be playing a major role. The authors concluded that the heritability of DD was approximately 80%.[12]

Basic science researchers continue to search for the genes responsible for DD. Thus far, no single gene has been implicated, and most scientists believe the exact etiology must be multifactorial. Genome-wide studies have suggested multiple loci are involved, including several genes in the Wnt signaling pathway and others related to the MafB oncogene. The Wnt signaling pathway is linked to a range of diseases; of the nine loci discovered in a genome-wide analysis of DD, six are related to this pathway.[13] The MafB oncogene has the ability to transform fibroblasts and is abundantly found in DD tissue, where it localizes to myofibroblasts.[14] Despite ongoing investigations into these genes, there is currently no genetic test for DD.

Although there is strong evidence supporting a genetic basis for DD, many environmental factors also appear to influence its development. As with studies of disease prevalence, reports of associations with various environmental factors often suffer from bias of one kind or another, which can result in studies that appear to contradict each other. For example, a population study in Iceland concluded an association between DD and manual labor,[15] whereas a large survey study in England found no such association.[16]

Both cigarette and alcohol consumption have been linked with increased prevalence of DD, but a causative factor is not known.[17] Despite the increased prevalence of DD in alcoholics, for example, patients with liver disease due to other causes do not have an increased risk of DD.[18] It is also well documented that there is an increased risk of DD in patients with seizure disorders. Some authors have argued that the association is not truly with epilepsy, but with the common antiseizure drug, phenobarbital.[19] Additional positive associations have also been reported with diabetes mellitus, human immunodeficiency virus, hypercholesterolemia, hypertriglyceridemia, frozen shoulder, and rock climbing, though many of these have not been validated in large, controlled studies. Interestingly, the only apparent *negative* risk factor for the development of DD is the presence of rheumatoid arthritis.[20]

PATHOPHYSIOLOGY

Regardless of the underlying etiologic factors, the common pathway for development of DD is the transformation of fibroblasts to myofibroblasts,[21] a process mediated by transforming growth factor beta.[22] Three stages of DD development have been described[23]:

- Proliferative stage: nodules form as fibroblasts proliferate
- Involutional stage: contractures form, collagen is produced, cellularity reduced
- Residual stage: nodules regress, hypocellular cords remain

One abnormality noted in Dupuytren tissue is the relative abundance of type III collagen compared with normal fascia. This increased ratio of type III to type I collagen in Dupuytren tissue does not appear to be related to a defect in collagen production, but rather a typical reaction to the increased fibroblast density in this disorder.[24]

As DD progresses, physiologic *bands* of fascia become diseased *cords*, causing contractures of the digits. The terminology used to describe bands and cords are presented in Figure 85.1.

In general, pretendinous cords cause metacarpophalangeal joint (MCP) contractures, whereas central and spiral cords cause proximal interphalangeal joint (PIP) contractures. Natatory cords can lead to webspace contractures; this may be referred to as a commissural cord at the thumb-index web. Deep retrovascular cords and extensions of lateral cords have been implicated in distal interphalangeal joint (DIP) contractures.[25] In DD, the DIP joint sometimes becomes contracted in hyperextension, as these cords are often dorsal to the axis of rotation of that joint.

Spiral cords are particularly notorious in that they displace the neurovascular bundle as they contract. Most authors describe the spiral cord as arising from four structures: the pretendinous band, spiral band, lateral digital sheet, and Grayson ligament. Because of these anatomic origins, the course of the spiral cord passes deep to the neurovascular bundle (spiral band) toward the lateral side of the digit, and then continues in Grayson ligament superficial to the bundle. Therefore, as the spiral cord contracts, it displaces the neurovascular bundle proximally, centrally, and superficially related to its native position.[illegible] More often than not, the digital nerve appears to be spiraling around the cord, leading some authors to prefer the term *spiral nerve* rather than *spiral cord*.[25] An ulnar spiral cord of the small finger is sometimes referred to as the *isolated digital cord*. This unique cord originates from the fascia or tendon of the abductor digiti quinti muscle, and it can cause PIP and sometimes DIP contractures of the small finger.

Dupuytren Diathesis

Dupuytren diathesis refers to the presence of certain patient and/or disease characteristics that may indicate a more aggressive form of DD. Specifically, research has tried to identify factors that might predict a greater risk of early recurrence and/or extension of DD following surgical management. Hueston originally coined this term in 1963 and pointed out four distinct factors[27]:

- Bilateral palmar disease
- Family history of DD
- Ectopic disease
- Ethnicity

Ectopic disease refers to other fibroproliferative conditions that are related to DD. Typically, three conditions are considered: Ledderhose disease (plantar fibromatosis), Garrod pads (knuckle pads over the dorsum of the PIP joints), and Peyronie disease (fibrotic disease causing curvature of the penis).

Based on his series of 65 patients, Abe et al. proposed the diathesis criteria should also include the presence radial-sided disease and the presence of surgical disease of the small finger.[28]

In larger series, Hindocha et al. pointed out that male patients and younger patients also tended to have increased risk of recurrence and/or extension. Furthermore, this study showed the risk associated with Garrod pads was higher than that associated with other forms of ectopic disease.[29] This has led us to a modern definition of Dupuytren diathesis to include these additional factors (Table 85.1).

- Male gender
- Bilateral disease
- Family history
- Garrod pads
- Age of onset less than 50

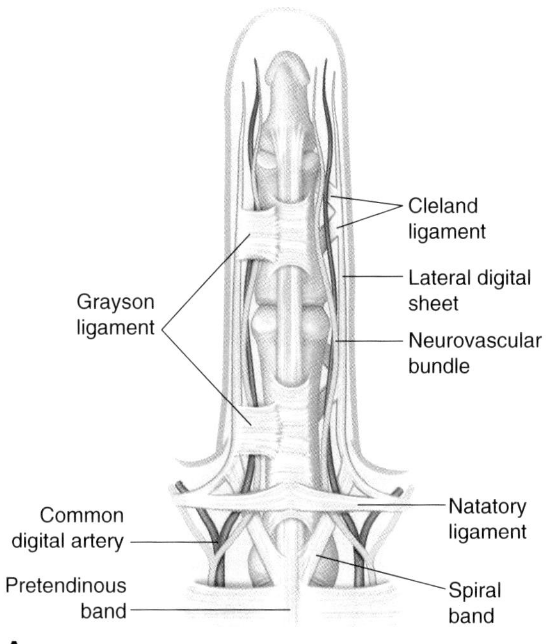

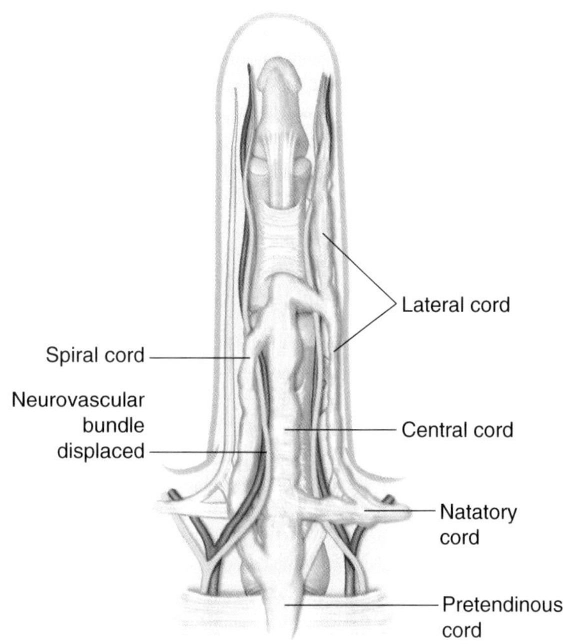

FIGURE 85.1. **A.** Anatomy of normal fascial bands, relative to the native position of the neurovascular bundles. **B.** Anatomy of diseased fascial cords, with consequent displacement of the neurovascular bundle.

TABLE 85.1. DESCRIPTIONS OF DUPUYTREN DIATHESIS
Hueston (1963)[39]
Bilateral palmar disease
Family history of DD
Ectopic disease
Ethnicity
Abe et al. (2004)[28]
Bilateral palmar disease
Small finger surgery
Early onset of disease
Plantar fibrosis
Knuckle pads
Radial side involvement
Hindocha et al. (2006)[29]
Male gender
Bilateral disease
Knuckle pads
Early onset (<50 years)
Family history

TABLE 85.2. NONOPERATIVE OPTIONS FOR DUPUYTREN DISEASE
Pharmacological Therapy
■ Intralesional steroid injection
■ Topical steroids
■ Oral steroids
■ Intramuscular steroids
■ Vitamin E
■ Topical aminosyn
■ Furazolidon injection
■ Hyperbaric oxygen
■ Dimethyl sulfoxide
Physical Therapy
■ Splinting
■ Frictional massage
■ Ultrasound
■ Heat treatment
Radiotherapy
■ External beam radiation

PATIENT EVALUATION

As with any hand surgery patient, evaluation should begin with a detailed history, with special attention to those factors identified earlier (Dupuytren diathesis). Assessing a patient's personal risk for disease recurrence and/or extension is important, especially when approaching a younger patient who will be dealing with this disease for the rest of his/her life. Family history of DD, age of onset, speed of progression, ectopic disease, environmental exposures, and significant comorbidities should all be documented in the medical record. Open-ended questions regarding the impact of the disease on the patient's daily life can be helpful to elucidate the amount of inconvenience and/or disability they are experiencing.

Physical exam should include notation of prominent nodules, cords, and careful measurements of each contracture, preferably made with a goniometer, for maximum accuracy. Staging systems have been developed based on degrees of contracture and joints involved, but these are rarely used in practice, as they are not really helpful in determining a course of treatment. Furthermore, most research studies on DD evaluate the degree of contracture correction at individual joints; the stage of disease is rarely documented.

Patients with mild disease with minimal or absent contractures can still easily place their palm flat on a tabletop. This tabletop test is often used as a simple tool to help patients monitor their disease: if their contractures progress to a point where they can no longer flatten their hand on a table, they should be reevaluated for additional treatment.

TREATMENT

The degree of contracture, chronicity of contracture, associated disability, likelihood of full correction, and chance of recurrence must all be considered before intervention. For example, isolated MCP contractures are easily corrected by many methods, partially because that the collateral ligaments do not become pathologically shortened when these joints are fixed in flexion for significant periods of time. However, PIP joints positioned in flexion for long periods of time develop intrinsic joint contractures, which limit the overall success rates of treatment. For these reasons, mild MCP contractures (less than 30°) can be observed safely, but progressive PIP contractures should have earlier intervention to obtain the best outcome.

Treatment options can be categorized into the following:

- Nonsurgical options
- Minimally invasive options
- Surgical options
- Adjunctive procedures
- Salvage procedures

Nonsurgical Options

A wide variety of nonoperative treatments have been considered for DD (**Table 85.2**).[30] A systematic review of the literature found that only steroid injection and radiotherapy appeared to offer some benefit. Unfortunately, the studies supporting these interventions were hampered by significant sources of bias, and lack of control groups.[31] Patients often ask whether hand therapy, steroid injections, or radiation can be of benefit, but there is no objective evidence for efficacy of these options. Furthermore, although radiation-induced cancers have yet to be reported following treatment for DD, this remains a potential risk after radiotherapy.[32]

Minimally Invasive Options

- Needle aponeurotomy
- Collagenase injection

Needle aponeurotomy, as the name implies, is a procedure that uses a hypodermic needle to disrupt the cord or cords responsible for Dupuytren contractures. This is typically an office-based procedure done with local anesthetic. It has the advantage of a rapid recovery, minimal discomfort, high patient satisfaction, and lower cost than more invasive procedures. However, there is a steep learning curve, and most studies have shown higher and faster rates of recurrence compared to other treatments. There is also a small risk of tendon and/or digital nerve injury.

Needle aponeurotomy can be considered for any symptomatic MCP or PIP joint contracture with a palpable cord, but is not a good choice for patients that have experienced rapid recurrence following treatment or in patients with severe scarring or skin shortening.[33] The effectiveness of needle aponeurotomy is increased by corticosteroid (triamcinolone) injection.[34]

Collagenase injection, specifically with collagenase *Clostridium histolyticum* (CCH) emerged in 2009 as a new option for the treatment of Dupuytren contractures with a palpable cord[35] (see Figure 85.2). Although this is also administered in the office setting with local anesthesia, it requires two separate visits: one for injection of CCH, and one for manipulation of the digit into extension. While the original recommendation was for these procedures to be done on consecutive days, many practitioners have had success with manipulation up to 7 days later.[36] In 2014, the FDA approved CCH for injection in two cords in the same hand simultaneously; this medication is also approved for use in the treatment of Peyronie disease.

CCH injection frequently causes localized bruising and pain, and occasional lymphadenopathy and manipulation-related skin tears. Rarely, tendon ruptures and allergic reactions have been reported. Although it is quite effective, this medication is expensive and is not available in much of the world.

Surgical Options

- Fasciotomy
- Limited fasciectomy
- Radical fasciectomy
- McCash open palm technique

Upon deciding to proceed with open surgery for Dupuytren contracture release, one must still decide on the extent of the procedure to be performed. Patient preference, severity of disease, prior surgical scarring, propensity for recurrence, and surgeon experience may all play a role in the choice of surgical procedure.

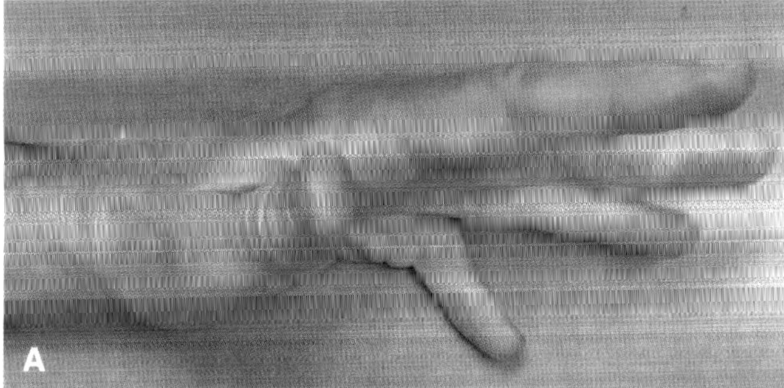

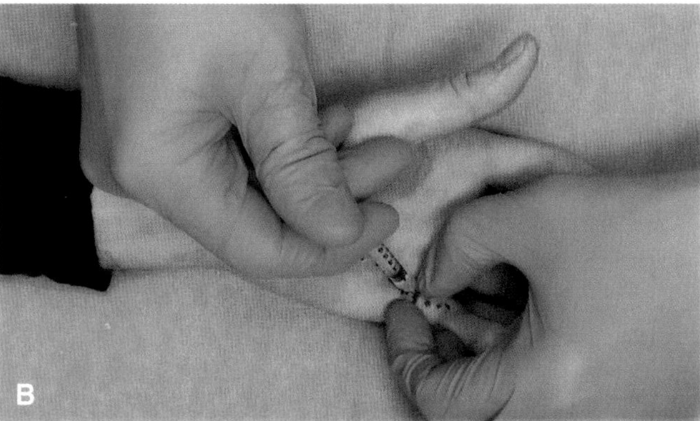

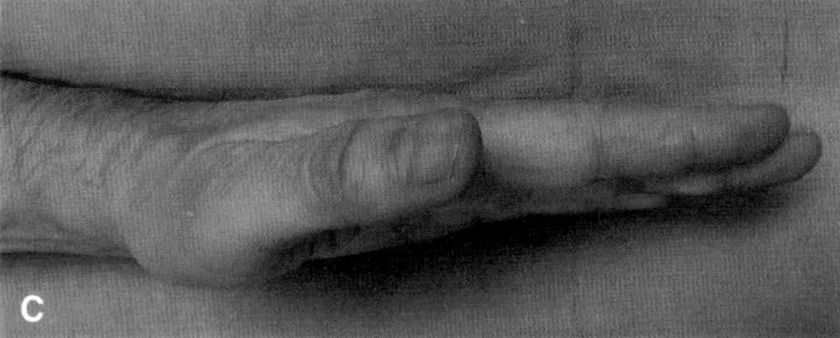

FIGURE 85.2. **A.** Before collagenase treatment, this patient has symptomatic pretendinous and central cords, resulting in contracture of both the MCP and PIP joints of the left small finger. **B.** The collagenase procedure is done in the office under local anesthesia. **C.** One month after treatment, the patient has full extension of both MCP and PIP joints.

Patients with severe comorbidities presenting with simple, narrow Dupuytren cords may be an ideal candidate for simple *fasciotomy* through small skin incision(s). While similar to needle aponeurotomy in some respects, making a small skin incision should afford better visualization of the neurovascular bundles.

Fasciectomy typically requires a more extensive exposure for resection of the diseased fascia and release of contracture. Skin incisions for exposure should be carefully designed, avoiding incisions that cross flexion creases at right angles during closure. This can be accomplished by using zigzag (Bruner) incisions, or by using a longitudinal midline incision that is converted to Z-plasties at each flexion crease at time of closure. Z-plasty closures can add length to the scar, and is very helpful in patients with shortened, scarred skin. Similarly, each of the points in a zigzag incision can be extended into a Y, allowing a Y-to-V closure for each flap, lengthening the incision (Figure 85.3).

At the time of fasciectomy, the surgeon can choose to remove just the diseased fascia (limited fasciectomy) or remove both diseased and nondiseased fascia (radical fasciectomy). In modern practice, radical fasciectomy is uncommonly performed due to its increased morbidity; most surgeons perform limited fasciectomy, concluding the operation once the contracture has been corrected.

The operation commences with elevation of the skin edges and/or flaps (Figure 85.4A and B). Whenever feasible, nondiseased subcutaneous tissue should be left on the skin flaps to preserve as much blood supply to the skin as possible. Dissection of the diseased cord proceeds from proximal to distal in most cases, starting in the proximal palm. At this location, the longitudinal fascial fibers may become diseased, but the deeper, transverse fascial fibers remain disease-free. If dissection remains superficial to these transverse fibers, the underlying superficial arch and common digital vessels and nerves are protected. Once dissection reaches the distal third of the palm, the transverse fascia is no longer present, and the neurovascular bundles should be identified before continuing the dissection into the distal palm and digit

Excision of diseased fascia should proceed until all contractures are released [illegible] If no palpable cords or nodules remain

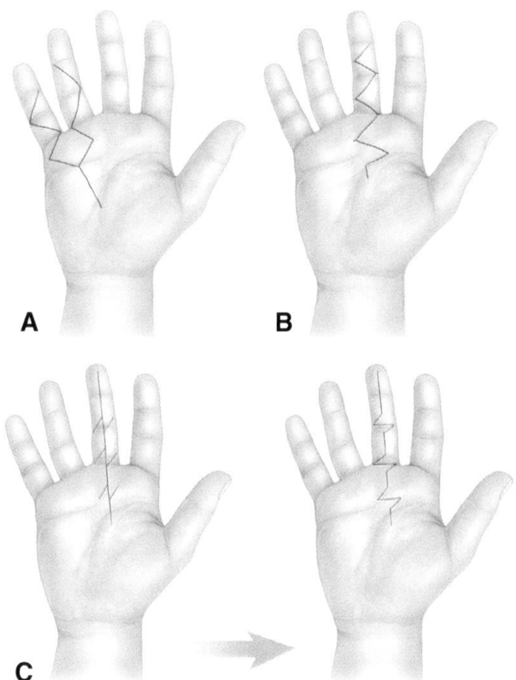

FIGURE 85.3. Incisions useful for Dupuytren fasciectomy. **A.** Classic Bruner (zigzag) incisions. **B.** Modified Bruner incisions, with transverse extensions that can allow for Y-to-V flap closure at each point along the incision. **C.** Longitudinal incision, which is broken up with Z-plasties at time of closure.

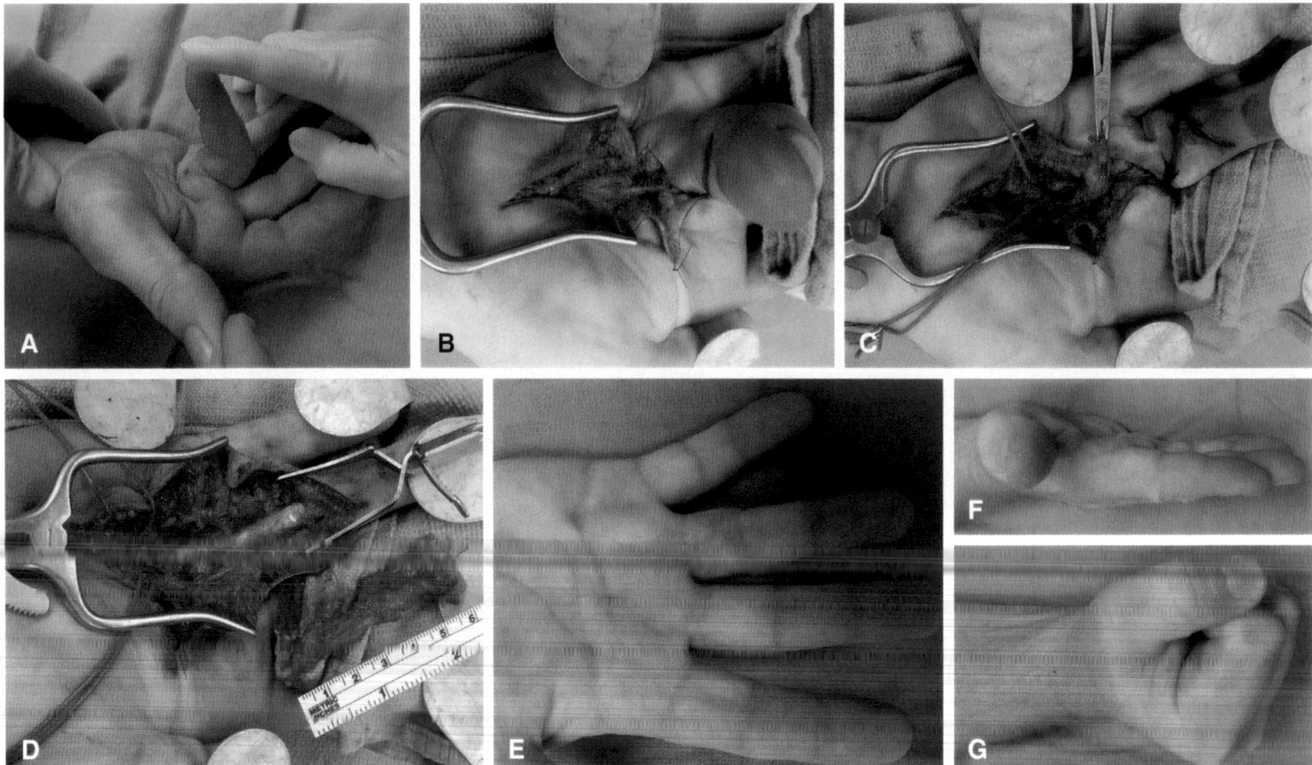

FIGURE 85.4. **A.** Before fasciectomy, this patient had progressive, symptomatic contractures of both the MCP and PIP joints of the right ring finger. **B.** Initial palmar exposure, revealing the pretendinous cord. **C.** The pretendinous cord has been divided and reflected distally, held with a hemostat. The neurovascular bundles have been identified (red vessel loops). **D.** The diseased pretendinous and central cords have been completely excised. **E–G.** Two months after surgery, the patient has well-healed incisions and restoration of normal range of motion.

and joint contractures persist, then some intrinsic joint contracture may be responsible. This is particularly common in cases of PIP joint contracture, and there is some debate as to the utility of additional PIP joint capsulotomy in these cases. Of note, the studies that report no difference in outcomes with capsulotomy were neither prospective nor randomized, and the lack of a control group makes drawing conclusions difficult.[37] In practice, it may be best to proceed with PIP joint capsulotomy and/or ligamentous release in select cases, counseling those patients that they are at higher risk for contracture recurrence.

At the conclusion of the case, skin closure is performed, incorporating Z-plasties or Y-to-V advancements where necessary to lengthen the skin in cases where skin shortening is present. If complete skin closure is not possible, skin grafting can be performed, or wounds can be left open to heal by secondary intention. The latter is certainly not a new concept; Baron Guillaume Dupuytren himself left his patient's wounds open in his well-publicized surgical demonstrations. This technique was popularized in the modern era by McCash, and is often referred to as the McCash open palm technique. McCash advocated transverse incisions in the palm and digits to perform the required fasciectomy, followed by weekly dressings with nonadherent gauze until healed.[38]

Adjunctive Procedures

- *Firebreak* skin grafts
- Dermofasciectomy
- Soft tissue distraction
- Lipofilling

Although McCash advocated leaving fasciectomy wounds open, other authors have encouraged the use of small full-thickness skin grafts when skin closure is not possible without tension. In fact, Hueston believed that full-thickness skin grafts could act as a *firebreak* in DD, as he observed no instances of recurrence in skin-grafted digits.[39] Ketchum reported a similar finding in 24 patients observed for about 4 years postoperatively: no recurrence was noted in any of the full-thickness skin grafts.[40] Based on these findings, Ketchum advocated wide excision of diseased fascia and involved skin (dermofasciectomy), especially in recurrent cases. Of note, Ketchum injected residual Dupuytren disease with triamcinolone as part of his standard surgical protocol.

This finding was challenged by Ullah, who performed a randomized prospective trial comparing patients closed with Z-plasty to those closed using small full-thickness skin grafts at the intended Z-plasty site. No difference in recurrence was noted between the two groups, although these patients did not have heavy skin involvement, nor did they have a shortage of skin at the time of closure.[41] In many ways, these patients were very different from those requiring large excisions of skin and fascia as were reported by Hueston and Ketchum, so direct comparison of these findings is difficult.

Because the fibers of the palmar fascia attach to the skin in multiple locations, it is not surprising that the skin can become directly involved with DD. Indeed, it is often difficult to find a plane of dissection between an adherent fascial nodule and the overlying dermis. This problem is worsened exponentially in cases of recurrent contracture, when postoperative scarring further complicates the dissection. In these cases, wide resection of involved skin and fascia, followed by resurfacing of the entire wound with a full-thickness skin graft, may be the best option to help reduce risk of further recurrence.[42]

Soft tissue distraction has been used to treat Dupuytren contractures, relying on slow steady stretch to help overcome problems with foreshortened skin and other soft tissues. Using devices such as the Digit Widget® (Hand Biomechanics Lab, Sacramento, California), gradual tissue lengthening can be accomplished slowly over a period of weeks or months, making subsequent surgery easier and more successful (Figure 85.5). Problems such as skin deficiency, vascular

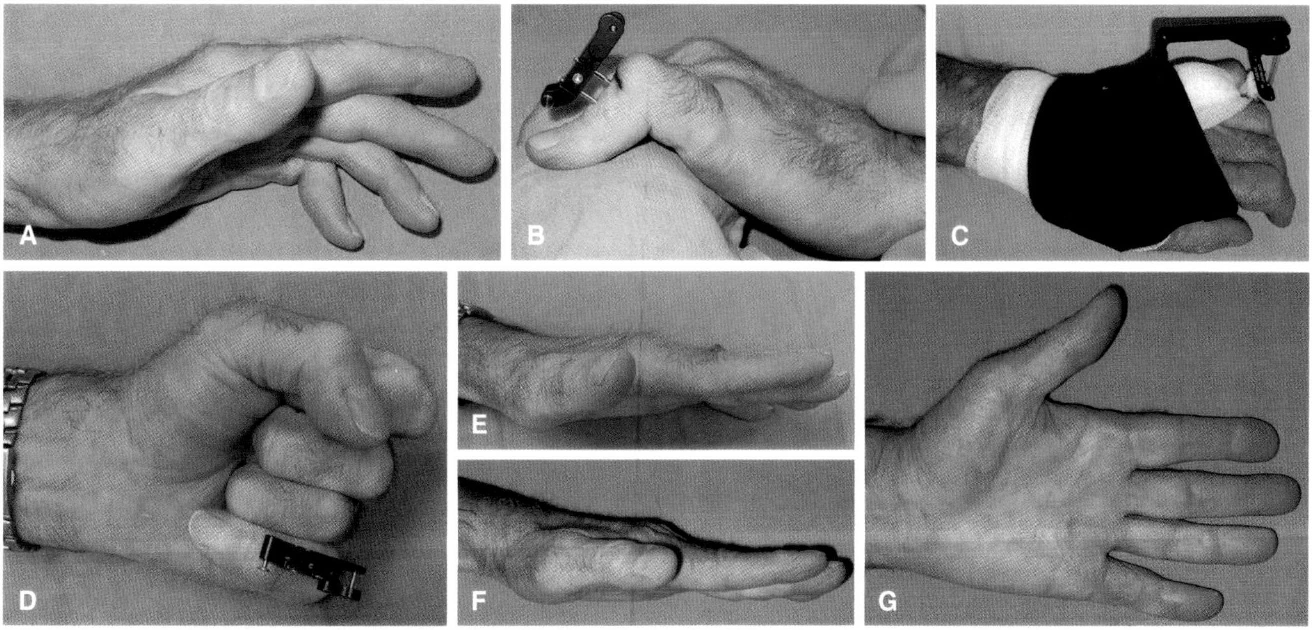

FIGURE 85.5. **A.** Before intervention, this patient had recurrent Dupuytren contracture of the left small finger, primarily affecting the PIP joint. **B.** The Digit Widget® installed on the middle phalanx. **C.** The device connects to a hand-based wrap, using rubberbands to generate constant extension force at the PIP joint. **D, E.** After 2 months of gradual distraction, the finger position is greatly improved. At this time, fasciectomy was performed. **F, G.** Eight weeks after revision fasciectomy, with restoration of normal range of motion.

compromise due to stretched arteries, and intrinsic PIP joint contractures can be overcome with the preliminary distraction. When compared to fasciectomy and checkrein ligament release, this approach was shown to provide a better degree of contracture correction.[43]

Percutaneous aponeurotomy and lipofilling (PALF) has been advocated by some as a viable alternative to standard limited fasciectomy. This procedure begins with a thorough percutaneous aponeurotomy to disintegrate the Dupuytren cord, followed by infiltration of the area with autologous lipoaspirate (lipofilling). Proponents of this technique believe that the fat graft may act in several ways:

- Reduction in myofibroblast density and cell-to-cell contact
- Inhibition of myofibroblast proliferation mediated by adipose-derived stem cells
- Prevention of recurrence by replacing the deficient subdermal fat

In a randomized study of 80 patients, comparing PALF to limited fasciectomy, no difference in recurrence was noted at 1 year. Although the two groups sustained complications at statistically identical rates, the authors report that the fasciectomy group sustained more *permanent complications*.[44] Although these results are encouraging, long-term studies are necessary to prove the effectiveness of this—or any—new technique for correction of Dupuytren contractures.

Salvage Procedures

- Arthrodesis
- Amputation

While salvage procedures are rarely discussed early in the course of this disease, patients who have experienced rapid recurrence after surgery, or complications related to surgery, may have to consider various salvage procedures. It is important for patients to understand that the risk of surgery dramatically increases for each subsequent surgery on a digit. For example, although the risk of nerve injury in a primary limited fasciectomy operation is around 3%, this number increases dramatically for subsequent operations. Roush and Stern reported 68% of patients had some disturbance of sensation at final follow-up after repeat fasciectomy; 11% of fingers had no sensibility.[45]

With this in mind, the overall goal should be to reduce the number of operations on any given digit with DD. For patients with early, severe recurrence, PIP *arthrodesis* is one option that can stabilize the finger position and preserve some finger function. In patients with severe contractures and strong diathesis, repeat fasciectomy with interphalangeal fusion has been shown to preserve total active motion similar to preoperative status, as motion lost from the arthrodesis is offset by motion gained at other joints.

Amputation is considered only as a last resort in DD. Patients with severely contracted digits may experience chronic pain, hygiene issues, and ongoing disability related to the troublesome digit. If multiple attempts at contracture correction are met with early, rapid recurrence, then amputation may be considered a reasonable option, especially in a patient with a strong Dupuytren diathesis, where recurrent contracture appears to be inevitable. Elective amputation should be performed with careful planning, especially in patients already suffering from chronic neuropathic pain. Phantom sensation and phantom pain after surgery cannot be predicted easily, and sometimes pain related to complex regional pain syndrome is not eliminated with an amputation of the involved digit.

OUTCOMES

The physical outcome most commonly reported in Dupuytren studies is range of motion. Specifically, it is important to accurately measure the contracture before an intervention, then define a point in time when it is appropriate to determine the end result after the intervention. Finally, because recurrence is an important concern, studies should consistently report the incidence of contracture recurrence over an appropriate time frame. When one reviews the existing literature on outcomes in DD, one quickly discovers that studies are very inconsistent in their reporting of range of motion, defining recurrence, and in the timing of these assessments.

To help establish consistency in Dupuytren outcome reporting, a consensus group used the Delphi method to establish a definition of recurrence in 2014. They defined recurrent contracture as passive extension deficit of more than 20° for at least one treated joint, in the presence of a palpable cord, compared to the result obtained at time 0. *Time 0* was further defined as between 6 weeks and 3 months after an intervention.[46]

Patient-reported outcomes are increasingly used to evaluate the benefits of one procedure over another from the patient's perspective. Traditional tools such as the disabilities of the arm, shoulder, and hand (DASH) questionnaire and the Michigan Hand Outcomes Questionnaire have both been found to be acceptable and validated for Dupuytren disease. A DD-specific assessment tool has also been developed and validated: the Unité Unité Rhumatologique des Affections de la Main (URAM) scale.[47]

Many published studies have sought to compare the results of common interventions, including surgery, needle aponeurotomy, and collagenase treatment. Not all studies use the same definitions and endpoints, and there is potential for bias, but a review of some of these results can inform the shared decision-making process. Although there are many large case series reported on each of these techniques, showing very optimistic results, the discussion here will focus on the small number of high-level studies that have been published to date.

Van Rijssen et al. performed a randomized controlled trial (RCT) comparing limited fasciectomy to needle aponeurotomy.[48] In their initial publication, the 6-week results were reported. Improvement in contracture was statistically better in the fasciectomy group compared to the needle aponeurotomy group (79% versus 63%). However, DASH scores were significantly lower in the needle aponeurotomy patients at all time points, reflecting less disability after the intervention. In a follow-up study, the 5-year recurrence rates were reported.[49] Patients who underwent limited fasciectomy had significantly fewer recurrences (9 of 78 rays) compared to the needle aponeurotomy group (45 of 88 rays). Fasciectomy patients were also significantly more satisfied with their outcomes, and this was significantly associated with recurrence. This study nicely demonstrated that the more invasive procedure (fasciectomy), while resulting in more short-term disability, has better long-term outcomes due to a lower recurrence rate.

In an effort to compare results among minimally invasive options, several studies have performed head-to-head comparisons of needle aponeurotomy and collagenase treatment. A single-blinded RCT was performed by Strömberg et al. to examine the effectiveness of these two procedures on contractures of the MCP joint of 20° or more.[50] Collagenase injection was found to have more procedural pain than needle aponeurotomy. Final results at 1 year showed no difference between treatment groups in terms of MCP contracture or URAM scores.

Another RCT performed by Scherman et al. looked at these two interventions in patients with involvement of the PIP joint.[51] Reduction of contracture was similar at 3- and 12-month time points between the groups, and collagenase was again noted to be more painful at the time of treatment compared with needle aponeurotomy. Although correction of MCP contracture was maintained at 1 year, PIP joint correction was not maintained in either group. These results were confirmed in a follow-up study reporting this group's 3-year follow-up.[52]

In summary, comparison studies show that needle aponeurotomy has early results equivalent to fasciectomy for cases of mild contracture, but may not be as effective for contractures involving the PIP joint. Although needle aponeurotomy has less disability and pain, it has higher recurrence rates than fasciectomy. At least three RCTs have compared needle aponeurotomy and collagenase; all three have failed to show any long-term difference in recurrence rates.

SUMMARY

Dupuytren disease is a benign—but incurable—fibroproliferative disease with a strong genetic component as well as several environmental associations. The concept of Dupuytren diathesis has helped define risk factors that can help distinguish patients who may have an unfavorable result after intervention (early recurrence or extension of disease). High-level studies to evaluate outcomes show that limited fasciectomy has better durability, but greater short-term disability, compared to the minimally invasive options of needle aponeurotomy and collagenase injection. A patient-centered, shared decision-making process is favored when deciding on interventions for individual patients.[53] Patient risk factors, severity of disease, physician experience, and available resources may all impact the choice of treatment.

REFERENCES

1. Elliot D. The early history of contracture of the palmar fascia. Part 1: the origin of the disease: the curse of the MacCrimmons: the hand of benediction: Cline's contracture. *J Hand Surg Br.* 1988;13:246-253.
2. Belusa L, Selzer AM, Partecke BD. Description of dupuytren disease by the Basel physician and anatomist Felix Plater in 1614. *Handchir Mikrochir Plast Chir.* 1995;27:272-275.
3. Elliot D. The early history of contracture of the palmar fascia. Part 2: the revolution in Paris: Guillaume Dupuytren: Dupuytren's disease. *J Hand Surg Br.* 1988;13:371-378.
4. Osterman AL, Murray PM, Pianta TJ. Cline's contracture: Dupuytren was a thief—a history of surgery for Dupuytren's contracture. In: Eaton CE, Seegenschmiedt MH, Bayat A, et al, eds. *Dupuytren's Disease and Related Hyperproliferative Disorders: Principles, Research, and Clinical Perspectives.* Heidelberg, Germany: Springer; 2012:195-206.
5. Ross DC. Epidemiology of Dupuytren's disease. *Hand Clin.* 1999;15:53-62, vi.
6. Lanting R, Broekstra DC, Werker PM, van den Heuvel ER. A systematic review and meta-analysis on the prevalence of Dupuytren disease in the general population of Western countries. *Plast Reconstr Surg.* 2014;133:593-603.
7. Dibenedetti DB, Nguyen D, Zografos L, et al. Prevalence, incidence, and treatments of Dupuytren's disease in the United States: results from a population-based study. *Hand (NY).* 2011;6:149-158.
8. Hindocha S, McGrouther DA, Bayat A. Epidemiological evaluation of Dupuytren's disease incidence and prevalence rates in relation to etiology. *Hand (NY).* 2009;4:256-269.
9. Thurston AJ. Dupuytren's disease. *J Bone Jt Surg Br.* 2003;85B:469-477.
10. Foucher G, Lequeux C, Medina J, Garcia RN, Nagel D. A congenital hand deformity: Dupuytren's disease. *J Hand Surg Am.* 2001;26:515-517.
11. Urban M, Feldberg L, Janssen A, Elliot D. Dupuytren's disease in children. *J Hand Surg Br.* 1996;21:112-116.
12. Larsen S, Krogsgaard DG, Aagaard Larsen L, et al. Genetic and environmental influences in Dupuytren's disease: a study of 30,330 Danish twin pairs. *J Hand Surg Eur Vol.* 2015;40:171-176.
Twin studies are an elegant way to try to differentiate the influence of genetics versus environment. In this large twin study on Dupuytren disease in the Danish population, the authors found increased concordance in monozygotic twins compared to dizygotic twins, meaning genetic factors must play a major role. Statistically, they concluded that the heritability of DD is approximately 80%.
13. Dolmans GH, Werker PM, Hennies HC, et al. Wnt signaling and Dupuytren's disease. *N Engl J Med.* 2011;365:307-317.
14. Lee LC, Zhang AY, Chong AK, et al. Expression of a novel gene, MafB, in Dupuytren's disease. *J Hand Surg Am.* 2006;31:211-218.
15. Gudmundsson KG, Arngrimsson R, Sigfusson N, et al. Epidemiology of Dupuytren's disease: clinical, serological, and social assessment: the Reykjavik study. *J Clin Epidemiol.* 2000;53:291-296.
16. Early PF. Population studies in Dupuytren's contracture. *J Bone Jt Surg Br.* 1962;44B:602-613.
17. Burge P, Hoy G, Regan P, Milne R. Smoking, alcohol and the risk of Dupuytren's contracture. *J Bone Jt Surg Br.* 1997;79B:206-210.
18. Noble J, Arafa M, Royle SG, et al. The association between alcohol, hepatic pathology and Dupuytren's disease. *J Hand Surg Br.* 1992;17:71-74.
19. Critchley EM, Vakil SD, Hayward HW, Owen VM. Dupuytren's disease in epilepsy: result of prolonged administration of anticonvulsants. *J Neurol Neurosurg Psychiatry.* 1976;39:498-503.
20. Arafa M, Steingold RF, Noble J. The incidence of Dupuytren's disease in patients with rheumatoid arthritis. *J Hand Surg Br.* 1984;9:165-166.
21. Gabbiani G, Majno G. Dupuytren's contracture: fibroblast contraction? An ultrastructural study. *Am J Pathol.* 1972;66:131-146.
22. Badalamente MA, Sampson SP, Hurst LC, et al. The role of transforming growth factor beta in Dupuytren's disease. *J Hand Surg Am.* 1996;21:210-215.
23. Luck JV. Dupuytren's contracture; a new concept of the pathogenesis correlated with surgical management. *J Bone Jt Surg Am.* 1959;41A:635-664.
24. Murrell GA, Francis MJ, Bromley L. The collagen changes of Dupuytren's contracture. *J Hand Surg Br.* 1991;16:263-266.
25. Leibovic SJ. Normal and pathologic anatomy of Dupuytren disease. *Hand Clin.* 2018;34:315-329.
Written by a knowledgeable expert in the field, this detailed description of the normal and pathologic fascial structures of the hand is truly a comprehensive review. Excellent illustrations make the anatomy easy to understand for both the medical student and the seasoned surgeon.
26. Hettiaratchy S, Tonkin MA, Edmunds IA. Spiralling of the neurovascular bundle in Dupuytren's disease. *J Hand Surg Eur Vol.* 2010;35:103-108.
27. Hindocha S. Risk factors, disease associations, and Dupuytren diathesis. *Hand Clin.* 2018;34:307-314.
28. Abe Y, Rokkaku T, Ofuchi S, et al. An objective method to evaluate the risk of recurrence and extension of Dupuytren's disease. *J Hand Surg Br.* 2004;29:427-430.
29. Hindocha S, Stanley JK, Watson S, Bayat A. Dupuytren's diathesis revisited: evaluation of prognostic indicators for risk of disease recurrence. *J Hand Surg Am.* 2006;31:1626-1634.

Knowing a patient's risk factors for recurrence and extension of disease is important for shared decision-making and patient-centered care. This "revisit" of the Dupuytren diathesis is a helpful review of the factors that are statistically associated with poorer outcomes (recurrence and extension) after treatment.

30. Hurst LC, Badalamente MA. Nonoperative treatment of Dupuytren's disease. *Hand Clin*. 1999;15:97-107.
31. Ball C, Izadi D, Verjee LS, et al. Systematic review of non-surgical treatments for early dupuytren's disease. *BMC Musculoskel Disord*. 2016;17:345.
32. Kadhum M, Smock E, Khan A, Fleming A. Radiotherapy in Dupuytren's disease: a systematic review of the evidence. *J Hand Surg Eur Vol*. 2017;42:689-692.
Although radiotherapy is not a common choice for Dupuytren treatment in the United States, it is still something that patients will ask about, as it is often mentioned on informational websites, which patients seek out. This systematic review is a great summary of the data, and reminds us that the studies that have shown some mild benefit were hampered by significant sources of bias.
33. Elzinga KE, Morhart MJ. Needle aponeurotomy for Dupuytren disease. *Hand Clin*. 2018;34:331-344.
34. McMillan C, Binhammer P. Steroid injection and needle aponeurotomy for Dupuytren contracture: a randomized, controlled study. *J Hand Surg Am*. 2012;37:1307-1312.
35. Badalamente MA, Hurst LC. Development of collagenase treatment for Dupuytren disease. *Hand Clin*. 2018;34:345-349.
36. Mickelson DT, Noland SS, Watt AJ, et al. Prospective randomized controlled trial comparing 1- versus 7-day manipulation following collagenase injection for dupuytren contracture. *J Hand Surg Am*. 2014;39:1933-1941, e1.
37. Weinzweig N, Culver JE, Fleegler EJ. Severe contractures of the proximal interphalangeal joint in Dupuytren's disease: combined fasciectomy with capsuloligamentous release versus fasciectomy alone. *Plast Reconstr Surg*. 1996;97:560-566.
38. McCash CR. The open palm technique in Dupuytren's contracture. *Br J Plast Surg*. 1964;17:271-280.
39. Hueston JT. 'Firebreak' grafts in Dupuytren's contracture. *Aust NZ J Surg*. 1984;54:277-281.
40. Ketchum LD, Hixson FP. Dermofasciectomy and full-thickness grafts in the treatment of Dupuytren's contracture. *J Hand Surg Am*. 1987;12:659-664.
41. Ullah AS, Dias JJ, Bhowal B. Does a 'firebreak' full-thickness skin graft prevent recurrence after surgery for Dupuytren's contracture?: a prospective, randomised trial. *J Bone Jt Surg Br*. 2009;91B:374-378.
42. Werker PMN, Degreef I. Alternative and adjunctive [illegible] ease. *Hand Clin*. 2018;34:367-375.
43. Craft RO, Smith AA, Coakley B, et al. Preliminary soft-tissue distraction versus checkrein ligament release after fasciectomy in the treatment of Dupuytren proximal [illegible] *Plast Reconstr Surg*. 2011;128:1107-1113.
44. Kan HJ, Selles RW, van Nieuwenhoven CA, et al. Percutaneous aponeurotomy and lipofilling (PALF) [illegible]
45. Roush TF, Stern PJ. Results following surgery for recurrent Dupuytren's disease. *J Hand Surg Am*. 2000;25:291-296.
This study is an honest, conscientious report of what surgeons can expect when operating on recurrent Dupuytren disease. Drs. Roush and Stern found that 68% of patients had some disturbance of sensation at final evaluation, and a surprising 11% of fingers had no sensibility. These sobering statistics can help us as we counsel patients about reoperation in DD.
46. Felici N, Marcoccio I, Giunta R, et al. Dupuytren contracture recurrence project: reaching consensus on a definition of recurrence. *Handchir Mikrochir Plast Chir*. 2014;46:350-354.
47. Beaudreuil J, Allard A, Zerkak D, et al. Unite Rhumatologique des Affections de la Main (URAM) scale: development and validation of a tool to assess Dupuytren's disease-specific disability. *Arthritis Care Res (Hoboken)*. 2011;63:1448-1455.
48. van Rijssen AL, Gerbrandy FS, Ter Linden H, et al. A comparison of the direct outcomes of percutaneous needle fasciotomy and limited fasciectomy for Dupuytren's disease: a 6-week follow-up study. *J Hand Surg Am*. 2006;31:717-725.
49. van Rijssen AL, ter Linden H, Werker PM. Five-year results of a randomized clinical trial on treatment in Dupuytren's disease: percutaneous needle fasciotomy versus limited fasciectomy. *Plast Reconstr Surg*. 2012;129:469-477.
This randomized trial represents some of the best available outcomes data on the procedures we use to treat DD. It helped confirm the superiority of fasciectomy over needle aponeurotomy with regard to recurrence, but also highlighted the increased disability in the short-term for the more invasive procedure.
50. Stromberg J, Ibsen-Sorensen A, Friden J. Comparison of treatment outcome after collagenase and needle fasciotomy for Dupuytren contracture: a randomized, single-blinded, clinical trial with a 1-year follow-up. *J Hand Surg Am*. 2016;41:873-880.
51. Scherman P, Jenmalm P, Dahlin LB. One-year results of needle fasciotomy and collagenase injection in treatment of Dupuytren's contracture: a two-centre prospective randomized clinical trial. *J Hand Surg Eur Vol*. 2016;41:577-582.
52. Scherman P, Jenmalm P, Dahlin LB. Three-year recurrence of Dupuytren's contracture after needle fasciotomy and collagenase injection: a two-centre randomized controlled trial. *J Hand Surg Eur Vol*. 2018;43(8):836-840.
This multicenter randomized controlled trial aims to answer one of the biggest questions in Dupuytren treatment: which minimally invasive procedure is best? As it turns out, the outcomes are very similar with regard to contracture correction (or lack thereof) between groups, but the collagenase group had more pain associated with treatment.
53. Haase SC, Chung KC. Bringing it all together: a practical approach to the treatment of dupuytren disease. *Hand Clin*. 2018;34:427-436.

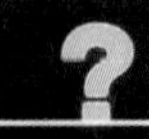

QUESTIONS

1. **Which of the following fascial structures, when diseased, is involved in the creation of a spiral cord?**
   a. Grayson ligament
   b. Cleland ligament
   c. Oblique retinacular ligament
   d. Retrovascular cord
   e. A1 pulley

2. **Which type of collagen is found in greater quantities in Dupuytren tissue as compared to normal fascia?**
   a. Type I
   b. Type II
   c. Type III
   d. Type IV
   e. Type V

3. **Which muscle is involved in the ulnar spiral cord of the small finger, sometimes known as the isolated digital cord?**
   a. Adductor pollicis
   b. Abductor pollicis longus
   c. Abductor pollicis brevis
   d. Abductor digiti quinti
   e. Extensor digiti minimi

4. **Which of the following disease characteristics has *not* been associated with increased risk of recurrence and/or extension of disease following treatment of Dupuytren contracture?**
   a. Male gender
   b. Cigarette smoking
   c. Ectopic disease
   d. Onset before age 50
   e. Family history of Dupuytren disease

5. **Which of the following has been established as a disadvantage of the use of CCH for the treatment of Dupuytren contracture, compared to other treatment options?**
   a. Allergic hypersensitivity
   b. Cost of the medication
   c. Poor wound healing
   d. Unacceptable rate of recurrence
   e. Increased risk of bacterial infection

1. **Answer: a.** The structures that contribute to the spiral cord include the pretendinous band, spiral band, lateral digital sheet, and Grayson ligament. The Cleland ligaments are not typically involved in Dupuytren contracture. The oblique retinacular ligament is a component of the extensor mechanism and is not involved in Dupuytren disease. The retrovascular cord, when present, tends to cause DIP contractures and is not involved in the spiral cord or in displacement of the neurovascular bundle. The A1 pulley is not a typical site of attachment of Dupuytren cords, but is rather the site of triggering in cases of trigger digit.

2. **Answer: c.** Type III collagen is increased in Dupuytren tissue above the levels present in normal fascia. Specifically, the ratio of type III to type I collagen is increased, which appears to be directly related to the increased fibroblast density present in this disorder. Of note, the enzyme CCH (collagenase ***Clostridium histolyticum***) preferentially targets collagen types I and III, but has less effect on collagen type IV. This is important because type IV collagen is a major structural component of the connective tissues surrounding arteries, veins, and nerves.

3. **Answer: d.** When present, the ulnar spiral cord of the small finger often originates from the fascia and/or insertional tendon of the abductor digiti quinti muscle, causing PIP and sometimes DIP contractures of the small finger. The adductor pollicis, as well as the abductor pollicis longus and brevis, all attach to the thumb ray, and are not involved in disease of the small finger. The extensor digiti minimi tendon inserts onto the dorsum of the small finger as part of the extrinsic tendon contribution to the extensor mechanism. The extensor mechanism is not involved in Dupuytren contracture.

4. **Answer: b.** Although cigarette smoking has been associated with increased prevalence of Dupuytren disease, it has not been linked to Dupuytren ***diathesis***, which describes the tendency for patients to experience recurrence and/or extension of disease after treatment. Each of the other factors listed earlier has been identified as part of the Dupuytren diathesis.

5. **Answer: b.** Allergic reactions to CCH have been extraordinarily rare in the case series reported so far. Despite the intent of the enzyme, skin tears sustained during manipulation generally heal within a few weeks; delays in wound healing have not been a problem in the reported series. The rate of recurrence after CCH treatment is comparable—and maybe somewhat better than—needle aponeurotomy. There has been no increased risk of infection after CCH treatment. The main barrier to widespread adoption of CCH treatment is cost: the medication still costs thousands of dollars per treatment, which is a serious barrier to worldwide implementation of this procedure.

CHAPTER 86 Hand Tumors

Mark E. Puhaindran

KEY POINTS

- Soft tissue sarcomas in the hand present early and are frequently mistaken for benign tumors. This has to be taken into account when assessing tumors of the hand.
- Magnetic resonance imaging should be performed for suspicious tumors, followed by an incision or needle biopsy before definitive treatment is decided.
- Epidermal inclusion cysts in the fingertip can mimic infective or malignant conditions—a definitive diagnosis should be made before ablative surgery is performed.
- Most ganglions can be managed conservatively. However, surgical management of mucous cysts of the distal interphalangeal joint should be considered due to the risk of rupture and subsequent infection and septic arthritis.

The hand is a compact structure, with nerves, vessels, muscles and tendons, bone and joints lying close together. Any tumor that arises there would quickly involve adjacent structures. It is also very *visible*, and most tumors are detected when they are small. Although the majority of tumors that arise in the hand and wrist are benign, malignant tumors will also be encountered occasionally.[1] These malignant tumors may not have the typical features of malignancy like a large size or overlying skin changes, and this may lead to a wrong diagnosis and management. Finally, the intricate anatomy and complex functions of the hand and wrist have significant implications on definitive resection and reconstruction. The aim of this chapter is to highlight the clinical assessment of hand masses, the role and limits of different imaging modalities, and principles of management of specific tumors that commonly affect the hand and wrist.

CLINICAL ASSESSMENT

The following points should be covered in the patient history:

- Age
- Onset and rate of progression of mass
- Associated symptoms (pain, numbness and/or weakness)
- Risk factors

In addition, a detailed medical and family history as well as information regarding occupational, recreational, travel, and sexual activity is useful when considering the various differential diagnoses. Other factors that may affect the functional outcome after surgery including the hand dominance, occupation, recreational activities, and general functional status should also be documented.

Tumors arising from the hand and wrist usually present as a painless mass. Skin and subcutaneous masses are often noticed early, particularly over the dorsum where the skin is thin and pliable, and may become painful if located over a bony prominence or if interfering with grip and pinch. Subungual tumors can cause pain, nail deformities, or bleeding. Deeper masses associated with nerves can produce sensory symptoms (e.g., numbness, paresthesia, and pain) or motor symptoms (e.g., weakness, muscle atrophy). Tumors that arise around joints can cause joint stiffness, and masses arising around the flexor sheaths can cause triggering. Finally, osseous tumors may present with acute pain and swelling following pathologic fractures.

During the physical examination, it is important to document the location of the mass, as well as the size, shape, overlying skin changes, temperature, consistency, adherence to adjacent tissues, and whether the mass is tender on palpation. Vascular lesions may be compressible and have an audible bruit and palpable thrill. Transillumination is an invaluable clinical sign when assessing for ganglions. A Tinel test is useful to evaluate masses that arise from, or are located adjacent to nerves. Tumors that arise from tendons or tendon sheaths are usually mobile sideways and move proximally and distally with tendon excursion. The passive and active range of joint motion should be assessed and documented. A vascular examination with Allen's test is essential, especially if the mass is near the radial, ulnar, or digital arteries. For lesions involving the nail complex, abnormal nail pigmentation and deformity (e.g., ridging, loss of adherence) should be looked for. Finally, examine the axilla and epitrochlear regions for lymphadenopathy.

There are many differential diagnoses for hand and wrist masses, and these include nonneoplastic pathologies such as infection (e.g., osteomyelitis, septic arthritis), trauma, autoimmune conditions (e.g., rheumatoid arthritis), and metabolic problems (e.g., gout, calcinosis, and Brown tumors) (Figure 86.1). A detailed history and physical examination as well as selective laboratory and radiologic investigations are required to exclude these possibilities.

INVESTIGATIVE METHODS

Imaging studies, starting with plain radiographs, are main modality for evaluating hand tumors. For soft tissue tumors, soft tissue calcification, bone scalloping, and erosion should be looked for. The following must be assessed for osseous lesions: the bone affected, location within the bone (diaphyseal, metaphyseal, epiphyseal), matrix of the tumor, margins, periosteal reaction, fracture, and presence of a soft tissue component.

Because of the complex skeletal anatomy of the carpus and distal radioulnar joint, CT scans, which provide better resolution and three-dimensional bone anatomy, are frequently needed to augment X-rays to properly assess bony changes.

Ultrasound is a low-cost and readily available modality that can help to assess the nature of the mass (solid versus cystic), the vascularity, and the relative location of the mass. It even has a higher resolution than magnetic resonance imaging (MRI) scans. However, it is operator dependent and is limited in its ability to evaluate more complex masses, and it is difficult to differentiate between benign and malignant masses on ultrasound alone.

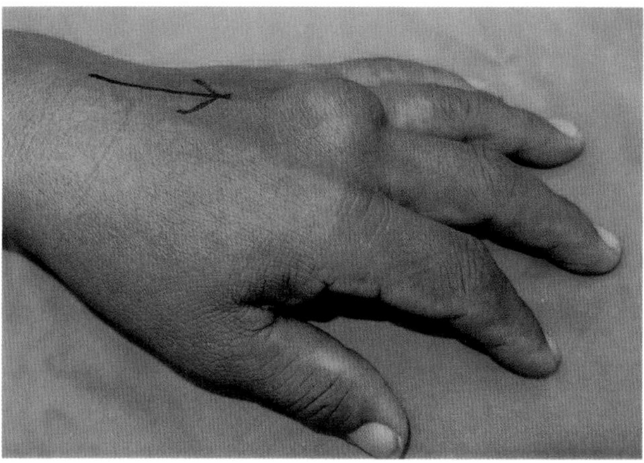

FIGURE 86.1. Solitary gouty tophus arising from the third MCPJ that was initially thought to be a soft tissue tumor.

MRI remains the main modality for imaging complex soft tissues masses. It plays an important role in characterization of tumor activity, with heterogeneous contrast enhancement as well as perilesional edema suggesting a locally aggressive tumor. In addition, MRI can be used to assess response to adjuvant therapy and look for local recurrence in a surgical bed. MRI can also delineate soft tissue compartments and relationship of the mass to neurovascular structures,[4] which is critical when planning surgical excision of the mass, especially in the hand.

Nuclear medicine scans are increasingly used in the evaluation of tumors. Bone scans are used to assess bone activity in the lesion, and can also help to assess for other sites of skeletal involvement. However, they are not specific and cannot differentiate between infection, trauma, and neoplasms. New radionuclides have been introduced in an effort to increase the diagnostic accuracy, with different radionuclides providing different information. For example, 18-FDG (18-flurodeoxyglucose), the most commonly used radionuclide for positron emission tomography scans, will be taken up preferentially by metabolically active tissue such as the brain, as well as a majority of aggressive tumors. This will reflect the metabolic activity of the primary tumour, and help in the detection of metabolically active distant metastases. When nuclear medicine scans are coupled with anatomical imaging such as CT and MRI scans, their utility is further enhanced. 18-FDG positron emission tomography scans can also help to monitor the response to neoadjuvant treatment such as chemotherapy, and can be used as a tool to help prognosticate patients.[5] However, some tumors, such as myxoid liposarcomas, may not be metabolic and have low 18-FDG uptake, which will limit the utility of these scans.

DIFFERENTIATING BENIGN AND MALIGNANT TUMORS

Patients with soft tissue sarcomas classically present with a mass that has been enlarging over weeks to mass. They often have a deep intramuscular location, firm consistency, attachment to surrounding structures, and overlying skin changes with prominent superficial vessels.[6] Many are large, with a size of more than 5 cm. In the hand, however, a majority (77%) of patients with soft tissue sarcomas present with tumors less than 5 cm in greatest dimension. Hence, size should not be the only criterion to rule out malignancy.[2]

Some of the imaging criteria used to differentiate benign from malignant soft tissue tumors include the size, depth of the lesion, and internal signal intensity.[4] However, again because a majority of malignant tumors in the hand are detected when they are small, size is not a useful criterion on imaging. Overall, it may be better to treat all *indeterminate* lesions as potentially malignant, and then an appropriate biopsy done to determine the diagnosis before definitive treatment is initiated (Figure 86.2).

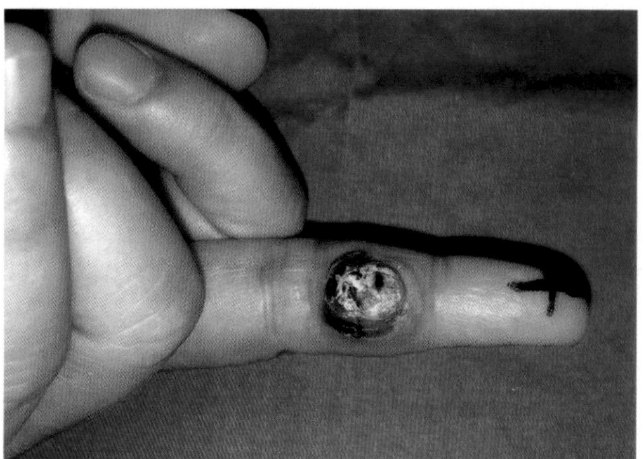

FIGURE 86.2. Fungating lesion arising from the middle finger with aggressive features. However, it was shown to be a pyogenic granuloma on biopsy.

Principles of Biopsy for Suspected Malignant Tumors

The standard for diagnosis is biopsy. A good biopsy helps to provide the diagnosis, and does not compromise the definitive treatment. Conversely, a poorly executed biopsy can have disastrous consequences, with either a wrong diagnosis, compromised definitive treatment, or both.[7] When performing a surgical biopsy for a tumor, the following factors need to be considered:

- The presumptive diagnosis
- The definitive treatment plan (limb salvage versus amputation)
- Who will perform the definitive treatment, and where should it be performed (and should the patient be referred there for the biopsy)
- Whether additional support services (e.g., frozen section, specialized pathology, immunohistochemistry, and molecular diagnostics) are required and available
- Core needle versus open incisional versus excisional biopsy

When performing an open incisional biopsy, the following steps should be observed:

1. Gravity exsanguination
2. Longitudinal skin incision
3. Minimize flaps
4. Avoid tumor spillage
5. Obtain a representative sample (verified with frozen section when necessary)
6. Avoid creating stress risers for bone lesions by creating ovoid bone windows
7. Meticulous hemostasis
8. Drain placement in line with incision
9. Sutures close to edges
10. Bulky, fitting dressings
11. Elevation for edema control
12. Early rehabilitation
13. Splint the affected extremity if required with protected weight bearing for bone biopsies

There are additional considerations when performing a biopsy of the hand, including placement of incisions in relation to skin creases, tendon sheaths, and neurovascular structures. The choice of biopsy incision has to consider the eventual plan for tumor resection, and may differ greatly from traditional operative approaches such as Bruner incisions. Because of this, it is imperative that a surgeon with experience in hand surgery and management of musculoskeletal tumors be involved in the planning and execution of biopsy of hand and wrist tumors. Ideally, the surgeon doing the biopsy should also be the surgeon who will carry out the definitive surgical treatment of the tumor.

MANAGEMENT

Benign Tumors

Marginal excision is sufficient for almost all benign soft tissue tumors. This is performed immediately around the capsule of the tumor, at the interphase with normal tissue. Wide excision, which involves excision of the tumor through a margin of normal tissue, may be required for some benign but locally aggressive tumors such as desmoid tumors.

Intralesional curettage and excision is performed for most benign bone tumors such as enchondromas, in an attempt to preserve as much bone as possible. For locally aggressive bone tumors such as giant cell tumors, local adjuvant treatment using techniques such as cryosurgery or phenol are added to reduce local recurrence rates.

Malignant Tumors

The main objective of surgical treatment for malignant tumors is to completely excise the tumor with negative gross and microscopic margins. For sarcomas, there is no universally agreed margin, but in general, 1 cm of soft tissue, or an appropriate anatomic layer such as fascia, is accepted.[8-10] Closer margins can be accepted to preserve critical neurovascular structures that are not involved by the tumor. In the hand, the margins are invariably narrow due to the closeness of critical structures.

Preoperative radiotherapy and/or chemotherapy can be considered for selected large and/or high-grade tumors, to downstage them and enable effective surgical resection.[11] However, there is a risk of tumor progression during neoadjuvant treatment, and higher wound infection rates are seen in patients that have undergone preoperative radiotherapy.

Postoperative radiotherapy should be considered for patients following resections with close margins or microscopically positive margins.[12,13] Postoperative chemotherapy can also be considered for selected patients with large, high-grade tumors.[14] The decisions on the type of treatment, and the timing that it is administered, should be individualized and made by a multidisciplinary tumor board.

The biopsy track should be excised en bloc together with the main tumor during the definitive resection. Dissection should be done through normal tissue that is not contaminated by tumor. Critical vessels and nerves that are not grossly involved by tumor can be preserved by dissecting through the adventitia or epineurium. Radical resection (resection of the entire anatomic compartment) is no longer routinely required for most patients. At times, amputation may still be required to achieve local tumor control, and should be considered when complete resection of the tumor would result in a limb that is nonfunctional and will be a liability to the patient.

Surgical clips can be used to mark the extent of resection to facilitate subsequent radiotherapy planning. Surgical drains should be inserted close to, and preferably in line with the surgical incision.

The surgeon and the pathologist should review the resection specimen, and mark the margins together, identifying the areas of concern. If a gross positive margin is identified, repeat resection to negative margins should be strongly considered. When a microscopic positive is identified on histological assessment, a repeat resection is advised. However, a microscopically positive margin can be accepted in situations where further resection will result in severe morbidity (e.g., when sacrifice of major vessels or nerves is required).

Hand preservation is possible for most patients with soft tissue sarcomas of the hand, even those with relatively large tumors.[15] At times, partial hand amputations—digit disarticulations or modified ray amputations—may be required.[16]

The final functional outcome depends on the amount of native tissue that can be preserved—the more extensive the resection, the poorer the functional outcome expected. Despite this, the priority of surgery is to remove the tumor, and this objective cannot be compromised in an effort to preserve limb function.

RECONSTRUCTION FOLLOWING TUMOR RESECTION

There is no fixed formula for functional reconstruction of the hand following tumor resection; these decisions have to be made on a case-by-case basis, tailoring treatment to the patient's functional requirements, goals, and expectations. For example, a well-performed ray amputation can result in a more functional hand than a reconstructed digit that is painful, poorly padded, and stiff.

Before planning any reconstruction, it is important to understand the *functional components* of the hand:

- The *radial component* comprises the thumb, index, and middle fingers. These are involved in precision tasks such as key pinch, pulp pinch, and tripod (chuck) grip. Important elements include a stable thumb metacarpophalangeal (MCP) joint, mobile trapeziometacarpal joint, and one or more opposing *posts* (index and middle fingers) that are sensate and of adequate length. Well-functioning thenar, first dorsal interosseous, and adductor pollicis muscles are also crucial.
- The *ulnar component* includes the ring and little fingers, and is principally involved in power grip. This requires painless flexion of the MCP and interphalangeal (IP) joints, intact long flexors, and mobile carpometacarpal joints for the hand to cup around an object.
- The *transverse component* of the hand is needed for activities that require reach as well as pronation and supination. This requires a wide span, provided by the border digits (thumb and little finger), stable MCP joints, a good thumb-index webspace, intact interosseous muscles, and a transverse arch maintained by the underlying palmar fascia.

Reconstruction after tumor reconstruction should follow this general approach[17,18]:

1. Skeletal reconstruction, with or without selective arthrodesis to establish a base for soft tissue support
2. Vascular reconstruction to reestablish distal perfusion, either through direct repair or through vein grafting
3. Soft tissue coverage with skin grafts and/or flaps that will closely replicate the tissue that has been removed. It needs to be durable and, when needed, able to withstand adjuvant treatment such as radiotherapy
4. Functional reconstruction to restore motor and sensory function through tendon transfers, nerve transfers, and free functioning muscle transfers. Functional reconstruction can be delayed until all other treatment has been completed.

SPECIFIC CONSIDERATIONS FOR COMMON HAND TUMORS

Ganglions

Ganglions are the most common soft tissue *tumors* seen in the hand—they are mucin-filled cysts and are not true neoplasms. Ganglions can occur at any age, though they are more commonly seen between the second to fourth decades. They can arise from any joint within the hand and wrist, as well as from tendon sheaths. The most commonly encountered are dorsal wrist ganglions (~70%), followed by volar wrist ganglions (~20%), then ganglions arising from the flexor tendon sheaths and mucous cysts arising from the distal interphalangeal joints.

The walls of ganglions are formed by compressed collagen fibers and lined by flattened cells, and the main constituents of the fluid include hyaluronic acid, glucosamine, albumin, and globulin.[19]

The exact cause of ganglions is not known—the most commonly accepted theory is that a small injury allows the mucin to dissect through the joint capsule and ligament, producing the cyst. The mucin is then prevented from returning to the joint because of the presence of a one-way valve.[20,21]

The diagnosis of a ganglion can be established on careful clinical evaluation—a cystic, occasionally multilobulated, mass that transilluminate (Figure 86.3). X-rays are helpful in evaluating underlying joint changes. MRIs can confirm the diagnosis, as well as identify occult ganglions that may be symptomatic but not clinically detectable.

There are many treatment options for ganglions—simple observation should be considered because up to 50% resolve without treatment,[22] with the rate of spontaneous resolution even higher in children.[23] Other options include aspiration and needle rupture, though this is associated with a high recurrence rate.[24] Various substances such as steroids[25] or hyaluronidase[26] have been injected following aspiration of the ganglion in an attempt to reduce the recurrence rate, albeit with limited success. Injection of sclerosants should be avoided due to the risk of articular cartilage damage.[27]

Excision of ganglions can be done using open or arthroscopic techniques. Open surgery traces the stalk of the ganglion down to the joint capsule and excises it together with a cuff of capsule. Recurrence rates between 0.6% and 40% have been reported following open surgery.[21,28] Arthroscopic resection, though technically more difficult, has the advantage of better visualization of the joint and a better surgical scar, with similar recurrence rates to open surgery.[29]

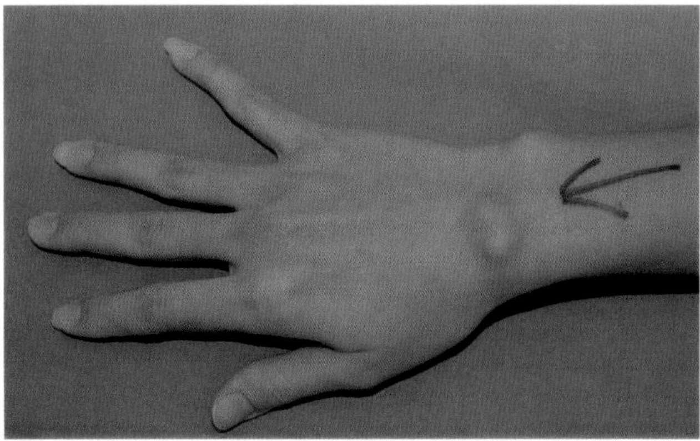

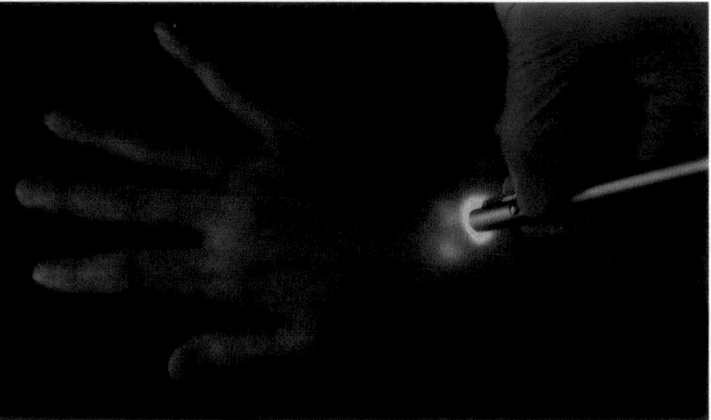

FIGURE 86.3. Patient with a dorsal wrist ganglion that transilluminates brilliantly.

Giant Cell Tumors of Tendon Sheath

Giant cell tumors of tendon sheath are known by various terms, including pigmented villonodular synovitis (PVNS), fibrous xanthoma, and localized nodular synovitis. They are the second most common soft tissue tumors seen in the hand after ganglions (Figure 86.4). Despite the name, these tumors do not always arise from the tendon sheath or contain giant cells.[30] The tumors are firm and nodular, and generally are nontender. They can cause pressure erosions of the underlying bone or rarely, actual bone invasion. These features can be detected on plain radiographs.[31,32]

Marginal excision is the treatment of choice, with recurrence rates of 9% to 27%[30,33] reported. Factors associated with local recurrence include the presence of degenerative joint disease, involvement of the distal interphalangeal joint, radiographic evidence of bone pressure erosion, as well as involvement of the flexor or extensor tendons, or joint capsule. The cause of local recurrence is thought to be due to satellite nodules that are not completely excised during surgery. Malignant transformation of giant cell tumors of tendon sheath has not been reported, though a malignant variant has been described.[34]

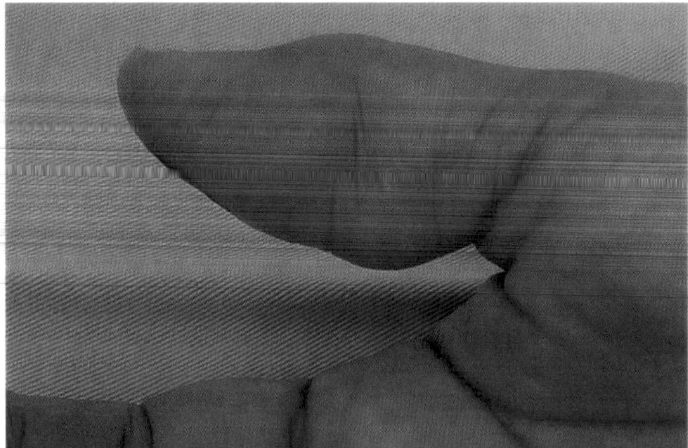

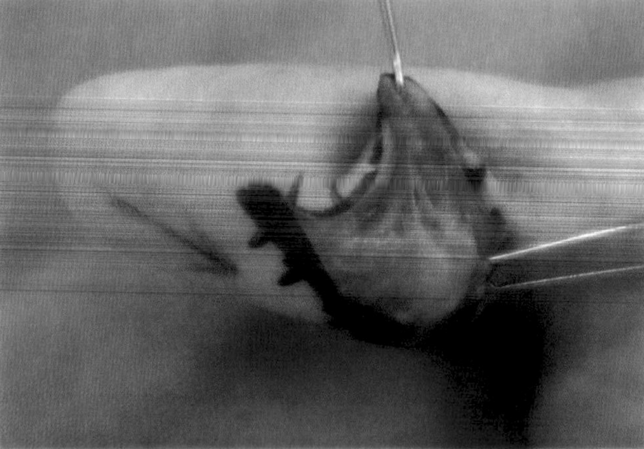

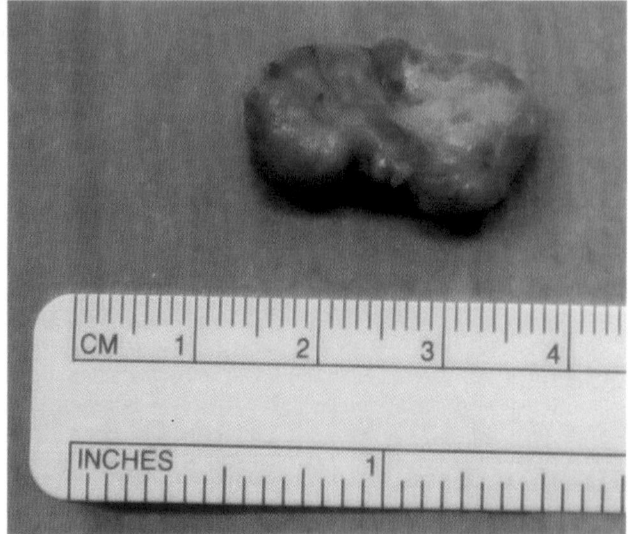

FIGURE 86.4. Patient with PVNS of the thumb that was associated with the ulnar digital nerve. Marginal excision of the mass was performed.

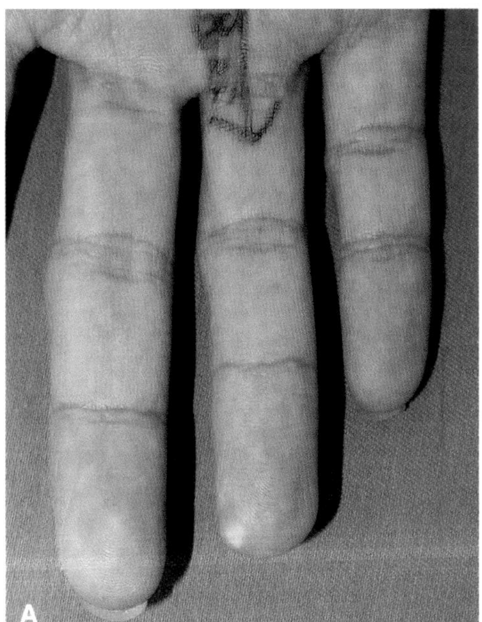

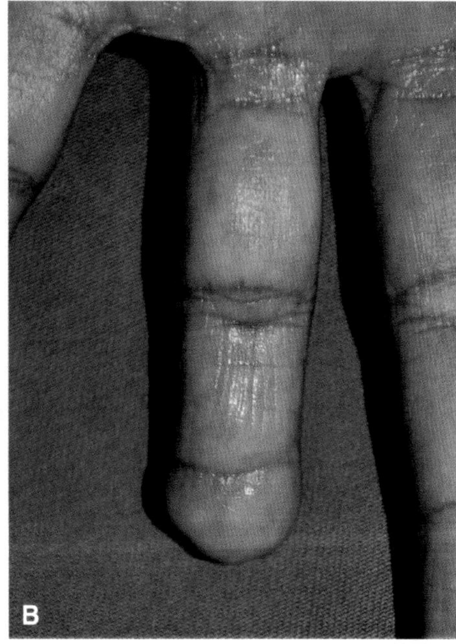

FIGURE 86.5. **A.** Epidermal cyst of the fingertip. **B.** Epidermal cyst in the stump of an amputated finger.

Epidermal Inclusion Cyst

Epidermal inclusion cysts or epidermal cysts are thought to result from the traumatic implantation of epithelial cells into the soft tissue, or even into bone.[35,36] Over a period of months to years, a painless lump forms as these cells grow. Epidermal cysts are frequently seen over the fingertips (Figure 86.5A) and at times even in the stumps of amputated fingers.

Patients most frequently present with a painless mass that has been growing slowly over months to years. Occasionally, the mass may be painful and erythematous. Often, the patient may not recall a prior history of trauma. On examination, cysts in the soft tissue will be firm, well circumscribed, and slightly mobile. Those that involve the bone will be fixed; and they may have a lytic appearance on X-ray. Because of this, epidermal cysts can be mistaken for an infectious or malignant process.[37] Hence, patients with lytic lesions involving the distal phalanx should undergo biopsy to confirm the diagnosis before any definitive surgical treatment is performed. Epidermal inclusion cysts can be treated with a marginal excision with a minimal risk of local recurrence.

Schwannoma

Schwannomas (also known as neurilemomas) are nerve tumors that are commonly seen in the upper extremity.[38-40] These benign tumors arise from the Schwann cells. They are slow-growing, well-circumscribed masses that often lie eccentrically within a peripheral nerve (Figure 86.6).

Patients often present with a painless mass, though they can occasionally present with radiating pain that occurs when the lesion is traumatized, or even neurological deficits. Examination will reveal a firm mass that is often mobile transversely (together with the nerve) and not longitudinally. MRI is the most useful investigation in delineating the lesion, and to identifying the nerve of origin. However, it is often difficult to differentiate a schwannoma from other nerve tumors such as neurofibromas, or even malignant peripheral nerve sheath tumors on MRI alone.[41]

It has been described that schwannomas can be easily dissected and *shelled out* from the nerve fibers. Magnification should be used to separate the nerve fascicles from the tumor mass. Even then, there are tumors that cannot be separated from the nerve fascicles even with the aid of a microscope. Postoperative loss of function has been reported in 2.5% to 30% of patients,[38,42,43] and patients need to be counseled on this possibility before surgery. Local recurrence following tumor excision is rare, and there have been cases of malignant transformation reported.[44]

Enchondroma

Enchondromas are the most common primary bone tumor seen in the hand. They are thought to develop from residual nests of cartilage originally arising from physis.[45] In the hand, enchondromas are most frequently seen in the proximal phalanges, followed by metacarpals and middle phalanges. The small finger ray is the most commonly involved, whereas carpal involvement is rare.[46] They are usually solitary, and are found in the diaphysis of the bone, though larger lesions can occupy almost the entire bone. Multiple enchondromas can be seen in patients with Ollier disease and Maffucci syndrome, where they are also associated with multiple soft tissue hemangiomas. Grossly, enchondromas have a lobulated appearance with a gray-white color. Microscopically, well-differentiated hyaline cartilage is seen surrounded by lamellar bone, with variable calcification of the matrix.

Patients are often asymptomatic, and present with pain and swelling due to a pathological fracture. Digital deformity can be seen in patients with multiple enchondromatosis. The diagnosis can usually

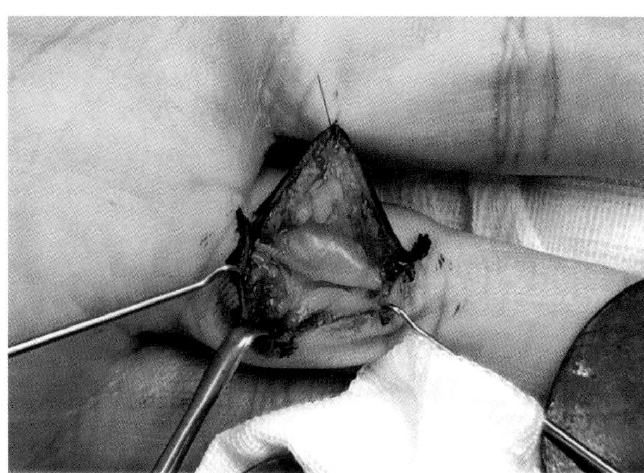

FIGURE 86.6. Schwannoma arising from the digital nerve of a finger.

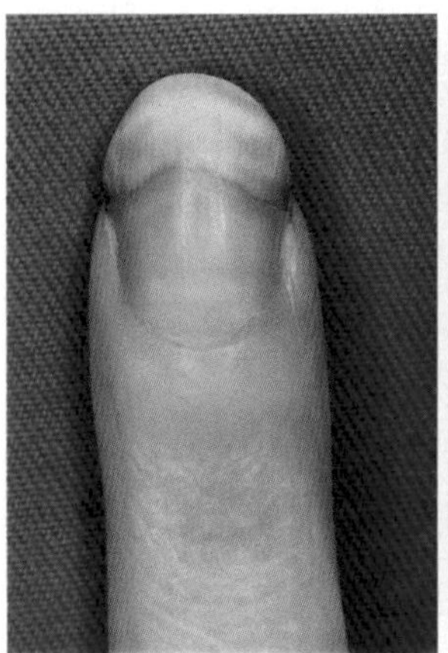
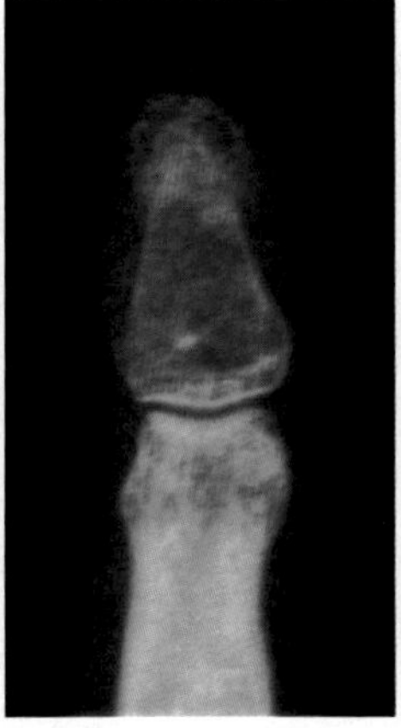
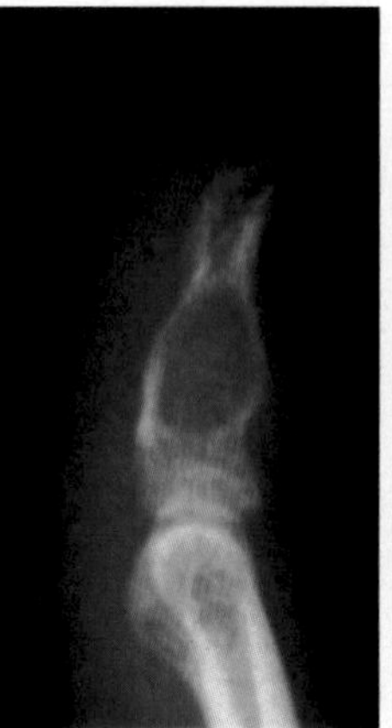
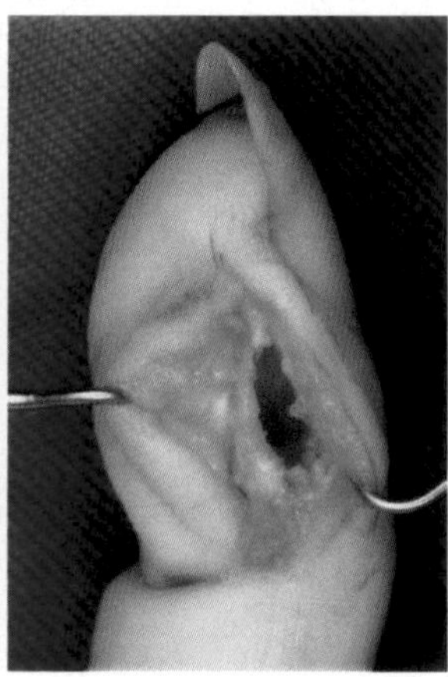
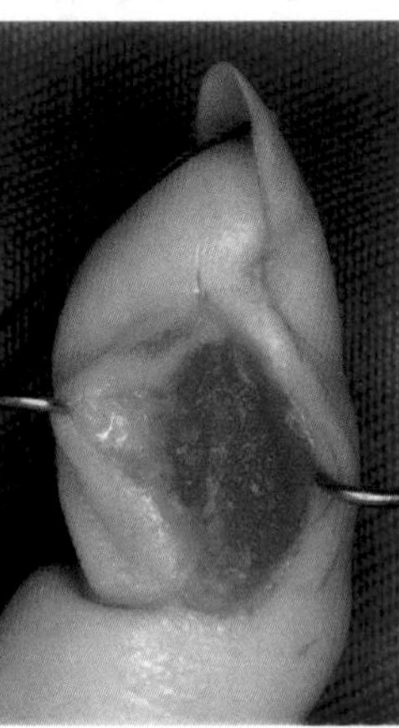

FIGURE 86.7. Patient with enchondroma of the distal phalanx causing nail plate deformity. X-ray showed a lytic bone tumor with expansion and thinning of the cortex. Curettage of the lesion was performed, and the defect was packed with autologous bone graft.

be made with plain radiographs, which will show a lytic diaphyseal lesion, with lobulated margins and endosteal scalloping; the matrix is clear with a chondroid calcification pattern.[45]

Increased pain and swelling may be a sign of malignant change, which is more frequently seen in patients with Ollier disease (25%) and Maffucci syndrome (100%). Features suggestive of malignant change include cortical destruction, loss of matrix mineralization, periosteal reaction, and a soft tissue mass.

Incidental lesions can be observed, with counseling with regards to the risk of pathological fracture. Surgical treatment of enchondromas generally involves intralesional curettage and burring of the cavity with or without local adjuvant treatment such as phenol or cryotherapy. Following removal of the tumor, the techniques for reconstruction of the bone defect that have been described include leaving it alone, cement, bone substitute, allograft, and autograft (Figure 86.7). For patients who present following pathological fractures, there is the option of early definitive treatment with intralesional curettage, bone grafting and internal fixation, or staged treatment with closed treatment of the fracture followed by delayed surgery once fracture union has occurred.[47] In the event of an atypical clinical presentation, or if there are suspicious radiographic findings, a biopsy should be considered before definitive treatment.

Soft Tissue Sarcomas

Sarcomas originate from the embryonic mesodermal layer, and there are more than 50 histological subtypes that have been described. The classification systems used continually evolve along with pathology diagnostic techniques (immunohistochemistry and molecular studies).

Soft tissue sarcomas of the hand were initially thought to have a poorer prognosis than tumors arising elsewhere in the extremities.[48] More recent publications suggest that the reverse is possibly true, with patients with hand sarcomas appearing to have a better prognosis.[2,49] Part of the reason could be that patients with hand tumors present earlier with small tumors. The balance between the need for complete excision of the tumor, with the desire to preserve maximum function in the affected limb, is even more challenging in the narrow confines of the hand. Continuing improvements in imaging techniques such as MRI allow better imaging and delineation of the tumor, and greatly assist surgical planning. This then results in better surgery that preserves more native tissue, while achieving the required negative resection margins, improving the overall outcomes for patients.

REFERENCES

1. Schultz RJ, Kearns RJ. Tumors in the hand. *J Hand Surg Am*. 1983;8(5 pt 2):803-806.
This article provides an overview on the types of hand tumors encountered in a hand surgery practice, This article provides an overview on the types of hand tumors encountered in a hand surgery practice. Ganglions are the most common, followed by PVNS. Malignant tumors are rarely encountered.
2. Puhaindran ME, Rohde RS, Chou J, et al. Clinical outcomes for patients with soft tissue sarcoma of the hand. *Cancer*. 2011;117(1):175-179.
This is the largest published series on soft tissue sarcomas of the hand. It showed that the majority patients with soft tissue sarcomas of the hand present early (<5 cm) and are misdiagnosed (large number of excision biopsies). Despite this, overall survival is good.
3. Miller TT. Bone tumors and tumorlike conditions: analysis with conventional radiography. *Radiology*. 2008;246(3):662-674.
4. Wu JS, Hochman MG. Soft-tissue tumors and tumorlike lesions: a systematic imaging approach. *Radiology*. 2009;253(2):297-316.
5. Kubo T, Furuta T, Johan MP, Ochi M. Prognostic significance of (18)F-FDG PET at diagnosis in patients with soft tissue sarcoma and bone sarcoma; systematic review and meta-analysis. *Eur J Cancer*. 2016;58:104-111.
6. Myhre-Jensen O. A Consecutive 7-year series of 1331 benign soft tissue tumours. clinicopathologic data: comparison with sarcomas. *Acta Orthop Scand*. 1981;52(3):287-293.
7. Mankin HJ, Mankin CJ, Simon MA. The hazards of the biopsy, revisited. Members of the musculoskeletal tumor society. *J Bone Joint Surg Am*. 1996;78A:656-663.
Second article on the hazards of biopsy published by members of the Musculoskeletal Tumor Society. Unfortunately, the first article did not have its desired impact, and a large number of the patients reviewed in this article still had poorly performed biopsies that compromised outcomes.
8. ESMO/European Sarcoma Network Working Group. Soft tissue and visceral sarcomas: ESMO clinical practice guidelines for diagnosis, treatment and follow-up. *Ann Oncol* 2012;23(suppl 7)vii92-vii99.
9. Grimer RJ, Athanasou N, Gerrand C, et al. UK guidelines for the management of bone sarcomas. *Sarcoma*. 2010;2010:317462.
10. von Mehren M, Randall RL, Benjamin RS, et al. Soft tissue sarcoma, version 2.2014. *J Natl Compr Canc Netw*. 2014;12:473-483.
11. O'Sullivan B, Davis AM, Turcotte R, et al. Preoperative versus postoperative radiotherapy in soft-tissue sarcoma of the limbs: a randomised trial. *Lancet*. 2002;359(9325):2235-2241.
12. Pisters PW, Harrison LB, Leung DH, et al. Long-term results of a prospective randomized trial of adjuvant brachytherapy in soft tissue sarcoma. *J Clin Oncol*. 1996;14(3):859-868.
13. Yang JC, Chang AE, Baker AR, et al. Randomized prospective study of the benefit of adjuvant radiation therapy in the treatment of soft tissue sarcomas of the extremity. *J Clin Oncol*. 1998;16(1):197-203.
14. Pervaiz N, Colterjohn N, Farrokhyar F, et al. A systematic meta-analysis of randomized controlled trials of adjuvant chemotherapy for localized resectable soft-tissue sarcoma. *Cancer*. 2008;113(3):573-581.
15. Puhaindran ME, Steensma MR, Athanasian EA. Partial hand preservation for large soft tissue sarcomas of the hand. *J Hand Surg Am*. 2010;35(2):291-295.
16. Puhaindran ME, Healey JH, Athanasian EA. Single ray amputation for tumors of the hand. *Clin Orthop Relat Res*. 2010;468(5):1390-1395.
17. Talbot SG, Mehrara BJ, Disa JJ, et al. Soft-tissue coverage of the hand following sarcoma resection. *Plast Reconstr Surg*. 2008;121(2):534-543.
18. Mehrara BJ, Abood AA, Disa JJ, et al. Thumb reconstruction following resection for malignant tumors. *Plast Reconstr Surg*. 2008;121(4):1279-1287.
19. Loder RT, Robinson JH, Jackson WT, Allen DJ. A surface ultrastructure study of ganglia and digital mucous cysts. *J Hand Surg Am*. 1988;13:758-762.
20. Jayson MI, Dixon AS. Valvular mechanism in juxta-articular cysts. *Ann Rheum Dis*. 1970;29:415-420.
21. Angelides AC, Wallace PF. The dorsal ganglion of the wrist: its pathogenesis, gross and microscopic anatomy, and surgical treatment. *J Hand Surg Am*. 1976;1:228-235.
22. McEvedy BV. The simple ganglion. *Lancet*. 1954;1:135.
Classic article on ganglions, reviewing the natural history, anatomy, pathogenesis, and options for treatment.
23. Rosson JW, Walker G. The natural history of ganglia in children. *J Bone Joint Surg Br*. 1989;71B:707.
24. Stephen AB, Lyons AR, Davis TR. A prospective study of two conservative treatments for ganglia of the wrist. *J Hand Surg Br*. 1999;24;104-105.

25. Varley GW, Needoff M, Davis TR, Clay NR. Conservative management of wrist ganglia: aspiration versus steroid infiltration. *J Hand Surg Br*. 1997;22:636-637.
26. Paul AS, Sochart DH. Improving the results of ganglion aspiration by the use of hyaluronidase. *J Hand Surg Br*. 1997;22:219-221.
27. Mackie IG, Howard CB, Wilkins P. The dangers of sclerotherapy in the treatment of ganglia. *J Hand Surg Br*. 1984;9:181.
28. Thornburg LE. Ganglions of the hand and wrist. *J Am Acad Orthop Surg*. 1999;7:231-238.
29. Rizzo M, Berger RA, Steinmann SP, Bishop AT. Arthroscopic resection in the management of dorsal wrist ganglions: results with a minimum 2-year follow-up period. *J Hand Surg*. 2004;29A:59-62.
30. Moore JR, Weiland AJ, Curtis RM. Localized nodular tenosynovitis: experience with 115 cases. *J Hand Surg Am*. 1984;9(3):412-417.
Broad overview on the presentation and management for PVNS of the hand.
31. Karasick D, Karasick S. Giant cell tumor of tendon sheath: spectrum of radiologic findings. *Skeletal Radiol*. 1992;21(4):219-224.
32. Uriburu IJ, Levy VD. Intraosseous growth of giant cell tumors of the tendon sheath (localized nodular tenosynovitis) of the digits: report of 15 cases. *J Hand Surg Am*. 1998;23(4):732-736.
33. Williams J, Hodari A, Janevski P, Siddiqui A. Recurrence of giant cell tumors in the hand: a prospective study. *J Hand Surg Am*. 2010;35(3):451-456.
34. Bliss BO, Reed RJ. Large cell sarcomas of tendon sheath: malignant giant cell tumors of tendon sheath. *Am J Clin Pathol*. 1968;49(6):776-781.
35. Carroll RE. Epidermoid (epithelial) cyst of the hand skeleton. *Am J Surg*. 1953;85(3):327-334.
Classic article on epidermal cysts of the hand. The discussion at the end of this paper between the author and authors of other articles in the journal (not included) is also interesting, particularly because it highlights that they had come across inappropriate management for epidermal cysts of the hand in their respective practices.
36. Lincoski CJ, Bush DC, Millon SJ. Epidermoid cysts in the hand. *J Hand Surg Eur Vol*. 2009;34(6):792-796.
37. Pagnano MW, Athanasian EA, Bishop AT, Rock MG. Intraosseous epidermoid cyst in a metacarpal mimicking malignancy. *Orthopedics*. 1997;20(8):719-721.
38. Kim DH, Murovic JA, Tiel RL, et al. A series of 397 peripheral neural sheath tumors: 30-year experience at Louisiana State University Health Sciences Center. *J Neurosurg*. 2005;102(2):246-255.
39. Phalen GS. Neurilemmomas of the forearm and hand. *Clin Orthop Relat Res*. 1976;(114):219-222.
40. Strickland JW, Steichen JB. Nerve tumors of the hand and forearm. *J Hand Surg Am*. 1977;2(4):285-291.
Classic article that reviews the nerve tumors that are encountered in the hand, and discusses the options of management.
41. Stull MA, Moser RP Jr, Kransdorf MJ, et al. Magnetic resonance appearance of peripheral nerve sheath tumors. *Skeletal Radiol*. 1991;20(1):9-14.
42. Knight DM, Birch R, Pringle J. Benign solitary schwannomas: a review of 234 cases. *J Bone Joint Surg Br*. 2007;89B:382-387.
43. Park MJ, Seo KN, Kang HJ. Neurological deficit after surgical enucleation of schwannomas of the upper limb. *J Bone Joint Surg Br*. 2009;91B:1482-1486.
44. Das Gupta TK, Brasfield RD. Solitary malignant schwannoma. *Ann Surg*. 1970;171(3):419-428.
45. O'Connor MI, Bancroft LW. Benign and malignant cartilage tumors of the hand. *Hand Clin*. 2004;20(3):317-323, vi.
This article provides an overview of the diagnosis and management for the cartilage tumors that are found in the hand.
46. Gaulke R. The distribution of solitary enchondromata at the hand. *J Hand Surg Br*. 2002;27(5):444-445.
47. Ablove RH, Moy OJ, Peimer CA, et al. Early versus delayed treatment of enchondroma. *Am J Orthop (Belle Mead NJ)*. 2000;29(10):771-772.
48. Brien EW, Terek RM, Geer RJ, et al. Treatment of soft-tissue sarcomas of the hand. *J Bone Joint Surg Am*. 1995;77A:564-571.
49. Buecker PJ, Villafuerte JE, Hornicek FJ, et al. Improved survival for sarcomas of the wrist and hand. *J Hand Surg Am*. 2006;31(3):452-455.

QUESTIONS

1. **A 30-year-old man presents with painless swelling of the right index fingertip. X-ray shows a lytic lesion involving the distal phalanx. MRI shows an indeterminate soft tissue mass scalloping of the bone. What is the next step of management?**
   - **a.** Ray amputation of the finger
   - **b.** Disarticulation of the finger at the distal interphalangeal joint
   - **c.** Staging CT scan of the thorax
   - **d.** Incision biopsy

2. **A 70-year-old patient presents with a firm swelling in the thenar muscles of the left hand. It has been progressively increasing in size over the past 3 months. Clinically, the mass is less than 5 cm in size and is nontender. What is the next step of management?**
   - **a.** MRI
   - **b.** CT scan
   - **c.** Incision biopsy
   - **d.** Excision biopsy

3. **A 30-year-old man presents with pain and deformity of the right index finger after minor trauma. X-ray shows a lytic lesion in the proximal phalanx, consistent with an enchondroma, with a pathological fracture. What is the next step of management?**
   - **a.** Bone scan to evaluate for multiple enchondromatosis
   - **b.** Immediate internal fixation of the finger for stability
   - **c.** Splinting of the fracture, with staged open biopsy, curettage, and bone grafting of the lesion
   - **d.** Ray amputation of the finger

1. **Answer: d.** Epidermal inclusion cysts are benign tumors that occur frequently in the distal phalanx. They can cause bone erosion and mimic malignant or infective conditions. Hence, a biopsy is advised so that a definitive diagnosis can be made before an ablative procedure is done.

2. **Answer: a.** MRI is the best imaging modality to evaluate soft tissue tumors, and should be performed before any surgery. Patients with soft tissue sarcomas in the hand often present early, when the tumor is less than 5 cm in size, hence there should be a lower threshold for requesting for imaging studies.

3. **Answer: c.** Most enchondromas are solitary, and routine bone scan is not required. If fixation of the fracture is to be performed, it should also be accompanied by curettage of the enchondroma. Because these lesions are benign and have a local recurrence rate, ablative procedures such as amputations are generally not required.

CHAPTER 87 Treatment of Vascular Disorders of the Hand

Brian C. Pridgen and James Chang

KEY POINTS

- Physical examination with Allen testing and pencil Doppler may be adequate for localization of obstructive arterial lesions, but angiography is the standard study for vascular imaging.
- Hand ischemia in the setting of chronic thrombosis typically is not responsive to medical management and requires surgical treatment.
- Arterial reconstruction requires careful preoperative planning with appropriate vascular imaging to identify suitable distal targets.
- Periarterial sympathectomy is a particularly effective treatment for patients with Raynaud phenomenon due to scleroderma who have failed treatment with behavioral modification and medical management.
- Following resection or ligation of diseased arterial segments, these defects should be reconstructed whenever possible with either direct repair if the defect is short enough or interposition vascular grafts.

Vascular disorders of the hand and associated hand ischemia may result in significant morbidity. Hand ischemia is caused by a diversity of conditions including local or systemic factors, acute or chronic processes, and occlusive, vasospastic, traumatic, or anatomic disorders. Proper treatment requires a detailed understanding of the complex vascular anatomy of the upper extremity, a comprehensive history and physical examination, appropriate use of diagnostic testing and knowledge of the various treatment options for each disorder.

ANATOMY

Arterial Anatomy

The primary blood supply to the hand is through the radial and ulnar arteries. The ulnar artery arises from the brachial artery in the proximal forearm and lies deep to the flexor carpi ulnaris along its course. Because of the distal muscle belly of the flexor carpi ulnaris, the underlying ulnar artery may be compressed in some instances and may not be palpable, in contrast to the more superficially located radial artery at the level of the wrist. Shortly after branching from the brachial artery, the ulnar artery gives rise to the common interosseous artery, which then forms the anterior and posterior interosseous arteries. The radial artery also arises from the brachial artery in the proximal forearm. It passes through the interval between brachioradialis and pronator teres proximally and between brachioradialis and flexor carpi radialis distally in the forearm. In the distal forearm, the radial artery often anastomoses with the anterior and posterior interosseous arteries. The interosseous arteries and a persistent median artery are possible sources of secondary collateral blood supply to the hand in cases of chronic ischemia.

In the hand, the radial and ulnar arteries form the deep and superficial palmar arches. As described in the classic anatomic study by Coleman and Anson in 1961[1] and in a more recent 2001 anatomic study by Gellman and colleagues,[2] the palmar arterial anatomy has significant variability.

The superficial palmar arch (Figure 87.1A and B) is formed from the ulnar artery as it crosses the wrist. It is located deep to the palmar fascia and distal to the deep palmar arch. There is significant variability in the superficial palmar arch, which can be described as either complete or incomplete depending on the presence or absence of anastomoses between the dominant ulnar artery contribution to the superficial palmar arch and the radial contributions to the superficial palmar arch. In Gellman's anatomic study, a complete superficial palmar arch was found in 84.4% of specimens and was subdivided into five variants initiated by the ulnar artery with various contributions from the superficial volar branch of the radial artery, the median artery, or communicating branches from the deep palmar arch. Branches from the superficial palmar arch typically include a branch to the deep palmar arch, a proper ulnar digital artery branch to the small finger, and common digital artery branches to the second, third, and fourth webspaces.

The deep palmar arch (Figure 87.1C) is formed from the dorsal branch of the radial artery after it has passed dorsally deep to the abductor pollicis longus and extensor pollicis brevis tendons and then returns volarly into the deep palm through the two heads of the first dorsal interosseous. Before returning volarly, the dorsal radial artery branch typically gives rise to the dorsal carpal rete and the princeps pollicis artery. The radialis indicis artery may arise either directly from the dorsal radial artery branch or from the princeps pollicis artery. As the deep palmar arch crosses the palm, it passes deep to the flexor tendons distal to the distal carpal row. A complete deep palmar arch was found in nearly all patients with anastomoses to one or both deep volar branches of the ulnar artery in all patients.

Venous Anatomy

Although the arteries of the hand are accompanied by two venae comitantes, the primary venous drainage of the fingers and hand is through the dorsal veins. These vessels drain into the basilic and cephalic veins in the forearm.

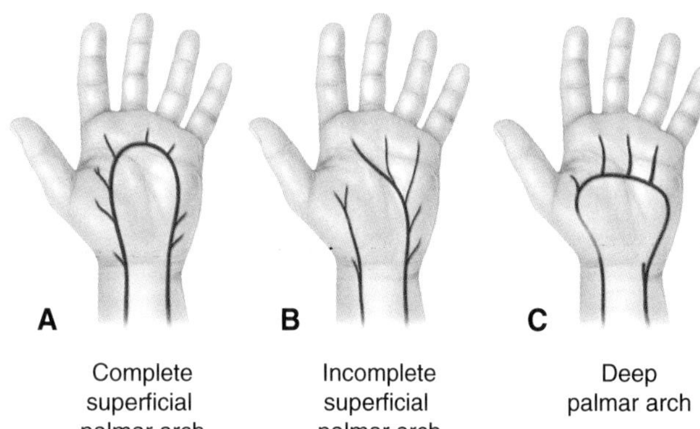

FIGURE 87.1. Most common variations of the palmar arterial anatomy as found by Gellman and colleagues. **A.** A complete superficial palmar arch, as defined by an anastomosis between the vessels constituting it, is most commonly formed by the dominant ulnar artery inflow and an anastomotic connection to the superficial volar branch of the radial artery. **B.** An incomplete superficial palmar arch is most commonly formed by the ulnar artery and the superficial volar branch of radial artery but without an anastomosis between these two vessels in the palm. **C.** The deep palmar arch is most commonly formed by the dorsal branch of the radial artery, which anastomoses with a deep volar branch from the ulnar artery.

EVALUATION

History

Accurate diagnosis of upper extremity vascular disorders requires a thorough history. Important details include a history of acute or repetitive trauma, known medical comorbidities including diabetes or cardiovascular disease, signs of systemic sclerosis or other rheumatologic conditions, drug or tobacco use, cold intolerance, prior digital ulcerations, and weakness or neurovascular changes. The history may be supplemented with the use of validated patient questionnaires for initial evaluation and longitudinal assessment, including the Cold Sensitivity Severity scale developed by McCabe and colleagues.[3]

Physical Examination

A thorough examination of the entire upper extremity should evaluate for prior scars or trauma, palpable masses, color changes including pallor or cyanosis, temperature differences, digital ulcers, and perfusion of the nail beds. The vascular examination may be supplemented by using a handheld pencil Doppler if evaluating for obstructive lesions. An Allen test may be used to evaluate for collateral inflow to the hand through the radial and ulnar artery. Ruengsakulrach and colleagues found the Allen test to be reliable when compared against Doppler ultrasonography, and when using the Allen test to assess patients for suitability for radial artery harvest, they had no ischemic complications following harvest of 1657 radial arteries over a 6-year period.[4] However, the reliability of the Allen test is controversial and has been questioned in case reports and studies, as reviewed by Brzezinski and colleagues.[5]

Capillaroscopy is a technique using high-powered light microscopy to evaluate the morphology and distribution of the nail bed microvasculature.[6] Visible spectrum evaluation may be augmented with the use of dynamic fluorescent angiography. Assessment of the nail bed capillaries using this technique is a useful screening tool to distinguish between patients with primary Raynaud phenomenon (RP) and secondary RP. These studies typically are performed by rheumatologists and dermatologists to document distal perfusion and are less commonly used by hand surgeons.

Diagnostic Studies

Vascular imaging often is necessary for diagnosis or surgical planning for vascular disorders of the upper extremity.[7] Duplex ultrasonography is most useful for providing real-time blood flow evaluation or larger blood vessels. Computed tomography angiography is a rapid and relatively noninvasive vascular imaging modality.[8] With recent improvements in image resolution with magnetic resonance angiography, this may be used when it is desirable to avoid ionizing radiation. However, the standard for vascular imaging is digital subtraction angiography owing to its superior spatial resolution, particularly for smaller vessels, and detailed temporal resolution allowing for real-time assessment of vascular inflow and outflow (Figure 87.2). Angiography also permits concomitant interventional procedures such as intra-arterial delivery of thrombolytics or thrombectomy. Risks of angiography include inherent risks of an invasive procedure such as aneurysm or hematoma, nephrotoxicity from higher doses of contrast, and higher doses of radiation. Surgeons treating vascular disorders of the upper extremity should be comfortable with proper selection and interpretation of the appropriate vascular imaging studies.[7]

ACUTE ISCHEMIA

Traumatic

Evaluation and management of traumatic injuries to the upper extremity requiring revascularization or replantation are reviewed in Chapter 83.

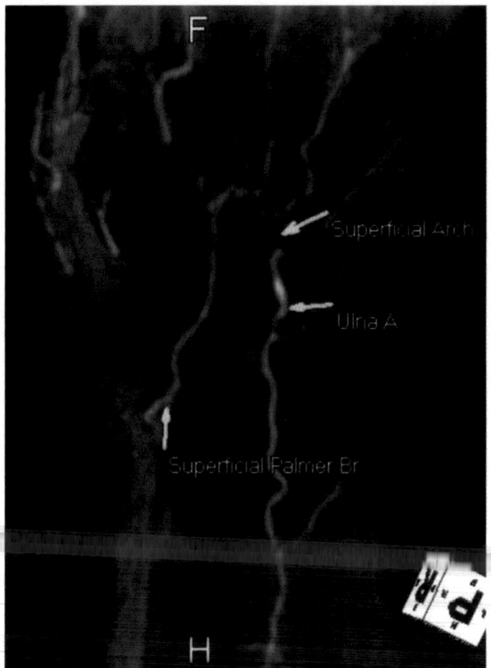

FIGURE 87.2. MR angiogram in a patient with scleroderma. Note the poor resolution of the common digital arteries.

Iatrogenic

Iatrogenic ischemia to the hand may result from arterial catheterization or harvest of the radial artery for either vascular reconstruction or with a radial forearm flap. Thrombosis of the radial and ulnar artery following catheterization may occur, but it rarely results in hand ischemia.[5,9] Similarly, in appropriately selected candidates for radial artery harvest, collateral flow and a compensatory increase in flow through the ulnar artery results in only rarely described cases of hand ischemia.[4]

In critically ill patients receiving vasopressors, peripheral vasoconstriction may result in digital ischemia in up to 2% of patients[10] (Figure 87.3). Treatment typically is limited to local wound care to prevent progression to wet gangrene followed by eventual amputation of the ischemic digits once the patient has recovered from their illness. One must, however, rule out concomitant radial artery injury from an arterial line that may rarely require repair or reconstruction to restore arterial inflow (Figure 87.4).

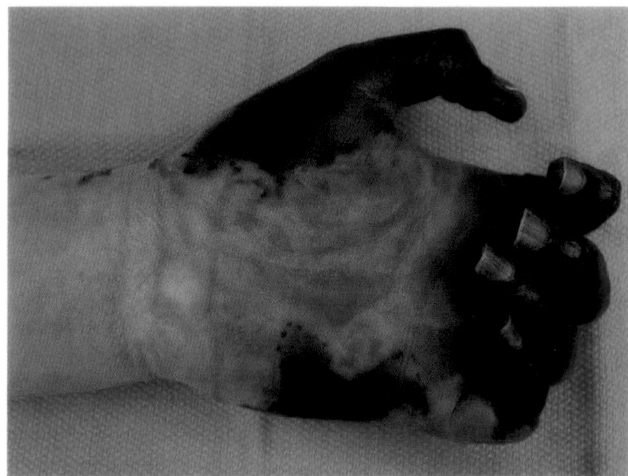

FIGURE 87.3. Patient who had been on high-dose vasopressors who developed tissue necrosis from hand ischemia with a clear line of demarcation.

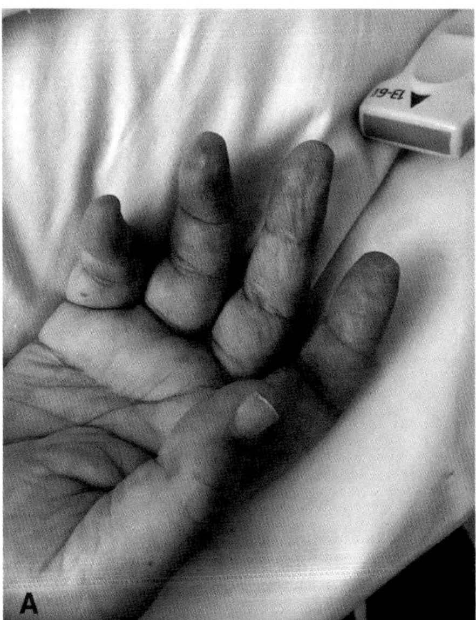

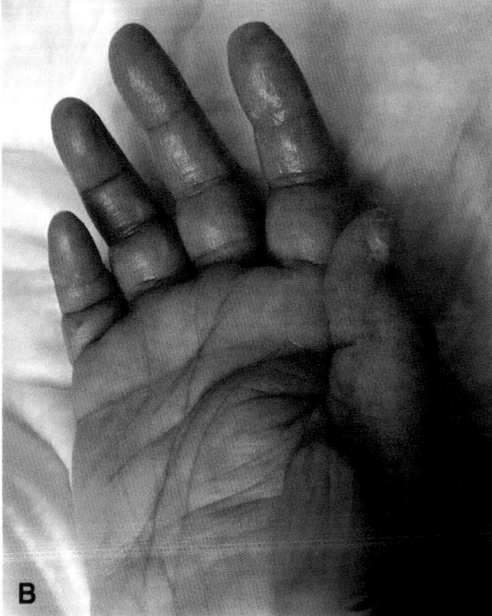

FIGURE 87.4. **A.** ICU patient on vasopressors with signs of hand ischemia, including cyanotic fingertips and poor turgor. **B.** Return of color and turgor without any surgical intervention after warming the patient and removing the radial artery catheter.

Creation of an arteriovenous fistula for hemodialysis access may result in decreased blood flow to the hand, but only rarely does it cause ischemic changes in the hand because of a steal phenomenon. In one series, the incidence of hand ischemia was 1.3% after placement of an arteriovenous graft and 1.8% after creation of an arteriovenous fistula.[11] A steal phenomenon was noted within 1 week in eight of the fifteen observed cases and within 1 month in twelve of the fifteen cases. Ligation of the arteriovenous access will improve the underlying steal phenomenon but leaves the patient without arteriovenous access for hemodialysis. Various treatments have been described for steal phenomenon, but in a recent large retrospective review from a single institution, distal revascularization with interval ligation (DRIL) was noted to have similar outcomes to ligation but with the benefit of preservation of arteriovenous access; the DRIL procedure had superior outcomes compared with other surgical treatments.[12]

Thromboembolism

Common causes of acute arterial occlusion from thromboembolism include embolism from a cardiac source because of an arrhythmia such as atrial fibrillation, endothelial injury from catheterization or local trauma, thrombus formation due to an aneurysm, intra-arterial injection of illicit substances, or hypercoagulable states.[13] Patients may present with pain, pallor, pulselessness, and coolness. Splinter hemorrhages in the nail beds, fingernail changes, or digital ulcers may be a sign of a more chronic etiology. Angiography is the study of choice to characterize the level of occlusion, sources of collateral flow, and possible proximal sources of emboli.

Treatment is directed at the underlying etiology. Proximal thromboembolism often is treated with embolectomy or surgical bypass as needed. However, more distal obstruction presents additional challenges owing to the small size of the vessels. Iannuzzi and Higgins reviewed treatment options for acute arterial thrombosis.[14] For the treatment of associated vasospasm, administration of vasodilators has had mixed results, and they instead recommend the use of local measures including warming and sympathetic blocks. Heparin and aspirin may be used to prevent progression of additional arterial thrombosis. In the absence of medical or surgical contraindications, intra-arterial delivery of thrombolytics such as tissue plasminogen activator often is considered as an initial treatment. However, there have been mixed results with thrombolysis, and it typically is most effective in cases of acute ischemia.[13,14] Thrombolysis may be used alone or as an adjunct to surgical revascularization. When treating patients with thrombolytics, they should be monitored closely for bleeding complications. Revascularization procedures should be reserved for cases in which there is a clear site of obstruction that either can be resected and reconstructed or bypassed to a patent distal target. If offered judiciously for appropriate indications, revascularization often has high rates of success.

Venous Thrombosis

Isolated deep venous thrombosis of the upper extremity is uncommon and rarely results in clinically significant problems in the upper extremity. However, in patients with total or near total thrombotic occlusion of the deep and superficial veins, they may develop ischemic thrombosis, also known as phlegmasia cerulea dolens. This is more frequently described in the lower extremity but has been observed in the upper extremity as well.[15] Following diffuse venous thrombosis, these patients can develop venous hypertension with resulting elevated interstitial pressures. Patients should be promptly diagnosed and treated before progressing from cyanosis to ischemia to venous gangrene. Described treatments include anticoagulation, thrombolysis, or thrombectomy. Additionally, signs of compartment syndrome should prompt consideration for surgical management with fasciotomies.

CHRONIC ISCHEMIA

Vasospastic Disease

Raynaud phenomenon (RP), first described by Maurice Raynaud in 1862, is characterized by episodic vasospasm of the digits. Classically, an episode of RP is triggered by cold exposure or emotional stress and is described as a triphasic progression of color changes from well-demarcated pallor (white) to cyanosis (blue) to reactive hyperemia (red) upon reperfusion. These episodes are associated with paresthesias and burning pain.

Owing to disagreement and conflicting diagnostic criteria described in the literature, a recent consensus panel of experts established a set of criteria for RP[16] (Figure 87.5). This panel agreed that a diagnosis requires cold sensitivity as a trigger and biphasic color changes from white to blue during an attack. Notably, although other triggers such as emotional stress have been described, and triphasic color changes were classically described, neither of these were

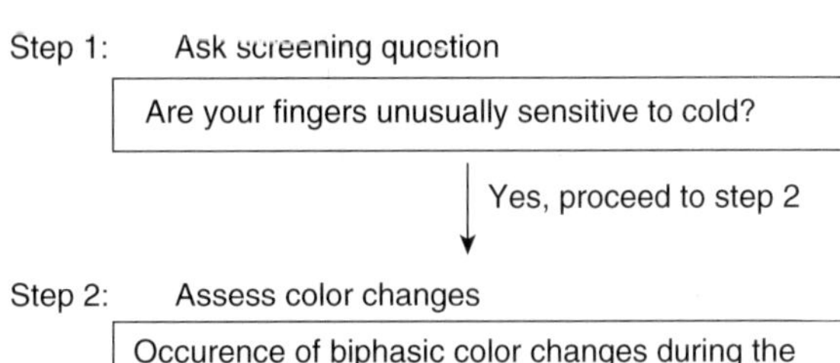

Step 1: Ask screening question
Are your fingers unusually sensitive to cold?
Yes, proceed to step 2
Step 2: Assess color changes
Occurence of biphasic color changes during the vasospastic episodes (white and blue)
Yes, proceed to step 3
Step 3: Calculate disease score
a) Episodes are triggered by things other than cold (i.e., emotional stressors)
b) Episodes involve both hands, even if the involvement is asynchronous and/or asymmetric
c) Episodes are accompanied by numbness and/or paresthesias
d) Observed color changes are often characterized by a well-demarcated border between affected and un-affected skin.
e) Patient provided photograph(s) strongly support a diagnosis of RP.
f) Episodes sometimes occur at other body sites (e.g., nose, ears, feet, and areolas).
g) Occurence of triphasic color changes during the vasospastic episodes (white, blue, red)

FIGURE 87.5. Three-step approach summarizing consensus criteria for diagnosis of Raynaud phenomenon. If three or more criteria are met from step 3, the patient has Raynaud phenomenon. (From Maverakis E, Patel F, Kronenberg DG, et al. International consensus criteria for the diagnosis of Raynaud's phenomenon. *J Autoimmun*. 2014;48-49:60-65, with permission.)

determined to be necessary for a diagnosis of RP. In addition to cold sensitivity and biphasic color changes, three of the following seven criteria must be met:

1. triggers other than cold,
2. bilateral involvement,
3. associated numbness or paresthesias,
4. well-demarcated areas of involvement,
5. photographic evidence of RP supplied by the patient,
6. involvement of areas other than fingers or toes, and
7. presence of the classic triphasic color changes from white to blue to red.

Other diagnostic criteria that had been previously described were not sufficiently agreeable among the panel members. Among patients who meet diagnostic criteria for RP, additional criteria for diagnosis of primary RP include normal capillaroscopy, no evidence of secondary causes or connective tissue disease, and negative or low antinuclear antibody titers.

RP may be subcategorized as either primary (Raynaud disease) if there is no underlying disorder or secondary (Raynaud syndrome) if there is an underlying systemic condition, including rheumatologic diseases such as systemic sclerosis (scleroderma), systemic lupus erythematosus, dermatomyositis, Sjögren syndrome, mixed connective tissue disease, or rheumatoid arthritis.[17,18] Other conditions that have been associated with RP include hematologic disorders, environmental exposures including mechanical injury from chronic vibrations, other vasospastic disorders such as migraines and Prinzmetal angina, and certain medications including serotonin agonists, beta-blockers, interferons, and certain chemotherapy agents.[17,18] Unlike in primary RP which is painful but typically has a benign course, secondary RP often is associated with significant morbidity including digital ulceration and gangrene.

Owing to regional variations and variable diagnostic criteria for RP, reported prevalence rates range from 1% in men to 30% in women across various studies.[19] A meta-analysis of epidemiology studies limited to primary RP among the general population demonstrated a prevalence of 1.6% to 7.5% for definite primary RP; the prevalence of possible primary RP was found to be 4.0% to 12.7%.[20] Risk factors included female gender, family history in a first-degree relative, smoking, and migraines. In two longitudinal studies of patients with primary RP who were screened at the onset of the study for associated underlying conditions, there were no cases of progression to secondary RP, and in many patients, their primary RP resolved.[21,22] However, other studies have found progression of primary RP to secondary RP in a small number of patients; the difference in these findings may be explained by careful screening for underlying conditions at the initial evaluation in the cited studies.

Although the mechanism of RP remains poorly understood, it is thought to be mediated by sympathetic alpha-adrenergic innervation, which often is cold induced.[23] This vasoconstrictive process may be exacerbated by endothelial cell dysfunction, including increased endothelin 1 activity and decreased nitric oxide activity.

Patients with primary RP often can be managed with behavior modifications such as cold avoidance, smoking cessation, and avoidance of certain medications such as sympathomimetics and migraine medications, without any additional medical or surgical intervention.[17] Treatment typically is reserved for patients with refractory primary RP or with secondary RP. A meta-analysis of medical treatments for RP demonstrated strong evidence supporting the use of calcium channel blockers and iloprost, limited evidence supporting the use of atorvastatin, and conflicting evidence for the use of ketanserin and bosentan.[24] Additional treatments evaluated include prazosin, cisaprost, cyclofenil, angiotensin-converting enzyme inhibitors, antioxidants, and tadalafil, but none were found in this meta-analysis to be of benefit. A more recent meta-analysis of randomized controlled trials evaluating phosphodiesterase-5 inhibitors including sildenafil and tadalafil demonstrated modest improvements in symptoms, duration, and frequency of attacks.[25] However, owing to the limited availability of high-quality clinical trials, treatment algorithms often are based on expert opinion and clinical experience.[17]

Injection of botulinum toxin for treatment of RP was first reported in 2004.[26] Additional work by Neumeister demonstrated improvements in symptoms and refinements of the injection technique.[27] A recent prospective, single-blind randomized trial of botulinum toxin B injections in patients with scleroderma, demonstrated improvements in symptoms, skin temperature recovery after cold immersion, and digital ulcers, in patients receiving higher dose treatments compared with untreated controls.[28] The mechanism of botulinum toxin for treatment of RP is not completely understood but is thought to be related to inhibition of sympathetic-mediated vasoconstriction and inhibition of substance P-mediated pain signaling.[27]

Surgical treatment with periarterial sympathectomy may be indicated in patients who fail medical management and have persistent digital pain or ulcerations, particularly in patients with systemic sclerosis (Figure 87.6). In the early 20th century, Leriche described his extensive experience with performing sympathectomies for a variety of indications, including periarterial sympathectomies for Raynaud disease and scleroderma.[29] Though more proximal procedures such as cervical or thoracic sympathectomies may be limited because of high recurrence rates, the digital artery sympathectomy described by Flatt in 1980[30] continues to be used for treatment of patients with refractory RP. A 2003 systematic review by Kotsis and Chung of patients undergoing digital sympathectomy for digital ischemia due to RP found that 14% of patients required digital amputation, 18% had ulcer recurrence or incomplete healing, and 37% experienced a postoperative complication.[31] They noted that their study was limited by heterogeneity and low quality of the published studies available for review. Subsequent reports by other groups have shown excellent results with periarterial sympathectomy in appropriately

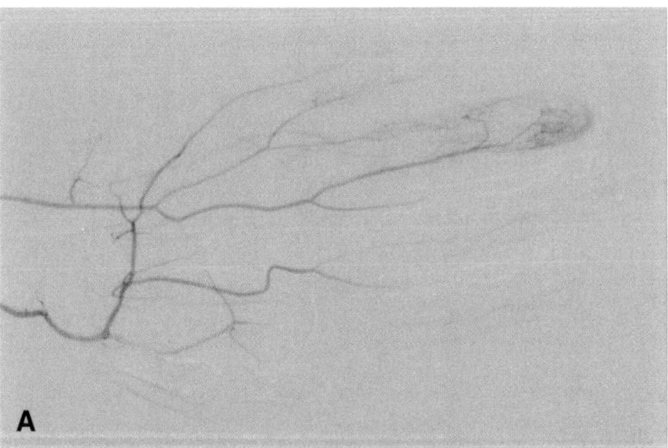

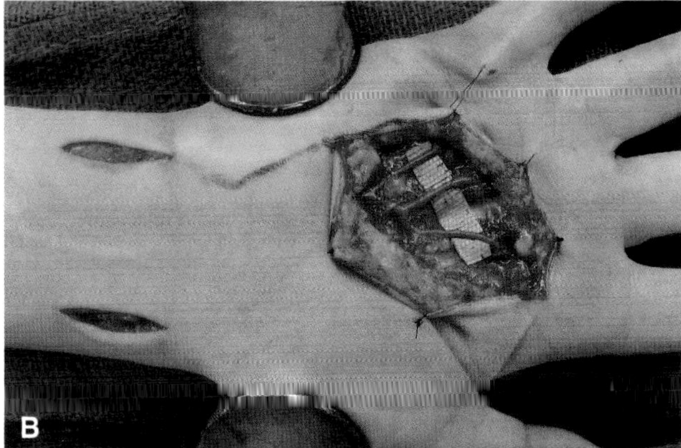

A: Angiogram of a patient with scleroderma with decreased flow in the common digital arteries and the proper digital arteries. B: The same patient underwent sympathectomy of the radial and ulnar arteries at the wrist and the superficial arch and common digital arteries in the palm. Note the dilated common digital arteries.

selected patients[32–35] and possibly decreased rates of ulcer recurrence in patients who undergo concurrent vascular bypass of occluded arterial segments.[33] Various techniques have been described by these groups and reviewed by others,[36] but the underlying principles and goals of the operation are to (1) disrupt sympathetic tone to the palmar and digital vessels by stripping the periarterial adventitia (Figure 87.7) and dividing the nerve of Henle arising from the ulnar artery,[37]

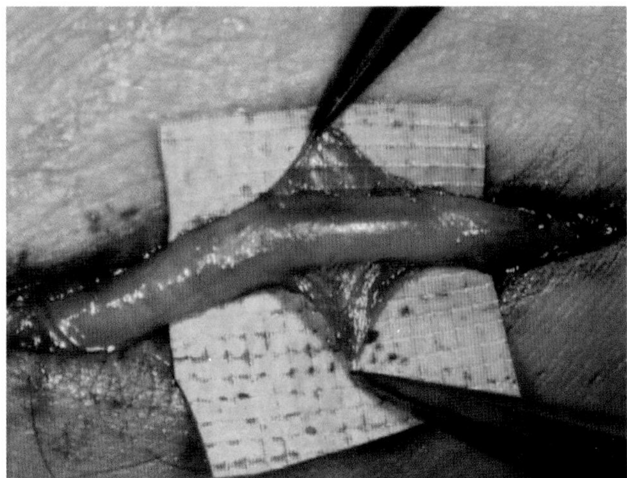

FIGURE 87.7. Patient with scleroderma who underwent sympathectomy 4 weeks earlier on the left hand. Note the improved color to the fingers (compared with the unoperated right hand), the healing left middle finger ulcer, and the healing incisions.

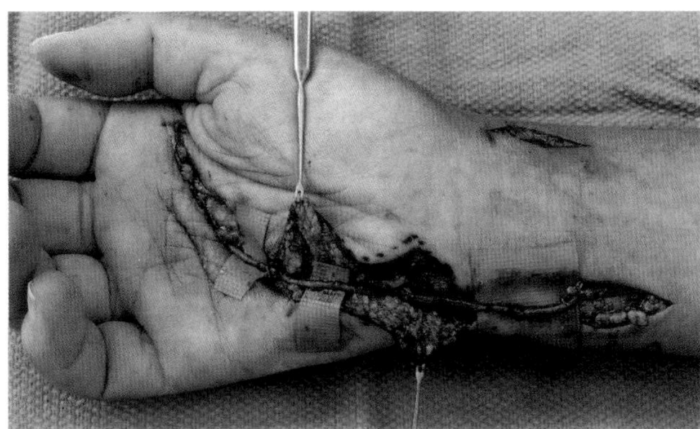

FIGURE 87.8. This patient with scleroderma had an occluded ulnar artery. She underwent interposition vein graft from the proximal ulnar artery to the common digital artery.

(2) perform distal revascularization if there is proximal occlusion and there are appropriate targets distally[33] (Figure 87.8), and (3) debride digital ulcers. However, for a variety of reasons including limited access to hand surgeons because of referral patterns from rheumatologists and surgeon availability, this operation is still not widely performed.[38]

Aneurysm and Thrombosis

True aneurysms result from dilation of all three layers of the arterial wall (Figure 87.9). False or pseudoaneurysms lack the intimal layer with endothelial cells and instead involve only the media and adventitia. Aneurysms often present as a painless, palpable, pulsatile mass that occasionally is associated with signs of local nerve compression. It is uncommon, however, that there is associated thrombosis and embolism.

Traumatic thrombosis of the ulnar artery was termed hypothenar hammer syndrome by Conn and colleagues in 1970.[39] It is classically described in patients who use the ulnar aspect of their hand as a hammer or are subject to repetitive trauma at this site, such as jackhammer operators, although it may also result from an isolated trauma. As the ulnar artery emerges from the Guyon canal, it is in a relatively superficial and unprotected position on the superficial aspect of the hamate where it is subject to trauma from external forces. This can result in formation of a true aneurysm or pseudoaneurysm. Patients are then at risk for thrombus formation, which can lead to secondary occlusion of the ulnar artery or distal embolization.

Among patients presenting to subspecialty clinics for evaluation of RP, 1.1% and 1.6% of patients in two separate studies were found to have hypothenar hammer syndrome upon further evaluation.[40,41] In these studies, nearly all patients were men, smokers, and had occupational or hobby-related exposures to repetitive hand trauma. Patients typically present with unilateral vascular insufficiency to the small, ring, or middle fingers; involvement of the thumb strongly suggests an alternative diagnosis. In some patients, the small finger is spared because of the proper ulnar digital artery to the small finger arises proximal to the Guyon canal. Symptoms may include pain, cold intolerance, and numbness or weakness due to local compression of the ulnar nerve. Examination findings may include a pulsatile mass at the level of the wrist, subungual splinter hemorrhages, ischemic changes in the fingers, or digital ulceration. Noninvasive diagnostic testing includes Allen test, handheld pencil Doppler to evaluate for the level of occlusion of the ulnar artery and digital blood flow, and duplex ultrasound. Angiography is the standard for diagnosis of hypothenar hammer syndrome and can be used to rule out more proximal embolic sources. The pathognomonic *corkscrew sign*, first described by Hammond and colleagues,[42] is an early sign of chronic damage to the intima and media leading to progressive fibrosis with ectasia. Additional angiographic findings include occlusion or

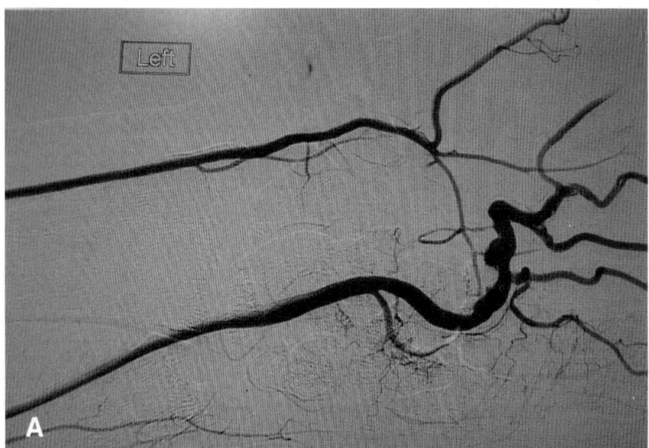

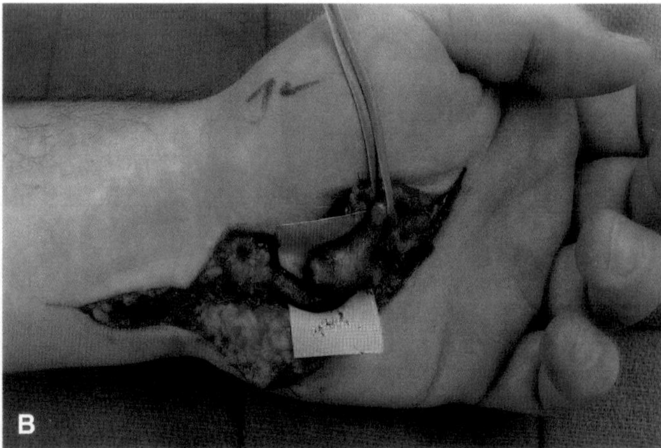

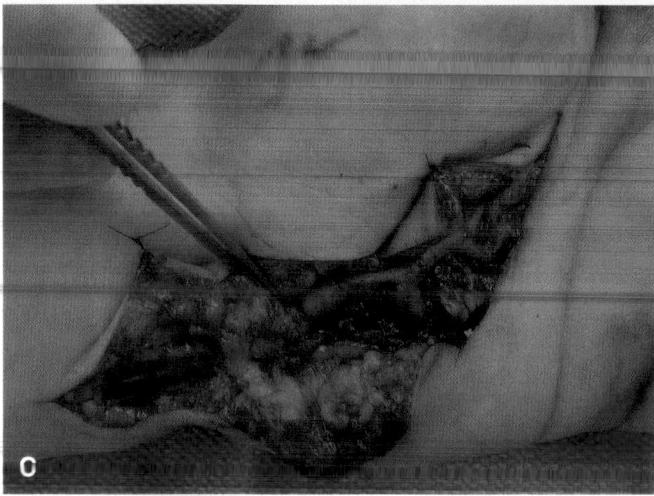

FIGURE 87.9 **A.** Angiogram of a patient with a true aneurysm extending from the ulnar artery into the common digital arteries. **B.** The entire aneurysm is dissected free. **C.** The ulnar artery and the common digital arteries were reconstructed with a Y vein graft.

aneurysm at the level of the hamate and multiple embolic occlusions of the digital arteries.[43] Angiography also facilitates operative planning by defining the level of involvement of the ulnar artery, evaluating for thrombotic occlusion and/or aneurysm, assessing perfusion and anatomy of the palmar arch, and determining inflow through the digital arteries.

Treatment of patients is guided by severity of symptoms and should restore inflow to the hand while reducing the risk of additional thrombotic or embolic events. Yuen and colleagues outline a comprehensive treatment algorithm[44] (Figure 87.10). Nonoperative treatment often includes behavioral modification, smoking cessation, and medical management with vasodilators and antiplatelet agents. In one series, 83% of patients were treated successfully with medical management alone.[41] For acute thromboembolic occlusion with associated ischemia, antiplatelet and thrombolytic therapy may be administered as described previously. If the thrombosis remains unresolved or if an aneurysm is present that may increase the risk of future thromboembolic events, surgical intervention is indicated. Rates of surgical intervention for patients presenting with hypothenar hammer syndrome range from 17% to 71% in two separate studies.[40,41] Surgical options include resection or ligation of the aneurysmal segment. Even if there is adequate distal flow with backfilling into the distal ulnar artery, the defect should be reconstructed with either direct repair if the defect is short enough or reconstruction with an interpositional vein or artery graft (Figure 87.11). Although vein grafts typically are longer, more easily harvested, and have less associated donor site morbidity, arterial grafts are more physiologic and may have improved long-term outcomes. A systematic review comparing venous and arterial grafts for upper extremity vascular reconstruction or bypass demonstrated 100% patency with arterial grafts at an average follow-up of 21 months compared with 82% patency of venous grafts at 40 months.[45] Arterial graft donor sites include the descending branch of the lateral femoral circumflex artery, deep inferior epigastric artery, thoracodorsal artery, or subscapular artery; the contralateral radial artery should not be harvested because of the high incidence of occlusion or ectasia of the ulnar artery seen in the contralateral asymptomatic extremity in a study of patients with hypothenar hammer syndrome.[40] Hui-Chou and McClinton suggest using arterial grafts in younger and more active patient populations.[46] In a systematic review of patients who underwent nonoperative treatment for hypothenar hammer syndrome, 12% of patients had a complete response to treatment and 70% had a partial response to treatment; among those who underwent operative treatment, 43% of patients had a complete response to treatment and another 43% had a partial response to treatment.[43]

Buerger Disease

Buerger disease, also known as thromboangiitis obliterans, is an inflammatory disease of the small- and medium-sized arteries of the upper and lower extremities.[47] Tobacco exposure is the primary risk factor, and it occurs most commonly in young men. Patients typically present with claudication and signs of limb ischemia including rest pain and ischemic ulcerations. Discontinuation of tobacco use is the only definitive treatment. Owing to the diffuse involvement of small caliber vessels that would serve as distal targets, bypass and revascularization procedures typically are not successful.

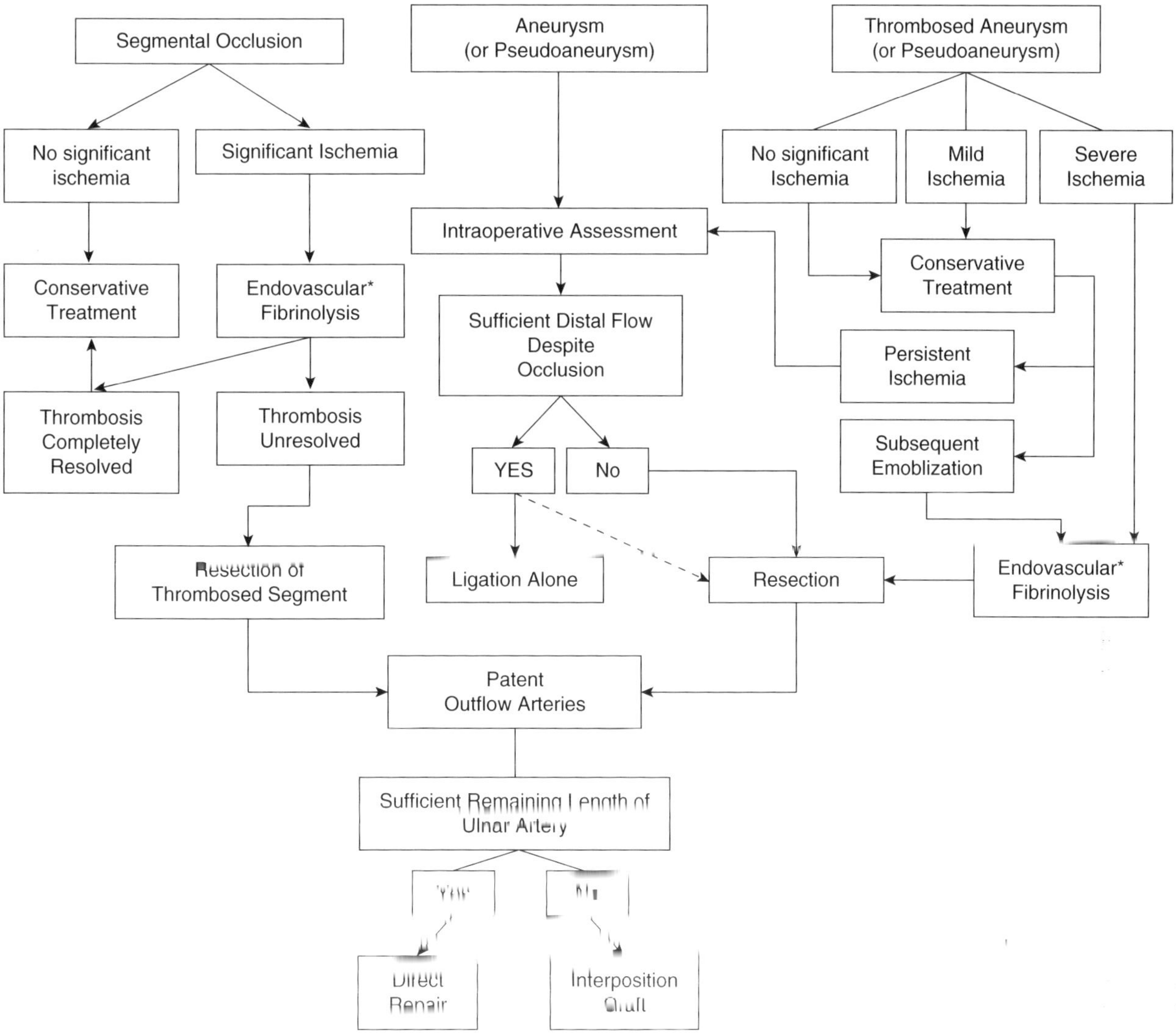

Segmental Occlusion
No significant ischemia
Significant Ischemia
Conservative Treatment
Endovascular* Fibrinolysis
Thrombosis Completely Resolved
Thrombosis Unresolved
Resection of Thrombosed Segment
Aneurysm (or Pseudoaneurysm)
Intraoperative Assessment
Sufficient Distal Flow Despite Occlusion
YES
No
Ligation Alone
Resection
Thrombosed Aneurysm (or Pseudoaneurysm)
No significant Ischemia
Mild Ischemia
Severe Ischemia
Conservative Treatment
Persistent Ischemia
Subsequent Emoblization
Endovascular* Fibrinolysis
Patent Outflow Arteries
Sufficient Remaining Length of Ulnar Artery
Yes
No
Direct Repair
Interposition Graft

FIGURE 87.10. Suggested treatment algorithm for management of hypothenar hammer syndrome. *Fibrinolysis (or thrombolysis) is advocated only for treatment in cases of acute onset of digital ischemia (less than 2 weeks). (From Yuen JC, Wright E, Johnson LA, Culp WC. Hypothenar hammer syndrome: an update with algorithms for diagnosis and treatment. *Ann Plast Surg.* 2011;67(4):429-438, with permission.)

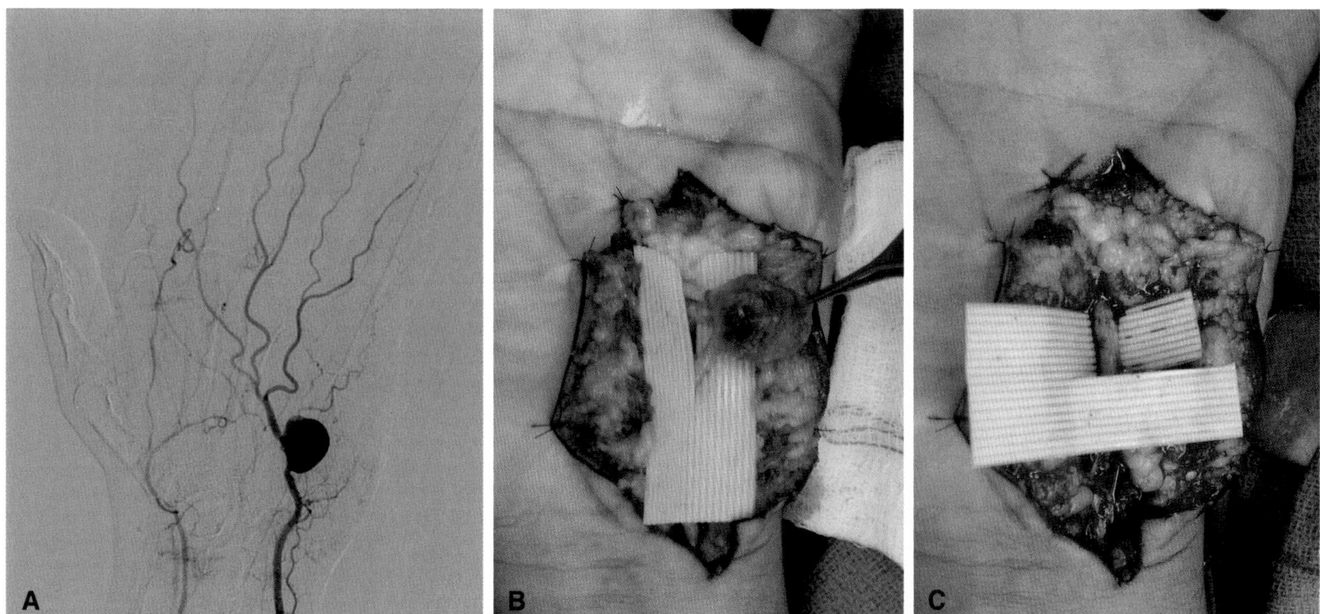

FIGURE 87.11. **A.** Angiogram of a patient with hypothenar hammer syndrome and aneurysm of the ulnar artery in the palm. **B.** The ulnar artery aneurysm is dissected free. **C.** Because the ulnar artery has some laxity, a direct end-to-end repair was performed after resection of the aneurysm. (From Galvez MG, Chang J. Upper extremity arterial reconstruction and revascularization distal to the wrist. In: Dalman RL, ed. *Operative Techniques in Vascular Surgery*. Philadelphia, PA: Wolters Kluwer; 2015, with permission.)

VASCULAR ANOMALIES

A comprehensive review of the diagnosis and management of vascular anomalies is beyond the scope of this chapter and is reviewed in more detail in Chapter 27. Upton and colleagues reviewed their 28-year experience in 270 patients with vascular anomalies of the upper extremity.[48] Although their descriptions of vascular anomalies predate the current naming conventions, they found that venous malformations comprised 46% of the patients in their series and that slow-flow venous, lymphatic, capillary, or combined malformations (Figure 87.12) comprised 88% of the patients in their series. They outline management algorithms and describe surgical principles for excision of slow-flow venous malformations, including delicate soft-tissue handling, meticulous dissection, ensuring complete excision, avoiding wide dissection planes resulting in devascularization, staged operations if necessary, and obtaining careful hemostasis. Complications after excision occurred in 22% of slow-flow lesions and 28% of fast-flow lesions; the most common complications included seroma/hematoma, amputation, neuroma, and wound healing complications.

Glomuvenous malformations (GVMs), previously known as glomus tumors, are a vascular anomaly most commonly found in the upper extremity. In one large series, all GVMs were located in the distal phalanx and 59% were in the subungual region.[49] This is due to the high concentration of glomus bodies in this region, which are neuromyoarterial cells important for peripheral thermoregulation. Patients typically present with a highly focal point of tenderness, which may be associated with cold intolerance and a bluish discoloration. Clinical examination alone may be sufficient for diagnosis, although ultrasonography and magnetic resonance imaging may be used as adjuncts for diagnosis (Figure 87.13). Surgical excision is the only known treatment, and in a retrospective review of 51 cases of GVMs treated with excision, there was a 3.9% recurrence rate.[49]

Pyogenic granuloma, also known as lobular capillary hemangioma, is a benign vascular tumor. Pyogenic granulomas are characterized by a small (typically <1 cm), rapidly growing, friable lesion of the skin or mucosal surfaces that may be either pedunculated or sessile. These may occur in the periungual region or elsewhere in the hand and upper extremity. Numerous treatments have been described owing to risk of recurrence. In a review of studies investigating the treatment of pyogenic granulomas, Lee and colleagues found that there was an overall recurrence rate of 2.94% with surgical excision (Figure 87.14) compared with 1.62% with cryotherapy with liquid nitrogen.[50] There was no statistical difference between the recurrence rates in these groups. Because cryotherapy often required multiple treatments in the reviewed studies and because surgical excision allows single-stage treatment with the opportunity to send the lesion for pathology, the authors recommended surgical excision except where a nonsurgical treatment is preferred, such as in cases where the lesion is located near cosmetically sensitive or vital structures.

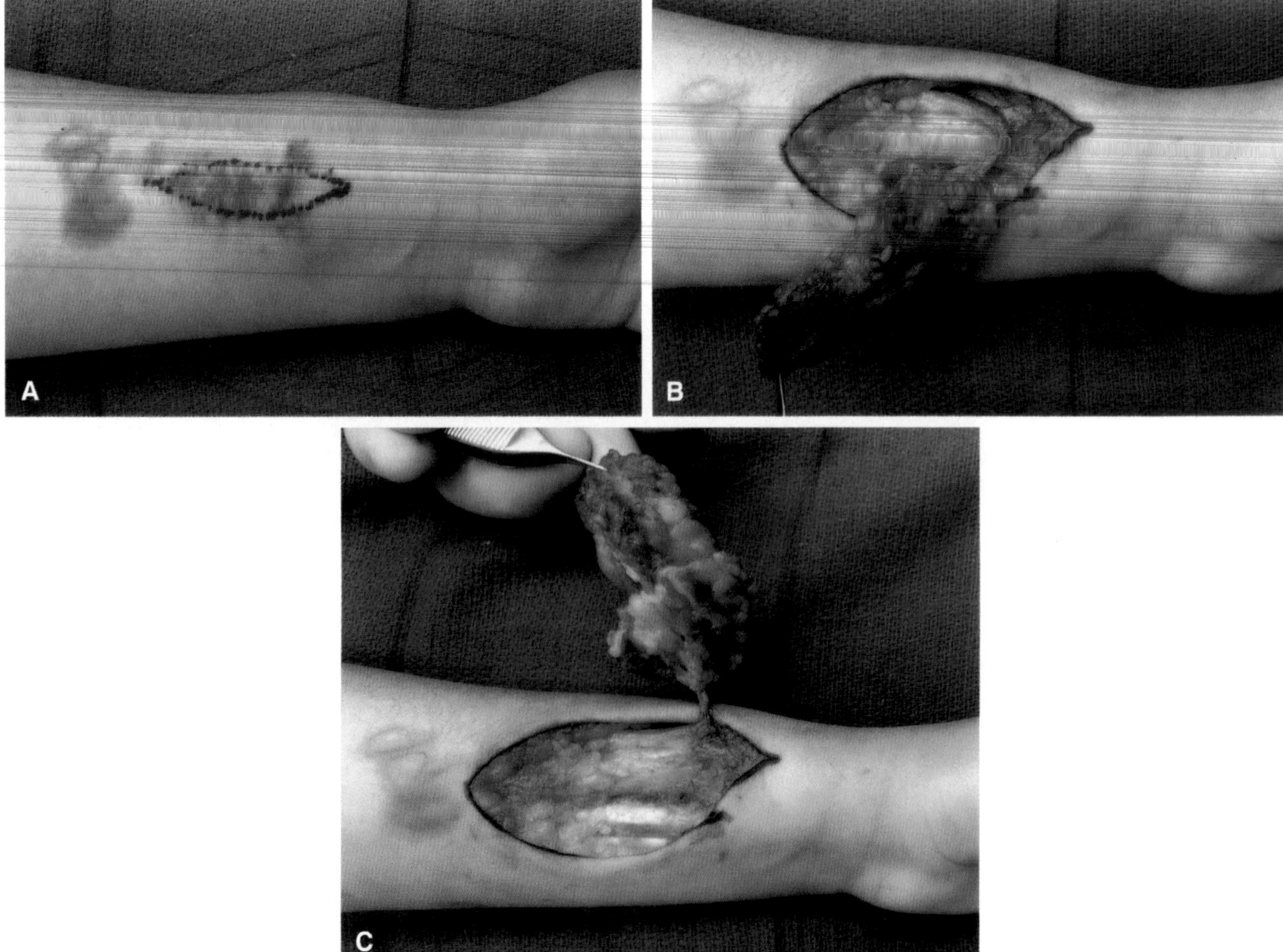

FIGURE 87.12. **A.** This patient had an arteriovenous malformation of the left wrist and forearm causing pain. **B.** The arteriovenous malformation was dissected free under tourniquet control. **C.** One arterial feeder from the radial artery was found and ligated.

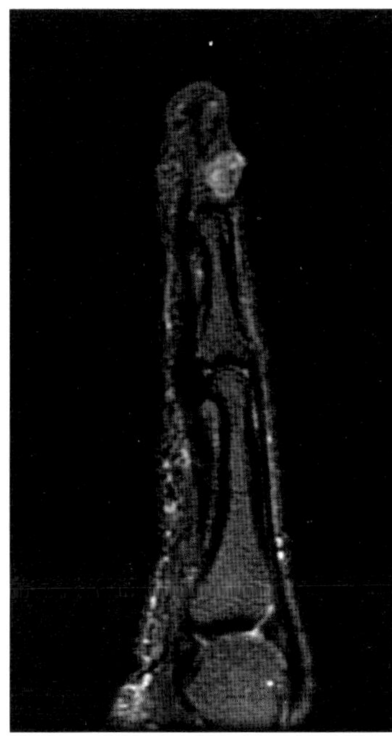

FIGURE 87.13. Magnetic resonance imaging demonstrating subungual glomuvenous malformation (glomus tumor).

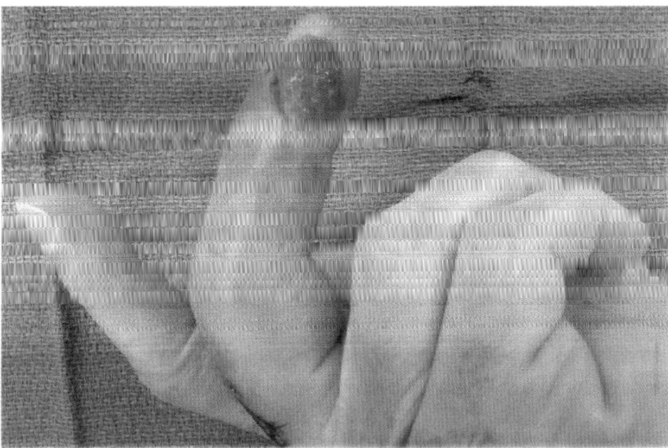

FIGURE 87.14. This patient had a pyogenic granuloma of the left middle finger that was treated eventually with resection and dressing changes.

REFERENCES

1. Coleman SS, Anson BJ. Arterial patterns in the hand based upon a study of 650 specimens. *Surg Gynecol Obstet*. 1961;113:409-424.
2. Gellman H, Botte MJ, Shankwiler J, Gelberman RH. Arterial patterns of the deep and superficial palmar arches. *Clin Orthop*. 2001;(383):41-46.
   This anatomic study of 45 fresh cadaver limbs investigated the arterial anatomy of the superficial and deep palmar arches. Consistent with the work of previous authors, they found highly variable anatomy of the superficial palmar arch, which included complete or incomplete arches with variable contributions from the ulnar, radial, and persistent median arteries. The deep palmar arch anatomy had less variability.
3. McCabe SJ, Mizgala C, Glickman L. The measurement of cold sensitivity of the hand. *J Hand Surg*. 1991;16(6):1037-1040.
4. Ruengsakulrach P, Brooks M, Hare DL, et al. Preoperative assessment of hand circulation by means of Doppler ultrasonography and the modified Allen test. *J Thorac Cardiovasc Surg*. 2001;121(3):526-531.
5. Brzezinski M, Luisetti T, London MJ. Radial artery cannulation: a comprehensive review of recent anatomic and physiologic investigations. *Anesth Analg*. 2009;109(6):1763-1781.
6. Cutolo M, Grassi W, Matucci Cerinic M. Raynaud's phenomenon and the role of capillaroscopy. *Arthritis Rheum*. 2003;48(11):3023-3030.
7. Wong VW, Katz RD, Higgins JP. Interpretation of upper extremity arteriography: vascular anatomy and pathology [corrected]. *Hand Clin*. 2015;31(1):121-134.
8. Bogdan MA, Klein MB, Rubin GD, et al. CT angiography in complex upper extremity reconstruction. *J Hand Surg Br*. 2004;29(5):465-469.
9. Chim H, Bakri K, Moran SL. Complications related to radial artery occlusion, radial artery harvest, and arterial lines. *Hand Clin*. 2015;31(1):93-100.
10. Russell JA, Walley KR, Singer J, et al. Vasopressin versus norepinephrine infusion in patients with septic shock. *N Engl J Med*. 2008;358(9):877-887.
11. Morsy AH, Kulbaski M, Chen C, et al. Incidence and characteristics of patients with hand ischemia after a hemodialysis access procedure. *J Surg Res*. 1998;74(1):8-10.
12. Leake AE, Winger DG, Leers SA, et al. Management and outcomes of dialysis access-associated steal syndrome. *J Vasc Surg*. 2015;61(3):754-760.
13. De Martino RR, Moran SL. The role of thrombolytics in acute and chronic occlusion of the hand. *Hand Clin*. 2015;31(1):13-21.
14. Iannuzzi NP, Higgins JP. Acute arterial thrombosis of the hand. *J Hand Surg*. 2015;40(10):2099-2106.
15. Bedri MI, Khosravi AH, Lifchez SD. Upper extremity compartment syndrome in the setting of deep venous thrombosis and phlegmasia cerulea dolens: case report. *J Hand Surg*. 2009;34(10):1859-1863.
16. Maverakis E, Patel F, Kronenberg DG, et al. International consensus criteria for the diagnosis of Raynaud's phenomenon. *J Autoimmun*. 2014;48-49:60-65.
    In a systematic fashion, the authors of this paper assembled an expert panel of physicians and researchers who treat patients with RP to define a set of diagnostic criteria. The agreed upon diagnostic criteria include cold intolerance and episodes with biphasic color changes.
17. Wigley FM, Flavahan NA. Raynaud's phenomenon. *N Engl J Med*. 2016;375(6):556-565.
18. Block JA, Sequeira W. Raynaud's phenomenon. *Lancet Lond Engl*. 2001;357(9273):2042-2048.
19. Fraenkel L. Raynaud's phenomenon: epidemiology and risk factors. *Curr Rheumatol Rep*. 2002;4(2):123-128.
20. Garner R, Kumari R, Lanyon P, et al. Prevalence, risk factors and associations of primary Raynaud's phenomenon: systematic review and meta-analysis of observational studies. *BMJ Open*. 2015;5(3):e006389.
21. Carpentier PH, Satger B, Poensin D, Maricq HR. Incidence and natural history of Raynaud phenomenon: a long-term follow-up (14 years) of a random sample from the general population. *J Vasc Surg*. 2006;44(5):1023-1028.
22. Suter LG, Murabito JM, Felson DT, Fraenkel L. The incidence and natural history of Raynaud's phenomenon in the community. *Arthritis Rheum*. 2005;52(4):1259-1263.
23. [illegible] nomenon. *Nat Rev Rheumatol*. 2015;11(3):146-158.
24. Huisstede BM, Hoogvliet P, Paulis WD, et al. Effectiveness of interventions for secondary Raynaud's phenomenon: [illegible]
25. Roustit M, Blaise S, Allanore Y, et al. Phosphodiesterase-5 inhibitors for the treatment of secondary Raynaud's phenomenon: systematic review and meta-analysis of randomised trials. [illegible]
26. [illegible] Raynaud's phenomenon: a pilot study. [illegible]
27. [illegible] *Hand Clin*. 2015;31(1):23-37.
28. Motegi S I, Uehara A, Yamada K, et al. Efficacy of botulinum toxin B Injection for Raynaud's phenomenon and digital ulcers in patients with systemic sclerosis. *Acta Derm Venereol*. 2017;97(7):843-850.
29. Leriche R. Surgery of the sympathetic system: indications and results. *Ann Surg*. 1928;88(3):449-469.
30. Flatt AE. Digital artery sympathectomy. *J Hand Surg*. 1980;5(6):550-556.
    Flatt introduces periarterial adventitial stripping for treatment of RP. He reviews his 20-year experience with this operation and reports durable results in nine patients.
31. Kotsis SV, Chung KC. A systematic review of the outcomes of digital sympathectomy for treatment of chronic digital ischemia. *J Rheumatol*. 2003;30(8):1788-1792.
32. Momeni A, Sorice SC, Valenzuela A, et al. Surgical treatment of systemic sclerosis – is it justified to offer peripheral sympathectomy earlier in the disease process? *Microsurgery*. 2015;35(6):441-446.
33. Shammas RL, Hwang BH, Levin LS, et al. Outcomes of sympathectomy and vascular bypass for digital ischaemia in connective tissue disorders. *J Hand Surg Eur Vol*. 2017;42(8):823-826.
34. Pace CS, Merritt WH. Extended periarterial sympathectomy: evaluation of long-term outcomes. *Hand (NY)*. 2018; 3(4):395-402.
35. Hartzell TL, Makhni EC, Sampson C. Long-term results of periarterial sympathectomy. *J Hand Surg*. 2009;34(8):1454-1460.
    This study of 28 patients who underwent periarterial sympathectomy for digital ischemia demonstrated that 75% of patients with an underlying autoimmune disorder had either complete healing or improvement in the number of digital ulcers at a mean follow-up of 90 months. Only one of eight (12.5%) patients with digital ischemia due to atherosclerotic disease had improvement at the end of the follow-up period.
36. Merritt WH. Role and rationale for extended periarterial sympathectomy in the management of severe Raynaud syndrome: techniques and results. *Hand Clin*. 2015;31(1):101-120.
37. Balogh B, Mayer W, Vesely M, et al. Adventitial stripping of the radial and ulnar arteries in Raynaud's disease. *J Hand Surg*. 2002;27(6):1073-1080.
38. Chiou G, Crowe C, Suarez P, et al. Digital sympathectomy in patients with scleroderma: an overview of the practice and referral patterns and perceptions of rheumatologists. *Ann Plast Surg*. 2015;75(6):637-643.
39. Conn J, Bergan JJ, Bell JL. Hypothenar hammer syndrome: posttraumatic digital ischemia. *Surgery*. 1970;68(6):1122-1128.

40. Ferris BL, Taylor LM, Oyama K, et al. Hypothenar hammer syndrome: proposed etiology. *J Vasc Surg*. 2000;31(1 Pt 1):104-113.
This 27-year retrospective review of 21 patients treated for hypothenar hammer syndrome describes the epidemiology and treatment outcomes in these patients. All patients were male and had an exposure to repetitive palmar trauma, and a majority (76%) of patients were smokers. Nearly all patients underwent segmental ulnar artery resection and reconstruction, which had an 84% patency rate at two years with no recurrent ischemia in patients with a patent vascular reconstruction.
41. Marie I, Hervé F, Primard E, et al. Long-term follow-up of hypothenar hammer syndrome: a series of 47 patients. *Medicine (Balt)*. 2007;86(6):334-343.
42. Hammond DC, Matloub HS, Yousif NJ, Sanger JR. The corkscrew sign in hypothenar hammer syndrome. *J Hand Surg*. 1993;18(6):767-769.
43. Vartija L, Cheung K, Kaur M, et al. Ulnar hammer syndrome: a systematic review of the literature. *Plast Reconstr Surg*. 2013;132(5):1181-1191.
44. Yuen JC, Wright E, Johnson LA, Culp WC. Hypothenar hammer syndrome: an update with algorithms for diagnosis and treatment. *Ann Plast Surg*. 2011;67(4):429-438.
The authors of this article provide a detailed review of the management of hypothenar hammer syndrome. Their review is supplemented by suggested algorithms for the diagnosis and treatment of hypothenar hammer syndrome.
45. Masden DL, Seruya M, Higgins JP. A systematic review of the outcomes of distal upper extremity bypass surgery with arterial and venous conduits. *J Hand Surg*. 2012;37(11):2362-2367.
46. Hui-Chou HG, McClinton MA. Current options for treatment of hypothenar hammer syndrome. *Hand Clin*. 2015;31(1):53-62.
47. Piazza G, Creager MA. Thromboangiitis obliterans. *Circulation*. 2010;121(16):1858-1861.
48. Upton J, Coombs CJ, Mulliken JB, Burrows PE, Pap S. Vascular malformations of the upper limb: a review of 270 patients. *J Hand Surg*. 1999;24(5):1019-1035.
The authors review their 28-year experience in which they treated 270 patients with upper extremity vascular malformations. They describe the frequency of each vascular malformation, treatment algorithms, and outcomes.
49. Van Geertruyden J, Lorea P, Goldschmidt D, et al. Glomus tumours of the hand: a retrospective study of 51 cases. *J Hand Surg Br*. 1996;21(2):257-260.
50. Lee J, Sinno H, Tahiri Y, Gilardino MS. Treatment options for cutaneous pyogenic granulomas: a review. *J Plast Reconstr Aesthet Surg*. 2011;64(9):1216-1220.

QUESTIONS

1. **In a patient with an arteriovenous fistula for hemodialysis access who develops steal phenomenon, what is the most effective treatment to improve hand ischemia while preserving arteriovenous access for hemodialysis?**
   a. Ligation and creation of a new arteriovenous fistula
   b. Banding
   c. Angioplasty
   d. DRIL
   e. Revision using distal inflow

2. **Which of the following is the preferred first-line agent for medical management of RP?**
   a. Statin
   b. Angiotensin-converting enzyme inhibitor
   c. Serotonin agonist
   d. Calcium channel blocker
   e. Aspirin

3. **Which of the following is not one of the key principles and goals of performing a periarterial sympathectomy for RP?**
   a. Periarterial adventitial stripping of the radial and ulnar arteries, the palmar arch, and the digital arteries
   b. Division of the nerve of Henle
   c. Reconstruction of occluded arterial segments
   d. Debridement of digital ulcers
   e. Local or distant flap coverage of surgical sites to reduce wound healing complications

4. **Which digit is least likely to be involved in hypothenar hammer syndrome?**
   a. Thumb
   b. Index
   c. Middle
   d. Ring
   e. Small

5. **What is the most effective treatment for thromboangiitis obliterans?**
   a. Anticoagulation
   b. Botulinum toxin injection
   c. Periarterial sympathectomy
   d. Cold avoidance
   e. Smoking cessation

6. **A 30-year-old woman presents with several months of severe pain in the distal phalanx of the right index finger. She notices the pain is exacerbated when immersing her hand in cold water. Physical examination is notable for a dark-blue subungual lesion with associated exquisite focal tenderness. What is the most likely diagnosis?**
   a. Melanoma
   b. Subungual hematoma
   c. Glomuvenous malformation
   d. Splinter hemorrhage
   e. RP

1. **Answer: d.** DRIL is a procedure in which an arteriovenous fistula is bypassed by a vein graft from proximal to the fistula to an artery distal to the fistula, followed by ligation of the recipient artery just distal to the fistula to prevent retrograde flow into the fistula. In patients with hand ischemia due to an arteriovenous fistula, the DRIL procedure results in similar improvements in hand ischemia compared with ligation. However, the DRIL procedure preserves access for hemodialysis.

2. **Answer: d.** In a systematic review of medical treatments for RP, calcium channel blockers were found to be the most effective. Aspirin typically does not have a role in medical management of RP.

3. **Answer: e.** Flap coverage of the surgical sites is not typically described when performing a periarterial sympathectomy for RP. Sympathetic tone to the vessels is disrupted by stripping the adventitial tissue and dividing the nerve of Henle. Any resected arterial segments should be reconstructed if distal targets are available. While these patients are under anesthesia, any digital ulcers should be debrided to facilitate wound healing.

4. **Answer: a.** Because of its typically radial-dominant blood supply and being most distally located from the ulnar artery relative to the other digits, the thumb is least likely to be affected by hypothenar hammer syndrome. The index finger is the second least likely digit to be affected.

5. **Answer: e.** Smoking cessation is the primary treatment for thromboangiitis obliterans or Buerger disease. Other treatments, including the ones listed, have shown either mixed results or no benefit in the management of Buerger disease.

6. **Answer: c.** The described scenario is a classic presentation for a GVM or glomus tumor. When presenting for evaluation, these malformations are nearly universally focally tender at a site of bluish discoloration and typically have associated cold sensitivity.

CHAPTER 88 Comprehensive Management of the Burned Hand

C. Scott Hultman and Mohammed Asif

KEY POINTS

- Any patient with a hand burn injury meets criteria, as defined by the American Burn Association, for transfer to a burn center, due to the overlapping and progressive goals of resuscitation, resurfacing, rehabilitation, reconstruction, and recovery.
- Resuscitation of the patient with hand burns includes establishing perfusion of the hand, including escharotomy for circumferential burns and fasciotomy for compartment syndrome, operative debridement of electrical burns, removal of the offending agent in chemical burns, topical and possibly intravenous antibiotics for infection, and skeletal stabilization for fractures.
- Resurfacing of the patient with hand burns involves tangential excision of partial-thickness injuries and suprafascial excision of full-thickness injuries, followed by coverage with temporary dressings, biologic matrices, xenograft, allograft, autograft, or vascularized tissues.
- Rehabilitation of the patient with the burned hand requires early mobilization, splinting, scar management, sensory reeducation, strengthening, and conditioning.
- Reconstruction in the patient with a hand burn restores form and function, which may include the following:
  - Release of dorsal/volar/web space contractures
  - Correction of intrinsic and extrinsic tightness
  - Nerve release and neuroma resection
  - Tendon, ligament, and joint revision
  - Thumb replacement
  - Revision of amputations
  - Identification and treatment of common hand disorders: trigger finger, tendon sheath and joint ganglions, basilar arthritis, de Quervain tenosynovitis, and exacerbation of Dupuytren disease
  - Photothermolysis and fractional laser ablation of hypertrophic scars
  - Fat grafting for chronic pain and pruritus
- Recovery of patients with a hand burn embraces the goals of return to work, school, and society, and often includes a final capacity evaluation, vocational rehabilitation, and a final impairment rating.
- The best outcomes after hand burn injuries occur through a coordinated, multidisciplinary approach that not only combines elements of hand, plastic, and burn surgery but also critical care, nursing, wound care, occupational therapy, chronic pain specialists, physical medicine, and rehabilitative counseling.

Comprehensive management of the severely burned hand begins with initial damage control interventions, proceeds through wound excision and coverage, enters a phase of rehabilitation and reconstruction, and extends to the final period of recovery, with the goal of returning to work, school, and social activity. The plastic surgeon leads a multidisciplinary and interprofessional approach that incorporates elements of critical care, nursing, wound care, occupational therapy, acute and chronic pain management, and physical medicine. Although the ultimate goal is to restore form and function, health care providers must individualize treatment plans and listen to their patients, as they articulate their concerns and needs. The best outcomes are achieved through a combination of art and science, by managing patient expectations, and by matching the needs of the patient with surgical solutions that are reliable and available.

RESUSCITATION

Just as patients with a large thermal injury (>20% total body surface area) must undergo formal resuscitation with a combination of intravenous fluids, colloids, vasopressors, and inotropes, the patient with a hand burn must receive *critical care* to maintain or restore perfusion and to avoid long-term stiffness through early range of motion (ROM). Furthermore, hand burns must get appropriate wound care to help prevent wound infection to avoid conversion of the burn to a deeper injury.

Obtaining a detailed history and physical examination creates a sound platform from which to make short- and long-term decisions about management of the burned hand. Mechanism needs to be established and can include the following types of injuries: scald, contact, flame, abrasion, electrical, chemical, radiation, cold, and infiltration. The burn should also be classified by depth of injury, as this impacts early care: partial thickness (which includes superficial, intermediate, and deep) and full thickness (which can extend past the dermis and affect fat, fascia, muscle, and bone). In addition to noting time since injury, the examination must include an assessment of the following:

- Perfusion—including presence of pulse and Doppler signals, and capillary refill distally
- Motor and sensory function
- Location of the burns—arm, elbow, forearm, wrist, palm, dorsal hand, and digits
- Distribution of the burns—circumferential or not

A *damage control* approach should be pursued to stabilize the acutely burned hand.[1] In addition to optimizing the patient's physiology, especially for large burns that cause global edema, the priority is restoring adequate perfusion to meet the metabolic demands of the upper extremity. Escharotomies may be carried out for circumferential deep partial-thickness and full-thickness burns, but the surgeon should proceed directly to fasciotomies, especially if the patient has diminished or absent Doppler signals, sensory changes, or clinical evidence of impending compartment syndrome. Key areas that must be released include the carpal tunnel, Guyon canal, hypothenar and thenar muscle groups, interosseous muscles accessed through the dorsal hand, the radial vessels in the distal forearm, the volar and dorsal compartments of the forearm, the cubital tunnel at the elbow (Figure 88.1), and the brachial vessels in the arm. Patients with electrical injury represent a special category because the pronator quadratus must also be decompressed, deep to the flexor tendons of the distal volar forearm.[2] Furthermore, these patients require multiple returns to the operating theater, as muscle necrosis is often progressive and must be debrided at each session. Finally, damage to underlying structures should be addressed early and may include debridement of clearly nonviable tissues, stabilization of fractures through open or closed reduction with percutaneous pinning, repairing tendons if possible, and tagging disrupted nerves.

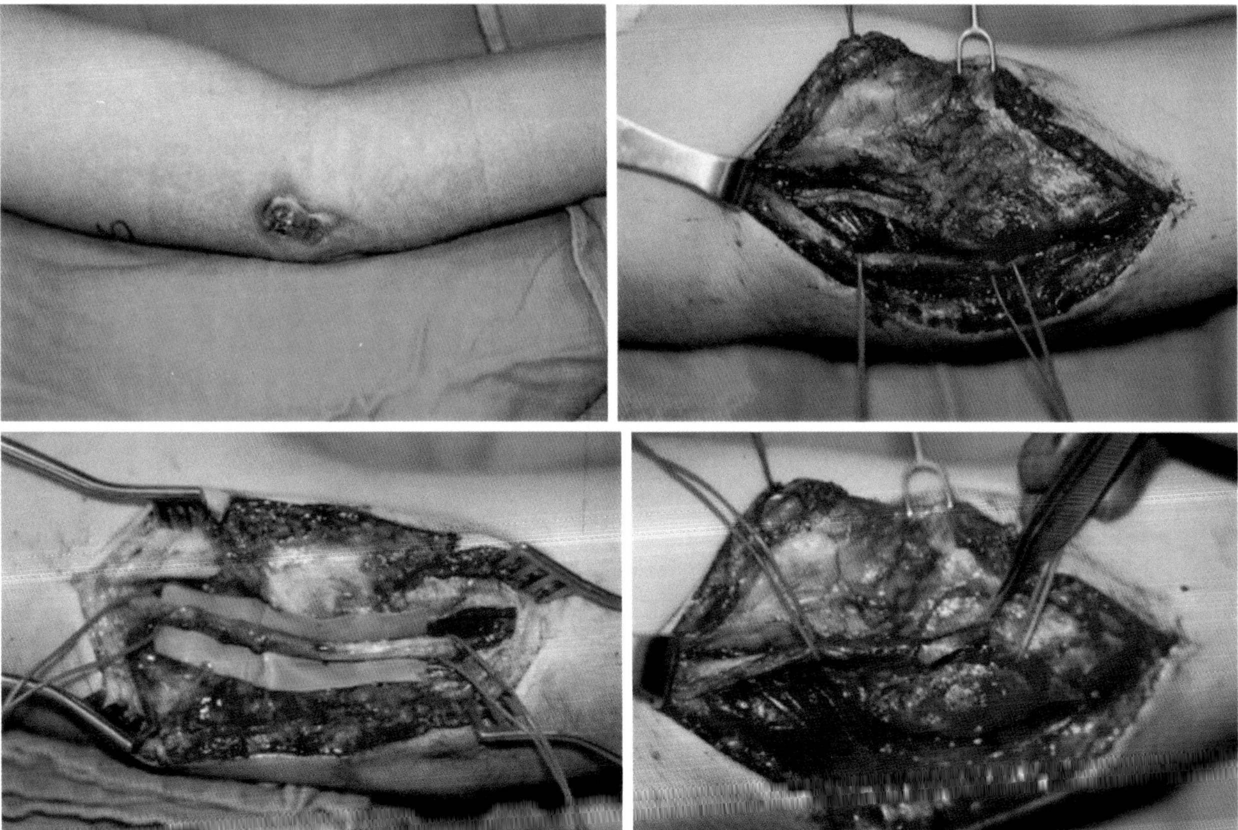

FIGURE 88.1. This patient is a 29-year-old construction worker who sustained a 1200 V electrical injury to the left elbow, with an exit wound at the right shoulder. He presented with a dense left ulnar nerve palsy. At exploration, after excision of the burn wound, the ulnar nerve was in continuity but had skip areas of coagulation extending proximally and distally from the cubital tunnel. The nerve underwent subfascial anterior transposition, with resection of the intermuscular septum. After complex closure of the burn wound, the ulnar nerve regained a Tinel sign 1 to 2 months later and the patient developed modest intrinsic motor function and protective sensation 10 months after his injury.

Wound care remains of paramount importance to help prevent desiccation of the wound, conversion to a deeper injury, and prevention of soft tissue infection.[3] In addition to elevation of the extremity, splinting in an intrinsic plus position, and keeping the ambient temperature warm, the surgeon must use a wound care algorithm that is consistent and incorporates depth of injury, time from injury, and location of injury, to maintain maximum viability of the wound bed. Our approach to management is as follows:

- First-degree burns (no disruption of epidermis): observation, moisturizing agent, mechanical protection from shearing, sunblock
- Second-degree burns, superficial partial thickness: topical bacitracin or mupirocin (if nasal swab is positive for methicillin-resistant *Staphylococcus aureus*), covered with xeroform or Vaseline gauze, consideration of early xenograft placement without the need for wound excision[4]
- Second-degree burns, indeterminate or intermediate: collagenase for 24 hours, followed by laser Doppler imaging to determine burn wound perfusion: if adequate, the wound should heal by secondary re-epithelialization; if not, the wound needs to be excised and autografted
- Second-degree burns, deep partial thickness: silver sulfadiazine, early excision, and autografting
- Third-degree burns, full thickness: silver sulfadiazine, early excision (<3 days after injury), allografting and sulfamylon slurry, and autografting when the wound and the patient are both stable
- Fourth-degree burns (involving fat, fascia, tendons, muscle, nerve, bone): immediate versus urgent debridement (<12–24 hours after injury), possible amputation, sulfamylon/nystatin slurry, staged allografting, consideration of vascularized coverage with regional flaps, distant flaps, or free tissue transfer[1]

RESURFACING

After initial stabilization of the acutely burned hand, timely wound excision and coverage should occur. For patients with scald injuries, a cost-effective option, which improves pain control and decreases length of stay, is superficial debridement of the wound with a soft scrub brush and xenografting, which permits the wound to heal by secondary re-epithelialization.[3] Furthermore, patients can begin early, aggressive ROM. For patients with deep partial-thickness injuries, preparation of the wound bed can be accomplished with tangential excision, using a Weck blade or the VERSAJET (Smith and Nephew, UK). Full-thickness injuries require full-thickness excision, often down to the level of the fascia. The authors do not routinely use tourniquets for excision of hand burns because the surgeon must identify the level at which the tissues exhibit fine, punctate, capillary bleeding. Once this level has been determined, with a blood loss approaching 1 cc per 1 cm^2 of excised tissue, the hand is wrapped with a compressive, epinephrine-soaked gauze for hemostasis.

For burns that are superficial partial thickness, such as scald injury, early xenografting (<36 hours after injury) permits rapid discharge from the hospital and more aggressive hand therapy. Although these burns most likely heal by secondary re-epithelialization, xenografting should be strongly considered, especially for children who may not tolerate dressing changes, for adolescents who are anxious to return to their social peer groups, and for adults who need to return to work sooner rather than later.[3] For patients who have deep partial-thickness or full-thickness injuries, the surgeon can proceed directly to autografting if all nonviable tissue has been excised from a stable burn wound. In this case, sheet grafts at a depth of 14/1000th

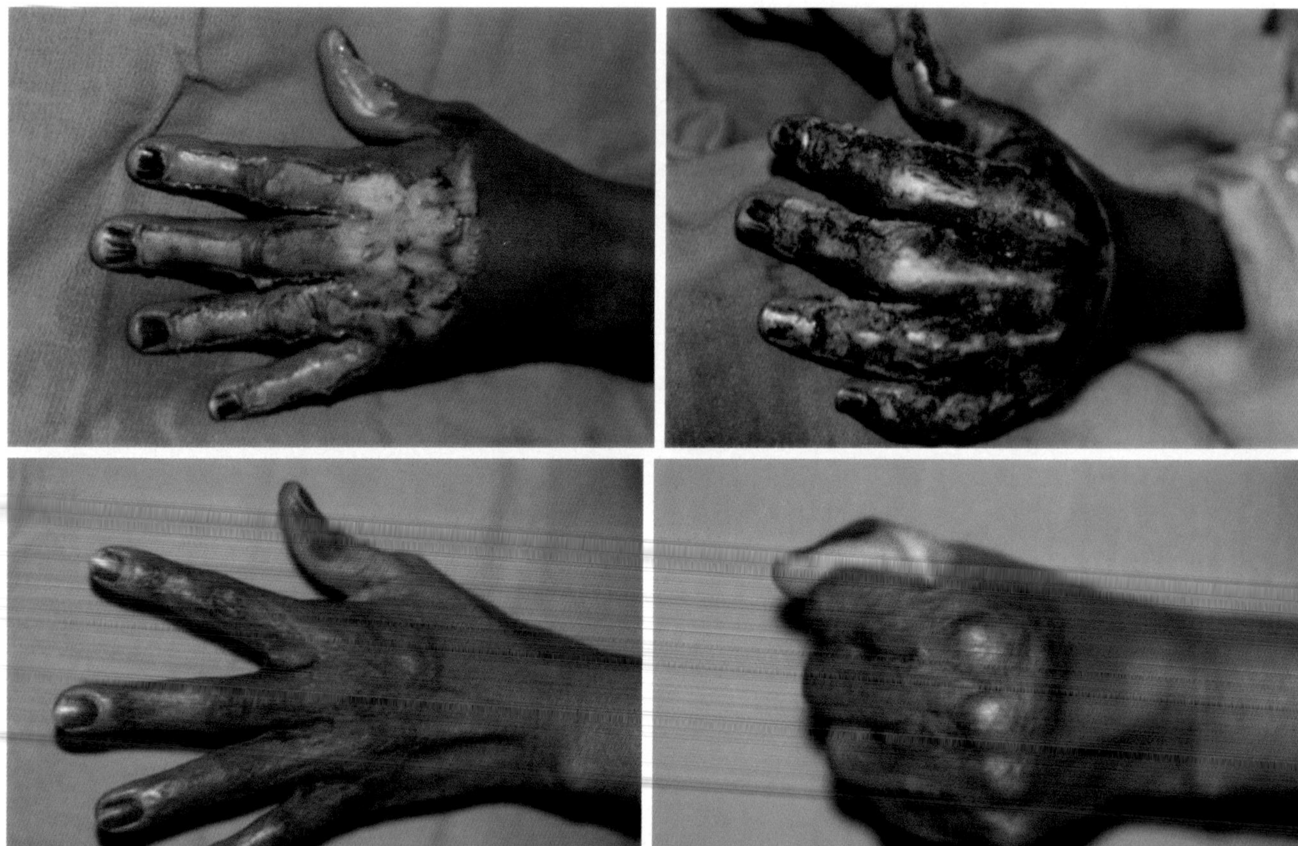

FIGURE 88.2. This patient is a 56-year-old woman who developed a full-thickness burn injury from a dry cleaning press. She underwent excision, staged closure with allograft, and split-thickness autografting. The patient did extremely well through hand therapy and underwent web space releases and full-thickness skin grafting. She has nearly normal hand function, as rated by her functional capacity evaluation, but she developed post-traumatic stress disorder and underwent vocational rehabilitation to work in a different setting, as a cashier.

of an inch are preferred to optimize long-term form and function. These grafts can be immobilized by circumferential fine mesh gauze, bolsters, or negative pressure wound therapy—whichever method permits safe, early mobilization by the occupational therapists. In addition, the digits are grafted with the metacarpophalangeal joints in flexion and the distal interphalangeal joint (DIPJ) and proximal interphalangeal joint (PIPJ) in extension, with an intrinsic plus splint protecting these fresh grafts from shear and disruption. For patients who have an evolving burn wound or whose depth and viability are uncertain at the time of excision, meshed allograft is indicated (Figure 88.2).

Patients with exposed vital structures, such as tendons, nerves, and bone, require either staged biologic coverage or definitive coverage with vascularized tissue. Biologic options include not only xenograft or allograft but also synthetic bilaminate skin substitutes—all of which will require autografting to achieve final wound closure. However, vascularized tissue will be needed for patients who have exposed hardware; open joints; tendon, nerve, or vascular repairs; or structures denuded of periosteum, paratenon, or epineurium. The following flaps are reasonably reliable, depending on the zone of injury, surface area requiring coverage, and technical expertise of the surgeon:

- Local flaps: kite, flag, heterodigital, Moberg, dorsal metacarpal artery, cross-finger, fillet
- Regional flaps: reverse radial or ulnar, adipofascial turnover (Figure 88.3), posterior interosseous (Figure 88.4)
- Distant random flaps: abdominal, infraclavicular
- Distant pedicled flap: groin (Figure 88.5), lateral thoracic
- Free flaps: rectus abdominis, anterolateral thigh, latissimus, serratus, omentum, and temporoparietal fascia

REHABILITATION

Once the hand burn has been excised and resurfaced, the patient can actively focus on the rehabilitative phase of healing, which involves restoring lost function and adapting to new challenges, which may include amputation, loss of sensation, and altered hand mechanics. During this period, the scar maturation will undergo several different phases to produce varying but significant degrees of stiffness, pain, and pruritus.

Hand therapy should begin shortly after injury, in the form of splinting, edema management, and ROM (active and passive), but after closure of the wound, the patient should become a more active participant. Nightly splinting may be necessary to retain gains in ROM, although the patient will need to work carefully with his or her therapist to further improve ROM. Both passive and active ROM exercises are critical to deal with the incessant pull of wound contraction, at both superficial (skin) and deep (ligament and tendon) locations in the hand. Strengthening and conditioning of intrinsic muscles, as well of flexors and extensors also remains critical goals of the rehabilitative period. Established contractures can have incremental gains in pliability, but ultimately surgical release may be necessary. However, as the scar softens, through critical components of occupational therapy, the degree to which the patient would need a release changes, allowing for less aggressive reconstructive efforts and the ability to achieve a more functional endpoint.

Scar management, from the early to late phases of wound healing, remains the focus of rehabilitation.[5] Skin care includes use of a moisturizing agent, sunblock, massage, and lymphedema management. As collagen matures and remodels, the previously burned hand can and should be treated with a variety of techniques designed to improve

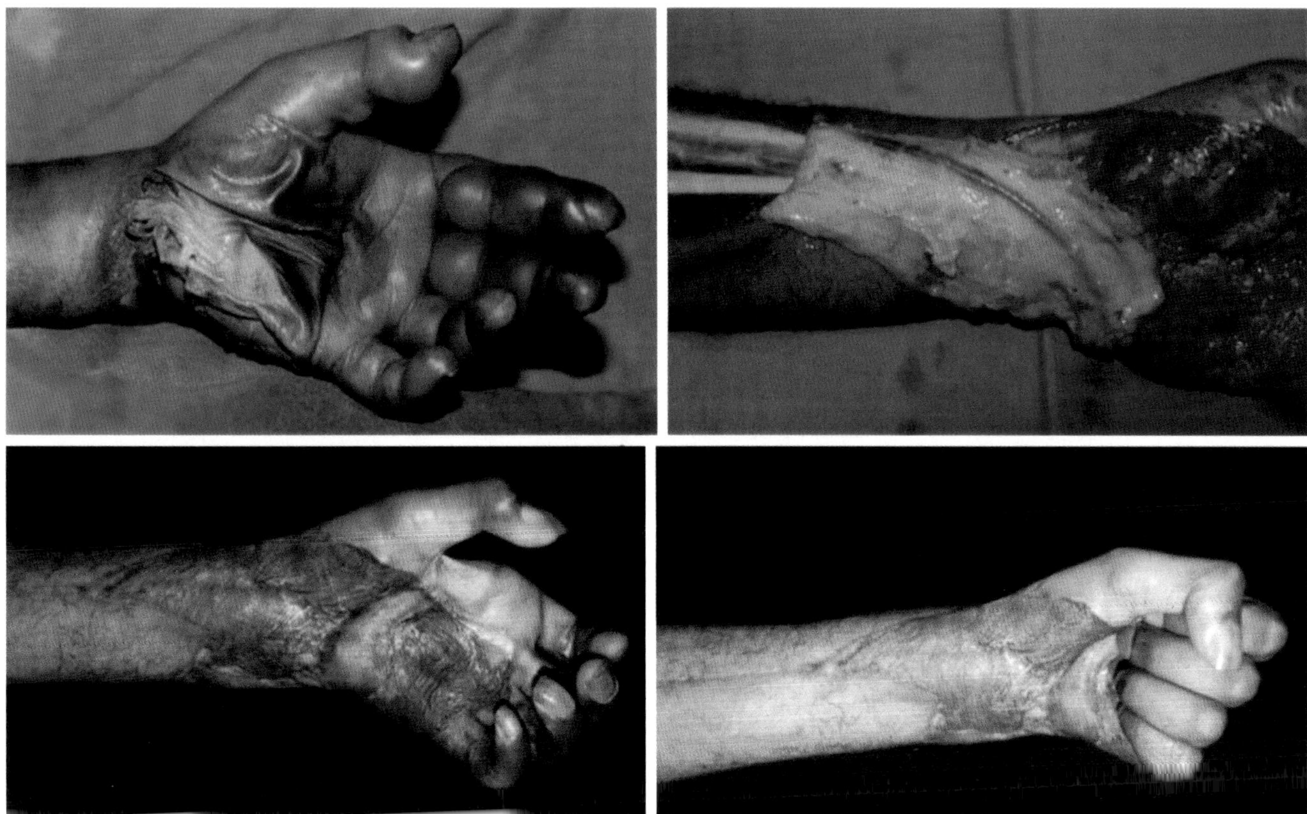

FIGURE 88.3. This patient is a 38-year-old assembly line manager who sustained a crush injury from an industrial press. He underwent emergent debridement, with release of the carpal tunnel and Guyon canal. An adipofascial turnover flap was used to cover exposed median and ulnar nerves, which was combined with negative pressure wound therapy, until the hand, wrist, and forearm were skin grafted. The patient regained use of his flexor and extensor tendons, with good gliding, but most of his intrinsic function did not return.

the pliability of the skin, mobility of ligaments, and balancing of the intrinsic and extrinsic tendons. Initially, successful edema management can yield impressive gains, as the patient transitions from the use of compressive dressings to compression garments. Areas of early hypertrophic scar formation can be treated through silicone sheeting. Paraffin application, fluidotherapy, and directed ultrasound can all improve ROM and pliability of tissues.[5]

By 6 months, patients may be candidates for laser remodeling of burned skin, grafted areas, and donor sites.[6-8] The authors prefer to use two or three rounds of pulsed dye laser photothermolysis first, targeting areas of persistent inflammation and increased vascularity of hypertrophic scars. The end points are reduction of erythema, with improvement of symptoms such as pruritus and pain. Once the areas of hypervascularity have been treated with pulsed dye laser, attention is then turned toward resurfacing with fractional CO_2 laser, targeting the thickness of the new scars, which have immature collagen. Although significant improvements can be achieved after one session, several rounds can yield dramatic gains in pliability. Because the fractional laser technology creates shallow and narrow channels within the skin, ranging from 100 to 2000 microns in depth and 20 microns in width, pharmacologic agents can be administered through vigorous massage, into these channels. Nearly all patients in our practice receive a maximum of Kenalog 1 mg/kg topically, applied in the operating theater after laser resurfacing, using semiocclusive dressings. Occupational therapy should begin immediately, although compression garments should be restarted only after these channels close, within 6 to 24 hours.

During occupational therapy, which may last weeks to months to years, adequate pain management is crucial to a successful outcome. Patients with preexisting substance abuse, large burns, narcotic habituation, and on multiple analgesics should receive ongoing care from a chronic pain specialist, from the fields of anesthesia, neurology, physiatry, or psychiatry, depending on the nature of the patient's type of pain. Premedication before therapy, as well as baseline control of symptoms, provides more comprehensive and compliant participation with the hand therapist. The plastic surgeon treating these patients does not need to have an exhaustive knowledge of potential pharmacologic agents, but the surgeon should be comfortable prescribing a regimen that includes nonsteroidal anti-inflammatory drugs, gabapentinoids, antipruritics, anticonvulsants, anxiolytics, and antidepressants. Opioids are tapered quickly, after wounds have closed, and used, sparingly, to premedicate prior to hand therapy sessions.

The treatment of chronic pain, which may present in the form of pruritus, paresthesia, allodynia, and dysesthesia, remains one of the most complex but important components to rehabilitation. In addition to pharmacologic approaches, the authors have increasingly relied on laser surfacing to modulate components of neuropathic pain, which may occur because of aberrant reinnervation of sensory nerves with damaged or absent sensory receptors within the burned of grafted skin.[6-8] Once baseline symptoms have improved through therapy, medication, and lasers, specific anatomic causes of pain may be identified, ranging from nerve compression to neuroma formation. The plastic surgeon must carefully reexamine patients during this period, as previously masked focal nerve pathology may become apparent and can respond well to surgical solutions. For patients who still have neuropathic pain, but require pharmacologic control, fat grafting can be considered as an adjunct and has had increasing success in our practice.[9,10] The authors harvest fat from a distant site, perform minimal mechanical manipulation *ex vivo*, take down adhesions through rigotomy, and inject volumes in increments of 0.05 to 0.10 cc in a radial, fanning manner, through different port sites, between the overlying skin and underlying structures, such as subcutaneous fat, fascia, or periosteum. Total volumes can range from 1 to 20 cc per region, although higher volumes are necessary to address structural volumetric deficiencies, with *take* rates higher than 90%.

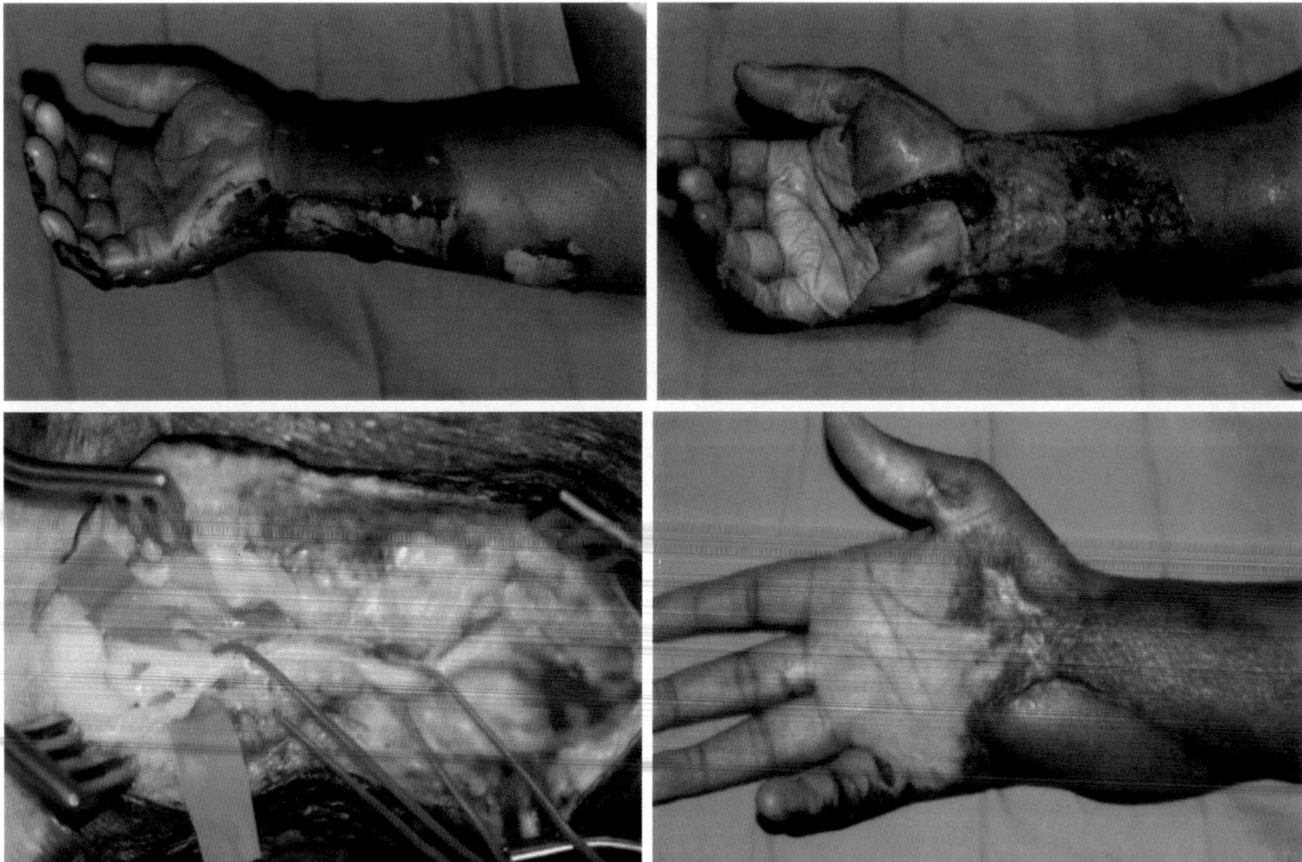

FIGURE 88.4. This patient is a 67-year-old woman with diabetes and rheumatoid arthritis, who had previously undergone carpal tunnel release, who sustained a seizure and fell onto the door of an open stove, which had been heated to 425°F. She underwent immediate extended carpal tunnel release for acute recurrent carpal tunnel syndrome, as well as excision of full-thickness burns, volar forearm fasciotomy, and staged autografting. Ten months after her injury, she developed rapid decline of her ulnar nerve function, with emergence of a Tinel sign over Guyon canal. She underwent excision of the hypertrophic scar at the level of the wrist, release of the ulnar nerve, including the deep motor branch and digital branches, and coverage with a posterior interosseous fasciocutaneous flap. Her sensation improved to be able to discriminate between light and deep touch, with improved strength of her interosseous muscles.

The mechanism by which fat grafting of burn scars improves neuropathic pain is not known but may include the following:

- Mechanical cushioning effects between the scar and underlying structures
- Disruption of aberrant innervation between sensory nerves and scar
- Release of growth factors and other cytokines from stem cells present in the mesenchymal stromal vascular fraction of adipose tissue

RECONSTRUCTION

Even after receiving appropriate care through the resuscitation, resurfacing, and rehabilitation phases, patients with hand burn injuries may still develop stigmata, deformities, and complications that require reconstruction to restore form and function. A helpful algorithm to follow is to ask two basic questions:

- What is the specific abnormality that the patient has identified?
- What intervention can be used to correct that abnormality?

General principles that should be followed include the fact that most patients with hand burns have deficient or abnormal tissue and benefit from the addition of tissues, through grafts, tissue rearrangement, or vascularized tissue. Serial contiguous Z-plasties can lengthen focal scar bands by 30% to 50%, and rhomboid-plasties (double opposing VY-plasties with double opposing YV-plasties) are especially effective for lengthening broad scar bands at the base of the thumb, over the snuffbox, and dorsal ulnar wrist. W-plasties do not add length to the original scar but can improve form, despite no gains in function.

The most frequent abnormalities that may be encountered are exacerbation or emergence of common hand conditions, such as ganglion of the joint or tendon sheath, basilar arthritis of the thumb carpometacarpal joint, trigger finger, de Quervain tenosynovitis, and worsening of Dupuytren disease. In general, normal incisions can be made through burn scars, to approach and correct these abnormalities, provided that the surrounding tissue is not extensively undermined, and perforators from major vessels are preserved when encountered. Wound healing may not be as robust as in unburned skin, so closure often requires multiple layers, plus sutures that are left in place for 10 to 14 days. Burn-specific conditions include volar and dorsal digital skin contractures, extrinsic and intrinsic digital tightness as determined by the Bunnell test, acquired syndactyly of the web spaces, first web space adduction contractures, and wrist contractures. Treatment involves release of the focal burn contracture, but also lysis of the scar tissue from the underlying structures, which may be tethered and shortened. A good example is the first web space reconstruction, which requires release of the transverse adduction contracture and tissue rearrangement with a five-flap jumping man Z-plasty, through which the surgeon can perform fasciotomies of the adductor pollicis and first dorsal interosseous muscles, neurolysis of digital nerves, tenolysis and A1 pulley release as needed, and manipulation of the joints with capsular or volar plate adhesions or contractures. Severe first web space contractures may even require placement of a full-thickness skin graft and skeletal fixation of the thumb metacarpal in abduction, with Kirschner wires for 1 to 2 weeks. Patients with focal contractures of the second through fourth web spaces can undergo

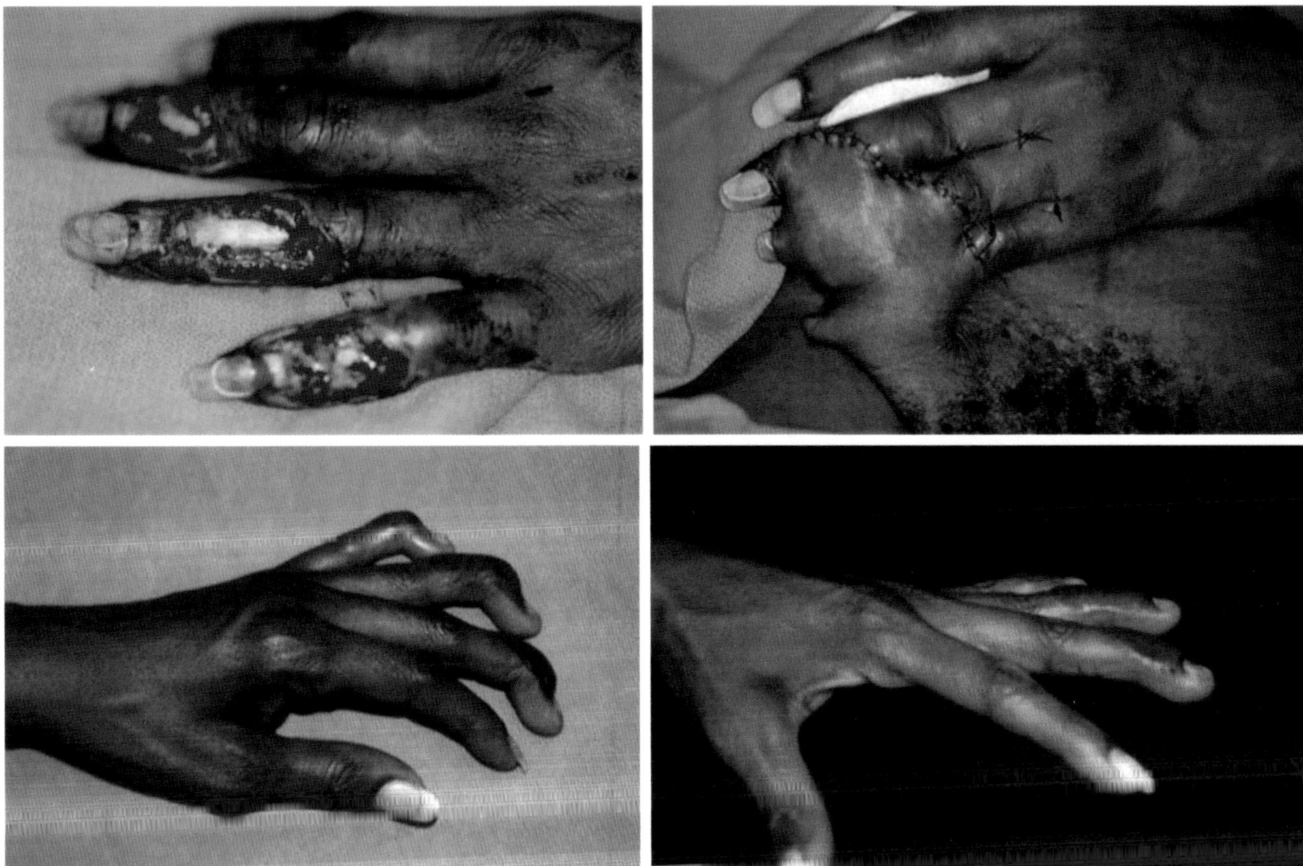

[illegible] This patient is a 23-year-old woman who sustained fourth-degree burn wounds, after getting her hand stuck in a hair straightener, destroying the extensor mechanism distal to the proximal interphalangeal joints of her middle, ring, and little fingers. After successful resurfacing of these digits with a thin groin flap, which was divided 3 weeks after coverage, she later underwent syndactyly release and arthrodesis in three unstable distal interphalangeal joints with percutaneous compression screws.

STARplasty, a technique that permits transverse, longitudinal, and oblique release, and utilize a robust local flap, with central blood supply, to correct the angle of inclination and resurface the web space.[11]

Patients with hand burns may have specific needs for repair of nerve, joint, and tendon abnormalities, due to the original injury or due to secondary effects of escharotomy/fasciotomy, excision, grafting, and immobilization. Perhaps the most frequently encountered condition is focal neuropathic pain due to anatomic compression or damage of underlying nerves and their branches.[12,13] Many patients will present with sensory and motor impairment that can be localized to an anatomic distribution, which can be diagnosed through careful physical examination that includes search for a Tinel sign at the point of suspected pathology. In almost all cases, the surgeon can identify the location and extent of nerve injury, if present. Nerve conduction studies, with electromyography, are only obtained if the patient's history and examination are not consistent, occult compression is suspected in another location, or if there are medicolegal concerns or requirements for preauthorization. The authors have a broad experience with nerve decompression of all nerves of the upper extremity, in the following order: median nerve at the carpal tunnel, ulnar nerve at Guyon canal, ulnar nerve at the cubital tunnel, antebrachial and dorsal cutaneous nerves of the forearm, superficial radial nerve and median nerve at the elbow and in the pronator tunnel, and anterior interosseous nerve. Increasingly, the authors have appreciated isolated cutaneous neuromas that benefit from excision and subfascial or intramuscular transposition and implantation. Finally, digital neurolysis is performed in almost all volar finger contractures to ensure integrity of the digital nerves, but also to release these nerves from any point of tethering or constriction.

In addition to neurolysis, neuroma resection, and occasional nerve grafting, patients may have underlying problems with tendons, ligaments, or bone that require reconstruction. Interventions that should be considered, depending on the clinical situation, include tendon transfer for specific nerve palsies, release of lateral bands for severe intrinsic tightness, repair of boutonniere deformities, extensor tenolysis for severe extrinsic tightness, volar plate release or division of checkrein ligaments for joint contractures, and capsulotomy or capsulodesis for joint pathology. For patients with unstable, painful joints that do not respond to the above interventions, arthrodesis can be performed with a variety of techniques, involving osteotomy and realignment of the joint, with compression from lag screws in the DIPJ and figure-of-eight dental wire over buried Kirschner wires in the PIPJ.

Management of the abnormal fingertip, which may be painful and have unstable tissue, includes a variety of techniques. For nail plate abnormalities, three approaches may be performed in isolation or combination: 1) sterile matrix grafting after excision of nail plate scars, 2) release of skin proximal to dorsal distal interphalangeal joint to help advance skin distally, and 3) harvest narrow skin flaps from the lateral and medial sides of the nail, to cover deficient eponychial skin. Damage to the germinal matrix is irreversible and, if symptomatic with nail fragmentation or splitting, is best treated with excision and/or destruction of the germinal matrix itself, to effect nail plate ablation. Finally, many burn patients with significant fingertip abnormalities may benefit from revision amputation that excises the nail apparatus and distal phalanx remnant, with closure using a volarly based, innervated fillet flap over the distal portion of the middle phalanx.

RECOVERY

After completing all reconstructive efforts to optimize form and function of the burned hand, attention turns toward final recovery. Depending on the goals of the patient, combined with his or her

TABLE 88.1. CRITERIA FOR RATING PERMANENT IMPAIRMENT DUE TO SKIN DISORDERS

Class 1 (0%–9% Impairment)	Class 2 (10%–24% Impairment)	Class 3 (25%–54% Impairment)	Class 4 (55%–84% Impairment)	Class 5 (85%–95% Impairment)
Signs and symptoms present or intermittently present *and*	Signs and symptoms present or intermittently present *and*	Signs and symptoms present or intermittently present *and*	Signs and symptoms constantly present *and*	Signs and symptoms constantly present *and*
No or few limitations in performance of activities of daily living (ADLs); exposure to certain chemical or physical agents may temporarily increase limitation *and*	Limited performance of some ADLs *and*	Limited performance of many ADLs *and*	Limited performance of many ADLs, including intermittent confinement to home or other domicile *and*	Limited performance of most ADLs, including occasional to constant confinement home or other domicile *and*
Requires no or intermittent treatment	May require intermittent to constant treatment	May require intermittent to constant treatment	May require intermittent to constant treatment	May require intermittent to constant treatment

prior vocational status, end points will vary considerably. At the very least, patients should work toward activities of daily living that will enhance their quality of life, allow for more independence, and provide a sense of competence that enhances self-worth and creates hope.[1,14] Specifically, patients should transform back into people, capable of taking caring of personal hygiene, clothing and feeding themselves, resuming activities that bring them joy, and reengaging with society through work and school.

Toward that end, patients often undergo a functional capacity evaluation, especially as they prepare to return to their previous job. These evaluations typically are quite extensive and measure the forces that patients can safely pull, push, lift, and carry; the degree to which patients put forth a consistent effort; their agility and balance; and finally, their conditioning and resistance to fatigue. Patients are then assigned low, medium, or high demand work levels, as defined by federal labor standards, with specific parameters recommended for their highest level of function. After receiving the results of the functional capacity evaluation, the plastic surgeon must then decide if the patient can safely return to work and determine limitations on work hours and restrictions on function. If employers do not have physical work that the patients can handle, then the employee enters a phase of vocational rehabilitation, in which old skills may be retaught or new skills must be learned.

For a patient who is cleared to work, the employee then begins a trial of work, typically for 3 months, until he or she reaches a steady state of performance. At this point, once the patient's physical condition and function are stable, the patient undergoes a final impairment rating. Although each state may have its own regulations regarding these assessments, most plastic/hand/burn surgeons use the *American Medical Association's Guides to the Evaluation of Permanent Impairment*.[15] We combine the rating criteria from both the skin and upper extremity sections to generate a percentage of impairment for the hand. Of note, these impairments can be extrapolated to impairment of the entire limb or even whole body, using tables provided by the guide. A few caveats will help simplify what can be a complex and subjective process in determining final ratings:

Digits: the thumb accounts for 40% of hand function, with the index and middle fingers contributing 20% each, the ring and little fingers contributing 10% each

Amputations: Loss of distal phalanges creates 45% impairment of the fingers and 50% impairment of the thumb; amputation at the metacarpophalangeal joint results in 100% impairment of that digit; complete loss of a hand yields 90% impairment of the upper extremity and 54% of the whole person

Nerve injuries: For the digits, total transverse sensory loss corresponds to 50% impairment of function of that digit

Range of motion: Given the challenges posed by the reproducibility of goniometric measurements (ROM is often not static, due to temperature, prior activity, and pain tolerance; and passive and active ROM may be quite different), the author does not utilize ROM criteria to calculate final impairment ratings

Condition of skin: Combining the signs and symptoms of the burn (which is considered a skin disorder by the American medical association guides), with limitations on activities of daily living and extent of treatment required to manage the skin disorder, the author can assign the patient a category of impairment (**Table 88.1**) that helps to generate a final impairment rating. Most significant burn scars require intermittent to constant treatment, which includes moisturizing agent, sunblock, massage, compression, and mechanical protection

ACKNOWLEDGMENTS

Dr Hultman thanks Damon Anagnos, MD, for his mentorship and inspiration for many of these cases. His influence on Dr Hultman's professional development is immeasurable and appreciated beyond what words can communicate.

REFERENCES

1. Hultman CS, Erfanian K, Fraser J, et al. Comprehensive management of hot-press hand injuries: long-term outcomes following reconstruction and rehabilitation. *Ann Plast Surg.* 2010;64(5):553-558.
   In this retrospective review, which remains the largest series to date, we analyzed the management and long-term outcomes of 56 patients with hot press hand injuries, which contain both a crush and thermal component. Over a 15-year period, 86% of patients required initial operative intervention and 50% of patients underwent secondary reconstruction. Final impairment rating was 22%, with 68% of patients returning to work, after a rehabilitative period of almost 18 months.
2. Kidd M, Hultman CS, van Aalst J, et al. The contemporary management of electrical injuries: resuscitation, reconstruction, rehabilitation. *Ann Plast Surg.* 2007;58:273-278.
3. Hultman CS, van Duin D, Sickbert-Bennett E, et al. Systems-based practice in burn care: prevention, management, and economic impact of healthcare-associated infections. *Clin Plast Surg.* 2017;44(4):935-942.
   In this retrospective cohort study of over 5000 patients admitted to a verified burn center, from 2008 to 2012, we observed that the development of a multidrug resistant bacterial infection was associated with an increase in mortality from 3% to 30%, an increase in length of stay from 12 to 94 days, and an increase in hospital charges from $57,000 to $325,000.
4. Diegidio P, Hermiz SJ, Ortiz-Pujols S, et al. Even better than the real thing? Xenografting for pediatric patients with scald injury. *Clin Plast Surg.* 2017;44(3):651-656.
5. Friedstat JS, Hultman CS. Hypertrophic scar management in burn patients: what does the evidence show? A systematic review of randomized controlled trials. *Ann Plast Surg.* 2014;72(6):S198-S201.

6. Hultman CS, Friedstat JS, Edkins RE, et al. Laser resurfacing and remodeling of hypertrophic burn scars: the results of a large, prospective, before-after cohort study, with long-term follow-up. *Ann Surg*. 2014;260(3):519-529.
   In this prospective, before-after cohort study of 147 patients who underwent laser resurfacing of hypertrophic burn scars, at a median of 16 months after injury, we demonstrated early response and lasting improvement in pruritus, paresthesias, pain, erythema, thickness, and pliability. Management of hypertrophic burn scars continues to involve massage, moisturizing agents, sunblock, silicone sheeting, and compression garments, but laser therapy should be strongly considered for patients who do not improve by 6 months after burn injury.
7. Hultman CS, Edkins RE, Cairns BA, Meyer AA. Logistics of building a laser practice for the treatment of hypertrophic burn scars. *Ann Plast Surg*. 2013;70:500-505.
8. Clayton JL, Edkins R, Cairns BA, Hultman CS. Incidence and management of adverse events after the use of laser therapies for the treatment of hypertrophic burn scars. *Ann Plast Surg*. 2013;70:606-612.
9. Fredman R, Edkins RE, Hultman CS. Fat grafting for chronic pain after severe burns. *Ann Plast Surg*. 2016;76(suppl 4):S298-S303.
   In this pilot study of seven burn patients with refractory, neuropathic pain, we demonstrated the safety and efficacy of fat grafting in patients with hypertrophic scars, who had previously undergone laser resurfacing. These patients demonstrated improvement by both patient reported outcome measures and their ability to wean from their complex pharmacologic regimen, which included narcotics, NSAIDs, gabapentinoids, antipruritics, anxiolytics, and antidepressants.
10. Fredman R, Katz AJ, Hultman CS. Fat grafting for burn, traumatic, and surgical scars. *Clin Plast Surg*. 2017;44(4):781-791.
11. Hultman CS, Teotia S, Calvert C, et al. STARplasty for reconstruction of the burned web space: introduction of an alternative technique for the correction of dorsal neosyndactyly. *Ann Plast Surg*. 2005;54:281-287.
12. Rapolti M, Wu C, Schuth OA, Hultman CS. Under pressure: applying practice-based learning and improvement to the treatment of chronic neuropathic pain in patients with burns. *Clin Plast Surg*. 2017;44(4):925-934.
   In this retrospective review of 223 symptomatic burn patients, who underwent nerve decompression from 2000 to 2015, most patients reported moderate to definitive improvement in sensory symptoms and motor function, with minimal morbidity, and a return to work rate that reached 65% by the end of the study period. Specific adaptations adopted by the senior author include the use of WALANT (wide awake local anesthesia no tourniquet) surgery, in situ decompression over nerve transposition, and increased resection of neuromas with subfascial implantation.
13. Wu C, Calvert CT, Cairns BA, Hultman CS. Lower extremity nerve decompression in burn patients. *Ann Plast Surg*. 2013;70:563-567.
14. Chudasama S, Goverman J, Donaldson JH, et al. Does voltage predict return to work and neuropsychiatric sequellae following electrical burn injury? *Ann Plast Surg*. 2010;64(5):522-525.
   In this retrospective review of 2548 patients admitted to a verified burn center from 2000 to 2005, including 115 patients with electrical injury, we observed that even patients with low voltage injuries (<1000 V) still demonstrated significant neuropsychiatric sequelae and may delay return to work, despite relatively low final impairment ratings.
15. Cocciarella L, Anndersson GBJ, eds. *American Medical Association Guides to the Evaluation of Permanent Impairment*. 5th ed. AMA Press; 2001.

QUESTIONS

1. **A 36-year-old electrician sustains a full-thickness hand burn from a low voltage arc flash, with an entry point over the volar aspect of the right thumb, which is insensate and has no active flexion at the interphalangeal joint. What is the best plan for management?**

   a. Exploration of the forearm and decompression of the anterior interosseous nerve
   b. Aggressive debridement of volar thumb, placement of integra, and wound vacuum-assisted closure
   c. Repair of the involved structures and coverage with an innervated kite flap
   d. Complete amputation of thumb and pollicization of index finger
   e. Partial amputation of thumb and toe-to-thumb free tissue transfer

2. **A 24-year-old woman sustains circumferential, full-thickness wrist and forearm burns from a propane explosion, after her long-sleeve blouse caught on fire. She has delayed capillary refill of all digits and no Doppler signal in her palmar arch. What is the best option for restoring perfusion?**

   a. Dorsal forearm escharotomy
   b. Volar forearm escharotomy
   c. Volar forearm fasciotomy
   d. Volar forearm fasciotomy with carpal tunnel release
   e. Volar forearm fasciotomy with carpal tunnel and Guyon canal release

3. **A 58-year-old petroleum engineer receives a hydrofluoric acid burn at work, to the dorsum of his hand. Immediate irrigation with water is performed as part of his first aid. Upon arrival to the burn center, he has a full-thickness burn that is painful. What agent should be administered to neutralize the fluoride ion and limit deeper tissue necrosis?**

   a. Calcium gluconate
   b. Calcium chloride
   c. Potassium chloride
   d. Potassium hydroxide
   e. Ferrous sulfate

4. **A 46-year-old presents with a boutonniere deformity of the middle finger, 8 months after sustaining a deep burn to the dorsum of the finger requiring excision and skin grafting. What is the primary mechanism for this sequelae?**

   a. Rupture of the extensor digitorum communis tendon
   b. Contracture of the volar plate of the PIPJ
   c. Displacement of the lateral bands volarly
   d. Adhesions of the flexor digitorum profundus
   e. Stenosing tenosynovitis of the A1 pulley

5. **A 12-year-old girl, who previously underwent excision and grafting to the hand for a grease burn, now has a first web space contracture, at the junction of the dorsal skin graft and the volar surface of the thumb and index finger. What is the mathematical gain in length of the contracture with a single two-flap Z plasty, set at 45-degree angles?**

   a. 10%
   b. 30%
   c. 50%
   d. 70%
   e. 90%

1. **Answer: c.** Following debridement of devitalized tissue, the best opportunity for achieving maximal function is repair of the injured structures, such as the flexor pollicis longus tendon and neurolysis versus nerve graft, which would require coverage of vascularized tissue. A kite flap, from the dorsum of the index finger, is particularly attractive because this flap is innervated. Decompression of the anterior interosseous nerve would not be indicated acutely, unless the patient had an exit/entrance wound in this location. Amputation during the early management is too aggressive, as the best long-term option is reconstruction of the current thumb, albeit injured.

2. **Answer: e.** Although escharotomies and fasciotomies of the forearm may improve perfusion to the hand, the ulnar vessels in the Guyon canal should also be decompressed, which can be performed through a carpal tunnel release. All attempts should be made to achieve a Doppler signal in the palmar arch, as well as digital vessels, before the patient can leave the operating room.

3. **Answer: a.** Hydrofluoric acid burns yield progressive tissue damage, with saponification of fat and liquefaction of fascia, due to interaction of the fluoride anions with calcium, magnesium, and potassium cations. In fact, extensive hydrofluoric acid burns can result in QT prolongation, hypotension, and ventricular arrhythmias. Calcium gluconate can help to neutralize the fluoride ion and can be delivered topically, subcutaneously, or intravascularly, depending on the extent of injury.

4. **Answer: c.** Although the other options can occur in the burned hand, the most common cause of a boutonniere deformity, with hyperextension of the DIPJ and flexion of the PIPJ, is disruption of the central slip over the capsule of the dorsal PIPJ and displacement of the lateral bands from a dorsal to volar position. This occurs because the dorsal skin over the PIPJ is very thin and the central slip is often involved in the original injury. Options for reconstruction of a boutonniere deformity depend on the quality of skin over the dorsal PIPJ but include plication of the lateral bands, a reverse tendon flap to replace the missing central slip, and figure-of-eight tendon grafting to realign the lateral bands.

5. **Answer: c.** Although the theoretical gain in length from a single 45-degree two-flap Z-plasty is 50%, in reality the gain is closer to 30%, due to decreased pliability of the previously injured volar skin and the dorsal skin graft. To increase the actual gain, especially in this location, a 5-flap ***jumping man*** Z-plasty is usually the best option for deepening and lengthening the web space. Critical to achieving full release of this adduction contracture is performing fasciotomies on the adductor pollicis and first dorsal interosseous muscles. The author also performs a digital neurolysis of the ulnar digital nerve to the thumb and the radial digital nerve to the index finger, to ensure integrity of the nerve and prevent any points of constriction or tethering.

CHAPTER 89 Compartment Syndrome of the Upper Extremity

Guang Yang and Kevin C. Chung

KEY POINTS

- Compartment syndrome is a group of the clinical symptoms and signs that are caused by sustained elevation of compartment pressure, and consequent circulatory impairment, tissue ischemia, and cell necrosis.
- Increased intracompartmental pressure due to increased compartmental content or decreased compartmental size is the central factor of pathophysiology of compartment syndrome.
- The diagnosis of compartment syndrome is primarily a clinical one based on careful history and physical examination.
- The standard clinical signs have been described as five Ps: pain out of proportion to the injury, pallor, paresthesia, pulselessness, and paralysis.
- Compartment pressure greater than 30 mm Hg or within 20 to 30 mm Hg of the diastolic blood pressure is considered to be indication for fasciotomy.
- Fasciotomy in a timely manner is the only management for compartment syndrome with good outcome expected.
- Some degree of permanent nerve and/or muscle function loss, and even Volkmann ischemic contracture may happen because of the extent of primary tissue damage at the time of injury, other comorbidities, or delayed management.

Compartment syndrome is a group of the clinical symptoms and signs that are caused by sustained elevation of compartment pressure, and consequent circulatory impairment, tissue ischemia, and cell necrosis. Good function of the affected upper extremity with only skin scarring is expected if compartment syndrome is treated correctly and promptly. On the contrary, delays in diagnosis and treatment will result in devastating complications, potentially limb or life threatening. It is critical for the surgeons to understand the relevant anatomy, etiology, pathophysiology, diagnosis, and management strategies of compartment syndrome.

HISTORY

Dr. Richard von Volkmann first described the consequences of untreated forearm compartment syndromes in 1881.[1,2] He and his coauthors emphasized that the cause of tissue ischemia was the prolonged blocking of arterial inflow due to tight bandages.[2] In 1906, O. Hildebrand commented that occlusion of small arteries and vein congestion caused by the pressure of the surrounding tissue could result in muscle necrosis.[3] Bardenheuer was the first to suggest fasciotomy as a preventive measure for Volkmann ischemic contractures in the forearm.[4] Based on a series of animal experiments, Paul N. Jepson further proposed that if the compartment underwent prompt surgical decompression, the patient would recover.[5] In 1940, Griffiths found that not only arterial injury but also reflex spasms of the collateral circulation caused the ischemic contracture.[6] Clinical manifestations including pain with passive stretch, painless onset, pallor, and pulselessness were first described by him to contribute to the diagnosis of a forearm compartment syndrome. In 1948, Bunnell and Doherty described their clinical findings of hand compartment syndrome.[7] In the 1970s and 1980s, a set of theories for compartment syndrome pathophysiology were proposed, and the concepts of compartment syndrome, Volkmann ischemic contracture, and crush syndrome were unified and generally accepted in the surgical field.[8]

EPIDEMIOLOGY

Although compartment syndrome can occur in any closed space in the body, it mostly occurs within fibro-osseous space in the upper and lower extremities. The most common site is the lower leg, followed by the forearm and hand.[9] Upper arm compartment syndrome is rare, with few reported cases.[10]

The true incidence of compartment syndrome of the upper extremities is difficult to identify because a variety of injuries may lead to this syndrome. The incidence of acute compartment syndrome was estimated by McQueen at 7.3 per 100,000 for men and 0.7 per 100,000 for women by collecting the data of an orthopedic trauma unit from 1988 to 1995.[11] In another report from Zuchelli, 2.5% of 3274 adults who had suffered a blunt trauma injury to an extremity and seen at a level I trauma center were diagnosed with compartment syndrome.[9] Branco reported approximately 1% patients who required a fasciotomy after extremity trauma out of 10,315 patients, of which about one-fifth received upper extremity fasciotomies.[12] Young men are at great risk for development of a compartment syndrome.[11] In McQueen's report, 71% of the patients were men in their thirties.[11] Besides being more likely to sustain high-energy injuries, the author suggested that less space for muscle swelling of the muscle after injury led to the higher incidence of acute compartment syndrome in young men.

RELEVANT ANATOMY

As the name implies, compartment syndrome occurs in the *compartment*, which is a closed space constructed by the skin or connective tissues, and bones. Knowledge of the components and contents of each compartment in the upper extremity is essential to comprehend the etiology, clinical signs, and treatment of compartment syndrome (**Table 89.1**).

The upper arm consists of two compartments around the humerus: the anterior and posterior compartments (Figure 89.1). They are divided by the lateral and medial intermuscular septae. The musculocutaneous nerve and median nerves run through the anterior compartment. The ulnar and radial nerves travel in one compartment first, and then pass through the intermuscular septum into another compartment at the level of distal third of the arm. Velmahos believed this is why symptoms of radial or ulnar nerve ischemia are not compartment specific.[15]

The forearm has three major compartments, and the radius, ulna, and rigid interosseous membrane constitute the stiff floor of the compartments. Volar, dorsal, and lateral (mobile wad) compartments are divided by three intermuscular septae, and there are some communications among them. The muscles in the volar compartments are usually divided into superficial and deep groups (Figure 89.2). The deep volar muscles are usually the most severely affected in forearm compartment syndrome, because they are close to the stiff floor of the compartment. The median nerve runs between the superficial and deep muscles and ends at the carpal tunnel. The median nerve is the most commonly affected nerve in forearm compartment syndrome. Its motor branch, the anterior interosseous nerve (AIN), goes deeper to innervate the deep volar muscles including the pronator

TABLE 89.1. THE CONSTITUTES AND CONTENTS OF EACH COMPARTMENT IN THE UPPER EXTREMITY

	Anatomical Boundaries	Compartments		Contents: Muscles	Contents: Nerves	Contents: Artery
Arm	Skin, fascia, lateral and medial intermuscular septae, and humerus	Anterior		Biceps, brachialis, coracobrachialis	Musculocutaneous and median nerves	Brachial artery
		Posterior		Triceps	Radial nerve and ulnar nerves	Profunda brachii artery
Forearm	Skin, fascial, three intermuscular septum, radius, ulna, and interosseous membrane	Volar	Superficial	Pronator teres, flexor carpi radialis, palmaris longus, flexor digitorum superficialis, flexor carpi ulnaris	Median, ulnar, and anterior interosseous nerves	Radial and ulnar arteries
			Deep	Flexor pollicis longus, flexor digitorum profundus, pronator quadratus		
		Dorsal		Extensor digitorum communis, extensor digiti minimi, extensor carpi ulnaris, abductor pollicis longus, extensor pollicis brevis, extensor pollicis longus, extensor indicis proprius, supinator	Posterior interosseous nerve	Posterior interosseous artery
		Lateral (Mobile wad)		Brachioradialis, extensor carpi radialis longus, extensor carpi radialis brevis	Sensory branch of the radial nerve	–
Hand	Palmar aponeurosis, thenar fascia, hypothenar fascia, and metacarpals	Thenar		Abductor pollicis brevis, flexor pollicis brevis, and opponens pollicis	Recurrent motor branch of median nerve	Digital arteries of the thumb
		Adductor pollicis		Adductor pollicis	Deep branch of ulnar nerve	–
		Dorsal interossei (4)		Dorsal interosseous muscles		–
		Volar interossei (3)		Volar interosseous muscles	–	–
		Hypothenar		Abductor digiti minimi, the flexor digiti minimi, and the opponens digiti minimi	Ulnar nerve	
Finger	Cleland's and Grayson's ligaments, and phalanx	–		–	Digital nerves	Digital arteries

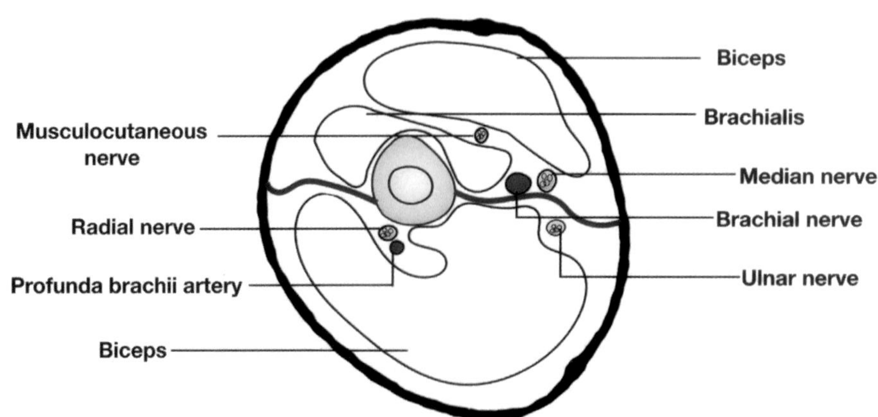

FIGURE 89.1. Cross-sectional anatomy showing two compartments of the upper arm.

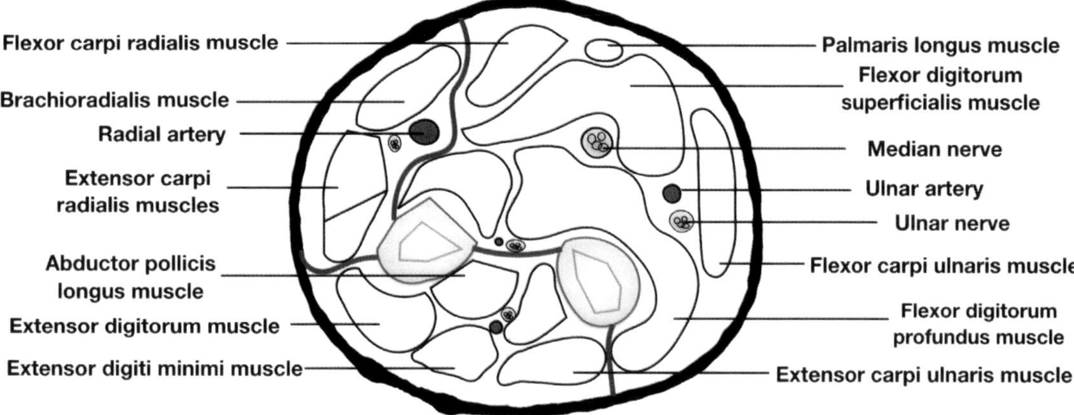

FIGURE 89.2. Cross-sectional anatomy showing three compartments of the forearm.

quadratus, the flexor digitorum profundus I and II, and the flexor pollicis longus. The AIN and the deepest portion of the flexor muscles are severely damaged when compartment syndrome involves the deep volar compartment.

The dorsal compartment contains the wrist and finger extensors, and the motor branch of the radial nerve (posterior interosseous nerve) that travels obliquely through and into the supinator muscle. The posterior interosseous nerve (PIN) then lies in a plane between the superficial and deep extensor muscles. In the distal forearm, the PIN lies on the interosseous membrane. The lateral compartment, also known as the mobile wad, is separated by [illegible] septum from the dorsal compartment. It is composed of brachioradialis, extensor carpi radialis longus, and extensor carpi radialis brevis muscles. The dorsal and lateral forearm compartments are usually affected along with volar forearm compartment syndrome, but also may develop isolated compartment syndrome.

There are at least 10 compartments in the hand that are usually divided into five groups; thenar, hypothenar, adductor pollicis, palmar, and dorsal interosseous [illegible]. Because of anatomic variations, these compartments may have two or more discrete subcompartments. The thenar, hypothenar, adductor pollicis, and interosseous compartments contain 14 intrinsic muscles of hand.

Although the finger has no muscle, compartment syndrome can still occur in the finger. The compartments of the finger are considered to be bounded by skin, and Cleland and Grayson ligaments.

PATHOPHYSIOLOGY

The pathophysiology of compartment syndrome is a multifactor process. Elevated intracompartmental tissue pressure in the myofascial compartment after injury is the central pathogenic factor.[8] Inadequate tissue perfusion within the compartment is the foundation, and progressive cell death is the final result of compartment syndrome.

Because the compartment is an enveloped space with limited elasticity, the intracompartmental pressure elevates because of increased compartmental content or decreased compartmental size after injury. Decreased arteriovenous gradient, declined arteriolar flow, and venous collapse result in decreased tissue perfusion within the affected compartment. The low tissue perfusion reduces the aerobic metabolism at the cellular level. As insufficient oxygen concentration decreases beyond the cell's intrinsic capacity to tolerate, toxic chemicals impinge the cellular membrane's function. The leak of the cellular membrane, especially the endothelium of a capillary,

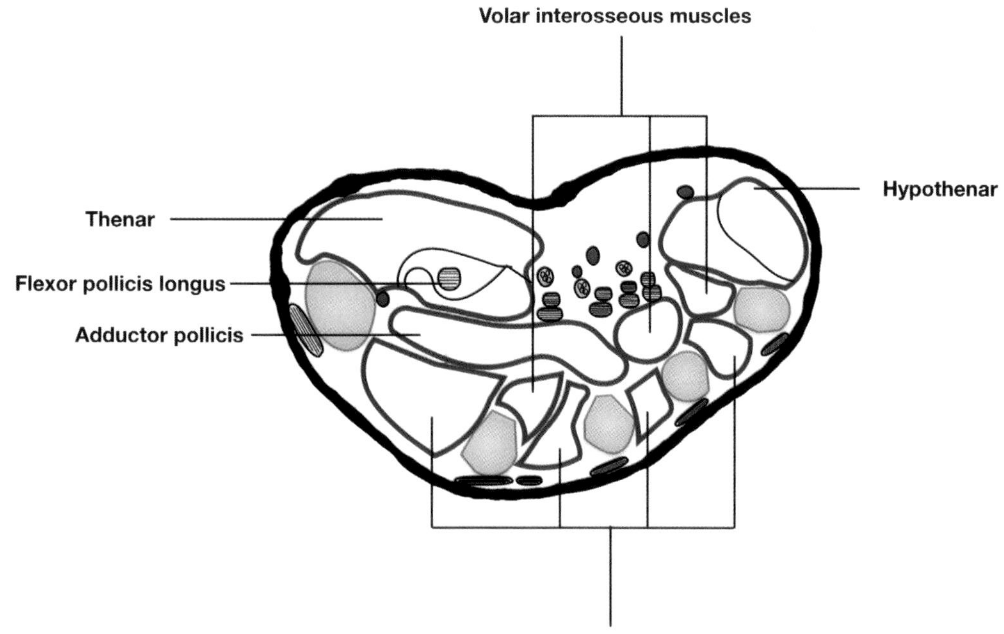

FIGURE 89.3. Cross-sectional anatomy showing 10 compartments of the hand.

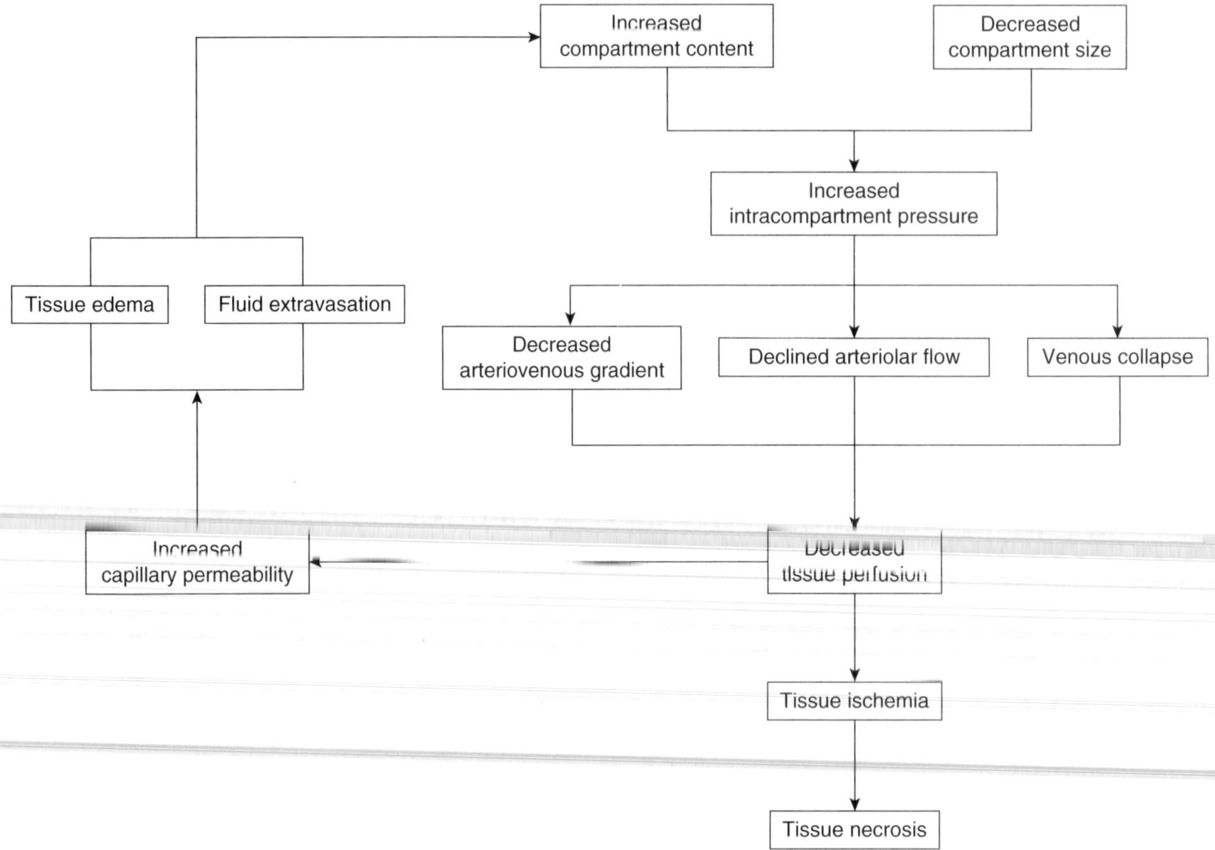

FIGURE 89.4. Compartment syndrome pathophysiology.

results in increased capillary permeability, causing the intravascular fluid to move into the interstitial space, and thus tissue edema develops. The increased compartment contents further deteriorate the tissues ischemia, which brings the pathological damage into a positive feedback loop (Figure 89.4). Without intracompartmental pressure relief, cell death presenting as muscular and neural fibrosis occurs.

Different tissues have different capacities to tolerate ischemia, and the clinical symptoms can arise simultaneously or following the initial trauma.[16] Skeletal muscle can tolerate up to 4 hours of ischemia, and can recover partially after 6 hours, but incurs permanent damage after 8 hours. Peripheral nerves are more sensitive to an ischemic change. Nerve conduction function is affected after 1 hour of ischemia, and peripheral nerves may undergo irreversible damage after 4 to 6 hours of ischemia.[17,18] Outcomes are determined by the extent of the damage and the level of the compartmental pressure. Volkmann ischemic contracture is used to term the final result of tissue ischemia following compartment syndrome, which is characterized by varying degrees of muscle fibrosis and neurologic deficiency. A severe local compartment syndrome can also arise the systemic manifestations, which is called crush syndrome. Rapid return of toxic muscle products into the circulatory system may lead to renal failure, cardiac failure, respiratory failure, and intravascular coagulation.[19]

ETIOLOGY

Theoretically, any factors that lead to increased compartmental pressure may account for compartment syndrome. Injuries that commonly cause compartment syndrome are categorized and listed in **Table 89.2**.

TABLE 89.2. THE ETIOLOGIES OF THE COMPARTMENT SYNDROME

Category	Examples
Fracture	Radius fracture, ulna fracture, both-bone forearm fractures, pediatric supracondylar humerus fracture, multiple metacarpal fractures
Vascular injury	Major vascular stab or rupture, ischemia-reperfusion after replantation or vascular repair, artery blood sampling
Crush injury	Closed blunt trauma, extremity crush resulting from coma or seizure
Iatrogenic compression	Tight dressing, splint or cast, constrictive bandages, tourniquet overuse, prolonged limb positioning, tight wound closure
Drugs or fluids extravasation and input	High pressure injection injury, drugs or contrast medium extravasation, peripheral parenteral nutrition extravasation
Burns	Electrical injury, thermal injury
Bleeding disorder and anticoagulation therapy	Hemophilia, heparin use
Infection	Tenosynovitis of the finger
Muscle overuse	Exercise, weight lifting
Others	Crotalid envenomation

Fractures are the most common cause for compartment syndrome in the extremities.[11,13,14] Fractured bones result in muscle injuries and hematoma formation may increase compartment contents.[20] The displaced bones can cause vascular injury. This is most commonly seen in pediatric supracondylar humerus fractures.[21] Multiple closed reduction attempts may make this worse. Open fractures do not necessarily prevent compartment syndrome because the wounds may not open the compartment completely. According to Branco's report, patients with open fractures had a higher incidence of fasciotomy than those with closed fractures.[12] Radius and/or ulna fractures were the most common cause of forearm compartment syndrome, followed by supracondylar fractures.[14] Hand compartment syndrome can be caused by multiple metacarpal fractures.

Vascular injury with subsequent reperfusion injury is another common cause of compartment syndrome.[22] Continuous bleeding from major arteries into a confined space can quickly lead to increased compartment pressure.[23] In addition, direct arterial injury leads to local tissue ischemic edema.[24] A delay in revascularization can aggravate ischemic edema that expands the compartment contents.

It is understandable that crush injury is one cause for the extremity compartment syndrome.[25] Iatrogenic compression, such as prolonged limb positioning, tight dressing or cast, and tourniquet overuse can also be responsible for a compartment syndrome. Surgeons should be aware that the ischemic condition after intramuscular perforator harvest may decrease pressure tolerance of the compartmental tissue.[26]

Except for a traumatic vascular stab injury or rupture, bleeding or inflowing into compartment from a high-pressure injection or iatrogenic fluid extravasation can also increase compartment pressure.[27–30] Thus, the patients who have a bleeding disorder or receive anticoagulation therapy have a higher risk for developing compartment syndrome.[10] Crotalid envenomation, infection, electrical injuries, and burns have also been considered to cause a cascade of events that leads to the rapid formation of vascular permeability and interstitial edema.[31] Rarer etiologies of compartment syndrome include muscle overuse, rhabdomyolysis, and systemic sclerosis.

DIAGNOSIS

The diagnosis of compartment syndrome is primarily clinical, and based on patient history, symptoms, and signs. Documenting the patient's history of any injuries that may increase compartment contents or decrease compartment volume is critical to identify compartment syndrome, which may be the only basis of the diagnosis and fasciotomy, for instance preventive fasciotomies after limb replantation.

Clinical Signs

The reliable physical sign is usually swelling or tightness in the extremity. The affected hand, forearm, or arm is hard to palpation, skin creases vanish, and overlying skin may become shiny and even develop blister (Figure 89.5). The fingers are often placed in flexion position in a forearm compartment syndrome, and in the intrinsic minus position in a hand compartment syndrome.

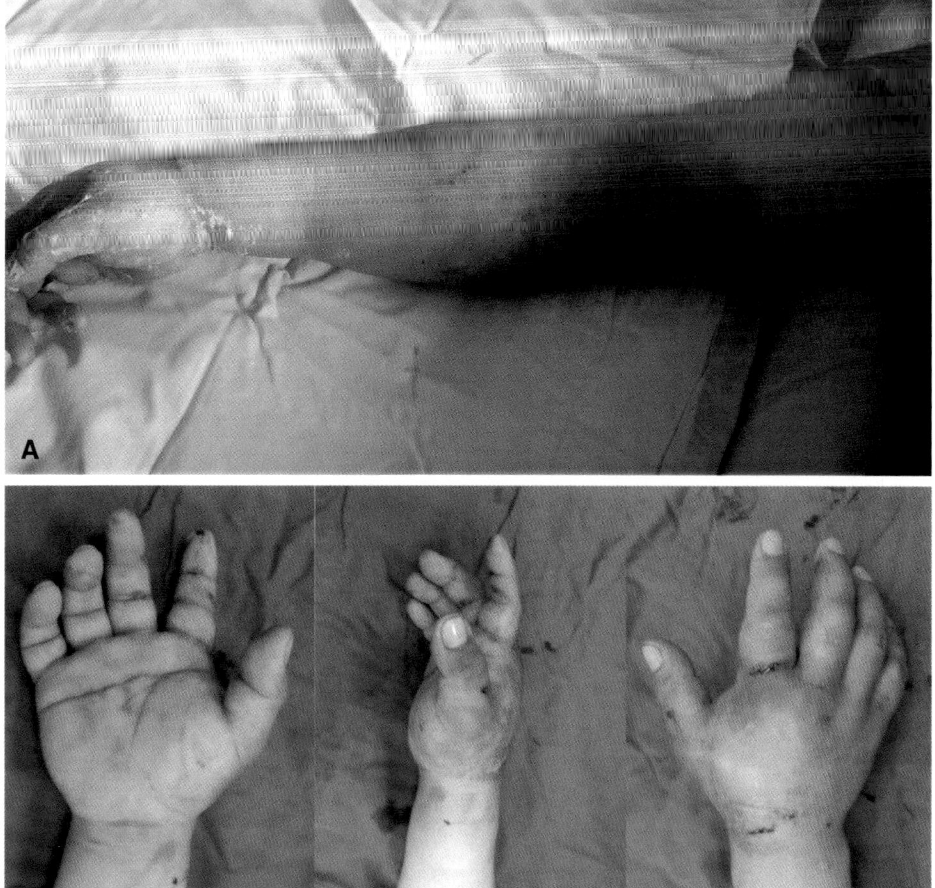

FIGURE 89.5. **A.** Acute forearm compartment syndrome in a patient who suffered a crush injury. **B.** Acute hand compartment syndrome in a patient presenting swollen appearance.

TABLE 89.3. CLINICAL SIGNS IN THE COMPARTMENT SYNDROME

Signs	Descriptions
Swelling	Reliable and nearly presented in all the patients
Pain	Severe and out of proportion to primary injury
	Worse as passive stretching of the compartmental muscles
	Early and sensitive finding
	Subjective, and difficult assess in children
Paresthesia	Indicates nerve ischemia in the affected compartment
	Early sign
	Very low sensitivity but high specificity
Paralysis	Often indicates the compartment syndrome in an irreversible injury
Pallor and Pulselessness	Late symptom
	Often exists with vascular injury
	May not presented in a compartment syndrome

The symptoms and signs of the compartment syndrome have been classically described as 5Ps: pain, paresthesia, paralysis, pallor, and pulselessness (**Table 89.3**). These nonspecific findings can be disclosed in the primary injury and can present from the first few hours after injury, to after the repair, or may not present at all. All five Ps are more commonly seen in a primary vascular injury rather than compartment syndrome.[32]

Pain is the early and sensitive finding before onset of ischemia, but it should be distinguished from the primary injury pain. The pain from high compartment pressure is usually out of proportion to the nature of the injury, especially on passive stretching of the compartment contents. For example, in the volar forearm compartment syndrome, the pain is often introduced by passive extension of the fingers and wrist, which increases the compartment pressure. Similarly, the pain on passive palmar abduction of the thumb, thus stretching the abductor pollicis brevis, is associated with a thenar compartment syndrome. Progressive pain often indicates increasing compartment pressure.

Paresthesia is another early sign, especially when a sensory nerve travels in the affected compartment. For example, in a patient with the volar forearm compartment syndrome, the thumb and index finger that are innervated by the median nerve may experience sensory changes.

Pallor and pulselessness are often present later and may not be confirmed even after irreversible tissue damage occurs.[33] Paralysis often suggests that the muscles in the affected compartment have undergone irreversible damage, which indicates that the compartment syndrome has reached the final stage.[34]

Compartment Pressure Measurement

When subjective physical examinations are not reliable or taking a history is not possible, the objective examination of compartment syndrome is to measure the intracompartmental pressure. Although normal intracompartmental pressures range dramatically, a pressure greater than 30 mm Hg is an indication for an urgent fasciotomy.[35-37] Additionally, a pressure difference within 20 to 30 mm Hg of the patient's diastolic blood pressure is an indication for compartment syndrome as well.[38,39]

Many measurement methods for compartment pressure have been described in the literature.[34,40,41] In 1975, Whiteside and colleagues proposed an apparatus for compartment pressure measurement.[35] After the needle is inserted into the compartment and stopcock is turned on, the compartment pressure is read on the manometer when the saline column moves by slowly depressing the plunger of the syringe. Currently, Whiteside's and other simply devices have been replaced by more convenient commercial monitor systems. Of them, the Stryker compartment pressure monitor system is the most commonly used in North America. It is easily accessible and found to be quite accurate if used properly.[42,43] The Stryker system involves the use of a side-ported noncoring needle, a syringe prefilled with 0.9% saline, and a digital pressure manometer with a display (Figure 89.6). To be measured, the compartment should be placed at the level of the heart. The site of the inserted needle is usually at the maximum swelling of each compartment. The needle is inserted perpendicular to the skin into the compartment space with a local anesthesia if necessary. At a proper needle depth, the pressure reading will increase when the affected compartment is compressed externally.[39]

Doppler ultrasound and radiography imaging have been used to evaluate the primary injury and identify the amount of tissue edema, but not helpful for diagnosis of compartment syndrome.

CHRONIC COMPARTMENT SYNDROME

Chronic compartment syndrome is characterized by exercise-induced and rest-relieved pain, and it rarely happens in the upper limb.[44,45] The pain is associated with moderately elevated compartment pressures due to muscular hypertrophy. Neurological symptoms such as tingling and hand numbness were found in some cases.[44] Negative findings of physical examination at rest can rule out other differential diagnoses including nerve compression syndrome, vascular claudication, and fascial herniation. Dynamic compartment pressure measurement is helpful to diagnose chronic compartment syndrome of the forearm.[44]

TREATMENT

If compartment syndrome is suspected, any external pressure including cast, bandage, or sutures should be immediately removed. The limb should be elevated at the level of the heart but not above this level.[46] When compartment syndrome is diagnosed, emergency fasciotomy is the only management with good expected outcomes.

Fasciotomy

Although subcutaneous and endoscopic-assisted fasciotomies have been reported, the traditional open technique remains the preferred method. There are several classic surgical approaches for upper extremity compartment syndrome. When the incision is designed, primary injury repair or late reconstruction should be considered. If there is an initial wound, the incision for compartment release will be carefully designed to avoid flap necrosis in the elevated flap. In cases of fracture, the incision must be considered to expose the underlying fracture for reduction and fixation. Fasciotomy procedures include not only dividing the skin and fascia to release the compartmental muscles and nerves, but also identifying and excising of nonviable muscles.

Upper arm fasciotomy is often performed via a medial incision and a lateral incision (Figure 89.7). The two incisions are used through the subcutaneous tissues and fascia to decompress the anterior and posterior compartments.

For the volar forearm compartment release, a wide extensile exposure starting at the medial epicondyle and extending to the proximal wrist crease is usually performed for fasciotomy (Figure 89.8). The incision must be made with adequate curving to avoid distal flexor tendons and median nerve exposure. Otherwise, these exposed deep tissues need a complex flap procedure rather than skin graft coverage. After the subcutaneous flap is elevated, careful inspection is carried out through the space

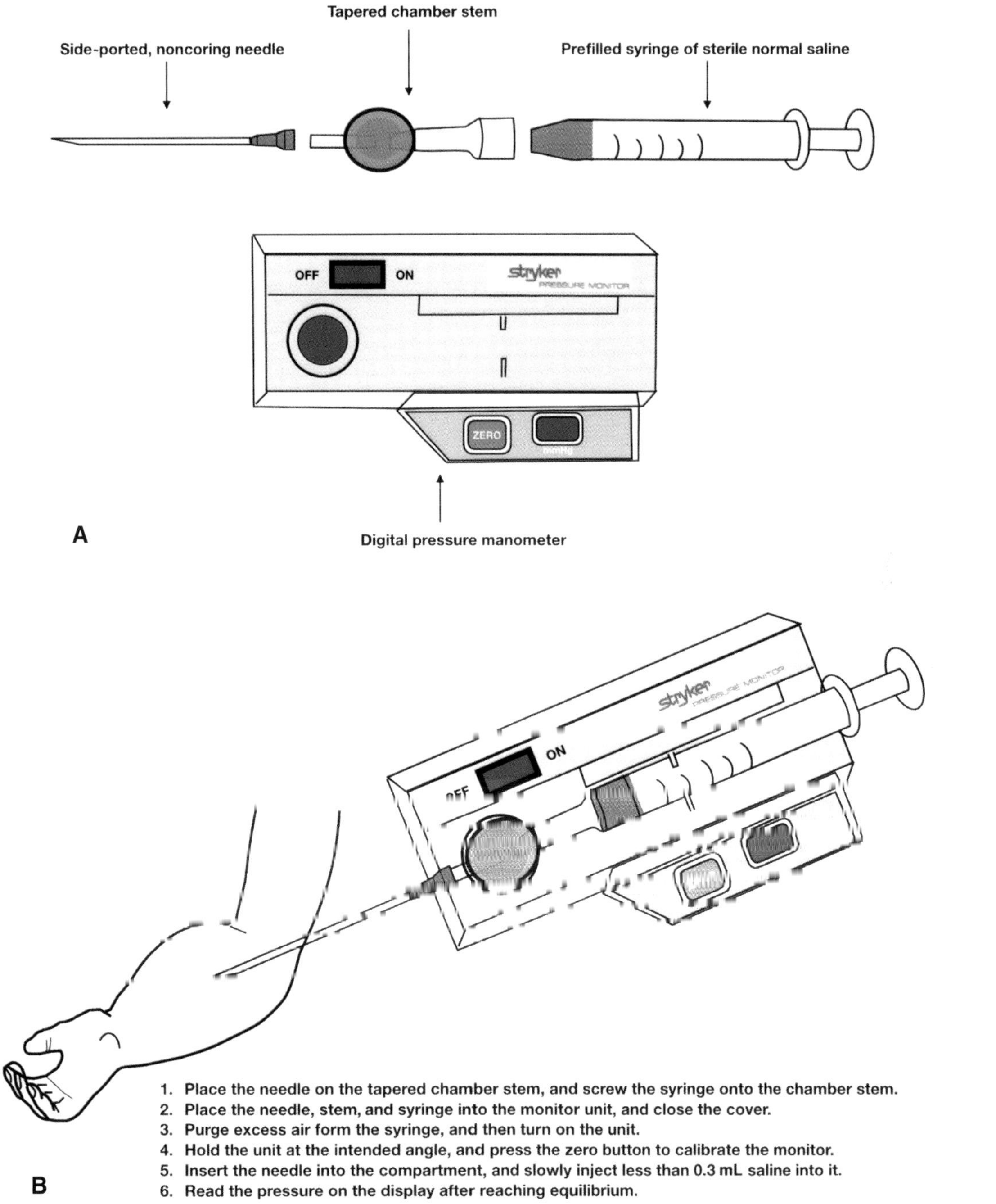

Tapered chamber stem

Side-ported, noncoring needle

Prefilled syringe of sterile normal saline

OFF ON

stryker PRESSURE MONITOR

ZERO

mmHg

A

Digital pressure manometer

OFF ON

stryker PRESSURE MONITOR

1. Place the needle on the tapered chamber stem, and screw the syringe onto the chamber stem.
2. Place the needle, stem, and syringe into the monitor unit, and close the cover.
3. Purge excess air form the syringe, and then turn on the unit.
4. Hold the unit at the intended angle, and press the zero button to calibrate the monitor.
5. Insert the needle into the compartment, and slowly inject less than 0.3 mL saline into it.
6. Read the pressure on the display after reaching equilibrium.

B

FIGURE 89.6. The Stryker intracompartmental pressure monitor system. **A.** The components of system. **B.** The steps of using Stryker device.

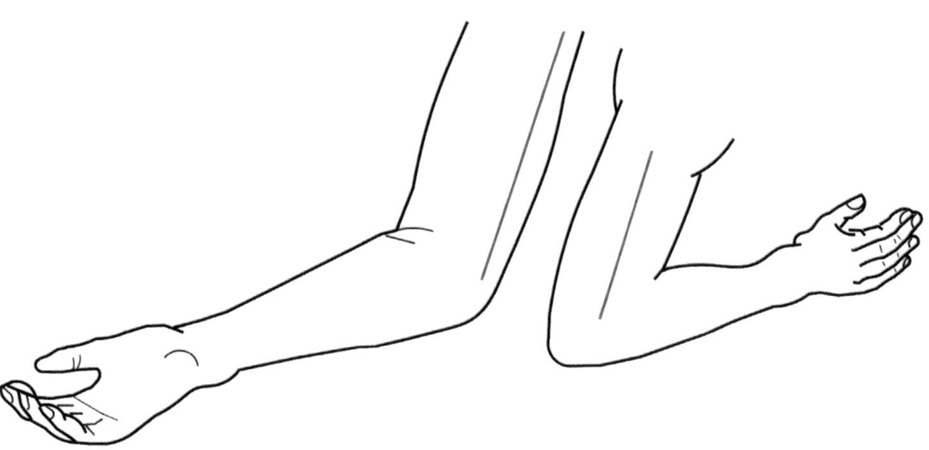

FIGURE 89.7. The incision design for the upper arm fasciotomy.

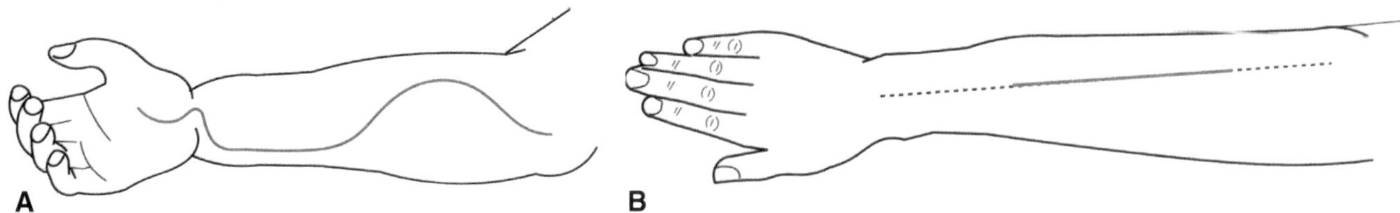

FIGURE 89.8. The incision design for forearm fasciotomy of the volar **(A)** and dorsal **(B)** compartments.

between the flexor carpi ulnaris and flexor digitorum superficialis to decompress the median nerve and deep group of flexor muscles. The median nerve in the carpal tunnel is susceptible to compressive pressures so that carpal tunnel decompression is often performed with forearm or hand fasciotomy.

If the pressure in the dorsal compartment does not decrease after volar compartment decompression, a dorsal compartment fasciotomy is indicated. For dorsal forearm compartment syndrome, a longitudinal incision is designed on the line between the distal radioulnar joint and the lateral epicondyle (see Figure 89.8). Usually, the incision is limited to the middle half of the forearm to avoid exposing the distal extensor tendons. The fascia is then divided and approached between the extensor digitorum communis and extensor carpi radialis brevis. The mobile wad can be released via the same incision by mobilization of the incision site.

Two longitudinal incisions are recommended by the authors to release the forearm compartment. One is along the ulnar edge of the radius over the flexor muscles, and the other is along the ulnar edge of the ulna over the extensor muscles. These two incisions are done above the muscle belly without the danger to expose the tendon.

Although there are more than 10 compartments in the hand, it is unnecessary to approach all the compartments. Except carpal tunnel release, hand compartments are usually released by four incisions (Figure 89.9). The dorsal two incisions parallel and radial to the second metacarpal and fourth metacarpal are made to access interossei and adductor compartments by either side of the bones (Figure 89.10). The standard approach for the thenar compartment requires a longitudinal incision along the radial aspect of the thenar eminence between the glabrous and nonglabrous skin. The standard approach for the hypothenar compartment is via a longitudinal incision along the ulnar aspect of the hypothenar eminence.

Finger decompression is performed with a midaxial lateral incision along the noncontact side of the finger to release the Cleland and Grayson ligaments (Figure 89.11). The dissection is carried out superficial to the flexor sheath carefully to avoid any injury to the neurovascular bundles.

POSTOPERATIVE MANAGEMENT

After fasciotomy, the incisions are left open to avoid recompression of the compartments due to muscular tissue edema.[36] However, the incision for carpal tunnel release is closed directly.[39] Usually, a couple of tacking sutures are used to approximate the skin over the wounds. The open wounds are covered by a bulky moist dressing, which requires regular dressing changes postoperatively. A vacuum-assisted closure system can also be used to cover the wound. A systematic review conducted by Jauregui et al found that vacuum-assisted closure could reduce the relative complications including wound edge necrosis, infection, and neurologic deficit.[25] The limb is then placed in a functional position by a removable splint with close observation after fasciotomy. Additional debridement may be performed for muscle necrosis and infection. Delayed primary closure or skin grafting to the open area is performed depending on the wound tension, which often requires 7 to 10 days. Early physical and occupational therapy exercises are helpful to prevent joint stiffness.

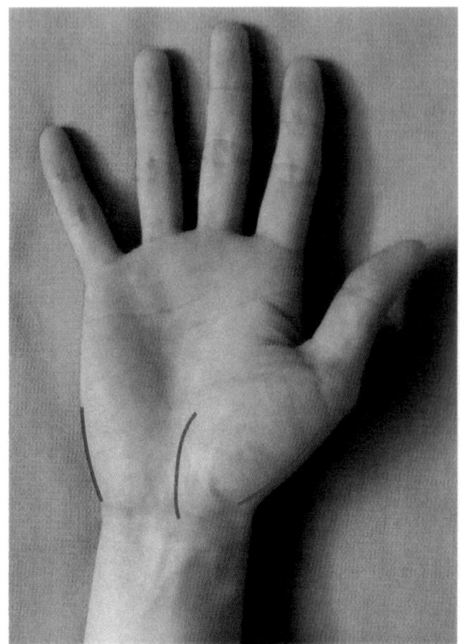

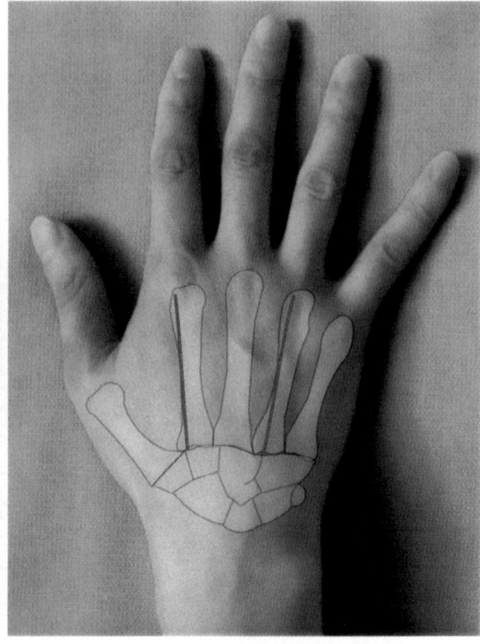

FIGURE 89.9. Volar and dorsal incisions for hand compartment releases.

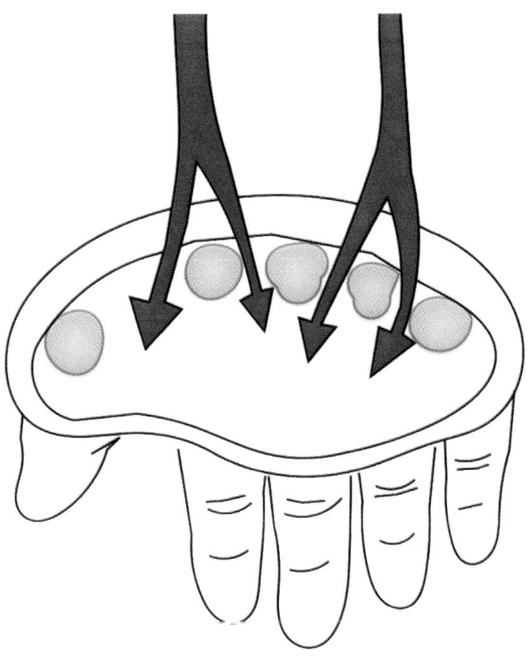

FIGURE 89.10. Interossei and adductor compartments are released by two dorsal incisions parallel and radial to the second metacarpal and fourth metacarpal.

OUTCOMES

The outcomes and complications of compartment syndrome mostly depend on primary injury severity and time from diagnosis to fasciotomy.[14] Only if fasciotomy is performed before irreversible cell death occurs (within 1 to 6 hours of compartment syndrome onset), the patient may regain full function and sensation from the compartment syndrome. Duckworth et al reported 90 patients who underwent fasciotomy for an acute forearm compartment syndrome.[14] Twenty-nine patients (32%) had complication associated with acute compartment syndrome. The patients who accepted fasciotomy more than 6 hours after presentation were more likely to develop complications, and the rate of complications increased with the time to fasciotomy. Ouellette and Kelly followed 17 patients with hand compartment syndrome at an average of 21-month follow-up period after fasciotomy.[47] Thirteen patients resumed almost normal hand function. Four patients whose primary injury or illness masked the compartment syndrome had poor results.

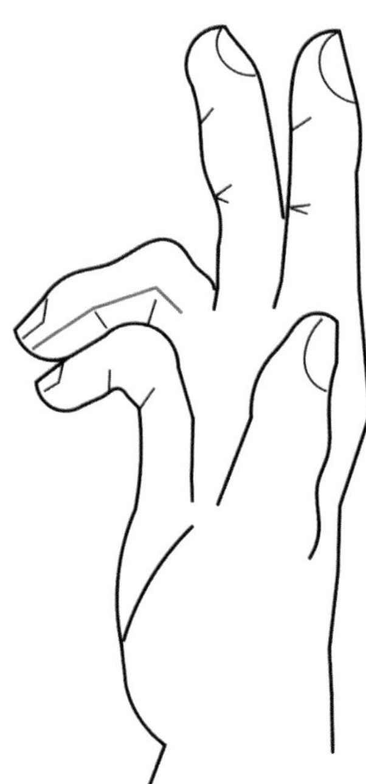

FIGURE 89.11. Incision design for digital compartment release.

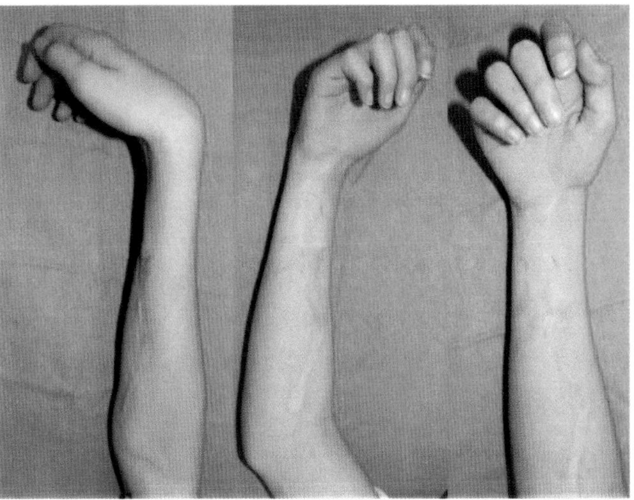

FIGURE 89.12. The patient with forearm Volkmann ischemic contracture presents as forearm pronation, wrist flexion, thumb adduction, MCP joints in extension, and IP joints in flexion.

Neurological deficit is the most common complication of the forearm compartment syndrome.[14,25] Other complications including infection, muscle necrosis, chronic pain, fracture nonunion, and even Volkmann ischemic contracture may happen because of the extent of direct trauma or delayed management.[illegible] The patients with Volkmann ischemia contracture present with muscle contracture deformities and nerve dysfunctions [illegible]. Function reconstruction strategy for these patients depends on the extent of the muscular necrosis and nerve damage.

ACKNOWLEDGMENTS

The work was supported by a Midcareer Investigator Award in Patient-Oriented Research (2 K24-AR053120-06) to Kevin C. Chung. The content is solely the responsibility of the authors and does not necessarily represent the official views of the National Institutes of Health.

REFERENCES

1. Ellis H. Richard von Volkmann: Volkmann's ischaemic contracture. *J Perioper Pract*. 2012;22(10):338-339.
2. von Volkmann R. Ischaemic muscle paralyses and contractures. 1881. *Clin Orthop Relat Res*. 2007;456:20-21.
3. Hildebrand O. Die Lehre von den ischamische Muskellahmungen und Kontrakturen. *Samml Klin Vortrage*. 1906;122:559-584.
4. Bardenheuer L. Die ischamische Kontraktur und Gangran als Folge der Arterienverletzung. *Leuthold's Gedenkschr*. 1906;2:87-131.
5. Jepson PN. Ischaemic contracture: experimental study. *Ann Surg*. 1926;84(6):785-795.
6. Griffiths D. Volkmann's ischaemic contracture. *Br J Surg*. 1940;28:239-260.
7. Bunnell S, Doherty EW, Curtis RM. Ischemic contracture, local, in the hand. *Plast Reconstr Surg (1946)*. 1948;3(4):424-433.
8. Matsen FA III. Compartmental syndrome: an unified concept. *Clin Orthop Relat Res*. 1975;(113):8-14.
   This is a classic review of the pathogenesis, pressure factors, time factors, physical findings, and treatment of compartment syndrome.
9. Zuchelli D, Divaris N, McCormack JE, et al. Extremity compartment syndrome following blunt trauma: a level I trauma center's 5-year experience. *J Surg Res*. 2017;217:131-136.
10. Thomas N, Cone B. Acute compartment syndrome in the upper arm. *Am J Emerg Med*. 2017;35(3):525.
11. McQueen MM, Gaston P, Court-Brown CM. Acute compartment syndrome: who is at risk. *J Bone Joint Surg Br*. 2000;82B(2):200-203.

12. Branco BC, Inaba K, Barmparas G, et al. Incidence and predictors for the need for fasciotomy after extremity trauma: a 10-year review in a mature level I trauma centre. *Injury*. 2011;42(10):1157-1163.
13. Grottkau BE, Epps HR, Di Scala C. Compartment syndrome in children and adolescents. *J Pediatr Surg*. 2005;40(4):678-682.
14. Duckworth AD, Mitchell SE, Molyneux SG, et al. Acute compartment syndrome of the forearm. *J Bone Joint Surg Am*. 2012;94(10):e63.
The authors retrospectively studied 90 patients who accepted fasciotomy for an acute forearm compartment syndrome from 1988 to 2010. Injury mechanism, presenting symptoms, time to fasciotomy, methods of wound closure, and long-term complications associated with fasciotomy were documented with a mean 11-month follow-up period. Younger patients were more likely to require split-thickness skin grafting for wound closure. The patients who accepted fasciotomy more than 6 hours after presentation were at a higher risk for development of complications.
15. Velmahos GC, Toutouzas KG. Vascular trauma and compartment syndromes. *Surg Clin North Am*. 2002;82(1):125-141.
16. Whitesides TE, Heckman MM. Acute compartment syndrome: update on diagnosis and treatment. *J Am Acad Orthop Surg*. 1996;4(4):209-218.
17. Malinoski DJ, Slater MS, Mullins RJ. Crush injury and rhabdomyolysis. *Crit Care Clin*. 2004;20(1):171-192.
18. Ugalde V, Rosen BS. Ischemic peripheral neuropathy. *Phys Med Rehabil Clin North Am*. 2001;12(2):365-380.
19. Bentley G, Jeffreys TE. The crush syndrome in coal miners. *J Bone Joint Surg Br*. 1968;50B(3):588-594.
20. [illegible] ment pressures in children with supracondylar fractures of the humerus. *J Pediatr Orthop*. 2002;22(4):431-439.
21. Cambon-Binder A, Jehanno P, Tribout L, et al. Pulseless supracondylar humeral fractures in children: vascular complications in a ten year series. *Int Orthop*. 2018;42(4):891-899.
22. Dente CJ, Feliciano DV, Rozycki GS, et al. A review of upper extremity fasciotomies in a level I trauma center. *Am Surg*. 2004;70(12):1088-1093.
23. Morin RJ, Swan KG, Tan V. Acute forearm compartment syndrome secondary to local arterial injury after penetrating trauma. *J Trauma*. 2009;66(4):989-993.
24. Suzuki T, Moirmura N, Kawai K, Sugiyama M. Arterial injury associated with acute compartment syndrome of the thigh following blunt trauma. *Injury*. 2005;36(1):151-159.
25. Kalyani BS, Fisher BE, Roberts CS, Giannoudis PV. Compartment syndrome of the forearm: a systematic review. *J Hand Surg*. 2011;36(3):535-543.
Twelve articles with 84 patients were included in this systematic review to discuss the etiology, diagnosis, treatment, fasciotomy wound management, complications, and outcome of forearm compartment syndrome. Skin grafting was required to close the fasciotomy wound in 61% cases, and the most common complication was neurological deficit.
26. Addison PD, Lannon D, Neligan PC. Compartment syndrome after closure of the anterolateral thigh flap donor site: a report of two cases. *Ann Plast Surg*. 2008;60(6):635-638.
27. Chinn M, Colella MR. Prehospital dextrose extravasation causing forearm compartment syndrome: a case report. *Prehosp Emerg Care*. 2017;21(1):79-82.
28. Funk L, Grover D, de Silva H. Compartment syndrome of the hand following intra-arterial injection of heroin. *J Hand Surg*. 1999;24(3):366-367.
29. Jue J, Karam JA, Mejia A, Shroff A. Compartment syndrome of the hand: a rare sequela of transradial cardiac catheterization. *Tex Heart Inst J*. 2017;44(1):73-76.
30. Elmorsy A, Nutt J, Taylor N, Kirk-Bayley J, Hughes S. Iatrogenic forearm compartment syndrome. *J Intens Care Soc*. 2017;18(1):63-65.
31. Leversedge FJ, Moore TJ, Peterson BC, Seiler JG III. Compartment syndrome of the upper extremity. *J Hand Surg*. 2011;36(3):544-559.
32. Oak NR, Abrams RA. Compartment syndrome of the hand. *Orthop Clin North Am*. 2016;47(3):609-616.
33. Willhoite DR, Moll JH. Early recognition and treatment of impending Volkmann's ischemia in the lower extremity. *Arch Surg*. 1970;100(1):11-16.
34. Dente CJ, Wyrzykowski AD, Feliciano DV. Fasciotomy. *Curr Probl Surg*. 2009;46(10):779-839.
35. Whitesides TE Jr, Haney TC, Harada H, et al. A simple method for tissue pressure determination. *Arch Surg*. 1975;110(11):1311-1313.
36. Kistler JM, Ilyas AM, Thoder JJ. Forearm compartment syndrome: evaluation and management. *Hand Clin*. 2018;34(1):53-60.
37. Kanj WW, Gunderson MA, Carrigan RB, Sankar WN. Acute compartment syndrome of the upper extremity in children: diagnosis, management, and outcomes. *J Child Orthop*. 2013;7(3):225-233.
The article was to retrospectively study 23 pediatric patients with acute compartment syndrome of the upper arm. Most patients developed compartment syndrome due to fracture. Pain and swelling were commonly seen in the patients. Seventeen patients (74 %) had no loss of function or sensation, and 5 (22%) obtained minor permanent change at the latest follow-up visit.
38. [illegible] syndrome of the hand: a little thought about diagnosis. *Case Rep Emerg Med*. 2016;2016:2907067.
39. Lipschitz AH, Litchez SD. Measurement of compartment pressures in the hand and forearm. *J Hand Surg*. 2010;35(11):1893-1894.
40. Matsen FA III, Winquist RA, Krugmire RB Jr. Diagnosis and management of compartmental syndromes. *J Bone Joint Surg Am*. 1980;62A(2):286-291.
41. Mubarak SJ, Hargens AR, Owen CA, et al. The wick catheter technique for measurement of intramuscular pressure: a new research and clinical tool. *J Bone Joint Surg Am*. 1976;58A(7):1016-1020.
42. Boody AR, Wongworawat MD. Accuracy in the measurement of compartment pressures: a comparison of three commonly used devices. *J Bone Joint Surg Am*. 2005;87A(11):2415-2422.
43. Hammerberg EM, Whitesides TE Jr, Seiler JG III. The reliability of measurement of tissue pressure in compartment syndrome. *J Orthop Trauma*. 2012;26(1):24-31.
44. Zandi H, Bell S. Results of compartment decompression in chronic forearm compartment syndrome: six case presentations. *Br J Sports Med*. 2005;39(9):e35.
45. Abe Y, Fujii K. Chronic compartment syndrome of the mobile wad: a case report. *J Hand Surg Asian Pac Vol*. 2017;22(4):516-518.
46. Chidgey LK, Szabo RM, Kolack B. Effects of elevation on nerve function in an acute upper extremity nerve compression model. *J Orthop Res*. 1989;7(6):783-791.
47. Ouellette EA, Kelly R. Compartment syndromes of the hand. *J Bone Joint Surg Am*. 1996;78A(10):1515-1522.
The retrospective study reported the outcomes of 17 patients after fasciotomy for hand compartment syndrome. Thirteen patients regained normal functions of the hand, but 4 patients whose compartment syndrome was obtunded by a serious illness or injury or anesthesia had poor results.

QUESTIONS

1. **Which of the following is the most common cause of a forearm compartment syndrome in children?**

   a. Vascular injury
   b. Crush injury
   c. Burn
   d. Fracture
   e. Snake bite

2. **Which of the following is the central pathogenic factor of compartment syndrome?**

   a. Inadequate tissue perfusion
   b. Increased compartment content
   c. Cell death
   d. Increased capillary permeability
   e. Increased intracompartmental pressure

3. **A 28-year-old man has an ulna-radius fracture after a car crash. The fractures are reduced and placed in a splint in the emergency room. What is considered the most important sign or symptom of a compartment syndrome of the forearm?**

   a. Pain out of proportion to the primary injury
   b. Numbness in the hand
   c. Loss of the movement of the fingers
   d. Decreased pulses
   e. Pallor appearance of the hand

4. **A 65-year-old man involves in a traffic incident. He had slipped into a coma by the time he reached emergency department. On physical exam, the right hand is severely swollen and feels firm. Which of the following is the most appropriate method to diagnose a compartment syndrome for this patient?**

   a. Doppler ultrasound
   b. CT scan
   c. Intracompartmental pressure measure
   d. X-ray
   e. Magnetic resonance image

5. **A young man, previously healthy, presents for evaluation of a painful and swollen left forearm approximately 3 hours after a crush injury. He complained that he did not have significant 10/10 pain until 40 minutes earlier. Physical exam reveals pain with extension of his fingers. Radial pulses are present and the skin color is normal. Radiographs demonstrate fracture of the distal radius. As a compartment syndrome is suspected, intracompartmental pressure is measured by the Stryker compartment pressure device. The pressure of the volar forearm compartment is 42 mm Hg. Which of following should be the next step?**

   a. Admission for observation and pain control
   b. Open reduction and fixation of the fracture
   c. Percutaneous pinning of the fracture
   d. Fasciotomy
   e. Physical and occupational therapy

1. **Answer: d.** Any factors that can elevate intracompartmental pressure by increasing compartment content or decreasing compartment size may lead to compartment syndrome. Fracture is the most common cause of forearm compartment syndrome in both children and adults in epidemiological studies. Fractured bones result in muscle injuries and hematoma formation, which increases compartment contents. Furthermore, displaced bones can injury the vessels, which may happen in pediatric supracondylar humerus fracture. The syndrome happens in not only close fractures but also open fractures. Vascular injury, crush injury, burn, and crotalid envenomation are also responsible for compartment syndrome, but not as common as fractures.

2. **Answer: e.** The pathophysiology of compartment syndrome is a multifactor-contributed process. Based on Matsen's arteriovenous pressure gradient and other theories, increased intracompartmental pressure introduces decreased arteriovenous gradient, declined arteriolar flow, and venous collapse. Elevated intracompartmental tissue pressure is the central pathogenic factor. These pathophysiological changes result in decreased tissue perfusion and ischemia. Increased capillary permeability followed by tissue ischemia deteriorates tissue edema. These bring the pathophysiological damage into a positive feedback loop. Cell death is the final stage of pathological change of compartment syndrome.

3. **Answer: a.** The most reliable and sensitive finding of compartment syndrome is pain out of proportion to the original injury. The pain is often deep and is worsened by passive stretch of the fingers. Paresthesia or numbness often occurs in the early phase but is not reliable. Paralysis is an unreliable finding, which may be related to pain. The true paralysis usually develops in a late stage of compartment syndrome. Distal circulation may not be blocked in spite of increased pressure in the deep forearm compartment, so the distal radial artery may still be palpable and pulseless may be not confirmed even when the irreversible tissue damage happens. The color of the hand may not change because of the patent of the arteries and the superficial veins.

4. **Answer: c.** When physical exam or taking a history is not available in an unconscious patient, the objective examination to diagnose a compartment syndrome is to measure intracompartmental pressure. Absolute pressure greater than 30 mm Hg or relative pressure within 20 to 30 mm Hg of the patient's diastolic blood pressure is an indication for a compartment syndrome. X-ray, CT scan, Doppler ultrasonography and magnetic resonance image can be used to identify the amount of tissue edema or assess primary injury, but not helpful for diagnosis of compartment syndrome.

5. **Answer: d.** Based on his history, symptoms, and signs, the forearm compartment syndrome is suspected. The pressure of 42 mm Hg confirms the diagnosis of compartment syndrome. Compartment pressure greater than 30 mm Hg is considered as an indication for fasciotomy, so the patient need fasciotomy for his compartment syndrome. Fasciotomy is to decrease the intracompartmental pressure so that it blocks the pathological way of compartment syndrome. Other choices are methods to treat his primary radius fracture but not compartment syndrome.

CHAPTER 90 Common Congenital Hand Anomalies

Paymon Rahgozar and Kevin C. Chung

KEY POINTS

- Congenital hand anomalies can be classified into seven categories based on the type of embryologic failure.
- Patients often have associated syndromes or systemic abnormalities that must be considered during the initial patient evaluation.
- Ideally, reconstruction is completed by school age to optimize hand function and growth, as well as to minimize self-conscious feelings around peers.
- The goals of syndactyly reconstruction include creation of an anatomically normal webspace, tension free closure of soft tissue, and return of function to the fingers.
- Ulnar polydactyly is common in African Americans and is frequently treated with an in-office ligation procedure.
- Patients with camptodactyly or clinodactyly frequently present with mild deformities and no functional deficits.
- Trigger thumb often presents with a palpable *Notta* nodule proximal to the A1 pulley.
- If severe enough, constriction ring syndrome can lead to critical lymphedema or compartment syndrome, requiring emergent release of the constricting bands.
- Pollicization is the preferred treatment for thumb hypoplasia that lacks a stable carpometacarpal joint.

Congenital hand anomalies are quite common with an incidence of 1 in 500 to 1900 live births.[1,2] Syndactyly, polydactyly, and camptodactyly are the most frequently encountered disorders. Approximately 60% of cases occur spontaneously, 20% are inherited, and 20% are secondary to an environmental cause.[3] Although inheritance patterns may be either autosomal dominant or recessive, congenital hand anomalies also present as part of a *sequence* or an *association*. A single in utero insult, such as a vascular thrombosis, may initiate a *sequence* of events with a series of subsequent anomalies. Poland syndrome, for example, occurs after a unilateral insult during embryogenesis, leading to a sequence of events resulting in a chest deformity and ipsilateral symbrachydactyly. On the other hand, an *association*, such as VACTERL association (vertebral abnormalities, anal atresia, cardiac defects, tracheoesophageal fistula, renal agenesis, limb anomalies) seen in patients with radial dysplasia, involves a series of nonrandom abnormalities that are not part of a syndrome nor the result from one specific event.

Management of the patient with a congenital hand anomaly requires many considerations. The surgeon may be one of the first practitioners to evaluate the patient, and the tendency will be to focus on the obvious defect. However, given the multitude of syndromes, sequences, and associations involved with hand anomalies, the surgeon must perform a comprehensive examination to rule out and appropriately treat any life-threatening conditions.

Unlike an adult, a child is not able to effectively communicate or follow instructions during an examination. Often, the most valuable historians are the parents, who observe the child regularly and can report on abnormal posturing or functional limitations. The in-office exam should focus on observing the child moving the extremity spontaneously, testing of the passive range of motion, and comparing the affected extremity with the contralateral side. The absence of flexion creases is suggestive of lack of motion, which may be due to a joint, soft tissue, or neurovascular cause. Plain films are an invaluable tool to determine the osseous anatomy as well as the presence of any abnormalities such as a triphalangeal thumb, complex syndactyly, or bracketed epiphysis.

The timing of intervention requires thoughtful planning. The hands double in length in the first 2 years of life. A digit that tethers another digit (syndactyly) will result in marked deformity during this rapid growth spurt and will require early release.[3] The cortical control for placing the limb in space and for strong grasping is developed by 1 year. Prehensile grasp and pinch between the thumb and fingers continue to become refined up to 3 years of age. Surgery is performed at an early age when the function of parts of the hand is to be altered by transposition (pollicization) to minimize the degree of cortical relearning required.

The major goals of surgery are to orient the hand in space and provide adequate prehension. The minimal prerequisites for a functional hand include the presence of a thumb, two ulnar sided digits, and a wide thumb webspace. Therefore, in cases where the child has acceptable hand function, as in many cases of cleft hand, surgery may not be indicated despite an *abnormal* appearance.[3] Operative intervention may also be contraindicated in an older patient who has already adopted alternative hand patterns for functional use of the extremity. Altering the hand position would require relearning how to use the hand entirely.[3] To minimize potential feelings of self-consciousness among peers, the goal should be to complete the reconstruction by school age, particularly if multiple procedures are necessary.

Classification of congenital hand anomalies not only requires a thorough understanding of normal anatomy, but also knowledge of embryology and development. To provide a unified system for the classification of congenital hand anomalies, the American Society for Surgery of the Hand (ASSH) and the International Federation of Societies for Surgery of the Hand (IFSSH) have adopted a system that groups anomalies into seven categories based on the type of presumed embryologic failure[4]:

Type I: Failure of formation of parts (e.g., radial dysplasia, phocomelia)
Type II: Failure of differentiation (separation) of parts (e.g., syndactyly, camptodactyly, clinodactyly, trigger digits)
Type III: Duplication (e.g., polydactyly)
Type IV: Overgrowth (e.g., macrodactyly)
Type V: Undergrowth (e.g., hypoplastic thumb)
Type VI: Congenital Constriction Band Syndrome
Type VII: Generalized skeletal abnormalities (e.g., dwarfism)

EMBRYOLOGY

Upper extremity development takes place between the fifth and eighth weeks of intrauterine growth. It begins with the outgrowth of the arm bud at approximately 30 days gestation, and by 37 days gestation the hand plate is well developed.[5,6] Concentration gradients of a variety of growth factors influence growth in three spatial axes: proximodistal, anteroposterior (radial-ulnar), and dorsoventral.

Proximodistal limb growth is controlled by a thickened ridge of ectodermal tissue known as the apical ectodermal ridge (AER). It is the last axis to develop and its function is dependent on the secretion of several fibroblastic growth factors that control the AER differentiation and growth.[6,7] Experimental removal of the AER leads to a truncated limb whereas implantation at another site leads to an ectopic limb.[6,8] The delineation of digital rays and finger separation occurs through apoptosis of specific portions of the AER between 47 and 53 days.[3,6] Aberrations in this process can lead to polydactyly or syndactyly.[3]

The zone of polarizing activity (ZPA) is responsible for anteroposterior or radio/ulnar growth and is driven by the expression of sonic hedgehog protein. It is the first axis to be established with its orientation predetermined before the start of limb bud growth.[6] Alterations in the ZPA can lead to the development of a mirror hand.[7,8] Experimental transplantation of the ZPA to the radial side of a developing limb will result in mirror duplication of the ulnar hand, or ulnar dimelia.[6] Finally, the dorsal ectoderm controls the dorsal/volar characteristics of the limb and is driven by the expression of wingless-type mouse mammary tumor virus integration site family member 7a (Wnt-7a). Disturbances of this axis of development may lead to palmar duplication syndrome.[7]

SYNDACTYLY

The term *syndactyly* is derived from Greek: *syn* = together and *dactylos* = digit. It occurs because of a failure of differentiation during embryogenesis with an incidence of 1 in every 2000 to 3000 births. Males are affected twice as often as females.[8,9] Although most cases are isolated occurrences, 10% to 40% of cases are familial, inherited in an autosomal dominant pattern with variable expressivity, incomplete penetrance, and less severe phenotypes compared to autosomal recessive cases.[3,10] The majority of inherited cases are associated with one of more than 300 distinct syndromic anomalies or sequences, such as Apert syndrome or Poland sequence.

Syndactyly may be classified into complete (extending through the fingertips with nail involvement), incomplete (webbing only partially along the length of the digit), simple (soft tissue involvement only), complex (bony or joint fusion), or complicated (multiple involved tissues including bones, joints, tendons, muscles, or neurovascular bundles). Complicated syndactyly is often seen in association with other conditions or syndromes such as polydactyly, constriction rings, toe webbing, brachydactyly, spinal deformities, heart disorders, or Apert Syndrome.[5] In cases of complete syndactyly, patients have a shared fingernail between the digits, known as synonychia. The most common webspace affected in nonsyndromic syndactyly is the middle/ring finger webspace (57% of cases) followed by the ring/little finger web space (27% of cases).[9,11] In syndromic cases, the thumb/index finger and index/middle finger webspaces are more commonly involved.[9,11]

The timing of surgical intervention is determined by the length discrepancy of the involved digits. For example, there is little length discrepancy between the long finger and ring finger. Therefore, there is less concern for digital tethering of the digits with growth and surgery may be delayed until approximately 12 months of age. Ideally, the release is timed so that it is done early enough to permit normal growth but late enough to avoid postoperative complications. Surgery before 1 year of age is associated with higher rates of scar contracture and potential anesthetic complications.

Syndactyly of the border digits (little/ring fingers, thumb/index fingers) results in a length discrepancy leading to growth and functional disturbances from asymmetric growth, flexion contractures, and rotation deformities. In these cases, surgical release should be considered earlier, specifically between 3 and 6 months of age.[9,12] Our preference is around 6 months when the infant is bigger and the anesthetic risk is minimal. Similarly, for complicated syndactyly, earlier intervention may be beneficial. With bilateral involvement, both hands should be corrected simultaneously in nonambulatory patients younger than 12 to 14 months.[9]

To avoid neurovascular compromise when multiple fingers are involved, staging of the releases is recommended, releasing one side of a digit at a time. Priority is given to the border digits, particularly the thumb and the little finger. Sequential surgery can be performed within 3 months of each other. It is ideal to complete the reconstruction before 24 months of age, when the patterns of function of the digits are established.[9]

The goals of syndactyly release include the following[9]:

- creation of an anatomically similar webspace,
- tension-free closure of soft tissue, and
- return of function to the fingers.

Normal function of the fingers requires proper webspace location and depth. The webspace has a dorsal to volar inclination of 40 to 45 degrees and it is reconstructed with a dorsal skin flap.[8] Because the circumference of the separated fingers is approximately 22% to 30% greater than the circumference of the conjoined digits, release often results in a skin deficit requiring skin grafting (Figure 90.1).[8,12] This can be demonstrated to the parents by measuring the circumference of a parent's ring and small fingers separately and comparing it to the measurement of the circumference when the fingers are held together. Full thickness skin grafts are preferable to minimize contracture but should be avoided in the webspaces and overlying PIP joints. Instead, these areas should be covered with carefully designed flaps. Skin grafts should be taken from the groin and not from the wrist or the forearm because these are exposed areas and the scars are aesthetically objectionable.

A dorsal rectangular or trapezoidal flap is designed approximately two-thirds the distance between the metacarpal heads and the PIP joints. As originally described by Cronin, dorsal and volar digital flaps are then designed in a zig-zag pattern to minimize scar contracture (Figure 90.2).[13] The dorsal zig-zag incision begins at the apex of the dorsal rectangular flap and extends to the midline of the PIP joint, then across to the neighboring middle phalanx, and back across to the midline of the DIP joint. The volar flap is designed as a mirror image with the proximal midline vertical incision extending to the level of the desired webspace, where a horizontal incision is made completing a T for inset of the dorsal webspace flap.[14] The triangular flaps are transposed and sutured in place ensuring flap coverage of the PIP joints. To reconstruct the nail folds, adequate skin and pulp are required. Transposition of pulp flaps described by Buck-Gramcko is elevated to create the paronychial folds (Figure 90.3).[15]

Postoperative dressings are important to a successful outcome. When skin grafts are used, compression and immobilization are the rule. In young children, the hand should be immobilized with an above-the-elbow cast with the elbow flexed at 90 degrees to prevent the cast from slipping down the arm. The cast is typically removed at 2 to 3 weeks and light dressings can be applied until all wounds are fully closed. Potential complications include graft loss or web creep (distal migration of the webspace) (Figure 90.4). Overcompensation of the webspace by positioning it more proximally may help minimize postoperative web creep deformities.[9]

In an effort to minimize or avoid the need for a skin graft, some surgeons advocate recruiting excess dorsal tissue with the design of a dorsal pentagonal flap. This requires more proximal dorsal hand incisions leading to a more conspicuous scar.[9,16] Defatting of the digits prior to flap closure is another method to minimize skin grafts. However, this must be done judiciously to avoid neurovascular injury, venous congestion, or a withered appearance. Younger patients (3–6 months) have the most digital fat amenable to defatting.[9]

Apert Syndrome: Acrocephalosyndactyly

Apert syndrome is an autosomal dominant congenital malformation that presents with craniosynostosis, midfacial malformations, and complex extremity malformations. It is associated with

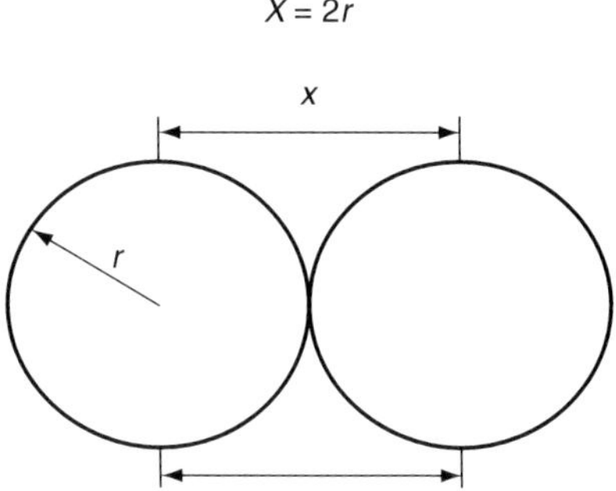

FIGURE 90.1. Diagram demonstrating the skin deficiency in syndactyly.

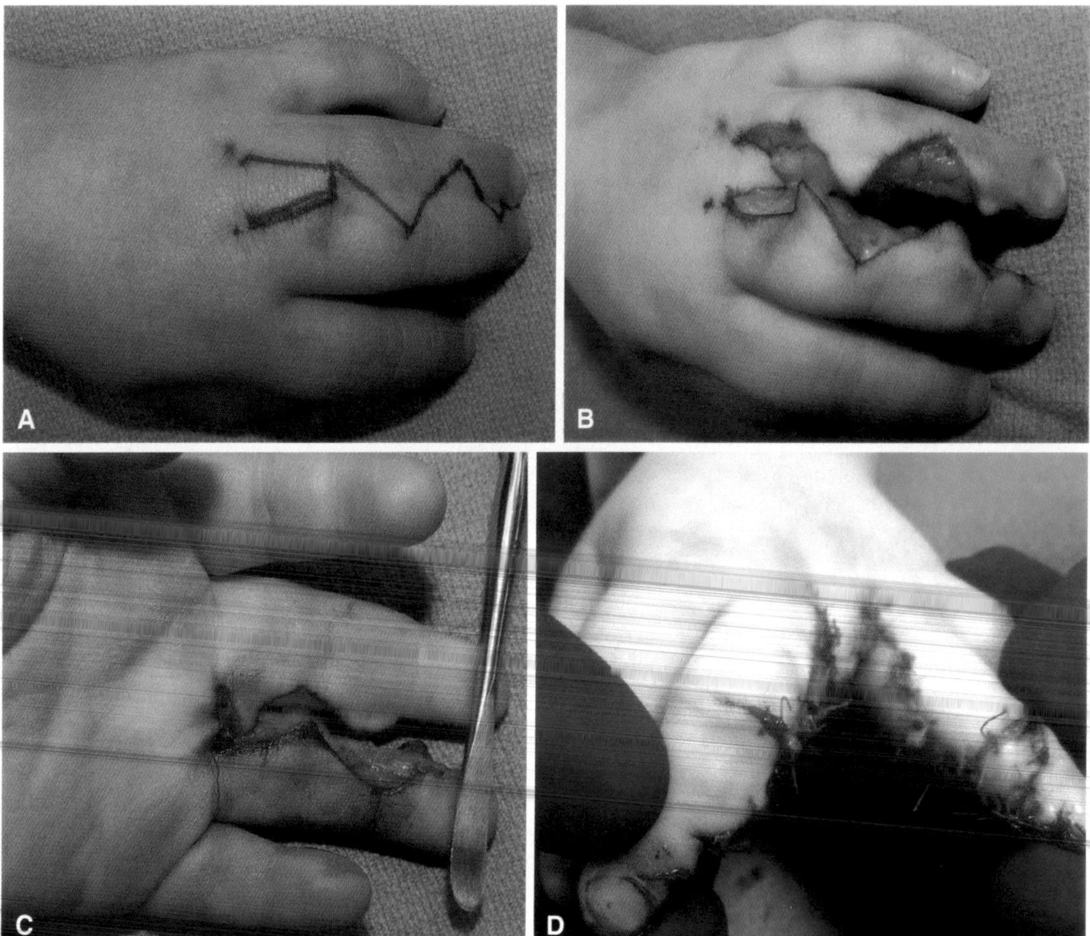

FIGURE 90.2. **A.** Skin markings for syndactyly release. A dorsal trapezoidal flap is designed two-thirds the distance between the metacarpal heads and the proximal interphalangeal joints to reconstruct the webspace. Zig-zag dorsal and volar flaps are utilized to separate the fingers. **B.** Dorsal release of the fingers. **C.** Volar release of the fingers. The volar flaps are drawn as mirror images of the dorsal flaps. Note that the flaps are designed so that they may cover the interphalangeal joints to minimize cicatricial contracture. **D.** Suturing of the flaps with an inset of full-thickness skin grafts.

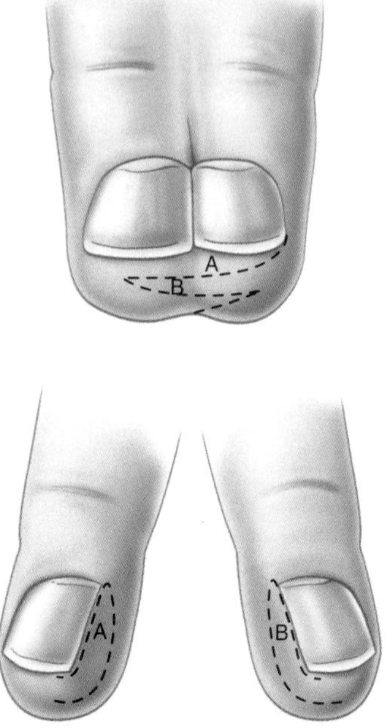

FIGURE 90.3. As described by Buck-Gramcko, *synonychia*, or fusion of the nails, is reconstructed by designing pulp flaps to create the paronychial folds. (Reproduced with permission from Bae D. Release of simple sundactyly. In: Hunt TRIII, ed. *Operative Techniques in Hand, Wrist, and Elbow Surgery*. Philadelphia, PA: Wolters Kluwer; 2016:1371. Figure 153-2.)

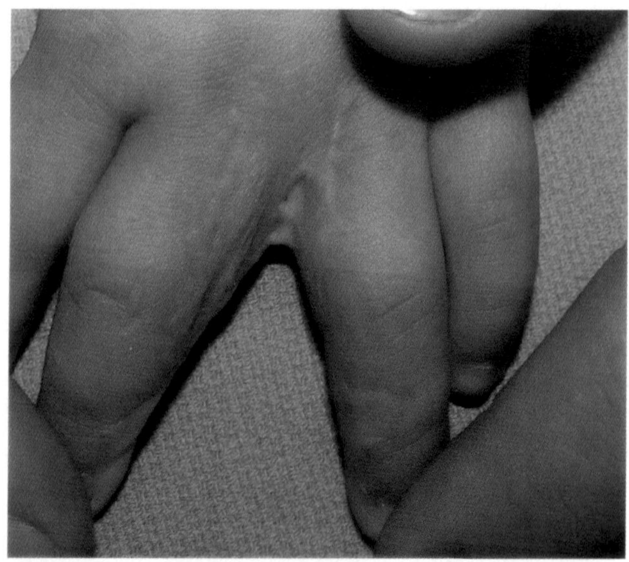

FIGURE 90.4. Web creep. Distal migration of the webspace may occur as the child grows. Positioning of the webspace more proximally at the time of syndactyly release may help limit the degree of web creep.

disturbance of the cell surface receptor for fibroblastic growth factor.[17] Apert syndrome represents the severe end of the syndactyly spectrum with involvement of bones, joints, tendons, and nerves. It can be classified into three types. Type 1 deformity, known as obstetrician's or spade hand, is characterized by a narrow first webspace and syndactyly of the four fingers without thumb involvement. This is the most common and least severe form. Patients with a type 2 deformity, also referred to as mitten or spoon hand, have syndactyly of all four fingers with a simple syndactyly of the thumb to the index ray. Finally, those with a type 3 deformity, also known as rosebud or hoof hand, have a tight osseous or cartilaginous fusion of the thumb, index, long, and ring fingers with conjoined nail plates. The little finger is often spared from an osseous union but is still joined to the other digits by a complete simple syndactyly.[17] Separation of the digits follows the principles of syndactyly reconstruction, requiring staged procedures starting at an early age. The staging principle is to separate the thumb and little finger bilaterally in the first stage, typically around the age of one when the child starts to use the thumb to provide a tripod pinch. Then in stage 2 separation of one of the central digits is done to give the child a four-digit hand. Because of skin shortage, it is not necessary for reasonable function to create a five-digit hand.

SYMBRACHYDACTYLY

Symbrachydactyly is caused by a disruption in embryonic formation and differentiation resulting in a hand with shortened or webbed digits, digital nubbins, or absent digits. It occurs in 0.6 per 10,000 live births, is more common in males, and is often unilateral, affecting the left extremity in two-thirds of cases.[18] When associated with Poland syndrome, it more commonly involves the right extremity and patients also present with an absent or hypoplastic pectoralis muscle.[19] Although symbrachydactyly may appear similar to amniotic band syndrome, the two can easily be distinguished from one another. Hands with symbrachydactyly often have small nubbins with fingernails, whereas with constriction bands the short digits occur as a result of intrauterine amputation and will lack nails.[18] Furthermore, patients with amniotic band syndrome will not only have a visible band on the hand but also on other locations of the body.

Surgical intervention is not always entirely straightforward and varies from patient to patient. It may require simple removal of nubbins to complex reconstruction with a microvascular toe transfer. Soft tissue reconstructions such as webspace releases must be done thoughtfully. Often the digits are hypoplastic and unstable, and separation may prove to be a detriment to function. The goal of reconstruction should be to improve pinch, grip, and single hand function. Reconstruction of one digit can provide a stable post to press a button. The presence of two digits permits pinch, and if one digit is positioned as a thumb it can provide opposition and improved prehension. A three-digit hand will further advance function by making a three-point pinch possible.[18]

POLYDACTYLY

Polydactyly, or the presence of an extra digit, occurs as a result of a duplication during development. It is one of the most common congenital hand anomalies and can be found on either the radial hand (preaxial) with duplication of the thumb, the ulnar hand (postaxial), or the central hand with involvement of the three central rays.

Preaxial polydactyly, or thumb duplication, has an incidence of 0.08 per 1000 live births (Figure 90.5A).[3] Although most cases occur sporadically, patients who present with a triphalangeal thumb exhibit an autosomal dominant inheritance pattern.[20] Thumb duplication is classified using the Flatt classification system, which sequentially describes the duplication from distal to proximal (Figure 90.6).[21] Even numbers represent complete phalangeal duplications and odd numbers describe incomplete duplications: type I deformity has a bifid distal phalanx; type II has a duplication

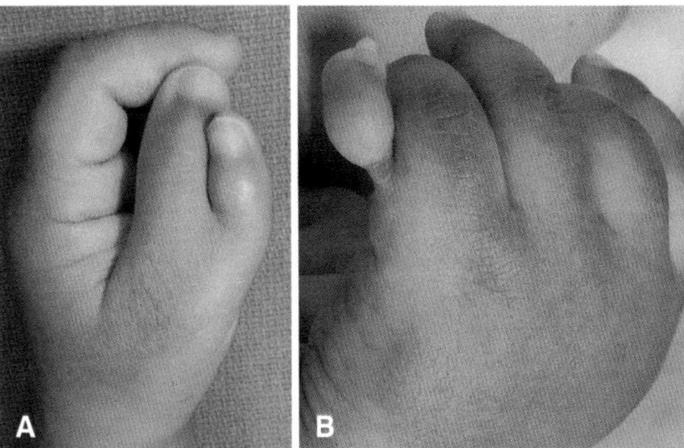

FIGURE 90.5. **A.** Preaxial polydactyly. Note that the radial thumb is more hypoplastic than the ulnar duplicate. **B.** Postaxial polydactyly.

at the level of the interphalangeal joint; type III is a bifid proximal phalanx; type IV (most common) describes duplication at the level of the MCP joint; type V is a bifid metacarpal; type VI describes duplication at the level of the carpometacarpal joint; and type VII involves a triphalangeal thumb.

Surgery for preaxial polydactyly is generally performed between 9 and 15 months of age, prior to the development of pinch grasp or progressive deviation of the duplicated thumbs. Reconstructive options include total ablation of one thumb, sharing of equal halves (Bilhaut-Cloquet procedure), or reconstruction using composite parts from each of the duplicated digits.[3] It must be recognized that none of the anatomic components of either duplicates is normal.[20] There may be varying degrees of hypoplasia, including abnormalities in osseous anatomy, tendon anatomy, or joint stability. Although both the ulnar and radial thumbs demonstrate a degree of hypoplasia, the ulnar thumb is usually larger. The ulnar duplicate is preferentially preserved, not only because of its larger size but also to preserve the native ulnar collateral ligament, which is essential to providing stability during thumb to index pinch. To maintain varus MCP joint stability, the radial collateral ligament of the ablated thumb is preserved and secured to the radial aspect of the retained ulnar thumb. Furthermore, the flexor and extensor tendons may be split with eccentric insertions, or may demonstrate fusion on the radial side of the thumb known as a *pollex abductus* deformity. The surgeon must carefully inspect the anatomy and realign or reposition tendons as necessary to ensure optimal function.

Postaxial polydactyly can present as a small skin *nubbin* on the ulnar aspect of the hand or as a fully formed digit (see Figure 90.5B). This is the most common type of polydactyly and is frequently found in African Americans with an incidence of 1 in 143 African American births compared to 1 in 1339 Caucasian births.[20] In African Americans, it has an autosomal dominant inheritance pattern with incomplete penetrance. However, in Caucasians it is more frequently associated with a syndrome and should prompt a genetics consultation.

Postaxial polydactyly can be classified into two main groups: type A describes a fully developed duplicate digit that articulates with the fifth or, at times, sixth metacarpal and type B represents a rudimentary poorly developed ulnar duplication with a thin, narrow stalk. Type B deformities require simple ligation of the skin bridge, which can be performed with surgical resection, or suture ligation. To avoid anesthesia, many prefer an in-office procedure that involves simple ligation of the base of the stalk with a vascular clip. We do not advocate suture ligation because it will leave a stump that eventually requires excision. A vascular clip can be placed at the base of the digit to leave no residual nubbin. This occludes the neurovascular supply to the duplicated digit leading to dry gangrene and autoamputation. Similar to duplicate thumb reconstruction, type A deformities require surgical reconstruction with consideration given to maintaining a stable, functional small finger with preservation of the ulnar collateral ligament and the adductor digiti minimi.[20]

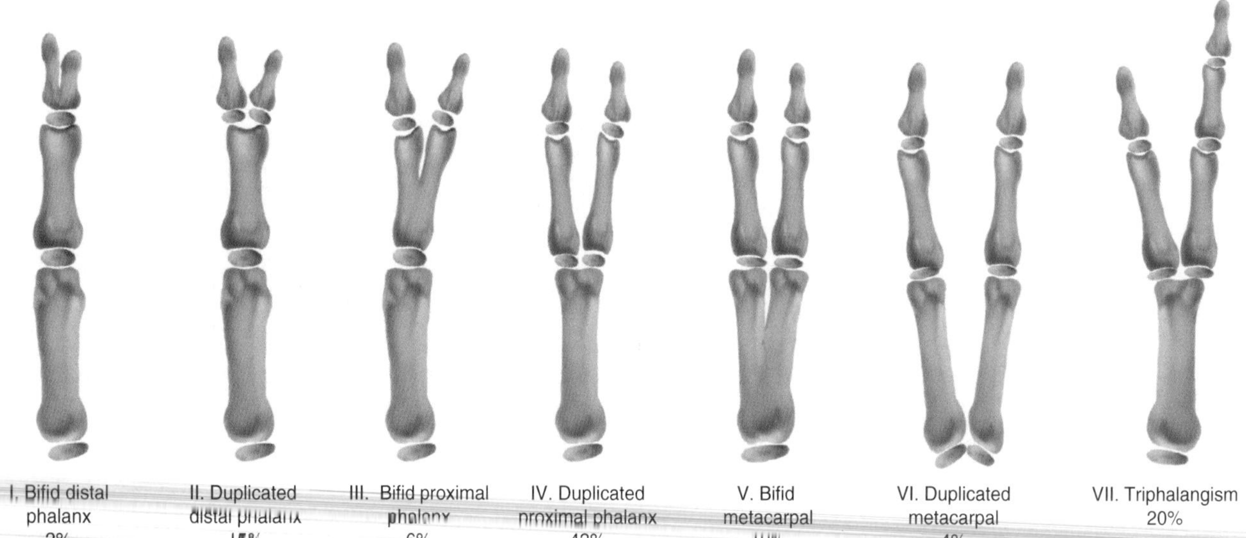

FIGURE 90.6. Flatt classification system of thumb duplication. (Reproduced with permission from Wassel HD. The results of surgery for polydactyly of the thumb. A review. *Clin Orthop Relat Res.* 1969;64:175-193. Figure 4-2.)

CAMPTODACTYLY

Camptodactyly is a nontraumatic irreducible flexion contracture of the proximal interphalangeal joint, most commonly involving the ring or small fingers. The term *camptodactyly* means *bent finger* in Greek.[22] It can be divided into simple and complex types. The simple type only has a flexion deformity of the PIP joint, whereas the complex type may have other associated deformities such as syndactyly or clinodactyly. Although hyperextension of the DIP or MCP joints may occur in camptodactyly, flexion contracture of these joints would instead suggest a post traumatic cause.[22]

Camptodactyly occurs in less than 1% of the population and typically presents in a bimodal pattern during the periods of most rapid growth: infancy and puberty.[23,24] The *early* type is often present at birth, involves the little finger, and affects boys and girls equally. The *delayed* type, which is more common, presents during adolescence, and affects girls more often than boys.[25] Although most cases occur sporadically, camptodactyly can be transmitted in an autosomal dominant fashion, or can be associated with Trisomy 13, oculodentodigital, orofacial digital, Aarskog, and cerebrohepatorenal syndromes.[25]

The etiology of camptodactyly has been the subject of much debate. Because of its presentation during periods of rapid growth, some believe that an inability of palmar tissues to grow and lengthen in proportion to skeletal growth causes abnormalities in the skin, soft tissue, or pericapsular tissue resulting in tethering of the finger.[22,25] Most commonly there is an anomalous or absent flexor digitorum superficialis or an anomalous lumbrical muscle.[23,26] Other potential causes include extensor mechanism laxity and anomalies of the interosseous muscles or the transverse or oblique retinacular ligaments.[22,23,27]

Patients may present with a loss of function that interferes with activities of daily living or with extracurricular activities such as inability to participate in sports, play musical instruments, or hold a brush.[23] However, because the involved ulnar digits are primarily involved in flexion and grasp, patients with mild camptodactyly (<30 degrees) have minimal impediment of hand function and can tolerate it quite well.[24] To differentiate between an intrinsic joint problem and extrinsic flexor tendon involvement, the examiner should assess the degree of flexion deformity with the MCP joint flexed and extended.[27] If the contracture improves with an MCP joint flexion, the tethering effect is most likely related to an extrinsic flexor tendon (i.e., flexor digitorum superficialis). More advanced cases may also present with an extensor lag from central slip laxity or a boutonniere deformity.

Camptodactyly can often be treated effectively with nonoperative management. PIP joint stretching exercises have been successful to improve contractures particularly in patients less than 3 years old.[28] Dynamic and static support splints as well as serial finger casting can be employed with gradual adjustments made as the finger contracture improves.[22,27] However, in patients with flexion contractures of 30 degrees or greater, impaired function, or unacceptable aesthetics, surgical treatment may be indicated if the deformity persists or progresses despite a 6 to 12 month trial of nonoperative therapy.[22–24]

During surgical release, one needs to avoid neurovascular injury from overaggressive extension of the contracted digit, or joint instability from overzealous release of the stabilizing joint structures.[24] Nearly all patients will at least require: (1) the release of skin pterygium with local transposition flaps or Z-plasties and possible coverage with full thickness skin grafts; (2) release of the fascia and subcutaneous tissues; and (3) tenotomy of the flexor digitorum superficialis tendon at the level of the Camper chiasm.[23,29] If a contracture persists despite the above maneuvers, a sliding volar plate release may also be necessary. In patients with a severe PIP joint extensor lag, an intrinsic transfer using the released FDS tendon can be performed. Additionally, a Fowler distal extensor tenotomy may be needed to treat a hyperextended DIP joint. Although in general, surgical intervention improves the degree of contracture, the amount of improvement is typically modest and prone to recurrence.[22,24,25,28]

CLINODACTYLY

Clinodactyly is a congenital radio-ulnar deviation of the fingers. Although all bones and all rays of the hand may be affected, bilateral small finger involvement with radial deviation of the middle phalanges is most common (Figure 90.7A). It occurs either sporadically or is inherited in an autosomal dominant pattern with variable expressivity and incomplete penetrance.[30] Clinodactyly can be found with other conditions of the hand and foot including polydactyly, cleft hand or foot, and mild tibial hemimelia.[31] It may also be seen in Down syndrome, Rubinstein-Taybi syndrome, Apert syndrome, and oculodental dysplasia.[32]

Patients often have an abnormal trapezoidal or triangular shaped middle phalanx referred to as a *delta phalanx*, or a longitudinally bracketed epiphysis. This C-shaped epiphysis is characterized by

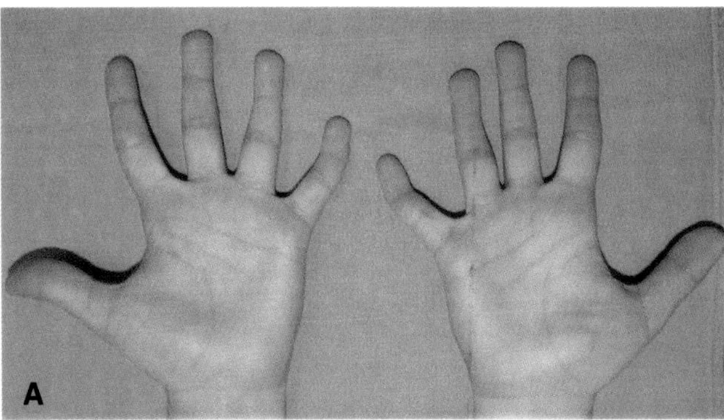

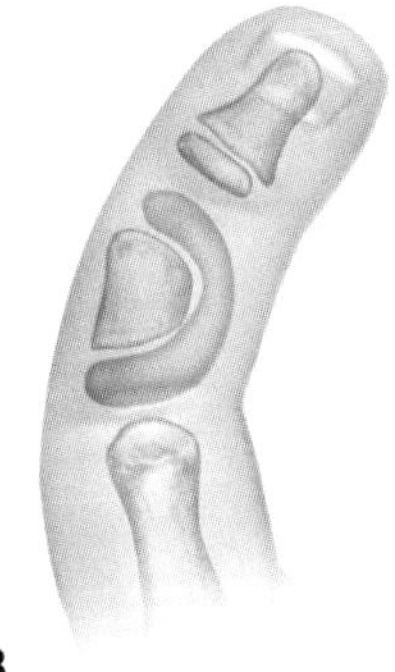

FIGURE 90.7. **A.** Bilateral small finger clinodactyly. **B.** Bracketed epiphysis with deviation of finger toward the epiphysis.

an irregularly shaped physis, or growth plate, that spans the axial length of the phalanx. Therefore, longitudinal growth is unilaterally restricted, leading to a progressive deviation of the digit toward the bracketed epiphysis (Figure 90.7B).[33] Although the exact etiology is not known, it is thought to result from incomplete development of primary ossification centers.[31]

Primary complaints with clinodactyly are either aesthetic or functional, such as difficulty with playing musical instruments. Treatment for clinodactyly is typically considered when there is more than 20 degrees of deviation.[32,33] Options for surgical treatment include a physiolysis or a corrective osteotomy. In a physiolysis the bracketed epiphysis is resected and tissue such as a fat graft is interposed to prevent recurrence.[30] This method does not immediately repair the deformity, but as the child grows, there is an increase in longitudinal growth and a decrease in angular deformity. This method is preferred in younger patients where an osteotomy of small bones may be technically more challenging and there is a longer propensity for growth and correction of the deformity.[32]

A corrective osteotomy is an alternative for patients who are older and have bone fragments that are large enough to permit accurate surgical manipulation. Although osteotomy options include closing wedge, opening wedge, and a reverse wedge osteotomy, the opening wedge osteotomy is preferred to maintain the finger length.[32] Osteotomy can also be used to treat older children who present after closure of the bracket epiphysis, or as a subsequent procedure after physiolysis, to lengthen or correct recurrent or persistent angulation.[31]

RADIAL COLUMN (PREAXIAL) ABNORMALITIES

Pediatric patients may present with a *trigger* thumb or a *clasped* thumb. These two entities can often be confused with one another, and at times patients may be referred by a pediatrician with an incorrect diagnosis of a fracture or dislocation.

Trigger thumb, also historically called congenital trigger thumb, has an estimated incidence of 3.3 children per 1000 live births by the first year of life.[34] The term *trigger* is a misnomer because it is uncommon to see snapping as in adult trigger finger. Instead, children typically present with a fixed flexion contracture of the IP joint averaging 25 to 35 degrees with inability or difficulty with active or passive thumb extension.[35,36] Furthermore, *congenital* trigger thumb is also a misnomer because studies of newborns have failed to show its presence at birth, suggesting an acquired etiology.[34,37] The average age of presentation is approximately 24 months.[35,36] It is thought to occur as a result of an enlarged flexor pollicis longus tendon proximal to a tight A1 pulley, leading to an area of thickening or a palpable *Notta* nodule.[35] The nodule obstructs the tendon's ability to glide through the A1 pulley maintaining it in a fixed position with a flexed posture.

Initial treatment involves a period of observation to assess for spontaneous resolution of symptoms. Baek et al. prospectively followed 87 trigger thumbs and found that within 5 years, approximately 75% had symptomatic improvement without residual deformity or compensatory hyperextension of the MCP joint.[36] Splinting has not been shown to be of any consistent benefit, and parents may find it difficult to keep the child from removing the splint. Candidates for surgery are those who fail to improve despite a period of observation, the exact timing of which is often surgeon dependent. Treatment is performed with a surgical release of the A1 pulley through an incision over the proximal flexion crease. Care should be taken to avoid the neurovascular bundles, which are found in a more central location on the volar surface of the thumb as compared to the fingers. The surgeon must demonstrate full extension of the thumb intraoperatively to confirm adequate release.

In contrast to trigger thumb, congenital clasped thumb deformity presents with contracture at the MCP joint. Clasped thumb can be divided into two subtypes: supple and complex. In the supple subtype, the extensor mechanism is hypoplastic or absent, and the contracture can be corrected with passive extension. Initial treatment involves a trial of splinting but may ultimately require tendon transfer if splinting fails. Patients with the complex subtype frequently have bilateral involvement and present with additional pathology such as joint or first webspace contractures, or abnormalities of the collateral ligaments and thenar musculature. This results in uncorrectable MCP flexion and thumb adduction contractures. Associated abnormalities such as arthrogryposis, digitotalar dysmorphism, or Freeman-Sheldon syndrome may also be present.[38] Treatment for the complex subtype requires reconstruction of the lax ligaments and appropriate correction of fixed contractures through a combination of Z-plasties for first web contractures, thenar and adductor muscle releases, flap coverage of the volar skin deficit, and flexor pollicis longus tendon lengthening.[38,39]

CONSTRICTION RING SYNDROME

Constriction ring syndrome, also known as amniotic band syndrome or constriction band syndrome, is a condition that results in distal limb malformation or deformation, lymphedema, acrosyndactyly, or amputation (Figure 90.8). The incidence has been described to range from 1/1200 to 1/15,000 live births with no known autosomal inheritance pattern or genetic predilection.[40] Factors that have been found to be associated with constriction ring syndrome include prematurity (<37 weeks), low birth weight (<2500 g), maternal drug exposure, and maternal illness or trauma during pregnancy.[40,41] Patients present with characteristic constriction rings, and if severe enough, may present with neurovascular impairment from direct compression or from compartment

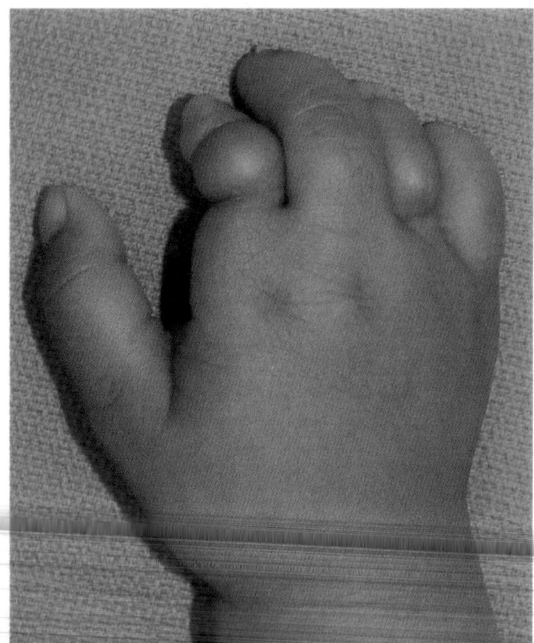

FIGURE 90.8. Patient with constriction ring syndrome. Note the shortened digits and the characteristic bands on the index and ring fingers.

syndrome. In cases of acrosyndactyly, digits that were at one point separated undergo refusion at the site of the band, resulting in an epidermal lined sinus tract that communicates from the dorsal side to the volar side.

The cause of constriction ring syndrome has long been debated. The intrinsic theory proposes that a teratogenic insult, viral infection, or vascular disruption results in an inherent defect during embryogenesis affecting mesodermal tissue, leading to the characteristic rings. The extrinsic theory suggests that an external *band* entangles, constricts, or amputates the limbs. Torpin theorized that early amniotic rupture followed by a period of oligohydramnios with torn cords of amnion results in extrinsic compression of the fetal appendages and the characteristic deformities.[42] Despite the debating theories, most contemporary authors believe the extrinsic theory to be more accurate, citing that the asymmetric clinical presentation of the limbs, the presence of a straight line across adjacent digits, and the occurrence of acrosyndactyly (refusion of previously separated digits) are better explained in an extrinsic cause.[40]

The goal of surgical treatment is to optimize function and appearance. The timing of surgery is dependent on the severity of the constriction band. Shallow bands may require no operative treatment other than for aesthetic purposes. However, more severe constriction bands that result in severe distal lymphedema, cyanosis, or circulatory compromise may lead to ischemia or compartment syndrome and should be treated urgently after birth.[40] In less acute cases, the treatment involves one or two stage releases beginning at around 3 months of age. Release is performed with a series of Z-plasties or W-plasties and excision of the bands. Given potential concerns of vascular interruption of the distal segment, some authors advocate a two-stage release where approximately 50% of the band is released at the first stage, followed by an interval of 6 to 12 weeks to reestablish cutaneous circulation across the scar before subsequent final release. To address the contour deformity that results from the subcutaneous deficiency under the constriction band, Upton and Tan published a technique describing separate advancement of subcutaneous adipose flaps to add bulk to the area underlying the constriction band. The skin flaps are then transposed as separate thin Z-plasty flaps resulting in superior aesthetic outcomes.[43]

RADIAL LONGITUDINAL DEFICIENCY

Radial longitudinal deficiency (RLD), or radial club hand, is a result of a congenital failure of formation of the radial column. The severity of presentation can vary from mild hypoplasia to complete absence of the radius, carpal bones, and radial digits. The radial musculotendinous units may be absent or hypoplastic and often form a fibrous tether at the wrist, contributing to the angled position of the hand.[44] It has an incidence of approximately 1 in 5400 live births.[2] RLD occurs because of an insult to the apical ectodermal ridge during the fourth to seventh weeks of intrauterine development.[45,46] The condition gained widespread attention in the 1960s with the thalidomide induced epidemic of phocomelia.[45]

Approximately one-third of patients have an associated syndrome such as Holt-Oram, Fanconi anemia, TAR (thrombocytopenia-absent radius), or VACTERL (vertebral abnormalities, anal atresia, cardiac defects, tracheoesophageal fistula, renal agenesis, limb anomalies). Furthermore, two-thirds of patients have an associated medical or musculoskeletal anomaly ranging from congenital heart malformations, blood dyscrasias, and renal or gastrointestinal dysfunction.[45] Often the limb abnormality may be the only outward manifestation of the underlying syndrome, necessitating the surgeon to perform an appropriate work-up including a renal ultrasound, echocardiogram, and complete blood count.[46] The Bayne and Klug classification divides the radial dysplasias into four types, based on the radiographic appearance[47]:

Type I: short distal radius,
Type II: hypoplastic radius,
Type III: partial absence of the radius, and
Type IV: total absence of the radius.

This classification system was further modified by James to include the presence of thumb hypoplasia, carpal anomalies, and radioulnar synostosis.[48]

Treatment for radial longitudinal deficiency initially involves passive stretching and serial splinting. In severe cases, some advocate distraction of the tight radial tissues with an external fixator device for at least 6-8 weeks before surgical reconstruction, a procedure we advocate. The goals of surgical treatment include the following[45]:

- straightening of the radial bowing of the forearm,
- correction of radial and volar subluxation of the carpus,
- improvement of the limb length to optimize function,
- improvement of aesthetic appearance, and
- treatment of the thumb hypoplasia.

The deformity is corrected by *centralizing* the carpal bones over the ulna and rebalancing the musculotendinous structures to alter the deforming forces on the wrist. Although centralization is commonly performed, it has been shown to result in recurrence of angulation and in limb shortening.[44]

All cases of radial longitudinal deficiency have an associated thumb hypoplasia, though thumb hypoplasia may exist without an abnormality of the radius.[48] Blauth developed a classification for thumb hypoplasia based on the size of the thumb, the thenar musculature, first webspace contracture, and stability of the carpometacarpal joint[49,50]:

Type I: minor thumb hypoplasia,
Type II: first webspace narrowing, hypoplastic or absent thenar intrinsic muscles, MCP joint instability,
Type III: first webspace narrowing, hypoplastic or absent thenar intrinsic muscles, MCP joint instability, extrinsic tendon abnormalities, skeletal abnormalities:
Type IIIA: hypoplastic metacarpal, stable CMC joint and
Type IIIB: partial metacarpal aplasia, unstable CMC joint,
Type IV: floating thumb (*pouce flottant*), and
Type V: absent thumb

Surgical treatment of thumb hypoplasia is most dependent on the presence and stability of the thumb carpometacarpal joint (CMC). In milder cases (Blauth types II and IIIA), reconstruction is focused on widening of the first webspace, an opponensplasty procedure, and

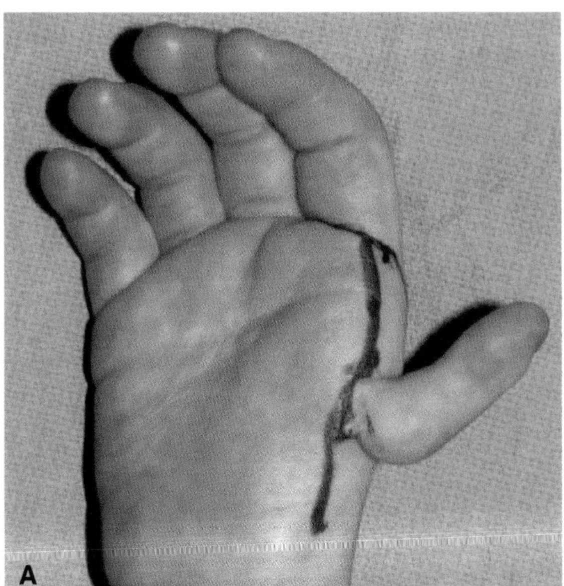

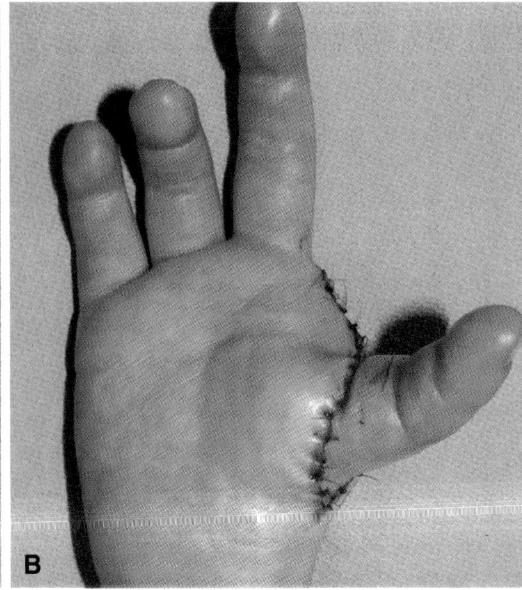

FIGURE 90.9. **A.** Preoperative image of patient with Blauth type IV thumb hypoplasia. **B.** Postoperative image after pollicization of the index finger.

metacarpophalangeal joint stabilization. However, in more severe cases that lack a stable CMC joint (Blauth types IIIB, IV, or V), the thumb, if present, cannot be effectively reconstructed. Treatment is best performed with thumb ablation and reconstruction with index finger pollicization, transferring the index finger to the thumb position (Figure 90.9). The principles include skeletal shortening of the index metacarpal shaft, rotation and stabilization of the index finger, and rebalancing of the musculotendinous units by transfer of the first dorsal and volar interossei muscles for abductor and adductor function.[46,51] Pollicization provides a pleasing aesthetic reconstruction of the thumb and successfully restores opposition and grasp functions.

CLEFT HAND (CENTRAL LONGITUDINAL DEFICIENCY)

Cleft hand or central longitudinal deficiency is characterized by varying degrees of growth suppression of the bones and soft tissue of the central hand, most frequently involving the central rays. The defect does not extend proximal to the wrist but may have associated carpal coalition or radioulnar synostosis.[44] It is frequently associated with central polydactyly or osseous syndactyly. Although the cleft itself causes little functional limitation, the main deficit is secondary to a narrowed thumb-index webspace. Many classification schemes exist, but arguably the most useful one that can help guide surgical treatment is that proposed by Manske and Halikis that characterizes the degree of first webspace narrowing.[52]

Surgical reconstruction is performed to improve functional limitations of the hand that may be related to a severe flexion contracture of one or more digits, a malpositioned index finger ray, or syndactyly involving the thumb. Because deformities may worsen with growth, patients are treated by 1 year of age with completion of any additional reconstructions by school age (5–6 years). Surgical repair involves: (1) preservation of a stable and mobile thumb; (2) transposition of the index ray to the ulnar side of the cleft; (3) creation of a wide and functional first webspace; (4) correction of any index finger malrotation or deviation; (5) preservation of an adductor pollicis muscle; and (6) creation of a satisfactory aesthetic appearance.[53]

CONCLUSION

The evaluation and treatment of a patient with a congenital hand anomaly can be both challenging and rewarding. The overall goal is to restore form and function, and this is typically achieved by the time the child is of school age. To be able to appropriately reconstruct the hand, the surgeon must not only have mastery of normal anatomy, but also must grasp the intricacies of the defect, which may involve bones, joints, tendons, muscles, and neurovascular structures. The potential to impact an individual for an entire lifetime makes treatment of congenital hand anomalies arguably one of the most fulfilling of all surgeries.

ACKNOWLEDGMENTS

The work was supported by a Midcareer Investigator Award in Patient-Oriented Research (2 K24-AR053120-06) to [illegible]. The content is solely the responsibility of the authors and does not necessarily represent the official views of the National Institutes of Health.

REFERENCES

1. Giele H, Giele C, Bower C, Allison M. The incidence and epidemiology of congenital upper limb anomalies: a total population study. *J Hand Surg Am.* 2001;26(4):628-634.
2. Koskimies E, Lindfors N, Gissler M, et al. Congenital upper limb deficiencies and associated malformations in Finland: a population-based study. *J Hand Surg Am.* 2011;36(6):1058-1065.
3. Netscher DT, Baumholtz MA. Treatment of congenital upper extremity problems. *Plast Reconstr Surg.* 2007;119(5):101e-129e.
4. Swanson AB. A classification for congenital limb malformations. *J Hand Surg.* 1976;1(1):8-22.
   This article describes the seven categories used to classify congenital hand anomalies and the rationale for its use. This classification has been adopted by the American Society for Surgery of the Hand and the International Federation of Societies for Surgery of the Hand and is still in use today.
5. Bates SJ, Hansen SL, Jones NF. Reconstruction of congenital differences of the hand. *Plast Reconstr Surg.* 2009;124(1 suppl):128e-143e.
6. Sammer DM, Chung KC. Congenital hand differences: embryology and classification. *Hand Clin.* 2009;25(2):151-156.
7. Al-Qattan MM, Yang Y, Kozin SH. Embryology of the upper limb. *J Hand Surg Am.* 2009;34(7):1340-1350.
8. Tonkin MA. Failure of differentiation. Part I: syndactyly. *Hand Clin.* 2009;25(2):171-193.
9. Braun TL, Trost JG, Pederson WC. Syndactyly release. *Semin Plast Surg.* 2016;30(4):162-170.
10. Malik S. Syndactyly: phenotypes, genetics and current classification. *Eur J Hum Genet.* 2012;20(8):817-824.
11. Oda T, Pushman AG, Chung KC. Treatment of common congenital hand conditions. *Plast Reconstr Surg.* 2010;126(3):121e-133e.
12. Kozin SH, Zlotolow DA. Common pediatric congenital conditions of the hand. *Plast Reconstr Surg.* 2015;136(2):241e-257e.
13. Cronin TD. Syndactylism results of zig zag incision to prevent postoperative contracture. *Plast Reconstr Surg.* 1946;18(6):460-468.
    The original description of the zig-zag dorsal and palmar flaps used in syndactyly reconstruction to minimize scar contractures and improve aesthetic and functional outcomes. The paper also reviews the early evolution of the treatment of syndactyly.

14. Adkinson JM, Chung KC. Release of finger syndactyly using doral rectangular flap. In: Chung KC, ed. *Hand and Wrist Surgery.* 3rd ed. Philadelphia, PA: Elsevier; 2018:811-818.
15. Golash A, Watson JS. Nail fold creation in complete syndactyly using Buck-Gramcko pulp flaps. *J Hand Surg Br.* 2000;25(1):11-14.
Seventy-five fingertips with nail fold reconstructions using the Buck-Gramcko pulp flaps were reviewed. There was one flap loss and six flaps with tip necrosis. However, all fingertips had adequate pulp fullness with a round appearance. The Buck-Gramcko flaps are an aesthetically pleasing and effective way to reconstruct the nail folds.
16. Yuan F, Zhong L, Chung KC. Aesthetic comparison of two different types of web;space reconstruction for finger syndactyly. *Plast Reconstr Surg.* 2018;142(4):963-971
17. Pettitt DA, Arshad Z, Mishra A, McArthur P. Apert syndrome: a consensus on the management of Apert hands. *J Craniomaxillofac Surg.* 2017;45(2):223-231.
18. Woodside JC, Light TR. Symbrachydactyly: diagnosis, function, and treatment. *J Hand Surg Am.* 2016;41(1):135-143, quiz 143.
19. Catena N, Divizia MT, Calevo MG. Hand and upper limb anomalies in Poland syndrome: a new proposal of classification. *J Pediatr Orthop.* 2012;32(7):727-731.
20. Watt AJ, Chung KC. Duplication. *Hand Clin.* 2009;25(2):215-227.
21. Wassel HD. Results of surgery for polydactyly of the thumb. *Clin Orthop Relat Res.* 1969;64:175-193.
The manuscript proposes the Flatt classification for preaxial polydactyly, placing the anomaly into one of seven categories. It also reviews, in detail, 22 duplicated thumbs in 18 patients, discussing the deformity classification, treatment, outcome, [illegible]
22. Siegert JJ, Cooney WP, Dobyns JH. Management of simple [illegible] *J Hand Surg Am.* 1990;15B(2).
23. Hamilton KL, Netscher DT. Evaluation of a stepwise surgical approach to camptodactyly. *Plast Reconstr Surg.* 2015;135(3):568e-576e.
The authors review 18 fingers treated for camptodactyly with resolution of flexion contracture to a mean of 3 degrees, at a mean follow-up of 11 months. The article lays out a simple step-wise approach to effectively treat camptodactyly.
24. Evans BT, Waters PM, Bae DS. Early results of surgical management of camptodactyly. *J Pediatr Orthop.* 2017;37(5):e317-e320.
25. Engber WD, Flatt AE. Camptodactyly: an analysis of sixty-six patients and twenty-four operations. *J Hand Surg.* 1977;2(3):216-224.
26. McFarlane RM, Classen DA, Porte AM, Botz JS. Anatomy and treatment of camptodactyly of the small finger *J Hand Surg Am.* 1992;17(1):35-44.
27. Netscher DT, Staines KG, Hamilton KL. Severe camptodactyly: a systematic surgeon and therapist collaboration. *J Hand Ther.* 2015;28(2):167-174.
28. Rhee SH, Oh WS, Lee HJ, et al. Effect of passive stretching on simple camptodactyly in children younger than three years of age. *J Hand Surg Am.* 2010;35(11):1768-1773.
29. Kamnerdnakta S, Brown M, Chung KC. Camptodactyly correction. In: Chung KC, ed. *Hand and Wrist Surgery.* 3rd ed. Philadelphia, PA: Elsevier; 2018:842-849.
30. Vickers D. Clinodactyly of the little finger: a simple operative technique for reversal of the growth abnormality. *J Hand Surg Br.* 1987;12(3):335-342.
Description of physiolysis of the bracketed epiphysis and interposition of fat graft in twelve fingers with clinodactyly. At a maximum follow-up of 6 years, all patients had excellent aesthetic results and range of motion. Only one patient required a later osteotomy due to premature closure of the radial component of the physis.
31. Choo AD, Mubarak SJ. Longitudinal epiphyseal bracket. *J Child Orthop.* 2013;7(6):449-454.
32. Goldfarb CA, Wall LB. Osteotomy for clinodactyly. *J Hand Surg Am.* 2015;40(6):1220-1224.
33. Medina JA, Lorea P, Elliot D, Foucher G. Correction of clinodactyly by early physiolysis: 6-year results. *J Hand Surg Am.* 2016;41(6):e123-127.
34. Kikuchi N, Ogino T. Incidence and development of trigger thumb in children. *J Hand Surg Am.* 2006;31(4):541-543.
35. Slakely JB, Hennrikus WL. Acquired thumb flexion contracture in children: congenital trigger thumb. *J Bone Jt Surg Br.* 1996;78B:481-483.
36. Baek GH, Lee HJ. The natural history of pediatric trigger thumb: a study with a minimum of five years follow-up. *Clin Orthop Surg.* 2011;3(2):157-159.
The study progressively followed 87 thumbs in 67 pediatric patients with trigger thumb, who had no treatment. At a mean follow-up of 87 months, 76% of patients had complete resolution. The median time from initial visit to resolution was 49 months. The authors concluded that most patients with trigger thumb can safely be observed for a period of time, effectively delaying or avoiding an operation.
37. Rodgers WB, Waters PM. Incidence of trigger digits in newborns. *J Hand Surg Am.* 1994;19(3):364-368.
38. Hisham Abdel G, El-Naggar A, Hegazy M, et al. Characteristics of patients with congenital clasped thumb: a prospective study of 40 patients with the results of treatment. *J Child Orthop.* 2007;1(5):313-322.
39. Serbest S, Tosun HB, Tiftikci U, et al. Congenital clasped thumb that is forgetten a syndrome in clinical practice: a case report. *Medicine (Balt).* 2015;94(38):e1630.
40. Kawamura K, Chung KC. Constriction band syndrome. *Hand Clin.* 2009;25(2):257-264.
41. Foulkes G, Reinker K. Congenital constriction band syndrome: a seventy year experience. *J Pediatr Orthop.* 1994;14(2):242-248.
42. Torpin R, Faulkner A. Intrauterine amputation with the missing member found in [illegible] *JAMA.* 1966;198(2):185-187.
Postulated a series of events that has led to the extrinsic theory of [illegible] *syndrome. An early amniotic rupture causes oligohydramnios and a string of chorion to encircle the extremity causing compression and growth suppression or physiologic amputation.*
43. Upton J, Tan C. Correction of constriction rings. *J Hand Surg Am.* 1991;16(5):947-953.
44. Manske PR, Goldfarb CA. Congenital failure of formation of the upper limb. *Hand Clin.* 2009;25(2):157-170.
45. Colen DL, Lin IC, Levin LS, Chang B. Radial longitudinal deficiency: recent developments, controversies, and an evidence-based guide to treatment. *J Hand Surg Am.* 2017;42(7):546-563.
46. Maschke SD, Seitz W, Lawton J. Radial longitudinal deficiency. *J Am Acad Orthop Surg.* 2007;15(1):41-52.
47. Bayne LG, Klug MS. Long-term review of the surgical treatment of radial deficiencies. *J Hand Surg.* 1987;12(2):169-179.
48. James MA, McCarroll HR, Manske PR. The spectrum of radial longitudinal deficiency: a modified classification. *J Hand Surg Am.* 1999;24(6):1145-1155.
49. Blauth W. Der hypoplastische Daumen. *Arch Orthop Unfallchir.* 1967;62(3):225-246.
50. Manske PR, McCarroll HR, James M. Type III-A hypoplastic thumb. *J Hand Surg Am.* 1995;20(2):246-253.
51. Buck-Gramcko D. Pollicization of the index finger: method and results in aplasia and hypoplasia of the thumb. *J Bone Jt Surg Am.* 1971;53(8):1605-1617.
52. Manske PR, Halikis MN. Surgical classification of central deficiency according to the thumb web. *J Hand Surg Am.* 1995;20(4):687-697.
53. Upton J, Taghinia AH. Correction of the typical cleft hand. *J Hand Surg Am.* 2010;35(3):480-485.

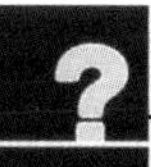

QUESTIONS

1. **A 2-year-old patient presents to the clinic with a left thumb duplication. Based on the Flatt classification system, which is the most common type of duplication?**

   a. Type I
   b. Type II
   c. Type III
   d. Type IV
   e. Type V
   f. Type VI
   g. Type VII

2. **A 14-year-old girl presents with progressive worsening of flexion deformities of the bilateral ring finger proximal interphalangeal joints. Which of the following diagnosis does she most likely have?**

   a. Clinodactyly
   b. Constriction ring syndrome
   c. Camptodactyly
   d. Syndactyly

3. **A 15-month-old girl is brought in by her mother who is concerned that she cannot fully extend the thumb. On examination, the thumb is in 20 degrees of flexion at the interphalangeal joint and cannot but passively corrected. What is the most likely diagnosis?**

   a. Triphalangeal thumb
   b. Trigger thumb
   c. Clinodactyly
   d. Camptodactyly
   e. Syndactyly

4. **A 4-month-old boy presents with syndactyly of all webspaces and decision is made to release his syndactyly in a staged fashion. Which of the following webspaces should be released at the first stage?**

   a. 1st and 4th
   b. 1st and 3rd
   c. 2nd and 4th
   d. 2nd and 3rd
   e. 3rd and 4th

5. **A 6-month-old girl presents to the office with syndactyly of the left middle and ring fingers. The fusion involves the entire length of the digits including the nails. An X-ray shows separate middle and ring finger phalanges. How is this syndactyly classified?**

   a. Complex, incomplete
   b. Complex, complete
   c. Simple, incomplete
   d. Simple, complete
   e. Complicated

1. **Answer: d.** The type IV deformity describes duplication at the level of the metacarpophalangeal joint and occurs 43% of the time. The next most common is type VII (20%), followed by type II (15%), type III ([illegible]), type V (10%), and types I and VI (6%).

2. **Answer: c.** Camptodactyly describes an irreducible flexion contracture of the proximal interphalangeal joints and most commonly involves the ring or small fingers. Patients frequently present either shortly after birth or during adolescence during periods of rapid growth spurts. Clinodactyly is most commonly found in the small finger and describes deviation of the digit in the radio/ulnar plane. Constriction ring syndrome presents with characteristic rings and often shortened digits. Syndactyly presents at birth and describes fusion of the digits involving soft tissue or bone.

3. **Answer: b.** Unlike adults, children who present with ***trigger thumb*** do not have triggering of the digit, but instead the thumb is maintained in a flexed position. Often there is a palpable ***Notta*** nodule proximal to the A1 pulley. A triphalangeal thumb may be found in patients with thumb duplication. Clinodactyly is most commonly found in the small fingers, and presents with radio-ulnar deviation of the digits. Camptodactyly describes flexion contractures of the PIP joints and is typically found in the ring or small fingers. Syndactyly describes fusion of the fingers and the digits typically are not held in a flexed position.

4. **Answer: a.** When syndactyly involves multiple webspaces, a thoughtful plan must be developed for its reconstruction. Border digits (thumb and small finger) should be released at an earlier age, typically 1 to 6 months, to minimize any growth disturbances. Furthermore, to avoid potential neurovascular compromise, both sides of a digit should not be released in the same operation. In this patient, the border digits should be released first (1st and 4th webspaces). The remainder of the webspaces can be released in subsequent operations.

5. **Answer: d.** Complex syndactyly describes bony fusion of the digits whereas simple syndactyly only has soft tissue involvement. When the syndactyly occurs along the entire length of the digits, including the nail bed, it is classified as complete. Incomplete syndactyly occurs when there is only partial fusion of the fingers. Complicated syndactyly is often seen with other syndromes, such as Apert syndrome, and may involve multiple structures including bones, joints, tendons, muscles, or neurovascular structures.

CHAPTER 91 Upper Limb Amputations and Prosthetics

Kate E. Elzinga and Kevin C. Chung

KEY POINTS

- Upper extremity amputations range from amputations of the soft tissue of the distal phalanx to shoulder disarticulation. As the injury becomes more proximal, there is greater patient morbidity and mortality.
- Durable, supple, sensate soft tissue coverage is important for all residual limbs. The level of amputation is determined based on the level of injury, the condition of the preserved tissues, the patient's overall health and goals, and the plan for prosthetic wear.
- Multidisciplinary care is essential after limb amputation. Collaborative care by plastic and orthopedic surgeons, physiatrists, physical and occupational therapists, nurses, social workers, prosthetists, engineers, and other professionals can optimize the function of an individual with amputation and minimize pain. The goal is to permit patients to return to work and recreational activities, albeit using modified techniques.
- Targeted muscle reinnervation (TMR) and regenerative peripheral nerve interfaces (RPNIs) are innovative techniques for neuroma management.
- Myoelectric prostheses permit movement of multiple degrees of freedom and, with targeted reinnervation, simultaneous movement of multiple joints. Cost and the limb-prosthetic interface are ongoing challenges that limit prosthetic use.
- Targeted muscle and sensory reinnervation techniques permit intuitive prosthesis control with the potential for sensory feedback.
- Many patients ultimately abandon the prosthesis owing to lack of comfort and/or lack of functionality.

Upper limb amputations are common, most often affecting the thumb and fingers. More proximal amputations, through the forearm, elbow, and upper arm, are less common but markedly more limiting in function. Most upper limb amputations are caused by trauma. With more proximal traumatic amputations, replantation success rates are lower because of the increased amount of skeletal muscle requiring revascularization and the longer regeneration distances for repaired nerves. Goals of upper extremity reconstruction include the following:

- Motion
- Length
- Sensation
- Durability
- Appearance
- Pain-free, prevention of symptomatic neuromas
- Prevention of joint contractures
- Eradication of disease
- Early prosthetic fitting, when appropriate
- Early return to work and recreational activities

After an injury, the primary goal is to maximize upper extremity function, with either limb salvage and reconstruction or amputation and prosthesis fitting. Other indications for amputation include malignancy, infection, vascular disease, high-pressure injection injury, burns, frostbite, and peripheral nerve injury. Following a burn, frostbite, thrombotic, or embolic injury, limb amputation is often delayed until tissue demarcation is complete in an effort to maintain functional length.

Patients with amputations are best managed by a multidisciplinary team that includes plastic and orthopedic surgeons, physical medicine and rehabilitation physicians, prosthetists, engineers, occupational and physical therapists, psychiatrists, psychologists, nurses, and social workers. The physical, mental, and emotional needs of the patient are addressed. The patient is taught how to perform their activities of daily living using their remaining limbs, various aids, and prostheses when appropriate.

Patient-specific management is a core component of care after amputation. Each patient's occupation and avocations are explored, their activities of daily living are observed, and their functional and esthetic goals are discussed. Despite similar amputation levels, patients with similar injuries can have vastly different desires regarding prostheses. For example, for a middle finger amputation through the midshaft of the proximal phalanx, some patients adapt to the function and appearance of the short proximal phalanx, others choose to wear a cosmetic prosthesis to maintain a five-fingered hand, and some undergo a ray amputation with or without the transposition of the index finger. If a patient is unsure of the treatment they would like to pursue, maintenance of tissue is recommended; further surgery can be performed later if the patient desires.

AMPUTATION VERSUS LIMB SALVAGE

Upper limb salvage has superior outcomes compared with lower limb salvage.[1] The main functions of the upper extremity are grip and prehension. This is typically achieved better with a salvaged upper extremity than an upper limb prosthesis.[2] The injured extremity maintains some sensory feedback, is more durable and convenient than a prosthesis, and requires less maintenance. Graham et al. determined that replanted upper extremities result in superior functional results compared to amputation and prostheses using the Carroll test.[3] Otto et al. reported that replantation is preferred with the advantages of sensation and psychological well-being compared to a prosthesis.[4]

For most upper extremity injuries, arm length preservation is the goal. Free tissue transfers can be performed to provide coverage over exposed bone, tendons, and neurovascular structures. Flaps permit stable and durable residual limb coverage for prosthetic fitting. Skin grafts are generally inadequate.

In contrast, the main functions of the lower extremity are weight-bearing and ambulation and can be well restored with a prosthesis. More than 15% of patients with salvaged lower extremities request elective amputation, but this is very rare in those with upper extremity salvage.[5] The upper extremity can tolerate shortening procedures to improve fracture, musculotendinous unit, nerve, and vessel repairs. Limb-length discrepancy is not well tolerated in the lower extremity. Most upper extremity amputations are caused by trauma, whereas most lower limb amputations are attributed to peripheral vascular disease.

For multitrauma patients, the "life before limb" principle applies. Damage control surgery principles are used to optimize the patient's chance of survival. Intracranial, intrathoracic, and intraabdominal injuries require emergent management. Extremity injuries are treated secondarily. Multiple surgical teams work in a coordinated fashion to address the patients' injuries, and then the patient is brought to the intensive care unit for monitoring and correction of hypothermia, coagulopathy, and acidosis.

AMPUTATION LEVEL

Preservation of upper extremity length is generally advocated, as long as stable soft tissue coverage can be achieved, the limb will be pain free, and the preserved muscles and nerves are functional. However, in some cases, the principle of length preservation is not applied. For example, a ray amputation can give better results than a partial finger amputation.

In non–life-threatening cases, management by a multidisciplinary amputation team permits optimal patient evaluation, education, and formulation of treatment recommendations. Amputation level and aptness for prosthetic wear are determined based on the patient's personal goals and lifestyle.

If surgery is indicated, the incisions for an amputation are planned in advance to ensure that the limb will be well padded with smooth and durable soft tissue to permit comfortable prosthetic wear (Figure 91.1). For the fingers, hand, and forearm, the thicker volar skin is preferred for coverage compared with the thinner dorsal skin. Sensory-innervated regional and free flaps are helpful adjuncts to provide sensate soft tissue coverage over exposed critical structures when preserving limb length.

Thumb Amputation

Thumb injuries are common and can result in significant morbidity. The thumb accounts for 40% of hand function; preservation of length is critical.[6] Length and position are more important than motion. The thumb functions well as a post.

Replantation is preferred but in cases when this fails or is not possible, options for increasing thumb length include first webspace deepening, metacarpal lengthening using distraction osteogenesis, osteoplastic reconstruction, pollicization (Figure 91.2), [illegible]

Digital Amputation

Following amputation of the index, middle, ring, or small finger, the patient's function is assessed. The length of the residual digit and the associated joint motion are evaluated. For example, if the amputation is through the middle phalanx, distal to the insertion of the flexor digitorum superficialis tendon, then preservation of the digital length is often recommended to maintain motion and strength through the proximal interphalangeal joint. However, if the amputation is through the middle phalanx, proximal to the insertion of the flexor digitorum superficialis, preserving the short middle phalanx stump is often a hindrance because there will be no active flexion through the proximal interphalangeal joint.

Proximal digital amputations through the proximal phalanx and more proximal can result in difficulty in holding small objects. For improved function and appearance, ray amputation may be preferred. This narrows the hand width, resulting in 40% less grip strength.[7,8] Digital transposition can be performed; for example, moving an intact second ray over to the base of the third metacarpal after ring finger ray amputation, to close the cleft and to improve the esthetic result (Figure 91.3).

Partial Hand Amputation

Toe to thumb transfers can be performed to restore sensation, durability, and function following a partial hand amputation (Figures 91.4 and 91.5). Prosthesis suspension is difficult at this level without impairing wrist motion. Prosthetic wear often makes the limb longer than the contralateral uninjured side to fit the required movable components.

Wrist Disarticulation

[illegible] to permit prosthetic wear without pressure points following a wrist disarticulation. The

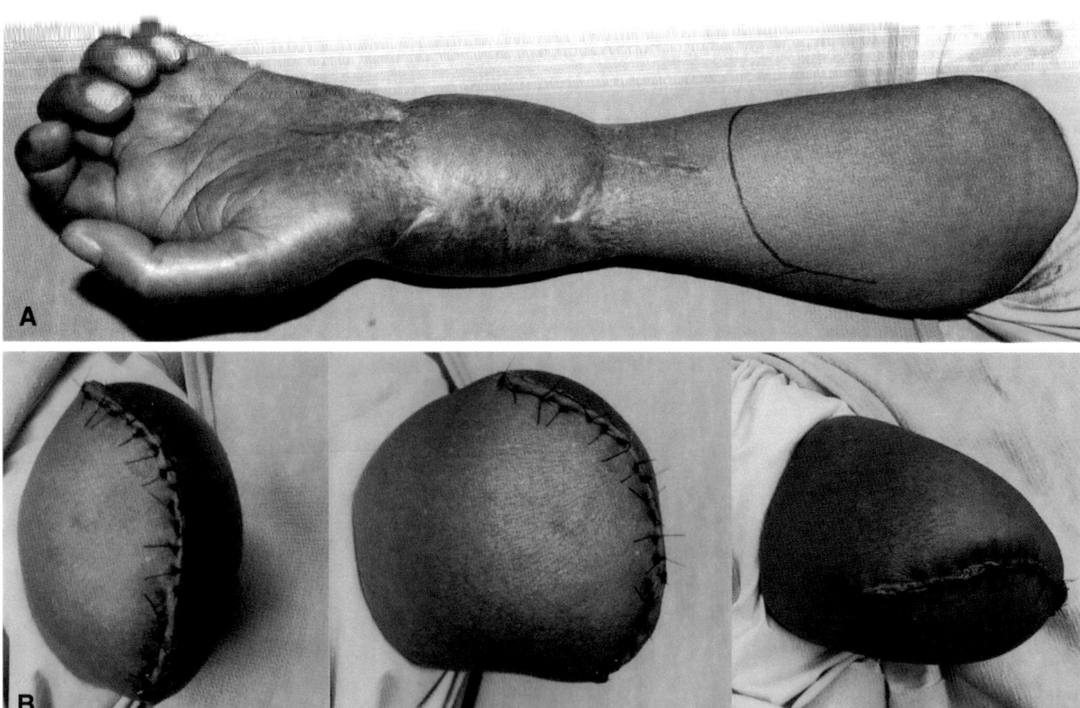

FIGURE 91.1. **A.** A transradial amputation was performed 5 years after a distal injury to the patient's median, ulnar, and radial nerves that had resulted in a nonfunctional hand. The patient found that the hand was in the way and often sustained traumatic injuries due to the lack of protective sensation. A fishmouth incision was used. A myodesis was performed. **B.** Fasciocutaneous skin flaps were elevated and closed over the residual limb to provide durable, supply soft tissue coverage, resulting in a good esthetic and functional result.

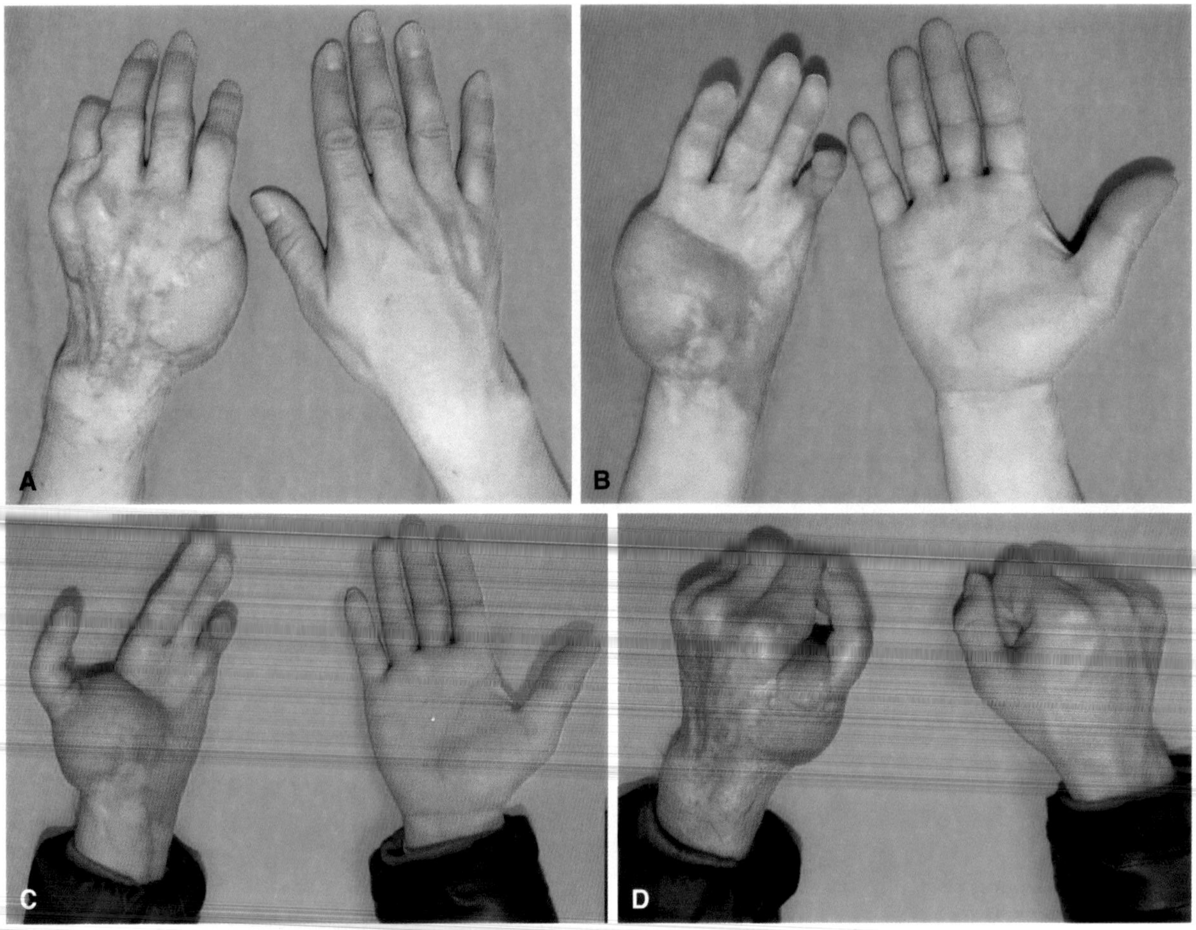

FIGURE 91.2. **A, B.** A pollicization was performed for this patient after a traumatic amputation of his left thumb. A groin flap was performed for initial wound coverage. **C, D.** After pollicization, the patient had improvement of his grip and pinch strength, shown here 6 months postoperatively.

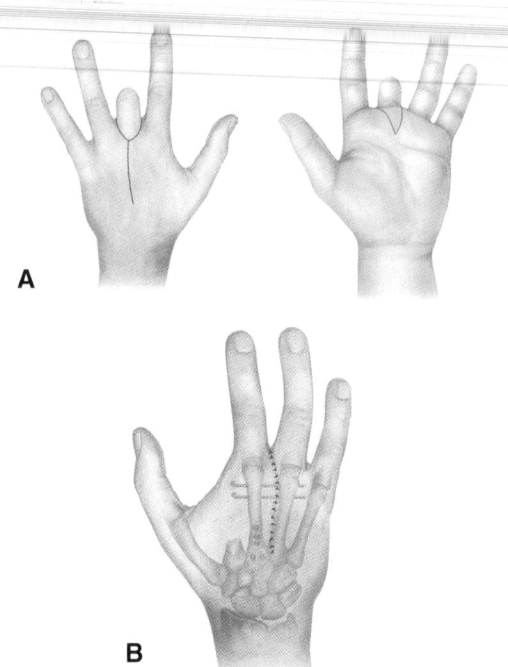

FIGURE 91.3. **A.** Ray amputation and transposition of the adjacent digit improves the esthetics of the hand. A transverse or a step-cut osteotomy is performed through the base of the adjacent metacarpal and the digit is mobilized and transposed into the site of the previous digital amputation. **B.** Internal fixation is performed at the metacarpal base. The intermetacarpal ligament is repaired at the distal metacarpal with sutures and reinforced with temporary K-wires if needed.

triangular fibrocartilage complex is preserved to maintain distal radioulnar joint (DRUJ) stability and forearm pronation and supination. At this level, with preservation of the DRUJ, radioulnar convergence does not occur.

Patients with unilateral amputations who do not want to wear a prosthesis are well served by a wrist disarticulation. However, if they want to wear a prosthesis, a transradial amputation may be preferred as this level permits space for prosthetic components and an improved appearance of the prosthesis.

Transradial Amputation

Transradial amputation is the most common level of upper extremity amputation. Myodesis (muscle sutured directly to bone, typically using bone tunnels) or myoplasty (muscle to muscle suture repair over the bone) is performed to provide durable soft tissue coverage over the distal bone, to stabilize the distal musculature, and to permit strong contraction of the distal musculature for prosthetic control. Proximal migration of the muscle mass impairs signal detection for a myoelectric prosthesis. Myodesis or a combined technique are preferred over myoplasty alone as they improve the stability of the amputated limb and result in less migration of the muscle with contraction, in turn permitting improved signal pick-up by a myoelectric prosthesis (Figure 91.6). With either myodesis and/or myoplasty, the muscles are repaired at their physiologic tension.

With the loss of the DRUJ, radioulnar impingement is common. Soft tissue interposition at the time of the amputation can help prevent this complication. Depending on the level of the amputation, the pronator quadratus or an extensor and a flexor tendon can be interposed.[5]

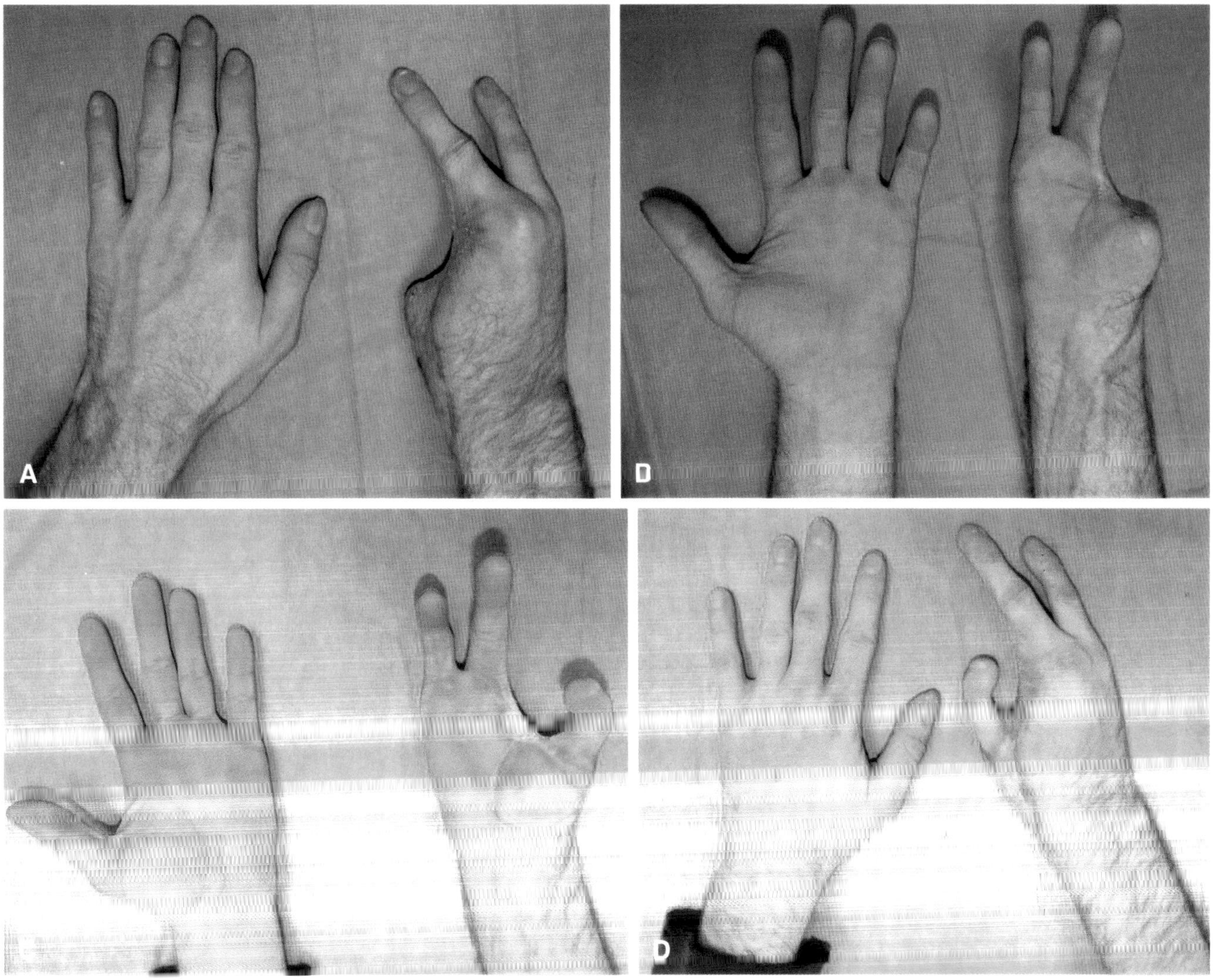

FIGURE 91.4. **A, B.** Toe transplantation provided a neo-thumb after a traumatic right radial hand amputation. **C, D.** Four months postoperatively, the toe transfer allowed the patient to grasp and manipulate objects.

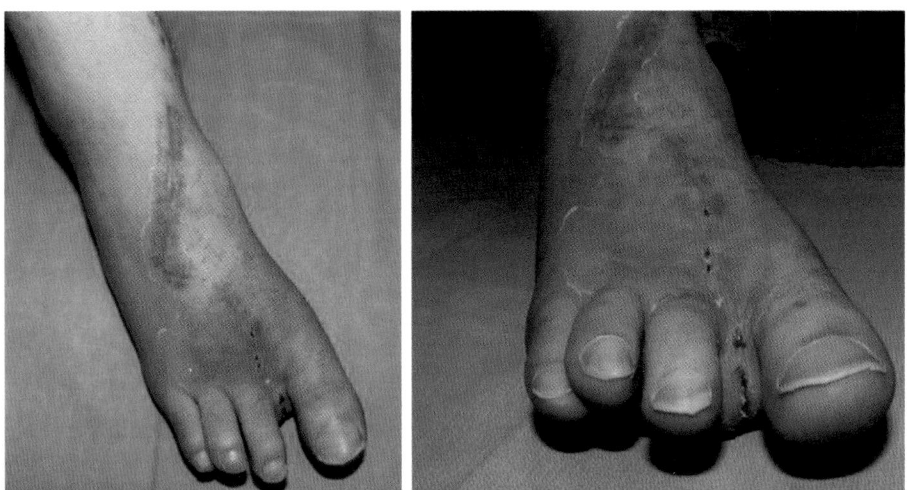

FIGURE 91.5. The donor site morbidity from a second toe transplant harvest, shown here with the toe harvested at the metatarsal phalangeal joint, is generally minimal.

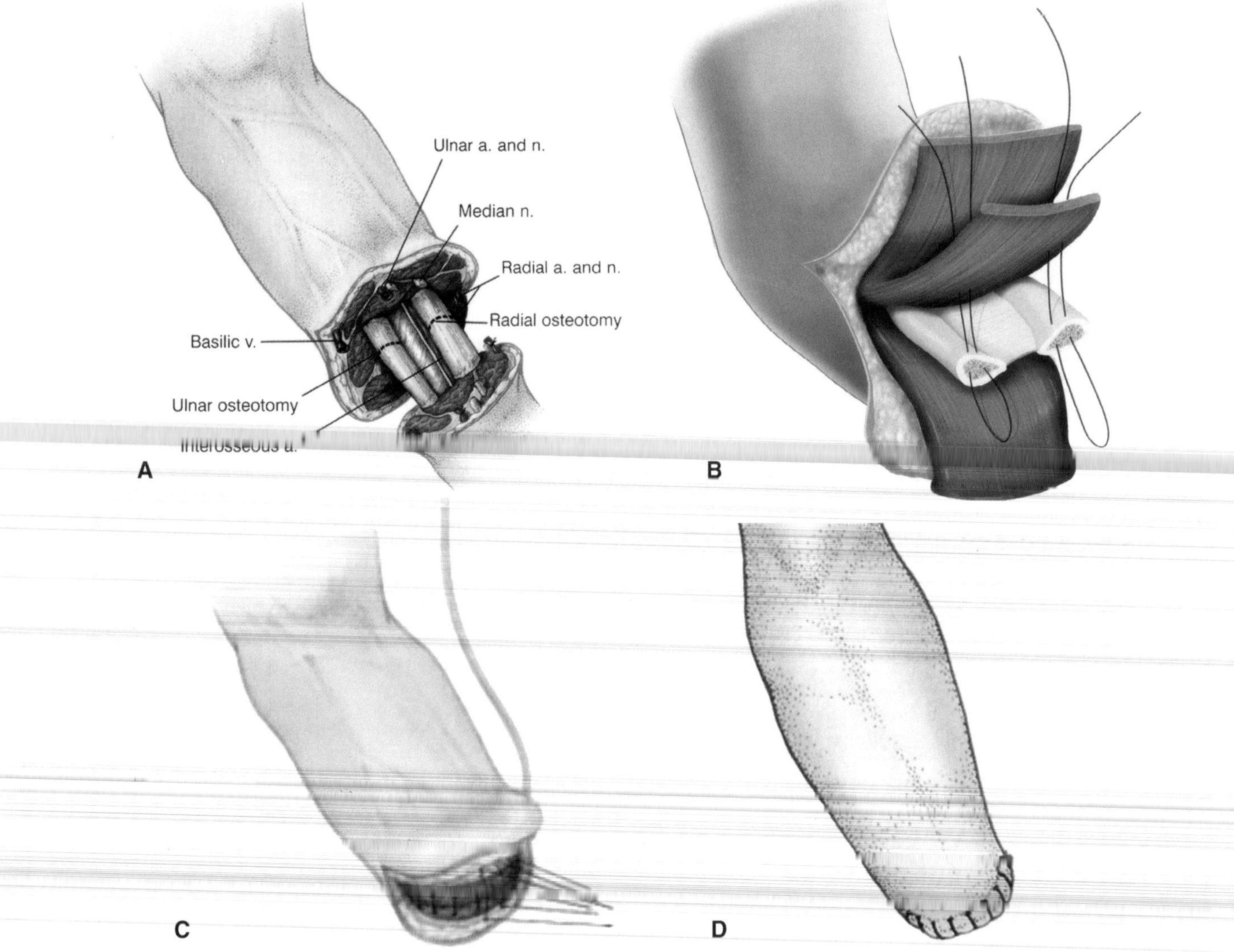

FIGURE 91.6. A transradial combined myodesis-myoplasty technique. The flexor compartment is elevated volarly and the extensor compartment is elevated dorsally from the radius and ulna. The muscle groups are secured to the bone, as well as to each other, distally over the bone to provide durable, stable soft tissue coverage and to create new insertions for the muscles. (**A,C,D** from Bickels J, Gortzak Y, Kollender Y, et al. Above-elbow and below-elbow amputations. In: Wiesel SW, ed. *Operative Techniques in Orthopaedic Surgery*. 2nd ed. Vol 2. Philadelphia, PA: Wolters Kluwer; 2016:2266. Figures 15-3B, 15-4B, 15-4D.)

Maintenance of two-thirds of the forearm length preserves pronation and supination. Amputations 10 cm or more proximal to the wrist permit increased prosthetic options; myoelectric prostheses can be considered.[9] Maintenance of a minimum of 5 cm of the ulna preserves elbow function and adequate fitting of a prosthesis. Patients with transradial amputations can wear harness-suspended body-powered prostheses or myoelectric prostheses suspended at their humeral condyles or using suction sleeves.

Patients with transradial amputations have greater function than those with transhumeral amputations. Pedicled and free tissue transfers should be performed to preserve the elbow and proximal forearm.

Elbow Disarticulation, Distal Transhumeral Amputation

For patients with unilateral amputations who do not want to wear a prosthesis, preserving the elbow permits for greater reach of the amputated arm to assist the uninjured arm in moving and stabilizing objects.

For patients who choose to wear a body-powered prosthesis, the elbow condyles permit suspension of the prosthesis. For those choosing a myoelectric prosthesis with a myoelectric elbow, a transhumeral amputation 5 to 6 cm above the olecranon can be performed.[10] Alternatively, a humerus shortening osteotomy can be performed to preserve the humeral condyles while elevating the elbow so that the elbow joint of the prosthesis will be at a similar level to that of the contralateral arm.[11]

For distal transhumeral amputations, a Marquardt angulation osteotomy at an angle of 70° to 110° at the distal humerus can be used to provide a lever arm for suspension when the epicondyles have been removed and for rotational control of the prosthesis (Figure 91.7).[12]

Proximal Transhumeral Amputation

Transhumeral amputations that preserve 5 to 7 cm of the proximal humerus are preferred compared with more proximal amputations to facilitate prosthetic suspension, proper maintenance of the function of the deltoid, and an acceptable shoulder contour.[5]

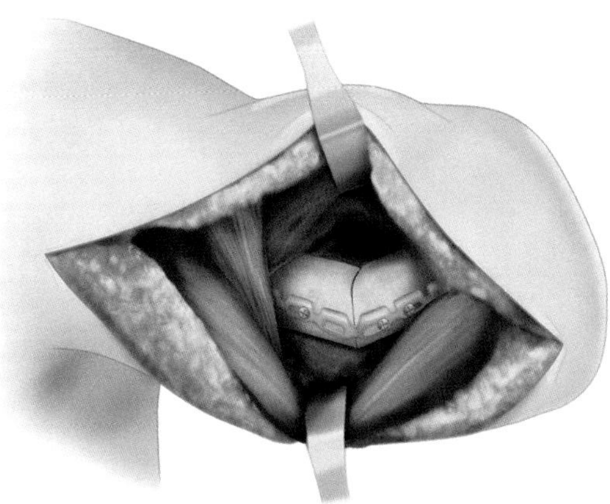

FIGURE 91.7. A distal humerus Marquardt angulation osteotomy can be performed to facilitate prosthesis suspension and rotational control when the humerus epicondyles have been removed in a distal transhumeral amputation.

More proximal amputations can be optimized for prosthetic fitting by maintaining length using a pedicled latissimus dorsi flap if the soft tissues are deficient or a free fibula flap if the humerus is deficient. Distraction lengthening using the Iliazarov technique is an alternative way of lengthening the residual limb for improved prosthetic fitting.

In a nonfunctional upper extremity, such as that following a pan-plexus preganglionic brachial plexus injury, transhumeral amputation at 25%-30% of humeral length is recommended by Dumanian and Kuiken to remove the weight of the arm while maintaining the shoulder and upper arm contour for clothing wear.[10]

Shoulder Disarticulation

Traumatic avulsion of the arm at the shoulder is a life-threatening injury, often presenting with associated thoracic and abdominal injuries due to significant trauma. Urgent surgical intervention is required to identify and stop bleeding from the axillary artery and vein. Blood transfusions are frequently required. Replantation is not attempted; these patients are hemodynamically unstable.

Once vascular control is obtained and the patient is stabilized, typically in a second operation, TMR can be performed using the terminal ends of the brachial plexus for both neuroma prevention and control of a myoelectric prosthesis. Preservation of the scapula and clavicle improves the shoulder contour and the appearance when the patient wears clothes. Flap coverage is often required to close the soft tissue defect at the disarticulation site, using regional or free flaps.

Pediatric Amputations

Preservation of length and physes is important.[9] Pediatric patients have greater healing ability than most adults. Tighter and more tenuous wound closure can be tolerated. Regional or free flaps are valuable adjuncts to maintain skeletal length.

Pediatric patients have a higher incidence of bony overgrowth than adults. Yearly follow-up is recommended with radiographs. Transhumeral amputations require revisions surgery for bony overgrowth most frequently, in up to 12% of pediatric patients.[13]

PROSTHESES

Upper extremity prostheses require more movement, control, and precision compared with lower extremity prostheses.[10] Unlike lower extremity prostheses, they do not need to support the weight of the body.

Despite significant advancements in the technology of prostheses, many patients reject their use. Rejection rates for esthetic and functional upper extremity prostheses are over 30%.[5] Commonly reported reasons for prosthesis rejection include the lack of sensation, poor training, delayed fitting, limited usefulness, weight, and socket discomfort.[14] Prostheses are more commonly worn by patients with more distal levels of amputations. Patients with transradial amputations wear prostheses more frequently than those with transhumeral amputations and shoulder disarticulation. Adequate training and early fitting encourage prosthetic use. Once the patients' edema has decreased following their injury and the incision is healed, prosthetic fitting begins.

Individuals with unilateral amputations generally return to work as they adapt to their amputation. Those with bilateral amputations have increased impairment and are less likely to return to their previous occupation, depending on the physical demands of the job. Patients with bilateral amputations are more likely than those with unilateral amputations to use a prosthesis.

Prostheses can be worn using self-suspended sockets, suction sockets, and harness suspension.[15] Osseointegration is an evolving technique that permits secure attachment of a prosthesis to the bone, with minimal irritation of the surrounding soft tissues. Advances in osseointegration may help increase prosthesis acceptability and use by eliminating socket-related problems (skin irritation, discomfort, pressure, perspiration, fit) and the need for harness devices to suspend the prosthesis to the body.

Types of Prostheses

Prostheses are classified as passive or active devices. Passive prostheses are worn primarily for esthetic improvement. Active prostheses are used to improve function. The two main categories of active prostheses are body-powered and myoelectric.

Body-powered prostheses use cables, pulleys, and hooks to transmit function from the patient's intact shoulder and scapular movement to the distal prosthesis. Generally, only one joint can be controlled at a time. For example, patients need to lock the elbow joint to transmit the cable excursion to open the hand. These prostheses are generally stronger, lighter, and less costly than myoelectric prostheses, but they are more cumbersome to operate and wear and have limited range of operation because of the harnessing. They are often preferred by patients who require a prosthesis for heavy labor.

Myoelectric prostheses are powered by small motors. They are more intuitive than body-powered prostheses, using electromyography signals from the residual limb for control. They require muscle activity of the residual limb and can therefore improve health of the limb, and also do not require harnessing or strapping for control. Myoelectric prostheses are larger and heavier as they require space for batteries and motors. They are difficult to place for distal amputations, for example, at the level of a wrist disarticulation. Most patients prefer the appearance of a myoelectric prosthesis compared with a body-powered prosthesis.[16] Newer devices provide options of multiple grasp patterns that are not possible with body-powered devices.

Hybrid prostheses can also be used, for example, body-powered for the elbow and myoelectric for the hand in a patient with a transhumeral amputation.[17]

Standard body-powered prosthetic function is poor for those with proximal amputations as patients cannot simultaneously control their elbow and hand.[18] Similarly, with conventional myoelectric prostheses the myoelectric elbow and hand cannot be controlled simultaneously, and the user must sequentially switch from one joint to the next. For this reason, typically for patients with amputations above the elbow, TMR is recommended.[18] TMR permits precise motor control of a myoelectric prosthesis, as well as simultaneous operation of multiple prosthetic joints. Amputated nerves are neurotized to nearby muscles. When the muscle contracts, its electromyogram (EMG) signal can be detected transcutaneously to direct the function of the prosthesis. A concurrent brachial plexus injury with an amputation typically precludes a TMR procedure.

NEUROMA MANAGEMENT

Prevention and treatment of symptomatic neuromas is a critical part of amputation management. Surgical technique, postoperative rehabilitation, and patient education are important.

Symptomatic neuromas develop in 25% of patients with major limb amputations, causing pain, difficulty with prosthesis wear, reductions in quality of life, and decreases in function.[19] Neuromas can be localized using Tinel sign. When pressure is applied over the neuroma, the patient will describe discomfort at the area and radiating dysesthesias in the area that the nerve had previously innervated. Diagnostic localized injections can be helpful. Phantom sensations are present when the patient feels that their amputated body part is still present following their amputation. Phantom pains are ongoing painful sensations felt coming from the amputated limb and may occur with or without neuromas.

Symptomatic neuromas can be treated surgically. Often, surgeons attempt to bury the nerve end by performing a traction neurectomy and positioning of the nerve end deep in the soft tissues, muscle, or bone. Other options include resection of the neuroma and then using the centro-centralization technique to divide the nerve 5 to 10 mm proximal to the neuroma and performing an additional repair as an autologous transplantation[20] or suturing the distal nerve to an allograft. However, TMR or RPNI techniques appear to be more reliable solutions, providing amputated nerves with new functions and preventing neuroma recurrence.

For amputations of the fingers, traction neurectomy is most commonly performed, resecting the digital nerves 5 to 10 mm proximal to the end of the preserved bone. For amputations at the wrist and more proximal, TMR or RPNI are recommended to prevent symptomatic neuromas at the time of the amputation or in a delayed fashion.[21] Small cutaneous nerves can be transposed deep to nearby muscle to protect them from pressure from a prosthesis.

Targeted Muscle Reinnervation

TMR was developed by Kuiken et al. at the Rehabilitation Institute of Chicago to create a new biological neural machine interface.[22,23] Residual nerves from an amputated limb, of the upper or lower extremity, are transferred to muscles that are no longer biomechanically functional owing to the loss of the limb. Over time, these muscles will be reinnervated by the transferred nerves. The muscles will amplify the amputated nerve motor commands. Success rates of 95% for muscle reinnervation with detectable EMG signals using the TMR nerve transfer technique have been reported.[24] Neuromas are prevented (primary TMR, performed acutely) or effectively treated with TMR (secondary TMR, can be performed years after the injury).[24] Phantom pain is improved. Phantom sensation is unchanged. The TMR technique is tailored to each individual patient, by a multidisciplinary team including a plastic surgeon, physiatrist, prosthetist, biomedical engineer, and therapist. TMR is useful for well-selected, motivated patients interested in using a myoelectric prosthesis and, on a much broader scale, to prevent and manage symptomatic neuromas.

For a patient with a transhumeral amputation, for example, the median nerve can be coapted to the medial head of the biceps and the ulnar nerve can be coapted to the brachialis (hand close signals). The distal radial nerve can be coapted to the lateral head of the triceps (hand open signal). The musculocutaneous nerve is left intact to the lateral head of the biceps (elbow flexion signal) and the proximal radial nerve is left intact to the long head of the triceps (elbow extension signal).

For a shoulder disarticulation patient, the musculocutaneous nerve can be transferred to the clavicular head of the pectoralis major (elbow flexion signal), the median nerve can be transferred to the upper sternal head of the pectoralis major (hand close signal), the radial nerve can be transferred to the lower sternal head of the pectoralis major (hand open signal), and the ulnar nerve can be transferred to the pectoralis minor (hand close signal) (Figure 91.8). The axillary

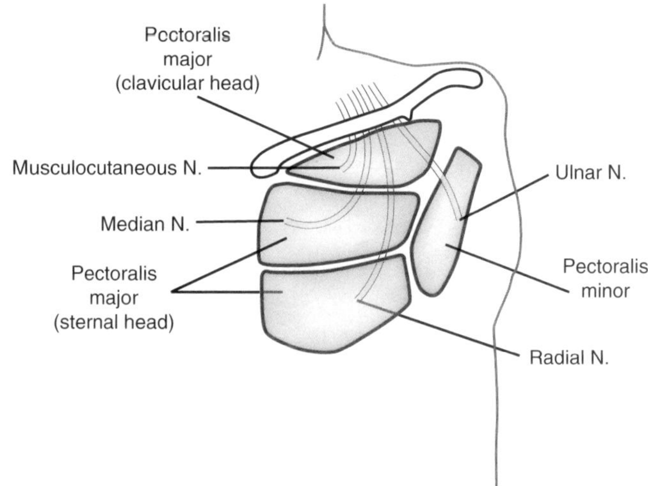

FIGURE 91.8. A common shoulder disarticulation targeted muscle reinnervation design is shown. The nerve targets are chosen based on each individual patient's injury.

nerve innervation to the deltoid and teres minor is kept intact. EMG signals from each of these muscles can be detected by a myoelectric prosthesis permitting intuitive, multidirectional, and simultaneous control of multiple joints of an advanced prosthesis. Alternative reinnervation targets have been described (**Table 91.1**).[25,26]

Patients can resume wearing their existing prosthesis 4 to 6 weeks after TMR. Three months after TMR, the first signs of muscle reinnervation are often noted and patients can be evaluated for a custom TMR prosthesis. Strong muscle contractions are visible and palpable 5 months postoperatively. Six months postoperatively, the EMG sites have begun to stabilize and EMG testing is performed to record and map out the signals at the nerve transfer sites. Strengthening of the amputated limb and control of the reinnervated muscles is guided by a therapist.

Targeted Sensory Reinnervation

Recent advancements in targeted sensory reinnervation (TSR) may permit sensory feedback back to the patient, with the goal of improving the ease of use and function of the prosthesis.[27-29] Rather than relying on visual and auditory clues, the patient can feel objects grasped, although the technology to integrate sensory feedback is not yet available as a commercial prosthetic system. TMR and TSR surgery can be performed acutely at the time of the patient's initial amputation or later in the subacute or chronic phase.

During TMR, the subcutaneous tissues under the skin overlying the anticipated EMG sites are thinned to minimize impedance and improve signal strength recording of the surface myoelectric signals. This results in local denervation of the skin. Competitive reinnervation of the skin then occurs from the underlying afferent nerve fibers. This process can be unpredictable and variable, resulting in intermixed skin sensations from the transferred nerves below and the native anatomic skin sensation.

To create distinct reinnervated sensory territories, cutaneous nerve end-to-side nerve transfers were developed by Kuiken et al.[28] In one patient with an amputation through the humeral neck, the supraclavicular cutaneous nerve was cut and coapted to the side of the ulnar nerve. The intercostobrachial nerve was cut and coapted to the median nerve. Six months later, the anterior chest skin had been reinnervated by both the median and ulnar afferents. However, a mixture of digit and native chest sensations were present.

To further refine TSR and to create the most discrete sensory patches of reinnervation for the ulnar and median nerves, Hebert et al. from the University of Alberta used a technique of sensory fascicle end-to-end TSR.[19,20] Somatosensory-evoked potentials are used intraoperatively to identify sensory fascicles of the main

TABLE 91.1. REINNERVATION MUSCLE TARGET EXAMPLES FOR SHOULDER DISARTICULATION TARGETED MUSCLE REINNERVATION[34]

	Example Reinnervation Target		
Nerve	**Case 1**	**Case 2**	**Signal/Function**
Axillary	Left intact to deltoid and teres minor		Shoulder abduction and external rotation
Musculocutaneous	Clavicular head of pectoralis major	Lateral half of the clavicular head of pectoralis major	Elbow flexion
Median	Upper sternal head of pectoralis major	Sternal head of the pectoralis major	Hand close
Ulnar	Pectoralis minor	Medial half of the clavicular head of pectoralis major	Hand close
Radial	Lower sternal head of pectoralis major	Inferior three slips of serratus anterior	Hand open

reinnervating nerves and target cutaneous nerves. Once a predominantly sensory fascicle is identified, it is cut and coapted to the cutaneous sensory target. The remainder of the main nerve is coapted to the motor branch of the target muscle. For example, in a transhumeral subject, a sensory fascicle of the median nerve is coapted to the intercostobrachial nerve and a sensory fascicle of the ulnar nerve is coapted to the cutaneous axillary nerve. This technique resulted in exclusive sensory patches in the designated territories, with no overlap.[30] Initial sensation was detected 4 to 8 months postoperatively and stable reinnervation occurred 1 year postoperatively.

Following TSR, experimental devices for providing feedback from the prostheses are being investigated. Specifically, touch and pressure sensors to convey object contact and grip can be matched to actuators over the reinnervated skin to apply proportional pressure stimuli back to the skin of the TSR site, providing the patient with matched sensory feedback. The sense of [illegible] has also been explored through vibration of the reinnervated muscles.[20] Further development of these techniques to clinical prostheses may allow the prosthesis user to "feel objects" with their prosthesis rather than having to rely on visual guidance and auditory cues.

Regenerative Peripheral Nerve Interfaces

Cederna et al., at the University of Michigan, developed the technique of RPNI to treat symptomatic neuromas and to permit myoelectric prosthesis control.[21,31,32] Motor RPNIs are fabricated by securing the distal end of a mixed or motor peripheral nerve within a small skeletal muscle graft. Dermal sensory interfaces are created by securing a sensory peripheral nerve fascicle within a small dermal skin graft.[33]

HAND TRANSPLANTATION

For select patients, hand transplantation is an alternative to prosthetic use, in particular for patients with bilateral amputations. The risks of immunosuppression must be weighed against the benefits of restoring appearance and function with a transplanted arm. Dumanian and Kuiken stated that patients with amputations at the transhumeral level and proximal would likely do better with TMR, and those with amputations at the transradial level and distal would do better with hand transplantation.[10]

ACKNOWLEDGMENTS

The work was supported by a Midcareer Investigator Award in Patient-Oriented Research (2 K24-AR053120-06) to Kevin C. Chung. The content is solely the responsibility of the authors and does not necessarily represent the official views of the National Institutes of Health. The authors would like to thank Dr. Jacqueline Hebert for her valuable review of this manuscript.

REFERENCES

1. Langer V. Management of major limb injuries. *Sci World J.* 2014;2014:640430.
2. Pet MA, Morrison SD, Mack JS, et al. Comparison of patient-reported outcomes after traumatic upper extremity amputation: replantation versus prosthetic rehabilitation. *Injury.* 2016;47(12):2783-2788.
   This multicenter study compared 9 patients who underwent successful replantation with 22 amputee patients who underwent prosthetic rehabilitation. Those in the replantation group reported better overall function and satisfaction and had higher DASH scores.
3. Graham B, Adkins P, Tsai TM, et al. Major replantation versus revision amputation and prosthetic fitting in the upper extremity: a late functional outcomes study. *J Hand Surg Am.* 1998;23(5):783-791.
4. Otto IA, Kon M, Schuurman AH, van Minnen LP. Replantation versus prosthetic fitting in traumatic arm amputations: a systematic review. *PLoS One.* 2015;10(9):e0137729.
   The outcomes of 301 replantation and 172 prosthetic patients were compared. Replantation patients had improved function and higher satisfaction scores compared to patients with amputations and prostheses. Sensation and psychological well-being were the two major advantages of replantation.
5. Tintle SM, Baechler MF, Nanos GP, et al. Traumatic and trauma-related amputations. Part II: upper extremity and future directions. *J Bone Joint Surg Am.* 2010;92(18):2934-2945.
6. Soucacos PN. Indications and selection for digital amputation and replantation. *J Hand Surg Br.* 2001;26(6):572-581.
7. Bhat AK, Acharya AM, Narayanakurup JK, et al. Functional and cosmetic outcome of single-digit ray amputation in hand. *Musculoskel Surg.* 2017;101(3):275-281.
   Forty-five patients were assessed after a single-ray amputation. There was a 43% decrease in grip strength (greatest after middle finger ray amputations) and a 34% loss of pinch strength (greatest after index finger ray amputations); 83% of patients reported good or excellent cosmetic outcomes.
8. Puhaindran ME, Healey JH, Athanasian EA. Single ray amputation for tumors of the hand. *Clin Orthop Relat Res.* 2010;468(5):1390-1395.
9. Marchessault JA, McKay PL, Hammert WC. Management of upper limb amputations. *J Hand Surg Am.* 2011;36(10):1718-1726.
10. Dumanian G, Kuiken T. Treatment of the upper extremity amputee. In: Neligan P, ed. *Plastic Surgery.* Vol. 6. 3rd ed. Philadelphia, PA: Elsevier; 2013:870-880.e872.
11. de Luccia N, Marino HL. Fitting of electronic elbow on an elbow disarticulated patient by means of a new surgical technique. *Prosthet Orthot Int.* 2000;24(3):247-251.
12. Marquardt E, Neff G. The angulation osteotomy of above-elbow stumps. *Clin Orthop Relat Res.* 1974(104):232-238.
13. Abraham E, Pellicore RJ, Hamilton RC, et al. Stump overgrowth in juvenile amputees. *J Pediatr Orthop.* 1986;6(1):66-71.
14. Wright TW, Hagen AD, Wood MB. Prosthetic usage in major upper extremity amputations. *J Hand Surg Am.* 1995;20(4):619-622.
15. Kistenberg RS. Prosthetic choices for people with leg and arm amputations. *Phys Med Rehabil Clin North Am.* 2014;25(1):93-115.
16. Carey SL, Lura DJ, Highsmith MJ. Differences in myoelectric and body-powered upper-limb prostheses: systematic literature review. *J Rehabil Res Dev.* 2015;52(3):247-262.
    This systemic review determined there is no significant advantage of a myoelectric prosthesis compared to a body-powered prosthesis. A patient's needs, preferences, and previous prosthetic experience should be considered. Body-powered prostheses are more durable, require less training time, and provide greater feedback. Myoelectric prostheses offer greater cosmesis, reduce phantom-limb pain, and are better for light-intensity work.
17. Lake C, Dodson R. Progressive upper limb prosthetics. *Phys Med Rehabil Clin North Am.* 2006;17(1):49-72.
18. Dumanian GA, Ko JH, O'Shaughnessy KD, et al. Targeted reinnervation for transhumeral amputees: current surgical technique and update on results. *Plast Reconstr Surg.* 2009;124(3):863-869.
19. Bowen JB, Wee CE, Kalik J, Valerio IL. Targeted muscle reinnervation to improve pain, prosthetic tolerance, and bioprosthetic outcomes in the amputee. *Adv Wound Care (New Rochelle).* 2017;6(8):261-267.

20. Gorkisch K, Boese Landgraf J, Vaubel E. Treatment and prevention of amputation neuromas in hand surgery. *Plast Reconstr Surg*. 1984;73(2):293-299.
21. Urbanchek MG, Kung TA, Frost CM, et al. Development of a regenerative peripheral nerve interface for control of a neuroprosthetic limb. *Biomed Res Int*. 2016;2016:5726730.
22. Kuiken TA, Dumanian GA, Lipschutz RD, et al. The use of targeted muscle reinnervation for improved myoelectric prosthesis control in a bilateral shoulder disarticulation amputee. *Prosthet Orthot Int*. 2004;28(3):245-253.
23. Cheesborough JE, Smith LH, Kuiken TA, Dumanian GA. Targeted muscle reinnervation and advanced prosthetic arms. *Semin Plast Surg*. 2015;29(1):62-72.
The TMR technique for transhumeral and shoulder disarticulation amputees is reviewed by the creators of this technique. Prosthetic arm technologies are discussed.
24. Souza JM, Cheesborough JE, Ko JH, et al. Targeted muscle reinnervation: a novel approach to postamputation neuroma pain. *Clin Orthop Relat Res*. 2014;472(10):2984-2990.
25. Kuiken TA, Miller LA, Lipschutz RD, et al. Targeted reinnervation for enhanced prosthetic arm function in a woman with a proximal amputation: a case study. *Lancet*. 2007;369(9559):371-380.
26. Gart MS, Souza JM, Dumanian GA. Targeted muscle reinnervation in the upper extremity amputee: a technical roadmap. *J Hand Surg Am*. 2015;40(9):1877-1888.
27. Hebert JS, Elzinga K, Chan KM, et al. Updates in targeted sensory reinnervation for upper limb amputation. *Curr Surg Rep*. 2014;2(3):1-9.
The evolution of TSR is discussed. The technique for sensory fascicle end-to-end is outlined.
28. Hebert JS, Olson JL, Morhart MJ, et al. Novel targeted sensory reinnervation technique to restore functional hand sensation after transhumeral amputation. *IEEE Trans Neural Syst Rehabil Eng*. 2014;22(4):765-773.
29. Schofield JS, Evans KR, Carey JP, Hebert JS. Applications of sensory feedback in motorized upper extremity prosthesis: a review. *Expert Rev Med Devices*. 2014;11(5):499-511.
30. Marasco PD, Hebert JS, Sensinger JW, et al. Illusory movement perception improves motor control for prosthetic hands. *Sci Transl Med*. 2018;10(432).
31. Woo SL, Kung TA, Brown DL, et al. Regenerative peripheral nerve interfaces for the treatment of postamputation neuroma pain: a pilot study. *Plast Reconstr Surg Glob Open*. 2016;4(12):e1038.
This is the first series to report on the outcomes of RPNI, in 16 patients. A reduction in neuroma pain, phantom pain, and narcotic use was observed. 75% of patients were satisfied or highly satisfied with their RPNI surgery. Minimal complications were reported.
32. Irwin ZT, Schroeder KE, Vu PP, et al. Chronic recording of hand prosthesis control signals via a regenerative peripheral nerve interface in a rhesus macaque. *J Neural Eng*. 2016;13(4):046007.
33. Sando IC, Gerling GJ, Ursu DC, et al. Dermal-based peripheral nerve interface for transduction of sensory feedback. *Plast Reconstr Surg*. 2015;136(4 suppl):19-20.
34. Kuiken TA, Marasco PD, Lock BA, et al. Redirection of cutaneous sensation from the hand to the chest skin of human amputees with targeted reinnervation. *Proc Natl Acad Sci USA*. 2007;104(50):20061-20066.

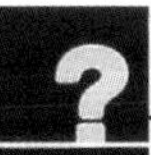

QUESTIONS

1. A 25-year-old male carpenter returns for follow-up 1 year after undergoing an amputation of his index finger at the level of the mid-proximal phalanx. He complains of difficulty grasping small objects (the objects fall out of the radial aspect of his hand) and holding a pencil and precision tools. What surgery would you recommend?

a. Revision amputation of the index finger at the metacarpophalangeal (MCP) joint
b. Ray amputation of the index finger at the metacarpal base
c. Fusion of the index finger MCP joint in 45° of flexion
d. Distraction osteogenesis of the index finger proximal phalanx
e. Toe transplant to the index finger

2. A 35-year-old man presents to the emergency department at 03:00 following an injury at a manufacturing plant at 02:15. He sustained a sharp, clean shoulder disarticulation. The amputated arm has been placed on ice and is with the patient. How would you treat the patient?

a. Pressure dressing, plan for exploration and possible closure in operating room at 07:30
b. Emergent angiogram
c. Emergent attempt at replantation
d. Emergent surgery for exploration with no attempt at replantation

3. An 8-year-old girl is brought in with a traumatic elbow disarticulation from a boating accident. The amputated arm was not recovered by the emergency medical personnel. How would you treat the patient?

a. Soft tissue closure over the distal humerus
b. Revision to a transhumeral amputation
c. Revision to a shoulder disarticulation amputation
d. Distraction osteogenesis of the humerus
e. Free fibula osteocutaneous flap to replace the forearm

4. A 40-year-old woman presents for a transradial amputation 10 years after sustaining a C8-T1 preganglionic brachial plexus injury, resulting in the loss of all hand function. She has intact elbow flexion and extension. What is the appropriate surgical management of distal amputation residual limb?

a. Permit the distal residual limb to heal by secondary intention. Place an antimicrobial dressing.
b. Perform tertiary closure of the residual limb. Place an antimicrobial dressing, permit time for tissue demarcation, and then return to the operating room for final closure.
c. Permit proximal retraction of the forearm musculature. Perform layered closure of the subcutaneous tissues and skin.
d. Perform a myodesis of the flexor and extensor musculature to the distal radius and ulna. Perform layered closure of the subcutaneous tissues and skin.
e. Perform a pedicled radial forearm flap, from the ipsilateral forearm, for closure of the residual limb.

5. A 28-year-old man presents with a symptomatic neuroma over his transradial amputation residual limb 1 year following his amputation. How would you manage this patient?

a. Perform a physical examination and a diagnostic local anesthetic block to confirm the site of the neuroma.
b. Refer the patient to a therapist to learn about scar desensitization and other nonoperative modalities to manage the neuroma pain.
c. Consider consultation with a multidisciplinary pain management team.
d. Discuss operative management of the neuroma with the patient, including traction neurectomy, burying the nerve, creation of a regenerative peripheral nerve interface, or targeted muscle reinnervation.
e. All the above

1. **Answer: b.** A ray amputation will functionally correct the patient's concerns and esthetically improve the appearance of the hand. A short amputated index finger often limits hand function. The residual digit is in the way, interfering with pinch between the thumb and middle finger. The index finger does not contribute to grip strength of the hand; this is provided by the middle, ring, and small fingers. Revision amputation at the MCP joint results in a less esthetically pleasing appearance than a ray amputation. A ray amputation provides increased soft tissue for tension-free closure and reconstruction of the first webspace. Fusion of the MCP joint would result in the index finger being even more limiting, blocking prehensile pinch between the thumb and middle finger. Distraction osteogenesis is a demanding, lengthy procedure for patients and would result in small gains in length but no additional joints to improve finger flexion and hand function.

A toe transplant should be reserved for restoration of a radial or ulnar post of the hand for prehension following complex hand injuries.

2. **Answer: d.** A traumatic shoulder disarticulation is a life-threating injury. Exsanguination can occur owing to lacerations in the axillary artery and vein. Advanced trauma life support protocols must be followed. Aggressive resuscitation with blood products is often required. The patient must be rapidly evaluated for other serious injuries, including thoracic and abdominal trauma. Hemorrhage can be temporarily controlled with hemostats and direct pressure in the emergency room, and then the patient should be emergently transferred to the operating room for definitive vascular control.

Postponing treatment or performing investigations such as an angiogram increases patient mortality. Replantation is contraindicated for shoulder disarticulation level amputations.

3. **Answer: a.** In children, preservation of length and physes is of utmost importance. Retention of the distal humeral physis will permit ongoing growth of the humerus, albeit at a decreased rate compared to the contralateral uninjured side. At skeletal maturity, the patient is likely to have a shortened humerus. This is ideal for a transhumeral prosthesis with replacement of the elbow joint and hand. If a transhumeral or a more proximal amputation was performed, at skeletal maturity, the humerus would likely be too short for a prosthesis because of the absence of distal physeal growth. An elbow prosthesis would be more functional than a long humerus without an elbow joint. Similarly, a free fibula flap would not restore the elbow joint.

4. **Answer: d.** A myodesis reestablishes an insertion for the amputated muscles. This permits the muscles to contract and to transmit a signal to a prosthesis. It provides soft tissue coverage over the distal bone. An elective amputation should be carefully planned with the patient and a multidisciplinary team, to determine the ideal amputation level for function, the best incision placement for comfortable prosthetic wear, and to permit

durable, tension-free soft tissue coverage over the residual limb. Secondary or tertiary healing is inappropriate. There is no zone of injury requiring time for demarcation in this case. Proximal retraction of the forearm musculature will cause the muscles to shorten and become fibrotic. Without an insertion, they will be nonfunctional. Flap closure is unnecessary in an elective transradial amputation. The local, sensate distal tissues are best used for closure. Flaps have a role in traumatic injuries with a loss of soft tissue and the need to preserve bone length.

5. **Answer: e.** Symptomatic neuromas are common following amputations. A multimodal treatment approach is best. Nonoperative management is typically recommended first, including desensitization therapy, neuropathic pain medications, prosthetic socket modifications, and occasionally psychiatric evaluation. If the neuroma is well localized and does not respond to nonoperative measures, surgery can be pursued.

CHAPTER 92 Rheumatoid Arthritis and Inflammatory Arthropathies

Brian P. Kelley and Kevin C. Chung

KEY POINTS

- Rheumatoid arthritis is a systemic disease affecting the synovium that may lead to multiple derangements of the hands and wrists.
- Inflammatory arthropathies are a spectrum of autoimmune diseases that require immunomodulatory medical treatment.
- For rheumatoid hand and wrist deformities, care should be taken to optimize the patient medically and to manage more proximal disease before correction of distal derangements to prevent disease flares and early recurrence.
- Synovectomy, joint balancing procedures, and joint stabilizing procedures are the mainstays of surgical treatment for rheumatoid arthritis.
- Radiographic changes of the hand, including erosions and decalcification.

RHEUMATOID ARTHRITIS

Rheumatologic and inflammatory arthroses are a broad spectrum of chronic, systemic diseases that often involve the joints of the upper extremity and the hand. The most prevalent of the rheumatologic conditions is rheumatoid arthritis (RA), but other diseases can result in an inflammatory arthritis of the hand or other issues that generate consultations for plastic surgeons. RA affects about 1% of adults based on population-level studies.[1-10] Importantly, the clinical presentation and severity can vary greatly among patients and populations, but upper extremity complaints are a hallmark of the disease. Over the past 30 years, the medical management of RA has improved dramatically and, therefore, small joint disease has also diminished in prevalence over those years. This is true of other diagnoses within the spectrum of inflammatory joint disease, including RA, psoriatic arthritis, juvenile idiopathic arthritis (JIA, formerly juvenile RA), or systemic lupus erythematosus (SLE). Despite a decrease in prevalence, upper extremity inflammatory joint disease can be debilitating and can drastically reduce the quality of life for patients due to recalcitrant pain and functional losses. Thus, hand surgeons and plastic surgeons should be aware of surgical management options because these remain an important adjunct to systemic therapy for these patients. Furthermore, in addition to a basic knowledge of typical RA, an understanding of other inflammatory arthropathies will help the surgeon to guide the patient through treatment.

Historic Background

Reconstructive surgery and hand surgery for patients with inflammatory arthritis have been established as a key component in the overall care of rheumatoid arthritis, specifically for improvement in physical deformity, ongoing functional loss, and pain. However, reconstructive procedures are not curative and should not be viewed as such. Instead, reconstructive hand surgery may serve a prophylactic, functional, or symptom-reducing role in managing the rheumatoid disease process. Before the 1950s, few surgeons advocated surgery due to the risk of wound-healing complications, and physicians feared that surgical intervention could reactivate the disease process.[11] However, the field became more prominent in the 1950s to 1960s. This coincided with surgical innovations in small joint surgery, improvements in systemic management, and a better understanding of the disease process. Over the next decade, surgeons began advocating prophylactic debulking of synovial nodules, small joint replacements, and tendon reconstruction. Early options for small joint arthroplasty were described as early as 1961 by Adrian E. Flatt.[12] The doctrines for management of RA-affected soft tissues, tendons, and joints have not changed significantly since then. In a review of the current principles of rheumatoid surgery in 1962, Dr. Flatt noted key factors in successfully navigating patients through rheumatoid surgery.

1. *Treat the Systemic Disease:* "No doubt drugs rather than the scalpel will ultimately conquer rheumatoid disease… Although rheumatoid arthritis of the hands cannot be cured by surgery, it seems wrong to stand aside and let crippling deformities develop."
2. *Prevent Progression of the Deformity:* "Treatment of rheumatoid hand should be prophylactic. Splinting, drug therapy, and physiotherapy have their place in the care of patients."
3. *Establish the Foundation Proximally:* "… to correct a deformity within the hand is profitless if the (wrist) elbow and shoulder are so badly afflicted that the hand cannot be moved …"
4. *Do Not Overcomplicate Simple Interventions:* "Simple mechanical problems such as tendon rupture, stenosing tenovaginitis, and trigger tendon can be solved by basic principles."

In addition to improvements in rheumatoid hand surgery, an awareness of historical advancements in systemic treatment is also necessary. Epidemiologically, the number of patients with RA seeking care for rheumatoid hand disease has slowly declined with the increase of disease-modifying antirheumatic drugs (DMARDs). The term *disease-modifying* drug has been used to describe both synthetic and biologic medications used to reduce the disease burden as adjuncts to glucocorticoid therapy.[13] Synthetic options, such as gold (1930s), hydroxychloroquine (1950s), azathioprine (1960s), methotrexate, or sulfasalazine (1980s), have been present for a long period. The newer of which still have roles in multimodal disease treatment. With the advent of biologic DMARDs in the 1990s, the prevalence of hand and wrist deformity began to fall more dramatically resulting in fewer patients with deforming hand disease.[14,15]

Epidemiology and Disease Impact

In the past decade, studies have shown a prevalence of rheumatoid arthritis of approximately 1%, ranging from 0.33% to 6.8%.[16] The overall trend, however, is a decreasing prevalence of RA since the 1960s.[17,18] In the United States, there is a growing population of elderly patients with RA compared with decreasing prevalence in younger age groups compared with the prevalence in prior decades.[18] A small percentage of patients with systematic disease advance to symptomatic hand deformity, and hand disease progression is often used as a marker of disease severity. In studies of Medicare beneficiaries with a diagnosis of RA between 2006 and 2010, hand and wrist joint procedures were performed at an annual rate of approximately 23.1 per 10,000 patients and tendon reconstruction occurred at a rate of 4.2 per 10,000 patients.[19] Therefore, surgical interventions for hand reconstruction, even in patients with a diagnosis of RA, remain infrequent. This result is likely a combination of variations in disease prevalence and availability of subspecialty care in different regions.[20,21] However, the true impact of RA includes loss of work production, loss of capital, higher healthcare costs, decreased quality of life, and opportunity costs. RA, like osteoarthritis, is associated with higher rates of depression than the general population. Pooled data from meta-analysis suggest depression in 16.8% of patients with RA.[22]

RA usually manifests in the third to sixth decade of life, but disease severity is commonly linked to the age of onset.[23] Earlier age of onset has also been associated with higher economic burden for both patients and health systems. There have been links to suggest high prevalence of RA in northern latitudes, but, interestingly, younger age of onset is associated with females and latitudes at the Tropic of Cancer.[24] The relationship to the tropics may represent geographic, environmental, or socioeconomic factors, and the causal relationship is unclear. Finally, certain ethnic groups such as the Pima Indians have demonstrated higher prevalence compared with the general population.[1]

There is a genetic component to RA, but a single, explicit hereditary etiology has not been found. A family history of RA increases the lifetime risk from three-fold to five-fold.[25] Furthermore, twin concordance rates also suggest genetic factors in inheritance.[26] Prior studies have estimated the genetic contribution to rheumatoid disease to be between 40% and 65% for rheumatoid factor (RF) seropositive disease, but less than 20% for RF seronegative disease.[illegible] This uncertainty is complicated by evidence from genome-wide analysis identifying more than a hundred gene loci associated with rheumatoid arthritis risk, many with overlapping loci for other inflammatory conditions.[27]

Diagnosis, Pathophysiology, and Medical Treatment

When untreated, RA may induce multiple pathologic abnormalities in the upper extremity. Other arthropathies are discussed in this chapter in brief, but rheumatoid arthritis will be covered in more detail because it is the most common presentation of inflammatory hand arthropathy. Appropriate diagnosis of joint pain can be difficult when patients present with symptoms but no prior medical workup. Surgeons should be prepared to recognize inflammatory conditions and make appropriate diagnoses in these cases. In patients with unexplained upper extremity joint pain and no clear history of trauma, laboratory evaluation and appropriate specialty referrals are critical to improving the patient's overall condition. In general, symmetric hand pain lasting 6 weeks or longer without a known etiology should prompt consideration of inflammatory arthropathy in the differential diagnosis.[28] **Table 92.1** lists common laboratory studies in the diagnosis of rheumatoid arthritis and other inflammatory arthropathies. Diagnosis requires consistent history and physical exam, a history of polyarthropathy for 6 weeks or more, laboratory analysis, and the exclusion of other causes of arthropathies.[29] **Table 92.2** provides diagnostic criteria used to confirm RA.

As a systemic disease, RA is classically associated with chronic polyarthritis; however, extra-articular manifestations should not be overlooked. These include, but are not limited to, vasculitis, pericarditis, pleural effusion, interstitial pulmonary disease, neuropathy, keratoconjunctivitis sicca, and osteopenia. Rheumatoid nodules are a common cause for referral to plastic surgeons but are present only in a minority of RA patients. Nodules are commonly located on extensor pads associated with synovitis but can appear in multiple extra-articular tissues including eyes, lungs, or vocal cords.

Medical management of RA is the cornerstone to both long-term disease control and surgical risk reduction. **Table 92.3** outlines common medications used in the management of inflammatory arthropathies, mechanism of action, and perioperative considerations. Medications used in the treatment of RA and other inflammatory arthropathies are not without risks. For instance, corticosteroids and DMARDs are typically used to halt synovitis and slow disease progression. However, these drugs target the patient's immune system and reduce their ability to respond to antigens and pathogens. Thus, these may predispose the patient to infections, malignancy, or

TABLE 92.1. COMMON LABORATORY TESTING FOR INFLAMMATORY ARTHROPATHIES

Test Name	Diagnosis[b]	Implications	Other Conditions[a]
RF	RA	Nonspecific, must correlate clinical history	MCTD (50%–60%), cryoglobulinemia (40%–100%), Sjogren's (75%–95%), SLE (20%–30%), healthy subjects (5%–10%)
		High titers (>50 IU/mL) 91%–96% specific, but low sensitivity (45%–54%). May suggest late disease severity	
ESR	Nonspecific	Acute phase reactant, inflammatory marker	Many
CRP	Nonspecific	Acute phase reactant, inflammatory marker	Many
ANA	SLE	High sensitivity (93%), but nonspecific	RA (41%), scleroderma (85%), polymyositis (61%), MCTD (100%), healthy subjects (up to 5% even with high titers)
		High ANA titer (>1:160) and positive RF, likely to develop RA over SLE	
		High ANA titer and negative RF, inconclusive	
		Low ANA titer (<1:80), low probability of SLE, but may develop other disease	
Anti-dsDNA	SLE	25%–85% sensitive, 99% specific	Drug-induced or infection-induced anti-dsDNA can occur in RA, but is not related to the disease
Anti-SSA/Ro	Sjogren's syndrome	Seropositive in 30% of SLE with skin involvement	SLE
Anti-SSB/La	Sjogren's syndrome		
Anti-CCP1	RA	44%–56% sensitive, 90%–97% specific	Used in combination are becoming standard for early RA diagnosis
Anti-CCP2	RA	64%–89% sensitive, 88%–99% specific	
Anti-Smith	SLE	26% sensitive, 99% specific	Confirmatory test for SLE
Anti-MCV	RA	62% sensitive, 92.9% specific	Psoriatic arthritis, spondyloarthropathy
Scl-70	Scleroderma	20%–43% sensitive, 90%–99.6% specific	Confirmatory test for scleroderma

[a]Denotes other conditions in which this test may be positive.
[b]Denotes most common diagnosis the test is ordered for or classically thought to imply.
RF, rheumatoid factor; ESR, erythrocyte sedimentation rate; CRP, C reactive protein; ANA, antinuclear antibody; anti-dsDNA, double-stranded DNA; anti-SSA/Ro, anti-Sjogren's syndrome antigen A; anti-SSB/La, anti-Sjogren's syndrome antigen B; anti-CCP, cyclic citrullinated peptides anti-MCV, anti-modified citrullinated vimentin; Scl-70, anti-topoisomerase 1; RA, rheumatoid arthritis; SLE, systemic lupus erythematosus; MCTD, mixed connective tissue disease.

TABLE 92.2. AMERICAN COLLEGE OF RHEUMATOLOGY/EULAR COLLABORATIVE DIAGNOSTIC CRITERIA FOR RHEUMATOID ARTHRITIS

Criterion/Symptom	Score[b] (0–10)
A. Joint involvement[a]	0–5
1 large joint	0
2–10 large joints	1
1–3 small joints	2
4–10 small joints	3
>10 joints (at least 1 small)	5
B. Serology (at least 1 necessary)	0–3
Negative RF *and* negative anti-CCP	0
Low-positive RF *or* low-positive anti-CCP	2
High-positive RF *or* high-positive anti-CCP	3
C. Acute-phase reactants (at least 1 necessary)	0–1
Normal CRP *and* normal ESR	0
Abnormal CRP *or* abnormal ESR	1
D. Duration of symptoms	0–1
<6 weeks	0
>6 weeks	1

[a]Large joints are shoulder, elbow, hips, knees, and ankles; Small joints are MCP, PIP, metatarsophalangeal, and wrist joints.
[b]Score ≥6 indicates definite RA. Score <6 may develop RA later, but cannot be diagnosed.

wound healing issues. Other medications, including over-the-counter antiinflammatory drugs or pain medications may be frequently used in the treatment of disease-associated pain. Nonsteroidal antiinflammatory drugs (NSAIDs) may predispose patients to gastrointestinal and renal adverse events. Narcotics are discouraged for chronic use given their risks for addiction/dependence, tachyphylaxis, and overdose.

Anatomy, Disease Progression, and Surgical Options

In the setting of poor systemic control, rheumatoid arthritis often progresses in a predictable pattern. Synovitis presents around multiple joints leading to bony erosions, joint instability, and tendon attrition. Synovium is the pathologic tissue affected in RA. In affected synovium, a pannus of proliferating synovitis expands. This can cause both a compressive and enzymatic joint injury. Ongoing growth and inflammation propagate the subsequent joint and soft-tissue destruction. Proteolytic enzymes released within the joint can directly damage bone, cartilage, and synovium. Any synovial joint may be affected, but hand involvement is often seen as a hallmark of disease development. The metacarpophalangeal (MCP) joint, proximal interphalangeal (PIP) joint, and wrist are often affected first, presumably due to the relatively high synovial surface area. Secondarily, large joints such as the elbows, knees, hips, shoulders are affected. Even small articular surfaces, such as the ossicles of the middle ear, can be involved.

Plastic surgeons are seldom called on to manage the orthopedic pathology of the large joints in RA but may be consulted if the soft tissues are tenuous. In these cases, wound-healing issues may prompt a need for flap coverage in elbow or knee operations. In other cases, patients may present with synovitic rheumatoid nodules around large joints. Rheumatoid nodules may be unsightly, painful, irritating to adjacent tendons, or cause nerve compression. In most cases, rheumatoid nodules can be simply excised alone or as part of a procedure to correct comorbid issues (Figure 92.1). For example, a cubital tunnel decompression may be necessary if the ulnar nerve is impinged at the elbow and may include removal of synovitis and osteophytes. Synovectomy should be combined with other joint and tendon repairs to prevent recurrence of the deformity due to continued attrition.

In contrast to large joint afflictions, most deformities associated with rheumatoid arthritis involve the hands and wrist. There are many pathologic abnormalities that can develop at each of the joints of the hands, but the distal interphalangeal joint (DIP) joint is often spared in RA (Figure 92.2). Bony erosions are first noted on radiographs at joint edges and vascular channels for nutrient vessels because of synovitis' direct access to the bone. On radiographs, early wrist erosions appear at the scaphoid waist, ulnar styloid, and the distal radioulnar joint (DRUJ). In RA, synovitis typically affects the radiocarpal joint more than the midcarpal joint. Eventually, as the severity worsens, the wrist demonstrates radiocarpal collapse, volar translation, and angulation of the lunate with compensatory midcarpal extension (Figure 92.3). End-stage arthritis of the wrist generally falls into one of three categories: ankylosis, arthritic stable, or arthritic unstable (which can be due to osteolysis or ligamentous attenuation). Ankylosis, or autofusion of the radiocarpal joint is often in acceptable alignment and intervention can be minimized. For arthritic stable or unstable joints, fusion or salvage procedures are often necessary to improve wrist stability and preserve function (Figure 92.4).

Synovitis around the wrist joint often involves the extensor compartments and may grow around the tendons within the extensor retinaculum. This can lead to attritional ruptures. This process is compounded by dorsal prominence of caput ulnae leading to progressive tendon ruptures from ulnar to radial along the dorsal wrist. This process is known as Vaughan-Jackson syndrome (Figure 92.5). Tendon ruptures are often sudden and are usually painless, though synovitis may be painful at the site before the rupture. Osteophytes on the radius or carpus can also lead to tendon attrition. For example, scaphoid osteophytes or synovitis can lead to attrition of the flexor pollicis longus (FPL) tendon, also known as a Mannerfelt lesion. Synovitis in this area may also contribute to carpal tunnel syndrome or triggering digits. Tendon reconstruction is most often

TABLE 92.3. MEDICAL TREATMENT OF INFLAMMATORY ARTHROPATHIES

Medication	Mechanism of Action	Perioperative Management
Corticosteroids	Steroid hormone	Continue at normal dosing
	Alters gene activation	Consider stress-dose corticosteroid at time of surgery
Methotrexate	Inhibition of dihydrofolate reductase (DHFR)	Continue at normal dosing
Synthetic DMARDs	Various	Discuss with rheumatologist, many are seldom used
Biologic DMARDs	Tumor necrosis factor alpha (TNF-α) inhibitor	Discuss with rheumatologist, in general consider holding 2–4 weeks
Etanercept, adalimumab, infliximab Anakinra	Interleukin-1 (IL-1) inhibitor	

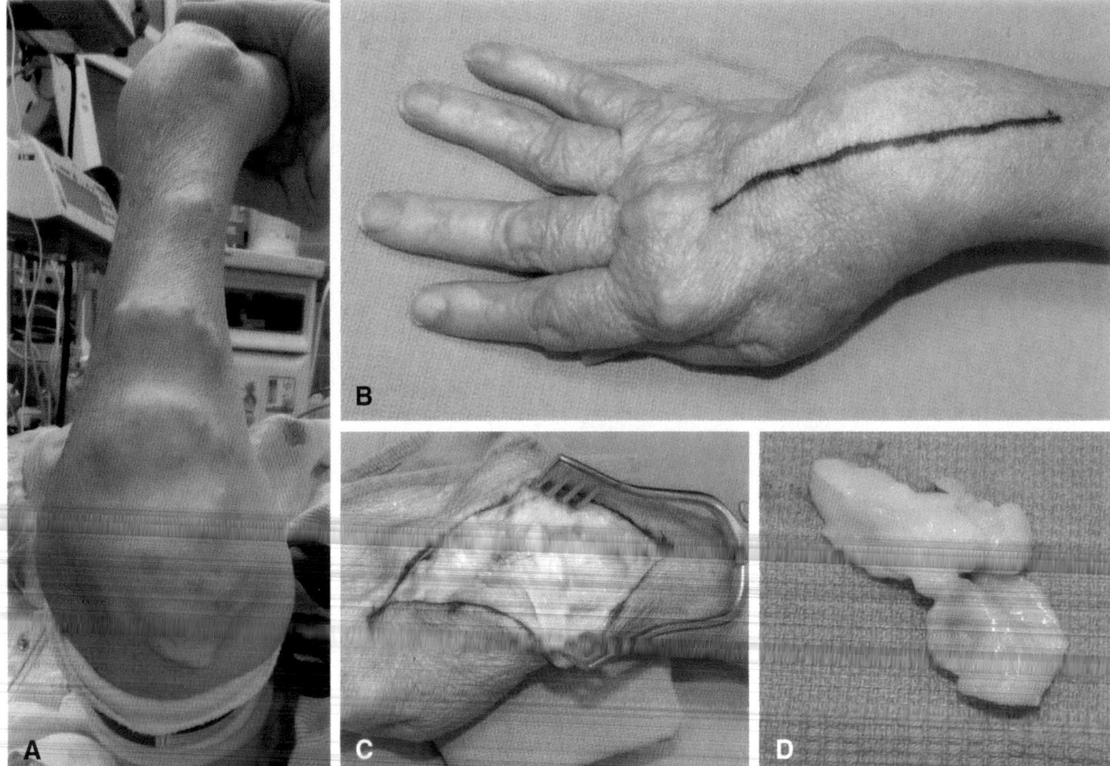

FIGURE 92.1. **A.** Rheumatoid nodules often affect the extensor surfaces or the elbow. **B–D.** Synovitis of the wrist and digits can often be surgical excised at the time of other procedures.

achieved through tendon transfers. In general, once a musculotendinous unit has ruptured, that muscle is no longer useful in the setting of RA. Therefore, tendon transfers offer reconstruction of the motor unit at the cost of some strength to the donor site. The principles behind tendon transfers are covered in more depth elsewhere, but the key points are to borrow tendons with redundancy and to progress along an algorithm with care to preserve options for future transfers (**Table 92.4**).

Deformity of the digits is common with involvement of the MCP and PIP joints and relative sparing of the DIP joints. At the MCP joint, patients often complain about the inability to fully extend their fingers. This can be secondary to ulnar subluxation of the extensor tendon due to attenuation of the radial sagittal band or due to progressive subluxation and volar translation of the proximal phalanx on the metacarpal head. A combination of ulnar forces during key pinch and radial deviation at the wrist often contribute to the ulnar vector on the tendons and digits. Very rarely, loss of extension can be due to compression on the posterior interosseous nerve that innervates all the extensor tendons. Ulnar subluxation of the tendon between the metacarpal heads causes a relative loss of mechanical advantage thus making full extension difficult. To rule out tendon ruptures, the digits can be passively reduced. If the patient can maintain the finger in extension once passively corrected, then the tendon must be intact. Before treating the acquired deformity, surgery to correct the wrist

FIGURE 92.2. In RA, there is progressive collapse of the upper extremity with joint deviation secondary to attenuation of supporting ligaments. Radial deviation and dorsal translocation of the ulna contribute to ulnar deviation at the MCP joints due to attenuation of the radial sagittal band. Attenuation of the volar plate and digital extensor apparatus may lead to boutonniere or swan-neck deformity. Rheumatoid nodules from synovitis may attenuate the radial sagittal band leading to ulnar deviation of the MCP joint and ulnar subluxation of the extensor tendons.

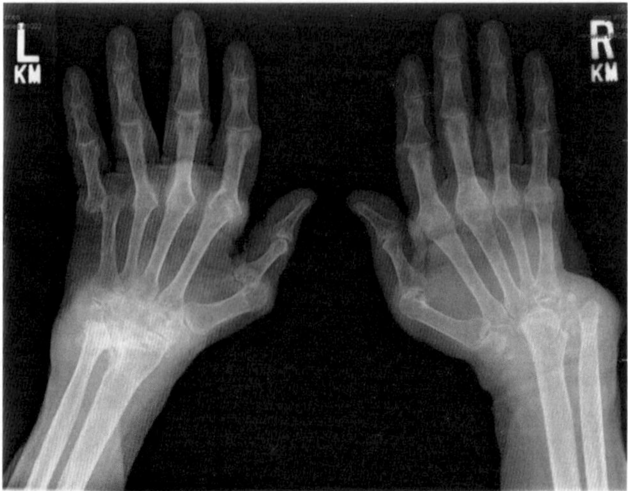

FIGURE 92.3. Wrist and hand plain PA radiographs demonstrating severe hand and wrist deformities associated with chronic, poorly controlled RA.

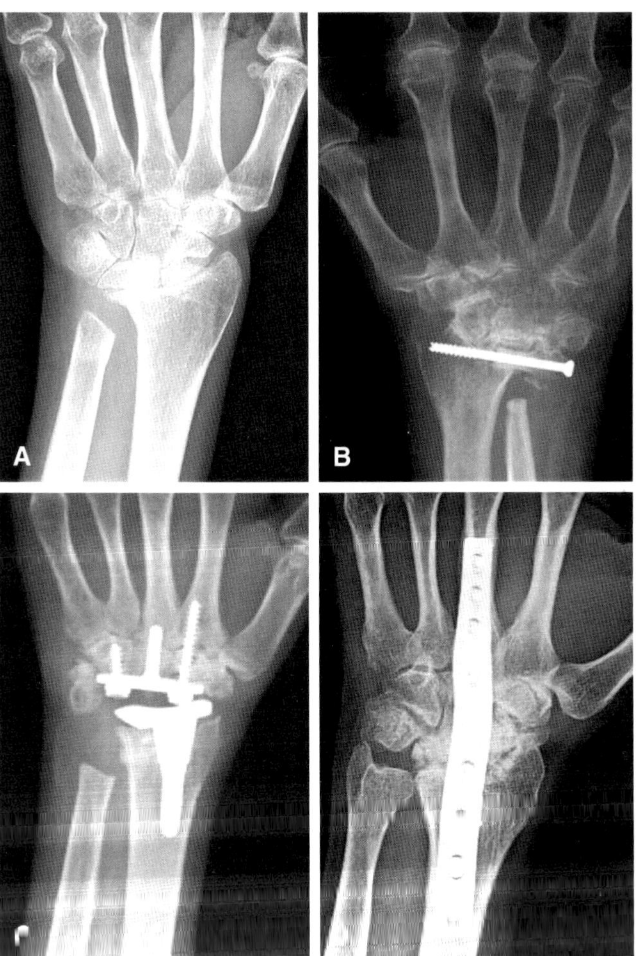

FIGURE 92.4. Radiographs for selected wrist salvage procedures for DRUJ and radiocarpal arthritis. **A.** Darrach procedure (ulnar head resection). **B.** Sauvé-Kapandji procedure (distal radio-ulnar fusion). **C.** Total wrist arthroplasty. **D.** Total wrist arthrodesis.

and extensor retinaculum synovitis should be performed to prevent early recurrence of the MCP deformities. Once the proximal issues are stabilized, surgery to correct MCP joint deformities depends on the state of the articular surface. Passively correctable ulnar translation of the joint or tendons can be corrected with soft-tissue surgeries such as extensor tendon centralization (typically a synovectomy and radial sagittal band imbrication) or a cross-intrinsic tendon transfer to apply more dynamic radial force. However, if the digit is shortened, irreducible, or the articular erosions are severe (Figure 92.6), first-line management is often joint replacements with silicone metacarpophalangeal arthroplasty (SMPA; Figure 92.7). In contrast, the PIP joint, wrist, and elbow are treated with joint replacement in only select cases.

The two most common intrinsic digital imbalances are the swan-neck and boutonniere deformities. Both deformities can occur in the same hand in different digits (Figure 92.8), but swan-neck is more common than boutonniere. A swan-neck deformity is characterized by flexion of the DIP joint, hyperextension of the PIP joint, and flexion of the MCP joint (Figure 92.9). In swan-neck, the anatomic derangement can occur at any of the three joints of the finger (MCP, PIP, or DIP joints), and **Table 92.5** lists possible etiologies for swan-neck deformity at each joint. Treatment depends on the severity of the deformity and whether the PIP joints are actively and passively reducible. Treatment options include figure-of-eight ring splints and therapy (actively reducible joints, mild deformity), soft-tissue reconstruction (passively reducible joints, minimal arthritic changes), and arthrodesis (PIP joint changes, irreducible joint).

In contrast to swan-neck, the boutonniere deformity is caused by pathology intrinsic to the PIP joint. In boutonniere, the most common cause of deformity is attenuation and rupture of the central slip of the extensor tendon leading to retraction of the proximal extensor apparatus and flexion of the PIP joint. Over time, the proximal and volar vector of force translates the collateral bands volar to the axis of the PIP joint. This [illegible] results in [illegible] tightening of the retinacular ligaments and hyperextension of the DIP joint.

Surgical correction of the boutonniere deformity also depends on the motion at the PIP joint and the suitability of the patient for reconstruction. In general, this is accomplished by a combination of central slip reconstruction and dorsal transposition of the lateral band/transverse retinacular ligament (passively reducible defect, minimal

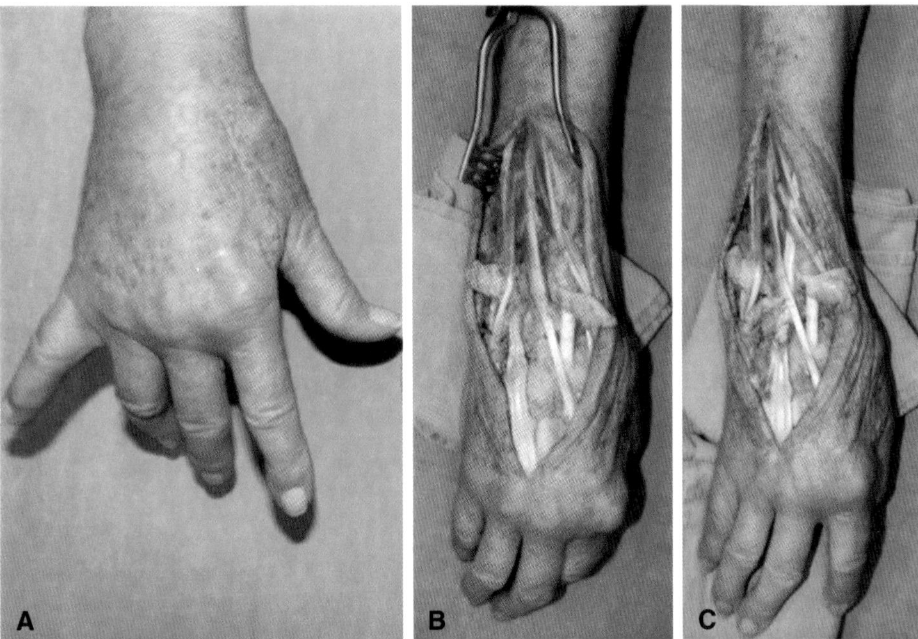

FIGURE 92.5. **A.** Vaughn-Jackson syndrome with progressive ulnar-to-radial rupture of extensor tendons. **B.** In this case, EIP and EDC to small, ring, and middle were ruptured. **C.** EDC to index was preserved, and ECRL was transferred to reconstruction small, ring, and middle extension.

TABLE 92.4. TENDON TRANSFERS FOR ATTRITIONAL RUPTURE

Finger Impairment	Diagnosis	First Line Transfer	Rescue
Small extension	Rupture of EDM/EDC to small	End-to-side EDM and SF EDC to EDC of ring	
Small, ring extension	Rupture of EDM and EDC to small and ring	EIP transfer to EDC of ring and small	
Small, ring, and middle extension	Rupture of EDM and EDC to small, ring, and middle	EIP transfer to EDM, EDC of ring and small End-to-side of EDC to middle to EDC index	
Small, ring, middle, and index extension	Rupture of EDM, EIP, and EDC to all digits	FDS middle to EDC index and middle FDS ring to EDM, EDC of ring and small	
Thumb extension	EPL rupture	EIP to EPL	ECRL to EPL EDM to EPL
Thumb, small, ring, middle, & index extension	EPL rupture	FDS middle to EPL & EDC index and middle	
	Rupture of EDM, EIP, and EDC to all digits	FDS ring to EDM, EDC of ring and small	
Thumb flexion	FPL rupture	BR to FPL	ECLR to FPL FDS long to FPL Thumb IP joint fusion
Independent PIP joint flexion	FDS rupture	PIP joint synovectomy to protect FDP No transfer	
DIP joint flexion	FDP rupture	DIP joint arthrodesis	Tenodesis of DIP joint
Loss of PIP and DIP joint flexion	FDP and FDS rupture	Staged flexor tendon reconstruction	

EDM, extensor digiti minimi; EDC, extensor digitorum communis; EIP, extensor indicis proprius; EPL, extensor pollicis longus; FDS, flexor digitorum superficialis; FDP, flexor digitorum profundus; BR, brachioradialis; ECRL, extensor carpi radialis longus; PIP, proximal interphalangeal joint; DIP, distal interphalangeal joint.

arthritic changes), or extensor tenotomy and volar plate release (intrinsic stiffness of PIP joint, minimal arthritic changes). Finally, arthrodesis can be considered for cases with more severe arthritic changes at the PIP joint.

Thumb deformities in RA are somewhat different than the phalanges. Derangements can be grouped into five general categories:

Type I: Boutonniere deformity (most common)
Type II: Boutonniere deformity with carpometacarpal (CMC) joint dislocation or subluxation
Type III: Swan-neck deformity with metacarpal adduction
Type IV: Gamekeeper's deformity (attenuation of MCP ulna collateral ligament)
Type V: Swan-neck deformity without metacarpal adduction deformity

Management for thumb anomalies is largely dependent on stabilization of the metacarpophalangeal (MP) joint and tendon reconstructions. Often, arthrodesis of the MCP joint is the best solution to establish stability of the MCP joint. CMC arthroplasty can be considered if the CMC joint is painful, but a focus should be placed on maintaining palmar abduction for grip using the first webspace.[30-34]

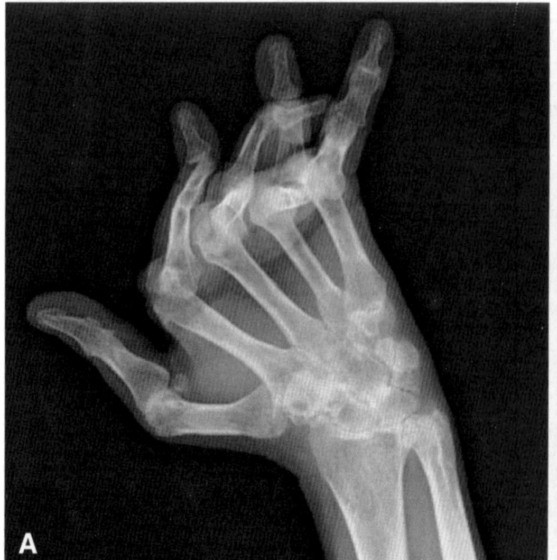

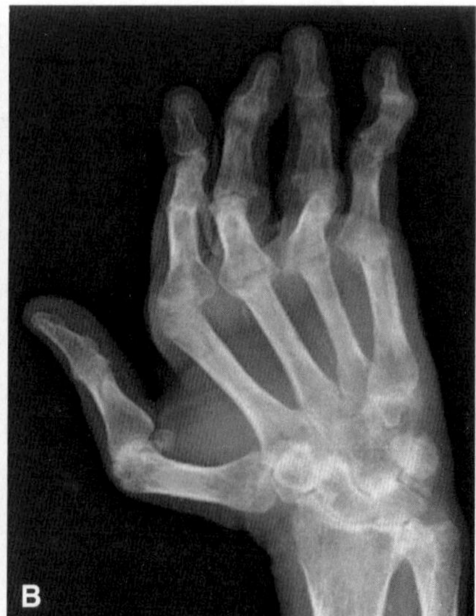

FIGURE 92.6. **A.** Patient radiographs with irreducible ulnar-volar subluxation of the MCP joint of multiple digits. **B.** After silicone implant arthroplasty, improvement is seen, with alignment of the MCP joint.

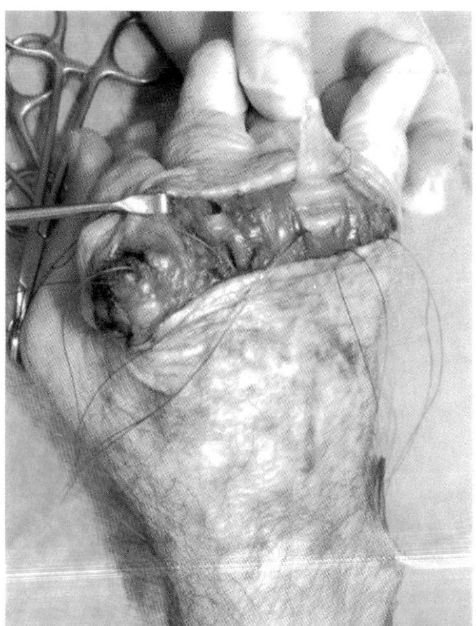

FIGURE 92.7. Silicone implant arthroplasty of the MCP joints demonstrating implant appearance and placement.

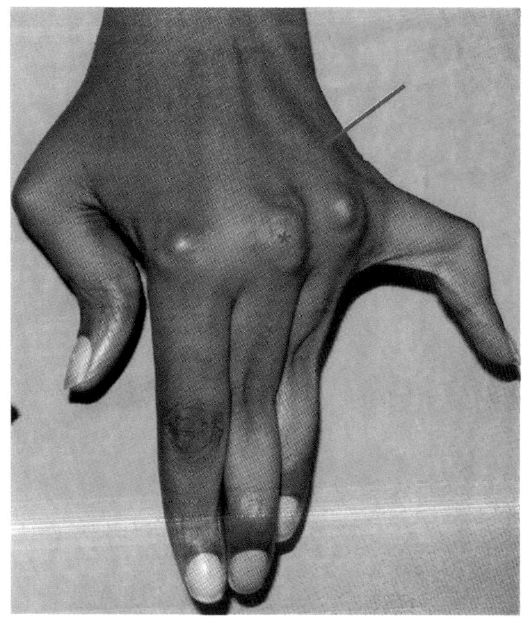

FIGURE 92.8. Patient with mixed finger deformities. There is swan-neck deformity of the middle and ring fingers. There is z-deformity of the thumb and a boutonniere of the index and small fingers. MCP joint synovitis (*) and ulnar subluxation of the extensor tendons (*arrow*) are also shown.

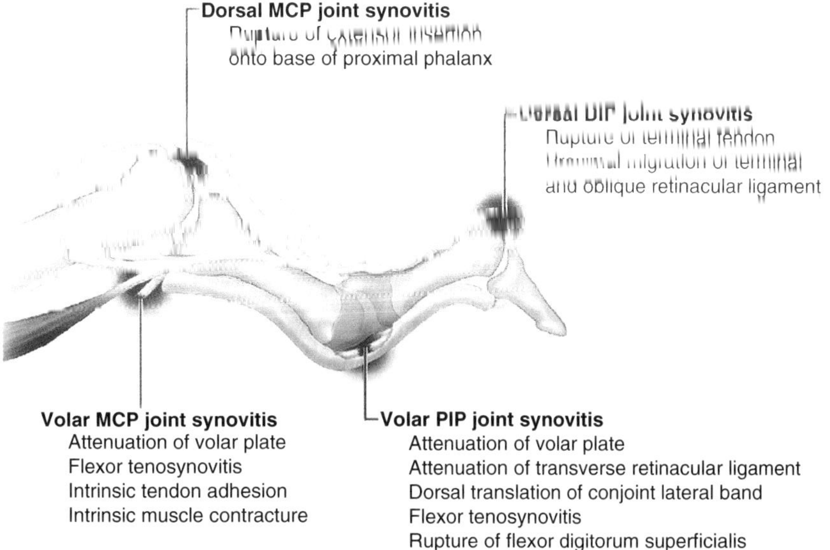

FIGURE 92.9. Swan-neck deformity is a disturbance of joint balancing that may result from changes at any of the joints of the finger. The finger is balanced by a combination of the intrinsic and extrinsic flexors and extensors. Specifically, the extensor apparatus acts to coordinate fine distal motion. With RA, the balancing forces are perturbed and a deformity can occur. At the MCP joint, flexion can result from tightness or flexion contracture on the volar surface or an extensor rupture at the level of the proximal phalanx. At the PIP joint, attenuation of the volar plate or rupture of the FDS tendon can result in hyperextension. At the DIP joint, classically a terminal tendon attenuation or traumatic mallet finger result in flexion. Any one of these, over time, can influence the joints around it resulting in the swan-neck appearance. (From Kelley BP, Chung KC. Correction of swan-neck deformity. In: Chung KC, ed. *Operative Techniques in Hand and Wrist Surgery*. 3rd ed. Philadelphia, PA: Elsevier; 2018:350.)

TABLE 92.5. CAUSES OF SWAN-NECK DEFORMITY BY JOINT LOCATION

MCP Joint	PIP Joint	DIP Joint
Dorsal Attenuation of extensor hood attachments at P1 base	Skin tightness Joint destruction	Rupture of terminal tendon Attenuation of the oblique retinacular or triangular ligaments
Volar Attenuation of volar plate Flexor tenosynovitis Tendon adhesions Intrinsic muscle contracture Skin tightness	Attenuation of volar plate Attenuation of transverse retinacular ligament Dorsal translation of conjoint lateral band Rupture of flexor digitorum superficialis	

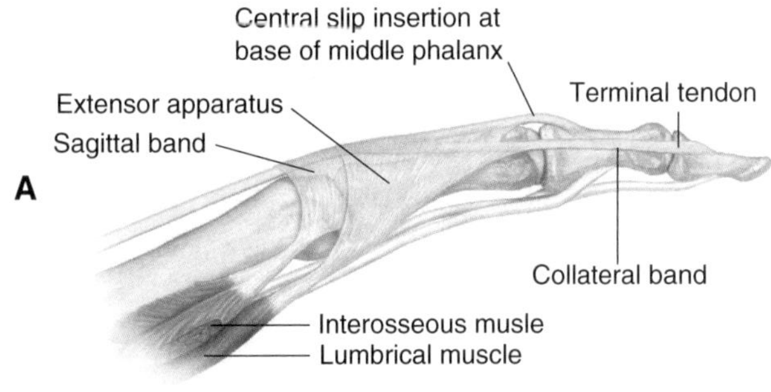

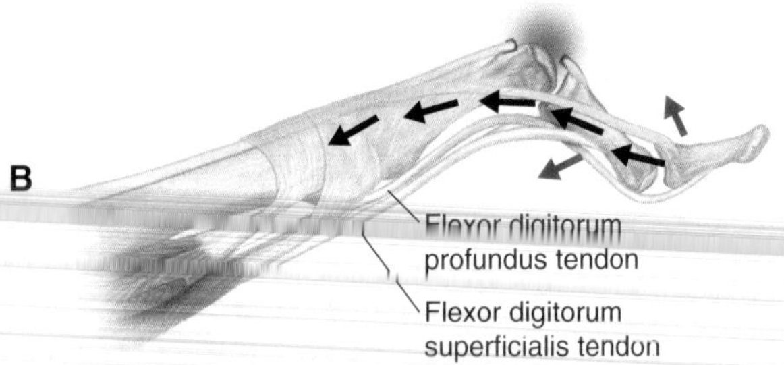

FIGURE 92.10. In contrast to swan-neck deformity, boutonniere deformity results from attenuation or rupture of the central slip of the extensor tendon at the PIP joint. This causes flexion of the PIP joint. Retraction of the central slip and proximal extensor apparatus tightens the collateral ligament and moves the axis of the joint volar. This tightening leads to DIP joint hyperextension.

NONRHEUMATOID INFLAMMATORY ARTHROPATHIES

Nonrheumatoid inflammatory arthropathies have a spectrum of diverse clinical findings, but often have similar effects on function and appearance. It is important to keep the underlying systemic disease in mind when developing a treatment plan, as subtle differences in pathophysiology may change surgical options. For example, patients with SLE-related arthritis may present with similar findings as RA, such as ulnar subluxation of the extensor tendons. However, SLE deformity is more likely to be the result of soft-tissue attenuation and laxity with sparing of the MCP joints. Most patients complain of pain with activities, but also note limited motion, dissatisfaction with appearance, and pain at rest.[35-37]

Epidemiology of Inflammatory Arthropathies

There are some epidemiologic differences in RA compared to other inflammatory arthropathies. For example, JIA has an incidence of around between 2 and 20 cases per 100,000 people per year, and a prevalence of around 16 to 150 cases per 100,000 in the general population.[38] The overall prevalence may have decreased over recent decades from the 1980s to 1990s.[39,40] JIA also appears to occur less frequently in African American and Asian populations compared to Caucasians.[17,41] JIA is a diagnosis made before the age of 16 years and may have environmental and genetic contributions unique from typical RA. Diagnosis of JIA includes a spectrum of similar conditions, including arthritis types: RF positive, RF negative, polyarticular, systemic, psoriatic, and others.[38]

SLE-related arthritis has an overall disease prevalence of between 40 and 103 per 100,000 with an estimated 9- to 10-fold higher rate in women.[17] In an Egyptian population, arthritis was present in about 77.8% of patients with SLE, whereas Raynaud phenomenon was present in 14.7%.[42] Retrospective studies estimate a rate of depression of approximately 13% in patients with SLE.[43] This compares to an estimated 6.7% prevalence of depression in the general population of the United States. This speaks to the propensity of patients with inflammatory arthroses to experience higher rates of depression-related disability.

Psoriatic arthritis, which is sometimes grouped with spondyloarthropathies, may affect about 101 per 100,000.[17] Approximately 5% of psoriatics may have a variation of inflammatory arthropathy, which can present before cutaneous manifestations 15% to 20% of the time. Psoriatic hand deformity can include nail deformities in about 80% of patients, but these are less frequent (15%) in patients with psoriatic arthritis variants.

Clinical Characteristics of Specific Conditions

Juvenile Idiopathic Arthritis (JIA; Juvenile RA)

Different from typical adult RA, JIA is not a single disease. JIA is a heterogenous group of related diseases with onset before the age of 16 years with a constellation of arthritic changes. Disease etiology is multifactorial, and the causal pathologic cell-type has been traced to multiple immunologic mediators, including T cells and macrophages. Classic variants, which are still poorly categorized, include polyarthritis, oligoarthritis, and systemic disease. Polyarticular disease is typically related to RF positivity and affects about 5% of JIA patients. RF-positive polyarthritis is similar to adult RF-positive RA in natural history and pathophysiology. However, JIA oligoarthritis can be subdivided into persistent oligoarthritis (affects <4 joints without increase) and extended oligoarthritis (initially affects <4 joints but increases to >4 joints after first 6 months from onset). The systemic characteristics of JIA, termed Still disease, are well characterized and include a constellation of features, such as fever, rash, and serositis. The adult variant of this is termed Adult Onset Still Disease and has a similar symptom pattern. Finally, about 35% to 40% of JIA patients will be HLA-B27 positive. Ongoing monitoring at up to 3 to 6 month intervals for functional loss and disease staging should be considered in cases of JIA,[44] but surgical interventions for should be delayed until medical management is initiated. A delay in surgical intervention may also be appropriate to allow patients to achieve skeletal maturity. However, in principle, specific anatomic pathology is managed by the same techniques as adult RA.

Psoriatic Arthritis

Psoriatic arthritis is an inflammatory arthropathy that affects around 30% of patients with psoriasis and is associated with obesity, positive family history, and HLA-B27 positivity.[45] Classic hand-related clinical features include fusiform swelling of fingers and toes, nail changes (pitting, thickening, or detachment), and psoriatic skin plaques (typically hyperkeratotic, red, scaly plaques over extensor skin). Psoriatic arthritis of the hands typically affects the DIP joint, in contrast to RA where the DIP joint is typically spared. A severe form of inflammatory arthropathy of the hands, known as arthritis mutilans (Figure 92.11), is common in psoriatic arthritis. Arthritis mutilans causes acroosteolysis of the phalanges, *pencil in cup* joint changes, and telescoping (*opera-glass hands*) of the digits. For arthritis of the DIP joint or in cases of arthritis mutilans, surgical options may be limited. In many cases, arthrodesis is the only surgical option that may maintain digit length and reduce pain.

Systemic Lupus Erythematosus

Multiple systems may be affected in SLE, but joints and skin are involved in up to 90% of patients with the disease. In fact, hand involvement is a common reason for patients to seek healthcare leading to the diagnosis.[37] Common deformities are similar to RA and include swan-neck deformity, ulnar deviation of digits, subluxation of the MCP joints, and boutonniere deformity of the thumb. In contrast to RA, erosive arthritis and loss of articular surfaces are not typical. This clinical constellation results in a classic Jaccoud arthropathy where the deformity is the result of soft-tissue laxity and ligamentous shortening rather than from direct destruction of the joints. Systemic signs of SLE include malar rash, sun sensitivity, nail deformity, kidney disease, gastrointestinal disease, nervous system complaints, and lymphadenopathy. Surgery for hand deformity in SLE is similar to RA, but there is less need for arthroplasty and arthrodesis as these

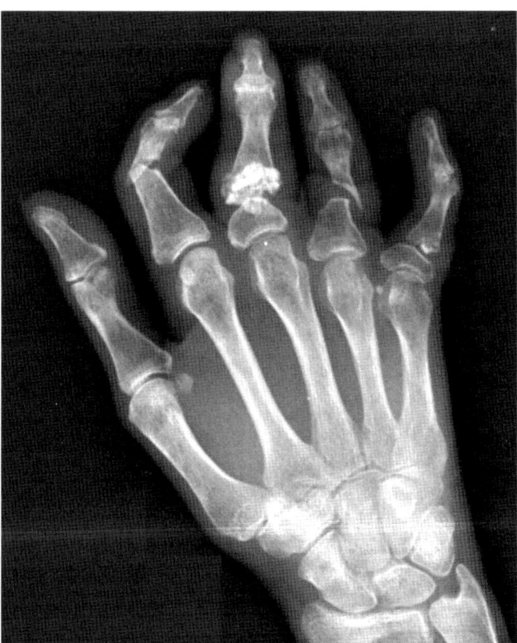

FIGURE 92.11. PA radiograph of patient with arthritis mutilans. Note acroosteolysis of PIP joints and calcinosis of the middle finger PIP joint. The telescoping of the ring finger notable on the soft-tissue silhouette is indicative of *opera glass* deformity due to the resemblance to classic opera binoculars.

patients may be spared joint destruction. Soft tissue surgery and joint balancing are the mainstay when joint degeneration is not present.

Scleroderma (Systemic Sclerosis)

Scleroderma is an autoimmune connective tissue disease affecting about 191 per 100,000 people and commonly presents with both [illegible] derma involves soft-tissue fibrosis with collagen deposition, and vaso-occlusive changes. However, multiple systems can be affected in the disease. For instance, CREST syndrome is an abbreviation for an expanded variant with calcinosis, Raynaud phenomena, esophageal dysmotility, sclerodactyly (sclerosis of digital skin causing flexion deformity), and telangiectasia. Surgical interventions for a plastic surgeon may include lipotransfer,[46] wound management, excision of calcinosis, temporomandibular joint reconstruction, and management of extremity effects of sclerosis and ischemia. Medical interventions may include DMARDs and myeloablative stem cell transfers[47]—not to be confused with the loose terminology of autologous fat graft as a stem cell source. Management of digital wounds may include botulinum toxin or sympathectomy to reduce vasospasm, amputation of nonviable digits, debridement of calcinosis, arterial bypass, or arterialization of the venous system in cases without distal targets. However, outcomes in scleroderma are often poor in the long term, and patient mortality is high with only a 70% to 80% 10-year survival rate.

Reiter Syndrome (Reactive Arthritis)

This *reactive* autoimmune arthritis is also related to patients with HLA-B27 positivity. The syndrome usually manifests 1 to 3 weeks after a known bacterial infection (common species include chlamydia, ureaplasma, salmonella, shigella, yersinia, and campylobacter). The classic triad involves urethritis, conjunctivitis/uveitis, and hand/foot arthritis. Dactylitis with fusiform swelling of a single digit (*sausage digit*) is a hallmark finding. About 10% of patients with chronic reactive arthritis may develop cardiac manifestations. Joints affected are typically monoarticular and often at the knees or sacroiliac joints. The glabrous skin on the plantar feet and palms of the hands may develop keratoderma blennorrhagicum (waxy, vesico-pustular skin lesions with a yellow-brown coloration or may appear similar to psoriatic plaques), which is pathognomonic for reactive arthritis even in the absence of the triad. Reactive arthritis may be self-limiting, but chronic changes and recurrent bouts of acute arthritis can occur in up to 15% to 30% of patients. Treatment is largely medical and can be similar to other inflammatory arthropathies.

Mixed Connective Tissue Disease

This inflammatory arthropathy is often a mixed variant of SLE and RA. Systemic pulmonary and gastrointestinal complaints are common. Compared to SLE, erosions do occur, but are often less severe than those encountered in RA. However, swan-neck deformity and ulnar subluxation can be severe when present and there is a connection with severe osteolysis leading to arthritis mutilans.

ACKNOWLEDGMENTS

The work was supported by a Midcareer Investigator Award in Patient-Oriented Research (2 K24-AR053120-06) to Kevin C. Chung. The content is solely the responsibility of the authors and does not necessarily represent the official views of the National Institutes of Health.

REFERENCES

1. Jacobsson LT, Hanson RL, Knowler WC, et al. Decreasing incidence and prevalence of rheumatoid arthritis in Pima Indians over a twenty-five-year period. *Arthritis Rheum*. 1994;37:1158-1165.
2. Boyer GS, Benevolenskaya LI, Templin DW, et al. Prevalence of rheumatoid arthritis in [illegible] populations. *J Rheumatol*. 1998;25:23-29.
3. Cimmino MA, Parisi M, Moggiana G, et al. Prevalence of rheumatoid arthritis in Italy: the Chiavari study. *Ann Rheum Dis*. 1998;57:315-318.
4. Saraux A, Guedes C, Allain J, et al. Prevalence of rheumatoid arthritis and [illegible] in Brittany, France. Société de Rhumatologie de l'Ouest. *J Rheumatol*. 1999;26:2622-2627.
5. Simonsson M, Bergman S, Jacobsson LT, [illegible] of rheumatoid arthritis in Sweden. *Scand J Rheumatol*. 1999;28:340-343.
6. Riise T, Jacobsen BK, Gran JT. Incidence and prevalence of rheumatoid arthritis in the county of [illegible]
7. [illegible] SE. The epidemiology of rheumatoid arthritis. *Rheum Dis Clin North Am*. 2001;27:269-281.
8. Symmons D, Turner G, Webb R, et al. The prevalence of rheumatoid arthritis in the United Kingdom: new estimates for a new century. *Rheumatol (Oxf)*. 2002;41:793-800.
9. Carbonell J, Cobo T, Balsa A, et al. The incidence of rheumatoid arthritis in Spain: results from a nationwide primary care registry. *Rheumatol (Oxf)*. 2008;47:1088-1092.
10. Gabriel SE, Michaud K. Epidemiological studies in incidence, prevalence, mortality, and comorbidity of the rheumatic diseases. *Arthritis Res Ther*. 2009;11:229.
11. Lam SJ. Surgery of the rheumatoid hand. *Br Med J*. 1965;1:1079-1080.
12. Flatt AE. The prosthetic replacement of rheumatoid finger joints. *Rheumatism*. 1960;16:90-97.
13. Buer JK. A history of the term "DMARD". *Inflammopharmacology*. 2015;23:163-171.
14. Shourt CA, Crowson CS, Gabriel SE, Matteson EL. Orthopedic surgery among patients with rheumatoid arthritis 1980–2007: a population-based study focused on surgery rates, sex, and mortality. *J Rheumatol*. 2012;39:481-485.
15. Gogna R, Cheung G, Arundell M, et al. Rheumatoid hand surgery: is there a decline? A 22-year population-based study. *Hand (NY)*. 2015;10:272-278.
16. Smolen JS, Aletaha D, McInnes IB. Rheumatoid arthritis. *Lancet*. 2016;388:2023-2038.
17. Helmick CG, Felson DT, Lawrence RC, et al. Estimates of the prevalence of arthritis and other rheumatic conditions in the United States. Part I. *Arthritis Rheum*. 2008;58:15-25.
18. Myasoedova E, Crowson CS, Kremers HM, et al. Is the incidence of rheumatoid arthritis rising?: results from Olmsted County, Minnesota, 1955–2007. *Arthritis Rheum*. 2010;62:1576-1582.
19. Zhong L, Chung KC, Baser O, et al. Variation in rheumatoid hand and wrist surgery among medicare beneficiaries: a population-based cohort study. *J Rheumatol*. 2015;42:429-436.
20. Alderman AK, Chung KC, Demonner S, et al. The rheumatoid hand: a predictable disease with unpredictable surgical practice patterns. *Arthritis Rheum*. 2002;47:537-542.
21. Alderman AK, Ubel PA, Kim HM, et al. Surgical management of the rheumatoid hand: consensus and controversy among rheumatologists and hand surgeons. *J Rheumatol*. 2003;30:1464-1472.
   Hand surgery is not always been well accepted in the field of rheumatology. This study clarifies the differences in opinions about the effectiveness of hand surgery and highlights the importance of working in interdisciplinary teams to treat this condition.
22. Sambamoorthi U, Shah D, Zhao X. Healthcare burden of depression in adults with arthritis. *Expert Rev Pharmacoecon Outcomes Res*. 2017;17:53-65.

23. Wolfe F, Cathey MA. The assessment and prediction of functional disability in rheumatoid arthritis. *J Rheumatol.* 1991;18:1298-1306.
24. GEO-RA Group. Latitude gradient influences the age of onset of rheumatoid arthritis: a worldwide survey. *Clin Rheumatol.* 2017;36:485-497.
25. Silman AJ, Pearson JE. Epidemiology and genetics of rheumatoid arthritis. *Arthritis Res.* 2002;4(suppl 3):S265-S272.
26. Silman AJ, MacGregor AJ, Thomson W, et al. Twin concordance rates for rheumatoid arthritis: results from a nationwide study. *Br J Rheumatol.* 1993;32:903-907.
27. Roberson ED, Bowcock AM. Psoriasis genetics: breaking the barrier. *Trends Genet.* 2010;26:415-423.
28. Farng E, Friedrich JB. Laboratory diagnosis of rheumatoid arthritis. *J Hand Surg Am.* 2011;36:926-927; quiz 928.
29. Aletaha D, Neogi T, Silman AJ, et al. 2010 Rheumatoid arthritis classification criteria: an American College of Rheumatology/European League Against Rheumatism collaborative initiative. *Arthritis Rheum.* 2010;62:2569-2581.
30. Chung KC, Kotsis SV, Burns PB, et al. Seven-year outcomes of the silicone arthroplasty in rheumatoid arthritis prospective cohort study. *Arthritis Care Res.* 2017;69:973-981.
The SARA trial involved a prospective cohort of patients with rheumatoid hand disease undergoing medical management and SMPA. This article at 7 years follow-up demonstrates low rates of implant fracture and deformity by patient reported outcomes.
31. Chung KC, Kotsis SV, Kim M, et al. Reasons why rheumatoid arthritis patients seek surgical treatment for hand deformities. *J Hand Surg.* 2006;31A:289-294.
This classic article is part of the SARA trial and prospectively enrolled patients were queried using the Michigan Hand Outcomes Questionnaire. Patients noted that impaired function and pain relief were the most common factors leading to surgery.
32. Flury MP, Herren DB, Simmen BR. Rheumatoid arthritis of the wrist: classification related to the natural course. *Clin Orthop Relat Res.* 1999;366:72-77.
The authors present a classification system for the rheumatoid wrist that is now commonly used and frequently referenced. This classification system uses radiologic indicators to divide wrists into those that are stable (types I and II) and those that are unstable (type III).
33. Mannerfelt L, Norman O. Attrition ruptures of flexor tendons in rheumatoid arthritis caused by bony spurs in the carpal tunnel: a clinical and radiological study. *J Bone Joint Surg Br.* 1969;51:270-277.
Describes the classic lesion involving flexor tendon rupture from bone spurs within the carpal canal.
34. Vaughan-Jackson OJ. Attrition ruptures of the tendons in the rheumatoid hand. *J Bone Joint Surg Am.* 1958;40A:1431.
This classic article describes attritional rupture of the extensor tendons in rheumatoid hand disease.
35. Bleifeld CJ, Inglis AE. The hand in systemic lupus erythematosus. *J Bone Joint Surg Am.* 1974;56:1207-1215.
36. Dray GJ. The hand in systemic lupus erythematosus. *Hand Clin.* 1989;5:145-155.
37. Malcus Johnsson P, Sandqvist G, Nilsson JA, et al. Hand function and performance of daily activities in systemic lupus erythematosus: a clinical study. *Lupus.* 2015;24:827-834.
38. Prakken B, Albani S, Martini A. Juvenile idiopathic arthritis. *Lancet.* 2011;377:2138-2149.
39. Towner SR, Michet CJ Jr, O'Fallon WM, Nelson AM. The epidemiology of juvenile arthritis in Rochester, Minnesota 1960–1979. *Arthritis Rheum.* 1983;26:1208-1213.
40. Peterson LS, Mason T, Nelson AM, et al. Juvenile rheumatoid arthritis in Rochester, Minnesota 1960-1993. Is the epidemiology changing? *Arthritis Rheum.* 1996;39:1385-1390.
41. Lawrence RC, Helmick CG, Arnett FC, et al. Estimates of the prevalence of arthritis and selected musculoskeletal disorders in the United States. *Arthritis Rheum.* 1998;41:778-799.
42. El Hadidi KT, Medhat BM, Abdel Baki NM, et al. Characteristics of systemic lupus erythematosus in a sample of the Egyptian population: a retrospective cohort of 1109 patients from a single center. *Lupus.* 2018;27:1030-1038.
43. Macedo EA, Appenzeller S, Costallat LT. Gender differences in systemic lupus erythematosus concerning anxiety, depression and quality of life. *Lupus.* 2016;25:1315-1327.
44. Farr S, Girsch W. The hand and wrist in juvenile rheumatoid arthritis. *J Hand Surg Am.* 2015;40:2289-2292.
45. Ritchlin CT, Colbert RA, Gladman DD. Psoriatic arthritis. *N Engl J Med.* 2017;376:957-970.
46. Griffin MF, Almadori A, Butler PE. Use of lipotransfer in scleroderma. *Aesthet Surg J.* 2017;37:S33-S37.
47. Sullivan KM, Goldmuntz EA, Keyes-Elstein L, et al. Myeloablative autologous stem-cell transplantation for severe scleroderma. *N Engl J Med.* 2018;378:35-47.

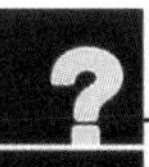

QUESTIONS

1. A 38-year-old woman presents with a 6-month history of bilateral hand and wrist pain with dorsal swelling. On examination, there is boggy swelling and extensor tenosynovitis. Laboratory analysis reveals elevated erythrocyte sedimentation rate and positive rheumatoid factor. Which of the following is most important for the patient's long-term outcome?

a. NSAIDs and splinting
b. Surgical synovectomy
c. Kenalog injection into the symptomatic area
d. Referral to rheumatology
e. Observation and repeated labs in 6 months

2. Biological DMARDs, such as etanercept (Enbrel), infliximab (Remicade), or adalimumab (Humira), used in treatment of rheumatoid arthritis work by what mechanism of action?

a. Binding of cell messenger protein IL-1
b. Antagonism of DNA modification
c. B-cell depletion
d. Blockade of T-cell activation
e. Tumor necrosis factor binding

3. A patient with known rheumatoid arthritis presents noting an inability to extend her right long and ring fingers actively. The joints are noted to be supple, and she can hold the finger in extension once passively extended to neutral. Which of the following is the most likely etiology of this complaint?

a. Rupture of the junctura tendinae
b. Extensor subluxation at the MP joint
c. Posterior interosseous nerve compression
d. Extensor tendon rupture
e. Caput ulnae

4. A patient with boutonniere deformity secondary to rheumatoid arthritis is being evaluated for extensor tendon reconstruction. Which of the following would be a contraindication to this procedure?

a. Rheumatoid nodules at the surgical site
b. Mild degenerative joint changes
c. History of silicone MP joint replacements
d. Stiffness at the DIP joint
e. Stiffness at the PIP joint

5. A 35-year-old female smoker with juvenile idiopathic arthritis presents with painful cold intolerance involving bilateral fingers and hands. On examination, there are ulcerations at the tips of multiple digits. An angiogram is ordered and reveals no occlusive disease proximal to digit vessels and no obvious bypass targets. Which of the following is the preferred initial treatment?

a. Oral calcium channel antagonist
b. Botulinum neurotoxin A
c. Avoidance of cold, tobacco, and vasoconstrictors
d. Surgical sympathectomy
e. Arterialization of the venous system

1. **Answer: d.** Wrist splinting, NSAIDs, and steroid injections are all conservative measures for tenosynovitis. In this case, however, the clinical picture and laboratory findings are specific for RA. Studies have shown that initiating DMARDs within 3 months of diagnosis leads to a significant decrease in disease morbidity. Options for medical treatment include anti-TNF alpha drugs or recombinant IL-1 antagonists. These, used in concert with methotrexate, can be effective in modifying the inflammatory response and subsequent joint destruction.

2. **Answer: e.** Multiple drugs can be used in combination to medically treat RA. DMARDs such as infliximab, etanercept, or adalimumab are all considered biologic DMARDs and modify the patient's immune system by binding tumor necrosis factor using engineered antibodies.

3. **Answer: b.** Patients with RA may be unable to actively extend the fingers for a variety of reasons and a clear understanding of the anatomy is necessary to make appropriate diagnoses in these cases. Possible causes include rupture of extensor tendons, posterior interosseous nerve palsy, subluxation of the extensor tendons over the metacarpal heads, and volar subluxation with contracture of the metacarpophalangeal joints. In this case, subluxation of the tendon is the appropriate choice because the other options can be ruled out. The extensor tendon is intact as the patient can maintain extension once the finger is positioned, the joints are supple without subluxation or contracture, and the muscles are functioning ruling out PIN nerve palsy. Caput ulnae can lead to tendon attrition or rupture but is not typically associated with extension lag.

4. **Answer: e.** Boutonniere deformity is a condition of the PIP joint and therefore reconstruction options are limited in cases where the joint is not supple. Typically, tendon reconstructions are not performed unless the joint has adequate range of motion. The other choices may add considerations to reconstructive procedures but are not contraindications.

5. **Answer: c.** This patient presents with Raynaud's phenomenon, and the initial primary treatment should include lifestyle modifications such as avoidance of cold, tobacco or vasoconstrictors. Medical therapy can be considered if symptoms persist or worsen beyond mild symptomatology. Botulinum neurotoxin A is recognized now for use in Raynaud's and is theorized to reduce perivascular sympathetic response. Surgical sympathectomy and arterial reconstruction can be considered when arterial occlusion is severe and bypass targets exist. Arterialization of the venous system is reserved for last-chance efforts if arterial bypass sites are not available and limitations in flow are significant.

CHAPTER 93 Osteoarthritis

Erin A. Miller and Jeffrey B. Friedrich

KEY POINTS

- First-line treatment of osteoarthritis (OA) is conservative management (rest, NSAIDs, steroid injection); surgery is only offered for refractory pain
- Surgical options for any hand arthritis relieve pain in exchange for loss of motion (fusion) or loss of strength (arthroplasty)
- Distal interphalangeal (DIP) arthritis is best managed with fusion in 10 to 20 degrees of flexion
- Refractory carpometacarpal (CMC) arthritis is most frequently treated with excision of the trapezium and surgeon's choice of stabilization of the metacarpal base
- Thumb metacarpophalangeal joint hyperextension and scaphotrapezoid arthritis must be treated to achieve successful outcome when treating CMC arthritis
- Treatment options for radiocarpal arthritis are dependent on the quality of the lunate fossa of the distal radius; proximal row carpectomy (PRC) and four-corner fusion (4CF) have equivalent outcomes in patients over 40 years of age

OA of the hand and wrist is a common reason for presentation to a surgeon. It is a disease of the articular cartilage in which progressive degeneration causes changes throughout the entire joint. The articular cartilage in joints is hyaline cartilage, and it is particularly susceptible to trauma given the slow turnover rate of chondrocytes and its inability to heal.[1] Although age, obesity, metabolic syndrome, and trauma are most commonly implicated in OA, current research demonstrates that the process is multifactorial and highlights the importance of occupational, hormonal, biochemical, metabolic, and genetic factors.[2–4] No link between hand dominance and OA has been proved. The disease begins with cartilage erosion and can progress to significant joint changes: thickening of adjacent bone (sclerosis), synovial inflammation, ligament instability (laxity), reactive bone formation (bone spurs), and subchondral bone erosion (cysts).[3]

The population impact of OA of any joint is huge, and it is the leading cause of disability in individuals over the age of 70 according to the World Health Organization.[1] Hand arthritis is most common in the DIP joint with a prevalence of 35%, followed by thumb CMC joint at 21% and the proximal interphalangeal joint (PIP) at 18%.[4,5] As expected, it has been shown that OA prevalence increases as age increases: at the age of 40, DIP involvement is seen in 35% of individuals as opposed to 65% of individuals over the age of 65.[3]

Conservative management of the OA is usually the first-line treatment. Unlike inflammatory arthropathies, such as rheumatoid arthritis, there are no known disease-modifying drugs. Antiinflammatory agents are often effective in early disease and activity modification is recommended with those of radiographic evidence of OA despite lack of level 1 evidence. Hand therapy yields short-term reduction pain scores in several randomized control trials. Splinting with either prefabricated or custom orthoses has been demonstrated to decrease pain but does not affect strength, function, or dexterity.[6] Steroid injections are commonly used for early stage arthritis in any joint. Although there is one trial suggesting they may provide permanent relief in early stage disease,[7] other randomized trials have found only temporary pain relief when compared to placebo and hyaluronic acid injections.[8] Patients should be counseled on potential side effects of steroid injection, including skin pigment changes and infection.

Assessment of the patient with hand pain suspected to be arthritic in nature should begin with a thorough history, physical examination, and subsequent radiographs. Hand dominance and occupation/leisure activities significantly direct treatment. Plain radiographs are the mainstay of diagnosis of hand and wrist OA; CT and MRI add little to the clinical diagnosis but are often used in research to further define the etiology and progression of OA. Imaging of the painful joint should be obtained in three views and assessed for joint space narrowing, sclerosis, subchondral cysts, angulation/subluxation, osteophytes, and bony collapse.[9] There are several grading scales available for OA in the hand, the most universal being the Kallman scale (**Table 93.1**).[10] Grading is primarily used to monitor the progression of OA over time, and it typically does not direct clinical decision-making. Instead, intervention is undertaken primarily for symptoms.

It is important to rule out other causes of joint pain—clinical and family history may distinguish OA from rheumatoid arthritis and crystalline arthropathies (gout and pseudogout) may be diagnosed with synovial aspiration and examination for crystals.[11] When presented with isolated arthritis of the index and middle finger metacarpal phalangeal (MCP) joints, care must be taken to rule out hemochromatosis with iron and liver function tests as hand pain may be the initial presentation of this life-threatening disease. The differential diagnosis of OA in the hand is shown in **Table 93.2**.

INTERPHALANGEAL/METACARPAL PHALANGEAL JOINT OSTEOARTHRITIS

The anatomy of the DIP and PIP joints is relatively similar, with a bicondylar hinge joint surface stabilized by strong collateral ligaments. In PIP joints, an extra degree of stability is added by the volar plate.[4] Nearly all arthritic DIP joints demonstrate abnormalities in the collateral ligaments, but further research is needed to determine

TABLE 93.1. KALLMAN GRADING SCALE FOR OSTEOARTHRITIS OF THE HAND[10]

Score[a]	Osteophytes	Joint Space Narrowing	Sclerosis	Cysts	Lateral Deformity	Collapse of Central Bone
0	None	None	Absent	Absent	Absent	Absent
1	Small	Definitely narrowed	Present	Present	Present	Present
2	Moderate	Severely narrowed				
3	Large	Joint fusion at one point				

A score of is assigned in each of the six categories, which are followed longitudinally over time to monitor for presence and progression of arthritis.

TABLE 93.2. DIAGNOSES TO CONSIDER WHEN WORKING UP OSTEOARTHRITIS

Diagnosis	Examination	Workup
Rheumatoid arthritis	Metacarpal phalangeal (MCP) involvement more than interphalangeal, ulnar deviation, swan neck deformity	Family history, serum rheumatoid factor, antinuclear antibody assay
Psoriatic arthritis	Nail involvement, psoriasis patches on skin, erosive lesions on radiographs	Dermatology referral, rheumatoid factor
Gout	Relapsing pain, multisite involvement	Joint aspiration—needle-shaped crystals
Pseudogout	Multiple joint involvement, pancarpal arthritis on imaging	Joint aspiration—rhomboidal crystals
Hemochromatosis	Isolated index and middle MCP arthritis	Iron studies, LFTs
Kienbock disease	Central wrist pain	MRI of the wrist
Septic arthritis	Sudden onset isolate joint pain, history of puncture	CBC, ESR, CRP, joint aspiration for cell count and Gram stain

CBC, complete blood count; CRP, C-reactive protein; ESR, erythrocyte sedimentation rate.

the inciting cause. MCP joints differ from the interphalangeal (IP) joints in that they are condyloid type, this allows for a greater range of motion that includes abduction, adduction, and circumduction in addition to the flexion seen at the IPs. The MCP collateral ligaments and sagittal bands are tight in flexion but lax in extension, allowing for the additional degrees of freedom.

Examination

On physical examination, it is important to assess and document the range of motion at each affected joint using a goniometer. Severe OA can lead to joint ankylosis and total loss of motion. Angulation in the coronal plane should be assessed to detect significant deviation. Herberden nodules may be seen at the DIP and may be lateral or dorsal midline swellings; they are related to osteophyte growth and extensor mechanism swelling, respectively.[12] Bouchard nodules are similar swellings found at the PIP. Mucous cysts are often present at the DIP and are unrelated to osteophytes but instead influenced by the synovium and tendon sheath and are amenable to treatment with excision.[3]

Imaging

Imaging should be ordered of the entire hand as well as the specific fingers in question. Osteophytes seen on radiographs are the first sign of IP OA.[3] Joint space narrowing coupled with lateral osteophyte proliferation may cause the classic "gull wing" appearance at the IP joints or a "sawtooth deformity" may be seen if there is erosion throughout the entire joint (Figure 93.1).[4] There are several grading systems regarding IP OA, most notably the Kellgren-Lawrence and the Ghent University Scoring System; however, they do not typically drive treatment recommendations.

Treatment

The patient's goals and occupation are considered when determining the treatment for IP and MCP arthritis as options must balance pain relief, stability, strength, and motion preservation. In general terms, surgical treatment of DIP degeneration consists solely of arthrodesis, and there are no commercially available arthroplasties for DIP joints. Implant arthroplasty is available for PIP and MCP joints, although they are not typically used for the index finger because of stresses from thumb-index pinch, and arthrodesis is usually recommended for this finger.

Fusion of the DIP joint is well tolerated, as only 15% of total digit motion occurs at the DIP. Grip strength has been found to decrease by 20% to 25% because of the effects of quadrigia; removing the excursion of the flexor digitorum profundus (FDP) tendon in the fused joint tethers the common FDP muscle belly. The angle of fusion that provides the most dexterity with least loss of grip strength is from 10 to 20 degrees and has been studied in several simulated fusion models.[13] The procedure is performed through a dorsal approach—the joint is excised and the bones fused with either 90-90 wiring or a compression screw. Recent retrospective reviews showed a decreased nonunion rate (0%–11%) with compression screws.[14] With any fusion, caution should be used in patients who consume nicotine products, as this will slow bony healing.

The PIP joint contributes more to the range of motion of the digit, but it may also be fused in patients with high demand. Although each surgeon has his/her preference for fusion angle, a fusion simulation study demonstrated an angle of 40 degrees was well tolerated with the least loss of power grasp.[15] The MCP is able to compensate for finger motion in the setting of DIP and PIP fusions; however, the converse does not hold true because MCP fusion severely limits hand function and is not routinely recommended. Fortunately, OA is more common in the IP joints and rarely seen in the MCP as opposed to rheumatoid arthritis which has widespread MCP involvement.[16]

Arthroplasty can be used to treat the PIP or MCP with good to excellent outcomes in proper candidates. Implant choice for OA is an important question that must be discussed with the patient and functional goals in mind as they demonstrate similar pain relief, range of motion, and patient satisfaction.[16,17] Silicone implants are constrained, designed to hinge in the sagittal plane for they act primarily as a spacer for the joint. They are held in place by the capsule formed around them, thus complications of synovitis and angulation are seen on top of the baseline risks of infection and implant fracture. Pyrocarbon implants are nonconstrained to allow greater motion but carry a higher reoperation rate and may dislocate, loosen, or squeak.[4,17] Srnec et al. recommend silicone use for the PIP and pyrocarbon at the MCP.[16] Patients should be counseled that joint range of motion is similar pre- and postoperatively regardless of implant choice. The risk of implant failure is real; in laborers or young active patients, an implant may not withstand the demands asked of it. Guidelines by joint for implant choice are seen in **Table 93.3**.

An isolated arthritic PIP joint is often posttraumatic and related to incongruity at the articular surface and additional options exist for treatment—volar plate arthroplasty, hemihamate arthroplasty, and vascularized toe joint transfer have all been described. In generalized OA of the hand, however, these techniques are less useful both for the lack of adequate donors (for example, each hand only has one hamate) as well as the soft tissue and synovial changes that make these options less reliable.

CARPOMETACARPAL JOINT ARTHRITIS

Basal joint or thumb CMC arthritis is one of the most widely studied and controversial topics in hand surgery. The anatomy of the thumb CMC is unique, permitting three degrees of freedom to precisely position the thumb tip in space. The joint comprises two saddles positioned perpendicularly to each other, allowing an average of 50 degree flexion/extension and 40 degrees adduction/abduction. Circumduction and opposition of 20 degrees are achieved with a

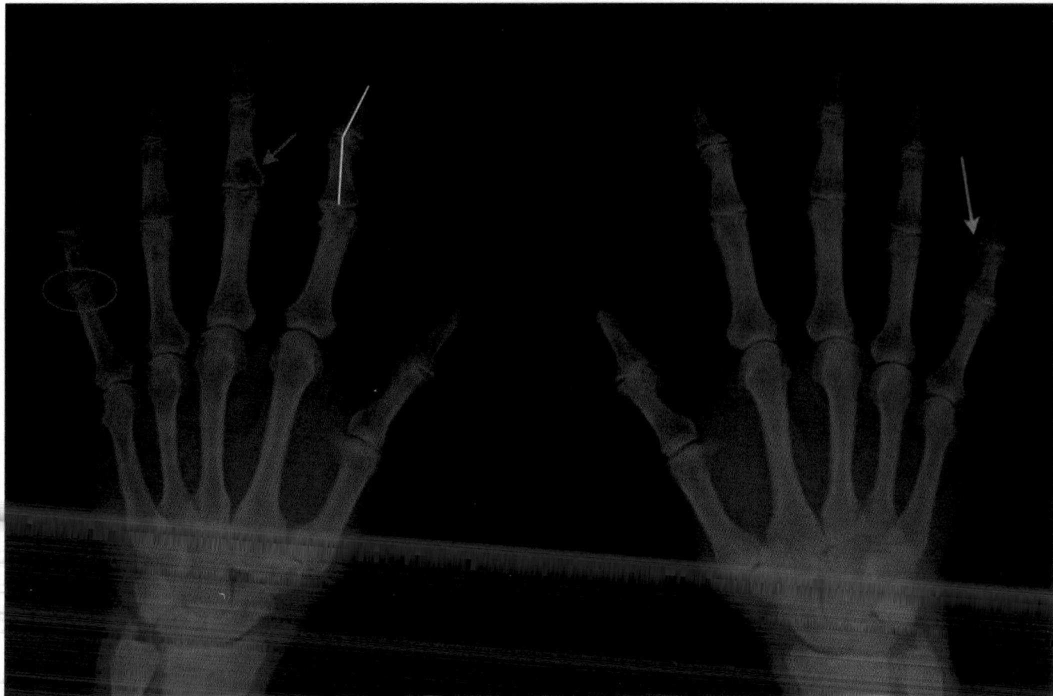

FIGURE 93.1. Pan IP arthritis with diffuse joint space narrowing. Red circle demonstrates an early gull-wing sign. Red arrow highlights a large subchondral cyst. The white lines accentuate coronal angulation. Blue arrow is representative of sclerosis. Green arrow demonstrates one instance of fusion.

twisting between the saddles and requires strong capsular and ligamentous support to prevent subluxation.[18] Ligament laxity of even 1 to 2 mm can disrupt the balance of the forces and predispose to cartilage injury.[18,19] In power grip, the CMC routinely experiences 120 kg of force, and in pinch the lever arm of the thumb multiples the force seen at the tip by 12 when translated to the CMC.[20] Given the demands placed on the thumb in routine activities, the high prevalence of OA in the CMC is not surprising.

Biomechanic knowledge is essential to understanding the pathology of CMC arthritis. Pinching the thumb against the fingers in a wide grip translates the force dorsally at the metacarpal base, and a restraint is needed to prevent dorsal subluxation. Many investigations have attempted to elucidate the ligamentous anatomy of the thumb. Early studies cited the anterior oblique or "beak" ligament as the primary stabilizer against dorsal translation and aimed treatment accordingly.[19,21] Recent landmark work, however, has demonstrated that the anterior oblique ligament is not the critical ligament to establish stability and it is laxed throughout motion.[22-24] Furthermore, these authors demonstrated the importance of the three dorsal ligaments in stabilization of the thumb. Although controversy still exists and recent reports describe between 3 and 16 different ligamentous contributions to the thumb CMC, most agree that the dorsal structures are of key importance.[20,22]

TABLE 93.3. TREATMENT OPTIONS AND RECOMMENDATIONS FOR FINGER ARTHRITIS

Joint	Options	Considerations
DIP	Arthrodesis	Fusion in 10–20 degrees of flexion
PIP	Arthrodesis	Fusion in 30–40 degrees of flexion
	Arthroplasty (not recommended for index)	Silicone implant preferred given constraint
MCP	Arthroplasty	Pyrocarbon implant preferred as nonconstrained

DIP, Distal interphalangeal; MCP, Metacarpal phalangeal; PIP, proximal interphalangeal.

Examination

Inspection of the thumb assesses for resting position; in end-stage disease, the webspace is contracted and the metacarpal is adducted. This adduction is compensation for dorsal subluxation of the metacarpal base. A palpable step off from the metacarpal to the trapezium may be present, termed a "shoulder sign" or "squaring." Pain on palpation over the volar metacarpal base is frequently present; however, the hallmark examination finding for CMC arthritis is a positive grind test, which is done with axial loading and rotation of the thumb.[9] It is important to note any MCP hyperextension on examination. Patients with a painful CMC will avoid thumb tip to index tip pinch and will instead use index tip to thumb pad, leading to chronic MCP hyperextension that should be addressed if greater than 30 degrees (Figure 93.2).[25,26] Range of motion and key and tip pinch strength should be documented as well.

Other pathologies to rule out during differential diagnosis are De Quervain tenosynovitis, intersection syndrome, flexor carpi radialis (FCR) tendonitis, and ulnar collateral ligament injury.

Imaging

Radiographs should include lateral, oblique, and anteroposterior (AP) views of the thumb. Obtaining a true AP view of the thumb, known as the Robert's view, is achieved with the forearm in maximal pronation with the dorsum of the thumb on the imaging table.[9] The Eaton stress view may be used as an adjunct to assess dorsal subluxation and compare to the contralateral hand. This is an AP view with the patient pushing the radial aspects of the thumb together.[19]

In addition to assessment of the CMC, the scapho-trapezial-trapezoid (STT) joint should be examined in every patient. As arthritis progresses, all surfaces of the trapezium become involved and failure to diagnose and address degenerative changes at the scaphotrapezoid articulation may result in treatment failure. Eaton proposed a radiographic classification of basal joint arthritis in 1973 that is still used today with minor modifications (**Table 93.4**; Figure 93.3).[9,19]

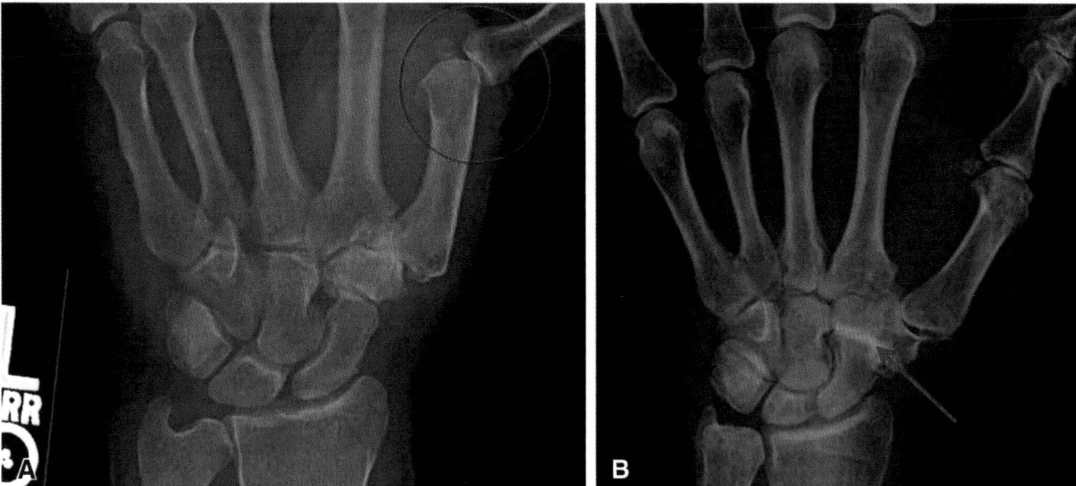

FIGURE 93.2. Additional pathology to watch for in patients with carpometacarpal arthritis. **A.** Concurrent metacarpal phalangeal hyperextension of 45 degrees (circle). **B.** Radiograph demonstrating severe STT arthritis with complete collapse of the scaphotrapezial joint space (arrow).

Treatment

Conservative treatment is typically the first step in basal joint arthritis. Splinting, hand therapy, activity modification, antiinflammatories, and hyaluronate or steroid injections all have short-term benefit.[6] When and if these measures fail to provide adequate pain relief, there are a variety of surgical options. Despite a multitude of studies, there has not been a method of treatment that demonstrates significantly improved outcomes. Metacarpal base osteotomy may be used as it is effective in early stage (I or II) disease by distributing the load of the metacarpal on the CMC joint. Studies have definitively shown that use of prosthetic material—silicone, Marlex, or Gortex—provides inferior results, and we recommend that if a spacer is [illegible] [illegible] fusion, and trapeziectomy.

Ligament reconstruction is the first [illegible] by Eaton and Littler in 1973, and there have been reports of using multiple different tendons (extensor carpi radialis longus, extensor pollicis brevis, extensor pollicis longus, abductor pollicis longus, and flexor carpi radialis) in an attempt to stabilize the CMC and prevent progression of arthritis. Ligament reconstruction has shown equivalent outcomes to other methods when used for stage I or II disease; in Eaton's 10 to 23 year follow-up series 71% of patients still reported mild pain despite all being satisfied with the procedure.[28]

TABLE 93.4. EATON STAGES OF THUMB CARPOMETACARPAL ARTHRITIS[9,19]

Stage	Joint Space	Osteophytes	Scapho-trapezial-trapezoid Joint	Other
I	Slightly widened	Absent	Preserved	<1/3 dorsal subluxation of metacarpal
II	Slightly narrowed	<=2 mm	Preserved	
III	Significantly narrowed	>2 mm	Preserved	Sclerotic of cystic changes in subchondral bone
IV	Significantly narrowed	>2 mm	Involved	Pantrapezial involvement

Arthrodesis of the CMC was pioneered by Muller in 1949,[25] and it is still recommended today for younger patients or laborers who rely on grip strength. Motion is well preserved in both subjective and objective measures; however, fusion carries a higher risk of complications than other procedures treating CMC. The only randomized control trial comparing arthrodesis to trapeziectomy and ligament reconstruction was halted as complications of delayed union, nonunion, complex regional pain syndrome and neuroma were significantly higher in the arthrodesis group despite functional outcomes being similar.[29] It is still a viable option, but the complications must be discussed with the patient and cessation of nicotine-containing products preoperatively until union is [illegible].

Trapeziectomy is the common component of [illegible] of CMC arthritis. There are many variations of this treatment. Each option follows the principle of [illegible] arthritic trapezium and prevention of metacarpal subluxation both dorsally and proximally onto the scaphoid. The simplest option is "hematoma distraction" where axial Kirschner wires are placed temporarily to maintain the space. The ligamentous reconstruction tendon interposition pioneered in 1986[30] is the most widely used in the United States with over 90% reporting this as the preferred method in 2010.[31] With the ligamentous reconstruction tendon interposition, the FCR is harvested proximally while the distal attachment to the index metacarpal base is maintained and tunneled through a drill hole in the base of the thumb metacarpal to prevent dorsal subluxation. The remainder of the tendon is interposed in the space formerly occupied by the trapezium to prevent proximal migration of the metacarpal.[30] Variations of this method include interposition only, suspension only, and use of abductor pollicis longus or half of FCR; a well-designed randomized trial as well as several systematic reviews have not been able to demonstrate superiority of any of these procedures.[27,32] A newer procedure is the "suspensionplasty" or tight-rope where a purpose-built permanent suture construct is passed through the index metacarpal to the thumb metacarpal base and back then tied over a button to help prevent proximal migration and decrease complications associated with the FCR donor site. These procedures are summarized in **Table 93.5**.

Complications specific to trapeziectomy procedures are primarily neuropathic: superficial radial or palmar cutaneous nerve dysfunction and complex regional pain syndrome.[32] Failure to identify and address concomitant thumb MCP hyperextension or STT arthritis can lead to persistent pain and poor outcome. STT arthritis may be managed surgically by excision of the proximal trapezoid at the time of trapeziectomy, as exposure is excellent. MCP hyperextension greater than 30 degrees should be treated. Although many surgeons temporarily pin the joint, there is a high rate of relapse, so MCP arthrodesis should be considered and is recommended if the MCP deformity exceeds 50 degrees.[26]

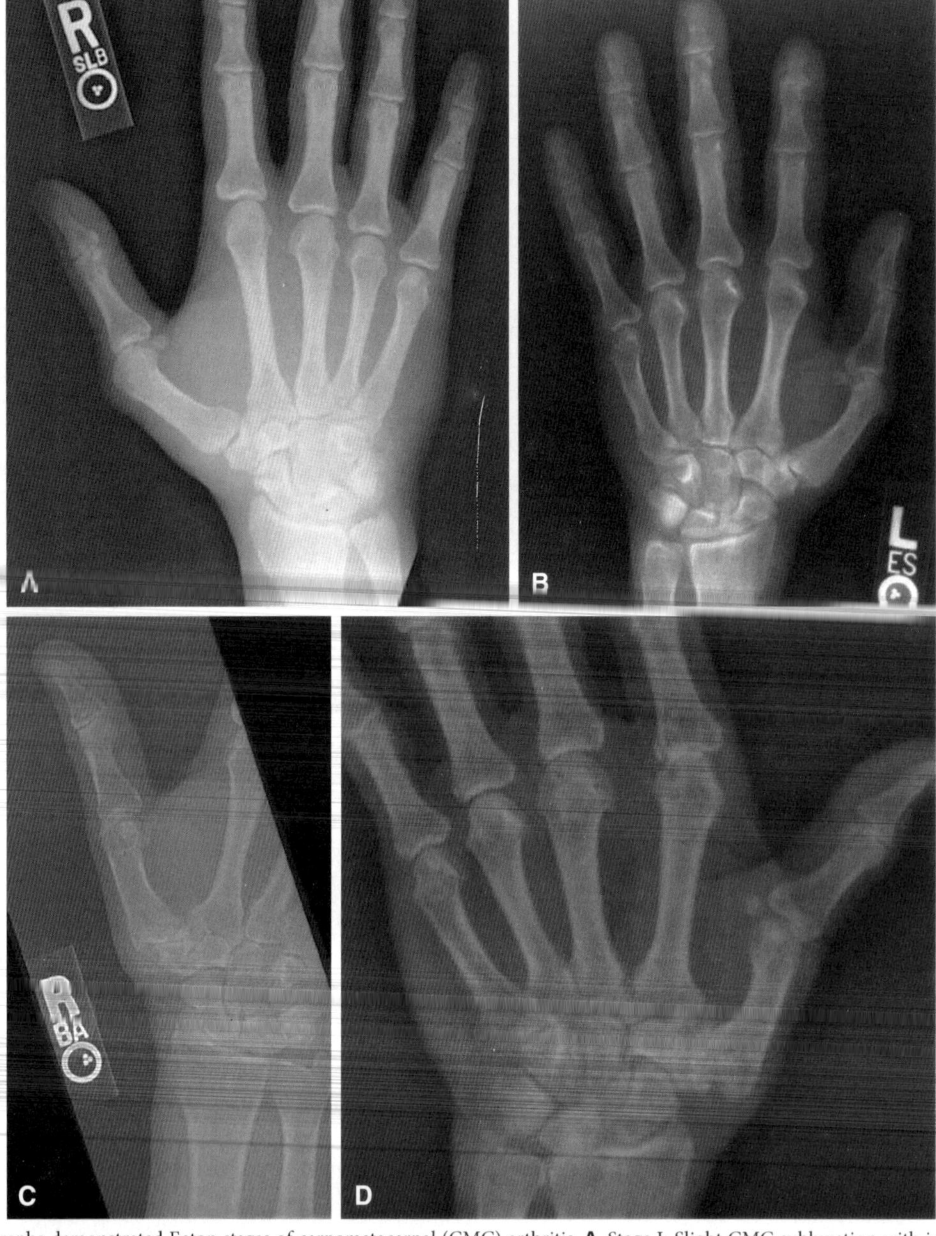

FIGURE 93.3. Radiographs demonstrated Eaton stages of carpometacarpal (CMC) arthritis. **A.** Stage I: Slight CMC subluxation with joint space widening, no osteophytes seen. **B.** Stage II: CMC subluxation of one-third with small osteophytes along the ulnar aspect of the trapezium, joint space narrowing. **C.** Stage III: Complete loss of joint space and large osteophytes seen throughout the trapezium. **D.** Stage IV: Demonstration of pantrapezial arthritis.

TABLE 93.5. SUMMARY OF CARPOMETACARPAL SURGICAL TREATMENTS

Procedure	Considerations
Ligament reconstruction	Used in Eaton Stage I or II
Metacarpal base osteotomy	Used in Eaton Stage I or II
Trapeziometacarpal arthrodesis	Higher complications reported than excision procedures (nonunion)
Trapeziectomy variations	
Hematoma distraction	Metacarpal pinned to prevent proximal migration
Tendon interposition	Frequently palmaris longus used
Ligament reconstruction tendon interposition	May be performed with FCR or abductor pollicis longus
Tight-rope suspension	Uses purpose-built suture suspension device

WRIST ARTHRITIS

Understanding of the anatomy of the articular surface of the distal radius is key to diagnosis and treatment of wrist arthritis. The wrist supplies the hand three degrees of motion: flexion/extension, radial/ulnar deviation, and rotation. Historically it was believed the majority of the load bearing was through the scaphoid fossa of the radius; however, recent in vivo pressure transduction determined the majority of the load passes through the lunate facet in all positions of the wrist, using a wide point of contact to transmit force through the triangular fibrocartilage complex to the ulna as well as down the intermediate column of the radius.[33] In contrast, greater motion occurs at the radioscaphoid articulation as the scaphoid flexes during radial deviation and extends with ulnar deviation, passing through a 40% range of motion arc.[34] The scaphoid drives the motion of the lunate and in turn the entire proximal carpal row; differential motion between the scaphoid and lunate or within the scaphoid, thus alters normal wrist kinematics and creates abnormal loading that predisposes to articular wear and injury. This process explains why 95% of wrist arthritis seen is periscaphoid.[35] Although Kienbock disease or idiopathic osteonecrosis of the lunate may lead to arthritic changes, it is a distinct process beyond the scope of this chapter.

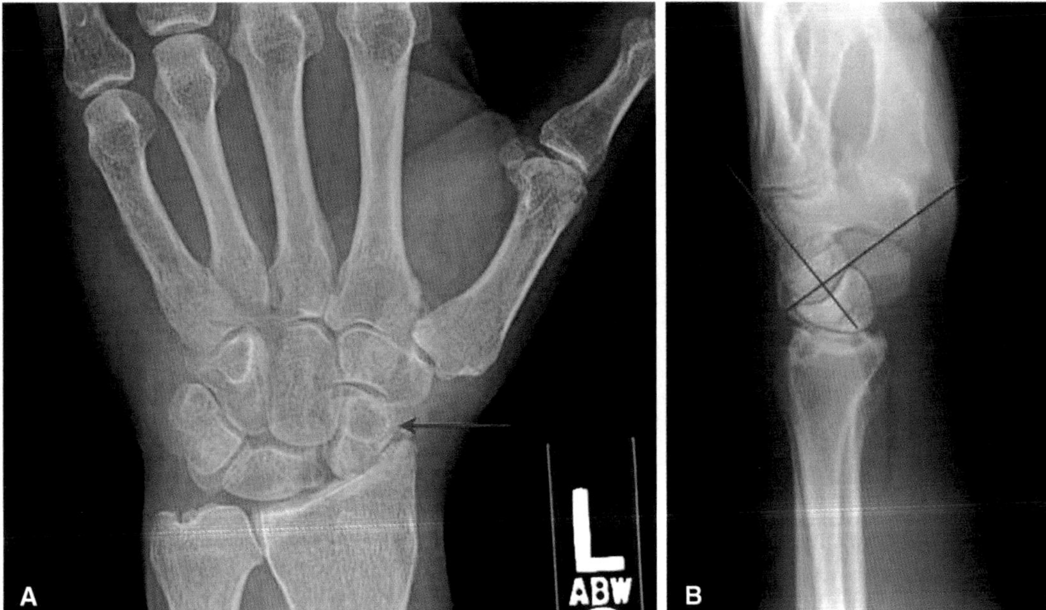

FIGURE 93.4. Radiographic findings in scapholunate advanced collapse. **A.** Scaphoid ring sign (arrow). **B.** Lateral view of a wrist with SL dissociation demonstrating dorsal tilt of the lunate and volar tilt of the scaphoid leading to an increased SL angle over 60 degrees. The lunate is highlighted in purple and the scaphoid in blue; the red lines allow visualization of the angle at almost 90 degrees.

Examination

A history of wrist trauma is common in wrist arthritis. Patients may have tenderness dorsally over the scapholunate (SL) interval. In those with a scaphoid nonunion triggering arthritis, a positive Watson's test may be present—a painful clunk when the wrist is brought from ulnar to radial deviation with volar pressure on the scaphoid. Range of motion is reduced and should be documented. Important conditions to rule out on examination are carpal tunnel syndrome, trigger finger, rheumatoid arthritis, basal joint arthritis, and pseudogout (the latter discussed below).

Imaging

Bilateral AP wrist views should be obtained in all patients with concern for radiocarpal arthritis. SL widening is an indicator of SL ligament compromise and may be seen only on a grip or clenched-fist radiograph view. A "ring sign" may be seen on an AP view with excessive flexion of the scaphoid (Figure 93.4A). Lateral views should be examined for SL angle. An angle greater than 60 degrees is abnormal and indicates scaphoid flexion with lunate extension (Figure 93.4B). This rotatory subluxation between the scaphoid and lunate causes abnormal wear and arthritis. Scapholunate advanced collapse (SLAC) is used to describe this spectrum of pathology (Figure 93.5), which constitutes 55% of radiocarpal arthritis[35,36] and is divided into three stages:

Stage I: Arthritis limited to the radial styloid.

Stage II: Radioscaphoid arthritis with preservation of the lunate facet.

Stage III: Progression to capitolunate arthritis.

Scaphoid nonunion advanced collapse (SNAC) is arthritis arising from a nonunited scaphoid fracture and demonstrates parallel stages to SLAC wrist. Similarly, there is abnormal rotation in the proximal row; however, the axis of this rotation is intrascaphoid instead of between the scaphoid and lunate (Figure 93.6).[37]

It is important to carefully assess the position of the scaphoid to rule out pseudogout. Scaphoid chondrocalcinosis advanced collapse due to pseudogout may be seen radiographically and is distinct from SLAC wrist in that the scaphoid *extends* and both the scaphoid and lunate facets are involved. Distinguishing scaphoid chondrocalcinosis advanced collapse is essential, as surgical treatment without addressing the underlying pseudogout will likely lead to failure.[11]

Treatment

The most conservative surgical option for wrist arthritis is denervation—this may be selective with excision of the posterior interosseous nerve only, or a total wrist denervation accomplished by excising both the anterior interosseous nerve and posterior interosseous nerve. It may be accomplished through a single incision and does not compromise any future reconstructive options. There have been variable results reported in the literature regarding success of this procedure, and it is accepted that more than 50% of patients experience some degree of improvement in pain score.[38] In early SNAC wrist, distal pole excision may be utilized if the fragment is less than half the scaphoid length. There is limited role for radial styloidectomy alone in wrist arthritis.

Later stage wrist arthritis with a preserved lunate fossa has two primary surgical treatment options. In reality, these are both considered salvage procedures and both lead to diminished range of motion that is hopefully pain-free. There is ongoing debate on the relative indications for PRC versus 4CF. PRC uses removal of the scaphoid, lunate, and triquetrum to convert the complex interactions between carpal bones into a simple hinge joint with the capitate articulating in the lunate fossa. As a result of the differential curvature radius of the capitate head and lunate, radiographic progression of arthritic change is frequently seen in the lunate fossa; however, this has not been clinically correlated with a return of pain.[39] Long-term results of PRC are acceptable, with a 14% to 35% conversion to wrist fusion. A capsular interposition flap has been suggested to improve pain scores.[38] When examining risk factors for failure, age less than 40 at the time of wrist fusion is strongly correlated and considered a relative contraindication for PRC.[39-41]

In the short term, 4CF has a higher complication profile, with increased risk of nonunion, infection, and hardware removal.[42] Nicotine cessation in the immediate pre- and postoperative periods should be advised. Performed by excising the scaphoid then removing the intercarpal articular surfaces of the lunate, capitate, hamate and triquetrum to allow fixation of these bones into a carpal fusion mass, this operation relies on an intact articular surface of the lunate to articulate with the distal radius.

The initial description uses Kirschner wires to hold the fusion; now fusion plates, compression screws and staples are all available. Fusing the lunate in slight flexion has been suggested to provide improved wrist extension as it prevents the fusion mass from impinging on the dorsal side of the radius.[43]

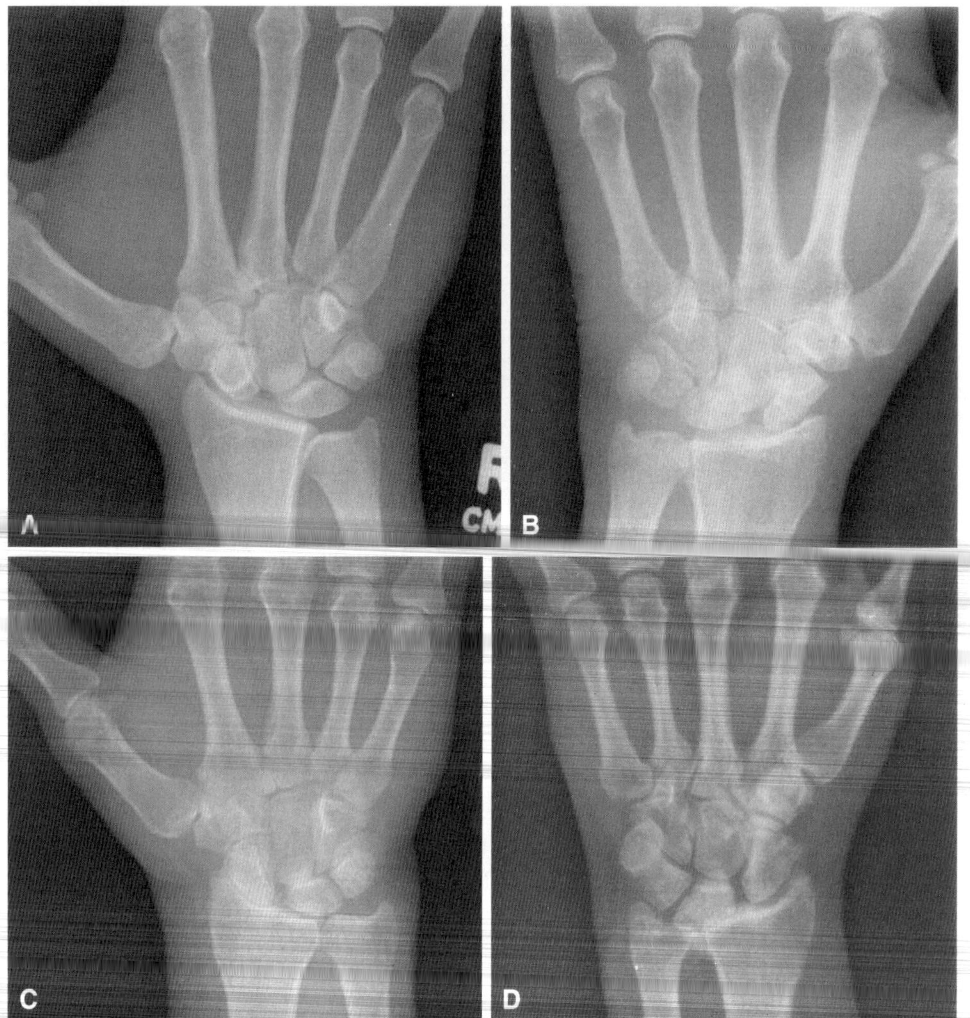

FIGURE 93.5. Radiographic progression of radiocarpal arthritis. **A.** The inciting injury in scapholunate advanced collapse (SLAC) wrist is a tear in the SL ligament that causes SL interval widening and proximal capitate migration; this image depicts a fairly acute injury prior to the onset of arthritis. **B.** SLAC stage I: Arthritic changes limited to the radial styloid. **C.** SLAC stage II: Severe arthritic changes in the scaphoid fossa with near complete loss of joint space. Note the preserved lunate fossa. **D.** SLAC stage III: Arthritis of the entire distal radius.

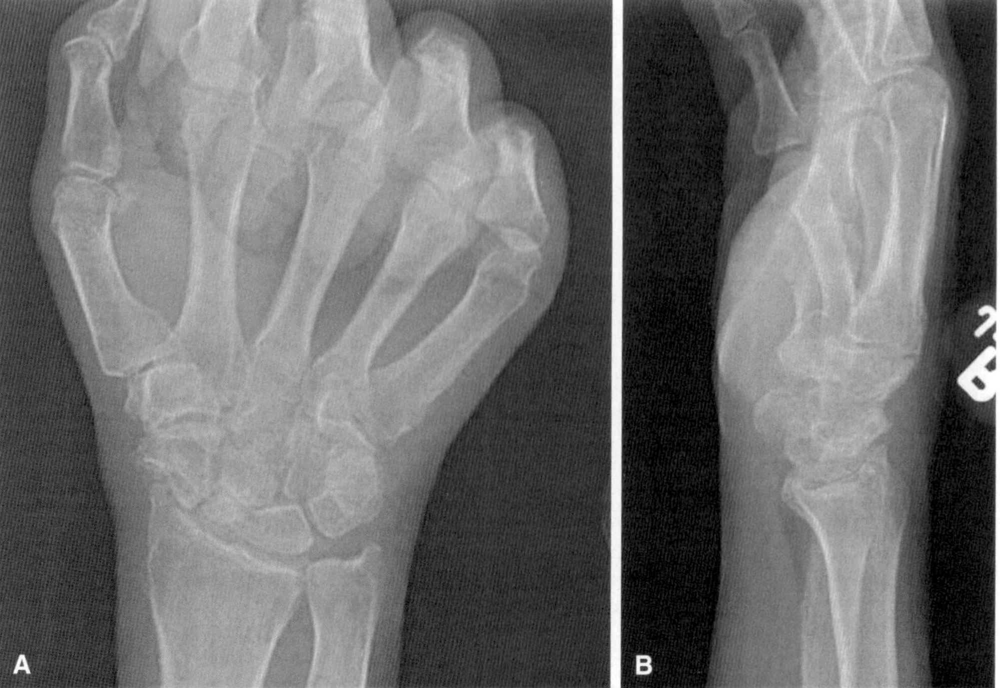

FIGURE 93.6. Scaphoid nonunion advanced collapse wrist in the anteroposterior **(A)** and lateral **(B)** radiographic views.

TABLE 93.6. COMPARISON OF PROXIMAL ROW CARPECTOMY (PRC) AND FOUR-CORNER FUSION (4CF)[a]

	Flexion Extension Arc	Radial-Ulnar Arc	Grip Strength	Functional Outcome	Pain Relief	Failure (Progression to Wrist Fusion)
4CF	64–76 degrees	13–30 degrees	70%–90% of contralateral	Minimal limitation	Significant	Rare
PRC	75–76 degrees	9–32 degrees	70%–90% of contralateral	Minimal limitation	Significant	Potentially increased in patients <40

[a]Ranges from 2009 metaanalysis by Mulford et al.[40] provided for patient counseling.

Historically, PRC was thought to decrease grip strength by shortening the wrist but provide a greater arc of motion, but multiple metaanalyses and a well-designed cohort study have demonstrated equivalence of the PRC and 4CF in range of motion, grip strength, and multiple subjective performance variables (**Table 93.6**).[38,42-44] When compared to the contralateral wrist, both procedures impart a 50% to 60% decrease in range of motion and maintain 80% of grip strength. The only significant difference is a greater arc of motion in radial-ulnar deviation with 4CF.[43] The insignificant difference in subjective measures may be explained by the fact that activities of daily living require an arc of 35 degrees flexion to 80 degrees of extension, and both 4CF and PRC typically provide this degree of motion.[41,42]

Small studies in the literature exist regarding limited intercarpal fusions—capitolunate fusion for example. These demonstrate similar outcomes to 4CF in range of motion and pain relief. A large metaanalysis of the available data indicates a greater propensity for nonunion when the fusion mass is smaller.[42] Because wrist fusion imparts an impairment on extremity function of 5% to 26%, total wrist arthrodesis is considered the ultimate salvage procedure. Once other options are exhausted, it can be effective. Despite overall acceptable outcomes, rates of pain relief vary widely, from 25% to 100% in the multitude of studies.[illegible]

Total wrist arthroplasty is typically used in older, low-demand patients and historically has played little role in the management of OA. These implants require a strict lifting restriction often less than ten pounds, and there has been scant investigation into the limits of this stipulation for the implants. There is a real risk of dislocation if the prosthesis is overstressed, and hardware loosening and infection are known complications. Recent retrospective reviews have demonstrated increasing success, ranging from 75% to 99% implant survival at 5 years,[46] and technological advances may make arthroplasty a more viable option in young, high-demand patients in the coming years.

CONCLUSIONS

OA affects the different joints of the hand and wrist in a variety of ways and treatment options vary accordingly. Common first-line treatment is nonoperative management, with splinting, hand therapy, antiinflammatories, and injections. Any surgical treatment of arthritis involves a tradeoff: in exchange for pain, patients lose either motion (in the case of arthrodesis) or strength (in the case of arthroplasty). Patient occupation and goals must be carefully considered before intervention, as many of our interventions have equivalent outcomes.

REFERENCES

1. Mobasheri A, Batt M. An update on the pathophysiology of osteoarthritis. *Ann Phys Rehabil Med.* 2016;59(5-6):333-339.
2. Martel-Pelletier J. Pathophysiology of osteoarthritis. *Osteoarthritis Cartilage.* 2004;12:31-33.
3. Kaufmann RA, Lögters TT, Verbruggen G, et al. Osteoarthritis of the distal interphalangeal joint. *J Hand Surg.* 2010;35(12):2117-2125.
4. Jacobs BJ, Verbruggen G, Kaufmann RA. Proximal interphalangeal joint arthritis. *J Hand Surg.* 2010;35(12):2107-2116.
5. Wilder FV, Barrett JP, Farina EJ. Joint-specific prevalence of osteoarthritis of the hand. *Osteoarthritis Cartilage.* 2006;14(9):953-957.
6. Spaans AJ, van Minnen LP, Kon M, et al. Conservative treatment of thumb base osteoarthritis: a systematic review. *J Hand Surg.* 2015;40(1):16-21, e1-6.
7. Day CS, Gelberman R, Patel AA, et al. Basal joint osteoarthritis of the thumb: a prospective trial of steroid injection and splinting. *J Hand Surg.* 2004;29(2):247-251.
8. Heyworth BE, Lee JH, Kim PD, et al. Hylan versus corticosteroid versus placebo for treatment of basal joint arthritis: a prospective, randomized, double-blinded clinical trial. *J Hand Surg.* 2008;33(1):40-48.
9. Tsai P, Beredjiklian PK. Physical diagnosis and radiographic examination of the thumb. *Hand Clin.* 2008;24(3):231-237.
10. Kallman DA, Wigley FM, Scott WW, et al. New radiographic grading scales for osteoarthritis of the hand: reliability for determining prevalence and progression. *Arthritis Rheum.* 1989;32(12):1584-1591.
11. Trehan SK, Lee SK, Wolfe SW. Scapholunate advanced collapse: nomenclature and differential diagnosis. *J Hand Surg.* 2015;40(10):[illegible].
12. Alexander CJ. Heberden's and Bouchard's nodes. *Ann Rheum Dis.* 1999;58(11):675-678.
13. Melamed E, Polatsch DB, Beldner S, Melone CP. Simulated distal interphalangeal joint fusion of the index and middle fingers in 0[illegible] of grip strength and dexterity. *J Hand Surg.* 2014;39(10):[illegible].
In this study of healthy volunteers, orthoses were used to simulate the degree of DIP fusion and effect of ADLs; 0 to 20 degrees was found to be acceptable, with the index providing the most limitation.
14. [illegible] Vaienti L. Distal interphalangeal joint arthrodesis for degenerative osteoarthritis with compression screw: results in 102 digits. *J Hand Surg.* 2012;37(7):1330-1334.
15. Woodworth JA, McCullough MB, Grosland NM, Adams BD. Impact of simulated proximal interphalangeal arthrodeses of all fingers on hand function. *J Hand Surg.* 2006;31(6):940-946.
16. Srnec JJ, Wagner ER, Rizzo M. Implant arthroplasty for proximal interphalangeal, metacarpophalangeal, and trapeziometacarpal joint degeneration. *J Hand Surg.* 2017;42(10):817-825.
17. Daecke W, Kaszap B, Martini AK, et al. A prospective, randomized comparison of 3 types of proximal interphalangeal joint arthroplasty. *J Hand Surg.* 2012;37(9):1770-1779, e1-3.
18. Cooney WP, Lucca MJ, Chao EY, Linscheid RL. The kinesiology of the thumb trapeziometacarpal joint. *J Bone Jt Surg Am.* 1981;63A:1371-1381.
19. Eaton RG, Littler JW. Ligament reconstruction for the painful thumb carpometacarpal joint. *J Bone Jt Surg Am.* 1973;55A:1655-1666.
Eaton and Littler first defined the classification of thumb CMC arthritis used today. Additionally, they describe their method of ligament reconstruction which is the basis of today's LRTI procedure.
20. Komatsu I, Lubahn JD. Anatomy and biomechanics of the thumb carpometacarpal joint. *Oper Techn Orthop.* 2018;28(1):1-5.
21. Napier JR. The form and function of the carpo-metacarpal joint of the thumb. *J Anat.* 1955;89(3):362-369.
22. Ladd AL, Lee J, Hagert E. Macroscopic and microscopic analysis of the thumb carpometacarpal ligaments: a cadaveric study of ligament anatomy and histology. *J Bone Jt Surg Am.* 2012;94A:1468-1477.
This anatomical study of the ligamentous stabilization of the thumb CMC overturned 50 years of dogma that the anterior oblique (aka beak) ligament is the primary stabilizer of the joint and instead demonstrated the importance of the dorsal ligaments as the key structural support at the CMC.
23. Pellegrini VD. Osteoarthritis of the trapeziometacarpal joint: the pathophysiology of articular cartilage degeneration. I. Anatomy and pathology of the aging joint. *J Hand Surg.* 1991;16(6):967-974.
24. Bettinger PC, Linscheid RL, Berger RA, et al. An Anatomic study of the stabilizing ligaments of the trapezium and trapeziometacarpal joint. *J Hand Surg.* 1999;24(4):786-798.
25. Muller GM. Arthrodesis of the trapezio-metacarpal joint for osteoarthritis. *J Bone Jt Surg Br.* 1949;31B:540-542.
26. Poulter RJ, Davis TRC. Management of hyperextension of the metacarpophalangeal joint in association with trapeziometacarpal joint osteoarthritis. *J Hand Surg Eur Vol.* 2011;36(4):280-284.

27. Vermeulen GM, Slijper H, Feitz R, et al. Surgical management of primary thumb carpometacarpal osteoarthritis: a systematic review. *J Hand Surg*. 2011;36(1):157-169.
28. Freedman DM, Eaton RG, Glickel SZ. Long-term results of volar ligament reconstruction for symptomatic basal joint laxity. *J Hand Surg*. 2000;25(2):297-304. doi:10.1053/jhsu.2000.jhsu25a0297.
29. Vermeulen GM, Brink SM, Slijper H, et al. Trapeziometacarpal arthrodesis or trapeziectomy with ligament reconstruction in primary trapeziometacarpal osteoarthritis: a randomized controlled trial. *J Bone Jt Surg Am*. 2014;96A:726-733.
A randomized, single-blind trial for treatment of basal joint arthritis comparing CMC arthrodesis to trapeziectomy with LRTI was designed and halted on midterm analysis due to the higher complication rate in the arthrodesis group. In those who completed the study, functional outcomes were equivalent.
30. Burton RI, Pellegrini VD. Surgical management of basal Joint arthritis of the thumb. Part II: ligament reconstruction with tendon interposition arthroplast. *J Hand Surg*. 1986;11(3):324-332.
Burton and Pellegrini's first description of the trapeziectomoy and ligament reconstruction tendon interposition, which remains the most widely used reconstruction for thumb CMC arthritis in the US today.
31. Yuan F, Aliu O, Chung KC, Mahmoudi E. Evidence-based practice in the surgical treatment of thumb carpometacarpal joint arthritis. *J Hand Surg*. 2017;42(2):104-112, e1.
32. Gangopadhyay S, McKenna H, Burke FD, Davis TRC. Five- to 18-year follow-up for treatment of trapeziometacarpal osteoarthritis: a prospective comparison of excision, tendon interposition, and ligament reconstruction and tendon interposition. *J Hand Surg*. 2012;37(3):411-417.
A randomized, single blinded trial for treatment of basal joint arthritis comparing trapeziectomy with temporary kwire fixation, trapeziectomy with palmaris interposition and trapeziectomy with LRTI. Five year follow-up was obtained, and no difference found in function (grip, key pinch, or tip pinch strength) or pain relief. Complications were equivalent.
33. Rikli DA, Honigmann P, Babst R, et al. Intra-articular pressure measurement in the radioulnocarpal joint using a novel sensor: in vitro and in vivo results. *J Hand Surg*. 2007;32(1):67-75.
A novel pressure transducer was verified in this study in cadavers and then introduced into the wrist of a human subject to properly quantify the distribution of forces in the wrist. Contrary to previous cadaver studies, they demonstrated that >50% of the load is transmitted through the lunate fossa and intermediate column of the forearm, which has important implications for reconstruction in the setting of wrist arthritis.
34. Palmer AK, Werner FW, Murphy D, Glisson R. Functional wrist motion: a biomechanical study. *J Hand Surg*. 1985;10(1):39-46.
35. Watson HK, Ryu J. Evolution of arthritis of the wrist. *Clin Orthop Relat Res*. 1986;(202):57-67.
36. Watson HK, Ballet FL. The SLAC wrist: scapholunate advanced collapse pattern of degenerative arthritis. *J Hand Surg*. 1984;9(3):358-365.
37. Vender MI, Watson HK, Wiener BD, Black DM. Degenerative change in symptomatic scaphoid nonunion. *J Hand Surg*. 1987;12(4):514-519.
38. Strauch RJ. Scapholunate advanced collapse and scaphoid nonunion advanced collapse arthritis—update on evaluation and treatment. *J Hand Surg*. 2011;36(4):729-735.
39. Wall LB, DiDonna ML, Kiefhaber TR, Stern PJ. Proximal row carpectomy: minimum 20-year follow-up. *J Hand Surg*. 2013;38(8):1498-1504.
40. DiDonna ML, Kiefhaber TR, Stern PJ. Proximal row carpectomy: study with a minimum of ten years of follow-up. *J Bone Jt Surg Am*. 2004;86A:2359-2365.
41. Mulford JS, Ceulemans LJ, Nam D, Axelrod TS. Proximal row carpectomy vs four corner fusion for scapholunate (Slac) or scaphoid nonunion advanced collapse (Snac) wrists: a systematic review of outcomes. *J Hand Surg Eur Vol*. 2009;34(2):256-263.
42. Siegel JM, Ruby LK. A critical look at intercarpal arthrodesis: review of the literature. *J Hand Surg*. 1996;21(4):717-723.
43. Cohen MS, Kozin SH. Degenerative arthritis of the wrist: proximal row carpectomy versus scaphoid excision and four-corner arthrodesis. *J Hand Surg*. 2001;26(1):94-104.
Cohen and Kozin present a well-designed cohort study comparing PRC to 4CF. Key in the selection of their cohort is the presence of two centers, each of which performed exclusively one of the two procedures, creating a "pseudorandomization." They found equivalent outcomes in grip strength, range of motion, pain relief and satisfaction
44. Wolff AL, Garg R, Kraszewski AP, et al. Surgical treatments for scapholunate advanced collapse wrist: kinematics and functional performance. *J Hand Surg*. 2015;40(8):1547-1553.
45. De Smet L, Truyen J. Arthrodesis of the wrist for osteoarthritis: outcome with a minimum follow-up of 4 years. *J Hand Surg Br*. 2003;28(6):575-577.
46. Sagerfors M, Gupta A, Brus O, Pettersson K. Total wrist arthroplasty: a single-center study of 219 cases with 5-year follow-up. *J Hand Surg*. 2015;40(12):2380-2387.

QUESTIONS

1. **A 60-year-old woman comes into the office complaining of 6 weeks of pain at the base of the thumb of the dominant right hand. It interferes with her leisure activities of knitting and cooking. On examination, she has a positive grind test and weak grip strength. There is mild MCP hyperextension of 15 degrees. Her X-rays demonstrate decreased trapeziometacarpal joint space and a 1 mm osteophyte. No cystic changes are noted. What is the next step in management?**

   a. CMC arthrodesis
   b. Trapezium excision and ligament reconstruction/tendon interposition
   c. Spica cast immobilization for 2 months
   d. Pinning of the MCP in neutral for 6 weeks
   e. Splinting, NSAIDs, and steroid injection

2. **A 40-year-old carpenter is seen in clinic complaining of base of thumb pain and difficult with grip strength in his right, dominant hand. His thumb ray is adducted, and there is a palpable step-off over the dorsum of the thumb MCP and pain with axial loading. Imaging demonstrates 50% subluxation of the metacarpal and a 4-mm osteophyte with severe subchondral sclerosis. He has previously seen two other surgeons and received different recommendations from each. Which of the following options along with trapeziectomy is *not* recommended?**

   a. Tight-rope reconstruction
   b. Hematoma distraction pinning
   c. Palmaris longus interposition
   d. [illegible]
   e. FCR ligament reconstruction tendon interposition

3. **A 66-year-old accountant returns to your office 1 year after undergoing trapeziectomy and ligament reconstruction tendon interposition [illegible] ongoing dull, aching pain in the wrist in a similar position to her presurgical pain. There is no thumb MCP hyperextension, Tinel sign is absent, and range of motion and grip strength are symmetric when compared to the contralateral side. X-rays of the wrist are obtained and do not demonstrate proximal migration of the first metacarpal. What is the most likely cause of her continued pain?**

   a. Untreated scaphotrapezoid arthritis
   b. Injury to the superficial branch of the radial nerve intraoperatively
   c. Noncompliance with hand therapy postoperatively
   d. Undiagnosed scaphoid injury
   e. Long duration of symptoms prior to surgery predisposing to chronic pain

4. **A 72-year-old man presents to clinic with a pain and a nodule over the lateral aspect of the index DIP on the nondominant hand. Active range of motion is absent at the DIP. Gull-wing sign and complete loss of the joint space are present on imaging. What is the best treatment option for a functional outcome?**

   a. Excision of the Heberden nodule to control pain
   b. Fusion of the DIP in 15 degrees of flexion
   c. Repair of the FDP tendon to improve range of motion
   d. Joint excision and pyrocarbon arthroplasty
   e. Arthrodesis in full extension

5. **A 42-year-old smoker is diagnosed with SLAC wrist. During the informed consent process, you review his treatment options and discuss the risks of both PRC and 4CF. Which statement is correct regarding the outcomes of the two procedures?**

   a. In his age group, PRC has a higher likelihood of conversion to wrist fusion
   b. 4CF will provide him a greater arc of flexion and extension than PRC
   c. His grip strength will be markedly decreased in 4CF when compared to PRC.
   d. PRC will more effectively relieve his pain than 4CF.
   e. He is at higher risk for nonunion with 4CF.

1. **Answer: e.** In this patient with fairly early CMC arthritis, conservative management is the first-line treatment. Her pain has been of relatively short duration and her X-rays demonstrate mild disease—Eaton stage II is described. Rest, splinting, antiinflammatory use and steroids are all described as first-line treatment. Splinting may be hand based and does not need to be rigid; it may take up to 12 months to resolve symptoms. Steroids have been demonstrated to provide short-term pain relief in 40% of patients with early CMC arthritis.

2. **Answer: d.** Over 90% of the CMC arthroplasties performed in the United States use the ligament reconstruction tendon interposition method despite four other well-described options. Multiple studies have attempted unsuccessfully to quantify the "best" procedure for basal joint arthritis. Both metaanalyses and randomized control trials have failed to find a difference in objective or subjective outcomes with various reconstructions after trapeziectomy with the exception of prosthetic spacer placement. Use of silicone, Marlex, or Gore-tex increases short- and long-term complications and does not provide any functional benefit. Any of the above-listed options are viable treatments for CMC arthritis with the exception of silicone spacer placement, which is not recommended.

3. **Answer: a.** Failure to diagnose and treat arthritis at the STT joint at the time of CMC arthroplasty may lead to persistent pain in the base of the thumb. This is preventable if specifically assessed on preoperative radiographs and should be part of the routine workup when planning basal joint surgery. Patients complain of pain in a similar location to their CMC pain with the same dull, aching quality. Temporary relief may be achieved with steroid injections.

4. **Answer: b.** This patient has a preoperative ankylosis of his DIP joint with severe OA and should receive a fusion. Although some patients may prefer the cosmetic appearance of a finger fused in extension, the index finger DIP is more functional with a 10- to 20-degree bend during routine activities of daily living. Fusion as more than 20 degrees would be bothersome to the patient. Although arthroplasty may be considered in specific patients, pyrocarbon is not designed for DIP joints. A silicone implant acts primarily as a spacer, and the pre- and postoperative motion is usually unchanged. With this patient's inability to flex the fingertip at baseline, he has significant inflammation of his synovium and surrounding structures that joint replacement would not solve; so implant replacement would not improve his result. Heberden nodules have not been shown to contribute to pain and excision is not recommended. There is no evidence of FDP injury in this patient—his absent range of motion is due to severe arthritis and ankylosis of the joint—thus repair of the FDP tendon is not indicated.

5. **Answer: e.** In this smoker, nonunion is the greatest risk during 4CF. It is well accepted that nicotine is a risk factor for delayed and nonunions. As PRC does not have any bony healing to complete, this risk is not present if the other procedure is chosen. The remaining outcomes of PRC and 4CF are equivalent. Multiple retrospective studies, metaanalyses, and a well-designed cohort study have demonstrated the same range of motion, grip strength, pain relief, and patient satisfaction. 4CF does have a consistently greater arc of radial-ulnar deviation; however, this has not been proven significant in day-to-day activities. There have been concerns raised about the progression of arthritis in PRC given the different radii of curvature in the capitate and lunate; however, this has only been found to be clinically significant in patients under the age of 40.

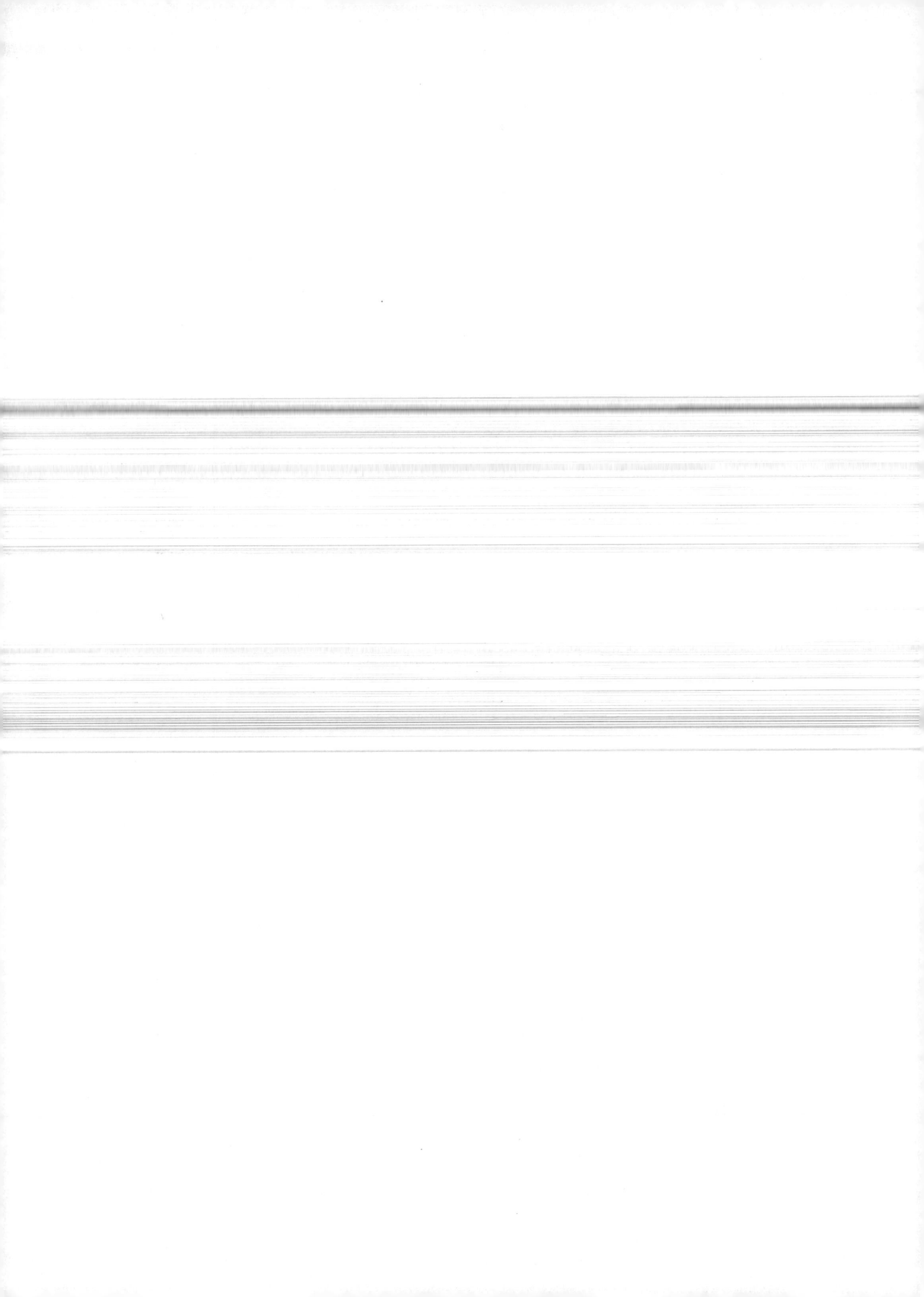

CHAPTER 94 Reconstruction of the Chest, Sternum, and Posterior Trunk

Alexander F. Mericli and Mark W. Clemens II

KEY POINTS

- A cohesive multidisciplinary approach is particularly important in thoracic reconstruction. A preoperative discussion with the thoracic surgeon should be made regarding the possibility of a latissimus-sparing thoracotomy.
- Anterior and lateral chest wall defects involving three or more adjacent ribs or that are 5 cm in width or greater will benefit from skeletal reconstruction. Posterior defects and resections in previously irradiated chest walls can tolerate a larger defect before skeletal reconstruction is necessary.
- Bioprosthetic mesh should be used for skeletal chest wall reconstruction in patients at high risk for wound healing complications, such as those with a history of radiation.
- Adequate treatment of a sternal wound infection includes adequate debridement, culture-directed antibiotics, and reconstruction with well vascularized soft tissue.
- The pectoralis major muscle flap is the workhorse flap for sternal and anterior chest wall reconstruction.
- Unlike other clinical scenarios involving infection and hardware, spinal instrumentation should be maintained at all costs in cases of acute wound infection.
- The paraspinous muscle advancement flap is the workhorse flap for midline posterior trunk wounds and is an adequate option at any spinal level.
- Prophylactic spinal wound reconstruction is prudent in high-risk situations, such as large resections/instrumentations, patients with multiple previous spinal surgeries, or a history or radiation, diabetes, obesity, or steroid use.

Defects of the chest wall and intrathoracic space can result from tumor resection, infection, radiation injury, or trauma, whereas sternal wounds are most frequently associated with infectious complications after cardiothoracic procedures, such as mediastinitis or sternal osteomyelitis. Soft tissue reconstruction of the posterior trunk is often related to tumor resection or infectious complications following spinal instrumentation. Thoracic and spinal wound reconstructions share a relatively unique distinction in plastic surgery in that the creation of a reliable, durable wound closure is truly a life-saving procedure. Therefore, an in-depth knowledge of and familiarity with these patients and surgical maneuvers are critical for all plastic and reconstructive surgeons. Although differing in anatomic location as well as etiology, the reconstructions of the chest, sternum, and posterior trunk share many of the same key principles, including adequate debridement, recruitment of well-vascularized soft tissue to fill dead space, and protection of vital structures and hardware using a durable external coverage.

CHEST WALL, STERNUM, AND INTRATHORACIC RECONSTRUCTION

Anatomy and Physiology

In addition to its role in protecting the heart, lungs, and mediastinum, the chest wall also serves an important physiologic function by harboring the muscles of respiration and maintaining a negative intrathoracic pressure.[1] The primary respiratory muscles include the diaphragm and the intercostal muscles. The intercostal muscles can be divided into three layers: the external, internal, and innermost. The intercostal neurovascular bundle runs along the interior surface of each rib, at the inferior border, between the internal and innermost muscle fibers; the nerve is most inferior, followed by the artery and then the vein. The thoracic skeleton serves to protect and contain the heart, lungs, and mediastinal structures and is an attachment point for the respiratory muscles. It comprises seven paired true ribs (which articulate with the sternum via costal cartilages), eight pairs of false ribs (which do not articulate with the sternum), and two pairs of floating ribs (11th and 12th), so called because they lack any connection to the sternum or the ribs superior to them (Figure 94.1). The sternum provides additional protection and structural support and consists of the manubrium, body, and xiphoid. The intrathoracic space, or pleural cavity, must remain intact to maintain a negative intrathoracic pressure. The parietal pleura lines the inner surface of the skeletal chest wall; a distinct structure termed as the visceral pleura lines the surface of the lungs and travels within each fissure, separating the lobes. Between the two pleurae is the fluid-filled pleural cavity.

Etiology

Chest wall defects can encompass soft tissue, skeletal structures, or both. The depth of the wound can involve only the skin and subcutaneous tissue or extend to full-thickness and into the intrathoracic space. A number of etiologies can contribute to these defects including neoplastic disease, infectious processes, osteoradionecrosis of the ribs and/or sternum, and trauma (**Table 94.1**).

The majority of chest wall wounds are the result of either the treatment or palliation of malignancy. Among these, the most common are locally invading tumors from adjacent structures, including breast cancer, lung cancer, mediastinal tumors, and mesothelioma.[2] A minority of chest wall lesions are caused by the hematogenous metastasis of solid tumors, most commonly sarcoma, followed by renal cell carcinoma, and gastrointestinal adenocarcinoma.[3] Adequate debridement of various infectious processes, such as mediastinitis, necrotizing fasciitis, or osteomyelitis, can result in a chest wall or sternal defect in need of reconstruction, as can trauma from ballistic, blunt-force, or blast injury. Lastly, osteoradionecrosis of the skeletal chest wall can emerge many years after the completion of radiation therapy, necessitating wide debridement and reconstruction with well-vascularized tissue.

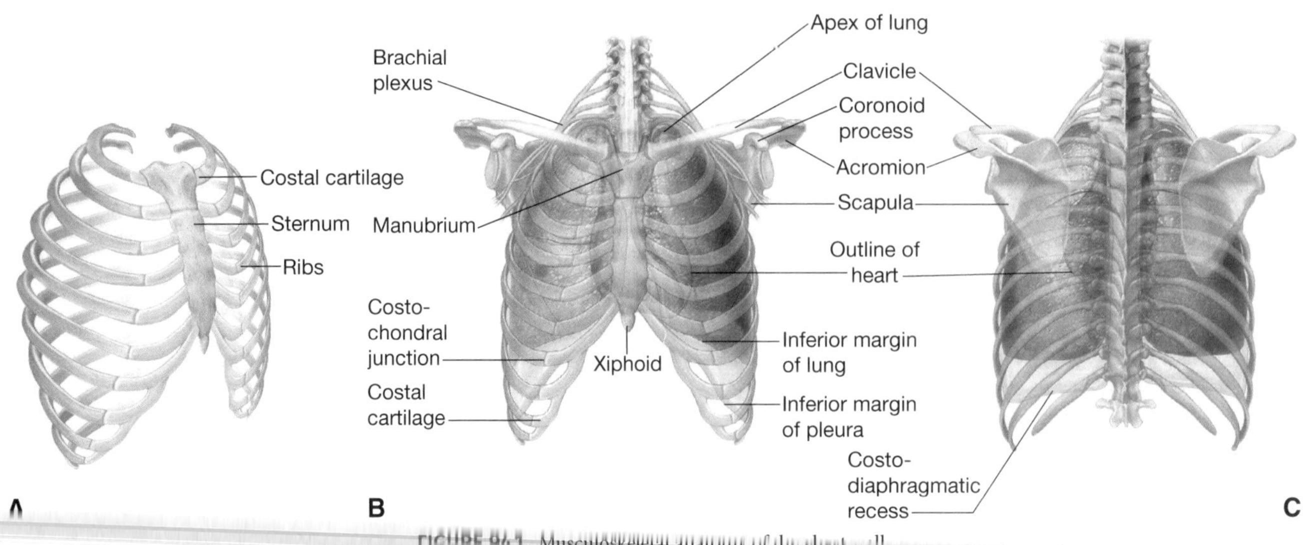

FIGURE 94.1. Musculoskeletal anatomy of the chest wall.

Preoperative Planning and Patient Selection

Compared to many other patient populations familiar to plastic surgery, those requiring thoracic reconstruction are often plagued with a multitude of comorbidities, such as obesity, diabetes, congestive heart failure, ischemic heart disease, and pulmonary disease. Patients must be optimized preoperatively to minimize potential complications. Glucose should be well controlled, nutrition and pre-albumin should be improved, and if possible, general deconditioning should be mitigated through preoperative physical therapy. For surgeries involving chest wall resection, partial, or complete lobectomy, preoperative pulmonary function testing is beneficial. Metrics such as forced vital capacity and forced expiratory volume in 1 second can help estimate the patient's ability to tolerate their extirpative surgery, which, in turn provides a more accurate prediction of their capacity for a complete recovery.[4]

TABLE 94.1. COMMON ETIOLOGIES OF THORACIC DEFECTS REQUIRING RECONSTRUCTION

Malignant Neoplasm
Locally advanced tumor Breast carcinoma Lung carcinoma
Primary tumor Soft tissue sarcoma Chondrosarcoma Ewing sarcoma
Metastatic tumor Sarcoma Renal cell carcinoma Gastrointestinal malignancy
Benign Neoplasm
Osteochondroma Chondroma Fibrous dysplasia Desmoid
Infection
Soft tissue Mediastinitis Osteomyelitis
Trauma
Osteoradionecrosis

A cohesive multidisciplinary approach is particularly important in thoracic reconstruction. A standard lateral thoracotomy will divide the latissimus dorsi muscle and a portion of the serratus anterior; both these muscles are workhorse flaps for the chest and must be preserved in case of their potential use. A preoperative discussion with the thoracic surgeon regarding the surgical approach and the possibility of a latissimus-sparing thoracotomy can be helpful. Regarding mediastinal defects after cardiac surgery, any reconstructive surgery or debridement should be performed in a cardiac surgery operating room, with the ability to accommodate a bypass pump if necessary, with a cardiac anesthesiologist and a cardiothoracic surgeon available. The plastic surgeon must have intimate knowledge of the coronary artery bypass grafts used, if any, so that well-vascularized flaps can be planned. Additionally, the plastic surgeon should be aware of any sternal wires or plating.

Chest Wall Skeletal Reconstruction

The goals of skeletal chest wall reconstruction include minimizing paradoxical motion, aiding pulmonary mechanics, protecting underlying thoracic viscera, and maintaining a normal chest contour. Functionally, reconstruction has been shown to decrease postoperative mechanical ventilation and length of stay.[5,6] The indications for chest wall skeletal reconstruction are controversial and should be determined on an individual basis. In general, guidelines suggest that defects involving three or more adjacent ribs along the anterior or lateral chest wall or defects with a diameter of 5 cm or greater will benefit from rigid reconstruction.[2,7,8] Posterior chest wall resections can typically tolerate a larger resection without the need for reconstruction given the additional stabilizing forces provided by the scapula and thoracic vertebrae. Similarly, defects in previously irradiated chest walls often do not require skeletal reconstruction because the radiation-related fibrosis will decrease chest wall compliance, which in turn, decreases the likelihood of paradoxical motion.

The ideal thoracic skeletal reconstruction promotes tissue ingrowth and is inert, malleable, and radiolucent.[9] Techniques using synthetic and biologic materials have been described. In general, synthetic materials are preferred in clean defects with minimal risk for complication (no history of radiation, few comorbidities, no current or past infection, nonfungating tumor, etc.). A variety of synthetic mesh materials have been described in chest wall reconstruction, the most common of which are polyethylene (Marlex; C.R. Bard, Inc., Bard Medical Division, Covington, GA), polypropylene (Prolene) (Ethicon LLC, Bridgewater, NJ), and expanded polytetrafluoroethylene (Gore-Tex; Gore & Associates, Newark, DE). Each material has its own advantages and disadvantages, summarized in **Table 94.2**. In general, all synthetic materials carry a risk of infection of up to 5% depending on the material and study.[5,10-12] Although not common, a

TABLE 94.2. MATERIALS USED FOR SKELETAL CHEST WALL RECONSTRUCTION

Material	Advantages	Disadvantages
Polyethylene	■ Inexpensive ■ Macroporous, permitting ingrowth	■ Prone to fraying and fragmentation ■ Contraindicated in contaminated/complex wounds ■ Infection necessitates removal
Polypropylene	■ Inexpensive ■ Macroporous, permitting ingrowth ■ Double-knitted; flexible in two dimensions	■ Contraindicated in contaminated/complex wounds ■ Infection necessitates removal
Expanded polytetrafluoroethylene	■ Watertight seal ■ Ease of handling	■ Encapsulates; no tissue ingrowth ■ Seroma formation ■ Contraindicated in contaminated/complex wounds ■ Infection necessitates removal
Methylmethacrylate	■ Used in combination with porous synthetic mesh ■ Can be molded to chest contour	■ Cures by an exothermic reaction, putting tissues at risk for thermal injury ■ May fracture ■ Rigidity is non-anatomic ■ No tissue ingrowth ■ Seroma formation
Bioprosthetic	■ Semi-rigid, dynamic ■ Incorporates into host tissues ■ Decreased risk of infection ■ Can be used in irradiated wounds	■ Expensive ■ Permeable ■ Will not maintain chest contour in large defects ■ Infection/exposure does not necessitate removal
Titanium rib plating	■ Anatomic design, recreating chest contour, and physiologic compliance ■ Improved pulmonary function	■ Expensive ■ Long term durability unknown ■ Requires an underlay synthetic or biologic mesh for pleural reconstruction ■ Requires specialty instrumentation ■ Radiopaque

wound infection in this situation can be a devastating complication, necessitating prolonged intravenous antibiotics, readmission, reoperation, and removal of the construct. In their extensive review of synthetic mesh chest wall reconstruction at M.D. Anderson Cancer Center, Spicer and colleagues identified a relatively low wound infection rate of 2.8%, and no significant association with the material used. In another study from the same institution, patients with and without Marlex chest wall stabilization were compared.[5] Patients with Marlex had 5% infection rate compared to 0% in those without Marlex. However, all patients with infection had coexistent necrosis of the overlying skin flaps; therefore, the authors recommend that any synthetic construct should be covered with a well-vascularized tissue, such as a muscle flap (Figure 94.2).

A bioprosthetic mesh is often favored in patients at high risk for wound healing complications (**Figure 94.2**). Due to their ability to incorporate into the patient and revascularize, these products have been shown to be resistant to infection and to function well in the irradiated defect.[13–15] Bioprosthetic meshes are classified by the source material—either xenograft or allograft. Initially human dermal allograft was most commonly used for chest wall reconstruction; however, more recent evidence suggests that porcine or bovine-derived material may be preferred for this application because of the lower amount of elastin compared to human dermis.[15,16] The decreased elastin content translates to a more anatomic, semirigid reconstruction, which better approximates normal chest wall biomechanics.

For large skeletal chest wall defects, synthetic and bioprosthetic meshes alone are unable to maintain the natural thoracic curvature. This has important implications not only for aesthetics, but also for pulmonary mechanics. Most commonly, sandwiching methylmethacrylate cement between two layers of porous synthetic mesh ameliorates this situation (**Figure 94.2**). Methylmethacrylate, however, has several disadvantages, including a tendency to fracture as well as an association with infection and seroma formation.[5,17] Because of these shortcomings, titanium rib plating osteosynthesis systems are gaining in popularity. These systems were initially utilized for the reconstruction of flail segments in the trauma patient. In flail chest injuries, rib osteosynthesis is associated with a decreased incidence of pneumonia, improved pulmonary function, faster return to work, and improved quality of life.[18] Recent design iterations have yielded spanning rib plates, which are useful for oncologic defects.[19,20] Spanning plate reconstructions have been associated with a low complication rate, good cosmetic result, and superior pulmonary function.[21,22] Rib spanning plates should always be combined with a synthetic or biologic mesh underlay for reconstruction of the parietal pleura and restoration of the negative intrathoracic pressure; and then should be covered anteriorly with a well-vascularized tissue, such as a muscle flap, to protect against possible exposure[20] (Figure 94.3).

Chest Wall Soft Tissue Reconstruction

Well-vascularized soft tissue coverage is vital to the success of any chest wall reconstruction. Adequate soft tissue is necessary for minimizing infection, protecting alloplastic implants, and promoting expeditious wound healing. This is especially critical after oncologic resection, in the setting of previous radiation or osteoradionecrosis, or in the presence of underlying prosthetic materials.

The principles illustrated by the reconstructive ladder can easily be applied to soft tissue chest wall reconstruction. Depending on the extent of the wound, patient comorbidities, and indications, reconstruction can be as simple as a skin graft or as complicated as a free tissue transfer.[23–27] Smaller defects can be reconstructed with a local flap or skin graft; a local flap may offer a superior cosmetic result, but its applicability is limited to smaller wounds. Alternatively, large partial thickness defects will require a skin graft. If the underlying rib, sternum, or hardware is exposed or if there is a history of radiation to the area, skin grafts or local random flaps are unlikely to be successful. In this scenario, a regional flap from outside the zone of radiation is a more appropriate choice; there are many options available, as the location of the chest is particularly conducive to regional reconstructive techniques (**Table 94.3**).[28,29] Many advocate for muscle flap coverage of underlying mesh or plates in patients requiring skeletal chest wall reconstruction.[5] Considering the devastating nature of a chest wall mesh infection or exposure, this technique is especially efficacious for patients at elevated risk for delayed healing (previous infection, high BMI, diabetes, history of radiation, smoking, etc).

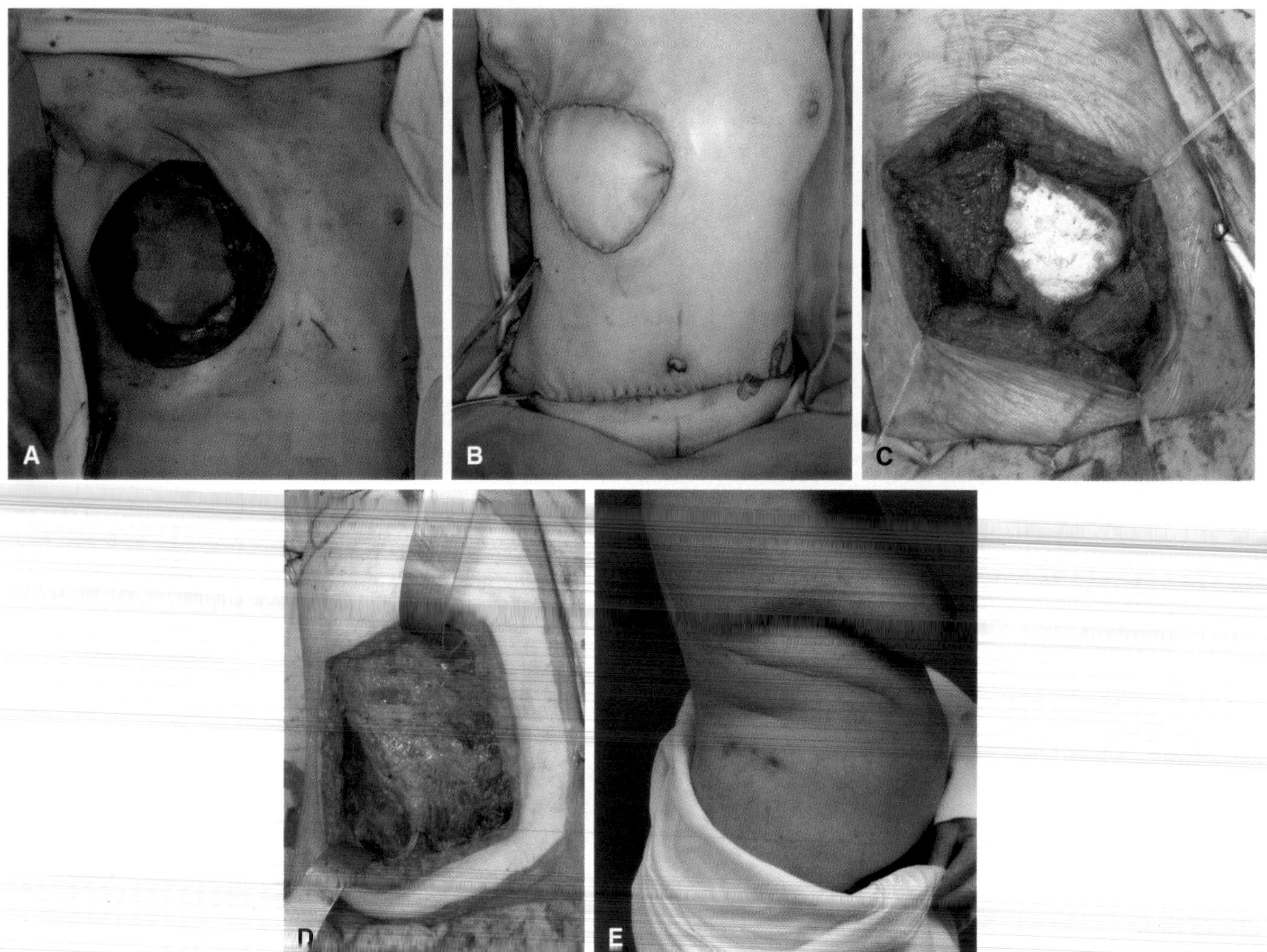

FIGURE 94.3 Skeletal chest wall reconstruction. **A.** A 56-year-old woman with locally advanced breast cancer invading the chest wall. She had been previously treated with radiation, and therefore a bioprosthetic mesh [illegible] the anterior chest wall after resection of four adjacent ribs. **B.** Postoperative result after coverage with a pedicled TRAM flap. **C.** A 58-year-old woman with metastatic colon cancer to the lateral right eighth rib. [illegible] resected and the defect was reconstructed with a polyethylene-methylmethacrylate sandwich. **D.** The synthetic chest wall construct was covered with a pedicled right latissimus dorsi muscle flap. **E.** Postoperative result.

Despite the numerous regional flap options, large chest wall defects such as those resulting from extensive oncologic resection, invasive infection, or osteoradionecrosis may require microsurgical techniques. Microsurgical tissue transfer provides great freedom in the reconstruction, as flap design and inset are not constrained by the length and positioning of the pedicle. Furthermore, provided that the anastomosis is technically excellent, the vascular supply of a free flap tends to be more robust and reliable than that of a pedicled flap, translating to a lower incidence of partial flap loss. Arya and colleagues report an extensive experience in microsurgical chest wall reconstruction, demonstrating a low complication rate and a 96% flap success rate.[30] Limiting the reconstructive indication to oncologic chest defects, Cordeiro et al. demonstrate a 100% free flap success rate.[27] Recipient vessel options in microsurgical chest wall reconstruction have been extensively described in the breast reconstruction literature and most commonly include the internal mammary or thoracodorsal vessels.

Radiation is commonly employed as part of the modern multimodality approach to thoracic malignancy. Neoadjuvant and adjuvant treatment plans may include radiation for the treatment of breast and lung cancers. Certain connective tissue tumors, such as Ewing sarcoma, are treated primarily with radiation therapy. Other sarcomas, such as angiosarcoma, may occur as a side effect of previous radiation therapy, necessitating wide resection in an irradiated field. Treatment of a radiation-related wound often requires a wide resection, by continuing tissue resection until a well-vascularized tissue is encountered (Figure 94.4). Given the blunted angiogenesis exhibited by irradiated tissue, skin grafts and local flaps have low utility, with most plastic surgeons preferring regional flaps instead.[2,31–35] The avoidance of synthetic materials in the irradiated chest wall is recommended; if skeletal reconstruction is necessary, bioprosthetic mesh is better tolerated due to its ability to revascularize. Unfortunately, despite an adequate debridement and reconstruction, wounds in an irradiated field are incredibly complex and continue to be prone to infection, wound dehiscence, and soft tissue fibrosis.

Sternal Wound Reconstruction

Most commonly, sternal wound reconstruction is required as part of the surgical treatment of an infected median sternotomy incision. A similar defect may be created after oncologic sternectomy, however this etiology is less common. Mediastinitis occurs in 0.25% to 5% of patients after cardiac surgery.[36–38] Risk factors include advanced age, chronic obstructive pulmonary disorder, smoking, diabetes, steroid use, immunosuppression, morbid obesity, reoperative surgery, and off-midline sternotomy. Pairolero and Arnold classified sternal wound infections into three distinct subtypes.[39] Type 1 infections are defined by faint erythema and serosanguinous incisional drainage within the first few postoperative days. These wounds are typically sterile and not infected, therefore their classification as a type 1

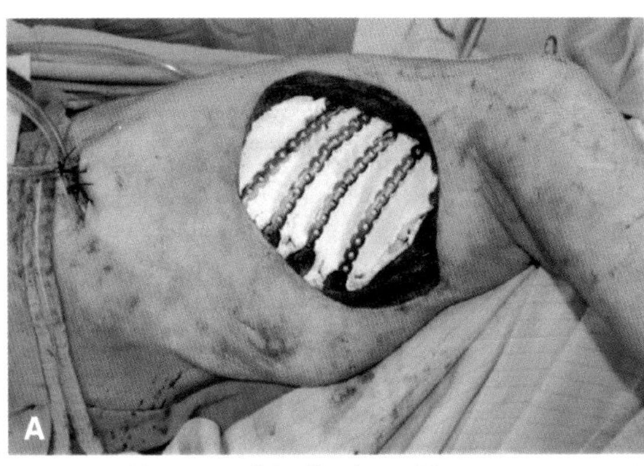

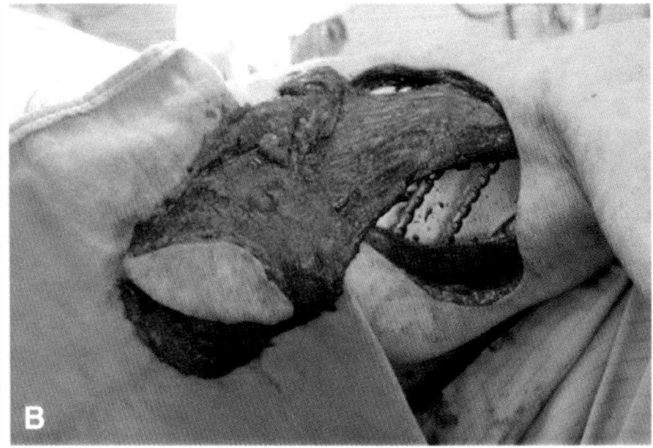

FIGURE 94.3. A 63-year-old woman with locally advanced lung cancer necessitating a latissimus-sparing thoracotomy, five-rib chest wall resection, and right lung lobectomy. **A,B.** Pleural defect reconstructed with Gore-Tex mesh, chest wall reconstructed with four titanium rib-spanning plates and pedicled latissimus myocutaneous flap.

infection is a misnomer. On the contrary, the type 1 wound is caused by mechanical failure of the sternal wire closure; in the absence of infection, these wounds can be treated effectively with conservative debridement and irrigation. If the type 1 patient proceeds to a symptomatic sternal nonunion, as defined by pain or a bothersome *click*, then the ineffective wires can be removed and the residual sternum can be rigidly fixated with titanium plates. Type 2 infections occur within the first few weeks and exhibit frankly purulent drainage and significant cellulitis. A type 3 infection is indicative of a chronic infection, due to osteomyelitis, costochondritis, or a retained foreign body. In general, type 2 and 3 infections require at least one significant debridement followed by a muscle flap wound reconstruction. Patients presenting with signs and symptoms of mediastinitis should have wound and blood cultures obtained. A CT scan of the chest can be helpful for identifying drainable abscesses. If osteomyelitis is suspected, an MRI permits visualization of the extent of disease and is useful in planning the debridement.

An adequate debridement is the cornerstone of the surgical management of mediastinitis. Such debridements are aggressive, including removal of all nonviable soft tissue, cartilage, and bone, until uniform bleeding is appreciated from the remaining tissues. All hardware and sternal wires should be removed. If definitive reconstruction is not possible after the first debridement, negative pressure therapy may be used to temporize the wound and stabilize the tissues. Negative pressure therapy decreases the number of days between the initial operative debridement and definitive closure, expedites the formation of granulation tissue within the wound, encourages angiogenesis, promotes wound contraction, and reduces the number and frequency of dressing changes.[40]

The need for rigid sternal fixation is controversial. Many believe that median sternotomy wound reconstruction is successful with soft tissue flaps only. This is based on the concept that limiting the number of foreign bodies within the wound (i.e., wires and plates) minimizes the risk of persistent infection. Other reconstructive surgeons prefer to adhere to the principles of osteosynthesis, which state that rigid skeletal fixation, such as titanium plating, reduces or eliminates micromotion at the osteotomy site, thereby promoting healing and decreasing infection. Titanium sternal plating systems may be best reserved for high-risk patients with multiple comorbidities contributing to poor healing. Indeed, in this patient population, prophylactic sternal plating may reduce or even prevent mediastinitis.[11,12]

Sternal wound soft tissue reconstruction is most commonly achieved with pectoralis major muscle flaps. Based on the thoracoacromial vessels, the pectoralis major muscle can be disinserted from its humeral attachment and advanced medially. Uni- or bilateral advancement flaps can resurface the superior two-thirds of the sternum. If the wound has a significant dead space component, or involves the inferior third of the sternum, a turnover pectoralis flap based on the internal mammary perforating vessels may be a better option. A turnover flap is contraindicated if the internal mammary

TABLE 94.3. COMMON REGIONAL FLAPS USED FOR CHEST WALL COVERAGE[28,29]

Flap	Included Tissues	Approximate Size (cm)	Vascular Supply	Common Applications
Pectoralis major	Muscle or myocutaneous	15 × 23	■ Thoracoacromial ■ Internal mammary perforators	■ Anterior chest ■ Sternal wound ■ Intrathoracic space
Serratus anterior	Muscle	15 × 20	■ Serratus branch of thoracodorsal ■ Lateral thoracic vessels	■ Intrathoracic space
Latissimus dorsi	Muscle or myocutaneous	25 × 35	■ Thoracodorsal vessels ■ Intercostal and lumbar perforators	■ Anterior, lateral, and posterior chest ■ Intrathoracic space
Rectus abdominis	Muscle or myocutaneous	25 × 6	■ Deep inferior and superior epigastric vessels	■ Anterior chest ■ Sternal wound
External oblique	Myocutaneous	15 × 30	■ Lumbar perforators	■ Inferior third of anterior chest
Omentum	Visceral adipose	Variable	■ Right or left gastroepiploic	■ Sternal wound ■ Intrathoracic space
Thoracodorsal artery perforator flap	Fasciocutaneous	8 × 35	■ Thoracodorsal	■ Anterior, lateral, and posterior chest
Intercostal artery perforator flap	Fasciocutaneous	5 × 15	■ Intercostal perforator	■ Small anterior chest wounds

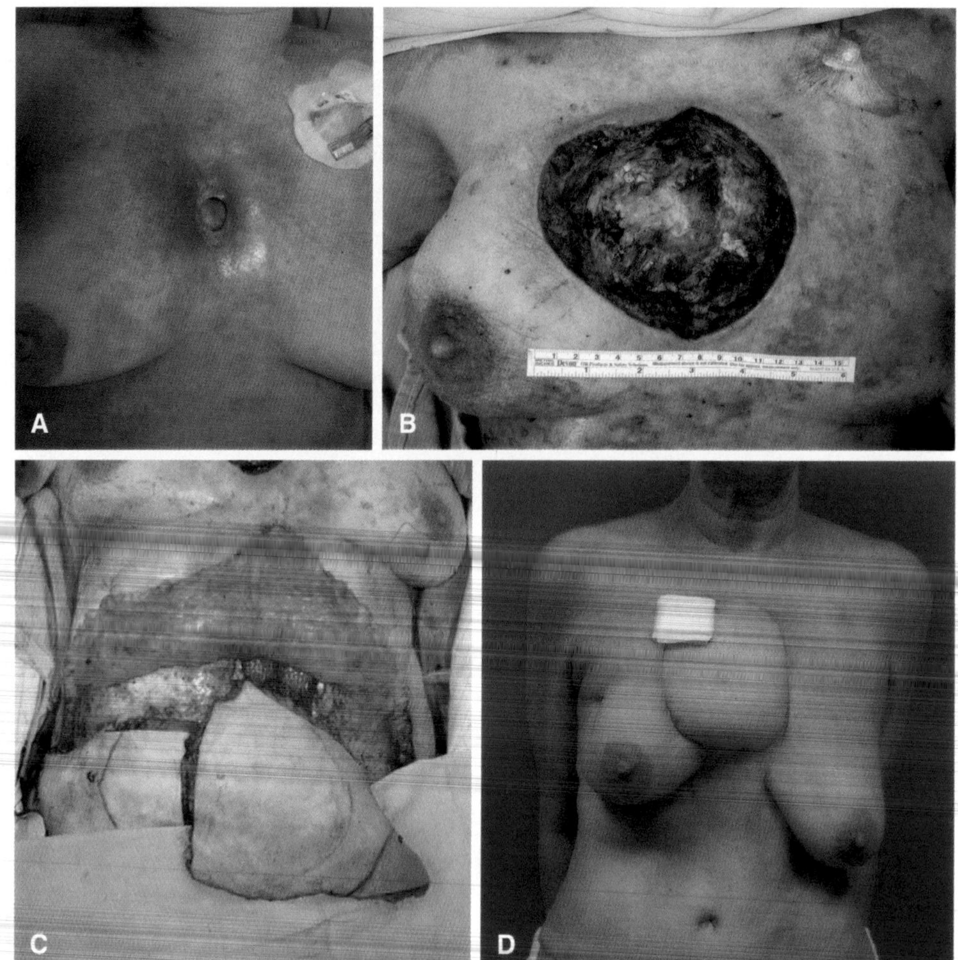

FIGURE 94.4. **A.** Osteoradionecrosis of the sternum and ribs presenting as a draining sinus. **B.** Resulting defect after adequate debridement, consisting of partial sternectomy. **C.** Right pedicled TRAM flap for reconstruction of the defect. **D.** Postoperative result.

artery has been used for coronary revascularization. Second-line options for soft tissue reconstruction of the median sternotomy wound include the superiorly-based rectus abdominis flap or an omentum flap. A vertically or transversely-oriented skin paddle can be included with the rectus abdominis muscle if additional volume or cutaneous resurfacing is needed. Although there are reports of designing a superiorly-based rectus abdominis flap on the eighth intercostal vessels when the internal mammary vessels have been disrupted, doing so is not advisable if other flap options are available. In such a scenario, the omentum flap can be designed on either the left or right gastroepiploic vessels and routed into the mediastinum either through the diaphragm or externally out through the epigastric abdominal wall and into the chest. The omentum provides a large surface area of well-vascularized tissue that can easily fill and resurface the entire mediastinum. Depending on the cutaneous requirement of the wound, the native chest skin can be closed over the omentum flap or, if skin coverage is limited, the flap can be skin grafted. Disadvantages of the omentum flap are the possibility of an epigastric or diaphragmatic hernia, the need to enter the abdomen, and the inherent complications of doing so (ileus, bowel obstruction, injury to viscera) and the unpredictable size and quality of the omentum in thin individuals or in those with previous abdominal surgery. To minimize abdominal donor site morbidity, the omentum flap may be elevated laparoscopically in select patients.

Midline sternal defects may also occur after partial or total sternectomy for oncologic purposes. Similar to the lateral chest wall, metastatic tumors are the most common indication for oncologic sternectomy, followed by primary bone or soft tissue tumor and osteoradionecrosis.[43] The pectoralis major muscle flap is a reliable option for soft tissue reconstruction unless there is a large cutaneous resection, in which case a free tissue transfer may be more appropriate[43] (Figure 94.5).

Intrathoracic Reconstruction

Intrathoracic, or pleural cavity, reconstruction is most commonly associated with the presence of an empyema or bronchopleural fistula. An empyema is a purulent infection between the visceral and parietal pleura. A bronchopleural fistula, often coexistent with an empyema, is a communication between the bronchiolar airway and the pleural cavity. If not appropriately treated, these complications are associated with a high mortality rate after pneumonectomy. Similar to the pelvis, the intrathoracic cavity is a bony, noncollapsible space. Therefore, deep space infections are unlikely to resolve unless the cavity is either collapsed down or filled with vascularized tissue. Historically, this was addressed via the thoracoplasty, in which multiple ribs were removed to collapse of the chest wall, or through the creation of an Eloesser flap, which is essentially a marsupialization of the pleural cavity to form a controlled fistula for spontaneous drainage.[44] Although still sometimes performed in certain clinical scenarios, these antiquated techniques have now largely fallen out of favor.

The omentum, latissimus dorsi, serratus anterior, rectus abdominis, and pectoralis major muscles are all options for filling the pleural cavity with well-vascularized tissue (Figure 94.6). After an adequate debridement, such flaps can help to heal an empyema cavity or seal a dehisced bronchial stump. Flaps can also be transferred prophylactically in patients thought to be at high risk for bronchial stump

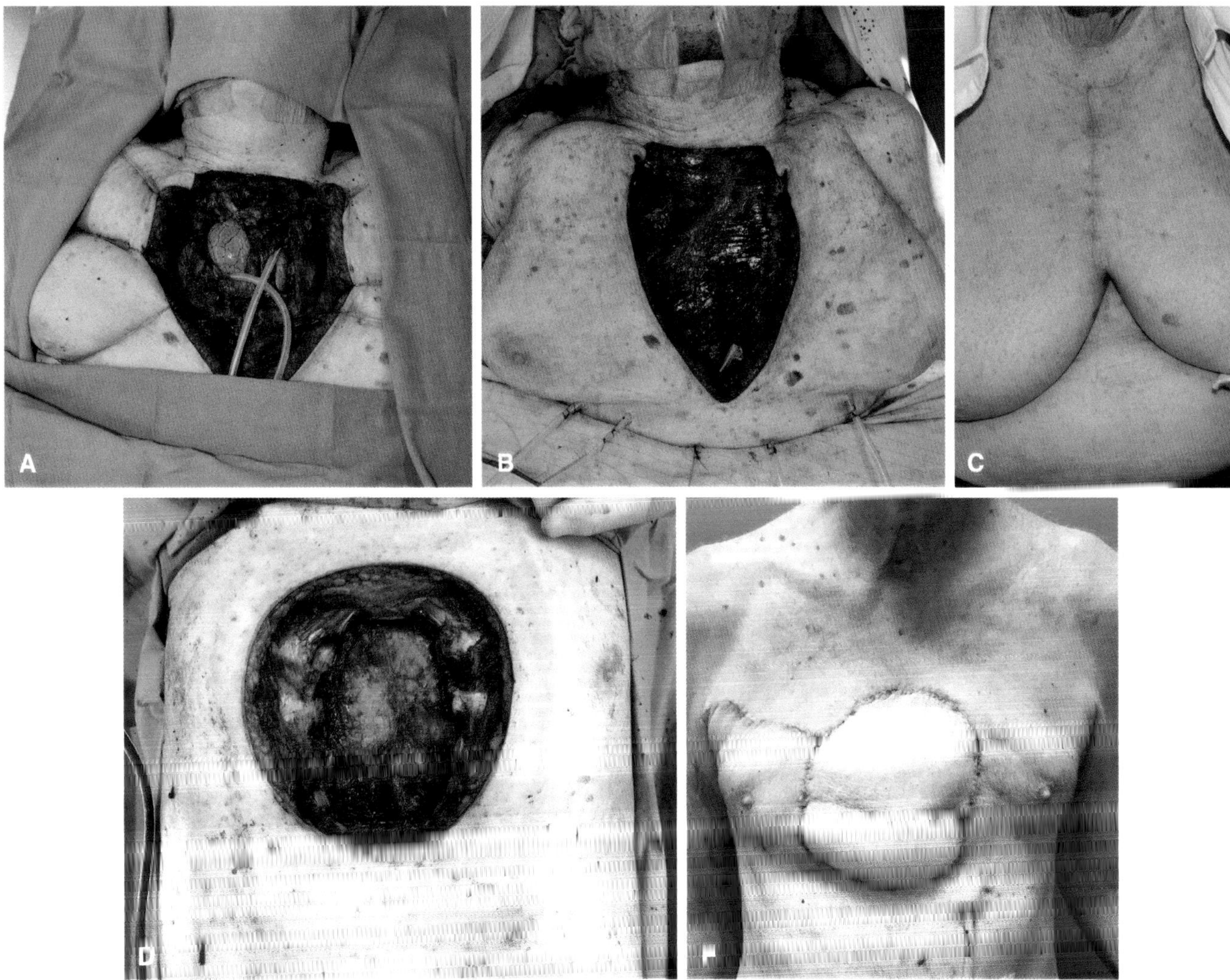

FIGURE 94.5. **A.** Partial sternectomy with exposure of right lung and great vessels after resection of metastatic thyroid cancer. **B.** Chest wall and great vessels covered with bilateral pectoralis major advancement flaps. **C.** Postoperative result. **D.** Total sternectomy after resection of locally advanced squamous cell carcinoma. The skeletal defect was reconstructed with a bioprosthetic mesh and, due to the significant skin resection, the cutaneous defect was reconstructed with a free TRAM flap. **E.** Postoperative result.

dehiscence after pneumonectomy such as those with previous radiation or multiple past thoracic procedures.[45] The latissimus, serratus, and pectoralis muscles are transferred into the chest cavity through the space created by a removal of a rib, whereas the rectus abdominis muscle and omentum are passed into the chest through a surgically created diaphragmatic window. Transposition of well-vascularized tissue into the pleural cavity for the treatment of empyema and bronchopleural fistula is an effective maneuver associated with a 73% resolution of infection in Arnold and Pairolero's landmark series.[46]

POSTERIOR TRUNK RECONSTRUCTION

Anatomy and Physiology

A thorough understanding of the cross-sectional musculoskeletal anatomy at the cervical, thoracic, and lumbosacral regions is essential in undertaking a posterior trunk reconstruction (Figure 94.7). The spinal cord travels through the vertebral foramen; the anterior wall of the foramen is the posterior aspect of the vertebral body; the posterior wall of the foramen consists of the bilateral lamina and spinal process, and the side walls are made up of the bilateral pedicles. The cord ends at L1/L2 and the dural sac terminates at S3. The paired paraspinous muscles, also known as the erector spinae, parallel the spine and function to stabilize and extend the vertebrae. The paraspinous muscles are made up of three distinct muscle bellies—spinalis, longissimus, and iliocostalis—and travel the length of the spine. The trapezius muscle is the most superficial muscle in the midline posterior trunk, extending from the occiput to the T12 spinous process and fanning out laterally to attach to the bilateral scapular spines. More inferiorly, the trapezius overlaps with the latissimus dorsi muscle from T7 to T12. The latissimus dorsi muscle transitions into the thoracolumbar fascia medially; this is most prominent in the lumbar region. The paraspinous muscles are immediately deep to the latissimus dorsi, except in the T10-L1 location, where the serratus posterior inferior muscle fibers may be found sandwiched between the paraspinous and latissimus dorsi.

Etiology

Reconstruction of the lateral posterior trunk is most commonly required after the surgical resection of soft tissue malignancy. Cutaneous malignancies such as melanoma or connective tissue tumors such as sarcoma often necessitate a wide local excision, making primary approximation of the resulting wound difficult.

Reconstruction of the midline posterior trunk wound is most commonly related to spinal instrumentation and fusion. Spinal hardware has evolved and improved tremendously over the past

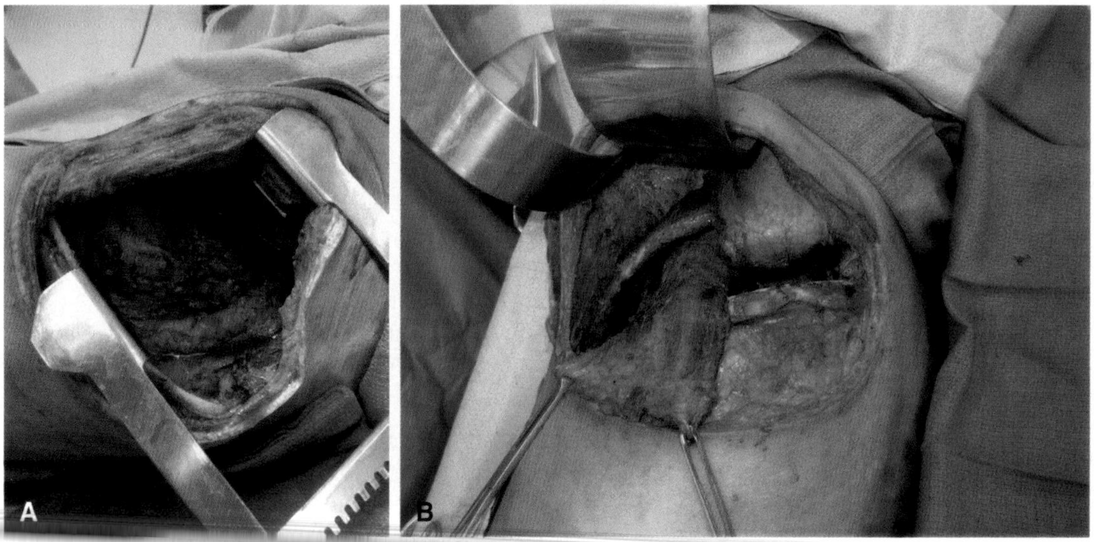

FIGURE 94.6. **A.** Intrathoracic defect in a 28-year-old woman after left pneumonectomy [illegible]. **B.** Bronchus stump closure reinforced with an intrathoracic pedicled serratus anterior muscle flap, passed into the thorax via a partial rib resection superior to the thoracotomy. Note the transected latissimus [illegible] as this was not a latissimus-sparing thoracotomy.

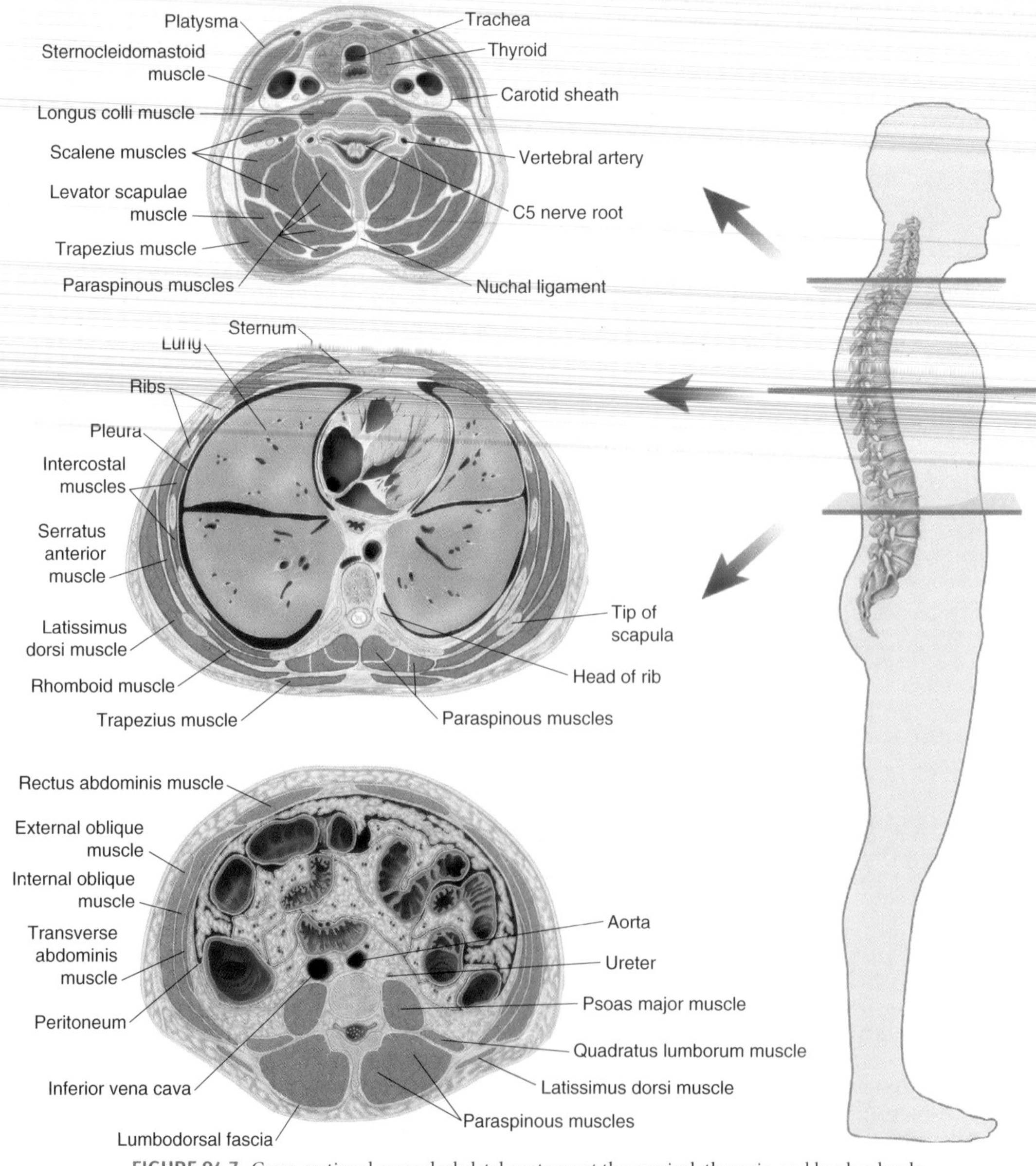

FIGURE 94.7. Cross-sectional musculoskeletal anatomy at the cervical, thoracic, and lumbar levels.

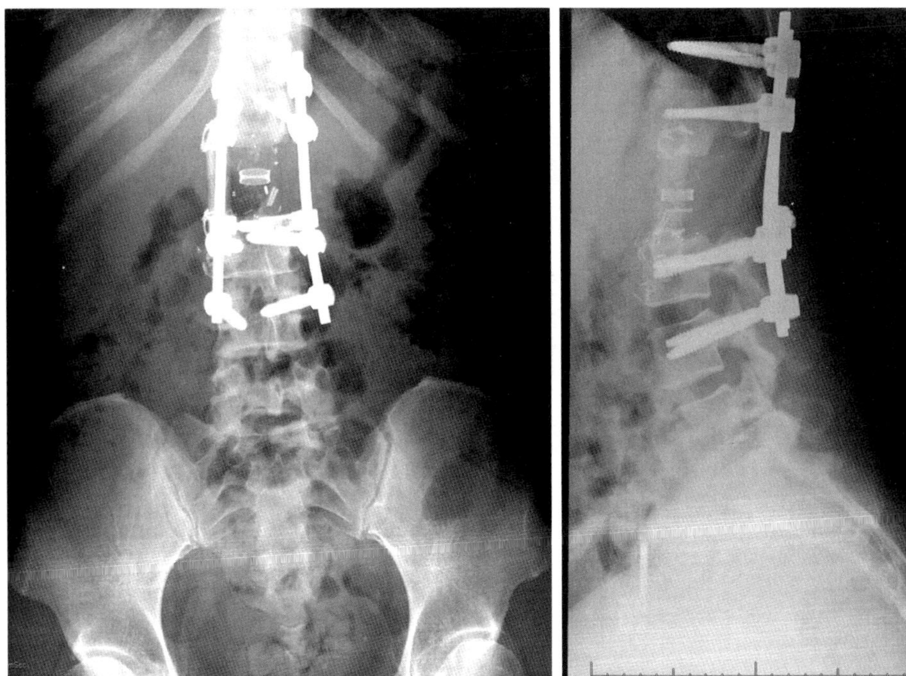

FIGURE 94.8. Six-month postoperative radiographs of a 36-year-old woman after L2 vertebrectomy for chordoma with free fibula flap plus polyetheretherketone expandable cage for vertebral body reconstruction.

two decades. Long posterior constructs spanning the length of the spine are now routinely performed for the correction of deformity. Simultaneous anterior and posterior spine exposures for multilevel oncologic vertebrectomies are possible, allowing for curative resection of what was previously considered unresectable disease. However, such extensive instrumentations come at a cost: to achieve the necessary exposure, the surrounding soft tissues are widely stripped and elevated away from the vertebrae, creating significant dead space and a challenging environment for normal wound healing.

Soft tissue reconstruction of the midline posterior trunk wound may be requested after the occurrence of a wound healing complication (infection, hematoma, seroma, skin edge separation, hardware exposure, etc.) following any variety of spine surgeries. In high-risk patients, such as those with a history of multiple previous spine surgeries, radiation therapy to the spine, neoadjuvant chemotherapy, obesity, or diabetes, the plastic surgeon may be asked to perform an immediate muscle flap reconstruction at the time of the index surgery to protect the hardware and obliterate dead space—with the intention of preventing a wound healing complication.[47-49] Although most reconstruction in the posterior trunk involves soft tissue, the plastic surgeon may play a role in skeletal reconstruction as well. The mainstay of bony fusion in spine surgery is a nonvascularized particulate bone graft in conjunction with rigid fixation; however, in spinal osseous defects >4 cm, up to 50% of patients fail to progress to fusion.[50] In these long constructs—often seen after vertebrectomy or sacroiliac joint resection—vascularized bone flaps can be a useful adjunct in addition to the standard instrumentation and particulate bone graft[51-53] (Figure 94.8).

Approach to Patient and Patient Selection

Wound healing complications after spinal instrumentation should be approached systematically and aggressively. Deep space infections, skin edge separations, seromas, and hematomas can easily lead to hardware exposure or loss—a devastating complication in spine surgery, associated with the possibility of paralysis and death. The plastic surgeon should communicate directly with the spine surgery team and have a thorough understanding of the surgical approach used and other important details. Is the hardware low profile? Was there a durotomy/is there concern for a cerebrospinal fluid leak? Was the spine approached anteriorly, posteriorly, or both? Has this patient had other spine surgeries? What disease process necessitated the spine surgery? Are there any fluid collections on imaging? The patient's wound healing physiology should also be optimized. A high protein diet should be initiated. If the patient is being treated with steroids, vitamin A supplementation should be considered. If the patient is paralyzed or otherwise immobile due to polytrauma or obesity, a low-pressure bed should be provided. In the paralyzed patient, involuntary muscle spasms and joint contractures that could result in additional wound closure tension should be ameliorated. Early infections (<6 weeks from the index procedure) are usually adequately treated with antibiotics, aggressive surgical debridement, and muscle flap reconstruction with maintenance of the spinal instrumentation. Chronic hardware infections, defined as a deep space infection at least 6 months after hardware placement, are difficult to effectively eradicate. In this situation, an MRI should be obtained to evaluate for vertebral osteomyelitis. In addition to debridement, the patient may require hardware removal and replacement for definitive treatment.

Lateral Defect

Nonmidline posterior trunk wounds are caused by a variety of pathologies, and therefore require a variety of solutions. Compared to midline spine wounds, the reconstructive approach to the lateral defect is more standard, following the typical dogma of plastic surgery. If the wound cannot be closed primarily, it can be skin grafted, provided there is a well-vascularized base. Aesthetically, some surgeons prefer local flap reconstructions in wounds that could be otherwise closed with a skin graft (Figure 94.9). Other wounds, due to exposed bone, hardware, or previous radiation, may not reliably heal with a skin graft, thereby necessitating a flap. Available regional flaps are the latissimus dorsi, trapezius, and lumbar perforator flaps. Free tissue transfer is complicated by the relative paucity of recipient vessels. The thoracodorsal vessels may be an option, but a vein graft or arteriovenous loop is needed.

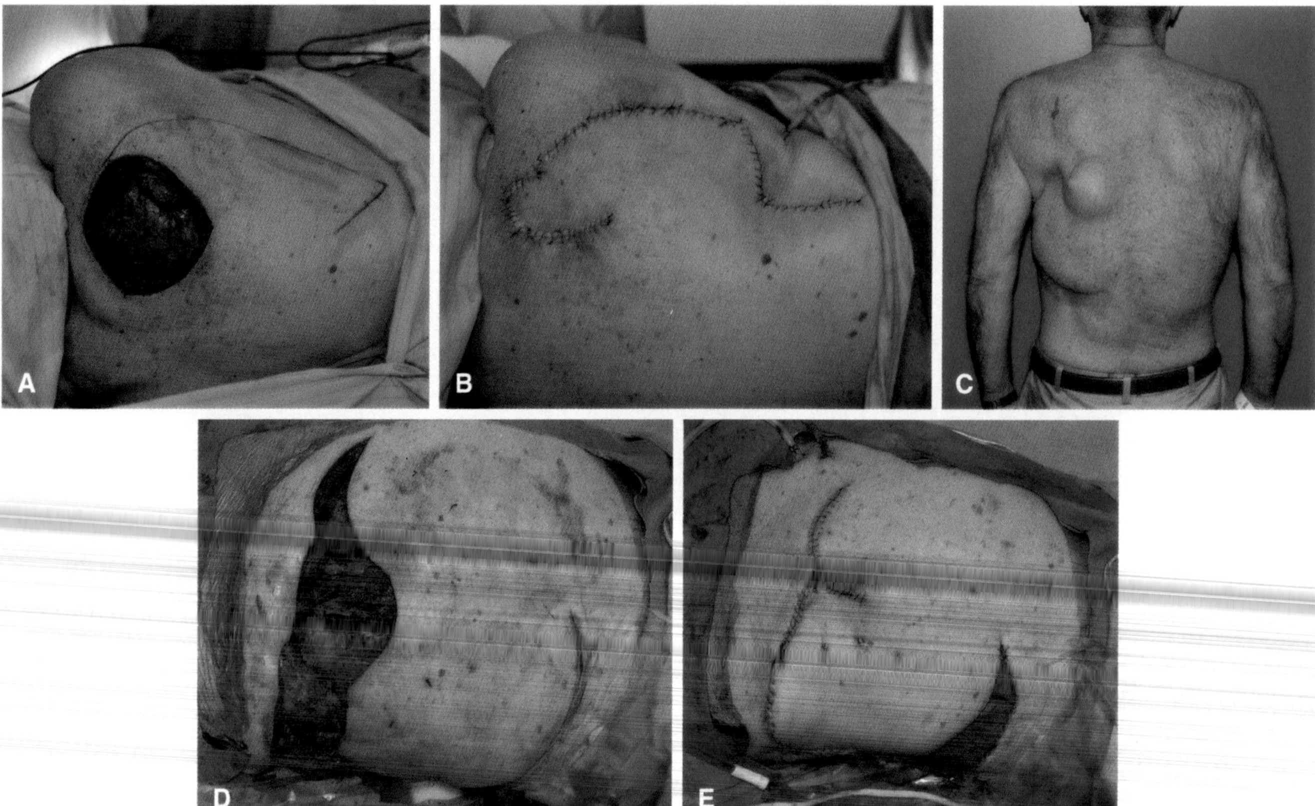

FIGURE 94.9. Defects of the lateral posterior trunk reconstructed with local flaps. **A,B.** Wide local excision of melanoma reconstructed with a hatchet flap. **C–E.** A 55-year-old man with recurrent posterolateral trunk sarcoma in an irradiated field. He was previously reconstructed with a fasciocutaneous rotation flap. Mass excised and defect reconstructed with readvancement of the rotation flap and split-thickness skin grafting of the donor site.

Midline Posterior Trunk Defects

A thorough debridement is a critical first step in the reconstruction of postsurgical back wounds. The entire incision should be opened in the operating room and all spine instrumentation exposed. The plastic surgeon should be knowledgeable about the initial spine surgery performed; if a laminectomy or partial/total vertebrectomy has been performed, the spinal cord and dura are vulnerable to injury during the debridement. All nonviable soft tissue and unincorporated bone graft should be removed. The wound should be copiously irrigated with antibiotic saline, and all purulent fluid should be drained. If the wound can be adequately debrided with a single procedure, then it should be fully closed over multiple drains, with the addition of a well-vascularized muscle flap for dead space obliteration, protection of the cord and hardware. If the wound is frankly purulent or still not clearly demarcated and therefore will require additional debridements, the drains should be placed in the deep space and the paraspinous muscles should be loosely approximated over the vertebra and hardware. The skin can be left open and a negative pressure wound dressing applied. Once the wound has declared itself and been fully debrided, it can be definitely closed with muscle flap transposition and skin reapproximation. Because of the proximity of the central nervous system, in this scenario it is advisable to return to the operating room and perform all dressing changes under general anesthesia.

Unlike the extremity, in which hardware present in an infected or dehisced wound is oftentimes removed, spine hardware should be maintained if at all possible.[54] Hardware maintains spinal stability, protects the spinal cord, and acts to stabilize the wound. Hardware that is well fixed promotes healing and prevents infection by eliminating micromotion and shearing of the fragile, traumatized soft tissues.

Paraspinous Muscle Flaps

As indicated by their name, the paraspinous muscles parallel the spine, traveling from the occiput and mastoid process down to terminate in the lumbosacral recess. These paired muscles represent the workhorse flaps for reconstruction of midline posterior trunk defects. On each side, the paraspinous muscles consist of three separate muscles: spinalis, longissimus, and iliocostalis. These muscle bellies can be indistinct, interdigitating, and creating the illusion of a single muscle on either side of the spine. The paraspinous muscles are perfused through a medial and lateral row of segmental perforating vessels from the lumbar, intercostal, or vertebral vessels, depending on the level, making them Mathes and Nahai type 4 flaps. Dissection must be performed immediately superficial to the paraspinous muscles until the lateral border is reached; at this point, the fascia is divided allowing for medial advancement. The muscles are then imbricated into the midline defect using a Lembert suture, which nicely directs the medial third of the flap into the dead space[55] (**Figure 94.10**). A summary of other common flaps for midline posterior trunk reconstruction can be found in **Table 94.4**.

Cervical Region

The most common indications for instrumentation of the cervical spine include cervical spinal stenosis and degenerative disk disease. In these situations, the cervical spine is most commonly instrumented anteriorly; these wounds rarely develop complications. Although more infrequent compared to the anterior approach, the posterior approach to the cervical spine is more likely to have a wound healing complication or infection. Posterior

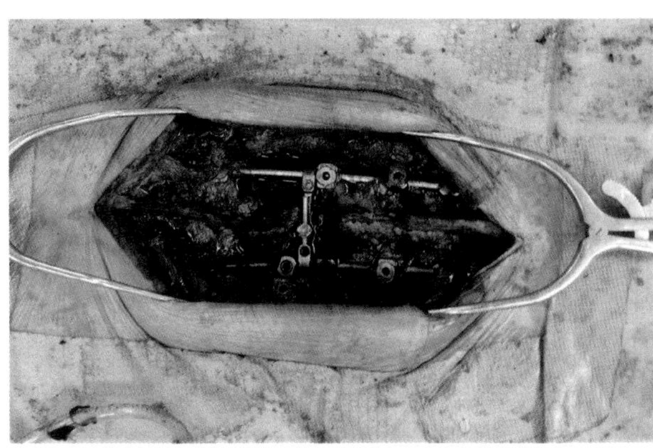

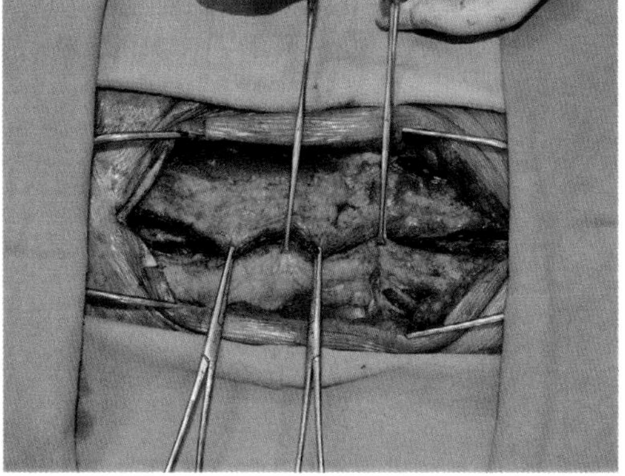

FIGURE 94.10. Bilateral paraspinous muscle advancement flaps for protection of exposed spinal cord and posterior instrumentation.

cervical wound complications involving instrumentation can be reliably reconstructed with bilateral paraspinous muscle flaps, despite their relatively thin caliber in this area.[56] Trapezius muscle flaps may also be used; however, they have a high seroma rate.[57] If cutaneous coverage is necessary, the trapezius muscle flap can be designed with a skin paddle. Fasciocutaneous perforator flaps are another option for cutaneous reconstruction in the midline posterior cervical spine.[58]

Thoracic Region

Midline posterior thoracic wounds after spine surgery can be treated with a variety of flaps. Bilateral paraspinous muscle advancement flaps are most commonly employed and should be considered a first-line option. However, there are situations in which the paraspinous muscles may be unavailable or inadequate for the obliteration of dead space and hardware protection. This could occur in patients who have had multiple previous spine surgeries, in patients whose paraspinous muscles have been resected in cases of spinal malignancy, or in patients who have been previously treated with radiation therapy, leaving the adjacent paraspinous musculature fibrotic and of poor quality. In these scenarios, the latissimus dorsi muscle can reach the superior midline thoracic back as an advancement flap. If the defect is along the inferior thoracic back or has a significant volumetric component, then a reverse latissimus dorsi flap—based on the thoracic and lumbar perforating vessels—may be a better option.[59] Yet another option, the omentum flap can be tunneled through the retroperitoneum to fill dead space along the thoracic spine.[60]

Locally advanced lung cancers and some primary bone tumors of the vertebra may necessitate a composite resection of the chest wall and thoracic spine. In this scenario, both anatomic areas will require soft tissue reconstruction. If a partial or total vertebrectomy has been performed and the pleural space has been entered, then the spinal cord and chest cavity are in continuity. The natural anatomic separation of the spinal cord, vertebral hardware, and chest cavity must be re-established by the interposition of healthy well-vascularized soft tissue.[61] This is usually achieved with a latissimus or trapezius muscle flap (Figure [illegible]). The thoracic spinal cord and hardware are typically protected by the imbrication of paraspinous muscle flaps. Despite the addition of a spine wound component to the defect, the standard parameters for skeletal chest wall reconstruction should be sufficient in restoring a normal chest wall contour and preventing paradoxical ventilation.

TABLE 94.4. COMMON FLAPS FOR MIDLINE POSTERIOR TRUNK RECONSTRUCTION

Flap	Included Tissues	Vascular Supply	Spinal Level
Paraspinous	Muscle	■ Thoracic and lumbar perforators	■ Cervical, thoracic, lumbar
Trapezius	Muscle or myocutaneous	■ Transverse cervical; dorsal scapular	■ Cervical ■ Upper thoracic
Latissimus dorsi	Muscle or myocutaneous	■ Thoracodorsal	■ Thoracic
Reverse latissimus dorsi	Muscle or myocutaneous	■ Thoracic and lumbar perforators	■ Lower thoracic ■ Lumbar
Omentum	Visceral adipose	■ Right or left gastroepiploic	■ Lower thoracic ■ Lumbar
Lumbar perforator	Fasciocutaneous	■ Lumbar perforator	■ Lumbar
Gluteal	Muscle, myocutaneous, or fasciocutaneous	■ Superior gluteal	■ Lumbosacral ■ Sacral

Lumbar and Lumbosacral Region

The paraspinous muscles are the largest and most mobile in the lumbar spine, making them ideally suited for reconstructions in this area. A second-line option for this area is the reverse latissimus dorsi muscle or myocutaneous flap, based on the lumbar perforating vessels. If additional dead space obliteration is needed, a lumbar perforator propeller flap can be dropped into the defect and de-epithelialized. Lumbar region reconstructions tend to have a higher rate of minor wound healing complications (seroma, skin edge separation, etc), owing to the more dependent location and lordotic spinal curvature, which may allow for seroma accumulation.[55] The liberal use of closed suction drains is encouraged to mitigate seromas.

Reconstructions of the sacral and lumbosacral spine are usually associated with a partial or total sacrectomy defect. These defects typically require obliteration of dead space for seroma and abscess prevention and to reduce the chance of a developing perineal hernia.[52] Some plastic surgeons prefer to place a bridging bioprosthetic mesh in the sacral defect to minimize perineal bulge development; however, this practice is controversial and has been associated with a higher complication rate.[62] Partial sacrectomies that are inferior to the sacroiliac joint are technically simpler from a reconstruction perspective because the entire resection and reconstruction can be performed from a prone, transperineal approach; these sacrectomies, in general, are at the S3 level or more inferior. Provided that the superior gluteal vessels are preserved, these defects

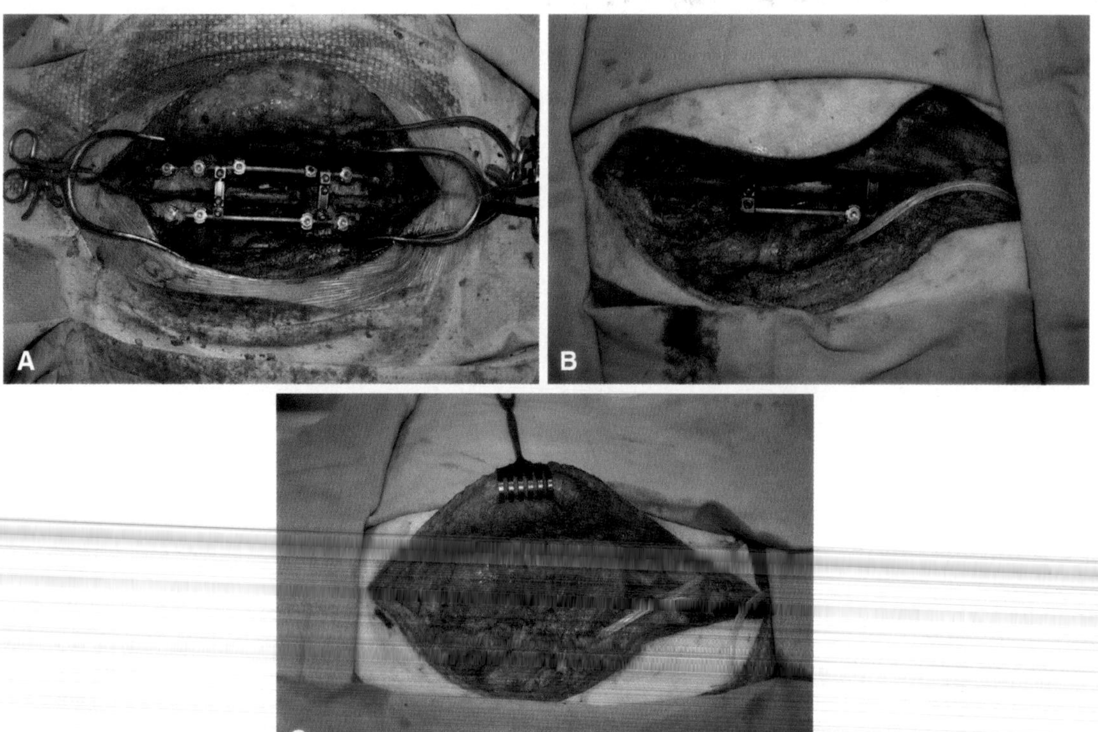

FIGURE 94.11. Posterior spine defect after partial vertebrectomy and composite chest wall resection for sarcoma. **A.** Defect with exposed spinal cord at base, posterior instrumentation, and exposed pleural cavity. **B.** Pleural cavity separated from spinal cord with a trapezius muscle flap. **C.** Right latissimus flap for coverage of spinal cord and instrumentation.

are reliably reconstructed with either V-Y or rotational fasciocutaneous advancement flaps or a superior gluteal perforator flap, depending on the mobility of the soft tissues and cutaneous requirement of the defect (Figure 94.12). A sacrectomy that includes the sacroiliac joint and/or the S1 or S2 level is much more complex. These resections require both a supine, trans-abdominal approach as well as a prone, transperineal approach. Moreover, if one or both of the S2 nerve roots are resected, then incontinence is likely. Because of the laparotomy requirement, trans-abdominal flaps based on the deep inferior epigastric vessels, such as a VRAM, are a good option to obliterate dead space and resurface the sacrum. Total sacrectomies and partial sacrectomies that include complete resection of one or both of the sacroiliac joints result in sacropelvic discontinuity. In this scenario, many surgeons believe that the longevity of the hardware construct may be improved with the addition of a vascularized bone flap.[52] The free fibula flap is the flap of choice and a variety of branches from the internal iliac artery and vein are often available for recipient sites.[51] The fibula flap may be used for large segmental defects, double barreled for added integrity, and as an A-frame strut with loss of the spinopelvic junction. Free fibula flaps will usually demonstrate radiographic signs of ossification at 6 weeks whereas fibula bone grafts may require 12 months or more for bony union.

Outcomes, Complications, and Management

Hardware Exposure

Acute hardware exposure is defined as occurring within 6 months of placement whereas a chronic exposure occurs more than 6 months after. In general, an acute exposure can be treated with aggressive debridement, irrigation, muscle flap closure, and culture-directed antibiotics. A chronic exposure is more difficult and requires removal of the exposed/involved hardware due to

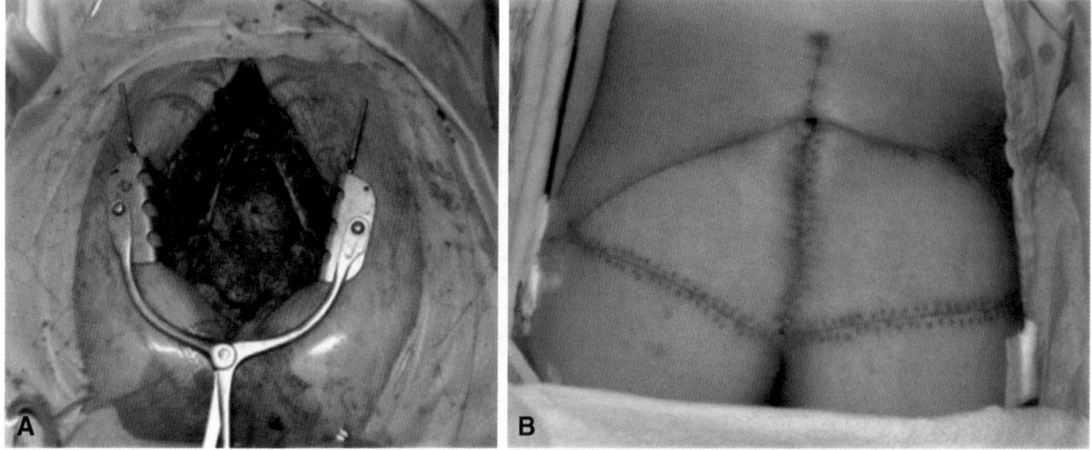

FIGURE 94.12. Posterior defect after partial sacrectomy for sarcoma. **A.** Defect with exposed spinal cord at base and exposed viscera of the peritoneal cavity. **B.** Bilateral gluteal advancement flaps for coverage of defect.

the likely presence of a bacterial biofilm. In chronic infections, all hardware bathed in purulent fluid should be removed; hardware encased in bone can be left in place. A muscle flap wound closure with numerous drains should be performed.

Cerebrospinal Fluid Leak

A CSF leak may become evident after persistent serous drain output from an epidural drain in combination with the subjective patient complaint of a postural headache. Drainage can be sent to the lab to test for beta-transferrin, the presence of which is indicative of a CSF leak. Most CSF leaks resolve with conservative management, such as restricting the patient to the supine or prone position and avoiding straining. If the leak persists, a lumbar drain or external ventricular drain can be placed to offload pressure on the leak site with the intention of promoting spontaneous healing. Occasionally, a chronic occult CSF leak will form a pseudomeningocele, which most often requires operative repair. The dura is either repaired primarily or with a patch; the repair site can then be reinforced with a muscle flap to help seal the leak.

Hematoma

When reconstructing any midline spine wound, drains should be placed deep to the muscle flaps in the epidural space as well as more superficially, between the skin and muscle closure. When laminectomies or vertebrectomies have been performed, the epidural drains are especially important because they help to drain away the excess serosanguinous fluid that, if allowed to accumulate, could cause a certain degree of cord compression. If a hematoma is suspected in the epidural space, deep to the muscle flap closure, the patient must be immediately returned to the operating room for evacuation and hemostasis; the pressure from an unaddressed expanding hematoma could easily injure the cord. Small superficial hematomas can be left to spontaneously resorb; however, if there is evidence of skin compromise, it must be drained.

CONCLUSION

Large defects of the chest, sternum, and back can result in significant functional impairment and present major challenges to the reconstructive surgeon. A cohesive multidisciplinary approach with preoperative communication facilitates and is essential for surgical planning and patient optimization. Adequate debridement, nutrition, rigid/semirigid stabilization of large defects, and soft tissue coverage are fundamental principles of this anatomy. A thorough knowledge of local pedicled and free flaps such as workhorses like the pectoralis major, paraspinous, and latissimus dorsi myocutaneous flap is critical for sternal and anterior chest wall reconstruction. Prophylactic reconstruction should be considered in high-risk situations, such as large resections/instrumentations, multiple previous surgeries, significant devascularization, and extensive patient comorbidities so as to avoid complications before they occur.

REFERENCES

1. Clemens MW, Evans KK, Mardini S, Arnold PG. Introduction to chest wall reconstruction: anatomy and physiology of the chest wall reconstruction. *Semin Plast Surg.* 2011;25:5-15.
2. Pairolero PC, Arnold PG. Thoracic wall defects: surgical management of 205 consecutive patients. *Mayo Clin Proc* 1986;61:557-563.
3. Hemmati SH, Correa AM, Walsh GL, et al. The prognostic factors of chest wall metastasis resection. *Eur J Cardiothorac Surg.* 2011;40:328-333.
4. Azarow KS, Molloy M, Seyfer AE, Graeber GM. Preoperative evaluation and general preparation for chest-wall operations. *Surg Clin North Am.* 1989;69:899-910.
5. Kroll SS, Walsh G, Ryan B, King RC. Risks and benefits of using Marlex mesh in chest wall reconstruction. *Ann Plast Surg.* 1993;31:303-306.
6. Netscher DT, Baumholtz MA. Chest reconstruction. I. Anterior and anterolateral chest wall and wounds affecting respiratory function. *Plast Reconstr Surg.* 2009;124(5):240e-252e.
7. Dingman RO, Argenta LC. Reconstruction of the chest wall. *Ann Thorac Surg.* 1981;32:202-208.
8. McCormack PM. Use of prosthetic materials in chest-wall reconstruction: assets and liabilities. *Surg Clin North Am.* 1989;69:965-976.
9. le Roux BT, Shama DM. Resection of tumors of the chest wall. *Curr Probl Surg.* 1983;20:345-386.
10. Spicer JD, Shewale JB, Antonoff MB, et al. The influence of reconstructive technique on perioperative pulmonary and infectious outcomes following chest wall resection. *Ann Thorac Surg.* 2016;102:1653-1659.
11. Hyans P, Moore JH Jr, Sinha L. Reconstruction of the chest wall with e-PTFE following major resection. *Ann Plast Surg.* 1992;29:321-327.
12. Hanna WC, Ferri LE, McKendy KM, et al. Reconstruction after major chest wall resection: can rigid fixation be avoided? *Surgery.* 2011;150:590-597.
13. Ouellet JF, Ball CG, Kortbeek JB, et al. Bioprosthetic mesh use for the problematic thoracoabdominal wall: outcomes in relation to contamination and infection. *Am J Surg.* 2012;203:594-597.
14. Butler CE, Langstein HN, Kronowitz SJ. Pelvic, abdominal, and chest wall reconstruction with AlloDerm in patients at increased risk for mesh related complications. *Plast Reconstr Surg.* 2005;116(5):1263-1275.
    This is the first report of the use of a bioprosthetic mesh in chest wall reconstruction. The authors demonstrate its efficacy in a contaminated environment with a low infection rate. The mesh can be placed in direct contact with the underlying lung without the development of adhesions.
15. Barua A, Catton JA, Socci L, et al. Initial experience with the use of biological implants of soft tissue and chest wall reconstruction in thoracic surgery. *Ann Thorac Surg.* 2012;94:1701-1705.
16. D'Amico G, Manfredi R, Nita G, et al. Reconstruction of the thoracic wall with biologic mesh after resection for chest wall tumors: a presentation of a case series and original technique. *Surg Innov.* 2018;25:28-36.
17. Thomas PA, Brouchet L. Prosthetic reconstruction of the chest wall. *Thorac Surg Clin.* 2010;20:551-558.
18. Bhatnagar A, Mayberry J, Nirula R. Rib fracture fixation for flail chest: what is the benefit? *J Am Coll Surg.* 2012;215:201-205.
19. Boerma LM, Bemelman M, van Dalen T. Chest wall reconstruction after resection of a chest wall sarcoma by osteosynthesis with the titanium MatrixRIB (Synthes) system. *J Thorac Cardiovasc Surg.* 2013;146:e37-e40.
20. Ng CS, Ho AM, Lau RW, Wong RH. Chest wall reconstruction with MatrixRib system: avoiding pitfalls. *Interact Cardiovasc Thorac Surg.* 2014;18:402-403.
21. Berthet JP, Canaud L, D'Annoville T, et al. Titanium plates and Dualmesh: a modern combination for reconstructing very large chest wall defects. *Ann Thorac Surg.* 2011;91:1709-1716.
22. [illegible] using titanium plates and mesh preserves chest wall function. *J Thorac Cardiovasc Surg.* 2010;140:476-477.
23. Arnold PG, Pairolero PC. Chest-wall reconstruction: an account of 500 consecutive patients. *Plast Reconstr Surg.* 1996;98:804-810.
    Seminal article with the largest series to date on chest wall reconstruction, spanning a period of 18 years. The authors describe various techniques for skeletal and soft tissue chest wall reconstruction.
24. Arnold PG, Pairolero PC. Chest wall reconstruction: experience with 100 consecutive patients. *Ann Surg.* 1984;199:725-732.
25. Mansour KA, Thourani VH, Losken A, et al. Chest wall resections and reconstruction: a 25-year experience. *Ann Thorac Surg.* 2002;73:1720-1725.
26. Villa MT, Chang DW. Muscle and omental flaps for chest wall reconstruction. *Thorac Surg Clin.* 2010;20:543-550.
27. Cordeiro PG, Santamaria E, Hidalgo D. The role of microsurgery in reconstruction of oncologic chest wall defects. *Plast Reconstr Surg.* 2001;108:1924-1930.
28. Althubaiti G, Butler CE. Abdominal wall and chest wall reconstruction. *Plast Reconstr Surg.* 2014;133:688e-701e.
29. Mathes SJ, Nahai F. *Reconstruction Surgery: Principles, Anatomy, and Technique.* St Louis, MO: Quality Medical Publishing; 1997.
30. Arya R, Chow WT, Rozen WM, et al. Microsurgical reconstruction of large oncologic chest wall defects for locally advanced breast cancer or osteoradionecrosis: a retrospective review of 26 cases over a 5-year period. *J Reconstr Microsurg.* 2016;3:121-127.
31. Arnold PG, Pairolero PC. Surgical management of the radiated chest wall. *Plast Reconstr Surg.* 1986;77:605-612.
32. Granick MS, Larson DL, Solomon MP. Radiation related wounds of the chest wall. *Clin Plast Surg.* 1993;20:559-571.
33. Samuels L, Granick MS, Ramasastry S, Solomon MP, Hurwitz D. Reconstruction of radiation induced chest wall lesions. *Ann Plast Surg.* 1993;31:399-405.
34. Hines GL, Lee G. Osteoradionecrosis of the chest wall: management of postresection defects using Marlex mesh and a rotated latissimus dorsi myocutaneous flap. *Am Surg.* 1983;49:608-611.
35. Kroll SS, Schusterman MA, Larson DL, Fender A. Long-term survival after chest-wall reconstruction with musculocutaneous flaps. *Plast Reconstr Surg.* 1990;86:697-701.
36. Sarr MG, Gott VL, Townsend TR, et al. Mediastinal infection after cardiac surgery. *Ann Thorac Surg.* 1984;38:415-423.
37. Jurkiewicz MJ, Bostwick J III, Hester TR, et al. Infected median sternotomy wound. Successful treatment by muscle flaps. *Ann Surg.* 1980;191:738-743.
38. Prevosti LG, Subramainian VA, Rothaus KO, et al. A comparison of the open and closed methods in the initial treatment of sternal wound infections. *J Cardiovasc Surg.* 1989;30:757-763.

39. Pairolero PC, Arnold PG. Management of infected median sternotomy wounds. *Ann Thorac Surg*. 1986;42:1-2.
Seminal article describing the three types of infected median sternotomy wounds and the associated management strategies for each.
40. Song DH, Wu LC, Lohman RF, et al. Vacuum assisted closure for the treatment of sternal wounds: the bridge between debridement and definitive closure. *Plast Reconstr Surg*. 2003;111:92-97.
41. Song DH, Lohman RF, Renucci JD, et al. Primary sternal plating in high-risk patients prevents mediastinitis. *Eur J Cardiothorac Surg*. 2004;26:367-372.
42. Lee JC, Raman J, Song DH. Primary sternal closure with titanium plate fixation: plastic surgery effecting a paradigm shift. *Plast Reconstr Surg*. 2010;125:1720-1724.
43. Butterworth JA, Garvey PB, Baumann DP, et al. Optimizing reconstruction of oncologic sternectomy defects based on surgical outcomes. *J Am Coll Surg*. 2013;217:306-316.
44. Langston HT. Thoracoplasty: the how and the why. *Ann Thorac Surg*. 1991;52:1351-1353.
45. Abolhoda A, Bui TD, Milliken JC, Wirth GA. Pedicled latissimus dorsi muscle flap: routine use in high-risk thoracic surgery. *Tex Heart Inst J*. 2009;36:298-302.
46. Arnold PG, Pairolero PC. Intrathoracic muscle flaps. An account of their use in the management of 100 consecutive patients. *Ann Surg*. 1990;211:656-660.
47. Garvey PB, Rhines LD, Dong W, Chang DW. Immediate soft-tissue reconstruction for complex defects of the spine following surgery for spinal neoplasms. *Plast Reconstr Surg*. 2010;125:1460-1466.
[illegible] complex wounds of the spine benefit from immediate soft tissue reconstruction. Despite 65% of patients having had previous radiation, there was only a 12% rate of major wound complications and no wounds required hardware removal.
48. Chang DW, Friel MT, Youssef AA. Reconstructive strategies in soft tissue reconstruction after resection of spinal neoplasms. *Spine (Phila Pa 1976)*. 2007;32:1101-1106.
49. Dumanian GA, Ondra SL, Liu J, et al. Muscle flap salvage of spine wounds with soft tissue defects or infection. *Spine (Phila Pa 1976)*. 2003;28:1203-1211.
50. Saraph VJ, Bach CM, Krismer M, Wimmer C. Evaluation of spinal fusion using autologous anterior strut grafts and posterior instrumentation for thoracic/thoracolumbar kyphosis. *Spine (Phila Pa 1976)*. 2005;30:1594-1601.
51. Clemens MD, Chang EI, Lewis V, Chang D. Composite extremity and trunk reconstruction with vascularized fibula flap in post-oncologic bone defects: a 10 year experience. *Plast Reconstr Surg*. 2012;129:170-178.
52. Houdek MT, Rose PS, Bakri K, et al. Outcomes and complications of reconstruction with use of free vascularized fibular graft for spinal and pelvic defects following resection of a malignant tumor. *J Bone Joint Surg Am*. 2017;99A:e69.
53. Moran SL, Bakri K, Mardini S, et al. The use of vascularized fibular grafts for the reconstruction of spinal and sacral defects. *Microsurgery*. 2009;29:393-400.
54. Mericli AF, Tarola NA, Moore JH Jr, et al. Paraspinous muscle flap reconstruction of complex midline back wounds: risk factors and postreconstruction complications. *Ann Plast Surg*. 2010;65:219-224.
Largest series to-date on paraspinous muscle flaps for spinal wound reconstruction. This article identifies several risk factors for wound healing complications after reconstruction, including a history of multiple previous spine surgeries, hardware removal, and lumbar location.
55. Mericli AF, Moore JH Jr, Copit SE, et al. Technical changes in paraspinous muscle flap surgery have increased salvage rates of infected spinal wounds. *Eplasty*. 2008;8:e50.
56. Mericli AF, Mirzabeigi MN, Moore JH Jr, et al. Reconstruction of complex posterior cervical spine wounds using the paraspinous muscle flap. *Plast Reconstr Surg*. 2011;128:148-153.
Article demonstrating the efficacy of paraspinous muscle flaps for reconstruction of posterior cervical wounds. The authors introduce their technique and report an acceptable complication rate.
57. Disa JJ, Smith AW, Bilsky MH. Management of radiated reoperative wounds of the cervicothoracic spine: the role of the trapezius turnover flap. *Ann Plast Surg*. 2001;47:394-397.
58. Sadigh PL, Chang LR, Hsieh CH, et al. The trapezius perforator flap: an underused but [illegible] of local and distant soft-tissue defects. *Plast Reconstr Surg*. 2014;134:449e-456e.
59. McGeorge DD, Stilwell JH. The use of the reverse latissimus dorsi flap in the closure of lower spinal defects. *Z Kinderchir*. 1988;43(suppl 2):30-32.
60. O'Shaughnessy BA, Dumanian GA, Liu JC, et al. Pedicled omental flaps as an adjunct in the closure of complex spinal wounds. *Spine (Phila Pa 1976)*. 2007;32:3074-3080.
61. Coon D, Calotta NA, Broyles JM, Sacks JM. Use of biological tissue matrix in postneurosurgical posterior trunk reconstruction is associated with higher wound complication rates. *Plast Reconstr Surg*. 2016;138:104e-110e.
62. Atkin G, Mathur P, Harrison R. Mesh repair of sacral hernia following sacrectomy. *J R Soc Med*. 2003;96(1):28-30.

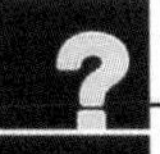

QUESTIONS

1. A 62-year-old woman with a history of disseminated breast cancer and spinal metastasis for which she received an external beam radiation therapy to her spine presents to the emergency room with a pathologic fracture of T8, and received an emergent titanium rod posterior stabilization by neurosurgery. Her postoperative course was complicated by incisional dehiscence with purulent drainage from her wound. Optimal initial management includes:

a. Infectious disease consultation and intravenous broad-spectrum antibiotics for 48 to 72 hours.
b. A bone scan with fluorescence-based leukocyte labeling to determine the extent of infection and presence of osteomyelitis
c. Operative debridement, irrigation, paraspinous muscle flap coverage of hardware, and wound specimens to allow for culture-directed antibiotic coverage
d. Neurosurgery consultation for removal of hardware
e. Application of vacuum-assisted closure with antibiotic instillation until demonstration of healthy granulation tissue and clearance of infection.

2. A 50-year-old woman is diagnosed with a 6 cm, fungating, locally advanced intraductal carcinoma of the right breast with direct invasion into the pectoralis major and intercostal muscles. A modified radical mastectomy is planned with resection of the underlying chest wall. The diameter of the musculoskeletal chest wall defect is 5 cm in diameter. What is the most appropriate reconstructive strategy?

a. Two-stage breast reconstruction with tissue-expansion followed by exchange for a permanent breast implant
b. Polyethylene mesh—methylmethacrylate construct for reconstruction of the skeletal chest wall followed by free deep inferior epigastric artery perforator flap for breast reconstruction.
c. Pedicled latissimus dorsi muscle flap followed by a split thickness skin graft
d. Bioprosthetic mesh for reconstruction of the skeletal chest wall followed by free anterolateral thigh flap for chest wall coverage.

3. A 75-year-old male patient requires a coronary artery bypass graft operation in which the left internal mammary artery and saphenous vein grafts were used. The operation is successful, however at his 3-week follow up appointment, the cardiac surgeon notes erythema overlying the sternum and purulent drainage from the incision. You are consulted for recommendations regarding treatment of this patient's wound. Optimal initial management includes:

a. Infectious disease consultation and intravenous broad-spectrum antibiotics for 48 to 72 hours.
b. A bone scan with fluorescence-based leukocyte labeling to determine the extent of infection and presence of osteomyelitis
c. Application of vacuum-assisted closure with antibiotic instillation until demonstration of healthy granulation tissue and clearance of infection
d. Operative debridement, irrigation, removal of all foreign bodies, followed by eventual reconstruction with bilateral pectoralis major advancement flaps.

4. A 33-year-old homeless woman is diagnosed with tuberculosis after having an episode of massive hemoptysis. The thoracic surgeon evaluates her and determines she will require an urgent pneumonectomy, as the disease is extensive and in danger of eroding into her hilum. A preoperative work up reveals severe protein malnutrition. You are consulted for immediate reconstruction. What is the most appropriate reconstructive option?

a. Immediate thoracoplasty after removal of the lung to reduce the size of the pleural cavity and encourage healing.
b. Latissimus-sparing thoracotomy followed by intrathoracic transposition of the latissimus dorsi muscle for reinforcement of the bronchial stump and filling the pleural cavity.
c. Trans-diaphragmatic transposition of a pedicled omental flap for reinforcement of the bronchial stump and filling the pleural cavity.
d. Respectfully explain to the thoracic surgeon that you do not believe that an immediate wound reconstruction is necessary.
e. Intrathoracic transposition of the pectoralis major muscle for reinforcement of the bronchial stump and filling the pleural cavity.

5. A patient undergoes a right partial sacrectomy at the S3 level for resection of a chordoma. What is the most appropriate reconstructive approach?

a. Elevation of a vertical rectus abdominis myocutaneous flap during the supine-positioned first stage followed by inset of the flap in the defect during the second prone-positioned stage
b. Right superior gluteal artery perforator flap
c. Left superior gluteal artery perforator flap
d. Bilateral paraspinous muscle flaps.

1. **Answer: c.** Surgical site infections are common after chest and spinal hardware procedures. The U.S. Centers for Disease Control and Prevention (CDC) recommends that surgical site infections be specified as superficial, deep, or organ space infections. The most common organism infecting is ***S. aureus***, seen in up to 81% of cases; this suggests skin flora contamination during hardware implantation. In general, hardware removal is not possible after immediate placement to stabilize a compression fracture. Treatment proceeds with wide operative debridement followed by elevation of paraspinous muscle flaps for hardware coverage. Wound specimens are taken to allow for culture directed antibiotic coverage; however, antibiotic treatment alone is insufficient to treat these complex wounds.

2. **Answer: d.** Because this chest wall defect is located on the anterior surface and is 5 cm in diameter, the patient will benefit from reconstruction to minimize paradoxical respiration and maintain a normal chest wall contour. The fungating nature of this patient's tumor qualifies her surgical wound as ***clean-contaminated*** according to the Centers for Disease Control. Because of this, she is at a higher risk for developing a postsurgical wound infection and so synthetic materials should be avoided; a bioprosthetic mesh is a good option in this situation. The size and locally advanced nature of her tumor will necessitate post-mastectomy radiation therapy, and so a tissue expander reconstruction would be inappropriate. Similarly, immediate reconstruction with an autologous abdominal flap should be reserved for after radiation and complete treatment of her malignancy.

3. Answer: d. Surgical site infections are a known complication after median sternotomy. Certain risk factors include diabetes, reoperative surgery, diabetes, obesity, and off-midline sternotomy. Treatment proceeds with wide operative debridement and irritation and removal of all sternal wires or plates. Wound specimens are taken for culture directed antibiotic coverage; however, antibiotic treatment alone is insufficient to treat these complex wounds. Once the wound has been adequately debrided—which may require multiple operations—it is reconstructed with well-vascularized soft tissue. Although the pectoralis turnover flap nicely fills the wound dead space, a left pectoralis major turnover flap is not possible in this patient because his left internal mammary artery has been used for coronary revascularization.

4. Answer: b. This patient is at high risk for developing a bronchopleural fistula after her pneumonectomy, considering her protein malnutrition, clean-contaminated wound classification, and severe disease. Therefore, immediate muscle flap reconstruction of the intrathoracic space is indicated for reinforcing the bronchial stump and filling the non-collapsible pleural cavity with well-vascularized tissue. The latissimus dorsi muscle provides the most bulk and is therefore the first choice, as long as it is preserved by the thoracotomy. Other options include the serratus anterior, rectus abdominis, pectoralis major, and omental flap.

5. Answer: c. A partial sacrectomy at the S3 level can be performed in a single stage, all from the prone position. Sacrectomies requiring resection at the S1 or S2 level will require an initial anterior, supine-positioned approach, making the VRAM flap a better option in that scenario. The superior gluteal vessels are often ligated on the side of the sacrectomy, therefore a right SGAP flap is not appropriate. The paraspinous muscles terminate at L5 and are not appropriate for sacral reconstruction.

CHAPTER 95 Abdominal Wall Reconstruction

Brett T. Phillips and Howard Levinson

KEY POINTS

- By addressing patient modifiable risk factors, such as hemoglobin A1C, obesity, nutrition, and tobacco preoperatively, postoperative outcomes are likely to be optimized.
- Hernia mesh reduces hernia recurrence by about 50%.
- Mesh and graft selection is a continuously evolving field with great controversy, but, in general, lightweight meshes and microporous meshes have lost favor because of their adverse effects.
- Surgical techniques vary widely, and with the exception of a few specific approaches, such as small bites 5 mm apart, 5 mm from the fascia edge to close laparotomy wounds, there are many reasonably good options for reconstructing the abdominal wall.
- Prophylactic hernia mesh or graft is an emerging field that will likely become a part of abdominal wall reconstruction.

DEFINITION OF HERNIA, BULGE, AND DIASTASIS RECTI

An abdominal wall hernia is defined as a defect in the abdominal wall fascia or musculature through which intra-abdominal contents protrude. In general, the goal of hernia surgery is to restore normal muscle anatomy and maintain the muscles in normal alignment. Common examples of hernia include ventral, inguinal, lumbar, Spigelian, umbilical, paraesophageal, diaphragmatic, and femoral (Table 95.1). Ventral hernia in adults is the most common hernia a plastic surgeon will typically manage, so it will be the focus of this chapter. An abdominal wall bulge is a weakness in the abdominal wall musculature where abdominal wall anatomy is normal but the muscles are denervated. Bulges typically form from previous surgery causing nerve injury or from an inability to restore normal muscle anatomy but may also be caused by neuromuscular disease. Diastasis recti is a widening of the linea alba fascia with lateralization of the rectus abdominis muscles but no fascial defect. Hernia, bulge, and diastasis recti are often differentiated by a combination of history, physical exam, and sometimes imaging.

EPIDEMIOLOGY

Approximately two million laparotomies are performed annually in the United States, with ventral hernia being a frequent complication in 10% to 30% of patients.[1–5] The timing of hernia recurrence is not well understood and there is likely a range of months to years from when they may recur.[6] The 10-year ventral hernia recurrence rate ranges from 63% without mesh to 32% when a mesh is added to a repair.[7–9] Approximately 350,000 ventral hernia repairs are performed each year in the United States and practically all include the use of a hernia mesh.[10] Given the above complication rate, incidence of ventral hernia repair, and average cost/patient for each hernia operation in the United States (in 2006, this amount was ~$15,899), an estimated $3 to $6 billion is spent annually on these operations.[10] However, these numbers underestimate recurrence rates in the rapidly growing morbidly obese population in the United States.[11,12] With significant increases in the morbidly obese population, ventral hernia formation is expected to significantly increase as well.[13] In fact, this industry is on the cusp of a giant boom as several publications, including a recent landmark paper in the Lancet, support the use of hernia mesh prophylactically in high risk undergoing laparotomy to prevent hernia occurrence.[14]

TABLE 95.1. ABDOMINAL WALL AND TRUNK HERNIAS

Hernia	Definition/Anatomic Location
Direct inguinal	Inguinal canal through direct fascial defect, medial to epigastric vessels
Indirect inguinal	Inguinal canal through deep inguinal ring, lateral to epigastric vessels
Femoral	Femoral canal, deep to inguinal ligament, medial to femoral vein
Umbilical	Fascial defect at umbilical stalk
Epigastric	General term for fascial defect in superomedial abdominal wall
Incisional	Fascial defect as a result of previous surgery
Ventral	General term for fascial defect of the abdominal wall
Parastomal	Enlarged fascial defect surrounding an ostomy site
Hiatal	Paraesophageal diaphragmatic defect or weakness
Reducible	Hernia defect in which contents can be manually relocated into the organ space
Irreducible	Hernia defect in which contents are fixed and cannot be manually relocated into the organ space
Incarcerated	Nonreducible hernia that may cause pain and bowel obstruction
Strangulated	Incarcerated hernia with compromised blood supply
Sliding	Hernia defect in which a portion of the hernia sac is formed by another viscus (i.e., colon, stomach)
Littre	Hernia that contains a Meckel's diverticulum, omphalomesenteric duct hernia
Amyand	Hernia that contains the appendix
Obturator	Pelvic floor hernia defect through the obturator foramen
Petit	Posterior lateral inferior lumbar triangle hernia; borders are external oblique, iliac crest, latissimus dorsi
Grynfeltt	Posterior lateral superior lumbar triangle hernia; borders are internal oblique, quadratus lumborum, 12th rib
Cooper	Femoral hernia with two sacs, one protruding through the superficial fascia
Pantaloon	Combined indirect and direct inguinal hernia; two sacs
Spigelian	Hernia defect along semilunar line, at the lateral border of the rectus muscle
Richter	Hernia defect that contains only the antimesenteric border of bowel

ANATOMY

Muscle/Fascia Anatomy

The abdominal wall is a multilayered structure composed of skin, subcutaneous fat, muscle, nerves, blood vessels, and fascia (Figure 95.1). Its function is to provide structural support and mobility of the trunk and to protect underlying abdominal organs.[15] In terms of musculofascial anatomy, the linea alba is central fascia between the paired recti and the semilunar line is the lateral border of the recti. The recti originate from the symphysis pubis and the pubic crest and insert onto the fifth, sixth, and seventh costal cartilages and the xiphoid process. They are encased in an anterior and a posterior rectus sheath. The arcuate line is a horizontal line below the umbilicus that demarcates the lower limit of the posterior rectus sheath, and it is also where the inferior epigastric vessels perforate the rectus abdominis. The anterior rectus sheath is composed of two overlapping fascia layers that are continuations of the external oblique aponeurosis and internal oblique aponeurosis, respectively. The posterior rectus sheath, superior to the arcuate line, is also composed of two overlapping fascia layers that are continuations of the internal oblique aponeurosis (the internal oblique aponeurosis splits into an anterior and a posterior layer at the semilunar line to envelope the recti) and the transversalis fascia. The muscular/fascial layers lateral to the semilunar line (from superficial to deep) include the external oblique aponeurosis, external oblique musculature, internal oblique aponeurosis internal oblique musculature, transversalis fascia, and transversus abdominis. External oblique flaps can be raised between the internal and external oblique muscles. Posterior to the transversalis fascia is the parietal peritoneum.

Nerve Anatomy

Understanding the path of nerves and preserving them during surgery is critically important to prevent postoperative denervation and bulges. If nerves are injured, bulges will occur and bulges are difficult to manage because adynamic fabric or scar underperforms innervated muscle. The rectus muscle is innervated by the lower intercostal and lumbar neurovascular bundles traveling between the internal oblique and transversus abdominis muscles and is a target for regional nerve blocks. They enter the rectus sheath laterally and pierce and innervate the rectus muscle and can be injured during dissection leading to bulges.

Vascular Anatomy

Blood supply of the abdominal wall comes from the distal internal mammary vessels and multiple perforating vessels from the iliac and femoral vessels. Understanding the blood supply of the abdominal wall and the superior thigh is important because it is the basis of local flap reconstruction. The deep inferior epigastric vessels are critical for blood supply of the abdominal wall and are often the donor vessel for abdominal autologous tissue reconstruction. The superior epigastric artery is the inferior extension of the internal mammary

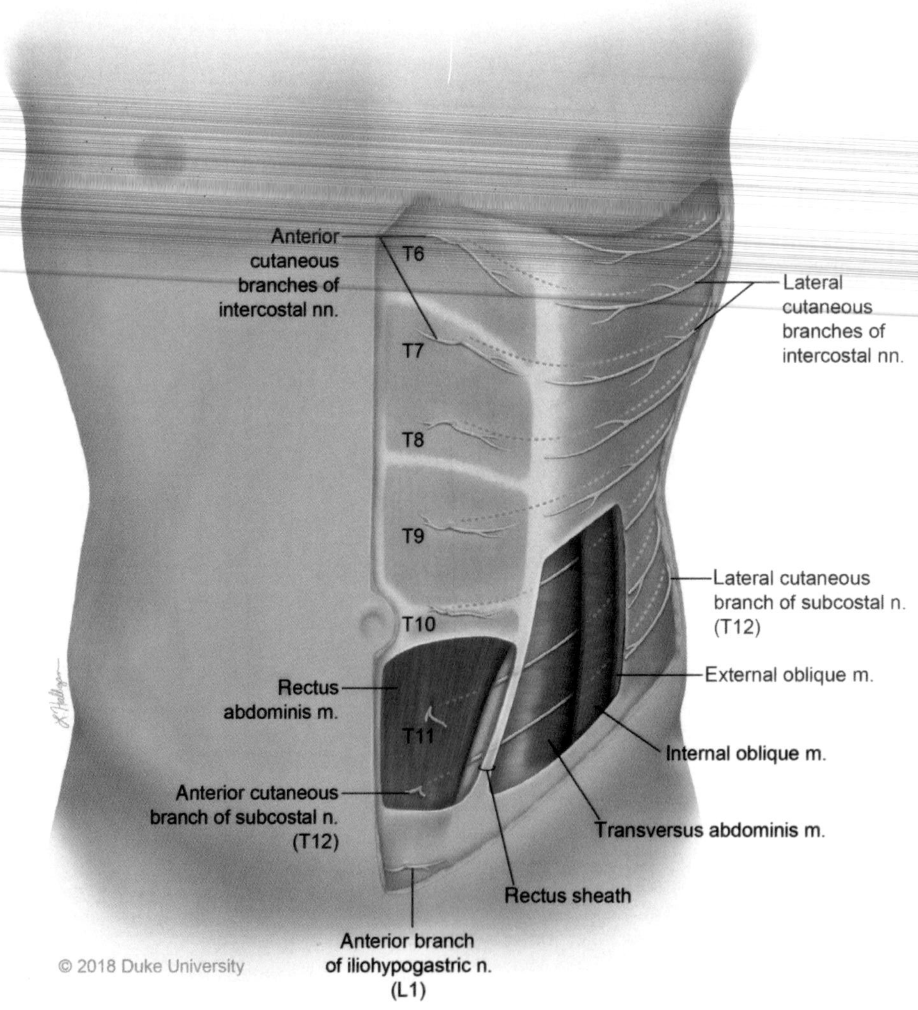

FIGURE 95.1. Abdominal wall anatomy and innervation.

artery and is critical for superior-based rectus pedicle flap that can be used for superior abdominal, back, and chest wall reconstruction. The superior artery runs the length of the rectus muscle and joins the deep inferior epigastric artery that originates from the external iliac artery superior to the inguinal ligament. Inferiorly based abdominal wall flaps can be used for breast (i.e., free transverse rectus abdominis myocutaneous), groin, thigh, and abdominal wall reconstruction. Branches of the common, superficial and profundal femoral arteries will supply options for superior thigh flaps that can be rotated superiorly to assist with middle and lower abdominal wall reconstruction.

PATHOPHYSIOLOGY

There are multiple risk factors that affect outcomes of ventral hernia repair, and these factors should be considered for each patient before surgery. Some of these risk factors are modifiable, in which case surgery may be delayed until after the risks have been managed. In many cases, the risks cannot be reduced but recognition of risk factors nonetheless helps predict outcomes and enhances informed consent. Below, risk factors are classified according to three areas: intrinsic factors, extrinsic factors, and technical factors.

Intrinsic Factors

Intrinsic factors are biologic factors specific to the patient such as collagen disorders; Ehlers Danlos and Marfan syndrome and neurologic diseases such as amyotrophic lateral sclerosis or shingles may weaken the abdominal wall musculature.[16] Although intrinsic factors are not necessarily modifiable, awareness may help with the decision to proceed to surgery. Some surgeons may use additional fixation techniques during repair to enhance outcomes.

Extrinsic Factors

Extrinsic factors are common conditions and medications that adversely affect wound healing. These include but are not limited to tobacco (modifiable), corticosteroids (potentially modifiable), abdominal aortic aneurysm, surgical site infection, chronic obstructive pulmonary disease, multiple surgeries, chemotherapy agents (potentially modifiable), immunodeficiency, radiation, uncontrolled diabetes (potentially modifiable), morbid obesity (potentially modifiable), parastomal hernias, and nutritional status (potentially modifiable).[17] The reader is referred to the literature for a deeper understanding of each factor because space is limited here.

Technical Factors

Technical factors are surgical performance, hernia mesh (graft or textile) selection, and anchoring techniques. Many of these technical factors are widely debated; yet, there are a few agreed upon principles listed below. In terms of surgical performance, a recent prospective, multicenter, double-blind, randomized controlled trial demonstrated that small tissue bites of 5 mm every 5 mm with 2-0 absorbable suture lead to fewer hernias (13%) versus large tissue bites of 1 cm every 1 cm (21%).[18–20] In terms of mesh selection, lightweight meshes have been associated with ventral hernia recurrence because of mesh tearing,[21] whereas moderate-weight and heavy-weight meshes do not appear to be at risk of tearing. Degradable meshes are significantly more expensive than nondegradable meshes but purportedly safer for use in clean-contaminated and contaminated cases, but these benefits are questionable,[22–24] particularly in bridging (rectus muscle cannot be reapproximated in the midline) repair. Mesh fixation technique is also critically important in preventing recurrence. An increased number of fixation points do not necessarily distribute tension across the abdominal wall. One study revealed that more than three fixation points along a 7-cm region does not increase bursting strength.[25] Therefore, sutures should be placed approximately 1 to 2 cm apart circumferentially around the mesh. A final point to consider is that, even with modification of technical factors, ~>20% of ventral hernia repairs recur and this is most often due to failure at the mesh, suture, and tissue interface from suture cheese wiring through the tissue or through the mesh.[26,27]

DIAGNOSIS

History

A thorough history and physical exam is helpful in diagnosing ventral hernias. The most common predictor of ventral hernia is previous abdominal surgery. Patients with signs and symptoms of a ventral hernia may present for elective or emergent repair. In general, surgery is indicated for all ventral hernias but not all patients are good candidates for surgery.[28] A special note is made for postpartum women who develop new onset abdominal bulges. These bulges are typically not hernias but rather diastasis recti from pregnancy. Although diastasis recti condition is an anatomic abnormality, there is no hernia so the disease is classified as cosmetic rather than reconstructive. Care should also be taken in the patient with a history of a pelvic malignancy because the patient may have received radiation through the abdominal wall—a fact can be overlooked in the history. Operating on an irradiated abdominal wall can lead to challenging complications.

Physical Exam

Abdominal Wall

Examination of the abdomen for surgical scars and obvious bulges is done during the initial evaluation. Common physical exam findings, which are typically best done with the patient lying flat yet flexing their abdominal wall muscles by raising their shoulders from midline hernia or twisting for flank hernias, are a separation of muscle edges and pain on palpation. Performing a Valsalva maneuver may also elucidate an incidental hernia. Of course, hernias may be difficult to ascertain in the morbidly obese patient where occult hernias may surprisingly be encountered at the time of panniculectomy if imaging has not been completed.

Laboratory Assessment

Depending on a patient's medical and surgical history, additional testing may be required. In a diabetic patient, hemoglobin A1C should be obtained to ascertain proper glycemic control. If nutrition is a concern, a nutrition evaluation can be obtained before elective surgery. Patients with respiratory disease may need pulmonary function tests to assess lung capacities. Patients with a history of tobacco use may be tested for cessation by assessing urine cotinine.

Imaging

Routine imaging surveillance, including CT scan, MRI, or ultrasound may identify asymptomatic ventral hernias or recurrences from previous abdominal surgery. Imaging is more reliable at diagnosing incisional hernias than physical exam. The caveat is that asymptomatic hernias not found on clinical exam require treatment.[19] The disadvantage to utilize CT scans is increased cost and radiation exposure. Ultrasound is user dependent but is more accessible and cheaper than CT and there is no radiation.

EMERGENCY VERSUS ELECTIVE SURGERY

Emergent need for ventral hernia repair is most commonly found in the setting of bowel obstruction or following abdominal trauma. Patients with bowel obstruction may complain of distension, abdominal pain, nausea, vomiting, absent flatus, or absent bowel movements. Abdominal findings include tenderness, distension, obvious mass or bulge, tympany, or overlying skin changes. Hernia contents can be reduced back through the fascial defect are considered reducible. An incarcerated hernia is a nonreducible hernia that may contain bowel but has no findings of vascular compromise. A strangulated hernia is a nonreducible hernia in which the blood supply to the hernia contents is obstructed and will result in necrosis if not repaired. Depending on the clinical situation, hernia repair may be performed during the initial surgery or in a delayed fashion. Obviously, trauma patients with an open, distended abdominal will have their hernia repaired in a delayed fashion, and these cases are typically complicated.

Elective ventral hernia repair is performed to relieve symptoms, improve abdominal wall appearance, prevent need for emergent surgical intervention, and improve quality of life. Hernia repair is often performed as a combined procedure with other surgical services, or it may be scheduled in a delayed fashion if the abdomen cannot be closed from the initial operation because of abdominal compartment syndrome, need for second look operation, or transplant mismatches, for example.

PATIENT-CENTERED OUTCOME TOOLS

Over the past decade, there have emerged several patient-centered areas of investigation and tool development to measure and improve surgical outcomes, including quality-of-life scales, patient registries, and preoperative risk assessment tools. These areas continually mature and rapidly evolve.

Quality of Life Scales

There are a number of validated scales to measure patient-related outcomes following ventral hernia repair, these include but are not limited to generic Short Form-36 (SF-36), and disease specific hernia-related quality-of-life assessment tool (HerQLes), and Carolinas Comfort Scale.[29] The generic SF-36 is useful to compare outcomes across different populations and interventions for cost-effectiveness studies, but it is less effective at assessing disease specific concerns. The Carolinas comfort scale is designed to measure quality of life after mesh implantation during hernia repair, so it cannot measure longitudinal outcomes because patients do not have mesh before surgery, whereas the HerQLes scale is meant to measure abdominal wall function pre- and postoperatively. The two scales complement each other.[29] This 12-question tool with questions related to activities of daily living found improvement in quality of life from preoperative to postoperative patients in as short as 4 weeks postoperatively.

Registries

The two best-known national registries are the National Surgical Quality Improvement Program from the American College of Surgeons, American Hernia Society Quality Collaborative from the American Hernia Society. These two widely used databases collect data from across the United States and the databases are available for inquiry. Each database has led to a number of publications, and this number is likely to increase exponentially over the years and *big data* systematically grows. Peer-reviewed studies have shown that both registries are effective in improving the quality of surgical care.

Risk Analysis

Risk analysis tools are intended to be used by patients and physicians preoperatively to inform both about predicted outcomes. Each of these tools calculates clinical outcomes from a database and the fidelity of the tools will obviously increase as the databases grow. From the Americas Hernia Society Quality Collaborative (AHSQC) registries come the outcomes reporting app for clinician and patient engagement (ORACLE). The AHSQC ORACLE uses preoperative and intraoperative information to estimate important 30-day and 1-year outcomes following elective ventral hernia repair using mesh. From the Charlotte Carolina group comes the Carolinas Equation for Quality of Life (CeQOL). The CeQOL predicts the chances of having chronic pain after inguinal hernia repair. The same group has also created the Carolinas Equation for Determining Associated Risks (CeDAR). This free app predicts a patient's risk for wound-related problems and associated costs following ventral hernia repair.

USE OF MESH IN HERNIA REPAIRS

Mesh and Graft Selection

There are a wide variety of hernia meshes or grafts that one can choose from for repair. They can be classified according to material (e.g., polypropylene, polyester, poly-4-hydroxybutyrate, poly-l-lactic acid, expanded polytetrafluoroethylene, or animal tissue), manufacturing approach (e.g., knitting or weaving of textiles versus tissue processing (allografts and xenografts)), presence of antiadhesive coating, physical characteristics (e.g., for textiles this includes pore size, filament diameter, thickness, areal density (this parameter differentiates light-weight, moderate-weight, and heavy-weight meshes)), and permanence (nondegradable versus degradable). For any given knitted or woven textile, the fabrics physical characteristics will vary according to the diameter of filament used to create the textile (typical filament diameters range between 100 and 150 μm) and the knit or weave structure. Physical characteristics, material selection, and manufacturing approach together affect the textiles mechanical performance (e.g., ball burst, suture retention strength, tear resistance, and stress strain). Current thinking on the clinical relevance of physical characteristics, material selection, manufacturing approach, and mechanical performance is briefly described later, with the understanding that the field is constantly advancing and concepts will become outdated.

The first consideration in choosing a product is whether to choose a textile or a graft. All hernia grafts degrade whereas many synthetic hernia textiles do not. Although each specific graft has its differentiating factors, it is difficult to state that any one graft has a clear competitive advantage over another graft. Hernia grafts were popularized in the 1990s as a means to overcome mesh infection because there was a belief that these were either resistant to infection or would degrade during an infection so there would not be a need to remove these at a second operation.[30] There was also a belief that grafts led to a more durable repair than a textile. These topics are still hotly debated. In 2010, a Ventral Hernia Working Group published consensus guidelines concluding that hernia grafts are appropriate for use in patients at high risk for a surgical site occurrence (e.g., clean-contaminated or contaminated cases) and most surgeons would probably agree with this approach.[31] The main disadvantages to using a hernia graft are that they are orders of magnitude more expensive than synthetic meshes and they lose their mechanical properties as they degrade. In general, the purpose of a synthetic degradable textile is to replace the use of grafts with a less-expensive textile.

The second consideration is whether to use a textile with an antiadhesive coating. Currently, mesh labeling contains warnings that meshes should not be placed in direct contact with the viscera because they may cause erosion, adhesion, fistula formation, or lead to sepsis. This labeling creates a surgical conundrum because meshes are often needed to treat bridging hernias defects. The purpose of an antiadhesive coating is to prevent viscera from adhering to mesh, so most surgeons would use a textile with an antiadhesive coating when bridging a fascia defect or when placing the mesh in a location where it could contact viscera.

Finally, when it comes to choosing a specific mesh for ventral hernia repair, all FDA cleared meshes have met mechanical performance metrics and these metrics appear to meet all clinical needs. There have been a few case reports of lightweight mesh tearing. So, many surgeons prefer moderate-to-heavy weight meshes.[32] In terms of which moderate- or heavy-weight mesh to choose, each mesh will have its specific advantages but it is difficult to state that any mesh is superior to another. In general, there is a belief that it is advantageous to choose a mesh with the largest pores because large-pore meshes have less material, which clinically related to less chance of infection and less pain because of reduced inflammation.[33] Oftentimes, mesh availability and surgeon preference lead to device selection. Perhaps, the greatest deficiency in mesh today is not which mesh to use but rather how to anchor mesh to tissue.[34] Many surgeons use suture, glue, tacks, or screws to anchor meshes; yet, despite these various approaches failure at the anchor point is common and ventral hernias recur in ~20% of patients. Some groups have invented novel sutures, meshes, and adjuncts in an attempt to overcome this problem, but these products are still under development.[27,35,36] Care should be taken in using permanent mesh in patients who grow show as children or women of child-bearing age.

Anatomic Mesh Placement

The most common locations for mesh placement are as follows[37] (Figure 95.2):

Onlay: anterior to the anterior rectus sheath
Retrorectus: between the recti and posterior rectus sheath
Preperitoneal: posterior to the posterior rectus sheath but anterior to the peritoneum
Intraperitoneal: within the abdomen

Care should be taken when placing a mesh intraperitoneally, because the bowel may come into contact with the mesh, leading to adhesions, erosions, sepsis, and fistula.

In almost all instances, the goal is to restore the recti to their normal anatomic position and to add mesh to bolster the repair, whichever tissue plane is chosen. In select patients, the rectus muscles may not be able to be reapproximated in the midline at the time of hernia repair, in which case a mesh or graft would bridge the defect. In a bridged repair, the mesh serves as surrogate abdominal wall to prevent evisceration. Because the mesh or graft is adynamic, it is inferior to an anatomic repair. Use of a degradable mesh in bridge repair has a high incidence of hernia recurrence.[38]

Mesh Controversies

Mesh type and location continue to be controversial to this day. Literature supports and contradicts itself and varies among geographic locations and patient populations. Because of this ongoing debate, specific recommendations for the location of mesh placement and in what clinical situations should specific mesh types be placed, continue to be based on personal experience and interpretation of the literature. The Ventral Hernia Working Group classified patients into four groups—clean, clean-contaminated, contaminated, dirty—based on contamination, complication risk, and mesh recommendations. They recommend the use of prosthetic mesh in all cases of incisional hernia repair except in situations of gross contamination. Bioprosthetic mesh was recommended in patients with medical comorbidities or any gross contamination.[31,39] Another recent multicentered retrospective review actually found that synthetic mesh when placed in a sublay position had decreased surgical site occurrences and decreased

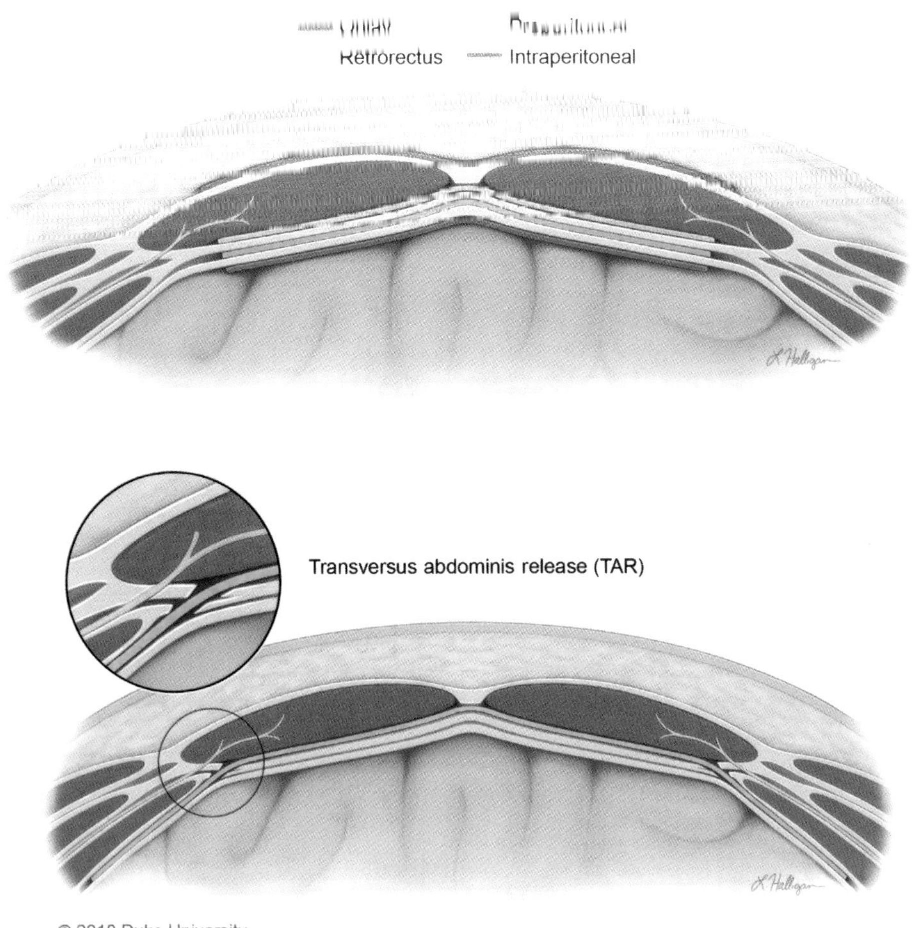

FIGURE 95.2. Anatomic mesh placement.

hernia recurrence rates compared with biologic mesh. High-level evidence with randomized prospective multicenter trials is needed to solve this ongoing debate.[22]

HERNIA REPAIR TECHNIQUE

Hernia repair techniques vary widely and there are oftentimes more opinions than surgeons. A few of the more commonly debated topics are listed below with evidence where applicable.

Suturing Techniques in Laparotomy Closure

A slowly absorbable or permanent monofilament running suture in small bite increments is recommended for primary fascial closure. Smaller bites that are <10 mm from the wound edge are obtained by using a smaller needle at smaller 5 mm intervals. Increased smaller bites and avoiding excessive suture tension will improve the suture length to wound length ratio to above 4.[20,40]

Mesh and Suture

Mesh placement is generally secured where the mesh overlaps the fascia by 3 to 5 cm in all directions. Of course, some studies suggest much wider overlap. There are a variety of techniques used to anchor the mesh including, glue, tacks, screws, and suture. Whichever technique is chosen, the surgeon should keep in mind that a durable repair is paramount. There are insufficient data to suggest that one type of suture is superior to another.

Component Separation

Ramirez described component separation in 1990 with the purpose of realigning the recti in the midline without the use of mesh or local flaps.[41,42] The rationale to the component separation is to release the lateral pulling or retracted oblique muscles, allowing the recti to centralize, without damaging the recti nerves or destabilizing the abdominal wall. The original paper describes relaxing incisions that are made 2 cm lateral to the rectus sheath through the external oblique fascia. The incision is made from costal margin to inguinal ligament. An avascular plane is developed between the external and internal oblique muscles. The posterior rectus sheath is released from the rectus muscles to obtain medialization of the recti 5 cm in epigastrium, 10 cm at the umbilicus, and 3 cm at the suprapubic region. Since the original publication in 1990, component separation has gained traction in the field and the addition of mesh further enhances the repair.[43] Previous stoma or surgery through the rectus muscle is not an absolute contraindication to component separation.[44]

Multiple adaptations of the original component separation have taken place since its original description, including general surgery laparoscopic and plastic surgery limited open approaches. The goal of these adaptations is to provide the same release while limiting dissection to reduce seroma formation and skin necrosis. Umbilical perforator sparing endoscopic techniques, creation of lateral tunnel incisions to provide external oblique aponeurosis release, and the laparoscopic transversus abdominis muscle release are a few examples of these approaches.[37,45]

Laparoscopic/Open Incisional Hernia Repair

Laparoscopic hernia repair with mesh was first reported in 1993 by Leblanc and colleagues.[46] A recent meta-analysis of several randomized controlled trials found that laparoscopic and open incisional hernia repairs with mesh had comparable outcomes including recurrence rates less than 10%.[47]

Local/Regional Flaps

Local and regional flaps for abdominal wall reconstruction are a special class of hernia cases that, in the adult, often occur following trauma or tumor resection. Fasciocutaneous, myocutaneous, and muscle flaps derive from the abdomen, back, and thighs. The most common flaps are listed in **Table 95.2**, where they have been categorized according to upper third, middle third, and lower third reconstruction. In general, lower and middle defects have thigh-based flaps available for reconstruction whereas the upper abdomen is limited to local tissue and the latissimus muscle. Defects of the epigastric and xiphoid regions pose the greatest challenges. In general, tissue expansion does not work well for abdominal wall reconstruction unless expanders are placed above a stable bone platform like ribs or pelvis.

Free Flaps

The same flaps that are listed as local rotational flaps can also be used as free tissue transfer. Typically, free flaps are indicated for very large epigastric defects that are difficult to cover with pedicled flaps. Recipient vessels could include superior and inferior epigastric vessels, and superficial or deep circumflex iliac vessels. If these vessels are not available, then vein grafts could be used to gain access to internal mammary recipient vessels. Intra-abdominal gastroepiploic vessels have also been used as recipient vessels when other vessels are not available. Functional free tissue transfer can also be done with an innervated chimeric anterolateral thigh, rectus femoris, and tensor fascia lata (TFL) flaps, but the long-term results of these approaches are unknown.[39]

Abdominal Wall Transplant

A special consideration in abdominal wall reconstruction is patients with massive abdominal wall defects who have lost most of their muscle. These patients may be considered candidates for composite tissue allotransplantation. To be a candidate for allotransplantation, the patient should be actively taking immunosuppressive therapy for other transplanted organs. The reason for this is that immunosuppression has been associated with de novo cancer formation and death. Abdominal wall transplantation is still considered experimental with less than 25 cases performed worldwide since 1994 and should only be performed in centers that have the necessary multidisciplinary teams in place.[39]

PROPHYLACTIC HERNIA PREVENTION

Recent studies suggest that there is a role for application of mesh or graft at the time of laparotomy closure in high-risk patients to prevent hernia formation. This is a relatively new concept that is gaining traction with a number of quality clinical trials. In a couple of meta-analyses of clinical trials of elective primary midline laparotomy patients, onlay mesh placement was found to have the least hernia occurrence rates compared to primary suture repair and sublay mesh placement. Onlay mesh repair was found to have higher seroma rates due to the increased subcutaneous tissue elevation.[14,48–50]

CONCLUSION

Incisional ventral hernia is perhaps one of the most common complications in all surgery. The field is ripe with intense debate and controversies and ongoing scrutiny of patient modifiable factors and risk mitigation strategies have lowered the complication rate, but in general better performing medical devices such as suture and mesh or graft are needed. A surgeon who is well versed in the hernia and abdominal wall reconstruction field and takes time to develop their skills appropriately will likely remain busy for a long time.

TABLE 95.2. PEDICLE FLAPS FOR ABDOMINAL WALL RECONSTRUCTION[37,39]

Location and Pedicle Flap	Blood Supply	Flap Characteristics
Upper Third		
Rectus abdominis	Superior epigastric	Inferior or superiorly based flap to cover wounds from chest wall, abdomen, groin, and perineum Vertical, horizontal, or oblique skin paddle orientations
External oblique	Lateral intercostal perforators	Ideal for lower chest wall and upper third abdominal defects due to arc of rotation
Latissimus dorsi	Thoracodorsal	Muscle or myocutaneous flap with large arc of rotation to reach superolateral abdominal wall defects
Omentum	Right gastroepiploic	May not be available in patients with previous intra-abdominal surgery or pathology Requires persistent abdominal wall defect to pedicle the flap Can provide soft tissue coverage for various abdominal wall defects, cover with skin graft
Middle Third		
Rectus abdominis	Superior or deep inferior epigastric	Inferior or superiorly based flap to cover wounds from chest wall, abdomen, groin, and perineum Vertical, horizontal, or oblique skin paddle orientations
External oblique	Lateral branches of posterior intercostal perforators	Ideal for lower chest wall and upper third abdominal defects due to arc of rotation Medial flap advancement for medial abdominal wall wounds
Tensor fasciae latae	Ascending branch of lateral circumflex femoral	Large skin paddle, distal flap prone to necrosis, fascial use for abdominal wall support
Anterior lateral thigh/vastus lateralis	Descending branch of lateral circumflex femoral	Large flap that usually reaches to umbilicus without difficulty, minimal donor-site morbidity Fascia can be used for abdominal wall fascial reconstruction
Anterior medial thigh/rectus femoris	Descending branch of lateral circumflex femoral	Muscle or myocutaneous flap that can be used alone or combined with anterolateral thigh flap or vastus lateralis
Lower Third		
Rectus abdominis	Deep inferior epigastric	Inferior or superiorly based flap to cover wounds from chest wall, abdomen, groin, and perineum Vertical, horizontal, or oblique skin paddle orientations
Internal oblique	Deep circumflex iliac	Limited arc of rotation, myocutaneous flap
Tensor fasciae latae	Ascending branch of lateral circumflex femoral	Large skin paddle, distal flap prone to necrosis, fascial use for abdominal wall support
Anterior lateral thigh/vastus lateralis	Descending branch of lateral circumflex femoral	Large flap that usually reaches to umbilicus without difficulty, minimal donor-site morbidity Fascia can be used for abdominal wall fascial reconstruction
Anterior medial thigh/rectus femoris	Descending branch of lateral circumflex femoral	Muscle or myocutaneous flap that can be used alone or combined with anterolateral thigh flap or vastus lateralis
Gracilis	Medial circumflex femoral	Small muscle or myocutaneous flap that could be used for inferior abdominal wall, groin, or perineal wounds

REFERENCES

1. Le Huu Nho R, Mege D, Ouaissi M, et al. Incidence and prevention of ventral incisional hernia. *J Visc Surg*. 2012;149:e3-e14.
2. Bhangu A, Nepogodiev D, Futaba K; West Midlands Research Collaborative. Systematic review and meta-analysis of the incidence of incisional hernia at the site of stoma closure. *World J Surg*. 2012;36:973-983.
3. Sanders DL, Kingsnorth AN. The modern management of incisional hernias. *BMJ*. 2012;344:e2843.
4. Wechter ME, Pearlman MD, Hartmann KE. Reclosure of the disrupted laparotomy wound: a systematic review. *Obstet Gynecol*. 2005;106:376-383.
5. Pauli EM, Rosen MJ. Open ventral hernia repair with component separation. *Surg Clin North Am*. 2013;93:1111-1133.
6. Parker SG, Wood CPJ, Butterworth JW, et al. A systematic methodological review of reported perioperative variables, postoperative outcomes and hernia recurrence from randomised controlled trials of elective ventral hernia repair: clear definitions and standardised datasets are needed. *Hernia*. 2018;22:215-226.
7. Peralta R, Latifi R. Long-term outcomes of abdominal wall reconstruction: what are the real numbers? *World J Surg*. 2012;36:534-538.
8. Luijendijk RW, Hop WC, van den Tol MP, et al. A comparison of suture repair with mesh repair for incisional hernia. *N Engl J Med*. 2000;343:392-398.
This landmark RCT studied the ideal closure technique for patients undergoing primary incisional ventral hernia or repair of a first hernia recurrence and compared suture versus mesh repair. Hernia repair with mesh was found to reduce recurrence by approximately 50%. Patients who already had a recurrence had an even more profound decreased rate of hernia development with the use of mesh.
9. Burger JW, Luijendijk RW, Hop WC, et al. Long-term follow-up of a randomized controlled trial of suture versus mesh repair of incisional hernia. *Ann Surg*. 2004;240:578-583.
10. Poulose BK, Shelton J, Phillips S, et al. Epidemiology and cost of ventral hernia repair: making the case for hernia research. *Hernia*. 2012;16:179-183.
11. Abo-Ryia MH, El-Khadrawy OH, Abd-Allah HS. Prophylactic preperitoneal mesh placement in open bariatric surgery: a guard against incisional hernia development. *Obes Surg*. 2013;23:1571-1574.
12. Cleveland RD, Zitsch RP III, Laws HL. Incisional closure in morbidly obese patients. *Am Surg*. 1989;55:61-63.
13. Sugerman HJ. Weight reduction after gastric bypass and horizontal gastroplasty for morbid obesity. *Eur J Surg*. 1996;162:157-158.

14. Jairam AP, Timmermans L, Eker HH, et al. Prevention of incisional hernia with prophylactic onlay and sublay mesh reinforcement versus primary suture only in midline laparotomies (PRIMA): 2-year follow-up of a multicentre, double-blind, randomised controlled trial. *Lancet*. 2017;390:567-576.
   This double-blind multicenter RCT examined the optimal abdominal closure pattern in elective midline laparotomy patients that were high risk for incisional hernia development. Patients were randomized to either prophylactic onlay synthetic mesh placement, sublay synthetic mesh placement, or primary fascial closure. Prophylactic onlay mesh placement had a significant reduction in hernia occurrence rate at 2 years compared to sublay mesh placement and primary fascial closure.
15. Punekar IRA, Khouri JS, Catanzaro M, et al. Redefining the rectus sheath: implications for abdominal wall repair. *Plast Reconstr Surg*. 2018;141:473-479.
16. Harrison B, Sanniec K, Janis JE. Collagenopathies: implications for abdominal wall reconstruction: a systematic review. *Plast Reconstr Surg Glob Open*. 2016;4:e1036.
17. Fink C, Baumann P, Wente MN, et al. Incisional hernia rate 3 years after midline laparotomy. *Br J Surg*. 2014;101:51-54.
18. Tolstrup MB, Watt SK, Gogenur I. Reduced rate of dehiscence after implementation of a standardized fascial closure technique in patients undergoing emergency laparotomy. *Ann Surg*. 2017;265:821-826.
19. Muysoms FE, Antoniou SA, Bury K, et al. European Hernia Society guidelines on the closure of abdominal wall incisions. *Hernia*. 2015;19:1-24.
20. Deerenberg EB, Harlaar JJ, Steyerberg EW, et al. Small bites versus large bites for closure of abdominal midline incisions (STITCH): a double-blind, multicentre, randomised controlled trial. *Lancet*. 2015;386:1254-1260.
   This article is a double-blinded multicenter RCT that addressed the optimal closure technique of midline laparotomies in an effort to decrease ventral hernia occurrence. They compared small-bite (every 5 mm) to large-bite (every 10 mm) closures in elective midline laparotomy patients. The article found that the smaller bite closure was more effective in preventing incisional hernia without increased adverse outcomes.
21. Lintin LA, Kingsnorth AN. Mechanical failure of a lightweight polypropylene mesh. *Hernia*. 2014;18:131-133.
22. Majumder A, Winder JS, Wen Y, et al. Comparative analysis of biologic versus synthetic mesh outcomes in contaminated hernia repairs. *Surgery*. 2016;160:828-838.
23. Purnell CA, Souza JM, Park E, Dumanian GA. Repair of recurrent hernia after biologic mesh failure in abdominal wall reconstruction. *Am J Surg*. 2014;208:788-793.
24. Giordano S, Garvey PB, Baumann DP, et al. Primary fascial closure with biologic mesh reinforcement results in lesser complication and recurrence rates than bridged biologic mesh repair for abdominal wall reconstruction: a propensity score analysis. *Surgery*. 2017;161:499-508.
25. van't Riet M, de Vos van Steenwijk PJ, Kleinrensink GJ, et al. Tensile strength of mesh fixation methods in laparoscopic incisional hernia repair. *Surg Endosc*. 2002;16:1713-1716.
26. Jamal K, Ratnasingham K, Shaunak S, et al. A novel technique for modified onlay incisional hernia repair with mesh incorporation into the fascial defect: a method for addressing suture line failure. *Hernia*. 2015;19:473-477.
27. Ibrahim MM, Poveromo LP, Glisson RR, et al. Modifying hernia mesh design to improve device mechanical performance and promote tension-free repair. *J Biomech*. 2018;71:43-51.
28. Evans KK, Chim H, Patel KM, et al. Survey on ventral hernias: surgeon indications, contraindications, and management of large ventral hernias. *Am Surg*. 2012;78:388-397.
29. Krpata DM, Schmotzer BJ, Flocke S, et al. Design and initial implementation of HerQLes: a hernia-related quality-of-life survey to assess abdominal wall function. *J Am Coll Surg*. 2012;215:635-642.
30. Slater NJ, van der Kolk M, Hendriks T, van Goor H, Bleichrodt RP. Biologic grafts for ventral hernia repair: a systematic review. *Am J Surg*. 2013;205:220-230.
31. Ventral Hernia Working Group; Breuing K, Butler CE, Ferzoco S, et al. Incisional ventral hernias: review of the literature and recommendations regarding the grading and technique of repair. *Surgery*. 2010;148:544-558.
   This systematic review provides recommendations on the repair of ventral hernia by the Ventral Hernia Working Group. Recommendations are made on repair techniques and on the use of biologic and synthetic mesh. A novel grading scale of hernias is also described in relation to patient risk factors and wound contamination.
32. Warren JA, McGrath SP, Hale AL, et al. Patterns of recurrence and mechanisms of failure after open ventral hernia repair with mesh. *Am Surg*. 2017;83:1275-1282.
33. Conze J, Rosch R, Klinge U, et al. Polypropylene in the intra-abdominal position: influence of pore size and surface area. *Hernia*. 2004;8:365-372.
34. Chatzimavroudis G, Kalaitzis S, Voloudakis N, et al. Evaluation of four mesh fixation methods in an experimental model of ventral hernia repair. *J Surg Res*. 2017;212:253-259.
35. Lanier ST, Fligor JE, Miller KR, Dumanian GA. Reliable complex abdominal wall hernia repairs with a narrow, well-fixed retrorectus polypropylene mesh: a review of over 100 consecutive cases. *Surgery*. 2016;160:1508-1516.
36. Harris HW, Hope WH, Adrales G, et al. Contemporary concepts in hernia prevention: selected proceedings from the 2017 international symposium on prevention of incisional hernias. *Surgery*. 2018;164(2):319-326.
37. Althubaiti G, Butler CE. Abdominal wall and chest wall reconstruction. *Plast Reconstr Surg*. 2014;133:688e-701e.
38. Blatnik J, Jin J, Rosen M. Abdominal hernia repair with bridging acellular dermal matrix an expensive hernia sac. *Am J Surg*. 2008;196:47-50.
39. Patel NG, Ratanshi I, Buchel EW. The best of abdominal wall reconstruction. *Plast Reconstr Surg*. 2018;141:113e-36e.
40. Israelsson LA, Millbourn D. Prevention of incisional hernias: how to close a midline incision. *Surg Clin North Am*. 2013;93:1027-1040.
41. Ramirez OM, Ruas E, Dellon AL. "Components separation" method for closure of abdominal-wall defects: an anatomic and clinical study. *Plast Reconstr Surg*. 1990;86:519-526.
   Anatomic and clinical study that introduced the concept of "components separation" in abdominal wall reconstruction. Release of anterior and posterior layers of the abdominal musculature provide medial advancement of myofascial layers to provide primary abdominal wall closure and improved hernia outcomes. This study provides detailed description on the surgical techniques and intricacies that are relevant to this day.
42. Heller L, McNichols CH, Ramirez OM. Component separations. *Semin Plast Surg*. 2012;26:25-28.
43. Ko JH, Wang EC, Salvay DM, et al. Abdominal wall reconstruction: lessons learned from 200 "components separation" procedures. *Arch Surg*. 2009;144:1047-1055.
44. Garvey PB, Bailey CM, Baumann DP, et al. Violation of the rectus complex is not a contraindication to component separation for abdominal wall reconstruction. *J Am Coll Surg*. 2012;214:131-139.
45. Pauli EM, Wang J, Petro CC, et al. Posterior component separation with transversus abdominis release successfully addresses recurrent ventral hernias following anterior component separation. *Hernia*. 2015;19:285-291.
46. LeBlanc KA, Booth WV. Laparoscopic repair of incisional abdominal hernias using expanded polytetrafluoroethylene: preliminary findings. *Surg Laparosc Endosc*. 1993;3:39-41.
47. Awaiz A, Rahman F, Hossain MB, et al. Meta-analysis and systematic review of laparoscopic versus open mesh repair for elective incisional hernia. *Hernia*. 2015;19:449-463.
48. Muysoms FE, Detry O, Vierendeels T, et al. Prevention of incisional hernias by prophylactic mesh-augmented reinforcement of midline laparotomies for abdominal aortic aneurysm treatment: a randomized controlled trial. *Ann Surg*. 2016;263:638-645.
49. Bhangu A, Fitzgerald JE, Singh P, et al. Systematic review and meta-analysis of prophylactic mesh placement for prevention of incisional hernia following midline laparotomy. *Hernia*. 2013;17:445-455.
50. Borab ZM, Shakir S, Lanni MA, et al. Does prophylactic mesh placement in elective, midline laparotomy reduce the incidence of incisional hernia? A systematic review and meta-analysis. *Surgery*. 2017;161:1149-1163.

QUESTIONS

1. **A 55-year-old man is undergoing a surgical repair of a recurrent ventral hernia. At the end of the case, the anesthesiologist asks the surgical resident whether or not they should provide a local anesthetic block to help with pain control. Where is the correct abdominal wall anatomic location to provide maximal local anesthesia in this patient?**
   a. 1 cm medial to the lateral border of the rectus sheath
   b. Lateral to the femoral artery on a line connecting the anterior superior iliac spine (ASIS) and pubic tubercle, superficial to the iliopsoas muscle
   c. Three fingerbreadths below the ASIS, between the sartorious and tensor fascia lata muscles
   d. 2 cm lateral to the rectus sheath, between internal oblique and transversalis muscle
   e. 2 cm medial and inferior to the ASIS

2. **In a standard component separation as described by Ramirez, where do you get the least advancement in a component separation?**
   a. Epigastric region
   b. Suprapubic region
   c. Umbilical region
   d. All regions are equal

3. **In a high-risk patient with an incisional midline hernia, which one of the following reconstructions is most likely to decrease the chance of hernia recurrence?**
   a. Bridge repair with mesh
   b. Primary fascial closure no mesh
   c. Bilateral component separation with mesh placement and primary fascial closure
   d. Unilateral component separation, primary fascial closure, no mesh
   e. Unilateral component separation with bridged mesh placement without primary fascial closure

4. **What is the primary blood supply to a vertical rectus abdominis muscle flap used to reconstruct a chest wall and xiphoid wound?**
   a. Superficial circumflex iliac artery
   b. Superficial epigastric artery
   c. Deep Inferior epigastric artery
   d. Musculophrenic artery
   e. Superior Epigastric Artery

5. **What is the optimal abdominal wall primary fascial closure technique?**
   a. Double looped 0-polydioxanone suture (PDS) continuous suture with 2-cm fascial bites every 2 cm
   b. #1 PDS interrupted simple sutures with 1 cm fascial bites every 1 cm
   c. #0 Polyester braided nonabsorbable continuous suture with 1-cm fascial bites every 1 cm
   d. #1 PDS continuous suture with 5 mm fascial bites every 5 mm
   e. #0 Prolene continuous suture with 2-cm fascial bites every 2 cm

1. **Answer: d.** Transversus abdominis plane block is a peripheral nerve block of T6-L1 intercostal nerves that has been shown to improve postoperative pain control in midline laparotomies and abdominal based breast reconstruction. The correct location of the sensory nerves is between the internal oblique and transversus abdominis muscles lateral to the rectus sheath. The femoral nerve is found lateral to the femoral artery along the inguinal ligament. The lateral femoral cutaneous nerve is found inferior to the ASIS between the sartorious and TFL muscles. The correct location for an ilioinguinal nerve block is 2 cm medial and inferior to the ASIS.

2. **Answer: b.** Components separation described by Ramirez et al. in 1990 states that approximately 5-, 10-, and 3-cm advancements can be made in a unilateral or 10-, 20-, and 6-cm advancements in a bilateral in the epigastric, umbilical, and suprapubic regions, respectively. Of note, to obtain these advancements, Ramirez described both anterior component release and release of the rectus muscle from the posterior sheath.

3. **Answer: c.** Although hernia reconstruction remains controversial, hernia recurrence is significantly reduced with the addition of mesh and the ability to obtain primary fascial closure. Component separation strives to advance the abdominal wall toward the midline to achieve primary fascial closure. The addition of mesh further decreases risk of recurrence.

4. **Answer: e.** In a superiorly based rectus abdominis flap, the primary blood supply is the superior epigastric artery which is a continuation of the internal mammary artery. The internal mammary branches into the musculophrenic and Superior Epigastric Artery, which is the primary blood supply to the superiorly based rectus abdominis muscle flap. The superficial epigastric artery is incorrect nomenclature. The superficial circumflex iliac artery supplies the superficial circumflex iliac artery perforator flap or groin flap and the deep inferior epigastric artery is the primary blood supply for an inferiorly based rectus abdominis muscle flap.

5. **Answer: d.** Midline laparotomy fascial closure has been shown to have the highest closure strength and resistance to hernia occurrence with the use of a slowly absorbable, monofilament suture with small fascial bites in smaller increments. This technique increases the suture to incision length ratio to greater than 4:1, which provides the additional strength of the closure.

CHAPTER 96 Lower Extremity, Foot, and Ankle Reconstruction

Jessica F. Rose, Stephen J. Kovach, and L. Scott Levin

KEY POINTS

- Lower extremity injury is commonly associated with other trauma, and therefore appropriate workup and patient stabilization (advanced trauma life support protocol) are necessary before determining reconstructive options.
- Primary amputation may sometimes be more beneficial than lower extremity salvage.
- When caring for patients with lower extremity injuries, timing of the reconstruction must be considered, and patients may benefit from initial external fixation and negative pressure therapy prior to staged definitive reconstruction.
- The reconstructive ladder may be a helpful guide to reconstructive options, although certain circumstances benefit from microsurgical intervention (reconstructive elevator).
- Reconstructing the leg can be thought of as a rule of thirds, with gastrocnemius being the classic option for the proximal third, soleus for the middle third, and free flap for the distal third.
- Appropriate care of these patients likely utilizes a combination of specialties including orthopedic, plastic, trauma, and vascular surgeons.
- The orthoplastic approach guides all treatments.
- Patients may have many confounding factors and comorbidities that need to be considered and appropriately managed, such as diabetes and vascular disease, in order to have a successful reconstruction.

ANATOMY

Vasculature

To effectively treat and reconstruct the lower extremity, extensive knowledge of the anatomy is when choosing flaps based on and understanding which muscles are viable options in different clinical scenarios the vascular supply of the leg. The blood supply to the leg begins at the common iliac vessels, as they branch from the aorta, and then divide into the internal and external iliac arteries. The external iliac artery and its branches supply the thigh, with the external iliac artery becoming the femoral artery below the inguinal ligament. The femoral artery branches into the superficial femoral artery and the profunda femoris artery, both giving off many muscular branches, but the superficial femoral artery continues as the popliteal artery after the adductor hiatus and the profunda gives rise to the circumflex femoral system. The popliteal artery gives off genicular branches at the knee and then divides into the anterior tibial artery and the tibioperoneal trunk. The anterior tibial artery continues as the dorsalis pedis artery in the foot, whereas the tibioperoneal trunk further divides into peroneal and posterior tibial branches, the later continuing into the foot to become plantar and then finally digital arteries. The venous anatomy, with the exception of the saphenous vein, mimics the arterial anatomy.

Bones

The lower extremity is a specialized structure, functioning exclusively for bipedal locomotion. The extremity itself comes off the pelvic girdle, becoming a free limb. The femur is the largest bone and stabilizes the thigh, whereas the bony structure of the leg is made up of the tibia and fibula, with the patella articulating between both to help form the knee joint and the tibia stabilizing the leg. The foot is made up of 26 bones (the tarsus has 7 bones, the metatarsus has 5 bones, and the forefoot has 14 phalanges). The blood supply to the long bones consists of a nutrient artery, metaphyseal vessels, and periosteal vessels. Proper healing requires an adequate blood supply.[1]

Neurosensory

The neurosensory anatomy is also important for reconstruction, particularly to design sensate flaps. Figure 96.1 shows neurosensory distribution in the lower extremity.

Muscles and Compartments

The muscles of the lower extremity are best understood by dividing them into compartments by location (**Table 96.1**). The thigh has three compartments, the anterior, posterior, and adductor compartments. The anterior compartment is made up of the extensors (sartorius and the quadriceps: rectus femoris, vastus medialis, vastus lateralis, vastus intermedius) and innervated by the femoral nerve. The posterior compartment is composed of the flexors (biceps femoris, hamstrings, semimembranosus, semitendinosus) and primarily innervated by the tibial nerve. The adductor group (adductor longus, adductor brevis, adductor magnus, adductor minimus, gracilis) is mainly innervated by the obturator nerve.

The compartments of the lower extremity are commonly affected by compartment syndrome. There are four compartments: anterior, lateral, superficial posterior, and deep posterior. Generally, the anterior compartment contains the extensors, the lateral compartment contains muscles that flex and evert the foot, and the posterior compartments contain muscles that flex the foot and the toes.

Compartment syndrome arises when pressures in osseofascial compartments are high enough to decrease the capillary perfusion and can be caused by trauma, intracompartmental bleeding, swelling, burns and venomous bites, and ischemic reperfusion,[1,2] but most commonly occurs because of tibial fractures. Typically, this is compartment pressure >40 mm Hg or 20 mm Hg below the diastolic pressure or 30 mm Hg below the mean arterial blood pressure, resulting in anoxia, ischemia, and muscle death.[1,2] It causes pain that is disproportionate to the injury, palpably swollen compartments, pain on passive stretch, diminished sensation, decreased muscle strength, and hypesthesia/anesthesia of the involved nerves.[1] The earliest and most important sign is increasing pain, particularly to passive stretch of the involved muscles. If compartment syndrome is suspected, rapid treatment should be initiated, and the involved compartments should be released with a fasciotomy[1,2] (Figure 96.2).

Many of the muscles of the foot can be used as local flaps to close small wounds of the foot. The muscles are separated into compartments by location and function. First are the dorsal intrinsic muscles, which include extensor digitorum brevis and extensor hallucis brevis, and are innervated by the deep fibular nerve. Next

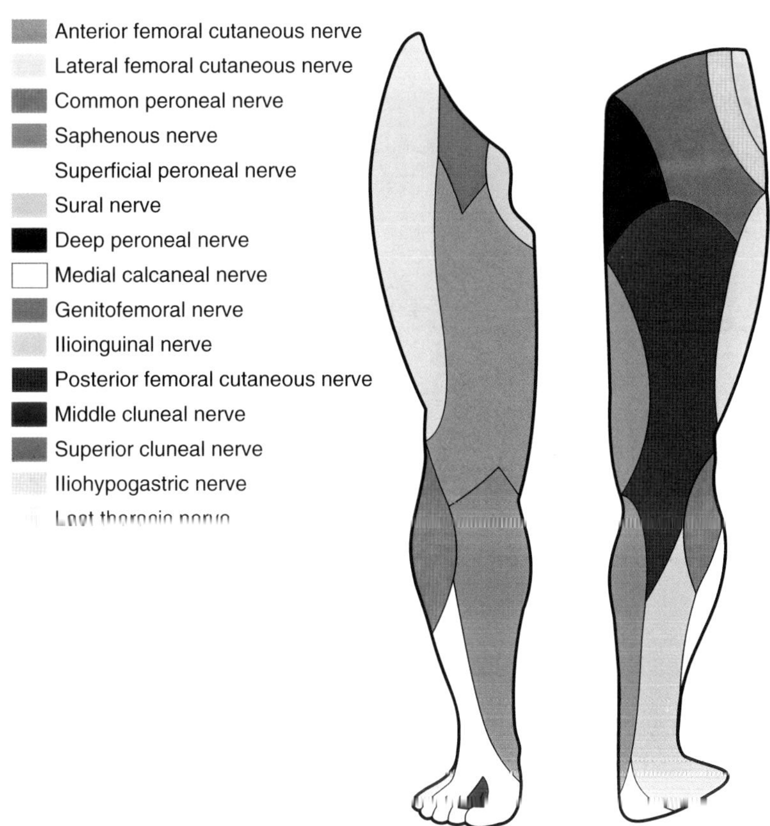

FIGURE 96.1. Sensory innervation of the lower extremity.

[illegible] lateral compartment, including the abductor digiti minimi, flexor digiti minimi, and opponens digiti minimi, all innervated by the lateral plantar nerve. The interosseous compartment (dorsal and planter interossei) is innervated by the lateral plantar nerve. The central compartment is made up of three separate levels. The first level contains adductor hallucis and is innervated by the lateral plantar nerve. The second level [illegible] lumbricals, and flexor digitorum longus, which are innervated by medial and lateral plantar nerves. The third level contains flexor digitorum brevis, supplied by the medial plantar nerve. The final compartment is the medial compartment, which contains abductor hallucis and flexor hallucis brevis, innervated by medial and lateral plantar nerves.

TABLE 96.1. COMPARTMENTS OF THE LEG

Compartment	Muscle	Function	Nerve	Artery
Anterior	Anterior tibialis	Extend, invert foot	Deep peroneal	Anterior tibial
	Extensor hallucis longus	Extend great toe, dorsiflex foot		
	Extensor digitorum longus	Extend toes II–V, extend foot		
	Peroneus tertius	Extend, evert foot		
Lateral	Peroneus longus Peroneus brevis	Flex, evert foot	Superficial peroneal	Anterior tibial, peroneal
Superficial posterior	Gastrocnemius	Flex foot, flex knee	Tibial	Posterior tibial, peroneal, sural
	Soleus	Plantar flex foot		Sural
	Popliteus	Flex knee, rotate tibia		Popliteal, genicular branches
	Plantaris	Flex foot		Peroneal
Deep posterior	Flexor hallucis longus	Flex foot, great toe	Tibial	Peroneal
	Flexor digitorum profundus	Flex foot, toes II–V		Posterior tibial
	Tibialis posterior	Flex, invert foot		Peroneal

Anterior compartment:
Tibialis anterior (TA)
Extensor hallicus Longus (EHL)
Extensor digitorum longus (EDL)
Peroneus tertius
Anterior tibial artery and vein
Deep peroneal nerve

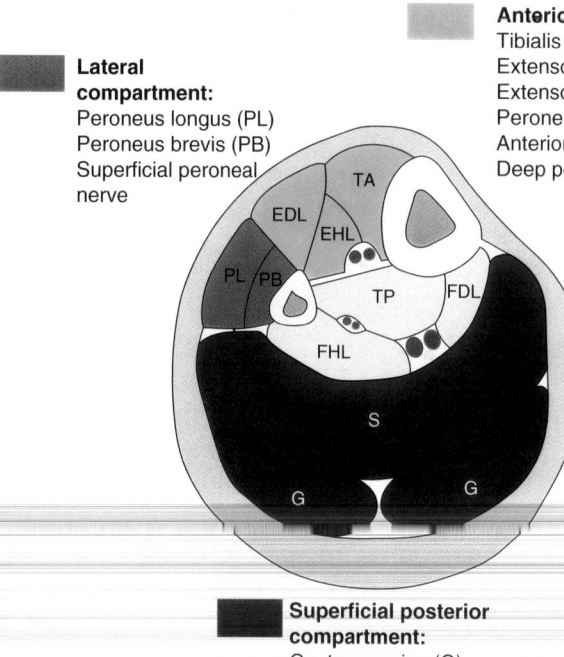

Lateral compartment:
Peroneus longus (PL)
Peroneus brevis (PB)
Superficial peroneal nerve

TA
EDL
EHL
PL
PB
TP
FDL
FHL
S
G
G

Deep posterior compartment:
Flexor hallucis longus (FHL)
Flexor digitorum profundus (FDP)
Tibialis posterior (TP)
Peroneal artery and vein
Posterior tibial artery and vein
Tibial nerve

Superficial posterior compartment:
Gastrocnemius (G)
Soleus (S)
Popliteus

FIGURE 96.2. Compartments of the lower extremity.

FRACTURE CLASSIFICATION

Many systems have been created to classify open tibial fractures, mostly to better describe the injury and prognosis. The most commonly used system is the Gustilo-Anderson classification[3]:

- **Grade I:** Open fracture, wound <1 cm in length
- **Grade II:** Open fracture, wound >1 cm in length without extensive soft-tissue damage
- **Grade IIIA:** Open fracture with extensive soft-tissue injury
- **Grade IIIB:** Open fracture with extensive soft-tissue injury, bone damage, periosteal stripping, massive contamination, often needs soft-tissue coverage
- **Grade IIIC:** Open fracture with extensive soft-tissue injury and arterial injury requiring vascular repair

This system is aimed to classify the soft-tissue injury related to the likelihood of development of infection.[1,3,4]. Plastic surgeons are most likely required to assist with patients who have Gustilo IIIB and IIIC injuries.

The next system is the Byrd classification, which was designed to classify open tibial fractures and to determine the usefulness of muscle flaps based on severity of injury[5] (Figure 96.3):

- **Type I:** Low-energy forces, spiral or oblique fracture, <2 cm laceration, relatively clean; healing process is prompt and uncomplicated
- **Type II:** Moderate-energy forces, comminuted or displaced fracture, skin laceration >2 cm, contusions, no devitalized muscle; also heal normally
- **Type III:** High-energy forces, displaced fracture with significant comminution or segmental with or without bone defect, skin loss, devitalized muscle; require vascularized coverage with debridement of nonviable muscle and closure and filling of dead space
- **Type IV:** High-energy forces or high-velocity gunshot, Type III fractures, crush or degloving, significant local damage, vascular injury requiring vascular repair; require free flaps to obliterate dead space and cover the wound

MANAGEMENT OF LOWER EXTREMITY TRAUMA

Traumatic injuries are the cause of more than 60% of lower extremity reconstructions.[6] Management of the mangled extremity is complex, as it involves a combination of injuries to the soft tissue, bone, vasculature, and nerves.[7] Appropriate trauma management is key to caring for this patient population. The first thing to assess is patient stability, focusing on the whole patient and following the advanced trauma life support guidelines.[8] Resuscitation and management of life-threatening injuries take priority to extremity salvage.[7] The extremity

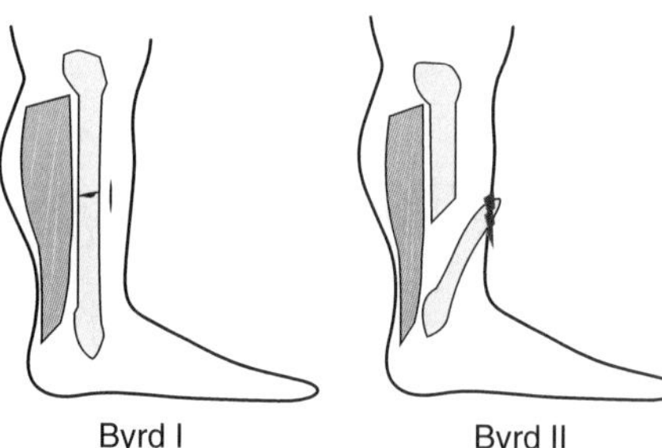

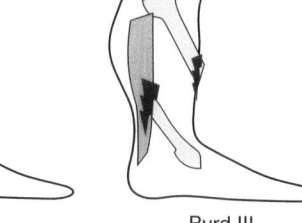

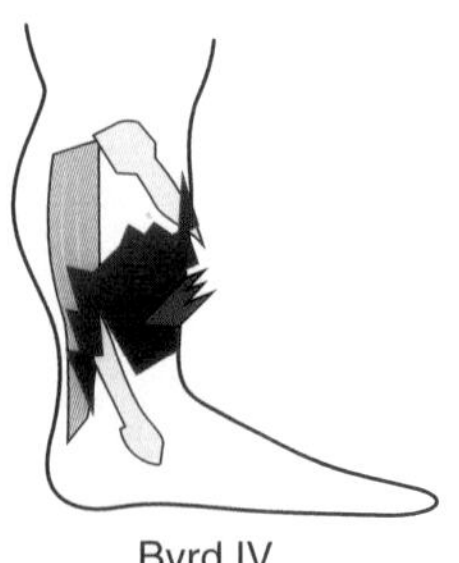

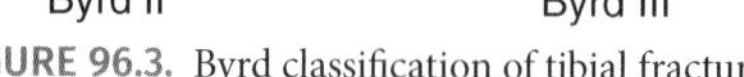

FIGURE 96.3. Byrd classification of tibial fractures.

examination should focus on the sensibility and vascularity of the extremity and include assessment of soft-tissue and bony trauma.[6,9] Compartment pressures and Doppler assessment of vascular signals may be necessary.[6] Patients are typically stabilized by the trauma and orthopedic surgeons first, including the management of compartment syndrome, open fractures, and arterial injuries.[10] Vascular injuries typically require management before fracture stabilization; however, sometimes temporary shunting and definitive repair after fracture fixation may be prudent.[7] Figure 96.4 is an algorithm for trauma management.

Once the patient is stable, care for the mangled extremity begins, which is often best done with a multidisciplinary approach including orthopedic and plastic surgeons.[8] Early management includes complete wound debridement and skeletal stabilization by either internal or external fixation.[8] Debridement is the most important step. Historically, serial debridement was performed, but it is better

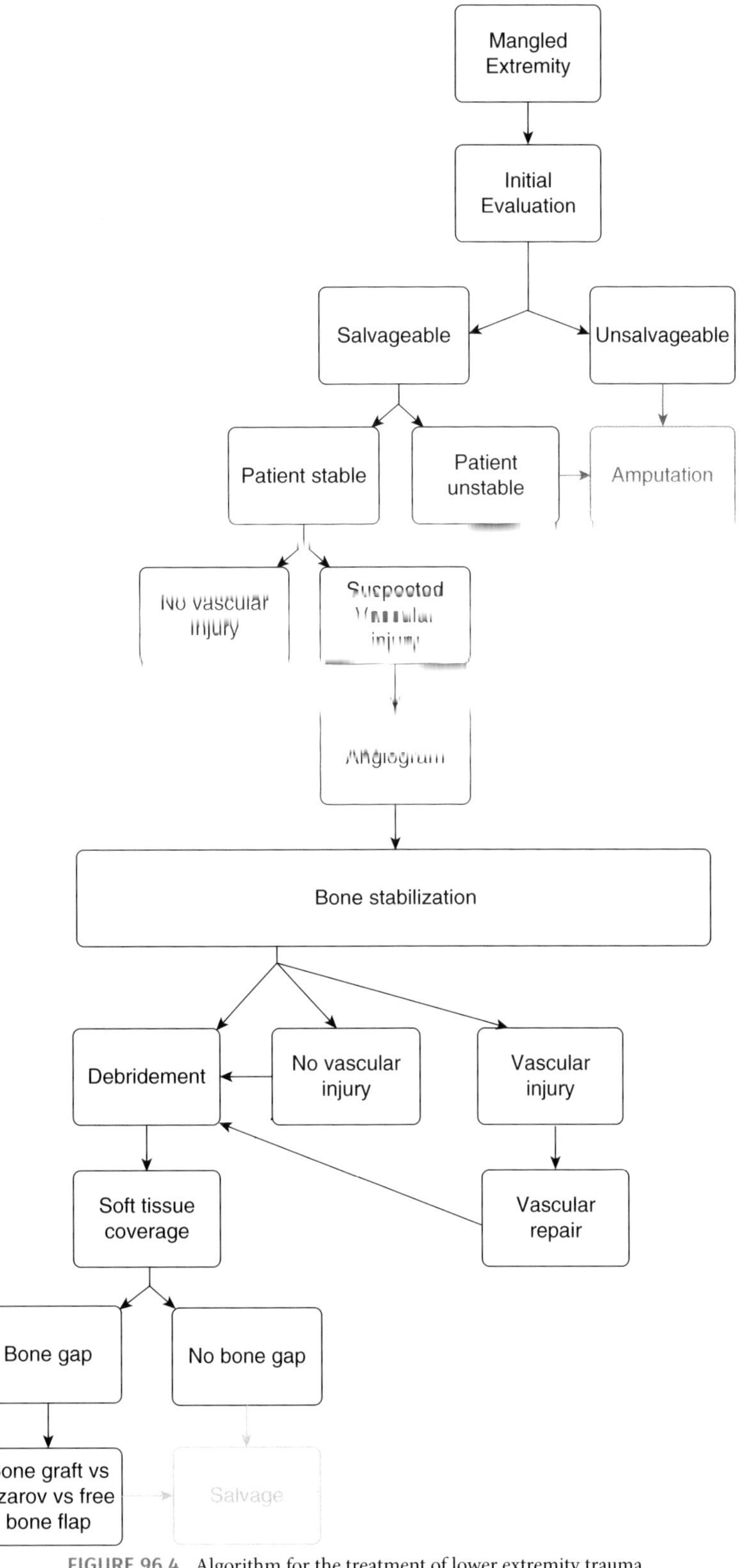

FIGURE 96.4. Algorithm for the treatment of lower extremity trauma.

to perform one thorough debridement (termed radical necrectomy) with early reconstruction and avoid desiccation of the wound bed.[8,11] However, if the wound is severely contaminated, an external fixator is beneficial for complete, staged, debridement, and coverage can be temporarily maintained with a wound vacuum during this phase.[4] Injured structures such as bone, tendon, blood vessels, and nerves should be reconstructed immediately for better and earlier functional rehabilitation.[8] External fixation was the traditional management of open fractures, to keep permanent hardware out a potentially contaminated field. It is still the preferred method if there is active wound infection or for infected nonunion or malunion. However, external fixation has increased healing times and higher rate of malunion and nonunion, along with the practicality of both the patient and surgeons working around the device. If infection is not an issue, internal fixation is recommended. This can be executed with plates, intermedullary nails, or minimally invasive plate osteosynthesis, all at the discretion of our orthopedic colleagues.[8]

ANGIOGRAPHY AND IMAGING STUDIES

For patients with possible or suspected vascular injuries, diagnostic studies may be necessary. Patients need imaging if there are abnormal pulses, Doppler signals, or ankle brachial indexes, the recipient vessels are located in the zone of injury, there is an extensive injury with a high-energy mechanism, or the patient has preexisting arterial disease.[10] Occasionally, imaging will elucidate injuries on patients who had a normal clinical examination.[10] Angiographic imaging can help determine which regional muscles are appropriately vascularized and usable for coverage and can determine which vessels are uninjured and available for free flap inflow.[10] This can be particularly useful if the anterior tibial artery might be needed, as it is superficial and has the highest rate of injury, so imaging would help determine its viability. The final and most important benefit of preoperative imaging is the ability to visualize the blood flow to the lower extremity.[10] If there is three vessel runoff, an end to end anastomosis is possible, whereas if there is only one vessel flow an end to side anastomosis is mandatory.

There are two options if imaging of the lower extremity vasculature is necessary—computed tomography angiogram (CTA) and formal angiography. The benefits of CTA are ease of imaging, cost-effectiveness, and low complication rate. It is less invasive and uses less contrast and radiation than traditional angiography. CTA also shows other anatomical information relative to the soft tissues, veins, and bones, while it also shows information about stenosis and obstruction. Formal angiograms are more expensive and invasive, but they may be necessary if CTA has too much scatter from hardware. Formal angiograms are particularly helpful in vasculopaths and patients requiring concomitant vascular reconstruction.[10]

COMORBIDITIES

Many patients have comorbidities that can compromise or complicate their care. Particularly in the case of the lower extremity, diabetes and vascular disease are important to understand and manage.

Diabetes

Twenty-four million Americans have diabetes mellitus, many of whom will end up with a wound or a foot ulcer during their lifetime. Major amputation is a risk factor for morbidity and mortality in this patient population. Using flaps for limb salvage can therefore affect their long-term survival. However, there is often nihilism surrounded reconstructing this population. This stems from high complication rates due to *small-vessel disease*, hyperglycemia, neuropathy, and noncompliance. Hyperglycemia inhibits white blood cell phagocytosis and increases postoperative complication rates. Diabetic patients need to have optimized glucose before and after surgical procedures.[4] Neuropathy leads to sensory loss, muscle atrophy, Charcot arthropathy, anhidrosis, and increased risk of wounding and ulceration. Reconstruction is a challenge because the wound bed tends to have decreased vascularization, making it difficult for skin graft take. Local flaps tend to be unreliable in this patient population as the area tends to be scarred. Pedicled flaps also have a higher complication rate in this population, although they also have a higher rate of success than extremity free flaps in these patients.[12] Microsurgery can be very difficult as local vessels are needed for inflow and tend to be calcified.[13]

Vascular Disease

Patients with vascular disease require imaging (either CTA or angiogram) to assess their vascular inflow before a reconstruction is attempted.[4] Ischemic limbs where no major vessel runoff is evident or those that are severely calcified cannot be used as recipient vessels.[13] These patients may require revascularization procedures first. Although they are higher risk, reconstruction has been successful even when performed simultaneously with a vascular bypass procedure.

Smoking

Smoking has a deleterious effect on perfusion and healing. Smokers have longer healing times and have higher rates of infection, nonunion, and osteomyelitis. Smoking also increases the rate of thrombosis with lower extremity reconstruction.[1,4]

Radiation

Radiation causes an inflammatory and vascular insult to tissues, which has a detrimental effect on donor vessels.[4] Radiated vessels are also technically challenging to use as donor vessels, as the walls are friable, inelastic, and difficult to suture.

Steroids

Steroids are [illegible] and have a negative impact on wound healing. These effects can be lessened with the use of vitamin A.

SALVAGE VERSUS PRIMARY AMPUTATION

In the trauma population, the decision to proceed with primary amputation versus proceeding with reconstruction can be very difficult to make. The decision should be made on an individual basis by considering the patient's occupation, age, associated injuries, and socioeconomic status.[8] Multiple scoring systems have been developed to attempt to make the decision clearer. The Lower Extremity Assessment Project was a randomized, prospective trial carried out at eight trauma centers, developed to determine who would benefit from salvage versus who would not. Microvascular techniques and external fixation can typically result in a successful salvage. However, patients who failed extremity salvage suffered more complications and some ultimately underwent amputation. Primary amputation in these patients would have avoided prolonged, costly, and futile procedures. The study evaluated existing injured extremity scoring systems but found that these scoring systems were effective in determining which limbs could be salvaged but could not predict who would fare better from primary amputation.[1,8,14,15] Lower Extremity Assessment Project showed that a patient's ability to function afterward was more attributed to their functional ability before trauma, regarding their social, economic, and personality disadvantages. Reconstruction does come with a higher rate of complication and rehospitalization rate than amputation, with 4% ultimately ending in amputation. Absent plantar sensation at presentation was not an indicator for amputation or functional outcome. Results 2 years after trauma show equivalent outcomes for those who underwent amputation versus those who underwent reconstruction, for patients with equivalent Sickness Impact Profiles.[14,15]

Making the decision to amputate on a case-by-case basis is also recommended. However, there are several prognostic factors for limb salvage to consider. There is a linear relationship between time to revascularization and limb loss (longer than 8 hours warm ischemia time is an indication for amputation). Patients with high-velocity penetrating injuries and blunt injuries have worse outcomes. Associated injuries and comorbidities should be considered. Those presenting with a cadaveric foot, severe tibial or sciatic nerve injury, severe polytrauma, shock, or extremis, and those with failed revascularization procedures will benefit from primary amputation.[1,4,7]

Replantation is usually not performed because prostheses can make a functional lower limb. However, replantation can be considered if there is minimal warm ischemia time and a durable, sensate, and painless foot seems possible.[8]

RECONSTRUCTIVE PLANNING

Plastic surgeons become necessary to aid in the reconstructive process in patients who have fractures with overlying soft-tissue loss.[10] Patients who have Gustilo IIIB and IIIC injuries necessitate lower extremity reconstructive surgery.[6] Early involvement by plastic surgeons helps in incision planning, or access to flaps or vessels necessary for the reconstruction. The so-called *orthoplastic* approach or the *fix and flap* approach may help decrease the wounds created for reconstruction and lead to earlier coverage.[9,10] Goals of the reconstruction are to promote fracture healing, prevent osteomyelitis, restore function, optimize aesthetics, and enhance conduct of sec[illegible][11]

Timing of Reconstruction

Marko Godina[11] showed that early flap closure (within the first 72 hours) of open tibial fractures leads to a lower flap failure rate, lower infection rate, quicker healing times, and shorter hospital stays.[11] His study grouped the patients according to when their reconstruction was performed:

- Early reconstruction: within first 72 hours
- Delayed reconstruction: between 72 hours and 3 months
- Late reconstruction: >3 months after injury

He then assessed infections, flap failure rates, number of anesthetics, hospitalization time, and time to healing. The early reconstruction group had the fewest flap failures and infections with shorter hospitalizations, decreased time to bone healing, and fewer anesthetics, indicating that this was the ideal time frame for flap closure (**Table 96.2**).[11]

Although Godina's work ushered in a new paradigm in lower extremity reconstruction, it is not always possible or necessary to obtain coverage in the first 72 hours. Wounds must be adequately debrided, and in some instances, this requires several serial operations.[4] If there is a question of tissue viability, a staged approach with a planned second operation or serial operations is warranted.[9] However, exposed critical structures (vessels and nerves) require immediate coverage.[4] Although early coverage decreases infection, fibrosis, and edema that make reconstruction more challenging, it is not always feasible because of concomitant injuries or delayed referral. In these patients, *damage control orthopedics* model with temporary fixation and secondary management can be useful. In this patient population, provisional closure can be obtained with a wound vacuum, which will decrease edema and fibrosis (and extremity circumference) and increase granulation tissue. Use of the vacuum device simplifies wound care until definitive closure, increasing sterility and decreasing the frequency of dressing changes. Use of this technology can allow for free flap reconstruction outside the 72-hour window with an acceptable complication rate.[16]

TABLE 96.2. HOW TIMING OF FREE FLAP COVERAGE AFFECT OUTCOME IN THE TREATMENT OF OPEN FRACTURES[11]

Timing	Failure Rate	Infection Rate	Bone Healing Time	Hospital Time
<72 h	1%	2%	68 mo	27 d
72 h to 3 wk	12%	18%	123 mo	130 d
>3 wk	10%	6%	29 mo	256 d

Management of Bone Gaps

Patients who have bone loss, as the result of trauma or tumor extirpation, have several treatment options, with the size of the bony defect predictive of the type of reconstruction used.[4,8] Patients with lesions less than 6 cm can be treated with traditional, or nonvascularized, bone grafts, whereas those with greater than 6 cm loss should undergo distraction osteogenesis or a vascularized bone graft (free flap).[4,6,9]

Conventional bone grafting heals by creeping substitution. As a result, it can be limited by significant graft resorption, even in a well-vascularized recipient site.[17,18] Cancellous grafts are preferred and are usually placed about 6 weeks after coverage to fill the bony defect or used to supplement osteosynthesis sites.[8] To mitigate graft resorption, the Masquelet, or induced [illegible] instituted. This is a two-stage technique that stimulates membrane formation for graft placement. A foreign body (in this case, an antibiotic impregnated cement spacer) is placed in the bony defect and left for several weeks causing a pseudosynovial membrane to form. This membrane is similar to a capsule around a breast implant, and it helps maintain length and space of the defect, prevents fibrous ingrowth and infection, and creates a vascularized space for the graft. At 4 to 12 weeks after spacer placement, the second stage is performed and the spacer is removed and a cancellous bone graft (likely from the iliac crest) is placed. This method gives the soft tissues or soft-tissue reconstruction time to heal before definitive bony reconstruction and provides vascularization and growth factors to aid in bone graft healing and prevent resorption. This method leads to union in 90% of cases.[4,17,19]

Intercalary transport was first successfully used by Ilizarov in 1943.[20] Intercalary transport can be used to correct malunion or nonunion, used immediately after shortening and corticotomy and coverage to regain length, or used as the definitive external fixator.[21] It is an alternative to free flaps for large bony defects and may be preferential in one-vessel extremities; however, its use is best tolerated in defects of 4 to 8 cm. Ilizarov transport works by placing a dynamic frame and using a combination of osteotomy and transport segment distraction osteogenesis. The transport segment is moved toward the defect to fill the space. An osteotomy can be created on both the proximal and distal bone segments, using two transport segments moving toward each other. The frame enables lengthening of the bone segments, while maintaining length and alignment of the extremity, and with simultaneous stretching of the soft-tissue envelope tissue.[1,8,22] The device requires long periods of treatment, pain with the transport, risk of pin site infections, and risks nonunion at the docking site.[19]

The final method of managing bone gaps, particularly those greater than 6 cm, is with vascularized bone grafts. These can be either pedicled (ipsilateral fibula), but are more commonly performed as free flaps[9] (**Table 96.3**). The free fibula graft was first described by Dr. Taylor in 1975.[23] This is an ideal reconstruction as the bone remains organized, does not resorb, and can hypertrophy to increase strength.[23] Large segments can be transferred with retaining osteocyte and osteoblast viability because the nutrient blood supply remains intact, creating a potential for primary

TABLE 96.3. COMMONLY USED BONE FREE FLAPS

Flap	Blood Supply/Pedicle	Size	Common Use/Advantages	Caveats/Disadvantages
Scapula	Thoracodorsal or circumflex scapular systems	10 × 1–2 cm	Multiple options to make chimeric flaps	Lateral positioning
Fibula (see Figure 96.5)	Peroneal artery	Long	Good length, pedicle Can have skin paddle and can take muscle Ability to hypertrophy	Requires use of uninjured leg
Iliac crest	Deep circumflex iliac vessels	15 × 6 cm	Large bone, has cancellous with it, can be uni or bicortical	Risk of hernia
Medial geniculate/medial femoral condyle (see Figure 96.6)	Descending genicular artery	3 × 2 cm	Good vascularized cancellous bone Good for nonunions	Not for bone gaps >4 cm

healing, with improved healing times and strength.[18,23] The fibula is ideal, as it can be taken from the contralateral leg, has a reliable blood supply from the peroneal artery and can be taken as a chimeric flap with a skin paddle or muscle as needed.[6] The pitfalls of using a free flap are flap failure (necrosis and anastomotic failure), donor site morbidity (operating on the uninjured or unaffected leg), and the risk of stress fractures.[19] Other options for bony free flaps can be taken from the iliac crest, scapula, or medial femoral condyle (Figures 96.5 and 96.6).

Soft-Tissue Management

Soft-tissue injuries are typically best managed with local available tissues; however, the nature of the defect and the state of the other local muscles (which may have also been traumatized) will dictate the reconstructive needs. The goal is to reconstruct with tissue that have similar properties.[4] As previously mentioned, all defects need to be adequately prepared and debrided before coverage is attempted and all associated fractures need to be stabilized. The reconstructive ladder is useful in guiding reconstructive choices because it is a stepwise technique for closure of wounds that mandates starting with the simplest possibility and moving to more complicated procedures only when required.[24] The first step of the reconstructive ladder is primary closure and the final rung of the ladder is free flap reconstruction, with skin grafts, local flaps, and regional flaps in between.[9] Occasionally *reconstructive elevator* should be utilized, using a more complex reconstructive option to maximize the final result, and may be a better way to describe it, and progression is based on what will offer the best form and function.[4,24]

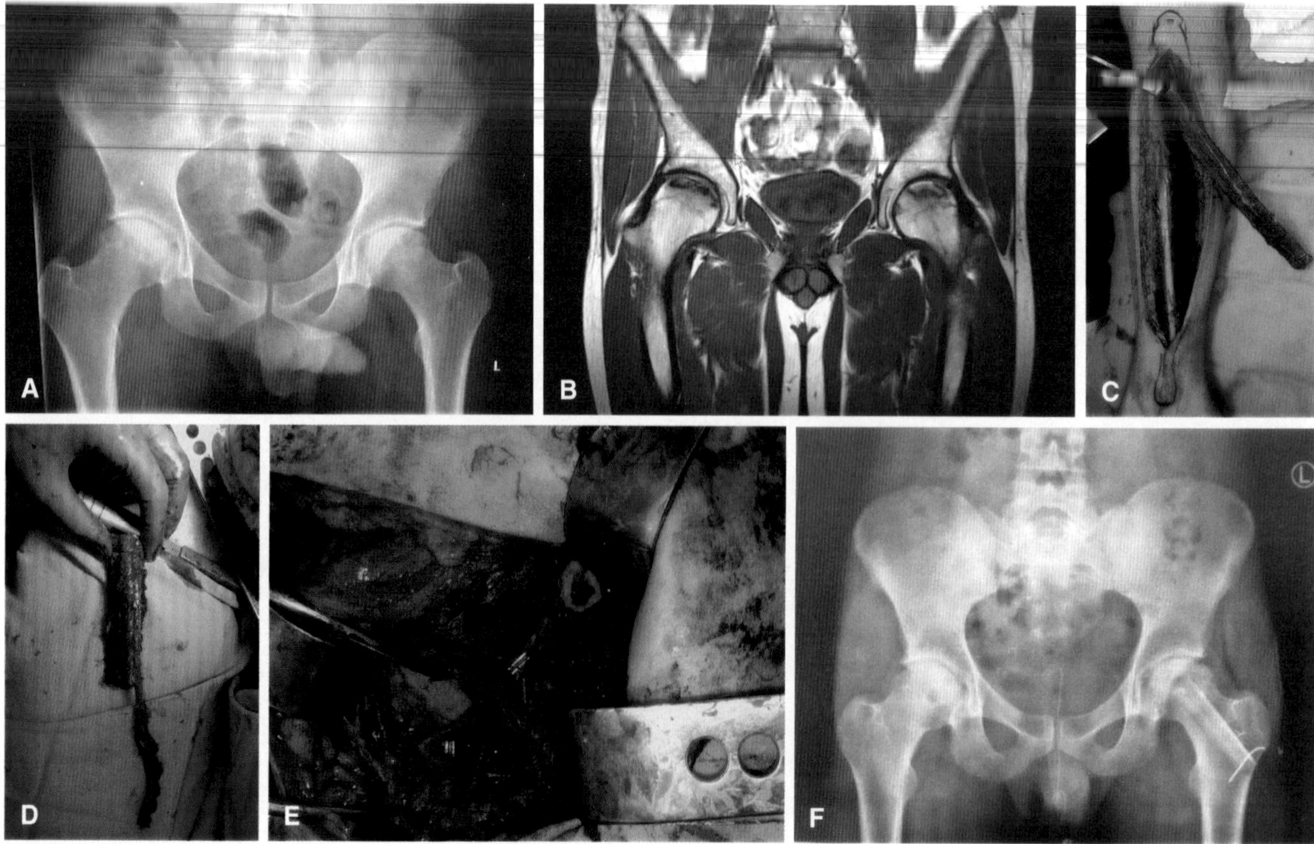

FIGURE 96.5. This is a patient with avascular necrosis of the head of the femur who was treated with a free fibula. **A.** Initial X-ray. **B.** Initial magnetic resonance imaging. **C.** Elevation of the fibula. **D.** Prepared fibula. **E.** Fibula in situ. **F.** Final X-ray showing fibula in situ.

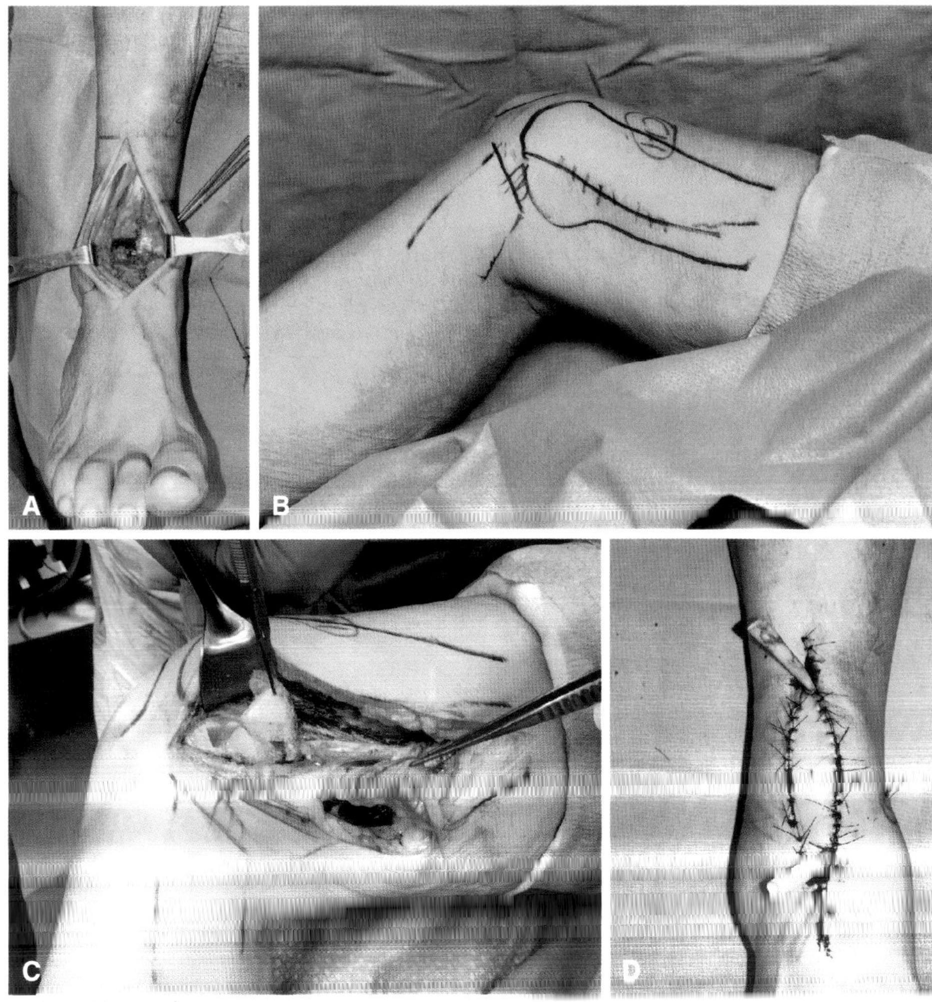

FIGURE 96.6. This is a patient with avascular necrosis of the tibiotalar joint. He was treated with a medial femoral condyle free flap. **A.** The defect after debridement of necrotic bone. **B.** Markings for the medial femoral condyle free flap. **C.** Elevation of the flap and skin paddle. **D.** On table result.

Skin Grafts

For many small wounds that cannot be closed primarily and do not have critical structures exposed, skin grafting can be a simple solution. Skin grafts are particularly useful for foot coverage, especially on the non-weight-bearing aspects of the foot.[1]

LOCAL FLAPS

A variety of local flaps can be used based on the location in the extremity. Fasciocutaneous flaps can be very useful for wound closure and offer the advantage of not risking functional loss with muscle use. The most commonly used fasciocutaneous flaps are described below.

Reverse Sural Artery Flap

The reverse sural artery flap is supplied by perforators from the peroneal artery and can be a sensate flap if the sural nerve is included with flap harvest.[1,10] The perforators are usually found about 5 to 6 cm above the lateral malleolus and are supplied by retrograde flow, so a design with a wide pedicle and a generous arc of rotation are needed to preserve flow[1,10,25] (Figure 96.7). The lesser saphenous vein needs to be included in the flap for venous outflow, and a delay procedure may improve viability in high-risk patients.[4] Maximal flap sizes can be 20 cm by 12 cm.[25] This flap can be good for heel coverage in high-risk patients. However, it has a high complication rate and lower aesthetic appeal.[1]

Lateral and Medial Calcaneal Artery Flaps

These are fasciocutaneous flaps good for small defects of the malleolar area or plantar heel region. They are based on terminal branches of the peroneal (lateral flap) and posterior tibial (medial flap) arteries (Figure 96.8). The sural nerve can be included for sensation, and the abductor hallucis muscle can be included with the medial flap.[1,25]

Keystone Flap

The keystone flap is a trapezoidal-shaped fasciocutaneous perforator flap, which is essentially made of two V-Y flaps on either end (Figure 96.9). It fits well into body contours and can reconstruct larger defects. The borders of the defect are extended on either side to 90° angles, the width of the flap is similar to the widest portion of the flap. The deep fascia is cut to allow advancement and superficial nerves and veins are incorporated into the flap design.[4,26]

Propeller Flap

Propeller flaps are a perforator-based local adipocutaneous flap. They can be designed off of a known source vessel or in a free-style fashion over a perforator found by Doppler. They can be rotated up to 180° to fill the defect.[27]

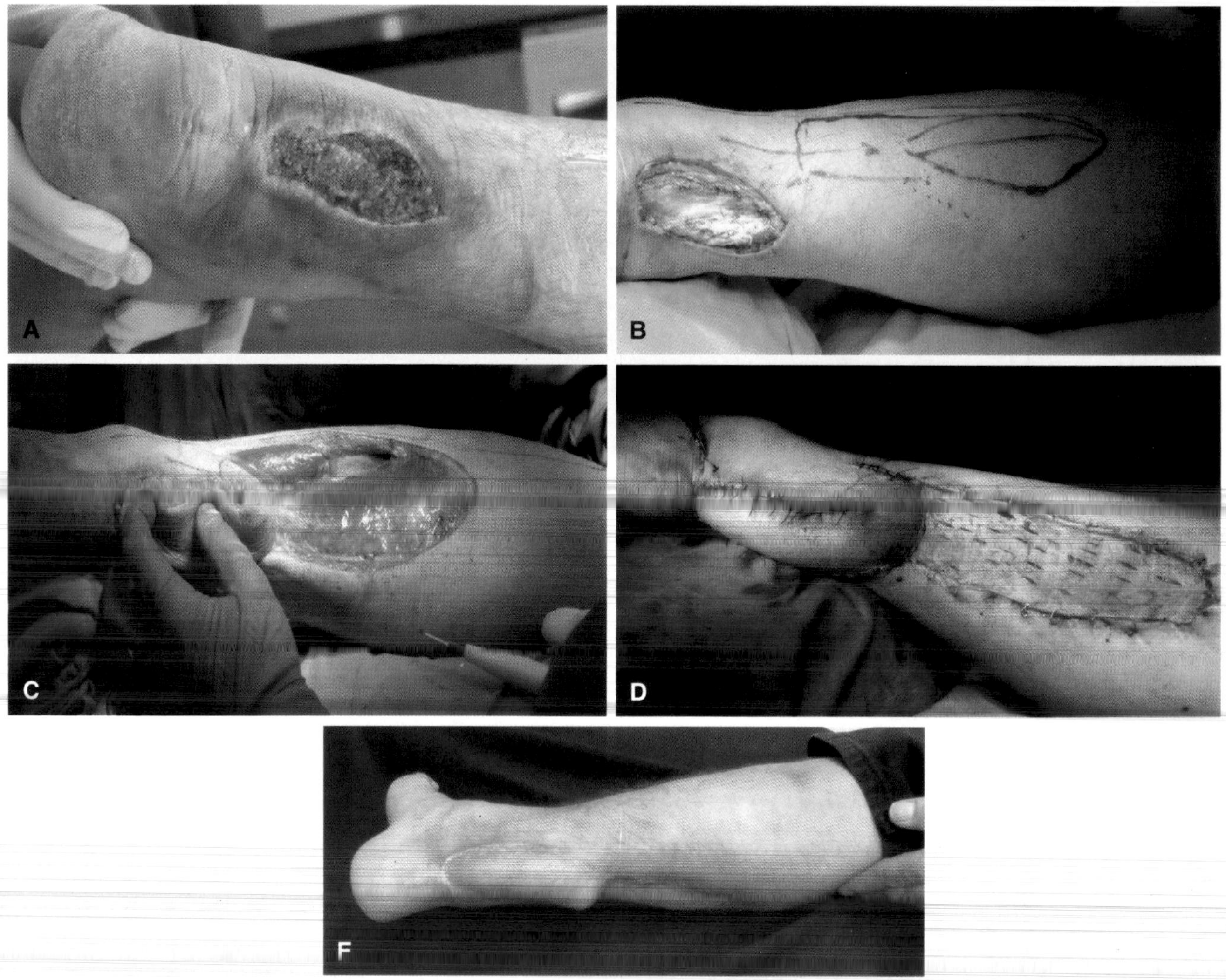

FIGURE 96.7. This is a patient with an exposed Achilles tendon treated with a reverse sural artery flap. **A.** Initial wound. **B.** After debridement. **C.** After flap elevation. **D.** After flap inset and skin graft. **E.** Final healed result.

Instep Flap

The plantar instep flap can be used as a fasciocutaneous island flap or as a free flap. It comes from the non-weight-bearing aspect of the plantar foot but provides similar tissue quality as the weight-bearing surface. It is most commonly based on the medial plantar artery (although laterally basing is possible as well) and can maintain sensation through the medial plantar nerve. This flap is ideal for plantar heel reconstruction.[28]

Cross-Leg Flap

With the widespread use of microsurgery, a cross-leg flap is rarely indicated. However, if the patient has no local donor sites, they lack appropriate inflow for a free flap, or are otherwise not a free flap candidate, a cross-leg flap is an option. The flap is fashioned on the opposite leg and transferred with a length-to-width ratio of 3:1. It requires prolonged immobilization and is not practical unless there are no other options.[29] Rarely, a free flap version of the cross-leg flap can be performed when there are no appropriate vessels for anastomosis in the injured leg.

Random Pattern

Other flaps can be used as well for smaller wounds. Standard V-Y advancement flaps or random pattern flaps can be utilized. Random pattern flaps should maintain a length-to-width ratio of 3:1.[1]

Muscle Flaps

Local muscle flaps tend to be preferable for lower extremity reconstruction; however, their viability must be confirmed before use.[1] They are highly vascularized, good for filling dead space, and improve local defenses to decrease infection.[6] Many muscles are available for lower extremity reconstruction and are listed in **Table 96.4** by location.

Free Flaps

The lower extremity can be a difficult area to reconstruct, as associated vascular injuries can make local tissues unusable, and there are increased rates of flap thrombosis (about 10%). It is always necessary to perform the anastomosis outside the zone of injury, which may require vein grafts or arteriovenous loops, and can be performed either proximal or distal to the injury.[1,4,8,30] However, the paucity of local tissues and functional requirement of the lower extremity frequently require bringing healthy tissue from a distant location, via free flap and microsurgery.[9] These techniques are applied for complex reconstructions, such as sensate flaps, functional muscle flaps, composite flaps with tendons, and flow through flaps for concomitant vascular repair, and are preferred if a large amount of tissue is required.[1,9] Because very large free flaps can be designed, they are also ideal for reconstructing a large tumor resection wound or after the removal of infected tissue.[6]

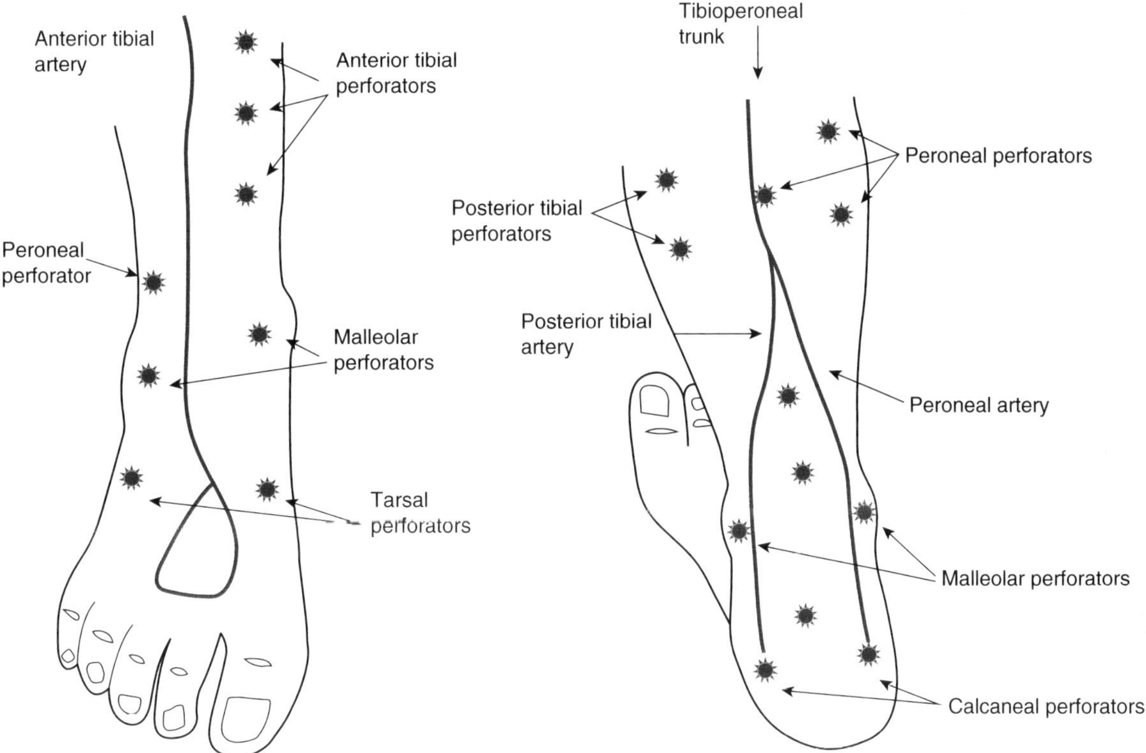

FIGURE 96.8. Location of perforators of the lower extremity

Anastomoses can be performed either end to end or end to side. Godina championed end to side anastomosis because it prevented disruption of the distal perfusion and thus remains the preferred choice in an extremity at risk for vascular insufficiency. When the recipient vessel is no longer in continuity from trauma, the anastomosis may be performed end to end. Importantly, the complication profile is similar with either type of anastomosis. Depending on the needs of the patient and the reconstruction, the patient can be positioned lateral decubitus, which is preferable for latissimus or subscapular flap access, or supine if other flaps are chosen. Positioning will determine which access is preferable to expose the donor vessels, whether it be posterior, lateral, or medial.[10]

Muscle/Myocutaneous Flaps

Historically, muscle flaps were the preferred treatment for lower extremity reconstruction. They are good at filling dead space, they bring additional blood supply, and they are flexible for ease of inset. It was thought that muscle was superior to fasciocutaneous flaps for fracture healing and infection prevention, but this theory has been disproven.[1,8,10]

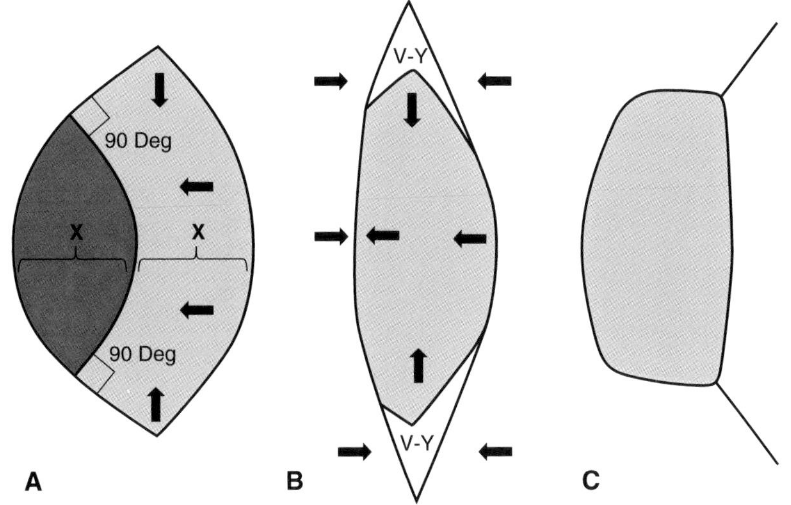

FIGURE 96.9. Keystone flap. **A.** *Red area* shows the defect, and the skin tone area is the flap design. The flap is cut only through the skin and subcutaneous tissues. If needed for mobility, the deep fascia of the far outer curve can be cut, with care taken not to sacrifice any perforators. **B.** The flap is advanced into the wound, with V-Y advancements used to close the superior and inferior positions. **C.** Appearance of closed wound.

TABLE 96.4. LOCAL MUSCLE FLAPS FOR FOOT AND ANKLE RECONSTRUCTION

Muscle	Blood Supply/Pedicle	Mathes and Nahai Type	Common Use/Advantages	Caveats/Disadvantages
Abductor digiti minimi (see Figure 96.12)	Lateral plantar artery	II	Useful for lateral ankle and calcaneal defects	Loss of abduction and flexion of fifth toe
Abductor hallucis	Medial plantar artery branches	II	Useful for medial midfoot, heel, and ankle defects	Loss of great toe abduction and foot spring
Extensor digitorum brevis	Dorsalis pedis	I	The malleoli, lateral and medial calcaneus, and pretibial region Only dorsal foot muscle	Requires sacrifice of the dorsalis pedis artery
Extensor digitorum longus	Anterior tibial artery	IV	Middle third	Requires care not to damage superficial peroneal nerve
Extensor hallucis longus	Anterior tibial artery	IV	Middle third	Cannot be completely sacrificed Requires care not to injure the extensor digitorum communis tendon
Flexor digitorum brevis	Medial plantar artery	II	Useful for plantar heel defects Minimal donor site morbidity	Very small volume and sometimes requires an additional flap
Flexor digiti minimi	Lateral plantar artery	IV	Useful for lateral foot	Small with limited arc of rotation
Flexor digitorum longus	Posterior tibial artery	IV	Middle third	Functional defect if taken with
Peroneus brevis	Peroneal artery	II	Distal third, fibula	Need to keep peroneus longus intact for eversion
Peroneus longus	Peroneal artery	II	Distal third, fibula	Need to keep peroneus brevis intact for eversion

Fasciocutaneous Flaps

Fasciocutaneous free flaps are preferable for many reasons; most notably, they minimize deficits by sparing muscles. These flaps are better for resurfacing as they restore contour without added bulk and can be treated with liposuction to improve contour. Fasciocutaneous flaps are easier to raise for secondary procedures.[8,10]

RECONSTRUCTIVE CHOICE BY LOCATION

The goal of reconstruction is to achieve soft-tissue coverage to aid the skeletal reconstruction, replacing *like with like* when possible. It is necessary to preserve both sensory and motor function in order to ambulate. To make the best reconstructive decision, the defect size, tissue deficit (types of tissues lost), location, length of vascular pedicle needed, and state of the wound have to be considered.[4,8,10] This is best approached by looking at the extremity by regions.

Thigh

The thigh is the least challenging area of the extremity to reconstruct. There is a large bulk of muscle to provide vascularized tissue. Typically, there are limited functional demands on the tissue other than coverage. In most cases, remaining muscle or fascia can be covered with skin grafts. Otherwise, a local muscle flap can be used to cover critical structures (like the femoral vessels) which then can be skin grafted.[1,4,10]

Knee and Proximal Third of Leg

Tissue in this area needs to remain thin for flexion at the knee. Generally, the upper third can be reconstructed with local flaps, minding the need to preserve the extensor function. The calf itself is mostly muscle in the upper third, so typically the only functional demand of the reconstruction is coverage. The tibia is just covered with skin, so the anterior part of the reconstruction needs to be thin. In this area, the gastrocnemius is the typical choice for reconstruction and is usually used as a muscle-only flap and covered with a skin graft. Secondary options include proximally based soleus (**Figure 96.10**), bipedicled tibialis anterior, and distally based pedicled anterolateral thigh (ALT) or vastus lateralis flap.[1,4,6,9,10]

Middle Third of Leg

The middle third of the leg is more difficult to reconstruct, as available options are likely to have been damaged by trauma. However, the classic option is a soleus flap. Other local flaps available include the gastrocnemius, flexor digitorum longus, extensor digitorum longus, extensor hallucis longus, tibialis anterior, and flexor hallucis longus. Large defects in this area require treatment with a free flap.[1,4,6]

Distal Third of Leg

The distal third of the leg is the most challenging part of the leg to reconstruct, as there is minimal available local tissue for coverage. Characteristically, this area requires a free flap for reconstruction. However, small volume closures can be treated with flexor hallucis longus, flexor digitorum longus, and tibialis anterior. In patients who are not free flap candidates, a distally based soleus or a reverse sural artery flap may be options, but both have high complication profiles. Flaps that are situated near the ankle and foot need to have appropriate contour so that the foot can still comfortably accommodate a shoe flap[1,4,6,25] (**Figure 96.11**).

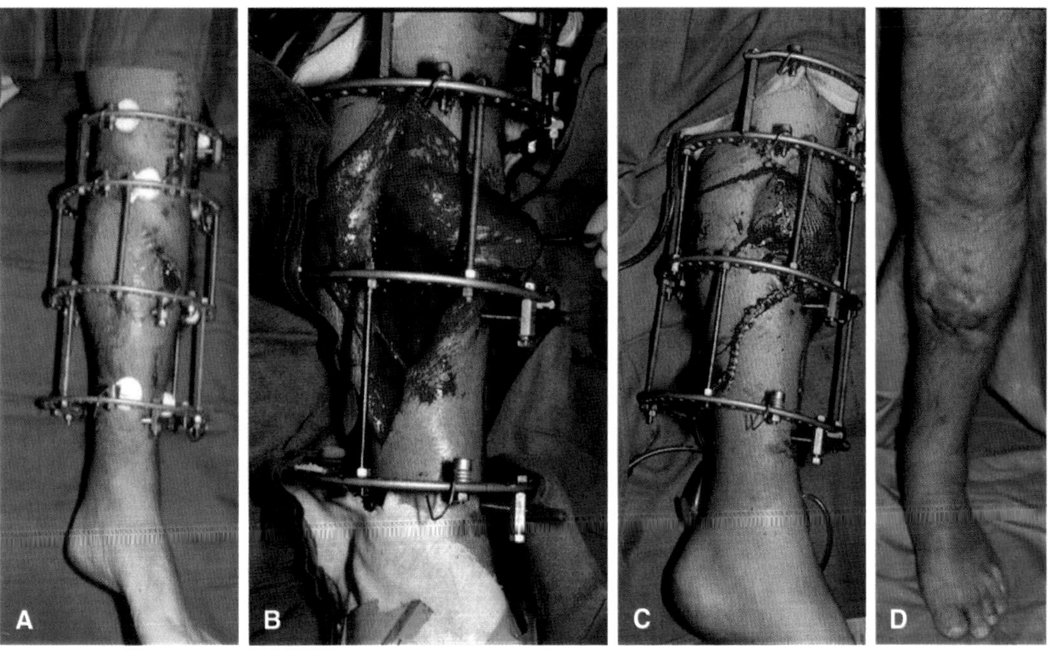

FIGURE 96.10. Open tibial fracture treated with soleus flap coverage. **A.** Initial wound. **B.** Soleus flap elevation. **C.** Immediate result after skin graft. **D.** Final healed result.

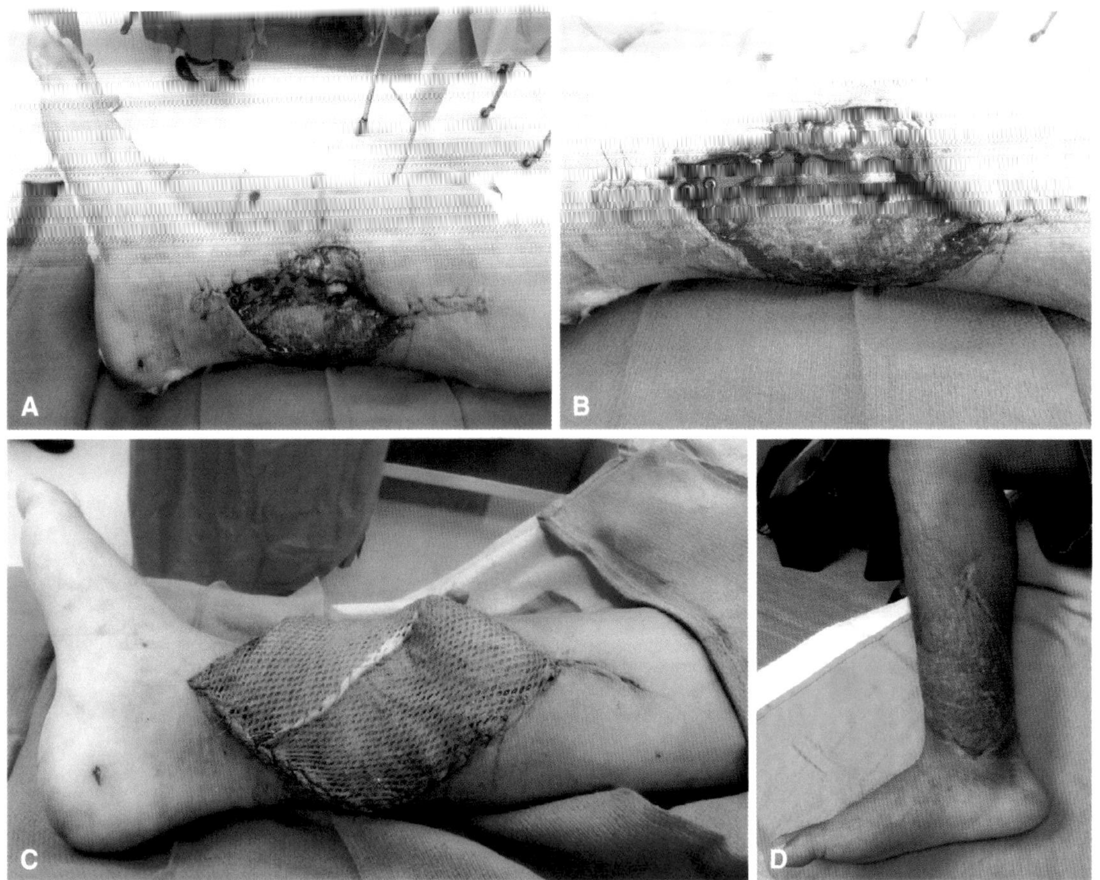

FIGURE 96.11. Example of a free latissimus with skin graft. This was a patient with an open tibial fracture treated with a plate. **A.** Image of the wound and plate. **B.** Zoomed in image of the wound. **C.** Immediate postoperative image of the latissimus flap with skin graft. **D.** Healed result at 6 months.

Foot

Like the distal lower leg, the foot is also a difficult area to reconstruct, and it is prone to injury and disease. It is best to think about foot reconstruction by subunits to obtain the best functional and aesthetic results. Generally, small wounds of the foot are best reconstructed with local muscle flaps (Figure 96.12). The whole plantar foot has glabrous skin and needs to withstand weight-bearing and shear. The dorsal foot needs to remain contoured to fit a shoe (Figure 96.13). Hollenbeck et al. created a subunit list and discussed flaps that best fit (Figure 96.14, Table 96.5).[6,10]

OTHER RECONSTRUCTIVE OPTIONS

Tissue Expansion

Tissue expansion is another modality available, although infrequently used, to aid with lower extremity reconstruction. It is typically used for skin resurfacing, coverage of wounds, removal of benign defects, and repair of contour abnormalities as it provides local tissue with appropriate skin match and similar quality. It is difficult to use in the acute setting and is more suitable for chronic conditions. The expanded tissue has a good blood supply from essentially being delayed, which can contribute to successful reconstruction. It is best to expand tissue transversely from the defect, as the tissue moves better in that plane. Large, crescent shaped expanders work best. They can be placed near the edge of a wound or with an endoscope to limit incisions. Expanders do have high infection rates (up to 30%). The more distal they are placed, the more common the complications and are infrequently successful below the knee, making the lower leg a relative contraindication to their use.[1,8,31]

Negative-Pressure Wound Therapy

The first commercially available negative pressure wound therapy device, or the wound vacuum-assisted closure (VAC), was available in 1990 (KCI, San Antonio, TX) and has transformed the practice of wound care.[30] The VAC uses an open-cell polymer foam in the wound bed, which is sealed and placed under negative pressure. In doing so, it promotes granulation tissue formation on a cellular level and increases blood flow, while grossly contracting the wound and decreasing bacterial contamination.[1,8,30]

The wound VAC is most useful as a temporizing measure before definitive closure and is not meant to be used as a definitive reconstruction.[8] It can safely be placed on soft tissue, bone, and tendon and produce adequate granulation tissue to take a skin graft or even achieve secondary healing in some cases[30] and will increase the survival of random pattern flaps.[8]

Dermal Regeneration Templates

A dermal regeneration template is a form of artificial skin (Integra, Life Sciences, Plainsboro, NJ) that can be used for the treatment of wounds. Integra is a layered product that is made up of bovine type I collagen with glycosaminoglycans that is covered with a silicone layer. The collagen matrix allows dermal regeneration, whereas the silicone is a temporary protective barrier. It is an immediate off-the-shelf product that can be used to close wounds and is particularly useful in patients who do not have adequate local donor tissue. Currently, Integra is most commonly used for burn wounds, but it can also be used for vascular ulcers, for wounds from lesion excision, and for tendon and bone exposure. It is placed on the wound bed and left in place for three or more weeks. Then, the silicone barrier is removed and a thin skin graft is placed over the Integra.[32,33]

OTHER PROBLEMS

Chronic Osteomyelitis

Chronic osteomyelitis is most commonly caused by retained necrotic bone, infected bone, ischemic tissue, dead space, and inadequate soft-tissue coverage. Treatment of chronic wounds and osteomyelitis require conversion to an acute wound again. This is best approached by thinking of the infected or necrotic area as a tumor and removing it in entirety, until healthy, viable tissue with punctate bleeding has been reached. Bacteria require eradication with antibiotics, typically those that cover *Staphylococcus* species, as those are most common. If present, hardware can harbor bacteria and should be removed. If the fracture is still not repaired and requires fixation, an external fixator is appropriate.[1,9]

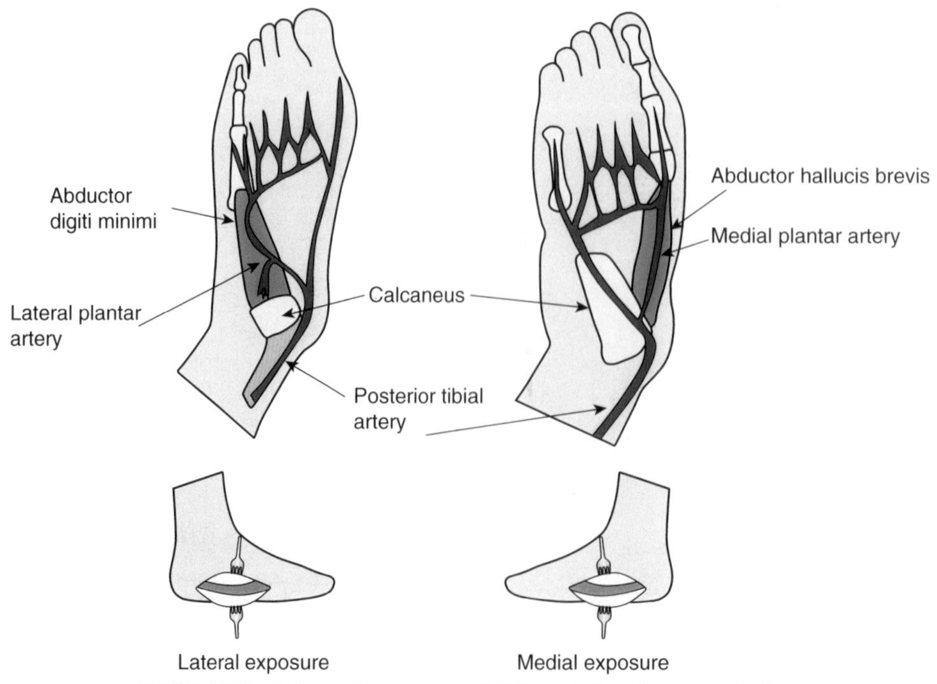

FIGURE 96.12. Abductor digit minimi and abductor hallucis brevis muscle flaps.

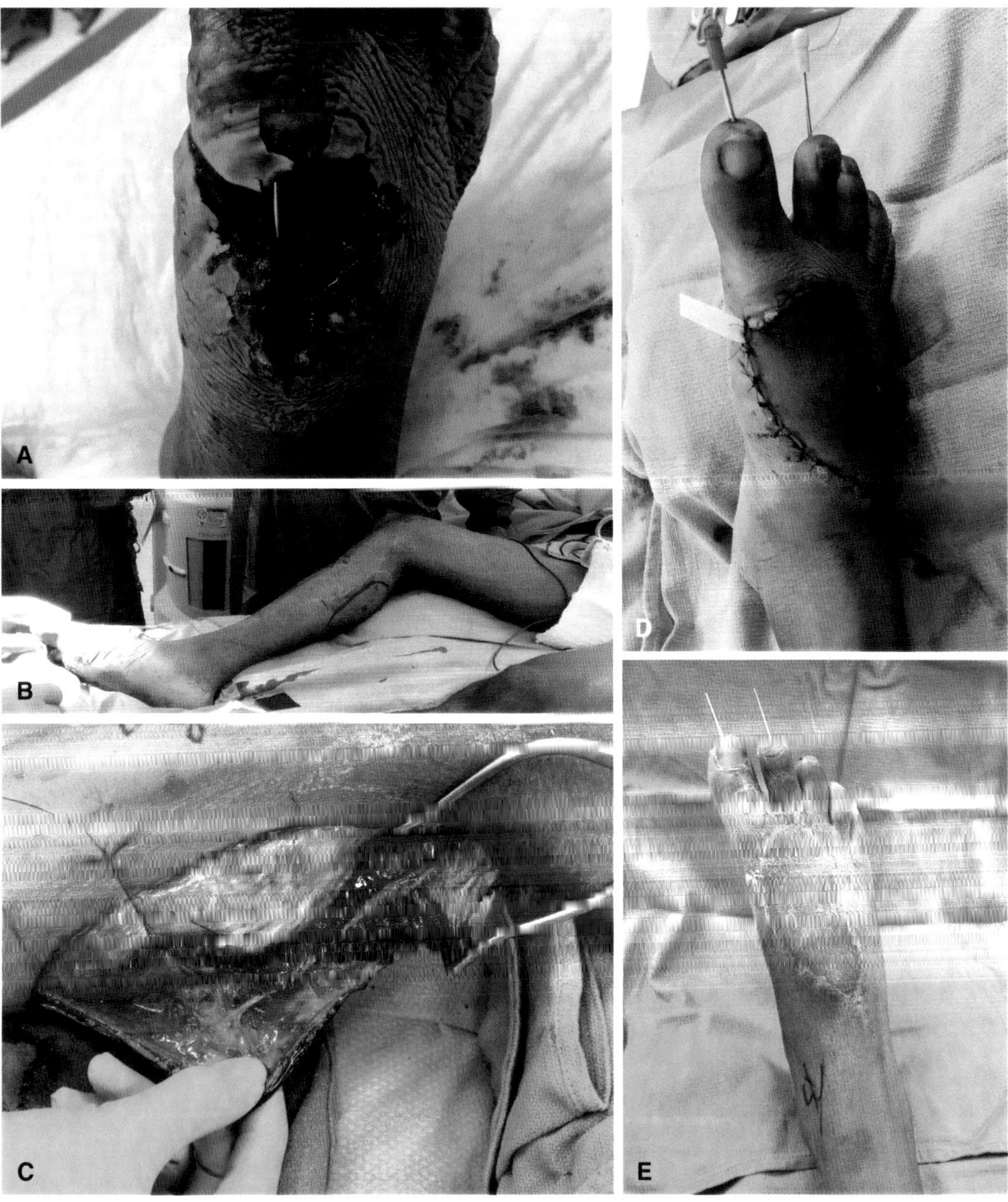

FIGURE 96.13. This patient with a gunshot wound to his foot was treated initially with an antibiotic spacer to preserve his metatarsal space and a medial sural artery perforator flap. **A.** Initial wound. **B.** Flap marking. **C.** Flap elevation showing the perforator. **D.** Immediate postoperative result. **E.** Healed result before final bone grafting.

Persistent Nonunion

Bony nonunions are more common in the foot because of the tenuous vascular supply of the talus and navicular bones. Some avascular necrosis is caused by trauma, whereas others are from damage from open approaches during fixation. Typically, this problem can be treated with arthrodesis. In patients who have had multiple revisions, infection, or significant osteonecrosis, vascularized bone flap is used. Large bone gaps require free fibula or free iliac crest. Smaller defects benefit from medial femoral condyle free flaps.[18] This flap is ideal because it contains a vascularized periosteum and cancellous bone and can be utilized to fix many different persistent nonunions. The donor site at the distal femur is well tolerated and does not cause any instability; the patient can be weight-bearing on the donor site immediately.[34]

Salvage of Below-Knee Amputation Stumps

Another important aspect of lower extremity reconstruction is salvage of amputation stumps. Patients are much more likely to use a prosthesis if they have a below-knee amputation versus an above-knee amputation. However, sometimes the trauma that cause the amputation creates a wound that is not amenable to primary closure without either shortening the stump, revising the amputation, or doing a free flap for coverage. About 14 cm of length is necessary to support a prosthesis for a below-knee amputation. If done during the inciting event, free flap with spare parts can be performed to preserve length, otherwise, traditional free flaps can be performed to make the amputation remnant amenable for a prosthesis[1,4,9]

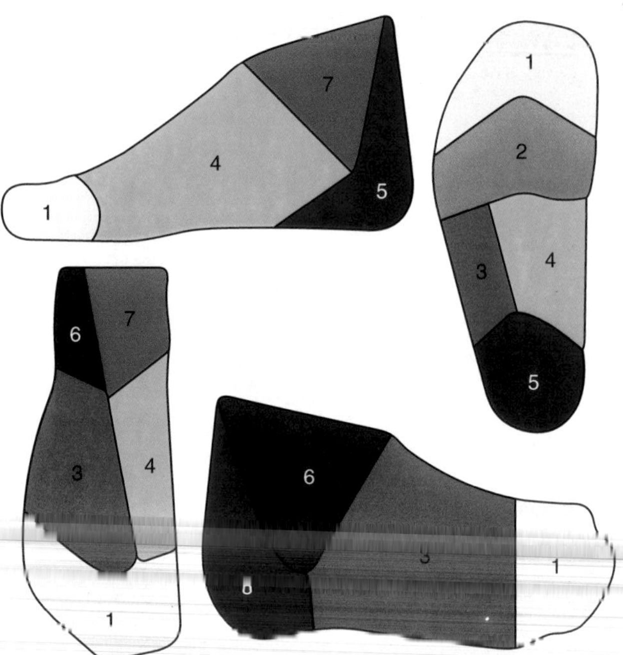

FIGURE 96.14. Four views of the foot and ankle demonstrate seven functionally and aesthetically different subunits.

Avascular Necrosis of the Femoral Head

Avascular necrosis of the femoral head is a progressive condition that initially affects patients between the ages of 20 and 50 years and is caused by alcohol consumption, steroids, trauma, and Perthes disease. It starts with osteonecrosis, which leads to cartilage destruction and secondary degenerative changes. Typically, this condition would be managed with total arthroplasty, but in this age group, it is fraught with a high rate of complications and a high rate of revisions. It can also be treated with core decompression, but this does not provide structural support. A good solution in this patient population is to use a vascularized free fibula graft. It requires core decompression of the dead sequestrum to create space for the fibula. The fibula is placed in this cored-out tunnel in the femoral head and brings both support and revascularization. Younger patients have a better outcome with free fibula grafting, although 20% of this patient population will still require a total joint replacement later in life.[1,35,36]

TABLE 96.5. SPECIFIC DEMANDS AND TISSUE NEEDS FOR EACH SUBUNIT[10]

Subunit	Demands: Tissue Needs	Optimal Flaps[a]
1	Low functional, moderate aesthetic: small, thin, and pliable	Radial forearm > lateral arm
2	High functional, low aesthetic: durable and minimal bulk	Radial forearm > lateral arm > gracilis with STSG > ALT[b]
3/4	Low functional, high aesthetic: smooth, thin, and pliable	Radial forearm > ALT > scapular > latissimus dorsi
5	High functional, low aesthetic: durable and moderate bulk	ALT > gracilis with STSG > latissimus dorsi > scapula > lateral arm > radial forearm[b]
6/7	Moderate functional, moderate aesthetic: may vary from smooth, thin, and pliable to large and bulky	Gracilis with STSG, latissimus dorsi, ALT, rectus abdominus, lateral arm, radial forearm, scapular

[a]Flap choices for each option are listed more to less optimal.
[b]Nerve coaptation may be considered.
ATL, anterolateral thigh flap; *STSG*, split-thickness skin graft.

Reconstruction of Peroneal Nerve Injuries

The common peroneal nerve is the most frequent nerve injury of the lower extremity, as it can be injured with penetrating trauma, fractures, knee dislocations, ankle sprains, or iatrogenically during a knee surgery. Traction injuries recover spontaneously, but patients who suffer irreversible damage benefit from surgical treatment, otherwise these patients are committed to wearing a foot drop brace. Treatment options include nerve grafting and tendon transfer. Nerve grafting has shown favorable results, particularly in small nerve gaps. Tendon transfer should be reserved for those who failed nerve recovery or repair. A posterior tibialis tendon to anterior tibial tendon transfer is the standard tendon transfer to treat foot drop. Garozzo et al had favorable results when combining nerve repair with grafting in a one-stage procedure, assuming that they felt tendon imbalance was part of the reason for poor recovery after nerve grafting alone.[37-39]

Oncologic Reconstruction

In cases of oncologic extirpation, extremity reconstruction can prevent an amputation. Most cases are caused by bony sarcomas, and removal of a large segment of bone requires a vascularized reconstruction, particularly in instances where the patient has been radiated. Most bony defects are amenable to reconstruction with a free fibula. However, the femur and tibia require strength, which can be accomplished with a double-barreled fibula or a fibula placed in an allograft (Capanna technique).[1,9]

Aesthetics of the Lower Extremity

Although the ultimate goal of lower extremity reconstruction is to create a functional result, appearance should not be ignored. The most important aspect of attaining an aesthetic result is proper flap choice. Muscle flaps covered by skin grafts tend to have a less aesthetic result. Over time, they remain bulky and frequently require revision for contouring. If a muscle flap is required, attention to inset and postoperative management can improve results. First, choosing a flap of appropriate dimensions for the defect can make the initial aesthetic result better. Then, insetting the flap with horizontal mattress sutures promotes a smoother junction between the flap and the native skin. Postoperative care with compression with an ACE wrap or compression sock can aid in shrinking the flap to fit the defect. If fasciocutaneous flaps are used, thinner flaps are better. This can be achieved by choosing a flap that is thinner to begin with (depending on the patient's body habitus), thinning the flap around the perforator intraoperatively, or performing revisions to thin the flap secondarily. Bulky flaps are not just an anesthetic problem in the lower extremity, those located distally can prevent proper footwear fit. If the cosmetic result after the initial reconstruction is poor, a revised reconstruction with a fasciocutaneous free flap may provide a better result.[40-42]

POSTOPERATIVE MANAGEMENT

Postoperative patient management is dictated by the reconstruction performed. For all free flaps, standard clinical free flap monitoring, including internal and/or external Doppler signal, color, capillary refill, and temperature are performed hourly by the nursing staff for the first 48 hours, then every 2 hours for the next 48 hours, and then every 4 hours for the remaining hospitalization. If the patient has a buried flap, an internal Doppler device is used.

All patients are initially on bed rest with the affected extremity elevated for 2 to 3 weeks. It is important to off-load pressure on the reconstruction, usually this can be achieved with positioning and splinting, but sometimes it requires an external fixator. Most acute reconstructions are prone to venous and lymphatic insufficiency early on. It is important to keep the extremity elevated and not dependent. After 2 to 3 weeks, a dangle protocol is started to give the reconstruction a gradual accommodation period. The patient is non-weight-bearing on that extremity until cleared by the orthopedic service.

CONCLUSION

Lower extremity reconstruction is a challenging area of surgery that requires consideration of a patient's occupation, other injuries, and comorbidities before a reconstructive plan is initiated. The best results are attributed to proper flap choice and timing, although the ability to incorporate microsurgery has significantly advanced orthoplastic extremity reconstruction.

REFERENCES

1. Griffin JR, Thornton JF. Lower extremity reconstruction. *Sel Read Plast Surg.* 2009;11(R1):1-59.
2. Olson SA, Glasgow RR. Acute compartment syndrome in lower extremity musculoskeletal trauma. *J Am Acad Orthop Surg.* 2005;13(7):436-444.
3. Gustilo RB, Mendoza RM, Williams DN. Problems in the management of type III (severe) open fractures: a new classification of type III open fractures. *J Trauma.* 1984;24(8):742-746.
   This is the article that introduced the most widely used classification system for open extremity fractures. This is important for plastic surgeons, as it is needed to help salvage and reconstruct the extremities on patients who have type IIIB and IIIC injuries.
4. Soltanian H, Garcia R, Hollenbeck ST. Current concepts in lower extremity reconstruction. *Plast Reconstr Surg.* 2013;130(6):813e-829e.
5. [illegible] *Reconstr Surg.* 1985;76(5):719-730.
   Classic article regarding classifying and treating open tibial fractures. Of particular [illegible] which types of injuries can be treated with local flaps, versus those that require distant tissue transfer.
6. Hollenbeck ST, Toranto JD, Taylor BJ, et al. Perineal and lower extremity reconstruction. *Plast Reconstr Surg.* 2011;128(5):551e-563e.
7. Pasquale MD, Frykberg ER, Tinkoff GH; ACS Committee on Trauma; Ad Hoc Committee on Outcomes. Management of complex extremity trauma. *Bull Am Coll Surg.* 2006;91(6):36-38.
8. Ong YS, Levin LS. Lower limb salvage in trauma. *Plast Reconstr Surg.* 2010;125(2):582-588.
9. Levin LS, Heitmann C. Lower extremity reconstruction. *Semin Plast Surg.* 2003;17(1):069-082.
10. Lachica RD. Evidence-based medicine: management of acute lower extremity trauma. *Plast Reconstr Surg.* 2017;139(1):287e-301e.
11. Godina M. Early microsurgical reconstruction of complex trauma of the extremities. *Plast Reconstr Surg.* 1986;78(3):285-292.
    Landmark article discussing the timing of treating lower extremity fractures with free flaps. The author broke patients into three groups—early, delayed, and late—and then assessed infections, flap failure rates, number of anesthetics, hospitalization time, and time to healing. This article is what led to more common treatment of open fracture with free flaps in the acute period.
12. Ducic I, Attinger CE. Foot and ankle reconstruction: pedicled muscle flaps versus free flaps and the role of diabetes. *Plast Reconstr Surg.* 2011;128(1):173-180.
13. Suh HS, Oh TS, Lee HS, et al. A new approach for reconstruction of diabetic foot wounds using the angiosome and supermicrosurgery concept. *Plast Reconstr Surg.* 2016;138(4):702e-709e.
14. Higgins TF, Klatt JB, Beals TC. Lower extremity assessment project (LEAP) – the best available evidence on limb-threatening lower extremity trauma. *Orthop Clin North Am.* 2010;41(2):233-239.
    The LEAP project is a landmark randomized, prospective trial performed at 8 trauma centers, developed to determine who would benefit from salvage versus who would benefit from primary amputation. While they were unable to make this determination, they did find that patient's ability to function afterward was more because of their functional ability before trauma, regarding their social, economic, and personality disadvantages. Whether treated with salvage or amputation, this patient population had equivalent 2-year outcomes.
15. Bosse MJ, MacKenzie EJ, Kellam JF, et al. An analysis of outcomes of reconstruction or amputation after leg-threatening injuries. *N Engl J Med.* 2002;347(24):1924-1931.
16. Steiert AE, Gohritz A, Schreiber TC, et al. Delayed flap coverage of open extremity fractures after previous vacuum-assisted closure (VAC) therapy – worse or worth it? *J Plast Reconstr Aesthet Surg.* 2009;62(5):675-683.
17. Wong TM, Lau TW, Li X, Fang C, Yeung K, Leung F. Masquelet technique for treatment of posttraumatic bone defects. *Sci World J.* 2014;2014:1-6.
18. Haddock NT, Wapner K, Levin LS. Vascular bone transfer options in the foot and ankle: a retrospective review and update on strategies. *Plast Reconstr Surg.* 2013;132(3):685-693.
19. Ronga M, Ferraro S, Fagetti A, Cherubino M, Valdatta L, Cherubino P. Masquelet technique for the treatment of a severe acute tibial bone loss. *Injury.* 2014;45(suppl 6):S111-S1115.
20. Wagels M, Rowe D, Senewiratne S, Theile DR. History of lower limb reconstruction after trauma. *AZN J Surg.* 2013;83(5):348-353.
21. Hollenbeck ST, Woo S, Ong S, Fitch RD, Erdmann D, Levin LS. The combined use of the Ilizarov method and microsurgical techniques for limb salvage. *Ann Plast Surg.* 2009;62(5):486-491.
22. Rozbruch SR, Weitzman A, Watson JT, Freudigman O, Katz HV, Ilizarov S. Simultaneous treatment of tibial bone and soft-tissue defects with the Ilizarov method. *J Orthop Trauma.* 2006;20(3):197-205.
23. Weiland AJ, Moore JR, Daniel RK. Vascularized bone autografts. Experience with 41 cases. *Clin Orthop Relat Res.* 1983;174:87-95.
24. Gottlieb LJ, Krieger LM. From the reconstructive ladder to the reconstructive elevator. *Plast Reconstr Surg.* 1994;93(7):1503-1504.
25. Parrett BM, Talbot SG, Pribaz JJ, Lee BT. A review of local and regional flaps for distal leg reconstruction. *J Reconstr Microsurg.* 2009;25(7):445-455.
    Good review article about options for reconstruction of the lower extremity.
26. Behan FC. The Keystone Design Perforator Island Flap in reconstructive surgery. *ANZ J Surg.* 2003;73(3):112-120.
27. D'Arpa S, Toia F, Pirrello R, et al. Propeller flaps: a review of indications and results. *Biomed Res Int.* 2014;2014:1-7.
28. Morrison WA, Crabb DM, O'Brien MB, Jenkins A. The instep of the foot as a fasciocutaneous island and as a free flap for heel defects. *Plast Reconstr Surg.* 1983;72(1):56-63.
29. Agarwal P, Raza H. Cross-leg flap: its role in limb salvage. *Indian J Orthop.* 2008;42(4):439-443.
30. Colon DL, Colon LB, Levin LS, Kovach SJ. [illegible] century and the evolution of lower extremity trauma reconstruction. *J Reconstr* [illegible]
31. Manders EK, Oaks TE, Au VK, et al. Soft tissue expansion in the lower extremities. *Plast Reconstr Surg.* 1988;81(2):208-219.
32. [illegible] JH, Nowygrod R, Marboe CC, et al. Artificial skin (Integra Dermal regeneration template) for closure of lower extremity wounds. *Vasc Surg.* 2000;34(6):557-567.
33. Lee LF, Porch JV, Spenler W, Garner WL. Integra in lower extremity reconstruction after burn injury. *Plast Reconstr Surg.* 2008;121(4):1256-1262.
34. Rodriguez-Vegas JM, Delgado-Serrano PJ. Corticoperiosteal flap in the treatment of nonunions and small bone gaps: technical details and expanding possibilities. *J Plast Reconstr Aesthet Surg.* 2011;64(4):515-527.
35. Urbaniak JR, Coogan PG, Gunneson EB, Nunley JA. Treatment of osteonecrosis of the femoral head with free vascularized fibular grafting: a long-term follow-up study of one hundred and three hips. *J Bone Joint Surg Am.* 1995;77(5):681-694.
36. Kawate KYH, Sugimoto K, Ono H, et al. Indications for free vascularized fibular grafting for the treatment of osteonecrosis of the femoral head. *BMC Musculoskelet Disord.* 2007;78:1-8.
37. Garozzo D, Ferraresi S, Buffatti P. Surgical treatment of common peroneal nerve injuries: indications and results: a series of 62 cases. *J Neurosurg Sci.* 2004;48(3):105-112.
38. Vigasio A, Marcoccio I, Patelli A, et al. New tendon transfer for correction of drop-foot in common peroneal nerve palsy. *Clin Orthop Relat Res.* 2008;466(6):1454-1466.
39. Sedel L, Nizard RS. Nerve grafting for traction injuries of the common peroneal nerve: a report of 17 cases. *J Bone Joint Surg Br.* 1993;75B:772-774.
40. Marek CA, Pu LQ. Refinements of free tissue transfer for optimal outcome in lower extremity reconstruction. *Ann Plast Surg.* 2004;52(3):270-275.
41. Ohjimi H, Taniguchi Y, Kawano K, et al. A comparison of thinning and conventional free-flap transfers to the lower extremity. *Plast Reconstr Surg.* 2000;105(2):558-566.
42. Jeon BJ, Lim SY, Pyon JK, et al. Secondary extremity reconstruction with free perforator flaps for aesthetic purposes. *J Plast Reconstr Aesthet Surg.* 2011;64(11):1483-1489.

QUESTIONS

1. A 27-year-old man had a previous fracture of the foot. He has been repaired operatively with open reduction internal fixation and bone grafting and has a nonunion of the talonavicular joint. What is the best option for treatment of this foot wound?

a. Repeat bone grafting
b. Vascularized fibular graft
c. Medial geniculate artery flap
d. Iliac crest osteocutaneous flap

2. An 88-year-old man with advanced heart failure has a chronic wound on his posterior heel with exposed tendon lacking paratenon. Which of the following is the best option for this patient?

a. Split-thickness skin graft
b. Reverse sural artery flap
c. ALT flap
d. Tissue expansion

3. Which is not true of the rule of thirds for lower extremity reconstruction?

a. Gastrocnemius is a good option for proximal third defects
b. Reverse soleus is a good option for middle third defects
c. Soleus is a good option for middle third defects
d. Free flaps are good options for distal third defects

4. A 65-year-old man just underwent an aortobifemoral bypass procedure. It was complicated by a ruptured pseudoaneurysm at the femoral anastomosis, and the patient now has an open wound with exposed graft. Which of the following is true?

a. The wound should be treated with a wound VAC until it granulates.
b. A sartorius flap should be placed over the exposed vessels.
c. Treatment for this patient's condition will require repeated laparotomy.
d. A skin graft should be adequate to obtain coverage.

5. Which half of the gastrocnemius flap is a better option for most knee wounds and why?

a. Medial because its blood supply is more robust
b. Lateral because the flap is larger with better reach.
c. Medial because there is no risk of peroneal nerve injury.
d. Lateral because the pedicle location is more consistent.

1. **Answer: c.** Having failed primary reconstructive options with hardware and bone grafting, likely from poor vascular supply, this patient needs a vascularized reconstruction, preferably a vascularized corticocancellous bone flap. Bone grafting did not correct his problem in the past. Although plausible, a vascularized fibular graft is essentially a cortical bone graft and is larger than necessary and more difficult to inset into the desired location. An iliac crest osteocutaneous flap creates a significant donor defect to the lateral abdominal wall.

2. **Answer: b.** This elderly patient with significant comorbidities is not a candidate for a free flap or any other prolonged operation, so an ALT flap is not an option for him. Exposed tendon lacking paratenon will not have good graft take, so a split-thickness skin graft is not an option. Tissue expansion in the distal lower extremity has a very high complication and failure rate and is therefore not advisable. Reverse sural artery flap is a good option in this patient as it can be harvested quickly and will provide stable coverage. If flap viability is a concern, a delay procedure could be performed. Although not an answer choice, Integra and then skin grafting later would also be a possibility in this scenario.

3. **Answer: b.** Reconstructing the leg can be thought of as a rule of thirds, with gastrocnemius being the classic option for the proximal third. Soleus for the middle third, and free flap for the distal third. Reverse soleus is indicated for distal third but is less ideal than a free flap since it is more prone to necrosis.

4. **Answer: b.** Exposed vascular structures should be covered with vascularized tissue, and a sartorius flap would fulfill this purpose. A wound VAC should not be placed directly onto vasculature. The wound is located at the distal part of the groin and should not require laparotomy for management. A skin graft would be inadequate to cover exposed vessels and would not take over a vascular prosthesis.

5. **Answer: c.** The peroneal nerve is at risk for injury if the lateral head of the gastrocnemius is used, and therefore the medial head is preferable.

CHAPTER 97 Perineal Reconstruction

Julie E. Park

KEY POINTS

- Perineal reconstruction may be required because of burns, infection, trauma, hidradenitis suppurative, or cancer.
- Reconstructive options can vary according to location of acquired defect.
- Reconstructive options include local, regional, and free flap reconstruction.
- Indications for specific reconstructive choice varies according to location and depth of acquired defect.
- Support of pelvic contents and obliteration of any dead space is essential in perineal reconstruction.

ANATOMY

The perineal region spans the pubic symphysis and the coccyx in the anteroposterior dimension and the ischial tuberosities in the transverse dimension. It is divided into anterior and posterior triangles by a hypothetical transverse line between the ischial tuberosities. The anterior triangle contains the urogenital structures, which include the vulva and vagina in females and the scrotum and penis in males. The posterior triangle includes the anorectal structures. The superior border of the perineum is the pelvic floor, which consists of the levator ani and coccygeus muscles (Figure 97.1). The pelvic floor, also referred to as the pelvic diaphragm, supports and separates the pelvic cavity from the perineum. The perineum refers to the area between the anus and vagina or scrotum. It has a superficial and deep fascial layer. The deep fascia is contiguous to Colles fascia.[1] The specifics of the anatomy of perineal structures are delineated in Table 97.1.

The perineum plays important roles in micturition, defecation, sexual activity, and body image, all of which need to be considered when planning reconstructive goals. Functional requirements include obliteration of any dead space, prevention of pelvic prolapse, and possible reconstruction of genitalia. The challenges of reconstructing the perineum consider dependent pressure during postoperative recovery, bacterial contamination from urogenital and perianal areas, and the propensity for radiation therapy to be used when oncologic resection is necessary.

CONSIDERATIONS BY ETIOLOGY

There are multiple scenarios in which the perineum requires reconstruction. Benign disease processes include burns, infection (such as Fournier's gangrene), trauma, and hidradenitis suppurativa. Oncologic resections include Paget disease; carcinomas of the vulva/vagina, penis, and/or scrotum; and anorectal cancer. Reconstruction of congenital defects is beyond the scope of this chapter while gender affirmation procedures are discussed in detail in Chapter 100.

Burns

The American Burn Association considers any perineal burn as a major injury and criteria for burn center referral.[2-4] Isolated perineal burns are unusual as the area is relatively protected by the thighs and abdomen. Perineal burns are typically part more extensive burns of trunk and lower extremity.[4] Adult etiology is typically due to flame, whereas pediatric etiology is usually due to scald burns from spills or immersion.[2,4] A third reason for perineal burns is the military cause.[3] The incidence of perineal burns ranges anywhere from 1.7% to 13% in adults and 1% in children.[4,5] Across adult, pediatric, and military cohorts, there is an increased male to female ratio.[3-5] The presence of a perineal burn is an independent risk factor for an increase in morbidity and mortality, although this is not from injuries to the urogenital structures, but is thought to be related to increased bacteremia and/or relationship to more extensive injuries.[2,3,5]

The presence of perineal burns is associated with increased hospital acquired infections and urinary tract infections.[2,5] Increased infection risks can convert partial-thickness burns to deeper tissue injury and can interfere with skin graft take.[4] There is consensus that urinary catheterization should be limited to resuscitation as much as possible, with some advocating its use to help hygiene and comfort.[2,4,5] Long-term catheterization risks infection and urethral stenosis. There is debate regarding the superiority of suprapubic versus urethral catheters.[2,4,5]

As with any other burn, the depth of the burn will determine need for excision and grafting. Unlike burns on other areas of the body, genitalia burns are typically not treated with early excision. The exception to this is the presence of extensive, deep necrotic tissue. Conservative treatment with topical antimicrobials and wound care is recommended. Most partial-thickness wounds heal by epithelialization. Perineal wounds heal well with secondary intention after eschar excision. If the perineal burn is part of more extensive burns, the other areas of burns have priority for skin grafts from available donor sites. Larger wounds may require excision and grafting to prevent deformities. Full-thickness injuries to genitalia may require full-thickness skin graft to prevent contracture and care must be taken with bolster dressings to secure the grafts. Internal vaginal burns can benefit from vaginal stents to help prevent stenosis.[2,4,5] Contracture of perineum can restrict the range of motion of hip and adversely affect micturition, defecation, and sexual activity. There are additional psychosocial complications of burns to genitalia that span loss of self-esteem and libido.[4]

Infections

Necrotizing soft tissues of the perineum is often referred to as Fournier gangrene. It can involve the skin, subcutaneous tissue, fascia, and muscle. Mortality rates range between 10% and 40%. There is a male predominance. The most common comorbidity is diabetes mellitus,[6] and other risk factors include the following[7]:

- Recent surgery to perineal structures
- Malignancy
- Alcoholism
- Morbid obesity
- Immunocompromise

The mainstay of treatment is prompt surgical debridement, broad spectrum IV antibiotics, and resuscitation. Surgical debridement should aggressively target any infected, ischemic, and/or necrotic tissues. Second look operations are often necessary. Antibiotic therapy should cover gram positive, gram negative, and anaerobic bacteria and then be adjusted to the antibiotic sensitivities as speciation of cultures return. Ideally, blood cultures should be drawn prior to antibiotic initiation. Common microorganisms involved in Fournier gangrene include the following[7-9]:

- Polymicrobial
- *Escherichia coli*
- *Staphylococcus aureus*
- *Streptococcus* species
- *Enterobacter*

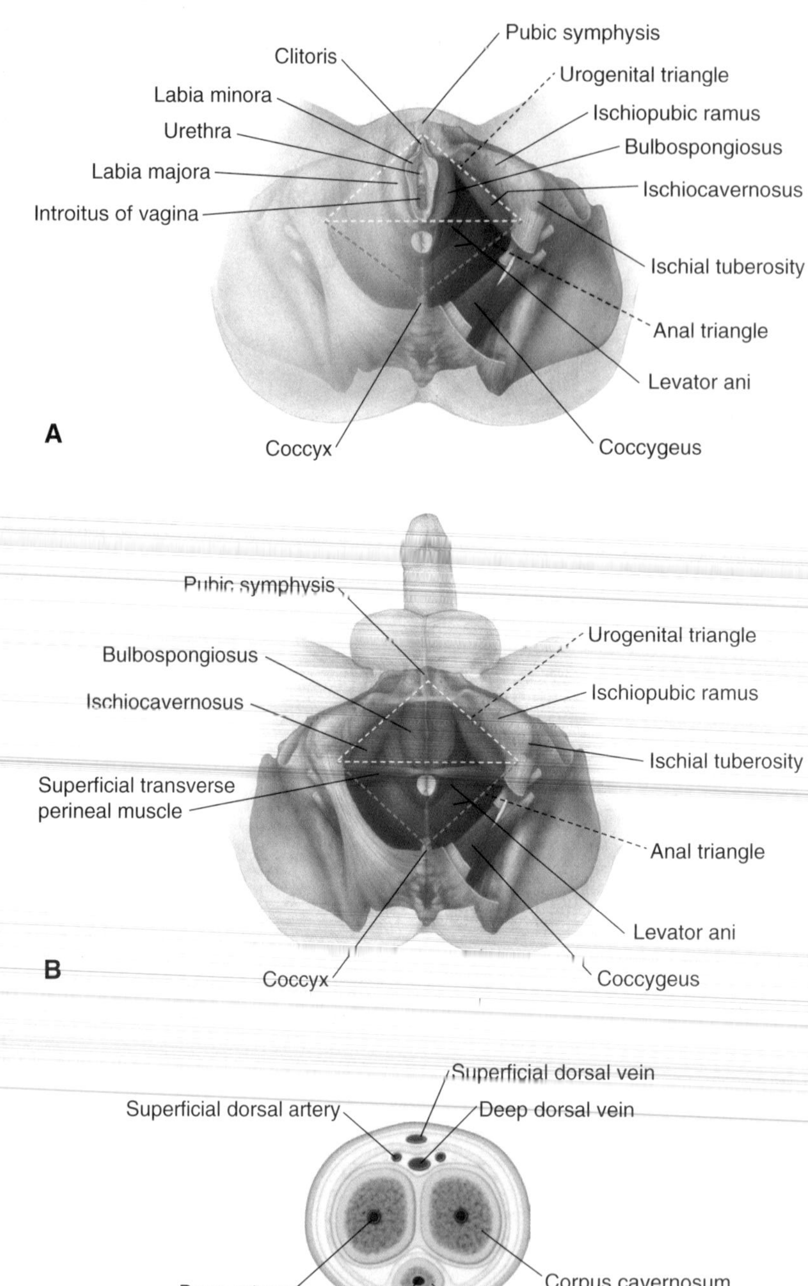

FIGURE 97.1. Structure of the female **(A)** and male **(B)** perineum. **C.** Cross section of penis.

- *Pseudomonas aeruginosa*
- Bacteroides
- *Proteus* species
- *Clostridia* species
- Klebsiella
- Corynebacteria
- *Acinetobacter baumannii*

There are conflicting reports on the benefits and cost-effectiveness of hyperbaric oxygen therapy.[7,8] Some patients may require urinary and/or fecal diversion.[7,8] Negative pressure wound dressings are helpful in controlling the wound once the infection is adequately debrided and treated.[7]

Orchiectomy should be performed only if the testicle itself is not viable.[8,9] In the event of total scrotal involvement and debridement, protection of the testicles from desiccation can be performed by placement in subcutaneous thigh pockets. However, as a long-term reconstruction, this is not well tolerated in younger patients and may decrease fertility owing to the increased temperature of the thigh pockets.[9] Testicular dressings should be designed to keep the testicle from desiccation and allow for granulation tissue to form. After granulation tissue is present, scrotal reconstruction can be performed with split-thickness skin grafts or thigh flaps.

Trauma

Perineal injuries from military trauma are typically involved in other traumas of the lower extremity and/or abdomen and pelvis and can be caused by blast injuries such as given by improvised explosive devices[10,11] or combat-related burns.[3] Military improvised explosive device injuries are further complicated by bacteria and soil particles that can be driven deep into the involved tissues.[10,11] In the civilian

TABLE 97.1. ANATOMY AND NEUROVASCULAR PEDICLES OF STRUCTURES OF THE PERINEUM[1,49]

	Vulva	Vagina	Penis	Scrotum
Anatomy	■ External aspect of female genitalia ■ Labia majora □ Bilateral, hair-bearing skin folds that fuse to form anterior/posterior commissures ■ Labia minora □ Bilateral folds within labia majora, superiorly forms clitoral frenulum and hood □ Flanks vestibule, which houses urethra and introitus	■ Muscular tube that connects vestibule to the uterus ■ Inferior to urethra ■ Introitus—opening ■ Approximate dimensions: □ Diameter 2.6–3.25 cm □ Length ● Anterior wall 6 cm ● Posterior wall 7.5 cm	■ Radix—root ■ Corpus—body □ Dorsal: two corpora cavernosa □ Ventral: corpus spongiosum ■ Glans penis—tip ■ Urethra passes through corpus spongiosum, meatus at tip of glans penis	■ Sack with two separate pockets that contain the testes, epididymis, ductus deferens ■ Protect testes, help maintain temperature of 35°C ■ Thin skin over dartos and cremaster muscles
Vasculature	■ Internal pudendal artery ■ Internal pudendal vein and vaginal venous plexus	■ Uterine and vaginal arteries, branches of internal iliac ■ Vaginal venous plexus	■ Dorsal penile artery ■ Deep artery of the penis ■ Both branches of internal pudendal artery ■ Dorsal veins of penis	■ Anterior scrotal artery, branch of deep external pudendal artery ■ Posterior scrotal artery, branch of internal pudendal artery ■ Testicular veins
Innervation	■ Anterior—branches of ilioinguinal (T12-L1) and genitofemoral (L1-2) nerves ■ Posterior—internal pudendal nerve (S2-4)	■ Pudendal nerve ■ Sympathetic and parasympathetic nerves of pelvic plexus	■ Dorsal nerve of penis	■ Posterior scrotal nerves ■ Anterior scrotal nerves ■ Genital branch of genitofemoral nerve ■ Perineal branch of posterior femoral cutaneous nerve

population, perineal trauma can be from straddle injuries, motor vehicle accidents, and anogenital penetration due to either accidental falls or sexual assault.[illegible]

Hidradenitis Suppurativa

Hidradenitis suppurativa presents as painful, recurrent nodules that progress to abscesses and malodorous, draining sinus tracts, which eventually lead to considerable fibrosis. Typically located in the axilla and/or groin, it can present in any area of the body with apocrine glands, such as the neck, breast, pannus, genito-anal region, and thighs. French surgeon Alfred Velpeau first described the clinical presentation of hidradenitis in 1839. However, it was another French surgeon, Aristide Verneuil, who linked the process to skin-bearing apocrine glands in 1857.[14,15] This gave rise to the term Hidradenitis Suppurativa, meaning suppurative sweat gland, and engendered its eponym Verneuil disease.

Hidradenitis suppurativa was once believed to be a disease arising from inflammation of apocrine glands with subsequent bacterial superinfection.[14,16,17] However, it is now understood to be a disease process of the terminal hair follicle, or the infundibulum.[18-20] A perifollicular lymphocytic infiltration results in inflammation, which prompts hyperkeratosis of the epithelium of the infundibulum. The resulting occlusion causes dilation of the follicle bulb and cyst formation. Eventually, the cyst ruptures, releasing keratin debris and other follicular contents, such as bacteria, into the dermis, resulting in an acute neutrophilic inflammatory response that progresses to a granulomatous stage with the presence of foreign body giant cells. If the inflammatory response is extensive, abscess formation occurs, creating further destruction of other follicles as well as apocrine and eccrine glands. Sinus tracts and fistulas form between ruptured follicles and the surface of the skin.[18,20,21] In reality, hidradenitis suppurativa is a misnomer based on historic clinical observations. Advances in understanding the pathophysiology of hidradenitis suppurativa has given rise to the term acne inversa.[14,15,22]

The incidence of hidradenitis is around 1%. There is a 3:1 female to male predominance and tends to manifest in the second or third decade. There may be a hormonal component associated with it, [illegible] after menopause. It is also associated with obesity, diabetes mellitus, metabolic syndrome, and nicotine use as well as other inflammatory disease processes, such as inflammatory bowel disease, pyoderma gangrenosum, arthritis, and [illegible] disease.[illegible] There are two commonly accepted scales describing the level of severity of hidradenitis, the Hurley Scale and the modified Sartorius Scale. These grade according to severity, location, and degree of scaring. The process can result in considerable physical and psychosocial disability.

A Cochran review of literature published up to 2015 found a paucity of high level evidence regarding the efficacy of definitive therapies for hidradenitis.[23] However, treatment modalities and algorithms have been suggested based on clinical practice, often graded to levels of classification or severity of disease.

Patient-focused life style modulations include smoking secession, weight loss, and avoidance of compression and friction in intertriginous areas. Intralesional triamcinolone has been described to decrease erythema, induration, pain, and lesion size in flare-ups, but long-term efficacy has not been established. Antibiotic therapies include topical treatments such as clindamycin gel and oral therapies such as tetracycline, ampicillin, ciprofloxacin, and rifampicin. Most advocate treatments ranging from 2 to 6 weeks. Chronic suppressive therapy may result in resistance. Though staphyloccocus species are predominant in many of the acute abscess, chronic lesions often are polymicrobial, in which anaerobic bacteria predominate.[20]

Antibiotic therapies do not treat the underlying problem, which is an abnormal inflammatory response. Several monoclonal antibody antiinflammatory therapies have been studied. Adalimumab, which targets and blocks TNF-α, is approved by the US Food and Drug Administration for treatment of hidradenitis.[21]

There have been several studies on laser therapy using either carbon dioxide (CO_2), 1064-nm neodymium-doped yttrium aluminum garnet (Nd:YAG), or Intense Pulse Light. Though improvement was noted, recurrence can still occur.[19]

Surgical excision is the only method at present to definitively treat the scars and sinus tracts of chronic hidradenitis. However, new areas of hidradenitis may still occur adjacent to the treated areas. Incision and drainage can relieve pain from fluctuant abscesses but should be avoided in firm, solid nodules that are not purulent. Repeated incision and drainage procedures can also add to the scar burden. Local excision procedure such as unroofing sinus tract or tangential excision may spare skin but are subject to higher recurrence rates compared to wide excision. These wounds are left to heal by secondary intention. Wide excision has a lower recurrence rate, but to resect the entire affected areas, large wounds can result. The smaller wounds can be closed primarily. Larger wounds can be covered with split-thickness skin grafting. Rotational flaps have been described to cover larger wounds. Care should be taken in designing flaps to minimize moving affected tissue into the wound.

Another option for treating these large wounds is healing by secondary intention. Unlike many other patients requiring perineal reconstruction, hidradenitis patients are uniquely accustomed to painful, malodorous drainage that requires assiduous dressing changes. Therefore, they are often willing to accept open, clean wounds that require dressing changes and, while still painful, are not malodorous and draining.[illegible] If hidradenitis is left to fester as chronic wound, over time, squamous cell carcinoma can arise in it, also known as a Marjolin ulcer.[25-28]

Oncologic Causes

Perineal reconstruction for oncologic defects has challenges specific to the nature of the cancer patient. Fibrosis from neoadjuvant radiation therapy can compromise local tissues available for reconstruction. The need to start adjuvant radiation therapy can limit the available time for postoperative healing as well as create the need for more durable coverage. Adjuvant radiation therapy can also cause stenosis of the perineal structures, such as the vagina. The need for creating stomas must be taken into consideration when planning flaps and possible rectus muscle harvest.

Cancer patients may also present with baseline nutritional deficits from either cancer cachexia and/or neoadjuvant chemotherapy.[1] Preoperative anemia may present via chronic blood loss from, for example, colon cancer, or from neoadjuvant chemotherapy. Optimization of nutrition and anemia may be limited owing to need for resecting the cancer. All of these things can adversely affect postoperative healing. Given the challenges of perineal reconstruction in oncologic patients, combination of closure with flaps decreases major wound complications compared to primary closure.[29,30]

Vulva and Labia

Malignancies of the vulva constitute 1% of female malignancies and 5% genital cancers.[1,31] Ninety-five percent of the cancers are squamous cell carcinoma (Bowen and Paget disease[32]), with melanoma, sarcoma, and basalioma comprising the remainder.[1] In younger patients, human papilloma virus is the leading cause of cancer, whereas in older patients, lichen sclerosus is often the culprit. Surgical excision is the first line of therapy and bilateral lymph node dissection is often warranted. Oncologic defects tend to be limited to skin and subcutaneous tissue. The reconstructive goals are tailored reestablishment of genitalia, body image, sexual health, and micturition.[1]

Vagina

Vaginal defects can result from primary vaginal malignancy, such as sarcoma. More often, acquired defects are due to colorectal, gynecologic, or urologic malignancies as part of abdominal perineal resections or pelvic exenterations. The anterior wall of the vagina is close to the urethra and bladder; the lateral wall is close to the pelvic muscles; whereas the posterior wall abuts the rectum. Defects involving the posterior wall need to maintain the separation of the rectum from the vagina. Oncologic resections of various areas of the vagina can include nearby structures and add to the complexities of reconstruction.[33,34] The resections can be partial or complete and have been classified according to location and extent.[33]

Cordeiro et al. described a classification of full-thickness vaginal defects from oncologic resection that is based on extent of resection and location after simplifying the vagina to a model of a cylinder that is closed superiorly (**Table 97.2**). Type I defects are partial, noncircumferential vaginal defects. This is further subdivided into type IA for anterior and lateral wall defects and type IB for posterior wall defects. Type II defects are circumferential defects and are subclassified as type IIA for the upper one-to two-thirds and type IIB for total vaginectomies.[33]

Scrotum and Penis

Most scrotal tumor resections are due to squamous cell carcinoma, Paget disease or human papilloma virus–related processes. Oncologic defects of the penis can be either partial or complete and are typically related to lichen sclerosus, carcinoma in situ, carcinoma of the penis, and neuroendocrine tumors.[1]

RECONSTRUCTION ACCORDING TO ANATOMY

The major goals of perineal reconstruction include a tension-free closure with well-vascularized tissue to restore or preserve sexual function, body image, micturition, and defecation. The pelvic cavity must be supported and any dead space must be obliterated in this noncompressible space. Tissue that matches the thickness of the reconstructed region and minimal donor site morbidity are other considerations.[1,34,35]

Multiple algorithms exist regarding the choices in perineal reconstruction, depending on the size and location of the defect.[31-37] Other factors that affect reconstruction choice include the presence or need for radiation therapy, need for pelvic support, and presence of a dead space.[35] Because the pelvis is generally noncompressible, inadequate obliteration of dead space with well-vascularized tissue can lead to collections, infection, and dehiscence. If the flap chosen for reconstruction lacks adequate volume, an omental flap can be added to obliterate pelvic dead space.

Patient-specific factors include amount of skin laxity, obesity, and other medical comorbidities that may restrict the extent of surgery the patient can tolerate. In obese patients, myocutaneous flaps such as the gracilis or rectus abdominus myocutaneous flaps may be converted to muscle flaps with skin grafting. In cancer patients, the potential for ostomy creation needs to be considered when planning abdominal-based flaps. Furthermore, pedicles such as the deep inferior epigastric artery may have been ligated in the cancer extirpation.

The perineum is rich in anastomosing vessels and perforators perfusing the region. There are multiple local, fasciocutaneous, island, perforator, and myocutaneous flaps that can be considered. Small defects can be closed primarily or with local undermining.

TABLE 97.2. CLASSIFICATION OF VAGINAL DEFECTS FROM ONCOLOGIC RESECTION[33,34]

	Defect	Associated Oncologic Resection
Type I	Partial, noncircumferential	
IA	Anterior or lateral wall defects	Bladder cancer Primary vaginal malignancies
IB	Posterior wall defect	Advanced colorectal cancer—abdominal perineal resection
Type II	Circumferential	
IIA	Upper one-third to two-thirds	Uterine or cervical cancers
IIB	Total vaginectomies	Pelvic exenterations

However, it is important that this can be achieved without distortion of the perineum, especially the urethra. Defects in which primary closure would cause perineal distortion or dehiscence require closure going up the reconstructive ladder. Perforator and muscle-sparing techniques have been applied to traditional myocutaneous flaps and advancement flaps to minimize donor site morbidity, improve arc of rotation, and provide thinner, better matching tissues.[37-42] The next section will discuss perineal reconstruction based on anatomic region. The flaps available for reconstruction by anatomy are summarized in **Table 97.3**. Because of the numerous flaps available to reconstruct the perineal region, the details of each flap are noted in **Table 97.4**, which also includes a citation in which specific, technical methods for harvesting the flap can be found.

Vulvar Reconstruction

Applying the subunit principle, the vulva can be divided into three zones. The upper-third spans the mons to the labia, the middle third consists of the labia minora and majora, and the lower third involves the vaginal introitus and perineum.[1]

Upper-third defects that are small (<20 cm) can often be closed primarily or with local flaps such as rhomboid and advancement flaps. Defect of patients who have not had radiation therapy and/or will not require radiation therapy, can often be reconstructed with a split-thickness skin graft. Defects larger than 20 cm or those that have been or will be radiated can be reconstructed with a pedicled anterolateral thigh flap. Middle-third defects can be reconstructed with Singapore flaps or lotus petal flaps if the field has not been radiated. Gracilis myocutaneous flaps or gluteal fold flaps are options if the field was previously irradiated or the pudendal perforators were ligated during the resection. Lower-third defects are well covered by gluteal fold flaps or VY-advancement based off of the internal pudendal artery perforators.[1] In the case of defect that crosses midline, bilateral flaps are recommended rather than crossing the midline with the reconstruction because this can lead to postoperative problems or distortion of the various orifices.

Vaginal Reconstruction

Partial-thickness defects may be amenable to split-thickness skin grafts or buccal mucosal grafts. Small defects may be closed primarily. Type IA flaps are most often addressed with the pudendal thigh flaps, also known as the Singapore flap. Type IB flaps are most typically reconstructed with rectus abdominus myocutaneous flap. The skin paddle can be oriented in a vertical or oblique manner depending on patient body habitus and size required for reconstruction. These flaps bring in well-vascularized tissue that can obliterate dead space as well as reconstruct the vagina. Perforator and muscle-sparing techniques reduce donor site morbidity by limiting the amount of rectus facia and muscle that are harvested.[40,41,43] This can spare rectus function, especially if multiple ostomies are necessary.

For type IIA reconstruction, a rolled transverse rectus abdominus myocutaneous is often used. For type IIB, option for total vaginal reconstruction is bilateral gracilis myocutaneous flaps, which would provide adequate tissue for obliteration of dead space as well as vaginal reconstruction. This is also a good choice if multiple ostomies are necessary.

In obese patients, in whom a myocutaneous flap would be too thick, or those with multiple medical comorbidities, a rectus abdominis or gracilis muscle flap paired with a split thickness skin graft may suffice. Vaginal stents to bolster the skin graft with or without negative pressure dressings can be useful in this area where prevention of shear is difficult.[5,34] In general, for total vaginal reconstruction, an inner diameter of about 4 cm is desired. In the rolled transverse rectus abdominus myocutaneous flap, this would translate to a flap width of about 12 to 15 cm depending on subcutaneous thickness.[34] Postoperative vaginal dilators help to prevent stenosis.

There are multifactorial physical and psychological barriers in the return to penile-vaginal penetrative sexual activity after reconstruction. These range from absence of pleasure, dyspareunia, dryness, discharge, lack of partner to body image concerns about [illegible] and/or ostomies.[illegible] Postoperative penile-vaginal penetrative sex is approximately 50%, and it is most correlated with preoperative activity. Those who were not sexually active prior to surgery did not become sexually active after surgery. Therefore, in this population, vaginal reconstruction may not be necessary. It is important to have a direct conversation about sexual activity and expectations prior to surgery to aid in the surgical planning as well as patients' psychological well-being. Postoperative counseling with a [illegible] may be beneficial.[illegible]

Perineal Reconstruction

Perineal defects typically occur after abdominal perineal resections for advanced colorectal cancers. In women, the vagina is often involved and the reconstruction is discussed in the previous section.

TABLE 97.3. FLAPS FOR RECONSTRUCTION BY ANATOMY

Vulva	Vagina IA	Vagina IB	Vagina IIA	Vagina IIB	Perineum	Scrotum	Penis
Pudendal thigh (Singapore)	Pudendal thigh	VRAM	Tubed VRAM	Rolled TRAM	RAM	SCIP	Radial forearm free flap
Lotus petal		ORAM	Tubed V-DIEP	Rolled DIEP	VY advancement of gracilis, gluteal, or perineal perforator +/− omental flap	ALT	Pedicled ALT
Gluteal fold rotational		V-DIEP	Tubed ORAM	Rolled ORAM/ms ORAM	Bilateral gluteal fold rotational	Internal pudendal perforator	
Gracilis-rotational or VY advancement		ms ORAM/VRAM	Tubed ms ORAM/VRAM	Bilateral gracilis	Internal pudendal perforator		
ALT					Perineal artery perforator		
Perineal artery perforator							
Internal pudendal perforator							

ALT, anterior lateral thigh; DIEP, deep inferior epigastric perforator; ms, muscle-sparing; ORAM, oblique rectus abdominus myocutaneous; SCIP, superficial circumflex iliac perforator; TRAM, transverse rectus abdominus myocutaneous; V-DIEP, vertical deep inferior epigastric perforator; VRAM, vertical rectus abdominus myocutaneous.

TABLE 97.4. FLAPS USED TO RECONSTRUCT THE PERINEUM

Flap	Type	Vasculature	Defect	Benefits	Limitations	Details on Harvest
Pudendal thigh flap (Singapore flap)	Rotational island flap	Posterior labial artery	Vulva Vagina	■ Thin skin ■ Erogenous sensation	■ Pedicle could be resected in defect or in field of radiation ■ Needs additional flap if significant pelvic dead space	Monstrey et al.[50]
Lotus petal flap	Rotational perforator flap	Perineal and internal pudendal artery	Vulva Partial vagina	■ Thin skin ■ Similar skin quality ■ Donor site well concealed	■ Perforators to Inner and intermediate petals may be resected in defect or in field of neoadjuvant radiation	Yii & Niranjan[51]
Gluteal fold flap	Rotational flap Lateral petal of the lotus petal flap	Internal pudendal artery	Vulva Vagina Perineum	■ Donor site well concealed ■ [illegible] of field of radiation therapy for vulvar cancers	■ Potential kinking of pedicle when rotated for inset ■ Donor site sensitive when sitting	Hashimoto et al.[52]
Gluteal VY advancement flap	Advancement flap	Internal pudendal artery perforators	Vulva Partial vagina	■ Thin skin ■ Similar skin quality ■ Well-concealed donor site ■ Avoids potential kinking of pedicle because not rotated	■ Donor site sensitive when sitting	Lee et al.[53]
Anterior lateral thigh flap	Rotational perforator flap	Descending branch of LCA	Vulva Scrotum Penis	■ Out of field of radiation therapy ■ May include muscle if needed ■ Can be sensate	■ Depending on patient BMI, tissue may be bulky ■ Sensation innervated by lateral femoral cutaneous nerve and not erogenous	Lin et al.[45] Xu & Watt[47]
Superficial circumflex iliac perforator flap	Rotational perforator flap	SCIA	Scrotum	■ Thin, durable tissue	■ Requires knowledge of perforator dissection	Han et al.[44]
Gracilis flap	Rotational myocutaneous flap	Medial femoral circumflex artery	Vagina Perineum	■ Out of field of radiation therapy	■ Skin paddle can be unreliable in obese patients	Pusic & Mehrara[34]
Rectus abdominus myocutaneous (RAM) flaps	Rotational myocutaneous flap	DIEA	Vagina Perineum			
VRAM	Rotational myocutaneous flap	DIEA	Vagina Perineum			Pusic & Mehrara[34]
TRAM	Rotational myocutaneous flap	DIEA	Vagina Perineum	■ Rolled for total vaginal reconstruction	■ Can have thick subcutaneous layer	Pusic & Mehrara[34]
ORAM	Rotational myocutaneous flap Perforator/muscle-sparing rotational flap	DIEA	Vagina Perineum	■ Thinner subcutaneous tissue ■ More rectus and fascia preserved	■ Pedicle of pure perforator dissection delicate and can be inadvertently avulsed; medial muscle-sparing strip of rectus is protective	Lee & Dumanian[43]

TABLE 97.4. FLAPS USED TO RECONSTRUCT THE PERINEUM (Continued)

Flap	Type	Vasculature	Defect	Benefits	Limitations	Details on Harvest
Vertical DIEP/ muscle-sparing	Perforator/ muscle-sparing rotational flap	DIEA	Vagina Perineum	■ More rectus and fascia preserved	■ Pedicle of pure perforator dissection delicate and can be inadvertently avulsed; medial muscle-sparing strip of rectus is protective	Wang et al.[54]
Internal pudendal perforator flaps	Rotational, propeller, or VY advancement flaps	Perforators of the internal pudendal artery	Vulva Scrotum Perineum	■ Free style–based perforator flap design based on defect and near by perforators found by Doppler.	■ Requires understanding of perforator flap dissection	Hong et al.[37]
Perineal artery Perforator Flaps	Rotational, propeller, or VY advancement flaps	Perforators of the perineal artery branch of pudendal artery	Vulva Perineum	■ Free style–based perforator flap design based on defect and near by perforators found by Doppler.	■ Flaps could be affected by neoadjuvant radiation therapy ■ Requires understanding of perforator flap dissection	Kim et al.[39]
Radial Forearm flap	Free flap	Radial artery	Penis	■ Thin ■ Sensate ■ Urethra reconstruction	■ Donor site visible ■ Requires microsurgery	Gottlieb[46]

DIEA, deep inferior epigastric artery; DIEP, deep inferior epigastric perforator; LCA, lateral circumflex artery; ORAM, oblique rectus [illegible] myocutaneous; SCIA, superficial circumflex iliac artery; TRAM, transverse rectus abdomin[illegible] myocutaneous; VRAM, vertical rectus abdominus myocutaneous.

In men, perineal reconstruction can be necessary without concurrent genital reconstruction. The same principles of obliteration of dead space and well vascularized tissue in the setting of radiation therapy are applicable. In addition to rectus abdominus myocutaneous flaps, reconstructive options include bilateral gluteal fold flaps and bilateral VY advancement flaps based on the gracilis, perineal, or internal pudendal perforators.[36,39] The presence of radiation may preclude flaps based on perineal perforators.

Scrotal Reconstruction

Many smaller defects can be closed after local tissue mobilization; larger defects can be reconstructed with split-thickness skin grafts with or without local tissue mobilization. In the event of previous irradiation or need for adjuvant radiation therapy, local flaps, such as pedicled pudendal thigh flaps are possible. Other flaps that have been described include anterior lateral thigh flaps and superficial circumflex iliac perforator flaps.[1,44,45]

Penile Reconstruction

Partial defects of the glans and/or distal corporectomy can be reconstructed with a split thickness skin graft. Partial or complete penectomy can be performed with phalloplasty techniques used for gender affirmation surgery (see Chapter 100). Basic principles include a tube within a tube design to reconstruct the urethra with the penis in a single flap. The radial forearm free flap provides thin, sensate tissue that allows for both urethral and penile reconstruction.[46] Rotational anterior lateral thigh flaps have also been described, but these can be bulky depending on the thickness of the patient's subcutaneous fat and more subject to urethral complications and revisions.[47] For total penile reconstruction, not in the setting of active oncologic therapy, new frontiers include composite tissue allotransplantation.[48]

POSTOPERATIVE PROTOCOLS

Although there are many postoperative protocols reported according to surgeon and institutional practices, several common themes exist. Suture line care to avoid maceration and to minimize bacterial contamination from urinary or fecal sources helps prevent dehiscence. Urinary catherization may be necessary depending on the location of the defect reconstructed. Avoidance of dependent pressure on the reconstruction can be tailored according to the location of the specific defect and flap by positioning the patient prone, supine, or lateral decubitus positioning. If the reconstruction crosses the ischial tuberosity, hip flexion and sitting are avoided in the immediate postoperative stage. Ambulation is important to avoid venous thromboembolic (VTE) events. However, some prefer to delay ambulation for several days. Most agree to avoid sitting and transition from a log roll to standing. Physical therapy is a useful adjunct to help patients remain mobile within their restrictions. In the event of restrictions in mobility, VTE prophylaxis is important. When sitting is allowed, it is introduced initially in limited periods followed with assessment of the flap for any hyperemia or compromise and gradually increased in frequency if the clinical examination remains stable.

REFERENCES

1. Weichman KE, Matros E, Disa JJ. Reconstruction of peripelvic oncologic defects. *Plast Reconstr Surg*. 2017;140(4):601e-612e.
   A good overview of reconstruction of acquired perineal defects in the setting of oncologic resection. Reviews anatomy and outlines methods to harvest various flaps.
2. Abel NJ, Klaassen Z, Mansour EH, et al. Clinical outcome analysis of male and female genital burn injuries: a 15-year experience at a level-1 burn center. *Int J Urol*. 2012;19(4):351-358.
3. Clemens MS, Janak JC, Rizzo JA, et al. Burns to the genitalia, perineum, and buttocks increase the risk of death among U.S. service members sustaining combat-related burns in Iraq and Afghanistan. *Burns*. 2017;43(5):1120-1128.
4. Weiler-Mithoff EM, Hassall ME, Burd DA. Burns of the female genitalia and perineum. *Burns*. 1996;22(5):390-395.

TRUNK AND LOWER EXTREMITY

5. Harpole BG, Wibbenmeyer LA, Erickson BA. Genital burns in the national burn repository: incidence, etiology, and impact on morbidity and mortality. *Urology*. 2014;83(2):298-302.
6. Demir CY, Yuzkat N, Ozsular Y, et al. Fournier gangrene: association of mortality with the complete blood count parameters. *Plast Reconstr Surg*. 2018;142(1):68e-75e.
7. Ferretti M, Saji AA, Phillips J. Fournier's gangrene: a review and outcome comparison from 2009 to 2016. *Adv Wound Care*. 2017;6(9):289-295.
8. Eke N. Fournier's gangrene: a review of 1726 cases. *Br J Surg*. 2000;87(6):718-728.
9. Bhatnagar AM, Mohite PN, Suthar M. Fournier's gangrene: a review of 110 cases for aetiology, predisposing conditions, microorganisms, and modalities for coverage of necrosed scrotum with bare testes. *N Z Med J*. 2008;121(1275):46-56.
10. Jacobs N, Rourke K, Rutherford J, et al. Lower limb injuries caused by improvised explosive devices: proposed "Bastion classification" and prospective validation. *Injury*. 2014;45(9):1422-1428.
11. Smith S, Devine M, Taddeo J, McAlister VC. Injury profile suffered by targets of antipersonnel improvised explosive devices: prospective cohort study. *BMJ Open*. 2017;7(7):e014697.
12. Jones JG, Worthington T. Genital and anal injuries requiring surgical repair in females less than 21 years of age. *J Pediatr Adolesc Gynecol*. 2008;21(4):207-211.
13. Csorba R, Engel JB, Wieg C. Surgical repair of an impalement genital injury from an inline skating accident in a 7-year-old prepubertal girl: a case report. *J Pediatr Adolesc Gynecol*. 2017;30(1):e11-e13.
14. Boer J, Weltevreden EF. Hidradenitis suppurativa or acne inversa: a clinicopathological study of early lesions. *Br J Dermatol*. 1996;135(5):721-725.
15. Dessinioti C, Katsambas A, Antoniou C. Hidradenitis suppurrativa (acne inversa) as a systemic disease. *Clin Dermatol*. 2014;32(3):397-408.
16. Elwood ET, Bolitho DG. Negative-pressure dressings in the treatment of hidradenitis suppurativa. *Ann Plast Surg*. 2001;46(1):49-51.
17. Shelley WB. The pathogenesis of hidradenitis suppurativa in man: experimental and histologic observations. *AMA Arch Dermatol*. 1955;72(6):562.
18. Prens E, Deckers I. Pathophysiology of hidradenitis suppurativa: an update. *J Am Acad Dermatol*. 2015;73(5 suppl 1):S8-S11.
19. Gulliver W, Zouboulis CC, Prens E, et al. Evidence-based approach to the treatment of hidradenitis suppurativa/acne inversa, based on the European guidelines for hidradenitis suppurativa. *Rev Endocr Metab Disord*. 2016;17(3):343-351.
20. Guet-Revillet H, Jais J-P, Ungeheuer M-N, et al. The microbiological landscape of anaerobic infections in hidradenitis suppurativa: a prospective metagenomic study. *Clin Infect Dis*. 2017;65(2):282-291.
21. Saunte DML, Jemec GBE. Hidradenitis suppurativa: advances in diagnosis and treatment. *JAMA*. 2017;318(20):2019-2032.
22. Sellheyer K, Krahl D. "Hidradenitis suppurativa" is acne inversa! An appeal to (finally) abandon a misnomer. *Int J Dermatol*. 2005;44(7):535-540.
23. Ingram JR, Woo P-N, Chua SL, et al. Interventions for hidradenitis suppurativa. *Cochrane Database Syst Rev*. 2015;(10):CD010081.
24. Humphries LS, Kueberuwa E, Beederman M, Gottlieb LJ. Wide excision and healing by secondary intent for the surgical treatment of hidradenitis suppurativa: a single-center experience. *J Plast Reconstr Aesthet Surg*. 2016;69(4):554-566. doi:10.1016/j.bjps.2015.12.004.
25. Maclean GM, Coleman DJ. Three fatal cases of squamous cell carcinoma arising in chronic perineal hidradenitis suppurativa. *Ann R Coll Surg Engl*. 2007;89(7):709-712.
26. Altunay IK, Gökdemir G, Kurt A, Kayaoglu S. Hidradenitis suppurativa and squamous cell carcinoma. *Dermatol Surg*. 2002;28(1):88-90.
27. Lin MT, Breiner M, Fredricks S. Marjolin's ulcer occurring in hidradenitis suppurativa. *Plast Reconstr Surg*. 1999;103(5):1541-1543.
28. Gur E, Neligan PC, Shafir R, et al. Squamous cell carcinoma in perineal inflammatory disease. *Ann Plast Surg*. 1997;38(6):653-657.
29. Devulapalli C, Jia Wei AT, DiBiagio JR, et al. Primary versus flap closure of perineal defects following oncologic resection: a systematic review and meta-analysis. *Plast Reconstr Surg*. 2016;137(5):1602-1613.
   A meta-analysis of primary versus flap closure for perineal defects in cancer patients. It shows a decrease in major wound complications in flap closure compared with primary closure without increase in hernia rate, unplanned reoperations, or length of hospital stay.
30. Crosby MA, Hanasono MM, Feng L, Butler CE. Outcomes of partial vaginal reconstruction with pedicled flaps following oncologic resection. *Plast Reconstr Surg*. 2011;127(2):663-669.
31. Tan B-K, Kang GC-W, Tay EH, Por YC. Subunit principle of vulvar reconstruction: algorithm and outcomes. *Arch Plast Surg*. 2014;41(4):379-386.
32. Mericli AF, Martin JP, Campbell CA. An algorithmic anatomical subunit approach to pelvic wound reconstruction. *Plast Reconstr Surg*. 2016;137(3):1004-1017.
33. Cordeiro PG, Pusic AL, Disa JJ. A classification system and reconstructive algorithm for acquired vaginal defects. *Plast Reconstr Surg*. 2002;110(4):1058-1065.
   Present the classification for vaginal defects from oncologic resections based on location and extent. Uses the classification to propose an algorithm for flap reconstruction.
34. Pusic AL, Mehrara BJ. Vaginal reconstruction: an algorithm approach to defect classification and flap reconstruction. *J Surg Oncol*. 2006;94(6):515-521.
   Presents algorithm for flap reconstruction of acquired vaginal defects based on the Cordeiro classification and describes the technical details of flap harvest.
35. Gentileschi S, Servillo M, Garganese G, et al. Surgical therapy of vulvar cancer: how to choose the correct reconstruction? *J Gynecol Oncol*. 2016;27(6).
36. John HE, Jessop ZM, Di Candia M, et al. An algorithmic approach to perineal reconstruction after cancer resection: experience from two international centers. *Ann Plast Surg*. 2013;71(1):96-102.
37. Hong JP, Kim CG, Suh HS, et al. Perineal reconstruction with multiple perforator flaps based on anatomical divisions. *Microsurgery*. 2017;37(5):394-401.
38. Sinna R, Qassemyar Q, Benhaim T, et al. Perforator flaps: a new option in perineal reconstruction. *J Plast Reconstr Aesthet Surg*. 2010;63(11):e766-e774.
39. Kim JT, Ho SYM, Hwang JH, Lee JH. Perineal perforator-based island flaps: the next frontier in perineal reconstruction. *Plast Reconstr Surg*. 2014;133(5):683e-687e.
40. Abbott DE, Halverson AL, Wayne JD, et al. The oblique rectus abdominal myocutaneous flap for complex pelvic wound reconstruction. *Dis Colon Rectum*. 2008;51(8):1237-1241.
41. Combs PD, Sousa JD, Louie O, et al. Comparison of vertical and oblique rectus abdominis myocutaneous flaps for pelvic, perineal, and groin reconstruction. *Plast Reconstr Surg*. 2014;134(2):315-323.
42. Huang J-J, Chang N J, Chou H-H, et al. Pedicle perforator flaps for vulvar reconstruction–new generation of less invasive vulvar reconstruction with favorable results. *Gynecol Oncol*. 2015;137(1):66-72.
43. Lee MJ, Dumanian GA. The oblique rectus abdominis musculocutaneous flap: revisited clinical applications. *Plast Reconstr Surg*. 2004;114(2):367-373.
44. Han HH, Lee JH, Kim SM, et al. Scrotal reconstruction using a superficial circumflex iliac artery perforator flap following Fournier's gangrene. *Int Wound J*. 2014;13(5):996-999.
45. Lin C-T, Chang S-C, Chen S-G, Tzeng Y-S. Reconstruction of perineoscrotal defects in Fournier's gangrene with pedicle anterolateral thigh perforator flap. *ANZ J Surg*. 2016;86(12):1052-1055.
46. Gottlieb LJ. Radial forearm. *Clin Plast Surg*. 2018;45(3):391-398.
   Describes the technical details in phalloplasty using a radial forearm free flap.
47. Xu KY, Watt AJ. The pedicled anterolateral thigh phalloplasty. *Clin Plast Surg*. 2018;45(3):399-406.
48. Tuffaha SH, Cooney DS, Sopko NA, et al. Penile transplantation: an emerging option for genitourinary reconstruction. *Transpl Int*. 2017;30(5):441-450.
49. Clerico C, Lari A, Mojallal A, Boucher F. Anatomy and aesthetics of the labia minora: the ideal vulva? *Aesthetic Plast Surg*. 2017;41(3):714-719.
50. Monstrey S, Blondeel P, Van Landuyt K, et al. The versatility of the pudendal thigh fasciocutaneous flap used as an island flap. *Plast Reconstr Surg*. 2001;107(3):719-725.
51. Yii NW, Niranjan NS. Lotus petal flaps in vulvo-vaginal reconstruction. *Br J Plast Surg*. 1996;49(8):547-554.
52. Hashimoto I, Nakanishi H, Nagae H, et al. The gluteal-fold flap for vulvar and buttock reconstruction: anatomic study and adjustment of flap volume. *Plast Reconstr Surg*. 2001;108(7):1998-2005.
53. Lee JH, Shin JW, Kim SW, et al. Modified gluteal fold V-Y advancement flap for vulvovaginal reconstruction. *Ann Plast Surg*. 2013;71(5):571-574.
54. Wang X, Qiao Q, Burd A, et al. A new technique of vaginal reconstruction with the deep inferior epigastric perforator flap: a preliminary report. *Plast Reconstr Surg*. 2007;119(6):1785-1790.

QUESTIONS

1. **What is the neurovascular pedicle for the Singapore flap?**
   - **a.** Deep inferior epigastric artery and lateral femoral cutaneous nerve
   - **b.** Posterior labial artery and posterior cutaneous nerve of the thigh
   - **c.** Inferior perineal artery and middle cluneal nerve
   - **d.** Superficial circumflex iliac artery and iliohypogastric nerve

2. **Which of the following best describes the etiology of hidradenitis?**
   - **a.** It is a dysfunction of eccrine glands of the skin, which cause cyst formation and abscesses.
   - **b.** It is a dysfunction of apocrine glands of the skin, giving rise to bacterial superinfection and abscess formation.
   - **c.** It is an abnormal neutrophilic infiltration of the follicular bulb, causing destruction of hair follicles and creating draining sinus tracts.
   - **d.** It is an abnormal lymphocytic infiltration of the follicular infundibulum, creating a keratin plug and rupture of the follicular bulb.

3. **A 14-year-old girl sustained deep second-degree scald burns on her bilateral inner thighs and labia from instant noodle soup that tipped over while she was holding it in her lap. She was admitted to a burn unit and on day 2 was taken to the operating room for excision of her bilateral inner thigh burns. Which of the following best describes the management for the second-degree burns of the labia while she is in the operating room?**
   - **a.** Full-thickness excision, covering with allograft, followed by autograft in 5 days
   - **b.** Tangential excision, covering with allograft, followed by autograft in 5 days
   - **c.** Mechanical debridement, leaving open to air
   - **d.** Mechanical debridement, covering with silver sulfadiazine

4. **A 62-year-old female with a T4N1M1 rectal adenocarcinoma was treated with neoadjuvant chemotherapy and 50 Gy of neoadjuvant radiation therapy. She was sexually active until her radiation therapy. An abdominoperineal resection with posterior vaginal wall resection and lymphadenectomy is planned. Which of the following is the most appropriate flap for reconstruction?**
   - **a.** Pudendal thigh flap
   - **b.** Vertical rectus abdominus myocutaneous flap
   - **c.** Perineal perforator VY advancement flap
   - **d.** Right gluteal fold flap

5. **A 58-year-old man had bilateral internal pudendal artery perforator VY advancement flaps to reconstruct the perineal defect after abdominoperineal resection. Which of the following postoperative activities should he avoid on postoperative day 7?**
   - **a.** Ambulation
   - **b.** Standing
   - **c.** Sitting
   - **d.** Laying supine

1. **Answer: b.** The Singapore flap is [illegible]. It [illegible] from the posterior labial artery and derives sensory innervation from the perineal branches of the posterior cutaneous nerve of thigh. The flaps are useful for vulvar or vaginal reconstruction because they are easily rotated into position and can provide sensate reconstruction that could be erogenous. Caution should be used if previous radiation therapy to the perineum has occurred, as the pedicle for this flap is often in the field of treatment.

2. **Answer: d.** Hidradenitis occurs as a dysfunction immune response. A perifollicular lymphocytic infiltration of the terminal shaft gives rise to overproduction of keratin in the epithelium, creating a keratin plug. The increased pressure forms a cyst in the bulb, which eventually ruptures, spilling keratin and bacteria into the dermis. This robust neutrophilic immune response over time becomes granulomatous with foreign body giant cells. Abscess formation causes further destruction of other follicles; sinus tract formation and dense fibrosis are common.

3. **Answer: d.** Unlike burns in other areas of the body, burns of the perineal region are not treated with early excision and grafting. They are initially treated conservatively with cleaning fibrinous exudate and topical antimicrobial drugs. They often heal primarily with this treatment.

4. **Answer: b.** Although a pudendal thigh flap (Singapore flap) could provide a sensate flap for partial vaginal reconstruction, its pedicle is likely in the zone of radiation therapy and it would provide insufficient tissue to obliterate pelvic dead space and support the pelvic floor. Perineal perforator VY advancement flaps would not provide adequate reconstruction for vaginal reconstruction. A unilateral gluteal fold flap would not provide enough volume for pelvic floor support and reconstruction of the vagina. A vertical rectus abdominus myocutaneous flap would provide well-vascularized tissue to prevent prolapse of pelvic contents, obliterate dead space, and reconstruct the vagina and the perineum in this radiated field.

5. **Answer: c.** The sitting position will put pressure on internal pudendal artery VY advancement flaps from the ischium and tension from the hip flexion. This could lead to flap compromise and/or suture line dehiscence. Ambulation is important for pulmonary toilet and prevention of VTE disease. Standing and laying supine should not put pressure on the flap.

CHAPTER 98 Diagnosis and Treatment of Lymphedema

Oluseyi Aliu, Jill P. Stone, and Ming-Huei Cheng

KEY POINTS

- Overweight/obesity (BMI >25), skin infections, axillary or pelvic node dissection, radiation, and genetic predisposition are known risk factors for secondary lymphedema.
- Patients should be counseled that there is *no cure* for primary and secondary lymphedema. Hence, nonsurgical and surgical treatments focus on symptom improvement and arresting disease progression.
- Prevention is the most effective intervention for lymphedema. Hence, at-risk patients should be closely monitored for any changes in limb volume to identify subclinical edema and implement early interventions.
- The first line treatment for lymphedema is compressive decongestive therapy, which consists of skin care, manual lymphatic drainage, and compression therapy.
- Lymphovenous anastomosis is indicated in the early stages of lymphedema with patent lymphatic vessels identified on indocyanine green lymphography. In this procedure, lymphatic fluid is bypassed into peripheral subdermal venules.
- Vascularized lymph node transfer is thought to restore physiologic lymphatic drainage either by reconstituting lymphatic channels or by soaking up excess lymphatic fluid and facilitating egress into the peripheral venous circulation.

The lymphatic system has three vital functions: support of the immune system, gastrointestinal lipid absorption, and fluid balance. Functionally, to accomplish fluid balance, the lymphatic system is structurally composed of a unidirectional circulatory network responsible for reabsorption and return of approximately 90% of interstitial capillary ultrafiltrate to the circulatory system.[1] Lymphedema is the result of derangements in fluid balance. Lymphedema is a chronic, progressive, and debilitating disease characterized by abnormal accumulation of protein-rich interstitial fluid resulting in swelling, inflammation, and irreversible tissue changes typically affecting the limbs[1,2] (Figure 98.1). The underlying mechanism is a drainage dysfunction due to a malformed or disrupted lymphatic system causing an insufficiency in reabsorption of ultrafiltrate and transport back to the circulatory system.[1]

Lymphedema profoundly impacts patient physical function, psychosocial well-being, and quality of life.[3-6] Lymphedema patients perform worse on objective tests of limb function and demonstrate greater functional impairment in recreational activities and tasks of daily living.[4-6] Psychosocial morbidity includes depressive symptoms such as helpless and hopelessness, poor body image, and social isolation to avoid scrutiny.[5,6] Finally, the economic burden of care is profound both to the patient and healthcare system as patients are typically afflicted with recurrent infections, open wounds, chronic pain and often require long-term intensive treatment for this chronic, progressive condition.[7,8] Current treatment options are largely palliative with the primary goals of providing symptom relief and preventing disease progression.

PRIMARY LYMPHEDEMA

Primary lymphedema is a result of intrinsic defects in lymphatic system development. Although genetic derangements underlie the disease mechanisms in primary lymphedema, the most commonly used classification of primary lymphedema is based on the time of onset of clinically apparent swelling. The types of primary lymphedema in this classification are congenital lymphedema, lymphedema praecox, and lymphedema tarda.[9,10] Congenital lymphedema presents at birth, and it accounts for 6% to 12% of primary cases. Women are affected twice as often as men, and the lower limb is involved three times as commonly as the upper limb. Lymphedema praecox presents most commonly as unilateral lower limb edema after birth up to age 35. It accounts for majority (77%–94%) of cases. Lymphedema praecox affects women four times as often as men. Finally, lymphedema tarda, also more common in women, presents after age 35. It accounts for 11% of primary cases.[10]

Although primary lymphedema is most commonly classified by time of onset, this classification is insufficient to account for phenotypic variations within categories. Additionally, time of onset alone as a feature of the disease provides no clear basis for clinical management. Recently, advances in molecular techniques have contributed to identifying causal mutations linked to specific phenotypes of primary lymphedema.[11,12] There are currently nine causal genetic mutations known for primary lymphedema and as more genes and causal mechanisms are identified, the classification of primary lymphedema based on phenotype will provide a better clinical structure for diagnosis and treatment.[11,12]

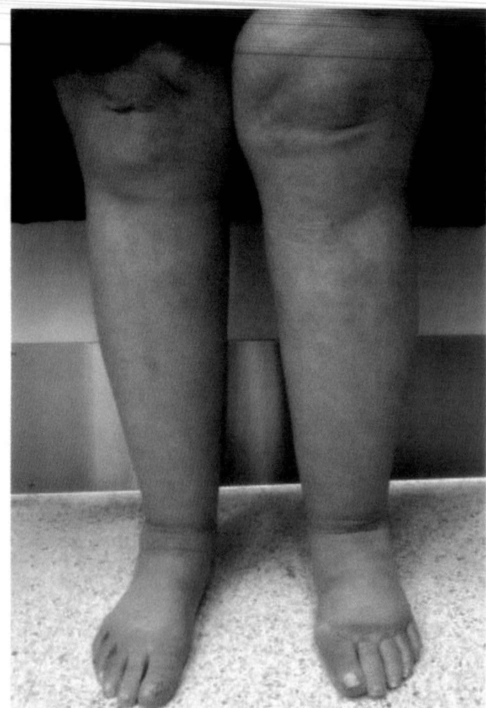

FIGURE 98.1. A patient with lymphedema of the left lower extremity.

SECONDARY LYMPHEDEMA

Secondary lymphedema is an acquired dysfunction of the lymphatic system from disruption by extrinsic factors. Disruption of the lymphatic system may be secondary to infection, malignancy, or as a consequence of tissue trauma most commonly from proximal lymph node dissection. The most common form of secondary lymphedema worldwide is caused by infection with *Wuchereria bancrofti*, a filarial nematode parasite that invades and obstructs lymphatic channels. The global burden of lymphatic filariasis is between 120 and 250 million people, largely affecting populations in low-income countries.[13] In middle and high-income countries, the most common cause of secondary lymphedema is tissue trauma from surgical procedures.[2] In the United States, the greatest burden of noninfectious secondary lymphedema is among the breast cancer patient population (breast cancer-related lymphedema (BCRL)) due to the relatively higher incidence of the disease compared to other solid malignancies. However, patients with other malignancies who undergo dissection of lymph node basins, including gynecological and genitourinary tumors, sarcomas, and melanoma, are also at risk for secondary lymphedema.[2,6,14] Among breast cancer patients, the risk of BCRL is strongly associated with axillary procedures.[15,16] The incidence of lymphedema following sentinel lymph node biopsy is between 5% and 7%.[16,17] The incidence for patients who undergo axillary lymphadenectomy is approximately 20% and that for patients who undergo a combination of axillary lymphadenectomy and radiation therapy reaches 25% to 40%.[16-19] Clearly, it appears that a higher degree of axillary intervention results in a higher risk of secondary lymphedema. Lymphedema incidence and prevalence data are not as robust for other solid malignancies. However, several large series in the gynecological patient population report up to 10% to 15% prevalence of clinically diagnosed secondary lymphedema.[2,9,14,20] Similar to the breast cancer population, pelvic lymphadenectomy and radiation treatment put patients at higher risk of lower limb lymphedema.[illegible]

Finally, there is a long list of widely debated risk-reducing behaviors proposed for patients at risk of developing secondary lymphedema. The most commonly cited of these risk-reducing behaviors include avoidance of venipuncture, blood-pressure monitoring, and resistance exercise involving at-risk limbs. The plurality of evidence has thus far not shown these risk-reducing behaviors as credible.[21] Moreover, there is evidence that both aerobic and resistance exercise, in addition to not increasing the risk of lymphedema, provide strength and physical function benefits.[21-23] The best evidence supported and widely acknowledged risk factors for secondary lymphedema include obesity, infections, radiation, and genetic predisposition.[24] Of these factors, obesity is perhaps the best recognized with robust evidence of its association with secondary lymphedema and equally good evidence that weight loss interventions can ameliorate symptoms of secondary lymphedema.[25] Thus, obesity and infections are potentially controllable risk factors that should be acted upon by clinicians who encounter high-risk patients.

NATURAL HISTORY AND PATHOPHYSIOLOGY

The natural history of primary lymphedema is widely variable within each of the currently defined categories (congenital, praecox, and tarda). The reason for this is that natural history perhaps depends more on underlying causal mutations and their penetrance rather than time of onset. Moreover, classification by underlying mechanism necessitates consideration of other associated features such as vascular anomalies and limb growth disturbances that manifest in several primary lymphedema phenotypes and can influence natural history.[11,12]

Patients who develop BCRL typically present an average of 8 to 12 months after surgery.[26] Up to 77% of patients who will develop BCRL do so by the third year after surgery and then the risk is approximately 1% per year.[27] Hence, some patients develop BCRL even decades after surgery. Most patients with lower limb secondary lymphedema have been treated for gynecological and genitourinary tumors.[illegible] Data from several large series showed that up to [illegible] of these patients who developed secondary lymphedema did so within the first year of surgery.[2,14,20] In the absence of interventions, secondary lymphedema is generally a progressive disease. However, the rate of disease progression is widely variable with some patients rapidly developing debilitating disease and others having an indolent course for several years.

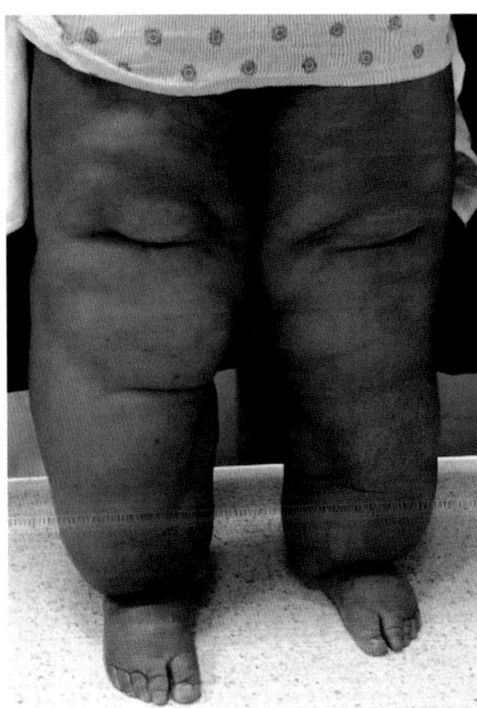

FIGURE 98.2. A patient with bilateral lower extremity elephantiasis characterized by severe limb hypertrophy and verrucous hyperkeratosis

With sustained disruption of lymphatic function by intrinsic defect or secondary influence, there is accumulation of protein-rich fluid within the affected tissues. The accumulated protein-rich ultrafiltrate triggers a pathological cytokine activation cascade that incites a profound inflammatory response.[1] Inflammatory cells, fibroblasts, keratinocytes, and adipocytes taxi to the involved tissues in response to proinflammatory messaging. The incoming cells induce a chronic inflammatory state, increased collagen deposition, fibrosis of skin and subcutaneous tissues, and excess adipose deposition.[1] The clinically overt manifestation of lymphedema begins with pitting edema that correlates with interstitial accumulation of protein-rich ultrafiltrate. Eventually, with fibrosis of lymphatic vessels, skin, and subcutaneous tissues, the edema is wooden and does not resolve with elevation. With these tissue changes, skin breakdowns and bouts of erysipelas are common and underlie a significant aspect of the morbidity of the disease. Lastly, severe limb hypertrophy and dysmorphia with a hyperkeratotic verrucous appearance otherwise known as elephantiasis ensues with further extracellular fibrosis and adipogenesis[10] (Figure 98.2).

DIAGNOSIS

Lymphedema is a clinical diagnosis that depends mostly on thorough history gathering and physical examination. Secondary lymphedema patients will have a history of antecedent trauma to the lymphatic system and report common symptoms such as limb swelling and heaviness, aching, fatigue, numbness, stiffness, and impaired mobility. Primary lymphedema patients in contrast, generally will not have an antecedent injury to the lymphatic system, will most likely be female, and may allude to a family history of idiopathic limb swelling. Clinicians must also consider that patients can present with a mixed picture of primary and secondary lymphedema.

Patient-reported outcome (PRO) instruments are increasingly gaining ground as part of the subjective assessment of lymphedema, especially in BCRL as this makes up a large proportion of secondary lymphedema population.[6] Data from PROs, as a complement to clinical symptoms, add information about functional impairment and psychosocial impact to capture a fuller picture of the patient's experience with lymphedema. The upper limb lymphedema-27 (ULL-27) questionnaire is currently the only validated condition-specific PRO for BCRL; however, most studies to date use generic functional, cancer and symptom-specific PRO instruments.[6,28] Regardless of the PRO instrument used, several studies demonstrate that lymphedema patients have poorer health-related quality of life with decreased physical functioning, psychological, and social well-being.[3-6,28]

In conjunction with the information gathered from the subjective history, patient-reported symptoms, and physical examination, objective measurements improve the accuracy and reliability of lymphedema diagnosis. Objective measurements also provide a means of interval assessments to track disease progression or the effects of interventions. There are several contemporary objective measurements used in clinical practice including bioimpedance spectroscopy, perometry, skin tonometry, tissue dielectric constant, water displacement, and circumferential measurement.[29] Ideally, an objective measure is easy to use, noninvasive, hygienic, cost-effective, reliable, reproducible, and quantifiable, and each of the above listed measures have merits and demerits with regards to these criteria. Water displacement (volume of water a limb displaces when immersed) is considered the most accurate measurement because of its high reliability.[29-31] However, significant challenges limit its use in clinical practice. For instance, water displacement cannot be used in patients with open wounds for hygiene reasons, and it cannot be used for severe lower limbs that do not fit in the water tank. Circumferential measurements are the most commonly used measures in clinical practice and if properly performed meet the desired criteria outlined earlier.[29,31] The measurement is performed with non elastic tape beginning from a fixed point on the limb and repeated at intervals. Using anatomical landmarks (e.g., radial styloid and elbow) as part of the intervals decreases measurement error. Lastly, having baseline measurements of ipsilateral and contralateral limbs are vital to account for potential differences between dominant and nondominant limbs. A 2 cm or greater increase in circumference is widely accepted as the definition of lymphedema.[29,31]

Radiographic tests also play a role in the objective assessment of lymphedema. Lymphoscintigraphy, the most commonly used radiographic test in lymphedema assessment, is a qualitative test based on detection of peripherally injected radiolabeled Technetium-99m colloid uptake by proximal nodal basins[31] Historically, lymphoscintigraphy has been mostly useful as a simple qualitative confirmatory test for lymphatic dysfunction. However, there is no standard protocol for quantifying radiocolloid uptake and transit time, making it difficult to standardize quantification of disease severity across centers and studies. Near-infrared fluorescence lymphography with indocyanine-green (ICG) has gained wider use, also as a qualitative test of lymphatic function. It shows superficial (up to 12 mm depth) lymphatic flow in real time, including the pattern of flow, that is, a linear pattern or various backflow patterns (splash, stardust and diffuse) that can be correlated with the severity of disease. Additionally, the ability to see flow in real time with this test is useful for intraoperative navigation in microsurgical lymphatic reconstruction.[32,33]

Finally, surveillance on at-risk patients is a new paradigm in the assessment of secondary lymphedema.[29,31,34] This paradigm originates in the knowledge that all modes of lymphedema treatment are palliative and not curative, thus making prevention the most effective intervention. Current surveillance guidelines propose preoperative and standardized interval postoperative subjective (patient-reported outcomes) and objective (e.g., circumferential measurement) assessments of ipsilateral and contralateral limbs for 3 to 5 years after surgery.[29,31] Lymphatic stasis and accumulation of protein-rich fluid trigger the cascade leading to disease progression. Hence, the objective of surveillance is to detect subclinical interstitial fluid accumulation manifested by as little as 3% to 5% limb volume changes.[34] Early detection permits time for implementing interventions to ameliorate fluid accumulation before the cascade of inflammation, fibrosis, and adipocytosis associated with chronic edema ensue.

STAGING

Although there is no universally accepted scheme, the most widely used staging classification for lymphedema is the International Society of Lymphology (ISL) staging system, which is based on the progression of clinical features of the disease[24] (**Table 98.1**). In this classification, early-stage disease is described as latent or subclinical edema. From latency, the disease progresses to clinically overt but reversible edema with or without pitting. Irreversible edema follows and finally, elephantiasis which is characterized by severe limb hypertrophy and dysmorphia with acanthotic hyperkeratosis and a cobble-stone appearance of the skin. However, more recently proposed staging schemes are based on the premise that objective results including imaging and limb circumference measurements are useful adjuncts to ISL staging to clarify diagnosis and disease severity. The MD Anderson classification defines stages of lymphedema based on flow patterns observed on ICG lymphography[33] (**Figure 98.3**). In this scheme, the severity of stages depends on a combination of the extent of patent linear lymphatic channels and extensiveness of dermal backflow seen on ICG lymphangiography. Cheng's lymphedema grading system in contrast bases its five-grade scheme on differential circumference at distinct anatomic landmarks (e.g., 10 cm above and below the elbow joint in upper limbs) between the affected limb and uninvolved contralateral limb[35] (**Table 98.2**).

TABLE 98.1. INTERNATIONAL SOCIETY OF LYMPHOLOGY LYMPHEDEMA STAGING CLASSIFICATION

Stage	Description	Pathophysiology	Clinical Features
0	Subclinical	Impaired lymph transport	Swelling not evident
I	Spontaneously reversible	Early lymph accumulation	Swelling relieved by limb elevation Pitting may be present
II	Not spontaneously reversible	Fat hypertrophy and deposition with tissue fibrosis	Swelling not improved by limb elevation Pitting edema present with fibrosis
III	Lymphostatic elephantiasis	Chronic lymphatic stasis and inflammation, further fibrosis and fatty deposition	Swelling not improved by limb elevation Edema nonpitting and wooden Hyperkeratotic and verrucous skin changes

From International Society of Lymphology. The diagnosis and treatment of peripheral lymphedema: 2016 consensus document of the International Society of Lymphology. *Lymphology*. 2016;49(4):170-184.

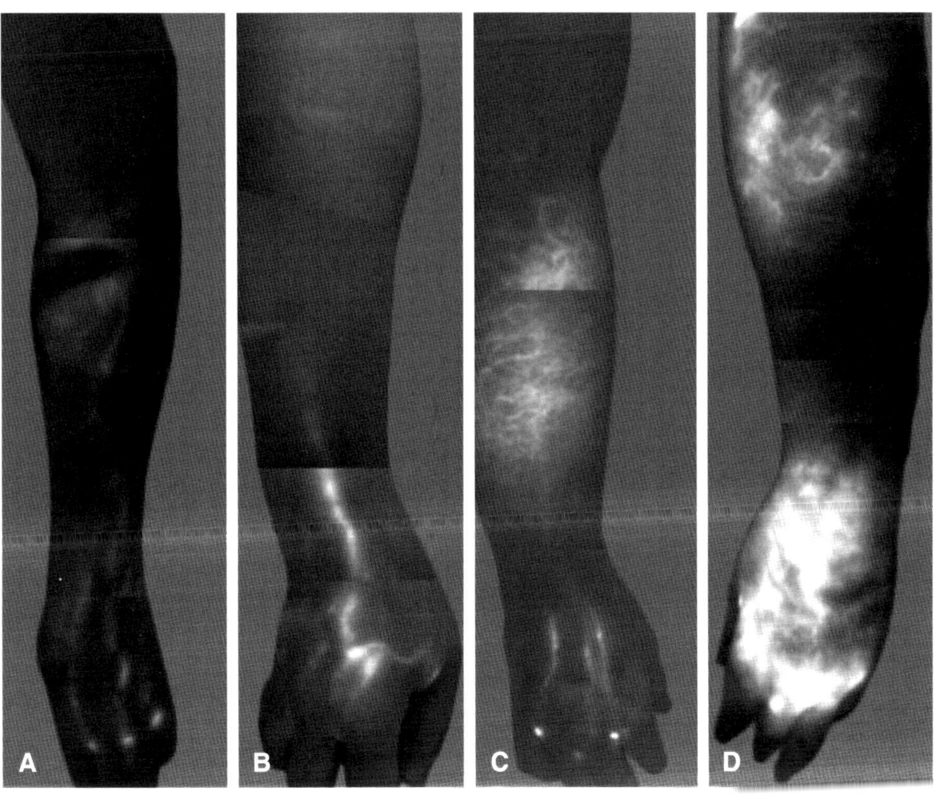

FIGURE 98.3. Lymphedema classification based on extent of patent lymphatics and lymphatic obstruction seen on indocyanine lymphography. **A.** Stage 1: many patent lymphatic vessels, with minimal, patchy dermal backflow. **B.** Stage 2: moderate number of patent lymphatic vessels, with segmental dermal backflow. **C.** Stage 3: few patent lymphatic vessels, with extensive dermal backflow. **D.** Stage 4: no patent lymphatic vessels seen, with severe dermal backflow involving the entire arm and extending to the dorsum of the hand. (Reproduced with permission from Chang DW, Suami H, Skoracki R. A prospective analysis of 100 consecutive lymphovenous bypass cases for treatment of extremity lymphedema. *Plast Reconstr Surg*. 2013;132(5):1305-1314.)

TREATMENT AND OUTCOMES

Nonsurgical Treatment

Generally, lymphedema treatment is palliative and not curative; therefore, the main objectives are preventing disease progression and ameliorating symptoms. Nonsurgical treatments are first line, including in situations when subclinical limb swelling is identified on lymphedema surveillance. Nonsurgical treatments also play an adjunctive role to preserve outcomes from surgical treatment of lymphedema. Finally, patient education is a crucial element of lymphedema care. Patients at risk of secondary lymphedema should be made aware of their lifetime risk, and they should be educated on early signs and symptoms to recognize. Additionally, clinicians should educate patients on practical and evidence based risk reducing strategies such as skin care, exercise, and weight loss.[24,29,31,34]

TABLE 98.2. CHENG'S LYMPHEDEMA GRADING SYSTEM

Grade	Symptoms	Circumferential Differentiation	Lympho-scintigraphy
0	Reversible	<9	Partial occlusion
I	Mild	10–19	Partial occlusion
II	Moderate	20–29	Total occlusion
III	Severe	30–39	Total occlusion
IV	Very severe	>40	Total occlusion

Reprinted by permission from Springer: Patel KM, Lin CY, Cheng MH. A prospective evaluation of lymphedema-specific quality-of-life outcomes following vascularized lymph node transfer. *Ann Surg Oncol.* 2015;22(7):2424-2430. Copyright © 2014 Society of Surgical Oncology.

Circumference differentiation: circumference of the lesioned limb subtracted from the circumference of the healthy limb and divided by the circumference of the healthy limb, which is measured at 10 cm above and below the elbow, 15 cm above and below the knee, and 10 cm above the ankle.

Complete Decongestive Therapy

Complete decongestive therapy (CDT) is considered the first line in lymphedema management. It is a multimodal approach that incorporates manual lymphatic drainage (MLD), compression bandaging, exercise, and skin care. This treatment involves a reductive phase (phase I) and a maintenance phase (phase II). In phase I, patients see a lymphedema specialist five times a week for up to 8 weeks and undergo MLD, compression therapy, and physiotherapy to achieve limb volume reduction. Phase II is largely patient-directed and includes meticulous skin and nail care, wearing compression garments or sleeves, self-lymph drainage massage and exercise to preserve gains in limb volume reduction. The drawbacks of CDT are that it is labor intensive, expensive, and time-consuming, making patient noncompliance an issue. Hence, a number of randomized trials have examined the effectiveness of less-intensive treatments such as compression bandaging alone and physiotherapy alone compared to CDT with mixed results. In 2015, the Cochrane Library published a systematic review of MLD for lymphedema treatment.[36] In that review, two similarly conducted trials comparing MLD with compression bandaging to compression bandaging alone reported equivalent additional volume reduction in favor of MLD and compression bandaging, especially for patients with mild to moderate disease.[37,38] However, other trials comparing MLD with compression to compression alone or compression with physiotherapy have shown no significant differences in volume reduction and subjective quality-of-life metrics.[36] Thus, in the absence of incontrovertible evidence that less-intensive therapy is superior or noninferior, CDT remains the first-line treatment for lymphedema.

Surgical Treatment

Surgical treatments are indicated when first-line conservative measures fail and when patients present with late-stage disease. There are two main categories of surgical treatment: excisional and physiologic procedures. Excisional procedures are essentially a surgical reduction of excess fibroadipose tissue in the affected limb whereas physiologic procedures reconstruct the lymphatic system to improve physiologic drainage. The goals of surgical treatment are to decrease the load of lymph production by excisional procedures or liposuction: to increase the drainage of the lymph by bypassing the lymph into subdermal venule or transfer of robust vascularized lymph node flap to restore the lymphatic drainage function.

Excisional Procedures

Liposuction

Chronic lymphedema induces excess adipose deposition in the subcutaneous tissues with subsequent limb hypertrophy and associated morbidities including limb heaviness, limited mobility, functional impairments, and cosmetically unappealing appearance. In patients with later stage disease who have failed conservative treatment and present with limb hypertrophy and nonpitting edema, liposuction combined with controlled compression therapy has been shown to be a safe and effective technique for significantly reducing limb volume.[39] Studies have also shown sustained limb volume reduction with this technique up to 15 years after surgery.[40] Albeit, postoperative care involves permanent use of compression garments and mandatory close follow-up to refit the garments periodically to maintain volume reduction gains from the procedure.[39,40]

Liposuction should be performed with tumescent technique and under tourniquet control to minimize blood loss and the need for transfusions. Moreover, fluid monitoring is imperative for patients who undergo large volume liposuction (>5 L), and these patients should be admitted for postoperative monitoring. Contraindications to liposuction include metastatic disease, open wounds, medical history of coagulopathy, patients unfit for surgery, or patients deemed unreliable to adhere to postoperative compressive therapy.[40] Complications of liposuction are generally minor and include small wound-healing problems, paresthesia, and contour irregularities. Rapid recurrence occurs if the patient is noncompliant with postoperative compressive therapy.[40]

Direct Excision

Direct excision techniques are not widely used and are generally reserved for patients with severe refractory lymphedema suffering significant morbidity with no other surgical options. For these patients, direct excision techniques offer limb debulking to improve function; however, outcomes are generally not ideal. The Charles procedure is one such technique for severe lower limb lymphedema. The Charles procedure resects skin and subcutaneous tissue to the level of the deep fascia[41] (Figure 98.4A). Split or full thickness skin grafts harvested from the resected specimen are then used as coverage for the open wounds. The procedure is fraught with risks including blood loss requiring transfusion, substantial skin graft failure necessitating reoperations or prolonged wound care, acute infections, recurrence of lymphedema, contour irregularities, and unaesthetic appearance of the limb in the long term. Another direct excision technique applies staged elliptical excisions of skin and subcutaneous tissues[42] (Figure 98.4B). Excisions may be targeted to specific sites to limit the morbidity of the operation; however, patients remain at significant risk of infections, delayed wound healing, contour irregularities, unaesthetic appearance, loss of limb function, and recurrence of lymphedema.

Physiological Procedures

Over the past century, surgeons have devised several techniques to treat lymphedema aimed at restoring the physiologic drainage function of the lymphatic system. The general basis of these techniques are bypassing lymph into venous system or using transferred tissue containing normal lymph nodes to reestablish functional drainage. Contemporarily, lymphovenous anastomosis (LVA) and vascularized lymph node transfer (VLNT) are the most commonly used physiological procedures in clinical practice.

Advances in imaging and surgical techniques have contributed immensely to the popularization of LVA and VLNT. Near-infrared fluorescence lymphography with ICG converted identifying patent lymphatic channels, for bypass techniques, from a somewhat speculative to a more precise process. Additionally, ICG lymphography has enhanced instructional studies on the function of the lymphatic system, patterns of obstruction underlying different stages of the disease, and lymphatic system response to surgical techniques.[32,33] The introduction of supermicrosurgery techniques that made it possible to perform anastomoses between submillimeter diameter lymphatic vessels and subdermal venules has also contributed immensely to the contemporary popularization of LVA.[43]

Lymphovenous Anastomosis

Peripheral collectors return lymphatic fluid to the venous circulation centrally via the thoracic duct. In lymphedema patients, the function of peripheral collectors is progressively impaired due to stasis-induced lymphatic channel fibrosis. LVA restores lymphatic fluid return

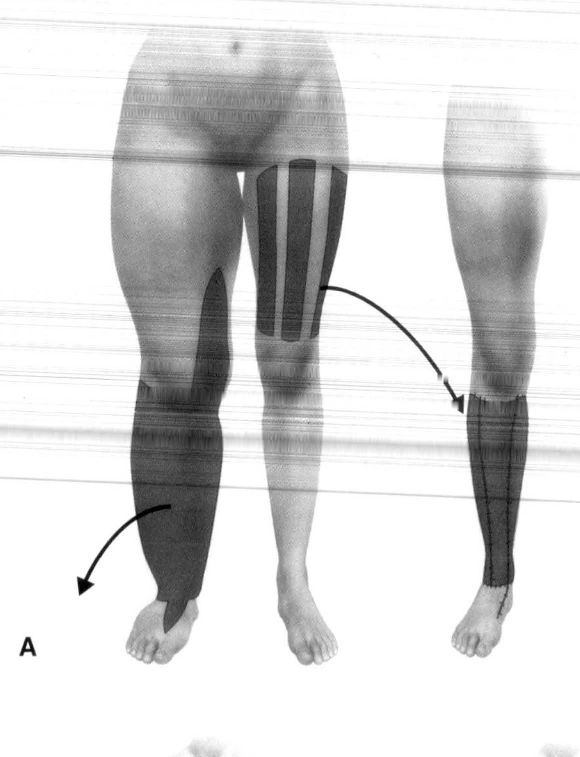

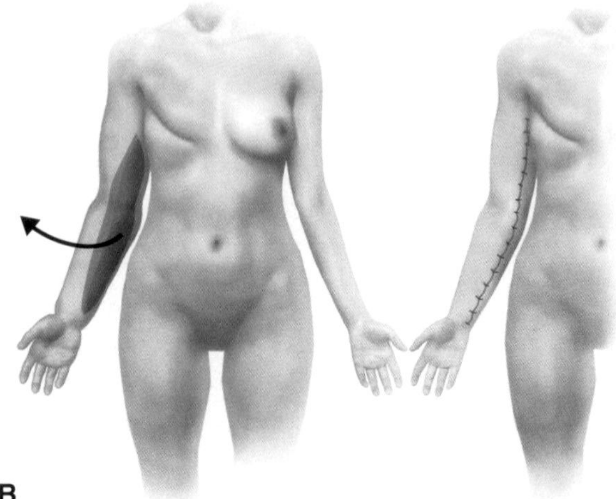

FIGURE 98.4. Excisional procedures for lymphedema. **A.** The Charles procedure: excision with skin grafting. **B.** Elliptical excision and primary closure.

to the venous circulation but does so peripherally with anastomosis of patent lymphatic channels to adjacent subdermal venules, to bypass lymph to the venous system (Figure 98.5). Although there are no clear evidence-based guidelines on indications for LVA, there is effectively wide agreement on conditions favorable to LVA. LVA is considered by most authors to be appropriate for patients with early-stage lymphedema. These patients generally exhibit partial lymphatic obstruction with residual patent lymphatic vessels on lymphoscintigraphy and ICG lymphography; moreover, they have not developed extensive fibrosis and adipose hypertrophy.[33,44]

ICG lymphography obviates the need for extensive dissection to find patent lymphatic channels. It enables intraoperative lymphatic mapping to identify target lymphatic collectors suitable for anastomoses. The ICG dye is injected intradermally in the webspaces of the hand or foot and binds to proteins transported in lymphatic fluid. Near-infrared light from an imaging source detects the ICG thus enabling real-time visualization of lymphatic fluid clearance.[32,33] Identifying patent collectors that demonstrate distal to proximal dynamic directional flow without dermal stasis is key to success of the anastomosis.[33,44]

A tourniquet is not necessary for a bloodless field if the surgical site is infiltrated locally with dilute epinephrine for vasoconstriction. A small transverse incision (2–3 cm) just through the dermis is all that is required, and dissection is performed in the superficial subcutaneous plane to isolate the lymphatic vessels identified on fluorescence lymphography. Injecting patent blue dye distal to the incisions helps with identifying otherwise clear lymphatic channels in situ. After identifying a suitable subdermal vein and collecting lymphatic vessel, end-to-end or side-to-end anastomosis is made and the passage of patent blue dye across the anastomosis serves an immediate patency test. Additionally, the passage of indocyanine green [illegible] confirms anastomotic patency. Most authors advocate several anastomoses to increase the likelihood of success with LVA. However, the basis of this practice is largely theoretical, as there is no evidence associating a threshold number of anastomoses with [illegible].

[illegible] LVA outcomes studies are small retrospective [illegible] with significant flaws in design. Study populations are often heterogeneous due to notable differences in criteria for patient selection for surgery and [illegible] patients with distinctly different conditions (e.g., primary and secondary lymphedema) are often mixed. This heterogeneity does undoubtedly confound findings. Moreover, variations in surgical technique(s) and adjunctive treatments, duration and adequacy of follow-up, and both objective and subjective outcome measurements used make high-level evidence difficult to obtain.[45]

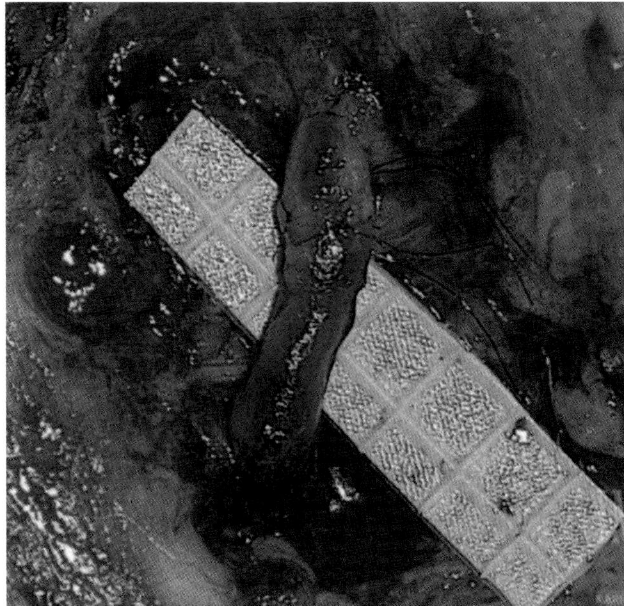

FIGURE 98.5. A patent lymphovenous anastomosis. Isosulfan blue dye passes through the anastomosis from the lymphatic vessel into the venule. (Reproduced with permission from Chang DW, Suami H, Skoracki R. A prospective analysis of 100 consecutive lymphovenous bypass cases for treatment of extremity lymphedema. *Plast Reconstr Surg*. 2013;132(5):1305-1314.)

With these shortcomings in mind, several reviews to date report objective limb volume reduction and subjective patient-reported symptom improvement after LVA.[45] In one of the larger and oft-cited case series consisting of 100 patients, Chang et al. demonstrated that 96% of patients who underwent upper limb LVA procedure reported symptom improvement.[33] Quantitatively, mean volume reduction varied depending on lymphedema stage. International Society of Lymphology classification stage I and stage II lymphedema patients had an average of 61% reduction in volume at 12 months, and stage III patients had only 17% volume reduction at 12 months. In another large series, Campisi et al. followed 843 LVA patients postoperatively (5–15 y) and reported that 73% had over 75% volume reduction and 24% had over 50% volume reduction.[46] In summary, LVA is a minimally invasive procedure that involves a low risk of morbidity to patients.[43,46] Although more rigorously conducted studies are necessary to establish LVA outcomes and better delineate patients who would most benefit from the procedure, a considerable plurality of current evidence demonstrates objective and subjective benefit for patients with early-stage lymphedema potentially eliminating the need for continued use of compression garments.[43,45,46]

Vascularized Lymph Node Transfer

VLNT is a transfer of lymphatic tissue including lymph nodes from one of several possible donor sites to proximal or distal recipient beds in the affected limb. There are two prevailing theories posited for the mechanism by which VLNT works. The first theory proposes that the transferred physiologically normal lymph nodes, through the action of growth factors and cytokines, induce reconstitution of lymphatic flow within the recipient bed.[47] The other theory is that vascularized lymph nodes behave like the motor of a pump, taking up interstitial fluid and [illegible] the fluid into the peripheral venous circulation. There is an accompanying [illegible] whereby the decrease in subcutaneous interstitial pressure in the lymphedematous limb due to the pump like action further directs lymph from surrounding tissues into the transferred lymph nodes.[48]

Vascularized lymph node flaps can be transferred to proximal or distal recipient sites in the affected limb. However, by the pump theory, the *gravity effect* resulting in interstitial fluid accumulating distally in lymphedematous limbs would maximize the drainage efficiency of flaps transferred to distal recipient sites. Other benefits of using a distal recipient site include an unscarred and nonoperated area with available recipient vessels. Lastly, the number of vascularized lymph nodes in the transferred flap is positively correlated with the degree of limb volume reduction. Therefore, choosing a flap with a high number of viable lymph nodes within it increases the chance of a successful outcome.[49]

There are a few donor sites described for VLNT, each with potential merits and risks.[44,50] The groin is the most commonly used donor site for lymph node harvest. Groin lymph node flaps offer the benefit of a concealed scar and the option to combine as a chimeric flap with abdominally based flaps for breast reconstruction. Groin lymph node flaps may be based on the superficial circumflex iliac, superficial inferior epigastric, or the deep inferior epigastric artery if combined with autologous breast reconstruction. Reverse lymphatic mapping and avoiding dissection below the inguinal crease improves the chances of including lymph nodes that drain the abdominal wall while leaving behind those that drain the lower limb to avoid iatrogenic lower limb lymphedema. The submental lymph node flap, based on the submental artery, includes lymph nodes from level Ia and Ib in the neck (Figure 98.6). Drawbacks of this flap include the potential for injury to the marginal mandibular branch of the facial nerve that can be avoided with dissection under microscope for better visualization. The merits of the submental lymph node flap are that it has a substantial number of lymph nodes that have been correlated with better outcomes with VLNT. Additionally, there is no risk of iatrogenic lymphedema. The supraclavicular flap is based on the transverse cervical artery and branches of the external jugular vein. This flap is commonly reported to have a variable

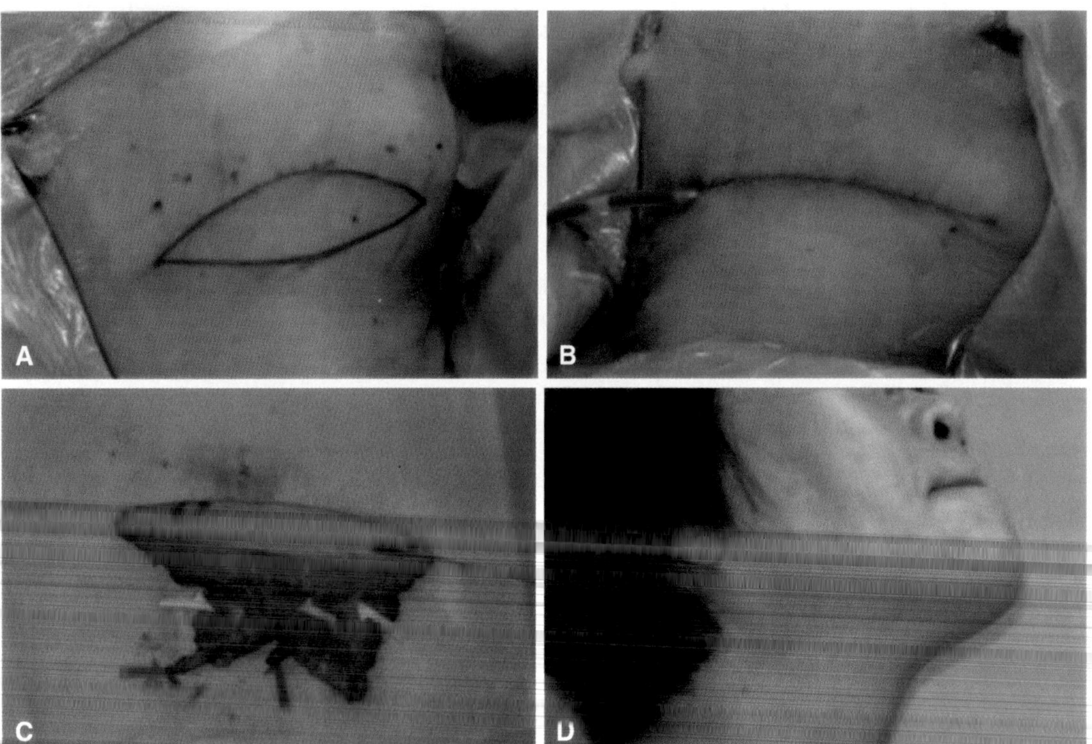

FIGURE 98.6. **A.** Design of the vascularized submental lymph node flap with a 2.5-cm elliptical skin paddle. **B.** The donor site was primarily closed and located below the mandibular edge, which allows the scar to be hidden. **C.** Sizable lymph nodes are evident at the base of the flap (*yellow arrows*) along the course of the submental artery (*red arrow*). A facial vein (*blue arrows*) was separated from the facial artery. **D.** Minimal donor site morbidity with an inconspicuous scar after the vascularized submental lymph node flap transfer at the 24-month follow-up. (Courtesy of Ming-Huei Cheng, MD.)

blood supply and an inconsistent skin paddle (if required) and also leaves a visible scar. In the lateral thoracic lymph node flap, axillary level I lymph nodes (inferior to lateral border of pectoralis minor) are harvested based on the lateral thoracic or thoracodorsal vessels. Harvesting these nodes carries the risk of iatrogenic upper limb lymphedema. Lastly, the omentum is a rich source of lymphatic tissue and can be harvested in open or laparoscopic fashion. The risks of omentum harvest include intra-abdominal solid and hollow viscus injuries and adhesions.[11]

VLNT is the most recent of surgical treatments for extremity lymphedema (Figure 98.7). Although studies are accumulating, there are yet no consistent objective and quality-of-life outcomes

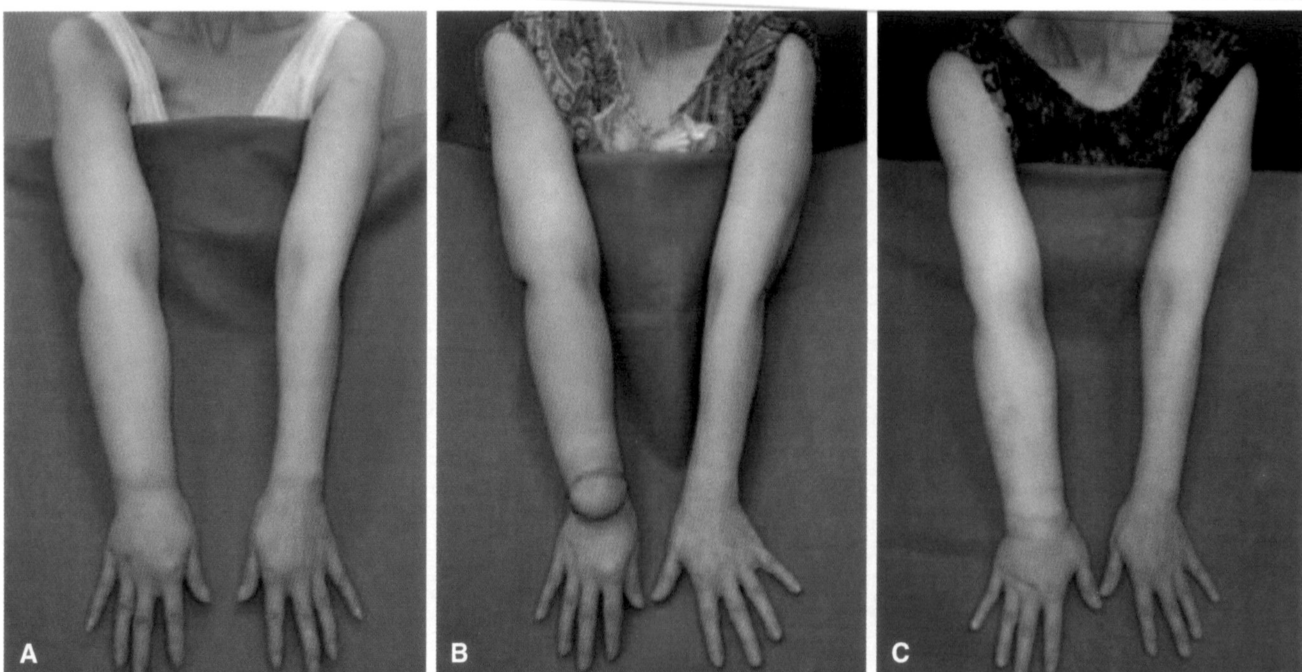

FIGURE 98.7. **A.** A 60-year-old woman with breast cancer-related lymphedema of the right upper extremity. **B.** She underwent left vascularized groin lymph node flap transfer to the right wrist. **C.** The skin paddle in the wrist was de-epithelialized, and the left upper medial arm was subjected to liposuction at 14 and 27 months. At the 36-month follow-up, the reduction rates of the affected limb circumference were 40% and 38% above the elbow and below the elbow, respectively, without the use of a compression garment. The improvements in circumferential difference were 25% and 18% above the elbow and below the elbow, respectively. (Courtesy of Ming-Huei Cheng, MD.)

data from which to draw definitive conclusions on efficacy.[50] However, the principal theories underlying the mechanism by which VLNT works are backed by clinical and laboratory evidence that offer a foundation with which to establish appropriate indications and produce higher level objective and subjective outcomes evidence of efficacy.

REFERENCES

1. Jiang X, Nicolls MR, Tian W, et al. Lymphatic dysfunction, leukotrienes, and lymphedema. *Annu Rev Physiol*. 2018;80:49-70.
2. Cormier JN, Askew RL, Mungovan KS, et al. Lymphedema beyond breast cancer: a systematic review and meta-analysis of cancer-related secondary lymphedema. *Cancer*. 2010;116(22):5138-5149.
3. Gärtner R, Jensen MB, Kronborg L, et al. Self-reported arm-lymphedema and functional impairment after breast cancer treatment – a nationwide study of prevalence and associated factors. *Breast*. 2010;19(6):506-515.
4. Fu MR, Ridner SH, Hu SH, et al. Psychosocial impact of lymphedema: a systematic review of literature from 2004 – 2011. *Psychooncology*. 2013;22(7):1466-1484.
5. Heiney SP, McWayne J, Cunningham JE, et al. Quality of life and lymphedema following breast cancer. *Lymphology*. 2007;40(4):177-184.
6. Pusic AL, Cemal Y, Albornoz C, et al. Quality of life among breast cancer patients with lymphedema: a systematic review of patient-reported outcome instruments and outcomes. *J Cancer Surviv*. 2013;7(1):83-92.
7. Basta MN, Fox JP, Kanchwala SK, et al. Complicated breast cancer-related lymphedema: evaluating health care resource utilization and associated costs of management. *Am J Surg*. 2016;211(1):133-141.
8. Boyages J, Xu Y, Kalfa S. Financial cost of lymphedema borne by women with breast cancer. *Psychoocology*. 2017;26(6):849-855.
9. Rockson SG, Rivera KK. Estimating the population burden of lymphedema. *Ann N Y Acad Sci*. 2008;1131:147-154.
10. Szuba A, Rockson SG. Lymphedema: classification, diagnosis and therapy. *Vasc Med*. 1998;3(2):145-156.
11. Mortimer PS, Rockson SG. New developments in clinical aspects of lymphatic disease. *J Clin Invest*. 2014;124(3):915-921.
12. Connell F, Gordon K, Brice G, et al. The classification and diagnostic algorithm for primary lymphatic dysplasia: an update from 2010 to include molecular findings. *Clin Genet*. 2013;84(4):303-314.
13. Lymphatic filariasis. World Health Organization. Available at http://[illegible]/lymphatic-filariasis. Accessed April 1, 2019.
14. Beesley V, Janda M, Eakin E, et al. Lymphedema after gynecological cancer treatment: prevalence, correlates, and supportive care needs. *Cancer*. 2007;109(12):2607-2614.
15. McLaughlin SA, Wright MJ, Morris KT, et al. Prevalence of lymphedema in women with breast cancer 5 years after sentinel lymph node biopsy or axillary dissection: patient perceptions and precautionary behaviors. *J Clin Oncol*. 2008;26(32):5220-5226.
16. DiSipio T, Rye S, Newman B, Hayes S. Incidence of unilateral arm lymphoedema after breast cancer: a systematic review and meta-analysis. *Lancet Oncol*. 2013;14(6):500-515.
17. Yen TW, Fan X, Sparapani R, et al. A contemporary, population-based study of lymphedema risk factors in older women with breast cancer. *Ann Surg Oncol*. 2009;16(4):979-988.
18. Ashikaga T, Krag DN, Land SR, et al. Morbidity results from the NSABP B-32 trial comparing sentinel lymph node dissection versus axillary dissection. *J Surg Oncol*. 2010;102(2):111-118.
19. Ververs JM, Roumen RM, Vingerhoets AJ, et al. Risk, severity, and predictors of physical and psychological morbidity after axillary lymph node dissection for breast cancer. *Eur J Cancer*. 2001;37(8):991-999.
20. Ki EY, Park JS, Lee KH, et al. Incidence and risk factors of lower extremity lymphedema after gynecologic surgery in ovarian cancer. *Int J Gynecol Cancer*. 2016;26(7):1327-1332.
21. McLaughlin SA, DeSnyder SM, Klimberg S, et al. Considerations for clinicians in diagnosis, prevention and treatment of breast cancer-related lymphedema, recommendations from an expert panel: part 2: preventive and therapeutic options. *Ann Surg Oncol*. 2017;24(10):2827-2835.
22. Schmitz KH, Ahmed RL, Troxel AB, et al. Weight lifting for women at risk for breast-cancer-related lymphedema. *JAMA*. 2010;304(24):2699-2705.
23. Kolden GG, Strauman TJ, Ward A, et al. A pilot study of group exercise training (GET) for women with primary breast cancer: feasibility and health benefits. *Psychooncology*. 2002;11(5):447-456.
24. International Society of Lymphology. The diagnosis and treatment of peripheral lymphedema: 2013 consensus document of the International Society of Lymphology. *Lymphology*. 2013;46(1):1-11.
25. Shaw C, Mortimer P, Judd PA. A randomized controlled trial of weight reduction as a treatment for breast cancer-related lymphedema. *Cancer*. 2007;110(8):1868-1874.
26. Norman SA, Localio AR, Potashnik SL, et al. Lymphedema in breast cancer survivors: incidence, degree, time course, treatment and symptoms. *J Clin Oncol*. 2009;27(3):390-397.
27. Petrak JA, Senie RT, Peters M, et al. Lymphedema in a cohort of breast carcinoma survivors 20 years after diagnosis. *Cancer*. 2001;92(6):1368-1377.
28. Launois R, Alliot F. Quality of life scale in upper limb lymphoedema – a validation study. *Lymphology*. 2000;33(suppl):266-274.
   The study describes the construction and validation of the Upper Limb Lymphedema—27 Questionnaire, currently the only condition-specific, quality-of-life, patient-reported outcome measure for upper extremity lymphedema. It improves the opportunity to design outcomes studies that provide informative conclusions about the effectiveness of lymphedema treatments.
29. McLaughlin SA, Staley AC, Vicini F, et al. Considerations for clinicians in the diagnosis, prevention, and treatment of breast cancer-related lymphedema: recommendations from a multidisciplinary expert ASBrS panel part 1: definitions, assessments, education, and future directions. *Ann Surg Oncol*. 2017;24(10):2818-2826.
30. Chen YW, Tsai HJ, Hung HC, et al. Reliability study of measurements for lymphedema in breast cancer patients. *Am J Phys Med Rehabil*. 2008;87(1):33-38.
31. Armer JM, Hulett JM, Bernas M, et al. Best practice guidelines in assessment, risk reduction, management, and surveillance for post-breast cancer lymphedema. *Curr Breast Cancer Rep*. 2013;5(2):134-144.
32. Ogata F, Narushima M, Mihara M, et al. Intraoperative lymphography using indocyanine green dye for near-infrared fluorescence labeling in lymphedema. *Ann Plast Surg*. 2007;59(2):180-184.
   This study introduced near-infrared lymphography with indocyanine green (ICG) for intraoperative lymphatic mapping during microsurgical lymphatic reconstruction. The practice obviates the need for extensive dissection to find patent lymphatics, essentially making LVA an easier minimally invasive procedure.
33. Chang DW, Suami H, Skoracki R. A prospective analysis of 100 consecutive lymphovenous bypass cases for treatment of extremity lymphedema. *Plast Reconstr Surg*. 2013;132(5):1305-1314.
34. International Society of Lymphology. The diagnosis and treatment of peripheral lymphedema: 2016 consensus document of the International Society of Lymphology. *Lymphology*. 2016;49(4):170-184.
35. Patel KM, Lin CY, Cheng MH. A prospective evaluation of lymphedema-specific quality-of-life outcomes following vascularized lymph node transfer. *Ann Surg Oncol*. 2015;22(7):2424-2430.
36. Ezzo J, Manheimer E, McNeely ML, et al. Manual lymphatic drainage for lymphedema following breast cancer treatment. *Cochrane Database Syst Rev*. 2015;21(5):CD003475.
37. Johansson K, Albertsson M, Ingvar C, et al. Effects of compression bandaging with or without manual lymph drainage treatment in patients with postoperative arm lymphedema. *Lymphology*. 1999;32(3):103-110.
38. McNeely ML, Magee DJ, Lees AW, et al. The addition of manual lymph drainage to compression therapy for breast cancer related lymphedema: a randomized controlled trial. *Breast Cancer Res Treat*. 2004;86(2):95-106.
39. Brorson H, Svensson H. Liposuction combined with controlled compression therapy reduces arm lymphedema more effectively than controlled compression therapy alone. *Plast Reconstr Surg*. 1998;102(4):1058-1067.
40. Brorson H. Liposuction in lymphedema treatment. *J Reconstr Microsurg*. 2016;32(1):56-65.
41. Dumanian GA, Futrell JW. The Charles procedure: misquoted and misunderstood since 1950. *Plast Reconstr Surg*. 1996;98(7):1258-1263.
42. Salgado CJ, Mardini S, Spanio S, et al. Radical reduction of lymphedema with preservation of perforators. *Ann Plast Surg*. 2007;59(2):173-179.
43. Koshima I, Inagawa K, Urushibara K, et al. Supermicrosurgical lymphaticovenular anastomosis for treatment of lymphedema in the upper extremities. *J Reconstr Microsurg*. 2000;16(6):437-442.
   In the evolution of LVA using larger caliber cutaneous veins, patency was a concern primarily because of backflow from the higher pressure cutaneous venous system. This study described supermicrosurgical LVA using subdermal venules with more favorable pressures, potentially improving patency rates.
44. Allen RJ, Cheng MH. Lymphedema surgery: patient selection and an overview of surgical techniques. *J Surg Oncol*. 2016;113(8):923-931.
45. Scaglioni FM, Fontein BYD, Arvanitakis M, et al. Systematic review of lymphovenous anastomosis (LVA) for the treatment of lymphedema. *Microsurgery*. 2017;37(8):947-953
46. Campisi C, Davini D, Bellini C, et al. Lymphatic microsurgery for the treatment of lymphedema. *Microsurgery*. 2006;26(1):65-69.
47. Shesol BF, Nakashima R, Alvavi A, et al. Successful lymph node transplantation in rats, with restoration of lymphatic function. *Plast Reconstr Surg*. 1979;63(6):817-823.
   The authors demonstrated, in laboratory experiments, that vascularized transplanted nodes established connections with local, open lymphatic channels after lymphadenectomy. This four-decade old finding forms a basis of contemporary VLNT techniques.
48. Cheng MH, Huang JJ, Wu CW, et al. The mechanism of vascularized lymph node transfer for lymphedema: natural lymphaticovenous drainage. *Plast Reconstr Surg*. 2014;133(2):192e-198e.
49. Lin CH, Ali R, Chen SC et al. Vascularized groin lymph node transfer using the wrist as a recipient site for management of postmastectomy upper extremity lymphedema. *Plast Reconstr Surg*. 2009;123(4):1265-1275.
50. Pappalardo M, Patel KM, Cheng MH. Vascularized lymph node transfer for treatment of extremity lymphedema: an overview of current controversies regarding donor sites, recipient sites and outcomes. *J Surg Oncol*. 2018;117(7):1420-1431.

QUESTIONS

1. **In using circumferential measurement as an objective diagnostic test, what is the minimum increase in limb circumference used to define lymphedema?**

   a. 1 cm
   b. 2 cm
   c. 3 cm
   d. 5 cm
   e. 10 cm

2. **Which of the following is *not* a risk factor for secondary lymphedema?**

   a. Cellulitis
   b. Resistance exercise
   c. Radiation
   d. Overweight

3. **A 45-year-old woman is suspected to have developed lymphedema of the right lower extremity 7 months after pelvic node dissection and radiation for uterine cancer treatment. Which of the following is the most appropriate diagnostic imaging test?**

   a. Magnetic resonance imaging
   b. Lymphoscintigraphy
   c. Fluorescence lymphography
   d. Lymphangiography

4. **A 52-year-old woman presents with swelling, heaviness, and soreness of the left upper extremity that began 12 months ago. Two years ago, she underwent bilateral mastectomies with right axillary lymph node sampling. You suspect secondary lymphedema. Which of the following is the most appropriate treatment?**

   a. Compression therapy
   b. LVA
   c. Diuretics
   d. CDT

5. **A 39-year-old woman describes a 20-year history of unilateral lower extremity swelling. She thinks her grandmother had a similar problem. On exam, her left lower extremity is severely enlarged with nonpitting wooden edema and verrucous hyperkeratosis. Which of the following is *not* an appropriate surgical option?**

   a. Excision
   b. Vascularized lymph node transplant
   c. Amputation
   d. LVA

1. **Answer: b.** Circumferential limb measurement is one of the most commonly used objective tools in lymphedema diagnosis generally, because it is inexpensive and convenient to use in clinical settings. The reliability of the test is high if it is administered properly: obtaining multiple circumference points along the limb using nonelastic tape measure. A 2 cm increase in limb circumference is most commonly used to define lymphedema.

2. **Answer: b.** Venipuncture, blood-pressure monitoring, and resistance exercise involving at-risk limbs are a few of several factors that have been largely discredited as risk factors for lymphedema. There also is robust evidence that both aerobic and resistance exercise, in addition to not increasing the risk of lymphedema, provide strength and physical function benefits. All of the other options ***are*** recognized risk factors for lymphedema. Radiation impairs lymphatic transport with fibrosis of lymphatic channels. Although the mechanism is not well understood, patients with overweight/obesity (BMI >25) have a higher incidence of lymphedema after exposure to risk (e.g., lymph node dissection). Moreover, excess adipose deposition is a key element of lymphedema pathophysiology. Cellulitis and other soft tissue infections also increase the risk of developing lymphedema. Overweight/obesity and soft tissue infections are potentially controllable risk factors.

3. **Answer: b.** Lymphoscintigraphy is the standard diagnostic test for lymphedema. The test requires injecting radiolabeled colloid into the dermis at the distal limb and observing the transit and proximal uptake of colloid in the nodal basin. Magnetic resonance imaging may show changes in the skin and subcutaneous tissues secondary to lymphedema; however, it is not a standard imaging technique used in diagnosis of lymphedema. In fluorescence lymphangiography, indocyanine green is injected in the dermis at the distal limb and a near-infrared light source is used to observe lymphatic drainage. It is a useful adjunct to lymphoscintigraphy for diagnosis and surgical planning for physiologic procedures but it is not the recognized gold standard diagnostic test. Lymphangiography involves injection of contrast dye directly into a lymphatic vessel to visualize the lymphatic system under fluoroscopy. Lymphangiography is not widely used because of concerns that the inflammatory reaction to intraluminal injection of contrast can damage lymphatic vessels.

4. **Answer: d.** CDT is the first-line treatment for lymphedema. It comprises several elements including MLD, compression therapy, and skin care, which in combination are effective in decreasing limb swelling and bouts of skin infections. Compression therapy is one of the elements of CDT, and several studies have compared its effectiveness as a lone measure, to CDT so far with mixed results. Hence, CDT remains the standard treatment for lymphedema. LVA is a surgical option for treating lymphedema in patients who have failed conservative treatments. Diuretics are not effective as primary treatment for lymphedema.

5. **Answer: c.** Staged elliptical excisions or excision of diseased tissue followed by wound coverage with skin grafts are surgical options for patients who present with late-stage lymphedema and elephantiasis causing functional limitations. Amputation is not a primary treatment for lymphedema and unnecessarily subjects the patient to significant loss of limb function. Vascularized lymph node transplant and LVA are surgical options to reconstruct the lymphatic system. These options are most appropriate in patients with earlier stage lymphedema (International Society of Lymphology stage I or II) with partial lymphatic obstruction and no severe hypertrophic limb changes.

CHAPTER 99 Pressure Injuries

Christi M. Cavaliere and Rachel E. Aliotta

KEY POINTS

- When external pressure exceeds capillary bed pressure (32 mm Hg), perfusion is impaired and results in ischemic tissue and pressure-related injuries.
- Relieving pressure over a bony prominence for 5 minutes every 2 hours will allow adequate perfusion and reduce the risk of soft tissue breakdown.
- Pressure injury resolution can only occur if infection is treated, pressure is relieved, and exacerbating spasms or contractures are controlled.
- Medical and nutrition optimizations are critical before reconstruction should be attempted.
- Because of the high risk of recurrence, the choice of soft tissue closure should always anticipate the need for future reoperations.
- Successful pressure injury treatment depends on multidisciplinary team efforts employing both medical and surgical management in a team-based approach.

Unrelieved prolonged pressure, commonly over a bony prominence such as the sacrum, can result in localized soft tissue injury. Although historically referred to as *bed sores* or *decubitus ulcers*, these wounds can occur anywhere on the body when there is increased pressure or friction, shearing forces, or limb spasticity.[1] [illegible] repositioning, is critical for prevention and healing of pressure-induced wounds. Wound management begins with identifying and aggressively managing the modifiable factors that contribute to pressure injury development such as positioning, incontinence, spasticity, nutrition, equipment, and medical comorbidities. Early interventions include dressing care and cleaning of the wound as well as appropriate support surfaces. Bedside debridement of nonviable or infected tissue may be appropriate in some cases; however, surgical management may be necessary in more severe cases or to promote patient comfort. Preoperative medical optimization, thorough debridement, and tension-free soft tissue coverage for closure of these defects remain the fundamental pillars of pressure injury management.[2] With increasingly complex patient populations suffering from these often-debilitating wounds, multidisciplinary specialty team care is essential for long-term success.

EPIDEMIOLOGY

An estimated 2.5 million pressure injuries are treated annually in the United States.[3] These patients are more likely to have increased hospital admissions and longer length of stay, and they are more likely to be discharged to a skilled nursing facility on discharge.[4] With costs over $11 billion, pressure injuries pose a significant burden to the health-care system.[5] The cost to treat one hospital-acquired pressure injury is estimated to be over $100,000.[6,7] Moreover, pressure-related injuries are now considered among the eight preventable conditions identified by the Centers for Medicare and Medicaid Services in 2008 as, *never events*. By this designation, the cost of treatment is no longer reimbursable for hospitals, no matter the inevitability or attempts made to prevent their occurrence.[8,9]

Certain populations have been identified as high risk for developing pressure-related injuries[2]:

- Patients with hip fracture or spinal cord injury (SCI)
- Patients with lower extremity trauma resulting in bone or soft tissue injury with fixation and casting
- Elderly patients with immobility and/or cachexia
- Intensive care unit (ICU) patients

The risk is even more pronounced in the SCI population, in which there is an estimated incidence of 20% to 30% in paraplegic and quadriplegic patients.[10] Patients may also present with more complicated risk factors, such as long-term use of pain medications, suicidal behavior, history of incarceration, smoking, and substance abuse.[2,11]

Multiple pressure injury risk assessment tools have been developed to stratify patient risk and may be used to guide prevention interventions, such as the Braden, Waterlow, and Norton scales. Patient characteristics are included in the scales, such as mobility, nutrition, incontinence, and mental status.[12-14] Predictive value of these scales is fair, but there is no significant effect of implementation of the scales on reducing the incidence of pressure injuries.[15]

The National Pressure Injury Advisory Panel is the authoritative voice for pressure injury prevention, treatment, and outcomes in the United States. In 2016 the National Pressure Injury Advisory Panel [illegible] injury staging system. Although there are some clinical exceptions, in general stage 1 and 2 pressure injuries are [illegible] require operative intervention [illegible]. Proper staging may require initial debridement of any [illegible] on initial clinical [illegible] (Table 99.1).

The economics of pressure injuries and prevention are astounding. Pressure-related injuries account for the second-most common hospital billing claim, and are estimated to cost $70,000 to $150,000 per patient for stage 3 or 4 injuries, at times resulting in over $250,000 in legal settlements.[6,17,18] Therefore, understanding common clinical situations and appropriate documentation and coding is essential in clinical practice management.

PATHOPHYSIOLOGY

Pressure

Pressure injures are caused by unrelieved mechanical pressure to soft tissue, most commonly over a weight-bearing bony prominence such as the sacrum, ischium, heel, or trochanter (Figure 99.1). When external pressure exceeds capillary bed pressure (32 mm Hg), perfusion is impaired resulting in both ischemic tissue injury and pressure-related injury. Relieving pressure over a bony prominence for 5 minutes every 2 hours will generally allow adequate perfusion and reduce the risk of soft tissue breakdown[19] (Figure 99.2). When the pressure exerted on the soft tissue becomes higher than that of the supplying blood vessels, edema and ischemia occur, metabolic waste products and free radicals accumulate, and with time permanent tissue destruction leads to significant defects[20]. Perhaps counterintuitively, the clear relationship between pressure and time is seen pathologically first in the muscle overlying the bone, followed by the superficial soft tissues and lastly the skin.[21] This distribution with less visible injury at the surface and the more extensive tissue injury deep, adjacent to the bone, is referred to as the *tip of the iceberg* (Figure 99.3).

TABLE 99.1. NATIONAL PRESSURE ULCER ADVISORY PANEL STAGING SYSTEM FOR PRESSURE INJURIES[16]

	Description	Treatment
Stage 1	Nonblanching erythema	Pressure relief
Stage 2	Partial-thickness loss of dermis	Pressure relief, wound care
Stage 3	Full-thickness loss; subcutaneous tissue visible (but no muscle or bone)	Pressure relief, wound care, possible surgical debridement
Stage 4	Full-thickness loss with exposed bone, tendon, or muscle	Pressure relief, wound care, possible surgical debridement
Unstageable	Full-thickness loss unknown depth due to eschar or slough	Wound care, removal of devitalized tissue for proper staging, possible surgical debridement
Deep tissue pressure injury	Purple/maroon colored intact skin with unknown true depth, or epidermal separation revealing dark wound bed or blood filled blister	Pressure relief, monitor wound over time, may go on to need surgical debridement
Mucosal membrane	Found on mucous membranes with a history of a medical device used at the location. These are not staged.	

Inflammation

Inflammation plays a key role in tissue injury, repair, and regeneration. Dynamic reciprocity, or the ongoing bidirectional interaction between cells and their surrounding environment, is an integral process in wound healing.[22] The lack of objective quantifiable biochemical and physiologic markers that can be used to assess wound status is still a major hurdle in the progress of improved treatment regimens.

Edema

Increased applied pressure leads to plasma extravasation and edema. Inflammatory mediators (e.g., prostaglandin E2) are released in response to compression and cause leakage through cell membranes, which increases the amount of interstitial fluid. With local denervation there is a loss of sympathetic tone to area vasculature, leading to vasodilation and vessel engorgement. This is exacerbated by circulatory disease (i.e., heart or renal failure, venous insufficiency) and further increases edema in dependent areas.

Other Factors

Additional factors contributing to or exacerbating soft tissue loss include friction, shearing forces, malnutrition, moisture, and neurologic injury. Perspiration, wound drainage, and incontinence can lead to an increased coefficient of friction between the wound and dressing or bed linens. This further potentiates contact damage and tissue breakdown.[23] Despite this, there is no known direct evidence linking urinary or fecal incontinence with the direct formation of pressure-related injuries themselves.

CLINICAL PREVENTION AND MANAGEMENT

Control Extrinsic Factors

- Behavioral modification: The mainstay of pressure injury prevention is the even distribution of pressure across the body in contact with any surface.
  - Mobilize and/or reposition
  - Avoid prolonged sitting
  - Encourage smoking cessation
  - Manage excess perspiration in and around wound and skin folds with appropriate dressings and clothing
  - Establish effective toileting routine to reduce/prevent soilage and maceration
- Pressure relief: No single specific device has been proven superior for prevention relative to others.[24]
  - Minimize head-of-bed elevation to reduce sacral shear forces (<45°)
  - Reposition every 2 hours, encourage mobility (if able)
  - Adjunct pressure offloading devices (i.e., foam wedge, pillows, boots)
  - In the operating room: *float heels*, intermittent scalp massage, pressure points padded
  - Pressure-relieving mattresses or seating surfaces (eg. Foam, low-air loss, or air-fluidized)
  - Consider prophylactic foam dressings on high-risk surfaces

Control Intrinsic Factors

- Medical optimization
  - Optimize other underlying medical comorbidities; congestive heart failure, respiratory failure, and complicated diabetes are the most common diagnoses in patients with pressure injuries.[25]
  - Optimize kidney function
  - Manage urinary and fecal incontinence—modify bowel routine or divert
  - Manage uncontrolled fistulas
  - Optimize blood glucose control, HgbA1c to <6%
  - Correct anemia
- Nutrition: Malnutrition correlates with development of primary injuries and poor wound healing.
  - Consult nutritionist for assessment and dietary modifications to meet caloric goals for wound healing (e.g., tube feed, high-calorie shakes).
  - Laboratory test results: serum albumin, prealbumin, and micronutrients: Zn, Ca, Fe, Cu, Vit A and C
  - Optimize healing potential with serum albumin ideal goal >3.0 g/dL before operating. Goal is to provide adequate protein for positive nitrogen balance.
  - Track inflammatory markers in conjunction with nutritional laboratory results (erythrocyte or Westegren sedimentation rate, or C-reactive protein) as inflammation may artificially suppress albumin and prealbumin levels.
  - May need colorectal diversion for wound hygiene, as well as to improve diet and nutritional health
  - Swallow evaluation with or without feeding tube
- Infection management
  - Septicemia, pneumonia, and urinary tract infections are the most common infection diagnoses in patients with pressure injuries.[25]
  - Laboratory test results: evaluate markers of inflammation and infection (white blood cell count, erythrocyte sedimentation rate, C-reactive protein)
  - Avoid bedside swab of wounds due to contamination; intraoperative deep cultures are superior for antibiotic tailoring (22%–36% concordance between superficial swab versus intraoperative cultures reported).[26,27]
  - Treat with pathogen-directed antibiotics when indicated
  - MRI may be indicated to evaluate extent of osteomyelitis (97% sensitive, 89% specific).[28]
  - Bone biopsy is gold standard for diagnosis.

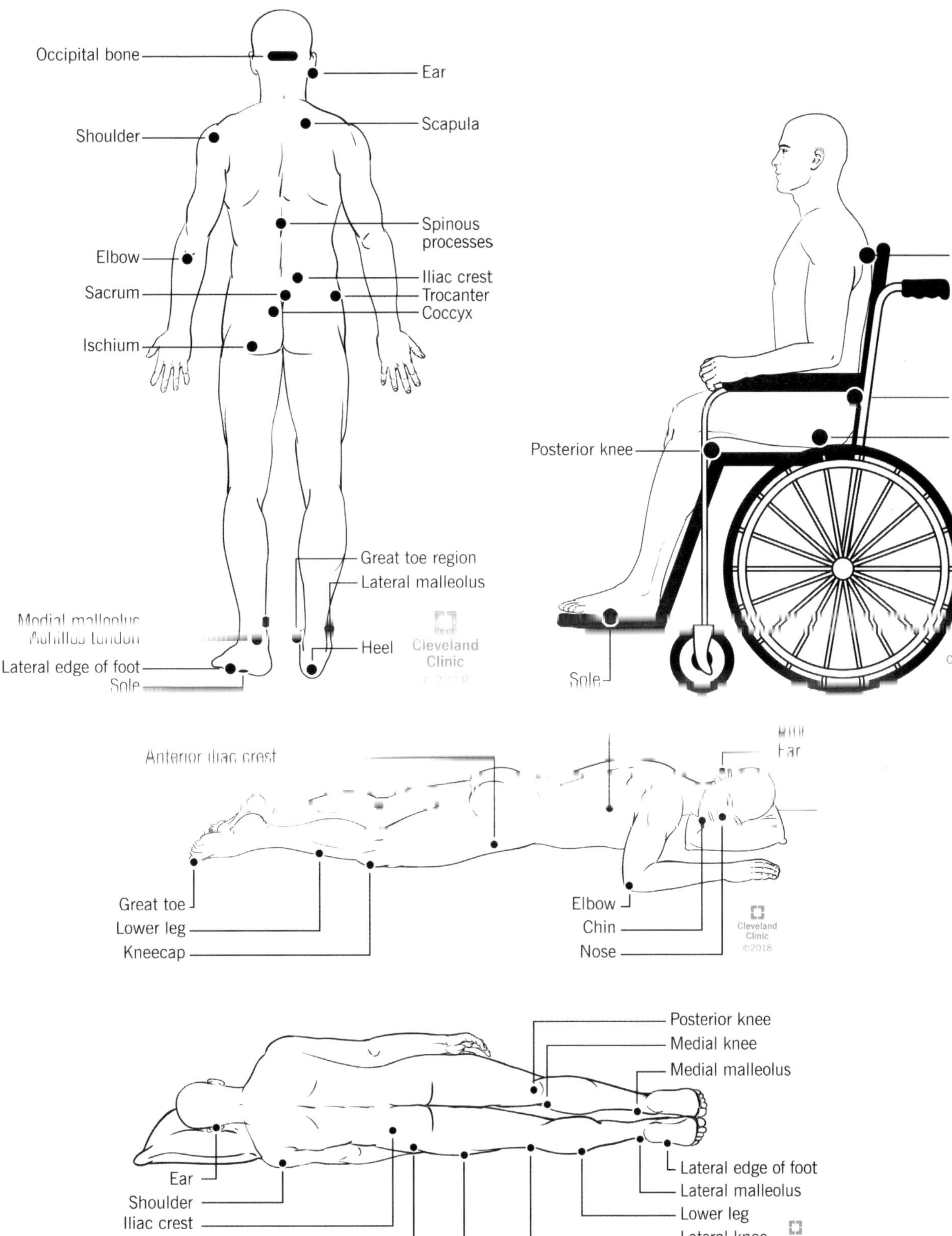

FIGURE 99.1. Common sites of pressure on the human body when seated, prone, and supine. (Reprinted with permission of Cleveland Clinic Center for Medical Art & Photography ©2018. All rights reserved.)

- Neurologic spasm and contracture management
  - Especially SCI: Incidence of spasm varies with level of SC injury (proximal lesion = higher incidence)
  - Spasm and contracture create shear forces contributing to pressure injury development
    - Common in hip and knee joints
  - Antispasmodic pharmacotherapy: baclofen, diazepam, dantrolene
    - Botulinum toxin improves function and reduces limb spasticity with minimal side effects.
- Procedural intervention if severe, after failed medical management
  - Peripheral nerve block, epidural stimulator, baclofen pump, rhizotomy
  - Surgical release of joint contracture or in severe cases amputation
  - Consider medical rhizotomy (phenol)

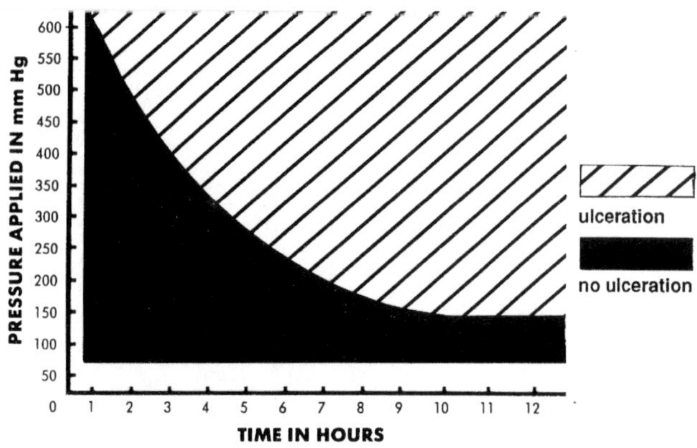

FIGURE 99.2. The inverse relationship between time and pressure in the formation of pressure injuries.

WOUND CARE

Make clinical assessment before choosing appropriate wound care dressing regimens for each patient and each wound. Be sure to diagram, use photographs, and document a comprehensive physical examination of all affected areas, including:

- Dimensions (length × width × depth)
- Presence of undermining, position (clock face location)
- Indicators of infection and/or systemic symptoms of infection
- Drainage, amount, and character
- Odor, possible source, or cause
- Deepest visible layer affected or seen in base of wound
- Condition of periwound skin (such as bruising or maceration)
- Vascular assessment of surrounding tissue or affected

Nonoperative Management

Dressings

Based on patient and wound assessment, select a dressing that will support a moist healing environment for the wound. Appropriate wound-healing agents include hydrocolloids, alginates and hydrofibers, hydrogels, paraffin gauze dressings, and many other dressings and topical agents.[29] However, there is little clinical evidence to aid the choice between different dressings. In general, the consensus opinion favors hydrogels during the debridement stage, foam and low-adherence dressings for the granulation stage, and hydrocolloid and low-adherence dressings for the epithelialization stage. Packing the wound cavity with moist gauze may be appropriate in some circumstances. Ultimately, the dressing chosen should be best suited to manage the moisture level in and around the wound.

- Preventive: A recent consensus panel recommendation concluded multilayered silicone dressing was effective as an adjunct for reducing pressure-related injuries to sacrum, buttocks, and heels in high-risk environments (the OR, ICU) when combined with traditional preventative measures. Silicone is elastic and therefore able to absorb the shear forces and reduce skin deformation.[30]
- For dry wounds, create a moist healing environment. Many are dressings appropriate.
    - Traditional wet to moist saline dressing, typically should be changed one or two times per day, depending on wound debridement needs
    - Use sodium hypochlorite solution or bleach-based solution if infection is suspected, particularly *Pseudomonas*. Diluted sodium hypochlorite solution has been shown to be bactericidal with fibroblast preservation.
    - Hydrogels—Used as tube of gel or sheet; water-based, nonadherent; changed daily
    - Hydrocolloid dressing has been associated with almost three times more complete healing compared with the use of saline gauze alone.[31] There is no evidence to support superiority of topical collagen versus hydrocolloid for pressure injury healing, and it is more costly.[32]
    - Honey—variable gel thickness and composition, minimal risk, and low cost, with possible autolytic and antimicrobial properties.[33]
    - Studies on sustained silver-releasing dressing demonstrated a tendency for reducing the risk of infection and promoting faster healing, but sample sizes have been too small for statistical analysis to draw formal conclusions.[34]
    - For wounds with large amount of drainage, use dressings that are absorbent.
        - Alginates (derived from seaweed) or synthetic hydrofibers. These dressings have a dry, felt-like texture and absorb several times their weight in moisture. There is evidence the use of alginates with hydrocolloid results in significantly greater reduction in the size of stage 3 and 4 pressure injuries compared to hydrocolloid alone.[35]
        - Hydrocolloid gel forming polymers
        - Foam dressings—can be used alone or as a cover dressing. Gentle on skin but can be more costly.
        - Wicking systems or salt-impregnated gauze

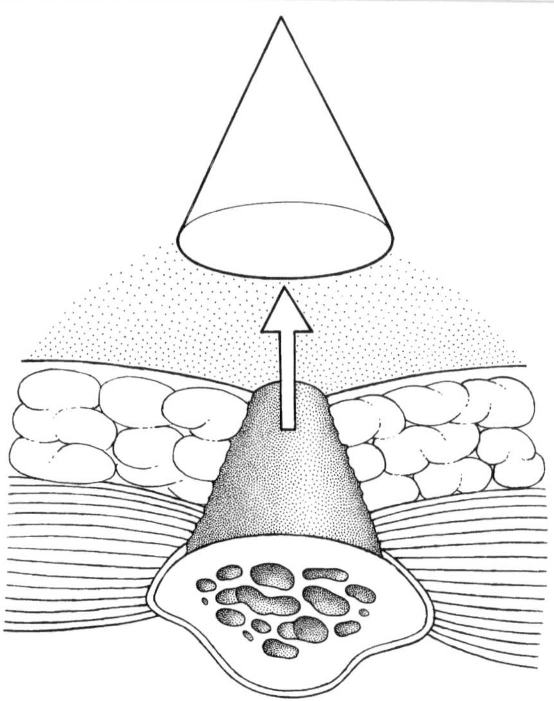

FIGURE 99.3. *Tip of the iceberg* cone-shape pattern of pressure-related injury from unrelieved pressure affecting the deepest structures adjacent to the bone with the greatest injury.

Negative-Pressure Wound Therapy

Negative-pressure wound therapy (NPWT), as well as NPWT systems with automated instillation capabilities and dwell time, is gaining popularity in the wound care armamentarium. In addition to the benefits of negative-pressure therapy the cyclic instillation and dwelling of topical wound solutions aided cleaning and granulation tissue formation. The proposed benefits include removal of infectious materials,[36] reduced risk of compromise due to contamination, the ability to solubilize necrotic tissue, reduced volume of exudate, increased granulation tissue, and decreased wound size.[37] However, the use of negative-pressure systems should be considered in light of the effect it may have on patient mobility and ambulation, as well as cost-to-benefit ratio given clinical and social scenario of each individual patient. Contraindications to the use of NPWT include exposed vessels or organs, nonenteric and unexplored fistulas, malignancy, and untreated osteomyelitis.[38]

Hyperbaric Oxygen Therapy

Hyperbaric oxygen therapy (HBOT) has been used as an adjunct to treat wounds for decades, proving to be safe and beneficial for selected patients. HBOT increases oxygen transport to the wound area, facilitates angiogenesis, reduces inflammation and swelling, improves lymphatic circulation, reduces infection by increasing the capacity of the leukocyte, and may relieve some pain.[39] A pressure injury itself is not an indication for HBOT; however, HBOT may be used as adjunctive treatment for chronic refractory osteomyelitis within a pressure injury or a failed graft or flap.[40]

Biologic Therapies

The efficacy of platelet-derived growth factors, fibroblast growth factor, and granulocyte macrophage colony stimulating factor in improving complete pressure injury healing has not been well established. There is limited low-quality evidence on skin matrix and tissue-engineered skin equivalents, with insufficient evidence to draw conclusions.[34]

Other Therapies

There is some evidence that electrotherapy[41] and whirlpool therapy[42] may help reduce the size and surface area of stage 2 to 4 pressure injuries. However, the efficacy of other therapy modalities such as electromagnetic therapy, low-level laser therapy, cold lasers, light therapy, or ultrasound therapy has not been found to promote superior healing of pressure injuries at present.[34]

Surgical Management

Indications

- Necrotizing infection
- Need for significant debridement
- Biopsy for malignancy, deep cultures
- Bone and/or hardware exposure
- Vasculature exposure
- Organ exposure
- Retained foreign body (i.e., packing)
- Small skin opening with area of large undermining
- Necessity due to medical complexity

Debridement and Wound Optimization

Soft Tissue

Infected and necrotic wounds require early and aggressive debridement of any infected or devitalized tissue. Goals are the following:

- Remove necrotic tissue
- Decrease the bacterial count and biofilm
- Convert a chronic wound to an acute wound

Bedside debridement may be limited by patient comfort and ability to secure hemostasis in both sensate and insensate patients. Consider the patient's risk of autonomic dysreflexia (AD) with pain stimulus. Intraoperatively, consider painting wound borders with methylene blue to ensure removal of the entire cavity. Send deep tissue for culture to tailor antibiotic choice because this has been shown superior to superficial swabs, which tend to have high rate of misdiagnosis and may lead to antibiotic over treatment.[26] Initiate wound care following debridement.

Bone

Some institutions advocate taking bone biopsy only in conjunction with soft tissue debridement as needed, as to avoid seeding deep bone with any overlying infectious processes.[2] There is a high reported rate of osteomyelitis, with 56% of primary injuries and 79% of recurrent injuries having positive bone biopsies for osteomyelitis.[43] Remove as minimal bone as possible. Avoid radical ostectomy for bony prominences, as this can lead to skeletal instability, excessive bleeding, and pressure point redistribution (as seen with unilateral ischiectomy with contralateral injury formation).

Contracture Release and Management of Spasticity

These strategies are important to optimize positioning before attempted final reconstruction.

- Peripheral nerve blocks, epidural stimulator, baclofen pumps, rhizotomy
- Consider medical rhizotomy (phenol) or surgical
- Tenotomy for limb contracture. Avoid hip release in wheelchair-bound patients because this will interfere with transfers if flail extremity occurs.

Reconstruction

When considering flap reconstruction, it is essential to take into account that flap coverage does not address the root cause of the pressure injury (i.e., the complex interplay between ischemia, nutrition, infection, and overall health of the patient). Careful patient selection with flap choice tailored to the individual patient is the most critical step in improving overall patient outcomes in these difficult cases.

- Avoid primary closure of pressure injuries due to high rates of breakdown and dehiscence.
- Skin grafts will likely fail in this area because of lack of adequate tolerance to repeated pressure and shear.
- There is no reported difference in success using myocutaneous compared to fasciocutaneous flaps[44,45] (Figure 99.4).
- Despite the use of risk assessment tools and preventative risk reduction practice, complications and recurrence rates for flap coverage are high.[46,47]

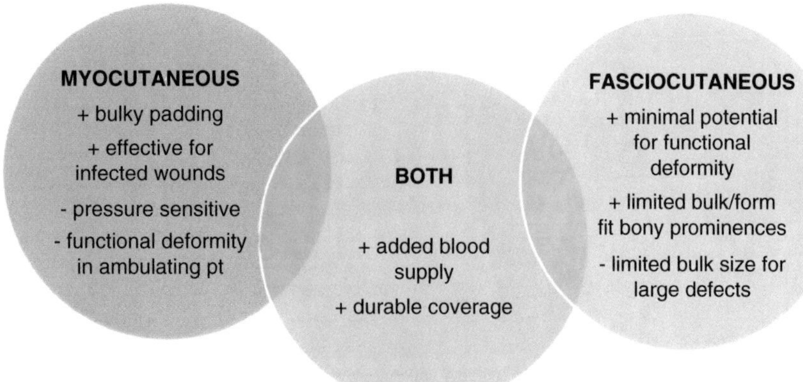

FIGURE 99.4. Considerations using myocutaneous versus fasciocutaneous flaps.

Management by Pressure Injury Location

Ischium

- These defects common in patients seated for prolonged periods (i.e., wheelchair-bound patients).
- High recurrence rates may be due to pressure and tension across joint while sitting. Recurrence rates of 19% to 33% have been reported for ischial pressure injuries after flap reconstruction.[47,48]
- Ischial flap design should take into consideration:
  - Ambulatory status
  - Possibility of future flaps due to high rate of recurrence
  - Avoid placing incisions over weight-bearing prominences
- Consider flaps that can be readvanced subsequently: for example gluteal rotation or V-Y hamstring.
- Avoid tension with these closures, as hip flexion can cause dehiscence.

Tensor fascia lata (TFL) may be considered, but it may be too thin distally.

Sacrum

- These defects are common in supine or bedridden patients (such as with an acute illness).
- Fasciocutaneous, musculocutaneous flaps are mainstay, with perforator flaps increasingly used.
- Recurrence rates 17% to 21% depending on flap choice.[49]
- Sacral flap design should consider the depth of wound and potential need to fill dead space.
- Most common musculocutaneous flap is based on gluteus maximus muscle. Can be superior or inferiorly based, with ability to rotate, advance, or turnover.
- A fasciocutaneous flap or partial gluteus muscle may be needed in ambulatory patient as gluteus maximus muscle is not expendable.

Trochanter

- These defects are common in patients positioned laterally for prolonged periods.
- Flap reconstruction most commonly TFL, but pedicled ALT flap is also an option.
- TFL blood supply consistent from underlying TFL muscle, but distal part of flap is random blood supply that may need to be delayed.
- If there is a SCI below L3, the TFL can be sensate via L1–L3 by way of the lateral femoral cutaneous nerve (Figure 99.5).

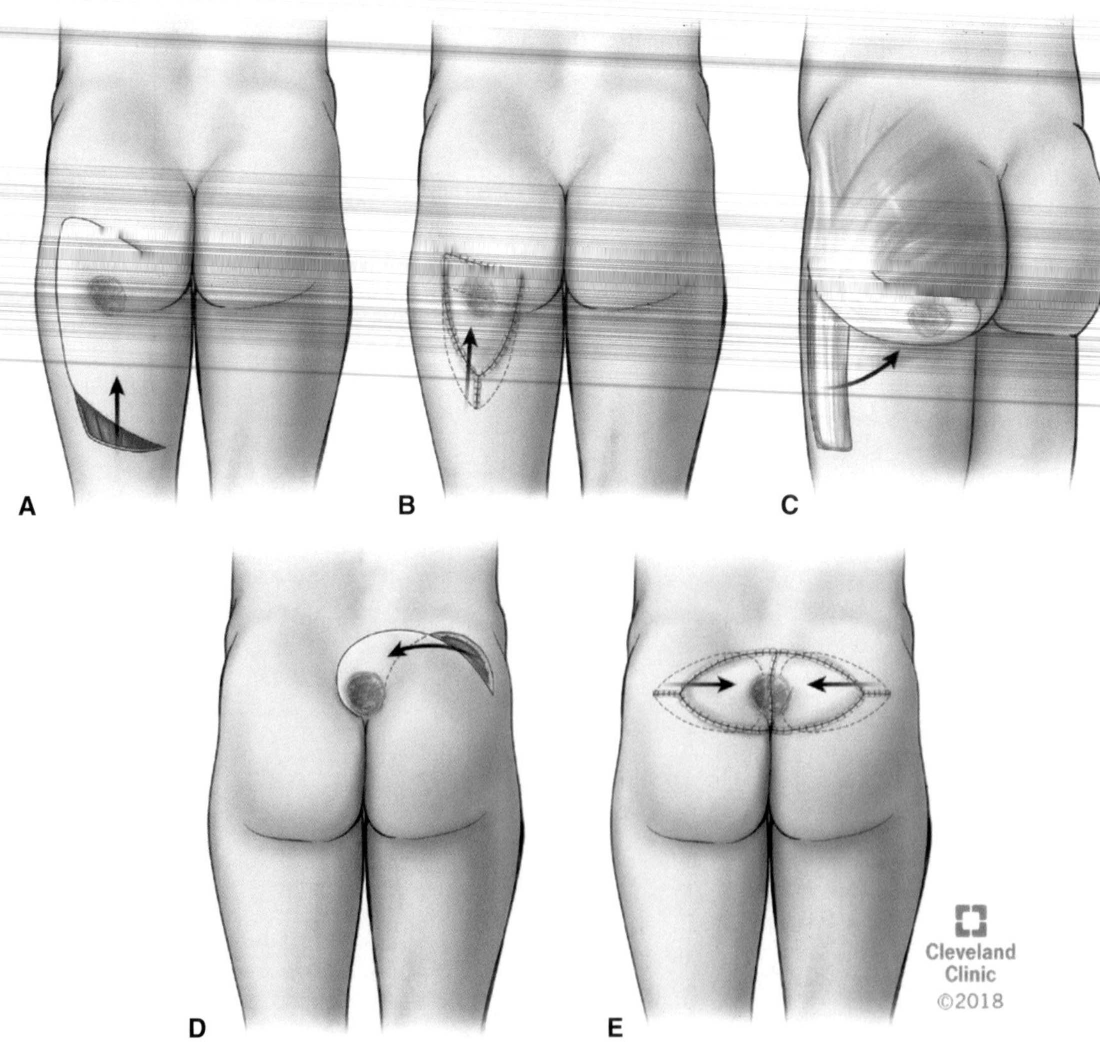

FIGURE 99.5. Flap options for pressure injury reconstruction. **A.** Local advancement of fasciocutaneous flap. **B.** V-Y advancement/hamstring flap. **C.** Tensor fascia lata flap. **D.** Gluteal rotation flap for sacral pressure injury can be elevated as myocutaneous or fasciocutaneous flap. **E.** Single- or double-opposing V-Y advancement flaps can be elevated as myocutaneous or fasciocutaneous flaps. (Reprinted with permission of Cleveland Clinic Center for Medical Art & Photography ©2018. All rights reserved.)

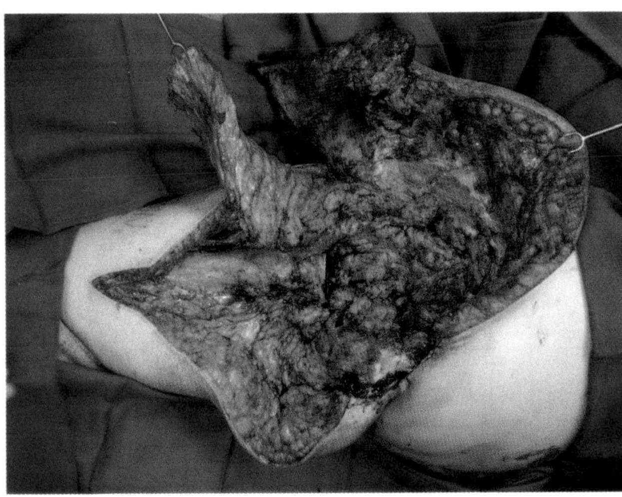
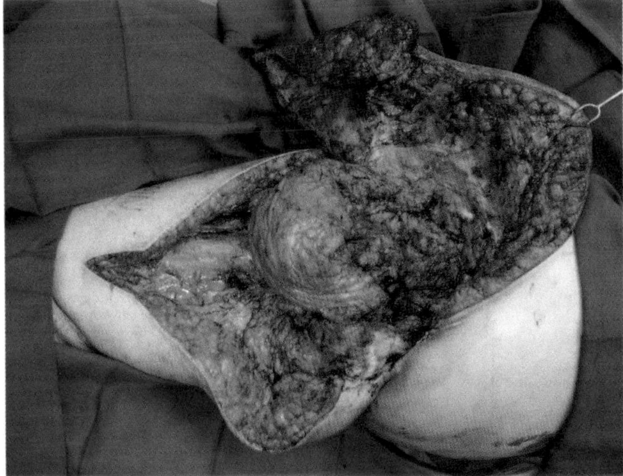

FIGURE 99.6. Tensor fascia lata with vastus lateralis for coverage of a resected femoral head (Girdlestone procedure). (Reprinted with permission of Cleveland Clinic Center for Medical Art & Photography ©2018. All rights reserved.)

Ears, Scapula, Heels

- Ears and scapula may be amenable to primary closure or local tissue rearrangement.
- Heels may require lifelong wound care, free flap coverage, or amputation depending on patient functional status and comorbid state.
- Lower-extremity pressure injuries require careful assessment of vascular status and treatment of underlying ischemia.

Massive or Multifocal Pressure Injuries

- It may not be technically feasible to cover with local or distant flap(s) because of overwhelming size, medical comorbidities, and ability to tolerate and comply with postoperative management.
- Local wound care indefinitely, with consideration of radical procedures such as Girdlestone resection and multiple flap reconstruction, or amputation with total thigh flap closure (Figure 99.6).

POSTOPERATIVE CONSIDERATIONS

Acute Management

- Continue behavioral modifications and multidisciplinary, team-based management of patient comorbidities and postoperative care to optimize wound healing.
- Place the patient on a pressure-relieving surface such as an air-fluidized bed or low-air loss mattress. A period of bedrest is beneficial to allow surgical incisions to heal without disruption; however, this must be considered in the context of the risks of bedrest such as pneumonia, VTE, and deconditioning. Recommendations vary from 2 weeks to approximately 6 weeks depending on surgeon preference, extent of the reconstruction, and location of the injury.
- Avoid sitting upright in bed. Resume sitting on a limited basis with gradual increase over several days. Ensure patient is seated on an appropriate pressure-reducing surface.
- DVT risk assessment: Patients with SCI are particularly susceptible to venous thromboembolism (VTE). Risk stratification such as the Caprini Risk Assessment Model may be useful to guide perioperative VTE prophylaxis. Although there is no evidence to suggest that there is higher risk of postoperative VTE in the plastic surgery population with chronic SCI, physicians are encouraged to exercise vigilance in monitoring for venous thromboembolic events, as the incidence of VTE has been reported as high as 11% in the acute SCI population, despite receiving VTE prophylaxis.[50]
- Awareness of potential AD in SCI patients: Caused by disordered response to stimuli below the level of the lesion, such as bladder and bowel distension. Clinical manifestations may include severe hypertension, increased intracranial pressure leading to seizures or hemorrhage, and cardiac complications including myocardial ischemic, arrhythmias, and pulmonary edema. Patients should be monitored for increase in blood pressure of >20%, headache, flushing, sweating, chills, nasal congestion, piloerection, and pallor. Patients with lesions above T6 are particularly susceptible.

Postoperative Complications

Complication rates are high, with recurrence and wound dehiscence as the most common complications. Recurrence rates as high as 80% are reported in some studies.[illegible] However, the literature examining complications and outcomes remains varied and is often limited to single-center retrospective analyses. Unfortunately, postoperative complications further raise the already substantial cost of surgery and care for these pressure-related injuries[51] (**Table 99.2**).

TABLE 99.2. RISK FACTORS FOR POSTOPERATIVE COMPLICATIONS

Recurrence/Reoperation
■ Young age (<45 yr) ■ Low albumin <3.5 g/dL ■ African American ■ Ischial location ■ Flap choice: V-Y thigh flap[a] ■ Smoking ■ Premature sitting ■ Anemia requiring perioperative blood transfusion
Infection
■ Diabetes ■ American Society of Anesthesiologists class >3 ■ Perioperative blood transfusion ■ Longer operative times
Wound Dehiscence/Flap Failure
■ Ischial location ■ Low albumin <3.5 g/dL ■ Anemia requiring perioperative blood transfusion ■ Longer operative time ■ Acute osteomyelitis ■ HgbA1c >6%

[a]Controversial because of tension on closure.

MORTALITY RISK

The association between pressure injuries and increased risk of mortality is well documented, especially among elderly patients.[52] Patients who develop a pressure injury in an ICU setting have in-hospital mortality rates as high as 48%.[53] Further, an Agency for Health Research and Quality report demonstrated a 4.2% in-hospital mortality rate for patients with a primary diagnosis of pressure injury, with an 11.6% in-hospital mortality rate in patients with secondary diagnosis of pressure injury, compared to only 2.6% mortality rate for all other diagnoses.[4] In a recent study examining the US-based National Surgical Quality Improvement Program, Kwok et al found that over 3% of all patients undergoing pressure injury surgery for closure die within 30 days of the operation.[25] Age above 65 years, diabetes, and total functional dependency were associated with increased mortality risk; however, given the data reporting style of the National Surgical Quality Improvement Program, exact cause of mortality could not be defined. Pressure injuries are a marker of other underlying disease processes, and the overall risks of surgery must be carefully discussed with patients and family members.

REHABILITATION AND PREVENTION

Recovery after surgical debridement and/or flap reconstruction may be best completed at a skilled nursing or rehabilitation facility to secure adequate assistance. Psychiatry and social services may need to be involved to assist with home environment, safety, compliance, and provide resources for access to services and supplies.

Prior to resuming sitting and returning to the home environment, the factors contributing to injury development must be addressed:

- Pressure injuries—depending on how much time is spent in bed versus chair, whether the patient has help at home, access to off-loading devices or a special bed, and the age of their wheelchair, may need referral to rehabilitation medicine and/or a homecare nurse for care.
- Extremity injuries—depending on whether the wound resulted from pressure from a brace or footwear, and what they plan to use moving forward, in addition to their weight-bearing status, may need referral to podiatry or orthotics for proper fitting.

LONG-TERM MANAGEMENT

Some patients may never be surgical candidates, in which case long-term nonoperative management is indicated. However, quality local wound care is labor-intensive, and social and financial considerations may limit long-term follow-up and compliance with regimen, ultimately leading to poor outcomes.

Chronic nonhealing injuries must be monitored for carcinoma (Marjolin ulcer). It is highly likely that the pathogenesis underlying malignant transformation is linked to multiple factors of environmental (unremitting irritation), immunological (avascular scar tissue interfering with lymphocyte mobility), and genetic nature (elevated protooncogenes). The most common malignancy is an aggressive form of squamous cell carcinoma, appearing anywhere from 2 to 25 years from time after the initial wound. With a 2-year survival rate of 66% to 80%, and metastatic rate of 61% (versus those occurring in burn scar 34%), treatment is wide surgical excision (lymph node dissection is not recommended unless clinical involvement).[54] If patients refuse surgery or the size location is deemed unresectable, chemotherapy and radiation may be used.

REFERENCES

1. Tchanque-Fossuo CN, Kuzon WM Jr. An evidence-based approach to pressure sores. *Plast Reconstr Surg.* 2011;127(2):932-939.
2. Ricci JA, Bayer LR, Orgill DP. Evidence-based medicine: the evaluation and treatment of pressure injuries. *Plast Reconstr Surg.* 2017;139(1):275e-286e.
3. Reddy M, Gill SS, Rochon PA. Preventing pressure ulcers: a systematic review. *JAMA.* 2006;296(8):974-984.
4. Russo CA, Steiner C, Spector W. *Hospitalizations related to pressure ulcers among adults 18 years and older, 2006: statistical brief #64. Healthcare Cost and Utilization Project (HCUP) Statistical Briefs.* Rockville, MD; 2006.
5. Cushing CA, Phillips LG. Evidence-based medicine: pressure sores. *Plast Reconstr Surg.* 2013;132(6):1720-1732.
6. Padula WV, Mishra MK, Makic MB, Sullivan PW. Improving the quality of pressure ulcer care with prevention: a cost-effectiveness analysis. *Med Care.* 2011;49(4):385-392.
7. Description of NPUAP. National pressure ulcer advisory panel. *Adv Wound Care.* 1995;8(4 suppl):93-95.
8. Zaratkiewicz S, Whitney JD, Lowe JR, et al. Development and implementation of a hospital-acquired pressure ulcer incidence tracking system and algorithm. *J Healthc Qual.* 2010;32(6):44-51.
9. Centers for Medicare and Medicaid Services. Medicare program: changes to the hospital inpatient prospective payment systems and fiscal year 2009 rates; payments for graduate medical education in certain emergency situations; changes to disclosure of physician ownership in hospitals and physician self-referral rules; updates to the long-term care prospective payment system; updates to certain IPPS-excluded hospitals; and collection of information regarding financial relationships between hospitals. Final rules. *Fed Regist.* 2008;73(161):48433-49084.
   The publication of these guidelines and changes in Medicare reimbursement for hospital acquired pressure related injuries changed the paradigm for pressure sore treatment and resulted in a drastically increased emphasis on the prevention and treatment of these wounds in all patients and facilities across the United States moving forward
10. McKinley WO, Jackson AB, Cardenas DD, DeVivo MJ. Long-term medical complications after traumatic spinal cord injury: a regional model systems analysis. *Arch Phys Med Rehabil.* 1999;80(11):1402-1410.
11. Stal S, Serure A, Donovan W, Spira M. The perioperative management of the patient with pressure sores. *Ann Plast Surg.* 1983;11(4):347-356.
12. Waterlow JC. Requirements for specialist training. *Lancet.* 1985;1(8428):576.
13. Wang LH, Chen HL, Yan HY, et al. Inter-rater reliability of three most commonly used pressure ulcer risk assessment scales in clinical practice. *Int Wound J.* 2015;12(5):590-594.
14. Braden BJ, Bergstrom N. Predictive validity of the Braden scale for pressure sore risk in a nursing home population. *Res Nurs Health.* 1994;17(6):459-470.
15. Moore ZE, Cowman S. Risk assessment tools for the prevention of pressure ulcers. *Cochrane Database Syst Rev.* 2014;(2):CD006471.
16. National Pressure Ulcer Advisory Panel. NPUAP Pressure Injury Stages. Available athttp://www.npuap.org/resources/educational-and-clinical-resources/npuap-pressure-injury-stages/ . Accessed November 8, 2018.
17. Lyder CH, Wang Y, Metersky M, et al. Hospital-acquired pressure ulcers: results from the national Medicare patient safety monitoring system study. *J Am Geriatr Soc.* 2012;60(9):1603-1608.
18. Bennett RG, O'Sullivan J, DeVito EM, Remsburg R. The increasing medical malpractice risk related to pressure ulcers in the United States. *J Am Geriatr Soc.* 2000;48(1):73-81.
19. Dinsdale SM. Decubitus ulcers: role of pressure and friction in causation. *Arch Phys Med Rehabil.* 1974;55(4):147-152.
20. Landis EM. The capillary pressure in frog mesentery as determined by micro-injection methods. *Am J Physiol.* 1926;75(3):548-570.
    In a series of landmark studies, the concept of the pressure-time relationship and soft tissue destruction was explored. As the pressure exerted on the soft tissue becomes higher than that of the supplying blood vessels, edema and ischemia occurs, metabolic waste products and free radicals accumulate, and with time permanent tissue destruction leads to significant defects.
21. Daniel RK, Wheatley D, Priest D. Pressure sores and paraplegia: an experimental model. *Ann Plast Surg.* 1985;15(1):41-49.
22. Schultz GS, Davidson JM, Kirsner RS, et al. Dynamic reciprocity in the wound microenvironment. *Wound Repair Regen.* 2011;19(2):134-148.
23. Gerhardt LC, Strassle V, Lenz A, Spencer ND, Derler S. Influence of epidermal hydration on the friction of human skin against textiles. *J R Soc Interface.* 2008;5(28):1317-1328.
24. McInnes E, Jammali-Blasi A, Bell-Syer SE, et al. Support surfaces for pressure ulcer prevention. *Cochrane Database Syst Rev.* 2011;(4):CD001735.
25. Kwok AC, Simpson AM, Willcockson J, et al. Complications and their associations following the surgical repair of pressure ulcers. *Am J Surg.* 2018;216(6):1177-1181.
    This 10-year examinated of the NSQIP database examined complications following repair of ulcers in 1243 cases, and showed mortality rates on par with hepatobiliary cancer and cardiac surgery risk for death. Elderly age, diabetes and dependency were associated with increased mortality following pressure ulcer surgery. Flap repair of these ulcers was found to be associated with decreased complications. The overall 30-day mortality for patients undergoing pressure ulcer surgery was found to be 3%.

26. Tedeschi S, Negosanti L, Sgarzani R, et al. Superficial swab versus deep-tissue biopsy for the microbiological diagnosis of local infection in advanced-stage pressure ulcers of spinal-cord-injured patients: a prospective study. *Clin Microbiol Infect*. 2017;23(12):943-947.
    This article examined the concordance rate between taking a superficial swab versus a deep tissue culture in the pressure sores of 116 spinal cord injury patients (a homogenous population not actively receiving antibiotics at the time of culture); they found a concordance rate of only 22%, with 27% false negative and 16% false-positives. Thus, concluding superficial swabs are not to be relied on for clinical diagnosis and treatment in advanced ulcers.
27. Heym B, Rimareix F, Lortat-Jacob A, Nicolas-Chanoine MH. Bacteriological investigation of infected pressure ulcers in spinal cord-injured patients and impact on antibiotic therapy. *Spinal Cord*. 2004;42(4):230-234.
28. Huang AB, Schweitzer ME, Hume E, Batte WG. Osteomyelitis of the pelvis/hips in paralyzed patients: accuracy and clinical utility of MRI. *J Comput Assist Tomogr*. 1998;22(3):437-443.
29. Ovington LG. Advances in wound dressings. *Clin Dermatol*. 2007;25(1):33-38.
30. Black J, Clark M, Dealey C, et al. Dressings as an adjunct to pressure ulcer prevention: consensus panel recommendations. *Int Wound J*. 2015;12(4):484-488.
31. Singh A, Halder S, Menon GR, et al. Meta-analysis of randomized controlled trials on hydrocolloid occlusive dressing versus conventional gauze dressing in the healing of chronic wounds. *Asian J Surg*. 2004;27(4):326-332.
32. Graumlich JF, Blough LS, McLaughlin RG, et al. Healing pressure ulcers with collagen or hydrocolloid: a randomized, controlled trial. *J Am Geriatr Soc*. 2003;51(2):147-154.
33. Molan P, Rhodes T. Honey: a biologic wound dressing. *Wounds*. 2015;27(6):141-151.
34. Health Quality Ontario. Management of chronic pressure ulcers: an evidence-based analysis. *Ont Health Technol Assess Ser*. 2009;9(3):1-203.
35. Belmin J, Meaume S, Rabus MT, Bohbot S; Investigators of the Sequential Treatment of the Elderly with Pressure Sores. Sequential treatment with calcium alginate dressings and hydrocolloid dressings accelerates pressure ulcer healing in older subjects: a multicenter randomized trial of sequential versus nonsequential treatment with hydrocolloid dressings alone. *J Am Geriatr Soc*. 2002;50(2):269-274.
36. Yang C, Goss SG, Alcantara S, et al. Effect of negative pressure wound therapy with instillation on bioburden in chronically infected wounds. *Wounds*. [illegible]
37. McKanna M, Geraci J, Hall K, et al. Clinician panel recommendations for use of negative pressure wound therapy with instillation. *Ostomy Wound Manage*. 2016;62(4):S1-S14.
38. Orgill DP, Bayer LR. Negative pressure wound therapy: past, present and future. *Int Wound J*. 2013;10(suppl 1):[illegible]
39. [illegible] *Lancet*. 1969;2(7617):405-409.
40. Worth ER, Tettelbach WH, Hopf HW. Arterial insufficiencies: enhancement of healing in selected problem wounds. In: Weaver LK, ed. *Hyperbaric Oxygen Therapy Indications*. 13th ed. North Palm Beach, FL: Best Publishing; 2014:25-46.
41. Adunsky A, Ohry A, Group D. Decubitus direct current treatment (DDCT) of pressure ulcers: results of a randomized double-blinded placebo controlled study. *Arch Gerontol Geriatr*. 2005;41(3):261-269.
42. Burke DT, Ho CH, Saucier MA, Stewart G. Effects of hydrotherapy on pressure ulcer healing. *Am J Phys Med Rehabil*. 1998;77(5):394-398.
43. Kenneweg KA, Welch MC, Welch PJ. A 9-year retrospective evaluation of 102 pressure ulcer reconstructions. *J Wound Care*. 2015;24(suppl 4a):S12-S21.
44. Thiessen FE, Andrades P, Blondeel PN, et al. Flap surgery for pressure sores: should the underlying muscle be transferred or not? *J Plast Reconstr Aesthet Surg*. 2011;64(1):84-90.
45. Bamba R, Madden JJ, Hoffman AN, et al. Flap reconstruction for pressure ulcers: an outcomes analysis. *Plast Reconstr Surg Glob Open*. 2017;5(1):e1187.
46. Sameem M, Au M, Wood T, et al. A systematic review of complication and recurrence rates of musculocutaneous, fasciocutaneous, and perforator-based flaps for treatment of pressure sores. *Plast Reconstr Surg*. 2012;130(1):67e-77e.
47. Keys KA, Daniali LN, Warner KJ, Mathes DW. Multivariate predictors of failure after flap coverage of pressure ulcers. *Plast Reconstr Surg*. 2010;125(6):1725-1734.
48. Schryvers OI, Stranc MF, Nance PW. Surgical treatment of pressure ulcers: 20-year experience. *Arch Phys Med Rehabil*. 2000;81(12):1556-1562.
49. Yamamoto Y, Tsutsumida A, Murazumi M, Sugihara T. Long-term outcome of pressure sores treated with flap coverage. *Plast Reconstr Surg*. 1997;100(5):1212-1217.
    Examining 45 ischial and 24 sacral sores in 53 paraplegic patients between 1990 and 1995, the types of flaps were categorized into fasciocutaneous or myocutaneous/muscle flaps. These investigators found that overall, the ischial sores had a higher recurrence rate than sacral sores; however, there was no significant difference in the percent pressure sore free survival (%PSFS) between the sites of sores. The group of the sores reconstructed with the fasciocutaneous flap demonstrated significant or marginally significant better results in the %PSFS compared with those reconstructed with myocutaneous or muscle flaps. These observations suggested the use of fasciocutaneous flaps provides just as durable, if not better longterm results in the surgical reconstruction of pressure sores compared to the myocutaneous or muscle flap.
50. Dakson A BD, Thibault-Halman G, Christie S. Venous thromboembolism and pressure ulcers in acute spinal cord injury: a retrospective review. *JSM Spine*. 2016;1(1):1001.
51. Brem H, Maggi J, Nierman D, et al. High cost of stage IV pressure ulcers. *Am J* [illegible]
52. Khor HM, Tan J, Saedon NI, et al. Determinants of mortality among older adults with pressure ulcers. *Arch Gerontol Geriatr*. 2014;59(3):536-541.
53. Manzano F, Perez-Perez AM, Martinez-Ruiz S, et al. Hospital-acquired pressure ulcers and risk of hospital mortality in intensive care patients on mechanical ventilation. *J Eval Clin Pract*. [illegible]
54. [illegible] wounds: review of available literature. *Contemp Oncol (Pozn)*. 2017;21(3):197-202.

QUESTIONS

1. A 56-year-old woman with a history of hypertension and depression, who sustained a pressure injury after prolonged immobilization following motor vehicle accident and bilateral femur fractures 14 months ago presents to your outpatient wound clinic for evaluation for closure of her healing right ischium stage 3 pressure sore. She has lost 7 kg since her accident but is now ambulating with assistance. On examination, her wound is 6 × 4 × 4 cm with a clean granulating soft tissue base with no bone exposed. Today's laboratory test results indicate a white count of 7000, hemoglobin 12.4, albumin 2.1, and prealbumin 13 mg/dL. Her final cultures show no growth. She is performing wet to dry packing with normal saline and gauze twice per day. She feels her wound is not progressing and would like to consider surgical closure. What is the next step?

    a. Schedule for surgery at the soonest for split thickness skin graft
    b. Obtain MRI to ensure no bone involvement suggesting osteomyelitis first
    c. Consult with nutrition for optimization prior to elective surgery
    d. Continue local wound care, as a flap in a patient of her position would most likely fail.
    e. Schedule for surgery for total ischiectomy to relieve pressure on overlying soft tissues before attempting soft tissue closure.

2. A 37-year-old man with history of traumatic SCI at T6 undergoes debridement of an ischial pressure injury with local wound care initiated. The patient spends appropriate time in the recovery room before being transported to the floor. Within 1 hour of the patient's arrival there, he complains of nausea and neck pain. His temperature is 37.4, blood pressure is 190/100, and HR is 59 bpm. What should be considered first in working up this patient?

    a. Increase pain medication postoperatively
    b. Add beta blocker as needed for systolic > 150 blood pressure control
    c. Add antiemetic
    d. Administer intravenous dantrolene
    e. Check urine output and place Foley catheter

3. A 54-year-old woman with paraplegia since age 24 comes to your clinic with a stage IV pressure injury of unknown time period; you suspect at least 6 months in duration based on your history and physical examination, in which you see denuded bone at the base of the wound and pink-granulating tissue on the periphery. She has been diligent with pressure offloading and wound care with moisture dressings, but it does not seem to be improving. Which of the following is the most appropriate next step?

    a. Order MRI of the pelvis
    b. Schedule for elective flap closure
    c. Order CT of the pelvis
    d. Schedule for debridement and bone biopsy
    e. Discuss long-term palliative care for this wound

4. A 38-year-old woman who works in accounting and spends most of her time in a wheelchair presents to your clinic with a trochanteric pressure-related sore. After appropriate medical workup and optimization of nutrition, you decide to cover her wound with a posterior thigh musculocutaneous flap. What is the chief disadvantage of this flap?

    a. Unreliable blood supply
    b. Limited amount of skin, fat, and muscle provided
    c. Limited upward mobility of the flap
    d. Inability to be readvanced if wound recurrence later
    e. High rate of donor site morbidity

5. You receive a consult for a 19-year-old boy who underwent a 13-hour liver transplant; following the case in the ICU, he was noted to have redness and skin breakdown on the left scapula and sacrum. When you roll him to assess the wounds, you note two well-demarcated areas of redness and blanching skin with minor skin breakdown involving the epidermis only overlying the tip of the scapula and the sacrum. There is no drainage or exposed structures. What is the most appropriate management of this pressure-related injury?

    a. Local wound care with placement of soft foam dressing and rigorous pressure offloading
    b. Excision of blanching area with placement of wet to dry gauze to be changed daily
    c. Excision of blanching area with placement of split thickness skin graft
    d. Excision of blanching area with local advancement flaps to close
    e. No intervention, encourage discharge from the hospital as soon as possible

1. **Answer: c.** This patient has a clean wound, which is not infected, and she does not have any systemic illnesses to preclude her from closure at this time. For wounds of this size and in this location a skin graft would not be a durable option. She is now ambulatory and the wound has soft tissue at the base indicating that a total ischiectomy is not required to get this wound healed. She has poor nutrition indicated by her recent laboratory test results, which will place her at increased risk for wound-healing complications, and she should have a nutrition consult to improve her nutrition prior to reconstruction first. Preoperative goals of albumin >3 g/dL and prealbumin >20 mg/dL should ideally be attained before performing elective flap closure for ischemic injuries, as studies have shown low serum prealbumin predicts a poor prognosis for wound healing. Although reasonable, there is no indication for MRI at this time given the duration and cause of her injury and that she does not have exposed bone on examination.

2. **Answer: e.** AD is a medical emergency characterized by severe hypertension. It can be brought on by wide array of stimuli below the level of the lesion. It can occur intraoperative or postoperatively. Commonly in a resting patient on the nursing floor, bladder or bowel distension can be the source of triggering an acute AD event. Therefore, bladder and bowel output should be monitored and considered when patients with SCI become acutely clinically unstable.

3. **Answer: d.** Patients with chronic nonhealing wounds in the face of adequate wound care and medical optimization must be examined and investigated for underlying condition. Any wound presenting with exposed bone, particularly in a chronic or nonhealing wound should be biopsied to rule out pathologic involvement and infection.

4. **Answer: c.** The posterior thigh flap has a very reliable blood supply (first perforating branch from the profunda femoris artery); it provides generous skin, fat, and muscle and retains the ability to readvance the flap if needed later. Additionally, medial and lateral donor sites and the gluteal muscles remain intact for additional flaps if needed later on. Depending on the size of the flap, the donor site can often be closed primarily, or with a skin graft if too large. The primary disadvantage is the limited upward mobility of the flap with only 10 to 12 cm of movement, which may necessitate additional flaps to be utilized if not adequate for larger wounds.

5. **Answer: a.** This early-stage pressure-related injury is acutely related to his recent surgery and will likely recover when he is no longer in a confined position for many hours. Iatrogenic pressure-related injuries such as these are considered *never events*, and hospitals are no longer reimbursed for treatments provided for their care when acquired in the hospital setting. The operating room and ICUs should follow strict guidelines for pressure-offloading surfaces during long operative cases or in patients who have high risk in critical care settings to avoid these from occurring.

CHAPTER 100 Gender-Affirming Surgery

William M. Kuzon, Jr and Katherine M. Gast

KEY POINTS

- Gender dysphoria, the incongruence between anatomic sex and gender identity, affects 0.6% of the population, 1.4 million people in the United States.
- Treatment of gender dysphoria including mental health, hormonal therapy, puberty suppression, and gender-affirming surgery is deemed medically necessary by nearly all expert led medical societies including the American Medical Association and the American Society of Plastic Surgeons. Chest and genital surgery is often covered by insurance, including Medicare.
- WPATH, the World Professional Association for Transgender Health, is an international society with universally adopted standards of care (SOC) for gender-expansive patients, including prerequisites prior to hormonal therapy and gender-affirming surgery.
- Transfeminine surgery for patients assigned male at birth but identified as women, includes facial feminization, thyrochondroplasty, breast augmentation, and vaginoplasty.
- Transmasculine surgery for patients assigned female at birth but identified as men, includes mastectomy, metoidioplasty, and phalloplasty.
- Multidisciplinary care inclusive of mental health for gender-expansive patients, much like a bariatric or transplant care model, is paramount for good patient outcomes.

Gender dysphoria is the incongruence between one's experienced and assigned gender,[1] estimated to affect 0.6% of the population.[2] It is now recognized that gender identity may be nonbinary and patients may identify as transmasculine, transfeminine, trans (without gender specification), gender queer, nonbinary, gender expansive, or agender.[3] **Table 100.1** provides helpful definitions of gender, sex, and other terms used throughout this chapter.

Patients with gender dysphoria have normal anatomy and hormonal physiology, distinguishing this patient population from those with disorders of sexual development. Notably, there is now substantial and accumulating evidence that an individual's gender identity is determined largely by biological factors, and sexual orientation is an independent characteristic not directly related to gender identity.[4-6] For gender dysphoric patients, management must be individualized for each patient. The timeline of care typically follows this order: mental health counseling, hormonal therapy, and lastly, surgery for patients who desire it.[7] Gender-affirming surgery is recognized as medically necessary and associated with quality of life and functional improvements by every professional-led medical association, including the American Society of Plastic Surgeons.[8]

Transgender and gender-expansive patients are an underserved and at-risk patient population within plastic surgery.[9] Patients have impaired access to care and experience discrimination in housing, employment, and social services.[10-12] Transgender patients have elevated rates of homelessness, joblessness, estrangement from their families and social support systems, interpersonal violence, suicide, HIV, and mental health comorbidities. Rates of comorbid mental illness and of suicidal ideation and suicide attempts greatly exceed those of the general population.[13-15]

OFFICIAL STANDARDS OF CARE

The WPATH, is an international society of patients, health-care providers, and advocates that issues a SOC document (current Version 7 is from 2011) to define best practices and to prevent patient harm and regret.[7] The WPATH SOC define recommended prerequisites prior to hormonal therapy and gender-affirming surgery procedures (**Table 100.2**). The SOC have been criticized as authoritative and paternalistic, and alternative "informed consent" models of care have been advocated.[16-20] Although we acknowledge that the SOC are a source of controversy, we also strongly support adherence to the WPATH SOC when providing surgical care to gender-dysphoric patients. This cannot be overemphasized; Plastic Surgeons cannot independently diagnose gender dysphoria, so the determination of surgical candidacy for any gender confirming procedure should be made in the setting of a multidisciplinary team and in accordance with WPATH SOC.

COMPREHENSIVE GENDER CARE

Ideal care for transgender patients requires close communication and collaboration among a diverse multidisciplinary team; centers for cleft lip and palate, bariatric, or transplant surgery are analogous models. This is a critical point: close collaboration between team members is vital to good patient outcomes.[21] Depending on where patients are in their transition, they may need mental health, social

TABLE 100.1. DEFINITIONS OF GENDER, SEX, AND OTHER TERMS USED IN THE CARE AND TREATMENT OF TRANSGENDER AND GENDER NONCONFORMING PATIENTS

Gender	Internal sense of being a man or woman as defined by culture norms and customs.
Cisgender	Patient with gender identity that matches anatomic sex. Nontransgender patients.
Sex	Physical anatomy, assigned at birth.
Gender dysphoria	Incongruence between gender identity and physical sex resulting in functional impairment: ■ Separate from sexual orientation ■ ICD 10 diagnosis code F64 ■ Included in the DSM V
Disorders of sexual development	Reproductive organs and genitals do not develop as expected. DSD patients may or may not experience gender dysphoria.
Sexual orientation	The emotional, sexual, romantic attractions one has with other people.
Gender-affirming surgery	Procedures to align a patient's body and features with their gender identity.
Transfeminine patient	Assigned male at birth, identifies as female or on the feminine end of gender spectrum.
Transmasculine patient	Assigned female at birth, identifies as male or on the masculine end of gender spectrum.

DSD, disorders of sexual development

work, pediatric or adult endocrinology, fertility services, and/or surgery if they choose. Patients also need access to "gender-friendly" providers who can provide permanent hair removal, speech therapy, and pelvic floor physiotherapy. Organized peer support is also valuable for patients and families. Centers performing gender-affirming surgery should have resources in all these areas available.

In addition, it is important to provide a supportive environment of care. This population is very sensitive to misgendering, so it is important to educate all staff who interact with patients to use preferred pronouns, and, especially if the patient has not yet made a legal name change, preferred first names. For patients undergoing surgical procedures and who are admitted to hospital, they should be identified and housed in their expressed gender.

CARE OF CHILDREN AND ADOLESCENTS

The care of children and adolescents with gender dysphoria requires specialized training and is also evolving rapidly. Preadolescent children may express gender dysphoria consistent with gender identity disorder of childhood.[1,22-24] In some studies, 60% or more of these children will "desist" and return to the gender consistent with their anatomy,[24] although there is not a clear consensus in the literature.[1] For this reason, surgery is never indicated in children nor advised in the WPATH SOC (see **Table 100.2**).[7]

If gender dysphoria persists into or appears in adolescence and is consistent with a diagnosis of gender dysphoria of adolescence and adulthood, patients may be candidates for puberty suppression therapy.[25] This typically consists of GnRH agonists that suppress the pulsatile stimulation of the gonads, which is safe and reversible; cross-hormone therapy at age 15 or 16 may then be initiated later. Hormonal therapy for transfeminine patients (assigned male at birth, identify as female), includes estrogen and spironolactone or finasteride (androgen blockers). Hormonal therapy for transmasculine patients (assigned female at birth, but identify as male) includes testosterone. On a case-by-case basis, with treatment decisions made among the adolescent, the family, and the multidisciplinary treatment team, surgical intervention in adolescents may be appropriate. For chest recontouring in transmasculine adolescents, WPATH SOC recommend a year of testosterone therapy before surgery.

TABLE 100.2. THE WORLD PROFESSIONAL ASSOCIATION FOR TRANSGENDER HEALTH STANDARDS OF CARE GUIDELINES[7, a]

Procedure	Specifications	Referral(s)[b]	Hormones
Transfeminine			
Breast augmentation (implants/lipofilling)	Persistent, well-documented gender dysphoria	One referral (letter) by a qualified mental health professional	Not an explicit criterion, but recommended that patients receive 12 mo postfeminizing hormone therapy.
Orchiectomy[d]	Persistent, well-documented gender dysphoria	Two referrals (letters) by qualified mental health professionals.	12 continuous months of hormone therapy as appropriate to patient's gender goals. Exception if the patient has medical or personal reasons to not take hormones.[c]
Vaginoplasty[d]	Persistent, well-documented gender dysphoria Must be living 12 continuous months in gender role that is congruent with gender identity	Two referrals (letters) by qualified mental health professionals	12 continuous months of hormone therapy as appropriate to patient's gender goals. Exception if the patient has medical or personal reasons to not take hormones.[c]
Transmasculine			
Mastectomy and creation of male chest	Persistent, well-documented gender dysphoria	One referral (letter) by a qualified mental health professional	Not a prerequisite
Hysterectomy and ovariectomy[d]	Persistent, well-documented gender dysphoria	Two referrals (letters) by qualified mental health professionals If one letter is from therapist, the other should be from evaluator	12 continuous months of hormone therapy as appropriate to patient's gender goals. Exception if the patient has medical or personal reasons to not take hormones.[c]
Metoidioplasty or phalloplasty[d]	Persistent, well-documented gender dysphoria Must be living 12 continuous months in gender role that is congruent with gender identity	Two referrals (letters) by qualified mental health professionals. If one letter is from therapist, the other should be from evaluator.	12 continuous months of hormone therapy as appropriate to patient's gender goals. Exception if the patient has medical or personal reasons to not take hormones.[c]

Reprinted by permission from World Professional Association for Transgender Health. Standards of Care for the Health of Transsexual, Transgender, and Gender Nonconforming People. 7th Version. Elgin, IL: The World Professional Association for Transgender Health; 2011. WPATH SOC Guidelines can be accessed at https://www.wpath.org/media/cms/Documents/Web%20Transfer/SOC/Standards%20of%20Care%20V7%20-%202011%20WPATH.pdf.

[a]Standards of care guidelines for the surgical treatment of gender dysphoria in transgender and gender-nonconforming adults, suggested by the World Professional Association for Transgender Health. Note that patients should be 18 years of age, able to legally give consent, and any comorbid psychiatric conditions must be "reasonably well controlled."

[b]Referral letters should include:

1. Patient's identifying characteristics
2. Diagnosis and other psychological evaluation results
3. Details of relationship to patient: duration of care, type of evaluation, type of counseling or treatment
4. Endorsing patient's application and explaining how they fulfill criteria for surgery
5. Confirmation of informed consent
6. Confirmation of availability for coordination of care
7. Confirmation of adequately controlled mental health concerns

[c]To introduce a period of reversible estrogen or testosterone suppression, before the patient undergoes irreversible surgical intervention.

[d]Though it is not an explicit criterion, it is recommended that these patients also have regular visits with a mental health or other medical professional.

Note that for all procedures, except when specific variance from the Standards of Care are justified, the patient should be 18 years of age and legally able to consent to the surgery on their own.

The decision to perform genital surgery on an adolescent, in addition to the WPATH SOC criteria for adults, is again a case-by-case decision by the multidisciplinary team. This remains a topic of active discussion by WPATH's SOC Committee, as poor psychosocial, body image, and mental health outcomes may manifest in late adolescence.

GENDER-AFFIRMING SURGERY

Gender-affirming surgeries generally fall within the scope of well-trained plastic surgeons. **Table 100.3** outlines the main surgical treatments of gender dysphoria. For transfeminine patients, gender-affirming surgery often includes facial feminization, thyroid chondroplasty or "tracheal shave," orchiectomy, breast augmentation, and vaginoplasty. For transmasculine patients, gender-affirming surgical procedures can include hysterectomy and oophorectomy, mastectomy, and genital reconstruction (i.e., phalloplasty, metoidioplasty).

Transfeminine Surgery

Facial Feminization

Human beings are accustomed to determining the gender of an individual simply by looking at them while clothed. This is possible because, in addition to obvious morphologic differences in the breasts and body, there are major differences in both skeletal and soft tissue morphology that distinguish the cis-female from the cis-male face.[26] An incongruence between their facial morphology and their feminine gender is a source of dysphoria for many transwomen who find it difficult to "pass" in society with a distinctly male face. The goal of facial feminization surgery is to alter the [illegible] bony skeleton and soft tissues of the face to achieve a facial appearance that is easily identified as female rather than male.

Female Facial Morphology

Masculine faces have been described as being square or rectangular, with a tall forehead, high hairline, a pronounced posterior sloping forehead contour, and prominent supraorbital ridges. Masculine faces tend to have wide and prominent mandibular angles, a square chin, a long upper lip, and a relatively acute nasolabial angle. In contrast, feminine faces have been described as oval-shaped, with a shorter, vertically oriented forehead and lower hairline, minimal supraorbital ridges, a shorter upper lip, narrower mandibular angles, a more obtuse nasolabial angle, and a more pointed chin. A masculine-appearing nose is generally larger and "less delicate" than the average feminine nose. There are multiple other differences between the masculine and feminine craniofacial skeleton and soft tissue envelope. To achieve optimal facial feminization, a careful analysis of each patient's facial features and a comprehensive, individualized surgical plan developed. Because the prominent male supraorbital ridge and robust mandible most often require significant bony resection and recontouring, surgeons performing facial feminization must be skilled in maxillofacial and craniofacial surgical procedures.[27]

TABLE 100.3. TRANSFEMININE AND TRANSMASCULINE GENDER-AFFIRMING SURGERIES THAT FALL WITHIN THE SCOPE OF PLASTIC SURGERY

Transfeminine Surgery	Transmasculine Surgery
Facial feminization surgery ■ Lower hairline ■ Shave brow bone +/− posterior reset of the anterior wall of frontal sinus ■ Rhinoplasty ■ Malar augmentation ■ Reduce angle of mandible Tracheal shave Laryngoplasty ■ Voice surgery performed by ENT	
Breast augmentation	Mastectomy ■ Periareolar ■ Circumareolar ■ Inferior pedicle ■ Double-incision free nipple graft
Orchiectomy	Hysterectomy ■ +/− Salpingo-oophorectomy
Vaginoplasty ■ Penile inversion (most common) ■ Sigmoid	Metoidioplasty Phalloplasty

Preoperative Evaluation

All of the sex-specific characteristics noted above should be carefully assessed on physical examination. Most importantly, a thorough discussion with the patients should define their perception of their facial features and their desired changes. For patients undergoing forehead recontouring, a lateral cephalograph or maxillofacial computed tomography scan should be obtained. This is essential to determine the thickness of the frontal bone over the frontal sinus and to gauge the degree of supraorbital reduction that will be necessary. If the frontal bone is sufficiently thick and the setback required is modest, burring of the supraorbital ridges may be performed. If the frontal bone is thin and/or if the setback required is significant, the surgeon must be prepared to do a formal frontal sinus recession, removing the anterior table of the frontal sinus in total, performing osteotomies on the excised segment of bone, and then replacing and rigidly fixing the bone segments in a [illegible] configuration. If rhinoplasty, brow lifting, or blepharoplasty are to be performed (Figure 100.[illegible]), the usual analysis of nasal airflow and anatomy, dry eye, negative orbital vector, and so on should be done. If mandibular recontouring or height reduction is planned, an analysis of occlusion and consideration of an X-ray to identify the mental foramen and inferior alveolar nerve position are important.

Forehead Feminization

Forehead feminization generally includes both lowering the hairline and reducing the prominence of and reshaping the supraorbital ridges. A pretrichial incision can be used to correct widow's peak and bring the hairline forward with posterior scalp advancement and forehead skin excision. This incision can serve as the access point for a bony brow reduction with lateral burring of the supraorbital rims, burring or formal recession of the anterior table of the frontal sinus, and brow lift. Hair grafting can help disguise the scar and contour the hairline.

Midface Feminization

Malar implants or fat grafting can help define the cheekbones and feminize the midface. A rhinoplasty should focus on correcting a dorsal hump, osteotomies to narrow the upper vault, cephalic trim to rotate the nasal tip and create a supratip break, and interdomal sutures to create more tip definition.

Feminization of the Mandibular Contour and Lower Face

An upper lip lift, done through a gull-wing excision of skin along the nasal sill, can provide incisal tooth show at rest and increase the fullness of the vermillion. A narrowing genioplasty, most commonly through a transverse and vertical wedge excision osteotomy, reduces the prominence of the chin. The mandible angles can be reduced through osteotomies or burring through intraoral access incisions. If appropriate, reduction of the total mandibular height can be performed via resection of the entire inferior border of the mandible.

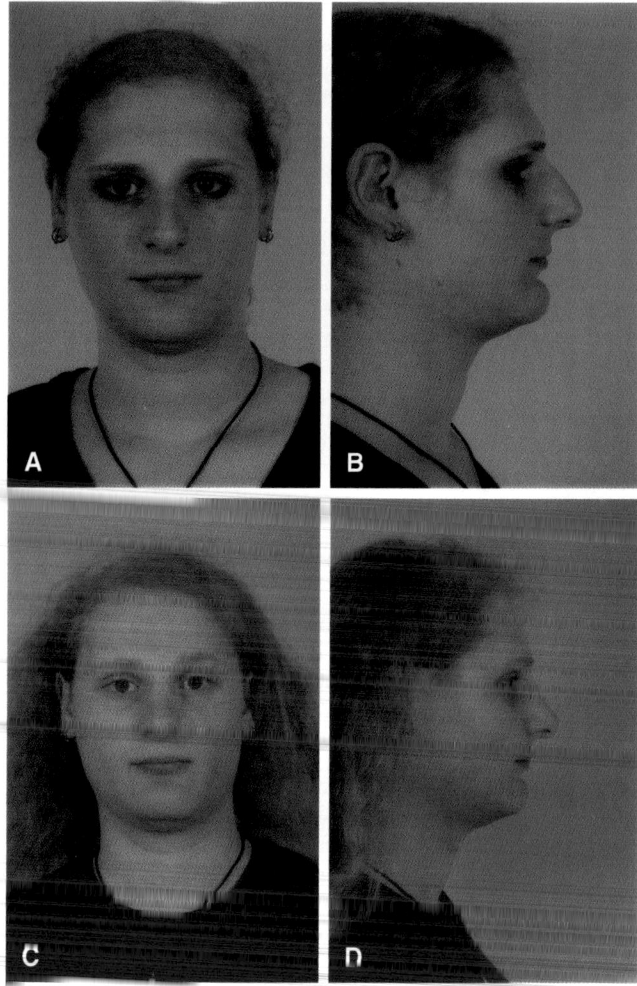

FIGURE 100.1. Facial feminization. Preoperative **(A, B)** and 6-month postoperative **(C, D)** photos of a patient [illegible] feminizing brow lift, forehead and supraorbital ridge recontouring, and septorhinoplasty.

Thyrolaryngoplasty

The laryngeal prominence of the thyroid cartilage, or Adam's apple, is a distinctly masculine feature that is often noticeable on profile of transfeminine patients. The thyroid cartilage is connected to the superior hyoid bone through thyrohyoid membrane and to the inferior cricoid cartilage through the cricothyroid ligaments. The thyroid cartilage consists of paired lamina with a central superior thyroid notch and midline laryngeal prominence. The cartilage is more prominent in men because of a more acute angle (90° versus 120°) between the paired lamina.

Reduction of the prominence of the thyroid cartilage, also erroneously referred to as a "trach shave" (Figure 100.2), should be performed through a submental incision to leave a scar that is not visible on frontal view. Dissection should expose the superficial surface of the thyroid cartilage and can be aided by lighted retractors or endoscopic instruments. The location of the anterior commissure of the vocal cords can be determined by passing a flexible laryngoscope, observing the emergence of a needle passed through the thyroid cartilage, and marking that location with methylene blue. The "Adam's apple" is then reduced by shaving the external surface of the thyroid cartilage down until a reasonable contour is achieved. In adults, the thyroid cartilage is frequently calcified, so the use of a bur or rongeurs may be necessary. The resection should be conservative to avoid vocal cord injury.

Voice Pitch Alteration

The average pitch of the female voice is higher than that of the male voice, so the field of vocal pitch alteration surgery is rapidly evolving. A number of procedures have been described,[28] but the most commonly performed contemporary procedures involve endoscopic, laser-assisted fusion of the anterior vocal cords. This moves the anterior commissure posteriorly and shortens vocal cord length, effectively raising the pitch of the voice. These specialized procedures require subspecialty training and are best performed by surgeons certified by the American Board of Otolaryngology/Head and Neck Surgery.

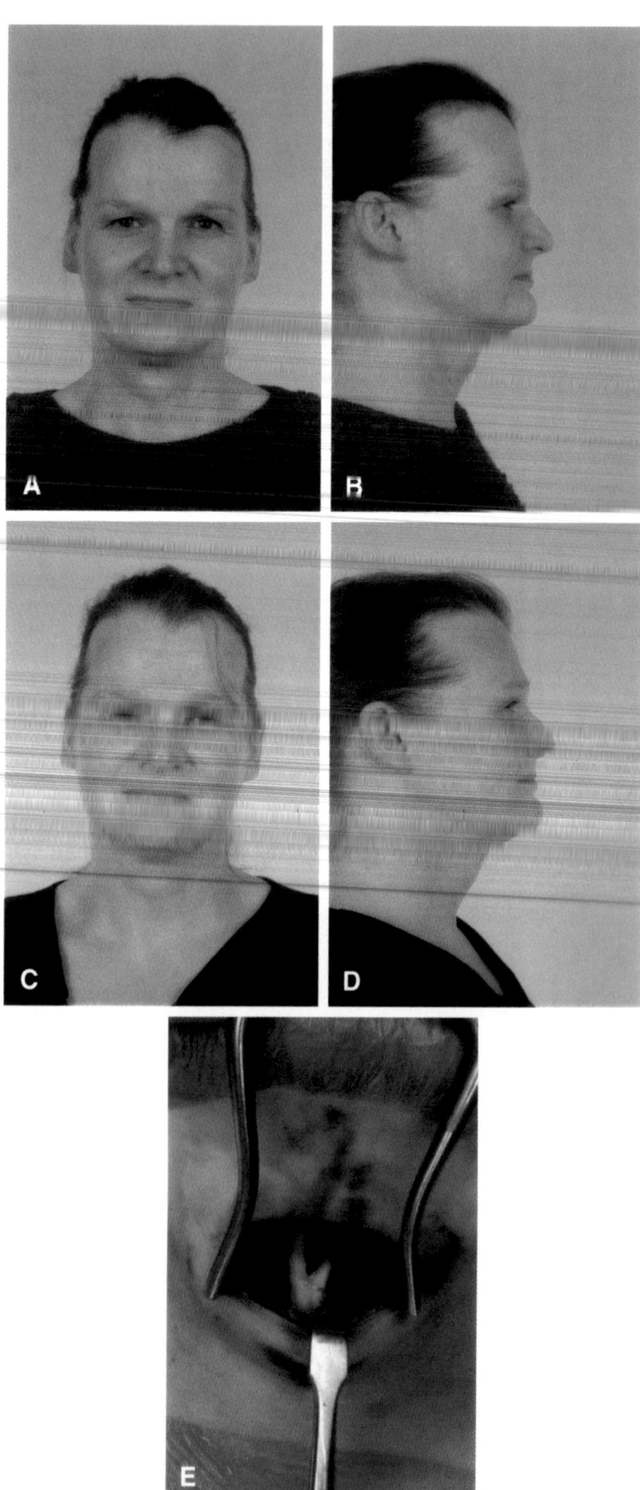

FIGURE 100.2. Thyroid chondroplasty, or "tracheal shave." Preoperative **(A, B)** and postoperative **(C, D)** photos of feminizing thyrochondroplasty to eliminate appearance of the Adam's apple, a commonly denoted masculinizing feature. **E.** Intraoperative photo of thyroid cartilage just after cartilage trim. Approach should be made through a submental incision to minimize scarring.

Breast Augmentation

Feminizing breast surgery in transfeminine patients most often requires augmentation with an implant. Fat grafting, or lipofilling, has been described and may be an option for modest augmentation, but patient goals and chest wall morphology usually requires an alloplastic device. Breast augmentation, as in cisgender women, involves placement of a silicone- or saline-filled device through an incision in the inframammary fold in either the subpectoral or subglandular position.

Preoperatively, patients over 40 years of age on feminizing hormones should have a screening mammogram and assessment of breast cancer risk with complete family history. WPATH SOC requires one letter of readiness from a mental health professional prior to surgery and 1 year of estrogen therapy for breast development is recommended. No duration of "real-life experience" or living full time in the female gender role is required. Holding estrogen prior to surgery is recommended to prevent perioperative venous thromboembolism (VTE) given the elevated risk of VTE in transfeminine patients on hormonal therapy.[29,30]

Preoperative physical examination should note the location of the nipples on the chest wall, which is often more lateral than cisgender women. The sternum and chest wall is also wider in transgender women. The implants must be placed with the nipple centered on the implant, so it is difficult to achieve cleavage in the midline in bras and clothing. Patients should be counseled about this at time of consultation. The inframammary fold is higher and more transverse in male chests; the patient's goals of size and shape should be discussed, and the surgeon should estimate the upper limit of implant size that is achievable with the existing skin envelope. Often, breasts are constricted and tuberous appearing, which may necessitate scoring of the parenchyma at time of augmentation to redrape the parenchyma over the implant. Choice of subpectoral or subglandular position is a choice between the surgeon and patient. The subpectoral plane creates a more natural slope of the breast mound superiorly but limits the medial extent of the implant, especially if the patient has a wide sternum. The subglandular plane, although carrying a higher risk of capsular contracture, provides greater definition of the breast mound and may be preferable in patients with a broad pectoralis major muscle.

Our preferred approach is through a 6-cm inframammary fold (IMF) incision at the location of the desired IMF, which may be lower than the existing fold. The new location of the IMF should be determined based on the diameter of the implant to be placed, placing the nipple at the most projecting aspect of the breast mound. Markings in the preoperative area should include sternal notch, midline, current IMF, desired IMF, breast base width, and limits of the pocket dissection. If subpectoral position is selected, complete release of the pectoralis major origin inferiorly should be performed with weakening of the medial sternal attachments.

Postoperative care following transfeminine breast augmentation is similar to that of cis-gender women. A superior strap can be considered to keep implants low in the pocket in subpectoral augmentations. If significant IMF work is done, a postoperative underwire bra can help reinforce that position to prevent dropping of the implant. Results of breast augmentation are presented in Figure 100.3.

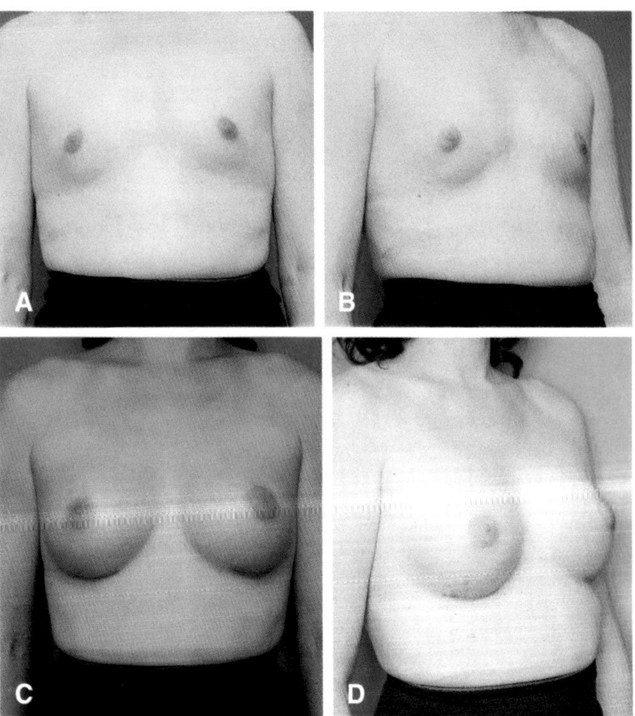

FIGURE 100.3. Breast augmentation. Preoperative **(A, B)** and Postoperative **(C, D)** photos of transfeminine breast augmentation via an inframammary approach placing smooth, round implants in the subpectoral position.

Vaginoplasty

Transfeminine gender-affirming bottom surgery creates a neoclitoris from the dorsal glans penis, labia minora from the prepuce or distal penile shaft skin, and labia majora from scrotal skin with removal of the erectile tissue of the penis, bilateral orchiectomy, and creation of a vagina (Figure 100.4). The vagina may be lined with inverted penile shaft skin (the penile inversion vaginoplasty technique, or Amsterdam procedure) or sigmoid colon (most often reserved as a rescue operation in cases of vaginal stenosis).[31]

Preoperative Considerations

The WPATH SOC guidelines dictate that prior to vaginopalsty surgery, patients must have two letters of readiness from independent mental health professionals, be on estrogen therapy for 1 year, and live in their congruent female gender role (formerly known as "real life experience") for 1 year (see Table 100.2). Vaginoplasty surgery is sterilizing, so discussion of preserving fertility through banked sperm must take place, especially for young patients. Patients should be 18 years old, with exceptions made when appropriate. Postoperatively, most patients are able to achieve orgasm with stimulation of the neoclitoris. Many also achieve orgasm with stimulation of the prostate with penetration.

Patients should perform permanent hair removal with either laser (most effective in patients with fair skin and dark hair) or electrolysis. Hair around the circumference of the base of the penis and the posterior scrotum must be cleared as this tissue will line the introitus and posterior vaginal wall. The duration of hair removal depends on patient's hair pattern and response to the hair removal sessions. Typically, this takes 3 to 6 months. Estrogen is held 3 weeks prior to surgery while the patient is on modified activity restrictions

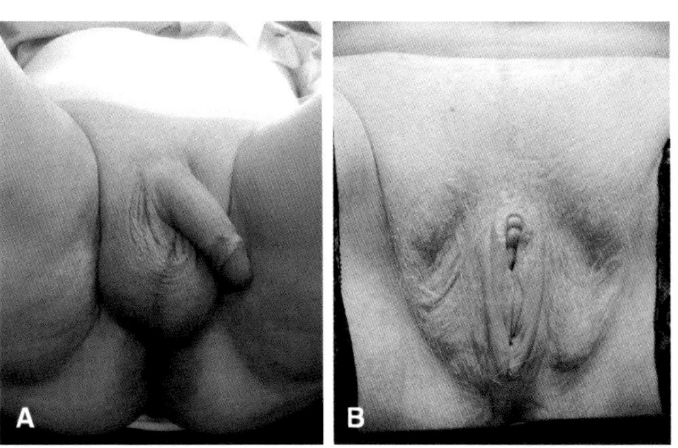

FIGURE 100.4. Penile inversion vaginoplasty. Preoperative **(A)** and postoperative **(B)** photos of transfeminine penile inversion vaginoplasty. Patients must continue to dilate or engage in penetrative intercourse to maintain depth and prevent neovaginal contraction.

postoperatively to lower the risk of VTE. And a bowel prep is performed the day before surgery to clear the rectum of stool and lower the risk of rectal perforation (2% incidence) and rectovaginal fistula (around 1%).[32]

Penile Inversion Vaginoplasty Technique

The penile inversion vaginoplasty procedure begins with elevation of a posterior perineal flap on skin that has previously been cleared of hair. The scrotal skin is split up the midline through the raphe to the base of the penis. A bilateral orchiectomy is performed with ligation of the spermatic cords at the level of the external inguinal ring; testicles should be sent to pathology for evaluation. A space for the vagina is dissected between the urethra and the rectum with sharp and then blunt dissection along the prerectal fascia. To be sure of not entering the rectum, the surgeon's left hand can be placed in the rectum while making the tunnel with the right, feeling the anterior wall of the rectum between their two hands. The neovaginal tunnel should be developed up to the peritoneal reflection. One can instill betadine into the rectum with a moist sponge in the neovagina. Any evidence of betadine on the sponge will indicate a rectal leak and rectal injury in need of repair. A circumferential incision is then made 2 cm proximal to the glans penis and the penis is then degloved superficial to Buck fascia. The penis is then pulled through the skin tube and the mons pubis is undermined for 8 to 10 cm to facilitate pullback of the penile shaft skin to line the neovagina. The neoclitoral flap is then raised from a W-shaped dorsal glans penis flap, incorporating the distal penile shaft skin as associated labia minora flaps. The neoclitoral flap is based on the dorsal penile artery, nerve, and associated veins. The neurovascular bundle is within Buck's fascia, and it is peeled off the tunica albuginea of the corpora distal to proximal with sharp dissection. The pedicle is dissected to the level of the pubic symphysis. A Foley catheter is placed in the urethra and the corpus spongiosum is separated from the paired corpora cavernosa. The corpora cavernosa are then separated, clamped, divided, and suture ligated in the midline. The neoclitoral flap is inset to the stumps of the corpora and the urethra is shortened and inset just posterior to the clitoris. The labia minora flaps are sutured around the neourethral edge to form a vulva. The central penile skin tube is inverted and pulled back. The scrotal skin is fashioned into labia majora with placement of incision in the groin crease. The penile skin tube is then lengthened with full thickness skin graft from the extra scrotal skin and finally a vaginal pack is placed with drains to remain in place for 5 to 7 days.

Postoperative Care and Management of Complications

Postoperative care includes modified activity of shuffling between chair and bed while the pack is in place and chemoprophylaxis for deep venous thrombosis (DVT). Following removal of the pack, drains, and Foley, the patient is taught to dilate and perform three times daily vaginal rinses. In addition to those seen with any major surgical procedure, complications of vaginoplasty include wound dehiscence and tissue loss (25%–39%), urethral stenosis and/or divergent urinary stream (20%–55%), vaginal or introital stenosis (6%–27%), pelvic floor spasm or dyspareunia (2%, which may require referral to a pelvic floor physiotherapist), and rectovaginal fistula (0.01%–2%).[32-34] Most series report a 20% or higher rate of revisionary surgery, especially for divergent urinary stream and aesthetics.[32] Speculum examinations should be performed in clinic to assess healing of the internal lining of the vagina. If areas of hypertrophic granulation tissue develop, then spot treatment with silver nitrate is helpful. If patients should develop malodorous vaginal secretions in the immediate postoperative period, suspicion must be high for a rectovaginal fistula. Imaging with per rectum contrast can help diagnose a fistula. If a fistula develops, the patient must have a temporary diverting ostomy for several months and keep dilating. If the patient stops dilating, the vaginal vault will completely contract down. A secondary gracilis flap may be considered in refractory cases of rectovaginal fistula.

Patients must dilate for life or the vagina will slowly contract and they will lose depth. Patients will need to use lubricant for penetrative intercourse and are at elevated risk for urinary tract infections with a shorter urethra. The prostate is not removed and patients will need prostate cancer screening with a per vagina prostate examination beginning at the age of 50.

Transmasculine Surgery

Mastectomy

Top surgery, or gender mastectomy, is a commonly requested operation among transmasculine patients. Patients often wear binders, very tight compressive garments, to flatten their chests and appear masculine in clothing. They report significant dysphoria related to their breasts, with resulting impairment in social and emotional function.[35] One letter of readiness is required per WPATH SOC, but no duration of testosterone therapy is needed prior to surgery in adults. Agender, gender fluid, or gender expansive patients who do not desire hormonal therapy may need top surgery owing to dysphoria related to their breasts.

Preoperative Considerations

Complete patient medical, surgical, social, and family histories should be obtained with emphasis on risk factors for breast cancer. Patients with strong family histories of breast cancer should be referred to a breast center for assessment of risk and potential imaging. If patients truly desire risk-reducing mastectomies for future breast cancer risk, this is a different operation and should be performed by a breast surgeon. Top surgery is a cosmetic mastectomy and breast tissue is left behind. Patients should be screened accordingly for cancer with clinical examinations and mammography after the age of 40 postoperatively. There is no need to discontinue testosterone therapy in the perioperative period as studies have not shown any effect on wound healing, bleeding, or DVT risk in cisgender men.[36]

Surgical Planning

Degree of breast tissue, volume of parenchyma to be resected, skin redundancy, and ptosis are all factors that determine optimal technique.[37] Algorithms have been published to help determine optimal surgical technique,[38] but modifications should be made based on surgeon and patient preference.

Periareolar Mastectomy

Patients with small breast volume with limited skin are candidates for a periareolar mastectomy with a small incision along the inferior areola border from 9 o'clock to 3 o'clock. The tissue is directly excised through this incision, first dissecting planes along the breast capsule to the inframammary fold, medial, lateral, and superior borders of the breast. The parenchyma is elevated off the pectoralis major muscle and removed. The inframammary fold is ablated and scored to remove any feminine definition of breast borders. Liposuction can be used to further contour the chest, including lateral chest side wall and preaxillary fat. Drains are placed through separate stab incisions and the patient is placed in a compression vest. This technique limits the ability to reposition the nipples to a more masculine location on the chest wall, but skin recoil slightly reduces the diameter of the nipple areolar complex (NAC). The advantage of this technique is a favorable inferior periareolar scar that may be unnoticeable when shirtless (Figure 100.5).

Circumareolar Mastectomy

In patients with modest skin excess who desire a limited scar technique, a concentric-circle, circumareolar approach, with resizing of the NAC, and small donut skin excision may be performed. The new diameter of the NAC should be measured with maximum skin resection width of 2 cm. The parenchyma is excised directly through a full thickness incision on the inferior areola border, and the intervening skin to be removed is deepithelialized. The NAC survives on a deepithelialized dermal pedicle based superiorly.

Following completion of the parenchyma resection along the breast capsule, liposuction is used through a separate stab incision along the inframammary fold to contour the chest wall superiorly and laterally. The inframammary fold is undermined and scored through the open incision.

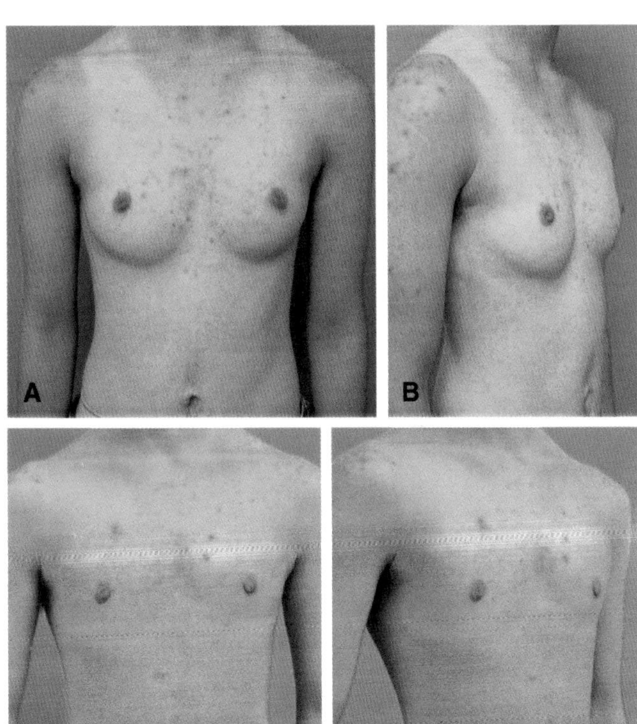

FIGURE 100.5. Periareolar mastectomy. Preoperative **(A, B)** and postoperative **(C, D)** photos of transmasculine gender mastectomy using the periareolar incision technique. Ideal candidates for this procedure have a small breast size (A cup), grade 0-1 ptosis, and good tissue elasticity.

Closure of the donut incision is achieved with a spoke wheel pattern of 2-0 polydioxanone suture to help distribute skin excess and relieve tension on the closure. The important thing is to prevent undue tension on this scar, as it tends to spread due to forces in all directions. As in the periareolar approach, the ability to relocate the nipple into a more lateral masculine position is limited.

Double Incision with Free Nipple Grafting

Most patients with significant breast volume and long-term use of a binder require a double-incision free nipple grafting technique to adequately remove excess skin and contour the chest (Figure 100.6). The first incision should be located just inferior to the IMF to prevent superior displacement in closure. The second incision is on top of the breast and generally designed to be straight across. In closure, the incision should be straight or, if the patient prefers, slightly curved downward. A lateral upward extension along the lateral border of the pectoralis may be used to help camouflage the lateral scar. The nipples are taken off as full thickness grafts either as a central piece around the nipple papule or as a two-piece graft of areola and small piece of papule if patient desires reduction of papule diameter. The nipple size should be approximately 2.4 cm × 2.0 cm and oval shaped.

The inferior incision is made first and the breast tissue is undermined superficial to the pectoralis major fascia to the superior border of the breast. The superior breast incision is then made and dissection carried down to the breast capsule. All subcutaneous fat should be preserved on the superior mastectomy flap and dissection carried up to the superior border of the breast. A small amount of parenchyma is left superiorly to retain some contour, which appears like pectoralis major development, and the remaining parenchyma is then resected. Drains are placed through separate stab incisions inferior and lateral on the chest wall. The IMF is then obliterated and scored to remove the feminine contour of the inferior breast. The incision is then closed in three layers, Scarpa fascia, deep dermal, and subcuticular. The patient is then placed in the seated position, and sterile stickers (labels for medications on the field) are used to estimate nipple position along the lateral inferior border of the pectoralis major muscle. The patient is then placed back in the supine position and the nipple inset area is marked as a transverse ellipse 2.4 × 2.0 cm. This area is deepithelialized and the thinned nipple graft sutured in place. A bolster dressing is then secured.

Postoperative Care

Drains are removed within 1 week and bolsters removed at 1 week. The patient is kept in a compression vest for 3 weeks postoperatively with modified activity restrictions. Aggressive scar management with massage and silicone sheeting at night at 3 weeks postoperatively helps prevent bothersome hypertrophic scars. The breast tissue should all be sent to pathology and results reviewed with the patient, regardless of age. Revisionary surgery is relatively common, with incidence approximately 40%[39] in general, any decision to revise the scar or perform liposuction to improve contour should be delayed until 4 to 6 months postoperatively for postoperative edema to completely resolve.

Phalloplasty

In properly selected transmale patients, phalloplasty may be indicated. Phalloplasty procedures have specific goals including constructing reasonable male anatomy to affirm gender identity, preservation of erogenous and orgasmic sensibility, the ability to stand to urinate, and the potential for penetrative intercourse. In reality, achieving all of these goals is challenging and, although current reconstructive strategies all employ similar principles, there is wide variation among surgeons in the specifics of phalloplasty procedures. The choice of a one- or multiple-staged approach, which specific flaps are used for phallic and urethral reconstruction, the methods for reconstruction of the pars fixa of the urethra, and strategies to restore or preserve

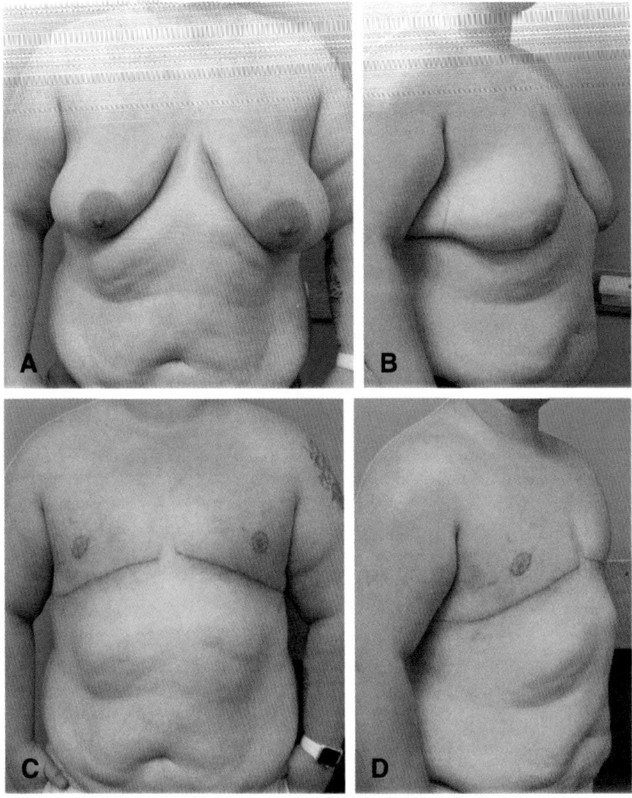

FIGURE 100.6. Double-incision mastectomy with free nipple grafting. Preoperative **(A, B)** and postoperative **(C, D)** photograohs showing transmasculine mastectomy using the double-incision with free nipple grafting technique. Candidacy selection for this method includes patients of various breast sizes, grade II ptosis and above, and moderate to poor tissue elasticity.

TABLE 100.4. PENILE RECONSTRUCTION: FREE-FLAP UTILIZATION METHODS[a]

Year	Donor Site	Described As	Description	Downfalls
1936	Abdomen	Classic method	Use of pedicled oblique to create tube for neophallus	No neourethra
1946	Abdomen	Tube within a tube	Neophallus with neourethra using a multistage approach.	Scarring; insensate neophallus
1972	Groin (+below waist)		Branches of femoral and saphenous systems are used for recipient free-flap vessels	Scarring, insensate neophallus, unsatisfactory cosmetic results
1982	Radial artery free flap	Updated tube within a tube design	Flaps from radial artery used for tube design.	Scarring, difficult to create sustainable corona ridge and shape neophallus, still relatively high complication rate
2006	Anterolateral thigh flap	Pedicled to groin	May be used as outer phallus with ulnar or radial artery flap for urethral reconstruction	May not be option in patients with thick thighs

[a]Historical account of donor-site location and free-flap reconstruction methods in the creation of the neophallus for transmasculine gender-affirming surgery.

erogenous sensibility vary considerably among surgeons and centers; there is no hard evidence supporting one specific approach for phallic construction.

This large variation in the specifics of phalloplasty procedures is principally related to the large cutaneous surface of the male phallus, necessitating a large cutaneous donor site and because of the complexity and difficulty of reconstructing the pars fixa and the penile urethra.[40]

Complications of urinary stricture and fistula are prevalent. Considerable variation among centers has resulted from attempts to improve on these high urologic, flap-related, and prosthetic complication rates, ranging from 33% to 77% in large case-series.[41,42] Regarding donor-site selection, an individualized discussion with each patient regarding the acceptance of, and the location of, a large cutaneous donor-site scar is essential. Because Plastic Surgeons are not trained in urethral reconstruction or the management of urethral strictures and fistulas, we believe it is mandatory that a qualified reconstructive urologist is involved in each phalloplasty that involves urethral reconstruction. It therefore becomes a shared decision between the Plastic Surgeon and the Urologist regarding urethral reconstruction. That, along with the lack of consensus in the literature, is the basis of the variation in methods for urethral reconstruction.

Transmasculine patients desiring a phalloplasty will also generally undergo hysterectomy, oophorectomy, and vaginectomy. This can be done at the time of phalloplasty or done as a separate procedure several months beforehand.

Surgical Staging

Reconstruction of the male external genitalia is always performed in multiple stages. There is, however, no "standard" sequence. Hysterectomy, oophorectomy, and vaginectomy are often performed as stand-alone procedures several months in advance of the phalloplasty. There is accumulating evidence that this may reduce the incidence of urethral leaks into the cavity left by the vaginectomy, but some centers will still do the vaginectomy at the time of phalloplasty. Many centers will perform a urethral lengthening or even a formal metoidioplasty (see below) to establish the pars fixa urethra in advance of formal phalloplasty, either synchronous with, or as a separate stage from the vaginectomy. The formal phalloplasty, usually a free tissue flap transfer procedure, is then performed. If a pars fixa reconstruction has not been done in a prior stage, it is done at the time of the formal phalloplasty. Reconstruction of the penile urethra can be done using the classic "tube within a tube" single-flap technique, using two separate flaps for urethra and for phallic skin, or by prefabricating a urethra within the penile flap in advance. Many centers perform a coronaplasty and begin scrotal construction at the time of phalloplasty, although this is not universal. Scrotoplasty and insertion of testicular prosthesis are done once the phalloplasty and urethral reconstruction are healed for several months. If penile prosthesis for erectile function are to be placed, this is always done in a delayed stage, typically no sooner than 1 year after the phalloplasty.

This myriad of approaches to staging underscores the difficult and the as yet imperfectly resolved challenge of reconstruction of functional male genitalia. Below, we will describe the general approach for a single-stage, one-flap phalloplasty, followed by a discussion of some specific alternatives. A brief description of historical flap design and utilization is outlined in **Table 100.4**.

Single-Stage, One-Flap Phalloplasty

This approach, using the radial forearm free flap, is arguably the most commonly employed strategy at the present time. It is also possible to perform phallic construction with an anterior-lateral thigh (ALT) flap, although the thickness of that flap in most patients makes it difficult to produce a tube-within-a-tube structure without constructing an unduly large phallus. Below, the radial forearm flap procedure is described; using ALT would be analogous.

The patient is prepared for surgery according to the general guidelines discussed above. Specific to this procedure, a suprapubic urinary catheter is required. For the portion of the flap that will become the urethra, permanent hair removal is mandatory preoperatively to prevent future strictures. Preoperative examination focuses on examination of the forearm and an Allen's test to ensure perfusion of the hand based on the ulnar artery alone. The flap is planned as a "tube-within-a-tube." The dimensions of the flap account for penile length (average erect length of the male penis is 5.75 inches [about 15 cm]), the inner circumference of the urethra (3–4 cm), and the external phallic skin (at least 15 cm). This therefore requires a very large skin flap, 15 × 18 cm minimum, on the forearm. The flap is based on the radial artery and its venae commitans, with the ulnar forearm becoming the urethral portion. The cephalic vein, and the medial and lateral antebrachial cutaneous nerves are harvested with the flap. A strip of the skin surface is deepithelialized to separate the urethra and phallic skin, and the urethral portion is tubed over a Foley catheter. The remaining flap skin is now sutured around the urethral portion and to the distal urethra. Some centers will also perform a primary glansplasty at this point, although reports of necrosis of the flap distal to the coronal incision argue for delaying the glansplasty for a later stage. After flap transfer, the donor defect is closed with a skin graft.

Preparation of the recipient site can occur synchronously with flap elevation. Again, there are multiple variations in the specifics, but the basic elements include the following:

1. Preparing recipient vessels for the free flap, typically in the groin using branches of the femoral and saphenous systems,
2. Lengthening the female urethra to create the pars fixa urethra of the male. Vaginal mucosal turnover flaps, labia minora flaps, and buccal mucosal grafts have all been employed in various combinations for this purpose

3. Deepithelializing the clitoris after release of the chordee and harvesting one of the clitoral nerves for coaptation to a flap nerve
4. Beginning scrotal reconstruction with V-Y and/or transposition flaps of the labia majora

The still-innervated clitoris at the base of the neophallus provides for erogenous sensation; tactile sensation on the phallus is provided through the medial and lateral antebrachial cutaneous nerve coaptations to the clitoral and ilioinguinal nerves. This approach preserves erogenous and orgasmic sensibility in nearly 100% of patients.

The radial forearm flap is then transferred to the recipient site and positioned so that the clitoris is at the base of the neophallus. The urethral coaptation is performed leaving a Foley catheter in place. The flap is reinnervated by coapting one of the flap nerves (typically the LABC) to the selected clitoral nerve and the other flap nerve to a local cutaneous nerve, generally the ilioinguinal nerve. The flap is revascularized via microvacular anastomoses, and the remaining local incisions are closed. Postoperative care is as for any free-tissue transfer with urinary drainage via the suprapubic catheter. The Foley catheter is left in the reconstructed urethra for 3 to 6 weeks before a cystoscopy and/or urethrogram verify urethral integrity.

The advantages of this approach are the reliable anatomy and robust vascularity of the radial forearm flap, the ability to perform a one-stage construction of the phallus and urethra, excellent return of tactile sensation in the phallic skin, and acceptable aesthetics of the phallus. The primary disadvantage is the very large cutaneous donor site on the forearm. Efforts to improve the aesthetics of the donor site by sparing the deep fascia over the majority of the forearm or by using Integra to generate a thicker base for skin grafting have been described.[43] As discussed above, the ALT flap can be used in an analogous fashion, as has the latissimus dorsi myocutaneous flap. Figure 100.7 demonstrates the result from a single-stage, radial forearm flap phalloplasty.

Single-Stage Phalloplasty With Two Flaps

Because of the very large donor defect on the forearm and concerns about reduced vascularity at the periphery of large free-flap skin paddles, the simultaneous use of two separate flaps, one for the urethra and one for the phallus have been described. Common combinations include a small radial forearm or ulnar forearm free flap for the urethral component and a pedicled ALT flap for phallic skin or a pedicled superficial circumflex iliac artery perforator flap for the urethra and an ALT flap for phallic skin. Multiple other permutations of flaps have been proposed and tried; this heterogeneity underscores the significant challenge of phallic construction.

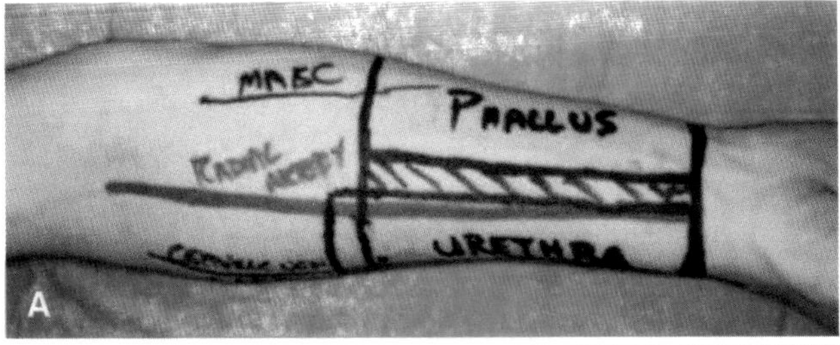

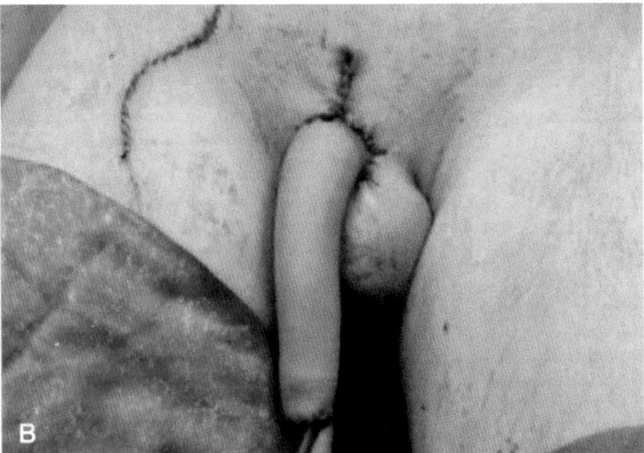

FIGURE 100.7. Phalloplasty using radial forearm free flap. **A.** Preoperative photo of radial forearm donor site. **B.** Immediate postoperative photo of neophallus. The patient had previously undergone a scrotoplasty with testicular implants.

Staged Phalloplasty

In an attempt to overcome the high urethral stricture and fistula rates observed after single-stage phalloplasty, staged procedures have been proposed. One strategy is to perform a urethral lengthening (a construction of the pars fixa urethra) or even a full metoidioplasty as a first stage, followed by the flap-based phalloplasty as a second stage. In this approach, the pars fixa urethra is constructed in the same way as for single-stage phalloplasty, but it is allowed to heal completely before the phalloplasty flap procedure is performed.

Another strategy has been to prefabricate the penile urethra prior to phalloplasty.[44] Several months in advance of the planned phalloplasty, the donor flap is partially raised; and vaginal mucosa, buccal mucosa, or skin grafts are tubed around a catheter within the substance of the flap. This neourethra is allowed to mature for several months before the entire donor flap is raised and transferred as the neophallus.

Scrotal Construction

Scrotal construction is generally begun at the time of phalloplasty using hair-bearing flaps from the labia majora. It is important to place the neoscrotum in its normal anatomic location, anterior to the perineum at the base of the phallus so as not to interfere with the legs while walking. Multiple specific designs for scrotal reconstruction have been described, with the most commonly used strategy likely being a V-Y plasty of the labia majora in combination with labial flaps rotated 90°, thereby recruiting additional skin anteriorly.

Prostheses for Erectile Function

Semirigid or hydraulic prostheses have been used to achieve erection in phalloplasty patients. The insertion of the prosthesis is always delayed, generally for at least a year, after phalloplasty. Multiple strategies to encase the prostheses in synthetic or biologic sheaths and to anchor the prosthesis to the pubis have been proposed to overcome the high complication rate associated with penile prostheses in phalloplasty patients. Because most centers still report a 30% or higher rate of extrusion necessitating removal within 2 or 3 years of prosthesis placement and because reoperation rates approach 100% at 5 years, some centers decline to place penile prostheses.[45,46] As an alternative, patients can be instructed on the use of external stiffening strategies to engage in intercourse. New prostheses, developed specifically for phalloplasty patients, may improve success rates in the future.

Complications and Outcomes of Phalloplasty

Because phalloplasty is a multistage, complex flap-based endeavor, patients should be informed that complications are common. In addition to all the complications attendant with any surgery and with free-flap surgery specifically, the rates of urinary strictures and fistulas and complications with penile implants remain, as noted above, high despite the multiple strategies employed to lessen the frequency of complications.[47,48]

There are no high level-of-evidence studies using validated instruments to accurately define patient-reported or health status outcomes in phalloplasty patients. However, the less rigorous data in the existing body of literature indicate that despite the high complication rate, the overall patient satisfaction and results of phalloplasty appear to be acceptable and that "regret" following phalloplasty is rare.

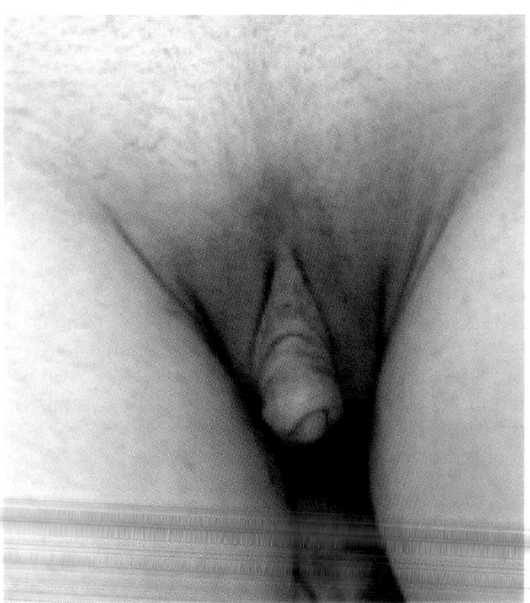

FIGURE 100.8. Metoidioplasty. A small phallus resulted from metoidioplasty in this patient.

Metoidioplasty

For patients who decline the complexity, multiple stages, and donor-site morbidity of a phalloplasty, metoidioplasty may be a reasonable option. Testosterone therapy will result in clitoromegaly, allowing conversion of the clitoris into a small phallus. The basic elements of the procedure include a release of the ventral chordee of the clitoris, a release of the clitoral suspensory ligament, and lengthening of the female urethra to exit the tip of the enlarged clitoris. The same techniques for urethral lengthening for phalloplasties are employed. Vaginal mucosal turn-over flaps, labia minora flaps, and buccal grafts, usually in combination. Because the most critical part of this procedure is the urethral lengthening, and because the complications of urethral strictures and fistulas are common, it is again our opinion that a reconstructive urologist should be involved unless the Plastic Surgeon has received additional specialized training.

The goal of metoidioplasty is to fashion a phallus to affirm male gender identity and to allow standing micturition, although not all patients achieve this latter goal. Metoidioplasty typically results in a phallus 4 to 8 cm in length so penetrative intercourse is not generally possible (Figure 100.8).

SUMMARY

Gender-affirming surgery is a broad and growing part of Plastic Surgery. For properly selected gender dysphoric individuals, appropriate surgical intervention can have significant, positive health and quality of life benefits. Because the diagnosis of gender dysphoria and the selection of candidates for gender-affirming surgical intervention are outside of the scope of expertise of Plastic Surgeons, it is essential that care is delivered in a multidisciplinary environment and especially in collaboration with the mental health team. The WPATH SOC should be the guiding principles for working with this patient population and for gauging a patient's readiness for surgery. As reviewed above, a very broad range of surgical procedures can be considered for both transfeminine and transmasculine individuals. Facial feminization surgery and transgender top surgery are within the scope of well-trained Plastic Surgeons. On the other hand, genital sex reassignment procedures, both vaginoplasty and phalloplasty, involve anatomy and may result in complications that are outside the scope of current Plastic Surgery training. Surgeons intending to become involved in these procedures must seek additional training and should work with gynecologic and urologic colleagues to assure appropriate patient outcomes.

REFERENCES

1. American Psychiatric Association. *Diagnostic and Statistical Manual of Mental Disorders*. 5th ed. Arlington, VA: American Psychiatric Publishing; 2013.
2. Flores AR, Herman JL, Gates GJ, Brown TNT. *How many Adults Identify as Transgender in the United States?* 2016. Available at http://williamsinstitute.law.ucla.edu/wp-content/uploads/How-Many-Adults-Identify-as-Transgender-in-the-United-States.pdf. Accessed August 17, 2018.
3. Richards C, Bouman WP, Barker M-J. *Genderqueer and Non-binary Genders*. London, UK: Palgrave Macmillan; 2017.
4. Gender and Genetics. Genomic Resource Centre: Gender and Genetics. http://www.who.int/genomics/gender/en/. Published December 1, 2010. Accessed August 27, 2018.
5. Swaab DF, Garcia-Falgueras A. Sexual differentiation of the human brain in relation to gender identity and sexual orientation. *Funct Neurol*. 2009;24(1):17-28.
6. Saraswat A, Weinand JD, Safer JD. Evidence supporting the biologic nature of gender identity. *Endocr Pract*. 2015;21(2):199-204.
7. World Professional Association for Transgender Health. *Standards of Care for the Health of Transsexual, Transgender, and Gender Nonconforming People*. 7th Version. Elgin, IL: The World Professional Association for Transgender Health; 2011.
8. American Society of Plastic Surgeons. *Comment Letter on Proposed Rule on Medicare Program: Hospital Inpatient Prospective Payment System for Acute Care Hospitals and the Long-term Care Hospital Prospective Payment System and Proposed Policy Changes and Fiscal Year 2018 Rates*. American Society of Plastic Surgeons; June 2017. https://www.regulations.gov/document?D=CMS-2017-0055-4304. Accessed August 17, 2018.
9. Weissler JM, Chang BL, Carney MJ, et al. Gender-affirming surgery in persons with gender dysphoria. *Plast Reconstr Surg*. 2018;141(3):388e-396e.
The authors describe a multidisciplinary approach for the treatment of gender dysphoria treatment, and the specific role of plastic surgeons within its collaborative, integrated care framework. They outline plastic surgery's advancement in transgender medicine and underscore the breath of positive health outcomes that follow gender-affirmation surgeries.
10. James SE, Herman JL, Rankin S, et al. *The Report of the 2015 US Transgender Survey*. Washington, DC: National Center for Transgender Equality; 2016. http://www.transequality.org/sites/default/files/docs/usts/USTS%20Full%20Re port%20-%20FINAL%201.6.17.pdf. Accessed August 17, 2018.
11. Bockting WO, Miner MH, Swinburne Romine RE, et al. Stigma, mental health, and resilience in an online sample of the US transgender population. *Am J Public Health*. 2013;103(5):943-951.
12. Grant J, Mottet L, Tanis J. *Injustice at Every Turn: A Report of the National Transgender Discrimination Survey*. Washington, DC: National Center for Transgender Equality and National Gay and Lesbian Task Force; 2011. Accessed August 17, 2018. https://www.hivlawandpolicy.org/resources/injustice-every-turn-a-report-national-transgender-discrimination-survey-jaime-m-grant.
13. Reisner SL, Greytak EA, Parsons JT, Ybarra ML. Gender minority social stress in adolescence: disparities in adolescent bullying and substance use by gender identity. *ML J Sex Res*. 2015;52(3):243-256.
14. Adams KA, Nagoshi CT, Filip-Crawford G, et al. Components of gender-nonconformity prejudice. *Int J Transgenderism*. 2016:17:185-198.
15. Fredriksen-Goldsen KI, Simoni JM, Kim HJ, et al. The health equity promotion model: reconceptualization of lesbian, gay, bisexual, and transgender (LGBT) health disparities. *Am J Orthopsychiatry*. 2014;84(6):653-663.
16. Deutsch MB. Use of the informed consent model in the provision of cross-sex hormone therapy: a survey of the practices of selected clinics. *Int J Transgend*. 2013(3):140-146.
17. Callen Lorde Community Health Center. *Transgender Health Program Protocols*. New York, NY: Callen Lorde Community Health Center; 2011.
18. Tom Waddell Health Center. Protocols for Hormonal Reassignment of Gender. http://www.sfdph.org/dph/comupg/oservices/medSvs/hlthCtrs/TransGendprotocols122006.pdf. Revised May 7, 2013. Accessed August 17, 2018.
19. Cavanaugh T, Hopwood R, Gonzalez A, Thompson J. *The Medical Care of Transgender Persons*. Boston, MA: Fenway Health; 2015. http://www.lgbthealtheducation.org/wp-content/uploads/COM-2245-The-Medical-Care-of-Transgender-Persons-v31816.pdf. Accessed August 17, 2018.
20. Cavanaugh T, Hopwood R, Lambert C. Informed consent in the medical care of transgender and gender-nonconforming patients. *AMA J Ethics*. 2016;18(11):1147-1155.
21. Coleman E, Bockting W, Botzer M, et al. Standards of care for the health of transsexual, transgender, and gender-nonconforming people, version 7. *Int J Transgenderism*. 2012;13(4):165-232.
22. Vance SR Jr, Ehrensaft D, Rosenthal SM. Psychological and medical care of gender nonconforming youth. *Pediatrics*. 2014;134:1184.
23. Shechner T. Gender identity disorder: a literature review from a developmental perspective. *Isr J Psychiatry Relat Sci*. 2010;47:132.
24. Steensma TD, McGuire JK, Kreukels BPC, et al. Factors associated with desistence and persistence of childhood gender dysphoria: a quantitative follow-up study. *J Am Acad Child Adolesc Psychiatry*. 2013;52:582-590.
Thirty-seven percent of adolescents (<12 years old) diagnosed with gender dysphoria at the Vrije Universiteit (VU) University Medical Center in Amsterdam, the Netherlands showed persistence of gender dysphoria into adulthood. Ethical treatment options for trans and gender-nonconforming youth is widely debated, emphasizing the current gap in the literature reporting childhood gender dysphoria persistence in adulthood. This study suggests predictors of gender dysphoria in adulthood, including differences between natal sex, familial management, social transitions in childhood, and cognitive representation of gender. Better understanding of gender dysphoria persistence can help develop improved models of care and health outcomes.

25. de Vries AL, Steensma TD, Doreleijers TA, Cohen-Kettenis PT. Puberty suppression in adolescents with gender identity disorder: a prospective follow-up study. *J Sex Med*. 2011;8(8):2276-2283.
26. Altman K. Facial feminization surgery: current state of the art. *Int J Oral Maxillofac Surg*. 2012;41(8):885-894.
27. Morrison SD, Vyas KS, Motakef S, et al. Facial feminization: systematic review of the literature. *Plast Reconstr Surg*. 2016;137(6):1759-1770.
28. Song TE, Jiang N. Transgender phonosurgery: a systematic review and meta-analysis. *Otolaryngol Head Neck Surg*. 2017;156(5):803-808.
29. Asscheman H, T'Sjoen G, Lemaire A, et al. Venous thromboembolism as a complication of cross-sex hormone treatment of male-to-female transsexual subjects: a review. *Andrologia*. 2014;46:791-795.
30. Hembree WC, Cohen-Kettinis P, Delemarre-van de Waal HA, et al. Endocrine treatment of transsexual persons: an endocrine society clinical practice guideline. *J Clin Endocrinol Metab*. 2009;9:3132-3154.
31. Horbach SE, Bouman MB, Smit JM, et al. Outcome of vaginoplasty in male-to-female transgenders: a systematic review of surgical techniques. *J Sex Med*. 2015;12(6):1499-1512.
32. Buncamper ME, van der Sluis WB, van der Pas RS, et al. Surgical outcome after penile inversion vaginoplasty: a retrospective study of 475 transgender women. *Plast Reconstr Surg*. 2016;138(5):999-1007.
Four hundred and seventy-five transgender women who underwent penile inversion vaginoplasty (PIV) at the VU University Medical Center between 2000-2014 were retrospectively reviewed for intraoperative and postoperative outcomes, including complications, risk factors, reoperation and revisions, and necessitated secondary surgical procedures. This is a high-case volume report concludes that PIV can be successfully implemented with minimal risk of intraoperative complications, and, though frequent (93%), easily managed postoperative complications.
33. Goddard JC, Vickery RM, Qureshi A, et al. Feminizing genitoplasty in adult transsexuals: early and long-term surgical results. *BJU Int*. 2007;100:607-613.
34. Rossi Neto R, Hintz F, Krege S, et al. Gender reassignment surgery: a 13 year review of surgical outcomes. *Int Braz J Urol*. 2012;38:97-107.
35. Wilson SC, Morrison SD, Anzai L, et al. Masculinizing top surgery: a systematic review of techniques and outcomes. *Ann Plast Surg*. 2018;80(6):679-683.
The authors identify eight masculinizing top surgery studies to compare techniques and outcomes of gender-affirming mastectomy. They report the most common technique as "inframammary fold skin excision with free nipple grafting" [illegible] responding to a significantly less acute reoperation rate compared to other gender mastectomy techniques; the highest rate of secondary operations occurred highest in the periareolar skin resection cohort (37.5%). Satisfaction outcome measures were [illegible] in all studies with [illegible] surgical technique.
36. [illegible] et al. [illegible] of testosterone replacement therapy and the incidence of a composite of postoperative in-hospital mortality and [illegible] events in men undergoing noncardiac surgery. *Anesthesiology*. 2017;127(3):457-465.
A major source of contention in current surgical practice [illegible] mone replacement therapy (HRT) in transmasculine men prior to surgery. This is not addressed in the WPATH SOC guidelines, and many patients are reluctant to stop testosterone due to undesirable side-effects. This study analyzes the instances of in-hospital mortality and cardiovascular events between patients who are and are not on HRT. Their report of nearly 50,000 patients (~1,000 on testosterone) does not indicate a significant association between preoperative testosterone use and an increased incidence of postoperative mortality and/or cardiovascular events, underscoring the need to re-evaluate the risks associated with stopping HRT prior to transmasculine gender-affirming surgery.
37. Ammari T, Sluiter EC, Gast K, Kuzon WM. Female-to-male gender-affirming chest reconstruction surgery. *Aesthet Surg J*. 2018. doi:10.1093/asj/sjy098. [Epub ahead of print].
38. Donato DP, Walzer NK, Rivera A, Wright L, Agarwal CA. Female-to-male chest reconstruction: a review of technique and outcomes. *Ann Plast Surg*. 2017;79(3):259-263.
39. Cregten-Escobar P, Bouman MB, Buncamper ME, et al. Subcutaneous mastectomy in female-to-male transsexuals: a retrospective cohort-analysis of 202 patients. *J Sex Med*. 2012;9:3148-3153.
40. Monstrey S. Penile reconstruction with the radial forearm flap: an update. *Handchir Mikrochir Plast Chir*. 2011;43:208-214.
41. Monstrey S, Hoebeke P, Selvaggi G, et al. Penile reconstruction: is the radial forearm flap really the standard technique? *Plast Reconstr Surg*. 2009;124(2):510-518.
The authors describe the results of a large-volume (287) gender-affirming phalloplasty patient series of one surgical team. Their main findings indicate that the radial forearm flap provides the best and most reliable outcome, though no technique fully satisfies construction of an aesthetically pleasing, sensate, and functional neophallus. This overview suggests that a two-stage technique provides the most satisfactory results, though high complication rates, scarring, and lack of long-term follow-up has yet to be eliminated with any existing technique.
42. Garaffa G, Christopher NA, Ralph DJ. Total phallic reconstruction in female-to-male transsexuals. *Eur Urol*. 2010;57(4):715-722.
43. Zuo KJ, Roy M, Meng F, Bensoussan Y, Hofer SOP. Aesthetic and functional outcomes of radial forearm flap donor site reconstruction with biosynthetic skin substitutes. *J Plast Reconstr Aesthet Surg*. 2018;71(6):925-928.
44. Salgado CJ, Fein LA, Chim J, et al. Prelamination of neourethra with uterine mucosa in radial forearm osteocutaneous free flap phalloplasty in the female-to-[illegible] transgender patient. *Case Rep Urol*. 2018;2018:8742531.
45. [illegible], et al. Erectile implants in female-to-male transsexuals: our experience in 129 patients. *Eur Urol*. 2010;57(2):334-340.
46. Scherzer ND, Dick B, Gabrielson AT, et al. Penile prosthesis complications: plan-[illegible] [Epub ahead of print].
47. [illegible] and radial forearm flap phalloplasty in female to male transgender genital reconstruction [illegible] *Plast Reconstr Surg Global Open*. 2016;4(12):e1131.
48. [illegible], et al. Phalloplasty: a review of techniques and outcomes. *Plast Reconstr Surg*. 2016;138(3):594-615.

TRUNK AND LOWER EXTREMITY

QUESTIONS

1. The neoclitoris is constructed from the dorsal aspect of the glans penis in a penile inversion vaginoplasty operation. The nerve supplying this flap that provides erogenous sensation and orgasmic function is the
   a. Dorsal penile nerve
   b. Ilioinguinal nerve
   c. Pudendal nerve
   d. Clitoral nerve

1. A patient presents requesting penile inversion vaginoplasty surgery. What are the prerequisites for transfeminine bottom surgery according to WPATH criteria?
   a. Two letters of readiness for surgery from mental health professionals
   b. One year of living full time in congruent gender (as a woman)
   c. One year of hormonal therapy including estrogen
   d. All of the above

3. During the preoperative consultation for radial forearm phalloplasty, a patient asks about postoperative urinary function. It is very important to him to be able to stand and use a urinal after surgery. What is the incidence of postoperative urinary stricture/fistula?
   a. 5%
   b. 10%
   c. 30%
   d. 80%

4. A patient presents to the office 3 weeks following penile inversion vaginoplasty surgery complaining of malodorous secretions from her neovagina. On examination, there is feculent smelling discharge. What should be ruled out?
   a. Vaginal candidiasis
   b. Menstruation
   c. Inadequate hygiene
   d. Rectovaginal fistula

5. To prevent perioperative VTE, what medication should be held 3 weeks prior to vaginoplasty surgery in transfeminine patients?
   a. Spironolactone
   b. Estradiol
   c. Testosterone
   d. Depo-provera

6. A patient desires a radial forearm phalloplasty for gender-affirming bottom surgery. Prior to the operation the operating surgeon must perform what test?
   a. Retrograde urethrogram
   b. Allen's test
   c. Speculum examination
   d. Angiogram of upper extremity

1. **Answer: a.** The dorsal penile nerve is invested between Buck fascia and the tunica of the corpus cavernosa and together with the dorsal penile artery and veins composes the pedicle of the neoclitoral flap.

2. **Answer: d.** The WPATH SOC are internationally accepted guidelines for transgender care including prerequisites prior to genital gender-affirming surgery.

3. **Answer: c.** Urinary strictures and fistula are common at the juncture of the urethral portion of the radial forearm and the pars fixa urethra.

4. **Answer: d.** Rectovaginal fistula is a rare (1% incidence) but serious complication of penile inversion vaginoplasty surgery. A temporary diverting ostomy is required to let the fistula heal in and the patient must continue to dilate the neovagina during this time. Failure to dilate will result in contraction of the entire neovagina.

5. **Answer: b.** Transfeminine patients are at elevated risk of VTE on estrogen therapy, over 14 times that of cisgender women after 9 years of therapy. Vaginoplasty is a major 5 hour operation with 1 week of modified activity restrictions. Holding estrogen therapy is socially and emotionally difficult for transgender women, but is necessary to prevent a postoperative pulmonary embolus.

6. **Answer: b.** An Allen test assesses the superficial and deep arches of the hand. Harvest of a radial forearm flap will potentially threaten the vascular supply of the hand in patients with an incomplete arch.

Note: Page numbers followed by "f" indicate figures and "t" indicate tables.